D1639740

Foundations of Respiratory Care

Foundations of Respiratory Care

Second Edition

Kenneth A. Wyka, MS, RRT, AE-C, FAARC
Center Manager and Respiratory Care Patient Coordinator
Anthem Health Services
Queensbury, New York and Healthcare Consultant
Lake George, New York

Paul J. Mathews, PhD, RRT, FCCM, FCCP, FAARC
Associate Professor
School of Allied Health
Department of Respiratory Care Education
University of Kansas Medical Center
Kansas City, Kansas
Honorary Professor University of Costa Rica,
San Jose Costa Rica
Honorary Professor National University of Medicine and Pharmacy,
Ho Chi Minh City Peoples Republic of Vietnam

John A. Rutkowski, MPA, MBA, FACHE, RRT
Director Cardiorespiratory Services
Bergen Regional Medical Center
Paramus, New Jersey
Adjunct Assistant Professor
University of Dentistry and Medicine of New Jersey
School of Health Related Professions
Newark, New Jersey

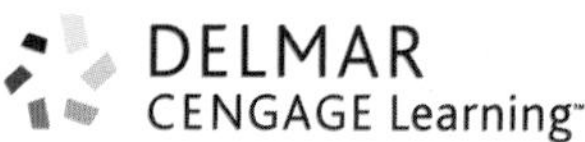

Australia • Brazil • Japan • Korea • Mexico • Singapore • Spain • United Kingdom • United States

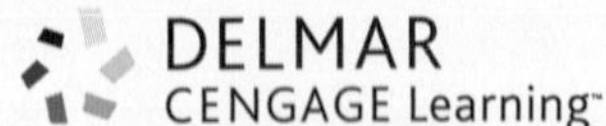

Foundations of Respiratory Care, Second Edition

Kenneth A. Wyka, Paul J. Mathews, John A. Rutkowski

Vice President, Career Education and Training Solutions: Dave Garza

Director of Learning Solutions: Matthew Kane

Associate Acquisitions Editor: Christina Gifford

Managing Editor: Marah Bellegarde

Senior Product Manager: Darcy M. Scelsi

Editorial Assistant: Nicole Manikas

Vice President, Career Education and Training Solutions: Jennifer Baker

Associate Marketing Manager: Jonathan Sheehan

Senior Production Director: Wendy Troeger

Production Manager: Andrew Crouth

Content Project Manager: Tom Heffernan

Senior Art Director: David Arsenault

Technology Project Manager: Patricia Allen

Production Technology Analyst: Mary Colleen Liburdi

Library of Congress Control Number: 2011934924

ISBN-13: 978-1-4354-6984-6

ISBN-10: 1-4354-6984-4

Delmar
5 Maxwell Drive
Clifton Park, NY 12065-2919
USA

Cengage Learning is a leading provider of customized learning solutions with office locations around the globe, including Singapore, the United Kingdom, Australia, Mexico, Brazil, and Japan. Locate your local office at: **international.cengage.com/region**

Cengage Learning products are represented in Canada by Nelson Education, Ltd.

To learn more about Delmar, visit **www.cengage.com/delmar**

Purchase any of our products at your local college store or at our preferred online store **www.cengagebrain.com**

Notice to the Reader

Publisher does not warrant or guarantee any of the products described herein or perform any independent analysis in connection with any of the product information contained herein. Publisher does not assume, and expressly disclaims, any obligation to obtain and include information other than that provided to it by the manufacturer. The reader is expressly warned to consider and adopt all safety precautions that might be indicated by the activities described herein and to avoid all potential hazards. By following the instructions contained herein, the reader willingly assumes all risks in connection with such instructions. The publisher makes no representations or warranties of any kind, including but not limited to, the warranties of fitness for particular purpose or merchantability, nor are any such representations implied with respect to the material set forth herein, and the publisher takes no responsibility with respect to such material. The publisher shall not be liable for any special, consequential, or exemplary damages resulting, in whole or part, from the readers' use of, or reliance upon, this material.

Printed in the United States of America
1 2 3 4 5 6 7 14 13 12 11

Dedication

To my wife, Kathy, in sincere gratitude for her continued encouragement, support, and love.

KAW

To my parents, Paul J. and Ruth Irene (O'Malley) Mathews. May they rest united and in peace. To the next generation Logan Elizabeth and Sydney Marie Rush - Grand kids extraordinare.

PJM

To my wife, Joanne, thank you for your unwavering patience, understanding, and most of all love.

JAR

BRIEF CONTENTS

EXTENDED CONTENTS

PREFACE

The field of respiratory care is continually growing and changing as new research, therapies, and theories about the causes and treatments of respiratory alterations emerge. *Foundations of Respiratory Care*, Second Edition provides a clear presentation of the concepts and issues in the field. Practitioners will find the book helpful as a review of interventions and therapeutics and as a tool to update their knowledge.

Conceptual Approach

The concept underlying *Foundations of Respiratory Care*, Second Edition was born of the need for a straightforward text that could be easily read and assimilated. Empowering readers as educated decision makers, helping them develop skills of analysis and critical thinking, and providing guidance for excellent clinical and patient care skills were all goals in writing this text. Chapters cover all the technical aspects of anatomy, physiology, and intervention while highlighting clinically relevant information. The text offers users a friendly approach that delivers a wealth of information in a consistent, easy-to-follow format with recurring pedagogical features. This text was written *by* respiratory therapists *for* respiratory therapists.

Organization

Foundations of Respiratory Care, Second Edition comprises 41 chapters organized into six sections.

Section I lays the foundation for understanding the respiratory care profession by outlining its history and scope of practice and discussing related legal and ethical principles.

Section II presents the applied sciences that underlie sound respiratory practice. Applied physics, chemistry, and microbiology are covered as they relate to respiratory care. Chapters on cardiopulmonary anatomy, physiology, pathology, and pharmacology give the reader the information needed to understand the chapters that follow.

Section III opens with a description of the comprehensive patient history, assessment, and documentation processes. Radiology and lab studies, including blood gases and noninvasive monitoring, are discussed in detail. Pulmonary function testing, polysomnography, and cardiac and hemodynamic monitoring round out this section.

Section IV outlines current therapies and approaches to managing patients with respiratory alterations. Oxygen and medical gas therapy, humidity and aerosol therapy, and hyperinflation therapy are all thoroughly discussed. Specifics on pulmonary hygiene and chest physical therapy, as well as techniques of airway management, are included. The chapters on invasive and noninvasive mechanical ventilation offer readers the most up-to-date information on these therapies.

Section V covers levels of delivery. Age-related considerations for neonatal, pediatric, and geriatric patients are discussed. Variations in approaches based on care setting are also covered; emergency medicine, critical care, subacute care, home care, and rehabilitation settings are each discussed in a separate chapter.

Section VI helps the reader assimilate and synthesize the wealth of information presented in the text. Specific guidelines and reminders for protecting the patient and health care provider are outlined. Health promotion and patient education receive thorough coverage. A final chapter on management of respiratory care services speaks to the administrative aspects of managing a service unit.

Chapter Format and Features

Innovative features in *Foundations of Respiratory Care*, Second Edition stimulate critical thinking and technical competence and encourage readers to synthesize and apply information presented in the text:

- **Objectives** open each chapter and introduce the main areas targeted for mastery in each chapter, providing a checkpoint for study and a tie-in to crucial skills.
- **Chapter Outlines** prepare the reader for study by indicating the content and order of material to be covered in each chapter.

- **Key Terms** are listed so the reader can become familiar with terms to be used and can research those that are unfamiliar. Key terms are boldfaced in text the first time they are used and are included in the end-of-text glossary.
- **Case Studies** present realistic scenarios, offering an opportunity for the reader to apply the chapter material, thereby encouraging analysis and critical thinking. Case studies include a sample patient or equipment troubleshooting scenario followed by several critical thinking questions requiring understanding and decision making on the part of the reader.
- **Spotlight On . . .** boxes describe new or upcoming approaches involving new therapies, new equipment, or technological innovations.
- **Best Practice** helps the reader to apply basic knowledge to real-life situations and offer hints and shortcuts useful to both new and experienced practitioners.
- **Age-Specific Competencies** outline skills that have variations based on the age of the patient or highlight considerations the reader should be sensitive to when managing the care of patients of different ages.
- A **Summary** concludes each chapter, offering a conceptual framework for chapter review and highlighting the main content points.
- **Study Questions** offer readers an opportunity to assess their understanding of the content and to define areas needing additional study. Questions are included in three formats (review questions, multiple choice questions, and critical thinking questions) to challenge the reader and to develop recall, analysis, and critical thinking skills.
- **References** and **Suggested Readings** at the end of the chapter document the theoretical basis of each chapter and provide additional resources for continued study.
- A **Glossary** at the end of the book defines all key terms used in the text and serves as a comprehensive resource for study and review.
- The **Index** facilitates access to material and includes special entries for tables and illustrations.

New to this Edition

CHAPTER 2

- Discussion of HIPAA
- Discussion of the ethical decision making model of Divine Command

CHAPTER 3

- Additional examples to demonstrate principles and formulas

CHAPTER 4

- New illustrations to demonstrate the concepts discussed in the chapter

CHAPTER 5

- Improved description of the immune system as a defense mechanism for fending off disease

CHAPTER 7

- Chapter 8 in the first edition
- Definitions of drug actions and interactions
- Addition of drugs used to manage COPD

CHAPTER 8

- New stand-alone chapter (Topics formerly covered in Chapter 7 have been placed in their own chapter with more well-rounded discussions: pneumonia, tuberculosis, nontuberculous *Mycobacterium* infections, and fungal pulmonary infections.)

CHAPTER 9

- New stand-alone chapter (Topics formerly covered in Chapter 7 have been placed in their own chapter with more well-rounded discussion: asthma, chronic bronchitis (COPD) and emphysema, and bronchiectasis.)

CHAPTER 10

- New stand-alone chapter (Topics formerly covered in Chapter 7 have been placed in their own chapter with more well-rounded discussions: diffuse parenchymal lung diseases.)

CHAPTER 11

- New stand-alone chapter (Topics formerly covered in Chapter 7 have been placed in their own chapter with more well-rounded discussions: atelectasis, pleural disorders, and lung cancer.)

CHAPTER 12

- New chapter with coverage of hemodynamic pulmonary edema, pulmonary heart disease, and noncardiogenic pulmonary edema

CHAPTER 14

- Fully updated with extensive images

CHAPTER 15

- Content on indirect ion-specific electrodes

CHAPTER 16

- Discussion and explanation of calculations and the significance of anion gap variations
- The differentiation of S_aO_2, S_pO_2, and O_2 content

CHAPTER 17

- Updated content and clarified procedural steps

CHAPTER 18

- Added discussions on insomnia, multiple sleep latency test, and maintenance of wakefulness test
- Updated and expanded discussions related to new manual for scoring sleep, sleep stages across the life span, and obstructed sleep apnea

CHAPTER 19

- Added discussion of combined disorders of automaticity and conductivity, nonparoxysmal junctional tachycardia, second degree/advanced heart block
- Updated discussion of atrial tachycardia and atrial fibrillation and hemodynamic monitoring

CHAPTER 20

- Added discussion of oxygen-conserving devices
- Discussion of new low-flow oxygen delivery devices the Oxy-Arm and the Oxy-View
- Updated uses of carbogen

CHAPTER 21

- Updated discussion of humidification devices
- Added discussion of heated humidification by nasal cannula
- Added discussion of breath-actuated devices

CHAPTER 22

- Discussion of glossopharyngeal breathing

CHAPTER 23

- Added discussion of the functions of airway mucous
- Added discussion of combined mechanical and acoustical vibration

CHAPTER 24

- Added discussion of use of stylet, elastic gum bougie, and lighted stylet
- Added discussion of fiberoptic intubation and blind nasotracheal intubation
- Added discussion of the management of the difficult airway
- Added discussion of patient safety and use of artificial airways

CHAPTER 25

- All new chapter on the physiological effects of mechanical ventilation

CHAPTER 26

- All new chapter on ventilator graphics, focusing on the interpretation of wave forms

CHAPTER 27

- Comprehensively revised and updated, focusing on the initiation and maintenance of invasive mechanical ventilation and including a discussion of a variety of modes of ventilation
- Discussion of the work of breathing

CHAPTER 28

- Updated information on newer forms of EPAP, CPAP, and BiPAP

CHAPTER 29

- Completely new chapter covering neonatal and pediatric respiratory care

CHAPTER 30

- Thoroughly updated
- Added discussion of increased costs of health care for the elderly
- Added discussion of improving communication with the elderly

CHAPTER 31

- Updated content on standards of care for BLS and ALS in both the adult and pediatric populations

CHAPTER 32

- Completely new chapter covering the timely topics of emergency preparedness

CHAPTER 33

- Updated discussion of the design and function of the intensive care unit
- Provides upgraded explanation of evidence-based scientific research
- Added discussion of ventilator-associated pneumonia under the quality improvement section

CHAPTER 34

- Discussion of long-term care

CHAPTER 36

- Addresses new evidence-based guidelines by the American College of Chest Physicians (ACCP) and the AACVPR recommending pulmonary rehabilitation for patients with COPD

- Discussion of HR 6331 (Medicare Improvements for Patients and Providers Act)

CHAPTER 37

- New chapter on the transport of the respiratory care patient

CHAPTER 38

- Expanded discussion on health care settings where the risk of hospital-acquired infection is increased
- Discussion of respiratory hygiene and cough etiquette
- Discussion of bioterrorism and pandemic influenza

CHAPTER 39

- Updated statistics throughout

CHAPTER 40

- Updated as relevant throughout
- Discussion of how to assess effectiveness of preprepared patient education materials

Ancillary Materials

The complete supplements package was developed to assist instructors in planning and implementing their programs for the most efficient use of time and other resources. Components of this package include the following:

INSTRUCTOR'S MANUAL

Order 1-4354-6985-2

The *Instructor's Manual* is designed to assist instructors in preparing for class lectures and examinations. Sections include objectives, introduction, outline, summary, activities, and answers to text review questions, multiple choice questions, and case study questions.

INSTRUCTOR RESOURCE CD-ROM

Order 1-4354-6986-0

This invaluable instructor tool consists of several components, an electronic version of the *Instructor's Manual*, a computerized test bank, and an electronic image library.

COMPUTERIZED TESTBANK

The electronic testbank contains more than 1000 multiple choice questions. The format follows that of the NBRC exams. The instructor can create and administer online tests that automatically correct and return the grades to the instructor via e-mail. Online testing allows exams to be administered online via a school network or stand-alone PC. Site license is included.

IMAGE LIBRARY

The Image Library is a software tool that includes an organized digital library of more than 700 illustrations and photographs from the text. With the Image Library you can:

- Create additional libraries.
- Set up electronic pointers to actual image files or collections.
- Sort art by desired categories.
- Print selected pieces.

The Image Library works in combination with standard presentation packages such as Microsoft PowerPoint for Windows.

WORKBOOK AND LAB MANUAL

Order 1-4354-6987-9

The workbook/lab manual provides a review of each chapter and additional exercises and activities to study and apply knowledge. Additional activities include short answer questions, multiple choice questions, lab exercises, just to name a few.

WebTutor on WebCT and Blackboard

Order 1-4354-6989-5 for Blackboard
Order 1-4354-6988-7 for WebCT

This resource is an online workbook that contains a variety of additional exercises and questions for study and review, flashcards, Web links, and discussion questions.

Acknowledgments

We gratefully acknowledge all of the reviewers for their hard work and all of our contributing authors for understanding our deadlines and insistence on quality. We also thank the following individuals for their help with this book.

CONTRIBUTORS

Dianne A. Adams, AS, BS, MA, RRT, NPS
Associate Professor and Program Director, County College of Morris Randolph, New Jersey

G. William Atkinson, MD, FACP, FCCP
Senior Associate Dean for Clinical Affairs
Professor, Pulmonary and Critical Care Medicine, School of Medicine
Medical Director, Respiratory Care Education
School of Allied Health, University of Kansas Medical Center
Kansas City, Kansas

Patricia Carroll, RRT, RN, BC, CEN, MS
Adjunct Professor, School of Health Sciences, Excelsior College
Albany, New York
Owner, Education Notebook, LLC
Meriden, Connecticut

William F. Clark, PhD, RRT
Dean of Health, Wellness and Sports Technology (Retired), Hillsborough Community College
Hillsborough, Florida

Glendon G. Cox, MD, MBA, MHSA, FCCP
Professor and Chair, Department of Health Policy and Management
Professor of Radiology, School of Medicine
University of Kansas Medical Center
Kansas City, Kansas

Robert DiBlasi RRT-NPS
Respiratory Research Coordinator, Seattle Children's Hospital, Research Foundation
Seattle, Washington

Raymond Edge, EdD, RRT
Former Dean, Maryville University
St. Louis, Missouri

Anthony Everidge, BA, RRT-NPS
Respiratory Therapy Program Director, Prima Medical Institute
Las Vegas, Nevada

Robert R. Fluck Jr, MS, RRT, FAARC
Associate Professor Emeritus, Upstate Medical University
Syracuse, New York

George W. Gaebler, MSEd, RRT, FAARC
Director, Respiratory Care, Upstate Medical University and Golisano Children's Hospital
Syracuse, New York

William F. Galvin, MSEd, RRT, CPFT, AE-C, FAARC
Assistant Professor, School of Allied Health Professions
Program Director, Respiratory Care Program
Administrative and Teaching Faculty, TIPS Program
Gwynedd Mercy College
Gwynedd Valley, Pennsylvania

Melaine (Tudy) Head Giordano, MS, RN, CPFT, RCP
Geriatric Consulting
Carrollton, Texas

David A. Gourley, RRT, MHA, FAARC
Executive Director of Regulatory Affairs, Chilton Hospital
Pompton Plains, New Jersey

Jodi B. Green, BS, RRT

Patient Care Coordinator, Home Therapy Equipment
Glens Falls, New York

Bethene Gregg, PhD, RRT

Associate Professor, Respiratory Care Education, School of Allied Health, University of Kansas Medical Center
Kansas City, Kansas

Joy Hargett, BS, RRT, RCP

Manager, Patient Care Services, Respiratory Care, St. Luke's Episcopal Hospital
Houston, Texas

Ken Hargett, MHA, RRT, RCP, FAARC

Director, Respiratory Care Services, Pulmonary Diagnostic Laboratory, The Methodist Hospital
Houston, Texas

Al Heuer, PhD, MBA, RRT, RPFT

Associate Professor, University of Medicine and Dentistry, School of Health Professions
Newark, New Jersey

Thomas J. Johnson, MS, RRT, EMT-B, RT

Program Director and Assistant Professor of Respiratory Care, Division of Respiratory Care, School of Health Professions, Long Island University, Brooklyn Campus
New York City, New York

Ingo S. Kampa, PhD

Director, Medical Multi-Specialty Associates, P.A.
Fair Lawn, New Jersey

Barbara Ludwig, MA, RRT

Assistant Professor and Chair, Respiratory Care Education, School of Allied Health, University of Kansas Medical Center
Kansas City, Kansas

L. Micky Mathews, BA, RN, CEN

Emergency Nurse Clinician, Menorah Medical Center
Overland Park, Kansas
Adjunct Assistant Professor, Respiratory Care Education, School of Allied Health
Nurse Preceptor, School of Nursing, University of Kansas Medical Center
Kansas City, Kansas

Doug McIntyre, MS, RRT, FAARC

President, Durable Medical Supply
Destrehan, Louisiana

Chad Pezzano, MA, RRT-NPS

Pediatric Clinical Instructor, Albany Medical Center
Albany, New York

John Salyer RRT-NPS, MBA, FAARC

Director Respiratory Therapy, Seattle Children's Hospital, Research Foundation
Seattle, Washington

Helen M. Sorenson, MA, RRT, FAARC

Associate Professor, Department of Respiratory Care, University of Texas Health Science Center
San Antonio, Texas

Gail Varcelotti, BS, RRT, FAARC

Vice President, Ganésco, Inc.
Venetia, Pennsylvania

Tina Wellman, BA, RRT, CPFT

Senior Sales Consultant, Carefusion
Yorba Linda, California

Robert Whitman, PhD, D.ABSM, RRT, RPFT

Director, Sleep Disorders Center
Director, Pulmonary Diagnostics Services, Cardiopulmonary Rehab and Neorophychology
Adjunct Assistant Professor, Pulmonary Medicine
University of Kansas Medical Center
Kansas City, Kansas

Kathleen S. Wyka, AAS, CRT, AE-C

Respiratory Clinical Specialist
Anthem Health Services
Queensbury, New York

ABOUT THE AUTHORS

Kenneth A. Wyka, MS, RRT

Kenneth A. Wyka has been in the field of respiratory care since 1970. He obtained his bachelor's and master's degrees from Fairleigh Dickinson University in Teaneck, New Jersey, and formal training in respiratory care from the Lenox Hill Hospital School for Respiratory Therapy in New York City. In 1972, he founded the respiratory therapy program at Passaic County Community College in Paterson, New Jersey. Since then, he managed the respiratory care department at Valley Hospital in Ridgewood, New Jersey, was the director of respiratory clinical education at the University of Medicine & Dentistry of New Jersey, started several pulmonary rehabilitation programs, worked in home care, and began a health care/respiratory care consulting practice. He is the author of *Respiratory Care in Alternate Sites* and coauthor of *Oakes' Respiratory Home Care: An On-Site Reference Guide.* In addition, he has been the president of both the New Jersey and New York Societies for Respiratory Care and has been actively involved in several voluntary health and professional organizations. Currently, Ken is the Center Manager and Respiratory Care Patient Coordinator for Anthem Health Services in Queensbury, New York.

Paul J. Mathews, PhD, RRT

Paul J. Mathews is associate professor of respiratory care, School of Allied Health; associate professor in physical therapy; and adjunct associate professor at the Center on Aging, University of Kansas. He received his respiratory therapy training at Yale–New Haven Medical Center in New Haven, Connecticut. He holds his undergraduate degree from Quinnipiac College, Hamden, Connecticut; a master of public administration degree from the University of Hartford in Connecticut; and EdS and PhD degrees from the University of Missouri in Kansas City, Missouri. He has published more than 160 articles in various national journals, has authored several books, serves on six editorial boards, and has lectured at many national and international meetings. In 1989, Dr. Mathews was president of the AARC, and, in 1990, he was selected for AARC Life Membership. He is also a Fellow of the American College of Critical Care Medicine and of the American College of Chest Physicians. Currently, he is a member of the New York Academy of Sciences and is listed in *Who's Who in America* and *Who's Who in the World.*

John Rutkowski, MPA, MBA, RRT

John Rutkowski is the director of Cardiopulmonary Services at Bergen Regional Medical Center in Paramus, New Jersey. He is also an adjunct assistant professor at the University of Medicine and Dentistry in Newark, New Jersey. His career in respiratory care includes over 40 years of clinical, managerial, and community outreach experience. He received his formal respiratory therapy training and certificate from St. Joseph Hospital School of Respiratory Therapy in Lancaster, Pennsylvania, along with an associate of science degree from York College of Pennsylvania. He has also earned an undergraduate degree in chemistry from Jersey City State College, a master of business administration from Fairleigh Dickinson University, and a master of public administration from Seton Hall University. In addition to his work as a respiratory therapist, he remains active in the American Association for Respiratory Care and its New Jersey affiliate. He has served as a board member and on many committees for the New Jersey Society for Respiratory Care, including president, and as the New Jersey representative to the AARC House of Delegates. He is a member of the American College of Healthcare Executives and its New Jersey affiliate, the Association of Healthcare Executives of New Jersey, and has earned the Fellow of the American College of Healthcare Executives (FACHE) credential. Throughout his career, he has been active in the American Lung Association. He is a member of the ALA's Nationwide Assembly, board member, and past chair of the American Lung Association in the Mid-Atlantic, advisory board member and past chair of the American Lung Association in New Jersey, and a member of the Pediatric/Adult Asthma Coalition of New Jersey.

HOW TO USE THIS TEXT

The following suggests how you can use the features of this text to gain competence and confidence in your respiratory care skills.

OBJECTIVES

Upon completion of this chapter, the reader should be able to:

- List the characteristics used to classify microorganisms.
- Describe disinfection and sterilization methods.
- Identify the beneficial roles of endogenous microflora.
- Describe the factors influencing bacterial growth.
- Identify human defenses against infectious diseases.
- Discuss infectious diseases of the respiratory system.

Objectives

Read this list before starting the chapter so that you are prepared for the material that will be presented. Ask yourself which goals you are already familiar with and which will require more investment on your part to master.

CHAPTER OUTLINE

Scope of a Profession
- Self-Regulation
- Union Status
- Discrete Body of Knowledge
- Patient Status
- Educational Requirements
- Historical Agreement on Professional Status

Respiratory Care as a Profession

History
- Early Foundations
- Twentieth-Century Developments

The Organizing of the Profession
- A National Professional Association
- The Late 1950s and the 1960s: Organizational and Clinical Maturation

Formal Education System
- Joint Review Committee for Inhalation Therapy Education
- American Registry for Inhalation Therapy

Certified Inhalation Therapy Technicians
- The 1970s: Growth and Unrest
- The 1980s: Change in Many Areas

Chapter Outlines

These outlines serve as your reference guide to reviewing material.

KEY TERMS

acute respiratory distress syndrome (ARDS)
anthrax
blast lung injury (BLI)
blast overpressure injuries
bronchopleural fistula
cidofovir
coccidioidomycosis
cytokine storm
Diplopia
disseminated intravascular coagulopathy (DIC)
dumbbells
high-order explosion (HE)
hospital emergency incident command system (HEICS)
incident command system (ICS)
interferon
interleuken-6, 7, 8
lewisite
live attenuated vaccine (LAV)
low-order explosion (LE)
mass casualty incident (MCI)
MetHb
multidrug-resistant tuberculosis (MDRTB)
Pirfenidone
primary blast injury
quaternary blast injury
racemic epinephrine
ribavirin
secondary blast injury
self-contained breathing apparatus (SCBA)
self-evacuation
spalling
staphylococcal enterotoxin B (SEB)
systemic inflammatory response

Key Terms

Glance over this list and identify the terms you need to look up in the Glossary. Keep a running list of terms and check them off as you master their meaning.

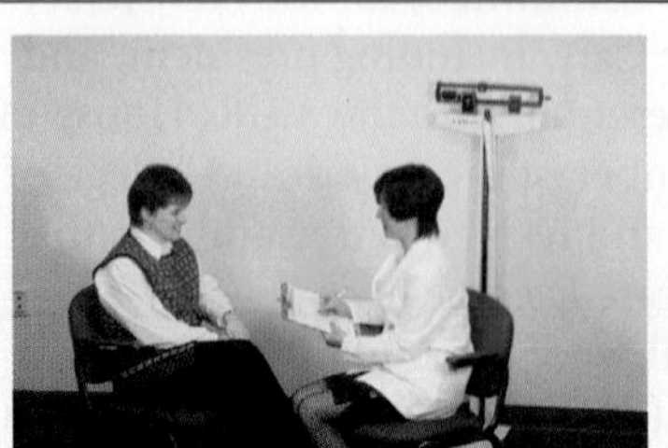

FIGURE 13-1 The patient interview.

final area, **intimate space** (less than $1^1/_2$ feet), is where the actual physical examination is performed.[2] The patient's privacy should be honored at all times.

In addition to space, other environmental factors influence the interview. Room lighting, noise, and temperature can be controlled to provide the best

CASE STUDY 13-1

William Smith is a 35-year-old male who has come to the clinic and who has been waiting for over 2 hours. Mr. Smith is finally called into a treatment room, and the practitioner enters to start the history and physical. As the practitioner enters the room, she observes an anxious Caucasian male sitting on a chair. The patient looks up as the practitioner approaches. (*Note:* Mr. Smith will be the patient throughout most of the chapter. For simplicity and clarity, the patient in the text will be assumed to be male, the practitioner female.)

Questions

1. How far away should the practitioner be when she makes her initial introduction?
2. When can the practitioner move into the room and enter the personal space?
3. What should the practitioner do to make the environment more comfortable for the patient?

Case Studies

Brief scenarios in selected chapters encourage you to approach situations with a critical eye and to assimilate the information presented in text. Use the related questions to apply the information you have learned in the chapter to actual clinical cases. Consider alternative solutions to the questions by discussing the cases with your classmates and colleagues.

Spotlight On

Pause when you come across one of these boxes and take time to research the innovation or therapy discussed. Search the Internet, visit the library, or ask your instructor for more information.

Spotlight On

The Logistics Service Branch of the ICS

- *Communication Unit.* Prepares and implements the Incident Communication Plan (ICS-205), distributes and maintains communications equipment, supervises the Incident Communications Center, and establishes adequate communications over the incident.
- *Medical Unit.* Develops the Medical Plan (ICS-206), provides first aid and light medical treatment for personnel assigned to the incident, and prepares procedures for a major medical emergency.

incident. The Unit orders, receives, stores, and distributes supplies, and services nonexpendable equipment. All resource orders are placed through the Supply Unit. The unit maintains inventory and accountability of supplies and equipment.

- *Facilities Unit.* Sets up and maintains required facilities to support the incident. Provides managers for the incident base and camps. Also responsible for facility security and facility maintenance services; sanitation,

Best Practices

In any profession, many helpful hints can help you perform more efficiently. The wide variety of hints, tips, and strategies presented here help you as you work toward professional advancement. Study, share, and discuss them with your colleagues.

Best Practice

In the Event of a Suit ...

During dispositions and court testimony, do *not* answer:

- Questions you do not understand.
- Compound questions.
- Questions with double negatives in them.

For each of these, ask the lawyer to simplify and restate the question.

Do not answer questions that were not asked. Answer only the question that was asked; do not expand on the answer. If the question can be

court) have a jury. Once the jury has been impaneled, the trial begins with the attorneys' opening statements, with the plaintiff's attorney leading. The opening statements outline the facts that the attorneys hope to establish in the trial process. The plaintiff has the burden of proving the case to the jury. The defendant does not have a burden of proof, has to prove nothing, and could, technically, remain silent. After each side has presented its case and cross-examined the witnesses, each is allowed time for a closing argument. After the closing argument, the judge instructs the jury of any applicable law and any presumptions the jury should consider in their deliberations. Then the jury is dismissed to deliberate. The trial usually ends with the verdict.

Age-Specific Competencies

After reading these boxes, ask yourself what other considerations would be appropriate when managing the care of patients at different ages. Make a list of approaches you could use when working with children or elderly people.

Age-Specific Competency

Preventing Injury and Death

Even more than for adults, for children, the key to minimizing injury and death is prevention.

- Because motor vehicle trauma causes nearly half of all pediatric injuries and deaths each year, it behooves adults to use appropriate restraints when children are in the car. Children should be buckled into an age-specific car seat that is properly fastened to the car. (Proper fastening of a child or infant seat may include a strap that fastens to the car floor.) They should
- Because drowning is a major cause of death in the younger population of children, adults should supervise these children closely when they are near water. Children should know how to swim and what to do in an emergency around water. Even such a seemingly innocuous "body" of water as a 2-gallon bucket can be fatal to the unsupervised child.
- Adults have the responsibility to minimize the danger from house fires, which result in the overwhelming majority of burns. Having

Summary

Read the summary. Then go back to the objectives and consider how well you have assimilated and understood the information in the chapter. Use the summary as a brief review when you study and prepare for an examination.

Summary

When transporting critically ill patients, safety is paramount. However, many patients are transported within or between health-care facilities because they are critically ill and need special services or procedures. The additional stress that may be imposed on such patients can be clinically challenging. However, through proper planning and execution and follow-up, these risks can be minimized. By following the procedures outlined in this chapter, including maintaining a state of readiness, properly prescreening patients, selecting the most appropriate means of transportation, and ensuring the proper personnel and equipment in

II. noise
III. motion
IV. temperature variations
a. I and II
b. I, II, III, and IV
c. I and IV
d. I, II, and III

4. It is recommended that all of the following equipment accompany all critically ill patients on transport, *except* which?
   a. oxygen source with sufficient duration of flow
   b. cardiac defibrillator
   c. manual resuscitator bag and mask
   d. cardiac pacemaker

Study Questions

After reading a chapter, read the study questions and identify areas in which you need to work on your understanding. Go back and reread those sections of the chapter; then answer the questions again until you are comfortable that you have grasped the material.

Study Questions

REVIEW QUESTIONS

1. List three major criticisms to the use of utilitarianism in making ethical decisions.
2. List four legal requirements for breaking patient confidentiality.
3. List three forms of intentional torts that a respiratory therapist might be involved with.
4. List three major criticisms to the use of Kantian ethics in making ethical decisions.
5. List and define the basic principles of health-care ethics.
6. List three major criticisms to the use of the divine command theory in making ethical decisions.
7. Define the basic function of normative ele-

c. retributive justice.
d. beneficence.

4. Informed consent flows mainly from the basic ethical principle of:
   a. autonomy.
   b. beneficence.
   c. justice.
   d. role duty.
5. In its best sense, paternalism is a contest between which of the following principles?
   a. autonomy and beneficence
   b. justice and role duty
   c. veracity and nonmaleficence.
   d. role duty and autonomy
6. Which of the following ethical decision-making formats is focused on the moral agent rather than on the decision?
   a. utilitarianism

HOW TO USE STUDYWARE™ TO ACCOMPANY *FOUNDATIONS OF RESPIRATORY CARE*, SECOND EDITION

The StudyWARE™ software helps you learn terms and concepts in *Foundations of Respiratory Care*, Second Edition. As you study each chapter in the text, be sure to explore the activities in the corresponding chapter in the software. Use StudyWARE™ as your own private tutor to help you learn the material in the textbook.

Getting started is easy. Install the software by downloading it to your computer's CD-ROM drive and following the on-screen instructions. To access the software, go to Cengagebrain.com, and log into your CengageBrain account. Search for the book by title, author, or ISBN. Click on the access now button for additional resources that accompany the book. When you open the software, enter your first and last name so that the software can store your quiz results. Then choose a chapter from the menu to take a quiz or explore one of the activities.

- **Menus.** You can access the menus from wherever you are in the program. The menus include quizzes and other activities.

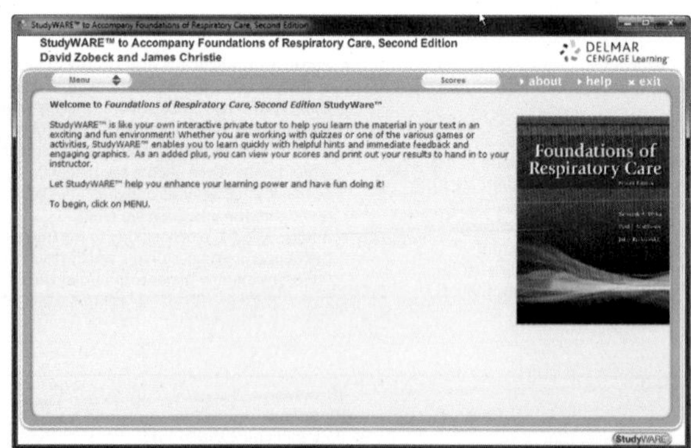

- **Quizzes.** Quizzes include multiple choice, true/false, word building, fill-in-the-blank, and case study questions. You can take the quizzes in practice or quiz mode. Use practice mode to improve your mastery of the material. You have multiple tries to get the answers correct. Instant feedback tells you whether you are right or wrong and helps you learn quickly by explaining why an answer was correct or incorrect. Use quiz mode when you are ready to test yourself and keep a record of your scores. In quiz mode, you have one try to get the answers right, but you can take each quiz as many times as you want.

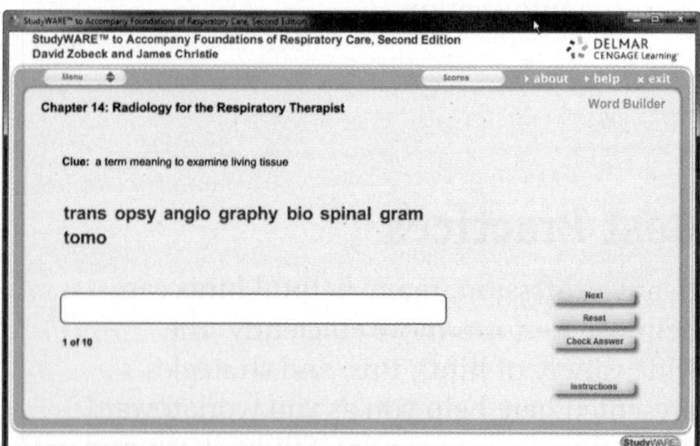

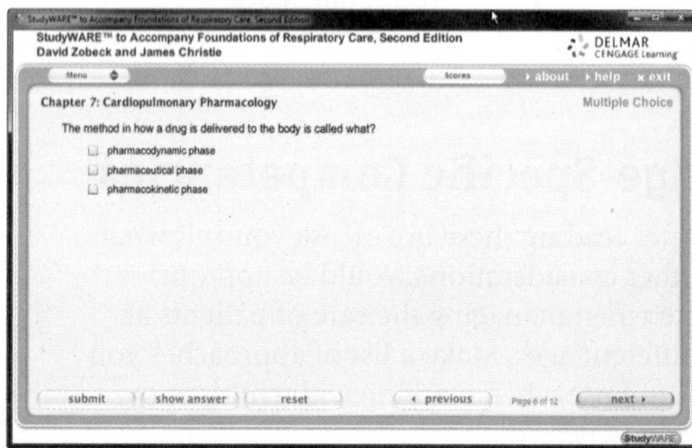

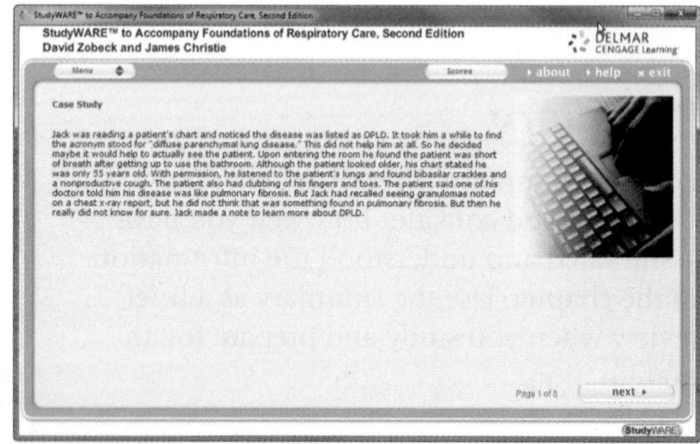

- **Scores.** You can view your last scores for each quiz and print your results to hand in to your instructor.

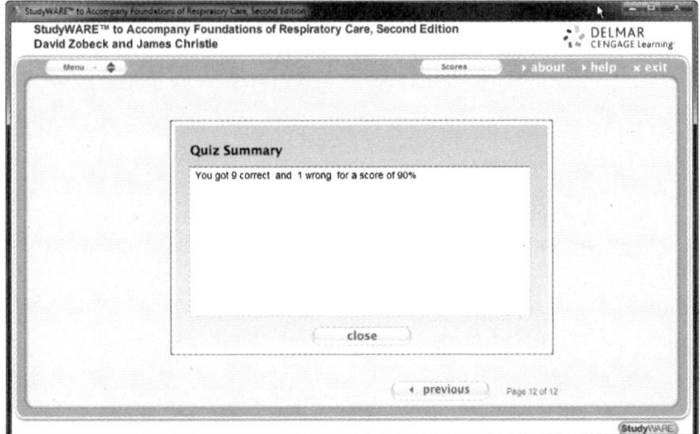

- **Activities.** Activities include hangman, concentration, and championship game. Have fun while increasing your knowledge!

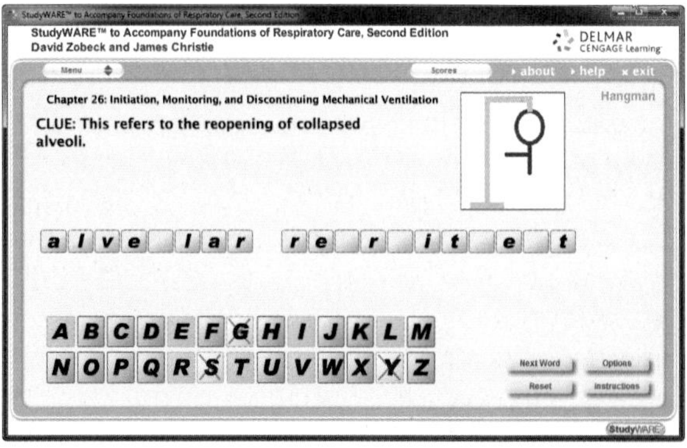

SECTION I

Scope of Practice

CHAPTER 1

The History and Scope of Respiratory Care

Raymond S. Edge and Paul J. Mathews

OBJECTIVES

Upon completion of this chapter, the reader should be able to:

- List the general criteria for a profession.
- Describe the contributions to the study of respiration made by the early foundational figures.
- Provide a synopsis of the pre–twentieth-century scientific foundations for respiratory care.
- Outline the contributions to the development of respiratory care provided by Thomas Beddoes, Joseph Priestley, and Robert Boyle.
- Provide a short, historical synopsis for the organizational development of the specialty, with attention to the AARC, CoARC, and NBRC.
- Identify and describe three of the "Allied" Professional Organizations who are aiding in advancing our professional status.
- Provide an analysis of the strengths of the allied health specialty and the challenges it will face in the twenty-first century.

CHAPTER OUTLINE

(continues)

(continued)

KEY TERMS

American Association for Respiratory Care (AARC)
Committee on Accreditation of Respiratory Care Programs (CoARC)
diagnosis-related group (DRG)
fee-for-service
FAARC
fellowship
fiduciary relationship
health care protocols
managed care
Medicaid
Medicare
National Board for Respiratory Care (NBRC)
outcome-oriented essentials
phlogiston theory
Pneumatic Institute
process-oriented essentials
product-oriented essentials
prospective payment system (PPS)
respiratory care practitioner
respiratory therapist
scope of practice
Sugarloaf Conference

This chapter addresses respiratory care's status as a profession and explores its development, history, and related organizations. Anyone launching a career as a **respiratory therapist** or **respiratory care practitioner** will find it helpful to understand the history of the profession. Knowing its historical foundations and place among the medical professions enables the entrant to better appreciate why training and certain skill sets are required to become a respiratory care practitioner.

Scope of a Profession

Any working person can function professionally. For example, we might comment that, "Our hair stylist is a real professional" or "The salesperson was very professional." Using the term "professional" in this sense is a reference to a person's work attributes, such as being knowledgeable and competent, showing up on time, providing fair prices, honoring one's word, providing good service, and having appropriate attitudes or exceptional skills. No one needs to be a member of a profession to function as a professional. The term "professional," used in this generic sense, describes an individual's personal work attributes and is very value laden.

However, the terms "profession" and "professional" are also used more discriminately to describe certain occupations and those who work in them. The individuals in many careers are considered professionals—physicians, lawyers, educators, and the clergy. (Of course, physicians, lawyers, educators, and the clergy are not the only professionals, but they are the four whose professional nature enjoys a high level of agreement.) Other careers are not thought of as professions, such as sales, carpentry, cosmetology, and taxi driving. This distinction does not mean that some occupations are better than others or even that one group acts more professionally than another. Rather, it means only that there is a generally recognized difference between professions and occupations.

The question is, What distinguishes some specialties from occupations in general? Is there a way to examine occupations, such as nurse, respiratory care practitioner, or pharmacist, to determine whether they may be considered professions? What separates professions from other occupations? One answer is based on an examination of the common attributes of professions.

SELF-REGULATION

Professional groups regulate their members in accordance with criteria for ethical behavior and standards of practice. These groups thus often play an important gatekeeping function; that is, they determine who may enter the specialty and practice within it. Self-regulation is considered a major attribute of a profession and a special obligation of its practitioners. Most professions hold their members to a code of ethical conduct. Typically, the relationship of professionals with their clients is based on trust, and they are held to a higher standard of behavior than in those who work in nonprofessional fields.

UNION STATUS

Unions serve their individual members whereas professional organizations serve the profession as a whole. Professional organizations concern themselves with such issues as standards of practice, the education of their members, service to the community, the maintenance and expansion of the body of knowledge, communication with government and other professional groups, and the mentoring of new practitioners. They generally do not take on the personal bread-and-butter concerns, such as working conditions and wages. However, in recent years, some professional groups, such as teachers and physicians, have begun to organize into true unions. So it is difficult to know whether neutrality on working conditions and wages will remain a distinctive feature of professional groups in the future.

DISCRETE BODY OF KNOWLEDGE

Medicine, education, law, and theology have discrete bodies of knowledge that other specialists or the lay public generally do not possess. Professionals often use terms and language—jargon—not commonly used by those outside the profession that may be confusing to the general public. Students of respiratory therapy learn not only the science and art of respiratory care but also its specialized language, most of which (but not all) is shared with fellow health care professionals. Advanced higher education and years of internships are often required to master the subject area.

In addition to a common language, colleagues in other health care professions also share much of the same knowledge base and skills sets. Even though the depth and breadth of these shared attributes vary, all health care practitioners have much in common. The variations in learning and experience are valuable to the overall quality of patient care because the different perspectives provide an enriched inventory of knowledge to draw on.

An interesting feature of a profession's body of knowledge is that it is directed toward doing away with the need for the practice. The practice of medicine is directed toward ending disease, the practice of law is directed toward ending injustice, and the practice of theology is presumably directed toward creating an ethical society. At the moment, no profession has managed to achieve its chief aim of ending society's need for its services, and none is likely to do so in the foreseeable future. Yet, that remains the goal of most professions.

PATIENT STATUS

Those who work in sales and commerce often say, "The customer is always right." In a client- or patient-focused situation, individuals come to the professional for information that they do not possess or for skills and services they cannot provide for themselves. Of course though, the professional does not circumvent the autonomy of the individual. (In simple terms, *autonomy* [or self-determination] means that the individual has a right to make his or her own decisions.) However, the patient or client is not always right; the concept just does not suit the relationship. Instead, professionals are thought to be in a **fiduciary relationship** with those they serve. A fiduciary is a trustee, one who holds something in trust. The central feature of a fiduciary relationship is some form of duty. Once the health care provider establishes a relationship with the patient, the provider has a duty to offer a proper standard of care. In fact, the provider can be held liable for failure to provide service in accordance with the established standards of practice.

EDUCATIONAL REQUIREMENTS

Since professional work is predominately intellectual and varied in character—as opposed to routine mental, manual, mechanical, or physical labor—professionals often have to undergo extended periods of specialty education. The prolonged course of intellectual study usually takes place in a specialized institution of higher education or hospital, as distinguished from a general academic institution or apprenticeship. This can be seen especially clearly in law, medicine, and theology.

HISTORICAL AGREEMENT ON PROFESSIONAL STATUS

What qualifies occupations as professions is somewhat dependent on societal agreement. In other words, to some extent, some occupations are professions because people believe they are. For instance, nursing is often thought of as a profession, even though it may not have all the attributes commonly associated with professional groups. Yet, given the historical context and the social climate at the time of the American Civil War, most ordinary citizens would not have considered nursing a profession in 1865. Over the last 140 years, however, nursing has come to be held in much higher esteem by everyday people and is now often regarded as a profession.

Respiratory Care as a Profession

Can as much be said of respiratory care and its practitioners? Clearly, respiratory care practitioners act professionally, but are they members of a profession? The history and development of respiratory care furnish evidence that the field fulfills most of the criteria for being a profession. Respiratory care has a distinguished history and a professional organization;

it is self-regulating; and practitioners have a professional relationship with the people they serve. However, in the areas of a discrete body of knowledge, advanced education, and societal acceptance, the field needs further development to meet all the basic criteria for a profession.

In large measure, the issue of professionalism lies more in perception than it does in classical definitions. The professionalism of respiratory therapists is determined by how their colleagues "see" them, how their patients perceive them, and, most importantly, how they view themselves individually and collectively. To be "seen" as professionals, they must act as professionals.

History

Some professions are based on a singular event such as the development of a certain technology. Most professions, however, have an historical context and roots. Most people think of respiratory care as a modern profession with roots that extend back only to the 1940s, but it has foundations that extend back much further in time.

EARLY FOUNDATIONS

> "And the Lord God formed man from the dust of the ground, and breathed into his nostrils the breath of life; and man became a living soul..." (Genesis 2:7).

The Bible contains a vivid description of mouth-to-mouth resuscitation. In II Kings 4:34,

> Elisha breathes life into his son: "And he [Elisha] went up, and lay upon the child, and put his mouth upon his mouth, his eyes upon his eyes, and his hands upon his hands and he stretched himself upon the child, and the flesh of the child waxed warm."

This and other early references are evidence of respiratory therapy having its origin thousands of years ago (as early as 2697 BCE). Table 1-1 lists some important early figures in the development of the practice of respiratory therapy.

TABLE 1-1 **Early foundational figures**

Early Figure	Area of Origin
Huang Ti (reigned from 2697 BCE)	China
Hippocrates (460–377 BCE)	Greece
Aristotle (384–322 BCE)	Greece
Galen (131–201 CE)	Rome
Maimonides (1135–1204)	Arabia
Leonardo da Vinci (1452–1519)	Rome
William Harvey (1578–1657)	England
Robert Boyle (1627–1691)	England
Joseph Priestley (1733–1804)	England
Antoine Lavoisier (1743–1794)	France
Thomas Beddoes (1760–1808)	England
John Dalton (1766–1844)	England

Hippocrates (460–377 BCE) and Aristotle (384–322 BCE) are credited with adding to the early foundation of the understanding of respiratory physiology and the therapeutic use of oxygen. Hippocrates is rightly recorded as the father of Western medicine because he rejected much of the mysticism surrounding the medical thinking of his time and emphasized the importance of clinical observation. In his treatise "On Air, Minerals, Waters, and Places," Aristotle influenced the early thinking regarding the therapeutic use of the so-called vital spirit (air).[1] In this period, before the age of science, most people recognized that air was an important vital spirit, but no one understood its physical properties. Aristotle concluded that air was one of four elemental substances; the others were earth, water, and fire. He recorded some of the first studies showing the effects of oxygen deprivation on animals. Like most of his contemporaries, Aristotle misunderstood the nature of respiration, believing that it served the purpose of cooling the system. When he placed animals in airtight chambers and observed their deaths, he concluded that they had lost the ability to control body temperature because they could not breathe. This conclusion is somewhat understandable given that persons who are ill and die often have a fever as part of the process.

Perhaps the most influential successor to the Hippocratic framework of medical thinking was Galen (131–201 CE). He was a Greek physician who synthesized a system of medicine that dominated Western thinking for the next thousand years. Galen did foundational work in cardiac physiology and taught that blood leaving the right ventricle passed through the lungs and, in doing so, mixed with air, which formed a necessary "Vital Spirit." Unfortunately, the early Greek idea regarding respiration as essentially a mechanism for cooling the blood continued in his writings. Galen's observations and writings cover every aspect of medicine, and much of his thinking went unchallenged until the Renaissance.[2] His work essentially framed the discussion of medicine in the West for over a thousand years.

Huang Ti, the Yellow Emperor of China who began his reign about 2697 BCE, had a similar impact on Eastern medical thought. In the classic work *Nei Ching (The Yellow Emperor's Book of Internal Medicine)*, Huang Ti outlined the tenets of traditional Chinese medicine. The text provides a coherent system of health care, diagnostic methods, and therapeutic regimes, and it extensively covers pulmonary diseases such as asthma.

The thinking regarding preventive care in this manual of health care bears a striking similarity to modern Western thought. The text calls for the physician to maintain the patient's health rather than to cure disease, on the premise that waiting for an illness to occur is like forging weapons after the battle has begun or like digging the well after you are already thirsty. As Galen's work did in the West, the *Yellow Emperor's Book of Internal Medicine* tended to freeze the discussion of medicine in the East, and it is still influential in the current practice of traditional Chinese medicine.[3]

In the West, advancement in medical thinking during the Dark Ages often came from non-Western physicians such as Maimonides (1135–1204), who brought new thinking from the Arabic culture. Maimonides, a Jewish physician and philosopher, was appointed physician to the court of the Egyptian sultan. His writings, particularly *Regimen Sanitatis* and *Medical Aphorisms*, exerted great influence on European medicine.[4] The drawings and writings of Leonardo da Vinci (1452–1519) clearly indicate that, by the late 1400s, he had come to understand the true nature and function of respiration. However, perhaps as a matter of pragmatism, he chose not to resist the dogma of the time.[5]

A rebirth, or Renaissance, of medical science was soon to come. By the early 1500s, the task of finally dispelling the ancient dogma regarding human anatomy waited for Vesalius and Michael Servetus. They not only came to know the truth by their dissections and studies, but also taught it. Unfortunately, Servetus paid a heavy price for his heretical beliefs; he was burned at the stake on orders of John Calvin. Vesalius published his *De Fabrica Humani Corporis* in 1543, which put to rest many of the false dogmas regarding human body structure.[6]

The Galenic system of medicine, along with the view that respiration was a means of cooling the blood, was finally put to rest by William Harvey (1578–1657). In his *De Motu Cordis* (1628), Harvey demonstrated blood circulation through the heart and provided the first estimations for the volume of blood pumped through the vascular system. The book was influential in founding the modern principles of physiology.[7]

In 1660, the work of scientist Robert Boyle (1627–1691) added to the understanding of air and the process of respiration. Boyle built a primitive barometer for the prediction of weather and speculated that the processes of combustion and respiration are due to a substance in air. During this time, he created what is now called *Boyle's law*, which states that the volume of a gas decreases as pressure increases.[8]

The discovery of oxygen offers an interesting problem of credit. In the middle of the eighteenth century, despite Boyle's speculations, scientists still held that air was inert and that it did not take part in combustion. Most scientists of the day accepted an erroneous assumption, which held that burning materials released an invisible gas known as phlogiston, which was associated with heating and was known as the **phlogiston theory**.

Joseph Priestley (1733–1804), an English cleric, discovered that plants consumed a gas that was harmful to animals and gave off another that rendered the air capable of supporting animal life. In 1774, by concentrating the sun's rays through a magnifying glass, Priestley heated red mercuric oxide and produced oxygen. As a follower of phlogiston theory, which held that during combustion phlogiston (a gas) was given off, Priestley called his new gas "dephlogisticated air." After a clinical trial with mice, he emptied a container of oxygen, breathed it, and noted the following effects:

> My reader will not wonder that, having ascertained the superior goodness of dephlogisticated air by mice living in it, and the other tests above mentioned, I should have the curiosity to taste it myself. . . . I have gratified that curiosity by breathing it, drawing it through a glass siphon, and by this means I reduced a large jar full of it to the standard of common air. The feeling of it to my lungs was not sensibly different from that of common air, but I fancied that my breath felt peculiarly light and easy for some time afterwards. Who can tell but that in time this pure air may become a fashionable article of luxury? Hitherto, only two mice and myself have had the privilege of breathing it.[9]

French chemist Antoine Lavoisier (1743–1794) duplicated Priestley's early experiments and thought that he had isolated pure air. Lavoisier later concluded that he had separated only a component of air but that it came into existence when air was heated. He named the gas *oxygen*, meaning "acid-maker." Lavoisier correctly described the basic physiology of respiration and demonstrated that the lungs absorb oxygen and that water and carbon dioxide are given off during exhalation.[10]

At approximately the same time as the work of Priestley and Lavoisier, Swedish scientist Carl Scheele (1742–1786 AD) had also been working on oxygen, isolating it from saltpeter. Although he had completed his studies earlier than Priestley or Lavoisier, he published his results in the treatise *Air and Fire* (1781)—after they had published their results—and has been given very little credit for his discoveries, proving once again that publication in science, like timing in investments, is everything.

Who should be given the credit for the discovery of oxygen? Priestley isolated oxygen but did not know what he had; Lavoisier understood that oxygen was a component of air and gave it its name, but he did not quite understand its nature. Scheele may have been first to isolate the gas but published his works only after others had received the credit. Maybe the credit belongs to none of them because oxygen could not truly be understood using the science of the day.

In this light, perhaps the credit should go to the British chemist and physicist John Dalton (1766–1844 AD), who, in his formulation of the atomic theory of matter, placed the final piece into the oxygen puzzle.

Thomas Beddoes (1760–1808), who established the **Pneumatic Institute** of Bristol, England, is credited with the first therapeutic use of oxygen. In the Institute, Beddoes and his colleagues used primitive oxygen masks made of oiled silk rags to treat heart disease, leprosy, asthma, opium addiction, venereal disease, and dyspnea. Although oxygen has no therapeutic effect on many of the diseases on which it was tried at the Institute, Beddoes is often referred to as the father of respiratory therapy because he was the first to use oxygen therapeutically.[11]

During the 1800s, several clinical attempts were made to use oxygen under ambient and positive pressure to effect some health benefit. In 1878, M. J. Oertel, using air compressed by 1/50 of an atmosphere to 775.2 mm Hg, was the first to try using positive pressure to treat asthma. In 1897, N. R. Norton attempted to treat acute pulmonary edema caused by carbolic acid poisoning with oxygen under positive pressure. Although these attempts were innovative and advanced for the time, truly therapeutic uses of oxygen required the technological advances of the 1900s.[10]

TWENTIETH-CENTURY DEVELOPMENTS

The development of the knowledge and technical base for respiratory therapy in the twentieth century can be divided roughly into halves. The first half is filled with scientists whose names all practitioners memorize as part of the principles and equations that are fundamental to our practices: Sir William Arbuthnot-Lane (1856–1943), Jack Emerson (1906–1997), Donald Dexter (1881–1973), Sir George Gabriel Stokes (1819–1903), and John Scott Haldane (1860–1936), to name a few. An important development of the period was that of Karl Von Linde (1842–1934), whose 1901 large-scale, commercial application of fractional distillation made compressed oxygen available in amounts suitable for large-scale use. Table 1-2 provides a chronology of other important clinical and research developments during the twentieth century.

The Early 1900s. The first half of the twentieth century is a fascinating period in which scientist-clinicians made the first serious attempts at mechanical ventilation. Heinrich Drager's portable pulmotor device allowed for resuscitation, and the 1909 Emerson pressure ventilator showed the efficacy of positive pressure in reducing pulmonary edema in rabbits.[13]

This same period saw a number of attempts to use oxygen therapeutically. Oxygen rooms and even hotels were established that had greater-than-ambient pressure. These rooms were very difficult to control, and, given the potential for fire, they were quickly replaced by smaller tents. There is a story about the eminent scientist Haldane, who entered an oxygen room after putting the pipe he was smoking into his pocket. The

TABLE 1-2 **Twentieth-century chronology**

Lane (1907)	Advised the use of oxygen via nasal catheter
Emerson (1909)	Demonstrated that artificial ventilation could successfully treat pulmonary edema in rabbits
Stokes (1917)	Reintroduced the idea that oxygen could be administered by nasal catheter
Haldane (1917)	Developed an oxygen mask for the treatment of pulmonary edema
Hill (1920)	Developed the first oxygen tent
Barcroft (1920)	Built the first oxygen chamber (in England) and created the oxygen deficiency classifications anoxic, anemic, and stagnant
Van Slyke (1931)	Added to the three Barcroft classifications a fourth type, histotoxic
Barach (1926)	Improved the oxygen tent by controlling heat and moisture buildup
Drinker and Shaw (1929)	Developed the first iron lung device, in which the patient's head extended from the ventilator
Boothby, Lovelace, and Bullbullion (1938)	Developed the BLB mask; Boothby established the use of oxygen postoperatively for bronchopneumonia

increased oxygen concentration and pressure restored his tobacco to a flame, and, as one can imagine, he quickly left the chamber.[14] Other early attempts at the use of therapeutic oxygen were Lane's 1907 advocacy for the administration of ambient oxygen through the nasal catheter and its introduction into the United States in 1931 by Waters and Wineland.[10]

Lawrence Joseph Henderson did preliminary work on blood gas analysis and delineated the basic relationships used in the acid-base studies used today.[14] Although World War I interrupted much of the research on pulmonary physiology, the war effort itself was a stimulus for developing additional modes of oxygen therapy to handle patients injured in poison gas attacks. During this period, tracheal intubation was begun, and masks to treat pulmonary edema were developed. There is little indication that any effective efforts were made toward positive pressure ventilation during World War I.

After the war, experiments in animal ventilation continued in American and British laboratories, with a great sharing of ideas and theories. Sir John Barcroft in England and Leonard Hill in the United States developed oxygen tents to treat edema, but these early tents had serious problems. Without a system for the control of humidity and temperature, they were incredibly uncomfortable.[14]

The first half of the twentieth century was a time of seminal scientific and clinical research. During this period, masks, catheters, tents, and basic ventilators—albeit crude—were first developed. However, to become a modern field of study, respiratory therapy needed to wait for the technological and therapeutic advances that followed World War II.

The 1940s and 1950s: Early Clinical and Organizational Growth. One of the important pioneers of the profession was Dr. Alvin Barach. His work in devising low-flow oxygen devices, nonrebreathing masks, and a postoperative device known as the *Cof-a-lator*, which simulated deep breathing and a cough, turned many of the early ideas of the first half of the twentieth century into practical therapeutic realities. In 1944, Barach authored the first textbook for what was then known as *inhalation therapy*.[12] Other pioneers whose clinical work extended into the second half of the century were Drinker and Shaw, who in 1929 modified the oxygen chamber into what was to become the iron lung. These devices were later to become the standard for treating polio patients during the epidemics of the 1940s and 1950s.[10]

World War II brought several important technological advances that were rapidly applied to medicine in the postwar period. Manufacturers that had developed oxygen systems and masks for the war effort quickly made the transition to a postwar economy and made these devices available for treatment and research. There had also been much war-related research into the measurement and recording of venous and arterial saturation and pressures and of pulmonary function through the use of spirometry. This knowledge quickly found its way into clinical practice.

One singularly important clinical practice that developed in the postwar period was intermittent positive pressure breathing (IPPB). After World War II, a simple valve that had been designed at the University of Southern California was redesigned as a device that allowed for the provision of positive pressure during inspiration and expiration to the atmosphere. This valve, which took the name of its engineer designer (V. Ray Bennett), became the basic equipment for providing intermittent positive pressure breathing treatments. Shortly after the commercial arrival of the Bennett IPPB device, Forrest M. Bird, MD, PhD, ScD (1921–) developed a series of devices (Bird Machines) that allowed for intermittent positive pressure breathing as well as for ventilation during anesthesia.[10]

The increased usage of oxygen and other types of modified atmosphere, as well as the rapid advances in new technologies and therapeutics, quickly went beyond the basic training of the nurse. Before long, a new technician was working at the bedside. At first, the new technicians were orderlies dispatched from central supply or maintenance to deliver the heavy oxygen cylinders to the patients' rooms and to put ice in the tent chambers. Often these orderlies were responsible for diverse tasks, such as oxygen therapy and orthopedic traction. Because their work was most closely associated with the delivery of oxygen, however, they became known as *oxygen orderlies*.

The physicians and nurses using the services of the oxygen orderlies were not particularly knowledgeable about the equipment. As a result, the on-the-job-trained orderlies who delivered, took down, cleaned, and repaired the equipment soon became the experts. They were assisted in becoming the experts by the commercial companies, such as Linde and Bennett, that would often provide classes, seminars, films, and handbooks on the use of the equipment. The new technicians began to see themselves as unique and separate from the other hospital orderlies and began to meet with other local technicians to share information about new practices.

The reliance of physicians on the technicians' understanding of the equipment formed strong professional bonds between the two groups. Many physicians gave of their time and knowledge to further the education of this new group of specialists. This generosity actually enlightened self-interest because the time spent by the physicians in educating the technicians translated into better care and improved bedside therapeutics for their patients.

The Organizing of the Profession

The close bond between physicians and technicians has been a hallmark of the field of respiratory therapy. Since its beginnings, the profession has had the recognition and support from the American Society of Anesthesiologists (ASA), the American Thoracic Society (ATS), and the American College of Chest Physicians (ACCP). Over time, these close associations proved to be a great strength for the developing allied health profession.

The growth of the early technician groups was uneven. There were small groups throughout the United States, with significant growth throughout California and in Chicago, Miami, Washington, D.C., and New York City. In Chicago, three exceptional physicians—Drs. Edwin Levine, Max Sadove, and Al Andrews—supported the technician groups. Recognizing that the orderly status of the technicians was not in keeping with the clinical requirements of their role, these physicians began to meet regularly with the Chicago technician group and to elevate their education from the bedside to the classroom.

In the mid-1940s, the technicians' groups in the various centers began to form organizations. The Miami group formed the Florida Inhalation Therapy Association. The Washington, D.C., group formed the American Society of Inhalation Therapy. However, the Chicago group formed the organization that was to evolve into the **American Association for Respiratory Care (AARC)** (Figure 1-1).[12]

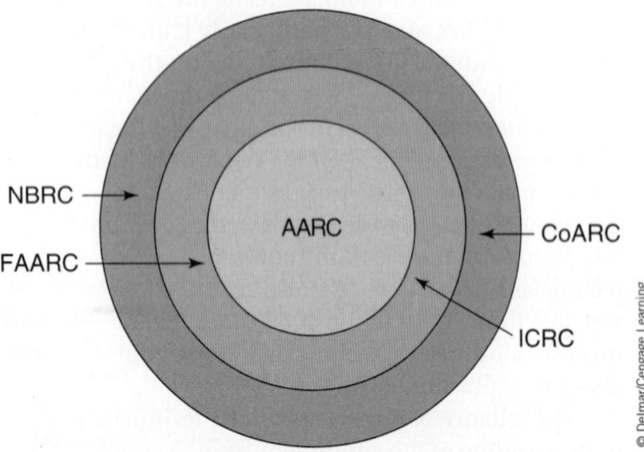

FIGURE 1-1 The AARC and its related organizations. Green entities are subsidiary organizations. Red entities are independent organizations that are closely related to the AARC and provide professional credentialing (NBRC) or program accreditation.

In 1947, the Inhalational Therapy Association (ITA) was established as an incorporated entity in the state of Illinois, with 59 members. George A. Kneeland, from the University of Chicago Hospitals, served as chair for the new organization, and Drs. Levine, Andrews, and Sadove served as medical advisers. The charter of the ITA clearly established it as a professional organization. Its goals were far-reaching and ambitious. It called on its members to:

- Promote high standards in methods and the professional advancement of association members.
- Create mutual understanding and cooperation among the technician, the physician, and all others who were employed in the interest of individual and public health through the Tri-State Hospital Assembly.
- Advance the knowledge of inhalation therapy through institutes, lectures, and other means given under the sponsorship of doctors of the American Society of Anesthesiologists and to grant certificates of qualification to individuals who successfully complete the prescribed requirements.[12]

The fledgling ITA continued to plan local seminars and institutes for the technician group. In 1948 the organization changed its name to the Inhalation Therapy Association, and George Kneeland was elected its president.

A NATIONAL PROFESSIONAL ASSOCIATION

In 1950, the Inhalation Therapy Association sponsored its first annual convention and began to publish its first newsletter, known as *Bulletin*. In 1953 the association again changed its name, this time to the American Association of Inhalation Therapy (AAIT). In 1955 the organization, which had by this time grown to 177 members, established a national office and employed Albert Carriere as its first executive director. Carriere provided dynamic managerial leadership to the organization, assisting in the establishment of local chapters across the nation.

In 1955, the *Bulletin* was revised in format and style and was published as the *AAIT Bulletin*, a name that continued in use until 1977, when the association began publication of the *AARC Times*.[10] The first editor of the *AAIT Bulletin* was James Whitacre, a distinguished early educator.[12] By 1956, the association had two publications. In addition to the *AAIT Bulletin*, a new scientific journal, known as *Inhalation Therapy*, was the forerunner to the current *Journal of Respiratory Care*.

Over time, the demand for services across the country was broadened to include such services as the administration of aerosolized medications, oxygen, carbon dioxide–oxygen mixtures, helium-oxygen mixtures, iron lungs, and intermittent positive pressure breathing and Cof-a-lator treatments. In 1953, Drs. Motley and Smart published an article describing a series of cases in which patients were treated with intermittent positive pressure breathing (IPPB). IPPB treatments, with or without bronchodilators (medications that increase the size of narrowed airways in the lungs), were given to asthma patients, patients suffering with chronic obstructive pulmonary disease (COPD), and preoperative and postoperative patients.[14] The demand for these services became such that specialty departments were established to facilitate the delivery of the services, and the oxygen orderlies became generally known as *inhalation therapists*. Although the overuse of IPPB was eventually to become an embarrassment to the profession, IPPB devices could be seen throughout most hospitals in the United States in the late 1950s and 1960s.

THE LATE 1950s AND THE 1960s: ORGANIZATIONAL AND CLINICAL MATURATION

Respiratory therapy started coming together as a discrete profession in the late 1950s. In 1957, the American Society of Anesthesiologists (ASA) began its official sponsorship of the AAIT. The ASA medical advisers to the AAIT were Drs. Vincent Collins, Edwin Emma, and Meyer Saklad. By 1958, the AAIT had grown to 600 members. It had two professional publications, it held a national convention, and it was sponsored and supported by physician groups. Inhalation therapy was becoming an important revenue center in hospitals and clinics. Perhaps most importantly, the AAIT's growing membership was young, hard-driving, creative, and eager to improve their education.

It was apparent early on that the training could not remain at the on-the-job level. The therapists were being called on to perform tasks well above their training level. Often the least trained technicians could be found on the evening and weekend shifts, when there was also the least supervision. Most of the training programs were hospital based. Although some were doing an excellent job in preparing practitioners, other programs were designed to acquire free labor under the guise of an educational program. The new field had a perplexing incongruence: Although the inhalation therapists dealt with some of the most critical medical situations, they often had the least formal education.

Formal Education System

In recognition of these problems, Emma and Collins began to work toward the development of legitimate schools of inhalation therapy. In April 1956, "Essentials of an Acceptable School of Inhalation Therapy Technicians" was published in the *New York State Journal of Medicine* and later reprinted in the August 1956 edition of the *AAIT Journal*. The so-called essentials were offered in the form of a recommendation to hospitals wishing to start training programs.[5]

In 1963, representatives from the American Medical Association (AMA), Council on Medical Education (CME), the American College of Chest Physicians (ACCP), the American Registry for Inhalation Therapy (ARIT), and the American Society of Anesthesiologists (ASA) came together in the Chicago headquarters of the AMA to create a Board of Schools for the new field. The board was to function under the AMA Council on Medical Education. In 1964, the Board of Schools, which later was renamed the Joint Review Committee for Inhalation Therapy Education (JRCITE), began its first site visits to evaluate inhalation therapy educational programs. The establishment of the AMA-sponsored accreditation process was an important step in the creation of the profession. Not only did it elevate the programmatic requirements and thus weed out the poor and exploitative programs, but it also legitimized the field with AMA's recognition of inhalation therapy as a true allied health occupation.

JOINT REVIEW COMMITTEE FOR INHALATION THERAPY EDUCATION

The Joint Review Committee for Inhalation Therapy Education played an important part in the development of the profession. Each approved program had to comply with the essentials, which were the general lists of processes and inputs that had been deemed necessary for the education of clinicians. Only graduates of approved programs could gain access to the specialty credentialing system (see "American Registry for Inhalation Therapy").

As the field developed, the essentials evolved, and the programs were moved from hospitals to academic institutions. The early essentials were process oriented, and programs were approved on the basis of such things as the types of equipment available, the books available, the level of medical support, and the types and numbers of classes. A real problem with **process-oriented essentials** (evaluation measures based on how things are accomplished) was justifying what was required: For example, are 50 books too many? Are 49 too few? Are they the right ones? In retrospect, these processes clearly were not appropriate criteria for judging the quality of the educational programs.

However, they did and still do have roles in terms of available resources.

Beginning in 1980, the Joint Review Committee began to question the validity of the old process-oriented essentials and to plan for new **product-oriented essentials** (evaluation measures based on the quality of the product—in this case, program graduates). The new essentials could also be described as **outcome-oriented essentials** (measures of the attainment of stated goals). A program would determine its goals and then give evidence that it was attaining them. Rather than allowing the essentials to determine what was necessary, the programs would be justified based on how well they achieved their goals. Compared to process-oriented essentials, outcome-oriented essentials are clearly more in the mainstream of modern programmatic evaluation and fairer to the programs.

However, the importance of passing Joint Review accreditation would seem to be a powerful incentive for educators to be modest in setting their programs' goals. Whether the new essentials will have a flattening effect on innovation in respiratory therapy education is yet to be determined. Nevertheless, the emergence of Web-based curricula, problem-based learning, and online outreach programs are all reasons to be optimistic that creativity and innovation will remain strong attributes of respiratory care education programs.

As of January 2011, there were 10 level-100 (entry-level) programs and 362 level-200 advanced practice (AS/AA, BS, or master's) programs, for a total of 372 accredited RC/RT programs in the United States. Of the advanced-level programs, 306 were at the associates level, 53 were at the BS level, and 3 were at the master's degree level. Of the 10 100-entry level programs, 6 were stand-alone programs with no affiliation with an institution of higher learning (community or 4-year colleges or universities). By 2012, five of the six stand-alones will have completed affiliation agreements with colleges or universities, and one has started the process to voluntarily withdraw its CoARC accreditation. The net effect of these moves is that all RC programs will be capable of offering two years of CoA RC education.

AMERICAN REGISTRY FOR INHALATION THERAPY

Concurrent with the development of AMA-approved schools for inhalation therapy was the start-up of a credentialing system to provide recognition for qualified inhalation therapists. The autumn 1959 *AAIT Bulletin* announced the development of a constitution and bylaws for a nonprofit corporation that would be created for registering individual practitioners.[12] The organizational meeting for the American Registry for Inhalation Therapy (ARIT) took place in November 1960, and 12 individuals successfully completed the examinations. Because the ARIT did not complete incorporation until January 1961, the new therapists did not officially receive their titles until the second examination, which took place in April 1961.

The first examination process consisted of two components, an objective written examination and an oral examination. The successful completion of both exams was required to obtain the coveted credential of American Registered Inhalation Therapist (ARIT), now called Registered Respiratory Therapist (RRT).

The written examination tested basic knowledge in areas such as gas laws, history, oxygen therapy theory, and infection control. The more controversial of the two test segments was the oral exam, which was divided into two tests. Usually, a physician in one room and a therapist team in another room administered the oral tests. In the physician's room, the candidate was questioned in areas concerning theoretical and professional matters. In the therapist team's room, the emphasis was on practical equipment matters; the candidate was asked to identify and troubleshoot equipment. The rationale for the orals was that, in the clinic, the candidates were not going to face multiple-choice situations and given time to ponder their answers. Rather, they would be required to function under pressure and to make quick decisions. The orals therefore provided a means of simulating the conditions under which the therapists would actually practice.

Oral Exams. The oral examination system was at first under the direction of Dr. Meyer Saklad, who worked to overcome the inevitable criticism of subjective examinations. After the death of Dr. Saklad, Dr. Robert Lawrence became the director and continued in that role until the orals were discontinued in 1978. Despite the tireless efforts of Drs. Lawrence and Saklad to make the oral examinations fair, the system was inherently flawed: The bar was not at the same level for all the candidates. Certain examiners were tough; others were lax. Thus, becoming registered in the profession was a matter of the luck of the draw. Ironically, the last oral examinations were given in November 1978 in Las Vegas.[12]

The orals hold an interesting place in the hearts and minds of those who went through them. In a sense, they became a badge of honor for the therapists who shared the not-altogether-pleasant experience. Therapist gatherings were often and still are peppered with stories of the orals, each more striking than the last.

Clinical Simulation Exam. The orals were finally replaced by a written clinical simulation, which resolved the inherent problem of unevenness in the oral testing system. The shift away from oral examinations enabled the Registry to review an essentially unlimited number of candidates each year. In its initiating trial in June 1979, the clinical examination was given to 3176 candidates—over six times the number of candidates who could be accommodated by the orals.

Certified Inhalation Therapy Technicians

In the early to mid-1960s, registered inhalation therapists were in short supply. The job market was in such a state of growth that therapists could move from position to position. They could pick the state, the city, and in many cases even the hospital they wanted. To fill the need for trained personnel, in September 1968, the AAIT announced the appointment of a committee for the establishment of a second level in the field: certified inhalation therapy technician (CITT), now called certified respiratory therapist (CRT). A pilot examination was provided for 99 candidates for the new certification at the annual meeting held in Kansas City in 1969.[14]

The recognition of certified inhalation therapy technicians (CITTs) was very successful in meeting the clinical needs for more practitioners. These practitioners graduated from programs that were about half the length of those for registered therapists. The CITTs, along with practitioners graduating from nontraditional, entry-level (correspondence) programs, quickly filled the available positions.

In 1974 the AART's Technician Certification Examination, and the ARIT's Registry examination were placed under a single credentialing entity: the National Board for Respiratory Therapy (NBRT), later renamed the **National Board for Respiratory Care (NBRC)**.

A problem associated with the establishment of certified inhalation therapy technicians was how to differentiate technicians from registered inhalation therapists in the clinics. One of the tasks accepted by the NBRC was to perform a national job analysis to identify the specific job tasks that were expected of the entry-level practitioners. The job analysis identified two distinct levels of practice. Compared to entry-level (certified technicians) staff, advanced practitioners (registered therapists) were expected to handle a different set of tasks, to have a more in-depth and diversified knowledge base, and to operate at a higher level of complexity and with less supervision.

Although it was easy to make such distinctions and even to write up a listing of job duties, the reality remains that whoever is on duty at the time is expected to do everything. Small clinical units could not afford to hire two sets of practitioners, and, given the difference in salary, the standard became entry level. Often, the two levels of qualifications became meaningless in the clinics, and in times of cost containment clinical units began to find the lower-paid, entry-level practitioners preferable.

THE 1970s: GROWTH AND UNREST

The AAIT entered the 1970s in a high-growth mode. Membership grew from 5147 members in 1969 to 7934 members in 1970. By 1975, the membership was 23,448. As of 2009, membership exceeded 47,000. During this high-growth period, strains appeared between the allied health practitioners and their physician supporters. As the field grew and the AAIT matured, the therapists' views began to diverge from and in some areas conflict with those of many of the supporting physicians, who had come to feel almost as if they owned the specialty.

These conflicts were unfortunate; physicians had played and continue to play an important role in the development of the specialty. By the 1970s, the needs and views of the physician groups were not always congruent with those of respiratory therapists in such areas as licensure, accreditation, and federal policy. Yet, even in the turbulent 1970s, physician colleagues lent remarkable support in helping respiratory care escape from some of the more stringent federal regulations directed toward hospital cost containment.

In the mid-1970s the National Heart and Lung Institute (NHLI) and the American Thoracic Society (ATS) cosponsored a conference on the scientific basis for respiratory therapy.[15] The meeting became known as the **Sugarloaf Conference**, after its meeting place in Philadelphia. Although the findings of the conference took several years to be felt, they were to have a profound effect on the types of therapy provided. By the mid-1980s the IPPB devices, which had been a standard for the profession, were generally replaced by volume-oriented postoperative devices.

THE 1980s: CHANGE IN MANY AREAS

Major advances in respiratory care in the 1980s were found in intensive care units, where the greater understanding of cardiopulmonary pathophysiology was matched by improved technologies for monitoring and supporting the systems. The 1980s saw the pneumatically controlled equipment evolve into microprocessor-controlled ventilators, monitoring systems, and diagnostic instruments such as blood gas analyzers. (See Chapters 16–19.)

To provide a comprehensive overview about a dynamic aspect of pulmonary physiology, pulmonary medicine, or clinical respiratory care, the AARC Program

TABLE 1-3 **Donald F. Egan Scientific Lectures**

1974	John F. Murray, MD: "Oxygen Transport: New Concepts, New Problems"
1975	Lynne Reid, MD: "New Perspectives in Pulmonary Hypertension"
1976	David Bates, MD: "Early Detection of Airway Obstruction"
1977	George Burton, MD: "How to Succeed in Respiratory Therapy by Really Trying"
1978	John Hedley-Whyte, MD: "Ventilatory Care"
1979	Albert Fishman, MD: "Changing Concepts of Pulmonary Edema and the Respiratory Distress Syndrome"
1980	Alan Pierce, MD: "Respiratory Therapy, State of the Art"
1981	John Severinghaus, MD: "Transcutaneous PO_2 and PCO_2 Monitoring"
1982	Reuben Cherniack, MD: "Pitfalls in Pulmonary Function Testing"
1983	Roger Bone, MD: "Adult Respiratory Distress Syndrome: Treatment in the Next Decade"
1984	Thomas Petty, MD: "Pulmonary Rehabilitation: Better Living with New Techniques"
1985	Irwin Ziment, MD: "Five Thousand Years of Attacking Asthma"
1986	Ronald Harrison, MD: "Ventilatory Support Techniques: A Resource for Discovery"
1987	David Dankzker, MD: "PEEP and Oxygen Consumption: Is O2 Delivery Really Our Goal?"
1988	John West, MD: "Severe Hypoxia: Lessons from High Altitude"
1989	Leonard Hudson, MD: "The Prediction and Prevention of ARDS"
1990	Mary Ellen Avery, MD: "Twenty-Five Years of Progress in Hyaline Membrane Disease"
1991	E. Regis McFadden Jr., MD: "Fatal Asthma"
1992	John Marini, MD: "Patient-Ventilatory Interaction: Rational Strategies for Acute Ventilatory Management"
1993	Lee Reichman, MD: "Tuberculosis: An Old Enemy Back"
1994	C. James Carrico, MD: "The Trauma Patient: Our Responsibilities in the ICU and in Society"
1995	Jerome Modell, MD: "What Have We Learned About Lung Injury from the Management of Near Drowning?"
1996	Luciano Gattinoni, MD: "How Does PEEP Work?"
1997	William Sibbaid, MD: "The Whys and Wherefores of Measuring Outcomes in Respiratory Critical Care"
1998	Gordon Bernard, MD: "ARDS: New Approaches to a Serious Respiratory Illness"
1999	Martin J. Tobin, MD: "Weaning from Mechanical Ventilation: What Have We Learned?"
2000	James K. Stoller, MD: "Are RTs Effective? Examining the Evidence"
2001	John E, Hefner, MD: "Chronic Obstructive Pulmonary Disease—On the Exponential Curve of Progress"
2002	John B. Downs, MD: "Controversial Aspects of Oxygen Therapy"
2003	Gordon D. Rubinfeld, MD: "MSc Translating Clinical Research into Clinical Practice"
2004	Arthur S. Slutsky, MD: "Ventilator Induced Injury: From Barotrauma to Biotrauma"
2005	Homer A. Boushey, MD: "Past and Future Therapies for Asthma"
2006	Bartolome Celli, MD: "COPD: From Unjustified Nihilism to Evidence Based Optimism"
2007	J. Randall Curtis, MD: "MPH Caring for Patients with Life-threatening Illness and for Their Families: The Value of the Integrated Clinical Team"
2008	David J. Pierson, MD: "FAARC The Cardiopulmonary Physiology of Dinosaurs"
2009	Bruce Ruben, MD: "Air and Soul—The Science and Practice of Aerosol Therapy"
2010	Robert Kacmarek, PhD, RRT: "The Mechanical Ventilator—Past, Present and Future"

Committee established the Donald F. Egan Scientific Lectures in 1974. Each year, the lectureship is extended to a prominent investigator, clinician, or academician in the arena of interest. The lectureship honors Dr. Donald F. Egan, an early champion and supporter of respiratory therapy and one of its first major educators and authors. Table 1-3 provides a chronological listing of the lectures. A review of the subjects provides insight into the developing growth and maturity of the scientific and clinical interests of the profession.

Effects of Governmental Programs

Important engines for growth of the new allied health field were the federal programs authorized in the mid-1960s to increase citizen access to health care. Two such programs were Medicare and Medicaid, authorized in 1965 under the Social Security Administration (SSA) of the U.S. Department of Health Education and Welfare (HEW). **Medicare** provides assistance to pay for health services for people 65 and older and for persons who have been receiving Social Security disability benefits for 2 years. **Medicaid** authorizes federal matching funds to assist the states in providing health care for certain income groups at or near the federal poverty line.[16]

In 1977 both programs were administered by the new Health Care Finance Administration (HCFA) of the U.S. Department of Health and Human Services. In 1980 HEW was split into two agencies, the Department of Education and the Department of Health and Human Services (HHS), the latter of which became HCFA's new supervising agency. By 2001 HCFA was renamed the Center for Medicare & Medicaid Services. The name change recognized the mandates to oversee not only Medicare and Medicaid but also the State Children's Health Insurance Program, as well as the Health Insurance Portability and Accountability Act (HIPAA) Standards and the quality standards for long-term care facilities (nursing homes) and clinical laboratories. (For details of Medicare and Medicaid payments for individuals 65 and older, see Chapter 35.)

In their original formulation, both Medicaid and Medicare were strictly **fee-for-service** systems. Hospitals and physicians were reimbursed for whatever they spent on qualified patients. In that health care is one of the few areas in which the sellers, not the consumers, make the buying decisions, health care providers had an immense incentive to provide more and more services. This is not to say that physicians and hospitals exploited the new programs. However, the physicians' and hospitals' desire to provide services coincided closely with the consumer's desire that all that could be done would be done. The result was an explosion in health care costs. Specialty areas such as respiratory care became highly profitable revenue centers for hospitals, and services expanded well beyond any justifiable need.

COST CONTAINMENT

In the early 1980s, the federal government again significantly changed how it provided health care services to the poor and elderly. As fee-for-service programs, Medicaid and Medicare were about to collapse under the weight of rises in costs. Early attempts at cost containment (actually wage and price controls) in the 1970s had proved disruptive and ineffective. In 1983, the government adopted a **prospective payment system (PPS)**, which was to have a dramatic impact on the respiratory therapy.

The basis of the Medicare prospective payment system is the **diagnosis-related group (DRG)**. For a given diagnosis, each institution is paid a set amount rather than the actual amount spent on the patient. This system allowed rates of payment to be determined in advance for a medical diagnosis. Because payments for an illness were predetermined and fixed, regardless of the amount of care or services actually rendered, health care facilities had a powerful incentive to contain costs and to curb the amount of therapy provided. The most common forms of cost containment were reduced services, decreased staff, and shortened lengths of patient stay. In effect, the patients were being sent home "quicker and sicker." Because the prospective payment system was initially focused on hospital costs, it caused a shift of services from the hospital to the physician's office, to external clinics, and to homes. This shift established a need for greater respiratory therapist activity in the homecare market and an increased **scope of practice** (the functions performed).

Thus, cost containment hinged on three major issues: patient acuity (how sick the patient's were), length of stay (how long the patients remained in the hospital), and manpower costs (wages and benefits costs for health care workers).

CHANGING ACUITY LEVELS

The general acuity level in the hospital increased as patients who were not critically ill were moved from the hospital to other service venues. Patients who required less technical, less complicated care were considered to be at the subacute care level (see Chapter 34). The heightened acuity level in the hospital shifted the emphasis of respiratory care services from the general patient floor to the intensive care units and to diagnostic areas, such as cardiology and pulmonary function.

The patients being released from the hospital earlier than in the past needed to be serviced in other venues, such as the home. As one of the major effects of governmental attempts at cost containment, subacute care (see Chapter 35) quickly became a specialty area for respiratory therapists. As of 1997, it was projected that 30,000 to 50,000 practitioners were providing respiratory care in practice sites outside the hospital.[17] Although this is a reasonable shift in respiratory care priorities, to be fully successful, respiratory care practitioners needed more complete governmental recognition of the value of their services. Over the past three decades, several bills have been introduced in Congress that addresses the issues of recognition and reimbursement for RTs who practice outside of hospitals in skilled nursing facilities (SNFs), in home care, and in subacute, intermediate, and acute long-term care facilities. None of these bills has successfully passed through the Congressional process, but support appears to be gathering in both the House and the Senate. As a result of the 2008–2009 worldwide financial crisis it appeared that the then-current initiative would be likely also to fail unless a compelling case can be made for significant increases in the quality of care and cost reductions associated with that care and RT reimbursement. In 2010 Congress passed a bill that provided RT reimbursement for BS-educated RRTs. Although the bill passed and was enacted, the rule-writing process by the administrative bodies is still ongoing.

The 1990s: A Maturing Profession

Cost control continues to be a major factor in how, when, and where respiratory care practitioners provide services. The advent of managed care and case management has greatly affected all facets of health care. **Managed care** is a system in which preventive services and volume purchasing are emphasized in hopes of providing quality care at lower costs. In the search for less costly ways to provide care, however, both access to care and the quality of it can suffer at times.

MANAGED CARE

Since the late 1990s, health care reform efforts have taken the form of managed care systems, which attempt to bring free-market restraint to spiraling health care costs. Essentially, managed care is an umbrella concept for plans that coordinate health care through primary care (generalist) physicians. Managed care systems use a variety of approaches to alter the practice behaviors of physicians and other health care providers. The use of case managers to coordinate care, financial incentives to conserve resources, and **health care protocols** to guide the delivery of care all seek to lower the expenditure of funds. Case managers review health care records and may deny payment for what they deem to be unnecessary services, and they seemingly ration certain services provided within the plan.

As a result, managed care activities have, in fact, lowered the rising costs of health care in the United States. However, it is unclear whether market forces can hold down health care costs in the long run without disrupting the quality of the services provided. The issue is that, for many practitioners, managed care seems to place others between them and the patients they serve. These others make the decisions about the type, length, and conditions of the care to be provided. At least some of the medical decision making seems to have been taken out of hands of the physician and given over to the clerks and accountants in the government and insurance companies.

CRISIS IN CARE

The crisis in U.S. health care will not go away soon. At the beginning of the twenty-first century, the costs of health care are too high and rising. Ways must be found to maintain quality, increase access, and control costs. Whether these changes occur as a result of government intervention or market forces is an issue that must be addressed.

The crisis will make for difficult times for respiratory care providers, as well as for most health care practitioners and certainly for patients. Despite the current practice dilemma, the respiratory care practitioner must remain committed to providing the best of care, in a system that is trying simultaneously to maintain provider and receiver choice and to contain cost. The crisis is exacerbated by the fact that higher survival rates and an aging population have resulted from improved (and more expensive) technologies and from heightened knowledge and understanding of the disease process and treatment. At the same time, health manpower (the workforce) and monetary resources have not kept pace with such improvements in care.

The look of the future system is unclear, but its requirements are not: It must contain costs without the loss of quality of care.

Respiratory Care in the Twenty-First Century

Respiratory care enters the twenty-first century with heightened professional maturity. Changes in the title of entry-level practitioners (individuals who complete the entry-level examination) reflect these changes. Certified Inhalation Therapist became Certified Inhalation Therapy Technician (CITT) and then Certified Respiratory Therapy Technician (CRTT). In recognition of the increases in responsibility over the decades, the National Board for Respiratory Care (NBRC) has recommended and approved that the name of the credential be changed again to Certified Respiratory Therapist (CRT). All respiratory care personnel are now expected to have the knowledge and skills to perform a common set of job duties, regardless of education level or whether they are referred to as technicians or therapists.[18]

The 2004 figures from the NBRC indicated that 172,113 professionals had received their CRT credentials and that 88,384 had also qualified for the RRT credential since the inception of the credentialing process. AARC data for 2004 indicated a membership of 36,995, and 2005 reports indicate 47,000 plus members. The AARC's 2010 membership report showed 51,343 as of December 2010. CoARC reported program enrollment of 6231 for the 2004 academic year with 3994 graduates in that year and an attrition rate of 35.9% and a 5-year attrition rate of 33–36%.[19]

EDUCATION

To accommodate the need for a more broadly based practitioner, the AARC and Joint Review Committee for Respiratory Therapy Education (JRCRTE) agreed to establish a new accrediting agency for respiratory care educational programs, the **Committee on Accreditation of Respiratory Care Programs (CoARC)**. CoARC has proposed a new set of standards for the education of practitioners, which requires a minimum of an associate's degree in respiratory care for entry-level practice.[20]

Also, a movement in RT education circles is afoot to promote an increased education level to bachelor's degree programs, and some programs are studying and implementing graduate degree (master's) programs for RTs. In a 2009 report, The Commission on Accreditation of Allied Health Education Programs (CAAHEP) lists 355 respiratory therapy education programs in the 50 states.[21] According to the AARC's Coalition Baccalaureate and Graduate Respiratory Therapy Education (CoBgRTE), as of 2009, 54 of these were colleges and universities offering respiratory therapy programs awarding baccalaureates (51) or master's degrees (3) with a major or concentration in respiratory therapy (care). One of the master's-level programs is an entry-level program requiring a previous bachelor's degree for admission.[22]

Additionally, on the education front, in 2004 the AARC Board of Directors approved a document titled "Standards for International Respiratory Care Education," which was developed in conjunction and cooperation with the International Council for Respiratory Care (ICRC). This 21-page document sets forth standards and evaluation criteria for three levels of AARC recognition for educational programs based on the quality and duration of the programs. This action recognizes the increasingly global interest in formal RT education.[23]

LICENSURE

The mid-1980s to the late 1990s saw a surge of legislative activity, with more than 40 states gaining licensure for the practice of respiratory care. These licensure acts varied significantly in many ways, but they did not restrict the growth of the profession or the scope of its practice. While protecting the scope of respiratory care practice, these laws allowed other health care professionals, with appropriate training, to perform some of the duties of the licensed respiratory therapist. As leaders in the field of respiratory care become more adept at drafting, amending, and enforcing legislation, the strength of the profession should continue to grow.

As of 2009, 48 states, Puerto Rico, and the District of Columbia have established licensure or an other form of legal credentialing. All of those jurisdictions utilize the NBRC CRT (entry-level) examination as their licensure requirement. Only Alaska and Hawaii have not passed a legal credentialing act at the time of this writing; although Hawaii has introduced legislation to do so.

SCOPE OF PRACTICE

In 1991, the leadership of the profession undertook the task of providing a vision of the roles and responsibilities of the practitioner in the twenty-first century. The resultant document was titled "Respiratory Care Practitioner 2001."[24] In addition to listing the clinical duties, required characteristics, attributes, nonclinical duties, and practice settings (Table 1-4), the group addressed the issues of medical direction and whether the future practitioner was to be a specialist or a generalist. Respiratory care scope of practice has been legitimized through the licensure laws of most of the states and other political bodies in the United States. Each of these states or territories (plus Washington D.C.) has included a scope of practice statement in its legislation or regulation, making it a legal or regulatory mandate. All of these bodies recognize and mandate that the NBRC Certified Respiratory Therapist credential is the minimum level of credentialing required to practice in their jurisdictions. None of these entities has enacted a restricted scope of practice, thereby allowing the growth of the profession's skills and practice. By the third quarter of 2010, the NBRC issued 11,677 new credentials and administered 29,119 examinations in seven areas:

- CRT
- RRT Written
- RRT, Clinical Simulations,
- Pulmonary Function Technician (CPFT)
- Pulmonary Function Technologist (RPFT)
- Neonatal Pediatric Specialist (NPS)
- Sleep Disorders Specialist (SDS)

TABLE 1-4 **Respiratory care practitioner 2001**

Clinical Duties	Characteristics	Attributes	Nonclinical Duties	Care Settings
Be involved in direct patient care. Furnish monitoring for cardiopulmonary and other systems utilizing sophisticated, high-tech devices. Be positioned on the health care delivery team in such a way as to have the responsibility for refining broad or general physicians' orders within the parameters of predesigned protocols. Administer medications via aerosol, parenteral, IV, and IM routes of delivery. Educate other caregivers, patients, and family caregivers on methods of self-administration and other related subjects such as wellness and equipment maintenance. Assess patients and their progress as it relates to the overall care plan. Render clinical interventions over and above the traditional scope of practice, including clinical interventions that rely on a qualified patient evaluator, competence with high-tech equipment, and interventions, both therapeutic and diagnostic, that could readily be mastered by qualified respiratory care practitioners. Perform invasive diagnostic and monitoring procedures.	Be a product of a multilevel educational system, with entry level residing at the associate's degree level and advanced at the baccalaureate degree level. Possess training and education in the following areas: Critical thinking skills Liberal arts Basic sciences Communication skills Affective skills (dependability) Computer science Have awareness of one's environment and an ability to be flexible and adaptable. Possess human relations skills in order to work as part of a team. Be a licensed professional.	Possess an ability to practice in all care settings. Have stamina, both physical and mental. Possess a holistic caregiver's perception. Be compassionate. Have an ability to move back and forth from high tech to high touch. Be an innovator and a creator. Be efficient and effective. Be able to respond to change as well as to be a change agent. Possess skills as a negotiator. Act as a mentor. Remain professionally dynamic as manifested by a commitment to being a lifelong student. Be compensated commensurate with skill level, responsibility, and authority. Refuse to be a captive of paradigms and be willing to create new ones as needed. Possess an awareness of cultural sensitivity and diversity.	Participate in discharge planning. Teach at both primary and secondary levels within the context of health care delivery. Be responsible for preventive medicine and wellness interventions. Expand involvement within the infrastructure of the health care delivery system. Possess a leadership role in allied health so as to bring about change in health care practices and health care policy. Expand role in each organization's quality improvement process and data collection in order to improve resource accounting and document efficiency and effectiveness. Expand managerial skill base. Enlarge role in research. Possess an in-depth familiarity with other allied health procedures and interventions.	Possess an ability to render care across the entire health care delivery spectrum, from critical care on one extreme to self-care in the home on the other and all points in between, such as transitional care settings, skilled nursing facilities, and all outpatient venues.

From American Association for Respiratory Care. Proceedings of a National Consensus Conference on Respiratory Care Education. *Dallas, Tx: American Association for Respiratory Care; 1992.*

The NBRC has issued over 350,000 professional credentials to more than 209,000 individuals since its beginning in 1960.

SPECIALTY PRACTICE AND CREDENTIALS

One conclusion of the group was that the historically solid bond between respiratory care and its physician supporters has been an integral component of the profession's past successes and is the framework in which the scope of practice should expand. Furthermore, the group agreed that the field needs both generalists and specialists. Generalists are felt to be necessary as the specialty continues to move into alternative practice settings.

The development and implementation in 2002 of the Asthma Educator Certification (AE-C) course, jointly sponsored with AARC, has opened another path for professional growth and recognition. Successful completion of the 12.5-hour course and its final exam results in certification as a Certified Asthma Educator (AE-C).

Clearly, respiratory care practitioners will need to increase their level of educational requirements to practice effectively as members of multidisciplinary teams and to assume the expanded roles demanded by current health care practice. If the graduate is to be able to survive and to work collaboratively on the health care team, curricula will need to focus on multiskilling and on a systems approach to the organization and delivery of health care. Critical thinking, problem solving, oral and written communication skills, and skills in interpersonal relations and information technology will all be needed by the respiratory care practitioner of the twenty-first century. RTs can no longer afford to be the practitioners who work with the most critical patients while having the least formal education.

Professional Recognition

Over the last decade, recognition by peers, colleagues, and the government has done much to elevate the professional status of respiratory care as a true profession. Consider the following examples:

- In 1998, the AARC established a professional recognition program. The purpose is to recognize RTs who have distinguished themselves in the professional practice of respiratory therapy. From 1998 to 2006, 178 individuals have been inducted as fellows of the AARC (**FAARC**). These individuals are RTs, physicians, clinicians, educators, medical directors, and researchers from the United States and several other countries.
- The American College of Chest Physicians (ACCP) has opened its active and associate membership rolls to respiratory therapists. Additionally, several respiratory therapists have been elected as fellows of the college (FCCP). This election represents recognition as an exemplary clinician, teacher, and/or researcher in the area of chest medicine.
- As of 2007, the Society of Critical Care Medicine (SCCM) has welcomed 172 RTs into membership and inducted 21 RTs into its **fellowship** program (FCCM). With more than 14,000 member, SCCM is an international, multidisciplinary, multi-professional organization dedicated to the advancement of critical care through excellence in patient care, education, research, and advocacy. This organization includes physicians, nurses, RTs, pharmacists, physician's assistants, architects, and veterinarians as well as research scientists. RTs have served at the highest levels of this organization and as chairs of major committees.
- The 50,000 plus members in the AARC represent about 30% of the RT population. The National Board for Respiratory Care (NBRC) is the credentialing body for respiratory care professionals. The NBRC offers credentialing exams for the entry-level Certified Respiratory Therapist (CRT) and advanced practice Registered Respiratory Therapist (RRT) level. Additional credentials include the Neonatal-Pediatric Specialist (NPS). NBRC has issued over 180,000 credentials to more than 198,000 individuals and currently tests nearly 18,000 candidates every year. In 2009, a new Sleep Disorders Specialty (SDS) exam was developed and released. In the last several years, preliminary planning and data gathering were done to examine the feasibility of developing a similar credentialing exam in Critical Respiratory Care, which will be given for the first time in mid-2012.
- Rapid Response Team (RRT) (also known as Medical Emergency Teams [METs]) and Critical Care Outreach Teams (CCOT) were developed to ". . . . rapidly identify and manage seriously ill patients at risk of cardiopulmonary arrest and other high risk conditions."[25] The adoption of the Rapid Response Team (RRT) concept in the United States in mid-2000 opened new doors for respiratory therapists. First developed in the 1990s in Australia and the United Kingdom, the systems have reported success in reducing deaths, ICU stays, overall hospital stays, and all of the costs associated with prolonged hospital and ICU stays. Their success made it easy for many U.S. hospitals to implement the system, even though debate is

ongoing as to whether the RRT system has all the benefits that its supporters claim. The majority of papers and news articles published on the subject include the respiratory therapist as a member of this three- or four-person team. Their inclusion in the system is recognition of RTs' specialized assessment skills and ability to rapidly apply appropriate emergency interventions and stabilization techniques and technology for fragile patients. RTs as a profession have thus enjoyed excellent publicity and public exposure as valued and vital members of the health care team.

- The Joint Commission (formerly the Joint Commission on Health Care Organizations [JCAHO], the body that inspects and accredits hospitals, long-term care facilities, and home care organizations) has appointed six RTs to serve on their Professional Technical Advisory Committees (PTACs). These therapists serve on the home care, laboratory services, and the ambulatory care PTACs. The PTAC's function is to advise, propose, and consult with the rule-making bodies in the Joint Commission. Several other RTs serve the Joint Commission as site visitors and inspectors for The Joint Commission accreditation process.
- In response to natural disasters, the federal government has enlisted the assistance of RTs to provide short-term respiratory care procedures as part of the Emergency Mass Critical Care (EMCC) initiative during the disaster period. A supplement to *Chest* details this program.[26] Respiratory Therapists act as part of a DMAT (Disaster Medical Action Team). DMAT is defined as:

  > a group of professional and para-professional medical personnel (supported by a cadre of logistical and administrative staff) designed to provide medical care during a disaster or other event. NDMS recruits personnel for specific vacancies, plans for training opportunities, and coordinates the deployment of the team. To supplement the standard DMATs, there are highly specialized DMATs that deal with specific medical conditions such as crushing injuries, burn, and mental health emergencies.[27]

  The federal officials responsible for this project specifically requested RTs as DMAT members.
- A long-awaited change in federal policy has resulted in the approval to award officer status in the U.S. Public Health Service (USPHS). The USPHS is a part of the U.S. Department of Health and Human Services and is the 5th Uniformed Branch of the U.S. government. Officers in the USPHS are also awarded reserve commissions in the United States Navy. To be granted commissioned status, therapists must be Registered Respiratory Therapists and hold a BS degree or higher, among other qualifications.[28]

Summary

Respiratory care practice is an emerging profession, but its roots extend back thousands of years to the works of Hippocrates, Aristotle, and Galen. Not until the 1600s did the role of oxygen begin to be understood. William Harvey demonstrated blood circulation. Robert Boyle elucidated the volume and pressure relationships of gases. Joseph Priestley experimentally produced oxygen. In the 1700s, Antoine Lavoisier gave oxygen its name and correctly described the basic physiology of respiration. Thomas Beddoes established the Pneumatic Institute of Bristol, England, and was the first to use oxygen therapeutically. Growth of the field of respiratory care burgeoned in the twentieth century with rapid advancements in science and technology, many of which resulted from research in World Wars I and II.

Over the years, the role of persons who delivered oxygen therapy changed from mere equipment technicians (oxygen orderlies) to fully accredited allied health care providers. A national professional organization developed a set of standards for requirements, education, and scope of practice.

Implementation of evidence-based practices and the refinement of protocol-based care methods will, without a doubt, continue to expand the scope of practice. They will lead to the advancement of the respiratory care practitioner's ability to provide timely and efficacious patient care with reduced morbidity and mortality. They will also enhance the potential for developing effective multidisciplinary care teams.

Future health care reform in the United States will pose many challenges to the field of respiratory care as the government attempts to contain rising prices while preserving and increasing access for citizens. The leadership of the specialty will need to be especially nimble in negotiating each of the legislative changes that affect practice sites.

Study Questions

SHORT ANSWER

1. Of the three individuals associated with the discovery of oxygen (Priestley, Scheele, and Lavoisier), to whom would you give the credit for the discovery of oxygen? Explain your answer.

2. Briefly state the purpose and effect of the Sugarloaf Conference.
3. What are some reasons for the close relationship between physician groups and respiratory care specialists?
4. It has been said that the lessons of war speed the development of medicine. Why is that?

MULTIPLE-CHOICE QUESTIONS

1. Which of the following is true?
   a. Much of the success of respiratory care is due to its close relationship with physician supporters.
   b. Respiratory care ranks on par with nursing in terms of professional status.
   c. The length of education or training is not an issue in obtaining professional status.
   d. Respiratory care can trace its roots to the mid-1960s.
2. Which of the following entities deals with professional credentialing?
   a. American Association for Respiratory Care (AARC)
   b. Committee on Accreditation of Respiratory Care (COARC)
   c. State Boards of Healing Arts Regulation (SBHAR)
   d. National Board for Respiratory Care (NBRC)
3. Which are the major challenges that face the profession in the twenty-first century?
   I. Determining the appropriate level of education
   II. Gaining government recognition
   III. Gaining recognition as an independent primary care provider
   IV. Determining the need for two levels of practitioner professional credentialing
   V. Delineating a standard scope of practice
      a. I, II, III only
      b. I, III, IV only
      c. I, II, IV, V
      d. All of the above
4. State licensure laws for the practice of respiratory care:
   a. are unified, with the same requirements and scope of practice.
   b. are in effect in all U.S. states and territories.
   c. generally restrict areas of practice and skills.
   d. allow nonrespiratory therapists to practice some respiratory therapist tasks.
5. From an organizational perspective, respiratory care had its beginnings
   a. in New York City in 1930.
   b. in Chicago in 1947.
   c. in San Francisco in 1963.
   d. in Washington, D.C., in 1999
6. Which of the following pre-twentieth century developments in science was the most important for the modern allied health profession of respiratory care?
   a. the development of the germ theory of disease
   b. the study of cardiopulmonary anatomy by Vesalius
   c. the development of the dephlogistication theory of respiration
   d. the discovery and publication of the gas laws
7. The first organized clinical use of oxygen as a therapeutic gas was carried out by
   a. Thomas Beddoes.
   b. Joseph Priestley.
   c. Robert Boyle.
   d. Galen.
8. Which of the following is the correct chronological sequence of the establishment of the listed agencies?
   a. AARC, CoARC, NBRT
   b. JRCRTE, NBRT, AARC
   c. AARC, CoARC, JRCRTE
   d. AARC, NBRT, CoARC
9. Which of the following would appear to produce a cost-effective care model?
   I. Evidence-based practice
   II. Integrated care teams
   III. Respiratory protocols
   IV. Function-based care
      a. I, II, IV
      b. II and IV only
      c. I, II, III
      d. All of them

CRITICAL-THINKING QUESTIONS

1. How has respiratory care addressed the extended education requirement for professional status?
2. Only about 30% of respiratory therapists belong to a professional organization. What can be done to increase the number of active members?
3. How can the profession gain the level of governmental recognition needed to ensure its place in the new collaborative health care team?
4. What is the value of aligning the profession with other groups such as the Society for Critical Care Medicine and the American College of Chest Physicians?

References

1. Byrne P. *Analysis and Science in Aristotle*. New York: State University of New York Press; 1917.
2. Brock A. *Greek Medicine, Being Extracts Illustrative of Medical Writing from Hippocrates to Galen*. New York: Library of Greek Thought; 1976.
3. Zhou C, Han Y. *The Illustrated Yellow Emperor's Canon of Medicine*. Beijing, PRC: Dolphin Books; 1995.
4. Bowman I. *Historical Vignettes Brochure for John P. McGovern Hall of Medical History*. Galveston, TX: University of Texas; 1986.
5. Burton G, Gee G, Hodgkin J. *Respiratory Care*. Philadelphia: JB Lippincott; 1977.
6. Hillar M. *The Case of Michael Servetus*. Lewiston, NY: E. Mellen; 1997.
7. Yount L. *William Harvey. Discoverer of How Blood Circulates*. Berkley Heights, NJ: Enslow Publishers; 1994.
8. Kaplan B. *"Divulging of Useful Truths in Physick": The Medical Agenda of Robert Boyle*. Baltimore, MD: Johns Hopkins University Press; 1930.
9. Priestley J. As quoted in Levine, Edwin, eds., *Effective Inhalation Therapy*. Chicago: National Cylinder Gas; 1953.
10. Eubanks D, Bone R. *Comprehensive Respiratory Care*. St. Louis: Mosby; 1990.
11. Porter R. *Doctor of Society; Thomas Beddoes and the Sick Trade in Late Enlightenment England*. Atlanta: Rodopi Publishers; 1992.
12. Personal communication CoARC and Paul Mathews, January 2011.
13. Motley H, et al. Observations on the use of positive pressure. *J Avia Med*. 1947;18:417.
14. Smith G. *Evolution of a Profession*. Lenexa, KA: Applied Measurement Professionals; 1989.
15. Conference on the scientific basis of respiratory therapy: final report, summaries and recommendations. *Am Rev of Respir Dis*. 1985;110:4–15.
16. Edge R, Krieger J. *Legal and Ethical Perspectives in Health Care*. Clifton Park, NY: Delmar Cengage Learning; 1998.
17. Dunne PJ. Respiratory care for the homebound patient. *Respir Care*. 1997;42:133–140.
18. Ross B. NBRC approves new entry level credential designation. *NBRC Bulletin*. June 5, 1998.
19. Mathews PJ, Drumheller L, Carlow JJ. Respiratory care manpower issues in Interface of Public Policy and Critical Care Medicine; Model and Workforce. *Critical Care Medicine*. Supp. March 2006;34,3: S32–S45.
20. COARC lives! . . . accreditation for respiratory care . . . questions about respiratory care program accreditation. *AARC-Times*. February 22, 1998;22–25.
21. Respiratory therapy programs search. Commission on the Accreditation of Allied Health Education Programs (CAÁHEP). http://www.caahep.org.
22. Barnes T, Beachy W, Black C. 2008 Roster: Respiratory therapy programs awarding a baccalaureate or masters degree. American Association for Respiratory Care. 2009. www.aarc.org/education/accredited_programs/bsrt_msrt_roster.pdf
23. Recognition guidelines for quality international respiratory care education. International Education Recognition System. http://www.aarc.org/iers/6/index.cfm.
24. American Association for Respiratory Care. *Proceedings of a National Consensus Conference on Respiratory Care Education*. Dallas TX: American Association for Respiratory Care; 1992.
25. King E, Horvath R, Shulkin DJ. Rapid response teams: a bridge over troubled waters. White paper. Irving, TX: Voluntary Hospitals of America; 2007. https://www.vha.com/Solutions/ClinicalImprovement/Pages/RapidResponseTeams.aspx
26. Definitive care for the critically ill during a disaster: from a task force for Mass Critical Care Summit Meeting, January 26–27, 2007 *Chest*. Supp. May 2008;133,5:66.
27. Public Health Emergency. http://www.hhs.gov/aspr/opeo/ndms/teams/dmat.html.
28. Questions and answers regarding PHS service for RTs. http://www.aarc.org/headlines/07/11/phs/siegal.cfm

Suggested Readings

Annas G, et al. *The Rights of Doctors, Nurses and Allied Health Professionals*. Cambridge, MA: Ballinger; 1981.

Eicher J. State overview. Pew Commission releases new report on professional regulation. *AARC Times*. December 1998:22:12–13.

Final draft report of the Advisory Panel for Allied Health to the Pew Health Professions Commission. *J Allied Health*. 1992;21:1–74.

Healthy America: Practitioners for 2005, an Agenda for Action for U.S. Health Professional Schools. San Francisco: Pew Health Prof Commission; 1991.

Van-Scoder LI, Johnson JC, Nyhuis AW. Frequency with which staff respiratory therapists perform selected entry-level tasks. *Respir Care Educ Annu*. 2000; 9:3–17.

CHAPTER 2

Legal, Professional, and Ethical Practice

Raymond S. Edge

OBJECTIVES

Upon completion of this chapter, the reader should be able to:

- Define the principle of *stare decisis* and state the benefits derived from it.
- List the major elements found in a practice act.
- Define the legal term *tort* and list the elements of a tort.
- Differentiate between libel and slander.
- Differentiate between intentional torts and negligent torts.
- Differentiate between morals and ethics.
- Identify the basic principles involved in health care ethics.
- List the legal requirements for breaking patient confidentiality.
- List the legal requirements found in HIPAA as it relates to patient access to medical records.
- Explain how the principle of informed consent is derived from the principles of autonomy and veracity.
- Differentiate among compensatory, procedural, and distributive justice.
- Differentiate between duty, consequence, divine command, and virtue as bases of ethical reasoning and list the major criticisms of each.
- Solve an ethical dilemma using the following decision-making formats: utilitarianism, Kantian, virtue, and divine command.

CHAPTER OUTLINE

(continues)

(continued)

KEY TERMS

administrative law
assault
autonomy
battery
beneficence
case law
common law
confidentiality
constitutional law
defamation
defendant
discovery
divine command ethics
divine command theory
double effect
ethics
false imprisonment
felony
harm principle
Health Insurance Portability and Accountability Act (HIPAA)
informed consent
interrogatory
invasion of privacy
justice
liability
libel
misdemeanor
morals
negligence
nonmaleficence
normative elements
plaintiff
practice acts
private law
respondeat superior
role duty
slander
stare decisis
statutory law
summary judgment
tort
utilitarianism
veracity
virtue ethics

Texts such as *The Foundations of Respiratory Care* are designed to assist individuals in the process of enculturation into the profession. The practice of respiratory care goes beyond the study of applied sciences, essential therapeutics, and technical competence. Important **normative elements** of professional conduct are found in rules of professional etiquette, legal requirements, and ethical codes. Members of the respiratory care profession are expected to accept a shared set of ideals, values, and standards of behavior and practice. This chapter is intended to assist the practitioner in:

- Understanding the legal and ethical environments of health care.
- Making appropriate legal and ethical choices in practice.

Defining a Profession

One of the definitional elements of all professions is that they are self-regulating. Professions provide guidance for their members in regard to a set of norms of behavior that go beyond technical or clinical expertise and are part of the ideology of the group. An important element of professional self-regulation is the creation of a professional code of ethics and professional conduct. Figure 2-1 provides the current AARC Statement of Ethics and Professional Conduct. These normative prescriptions are intended to reflect and promote the values and aspirations of the group.

Rules of professional etiquette are generally based on traditions of good practice and good manners. Rules of professional etiquette are standards of behavior that are socially approved but not generally ethically or

AARC Statement of Ethics and Professional Conduct

In the conduct of professional activities the Respiratory Therapist shall be bound by the following ethical and professional principles. Respiratory Therapists shall:

- Demonstrate behavior that reflects integrity, supports objectivity, and fosters trust in the profession and its professionals. Actively maintain and continually improve their professional competence and represent it accurately
- Perform only those procedures or functions in which they are individually competent and which are within their scope of accepted and responsible practice
- Respect and protect the legal and personal rights of patients they treat, including the right to privacy, informed consent and refusal of treatment
- Divulge no protected information regarding any patient or family unless disclosure is required for responsible performance of duty, or required by law
- Provide care without discrimination on any basis, with respect for the rights and dignity of all individuals
- Promote disease prevention and wellness
- Refuse to participate in illegal or unethical acts
- Refuse to conceal, and will report, the illegal, unethical, fraudulent, or incompetent acts of others
- Follow sound scientific procedures and ethical principles in research
- Comply with state or federal laws which govern and relate to their practice
- Avoid any form of conduct that is fraudulent or creates a conflict of interest, and shall follow the principles of ethical business behavior
- Promote health care delivery through improvement of the access, efficacy, and cost of patient care
- Encourage and promote appropriate stewardship of resources.

Effective 12/94

Revised 12/07

FIGURE 2-1 American Association for Respiratory Care Statement of Ethics and Professional Conduct.
Courtesy of American Association for Respiratory Care, Irving Texas

morally significant. These rules help the specialty maintain order and civility and create an environment that promotes professional conduct and practice. They often involve matters such as respect for persons, such as the need to avoid talking ill about other members of the health care team. Most often the new practitioner is mentored into an understanding of the etiquette requirements of the health care environment. These rules of social behavior are often not formally written and, when broken, do not generally evoke the same level of negative response to infractions as do legal or ethical lapses. However, a practitioner who continues to break the rules of professional etiquette can face serious consequences, not the least of which is that one is considered boorish by ones colleagues and, when possible, avoided.

Legal requirements are the formal body of rules or principles enacted and backed by the power of the state. Therapists can think of legal requirements as being a set of principles and rules that command us or restrain us from doing or not doing certain things. Legal requirements can be considered to be the minimal standard of expected behavior. To ensure that practitioners abide by this lowest standard of behavior, many professional codes of ethics contain rules that require the practitioner to stay within the law in their professional conduct. The following statement from the AARC Statement of Ethics and Professional Conduct speaks to the need for practitioners to be law abiding in their practice. According to the AARC statement a practitioner shall:

> Refuse to participate in illegal or unethical acts, and shall refuse to conceal illegal, unethical or incompetent acts of others.

Ethical standards and legal requirements are usually closely related, with our ethical obligations typically exceeding our legal duties. If a situation occurs where a practitioner believes a legal requirement is unjust or unethical, there is an obligation to work within the system to change the law or remove oneself from the process.

Like rules of professional etiquette, the rules of ethics are also designed to promote order and civility. However, professional ethics generally doesn't deal with something considered to be bad manners; professional ethics deals with the rights and welfare of another person. As a result, the sanctions for ethical failure are more severe than for matters of etiquette. It should be noted that a single act could have consequences that involve an individual's ethical, legal, and etiquette standing in the profession.

Appropriate ethical, legal, and etiquette behaviors are necessary components of practice for every health care provider. In their daily activities, respiratory therapists (RTs) serve clients and patients whose condition has placed them in a position of high need and vulnerability. As a result of their trust, RTs have available a great deal of personal and confidential information. They are entrusted with expensive instruments, have access to controlled substances, and perform duties that are essential to patients' health and well-being. Their patients and clients come to them for their clinical skills and for their commitment to professional standards. It is a special relationship where all patients or clients have the right to expect compassionate and competent care of the highest quality, indeed the very best RTs have to offer.

Our decisions involving professional etiquette, ethical conduct, and legal matters have real consequences for our patients, ourselves, our profession, and the community at large.

TABLE 2-1 **Common legal and ethical issues**

Common Legal Issues	Common Ethical Issues
Falsification of credentials	Indiscriminate and unnecessary use of resources
False or incomplete patient records	Failure to protect patient confidentiality
Performing duties beyond scope of practice	Failure to report incompetent, unethical, or illegal activities of colleagues
Performing nonprescribed services	Failure to provide equal care to all
Practicing under the influence of alcohol, drugs, or narcotics	Issues involving patient advocacy (e.g., inadequate staffing for patient safety)
Conflicts of interest	Use of inappropriate research procedures
Failing to practice at an appropriate standard	Issues involving the dying patient (e.g., DNR orders, advanced directives, organ donations)

Professional Obligations

To enter into the practice of respiratory care is to enter into a social agreement not only with the patients being served but also with the greater community at large and with all other health care providers. This social agreement will require a high level of personal commitment to excellence of practice, continuing education and lifelong learning, and the acceptance of a set of appropriate moral, legal, and social behaviors.

Often the answers to the important questions that face respiratory care practitioners are the product of evaluating, understanding, and utilizing scientific information. Most practitioners see their clinical competence as the measure of their professional competence. It is these clinical competency skills that are judged in the teaching laboratories and clinical portions of our educational programs. Although respiratory care education programs make reference to ethical, professional, and legal behaviors as being important to practice, unless a student strays far from the path, grades are primarily given on the basis of perceived clinical knowledge and skills quickness. Yet, when they enter practice, the clinical questions are often the easy area, the area in which there is the highest level of agreement among the health care team. In the areas of professionalism, legal practice, and ethical conduct there is often less consensus, often no clear right answer, and yet, wrong decisions can be devastating to the patients, the reputation of the profession, and personal careers. Although the professional, legal, and ethical arena in which respiratory therapists (RTs) practice abounds with problems that have no clear right answer, there are clearly wrong decisions that must never be made. Table 2-1 lists common legal and ethical issues that often confront the respiratory therapist.

To avoid the legal and ethical pitfalls of professional life, one must have some understanding of the basics of law and ethical conduct as they relate to our practice. For most of us, information regarding how to avoid legal, ethical, and professional pitfalls will be at least as important as having liability (malpractice) insurance.

The ability to reason to a right ethical or legal decision is a real strength for a practitioner. As health care professionals, RTs are responsible to their colleagues for appropriate professional conduct and etiquette and for the maintenance of lawful and ethical standards. Table 2-2 compares the sanctions imposed for inappropriate legal, ethical, and professional behavior. As can be seen, the adoption of illegal, unethical, or unprofessional behavior is no small matter and can end a career.

TABLE 2-2 **Comparison of sanctions for illegal, unethical, and unprofessional behavior**

Area	Judgment	Sanctions
Legal	Legal or illegal	Loss of professional reputation, loss of professional affiliations, punishments determined under law
Ethics	Right or wrong	Loss of professional reputation, loss of professional affiliations, personal remorse
Professional etiquette	Proper or improper	Professional condemnation

Legal Aspects of Respiratory Care Practice

This chapter's discussion of the legal aspects of the profession is not an attempt to provide all the necessary information that the respiratory therapist may need to know. It is certainly not intended to provide legal advice. Many activities of practice require legal knowledge, and it is hoped that the basic knowledge provided here will help the practitioner avoid performing illegal acts.

Perhaps the most fundamental principle of law is a concern for justice and fairness. An important secondary principle is plasticity and change. Although the law appears to be a complete and solid structure from the outside, it is a shifting process that reacts to its environment. The third principle is that acts are judged on the universal standard of the reasonable person. What would a similarly trained, reasonable, and prudent person have done in the particular situation? The doctrine of personal responsibility is fundamental to the rule of law. Every practitioner is liable for his or her own actions.

The Foundations of U.S. Law

We can think of laws as a set of principles and processes by which people in a society seek to settle disputes and problems without resorting to force or violence. In some sense, law can be considered the minimum standard of expected performance by individuals in a society. Laws can be thought of as general rules of conduct whose compliance is enforced by government-imposed penalties.

The U.S. system of law was generally derived from that of Great Britain. Common elements of law that have come to us from the English system are the concept of trial by jury, the use of grand juries, the appellate review of lower court decisions, and a professional judiciary.

The basic sources of modern law are common law, which emanates from judicial decisions; statutory law, which arises from legislative bodies; and administrative law, which flows from the rules, regulations, and decisions of administrative agencies.

COMMON LAW

Common law, as distinguished from law created by the enactment of legislatures, derives its authority solely from usages and customs. The source of common law is primarily **case law** (law resulting from judicial interpretation of statutes). The set of common principles entailed in common law has evolved from the practices of the past and continues to evolve and expand from judicial decisions that arise from court cases. These decisions are often based on long-term custom or are guided by ethical principles such as fairness. One example of how the law changes over time can be seen in modern cases involving victims' rights and restitution, in which fines collected are paid to the victim rather than retained by a government agency, as they once were.

Common law represents the gradual accumulation of decisions. Cases arise out of disputes between individuals and, in adjudicating these cases, the judge examines earlier cases involving similar problems and circumstances to discover general principles that can be applied to the case at hand. This process has given rise to the principle of ***stare decisis***, which translated means "let the decision stand." The use of the principle *stare decisis* has provided the system with needed stability and yet has allowed for the creation of new principles as new or changing patterns of facts have emerged. In addition to classification by source, the law has been classified as being either public or private.

STATUTORY LAW

Under our federal constitution and the various state constitutions, legislative bodies are given the power to enact laws to govern the people. The U.S. Constitution is the supreme law of the land.

- **Constitutional law** deals with the organization, granted powers, and framework of government and sets limits on what the federal and state governments may do.

- **Statutory law** consists of the rules and regulations (statutes) set down in printed form by a legislative branch of the government. Congress establishes federal statutes, whereas state statutes are established by the various state legislatures. Examples of statutory law at the federal level include the creation of such agencies as the Centers for Disease Control and Prevention, the Social Security Administration, and the National Institutes of Health. Examples of important state statutes that affect the provision of health care include health providers practice acts, Good Samaritan laws, and child abuse laws.

Practice Acts. Respiratory care **practice acts** are examples of statutory law that seek to regulate the practice of respiratory care. Practice acts will vary in emphasis, but the majority will address the following elements:

- Scope of professional practice
- Exemptions
- Grounds for administrative action
- Creation of an examination board and processes
- Penalties for unauthorized practice

A board or council usually is designated to administer and enforce the statute that created the practice act.[1]

Criminal Law. Criminal law is an important aspect of statutory law. It defines and prohibits conduct deemed injurious to public order and safety and provides for punishment of persons found to have engaged in criminal practices. In general this includes the definition of specific offenses and general principles of **liability** (a responsibility or an obligation).

Crimes are divided by their seriousness and level of punishment.

- A **misdemeanor** is a crime punishable by less than a year's incarceration in jail or house of correction. Examples of common misdemeanors are the theft of small amounts of money, disorderly conduct, and breaking into an automobile.
- A **felony** is the far more serious breach of law and is punishable by death or imprisonment in a state or federal penitentiary.

Legislatures enact laws that determine whether an act is a crime and whether it will be considered a felony or a misdemeanor. Examples of felonies are fraud and forgery. Some activities, such as murder, rape, sodomy, larceny, manslaughter, burglary, robbery, and arson have been determined by common law to be felonies.

Sometimes practitioners engage in illegal activities that have criminal penalties, such as falsifying their application when applying for a state license to practice or placing false information on the medical record. All practitioners have a legal and ethical obligation to protect themselves and others in the professions. The general thrust of public law, in all of its forms, is to assist the society in attaining its public goals.

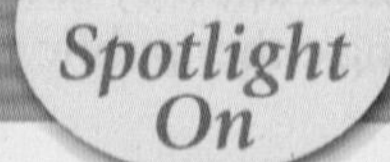

Licensure

As of January 2011 49 states have adopted licensure or other legal requirements for the practice of respiratory therapy in their jurisdictions. Only Alaska has not passed a law regulating respiratory therapy practice. In addition to the 49 states, the District of Columbia and the U.S. territory of Puerto Rico have established regulations governing these practices.

ADMINISTRATIVE LAW

Administrative law is the body of rules and regulations promulgated by administrative agencies of the federal government and state governments. Medicare, Medicaid, and OSHA, for example, are created by statutory law, but their rules and regulations are examples of administrative law. Violation of a regulation generally carries with it the imposition of a penalty in the form of restricting or restraining the professional's right to practice. As an example, a clinic that fails to comply with Medicare or Medicaid regulations may lose the right to claim compensation from these programs for services provided. A more relevant example for RTs is the failure of the therapist to earn the minimum number of required continuing education units (CEUs) over the licensing period. This lapse breaks the RT-administrated regulations and may result in suspension or revocation of the individual's license and perhaps right to work as an RT.

PRIVATE LAW

Private law, or civil law, deals with definition, regulation, and enforcement of rights in cases between citizen and citizen or between citizens and organizations. Two basic types of private law are torts and contract law.

Torts. A **tort** is a legally defined wrong committed upon a person or property independent of contract that renders the individual who commits it liable for damages in a civil action. Torts are the violation of some private duty by which damages accrue to the

CASE STUDY 2-1

An intensive care nurse who was planning to move to North Carolina had a stroke and died before she could make all the arrangements. A respiratory therapist who had worked with the nurse discovered the paperwork that she had planned to send to the North Carolina Board of Nursing. In that the paperwork was complete, the therapist forwarded the materials to North Carolina, resigned from the respiratory therapist position, and moved, assuming the name and credentials of the nurse.

Unfortunately the preparation of a nurse is very different from that of a respiratory therapist, and the therapist soon had numerous incidents of incompetence on her records in North Carolina. These records eventually aroused suspicion that this person was not what she said she was. Her supervisor called the hospital from which the new "registered nurse" had come. During the conversation, the supervisor discovered that the nurse in question had recently died.

Questions

1. Who bears responsibility for the risks to patients due to the respiratory therapist being employed as a nurse?
2. What actions should be taken by the state board of respiratory care?
3. What message does this case send to employers?

individual and for which the courts will provide a remedy in the form of an action for damage. The legal wrong committed upon the person may be a direct invasion of some legal right of the individual, the infraction of some public duty by which special damages accrue to the individual, or the violation of some private obligation by which the damages accrue to the individual.

Every tort action has three basic elements:

- A legal duty owing from defendant to plaintiff
- A breach of that duty
- Damages that are a proximate result of the breach of duty

Torts are usually classified into three broad categories: intentional torts, negligent torts, and torts in which the liability is assessed irrespective of fault (strict liability), such as claims against the manufacturers of defective medical products. Tort law is often used by the courts to influence the behavior of companies and to encourage them to behave responsibly. As an example, if a medical product harms an individual and the customer sues the manufacturer, the company is likely to provide additional instructions and warning labels on the products in the future. Common forms of intentional torts that have implications for respiratory therapists are:

- Assault and battery.
- Defamation of character.
- False imprisonment.
- Invasion of privacy.

Common Forms of Intentional Torts Assault and battery are tantamount to tort action, giving rise to civil liability, but they also may be considered, under certain circumstances, criminal activity. **Assault** is defined as the unjustifiable attempt to touch another person or threat to inflict injury on another, coupled with an apparent present ability to inflict such injury. **Battery** is the intentional touching of another person without that person's consent. Harmful or offensive touching or contact by another person is the essence of battery. It would be a rare instance in which the respiratory therapist was involved in an assault; battery is a more common offense. Any unnecessary mishandling of the patient during a treatment may amount to a battery.

Defamation is an injury to a person's reputation or character caused by false statements made by another to a third party. Defamation includes both libel and slander. **Libel** involves false or malicious writing that is intended to defame or dishonor another. The libel must be published in such a way that someone else other than the one defamed will observe it. Along with written statements, libel can also be presented in signs, cartoons, photographs, e-mails, and so on. **Slander** is the spoken form of defamation. It is defined as false oral statements that injure the character or reputation of another and that are made in the presence of a third person. Defamatory statements communicated only to the injured party and to no one else, while potentially hurtful, are not grounds for action. As practitioners, therapists must always be especially cautious about comments made about other members of the health care team, as hasty, and inappropriate actions or comments may subject us to a defamation action.

Normally for a case of slander or libel to be actionable, injury must result. However, there are four classes of exceptions in which the courts have held that no proof of actual injury is required to recover damages:[2] When statements fall in these categories, the law presumes that damages will result and they need not be proven:

- Accusing someone of a serious crime.
- Using words that tend to injure another in his or her trade, business, or profession.
- Imputing unchastity to a woman.
- Accusing the plaintiff of having a loathsome disease.

Truth and privilege are the two main defenses against a charge of defamation of character. When someone is charged with defamation, after making statements that harmed another's reputation, that person cannot be held for slander if indeed the statements can be proved to be true. The defense of privilege is used in cases in which the statements, which ordinarily may be considered defamatory, are made in circumstances under which the individual is charged with a higher duty. For example, practitioners may be required under law to report certain health problems or a state may have provided immunity for persons involved in peer-review processes.

False imprisonment, the unlawful restriction of another's freedom of movement, is a tort. Actual physical force is not necessary to prove this claim. A reasonable fear that force, which may be applied by words, threats, or gestures, will be used to detain a person is often sufficient. The health care provider who forces a patient to remain until a bill is paid or forms are signed may be liable under the tort of false imprisonment. Certain state statutes have allowed the detention of mental patients who were considered a danger to themselves, to property, or to others and of persons with a contagious disease. The mentally ill or contagious may be restrained only to the degree necessary to protect themselves from harm or to prevent them from harming others (minimum necessary restraint). In these cases it is wise for the practitioner to document clearly and carefully the reasons for the detention, the harm that would arise from the patient's leaving, and the patient's insistence on leaving.

The right to be left alone, free from unwarranted publicity, is considered an important freedom in American society and has found its way into both state and federal statutes. The phrase *right to privacy* is a generic concept encompassing a variety of rights thought to be necessary for an ordered democracy. The standard to determine whether an invasion of privacy has taken place is that of a "person of ordinary sensibilities." If such a hypothetical individual would find that the appropriation or exploitation of one's personality, the publicizing of one's private affairs, or wrongful intrusion into one's private activities was unwarranted and brought mental suffering, shame, or humiliation, then there would be grounds for action on invasion of privacy. Tort actions involving **invasion of privacy** issues generally involve one or more of four classes:[3]

- *Misappropriation* usually deals with the unpermitted use of an individual's name or likeness for another's benefit or advantage.
- *Intrusion* usually involves encroachment upon another's solitude or seclusion: for example, invasion of an individual's home, persistent unwanted telephone calls, or eavesdropping.
- *Public disclosure of private facts* of an objectionable nature may give rise to legal action even if the information is essentially true.
- *Presenting someone in a false light to the public* usually involves the publication of information that misleads the public. An example might be an article about Medicare fraud that includes a respiratory care team who were not involved in the case.[3]

In general, respiratory therapists have the right to make fundamental choices involving their families, ourselves, and our relationships with others. These activities should under most circumstances be free from the scrutiny of others, so long as our assertion of these rights is consistent with law or public policy. RTs have the right to maintain their private lives and to restrict the collection, processing, use, and dissemination of data about their personal attributes and activities. The law provides legal redress against those who would infringe upon our legitimate privacy from motives of malice, greed, curiosity, or gain.

Negligent Torts The salient difference between intentional torts and **negligence** is the element of intent, which is present in intentional torts and absent in negligence. A second important difference is that intentional torts involve a willful act that violates another's interest, whereas in negligence, the problem is likely to be an omission of an act that is deemed reasonable. The most common forms of negligence are:

- *Malpractice*. Carelessness or failure to act with due care on the part of a professional.
- *Malfeasance*. Execution of an unlawful or improper act.
- *Misfeasance*. Improper performance of an act that leads to injury.
- *Nonfeasance*. Failure to perform an act, when there is a duty to act.

- *Criminal negligence.* Reckless disregard for the safety of another.

Sustaining a claim of negligence requires the following forms of evidence, often called the four Ds of a negligence claim:

- *Duty.* A provider-patient relationship must be established. A duty to care must exist.
- *Dereliction of duty.* There must have been a breach of duty; that is, the provider failed to act as an ordinarily competent provider would have acted in a similar situation.
- *Direct cause.* The breach of duty must have been the direct (proximate) cause of the injury, damage, or loss.
- *Damages.* An injury or loss must actually have taken place.

Respondeat Superior Respiratory care is a specialty that in its development has had a close and positive association with physicians, especially those involved in anesthesiology and pulmonary medicine. Practice by respiratory therapists has traditionally been under the authority of the local state medical practice act of the physician. The movement toward state licensure for the profession has somewhat changed the relationship and shifted the responsibility more toward the respiratory care practitioner.

In the early years of the profession, many respiratory care practitioners felt that there was no need to seek licensure for the profession, given that they worked under the license of the physician. In that the therapist performed only those duties prescribed by the physician it was felt that the physician was the one who had the legal liability under a doctrine known as ***respondeat superior***, which means "let the master answer." The original intent of the doctrine, under English common law, was to make the Landed Lords of the land liable for the acts of their servants. The doctrine has evolved to include liability assessment against employers for negligent acts committed by employees, if the negligent conduct occurred in the course and scope of their employment duties. Liability is often assessed against hospitals and physicians for the negligent actions of allied health personnel on the basis of the fact that the employer placed these individuals in a position and gave them the apparent authority to act on their behalf.[4]

Although *respondeat superior* allows for the assessment of vicarious (indirect) liability to be assessed against those with whom RTs have a master-servant relationship, it in no way exempts respiratory therapists from responsibility for their personal acts. Health care is practiced on many levels, from simple tasks requiring almost no training to complex tasks requiring years of education and intensive internships. Physicians, therapists, nurses, and aides are all held to the level of practice that meets the prevailing standards for their group. For example, respiratory therapists are not held responsible for the level of care expected of the physician. They are, however, held responsible for the level of knowledge, skill, and care ordinarily possessed and exercised by other respiratory therapists. In the case of *State University of New York v. Young*,[5] the therapist was suspended for using the same syringe for drawing blood from a series of critically ill patients even after having been warned that the practice fell below the standard of care.

Often in cases of negligence more than one person may be involved in causing a patient's total injury. Under the doctrine of joint liability, several individuals may be held responsible for contributing to the injury. In these cases the plaintiff may recover damages from one or all.

Contracts. A contract comes into being when one party makes an offer that is accepted by another party and consideration passes between them. In a contractual arrangement, each party gives or does something for what is exchanged; the thing given or action performed is known as consideration. Most often in

CASE STUDY 2-2

A therapist in a hospital was called upon to set up a ventilator for a nonbreathing patient. The therapist managed to hook the patient to the ventilator without an expiratory valve in place. The alarm began to sound with each attempted cycle, and the therapist began to troubleshoot the device without taking the patient off the ventilator. After 7 minutes of troubleshooting, the therapist figured the problem out. However, the patient, who had been apneic for the 7 minutes, had suffered irreversible brain damage. The patient's family claimed that the injury was due to the therapist's negligence.

Questions

1. How does this case satisfy the four elements of a negligence claim?
2. What would an ordinarily competent provider have done?
3. Under the doctrine of *respondeat superior*, can the hospital be held responsible for the therapist's actions? Explain your answer.

medical practice, the consideration is the fee for service. Contracts are relationships of mutual consent; the party who makes the offer and the one who accepts it must be saying and thinking the same thing.

In a breach of contract, there is a failure, without legal excuse, to perform any promise that constitutes the whole or part of the contract. The formal contract is established when both parties have promised to be bound in the agreement. Thus, when one party offers to do something in exchange for the other party's agreement to do something, the contract is formed by the acceptance of the offer.

Contractual duty can occur as the result of signing formal documents, or it can arise out of implication. For example, if a patient shows up at the blood gas laboratory and is met by the receiving therapist, fills out the paperwork, and allows the therapist to palpate the vessel, it can be inferred that the patient is willing to allow the blood to be taken and also to pay for the services.[6]

The Civil Lawsuit

When a claim goes to court, the first stage is complaint and answer. The individual who begins the lawsuit or action, claiming damage or harm, is the **plaintiff**; the party against whom the suit is brought is the **defendant**. It is hoped that the respiratory therapist would never be involved in a lawsuit, but it is useful to explore the process by which a case proceeds through the legal system.

INITIATING THE SUIT

It is the duty of the plaintiff to establish the elements of a case, consistent with case law or statute. To initiate the legal process, the plaintiff files a complaint with the court that addresses the elements of the prima facie case and the number of offenses (counts) the plaintiff alleges the defendant is guilty of violating. (*Prima facie* means legally sufficient to establish a case.) The common elements of a complaint are:

- A short statement laying out the grounds on which the court's jurisdiction depends. In essence, the plaintiff tells the court why he or she thinks it has the authority to rule on the suit.
- A statement of the claims that call for relief for the plaintiff. In this part of the filing, the plaintiff states how he or she was wronged.
- A demand for judgment for a relief to which the plaintiff feels entitled. Here the plaintiff states what he or she wants done to resolve the wrong.

In federal courts, this filing is called the *complaint;* in most state courts it is called a *petition*.

A copy of the complaint, along with a summons, is served on the defendant. The complaint must be served on the defendant to give notification that a suit has been initiated against him or her. There generally is a statutorily required period in which the complaint must be answered. In that the answer to the complaint will become part of the court's record and the defendant will be held for anything stated therein, it is important that the therapist gain the assistance of an attorney before answering the complaint. The defendant, in the response to the complaint, will admit, deny, or plead ignorance to each allegation in the complaint. This is a period in which there is often anger and fear on the part of the defendant, but it is also important to understand that being "served with process" is just a notice of a lawsuit and nothing more.

Once the answer to the complaint has been filed, the defendant may file a motion to dismiss or motion for summary judgment, also known as a *demurrer*. A **summary judgment** is one made by a judge without there being a trial. The motion for summary judgment may be directed at all or part of the claim. In that a summary judgment is asking the judge to make a ruling on a dispute of law, it is important that there be agreement between the parties as to the facts in the case. If there is a dispute in regard to facts, then a motion for summary judgment will not stand. The defendant may also bring a motion to dismiss based on the belief that the plaintiff has not established a prima facie case in the complaint or that the complaint does not state a remedy for which the law provides. Either the motion for summary judgment or the motion to dismiss can be brought any time before the trial begins.

DISCOVERY

The discovery period is usually the longest part of a suit and is the stage at which most lawsuits end because often information is discovered that is detrimental to one party. Once the defendant has been notified of the complaint, and certain statutory procedures have been complied with by both parties (e.g., scheduling conferences to determine deadlines for discovery and trial), the process of discovery can be begun by either party.

Discovery is basically the fact-finding phase, during which each party has the opportunity to discover the strength of the other party's case. Information that is normally private may be brought to light (e.g., patient records, departmental records, and personal histories). Because discovery is the only opportunity that both sides have to discover information that will help their case, great latitude is given to both parties in their discovery efforts.

The major elements in discovery usually involve interrogatories, document requests, and depositions. Each of these elements should be posted and answered

Best Practice

In the Event of a Suit ...

During dispositions and court testimony, do *not* answer:

- Questions you do not understand.
- Compound questions.
- Questions with double negatives in them.

For each of these, ask the lawyer to simplify and restate the question.

Do not answer questions that were not asked. Answer only the question that was asked; do not expand on the answer. If the question can be answered with yes or no, answer with a yes or no.

As soon as the RT receives notice that a suit is being contemplated, he or she should get an attorney. It can get complicated very quickly. The therapist will need a lawyer. The hospital's lawyer's primary job is to protect the hospital, not the RT.

Professional liability (malpractice) insurance is not only a good idea, but it is a necessary action. RTs are more likely to be included in legal action now that licensure is the common practice nationally, and they are becoming more visible to the public.

with the assistance of an attorney in that they will become a permanent part of the court record.

Depositions are the most common and effective methods of discovery because they provide an opportunity for each side to question witnesses and parties to a suit in order to elicit information about the case. In the deposition, the witness testifies under oath before a reporter, who transcribes the testimony. In that the deposition can be used to impeach later testimony given in the trial, it is important that witnesses answer the questions exactly as if they were testifying in court.

An **interrogatory** is a series of questions sent by one side to the other. Document requests are just that—requests for documents. Document requests are often important in health cases because they provide access to medical records. The resulting information may provide overwhelming evidence for the plaintiff or may show that the plaintiff cannot establish the elements of a case. After discovery, either the case is dropped or the parties proceed to trial or arbitration.

THE TRIAL PROCESS

A case may be tried before a judge only or before a judge and jury; most trials (except in small-claims court) have a jury. Once the jury has been impaneled, the trial begins with the attorneys' opening statements, with the plaintiff's attorney leading. The opening statements outline the facts that the attorneys hope to establish in the trial process. The plaintiff has the burden of proving the case to the jury. The defendant does not have a burden of proof, has to prove nothing, and could, technically, remain silent. After each side has presented its case and cross-examined the witnesses, each is allowed time for a closing argument. After the closing argument, the judge instructs the jury of any applicable law and any presumptions the jury should consider in their deliberations. Then the jury is dismissed to deliberate. The trial usually ends with the verdict.

THE APPEAL

The losing party may appeal a trial court decision to a higher court in that particular jurisdiction, but only a final judgment may be appealed. The higher court will accept appellate arguments from both parties, but an appellate court will not entertain any new issues. Essentially, an appellate court is a trier of law, reviewing the processes of the lower court and the applicable decision of law rendered by the lower court.

ARBITRATION

A recently applied process for settling legal disputes is the process of arbitration. In arbitration, the parties to the potential suit meet with a mutually agreed-upon third party, the arbitrator. The arbitrator listens to statements, reads documents, reviews evidence presented by each party, and proposes a compromise settlement. It is felt that the arbitrator, as an unbiased party, can substitute for judge and jury. Arbitration can be either binding or nonbinding. With binding arbitration the arbitrator's findings are final and not appealable. Nonbinding arbitration leaves the door open for appeals and refusal to comply with the arbitrator's findings.

Because arbitration generally is less time consuming and less expensive than suit and trial proceedings, it is more appealing to both the legal system and the parties in dispute. This process will likely be used more often as both civil and criminal courts become more crowded.

The Duty of Ethical Practice

Moral and ethical decisions can be seen as a less prescriptive standard of conduct than just obeying the law. It is perhaps important in the beginning of this section to distinguish between **morals** and **ethics**.

According to the ethicist Joseph Fletcher, "Morals are what people believe to be right and good. . . . Ethics is the critical reflection about morality and the rational analysis of it."[7] Van Rensselaer Potter, who is credited with coining the term *bioethics*, explained that this new discipline had as its focus the traditional task of medical ethics, that of aiding the individual practitioner in making value-laden decisions and living by them.[8] *Ethics*, then, is nothing more than a generic term for the study of how people make judgments with regard to right and wrong. Ethics provides us with the framework to examine the moral life and the moral practice of health care professions.

Human babies are not born with a set of prescribed value rules or moral standards as to what they should do in any given situation. They draw from their cultural environment a set of beliefs, attitudes, feelings, and opinions that we develop into a rather consistent worldview, and it is with this that they judge the world around them—good, bad, right, wrong, positive, negative. Although each of us—in accordance with our varying beliefs, experiences, and upbringing—has a unique overall view of the world, most people in a society hold similar sets of values and moral beliefs. These reflections from our worldview are all part of the individual's personal values; they are reflections of the individual's moral life.

The capacity to become ethical beings and to conform to some universal principles of cooperation and altruism seems as old as the human species itself. One of the earliest anthropological findings of Neanderthal remains was of an individual about 50 years of age. The skeletal remains showed that the individual suffered from several debilitating conditions including arthritis and could not have survived in the rough-and-tumble environment of his time without the care and support of his group. Neanderthals may not have had the words to express such concepts as love, individual respect, and altruism, but they certainly shared the behaviors by which people would describe such values.

The philosopher Friedrich Nietzsche (1844–1900) was correct in his assessment that humans are valuing animals. However, in regard to our values, humans are not programmed, as are the beasts of the field, to a proscribed set of correct actions but are condemned to lives of freedom and choice. There are a few people in any society who use this freedom of choice to subscribe to a philosophy of moral nihilism. Adherents to this philosophical position believe that there are no moral truths, no moral laws, no moral facts, no moral knowledge, and no moral responsibilities. In this sense nothing can truly be right or wrong in a moral sense. For the moral nihilist, morality, like religion, is a mere illusion. If one followed this philosophical position to its conclusions, heinous acts such as child abuse, rape, and torture would not necessarily be wrong. Fortunately for the rest of us, this is not a position that most in society feel comfortable adopting.

Slightly less troubling but far more common are those who ground their personal philosophy solely in a hedonistic worldview. In this worldview, the guideposts for decision making are personal desire and aversion, and nothing can be right or wrong apart from them. This attitude of total self-absorption is somewhat captured in the bumper sticker slogan, "He who dies with the most toys wins" Or "Its all about me." Gross personal self-absorption provides an inadequate framework for ethical decision making in health care. In the provision of health care, RTs are often called on to make decisions in accordance with our better selves; an attitude of "anything goes" is unacceptable.

As health care providers, when RTs involve themselves in unethical practices, they not only harm their patients, careers, and personal reputations, but also, by association, they harm all their fellow practitioners. Insofar as unethical practice lowers the general esteem in which health care providers are held, it harms the community at large. One analogy that is often used to describe the provision of health care is the community commons. In earlier times, often, each small town had a common shared field in which to keep the animals. This community commons was the shared responsibility of all the townspeople. In this sense the health care environment where we practice is the shared responsibility of all practitioners, and each of us has an obligation for its maintenance and upkeep. It is unthinkable and unwise to believe that maintenance of the health care commons is the responsibility of some other group, such as a state legislature or physicians. Providing ethical care, refining the quality of our practice, and providing community service are not the obligations of a few; they are the obligations of all. It is a privilege to be a health care provider; it is a duty to conduct ourselves in practice in such a manner that we can come again, and when we finally leave, to leave the commons healthy so that others can replace us in the labor. Nothing damages the community commons of health care as badly as does unethical practice.

Basic Principles of Health Care Ethics

Health care in the United States is aggressively patient centered but has ancient roots. Two models of health care from the ancient Greeks that have significance for our times are the cults of Aesculapius and Hygieia. The cult of Hygieia was developed on a broad public health and social model of prevention. The origin of the term *hygiene* means "good for health," and the cult of

I swear by Apollo, the Physician, by Asclepius, by Hygieia, Panacea, and the gods and goddesses, making them my witnesses, that I will fulfill according to my ability and judgment this oath and covenant.

To hold him who has taught me this art as equal to my parents and to live my life in partnership with him, and if he is in need of money to give him a share of mine, and to regard his offspring as equal to my brothers in male lineage and to teach them this art—if they desire to learn it—without fee and covenant; to give a share of precepts and oral instructions all the learning to my sons and to the sons of him who has instructed me and to pupils who have signed the covenant and have taken an oath according to the medical law, but to no one else.

- I will apply dietetic measures for the benefit of the sick according to my ability and judgment; I will keep them from harm and injustice.
- I will neither give a deadly drug to anybody if asked for it, nor will I make a suggestion to this effect. Similarly I will not give to a woman an abortive remedy. In purity and holiness I will guard my life and my art.
- I will not use the knife, not even on sufferers from stone, but will withdraw in favor of such men as are engaged in this work.
- Whatever houses I may visit, I will come for the benefit of the sick, remaining free of all intentional injustices, of all mischief and in particular of sexual relations with both male and female persons, be they free or slaves.
- What I may see or hear in the course of the treatment or even outside of the treatment in regard to the life of men, which on no account one must noise abroad, I will keep to myself holding such things shameful to be spoken about.
- If I fulfill this oath and do not violate it, may it be granted to me to enjoy life and art, being honored with fame among all men for all time to come; if I transgress it and swear falsely, may the opposite of all this be my lot.

FIGURE 2-2 The Hippocratic Oath.

Hygieia was directed toward the prevention of disease rather than therapy. In this sense it was more closely related to the traditional practices of Chinese medicine than those of the West, although the modern HMO system was originally based on a supposition that preventive care (preventing injury and illness) was less costly and more effective than curing illness and the effects of injury.

The cult of Aesculapius (introduced in Rome from Greece 293 BCE) was strictly a patient–health care practitioner affair aimed at getting the particular individual patient physically well. In this light, health care would be patient centered and the practitioner would not mix social, political, or economic considerations with the care of the patients. It is clear that the current health care model in the United States is more based on the traditions of Aesculapius than on those of Hygieia, although our public health and wellness efforts are more in keeping with the latter. The Hippocratic Oath (Figure 2-2) provides an early Aesculapian model for professional ethics.

A professional system of ethics, such as that found in respiratory care practice and health-related law, can be considered applied ethics. It is designed to promote ethical and legal practice in the profession and to promote the major purposes of the specialty. In health care, the major good or purpose is usually expressed as the pursuit of good health, with the prevention of death and the alleviation of suffering as secondary goals. The basic operative principles that have been developed to assist health care providers in determining right from wrong in value decisions are respect for persons, beneficence, nonmaleficence, justice, and role duty. Refer to Figure 2-1 for the AARC Statement of Ethics and Professional Conduct.

RESPECT FOR PERSONS

The principles that speak to the patient-centeredness of our ethical practices are gathered under the general principle of respect for persons. These include patient confidentiality, veracity, and personal autonomy.

Confidentiality. **Confidentiality** (the keeping private of information) is a principle that is perhaps the easiest to understand and the hardest to honor given the problems associated with modern health care. Any breach of confidentiality, in essence an invasion of privacy, can create a wide gulf of distrust between a patient and a respiratory therapist. Using knowledge of a patient's condition as grist for the cafeteria gossip mill is an inexcusable abuse of patient trust. Yet it is important to understand that society has determined that there are conditions under which confidentiality must be breached for the public good. The following are some situations in which there is a legal requirement to break confidentiality:

- Child abuse
- Elder abuse

- Communicable disease
- Births and deaths
- Wounds made with knives and guns
- Criminal acts (e.g., attempted suicide, rape, drug abuse)
- Communicable disease in newborns (e.g., diarrhea and staphylococcal infections)

Beyond legal requirements that overcome our duty to provide confidentiality, there are situations in which confidentiality is overridden by more compelling obligations. The personal protective privilege of confidentiality is limited by the **harm principle**. This principle requires that health care providers report information that is necessary to protect others who are vulnerable to grave health and safety risks. As an example, if the practitioner knew that someone was HIV-positive, and that the patient was unwilling to inform his sexual partners while still determined to continue sexual relations, there would be a duty to inform the vulnerable individuals. It would be unlikely that the respiratory therapist would have the direct obligation to tell the partners of their danger, but someone in the health care system would have that duty. The breaching of the obligation to maintain confidentiality is recognized and is stated in certain specialty codes of ethics, such as the 1992 Principles of Medical Ethics of the American Medical Association statement: "A physician may not reveal the confidences entrusted to him in the course of medical attendance . . . , unless he is required to do so by the law or unless it becomes necessary in order to protect the welfare of the individual or of the community."[9]

With health care information being available to great numbers of individuals throughout the hospitals via computer screens, confidentiality is very difficult to maintain. Because of the difficulty to maintain confidentiality in modern health care, confidentiality has been called the *decrepit concept*. On the other hand, perhaps confidentiality has become more important as a personal duty of providers, requiring an extra effort, precisely because it has become so much more difficult to maintain. Recognizing the growing problem in 1996, Congress enacted the **Health Insurance Portability and Accountability Act (HIPAA)** designed to encourage the use of electronic transmission of health information (to assist in cost containment) and provide new safeguards to protect the security and confidentiality of the information.[10] Under HIPAA, individuals have a right to:

- Request restrictions as to what information can be given out and to whom
- Receive notice of the health provider's privacy practices
- Access to see, and get copies of their records and request amendments
- Request an accounting of all disclosures of their health information

All health care providers have a duty to provide security for both paper and electronic transmission of individual health information: to become knowledgeable in regard to the requirements of HIPAA, to understand and comply with the institutions, policies in regard to the complaint process, and to assist in investigations. Failure to comply with HIPAA regulations is not only a breach of ethical conduct but also allows for both civil, monetary, and criminal penalties.

Veracity. Although we are taught that honesty is the best policy, the principle of **veracity** (truth telling), as an absolute, is difficult to fulfill. Yet veracity is an important principle in health care provision because telling lies cuts at the very heart of the patient-provider relationship. If the patient lies to the therapist, then the therapist has difficulty figuring out what is best for the patient. If the therapist lies to the patient, then the patient, not having appropriate information, will have a hard time making appropriate decisions. Although it is conceivable that lying to the patient may become necessary to avoid some greater harm, it cannot be entered into lightly because it interferes directly with the patient's autonomy. Tolerance for lying damages health care delivery. Patients believe lies only because truthfulness is the anticipated standard from health care providers. If patients begin to expect deceit an essential element of good health care delivery will have been lost.

Autonomy. Patient **autonomy** is perhaps the most important element under the respect for a person's principle. The word *autonomy* comes from the Greek *autos* ("self") and *nomos* ("governance"). In health care, autonomy has come to mean a form of personal liberty, where the patient is free to choose and implement his or her own decisions, free from deceit, coercion, duress, or constraint. **Informed consent** (a patient's authorization of medical intervention) flows directly from the principles of autonomy and veracity; patients can exercise self-determination in decision making only after they have appropriate information. The common elements of informed consent are:

- *Disclosure*. The nature of the condition, the various options, associated material risks, the professional's recommendation, and the nature of consent as an act of authorization.
- *Understanding*. Most states require that the physician provide information at the level that a hypothetical reasonable person could understand.
- *Voluntariness*. No effort toward coercion, manipulation, or constraint is allowed. The patient

must be in a position to make an authentic autonomous decision.

- *Competence.* Decisions in regard to competence usually take into account experience, maturity, responsibility, and independence of judgment.
- *Consent.* An autonomous, authentic authorization of medical intervention.

Legal exceptions to the rule of informed consent have been allowed under considerations of therapeutic privilege, especially in cases of emergency, of incompetence, of waiver, and in which there is implied consent. One ethically problematic use of therapeutic privilege is in cases in which benevolent deception is used. In such a case, the practitioner intentionally withholds information because of his or her "sound medical judgment" that to divulge the information would harm the depressed or unstable patient. Benevolent deception is a form of paternalism; the attitude that something is done for the patient's own good. Informed consent binds the physician to an adequate disclosure and explanation of the treatment and its various alternatives and consequences. It is the duty of the physician to obtain informed consent; other health professionals may assist in the process, but it is the doctor who must fully explain the procedures and treatment options.

Emphasis on patient autonomy over practitioner paternalism is a relatively new, but expanding, phenomenon in health care. The evolving body of information regarding this subject has been away from practitioner paternalism and toward patient autonomy. As stated in the AMA's 1992 Fundamental Elements of the Patient-Physician Relationship, the "patient has the right to make decisions regarding the health care that is recommended by his or her physician. Accordingly, patients may accept or refuse any recommended treament."[11]

BENEFICENCE

The common English usage of the term **beneficence** suggests mercy and charity. In health care usage the term is more in keeping with the Hippocratic Oath statement that the practitioner will "apply measures for the benefit of the sick." The obligation to benefit the sick imposes upon the practitioner a duty to promote the health and welfare of the patient above other considerations. Patients' assumption that their providers are struggling incessantly on their behalf is of great importance to their morale, especially those who are summoning all their energies to fight illness.

NONMALEFICENCE

Whereas statements involving beneficence are usually stated in active terms, as actions to prevent or remove harm, those involving **nonmaleficence** are stated in passive terms, as a duty to refrain from inflicting harm. Although it would seem only common sense that the therapist would not inflict harm on patients, when stopping to consider how often in the use of modern technology there are serious side effects, at times doing some degree of harm seems inevitable. As an example, morphine used as an analgesic will often suppress respiration.

Some scholars have advocated the principle of **double effect** when the practitioner is faced with an ambiguous situation in which there are multiple effects to an action. The following guiding elements are used in determining if an action is ethical when there are unintended but foreseeable negative side effects:

- The course chosen must be good or at least morally neutral.
- The good must not follow as a consequence of the secondary harmful effects.
- The harm must never be intended but merely tolerated as causally connected with the good intended.
- The good must outweigh the harm.

To examine the complexity and limitations of the principle of double effect, consider the case of conjoined twins. If the twins are not separated, both will die. If they are separated, one will die because she does not have lungs or adequate circulation and is dependent upon the other. Can the one twin be ethically sacrificed to save the other? Must both die? The guiding elements of the principle of double effect would seem to suggest that the surgery to separate the twins could not be ethically justified because the perceived good (the life of one) would be the direct result of the death of the other. A court might allow the separation of the twins, but it would not be able to do so on the basis of the principle of double effect.

There is no clear consensus as to the value of the principle of double effect. Many scholars feel that if a side effect is foreseen, then it has become part of the intended effects. Although there are arguments against the double effect principle, it still provides a manner in which to examine these difficult decisions.

JUSTICE

As are many of the basic principles of health care ethics, the principle of justice is seemingly very simple in the abstract and complex in application. **Justice** is the principle that deals with issues of fairness, just deserts, and entitlements. In a just society, what is due the individual?

Procedural justice, often known as *due process,* is the category of justice used in cases in which there is a dispute between individuals. For instance, if a practitioner is accused of falsifying a patient record, what due processes need be in place to ensure that the practitioner is treated fairly, or justly?

Distributive justice answers the question of how resources are to be distributed. Some common formulas for distributive justice are:

- To each an equal share.
- To each according to need.
- To each according to merit.
- To each according to contribution.
- To each according to effort.
- To each according to social worth.

Which of the categories is best suited to distribute health care fairly? Is there justice in having the rich receive better care than the poor? Is there justice in having children receive less of the health care dollar than the elderly?

Another category of justice is compensatory justice, in which individuals seek compensation for a wrong that has been done. This has become a major issue as the courts have struggled to provide justice to those who have claimed harm from breast implants, asbestos, and tobacco. If one considers the costs associated with lung cancer, chronic obstructive lung disease, and other problems directly related to cigarette smoking, how much money would be required to adequately compensate the individuals or the society? Does the warning label on the package overcome the claims, and therefore no compensatory justice is due?

ROLE DUTY

A **role duty** is a duty that exists owing to a person's job or position. In many cases, role duties are delineated in the scope of practice section of the state legislation that governs respiratory care practice in the state. The nature and traditions of the specialty are what define the role. As an example, the respiratory therapist and the physician are often both at the scene when patients are acutely ill or have died. Yet, by tradition and duty, it is the physician's role to explain to the patient's family the level of acuity of the patient. It is ethically and legally important that specialists practice faithfully in the constraints of our role. There is no excuse for respiratory therapists to overreach their scope of practice. When they do, the patients are poorly served and the whole profession is brought into a poor light.

Often, failures in the observance of role duty, such as sexual improprieties with patients, will have not only professional sanctions but also legal ramifications. A significant number of health professionals have been involved in litigated cases. Therapists who find themselves sexually attracted to their patients must seek personal help for themselves and must refer the involved patients to other therapists. Sexual misconduct represents a violation of patient trust, exploitation of vulnerability and use of undue influence.[12] In *Heineche v. Department of Commerce*,[13] a male nurse lost his license for having had a consensual sexual relationship with a patient, even though he had already resigned from the hospital where he had met her and she was no longer a patient.

Basic Decision-Making Models

Our societal morals and legal rights develop from our general worldviews. Ask almost anyone on the street to name some positive values, and the list would most likely contain the following:

- Honesty
- Love
- Lawfulness
- Equality
- Justice
- Charity
- Benevolence

Although few humans manage in their lives to uphold all of these values all of the time, we generally agree on them or at least agree that some things *are* right and some things are wrong. A morally neutral society could not keep social order and would probably never progress.

We can gain an understanding of how value decisions are made by examining how we talk about any controversial issue. Consider the following justifications of conflicting positions regarding abortion:

1. I have a right to my body, I can make whatever choice I want.
2. Life is sacred; the Bible tells us that abortion is wrong.
3. Abortion trivializes life. You start with the preborns, and then it will be the elderly and helpless.
4. People are breeding like rabbits; abortions are environmentally necessary to stabilize world population.
5. Abortion is acceptable only in the case of rape or incest; no baby should be born to someone who did not ask for it or want it.
6. Abortion is acceptable only to protect the health of the mother or if the baby would be grossly defective.
7. I don't want this baby because it interferes with my life plans.
8. A fetus is a human, and humans have the right to life, liberty, and the pursuit of happiness.

Examination of these arguments shows that most of them are based on the effects or consequences of the actions (teleological, or consequence-oriented, arguments). The others are based on an appeal to some rule or principle (deontological, or duty-oriented, arguments). Statements 3, 4, 5, 6, and 7 are not appeals to principles or rules but rather are justified on the basis of consequences, of what will happen if the decision to allow abortion is made. These arguments are generally designed to increase general happiness and avoid pain. Statement 1 appeals to the principle of the right of any individual to personal autonomy in making decisions regarding her body. Statement 2 makes an appeal to the religious principle of the sanctity of life, and statement 8 appeals to the principle of human rights.

CONSEQUENCE-ORIENTED THEORIES

The term *teleological* comes from the Greek word *telos*, which means "end." Teleological (consequence-oriented) theory then is the study of how things end, a study of outcomes. Consequence-oriented theories judge the rightness or wrongness of a decision by the outcomes or predicted outcomes. Individuals following a consequence-oriented theory would decide that the right decision was one that maximized some good. The right thing to do, then, is that which brings about the best outcome.

The most common form of consequence-oriented reasoning is **utilitarianism**, which is a philosophical position first described by Jeremy Bentham (1748–1832) and John Stuart Mill (1806–1873). To the utilitarian the good resides in the promotion of happiness or the greatest net increase in pleasure over pain.

The purest form of utilitarian reasoning is act utilitarianism, where the decision is made by listing all the potential alternatives for action and then weighing each in regard to the amount of pleasure or utility it provides and then selecting the choice that maximizes the pleasure. Figure 2-3 provides a format for decision

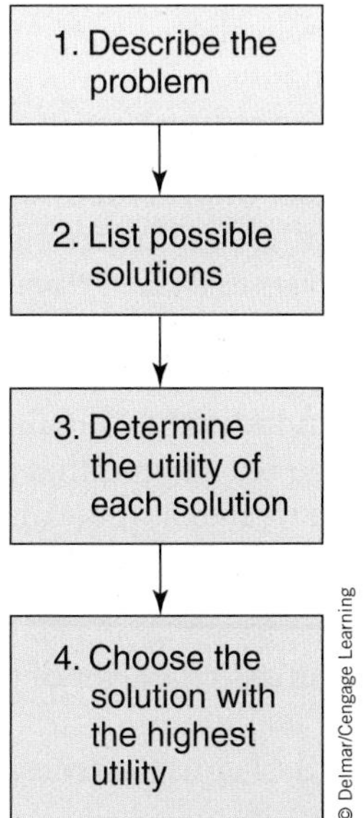

1. Describe the problem
2. List possible solutions
3. Determine the utility of each solution
4. Choose the solution with the highest utility
© Delmar/Cengage Learning

FIGURE 2-3 A flowchart for making consequence-oriented decisions.

making using utilitarian reasoning. Perhaps the greatest difficulty to problem solving using act utilitarianism is that the individual must somehow predict and calculate all the various levels of pleasure gained and pain avoided for each potential action.

On its surface, utilitarianism appears to be a rather hedonistic method of decision making as it might lead to the majority group's deriving pleasure from the pain of a minority and justifying the decision on the basis of the utility of the most good for the most people. To overcome these problems, most modern formulations of consequence-oriented reasoning have inserted the principle of "equal consideration of interest," which holds that each individual must be considered equally in the process. The basic formulation for act utilitarianism then can be captured in the principle that one should act in such a way as to produce the greatest balance of happiness over unhappiness, everyone considered. Another interesting problem with utilitarianism is that if all one considered in the decision was maximizing happiness and avoiding unhappiness, then it would be possible to consider that a happy, satisfied pig might be on a higher moral plane than a dissatisfied Socrates. In order to overcome this criticism that utilitarianism was a "pig philosophy," Mill defined happiness as a set of higher moral pleasures such as intellectual, aesthetic, and social enjoyments rather than just sensual pleasure.[14]

Rule utilitarianism overcomes some of the difficulties of act utilitarianism in that it does not require the exact quantification of all the pleasure gained and pain avoided with each option before making a decision. Rule utilitarianism is a theory that allows for rules to be prejudged using a measurement of utility. Utility would require that the rule would bring about positive results when generalized to a larger context. As an example, let us consider the rule regarding the freedom of speech. No one thinks that free speech brings about happiness and avoids pain in all cases, but, in general, free speech has a high utility in that under most circumstances a rule that allowed free speech would bring about positive results.

Consequence-oriented reasoning is often very persuasive in that it seems to support our modern skepticism regarding absolute truths and rules and speaks to our better selves in regard to tolerating the values and cultures of others. Although consequence orientation appears persuasive, it is not altogether free from problems in its usage. Several problems associated with utilitarian reasoning are:

- The calculation of all possible consequences of our actions, or worse, our inactions, appears impossible.
- The theory does not give enough respect to persons. Under the theory, the ends justify the

CASE STUDY 2-3

A certified therapist wished to pass himself off as a registered therapist in order to move up in the department. After considering falsifying his documents for a period of time, he decided not to because he feared sanctions and the loss of his position.

Questions

1. On the basis of consequence-oriented reasoning, is this therapist any different from another therapist who never considered fraud? Why?
2. On the basis of virtue-oriented reasoning, are they different? Why?
3. On the basis of duty-oriented reasoning, are they different? Why?

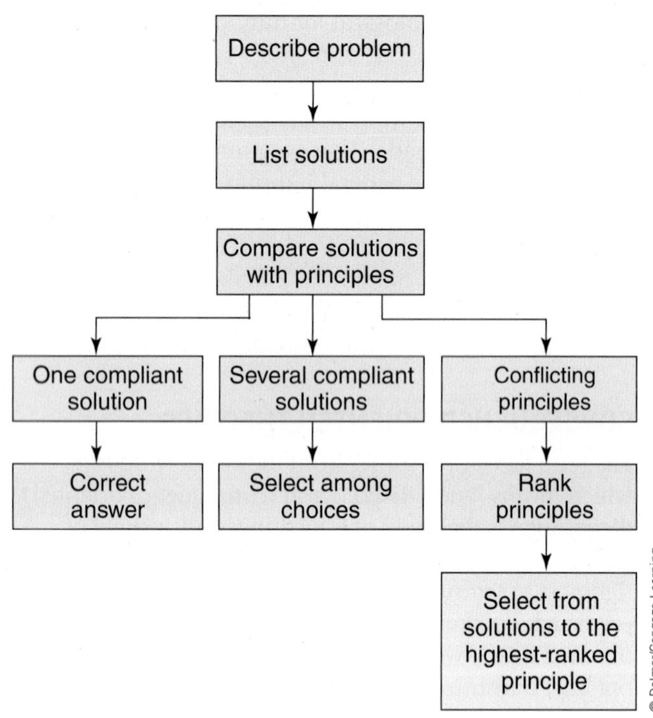

FIGURE 2-4 A flowchart for making duty-oriented decisions.

means so it may be moral to use a person as a means to our ends.

- Using the theory it could be justifiable to interfere with the personal liberty of others especially to prevent them from harmful acts to themselves. If smoking is bad, for the good of all legislators could ban it. Such a paternalistic view could justify unacceptable governmental intervention into the lives of individuals.
- Utilitarianism is not sensitive to the agent relativity of duty. As an example, we generally believe that parents have special duties to their children and that physicians have special duties toward their patients and that these special duties should prevent them from purposefully harming them. One could imagine a scenario in which harming patients and abusing children would have a high utility.

DUTY-ORIENTED THEORIES

Deontological (duty-oriented) ethicists feel that the basic rightness or wrongness of an act does not depend upon consequences or results but rather is part of its intrinsic nature. Figure 2-4 provides a format for decision making using a duty-oriented system. In this light, an act itself would be either right or wrong; it could not be both. This particular worldview is codified in several major ethical systems and by many religions.

Perhaps the foremost formulation of duty-oriented reasoning is Kantian ethics, based on the work of Immanuel Kant (1724–1804). Kant held that morality is derived not from human nature or from the consequences of actions but rather from pure reason. He held that as rational beings we could derive principles that are universal. These universal truths would be true for all people, for all situations, and for all times. An action could be known to be true when it conformed to one of these universal principles, which he called categorical imperatives. By "categorical" he meant that the rule did not permit exception, and by "imperative" he meant that it was a command derived from a principle. These rules have three major components:

- Universal application
- Unconditionality
- Demanding an action

Perhaps the most important of these categorical imperatives relevant to health care ethics is that "*one must always treat others as ends in themselves and not as means only.*" According to Kant all people have an absolute value, based on their ability to make rational choices. He felt that individual dignity was derived from our capacity to reason and that it was violated when a person was treated as a means (a thing) and not as a person.[15] Kantian ethics has many detractors. Several criticisms of Kantian reasoning are:

- The exceptionless character of the philosophy is too rigid for real life.
- The disregard of consequences can lead to disastrous results.
- The fact that people feel pain and pleasure is central to morality and the human experience. It

is unlikely that morality flows from pure reason alone.

- It is possible to be in a situation in which two duties conflict, yet are both equally supported by an imperative.

Duty-oriented theorists obviously wish to promote a good result; however, they believe that merely serving the good is not an adequate foundation for ethics. For these theorists, the right action is one based on a correct principle regardless of results. As an example, if we choose a principle such as the sanctity of life, then murder is wrong, and its wrongness cannot be modified by the situation leading to the action. Duty-oriented theorists argue among themselves as to how the principles are derived. Some claim they are based on reason; others, on natural law, intuition, social contract, or religious dictate. The individual who believes that murder is wrong in all cases and the priest who maintains the confidentiality of the confessional even in cases of unreported criminal activity are both following a duty-oriented form of reasoning.

VIRTUE ETHICS

It is clear that neither consequence nor duty ethics has produced a system that has been able to overcome its major criticisms. Since the 1970s, several theorists have begun to explore ethics not as a set of rules to guide actions but rather as an attribute of character.[16]

In consequence-oriented reasoning the focus is on reasoning to an appropriate action rather than on the intent of the agent. In **virtue ethics** the focus is not on the action but rather upon the moral agent. The Greek philosopher Aristotle posed the problem in his *Nicomachean Ethics* when he avoided both duty- and consequence-oriented reasoning and focused instead on the intent and the heart of the moral agent. "We may go so far as to state that the man who does not enjoy performing noble actions is not a good man at all. Nobody would call a man just who does not enjoy acting justly, nor generous who does not enjoy generous action, and so on." In this light it is not the weak person who is tempted and finally makes the right choice who is to be admired but rather the person who by virtue of his character is not tempted in the first place.

Virtue-based decisions are motivated by what the actor believes to be good and true. Duty- or role-based ethical decisions are motivated by stated or implied rationales that say, "In my role as a [whatever specialty]. I have a duty to do____." For example, "In my role as a respiratory therapist, I have a duty to make vigorous attempts to treat all patients with equal care regardless of my personal feelings for or about them."

The question then is how to gain the level of character at which one would, without analysis, make a virtuous decision. The answer according to Aristotle is practice. Virtue is not the natural state of humans but is rather gained by the habit of doing virtuous acts. Goodness of character is brought about by the practice of such virtues as courage, honesty, and justice. One becomes just and temperate by doing just and temperate things until justice and temperance become part of one's natural character. In this sense Shakespeare's Hamlet was correct: "If one would have virtue, one must first assume it."

Every profession has its set of ideal practices or virtues of practice. This set of virtues is gained from the practices of the past, especially from specialists who have expanded the profession. For nursing it would be individuals such as Florence Nightingale and Clara Barton; for respiratory care, it would be individuals such as Jimmy Young, Wilma Bright, and James Whitacre, who had distinguished careers and who helped establish the foundations of the profession and virtuous practices associated with what the good respiratory therapist does in a value-laden situation.

With virtue ethics, if current respiratory therapists found themselves in situations in which they needed to make a value-laden professional decision, they would not need to find a duty-oriented principle to apply or attempt to perform the mathematical calculations of all the potential pleasures gained and pains avoided. Rather, the process would require that the practitioner rely on the traditions of earlier good practitioners to guide the decision. In some sense, it is asking oneself, "What would a good respiratory therapist do in this situation?" Figure 2-5 provides a decision-making format for virtue ethics.

A major problem with using virtue ethics in making value-laden decisions in respiratory care practice is that the field is changing so rapidly. Many of the issues surrounding managed care, organ donations, and genetic technologies are new to the health care scene and therefore there is no precedence of good

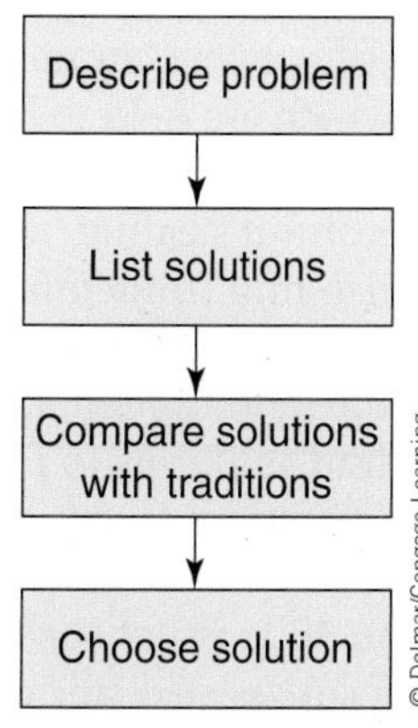

FIGURE 2-5 A flowchart for making virtue-oriented decisions.

practice that can be brought forward. It is quite possible that responsible good practice under managed care is significantly different than in previous times. Some major criticisms of virtue ethics are:

- Virtue ethics does not in general provide specific directions in regard to decision making.
- In that virtue ethics is based on traditional practice, it does not respond quickly to new situations.
- A traditional emphasis makes morality depend on past experience rather than on reason. This environment provides little respect for creative solutions or personal autonomy.
- Practitioners often find themselves attempting to address more than one set of idealized traditions, which may come into conflict (e.g., the need to be a team player versus the need to be a whistle-blower, as in a case of negligent care by a colleague).

Even with the problems associated with virtue ethics decision making there is something persuasive about the process. Examination of how we make decisions as practitioners shows how we often find ourselves following the dictates of an idealized role. What would a good respiratory therapist do in this situation?

To understand the difference between virtue ethics and consequence oriented theories, consider that focusing on consequences only would create the decision that a therapist who contemplates fraud, but did not carry it out, is no different from one who never considers it. Virtue-oriented reasoning would hold that because their intents, or hearts, were different the two therapists were different.

DIVINE COMMAND THEORY

An additional theory for ethical decision making, and one often used in ethical discourse, is **divine command theory**. The idea is relatively simple and straight forward. Divine command theorists hold that a divine being has given a finite set of rules that adherents can use to resolve most, if not all, moral dilemmas. One of the great examples of a divine command is the Ten Commandments, which are held to be moral imperatives by followers of Judeo-Christian faiths. The Ten Commandments prohibit stealing, murder, adultery, and so on, which also find condemnation in most of the world's cultures. In that a set of finite rules are by their very nature finite and limited, adherents attempt to extend them to find solutions to problems that seem related but are not directly covered, or covered only by implication. Hence, some extend the prohibition against murder to include issues such as abortion, stem cell research, physician assisted suicide, and euthanasia. Obviously, many others believe that the basic rules cannot be extended in this matter.

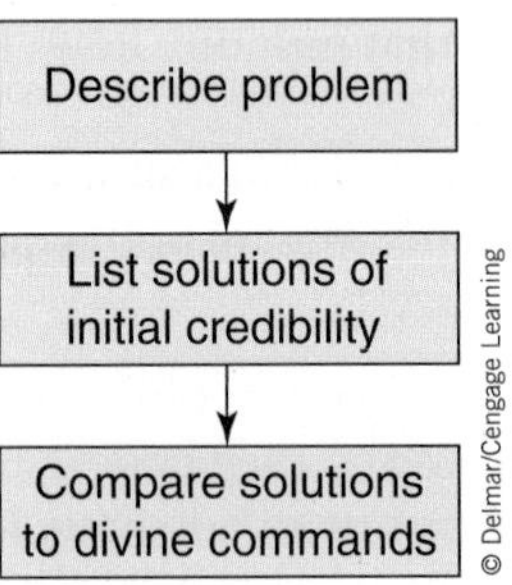

FIGURE 2-6 Divine command decision flowchart.

An important variant to divine command theory is the teachings of nondivine beings that are considered exemplary. Nondivine, but morally exemplary beings such as Siddhartha Gautama (Buddha) have also provided adherents with formal sets of rules that guide conduct. Rules such as The Noble Eight Fold Path, as found in Buddhism, function with the same logic as the divine command theory, with the important difference being that their origin is the teaching of a nondivine being.

For followers of rules set forth by a divinity, or exemplary but not divine individual, the logic of Divine Command theory works the same. Both groups follow rules that provide moral injunctions that believers are to obey upon pain of divine retribution in cases such as Judeo-Christian rules, or failure to achieve Nirvana for followers of Buddhism. Figure 2-6 provides a flowchart for making decisions using divine command theory. Divine command theory is similar to most deontological theories with the exception that the answer is gained not from an appeal to reason but rather to revelation. Like theories such as Kantian Ethics, divine command rules generally have three major components.

- Universal application
- Unconditionality
- Demanding of an action

There is no question that followers of divine command theory, whether derived from Judeo-Christian, Islamic, Buddhist, Hindu or other religious frameworks, often find in their traditions a meaningful system for decision making. However, as health care providers, we find ourselves in an increasingly complex world of believers and nonbelievers, in a world where new questions, seemingly unimaginable by earlier generations, arise. It is difficult to see how ancient texts can provide answers with a high degree of certainty involving questions such as cloning, or acceptable limits to posthumanism, or whether a child should be conceived using frozen sperm taken from a deceased spouse. These new questions associated with the continued development of science and technology threaten to stretch any absolutist theory such as divine command, to its very limit. Yet as seen in Figure 2-7,

AME and AME Zion – Donation is viewed as an act of neighborly love and charity. They encourage all members to support donation as a way of helping others.

Amish – The Amish consent to donation as they know it is for the health and welfare of the transplant recipient. They believe that since God created the human body, it is God who heals. However, they are not forbidden from using modern medical services, including surgery, hospitalization, dental work, anesthesia, blood transfusions, or immunizations.

Assembly of God – Donation is highly supported.

Baptist – In 1988, the Southern Baptist Convention passed a resolution supporting donation as a way to alleviate suffering and have compassion for the needs of others. Donation is advocated as an act of charity.

Buddhism – Donation is a matter of individual conscience and high value is placed on acts of compassion. Organ donation is a gift to help humanity and as such benefits the donor's karma. The importance of letting loved ones know your wishes is stressed.

Christian Scientist – Christian Scientists normally rely on spiritual means of healing rather than medical. They are free, however, to choose whatever form of medical treatment they desire, including a transplant. The question of donation is left to the individual member.

Episcopal – In 1982, a resolution was passed that recognizes the life-giving benefits of organ, blood, and tissue donations. All Episcopalians are encouraged to become donors.

Evangelical Lutheran Church of America – The Evangelical Lutheran Church in America passed a resolution in 1984 stating that donation contributes to the well-being of humanity and can be "an expression of love for neighbor in need."

Greek Orthodox Church – Donation is supported as a way to better human life through transplantation or research, leading to improvements in the treatment and prevention of diseases.

Hinduism – According to H.L. Trivedi in the scientific journal *Transplantation Proceedings,* "There is nothing in the Hindu religion indicating that parts of humans cannot be used to alleviate the suffering of other humans."

Islam – The principle of saving human lives is of utmost importance. According to A. Sachedina in *Transplantation Proceedings.* "The majority of the Muslims scholars belonging to various schools of Islamic law have invoked the principle of priority of saving human life and have permitted the organ transplant as a necessity to procure that noble end."

Jehovah's Witness – According to the Watch Tower Society, donation is a matter of individual decision. Members are often assumed to be against donation because of opposition to blood transfusions. However, this means only that all blood must be removed from the organs and tissue before being transplanted.

Judaism – All four branches of Judaism support and encourage donation. Numerous resolutions have been passed encouraging donation.

Mennonite – Mennonites have no formal position on donation, but are not opposed to it, leaving the decision to donate up to the individual and/or his or her family.

Mormon – The Church of Jesus Christ of Latter-Day Saints does not oppose donation. The church believes that the decision to donate is an individual one made in conjunction with family, medical personnel, and prayer.

Pentecostal – Pentecostals believe that the decision to donate should be left up to the individual.

Presbyterian – Presbyterians encourage and support donation. They respect a person's right to make decisions regarding his or her own body.

Roman Catholic Church – Donation is viewed as an act of charity and love. Transplants are morally and ethically acceptable to the Vatican.

Seventh-Day Adventist – Donation and transplantation are strongly encouraged and many of the church-run hospitals such as Loma Linda in California offer these services.

Shinto – In Shinto, the dead body is considered impure and dangerous, and thus quite powerful. Injuring a dead body is a serious crime. It is difficult to obtain consent from bereaved families for organ donation or dissection for medical education. Members relate donation to injuring a dead body. Families are concerned that they not injure the itai, the relationship between the dead person and the bereaved people.

Unitarian Universalist – Donation is widely supported and viewed as an act of love and giving.

United Methodist – A 1984 policy statement regarding organ and tissue donation states that the church "recognizes the life-giving benefits of organ and tissue donation, and thereby encourages all Christians to become organ and tissue donors . . . ."

FIGURE 2-7 Religious positions regarding organ donations.

Reprinted with permission of UNOS, from An Organ Donation Guide for Faith Leaders and Health Care Professionals[17]

when one examines the decisions by a variety of religions with regard to organ donation, it is clear that divine command reasoning can be very adaptive.

As with the other systems of ethical decision making, the **divine command ethics** format has not satisfied all scholars and critics. Some major criticisms of divine command ethics are:

- Divine command theories assume a belief in either divine or exemplary individuals. To the extent that these beliefs can be questioned, so can the theory.
- Divine command theories generally have a "no exception" clause, either explicit or implicit. This is a problem for individuals living in morally complicated times.
- It is difficult to imagine that any set of religious traditions could cover all possible cases of moral decision. This leads either to a fundamentalism, in which one states that the extension of the basic rules to other cases is unproblematic, or to differences in interpretation, and therefore differences in people's decisions regarding these issues.
- Divine command theory has been questioned by what is known as the *Euthyphro Problem*, taken from the Platonic dialogue from which it originated. The problem resides in how the divine or exemplary being came to the original decision for the rule. Did the divine or exemplary being decide arbitrarily that the rule was correct, or is the divine or exemplary being basing the decision on some justifying reason beyond "I told you so." If it is just "I told you so," then it is difficult to imagine why we should obey a rule so arbitrarily chosen. If it is based on some other underlying justifying reason, then perhaps we could refer directly to the justifying reason without reference to the deity. In either case, one could question assenting to divine command rules.

Regardless of the criticisms, divine command theory seems to be very useful for personal decision making and perhaps is an enhancement to the process of ethical reasoning. Given that the answers provided are from divine or exemplary sources, they are also very effective in reaching agreement among the community of believers. The real problems arise when one is reasoning toward an answer with a follower of a different belief system. If, after a person consults his or her particular belief system and an answer is gained, how does the person explore or value other options? Individuals, who perceive that they have revealed truth, often find it difficult to explore options from other sources. Another unfortunate side effect of divine command theory is that the true believer often sees his or her answer as not only being correct, but also good, which leaves the non-believer holding a position that is not only incorrect but perhaps bad.

CASE STUDY 2-4

Recently there has been a spate of cases where health care providers have refused to provide services based on their religious beliefs:

- Does a pharmacist have a duty to provide "day-after pills"?
- Does a Catholic hospital have a duty to permit obstetricians to perform sterilizations immediately after giving birth? Would the answer be different if they accepted any federal money?
- Can a physician be sued for violating state anti discrimination laws due to his refusal to artificially inseminate a patient involved in a lesbian relationship?
- Can health care providers be required to remove hydration and nutrition from patients for whom these seemingly ordinary and standard procedures have been deemed "extraordinary care"?
- If no other physician is available, can a physician refuse to participate in a request for physician-assisted suicide where state law permits the practice?

Questions

In order to answer the preceding questions, the two freedoms at stake must be examined. For the patient, the case will most often be presented in terms of personal autonomy, or relief of suffering. For the health care provider the issue will be a right to act in accordance with his or her conscience. Can a just society force people to violate their personal consciences?

1. Think of how you might answer these questions, using whatever ethical decision-making format you choose. Then consider them using divine command.
2. How would you handle a work situation where you were asked to perform a service that went against your personal conscience?

The Decision-Making Process

Whatever ethical framework chosen, whether duty, consequence, divine command, or virtue, the respiratory therapist will find he or she will need to proceed through certain steps as decisions are made. There are several problem-solving formulas from which to choose; however, most will include the following six steps:

1. *Identify the characteristics of the problem.* Describe the problem, identify the principles involved. Who are the concerned parties? Who is charged with making the decision?
2. *Gather the facts of the case.* What is fact? What is opinion? What are the legal ramifications? Has the issue been decided by the courts before? What documentation exists that outlines the problem?
3. *Examine and list the options of initial credibility.* One of the real problems with decision making in the area of values is a rush to judgment. The more options considered, the more likely the respiratory therapist is to find one to support and defend.
4. *Weigh and evaluate the potential options.* What will happen to the individuals involved, given each option? Has everyone been considered equally? What basic principles were favored? Were any sacrificed? What basic system is being used to make the decision—duty, consequence, divine command, or virtue?
5. *Make the decision and act on it.* In that these are decisions regarding values with which others may disagree, prepare a defense for the decision should it be questioned.
6. *Assess and evaluate the results.*

CASE STUDY 2-5

Dr. S. is a very senior surgeon at a hospital. It is common talk around the hospital that Dr. S.'s patients have a higher level of hospital-borne infection after surgery than do other doctors' patients. In this case, the patient is a 38-year-old female who has undergone a full mastectomy for breast cancer. During postoperative care, you have found her to be very quiet, seemingly depressed, and not talkative with you or the family members who come to visit. She seems to be in some pain during the treatments and has a low-grade fever. After a treatment, she asks you, "Is Dr. S. a good surgeon?"

Questions

1. What are some answers you could give?
2. What principles are involved?
3. Which of the ethical systems will you use—consequence, duty, or virtue?
4. Which answer will you give?

Some Practical Advice

Ethical, legal, and professional practice is something that is gained by serious reflection, constant vigilance, continued study, and honest self-evaluation. It is an area of practice that calls upon the practitioner to be a critical thinker and a systematic decision maker. Here is some practical advice on issues that have both legal and ethical implications.

- Practice in your comfortable scope of practice. Seek consultation when you have questions.
- Provide care in accordance with good medical practice and national standards.
- Maintain accurate and complete records. Verify all telephone medical orders.
- Maintain the confidentiality and privacy of patients.
- Do not disparage the professional skills of colleagues. When the practice of another warrants criticism, use appropriate reporting mechanisms.
- Investigate all patient complaints thoroughly and promptly. Allow the patient to fully explain the nature of his or her concerns.
- Remain current in your practice. Continue professional growth and development through continuing education and association with your professional organization.

Summary

Respiratory care is a clinical practice and for the most part our careers are involved with technical and scientific issues. However, in order to truly be successful in practice, RTs must ensure that our performance is not only technically correct but also legally, ethically, and professionally correct. As health care providers, RTs draw from a vast well of trust that has been formed by the past practices of the specialists who have come before us. The patient's trust—that the provider is working single-mindedly on his or her behalf, that there are no conflicts of interest, that no secrets are being hidden, and that the provider's behavior is both ethical and legal—is an important part of the therapeutic relationship.

The provision of ethical and legal practice is not negotiable; it cannot be set aside because of schedules or personal preference or in an effort to be more efficient or productive. Performing ethically and legally is not just a nice way to practice; it is the only way to practice. In some sense, ethical, lawful behavior lies at the very heart of what is meant by being professional.

Study Questions

REVIEW QUESTIONS

1. List three major criticisms to the use of utilitarianism in making ethical decisions.
2. List four legal requirements for breaking patient confidentiality.
3. List three forms of intentional torts that a respiratory therapist might be involved with.
4. List three major criticisms to the use of Kantian ethics in making ethical decisions.
5. List and define the basic principles of healthcare ethics.
6. List three major criticisms to the use of the divine command theory in making ethical decisions.
7. Define the basic function of normative elements (as found in our rules of professional etiquette, legal requirements, and ethical codes) as they relate to the practice of respiratory care.
8. What were the two general goals of the 1966 HIPAA legislation?
9. Take the common ethical dilemma faced by all practitioners (Should I take a gratuity from a patient?) and using the flowcharts for decision making provided in the chapter work out the solution using utilitarian, Kantian, virtue ethics, and divine command reasoning.

MULTIPLE-CHOICE QUESTIONS

1. According to the philosopher Joseph Fletcher, "[M]orals are what people believe to be right and good," whereas ethics is concerned with:
   a. critical reflection and rationales for judging value problems.
   b. legal policies and procedures.
   c. professional issues only.
   d. both legal and moral issues.
2. A respiratory therapist who refuses to accept a gratuity is attending to which of the following basic principles?
   a. autonomy
   b. justice
   c. beneficence
   d. nonmaleficence
3. When the large tobacco companies are forced to pay the health costs for smokers, the ethical principle being applied is:
   a. compensatory justice.
   b. nonmaleficence.
   c. retributive justice.
   d. beneficence.
4. Informed consent flows mainly from the basic ethical principle of:
   a. autonomy.
   b. beneficence.
   c. justice.
   d. role duty.
5. In its best sense, paternalism is a contest between which of the following principles?
   a. autonomy and beneficence
   b. justice and role duty
   c. veracity and nonmaleficence
   d. role duty and autonomy
6. Which of the following ethical decision-making formats is focused on the moral agent rather than on the decision?
   a. utilitarianism
   b. duty-oriented theories
   c. virtue ethics
   d. divine command theories
7. The criticism that it is exceptionless is most meaningful in which ethical decision-making format?
   a. Kantian ethics
   b. utilitarianism
   c. virtue ethics
   d. situation ethics
8. Which form of law would not include a state's respiratory care scope of practice?
   a. constitutional law
   b. statutory law
   c. administrative law
   d. common law
9. The highest form of public law in the United States is:
   a. administrative law.
   b. criminal law.
   c. constitutional law.
   d. legislative law.

10. The legal principle *stare decisis* means:
    a. "Let the buyer beware."
    b. "Let the master answer."
    c. "The thing speaks for itself."
    d. "Let the decision stand."
11. You are trying to give a patient a treatment, and he tells you to leave him alone. Because the doctor has ordered the treatment, you push the patient's hands away and apply the mask. What tort might you just have committed?
    a. assault
    b. battery
    c. defamation of character
    d. false imprisonment
12. Morals pertain to:
    a. beliefs about right and wrong.
    b. legal policies and procedures.
    c. professional issues only.
    d. legal and value issues.
13. Which of the following is not among the basic principles involved in health care ethics as applied to respiratory care?
    a. nonmaleficence
    b. autonomy
    c. polymorphism
    d. beneficence
14. In which of the following cases is one likely to receive compensatory justice?
    a. a criminal case regarding bank robbery
    b. a suit for slander
    c. a case involving traffic tickets
    d. an administrative hearing regarding application of rules
15. An indication that informed consent is derived from the principle of autonomy is:
    a. the patient's right to refuse.
    b. the patient's being asked to sign the forms.
    c. the presence of witnesses.
    d. the institutional representative's power to make agreements.
16. In order to differentiate between duty, consequence, divine command, and virtue as forms of ethical reasoning, one must:
    a. look at the outcomes of the situation.
    b. project the distribution of costs among those affected by the action.
    c. determine the philosophical grounding of the decision maker.
    d. determine the legality of an action.
17. Which of the following statements reflects a virtue ethics format?
    a. If it is good for me, I should do it regardless of what others think.
    b. Only actions that are desired by a consensus of the group are good.
    c. The outcome will be good if the agent making the choice is good.
    d. Situations change what is good or bad: What I am allowed to do today I might not be allowed to do tomorrow.
18. In which of the following situations could you legally break patient confidentiality?
    a. A child is brought into your ER with many bruises, both old and new.
    b. A father wants the results of his 18-year-old daughter's pregnancy test.
    c. A researcher wants the names, ages, and diagnoses for a sequential group of patients visiting your clinic.
    d. The police request the medical records of a suspected hit-and-run driver.
19. Which is an intentional tort?
    a. An automobile accident is caused by an oil spill during a violent thunderstorm.
    b. A neighbor's tree has fallen across your driveway, preventing you from attending a World Series baseball game.
    c. In order to save money, your car dealer substitutes used tires for new ones on the car you just bought. The tires fail, causing damage to your car.
    d. Because of mail delays, you miss your invitation to a free cruise. Now your vacation will be at the local mall.
20. All of the following are major elements found in a practice act except for:
    a. setting of reimbursement rates.
    b. description of scope of practice .
    c. reasons for administrative action.
    d. exemptions from the act.
21. Which is a benefit derived from the principle of *stare decisis*?
    a. Provides the system with stability and allows for the creation of new principles.
    b. Does not require judicial input or action.
    c. No one is found to be at fault.
    d. Only a six-person jury is required.

22. Which of the following is a tort?
    a. I contract with another health professional to share an office; she never pays her share of the rent.
    b. While caring for a ventilator case, I fail to drain the ventilator tubing and the patient aspirates and dies.
    c. Owing to a programming fault, the record function of the IV controller reads high under certain conditions. No patients have been harmed because the company warned all customers.
    d. John goes to a bookie each week and bets $200. After 2 years he finds that Joe, the bookie, was cheating him.
23. If I speak falsely and badly about you to others, which of the following statements is true?
    a. I have both libeled and slandered you.
    b. I have defamed and libeled you.
    c. I have not libeled, slandered, or defamed you.
    d. I have defamed and slandered you.
24. Divine command theory seems to be *least like* which of the following ethical decision-making systems.
    a. Kantian ethics
    b. utilitarian ethics
    c. virtue ethics
    d. deontological ethics
25. HIPAA requirements enhance and provide duties in regard to which of the basic principles of health care ethics?
    a. veracity
    b. justice
    c. confidentiality
    d. autonomy

CRITICAL-THINKING QUESTIONS

1. When you are moving between two beds you knock a carafe of water onto a patient. The patient is wet but otherwise unhurt. Have you created the situation of an actionable tort? Defend your answer.
2. You wait in an empty parking lot for a therapist who is giving you trouble to get off shift. As he approaches his car, you walk over to him and tell him off; you call him a "backbiting ###" who gossips about the patients and other staff members. Have you committed either libel or slander? Defend your answer.
3. An FBI agent comes into the clinic, shows his credentials, and demands that he be allowed to make copies of a patient's records. The practitioner should ___________.
4. You are a student in a clinic and make a grave error. To what extent does *respondeat superior* relieve you of your personal responsibility in the matter? Explain your answer.
5. Examine the following moral dilemma using a duty, a consequence, divine command, and then virtue ethics format: Joe is a therapist on the evening shift. In a bit of horseplay with his colleague, Jim, he pushes a standby ventilator over and breaks the device. He quickly changes the device and tags the broken device for repair. Joe asks Jim to keep the cause of the broken device confidential because he does not want to get into trouble. In the morning the supervisor notices the broken device and asks Joe what happened. Joe says that he does not know, and then the supervisor turns to Jim and asks the same question. What should Jim say?
6. In what ways do HMO and managed care systems follow the precepts of the Hygieian system of the ancient Greeks? In what ways do they differ from the Hygieian system?
7. How might telling a small child that an injection "won't hurt" affect the child's future interactions with health care providers? What approach to this situation should be taken?
8. Generally for every set of rights there is a concurrent set of obligations. Review the patient's rights to their health care information as outlined in the HIPAA regulations, and create a set of practitioner obligations that support those rights.
9. Compare and Contrast the early Hippocratic Code with that of the AARC statement of ethics and professional conduct as found in the chapter.
10. Review the AARC statement on ethics and professional conduct. List those that you think promote a more Hygieian form of health care provision.

References

1. Roach W, Chernoff S, Eslley C. *Medical Records and the Law.* New York: Aspen Publications; 2006.
2. Pozgar G. *Legal Aspects of Health Care Administration.* New York: Aspen Publications; 2006.
3. Edge R, Krieger J. *Legal and Ethical Perspectives in Health Care.* Clifton Park, NY: Delmar Cengage Learning; 1998.
4. Smith G. *Respiratory Care.* Lenexa, KA: Applied Measurement Professionals; 1989.
5. *State University of New York v Young,* 170 AD2d 510.
6. Flight M. *Law, Liability, and Ethics for the Medical Office Professional.* 4th ed. Clifton Park, NY: Delmar Cengage Learning; 2004.
7. Fletcher J. *The Ethics of Genetic Control.* Garden City, NY: Anchor Books; 1988.
8. Potter VR. *Bioethics: Bridge to the Future.* Englewood Cliffs, NJ: Prentice Hall; 1973.

9. Council on Ethical and Judicial Affairs. *Code of Medical Ethics, Current Opinions*. Chicago: American Medical Association; 1992.
10. U.S. Department of Health and Human Services. *Fact Sheet: Protecting the Privacy of Patient's Health Information*, May 9, 2001.
11. Council on Ethical and Judicial Affairs. American Medical Association.
12. American Dental Association. Licensing boards confront sexual misconduct. *Am. Dent. Assoc.* 2004;135,9:1326–1329.
13. *Heineche v Department of Commerce*, 810 P2d 459 (Utah App 1991).
14. Pojman L. *Ethics: Discovering Right and Wrong*. Belmont, CA: Thompson, Wadsworth Publishing Co; 2004.
15. Johnson O, Reath A. *Ethics*. Philadelphia: Harcourt Brace College Publishers; 2006.
16. Edge R, Groves R. *The Ethics of Health Care*. Clifton Park, NY: Delmar Cengage Learning; 2006.
17. Bolton DL and Mock K, (eds). An Organ Donation Guide for Faith Leaders and Health Care Professionals. Theological Perspective on Organ and Tissue Donation. 2007;114–151. UNOS: Richmond Virginia.

Suggested Readings

AARC Position Statement: Respiratory Care Education.

AARC Position Statement: Requirements for the Provision of Respiratory Care.

AARC Position Statement: Scope of Practice.

AARC Position Statement: Role of the Respiratory Therapist in the Hospital and Alternate Sites.

Carroll C. *Legal Issues and Ethical Dilemmas in Respiratory Care*. Philadelphia: F.A. Davis; 1996.

Edge, R, Groves, R. *Ethics of Health Care: A Guide for Practitioners*. Clifton Park, NY: Delmar Cengage Learning; 2006.

Pozgar, George. *Legal and Ethical Issues for Health Professionals*. Boston: Jones & Bartlett Publishers; 2005.

SECTION II

The Applied Sciences

CHAPTER 3

Applied Physics

Paul J. Mathews

OBJECTIVES

Upon completion of this chapter, the reader should be able to:

- Understand each of the physical laws presented in this chapter and relate its application in the practice of respiratory care.
- Perform simple physics calculations.
- Provide the correct formula for each of the gas laws.
- Calculate solutions to gas law problems.
- Define each physical law discussed in the chapter, and give its correct mathematical formula.
- Perform conversions from one measurement system to another.
- Convert data from ordinary numbers into scientific notation or vice versa.
- Apply physical laws to clinical situations using clinical case study data.

CHAPTER OUTLINE

(continues)

(continued)

Light Waves

Fluid Physics

- Viscosity
- Pressure Gradient
- Driving Pressure
- Types of Flow
- Bernoulli's Principle
- The Coanda Effect

Gas Laws

- Boyle's Law
- Charles's Law
- Gay-Lussac's Law
- The Combined Gas Law
- Dalton's Law
- Henry's Law
- Avogadro's Law
- Graham's Law

Surface Tension

- Laplace's Law

Thermodynamics

- Conservation of Matter and Energy
- Heat and Other Forms of Energy

KEY TERMS

acceleration
Boyle's law
Charles's law
Dalton's law
derived units
dimensional analysis
dimensionless number
distending pressure
equal reactions
exponent
flow
fluid physics
fractional concentration
Gay-Lussac's law
Hooke's law
inverse square law
law
mass effect
mathematical coupling
MKSD
physics
Poiseuille's law
principle
quantity equations
Reynolds number
scientific notation
specific gravity (SG)
sublimation
Système International d'Unités (SI system)
theory
triple point
vector

This chapter introduces the physical laws, principles, and theories especially pertinent to the scientific foundations of respiratory care, pulmonary anatomy and physiology, and pulmonary pathology. Physics is the science of how and why energy and matter interact to produce what we see and experience in our universe. The preceding words are chosen very carefully because modern physics suggests the possibilities of other universes in which physics may not work quite the same way as we think it does here. This chapter explores the physical principles governing the condition of the patient and affecting the equipment and procedures used in respiratory care, as well as the relevant general mathematical concepts, measurement systems, and analysis methods.

The art and science inherent in the practice of respiratory care are based on the principles of physics, chemistry, and mathematics. These principles act within the human body and within the equipment and techniques we use to maintain or alter the body's physiological balance. A thorough understanding of these basic sciences is necessary for an understanding of the practice of respiratory care.

Distinctions among the basic sciences have become, and will continue to be, blurred in modern scientific society. The overlaps between biology and chemistry (biochemistry), physics and chemistry (physical chemistry), and physics and biology (biophysics) have become more pronounced as our knowledge of the structure and function of the body systems has improved. Regardless of the complexity and diverse interactions among the sciences, however, having a strong grasp of the elemental truths of the basic sciences is still a necessity.

Scientific Discovery and Belief

There is a general hierarchy of thinking in any science, and physics is no exception. The highest order of thought is the scientific **law**, which, in science, is a statement that describes a scientific truth—something that has never been disproven either in the past or at the current state of knowledge. This definition should not be taken to mean that the description will never be disproven but only that the possible proof has not been yet discovered. **Theories** are statements that are believed to be true but that are still being tested or are doubted in some scientific circles. **Principles** are statements of perceived truths about defined situations. An example is the Munroe-Kellie principle (or hypothesis, or sometimes doctrine), which states that, in a confined or closed space changes in the size or mass of one component of the contents of the space will cause a reciprocal change in the sizes of the other contents. This principle is sometimes referred to as the **mass effect**.

Measurements and Nomenclature

The language of science and mathematics by necessity must be precise, understandable, and easily communicated across a broad spectrum of fields and in a multitude of languages. The language of physics is mathematics. For clarity and understanding, concepts in physics must be expressed mathematically. To do this in a comprehensive and coherent manner, we speak a common mathematical language. Based on mid-eighteenth-century work, the medical and scientific community has accepted and adopted the International System of Units.

THE INTERNATIONAL SYSTEM OF UNITS

To ensure that the mathematical expressions of physical and other scientific concepts are identical throughout the scientific and medical communities, a unified system of mathematical and measurement systems was introduced and accepted by the world's scientific community (with some local exceptions). This system is called the **MKSD** (meter, kilogram, second, degree) system, or metric system. A more proper name is the **Système International d'Unités** (French for International System of Units). The abbreviation "SI" units is commonly used.

Units of Measure. All measurements should be referred to in SI units. There are seven base units on which all other measures depend and from which all other measures are derived (Table 3-1). The seven base units are length, mass, time, electrical current, temperature (based on absolute zero), amount of a substance, and luminous (light) intensity. These units are further defined in this chapter.

Derived Units. In addition to the base SI units, other units are called **derived units**. Derived SI units are obtained by using the base units in specific formulas called **quantity equations**. Examples of these units and formulas are shown in Table 3-2. A derived unit consists of two or more base units or, more properly, the interactions of the expressions of two or more of the base unit properties.

TABLE 3-1 **SI base units**

Base Quantity	Name	Symbol*
Length	Meter	m
Mass	Kilogram	kg
Time	Second	s
Electrical current	Ampere	A
Thermodynamic temperature	Kelvin	K
Amount of substance	Mole	mol
Luminous intensity	Candela	cd

**Both the symbol and whether it is uppercase or lowercase are critical when using the SI system. Failure to use the right symbol and case can lead to serious errors and misunderstandings.*

SI PREFIXES, DIMENSIONAL ANALYSIS, AND SCIENTIFIC NOTATION

Because the numbers and units can get very large or very small, they can be difficult to refer to, use, and manipulate in their original state. Three systems have been developed to make them easier to use and comprehend: SI prefixes, dimensional analysis, and scientific notation.

SI Prefixes. Table 3-3 presents a series of prefixes that modify the magnitude of the base or derived SI units. Units whose magnitudes (sizes) are larger than the base are labeled with Greek prefixes; those whose sizes are smaller than the base are labeled with Latin prefixes. These prefixes can be used with any of the SI base units *except the kilogram (mass)*, because that unit already has the descriptor kilo as part of its name and symbol. For units of mass, we use the prefixes with the symbol "g" for gram.

Best Practice

Role of Physics

Physical phenomena occur because of the interaction of the basic properties of matter and energy. The business of physics is to express those interactions in meaningful and understandable terms.

TABLE 3-2 Examples of derived SI units

Derived Quantity	Name	Symbol	Formula
Area	Square meter	m^2	m·m
Volume	Cubic meter	m^3	m·m·m
Speed, velocity	Meter per second	m/s	m/s
Acceleration	Meter per second squared	m/s^2	m/(s·s)
Mass density	Kilogram per cubic meter	k/m^3	k/(m·m·m)
Specific volume	Cubic meter per kilogram	m^3/kg	(m·m·m)/kg
Substance concentration	Mole per cubic meter	mol/m^3	mol/(m·m·m)
Special Derived Units			
Frequency	hertz	Hz	s^{-1}
Force	newton	N	$m{\cdot}kg{\cdot}s^{-2}$
Pressure, stress	pascal	Pa	N/m^2
Energy, work	joule	J	n·m
Power	watt	W	J/s
Quantity of electricity	coulomb	C	s·A
Electrical potential	volt	V	W/A
Electrical resistance	ohm	Ω	V/A
Celsius temperature	degree Celsius	°C	K – 273.15

TABLE 3-3 SI prefixes

Increasing Magnitude			Decreasing Magnitude		
Factor	Name	Symbol	Factor	Name	Symbol
10^9	giga	G	10^{-9}	nano	n
10^6	mega	M	10^{-6}	micro	μ
10^3	kilo	k	10^{-3}	milli	m
10^2	hecto	h	10^{-2}	centi	c
10^1	deka	da	10^{-1}	deci	d

Dimensional Analysis. Mathematics in and of itself can be a source of anxiety for many people. Couple that feeling with the need for mathematical values to have defining labels, and the difficulty level seems to rise rapidly. Because many of the physics and physiological formulas used in respiratory care contain specific measured variables, labeling can be problematic. This is where **dimensional analysis** (the reduction of units of measure) comes into play to minimize confusion and to provide a clue as to the outcome of the mathematical formulas. For instance, consider the following hypothetical example of a mathematical equation that involves various forms of measured data:

$$\frac{9.765 \text{ kg} \times 1.056 \text{ m}}{5.0 \text{ s}}$$

In what unit of measurement will the outcome be? To perform the dimensional analysis, use the following process:

Where kg = kilogram, m = meter and s = second

1. Write down the formula or equation:

$$\frac{9.765 \text{ kg} \times 1.056 \text{ m}}{5.0 \text{ s}}$$

2. Cross out the numbers, retaining the units and mathematical symbols:

$$\frac{\text{kg} \times \text{m}}{\text{s}}$$

3. After determining the correct units for the outcome, simply perform the mathematical functions:

$$9.765 \times 1.056 = 10.31184$$

$$\frac{10.31184}{5.0} = 2.0624$$

4. Merge the mathematical results and the unit results to complete the problem and the dimensional analysis:

2.0624 kg/m/s

When the values are divided, so are the labels: for example, meters/second. When the values are multiplied, the labels are merged: for example, kilogram-meter.

This equation indicates that a force is capable of moving a mass of 2.0624 kilograms 1 meter in 1 second, but in some cases, dimensional analysis can result in the cancellation of all unit values.

In some cases, dimensional analysis results in the cancellation of all unit values. These cases yield what are termed **dimensionless numbers**, or dimensionless variables. An example is the Reynolds number, a description of fluid flow characteristics, described later in this chapter.

Scientific Notation. The third system designed to make the SI system easier and more convenient to use is **scientific notation**. This is a system of recording numerical data in a shorthand format, similar to an abbreviation. The notation is based on two simple rules: first, only numbers from 1 to 10 are allowed; second, an exponent of 10 indicates the magnitude of a number. These exponents may be either positive or negative depending on the size of the numerical data. This system allows scientists to express both very large numbers (e.g., 1,984,000,000) and very small numbers (e.g., 0.00000000014686) logically, efficiently, and precisely. Scientific notation allows mathematical operations involving large or small numbers or combinations of both to be performed simply and clearly.

Consider the preceding examples. The first is a very long and large number: 1,984,000,000. The first step is to reduce the number to a value between 1 and 10; so the number becomes 1.984. Next, the magnitude, or size, of the number is shown as an exponent of 10. In this case, the number is larger than 1. Therefore, to determine this exponent, count the number of places *before*, or to the left of, the decimal point. (In the next example [0.00000000014686], we move the decimal to the right until the number is between 1 and 9. Because the original number was less than 1; so the places *after* the decimal point are counted.)

1,984,000,000

There are 10 places to the left of the decimal, but the number must be from 1 to 9 because the exponent shows the number of places the decimal has to move in order to increase or decrease the written value to the original number. In this case, the exponent is 9; the decimal has to move 9 places to the left.

A positive exponent means the decimal moves to the right (increasing the value), and a negative exponent means that the value of the number must decrease by moving the decimal to the left. For 1,984,000,000, the scientific notation is 1.984×10^9. The multiplication sign indicates that we are multiplying the value (1.984) by the exponent (power) of 10, or raising 10 to the ninth power.

TABLE 3-4 **Examples of scientific notation**

	Scientific Notation		
Number	**Root**	**Exponent**	**Notation**
0.00987	9.87	10^{-3}	9.87×10^{-3}
1.007	1.007	—	1.007*
1,230,000	1.23	10^6	1.23×10^6
0.01	1.00	10^{-2}	1.00×10^{-2}
230	2.3	10^2	2.3×10^2

Numbers such as this cannot be further reduced by scientific notation.

The same procedure and rules can be applied in the second example involving a very small number: 0.00000000014686. Convert the number to a value between 1 and 10. To do that, move the decimal point to the right until only a single digit remains to the left of the decimal point: 1.4686. The original number had 10 places after the decimal point.

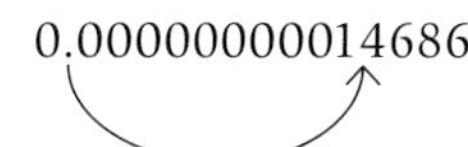

So the scientific notation is 1.4686×10^{-10}. In other words, to get the original number back, move the decimal 10 places to the right as indicated by the minus sign. Table 3-4 presents further examples.

Mathematical Operations

Most of the mathematics used in respiratory care involves the four basic *mathematical operations*—addition, subtraction, multiplication, and division—and a few formulas that require the use of exponents (powers and roots). Fortunately, these operations are familiar ones, and we need only review a few simple rules. Addition, subtraction, multiplication, and division have four rules in common:

1. Use only like entities (e.g., meters plus meters, not meters plus centimeters).
2. Reduce measurements to the lowest common denominator.
3. After completing the operation, restate the answer in the most reasonable form for the task at hand.
4. Line up decimals one over the other.

Multiplication is essentially a shorthand form for addition, and it follows the same basic rules as addition. However, here are six helpful hints for multiplication problems:

1. When positive values are multiplied by positive values or negative values are multiplied by negative values, the results are always a positive number: for example, $(+) \times (+) = (+)$, $(-) \times (-) = (+)$.

Best Practice

Use of Signs

By convention, positive signs (+) are not generally used; only negative values are signed (−).

Best Practice

Leading Zero

Always write decimals with a leading zero (0.xxx). Use of the leading zero can prevent tragic drug errors in the case of medication calculations. The leading zero is much more than a placeholder; it is a very important safety tool.

2. When negative values are multiplied by positive values, the results are always a negative number: for example, $(-) \times (+) = (-)$.
3. When numbers containing decimals are multiplied, the results should have at least as many decimals as the original number with the most decimal points: for example, $2.4 \times 3.34 = 8.016$.
4. When whole numbers are multiplied, their absolute value (the plus and minus signs are disregarded) are always equal to or larger than either of the numbers multiplied.
5. Multiplying decimal numbers always results in a number that is smaller than either of the original numbers: for example, $0.4 \times 0.3 = 0.12$.
6. If a whole number and a decimal number are multiplied, the result is always a number smaller than the whole number and larger than the decimal: for example, $14 \times 0.5 = 7.0$.

Division is essentially a sophisticated form of subtraction, so it follows the four basic rules. The hints for multiplication also apply, with one additional hint:

> Answers in division have at least one more decimal place than the longest number in the problem: for example, $285.68 \div 1334.379 = 0.214092$.

Exponents, or powers, are shown as superscripts. The superscript represents the number of times that the number (or base) is multiplied by itself (i.e., raised): for example, $2^4 = 2 \times 2 \times 2 \times 2 = 16$. The rules that apply to mathematical operations involving exponents are:

- When adding numbers with exponents, find the value of each number; then add the results: for example:

$$(3^2) + (4^3) = (3 \times 3) + (4 \times 4 \times 4) = (9) + (64) = 73$$

- When subtracting numbers with exponents, find the value of each number; then subtract the results: for example:

$$(3^2) - (4^3) = (9) - (64) = -55$$

- When multiplying numbers with exponents, multiply the numbers; then add the exponents: for example:

$$(2^4) \times (5^2) = (2 \times 5)^{4+2} \text{ or } (10)^6$$

- When dividing numbers with exponents, divide the numbers and subtract exponents: for example:

$$(6^3 \div 2^2) = (6 \div 2)^{3-2} = (3^1) = 3$$

ORDER OF OPERATIONS

The *order of operations* relates to the approach to mathematical formulas. Complex formulas contain numbers that must be added, subtracted, multiplied, and divided in various sequences and combinations. The general approach is to work from the inner elements of the formulas to the outer elements. Parentheses ( ), brackets [ ], and braces { } are used to separate portions of the formula and are used in that order from the inside out. For example, a formula with the numbers removed might look like this:

$$\{ [( )] + [( )] \} - ( )$$

Let's put some numbers in the formula and see how it works:

$$\{[4(3 + 2)] + [2(5 - 1)]\} - (7 + 2)$$

First, solve, or clear, the ( ):

$$\{[4(3 + 2)] + [2(5 - 1)]\} - (7 + 2)$$

Next, clear the [ ]:

$$\{[4(5)] + [2(4)]\} - 9$$

Then clear the { }:

$$\{20 + 8\} - 9$$

Finally, solve the problem:

$28 - 9$ Solve the problem.

19 This is the answer.

MATHEMATICAL COUPLING

Mathematical coupling deals with errors and their effect on subsequent measurements and calculations. The effects of undetected errors or inappropriate rounding in calculations move down the chain of subsequent calculations that use the result of the erroneous calculation. The effect of the error grows larger with each step in the flawed sequence of calculations. For example, if an exponent of 3 (e.g., 5^3) is mistakenly used instead of 2 (5^2) early in a series of calculations, all subsequent calculations will be based on the wrong number (125 instead of 25). For instance, one of the National Aeronautics and Space Administration's (NASA) Mars probes missed the planet Mars! An early error in converting from miles to kilometers caused a coupling effect that multiplied a small error in angle of flight into a planet-missing error.

HEISENBERG'S UNCERTAINTY PRINCIPLE

The work of Werner Heisenberg in atomic physics during the closing years of World War II led to important understandings about energy, materials, and measurement. Heisenberg was a German-American physicist and a member of the World War II Manhattan Project, which developed the first nuclear weapon. In the process of studying radioactivity, Heisenberg needed to determine and understand the atomic structure and activity level of high-energy radioactive substances. After many failed attempts to determine the speed of movement and the position of electrons in the substances being studied, Heisenberg made a very enlightened observation that has had implications far beyond nuclear physics.

The following is a paraphrase of what Heisenberg said: "The mere act of observing something changes the nature of the thing observed."[1] Known as *Heisenberg's Uncertainty Principle*, the statement means that a given instrument can tell you either the speed or the position of an electron—but not both simultaneously. The Heisenberg principle has shown that the observations themselves change the properties of matter; the measure becomes part of the measurement. In other words, the very act of introducing a measurement instrument into a system changes the system from what the scientist wishes to measure.

The keys to the accuracy of measurement are twofold. First, choose the instrument or method with the least likelihood of altering the system to be measured. Second, choose the method of data collection that is capable of providing the data desired within an acceptable degree of accuracy.

An example is the drawing of an arterial blood gas (ABG). For this test, an artery has to be punctured with a needle to obtain a blood sample. Patients may tend either to hold their breath or to breathe deeply and quickly in anticipation of or in response to pain or anxiety. Any of these actions can affect the blood gases (see Chapters 4 and 16) by altering the carbon dioxide levels in the arterial blood. So the instrument used to get the arterial blood can alter the results of the test. In other words, the ABG values are not as they existed before the arterial puncture, but rather they have been altered by the test. (Of course, there are remedies to offset this effect.)

OCCAM'S RAZOR

Occam's razor, so named because the Razor was held to "cut the truth finely," is another rule of science and math. It was named after a late Middle Ages English theologian, philosopher, and mathematician named William of Ockham (an alternate spelling) (1285–1349). The paraphrased rule states, "When given a choice of solutions, select the obvious (or simplest) one." In other words, do not complicate matters. Put another way, the simplest explanation or solution for a problem is often the best one. The Razor is popularly called the KISS principle: Keep it simple, stupid.

Physics

Physics is a scientific discipline that studies the relationships between matter and energy. Classical physics was devoted to describing how things work (descriptive physics) and to the interactions of matter and energy (theoretical physics). In fact, the ancient Greek and Roman schools of philosophy devoted much time and effort to describing how the world functioned and how things interacted. This inquisitive activity eventually resulted in the rise of all modern-day science.

From a clinical standpoint, the application of physical laws to diagnostic and therapeutic problems has led to today's highly sophisticated and functional biomedical technology. This technology is spread across the entire spectrum of medicine, affecting patients of all ages and with every injury or disease. Without an in-depth understanding of technology and its effects on the patient, the care provided would be ineffective and even dangerous. The interaction of physics and biology (both normal and abnormal) must be understood and utilized correctly to provide the best possible patient care.

Examples of the presence of classical physics in medicine and respiratory care are the gas laws and the concepts governing flow through tubes (such as blood vessels and airways). Examples of clinical physics are blood pressure measuring devices, thermometers, oxygen supply equipment, heart-lung machines, and radiology equipment. Largely due to the understanding and utilization of physical concepts has progress in the diagnosis and treatment of disease and injury been made possible.

TABLE 3-5 Equivalent pressures for one standard atmosphere

760 mm Hg: 1 standard atmosphere at 0°C
29.92 inches of Hg
10.332 meters of H_2O
406.78 inches of H_2O
33.899 feet of fresh water, 33 feet of sea water
14.696 pounds per square inch (psi) or pounds per square inch gauge (psig)
1.033 kilograms per square centimeter
101.325 kilopascal

MECHANICS

Mechanics is the branch of physics that studies force and movement, that is, all the phenomena that can influence, by retarding or augmenting, the application of force and the inception of motion. Mechanics includes such diverse variables as the flow of fluids through tubes, the resistance of the chest wall to movement, and the causes of injury in falls and automobile accidents.

Force and Motion. Issues of pressure and flow are determined by reference to force and motion equations, which are direct descendants of Sir Isaac Newton's observations and the natural laws he developed from them. Air (gas) pressure is measured in many units, which are listed in Table 3-5.

Force is defined as the energy that originates or arrests motion or other activities. Force can further be defined according to its type or source, such as electromotive force (EMF, the difference in electrical potential across an electrical circuit) and mechanical force. Other types of force are more commonly referred to as *energy*. The equation for force (F) is mass (M) times acceleration (a):

$$F = Ma$$

Acceleration is the change in velocity over time. Velocity is defined as distance (d) per unit of time (t). Force units, then, are $M(d/t)$ for simple constant linear acceleration. Examples are units such as kilogram-meter per second (kg-m/s), gram-centimeter per minute (g-cm/min).

Work (W) is the amount of energy expended to move a mass a given distance. It is the transfer of energy that occurs when a force is exerted on a moving body in the direction of the body's movement. Classically, the unit used to describe work is the kilogram-meter (kg-m). The kg-m describes the mass (kg) and the distance moved (m).

Power is the time or rate of doing work (W/s); that is, it expresses the amount of work done over a given period of time. Power units include the watt (1 joule of work per second) and the horsepower (550 foot-pounds of work per second).

Energy, another term used to represent power or force, is the power that can be used to do work. Energy exists in one of two states: kinetic or potential. *Potential energy* is the energy that can be translated into work of some type—moving an object, overcoming resistance, or affecting a chemical or physical energy change—but that is not doing so at present. An example of potential energy is a 20-lb rock sitting at the edge of a 50-ft-high cliff. Despite the conditions of mass (200 lb) and distance (50 ft), there is no active energy until some outward force makes the rock topple and fall the 50 feet, turning the potential force into a kinetic force.

Kinetic energy is energy in motion—energy that is doing something (like the rock falling off the cliff). Kinetic energy can assume several forms, such as electrical, thermal (heat), mechanical, chemical, or radiant.

Energy used to do work can be defined in terms of many descriptive units. Derived from combinations of force units and distance units, some commonly used energy units are joules, ergs, and foot-pounds. Likewise, combinations of power and time units are commonly used to indicate work or work potential. Examples of these units are horsepower-hours, watt-hours, and kilowatt-hours.

As energy changes form, some of it becomes "lost" to the system and cannot be used again. The loss is generally in the form of heat. Therefore, any calculations of energy, work, or force equations in terms of energy expenditure must account for heat loss or the equations will not balance.

$$\text{energy in} = \text{energy out} + \text{heat loss or}$$
$$\text{energy out} = \text{energy in} - \text{heat loss}$$

To demonstrate this concept, briskly rub one hand against the other. Work (the movement of the hands) is produced, but also produced is a significant amount of heat, which is absorbed by the skin. The heat represents energy loss due to friction.

Newton's Laws of Motion. Sir Isaac Newton (1642–1727), an English scientist and mathematician, was a prolific discoverer. Not only did he develop the field of differential calculus, but he also was responsible for the discovery that white light is composed of many colors. Newton also discovered the three *laws of motion*.[1]

Newton's First Law of Motion (Inertia) The *law of inertia* or Newton's first law of motion, states that "a body at rest tends to stay at rest and a body in uniform motion tends to stay in motion unless acted upon by an

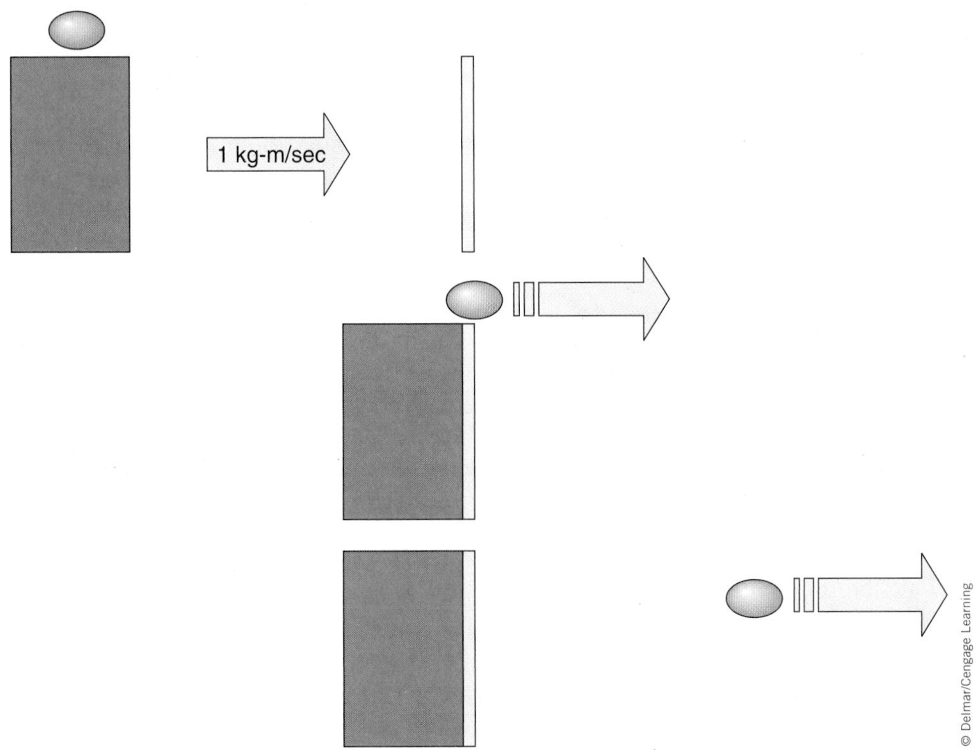

FIGURE 3-1 Newton's first law of motion: A body in motion tends to stay in motion unless it is acted upon by an outside force.

outside force." The assumption is that an ideal state exists when forces do not act on objects unless imposed by the observer. Intuitively, the first statement in the law is easy to grasp. If an object is securely positioned in a certain place, it remains there unless someone or something moves it.

The second statement in the law is not as intuitive and, in fact, may be counterintuitive. Casual observers of nature know that everything that moves eventually comes to a stop. The reason, however, is that all movement is affected by an outside retarding or resistive force—friction. Friction is a type of resistance or counter movement force (Figure 3-1).

The next logical question is, "If there are forces that slow and stop movement, do other forces promote or increase movement?" Newton addressed that question in his second law of motion.

Newton's Second Law of Motion (Acceleration) The law of **acceleration** (Newton's second law) states that "if a net force acts upon an object that object will accelerate." If the sum of the pushing and the pulling forces is other than zero, the object moves, and the movement is in the same direction as that of the greatest force (i.e., toward the lesser force). This quality of direction is called a **vector**. These concepts are shown in Figure 3-2.

The formula for this law is $F = Ma$, where F = force, M = mass, and a = acceleration. Force is measured in units called *Newtons*, abbreviated N in the SI system. More commonly, force is expressed in terms of the mass equivalent per unit of area affected, such as kilograms times meters per second squared (kg·m/s^2) or grams times centimeters per second squared (g·cm/s^2).

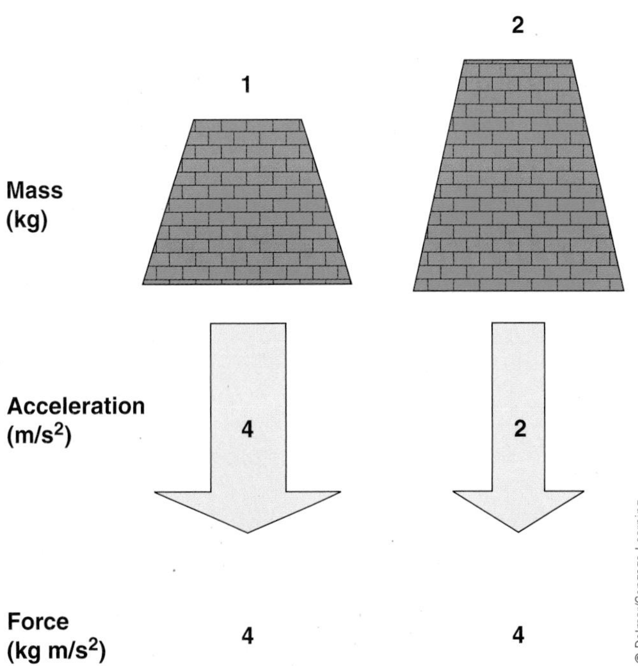

FIGURE 3-2 Newton's second law of motion: The force acting on an object is equal to its mass times its acceleration.

CASE STUDY 3-1

Think of a car parked on a hill. With the car in neutral and the brake off, a little shove starts it rolling down the hill. The tendency of the car is to keep rolling downhill until it hits something or has to go uphill and loses its forward momentum.

Questions

1. Given no crashes, what happens if the next hill is as high or higher than the hill the car started on?
2. What happens after that?
3. What is the final outcome?

Newton's Third Law of Motion (Equal Reactions) The law of **equal reactions** (Newton's third law) states that "for every action there is an equal and opposite reaction." If a weight is pushed with a given amount of force, an equal and opposite force will resist that push. These forces are in the form of friction, resistance, and heat, among others. Figure 3-3 illustrates the principle. The helium in the blimp is less dense than air and causes the blimp to rise (lift) to the altitude where the gas is at the same density as the surrounding atmosphere, the blimp is held at that altitude by the balance of the downward force of gravity and the upward lift force. Adding an engine and a propeller at the rear of the blimp gives a propulsive force to push the craft forward, through the atmosphere's gases, thus causing a resistance to the forward motion.

Here is a question for thought and discussion: What would the effect be if the blimp was shaped not like a bullet but like a railroad boxcar?

Momentum. Momentum relates the part of Newton's first law that says that a body in uniform motion tends to stay in motion. *Momentum* is the object's tendency to continue to stay in motion in the same direction (vector) unless or until it is acted on by outside forces. As Figure 3-4 illustrates, mass, vector (direction), and energy (force) are not changed; only their distribution in the system is altered. Note the effect of the small force on the mass accelerated by the large force in the figure (we will talk about his further when we discuss conservation of matter and energy). Can you think of some common applications of this law?

Gravity. *Gravitation* relates to the forces of attraction between objects. The theory of gravitation holds that all objects are attracted to all other objects. The force of attraction is a factor of the product of their masses ($M_1 \times M_2$) and the inverse of the square of the distance between the objects (d^{-2}). The complete formula for the force (F) of gravitation (G) is:

$$F = G(M_1 \times M_2) \div d^2$$

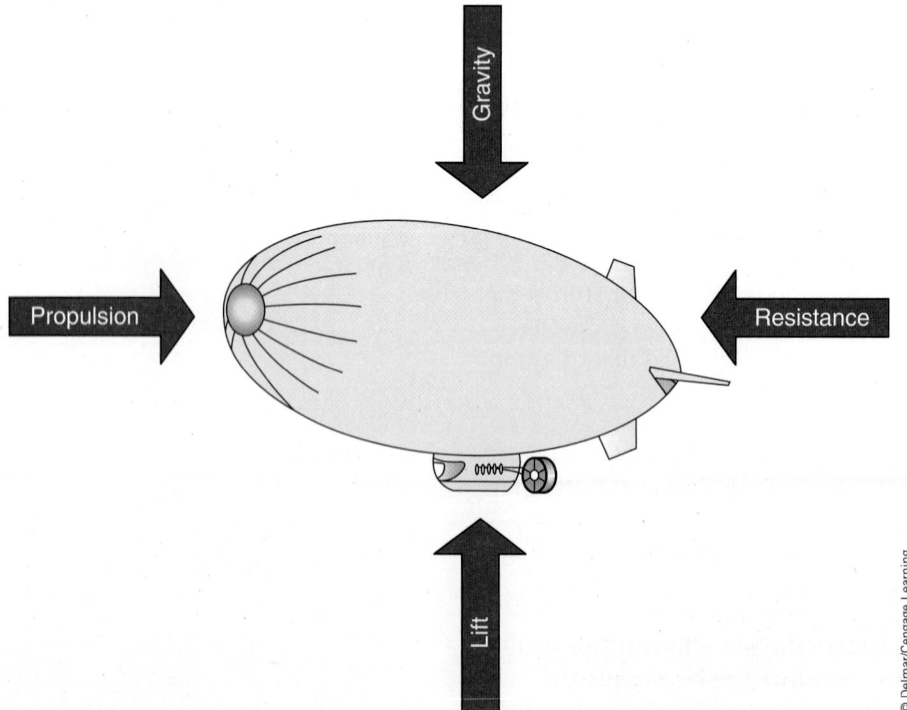

FIGURE 3-3 Newton's third law of motion: For every action, there is an equal and opposite reaction.

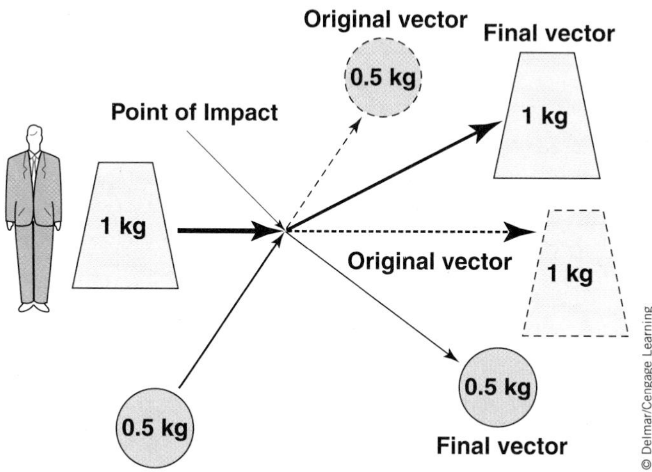

FIGURE 3-4 Newton's law of conservation of momentum: At the point of impact, the first object changes direction (vector), as does the second object, imparting its force acting on the first object. In the absence of friction or gravity, the sum of the forces remain unchanged, and the net deviation in the sum of the pre- and post-impact vectors are constant.

The gravitational constant, *G*, can be safely ignored because it is constant within the environment. The equation thus takes the form:

$$F = (M_1 \times M_2) \div d^2$$

This formula, sometimes referred to as the **inverse square law**, tells us two things.

- First, *the force of attraction decreases inversely with the square of the distance between objects*. If the energy or force exerted by one object on another has a value of, say, 10 units and the objects are moved twice as far apart, the force exerted decreases by a factor of 4 to 2.5 units. This fact also applies to bacterial contamination, radiation, and many other physical phenomena.
- Second, small objects are more strongly attracted to large objects than large objects are to small ones. This is why something that is dropped falls to the ground. The ground (the Earth) does not rise to meet the dropped object. This second effect also explains why some aerosol particles remain suspended for long periods of time while others rain out relatively quickly. This concept of fallout or sedimentation occurs in response to gravitational attraction.

The effects of gravity you are in play when the respiratory therapist chooses appropriate devices to ensure that aerosols will not only be in the therapeutic size range but also control particle retention in the lung. The particle must be respirable (small enough to penetrate the lung) and large enough to rain out in the lung before being exhaled.

Elasticity. Elasticity is an important topic. For example, suppose a person takes in a big breath, holds it, and then exhales. While breathing in and holding the breath, the body was actively using its respiratory muscles. When air is exhaled, the body only has to stop using those muscles, and the muscles relax into a resting state. That is the elastic recoil of the lungs and chest in action. Exhalation is normally a passive, non-energy-consuming function.

Diseases that modify the tissues of the chest wall and the lungs can adversely affect this elastic recoil mechanism. The effect can lead to inadequate emptying of the lungs, trapping of air in the lungs, and increased energy use for breathing. This is referred to as an increased *work of breathing* (*WOB*). Exhalation may become an active rather than a passive function. Loosely defined, elasticity might be seen as a form of stored or potential energy.

Hooke's law, named after Robert Hooke (1635–1703), an English physicist, describes the effects of elastance. It states that *the stretching of a solid is proportional to the force exerted on it*. Figure 3-5 shows that an elastic (distensible) structure stretches linearly with increasing force until, at its elastic limit (tensile limit), stretch is no longer possible, and the structure breaks. A simple example is an elastic band that snaps when stretched too far.

Figure 3-6 depicts the linear relationship between pressure change and volume change in a lung model. This is termed *elastance* ($\Delta P/\Delta V$). Its reciprocal, volume change per unit of pressure change ($\Delta V/\Delta P$) is called *compliance*. At the limits of elastance, the application of more pressure does not result in increased volume change (stretch) but does risk rupture of the lung unit.

CASE STUDY 3-2

Ms. T. S., age 25, fell while attempting a Waldo on her inline skates. Among her considerable injuries were a fractured right wrist, three fractured ribs, and four amputated artificial fingernails. Because of the fractured ribs, she is having difficulty breathing.

Question

Explain why fractured ribs (other than for reasons of pain) would interfere with breathing.

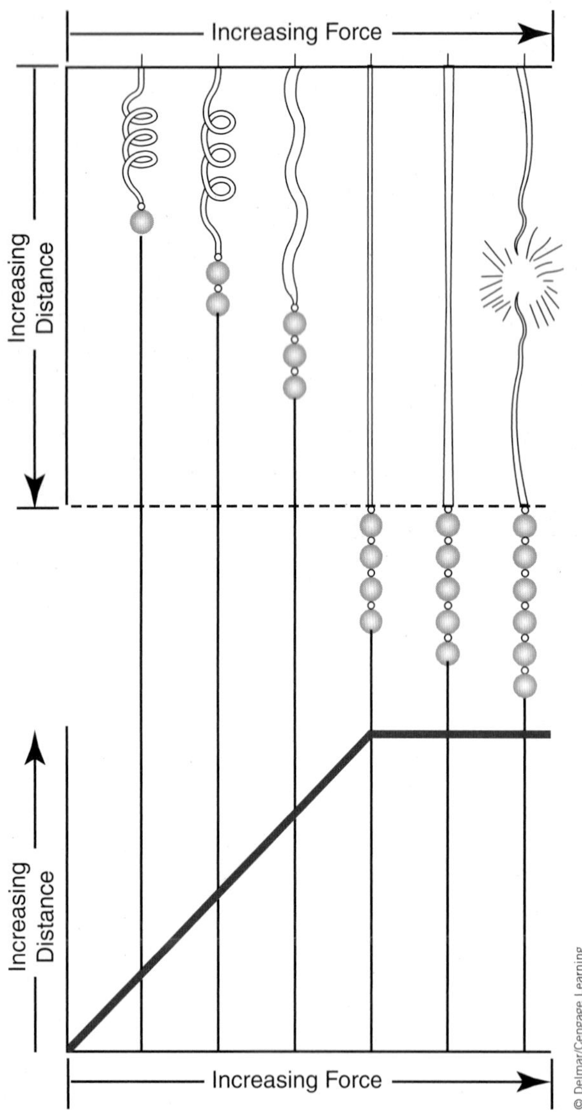

FIGURE 3-5 Hooke's law: Within the elastic limits of an elastic structure, the amount of stretch produced is directly and linearly proportional to the force exerted on the object. Beyond the elastic limits, stretch quickly declines until a breaking point (tensile limit) is reached.

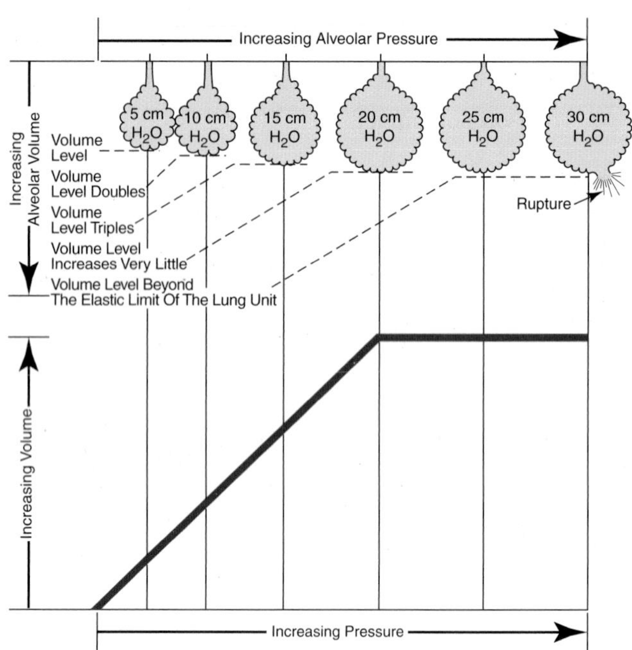

FIGURE 3-6 Hooke's law related to the elastic properties of the lung: Note the linear relationship between pressure change and volume change. Beyond the limits of stretch, the system breaks down and ruptures.

Age-Specific Competency

Elasticity

Elasticity of the chest wall varies considerably over the life span. The ribs of infants are mainly cartilage. Those of older children and of adults to late middle age retain flexibility, but flexibility deceases with age, and the ribs become rigid and brittle. When evaluating chest wall injuries, performing assessments, and initiating treatment regimes, be mindful of the elastic properties of the chest wall relative to the patient's age.

States of Matter

Matter exists in one of three states: solid, liquid, or gas. Each state imparts specific characteristics to the material. In addition to those three states, a transition state, called *plasma,* exists between solids and liquids. Also, some people consider vapors to be a transition state between liquids and gases. Plasmas, liquids, vapors, and gases can all be classified as fluids, and the laws of **fluid physics** (the physical properties of materials that flow) apply to these substances to a greater or lesser degree. These laws, however, do not apply to solids under circumstances we are likely to encounter.

Respiratory caregivers are often concerned with the transition of matter from one state to another. Figure 3-7 presents a conceptual view of the bond strength of each of the three main types of matter. The therapeutic use of humidifiers, vaporizers, liquid and gaseous oxygen, mists, and aerosols all demand a sound grasp of the general attributes of matter in each of its states, of the changes that occur when matter changes form, and of the factors that influence or cause changes of state.

SOLIDS

Solids are substances in which the molecules are very close to one another. The forces that cause the molecules

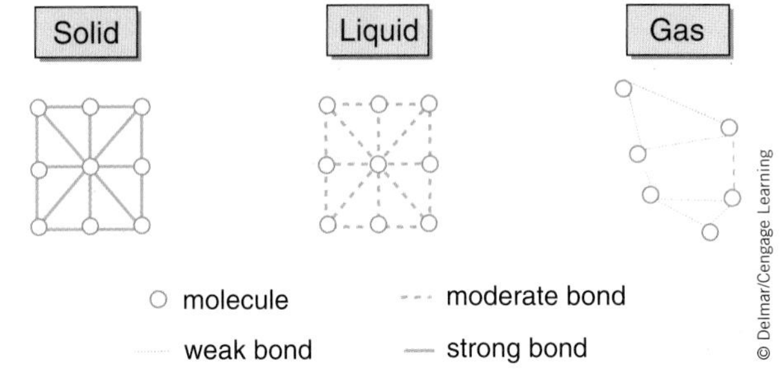

FIGURE 3-7 States of matter: States in which matter exist are in large measure determined by the type and strength of the bonds between atoms of the components of the substance and the strength of the intermolecular forces of attraction.

to become closely positioned are called *van der Waals forces*. Solids are not compressible; they retain their shape and mass unless acted on by outside forces. Solids are thought to be the densest form of matter (density is mass per unit volume, for example, grams per liter or mg/cc). Examples of solids are rocks, blocks of wood, steel beams, and ice.

PLASMA

Plasma is a type of matter that can be said to be transitional; that is, it exists in a state between a solid and a liquid. It has some of the properties of a solid and some of the properties of a liquid. In plasmas, the van der Waals forces of attraction are a bit less intense, allowing some adjustment of shape and position. The density of a plasma is a little lower than that of a solid. An example of a plasma is glass, which, over time, deforms and flows to its lowest point. Another example is an egg yolk, which deforms but does not flow unless broken.

LIQUIDS

Liquids are substances that have moderate molecular forces of attraction and that can take the shape of a container in which they are placed. They are denser than gases but less dense than plasmas or solids. Examples of liquids are water, gasoline, and blood plasma.

Liquids are also known as *fluids*. When liquids are given an opportunity to move from one place to another, the molecular attraction is great enough that they tend to move in mass quantities. This movement is called **flow**. Flow is defined as volume moved per time period: for example, gallons per minute, cubic centimeters per second, or liters per minute: The formula for calculating flow is:

$$\text{flow} = \text{volume} \div \text{time}$$

CASE STUDY 3-3

Ms. I. R. presents to the emergency room complaining of shortness of breath, fever, and headache. Tests indicate that her blood oxygen level is down, as is her blood carbon dioxide level. (Chapters 14–19 provide more detailed information on laboratory tests.) She needs oxygen delivered by as accurate a means as possible. This means her peak (maximum) inspiratory flow rate (PIFR) must be determined.

Questions

1. How will PIFR help the respiratory therapist decide how to deliver oxygen to Ms. R.?
2. What other information regarding Ms. R. does the therapist need to solve this problem?

Because gases are also fluid, we can refer to the movement of gases in terms of flow also. For example, in the calculation of respiratory flow, it is customary to differentiate between inspiratory (I) and expiratory (E) flow. Calculating these variables requires determination of the respiratory rate (RR), which is breaths per minute (bpm), and of the duration of the average breath in seconds. The duration of a breath is then subdivided into inspiratory (I-time) and expiratory (E-time) components. Combined and expressed as a ratio of total breath time, this information, when reduced to its lowest common denominator, provides us with the inspiratory-to-expiratory ratio, or the *I/E ratio*. The normal value is 1:2. Once the I/E ratio has been determined, finding the inspiratory flow is a simple matter.

VAPORS

Vapors are seen as either gases that act as liquid or as liquids that act as gases. Water vapor is the most common vapor, but others exist. They may flow coherently or have high resistance to compression, or they may not mix freely with other fluids.

GASES

A *gas* has the lowest density and the lowest strength of attraction of the three classical, or standard, states of matter. Like liquids, gases can take the shape of a container into which they are placed, and they are fluid. Examples of gases are helium (He), hydrogen (H), oxygen (O), nitrogen (N), and water vapor (H_2O). Air is a mixture of gases (Table 3-6). Gas mixtures have

TABLE 3-6 **Constituents of air at standard temperature and pressure (to 0.00 decimals) in the lungs**

Substance	Symbol	Vol% Composition	Pressure (mm Hg)
Nitrogen	N_2	78.084	556.74
Oxygen	O_2	20.947	149.35
Argon	Ar	0.934	6.66
Carbon dioxide	CO_2	0.033	0.24
Subtotal of air		99.998	712.99
Water (vapor)	H_2O	47.00	759.99
Trace gases		~0.002	760.00

certain characteristics that are discussed elsewhere in this chapter.

CHANGES OF STATE

Each material is capable of changing its state given an appropriate temperature (critical temperature) and an appropriate pressure (critical pressure). For each substance, a phase diagram can be constructed to illustrate this capability (Figure 3-8). The *phase diagram* is a graph that plots temperature versus pressure. It shows the effects of changing pressures and temperature on the state of matter in which a given material can exist. At any given point where temperature and pressure intersect, the material will be liquid, solid, or gaseous form or in a state of equilibrium between the various states of matter. This fact comes into good use in the fractional distillation of air to create gaseous oxygen (O_2). The theory is also applied in medical and

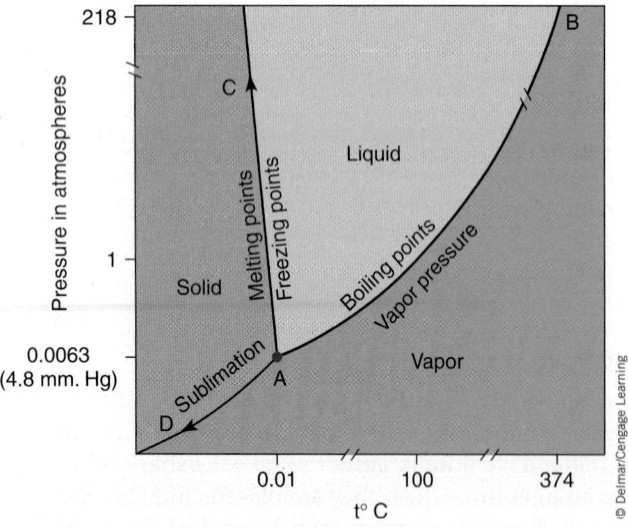

FIGURE 3-8 Example of a phase diagram. Point A is the Triple Point of this substance.

CASE STUDY 3-4

On a hot, hot summer day, a tall, cold drink of iced tea, with lots of ice in a sweaty glass, is very welcome. Thank the triple point of water for that pause that refreshes. Ice (solid water), tea (mostly liquid water), and a sweaty glass (condensed gaseous water vapor) all existed at once.

Questions

1. What is the value of knowing a substance's critical temperature, critical pressure, and triple point?
2. Name three devices used in respiratory care that take advantage of the transition points of materials.

industrial gas delivery systems. Both the large-capacity liquid systems used to supply oxygen to hospitals and industry and the smaller nitrous oxide (NO_2) cylinders depend on using pressure and temperature changes to turn liquid oxygen and nitrous oxide into their gaseous states.

The transition points have special but familiar names. The point of transition from solid to liquid is the *melting point*. The point at which a liquid turns into a solid is its *freezing point*. The point of transition from liquid to gas is called the *vapor point*, or point of vaporization, and the point of change from gas to liquid is the *dew point*. Some materials skip the liquid phase and go directly from solid to gas; this type of change is called **sublimation**. Dry ice is a good example. Dry ice is solid carbon dioxide (CO_2), which, at normal room temperature and pressure, turns from its solid (ice) state directly into gaseous CO_2.

Another important point on the graph is the place where all three curves come together, the so-called **triple point**. The triple point is significant because at that point a substance can exist in all three states of matter simultaneously. Water is one of the few materials that can do this within our preferred temperature and pressure range.

Mass, Weight, and Density

Mass, weight, and density are separate but interrelated concepts that, in some conditions, can be difficult to distinguish.

MASS

Mass is a difficult concept to define. One definition is that *mass* is the quality of matter that defines the amount of matter in an object. If this definition is accurate, then mass is an expression of the number of molecules or atoms that make up an object or substance. Until relatively recently, mass and weight have been treated and thought of as essentially identical concepts. However, it is now known that mass is independent of the location of the substance, whereas weight is dependent on the substance's location. Mass is said to be an invariant quantity; if we do not add or remove a quantity of matter, mass remains constant. Mass is measured in units of kilograms. The force needed to move one kilogram of matter 1 meter per second per second is called a *newton* ($N = kg \times m/s^2$).

WEIGHT

Weight on the other hand is a variable quantity whose value is dependent on position or location. Weight (W) is the quality of matter expressed by its mass (M) and the force of gravity (G) acting on the mass:

$$W = MG$$

The relationship between mass and weight is illustrated in Figure 3-9. An object with a mass of 70 kg on the Earth will also have a weight 70 kg on the Earth. On the moon, however, although its mass remains 70 kg, its weight is only 11.9 kg. The difference is due to the effects of gravity. Thus mass is invariable, and weight is location dependent, positional, and variable. In space, the weight of an object is even lower, although the mass remains constant. According to inverse square law, the farther two masses are from each other, the less the attraction (the effect of gravity) is of one mass for the other. How much less depends on the distance between them.

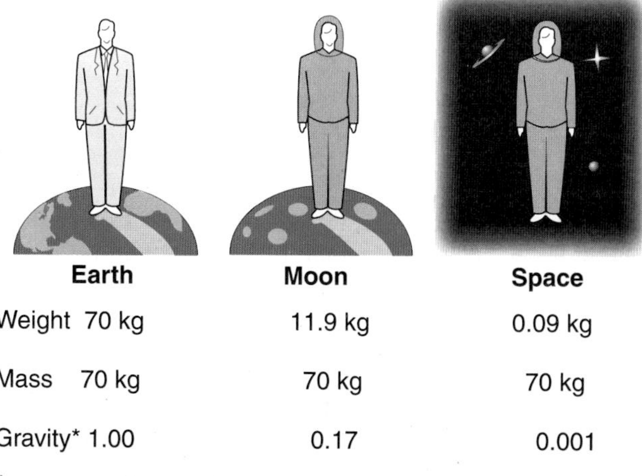

	Earth	Moon	Space
Weight	70 kg	11.9 kg	0.09 kg
Mass	70 kg	70 kg	70 kg
Gravity*	1.00	0.17	0.001

*Relative to the earth.

FIGURE 3-9 Mass versus weight: Weight is gravity dependent, whereas mass is independent of gravity. As the force of gravity decreases, so does weight, but mass remains constant.

DENSITY

Density is the expression of a substance's weight per unit of volume. To determine a substance's density, weigh a given volume of the material. This is not difficult for liquids or gases because they adopt the shape of the container they are in. For solids (and plasmas), getting a weight is a bit more complex; that is, it might be difficult to measure the volume of an irregularly shaped solid or plasma. The problem was solved by a Greek philosopher named Archimedes (c. 287–212 BCE), who discovered that, when a solid body is immersed in water, it displaces an amount of water equal to the volume of the immersed solid. This is called *Archimedes' principle*. Determining the volume of the displaced water, an easy determination to make, indicates the volume of the solid in question. Given the volume and the weight of the substance, its density can be calculated.

Specific gravity (SG) is a ratio of the density of one substance to the density of a standard substance. For solids and liquids, the standard substance is water. For gases, the standard substance is air. For example, the specific gravity of oxygen can be calculated as

$$\begin{aligned}\text{specific gravity of oxygen} &= \text{density of oxygen} \div \text{density of air}\\ &= 1.429\ \text{g/L} \div 1.293\ \text{g/L}\\ &= 1.105\end{aligned}$$

Note that the units canceled. Because the units are the same for both substances, they cancel out, and the values for specific gravity are dimensionless, that is, have no units.

Basic Electrical Theory

Knowledge of electrical theory is important for several reasons. First, many of the respiratory therapist's tools are powered by electricity. Second, the theories and behaviors of electrical circuits and the laws that govern those behaviors are in many cases identical to the laws and application in fluid physics. Several facts about electrical charges are important to keep in mind:

- *Like charges repel.* Two positively charged objects attempt to move away from each other. Conversely, unlike charges attract each other. Thus, a positively charged object is attracted to a negatively charged one, and vice versa.
- *Charge is conserved.* In a closed system, the total amount of charge is stable and neutral. The number of positive charges equals the number of negative charges. Therefore, the system is both at equilibrium and electrically neutral.

ELECTRICITY

Electricity is the movement of electrons (negatively charged subatomic particles) from one portion of space to another. Electricity, like other forms of energy, exists in one of two states: active (kinetic) and resting (potential). Electricity changes from the passive to the active state when two conditions are met:

1. There is an electrical potential, also known as a *charge difference*. In this case, *potential* means that there is a difference between the number of electrons (negatively charged particles) at one part of a circuit and the number of electrons at another part. So, if one area (D) has 1000 electrons and another area (H) has only 500 electrons, there is a net electron difference between D and H of 500 electrons. Electricity always moves from areas of high electron concentration to areas of low concentration.
2. A conductor connects D and H. A *conductor*, or medium, allows electrons to flow through it without altering it. This flow of electrons occurs with varying degrees of ease through different materials. Factors that impede the movement of electrons are said to cause increased electrical *resistance* in that material. The opposite of a conductor is an *insulator*, which is a substance through which electricity cannot easily flow.

CIRCUITS

Electrical *circuits* are devices designed to carry an electrical charge from one site to another. Circuits can be very simple or exceedingly complex. A simple circuit might consist of an electrical source, two lengths of insulated copper wire, a switch, and a light bulb. Figure 3-10 illustrates a simple electrical circuit. The movement of electricity depends on the power and resistance to flow in the circuit. Power in this sense refers to the difference between the electron concentration (charge) at the source of power and the concentration at the receiver (the light bulb in this case).

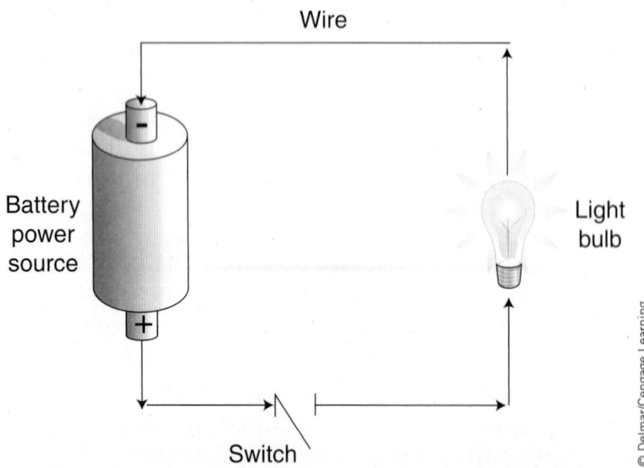

FIGURE 3-10 A simple electrical circuit consists of a power source, a conductor, a device to use this power, and a switch to control the flow of electrons.

OHM'S LAW

The movement of electricity through the electrical circuit is summarized by *Ohm's law*, which states that current (I) is equal to power (E) divided by resistance (R):

$$I = E \div R$$

Current (I) is the amount of electrical flow per unit of time passing a given point in the circuit. Flow is influenced by the difference in electrical charge (pressure) at each end of the circuit. This charge difference is directly proportional to the resulting flow (or current) and is inversely proportional to the resistance of the circuit to the flow. The charge difference is measured in volts (V). A *volt* is the amount of charge differential needed to send 1 ampere (A) of current through a circuit having 1 ohm (Ω) of resistance.

Power, or *electromotive force* (E), is the ability to do work. It is usually rated in base units of watts (W) or the more common kilowatts (kW).

Resistance (R) is an expression of the forces that impede or restrict current flow. It is measured in ohms (Ω). Electrical circuits use the inherent resistance of certain materials to electrical flow to perform desired tasks: for example, toasters, incandescent lights, space heaters, and soldering guns. All these examples depend on electrical resistance to produce heat—and, in the case of light bulbs—light plus heat, in response to current flow.

CAPACITANCE

Capacitance is the ability of a device to store an electrical charge for later use or to stabilize power in a circuit. This term is also used to refer to the potential difference between the two sides of a circuit.

FREQUENCY

Frequency is another factor to be considered when dealing with electricity or electrical devices. In circuits like the simple one in Figure 3-10, frequency is not a problem because the battery power is consistent, within reason. This type of current is called *direct current (DC)*. Direct current is mostly reserved for low-power, low-duration needs such as flashlights,

Best Practice

AC Versus DC

Equipment to be connected to AC or DC circuits must be rated—that is, approved—for use on these types of circuits. Devices designed for use with AC circuits must be matched to the frequency and power output of the circuit. Failure to match the type of equipment with the circuit can result in damage to both the circuit and the device and, in some cases, in injury to patients or staff.

CD players, or car starters. However, the current we use to run our household appliances, medical devices, and electric lights is *alternating current* (AC), that is, power is turned on and off many times a second. It is described in terms of cycles per second, or hertz (Hz). Although not important to our discussion, alternating current is used to reduce resistive forces and thus strain on the system.

The concepts embodied in Ohm's law are critical both to electrical flow and to the movement of gases in respiratory care equipment and the lung. Additionally, Ohm's law plays a large role in how blood circulates in the body. Ohm's law is another critical theory that the RT must master.

CASE STUDY 3-5

Different areas of the world use different mixtures of power and frequency. At some power levels, motors and electrical devices operate at faster or slower rates than at others. Some countries use higher-frequency power than is used in the United States.

Questions

1. What advice would you give your boss, who wants to donate some old ventilators to a medical mission in another country?
2. What would be the effect if a lower-power level were applied to a heater that worked on a resistor system?
3. How might you check to see whether equipment you wanted to donate would work where they would be sent?

Light Waves

The respiratory therapist needs to be familiar also with light wave characteristics. Several monitoring and analysis instruments depend on the ability to differentiate various types of light waves (see Chapter 16).

Light waves range from ultraviolet to infrared. A particular light wave's position in the light spectrum is a result of its wavelength, its amplitude, its period, and its frequency.

- *Wavelength* (lambda, λ) is the distance from the peak of one wave to the peak of the next wave. Wavelength is measured in nanometers (10^{-9}).
- *Amplitude* (A), the displacement of the wave particles, is the height of the wave from top to bottom. It represents the strength, energy, intensity, or power of the wave.
- *Period* (T) is the time it takes a wave to travel a given distance (i.e., the time between two peaks). Another more common term for this characteristic is "cycle."
- *Frequency* (Hz) is the number of waves that pass a given point per period of time or the number of periods divided by the time period. Frequency is generally expressed in terms of hertz (Hz). One hertz equals 1 cycle per second (cps).

Figure 3-11 illustrates these characteristics.

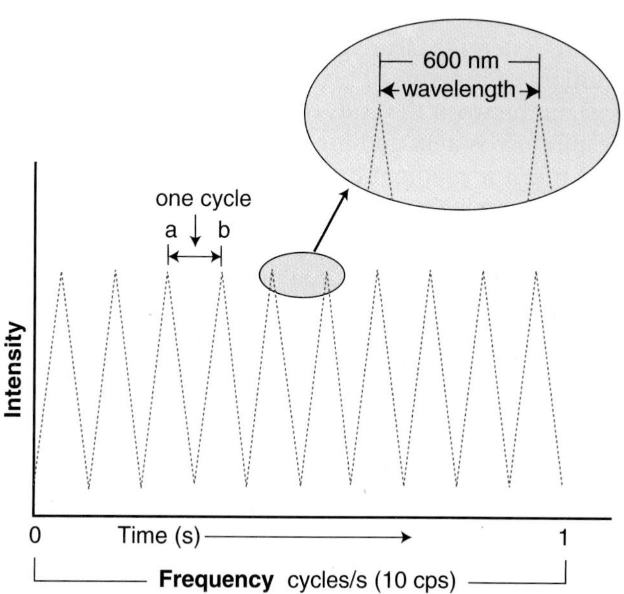

FIGURE 3-11 Characteristics of light waves: Intensity is essentially a power rating. Frequency is the number of cycles per time period, usually measured in seconds, and wavelength is the distance from one wave crest to the next.

From Mathews PJ. Co-oximetry. Respir Care Clin N Am. *1995;1:61*

Fluid Physics

Fluid physics is the study of why fluids (matter that flows) act as they do and of the forces that prompt those actions. Fluids include gases, liquids, and plasmas. The factors that influence or cause flow are varied both in effect and in strength.

VISCOSITY

Viscosity is a primary factor influencing the flow of fluids. Viscosity is often thought of as thickness (e.g., ketchup is thicker—has a higher viscosity—than water). The formal definition in a sense reinforces this commonly held conception. Formally, *viscosity* is the resistance that a gaseous or liquid system offers to flow when subjected to a shear stress. (A shear stress is what occurs when two or more parts of a system are moving at different speeds or in separate directions or both.) As a result, fluids become less viscid (thick) as they are stretched and pulled. Once rendered less viscid—having a lower viscosity—they flow more easily.

Viscosity is measured in SI units called *poises*. Simple gases have a low viscosity, ranging in the area of 100–200 micropoise at STP (standard temperature and pressure). Simple liquids have viscosities two orders of magnitude higher, in the centipoise range.

PRESSURE GRADIENT

The pressure gradient in the fluid system is another primary factor in flow dynamics. A *pressure gradient* is the difference in pressures from one area to another in the system. Pressure gradients are commonly thought of in terms of two areas of the respiratory system: between the ends of a tube or between the respiratory system and the external environment. The pressure gradient has both quantity and vector components; that is, pressure gradients are forces applied in a direction. The formula for pressure gradient (ΔP) is

$$\Delta P = P_1 - P_2$$

where P_1 is the higher pressure and P_2 is the lower pressure. For example, the pressure at end A of a tube is greater than the pressure at end B. As an example, calculate the pressure gradient if A equals 70 mm Hg and B equals 42 mm Hg. Indicate the direction (vector) of force.

$$\Delta P = P_1 - P_2$$
$$\Delta P = 70 - 42 \text{ mm Hg}$$
$$\Delta P = 28 \text{ mm Hg (A to B)}$$

Fluids therefore exhibit directionality (vectors)—movement—from high-pressure areas to low-pressure areas.

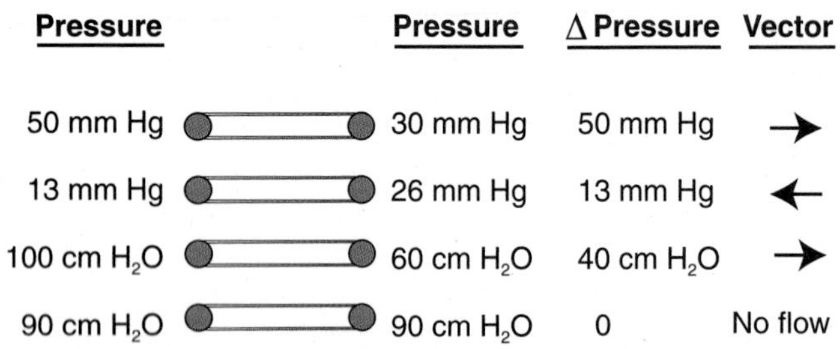

Pressure	Pressure	Δ Pressure	Vector
50 mm Hg	30 mm Hg	50 mm Hg	→
13 mm Hg	26 mm Hg	13 mm Hg	←
100 cm H_2O	60 cm H_2O	40 cm H_2O	→
90 cm H_2O	90 cm H_2O	0	No flow

FIGURE 3-12 Driving pressure gradients and flow: Three of the pipes have different pressures on their ends, resulting in a pressure gradient (ΔP) and flow in one direction (vector). Note that equal pressures result in $\Delta P = 0$ and no flow.

DRIVING PRESSURE

Driving pressure is another term used to refer to pressure gradient. Figure 3-12 provides several examples of pressure gradient, or driving pressure. The term "driving pressure" is used when the pressure provides the force, or drive, to overcome all the resistive forces that impede movement or, in the case of fluids, flow. Driving pressure is also a vector force, having both magnitude and direction.

Hagen-Poiseuille's law, better known as **Poiseuille's law**, describes in mathematical terms the factors that influence the flow of fluids through tubes. It explains the effects of tube geometry on resistance and flow in tubes. The formula for this description is:

$$\dot{V} = \frac{\Delta P r^4 \pi}{\eta 8L}$$

where $\dot{V}$ = fluid flow rate (volume per unit of time).

ΔP = driving pressure
r^4 = radius of the tube to the fourth power
η = viscosity of the fluid
$\pi/8$ = mathematical constant ($\pi = 3.14$)
L = length of the tube

This formula states that flow is directly proportional to the driving pressure and the radius of the tube and inversely proportional to the length of the tube and the viscosity of the fluid. For clinical purposes, the mathematical constant $\pi/8$ and the viscosity constant η can be eliminated. The restated formula is:

$$\dot{V} = \frac{\Delta P r^4}{L}$$

The restated formula now relates flow ($\dot{V}$) directly to the pressure gradient and to the radial size of the tube and inversely to the tube's length. The formula can be further rearranged to find ΔP:

$$\Delta P = \frac{L\dot{V}}{r^4}$$

One more step reveals an interesting conclusion. Move $\dot{V}$ to the other side of the equation so that

$$\frac{\Delta P}{\dot{V}} = \frac{L}{r^4}$$

but

$$\frac{\Delta P}{\dot{V}} = \text{resistance } (R)$$

So resistance (R) is directly related to length of the tube (l) and inversely related to the fourth power of the tube's radius (r^4). This conclusion suggests that short, wide tubes have lower resistance to flow than do long, narrow ones.

TYPES OF FLOW

Flow is dependent on the density and viscosity of the fluid and on the pressure gradient in the system.[2] The three most common types of flow are laminar, turbulent, and transitional or tracheal-bronchial (Figure 3-13).

Laminar Flow. *Laminar flow* is flow that runs parallel to the walls of smooth tubes. It is a smooth, relatively low-resistance flow. Laminar flow requires less force to move a given quantity of fluid through the tube than do the other two types of flow. Laminar flow is enhanced if low pressure gradients and low flow rates are used. Think of a garden hose with the spray attachment removed; when the water is turned on at a low flow, it comes out of the hose in a smooth clear stream. In fact, laminar flow is also called streamlined flow.

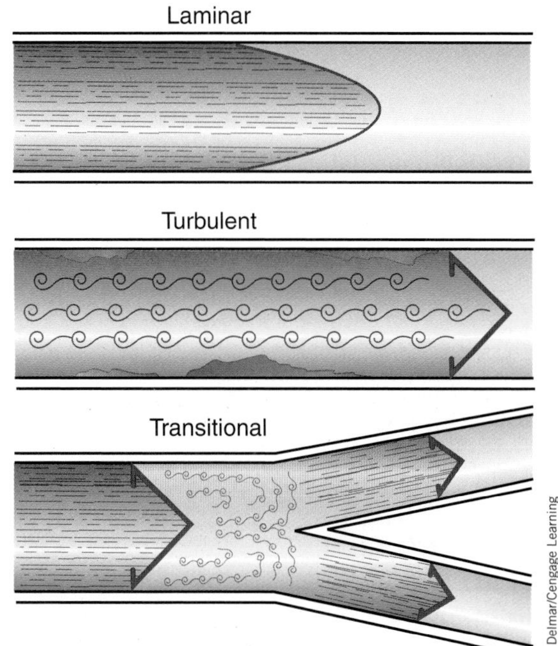

FIGURE 3-13 Flow types: The three basic types of flow are laminar (smooth), turbulent (rough), and transitional or tracheobronchial (a combination).

Turbulent Flow. *Turbulent flow*, on the other hand, is a type of flow that swirls and eddies, causing increased resistance and requiring increased pressure gradients to move the same amount of fluid as laminar flow would. In Figure 3-13, turbulent flow is caused by sidewall obstruction and changes in both the velocity and direction of flow caused by the obstructions.

Transitional Flow. *Tracheal-bronchial*, or *transitional*, flow has elements of both laminar and turbulent flow. Figure 3-13 illustrates transitional flow in a branching tube. The branch causes a slowing of flow and a change of vectors in parts of the flow while other parts of the flow remain laminar. For example, if a finger is placed into the water stream about an inch from the hose outlet, the stream splits in two. However, there is also some spray to the top and bottom as the turbulence from the finger takes effect. Another example is water running over a smooth stretch of streambed and then coming upon a rocky bottom with a few obstructions leading to rapids. The flow of the smooth-running stream is laminar, the rocks on the bottom cause transitional (tracheal-bronchial) flow, and the rapids produce turbulent flow.

Type of flow is determined by the **Reynolds number**, a dimensionless factor determined mathematically and based on density, velocity, viscosity, and the inertial force applied on the fluid. Flows with a Reynolds number greater than 3000 are turbulent; those with a Reynolds number below 2000 are laminar. Flows with a Reynolds number between 2000 and 3000 are transitional.

BERNOULLI'S PRINCIPLE

Bernoulli's principle is based on the law of continuity. The *law of continuity*, in effect, says that the product of flow ($\dot{V}$) times the cross-sectional area (A) of a tube is constant if the flow is constant. Therefore, at a given flow rate (indicated by $\dot{V}$, which means volume per unit of time—the definition of flow), if the size of the tube is increased, the velocity of the flow must decrease. For the net product of flow times cross-sectional area to remain unchanged, a change in cross-sectional area somewhere along the tube requires a change in velocity (distance in some direction in a period of time). This principle is diagrammed in Figure 3-14. The Bernoulli equation allows the approximation of the effect of changing one or more of these factors.

$$\dot{V}_1 \times A_1 \approx \dot{V}_2 \times A_2$$

where $\dot{V}$ is velocity and A is the cross-sectional area of the tube. The approximation symbol ($\approx$) is used to

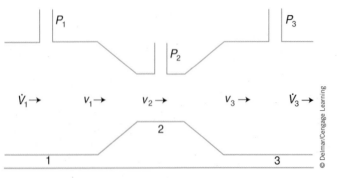

FIGURE 3-14 Bernoulli's principle: A system with constant flow ($\dot{V}_1 = \dot{V}_3$) exerts a side (lateral) wall pressure (P_1) and has a velocity (v_1) along segment 1. If the tube cross-sectional area (segment 2) decreases, the pressure (P_2) also decreases and the velocity (v_2) increases. As the cross-sectional area increases again (segment 3), the pressure (P_3) once more increases and the velocity (v_3) decreases. If the changes in cross-sectional areas are equal, the implied relationship is that $Pv = k$ (k is constant).

recognize that frictional and other resistance forces act to slow velocity and to remove energy from the system. Therefore, if the flow $\dot{V}$ through the tube is constant, then, when the cross-sectional area (A) decreases, the velocity (v) must increase to allow the equation to work. When applied to the Bernoulli equation (the lateral pressure of flowing fluid or gas is inversely proportional to the velocity), as the velocity increases due to the decrease in cross-sectional area, the lateral pressure also decreases.

An application of Bernoulli's principle and its effect is a device called a *Venturi*. The Venturi uses the sidewall pressure drop to add a secondary entrained gas to the system, as shown in Figure 3-15.

THE COANDA EFFECT

Closely related to Bernoulli's principle is the Coanda (or sidewall attachment) effect. In the *Coanda effect*, at

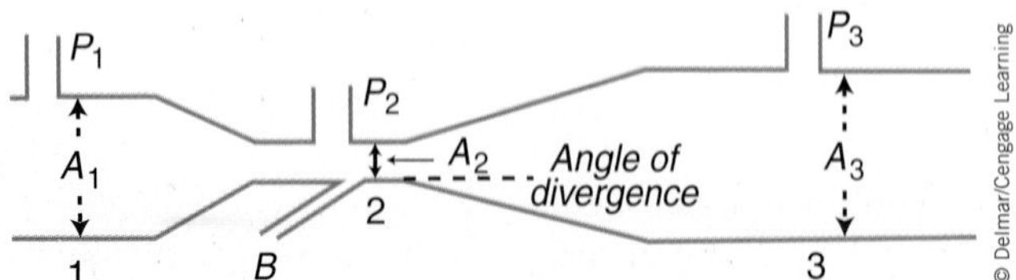

FIGURE 3-15 A Venturi device: The Venturi device makes air entrainment possible by the pressure drop in segment 2. Three factors are critical in the design. There must be a gradual tapering from segment 1 to segment 2; the angle of divergence from segment 2 to segment 3 must be less than 15°; and the cross-sectional area of segment 3 must be large enough to accommodate the increased volume of gas introduced from the entrainment port (B).

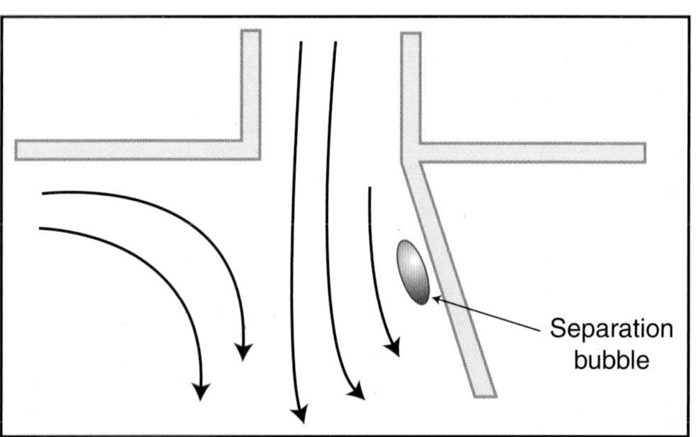

FIGURE 3-16 The Coanda effect: Given a high enough flow through a tube, the lateral wall pressure drop forms a separation bubble, which permits the flow to attach to one wall of the tube. Unless acted on by another force, the flow remains attached to that wall.

high velocities through tubes, fluids attach to one of the sidewalls due to the formation of a high-pressure fluid separation bubble on one wall. The result is the formation of a low-pressure boundary layer with slower flows at the walls and faster laminar flow in the center of the tube. See Figure 3-16. This attachment persists until another force acts on the flow.

Another effect of the Coanda or boundary layer phenomenon is that, in smooth tubes, the laminar flow forms a ballistic or bulletlike profile, as shown in Figure 3-17. Ballistic, or parabolic, flow patterns are known to reduce resistance to flow because of their wedgelike shape, which can be thought of as opening a path in the opposing material.

Gas Laws

The area of physics that is perhaps of greatest concern and interest to respiratory therapists is that of the gas laws. The *gas laws* are a series of equations that explain,

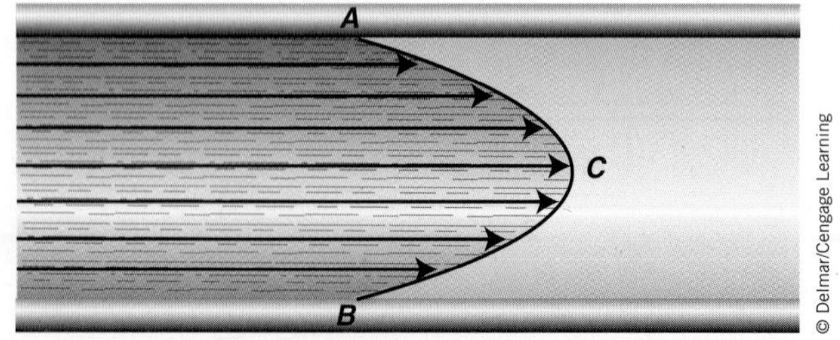

FIGURE 3-17 Ballistic flow profile: The characteristic laminar flow forms a bulletlike, or ballistic, velocity profile. In this profile, A and B (called *boundary layers*), are slower-moving gas streams than those of section C (axial flows) because of the relatively higher resistance to flow on the wall surfaces compared with the center of the lumen.

TABLE 3-7 **Gas law symbols and units**

Name	Symbol	Unit
Volume	V	mL
Pressure	P	mm Hg
Temperature	T	degrees Absolute (°A) or Kelvin (K)*
Moles of gas	η	η
Gas constant	R	J/η°A
Initial value (subscript)	1	
Final value (subscript)	2	

*K = °C + 273.15; no degree symbol is used with the unit K.

through the use of physics and mathematical formulas, the manner in which gases act under normal environmental conditions. Gas physics forms the groundwork and is the supporting structure of the art and science of modern respiratory care. Without a strong command of these principles, the respiratory therapist's success in the care and treatment of patients is severely limited.

In gas law problems, certain conventions, standard symbols for physical values, and specific units are used (Table 3-7). These units and conventions are frequently used in respiratory therapy and should become very familiar to therapists before long.

There are three major gas laws: Boyle's law, Charles's law, and Gay-Lussac's law. Memorize them and the combined gas law, which is a modification of the ideal gas law. The combined gas law allows the examination of all of the variations in the other three gas laws. These modifications take into account the fact that we generally work and live in a relatively constant physical environment. The major variables in the gas laws are gas pressure, gas volume, and gas temperature (Figure 3-18).

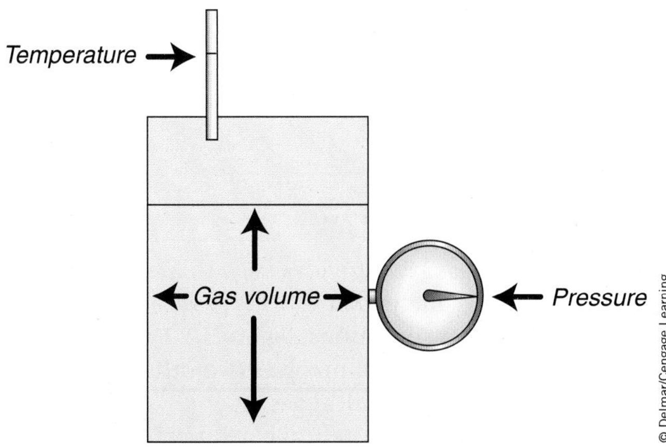

FIGURE 3-18 Elements of the gas laws: At physiological conditions, all gas laws can be stated as equations involving pressure (the gauge), temperature (the thermometer), and volume (the box).

BOYLE'S LAW

Boyle's law, developed by Robert Boyle in 1662, states that if the temperature of a gas is constant in a sealed container, its pressure (P) varies inversely with its volume (V). In other words, at any given temperature, if a gas is pressurized, its volume will be reduced proportionately to the pressure change; if we increase the volume of a gas, its pressure will increase. Figure 3-19 illustrates this law. The formula representing for Boyle's law is:

$$P_1 \times V_1 = P_2 \times V_2$$

Another way to express Boyle's law is:

$$PV = k$$

where k is a constant. Any increase in V must be offset by a reduction in P, and any reduction of V must be offset by an increase in P. For example, at a constant temperature, and with three known values, we can solve for the unknown value:

$$P_1 = 25 \text{ mL}$$
$$V_1 = 100 \text{ mm Hg}$$
$$V_2 = 50 \text{ mm Hg}$$
$$P_2 = ?$$

Thus:

$$P_1 \times V_1 = P_2 \times V_2$$
$$25 \times 100 = 50 \times V_2$$
$$V_2 = \frac{25 \times 100}{50}$$
$$V_2 = \frac{2500}{50}$$
$$V_2 = 50 \text{ mL}$$

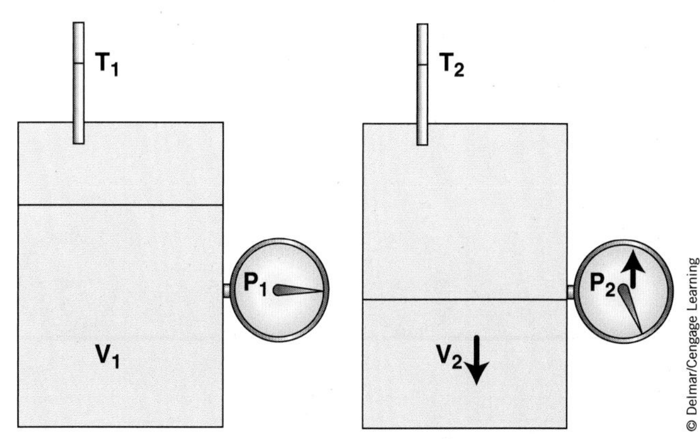

FIGURE 3-19 Boyle's law: If the temperature is kept constant, the volume of a gas varies inversely with the pressure of the gas.

Best Practice

Temperature

All temperatures in gas law equations must be stated in absolute (A) temperatures or kelvins (K).

CHARLES'S LAW

Charles's law, developed in the 1760s by Jacques Charles, is an extension of Boyle's law. Charles performed a series of experiments designed to test Boyle's law and to determine the effect that temperature changes have on gases. Charles found that, if pressure (*P*) is held constant, volume (*V*) changes directly with temperature (*T*). Therefore, if a volume of gas is heated while the same pressure is maintained, the volume (*V*) of that gas will increase or expand (Figure 3-20). The relationship between *T* and *V* is direct and equals a constant such that $V/T = k$. The formula representing Charles's law is:

$$\frac{V_1}{T_1} = \frac{V_2}{T_2}$$

For example, if *P* is constant, $V_1 = 1200$ mL, $T_1 = 320°A$, and $T_2 = 290°A$, then we can solve for V_2:

$$\frac{V_1}{T_1} = \frac{V_2}{T_2}$$

$$\frac{1200\text{ mL}}{320°} = \frac{V_1}{290°}$$

$$V_2 = \frac{1200 \times 290}{320} = \frac{348000}{320} = 1087.5\text{ mL}$$

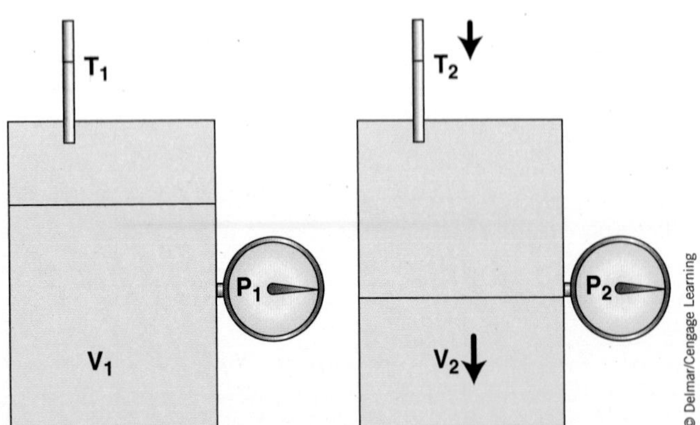

FIGURE 3-20 Charles's law: If the pressure is kept constant, the temperature of a gas varies inversely with the gas's pressure.

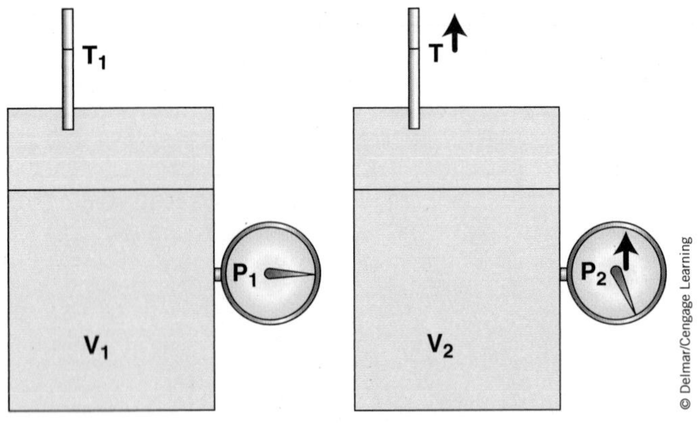

FIGURE 3-21 Guy-Lussac's law: Given a constant volume, pressure varies directly with temperature.

GAY-LUSSAC'S LAW

Gay-Lussac's law states that, if the volume (*V*) of a gas is kept steady, temperature (*T*) will change in the same direction as pressure (*P*). That is, the change in pressure of a given volume of gas is directly related to the change in temperature (Figure 3-21). This law can be expressed symbolically as $P \div T = k$. The equation illustrating Gay-Lussac's law is:

$$\frac{P_1}{T_1} = \frac{P_2}{T_2}$$

For example, letting $P_1 = 780$ mm Hg; $T_1 = 310°A$; $T_2 = 315°A$; and $V =$ a constant, solve for P_2.

$$\frac{P_1}{T_1} = \frac{P_2}{T_2}$$

$$\frac{780}{310°A} = \frac{P_2}{315°A}$$

$$\frac{780 \times 315}{310} = P_2$$

$$\frac{245700}{310} = P_2$$

$$P_2 = 792.58\text{ mm Hg}$$

THE COMBINED GAS LAW

The combined gas law provides us with a method of comparison and analysis of various gases at widely varying times and conditions. Figure 3-22 depicts the combined gas law, which involves two other laws: the ideal gas law and the clinical gas law.

Ideal gases are a theoretical construct used to analyze the mathematical relationships among the physical forces acting on gases. Ideal gases do not exist in nature. Nevertheless, they serve an important function because they allow us to imagine what would

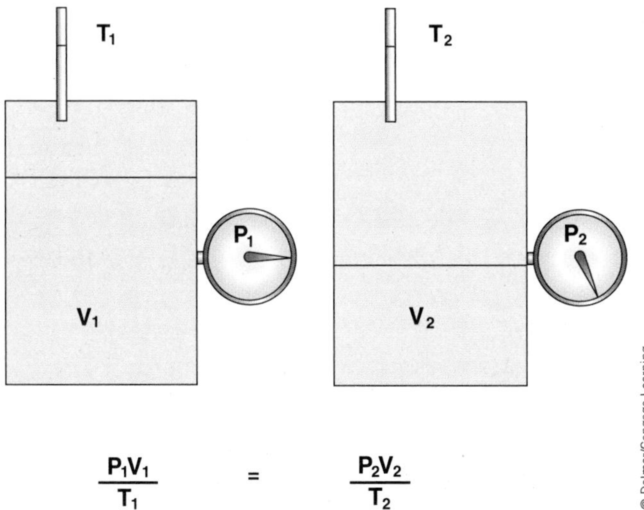

FIGURE 3-22 Combined gas law: The combined gas law illustrates the interrelationship among three variables. By using the formula presented, we can solve any gas law problem for which we know any five of six possible variable values.

happen to a gas or a mixture of gases if we altered the physical conditions acting on them.

The Ideal Gas Law. The *ideal*, or *perfect, gas law* states that the product of a gas's pressure (P) and its volume (V) is equal to the product of its temperature (T) and the number of moles (η) of the gas times the universal gas constant (R):

$$PV = \eta RT$$

The Clinical Gas Law. The molar concentration η of an ideal gas is constant (22.4 L; see the discussion of Avogadro's number later in the chapter). The energy value of gases (universal gas constant, R) within physiological ranges is also constant ($R = 8.31$ joules/mole/°A). That is the number of energy units released or absorbed per mole per degree of temperature change. Thus, molar concentration and energy value can be ignored. So, the combined gas law is used.

The Combined Gas Law. The combined gas law combines the laws of Boyle, Charles, and Gay-Lussac with the definition of a mole in a single equation that describes the actions of gases when one or more of the gas's physical characteristics undergo change.

$$\frac{P_1 V_1}{T_1} = \frac{P_2 V_2}{T_2}$$

This formula can be solved for an unknown of any of the incorporated factors. For this equation, no constant is needed, although, if a factor is constant, we can use it.

For practice with this concept, solve the following problem for T_2:

$P_1 = 770$ mm Hg

$V_1 = 500$ mL

$T_1 = 312$°A

$P_2 = 750$ mm Hg

$V_2 = 550$ mL

$$\frac{P_1 V_1}{T_1} = \frac{P_2 V_2}{T_2}$$

$$\frac{(770)(500)}{312} = \frac{(750)(550)}{T_2}$$

$$T_2 = \frac{(750)(550)(312)}{(770)(500)}$$

$$T_2 = \frac{128700000}{385000}$$

$$T_2 = 334.29$$

As shown, even complex problems with many changing variables can be solved using the combined gas law.

DALTON'S LAW

Air is a mixture of several gases, each of which imparts its own characteristics to the inhaled volume. Because respiratory therapists alter the mixture's composition for therapeutic reasons, it is important to know how the characteristics of the mixture are influenced by changes in composition and by changing conditions. **Dalton's law** describes the effect of gas composition on the pressures that the gas exerts on its surroundings.

Dalton's law of partial pressures states that the total pressure of a mixture of gases is equal to the sum of the pressures exerted by the individual gases. Each gas in the mixture exerts a pressure equal to the **fractional concentration** of that gas. Fractional concentration means the percentage of the total gas volume made up of a given gas. In other words, if a gas mixture is made up of four gases (A, B, C, and D), the pressure of the gas mixture (p_T) equals the total of all the gas pressures: Pressure A (p_A) + pressure B (p_B) + pressure C (p_C) + pressure D (p_D) equals p_T.

However, the law is not quite that simple because we have to account for the amount of each gas in the mixture. This is easy if the proportion or percentage of each gas is known. For example:

$$p_T = 200 \text{ mm Hg}$$

Gas A is 30% of the mixture: $200 \times 0.3 = 60$ mm Hg
Gas B is 10% of the mixture: $200 \times 0.1 = 20$ mm Hg
Gas C is 40% of the mixture: $200 \times 0.4 = 80$ mm Hg
Gas D is 20% of the mixture: $200 \times 0.2 = 40$ mm Hg
Total % = 100% Total pressure (p_T) = 200 mm Hg

The pressure exerted by each gas in the mixture is called its *partial pressure* (p or P). So gas A has a partial pressure of 60 mm Hg, and gas C has a partial pressure of 80 mm Hg.

A refinement of this technique is to determine the composition of the mixture of gases and then multiply the total pressure by the percentage concentrations of the individual gases to arrive at the fractional concentration of the gas (F). In the example, gas B has a fractional concentration of 10.0%, or more properly $F_B = 0.100$, where F = fractional concentration and B = gas B. Likewise, gas D has an F_D of 0.20, or a concentration of 20.0%, and gas A has a concentration of 30.0%, with an F_A of 0.30. Note that the F values for the gases are simply decimal equivalents of the percentage concentrations of each gas; that is, 15% equals 0.15, 6% equals 0.06, and 99% equals 0.99. Of course, 100% equals a fractional concentration of 1.00. Knowing the fractional concentrations of the gases and the total pressure of the mixture, we can determine the partial pressure of each gas.

The composition of the Earth's atmosphere is fairly constant. The fractional concentrations of the gases change little over the surface of the earth. What does change is the total pressure of the atmosphere and therefore the partial pressures of the gases making up the atmosphere. Table 3-8 lists the partial pressures of the four gases that account for 99.9% of the total volume of atmospheric gases. Table 3-9 lists the changes in atmospheric pressure and oxygen pressure as elevation changes from 1000 m (3280 ft) below sea level to 3500 m (11,483 ft) above sea level. The temperatures are the standard temperature of air at these altitudes.

Note that water vapor pressure is not affected by its fractional concentration. Water vapor, within physiological ranges, changes only in response to temperature changes. Water vapor pressure at normal body temperature (98.6°F, 37°C) and sea-level atmospheric pressure (760 mm Hg) is 47 mm Hg. To account for the water vapor in the saturated gases in the respiratory system, we must subtract p_{H_2O} (47 mm Hg) from the total pressure (760 mm Hg) before calculating the partial pressure of the other gases. This subtraction results in an adjusted partial pressure (p_{adj}).

$$p_{bar} - p_{H_2O} = p_{adj}$$

$$760 \text{ mm Hg} - 47 \text{ mm Hg} = 713 \text{ mm Hg}$$

So, assuming a gas mixture that is 20.93% O_2, 78% N_2, 0.3% CO_2, and 0.1% trace gases, what are the fractional concentrations (F_I) and partial pressures (P_I) of this inspired gas mixture at body temperature and 100% body humidity? The fractional concentrations are:

$$F_IO_2 = 0.2093$$

$$F_IN_2 = 0.78$$

$$F_ICO_2 = 0.003$$

$$F_{Itrace} = 0.001$$

TABLE 3-8 **Partial pressure (in mm Hg) of gases in the air, alveoli, and arterial blood at STP**

Gases	Dry Air	Alveolar Gas	Arterial Blood	Venous Blood
PO_2	159.0	100.00	95.0	40.0
PCO_2	0.2	40.0	40.0	46.0
pH_2O (vapor)	0.0	47.0	47.0	47.0
pN_2 (and trace gases)	600.8	573.0	573.0	573.0
Total	760.0	760.0	755.0	706.0

TABLE 3-9 **Standard temperatures and partial pressures of oxygen at selected elevations**

Elevations m	Elevations Ft	U.S. Std. Temp. (°C)	Atmosphere (mm Hg, dry)	Oxygen (mm Hg)
-1000	-3280	70.7	854.08	179.36
-500	-1640	64.9	806.00	169.89
0	0	59.0	759.99	160.00
250	820	56.1	737.24	154.82
500	1640	53.2	715.53	150.26
750	2461	50.2	694.85	146.92
1000	3281	47.3	673.65	141.47
1500	4921	41.5	633.84	133.11
1750	5742	38.5	614.71	129.10
2000	6562	35.6	595.58	125.07
2500	8202	29.8	559.91	117.58
3000	9843	23.9	525.79	110.42
3500	11483	18.1	493.22	103.58

From Glover TJ. Pocket Ref. *Littleton, Colo: Sequoia Publishing Inc; 1997*

where F_I is fraction of inspired. The partial pressures are:

$$(713 \times 0.2093) = 149.2309 \text{ mm Hg} = P_IO_2$$
$$(713 \times 0.7800) = 556.14 \text{ mm Hg} = P_IN_2$$
$$(713 \times 0.003) = 2.139 \text{ mm Hg} = P_ICO_2$$
$$(713 \times 0.0001) = 0.713 \text{ mm Hg} = P_{Itrace}$$

As these atmospheric gases travel down to the alveoli, they mix with a combination of end-expiratory gases and deadspace gases, which modify the actual alveolar gas concentrations and therefore the alveolar partial pressures. The actual alveolar partial pressures depend in part on the amount of ventilated but nonperfused alveoli (deadspace units) and on the number of perfused but not ventilated alveoli (shunt units). Also, the amount of carbon dioxide production plays a role in the final alveolar and arterial partial pressures of inhaled gases.

Dalton's law has many applications and is one of the most important biophysical concepts to master in the study of pulmonary physiology, medical gas administration, ventilator care, arterial blood gas and acid-base analysis and interpretation, and pulmonary pathophysiology.

HENRY'S LAW

Henry's law (of solubility) states that, given a constant temperature and a state of equilibrium between the gas pressures within and outside the liquid, the amount of gas dissolved in a liquid is directly proportional to the pressure of the gas on the surface of the liquid. In other words, if the pressure of a gas A, which is in contact with a liquid surface, is double, then the amount of the gas A dissolved in the liquid increases. If the original value is halved, the dissolved gas decreases proportionally.

Remember two things. First, dissolved gases are not chemically bound to their carrier mediums.

Second, dissolved gases exert a partial pressure equal to their gaseous partial (fractional) concentration. This is the case with oxygen in the alveolus and in the blood plasma. (Although no direct contact takes place across the alveolar-capillary membrane, the 2- or 3-cell separation has only a small and, in most cases, clinically insignificant effect.) As F_IO_2 changes, the dissolved oxygen in the plasma (P_aO_2) should undergo changes that are proportional to and in the same direction as the change in F_IO_2.

Another way of stating this principle is as follows: The amount of dissolved gas in a mixture is proportional to the pressure of that gas on the liquid surface. The proportionality is defined in terms of the solubility coefficient of the gas, and the solubility coefficient depends on the interaction of three factors:

- The nature of the solvent (the median in which the gas dissolves)
- The temperature of the solvent (and to a very small extent that of the gas)
- The pressure of the gas

The solubility coefficient, then, is the amount of gas that dissolves in 1 mL of a given solvent at standard pressure (760 mm Hg) and a given temperature (37°C). As temperature increases, so does the solubility coefficient; as temperature falls, so does the solubility coefficient.

AVOGADRO'S LAW

Avogadro (1776–1856) formulated what became his famous law in 1811. *Avogadro's law* states that equal volumes of gases contain equal numbers of molecules at the same temperatures and pressures regardless of their masses. Further investigations of this statement proved it to be true. It was shown that, at STP, each gram molecular weight (gmw) of an ideal gas consists of a volume of 22.4 L and contains 6.02 × 1023 molecules (Avogadro's number). Further, this was a constant across all gases tested.

GRAHAM'S LAW

Graham's law of diffusion deals with the movement of gases from one part of a system to another. This process is random; that is, where any given molecule will go is unpredictable. Because gas molecules move quickly (over 1000 mph) and independently, there are many collisions, resulting in random vectors and accelerations. The tendency over time is for the gases to become evenly distributed (homogeneous) throughout the area.

General Movement of Gases. The general movement of the gases is from areas of high concentration to areas of low concentration. A moment's reflection makes it clear that the areas of high concentration allow more collisions and direction changes, thus spreading the gas molecules out. Graham's law of diffusion, as it applies to gas mixtures, says that the rate of diffusion (r) is inversely proportional to the density of the gases. Specifically, Graham determined that the rate was inversely related to the square root of the density. Mathematically, this relationship is represented by the equation:

$$r = \frac{1}{\sqrt{D}}$$

As you can see, each gas has its own value for *r*, called its *diffusion coefficient*. A comparison of these coefficients indicates which gases diffuse most rapidly and by what amount. For example, assume that gas A has a density of 1.5 g/L and that gas B's density is 1.46 g/L. An equation (a proportionality) can then be set up:

$$\frac{rA}{rB} = \frac{\sqrt{DA}}{\sqrt{DB}}$$

$$\frac{rA}{rB} = \frac{\sqrt{1.5\ g/L}}{\sqrt{1.46\ g/L}}$$

$$\frac{rA}{rB} = \frac{1.225}{1.208}$$

$$rA = 1.014$$

This shows that gas A diffuses 1.014 times as fast as gas B.

Brownian Movement. The diffusion of gases in other fluids is erratic and seemingly random. This statement is especially true in the case of gas-to-gas diffusion systems, in which the molecules of the two gases randomly strike each other and thus alter the other molecules' path or trajectory. This random motion is called *Brownian motion* or *Brownian movement*. Because of the erratic and unpredictable movements of the molecules of gas, this process is sometimes referred to as the "drunkard's walk."

Diffusion through Liquids. For the diffusion of gases through liquids, one must consider the solubility coefficient (C_s) of the gas. This requires only a simple modification of the formula:

$$\frac{rA}{rB} = \frac{\sqrt{DA(C_{s_A})}}{\sqrt{DB(C_{s_B})}}$$

Simply solve the square root terms and multiply them by the respective solubility coefficients and then solve the proportionality as in the earlier problem.

Surface Tension

Surface tension is why bubbles form, why water collects in droplets, and why rain is globular or shaped like teardrops. The water or other fluid forms tight bonds between molecules where the gas and fluid meet. These bonds have the effect of a skin covering the liquid. The tighter the bonds get, the stronger the skin is, and the harder it is to disrupt the bubble, or skin, effect. The cohesive forces of the liquid tend to want to shrink the size of the liquid. Surface tension is a strong cohesive force. Disruptive forces are forces that tend to expand and eventually break the skin, allowing the liquid to move in any direction.

LAPLACE'S LAW

Pierre-Simon Laplace (1749–1827) found that the interrelationship of the surface tension forces and the forces acting to disrupt or break the liquid sphere varied inversely with the radius of the sphere. This came to be known as *Laplace's law*, which describes surface tension in relation to liquid spherical bodies. In other words, the smaller the sphere is, the higher the surface tension is and the smaller the sphere wants to get. Laplace's law says that the **distending pressure** (*P*, the pressure required to expand volume by a given amount) is directly related to the surface tension (*ST*) and inversely related to the radius (*r*) of the sphere. Distending pressure is defined in units of dynes per square centimeter, the surface tension in dynes/per centimeter, and the radius in centimeters. Stated as an equation, the law reads:

$$P = \frac{2ST}{r}$$

As an example, assume a liquid has a surface tension of 250 dynes/cm and a radius of 0.3 cm. What is the distending pressure?

$$P = \frac{2ST}{r}$$

$$= \frac{2(250\ \text{dynes/cm})}{0.3\ \text{cm}}$$

$$= \frac{500\ \text{dynes/cm}}{0.3\ \text{cm}}$$

$$P = 150\ \text{dynes/cm}^2$$

Thermodynamics

Thermodynamics is the study of the interrelationship between matter and energy. Familiarity with basic thermodynamic concepts aids in the understanding of

Age-Specific Competency

Laplace's Law

Laplace's law explains why newborns need higher ventilating pressures than adults do. Their alveoli are bubblelike and very small compared with those of a child or an adult. Surfactant is a biochemical, surface-active compound that alters the surface tension of the alveoli. The addition of surfactant by direct instillation reduces the collapsing forces, allowing better alveolar expansion. Commonly used in neonatal patients, surfactant may prove valuable in the treatment of adults with severe lung disease.

metabolic processes, both normal and abnormal. In addition, concepts such as entropy relate to the degradation of biological and electromechanical systems over time.

CONSERVATION OF MATTER AND ENERGY

According to Einstein's famous equation $E = MC^2$, if the speed of light (C) is a constant, then the ratio of energy (E) to matter (M) must always remain constant ($C^2 = E/M$). This statement suggests that, in any system where C is constant, changes in the amount of energy must be offset by proportional changes in matter. Hence the conservation of matter and energy. The total amount of energy and matter in a system must remain constant, although their proportions may change.

Law of Entropy. Entropy is a concept that at first glance appears to be at odds with the law of conservation of matter and energy. The *law of entropy* states that, in a closed system, everything moves toward a state of equilibrium. In other words, the entropy (entropic condition) is such that everything (matter and energy) is equally distributed. On the largest possible scale, the implication is that, at some far future date, all of the matter and energy in the universe will be evenly distributed. And if all things are evenly distributed, there will be no movement of either matter or energy. Carried further, without any movement or potential for movement, there is no energy. If there is no energy, there can be no matter—for energy is needed to hold matter together. Therefore, at the moment of total entropy, the universe will cease to exist.

HEAT AND OTHER FORMS OF ENERGY

As seen earlier in this chapter, heat is a product of molecular movement and a by-product of biochemical physiological processes. The process of measuring and recording temperature is not as simple as one would think.

Physiological Temperature. Human beings—and all living things for that matter—live and survive in a very narrow temperature range. Slight variations of that range cause havoc not only with biological systems but also with social and economic systems. Just think of heat waves and blizzards to realize how poorly equipped humans are at surviving outside their comfort range.

Temperature Scales. Globally, the vast majority of nations, as well as the entire scientific and medical community, have two common temperature reference systems: the Celsius scale (C) and the Absolute (°A) or

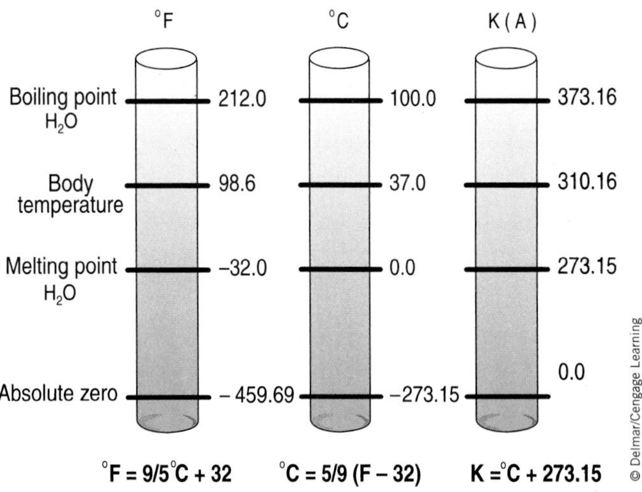

FIGURE 3-23 Comparison of temperature scales.

Kelvin (K) scale. The United States and, to a lesser degree, Great Britain commonly use a third system: the Fahrenheit system (°F). The presence of this third scale causes confusion and error when people are trying to communicate effectively in scientific and medical communities. The respiratory therapist must become familiar with and fluent in the Kelvin and Celsius temperature scales.

Figure 3-23 illustrates the three scales in reference to some important conditions. Note that the numbers associated with these events vary widely depending on the temperature system referenced. Points of special interest are body temperature, the boiling point of water, the freezing (or melting) point of water, and the point at which molecular activity ceases (absolute zero). Table 3-10 shows the calculations used to convert from one scale to another.

Radiation. Because radioactive substances are widely used in both therapeutic and diagnostic procedures, all health care workers should have at least a basic comprehension of them. Radiation exists in two forms: ionizing and nonionizing. Sunlight, heat, and radio waves are forms of *nonionizing radiation*, and they are generally no threat to humans. *Ionizing radiation*—X-rays, radioactive isotopic implants, and certain radioactive markers (contrast media)—are helpful in our practice of patient care. However, ionizing radiation can be hazardous if improperly used.

A *radioactive material* is a material that emits particulates of electromagnetic radiation as a consequence of nuclear decay. This decay results in the release of high-energy electrons (beta particles), electromagnetic energy (photons), or helium ions (alpha particles). The unit of measurement for radiation is the curie (Ci), which equals 37 billion disintegrations per second. One-millionth of a curie is a

TABLE 3-10 **Temperature scales and conversion formulas**

Scale	Description	Formula
°F (Fahrenheit)	1/180th of the difference between the melting point of water and its boiling point at standard pressure and temperature.	°F = 9/5 (°C + 32)
°C (Celsius)	1/100th of the difference between the melting and boiling points of water at standard pressure and temperature.	°C = 5/9 (°F − 32)
K (Kelvin)	Based on the average kinetic energy per molecule of a perfect gas. Zero on this scale is the temperature at which a perfect gas loses all its energy. Sometimes called *Absolute temperature.* The degree sign (°) is not used in this scale.	K = °C + 273.15

microcurie, which is the unit used to calculate dosage and exposures.

The emission of these radioactive particles diminishes over time. A critical piece of knowledge about a radioactive substance is its half-life: the amount of time it takes for the substance's radioactivity to be halved.

Best Practice

Radiation

Persons who work in areas where the potential for exposure to ionizing radiation sources is great and prolonged should wear *dosimeters,* which are devices that measure and record exposure levels. Persons who work in intensive care units, emergency rooms, and radiology departments are among those who should have dosimeters.

Summary

Physics, especially of fluids and gas, is among the most useful studies a respiratory therapist can undertake. An in-depth understanding of the principles of physics enables the respiratory therapist to understand the interactions among physics, physiology, and pathophysiology. In addition to the gas laws, the laws governing electricity, elasticity, force, and motion are all relevant to respiratory care. The respiratory therapist must be competent in the use of scientific notation, the metric system, and dimensional analysis because the solving of physiological equations plays a large part in the science of respiratory care.

As experts in the application of technology to the seriously ill or recovering patient, respiratory specialists must understand how both patient and equipment work and interact if they are to be at the peak of their profession. Having a grasp of physical principles and their application to both technology and humanity is a never ending duty owed to patients. Many people understand physics and many understand patients, but relatively few understand how to manage the interface where patient and technology meet. That is a respiratory therapist's skill.

Study Questions

REVIEW QUESTIONS

1. Name the traditional and transitional states of matter.
2. Write the formula for the combined gas law and the ideal gas law. Why are they different?
3. Explain Dalton's law.
4. Cite two uses for Boyle's law.
5. Convert 2 yd to meters and 3 lb to kilograms.
6. Change the following numbers into scientific notation: 195,000, 0.0085, 0.012.
7. Change the following scientific notations into numbers: 1.45×10^3, 2.568×10^{-3}, 7.16×10^5.

MULTIPLE-CHOICE QUESTIONS

1. Which of the following formulas would you use to determine volume changes at various pressures and temperatures?
   a. Boyle's law
   b. Charles's law
   c. Hagen-Poiseuille's law
   d. the combined gas law
2. To determine the water vapor pressure of a gas mixture, what information do you need?
   a. identity of the gases in the mixture
   b. pressure of the mixture of gases
   c. temperature of the mixture
   d. volume of the mixture

3. Which of the following measures would lower resistance to flow in a linear tube such as an airway?
   a. using a ballistic flow pattern
   b. employing a square-wave flow pattern
   c. Flow pattern is not a factor in resistance.
   d. using a ramp-shaped flow pattern
4. Why is the ideal gas law different from the clinical and combined gas laws?
   a. The combined gas law assumes that water vapor is inconsequential.
   b. The clinical gas law assumes that the number of molecules remains constant.
   c. There is no difference between the two laws other than their names.
   d. The ideal gas law fails to account for temperature changes over the narrow physiological range.
5. In a gas mixture with a pressure of 200 mm Hg at 37°C 100% saturated with water vapor, what is the water vapor pressure?
   a. 47 mm Hg
   b. 100 mm Hg
   c. 35 mm Hg
   d. 760 mm Hg
6. A gas mixture has a pressure of 300 mm Hg at 37°C 100% saturated. What is the pressure of gas A, one of the gases in the mixture, if its fractional concentration is 30%?
   a. 90 mm Hg
   b. 100 mm Hg
   c. 76 mm Hg
   d. 47 mm Hg
7. As the oxygen in a liquid O_2 storage vessel evaporates and turns into a gas, heat is extracted from the surrounding environment. What happens to the pressure in the storage vessel during this process as gas is formed?
   a. Pressure is not affected.
   b. Pressure decreases.
   c. Pressure fluctuates randomly.
   d. Pressure increases.
8. If we consider roads as airways and cars as gas molecules, which of the following is most likely to represent a situation demonstrating transitional flow?
   a. An interstate highway passing through sparsely settled land
   b. Entrance ramps and an adjacent interstate highway at midday
   c. Streets in New York City during rush hour
   d. Traffic stalled by gridlock or an auto accident
9. The triple point is defined as
   a. the point at which the freezing, boiling, and vaporization temperatures of two substances coincide.
   b. the time when the values of temperature, pressure, and volume are at equilibrium.
   c. the point at which a substance can exist as solid, liquid, and gas at the same time.
   d. the partial pressure of a gas when the fractional concentration passes 100.
10. Which is the correct and safest way to write the number nine-tenths?
   a. 0.9
   b. .9
   c. 009
   d. 9.0

CRITICAL-THINKING QUESTIONS

1. How does the science of physics specifically apply to respiratory therapy?
2. Look up the relationship between the terms "physics" and "physician" and between "physics" and "physic."
3. Why should a respiratory therapist have a solid understanding of physical principles?
4. What area of physics is most applicable to respiratory care?

References

1. *Macmillan Visual Desk Reference*. New York: Macmillan Publishing Co; 1993.
2. Eckhardt B. A critical point for turbulence. *Science*. July 8, 2011;333:165–167.

Suggested Reading

Branson RD, Hess DR, Chatburn RL. *Respiratory Care Equipment*. 2nd ed. Philadelphia: Lippincott, Williams & Wilkins; 1999.

CHAPTER 4

Applied Chemistry

Ingo S. Kampa

OBJECTIVES

Upon completion of this chapter, the reader should be able to:

- Understand the physiological applications of acids and buffers.
- Define physiological acids, bases, and buffers.
- Explain the regulation of pH (hydrogen ion concentrations) in various cellular and intracellular compartments.
- Describe the functions of various physiological buffers.
- Calculate pH and use the Henderson–Hasselbalch equation.
- Outline the physiology of acid–base disturbances.
- Recognize and understand the causes of acidosis and alkalosis.

CHAPTER OUTLINE

KEY TERMS

bicarbonate buffer system
hemoglobin buffer system
isohydric principle
metabolic acidosis
metabolic alkalosis
nonvolatile acid
pH
phosphate buffer system
physiological acid
physiological base
physiological buffer
protein buffer system
respiratory acidosis
respiratory alkalosis
strong acid
weak acid

This chapter begins with a review of certain aspects of atoms and molecules relevant to respiratory therapy. It also provides the basic concepts of chemistry that will help the reader learn and integrate the information throughout the book. The respiratory therapist must have a basic understanding of chemical structure, molecular bonding, and the four major groups of biological compounds and their interaction in a physiological organism.

All body fluids contain hydrogen ions (H^+). To sustain life, the hydrogen ion concentration (pH) in body fluids (which is a result of the acid–base balance) must be maintained within a relatively narrow range. Optimal metabolic function requires a pH in an even smaller range.

When hydrogen ions accumulate or are significantly decreased, the functioning of a multitude of metabolic pathways deteriorates. Physiological compensatory mechanisms are initiated to avert potentially disastrous consequences. Physicians, assisted by respiratory therapists, laboratory scientists, and technicians, must assess the acid–base status and take steps to correct any imbalance. This chapter defines acids, bases, and buffers and discusses the concept of pH. It will also show how these concepts apply to respiration and discuss common acid–base balance disturbances.

Review of Atoms and Molecules

In the nineteenth century, scientists looked for order in the chemical information gathered about elements. In 1869, two scientists, Dmitry Mendeleyev and Julius Lothar Meyer, independently produced a classification scheme for the elements. The scheme was based on the periodic law, which in its present form is an arrangement of all the elements in order of increasing atomic number. The result is that elements with similar properties occur at regular (periodic) intervals. A convenient way to compactly represent such behavior on the basis of the periodic law is in a table, which is called the *periodic table* (Figure 4-1). The periodic table is organized into groups that consist of representative elements, transition elements, inner-transition elements, and noble gases. The information provided for each element consists of the atomic number, symbol, name, and mass number.

ATOMS

An *atom* consists of a nucleus and one or more electrons (Figure 4-2). The *nucleus* consists of two different kinds of particles, protons and neutrons. The major difference between these two particles is that the *proton* has a positive electrical charge and the *neutron* has no electrical charge. *Electrons* are negatively charged particles located outside the nucleus. Protons and electrons carry opposite charges; so a neutral atom has the same number of protons and electrons. The electrons move around the nucleus in specific volumes of space called *atomic orbitals*, which have different shapes depending on the energy of the electrons they contain. The lowest-energy orbital in any atom is spherical and is called a *1s orbital*. Other spherical orbitals are also called s but have higher energies and thus are designated as 2s, 3s, 4s, and so on. Orbitals with characteristics different from s orbitals are designated as p, d, and f. The shapes of these are different from the shape of s orbitals. For example, p orbitals have a dumbbell shape, and d orbitals look like three-dimensional four-leaf clovers.

The number of electrons in a neutral atom determines the chemical properties of an element. The *atomic number* is identical to the number of protons in the nucleus of an element and to the number of electrons outside the nucleus. For example, hydrogen (H), which has the atomic number 1, has one proton and one electron; sodium (Na) has the atomic number 11 and contains 11 protons and 11 electrons. Protons and neutrons have approximately the same mass. The mass of electrons is negligible and does not add to the total mass of an element. As a result, the total mass of an element is approximately the total mass of the protons and neutrons.

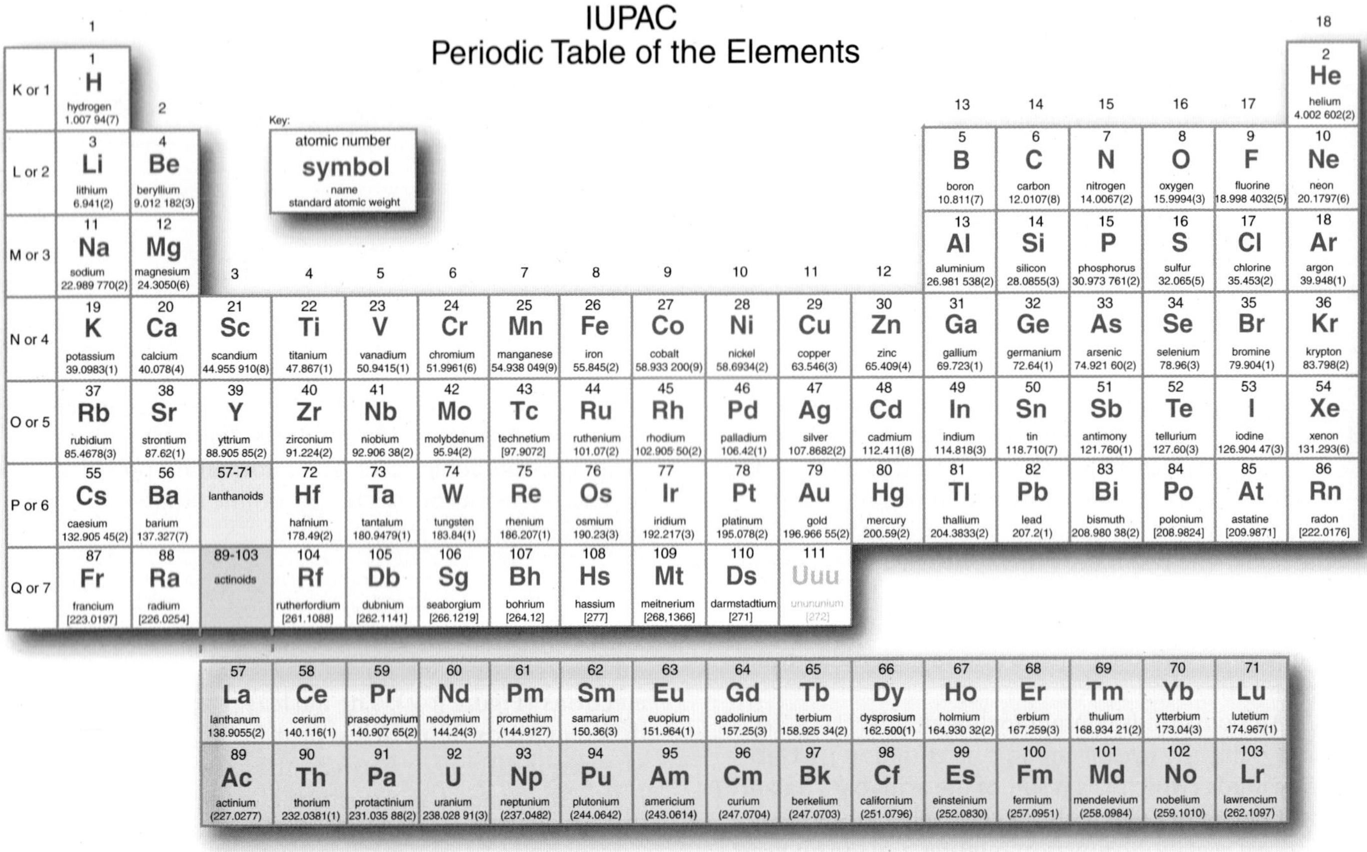

IUPAC
Periodic Table of the Elements

Key:

atomic number
symbol
name
standard atomic weight

	1	2	3	4	5	6	7	8	9	10	11	12	13	14	15	16	17	18
K or 1	1 **H** hydrogen 1.007 94(7)																	2 **He** helium 4.002 602(2)
L or 2	3 **Li** lithium 6.941(2)	4 **Be** beryllium 9.012 182(3)											5 **B** boron 10.811(7)	6 **C** carbon 12.0107(8)	7 **N** nitrogen 14.0067(2)	8 **O** oxygen 15.9994(3)	9 **F** fluorine 18.998 4032(5)	10 **Ne** neon 20.1797(6)
M or 3	11 **Na** sodium 22.989 770(2)	12 **Mg** magnesium 24.3050(6)											13 **Al** aluminium 26.981 538(2)	14 **Si** silicon 28.0855(3)	15 **P** phosphorus 30.973 761(2)	16 **S** sulfur 32.065(5)	17 **Cl** chlorine 35.453(2)	18 **Ar** argon 39.948(1)
N or 4	19 **K** potassium 39.0983(1)	20 **Ca** calcium 40.078(4)	21 **Sc** scandium 44.955 910(8)	22 **Ti** titanium 47.867(1)	23 **V** vanadium 50.9415(1)	24 **Cr** chromium 51.9961(6)	25 **Mn** manganese 54.938 049(9)	26 **Fe** iron 55.845(2)	27 **Co** cobalt 58.933 200(9)	28 **Ni** nickel 58.6934(2)	29 **Cu** copper 63.546(3)	30 **Zn** zinc 65.409(4)	31 **Ga** gallium 69.723(1)	32 **Ge** germanium 72.64(1)	33 **As** arsenic 74.921 60(2)	34 **Se** selenium 78.96(3)	35 **Br** bromine 79.904(1)	36 **Kr** krypton 83.798(2)
O or 5	37 **Rb** rubidium 85.4678(3)	38 **Sr** strontium 87.62(1)	39 **Y** yttrium 88.905 85(2)	40 **Zr** zirconium 91.224(2)	41 **Nb** niobium 92.906 38(2)	42 **Mo** molybdenum 95.94(2)	43 **Tc** technetium [97.9072]	44 **Ru** ruthenium 101.07(2)	45 **Rh** rhodium 102.905 50(2)	46 **Pd** palladium 106.42(1)	47 **Ag** silver 107.8682(2)	48 **Cd** cadmium 112.411(8)	49 **In** indium 114.818(3)	50 **Sn** tin 118.710(7)	51 **Sb** antimony 121.760(1)	52 **Te** tellurium 127.60(3)	53 **I** iodine 126.904 47(3)	54 **Xe** xenon 131.293(6)
P or 6	55 **Cs** caesium 132.905 45(2)	56 **Ba** barium 137.327(7)	57-71 lanthanoids	72 **Hf** hafnium 178.49(2)	73 **Ta** tantalum 180.9479(1)	74 **W** tungsten 183.84(1)	75 **Re** rhenium 186.207(1)	76 **Os** osmium 190.23(3)	77 **Ir** iridium 192.217(3)	78 **Pt** platinum 195.078(2)	79 **Au** gold 196.966 55(2)	80 **Hg** mercury 200.59(2)	81 **Tl** thallium 204.3833(2)	82 **Pb** lead 207.2(1)	83 **Bi** bismuth 208.980 38(2)	84 **Po** polonium [208.9824]	85 **At** astatine [209.9871]	86 **Rn** radon [222.0176]
Q or 7	87 **Fr** francium [223.0197]	88 **Ra** radium [226.0254]	89-103 actinoids	104 **Rf** rutherfordium [261.1088]	105 **Db** dubnium [262.1141]	106 **Sg** seaborgium [266.1219]	107 **Bh** bohrium [264.12]	108 **Hs** hassium [277]	109 **Mt** meitnerium [268,1366]	110 **Ds** darmstadtium [271]	111 **Uuu** unununium [272]							

57 **La** lanthanum 138.9055(2)	58 **Ce** cerium 140.116(1)	59 **Pr** praseodymium 140.907 65(2)	60 **Nd** neodymium 144.24(3)	61 **Pm** promethium (144.9127)	62 **Sm** samarium 150.36(3)	63 **Eu** euopium 151.964(1)	64 **Gd** gadolinium 157.25(3)	65 **Tb** terbium 158.925 34(2)	66 **Dy** dysprosium 162.500(1)	67 **Ho** holmium 164.930 32(2)	68 **Er** erbium 167.259(3)	69 **Tm** thulium 168.934 21(2)	70 **Yb** ytterbium 173.04(3)	71 **Lu** lutetium 174.967(1)
89 **Ac** actinium (227.0277)	90 **Th** thorium 232.0381(1)	91 **Pa** protactinium 231.035 88(2)	92 **U** uranium 238.028 91(3)	93 **Np** neptunium (237.0482)	94 **Pu** plutonium (244.0642)	95 **Am** americium (243.0614)	96 **Cm** curium (247.0704)	97 **Bk** berkelium (247.0703)	98 **Cf** californium (251.0796)	99 **Es** einsteinium (252.0830)	100 **Fm** fermium (257.0951)	101 **Md** mendelevium (258.0984)	102 **No** nobelium (259.1010)	103 **Lr** lawrencium (262.1097)

FIGURE 4-1 The Periodic Table of Elements

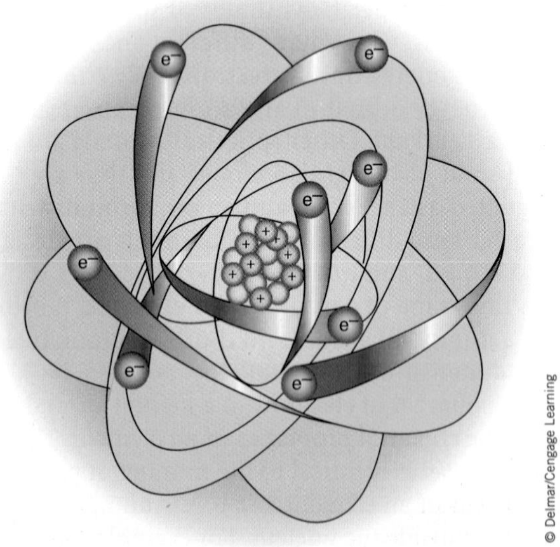

FIGURE 4-2 A three-dimensional diagram of an atom of oxygen, which contains eight protons, eight neutrons located in the center nucleus, and eight electrons in the orbital shells moving around the nucleus.

The number of neutrons in the nucleus of an element may be different. Thus, the same element may have different mass numbers (i.e., different number of neutrons). Atoms of the same element with different mass numbers are called *isotopes*. For example, carbon exists as three isotopes containing six, seven, and eight neutrons. Because these isotopes exist in various quantities, carbon has an average mass number of 12.011.

ATOMIC BONDS

Substances consist of atoms that are held together by bonds. The type of bond that holds atoms together determines in part the chemical property of a substance. A *bond* is an attractive force that exists between two atoms. The two most common types of bonds are ionic and covalent bonds.

The *ionic bond* is formed by the electrostatic attraction between a positive and a negative ion. A positive ion results from an element losing one or more electrons, giving it a positive charge. Such an ion is referred to as a *cation*. A negative ion results from an element gaining an electron, giving it a negative charge. It is referred to as an *anion*. For example, sodium and chloride exist in tissue fluids as ions (Nav^+ and Cl^-). When they are allowed to combine, however, they form an ionic bond, and sodium chloride (NaCl), a salt, is formed (Figure 4-3).

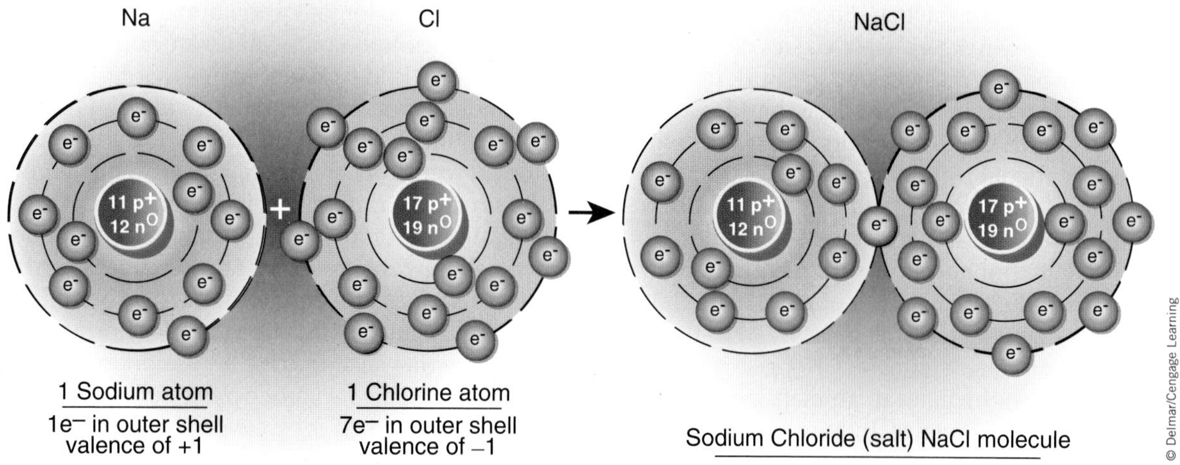

FIGURE 4-3 An ionic bond is formed between sodium (Na) and chlorine (Cl) to form table salt, sodium chloride (NaCl).

Covalent bonds are the result of sharing electrons between atoms. There are two types of covalent bonds: nonpolar and polar. For example:

- In hydrogen gas (H_2), the two atoms share the electrons equally. The attraction between the two atoms results in a molecule held together by a *nonpolar* covalent bond.
- In a water molecule (H−O−H), the electrons between the hydrogen and the oxygen are shared unequally and are closer to the negatively charged oxygen atom (Figure 4-4). This arrangement results in a net negative charge on the oxygen and a net positive charge on the two hydrogens, resulting in a *polar* covalent bond. The H_2O molecule is a dipole.

MOLECULES

Biological molecules are usually classified into four groups: carbohydrates, lipids, proteins, and nucleic acids. Many important biological molecules are very large and are called *macromolecules*.

Carbohydrates. *Carbohydrates* are complex organic compounds that can be further classified into monosaccharides, disaccharides, and polysaccharides.

- *Monosaccharides* are single polyhydroxy aldehydes or ketones.
- *Disaccharides* are two monosaccharides linked together.
- *Polysaccharides* are long chains of monosaccharides.

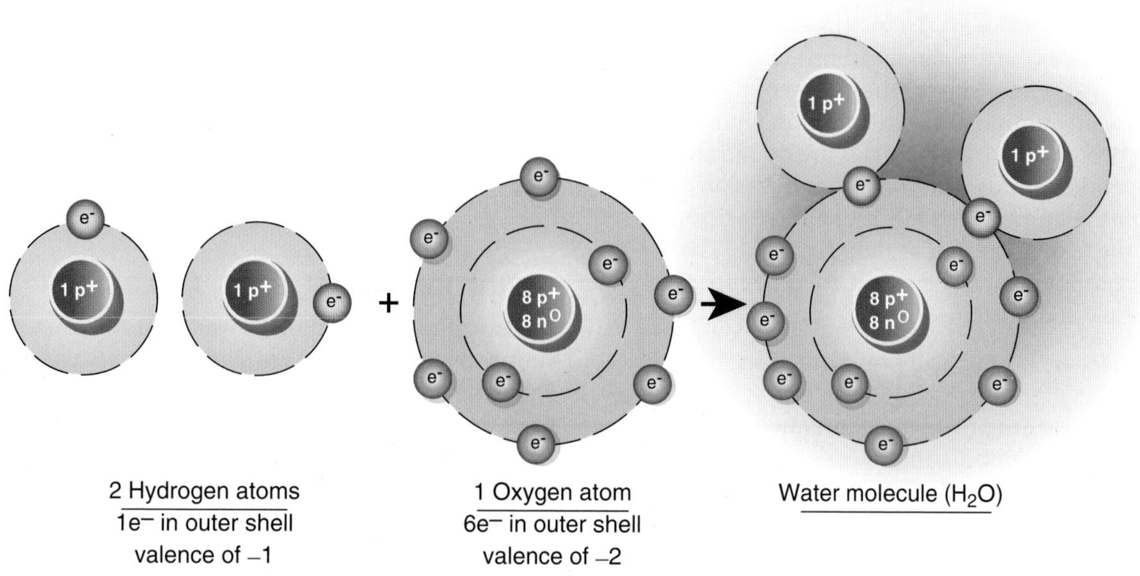

FIGURE 4-4 A covalent bond is formed between two hydrogen atoms and one oxygen atom to form water (H_2O).

The most important monosaccharides are glucose, fructose, and galactose, which are important energy sources in living organisms. Disaccharides are hydrolyzed to yield monosaccharides and are important energy sources as well. Important disaccharides are sucrose, lactose, and maltose. [Hydrolysis occurs when a compound is altered by the breakdown of a water molecule into H^+ (hydrogen) and OH^- (hydroxide ions).] Important polysaccharides are starch and glycogen. Both are polymers consisting entirely of glucose. Starch is the storage form of glucose in plants. When animals digest starch, it is hydrolyzed to produce the monosaccharide glucose. Glycogen is the storage form of carbohydrates in animals, and it is abundant in liver and muscles. In humans, stored liver glycogen maintains a normal blood glucose level for several hours after a meal. In a process known as *gluconeogenesis*, the liver produces glucose from nonglucose substances and maintains long-term normal blood glucose levels.

Lipids. *Lipids* can be simple or complex. *Simple lipids* contain only two types of components. For example, the simple lipid triglyceride consists of fatty acids and an alcohol. Waxes are another group of simple lipids. *Complex lipids* contain more than two components. Phospholipids and spingolipids are typical examples. Under basic conditions, these compounds can be saponified [i.e., hydrolyzed to an ester, a class of organic compounds that react with water to produce alcohols and organic or inorganic acids (see anion gap in Chapter 16)]. Typical classes of lipids that cannot be saponified are steroids and prostaglandins.

Proteins. *Proteins* are polymers consisting of amino acids. *Amino acids* are compounds consisting of an amino group (NH_3^+), the carboxylate group (COO^-), and a side chain (R group). These three groups are attached to a carbon (the alpha carbon). The properties of the amino acids depend on the nature of the R group. Twenty amino acids are found in naturally occurring proteins. The amino acids are bound to each other by peptide bonds. The properties of the protein depend on the number and kinds of amino acids found in the protein as well as their sequence. The resulting compounds can be classified as peptides, polypeptides, and proteins.

- *Peptides* are amino acid polymers of short-chain length.
- *Polypeptides* are polymers of intermediate lengths of up to 50 amino acids.
- *Proteins* are very large polymers of amino acids consisting of more than 50 amino acids, with molecular weights up to several millions.

Probably more than 200 peptides are essential for the proper functioning of an animal or human body. Many of the important peptides are hormones—such as insulin, prolactin, and glucagon—that regulate various metabolic processes essential for survival. Proteins or polypeptides have many functions, including structural, storage, regulatory, transport, and movement functions. The structural components in animals other than inorganic substances (e.g., calcium in bones or iron in hemoglobin) are proteins. Many essential stored substances, such as iron and hormones, are bound to proteins. Regulatory functions involve hormones (protein hormones such as growth hormone and thyrotropin) that regulate metabolic processes in the body. Many substances—such as ions, oxygen, and carbon dioxide—are transported while bound to proteins and are released from proteins at specific sites. Proteins also function in catalysis (enzyme activities), protection (antibody formation), and the transmission of nerve impulses.

Nucleic Acids. *Nucleic acids* consist of two major classes: ribonucleic acid (RNA) and deoxyribonucleic acid (DNA). RNA is found in the cytoplasm of cells; DNA is found in the nuclei. Nucleic acids are involved in the transfer of genetic information from existing cells to new cells. Nucleic acids are composed of nucleotides. Nucleotides consist of either a purine or a pyrimidine, either ribose or 2-deoxyribose, and phosphate. There are three types of RNA: messenger RNA (m-RNA), ribosomal RNA (r-RNA), and transfer RNA (t-RNA).

- Messenger RNA transfers genetic material from the nucleus of a cell to the cytoplasm, where protein synthesis occurs.
- In the cytoplasm, protein synthesis involves the r-RNA.
- Specific t-RNA molecules bind with amino acids and are transferred to the r-RNA site.

Acids, Bases, and Buffers

Key to understanding many of the body's metabolic functions is knowledge of the role of acids, bases, and buffers.

DEFINITIONS OF pH, BASE, AND BUFFER

Historically, acids and bases were first recognized simply by taste: Acids were sour and bases were bitter. Since the late nineteenth century, acids and bases have been defined according to their molecular characteristics. Organic chemists have embraced the definitions offered by American chemist Gilbert Lewis because they are the most useful in organic chemistry. According to Lewis, an *acid* is an electron pair acceptor, whereas a *base* is an electron pair donor. This concept is useful to the organic chemist because it adequately describes sharing electrons in an acid–base reaction in nonaqueous solvents.[1] Very simply, acids can be defined as a substance that gives off hydrogen ions, and bases are substances that absorb or neutralize hydrogen ions. An increase in hydrogen ions results in changes in the *pH*. *Buffers* are substances that resist changes in pH whenever hydrogen ion concentrations change.

Another definition is the *Bronsted–Lowry concept*, which defines acids as proton (H^+) donors and bases as proton acceptors.[2] In this context, a proton is a hydrogen atom without orbital electrons. According to this definition, a variety of compounds, including glucose, ethyl alcohol, and triglycerides, are classified as acids because of their potential to donate protons. In physiological systems, however, for a substance to be considered an acid or a base, it must donate or accept protons in an aqueous system. These conditions exclude glucose, ethyl alcohol, triglycerides, and many other compounds. Thus, the Bronsted–Lowry concept of acids and bases is restricted to compounds that can donate or accept electrons in an aqueous body and buffer system.

Therefore:

- A **physiological acid** is a substance that can donate electrons in a living physiological system.
- A **physiological base** is a substance that can accept electrons in a living physiological system.

In simple terms, **physiological buffers** are substances that resist changes in the hydrogen ion concentration when an acid or a base is added. Most buffers consist of a weak acid (HA) and its unprotonated form (where some protons are not present and the weak acid is transformed into a base), known as a *conjugate base* (A^-). Buffer actions can best be explained using the Henderson–Hasselbalch equation (Chapter 16) and the isohydric principle (discussed in the section "Concept of Buffers"). The important physiological buffers are the bicarbonate and phosphate buffers, hemoglobin, and plasma proteins.

CONCEPT OF pH

The **pH** is the measure of the acidity or alkalinity (baseness) of a solution. More technically, it is the negative log of the hydrogen ion concentration, ranging from $0–10^{-14}$ M, and it is commonly expressed as a range from 0 to 14.[3] Neutral solutions have a pH of around 7. Lower numbers indicate increasing acidity, and higher numbers indicate increasing alkalinity (Figure 4-5). Mathematically, pH is calculated as $pH = -\log [H^+]$ where [ ] indicates concentration.

Because pH is an approximation, not an absolute measure, of hydrogen ion concentrations in physiological fluids, it has been suggested that the hydrogen ion concentration of blood be expressed in terms of millimoles per liter (mmol/L). The pH concept, however, is widely used in physiology and medicine.

CONCEPT OF ACIDS AND THEIR PHYSIOLOGICAL APPLICATION

Body fluids are contained in two main fluid compartments: the intracellular and the extracellular compartments.[4] The extracellular compartment can be

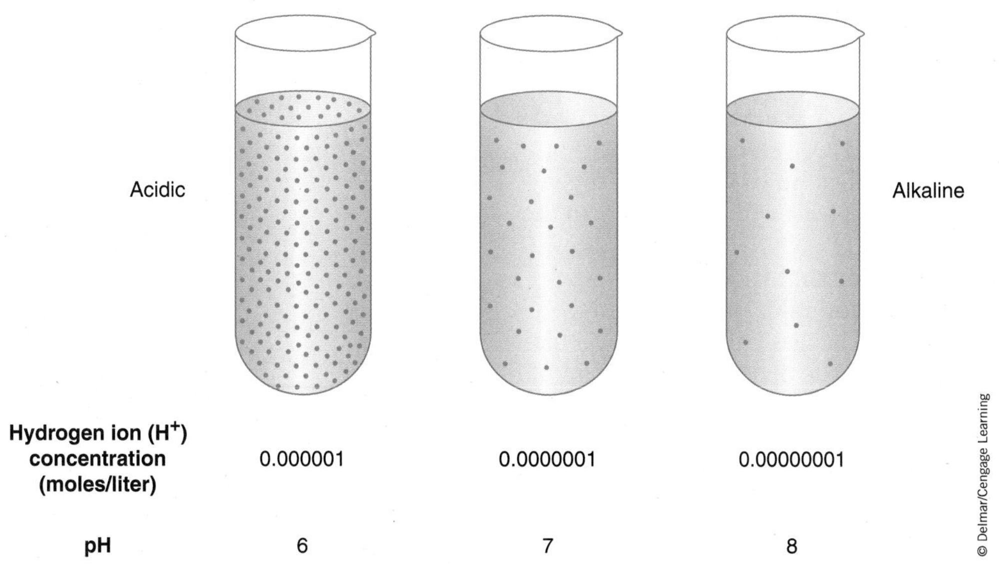

FIGURE 4-5 Schematic illustration of the relationship between hydrogen ion concentration, pH, and acidity and alkalinity. Dots represent hydrogen ions.

subdivided into plasma and interstitial fluid. The concentrations of electrolytes, acids, buffers, and water differ significantly in each of these compartments. For example, plasma and interstitial fluid have high concentrations of Na^+ and bicarbonate (HCO_3^-) ions, whereas intracellular fluids have high concentrations of potassium (K^+) and phosphate (PO_4^-) ions. Plasma, approximately 1300–1800 mL/m^2, represents about 15% of the total fluid volume.

Acids are classified as strong or weak depending on their degrees of ionization. **Strong acids** are represented by the following equations:

$$HA + H_2O \rightarrow H_3O^+ + A^-$$
$$H_3O^+ \rightarrow H^+ + H_2O$$

The hydronium ion (H_3O^+) results from the reaction of a hydrogen ion (H^+) with water in an aqueous solution. Thus a strong acid such as HCl ionizes completely as follows:

$$HCl + H_2O \rightarrow H_3O^+ + Cl^-$$
$$H_3O^+ \rightarrow H^+ + H_2O$$

A **weak acid** is only slightly ionized in an aqueous solution. Weak acids are represented by the following equation:

$$HA + H_2O \leftrightarrow H_3O^+ + A^-$$
$$H_3O^+ \rightarrow H^+ + H_2O$$

All gradations can be found between a strong and a weak acid. The tendency of acids to dissociate or ionize into H_3O^+ is expressed as the *dissociation constant* (k). At equilibrium, when the hydrogen ion and conjugated base pair are present in equal concentrations, the hydrogen ion concentration is equal to the dissociation constant. Thus, the dissociation constant is related to the hydronium ion concentration (H_3O^+). In the remainder of this chapter, the term "hydrogen ion" and the symbol H^+ will be used for the hydronium ion (H_3O^+) since H^+ is more commonly used. Remember, however, that hydrogen ions in aqueous solutions react with water to form the hydrated hydronium ion.

At equilibrium, the constant k_1 [HA] [H_2O] = k_2 [H^+] [A^-]. The numerical value of k is defined for a specific temperature and changes if the reaction occurs at a different temperature. The dissociation constant of an acid can then be expressed as

$$K = \frac{k_1}{k_2}$$

or

$$= \frac{[H^+]\,[A^-]}{[HA]\,[H_2O]}$$

Since more H_2O is present, as compared with H^+, A^-, and HA, its concentration remains constant, resulting in

$$k' = \frac{[H^+]\,[A^-]}{[HA]}$$

Acids of Physiological Importance. Physiologically important acids fall into two categories: bicarbonic acids and noncarbonic acids. The first group consists only of carbonic acids, which can readily permeate cell membranes, thus affecting hydrogen ion concentrations and cellular pH.

The noncarbonic group consists of a variety of acids, including sulfuric, lactic, and acetoacetic acids. Noncarbonic acids are often referred to as *fixed acids*. **Nonvolatile acids** (fixed acids), or nonvolatile acids, such as sulfuric and phosphoric acids, which are produced at a rate of 70–100 mmol daily and are eliminated through the kidneys.

Hydrogen ions are continuously produced in a living organism from the formation of carbon dioxide (CO_2) and must be eliminated in a manner that leaves the living organism unharmed. An individual weighing 70 kg produces approximately 15–20 moles (weight in grams/molecular weight) of carbon dioxide daily that need to be eliminated through the lungs. When elimination is not accomplished, the physiological acid–base balance is disturbed.

The main hydrogen ion production results from the metabolism of carbohydrates, fats, and proteins, forming large quantities of CO_2: for example, when glucose is converted to CO_2. The resulting CO_2 transfuses across cellular membranes into interstitial fluid to blood plasma and red blood cells and is finally eliminated in alveolar air. The reaction of CO_2 with H_2O in these compartments results in hydrogen ion production.

$$CO_2 + H_2 \leftrightarrow H_2CO_3 \leftrightarrow H^+ + HCO_3^-$$

Hydrogen ions produced in the various tissues must be buffered in a physiological organism. The overall process of these reactions is illustrated in Figure 4-6.

Noncarbonic acids, such as lactic acid, beta-hydroxybutyric acid, and acetoacetic acid are intermediate products of carbohydrate metabolism. These hydrogen ions are normally converted to carbon dioxide and water before excretion.

CONCEPT OF BASES

Bases are substances that accept electrons under physiological conditions. A base can also inactivate

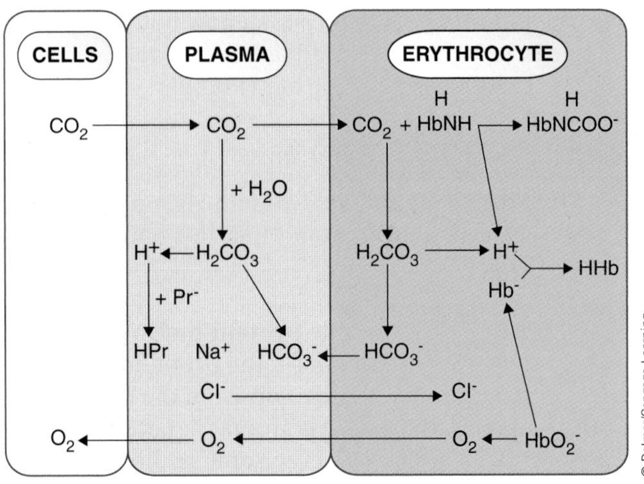

FIGURE 4-6 Transport of carbon dioxide.

an acid. In nonphysiological conditions, substances like the dihydrogen phosphate ($H_2PO_4^-$) ion theoretically can act as acids or bases; that is, they are able to donate or accept electrons. Under physiological conditions, however, body fluids such as blood would have to have a pH of 4 or less to act as a base. Clearly, $H_2PO_4^-$ cannot act as a base in blood. Two key physiological bases are bicarbonate and hemoglobin, which are discussed here as they function in buffer systems.

CONCEPT OF BUFFERS

A *buffer* is any substance that resists change in pH[5] and usually consists of a weak acid and its conjugate base. In a physiological system, a number of buffers in the plasma compartment, body fluids, and red blood cells maintain and regulate the pH.

Calculating the pH of a Buffer. The Henderson–Hasselbalch equation can best calculate the pH of buffers. Beginning with the equation

$$[HA] \rightarrow [H^+] + [A^-]$$

the dissociation factor for a weak acid can be calculated:

$$k_a = \frac{[^+H]\,[A^-]}{[HA]}$$

Solving for $[H^+]$ results in

$$[H^+] = k_a \times \frac{[HA]}{[A^-]}$$

Converting the equation into a log form yields

$$\log[H^+] = \log k_a + \log \frac{[HA]}{[A^-]}$$

The mathematical relationship between pH and hydrogen ion concentration can be expressed by the equation

$$pH = -\log[H^+]$$

The $\log[H^+]$ in the equation can be converted to $-\log[H^+]$ by multiplying each term by -1. Substituting pH for $-\log[H^+]$ and pk_a for $-\log k_a$ results in the following equation:

$$pH = pk_a + \log \frac{[A^-]}{[HA]}$$

(The pk_a is a physiologic constant for each species hemoglobin; for humans, $pk_a = 6.3$. It is essentially the dissociation constant for the physiologic acid/base pairs.) The Henderson–Hasselbalch equation is extremely useful for calculating the pH of a buffer system. Since [HA] represents undissociated acid and $[A^-]$ represents the completely dissociated salt (for example, A^-), the equation can be rewritten as

$$pH = pk_a + \log \frac{[\text{salt}]}{[\text{undissociated acid}]}$$

Buffers of Physiological Importance. Buffers in a physiological system can be divided into two broad categories: bicarbonate and nonbicarbonate. A series of buffer "events" is often referred to as a *buffering, or buffers, system*. The bicarbonate system consists of a single member, the bicarbonate–carbonic acid pair. This is the most important buffer of plasma. The nonbicarbonate buffer systems consist of the phosphate buffer system ($HPO_4^{2-}-H_2PO_4^-$), the plasma protein buffer system ($Pr^- - HPr$), and the hemoglobin ($Hb^- - HHb$ and $HbO_2^- - HHbO_2$) buffer system.

Bicarbonate Buffer System. The **bicarbonate buffer system** is unique in a variety of ways. Continuously being formed, HCO_3 thus exists in high concentrations and can readily be controlled by the lungs by either eliminating or retaining carbon dioxide. In addition, concentrations are regulated in the kidney by increasing or decreasing reclamation of bicarbonate ions from the glomerular filtrate. Carbon dioxide is continuously formed in the cells as a result of carbohydrate, fat, and protein metabolism. As it passes through different cell membranes, it reacts with water to form H^+ and HCO_3^-. This process is summarized in the following equation:

$$\underset{(gas)}{CO_2} \leftrightarrow \underset{(aqueous)}{CO_2} + H_2O \leftrightarrow H_2CO_3 \leftrightarrow H^+ + HCO_3^-$$

Since this reaction is bidirectional, CO_2 is released in the lungs and expelled, thus eliminating the continuously produced CO_2. If more hydrogen is retained, then the substance becomes more acidic.

The carbonic acid (H_2CO_3) exists only in trace quantities because it readily dissociates into the dissolved CO_2 and HCO_3^-, which are in equilibrium with each other.

$$k = \frac{[H^+] + HCO_3^-]}{\underset{\text{(aqueous)}}{[CO_2] + [H_2CO_3]}}$$

The equation can be restated as follows:

$$pk = pH + \log \frac{\underset{\text{(aqueous)}}{[CO_2] + [H_2CO_3]}}{[HCO_3^-]}$$

This equation can be rewritten using the Henderson–Hasselbalch equation to yield

$$pH = pk_a + \log \frac{[HCO_3^-]}{\underset{\text{(aqueous)}}{[CO_2] + [H_2CO_3]}}$$

The concentrations of both CO_2 and H_2CO_3 are easily obtained from the PCO_2 measurement multiplied by 0.03 at 38°. The pk_a under these conditions is 6.1. Substituting these values into the equation results in the following:

$$pH = 6.1 + \log \frac{[HCO_3^-]}{0.03 \times [PCO_2]}$$

In a normal individual, the average HCO_3^- concentration is approximately 24 mmol/L, and the PCO_2 is 40 mm Hg, resulting in the following pH:

$$pH = 6.1 + \log \frac{24\text{mEq/L}}{0.03 \text{ (conversion constant)} \times 40 \text{ mm Hg}}$$

$$= 6.1 + \log \frac{24}{1.2}$$

$$= 6.1 + \log 20$$

$$= 6.1 + 1.30 = 7.40$$

The PCO_2 is maintained at approximately 40 mm Hg by the lungs' regulating the loss of CO_2.

The continuous internal respiration of tissue cells consumes O_2 and produces CO_2. The CO_2 reacts with water to produce hydrogen ions (H^+). These acids need to be buffered to maintain the narrow range of pH in living organisms. When hydrogen ions are added to body fluids, the following reaction occurs:

$$H^+ + HCO_3^- \leftrightarrow H_2CO_3 \leftrightarrow CO_2 + H_2O$$

The following equation shows how buffers resist a change in pH when acid is added. If 2 mmol/L of H^+ is added, the following change of pH occurs:

$$7.36 = 6.1 + \log \frac{22}{0.03 \times 40}$$

Since the PCO_2 is kept at 40 mm Hg, only a minimal change in pH occurs. Thus, this buffer resists changes in pH.

Protein Buffer System. The **protein buffer system** acts as a physiological buffer for the pH of body. The more effective protein buffers consist of the immidazolium group because the pk_a is around 7. Because of their protein structure, however, some of these buffers have a pk_a as low as 5 and as high as 8, and their physiological-buffering ability deteriorates quickly as the pk_a deviates from 7. The pk_a of the protein buffers, consisting of alpha amino groups, ranges from above 7 to greater than 10. Only the buffers with a pk_a near or below 8 have physiological-buffering capabilities.

$$pH = pk_a + \log \frac{[\text{protein}^-]}{[\text{protein}]}$$

When an acid (H^+ ions) is added, the following reaction occurs:

$$H^+ + \text{protein}^- \leftrightarrow \text{HProtein}$$

Phosphate Buffer System. The **phosphate buffer system**, which consists of the dihydrogenphosphate (H_2PO_4) and monohydrogenphosphate (HPO_4^{2-}) ions, has a pk_a of 6.8. In addition, many organic phosphate compounds, such as adenosine monophosphate and nucleoside phosphate, have pk_a values between 6.5 and 7.5 and thus readily function as buffers in a physiological system. The following equations can be written:

$$H_2PO_4^- \leftrightarrow HPO_4^{2-} + H^+$$

$$pH = pk_a + \log \frac{H_2PO_4^{2-}}{HPO_4^{2-}}$$

Hemoglobin Buffer System. The **hemoglobin buffer system** consists of two buffering systems: nonoxygenated and oxygenated hemoglobin. The oxygenated hemoglobin buffer system differs from the nonoxygenated type due to the difference in the pk_a value. In these two systems, the weak acids consist of the nonoxygenated (HHb) and oxygenated hemoglobin ($HHbO_2$); the conjugate bases are Hb^- and HbO_2^-. The nonoxygenated hemoglobin buffer pair can be symbolized as follows:

$$HHb \leftrightarrow H^+ + Hb^-$$

The oxygenated hemoglobin can be symbolized as

$$HHbO_2 \leftrightarrow H^+ + HbO_2^-$$

The Isohydric Principle. The various fluid compartments in a physiological system contain a variety of buffers that interact with each other to form a single pH. For example, the plasma compartment is a homogeneous solution that contains several buffers, mainly the bicarbonate buffer, the phosphate buffer, and a variety of protein buffers. The plasma compartment is well mixed because of rapid blood circulation. In the plasma compartment is a single hydrogen ion concentration, as determined by pH measurements, that require various buffer pairs to be in equilibrium. This balance is referred to as the **isohydric principle** and is expressed as

$$pH = pk_{a1}\frac{[HA_1]}{[A_1^-]} = pk_{a2}\frac{[HA_2]}{[A_2^-]} = pk_{a3}\frac{[HA_3]}{[A_3^-]} = pk_{an}\frac{[HA_n]}{[A_n^-]}$$

How Acids, Bases, and Buffers Affect Respiration

The intracellular pH and the fluid pH are held at a steady concentration mainly because of the various buffers in these compartments. The interactions of acids, bases, and buffers are key to understanding how respiration works.

TRANSPORT OF CARBON DIOXIDE TO THE ALVEOLI

Respiration is a continuous interchange of oxygen and carbon dioxide between a living organism and its environment. Tissue cells continuously require oxygen for their metabolic processes, which form carbon dioxide that must be continuously eliminated. Respiration has two components: external and internal. *External respiration* is the exchange of oxygen and carbon dioxide in the lungs between blood and alveolar air. *Internal respiration* is the exchange of these gases at the tissue level.

Oxygen is carried from the lungs to the tissue by the blood. Normally, about 97–98% of the oxygen is carried in reversible combination by the hemoglobin (Hb) molecule. This relationship can be presented as

$$\text{Hb (deoxygenated)} + O_2 \leftrightarrow HbO_2 \text{ (oxygenated)}$$

The carbon dioxide produced by the tissue's metabolic processes enters the interstitial and plasma compartments. In the plasma compartment, a small portion of the carbon dioxide remains dissolved in the blood. Another small portion reacts with water to release hydrogen ions. Plasma protein buffers buffer this acid. Some carbon dioxide reacts, very slowly, with the carbamino groups of proteins to form carbamino compounds. Most of the carbon dioxide is transported as the bicarbonate ion, formed when carbon dioxide enters the red blood cells and reacts with water to form carbonic acid. This reaction is very fast because of the presence in the red blood cells of carbonic anhydrase, which rapidly catalyzes the formation of carbonic acid and brings the reaction to a quick equilibrium. The reaction quickly becomes 99.9% complete, forming hydrogen and bicarbonate ions.

Most of the hydrogen ion generated in the red blood cells reacts with deoxyhemoglobin. This process facilitates the release of oxygen from the oxygenated hemoglobin. A small amount of carbon dioxide remains dissolved, and some is carried by hemoglobin in the form of carbamate ($R\text{-}NHCO_2^-$). The unionized form of the alpha-amino groups of hemoglobin can react reversibly with carbon dioxide. The released oxygen from hemoglobin in the red blood cells is transported to the tissue cells. This process of exchanging oxygen and removing carbon dioxide occurs normally without changing the hydrogen ion concentrations in the various compartments. The overall process is known as the *isohydric shift* because the pH remains constant.

These reactions in the red blood cells form a bicarbonate ion, which diffuses rapidly out of the red blood cell into the plasma compartment. Since there is a substantial loss of anions as the bicarbonate ions leave the red blood cells, chloride ions enter the red bloods cells to maintain electrochemical balance. The exchange of chloride and bicarbonate ions across the red blood cell membrane is called the *chloride shift*. The reactions involved in the isohydric and chloride shifts are illustrated in Figure 4-7.

At the lungs, the reverse process occurs. The binding of oxygen to hemoglobin releases hydrogen ions from the hemoglobin. The reaction of hydrogen

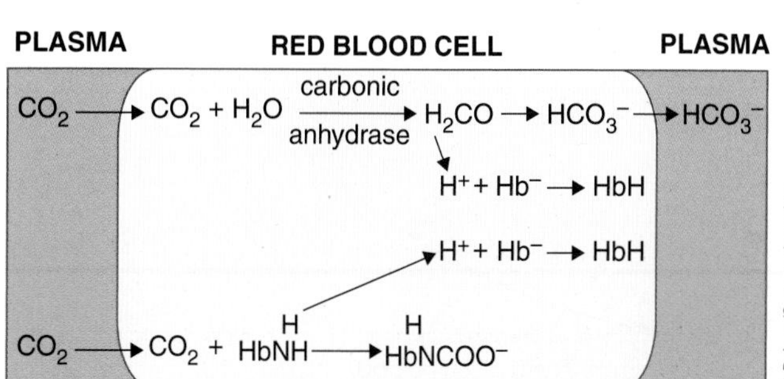

FIGURE 4-7 Carbon dioxide reactions in the red blood cell.

ions with the bicarbonate ions results in the formation of carbon dioxide, which is released by the lungs. These processes are aided by the *Haldane effect* (the binding of oxygen facilitates the displacement of carbon dioxide). The more acidic oxyhemoglobin has a reduced capacity to form carbamino hemoglobin; the facilitation of carbonic anhydrase in the presence of carbonic acid forms carbon dioxide. Maintaining the PCO_2 at approximately 40 mm Hg keeps the bicarbonate ion and pH at a steady level.

In a typical individual at rest, the bicarbonate ion concentrations in arterial and venous blood are approximately 24.0 and 25.1 mmol/L, respectively, resulting in a difference of approximately 1.1 mmol/L. Arterial blood and venous blood differ by approximately 0.15 mmol/L of dissolved carbon dioxide and 0.5 mmol/L of carbamino carbon dioxide. Thus, approximately 1.75 mmol/L of carbon dioxide is exchanged at each pass through the lungs at normal respiration. As the PCO_2 increases, an almost linear increase in alveolar ventilation occurs to remove the increased carbon dioxide produced and to maintain normal pH (Figure 4-8).

PROCESSING OF NONCARBONIC ACIDS

In humans, the most common noncarbonic acids are sulfuric and phosphoric acids, produced as a result of protein metabolism and the catabolism of phospholipids. Other noncarbonic acids produced in humans are beta-hydroxybutyric acid, acetacetic acid, lactic acid, and pyruvic acid. In addition, a variety of foods may contain organic acids. The acids other than sulfuric and phosphoric are of little consequence in the normal person

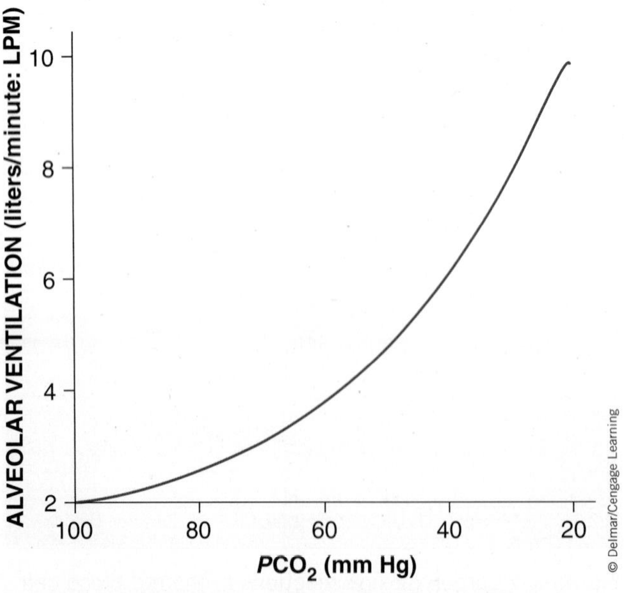

FIGURE 4-8 PCO_2 removal with increasing alveolar ventilation.

because they are present in small amounts and transient in nature. When present in small quantities, they are usually metabolized to carbon dioxide and water. For example, lactic acid accumulation due to exercise and beta-hydroxybutyric and acetic acids present after fasting are transient because they are metabolized to carbon dioxide and water. When these acids are present in very large amounts, however, perhaps as a result of diabetes or other pathological conditions, the kidney must eliminate them. The major noncarbonic acids (sulfuric and phosphoric) are eliminated by the kidney in amounts of 50–150 mmol per day.

REGULATION OF ALKALI IN THE BODY

In humans and other mammals, the major source of alkali production is the formation of CO_2 and H_2O, resulting in the bicarbonate ion. Often, increased alkali is not directly the result of alkali production but rather results from the consumption of hydrogen ion (usually in fruits and vegetables), increasing bicarbonate ion concentration. Dietary habits that include the consumption of significant amounts of meat result in the production of sulfuric and phosphoric acids, which provide adequate amounts of hydrogen ions and maintain plasma bicarbonate levels around 24 mmol/L. Thus, alkali is eliminated from the body mainly as expired air in the alveoli. Excessive amounts of carbonate ions must then be excreted by the kidneys, resulting in urine having an alkaline pH.

Disturbance of the Acid–Base Balance

Metabolic changes, as well as many pathological conditions, result in changes in electrolyte balance and acid–base disturbances that can be identified and monitored by examining extracellular fluids such as blood.[6,7] Common measurements include electrolyte, pH, PCO_2, bicarbonate, and total carbon dioxide. Theoretically, it should be relatively easy to characterize disturbances in acid–base status as either acidosis or alkalosis, which can be further differentiated into those having respiratory causes and those having metabolic causes.

- *Respiratory acidosis* is caused by an increase in carbonic acid relative to bicarbonate.
- *Respiratory alkalosis* is characterized by a decrease in carbonic acid with no change in bicarbonate.
- *Metabolic acidosis* is characterized by a decrease in bicarbonate without any significant change in carbonic acid.
- *Metabolic alkalosis* is an increase in bicarbonate without a significant change in carbonic acid.

This theoretical simplicity is complicated by various compensatory mechanisms. For example, compensation can occur by altering the carbon dioxide concentration through hyperventilation (eliminating more carbon dioxide) or through hypoventilation (retaining more carbon dioxide). Also possible is renal compensation by either retaining more bicarbonate ion or increasing its elimination. In addition to simple causes of any of these conditions, mixed causes can exist.

RESPIRATORY ACIDOSIS

Respiratory acidosis is caused by an increase in carbon dioxide retention, resulting in an increase in carbonic acid and in PCO_2 (Figure 4-9). Respiratory acidosis is caused by a variety of conditions, including impaired respiration as a result of diseases such as emphysema, asthma, pneumonia, chronic bronchitis, congestive heart failure, and hypoxia. Another cause is depression of the respiratory center in the medulla, as a result of the administration of anesthesia or the use of narcotics or sedatives. Exposure to sedatives and hypoxia can also cause decreased ventilation, resulting in respiratory acidosis.

An increase in carbonic acid results in a variety of compensatory mechanisms. In blood, an increase in carbonic acid is initially and immediately buffered by both the hemoglobin and protein buffer systems, resulting in a slight increase in bicarbonate ion. Renal compensation, on the other hand, requires more time. The resulting rise of PCO_2 in respiratory acidosis causes increases in bicarbonate ion reabsorption and ammonia formation by the kidney. The increase

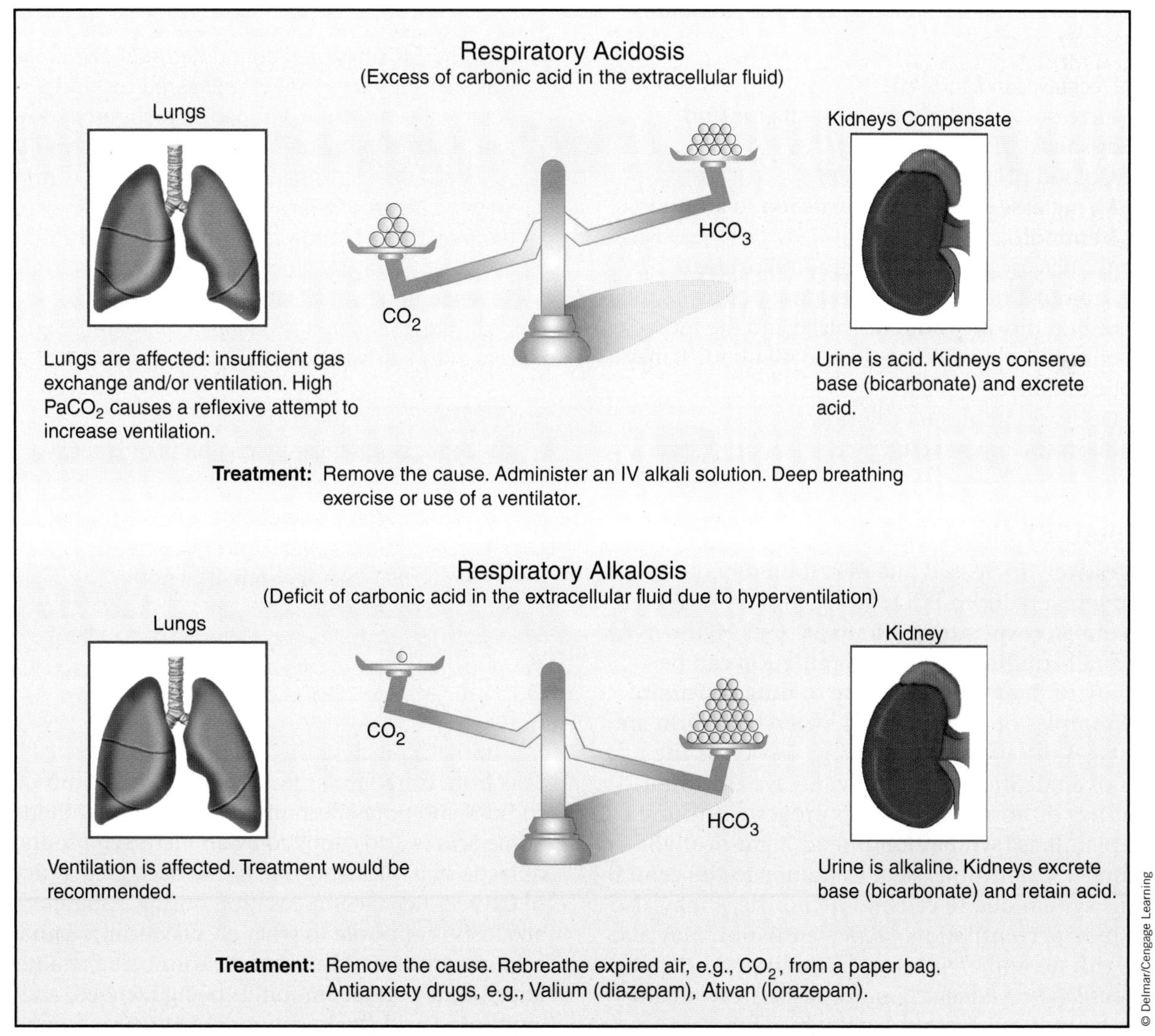

FIGURE 4-9 Body's defense action and treatment for respiratory acidosis and respiratory alkalosis.

Best Practice

Respiratory Acidosis

The renal response to respiratory acidosis is a slow process, requiring several days.

in bicarbonate retention is directly related to PCO_2 but not to pH. As a result, in the early stages of respiratory acidosis, significant increases in arterial PCO_2 can be expected. Once renal compensation is fully developed, it becomes more efficient than the initial rapid response of the buffer system. Once full compensation has occurred, the increased resorption of HCO_3^- reduces the extracellular H^+ concentration to normal or near-normal blood pH.

In uncomplicated respiratory acidosis, laboratory findings consist of:

- Decreases in blood pH.
- Increases in both the bicarbonate ion and dissolved bicarbonate.
- A blood pH of less than 7.35.
- An increase of the bicarbonate ion to around 30 mmol/L.
- An increase of dissolved carbon dioxide to 2 mmol/L. Since most laboratories measure total carbon dioxide (both dissolved and the bicarbonate ion), results of close to 40 mmol/L may be obtained.
- Decreases in plasma chloride.
- Increases in potassium.

CASE STUDY 4-1

A 54-year-old male patient, C. S., was admitted to the emergency room (ER) exhibiting speech and gait disorders, irritability, and mental confusion. A chemistry profile, including electrolytes, was performed. The chemistry profile was essentially normal with the exception of glucose (47 mg/dL; normal range 70–110 mg/dL) and a total CO_2 concentration of 51 mmol/L (normal range 22–32 mmol/L). The ER physician subsequently requested a blood gas determination, which yielded the following results:

PO_2 = 65 mm Hg

PCO_2 = 71 mm Hg

pH = 7.18

HCO_3^- = 22 mEq/L

The ER physician concluded that the patient was suffering from uncompensated respiratory acidosis as a result of impaired respiratory drive caused by a metabolic condition (hypoglycemia).

Rationale for diagnosis: Since there were no known causes of overproduction of CO_2, elevations of PCO_2 are the result of defects in PCO_2 excretion. The low glucose level, along with the absence of airway obstructions or impaired respiratory mechanics, suggested an impaired respiratory drive caused by hypoglycemia.

Questions

1. What compensatory mechanism is likely to occur in this patient?
2. What is the likely compensatory mechanism in a patient suffering from respiratory acidosis when the defect is not in the respiratory center?

RESPIRATORY ALKALOSIS

An excessively increased rate of carbon dioxide loss resulting in a reduced PCO_2 along with an increased pH results in **respiratory alkalosis**. (See Figure 4-9.) The overall condition of hyperventilation can be voluntary or the result of disease or drug consumption. Examples of drug-induced hyperventilation are early stages of salicylate poisoning, as well as the effects of analeptic (central nervous system stimulant) drugs or hormones such as progesterone and catecholamines (sympathomimetic "fight-or-flight" hormones). Conditions such as trauma to the central nervous system due to cerebral hemorrhage may also result in hyperventilation. Hyperventilation may also occur with no apparent cause, a condition known as *hyperventilation syndrome*. Finally, respiratory alkalosis can be induced experimentally by deliberate hyperventilation.

Initially, much of the lost acid is replenished by ions from extracellular fluids, along with a shift of sodium and potassium into the intracellular fluid. Some acid is also supplied by an increased production of lactic acid, probably due to the decreased availability of oxygen. Renal compensation during respiratory alkalosis is opposite to what occurs during respiratory acidosis. Instead of bicarbonate ions being retained, a larger-than-normal amount is being excreted, and the amount of acid (hydrogen ions) in the urine significantly decreases.

Laboratory findings in respiratory alkalosis include.

- Increased lactic acid levels.
- Significantly reduced bicarbonate ions and dissolved carbon dioxide.
- Dissolved carbon dioxide that is generally less than 50% of normal.
- Total carbon dioxide analysis (the sum of dissolved carbon dioxide and bicarbonate ions) of less than 20 mmol/L.
- Lowered concentrations of both sodium and potassium.

Best Practice

Respiratory Alkalosis

Respiratory hyperventilation is a compensatory response to metabolic acidosis. Compensation for respiratory alkalosis consists initially of buffering by erythrocytes and tissues. Subsequently, renal buffering becomes a major factor if hyperventilation persists for several days.

METABOLIC ACIDOSIS

Metabolic acidosis is the result of increased hydrogen ion concentration (a decrease in blood pH) (Figure 4-10). It can occur as the result of excessive production of acids, increased transfer of hydrogen ion from intracellular to extracellular fluid, the ingestion or infusion of organic acids into the blood, kidney failure resulting in the reduced excretion of acid, and excessive loss of bicarbonate as the result of diarrhea and loss of duodenal fluid.

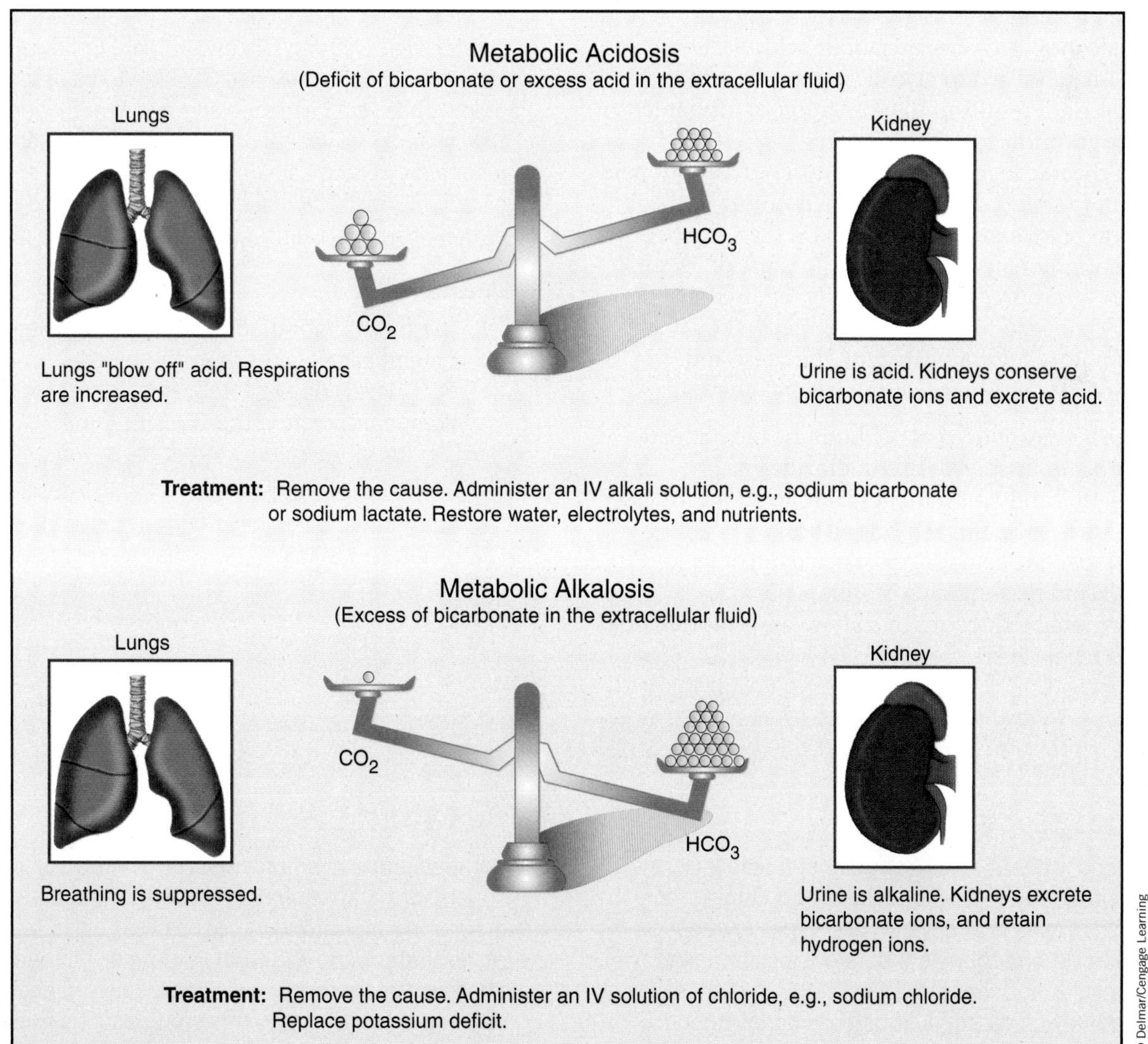

FIGURE 4-10 The body's defense action and treatment for metabolic acidosis and metabolic alkalosis.

A common cause of metabolic acidosis is diabetic ketoacidosis. Excessive mobilization of triglyceride results in the excessive formation of beta-hydroxybutyric and acetoacetic acid. The resulting severe metabolic acidosis can lead to coma and death if the patient is not treated with insulin. Before the availability of insulin, diabetic ketoacidosis was a common cause of death in juvenile diabetics.

Milder forms of metabolic acidosis can also be observed in cases of severe starvation, such as anorexia, in which ketoacids are produced in excessive amounts to meet the individual's energy needs.

Severe hypoxia can lead to significant increases in lactic acid, causing metabolic acidosis. Oxygen deprivation of tissue results in a significant increase in the blood lactate/pyruvate ratio. Hypoxia can be the result of pulmonary insufficiency or oxygen deprivation, initiating a chain of reactions that can culminate in coma and death. Increases in lactic acid can be the result of the patient's receiving large doses of drugs such as phenformin and streptozotocin.

The ingestion of antifreeze (ethylene glycol) or methyl alcohol can cause metabolic acidosis. Ethylene glycol is metabolized to glycolic and oxalic acid, and methyl alcohol results in the formation of formaldehyde and formic acid.

The chronic ingestion of high doses of salicylic acid can result in salicylate intoxication, resulting in the formation of excessive organic acids.

The bicarbonate buffer system, because of its ample supply of bicarbonate ion, is initially involved in resisting change in pH as a result of metabolic acidosis.

Laboratory findings vary with the cause and severity of metabolic acidosis. In general, they are:

- A significant decrease of both the bicarbonate ion and dissolved carbon dioxide.
- Significantly increased organic acids, regardless of the cause of metabolic acidosis.
- In diabetic ketoacidosis, large reductions in plasma sodium and chloride.
- Minimal reductions in sodium and chloride due to renal causes.

CASE STUDY 4-2

G. R., a 27-year-old female, was admitted to the emergency room (ER). She was in a state of hysteria, had a severe headache, and was hyperventilating. The ER physician requested a chemistry profile including electrolytes, a urine toxicology screen, and blood salicylate level and blood gas studies. The chemistry profile was essentially normal. The electrolyte studies and blood gas studies indicated significant depletion of total carbon dioxide (16 mmol/L; normal 22–32 mmol/L), a decreased PCO_2 of 29 mm Hg, a pH of 7.50, a PO_2 of 99 mm Hg, and HCO_3^- of 18 mEq/L. The urine toxicology screen was negative, but the blood salicylate level was 450 mg/L.

The ER physician concluded that the patient most likely was suffering from respiratory alkalosis brought on by hysteria and an overdose of salicylate.

Rationale for diagnosis: A salicylate level of greater than 200 mg/L is uncommon. Salicylate concentrations that exceed 300 mg/L are associated with severe headache and hyperventilation. Salicylate and a variety of other drugs stimulate the respiratory center, causing an excessive loss of carbon dioxide. The resulting uncompensated loss of the bicarbonate ions results in an alkaline pH.

Questions

1. The hyperventilation in this case resulted in a significant decrease in the blood PCO_2 level. As expected, this decrease significantly alters the 20:1 ratio of HCO_3^-/CO_2. What compensatory system will attempt to reestablish this 20:1 ratio?
2. Subnormal levels of PCO_2 can result in respiratory alkalosis. Discuss a mechanism for this occurrence.

Best Practice

Laboratory Tests

Many conditions, such as metabolic acidosis caused by diabetic ketoacidosis and chronic renal diseases that develop over a prolonged period, will alter classic laboratory results. Laboratory tests that determine the severity of diabetes and kidney diseases must be considered. Blood urea nitrogen (BUN), creatinine, and glucose levels provide important clinical information.

Best Practice

Metabolic Acidosis

Compensatory mechanisms in metabolic acidosis consist of both respiratory and renal mechanisms. In respiratory compensation, both the rate of ventilation and the tidal volume are increased. The respiratory response to metabolic acidosis is very rapid, occurring within minutes. Renal compensatory mechanisms are slower, taking place over a period of hours and days.

CASE STUDY 4-3

S. C., a 13-year-old female student who was complaining that she was ill, was transferred by ambulance from her junior high school to the emergency room (ER). The patient stated that she was feeling weak and was constantly thirsty. She had been urinating frequently for the past few weeks. A chemistry profile, including electrolytes, was performed. The chemistry profile revealed a very high glucose level of 782 mg/dL (normal range 70–110 mg/dL), along with a low total carbon dioxide concentration of 18 mmol/L (normal range 22–32 mmol/L) and an increased chloride concentration of 110 mmol/L (normal range 95–106 mmol/L). The physician subsequently requested a urinalysis, a blood lactic acid determination, and blood gas studies. The urinalysis was positive for ketones, and the blood lactic acid level was a normal 1.1 mmol/L (normal range 0.6–2.2 mmol/L). The blood gases yielded the following results:

PO_2 = 97 mm Hg
PCO_2 = 24 mm Hg
pH = 7.29
HCO_3^- = 16 mEq/L

The ER physician concluded that the patient most likely was suffering from metabolic acidosis as a result of type I diabetes. Upon consultation with the pediatric endocrinologist, the patient was admitted, and insulin administration was initiated.

Rationale for diagnosis: Diabetic ketoacidosis in children is a common cause of metabolic acidosis. The very high blood glucose levels with urine ketones and a normal blood lactate level are consistent with this diagnosis. Diabetic ketoacidosis results in large increases in ketoacid production, which, if not treated, overwhelm the buffering capacity. It is essential to administer insulin to facilitate the use of glucose by the cells. Failure to treat diabetic ketoacidosis could have fatal consequences.

Questions

1. The primary cause of metabolic acidosis is the production of organic acids at a rate exceeding that of their breakdown. Indicate possible causes of metabolic acidosis besides diabetes mellitus.
2. A patient who has been taking large doses of aspirin for a prolonged period developed symptoms of metabolic acidosis. What could be the cause of the patient's condition?

METABOLIC ALKALOSIS

Metabolic alkalosis has a number of causes:

- A decrease in hydrogen ion concentration due to decreased noncarbonic acid or increased bicarbonate ion or other conjugate base. (See Figure 4-10.)
- The excessive loss of hydrochloric acid from the stomach after sustained vomiting.
- Certain types of external fistulas and gastric suction.
- Prolonged administration of diuretics, as well as the administration of excessive alkali and therapies used to treat chronic pulmonary insufficiency.
- Excessive adrenal steroids, as in patients with Cushing's syndrome and hyperaldosteronism.

Laboratory findings in metabolic alkalosis include:

- Increases in bicarbonate ions and dissolved carbon dioxide.
- Decreases in chloride and potassium level.

Best Practice

Metabolic Alkalosis

Respiratory compensatory mechanisms in metabolic alkalosis are not clear and occur mostly by decreasing the resting tidal volume. Renal responses include decreased sodium–hydrogen ion exchange, formation of ammonia, and reabsorption of bicarbonate.

CASE STUDY 4-4

E. S., a 61-year-old female, was seen in the emergency room (ER). She was complaining of prolonged vomiting. A chemistry profile, including electrolytes, was performed. The chemistry results were essentially normal with the exception of chloride 82 mmol/L (normal range 95–106 mmol/L), potassium 3.2 mmol/L (normal range 3.5–4.5 mmol/L), and total carbon dioxide 38 mmol/L (normal range 22–32 mmol/L). The attending physician requested a blood gas determination that yielded the following results:

PO_2 = 98 mm Hg
PCO_2 = 38 mm Hg
pH = 7.46
Positive base excess

The ER physician concluded that the patient was suffering from metabolic alkalosis as the result of prolonged vomiting.

Rationale for diagnosis: Metabolic alkalosis is characterized by a decrease of chloride ion, or chloride depletion. The patient's prolonged vomiting resulted in the loss of fluid and a greater Cl^-/Na^+ ratio than is normally present in plasma. This condition caused the excessive reabsorption of HCO_3^-. Vomiting also resulted in the excessive loss of acid. Prolonged diuretic use may have further reduced the plasma potassium concentration.

Questions

1. Hyperaldosteronism causes the kidney secretion of K^+ and H^+ ions. How can hyperaldosteronism result in metabolic alkalosis?
2. Diminished levels of extracellular potassium can result in moving potassium ions from the cells into the extracellular space. How could this shift result in metabolic alkalosis?

Summary

In a living system, acids are substances that can donate electrons, and bases are substances that can receive electrons. The balance between acids and bases in body fluids, usually measured in terms of hydrogen ion concentration (pH), must be maintained for body systems to function.

Acids are categorized as strong or weak, depending on their degree of ionization. They are also further divided into bicarbonic (carbonic) and noncarbonic (fixed) acids. Fixed acids are eliminated daily by the kidneys, but carbonic acids can permeate cell membranes and affect cellular pH.

Buffers are substances that resist changes in pH when an acid or a base is added. Buffers are also divided into two broad categories: bicarbonate and nonbicarbonate. The bicarbonate–carbonic acid pair is the most important buffer in plasma. The nonbicarbonate buffering systems include the phosphate, plasma protein, and hemoglobin buffer systems. Buffers are crucial for transporting carbon dioxide to the alveoli during respiration.

The body closely regulates the acid–base balance, but several factors can disturb it. Disturbances in the balance can be categorized as acidosis or alkalosis. Each can be further categorized according to its cause: respiratory or metabolic.

The respiratory system responds immediately to a change in the acid–base status and becomes maximal in 3–6 hours. In comparison, the renal response is slow and prolonged. The renal response is important because of its ability to conserve or increase acids or bases depending on whether the patient is in acidosis or alkalosis.

Study Questions

REVIEW QUESTIONS

1. A solution contains 180 mmol/L of hydrogen ions. What is the pH of this solution?
2. What is the hydrogen ion concentration in millimoles per liter of a solution with a pH of 7.2?
3. To make 1000 mL of a 0.5-M acetate buffer solution of pH 4.6 at 25 °C from glacial acetic acid and sodium acetate, how many millimoles of each buffer pair is needed? The pk_a of acetic acid at 25 °C is 4.7.
4. If the pH of a solution is 8.0, what is the approximate concentration of the OH^-?
5. What is the HCO_3^- concentration of a plasma sample with a pH of 7.4 and a PCO_2 of 34 mm Hg? Under these conditions, the pk_a is 6.1.

MULTIPLE-CHOICE QUESTIONS

1. Respiratory acidosis may be caused by
   a. salicylate intoxication.
   b. vomiting.
   c. pulmonary obstruction.
   d. sodium bicarbonate infusion.

2. The concentration of bicarbonate in blood can be determined from the measurement of pH and PCO_2 by the relationship
   a. pH = $[HCO_3^-]/pk_a$
   b. pH = $pk_a + \log([HCO_3^-]/[PCO_2\ 3\ 0.03])$
   c. pH = PCO_2/HCO_3^-
   d. pH = PCO_2/pk_a
3. Which of the following would provide the best information to evaluate a disturbed acid–base balance?
   a. total PCO_2 capacity and total H_2CO_3
   b. pH and total carbon dioxide
   c. pH and PCO_2
   d. total H_2CO_3
4. In the tissues, most of the carbon dioxide that enters the erythrocytes is hydrated to form H_2CO_3, which dissociates to form H^+ and HCO_3^-. The H^+ thus produced is buffered by
   a. imidiazole groups of deoxygenated hemoglobin.
   b. histidine groups of carbonic anhydrase.
   c. carbamino groups of oxygenated hemoglobin.
   d. the phosphate buffer system.
5. Metabolic acidosis, with an increased concentration of acetoacetate, beta-hydroxybutyrate, may be associated with
   a. renal tubular defects.
   b. diabetes mellitus.
   c. ethanol consumption.
   d. diarrhea.
6. An increase in the plasma bicarbonate concentration without a change in the dissolved CO_2 will result in
   a. no change in the acid–base balance.
   b. metabolic alkalosis.
   c. metabolic acidosis.
   d. respiratory alkalosis.
7. Respiratory acidosis is characterized by
   a. an excess of dissolved carbon dioxide.
   b. an excess of bicarbonate.
   c. an excess of total carbon dioxide.
   d. a reduction in disolved carbon dioxide.
8. The bicarbonate ion concentration can be calculated from the PCO_2 and total carbon dioxide level using which equation?
   a. total carbon dioxide $-$ (0.03 × PCO_2)
   b. (total carbon dioxide + 0.03) × PCO_2
   c. cannot be calculated from carbon dioxide and PCO_2 values
   d. 0.03 × (PCO_2 $-$ carbon dioxide)
9. Respiratory alkalosis is characterized by
   a. a reduction in PCO_2.
   b. an increase in PCO_2.
   c. hypoventilation.
   d. an excess of dissolved carbon dioxide.
10. The Henderson–Hasselbalch equation can be used to calculate
    a. blood PCO_2 only.
    b. blood CO_2 only.
    c. pk_a of buffers only.
    d. blood PCO_2, blood CO_2, and pk_a of buffers.
11. The bicarbonate/carbonic acid ratio is calculated from the equation devised by
    a. Gilbert Lewis.
    b. Dmitry Mendeleyev.
    c. Bronsted–Lowry.
    d. Henderson–Hasselbalch
12. Maintaining a normal pH at 7.4 in plasma requires maintaining a
    a. 20:1 ratio of bicarbonate to dissolved carbon dioxide.
    b. 10:1 ratio of bicarbonate to dissolved carbon dioxide.
    c. 20:1 ratio of dissolved carbon dioxide to bicarbonate.
    d. 10:1 ratio of dissolved carbon dioxide to bicarbonate.
13. The chloride shift refers to
    a. an abnormally high concentration of plasma chloride.
    b. the shift of plasma chloride to the red blood cells.
    c. an abnormally low concentration of plasma chloride.
    d. the irreversible binding of chloride ions with the protein base.
14. The total CO_2 is defined as the sum of
    a. HCO_3^- + dissolved CO_2.
    b. HCO_3^- $-$ dissolved CO_2.
    c. PCO_2 + carbamino compounds.
    d. HCO_3^- + dissolved CO_2 + carbamino compounds.
15. Which is not a buffer system found in plasma?
    a. HPr/Prhr $^-$
    b. $H_2PO_4^-/HPO_4^{2-}$
    c. bicarbonate buffer system
    d. $HHbO_2/HbO_2^-$

CRITICAL-THINKING QUESTIONS

1. Metabolic acidosis can occur because of uncontrolled diabetes mellitus and renal failure. Identify what causes metabolic acidosis in these conditions.
2. Explain the differences among acids, bases, and buffers in a physiological environment and in a nonphysiological environment.

3. Explain how the body manages to eliminate the large quantities of carbon dioxide formed continuously without significantly changing the pH (hydrogen ion concentration).
4. Explain the different functions of the various buffer pairs in the body.
5. Using the bicarbonate buffer system, determine the pH of a plasma sample that has a PCO_2 of 50 mm Hg and a bicarbonate (HCO_3^-) concentration of 38 mmol/L. Assume that the value of the pk_a is 6.1.
6. Differentiate between respiratory and metabolic acidosis and between respiratory and metabolic alkalosis.
7. Provide specific causes for respiratory and metabolic acidosis.

References

1. Masoro EJ, Siegel PD. *Acid–Base Regulation: Its Physiology and Pathophysiology*. Philadelphia: WB Saunders Co; 1971.
2. Bronsted JN. The conception of acids and bases. *Rev Trev Chim*. 1923;42:718.
3. National Committee for Laboratory Standards. *Definitions of Quantities and Conventions Related to Blood pH and Gas Analysis: Approved Standards. C12-A*. Wayne, PA: National Committee of Laboratory Standards; 1994.
4. Heusel JW, Siggaard-Anderson O, Scott MG. Physiology and disorders of water, electrolyte, and acid–base metabolism. In: Burtis CA, Ashwood ER, eds. *Tietz Textbook of Clinical Chemistry*. 4th ed. Philadelphia: WB Saunders Co; 2005.
5. Scott MG, Heusel JW, LeGrys VA, Siggaard-Anderson O. Electrolytes and blood gases. In: Burtis CA, Ashwood ER, eds. *Tietz Textbook of Clinical Chemistry*. 4th ed. Philadelphia: WB Saunders Co; 2005.
6. Lippmann BJ. Fluid and electrolyte management. In: Edwald GA, McKenzie CR, eds. *Manual of Medical Therapeutics*. 32nd ed. New York: Little Brown & Co; 2007.
7. Dufour DR. Acid-base disorders. In: Dufour DR, Christenson RH, eds. *Professional Practice in Clinical Chemistry: A Review*. Washington, DC: AACC Press; 1999.

Suggested Readings

Bennett JC, Carpenter CJ, Andriole TE, eds. *Cecil Essential of Medicine*. 8th ed. Philadelphia: WB Saunders Co; 2010.

Brueckner PJ. Water, electrolyte, and hydrogen ion disorders. In: Gornall AG, ed. *Applied Biochemistry of Clinical Disorders*. 2nd ed. Philadelphia: JB Lippincott Company; 1986:99–128.

Dufour R. *Acid–Base Disorders and Blood Gas Analysis*. In: Clarke W, Dufour DR, eds. *Contemporary Practice in Clinical Chemistry*. Washington DC: AACC Press 2006:309–318.

Fall PJ. A stepwise approach to acid-base disorders. Practical patient evaluation for metabolic acidosis and other conditions. *Postgraduate Med*. 2000; 107–258.

Scott MG, Heusel JW, LeGrys VA, Siggaard-Anderson O. Electrolytes and blood gases. In: Burtis CA, Aswood ER, eds. *Tietz Textbook of Clinical Chemistry*. 3rd ed. Philadelphia: W.B. Saunders Co; 1999:1056–1092.

Siggaard-Anderson O. *The Acid–Base Status of Blood*. 4th ed. Copenhagen: Munsgaard; Baltimore: Williams & Wilkins; 1974.

Woolf CR. Respiratory disorders. In: Gornall AG, ed. *Applied Biochemistry of Clinical Disorders*. 2nd ed. Philadelphia: JB Lippincott Co; 1986:129–138.

CHAPTER 5

Applied Microbiology

Janet Hudzicki and Stephen F. Wehrman

OBJECTIVES

Upon completion of this chapter, the reader should be able to:

- List the characteristics used to classify microorganisms.
- Describe disinfection and sterilization methods.
- Identify the beneficial roles of endogenous microflora.
- Describe the factors influencing bacterial growth.
- Identify human defenses against infectious diseases.
- Discuss infectious diseases of the respiratory system.

CHAPTER OUTLINE

KEY TERMS

antigen
antiseptic
bacteria
disinfectant
disinfection
endemic
endogenous
epidemic
fomite
fungi
nosocomial infection
opportunistic
pandemic
pathogen
pathogenicity
resistant
sterilization
vector
virulence
virus

Respiratory therapists frequently work with patients with lung infections. Pneumonia, tuberculosis, AIDS, secretion management, and ventilator care are just a few of the situations in which they are called on to apply their knowledge of microbiology and infection control. In addition, between 5% and 10% of all patients who enter a hospital acquire an infection during their stays. Up to 40% of these hospital-acquired infections (formerly known as **nosocomial infections**) involve the respiratory system.

This chapter reviews how microorganisms are classified and explains the relationship between these organisms and health or disease. Methods for preventing and treating infection, including the proper cleaning and disposal of equipment, maintaining host defenses, and pharmacologic and therapeutic interventions, are presented. A strong foundation in microbiology will provide you with the skills needed to protect yourself and your patients.

Classification of Microorganisms

Taxonomy, or the science of classifying living things, recognizes five kingdoms: Plantae (plants), Animalia (animals), Myceteae (**fungi**), Protista (microscopic algae and protozoans), and Prokaryotae (bacteria). Each kingdom is subdivided into phyla, which are further divided into classes, orders, families, and finally genera and species. To identify the species, each organism is given two names: the genus name and the species name, usually a descriptive adjective or noun. Human beings, for example, are known as *Homo* (genus name) *sapiens* (species name); the bacterium that causes syphilis is *Treponema pallidum*.

Viruses are not included in the five-kingdom classification scheme. They are noncellular particles that do not exhibit most of the life processes of cells and that are unable to function independently of a host cell. They basically consist of a protein capsid (outer shell) and nucleic acid.

Bacteria make up the kingdom known as Prokaryotae. An important characteristic that distinguishes prokaryotes from other microorganisms is their lack of a nuclear membrane and organelles such as mitochrondria. In other words, they are very simple organisms. Scientists have described about 3000 species of bacteria, but this number probably represents less than 1% of the total types of bacteria. Bacteria are classified and identified according to nine characteristics: morphology, staining, motility, atmospheric requirements, nutritional requirements, metabolic activities, pathogenicity, growth, and genetic composition.

The sizes, shapes, and cell arrangements (morphology) of bacteria are easily observed under an ordinary light microscope. The three basic shapes are *cocci* (spherical), *bacilli* (rod-shaped), and *spirochete* and *spirillum* (curved or spiral-shaped). *Treponema pallidum* is spiral shaped. A short, plump, gently curved rod is a *Vibrio*. In addition to shape, the arrangement of bacilli may help with identification. For example, *Streptococci* are round bacteria arranged in chainlike groups. *Staphylococci* occur in clusters. *Corynebacterium diphtheriae* cells stack up next to each other like a fence or palisade. Figure 5-1 illustrates these shapes.

Staining Methods

Various staining methods are used to identify organisms.

GRAM STAIN

The *Gram stain* uses crystal violet (purple) as the primary stain and safranin (pink) as the counterstain.

> *Best Practice*
>
> **Scientific Nomenclature**
>
> The genus name is always capitalized, and the species name is always lowercased. Both are always in italics: for example, *Corynebacterium* [genus] *diphtheriae* [species].

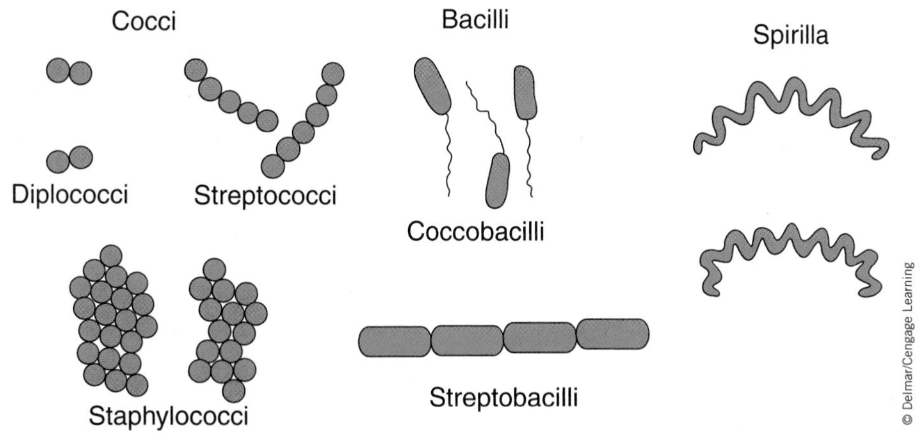

FIGURE 5-1 Various shapes of bacteria.

Figure 5-2 illustrates the Gram stain procedure. Organisms that retain the primary stain throughout the fixing, decolorizing, and counterstaining steps are considered gram-positive (purple). *Streptococcus pneumoniae* is a gram-positive organism that is seen in pulmonary infections. Bacteria that do not retain the primary stain are identified as gram-negative (pink). *Klebsiella pneumoniae, Pseudomonas aeruginosa,* and *Legionella pneumophila* are gram-negative pulmonary **pathogens**, or disease-producing organisms.

ACID-FAST STAIN

To identify bacteria that do not consistently take up the dyes used in the Gram stain, the *acid-fast stain* is another technique that may be useful. The genus

STEP	TIME	PROCEDURE	RESULT
1	one minute	Primary stain: Apply crystal violet stain (purple) ↓ Rinse slide	All bacteria stain purple
2	one minute	Mordant: Apply Gram's iodine ↓ Rinse slide	All bacteria remain purple
3	three to five seconds	Decolorize: Apply alcohol ↓ Rinse slide	Purple stain is removed from Gram-negative cells
4	one minute	Counterstain: Apply safranin stain (red) ↓ Rinse slide	Gram-negative cells appear pink-red; Gram-positive cells appear purple

FIGURE 5-2 Steps in the Gram stain procedure.

Mycobacterium, whose members cause tuberculosis and Hansen's disease (leprosy), are commonly identified by this method.

SPECIALIZED TESTS

Many specialized tests are used to identify specific organisms. *Fluorescent antibody techniques* can be used to detect pathogenic organisms directly in a patient's specimen. The dye-antibody complex will adhere to the organism in the specimen and can be viewed under an ultraviolet microscope. This test is often used to make a positive identification of *Legionella pneumophila*, *Bordetella pertussis*, rabies virus, and many other pathogens. Fluorescent techniques can also be used to detect antibodies in the patient's serum.

ELISA

Enzyme-linked immunosorbent assays (*ELISA*) are sensitive immunochemical techniques that use an enzyme-antibody-antigen combination placed in a test well. When a substrate for the enzyme is added, a color change develops if the antibodies or antigens are present.

Specimen Collection

Respiratory therapists are often called on to collect and handle sputum specimens that are to be examined for the presence of microorganisms. Proper techniques are essential to obtaining valid results. General guidelines should be followed for all specimen collection:

- Specimens should be collected in a sterile manner.
- Specimens should be collected before antimicrobial therapy is started.
- Specimens should be protected from heat and cold and delivered promptly to the laboratory.
- Specimens should be properly sealed in a plastic bag to avoid exposing other health care practitioners.
- Containers must be properly labeled to identify the patient, time of collection, date, source of specimen, and requested tests.
- Specimen collection should be performed with care and tact to avoid harming the patient or causing undue discomfort or embarrassment.

SUCTIONING

Specimens are obtained via suctioning with a sputum or Luken's trap. The technique is simple but requires the same safety precautions for the patient and practitioner as standard suctioning procedures.

Best Practice

Sputum Collection

Sputum may be obtained by allowing the patient to spit the coughed-up material into a wide-mouthed sterile bottle, by suctioning the airway, or via bronchoscopy. A possible problem with expectorated sputum is oral contamination of the sputum with saliva containing epithelial cells. The laboratory personnel will discard a specimen containing numerous epithelial cells. Directing the patient to remove dentures and to thoroughly rinse or gargle with water before trying to produce the specimen may reduce oral contamination. Special attention to safety should be given when collecting specimens for suspected tuberculosis.

BRONCHOSCOPY

Bronchoscopy is the best method for collecting specimens directly from the lung. Unfortunately, it is also the most expensive and invasive collection technique. It should be reserved for obtaining anaerobic specimens for:

- Cytology (the study of cells, such as for the diagnosis of cancer).
- Diagnosis of *Pneumocystis jiroveci* (also known as *Pneumocystis carinii*) pneumonia.
- Bacterial, fungal, and viral pathogens when simpler methods have failed.

The collected specimen is processed in the laboratory. The Gram stain technique is the usual first step in evaluating sputum. The Gram stain reaction (positive or negative), the shape of the bacteria present (rod, sphere, spiral, or curved), groupings (pairs, chains, or clusters), and the presence of spores are all noted. This information helps provide a presumptive diagnosis. For example, a patient may present with a cough, fever, and abnormal chest radiography typical of pneumonia. Analysis of the sputum reveals gram-positive diplococci. These findings are typical of *Streptococcus pneumoniae*, a common organism responsible for community-acquired pneumonia. On the basis of this information, the physician can initiate a course of antimicrobials appropriate to the organism and site of infection.

Culturing

Simple biochemical tests may be performed to further identify the genus and species of the organism. A definite diagnosis is made only after the organism has been *cultured*, or grown, on a special medium. The surface of an agar plate is inoculated with the pathogen, which is allowed to reproduce. Culturing may take several days or longer, depending on the type of organism.

Once the culture has grown, *sensitivity* (or *antimicrobial susceptibility*) *testing* is performed. Small paper disks are impregnated with various antimicrobials and placed on the culture to test whether the organism is susceptible or resistant to the battery of antimicrobials. Susceptibility testing is very important when dealing with organisms that have become **resistant** (i.e., that do not respond) to standard antimicrobials. The process of making a definitive identification of the organism and conducting susceptibility testing may take several days.

Human-Microbe Interactions

Microorganisms that are found in or on the body of normal individuals are referred to as **endogenous** microflora (also called *normal*, or *resident, flora*). These microorganisms include bacteria, fungi, viruses, and protozoa. After birth, both harmless and helpful organisms take up residence on the skin, in body openings, on mucus membranes, and in the gastrointestinal and genitourinary tracts. Microorganisms that are not normally found in or on the body are called *exogenous* or *transient flora*.

MUCUS MEMBRANES

The mucus membranes provide a warm, moist environment that is particularly suitable for the growth of organisms. In contrast, blood, lymph, spinal fluid, and most internal organs, including the lungs, are normally free of microorganisms. In addition to normal resident organisms, transient microflora may take up temporary residence in the body or on the body surface. These microbes are usually temporary for many reasons: They may be washed away during bathing; they may be unable to compete with resident organisms and fail to survive; or they may be flushed out by secretions.

NORMAL FLORA

When the number of normal resident organisms is reduced, such as by the administration of broad-spectrum antimicrobials, the delicate balance of resident flora organisms may be disrupted, allowing a normally nonpathogenic organism to cause an **opportunistic** infection. Opportunists are microbes with the potential to cause disease when the physiological state of the host is altered. *Candida albicans*, a yeast that lives near many body orifices, is a good example. This opportunistic organism may become pathogenic if competing flora are eliminated by antimicrobials or if the immune response of the host is impaired by HIV infection. Normal flora may also result in an infection if they migrate to a normally sterile organ system.

Humans benefit from their relationship with normal flora. For example, nutrients such as vitamins K, B_{12}, and pantothenic acid are obtained from the secretions of the coliform bacteria. These resident organisms also appear to stimulate the immune system, producing a more rapid, powerful response to foreign invaders. Resident microorganisms also compete with invading organisms for nutrients, thereby reducing the likelihood of harmful infection by the invaders.

Human Defense Mechanisms

Normal, healthy individuals have specific and general defenses that constantly safeguard against microbial infection; the disruption or derangement of these protective systems allows pathogens to gain a foothold for infectious disease. Our immune system defenses consist of two major arms: the innate and the adaptive arms.

- The *innate arm* includes our mechanical barriers (skin, mucus membranes), specific chemical compounds (complement, proteins that assist in the destruction of foreign particles), and the cells involved in phagocytosis (engulfing of foreign bodies).
- The *adaptive arm* has two branches: the cell-mediated and the humoral.

  The *cell-mediated branch* is made up of the responses by different types of white blood cells toward organisms that have invaded human tissues or that have been phagocytized by white blood cells.

  The *humoral branch* is responsible for the production of soluble antibodies, which includes the short-lived IgM class of antibodies and the long-lived IgG antibodies. Antibodies are formed in response to the presence of **antigens** (substances such as pollen and bacteria). Although described as separate parts of the immune system, the humoral and cell-mediated systems are intricately connected in the fight against infectious disease.

MUCUS MEMBRANES

The orifices of the body are lined with mucus membranes that are designed to entrap invaders. Because the respiratory system is constantly exposed to inhaled particles, it has a number of defensive mechanisms.

The hairs, mucus membranes, and irregular shape of the nose trap most of the inhaled debris. Mucus lining the pharynx and large airways traps particles so that the cilia can sweep them up and out of the system. Reflexes such as sneezing and coughing also assist in clearing particles. Microflora, phagocytic white blood cells, and enzymes in secretions add to the general protective functions.

CELL-MEDIATED RESPONSES

Cell-mediated responses involve cellular and chemical reactions to microbial invasion:

- Fever production.
- Cellular secretions (interferon, prostaglandins, interleukins) (Prostaglandins are hormone-like substances that have varied effects on organs and tissues. They derive from natural fatty acids in the body, reducing swelling and inflammation, increasing or decreasing blood flow depending on type.)
- Activation of blood proteins (complement), phagocytosis, neutralization of toxins, and the inflammatory response.

The fever that an ill person develops, for example, stimulates the white blood cells to increase their response. The reduction of free iron in the plasma helps to limit the production of bacterial toxins. Fever itself raises the body temperature above the preferred range of many bacterial strains, causing them to die off.

A variety of cellular secretions are increased during infection.

- *Interferons* are small particles of protein that enter cells and interfere with the protein synthesis necessary for the reproduction of pathogenetic viruses and bacteria. In the laboratory setting, human interferons are now being produced by bacteria containing recombinant DNA. This manufactured interferon is being used experimentally to treat viral infections, cancers, and immunodeficiency diseases.
- *Interleukins* are also secreted during infections; they serve to enhance the activation of T-lymphocytes during the immune response.

Phagocytosis is a process by which certain white blood cells surround and ingest foreign materials (Figure 5-3). *Neutrophils* are the most common and efficient phagocytes. *Eosinophils* play an important phagocytic role in allergic responses. *Macrophages* wander through the bloodstream and are attracted toward sites of infection.

Inflammation is a complex series of events triggered by irritation, injury, or microbial invasion. The inflammatory response occurs as the body attempts to localize infection and prevent the spread of microbes or toxins. Physiological reactions at the site of the inflammatory response are edema, redness, heat, pain, and often pus formation. The inflammatory response starts with some type of injury. Injured cells (mast cells, basophils, platelets) release powerful chemicals (histamine, heparin, bradykinin) that increase capillary permeability, allowing blood and cells to enter the affected area. Macrophages are attracted to the site. Fluid and cells may accumulate to form an exudate. As the exudate becomes filled with dead leukocytes and bacteria, it becomes thick and appears yellow or green; it is then referred to as pus. Figure 5-4 illustrates various cells of the immune system.

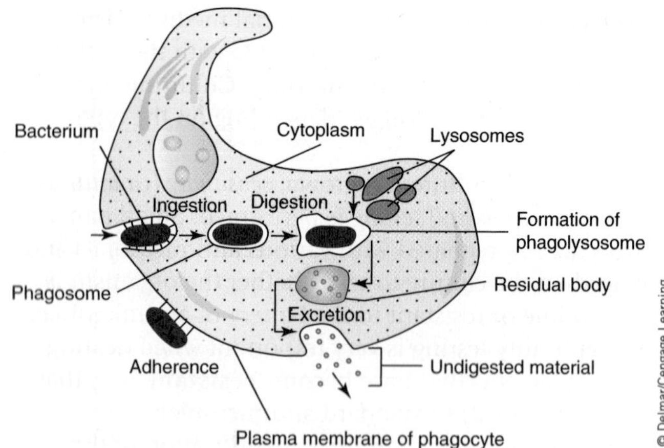

FIGURE 5-3 The phagocytic process.

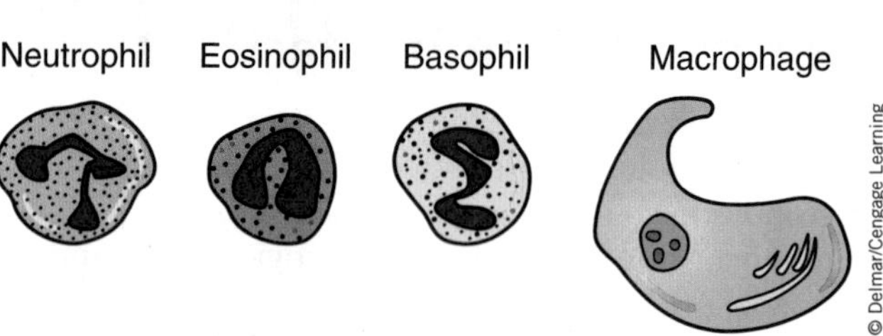

FIGURE 5-4 Cells of the immune system.

THE HUMORAL IMMUNE RESPONSE

The humoral immune response is the third line of defense against pathogens. Unlike our other body defenses, this response is usually specific in nature. Lymphocytes produce antibodies that recognize, attach to, inactivate, and destroy particular antigens. Antibodies are found circulating throughout the blood, lymph, and body secretions.

Immunity may be acquired naturally; for example, when you are initially exposed to a disease-producing organism, antibodies are produced that protect you in the event of re-exposure. Immunity may also be

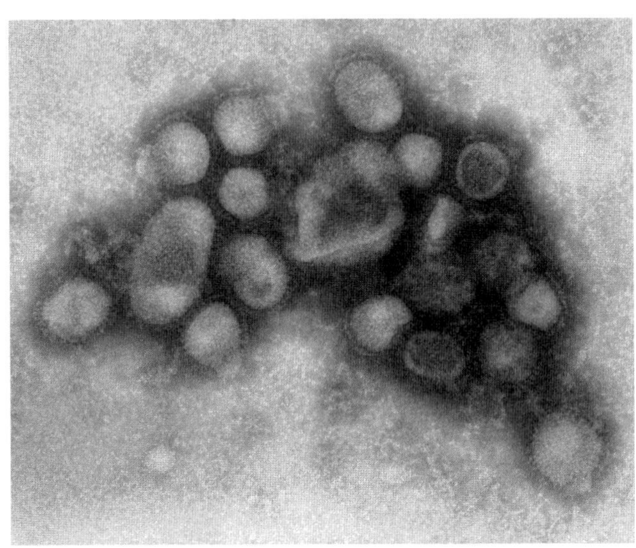

FIGURE 5-5 A negative-stained transmission electron micrograph (TEM) showing the morphology of the swine flu virus.

Courtesy of the Centers for Disease Control Public Health Image Library/ C. S. Goldsmith and A. Balish

acquired artificially through the administration of vaccines. *Vaccines* are made from living or killed pathogens or their toxins, and they play an important role in public health medicine, specifically in the prevention of serious illness. An important vaccine that benefits respiratory therapists, the elderly, and patients with chronic lung disease is the annual vaccine that is active against the A and B strains of the influenza virus (Figure 5-5). Vaccination against the hepatitis B virus is recommended for all health care workers who may be exposed to blood or body fluids in the course of their work. Vaccination against pneumococcal pneumonia is recommended for individuals over the age of 65 and for those with a chronic illness such as congestive heart failure, lung disease, or any condition associated with impaired immunity. The Centers for Disease Control and Prevention (CDC) recommends a wide variety of vaccines for all children before entering school: diphtheria, pertussis, polio, tetanus, mumps, hepatitis, and rubella. Although new vaccines are constantly being developed, there has been little success as yet in developing a vaccine for the common cold because the infection is caused by a large variety of viruses.

Antibodies. *Antibodies* belong to a class of proteins known as immunoglobulins (abbreviated Ig), a group of glycoproteins that participate in the immune response. They are called antibodies because they are generated in response to specific antigens. Five classes of immunoglobulin are identified (Table 5-1).

Immunoglobulin E is of special interest to respiratory therapists because it is most abundant in people with allergies and allergic forms of asthma. It is responsible for the immediate hypersensitivity seen with skin testing and for the shock reaction of anaphylaxis. The allergic reaction occurs when IgE antibodies, bound to basophils in the blood or mast cells in tissue, react to the presence of the allergen. The mast cells respond by releasing powerful chemical mediators such as histamine, prostaglandins, and leukotrienes. In asthma, the release of these mediators results in bronchospasm and airway edema.

B Cells and T Cells. B cells and T cells are other important cells of the immune system. *T cells* (named for the thymus gland) aid in the control of antibody production and are involved in cell-mediated responses. An HIV infection gradually destroys a specific type of T cell, eventually resulting in a deficient immune system. *B cells* (named for bursa) migrate to lymphoid tissue where they are responsible for the production of antibodies.

TABLE 5-1 **Classes and characteristics of immunoglobulins**

Ig Class	Percentage in Serum	Functions/Sites
IgA	10–15	Protects the mucus membranes; found in tears, saliva, and other secretions
IgD	0.2	Controls stimulation of B cells; found in blood and on lymphocytes
IgE	0.002	Causes allergic responses such as immediate hypersensitivity and anaphylaxis; high proportion in secretions
IgG	80	Secondary immune response; long-lived antibodies provide protection upon re-exposure to the pathogen; major systemic immunoglobulin; produces antimicrobial antibodies; found in extracellular fluids and blood
IgM	5–10	Primary immune response; short-lived; indicates an acute infectious process; produces antimicrobial and blood group (ABO) antibodies; bactericidal to gram-negative bacteria; found in lymph, blood, and extracellular fluid

Control of Microbial Growth

Important environmental factors that may affect the growth of microorganisms are moisture, pH, temperature, gases, and the presence of neighboring organisms. Virtually all organisms require water to survive. Since the human body contains a high proportion of water, the inadequacy or failure of immune mechanisms facilitates the growth of organisms. Although microbes can grow throughout a wide range of pH, most of the medically important pathogens grow best at a pH around 7.0, similar to that of the human body. The same is true of temperature. Both pathogens and normal flora tend to thrive at body temperatures.

The gaseous environment is so specific and important for the survival and growth of organisms that special terms are used to designate these requirements. Species that require oxygen are called *obligate aerobes*. Those that cannot survive in the presence of oxygen are known as *obligate anaerobes*. Gas gangrene, caused by infection with the obligate anaerobe *Clostridium perfringens,* may be treated by placing the patient in a hyperbaric chamber to increase the amount of oxygen to a level that kills the organisms. Bacteria that can adapt and live with or without oxygen are called *facultative organisms*.

Best Practice

Pasteurization

Pasteurization is used by many respiratory care departments for the disinfection of equipment. It is an efficient, cost-effective method that destroys most organisms except for spores. Although spore-formers such as *Clostridium* species are pathogenic to humans, they are obligate anaerobes and not found as contaminants of respiratory care equipment. The inability of pasteurization to kill spores is therefore of minor concern in respiratory care departments. In the batch process of pasteurization, equipment is immersed for 30 minutes in a water bath at 63°C. Aseptic techniques must be carefully followed to avoid recontamination of equipment during drying and packaging.

Sterilization and Disinfection

A variety of physical and chemical methods are used to achieve disinfection or sterilization of equipment in the hospital and home settings. **Disinfection** is the inhibition or destruction of pathogens; **sterilization**, or asepsis, is the complete absence or destruction of all microorganisms.

PHYSICAL METHODS

The five physical methods of sterilization and disinfection involve heat, pressure, radiation, sonic disruption, and filtration. Because heat is both efficient and inexpensive, it is commonly used for disinfection and sterilization. Boiling for a period of 10–30 minutes works well as a disinfection technique; however, some organisms, such as hepatitis viruses and spore-formers such as the *Clostridium*, are relatively resistant.

Autoclaving. An *autoclave* is a metal pressure cooker that uses steam under pressure to achieve sterilization. Steam at a pressure of 15 psi (pounds per square inch) and at 121 °C kills organisms on properly prepared and packaged equipment in about 20 minutes. Before autoclaving, equipment must be correctly processed by careful washing to remove debris. An indicator tape that is used to seal each package changes color when conditions for sterilization have been met. However, tape color change does not necessarily mean that an item is actually sterile if it was not properly prepared for autoclaving. Autoclaves should also be tested periodically, usually weekly, with biological indicators such as cultures of *Geobacillus* (formerly *Bacillus*) *stearothermophilus* to ensure proper functioning. This method of sterilization works well for many metal and glass items, but it is not acceptable for rubber, plastics, and equipment that would be damaged by high temperatures.

Dry Heat. *Dry heat* can be used to sterilize materials that do not tolerate moisture, such as powders and oils. Incineration, or burning, is a very effective way to destroy contaminated disposable items. Although it is important to know that refrigeration and freezing may slow the growth of bacteria, these processes do not kill all organisms.

Radiation. *Radiation* is another method used to kill microorganisms.

- *Ultraviolet (UV) rays* are useful in killing airborne and surface bacteria. Ultraviolet lamps help reduce the number of bacteria in the air, and so these lamps may be found in nurseries, operating rooms, and isolation rooms. *Caution:* Prolonged, direct exposure to UV light is harmful to skin and eyes, and it must be avoided.
- *X-rays* and *gamma rays* in certain wavelengths are also useful in disinfection and sterilization. Produced in special facilities, radiation is used to prevent food spoilage and to sterilize

heat-sensitive equipment. Plastic articles such as endotracheal tubes, tubing, and syringes may be sterilized with gamma radiation because it penetrates the prepackaged materials.

- In many areas of the world, food—including meats, milk, and milk products—and consumables are sterilized by *irradiation*. The method is so effective that refrigeration is not necessary for these products.

Ultrasonic Waves. *Ultrasonic waves* are useful for disinfecting delicate equipment. High-frequency sound waves, passed through a water bath, mechanically dislodge organic debris from instruments and glassware. The equipment is then usually sterilized by another method.

Filtration. *Filters* have long been used to separate bacteria and liquids.

- Filter masks can be worn to prevent the passage of microbes from the patient and to protect health care workers from inhaling bacteria, but they must fit very tightly for adequate protection. Unfortunately, most filters do not prevent the passage of viruses.
- *High-efficiency particulate air (HEPA) filters* are used in negative-pressure clinical devices, biological safety cabinets, and laminar flow hoods to protect health care workers from contamination.
- Powered, air-purifying respirators may be used to provide additional protection to practitioners in certain situations.

CHEMICAL METHODS

Chemical methods are commonly used for both disinfection and sterilization (Table 5-2). The effectiveness of chemical agents depends on many factors: the concentration of the agent; the duration of exposure; the temperature; and the presence of blood, mucus, pus, or other debris. Most chemical agents are too harsh to use directly on human tissue. An **antiseptic** is a solution that can be used on the skin and that is commonly used to reduce the number of organisms present on the skin.

Alcohols and Hydrogen Peroxide. *Alcohols* (ethyl and isopropyl) are good skin antiseptics. *Ethyl alcohol* is the most effective in a 70% solution; *isopropyl alcohol* should be used in a 90% solution. Alcohols are commonly used to disinfect stethoscopes, oximeter probes, and the surfaces of some respiratory care equipment. *Hydrogen peroxide* is another useful skin disinfectant. Respiratory care personnel use hydrogen peroxide for the stoma sites during tracheostomy care.

Disinfectants. Disinfectants are chemical agents that are used to clean the surfaces of equipment and countertops and that are too harsh to use on skin. *Phenols*, such as Lysol, are good examples of chemical disinfectants. Phenols are effective even in the presence of organic material, but they may not kill all viruses. A weak solution of *sodium hypochlorite* (bleach, 1:10 solution) has also been advocated for disinfecting areas where blood has been spilled. Equipment or surface areas must be cleaned before hypochlorite disinfection because the presence of organic matter will inactivate the solution. Also, bleach solutions can be corrosive and must be used carefully to avoid harm to personnel or equipment.

Ethylene Oxide and Glutaraldehydes. Two chemical agents that are often used to sterilize respiratory care equipment in the hospital setting are ethylene oxide (ETO) and glutaraldehydes.

Ethylene oxide is a highly penetrating toxic gas. Ethylene oxide sterilization chambers are carefully controlled for temperature (50–56°C) and humidity (30–70%) to ensure optimum conditions for sterilization. The gas mixture contains 1000 mg ETO/L, with a

TABLE 5-2 **Characteristics of chemical agents of sterilization and disinfection**

Agent	Mode of Action	Advantages	Disadvantages
Alcohols	Denature proteins	Easy to use, not toxic	Concentration is important; not effective against spores
Ethylene oxide (ETO) gas	Lethally disrupt cell metabolism	Can be used for items sensitive to heat	Requires safety precautions; carcinogenic and explosive
Glutaraldehydes	Attack lipoproteins in bacteria cell membrane and cytoplasm	Will kill all living material (sterilizing agent)	Toxic effect on human mucus membranes and eyes
Phenolic compounds	Coagulate proteins, lyse cells	Powerful bactericide at proper concentrations	Toxic, strong odor

Best Practice

Ethylene Oxide Sterilization

Once the sterilization process has been completed, items must be aerated sufficiently to ensure that all ETO is removed from them. Aeration times vary according to the composition of the sterilized items and the method and temperature of the mechanical aeration chamber. An IPPB machine used for the treatment of a patient with active tuberculosis is an example of respiratory care equipment that should be gas sterilized.

balance of carbon dioxide and nitrogen or other inert gas to decrease flammability.

Items are placed in the ETO chamber. They must be dry to prevent the formation of toxic ethylene glycol and packaged in a moisture-permeable package. Special indicator tape is used to seal the package. As in autoclaving, the indicator tape changes color when the proper conditions are met. The effectiveness of the sterilization process should also be checked with indicator strips containing *Bacillus subtilis* organisms.

Glutaraldehydes are liquid sterilizing agents commonly used in health care and by respiratory care departments. Bronchoscopes, resuscitation equipment, tubing, circuits, masks, and many other equipment items can be sterilized by this method. Glutaraldehydes are available in alkaline and acidic forms. Cidex is an example of an alkaline product; Sonicide is an acidic solution.

- *Alkaline glutaraldehydes* kill viruses, bacteria, and *Mycobacterium* species in about 10 minutes, spores in 10 hours. The alkaline solution remains active for approximately 2 weeks.
- *Acid glutaraldehydes* are bactericidal in 20 minutes, but they can be ready in about 5 minutes if the solution is heated to 60°C. Spores may be killed in 1 hour with the heated solution. Acid glutaraldehyde is considered effective for 28 days.

Glutaraldehydes are now available for home use and are recommended by the American Association for Respiratory Care for the disinfection of respiratory care equipment in the home. Thoroughly washed home equipment can also be disinfected by soaking it for 30 minutes in a white vinegar solution (1:3 dilution). This method is simpler but may not kill all organisms.

Several factors must be considered when using liquid sterilizing agents.

- Equipment must be washed carefully with soap (or detergent) and water to remove proteinaceous material such as mucus or blood.

Best Practice

Disinfection in the Home

When teaching families or caregivers to disinfect respiratory care equipment in the home setting, consider cost, infection risk, the skills of caregivers, and safety.

- The equipment must then be rinsed well and excess water drained to avoid diluting the glutaraldehyde solution.
- Glutaraldehyde is toxic to human tissue; so gloves and eye protection should be worn during equipment processing.
- After the equipment has been soaked in the glutaraldehyde solution for the proper length of time, it must be rinsed well to remove all of the chemical solution.
- Finally, the equipment must be air-dried, reassembled, and packaged under sterile, or at least aseptic, conditions.

Antimicrobials

Despite careful disinfection and sterilization procedures, some patients become infected with microorganisms. A wide variety of chemotherapeutic agents, known as *antimicrobials*, are used to treat infections. The goal of antimicrobial chemotherapeutics is to selectively kill the desired organism without seriously harming the human host.

HISTORY

The era of modern chemotherapy began in 1909, when Paul Ehrlich developed an arsenic compound for the treatment of syphilis. In 1928, Alexander Fleming found that a substance produced by the mold *Penicillium notatum* inhibited the growth of *Staphylococcus* in the laboratory (Figure 5-6). In 1935, Gerhard Domagk discovered a red dye that killed *Streptococcus* in mice. Further research showed that the dye was broken down in the body into the active agent sulfanilamide.

During World War II, Sir Howard Florey and Ernst Chain purified penicillin for use on humans. By 1942, the U.S. drug industry was producing penicillin in sufficient quantities for public use. However, not until after World War II did medicine begin to build an arsenal of drugs that would effectively treat infections, a technique that we now take for granted. Anti-infective drugs are usually called *antibiotics*, although this term

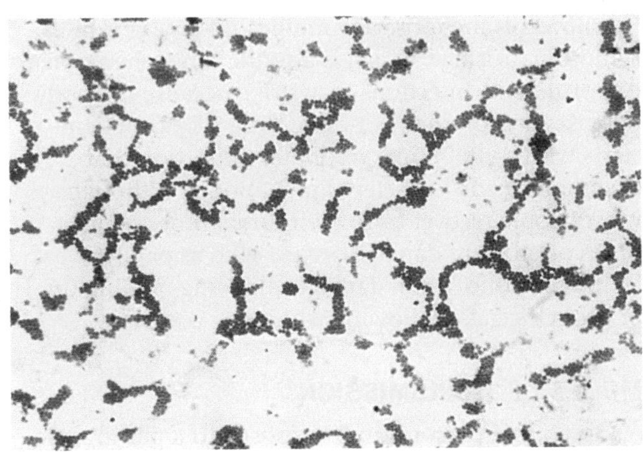

FIGURE 5-6 Gram stain of staphylococci.

Courtesy of the Centers for Disease Control Public Health Image Library/ Dr. Richard Facklam

TABLE 5-3 **Methods of antimicrobial action of selected agents**

Method	Examples
Inhibition of cell wall synthesis	Penicillins, cephalosporins
Disruption of cell membrane	Amphotericin B, nystatin
Inhibition of nucleic acid synthesis	Ciprofloxacin, rifampin, pentamidine, zidovudine (AZT)
Inhibition of protein synthesis	Erythromycin, tetracycline
Inhibition of metabolism	Sulfonamides, ribavirin

specifically refers to substances produced by microorganisms to kill other microorganisms.

MECHANISMS

Most antimicrobial drugs work by disrupting the structure or metabolism of the pathogen in a way that does not affect human cells. Sulfonamides, for example, kill bacteria because they are shaped like the molecule of para-aminobenzoic acid (PABA). Bacteria convert PABA into folic acid, which is needed to produce essential proteins. The attempt by bacteria to convert the sulfonamide into PABA fails, resulting in their death. Humans are not harmed by the drug because we must obtain our folic acid from food and are not able to synthesize it. Penicillin, on the other hand, interferes with the synthesis of peptidoglycans (chains of sugar and peptide) that make up the bacterial cell wall. The bacterial cell is unable to generate a wall and dies. Because human cells do not have walls, penicillin does not damage them.

RESISTANCE

Frequently, a single antimicrobial drug is not adequate to kill all the pathogens. In cases of tuberculosis, for example, three or more drugs are used in combination. The problem of drug-resistant bacteria, or so-called superbugs, has become important in the treatment of infectious disease. These organisms have mutated so that either the antimicrobials that were once able to destroy them are no longer effective or larger and more toxic doses must be given to kill the bacteria. (For ways that superbugs emerge and spread, see Chapter 38.)

Methicillin-resistant Staphylococcus aureus (*MRSA*), the causative agent of toxic shock syndrome, food poisoning, and other diseases, is a resistant organism frequently encountered in the health care setting. Vancomycin, a very expensive and toxic antimicrobial, must be used to treat MRSA. Because vancomycin is now used frequently, there is great concern that the *Staphylococcus* species will become resistant. Of the many theories as to why drug-resistant organisms are increasing so rapidly, the overuse of antimicrobials and their misuse by patients are commonly cited ones.

CLASSIFICATION

Antimicrobial agents can be classified by how they kill bacteria. Table 5-3 shows five general methods of antimicrobial action, with accompanying examples. For the ways in which microbes overcome these methods, see Chapter 38.

Antituberculosis Agents. Tuberculosis, caused by the bacterium *Mycobacterium tuberculosis*, is one of the most prevalent and important infectious diseases. Worldwide, millions of new cases and millions of deaths are reported each year. One problem in the control of tuberculosis is the development of drug-resistant bacteria. Outbreaks of *multi-drug-resistant tuberculosis* (*MDR-TB*) have been reported in most of the states. The most common drugs used to fight tuberculosis are ethambutol, isoniazid, pyrazinamide, rifampin, and streptomycin.

Antifungal and Antiprotozoan Agents. Fungal and protozoan pathogens are more difficult to eradicate than are bacteria because, unlike bacteria, fungi and protozoans are *eukaryotic* (i.e., they have a defined nucleus and organelles). Drugs that are used against these organisms are more toxic to human cells than are drugs used to kill bacteria. Amphotericin B and nystatin are examples of antifungal agents. Pentamidine is an antiprotozoan agent used to prevent and treat *Pneumocystis jiroveci* pneumonia (PCP) in HIV-infected or immunodeficient patients.

Antiviral Agents. Effective antiviral drugs are difficult to create because viruses replicate inside host cells. Acyclovir is used against herpes. Zidovudine (AZT) is one of several agents developed to slow the progression of HIV infection. Ribavirin was developed for treatment of respiratory syncytial virus (RSV) infections in fragile infants. Its effectiveness is now being questioned, and the use of RSV-immune globulin (RespiGam) or palivizumab (Synagis) monoclonal antibody prophylaxis is recommended.

Microbial Pathogenicity

An *infection* occurs when a pathogenic microbe is able to invade tissues in the body and multiply. **Pathogenicity** is the ability of an organism to cause disease. The relative ability of a pathogen to invade, infect, and cause damage or disease is called **virulence**. In other words, virulence is the strength of pathogenicity. Some pathogens are more virulent than others and thus are more likely to result in infection and disease. Infections that can be transmitted from one person to another, such as *Varicella* (chickenpox) or HIV, are called *communicable diseases*. Communicable diseases that are easily transmitted from person to person, such as colds or influenza, are called *contagious diseases*.

Infection occurs when pathogens are able to enter the host, attach, multiply, and cause damage to the tissues. *Clinical disease* occurs when the body's primary defenses lose the battle with a pathogen. The disease may be a local infection, such as a boil, strep throat, or tuberculosis. If the organism is not stopped at the local level, a systemic infection may develop as the pathogen is spread throughout the bloodstream.

DISEASE TYPES AND STAGES

An *acute* disease has a rapid onset and usually a rapid recovery. Influenza and measles are good examples. A *chronic* disease has a slow onset and a long duration. Tuberculosis and Hansen's disease (leprosy) are examples of chronic infectious diseases.

Once a person has been exposed to a pathogen, the course of an infectious disease progresses through four stages:

- An incubation period with no symptoms
- A prodromal, or preacute, phase in which the person feels unwell but has no symptoms
- Acute illness with symptoms
- Recovery, disability, or death

Illness is the most communicable to others in the symptomatic stage, which is also the time when other, opportunistic, infections may strike because the body defenses are lowered. For example, a COPD patient starts with a viral upper respiratory infection that eventually leads to bacterial pneumonia. Although most people recover from their initial illness, sometimes permanent damage occurs, such as paralysis following polio, brain damage following meningitis, or bronchiectasis following whooping cough.

MODES OF TRANSMISSION

A susceptible person can be exposed to a pathogenic organism by means of seven primary modes of transmission:

- Person-to-person contact via the skin
- Direct mucus membrane contact such as kissing or sexual intercourse
- Airborne droplets of liquid or dust that contact the skin, eyes, or lungs
- Contamination of food or water by fecal material, soil, or other impurities
- Blood contamination from injections, transfusions, or invasive medical devices
- Contact with vectors, such as the bites of insects—mosquitoes, ticks, or biting flies
- Contact with inanimate objects that carry a pathogen (*fomites*)

Diseases transmitted directly via the mucus membranes include sexually transmitted diseases such as herpes, syphilis, gonorrhea, and *Chlamydia*.

Respiratory pathogens in particular are known to be spread by contaminated dust particles or droplets of moisture. Diseases that can be transmitted in this

Best Practice

Disease Transmission Prevention

Many diseases are transmitted by direct contact with organisms carried on the skin. The pathogen is then transferred via the hands to the mouth, nose, or eyes. In the hospital setting, hands are frequently the means of transfer of colds, influenza, and staphylococcal, streptococcal, and gastrointestinal tract organisms. For this reason, frequent and proper handwashing is the most important infection control process in health care. See Chapter 38 for detailed discussions of this and other personnel and patient protection issues.

manner include colds, measles, mumps, and chickenpox, to name a few. Legionnaire's disease is spread through contaminated air conditioning systems or shower heads.

Fungal respiratory diseases such as histoplasmosis may be spread via dried bird or bat droppings or, in the case of coccidioidomycosis, by dust from dried soil. In the hospital or home setting, improperly cleaned respiratory care equipment, especially aerosol generators, can transfer pathogens.

Organisms can easily contaminate food and water supplies. Human feces may get into the water from outhouses, cesspools, and sewer line breaks; animal contamination can occur from feedlots and processing plants. Improper handling or storage may result in contaminated food supplies. Botulism, *Salmonella* poisoning, typhoid fever, hepatitis A, and giardiasis are all diseases transmitted via food or water. Hanta virus respiratory disease is an example of disease spread by the droppings of field mice.

Because blood is normally sterile, special methods are usually required to cause the transmission of organisms directly into the bloodstream. A **vector** (an intermediate host) is needed to transmit the pathogen. Many vectors are arachnids (ticks) or insects (fleas, lice, flies, and mosquitoes). In most cases, the organisms live in the vector itself. Fleas, for example, may carry plague or typhus organisms. Mosquitoes transmit malaria, yellow fever, and encephalitis. In the United States, there is great concern over ticks, which are known to transmit Rocky Mountain spotted fever and Lyme disease. The vector merely transports the organisms from one person to another in the blood.

Pets and wild animals may serve as reservoirs of *zoonoses*, or animal infections that can be transmitted to humans. Dogs, cats, skunks, and bats are well-known vectors for rabies. Turtles and chickens commonly transmit *Salmonella*. Toxoplasmosis, a protozoan disease that can cause birth defects, may be acquired by contact with cat feces in litter boxes.

Inanimate objects through which pathogens are transmitted are called **fomites**. Hospital instruments and equipment can be fomites. Needles, syringes, surgical devices, solutions, and blood-processing equipment such as kidney dialyzers are all possible culprits. As an example, the suctioning procedure in respiratory care has a high potential for mechanically introducing organisms into a patient's lungs. A good way to decrease the risk of cross-contamination among patients is to adopt single-use disposable equipment.

Epidemiology

Epidemiology is the science that deals with the frequency and distribution of diseases and factors leading to the spread of infection. Respiratory caregivers should be familiar with the terms that epidemiologists use.

Endemic diseases are those that are constantly present in a population, usually involving only a few people. The number of infected individuals may increase or decrease from year to year, but the disease never goes away completely. Endemic infections in the United States include streptococcal infections, influenza, tuberculosis, and plague. Plague (caused by the bacterium *Yersinia pestis*) is endemic in rats, prairie dogs, and squirrels in certain parts of the United States. Periodically, humans become infected. How many people are sick from an endemic disease at any one time depends on environment, behavior, the reservoir or source of infection, and the number of immune people.

An **epidemic** occurs when a greater-than-normal number of cases of an endemic disease occur in an area at a specific time. For example, a modern respiratory epidemic occurred in 1976 in Philadelphia, Pennsylvania. Many of the large number of members of the American Legion who met for a convention became severely ill and were hospitalized. Some even died from severe lung infections. The causative organism was extremely difficult to isolate and grow. When it was finally identified, the bacterium was given the name *Legionella pneumophila*.

Epidemics may also break out in communities where the pathogen was not previously present. Travelers can easily bring organisms into an area. Natural disasters and poverty lead to epidemics when sanitation practices decline, resulting in food and water contamination. Outbreaks of cholera, typhoid, giardiasis, and dysentery result.

The CDC is responsible for monitoring potential and actual epidemics in the United States.

When an epidemic reaches worldwide proportions, it is called a **pandemic**. Pandemics of the flu were recorded in 1898, 1917, 1955, 1968, 1972, 1975, 1978, and 2009. Influenza pandemics are usually named after the point of origin, such as the Hong Kong flu or the London flu. The best-known pandemics in the world today are human immunodeficiency virus (HIV) infection and acquired immunodeficiency syndrome (AIDS). An important outcome of the AIDS pandemic is increased attention to sexually transmitted diseases in general and to methods of prevention in particular.

Important Respiratory Pathogens

Infection is a common cause of respiratory disease. Microorganisms responsible for significant upper and lower respiratory tract infections are viruses, bacteria, fungi, and protozoans. Even given today's effective antimicrobial therapies, pneumonia remains a significant cause of morbidity (disease) and mortality (death). As the scope of medical care has expanded, the range of microorganisms being seen with both

Age-Specific Competency

High-Risk Populations

Infants and children under age 7 are at particular risk of infectious disease because of immature immune systems. The elderly are also susceptible owing to failing immune function. Prevention and control efforts have their greatest effect when targeted toward these populations.

community- and hospital-acquired pneumonias has increased.

PNEUMONIAS

Pneumonias have many causes.

- A high percentage of the pneumonias occurring in otherwise healthy individuals result from infection with *Streptococcus pneumoniae, Hemophilus influenzae, Chlamydia pneumoniae, Mycoplasma pneumoniae*, or common viruses, such as influenza in adults.
- Respiratory syncytial virus and parainfluenza virus are causative microorganisms in infants and children.
- Less common causes of pneumonias in normal adults are *Legionella pneumophila*, group A beta-hemolytic *Streptococcus*, and *Mycobacterium tuberculosis*.
- Fungal infections, or *mycoses*, cause respiratory disease, the particular agents being geographically endemic. *Histoplasma capsulatum* is found in the soil of the Mississippi valley. *Coccidioides immitis* is a common fungus found in the arid and semiarid areas of New Mexico, Utah, California, Texas, and Arizona.

INFLUENZA

Exacerbations of *chronic obstructive lung disease* (COPD) are often caused by infections with viral agents such as influenza viruses. The most common bacterial organisms associated with pneumonia in chronic lung patients are *Streptocococcus pneumoniae, Hemophilus influenzae*, and recently *Moraxella catarrhalis*. Because the airways of some COPD patients may be colonized with these microbes, determining whether the symptoms of exacerbation are related to their presence can be difficult.

Predisposition

Especially susceptible to pneumonias from unusual organisms are individuals with compromised immune systems, such as those with HIV infection or AIDS, alcoholism, ARDS, or diabetes, as well as persons undergoing cancer chemotherapy, immunosuppressive therapy, or prolonged endotracheal intubation.

Common microorganisms causing infections in compromised hosts are *Staphylococcus aureus*, gram-negative bacilli such *Pseudomonas aeruginosa* and *Klebsiella pneumoniae*, and anaerobic bacteria such as *Bacteroides*. *Aspergillus* species are ubiquitous fungi that can cause bronchopulmonary infection, fungus balls (aspergilloma), or disseminated disease in compromised hosts. Because of their impaired immunity, patients with HIV infection or AIDS often are infected with *Pneumocystis jiroveci*, an atypical fungus (sometimes classified as a protozoan) that can cause severe pneumonia. *Mycobacterium tuberculosis* is also often the first infectious agent to appear in AIDS patients. Persons with AIDS may also have multi-drug-resistant forms of the infection and are also susceptible to a noncommunicable type of tuberculosis caused by *Mycobacterium avium* complex.

Summary

Respiratory therapists work with many patients either who are susceptible to pulmonary infections or who have already developed pneumonia. An understanding of the types, identification, and management of pathogens capable of causing pulmonary disease can help practitioners minimize the occurrence and transmission of respiratory infections.

Organisms that can infect the lung include bacteria, viruses, fungi, and protozoa. Specific microorganisms are identified in the laboratory through a process that may use Gram staining, acid-fast testing, enzyme-linked immunosorbent assays, and cultures. Specimens may be obtained by having the patient cough, by suctioning, or by bronchoscopy. The specimens must be carefully collected and handled to avoid contamination and to provide accurate information.

Host defense mechanisms are the skin, the mucus membranes, and cellular and chemical responses to invasion. The immune response specifically generates protective antibodies in response to antigen challenges. Vaccines artificially stimulate antibody production to protect people from disease.

Disinfection and sterilization may be accomplished by means of physical methods, such as heat, pressure, radiation, sonic disruption, and filtration. The autoclave is an example of a device that incorporates both heat and pressure to sterilize medical items and equipment. Disinfection using the process of pasteurization is appropriate for many types of equipment used in respiratory care. Chemical agents may also be used for sterilization; ethylene oxide gas and gluteraldehyde solutions are two examples.

Antimicrobial drugs are key in the management of infections. However, because many pathogens have become drug-resistant as they mutate, the development of new agents is now of grave importance.

Infections may be transmitted by skin or mucus membrane contact, by airborne droplets, by contaminated food and water, by blood that has been contaminated by vectors, or by contact with contaminated inanimate objects. Thorough and frequent handwashing remains the most important procedure for limiting the transmission of infection.

Study Questions

REVIEW QUESTIONS

1. Name five of the nine characteristics used to classify or identify bacteria.
2. List the five physical methods used for sterilization and disinfection.
3. Name the three benefits that humans receive from their endogenous flora.
4. List the environmental factors that affect the growth of microorganisms.
5. Name the three lines of defense that humans have against infection.
6. List the four types microorganisms responsible for infectious diseases of the respiratory system.

MULTIPLE-CHOICE QUESTIONS

1. Which of the following microorganisms does not flourish in an oxygen environment?
   a. *Streptococcus pneumoniae*
   b. *Clostridium perfringens*
   c. *Hemophilus influenzae*
   d. *Candida albicans*
2. Which of the following microorganisms is a part of endogenous flora that can become pathogenic, especially in the mouth and throat, if the immune system is impaired by the use of inhaled steroids?
   a. *Streptococcus pneumoniae*
   b. *Clostridium perfringens*
   c. *Hemophilus influenzae*
   d. *Candida albicans*
3. Which of the following vaccines is not recommended by the CDC for all children before entering school?
   a. hepatitis B
   b. diphtheria
   c. human papillomavirus
   d. rubella
4. Which of the following immunoglobulins is associated with an allergic response in the body?
   a. IgA
   b. IgD
   c. IgE
   d. IgG
5. To increase the effectiveness of acid glutaraldehydes, the respiratory therapist should do which of the following?
   a. Mix it with another agent such as alcohol.
   b. Heat the acid glutaraldehyde to 60°C.
   c. Do not rinse the equipment after immersion in the acid glutaraldehyde.
   d. Chill the acid glutaraldehyde to 0°C.
6. How does the antimicrobial amphotericin kill bacteria?
   a. inhibiting cell wall synthesis
   b. inhibiting nucleic acid synthesis
   c. inhibiting metabolism
   d. disrupting cell membrane

CRITICAL-THINKING QUESTIONS

1. With more and more immunosuppressed patients, what precautions should the respiratory therapist take? How do these precautions affect the efficiency of the practitioner while performing procedures?
2. More and more physicians are prescribing broad-spectrum antibiomicrobials. What are some of the hazards of this practice? What changes would you recommend? How can respiratory therapists help to change this practice?
3. *Mycobacterium tuberculosis* and *Staphylococcus* are currently the most common drug-resistant microorganisms that a respiratory therapist must deal with. What can respiratory therapists do to decrease the likelihood that other pathogens will become drug resistant?

Suggested Readings

Centers for Disease Control and Prevention, Hospital Infections Program. *Bloodborne Pathogens: Worker Protection.* http://www.cdc.gov/ncidod/hip/Blood/uni

Kacamarek RM. *The Essentials of Respiratory Care.* 4th ed. St. Louis: Mosby-Yearbook; 2005.

Winn Jr, W, Allen S, Janda W, Koneman E, Procop G, Schreckenberger P, Woods G. *Koneman's Color Atlas and Textbook of Diagnostic Microbiology.* 6th ed. Philadelphia: Lippincott Williams & Wilkins; 2006.

CHAPTER 6

Cardiopulmonary Anatomy and Physiology

Oliver J. Drumheller

OBJECTIVES

Upon completion of this chapter, the reader should be able to:

- Name the respiratory system's structures and functions.
- Describe ventilation principles for the lung.
- Review pulmonary gas diffusion properties.
- Summarize the structure and functions of the circulatory system.
- Discuss the body's oxygen transport mechanisms.
- Describe carbon dioxide transport and acid-base balance.
- State the effects of the renal system on the cardiopulmonary system.
- Summarize ventilation/perfusion relationships.
- Explain the principles of the control of ventilation.
- Describe the cardiopulmonary physiology of the fetus and newborn.
- List the effects of aging on the cardiopulmonary system.
- Summarize the effects of exercise and high-altitude and high-pressure environments on the cardiopulmonary system.

CHAPTER OUTLINE

(continues)

(continued)

KEY TERMS

alveolar-capillary membrane
atelectasis
automaticity
autonomic nervous system (ANS)
Bohr effect
cardiac output (CO)
compliance
conducting zone
contractility
diffusion
elastance
epithelium
Frank-Starling principle
Haldane effect
lower airways
lung-thorax relationship
mucociliary escalator
oxygen content
oxyhemoglobin
pulmonary shunting
pulmonary surfactant
respiratory zone
stroke volume (SV)
trachea
tracheobronchial tree
upper airway
Valsalva maneuver
ventilation
ventricular afterload
ventricular preload
vibrissae

The practice of respiratory care is based on thorough preparation in normal cardiopulmonary anatomy and physiology. Grounding in these areas allows the respiratory therapist to compare, analyze in-depth, and diagnose abnormalities brought about by disease processes, and it fosters objective treatment planning and patient management.

The cardiopulmonary system brings atmospheric gas into the lungs, through successively smaller airways to the alveoli. There, the gases are brought into close contact with pulmonary capillary blood (mixed venous blood) from the pulmonary vascular system. Oxygen diffuses from gas exchange units into the blood, as carbon dioxide diffuses from the blood into the gas exchange units.

This chapter presents the structures and functions of the cardiopulmonary system. Breathing and circulation are regulated efficiently, and benefit and energy expenditure are continually balanced to meet the body's always-changing needs. General science principles are applied throughout the chapter to explain lung ventilation, gas diffusion, perfusion of blood, gas transportation, and cellular delivery mechanisms. The wonders of the fetus and newborn, the effects of aging, exercise, and high-altitude and high-pressure environments are also described.

Upper Airway: The Nose, Oral Cavity, and Pharynx

The respiratory system is divided into the upper airway and the lower airways. The **upper airway** contains the nose, oral cavity, and pharynx (Figure 6-1), and it:

- Conducts air from the atmosphere to the lower airways.
- Prevents foreign objects from entering the **tracheobronchial tree**.
- Serves as sites for speech and smell.

NOSE

The nose filters foreign materials to prevent them from entering the lower airways, and it humidifies (attaining 100% relative humidity) and warms the inspired air to body temperature (98°F; 37°C). The outer nose consists of bone and cartilage (connective tissue). The internal portion, the nasal cavity, is divided into two equal chambers by the nasal septum (Figure 6-2). Air enters the nose through two external openings called the *nares*, or nostrils. The air passes through vestibules, which contain coarse hairs, called **vibrissae**, that filter out foreign materials and are the respiratory system's first line of defense.

The respiratory system has a complete epithelial lining consisting of ciliated and nonciliated cells (Figure 6-3). Mucus is transported from the lungs by the ciliated cells toward the larynx for elimination by swallowing or coughing.

Turbinates, or *conchae*, are three bony projections from the lateral walls of the nasal cavity (see Figure 6-1). They divide the inhaled gas into different gas streams, thereby increasing the contact area between the inhaled gas and the nasal **epithelium**. In the turbinates, the gas is warmed and humidified before it enters into the lower airways.

The *paranasal sinuses* are air-filled cavities in the cranium that communicate with the nasal cavity, produce mucus, and provide resonation for speech (Figure 6-4). The *olfactory (smell receptors) region* is located near the superior and middle turbinates.

ORAL CAVITY

The oral cavity (mouth) is primarily the beginning of the digestive system, but it also is an accessory respiratory passage that participates in speech and sometimes in breathing. It extends from the teeth back to the oropharynx (Figures 6-1 and 6-5). The tongue is

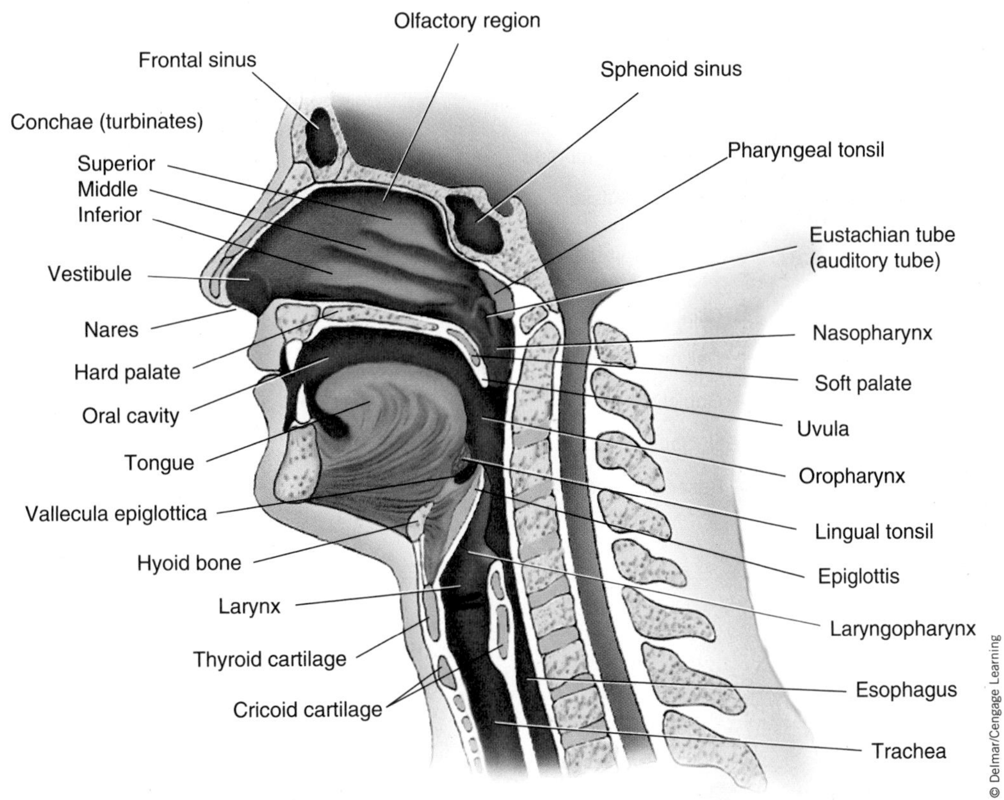

FIGURE 6-1 Structures of the upper airway.

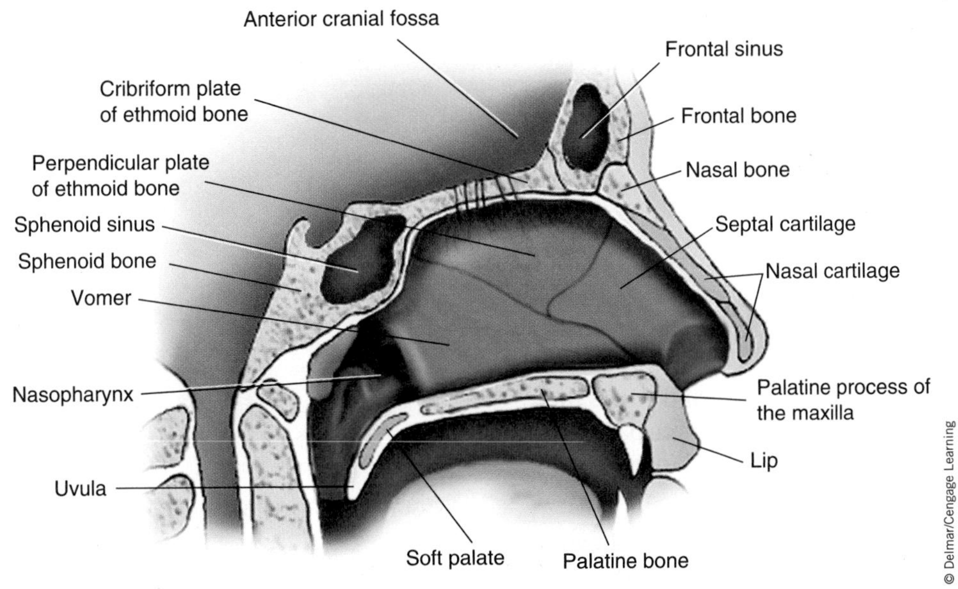

FIGURE 6-2 The nose and parts of the nasal septum.

attached posteriorly (toward the back, dorsally) to the hyoid bone and mandible. The roof of the mouth is formed by the hard palate and soft palate. The soft palate projects backward and downward, ending in the soft, fleshy structure called the *uvula,* which is responsible for the gag reflex. The soft palate closes the opening between the nasopharynx and oropharynx (described next). It moves upward and backward during swallowing, sucking, blowing, and speech. The palatine tonsils, located on each side of the oral cavity, are lymphoid (or lymphatic) tissues with immunological functions.

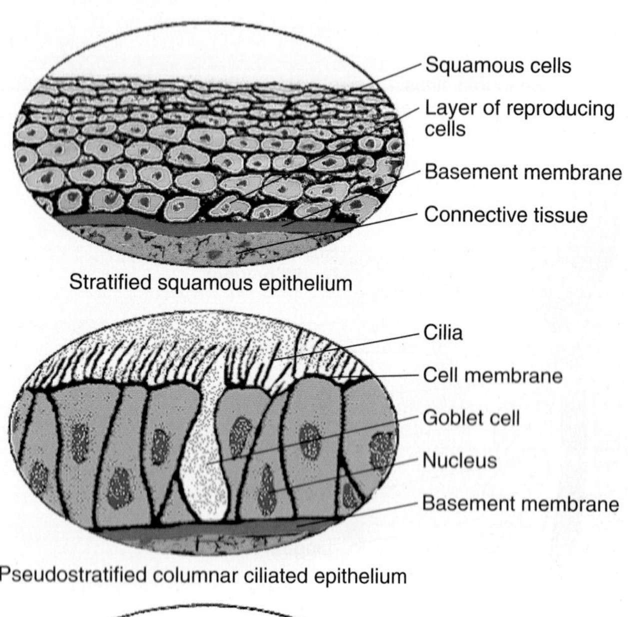

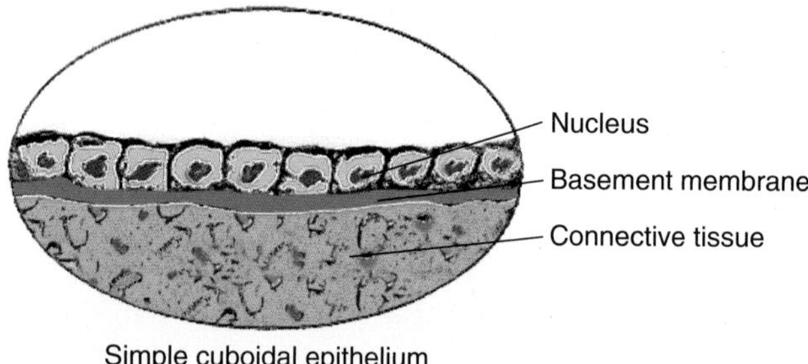

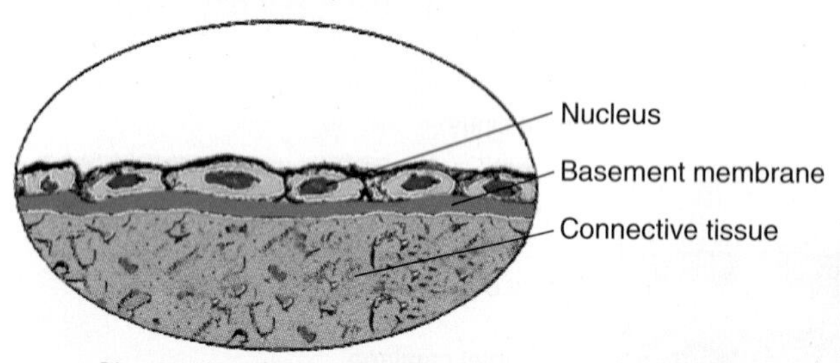

FIGURE 6-3 Epithelial cell types of the respiratory system.

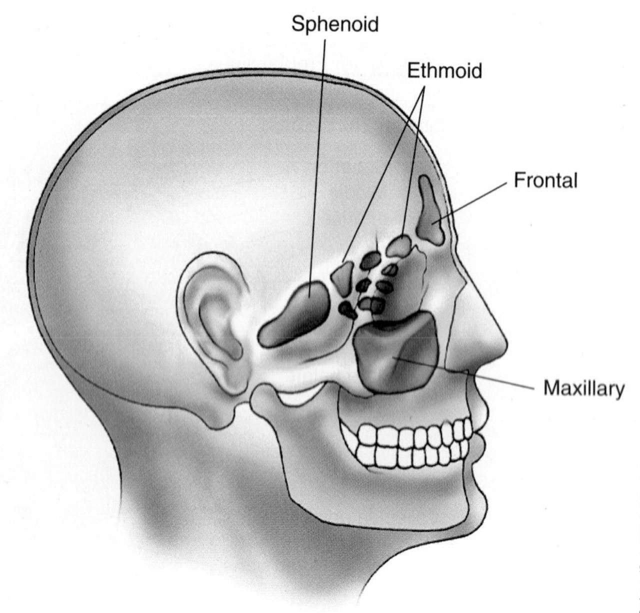

FIGURE 6-4 A lateral view of the head showing the sinuses.

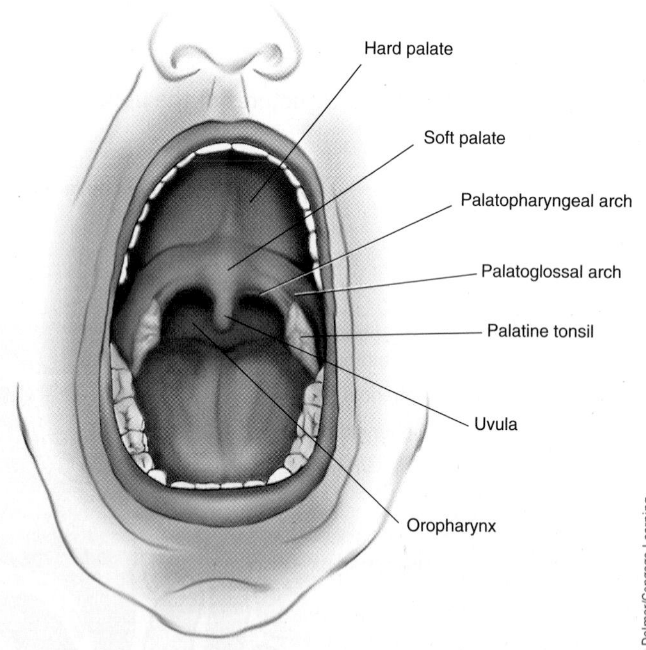

FIGURE 6-5 The oral cavity.

PHARYNX

The inspired air passes from the nose and enters the pharynx. The pharynx is divided into three parts: the nasopharynx, the oropharynx, and the laryngopharynx (see Figure 6-1).

- The *nasopharynx* is posterior to the nasal cavity and above the oral cavity. Lymphatic tissues, called *pharyngeal tonsils* or *adenoids*, are in the posterior nasopharynx. The *eustachian tube* (also called the *auditory canal*) connects the nasopharynx to the middle ear and functions to equalize pressure in the middle ear.
- The *oropharynx* lies between the soft palate and the base of the tongue. The lingual tonsil (lymphatic tissue) is located at the root of the tongue.
- The laryngopharynx is between the base of the tongue and the entrance to the esophagus. The epiglottis is directly anterior (toward the front, ventral) to the laryngopharynx and covers the glottis during swallowing.

Lower Airways

The **lower airways** begin in the area below the larynx.

LARYNX

The *larynx*, or voice box, located between the base of the tongue and the upper part of the **trachea**, serves three functions. It:

- Acts as a passage between the pharynx and the trachea.
- Protects against aspiration (inhaling materials).
- Generates sounds for speech (phonation).

The larynx consists of cartilages that are held together by ligaments, membranes, and intrinsic and extrinsic muscles (Figure 6-6). The body of the larynx consists of three large unpaired cartilages: the thyroid cartilage, the epiglottis, and the cricoid cartilage. It also has three pairs of smaller cartilages: the arytenoid, corniculate, and cuneiform cartilages.

The *thyroid cartilage*, or Adam's apple, is the largest cartilage and covers the anterior part of the larynx (see Figures 6-1 and 6-6); its superior border is V-shaped (thyroid notch). The upper thyroid is suspended from the hyoid bone by the thyrohyoid membrane (Figure 6-6).

The *epiglottis* is a broad fibrocartilaginous structure attached to the medial (toward midline of the body) aspect of the thyroid cartilage and is connected to the tongue by mucus membrane. The epiglottis prevents the aspiration of liquids and solids by covering the larynx during swallowing.

The *cricoid cartilage*, located below the thyroid cartilage, is ring-shaped and attached to the first C-shaped tracheal cartilage. The arytenoid cartilages are three-sided, with their base resting on the cricoid cartilages' superior surface; they are attached to the vocal cords.

The interior of the larynx is lined by a mucus membrane that forms the false vocal cords (having no role in speech) and true vocal cords (producing speech) (Figure 6-7). The vocal cords attach to the thyroid cartilage and to the arytenoid cartilages, which loosen or tighten the vocal cords. The glottis, the opening

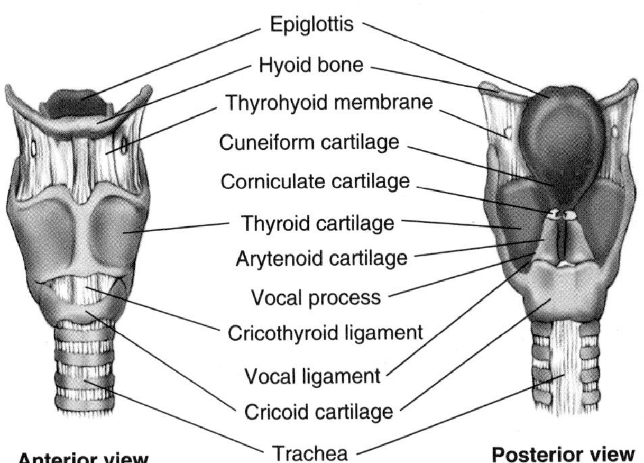

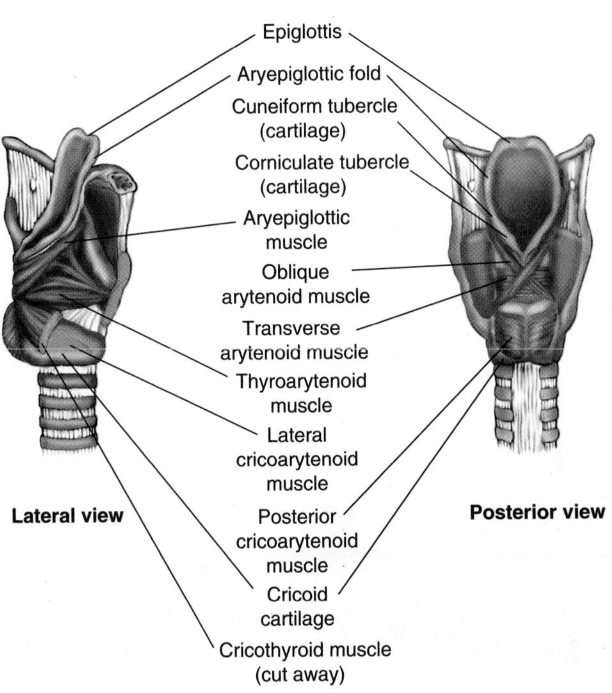

FIGURE 6-6 Cartilages and intrinsic muscles of the larynx.

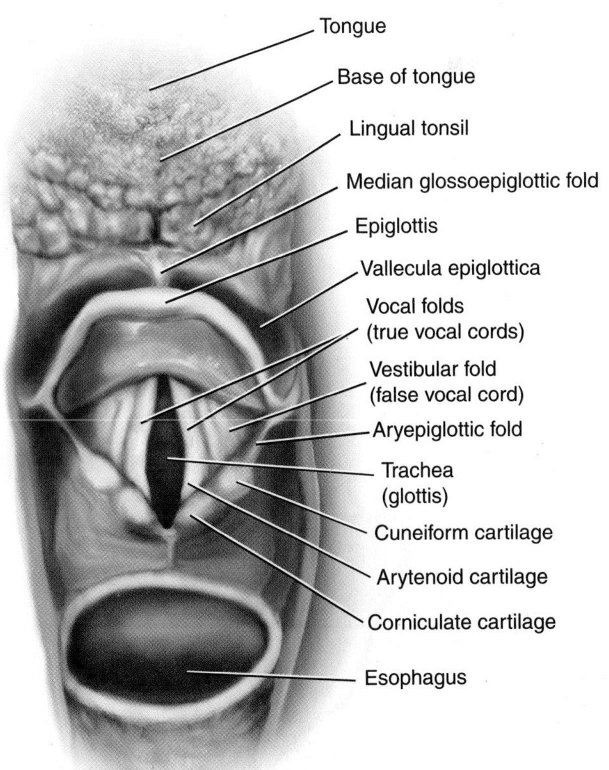

FIGURE 6-7 View of the vocal cords.

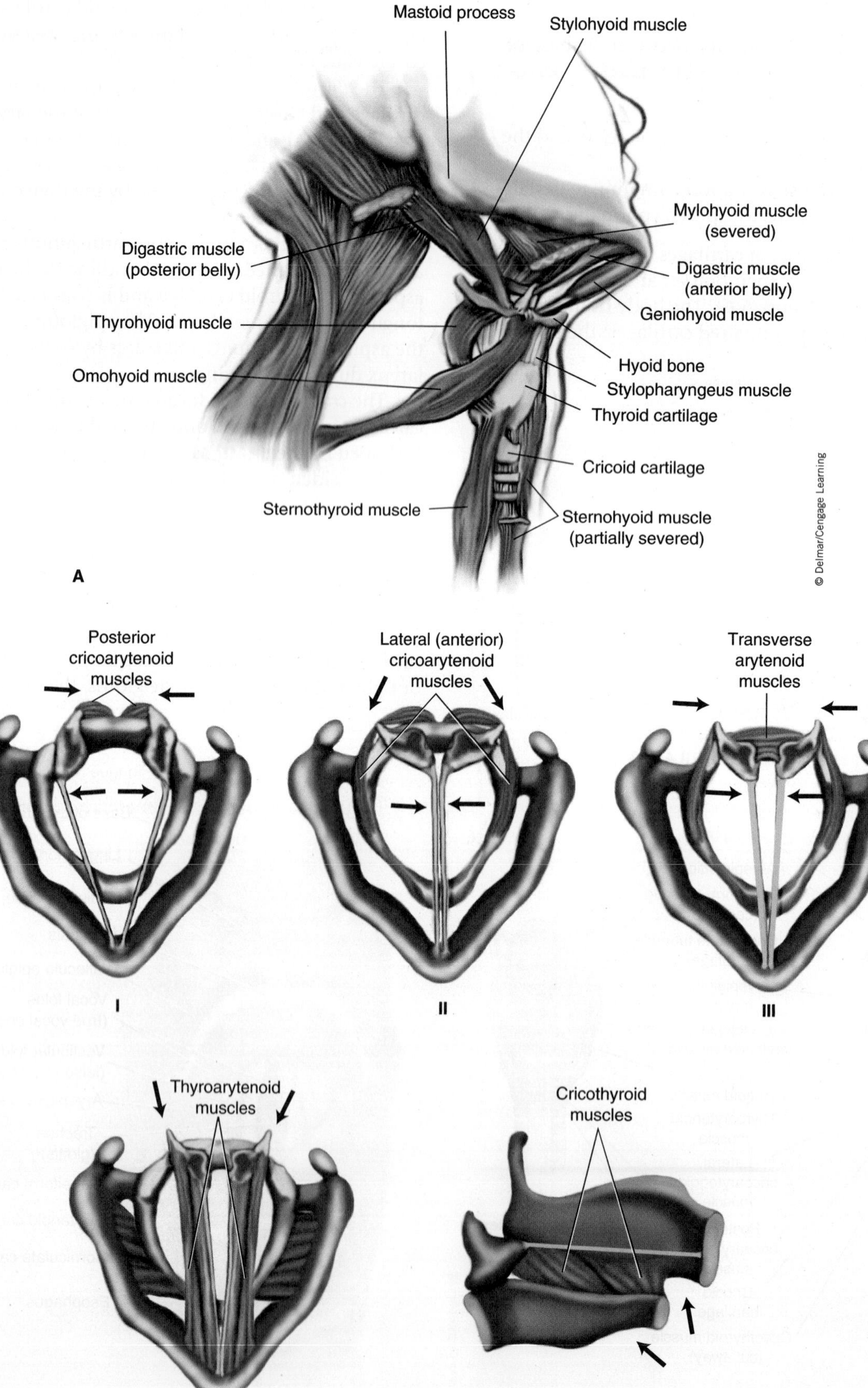

FIGURE 6-8 (A) Extrinsic laryngeal muscles. (B) Intrinsic laryngeal muscles I–V.

between the vocal cords, is the narrowest point in the adult larynx (Figure 6-7). The cricoid cartilage is the narrowest place in the newborn airway. Above the vocal cords, the larynx is lined with nonciliated stratified squamous epithelium; below the cords the covering is pseudostratified columnar epithelium. The musculature of the larynx consists of the extrinsic muscles (Figure 6-8A) and intrinsic muscle groups (Figure 6-8B), which control the vocal cords.

The larynx has two primary ventilatory functions. In quiet breathing (breathing at rest), the vocal cords abduct (move apart) during inspiration and adduct (move closer together) on expiration. The glottis is always open to allow a free flow of air into and out of the lungs. The **Valsalva maneuver** is the tight closing of the larynx during exhalation, with an increase in pressure in the lungs. It is while a person is performing physical work such as lifting, coughing, vomiting, and defecating. During scuba diving and flying, the use of the Valsalva maneuver can help to equalize the pressures in the sinuses and ears, which become unequal during environmental pressure changes.

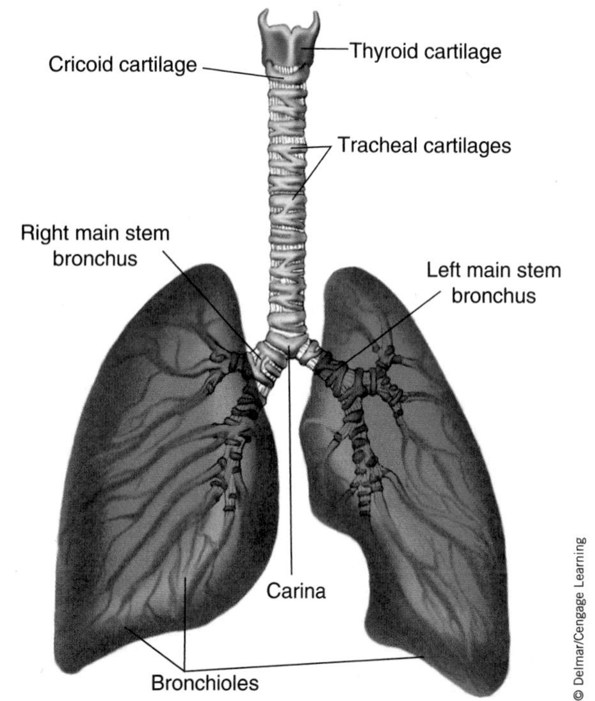

FIGURE 6-9 Tracheobronchial tree.

TRACHEOBRONCHIAL TREE

The *tracheobronchial tree* is a series of airways that begins at the trachea (the windpipe) and branches into the right and left bronchi, which in turn divide into progressively smaller, shorter, and more numerous airways (*bronchioles*) throughout the lungs (Figure 6-9). These divisions are called *airway generations* (Table 6-1). Although at each division, the individual airways become smaller, the total cross-sectional area inside the airways greatly increases. The large cross-sectional area promotes smooth (laminar) airflow (see Chapter 3). The smallest and most numerous bronchioles, the respiratory bronchioles, connect to the alveoli. Together, the respiratory bronchioles and the alveoli provide the sites for gas exchange.

There are two major types of airway: cartilaginous and noncartilaginous. The cartilaginous airways' only

TABLE 6-1 Major structures and corresponding generations of the tracheobronchial tree

	Structures	Generations	
Conducting zone	Trachea	0	Cartilaginous airways
	Main stem bronchi	1	
	Lobar bronchi	2	
	Segmental bronchi	3	
	Subsegmental bronchi	4–9	
	Bronchioles	10–15	Noncartilaginous airways
	Terminal bronchioles	16–19	
Respiratory zone*	Respiratory bronchioles	20–23	Sites of gas exchange
	Alveolar ducts	24–27	
	Alveolar sacs	28	

Note: The precise number of generations between the subsegmental bronchi and the alveolar sacs is not known.

**These structures collectively are referred to as a primary lobule or lung parenchyma; they are also called terminal respiratory units and functional units.*

function is to conduct air between the external environment and the noncartilaginous airways. The noncartilaginous airways serve to conduct air between the cartilaginous airways and the sites of gas exchange. The number of airway divisions varies markedly within the lungs.[1] Notice from Table 6-1 that the lung **conducting zone** consists of both cartilaginous and noncartilaginous airways, starting at generation 0 (trachea) and ending with generations 16 to 19 (terminal bronchioles). The **respiratory zone** is the gas exchange area; it starts at generations 20 to 23 and ends in generation 28 (alveolar sacs).

The tracheobronchial tree is made up of three layers: an epithelial lining, the lamina propria, and a cartilaginous layer (Figure 6-10). The epithelial lining is primarily pseudostratified ciliated columnar epithelium with numerous mucus glands interspersed, separated from the lamina propria by a basement membrane (Figures 6-3 and 6-10). The basement membrane contains basal cells that replace the ciliated and mucus cells as needed (Figure 6-11). The pseudostratified ciliated columnar epithelium extends from

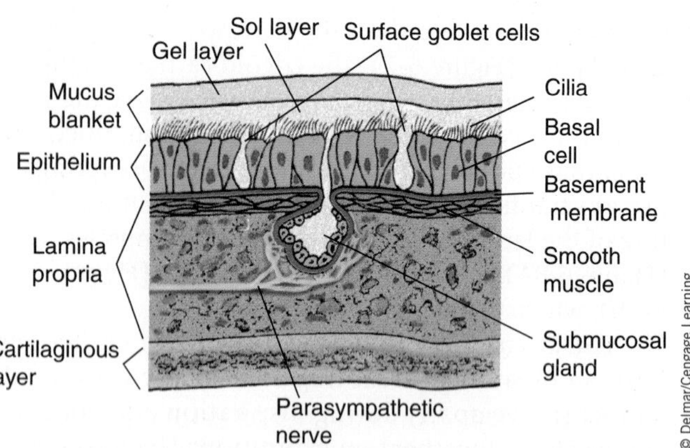

FIGURE 6-11 Epithelial lining of the tracheobronchial tree.

the trachea to the respiratory bronchioles, slowly decreasing in height and becoming cuboidal. Each cell has about 200 cilia, and each cilium is about 5–7 μm long. The cilia disappear in the respiratory bronchioles.

The mucus blanket covers the epithelial lining of the tracheobronchial tree (Figure 6-11). Mucus is

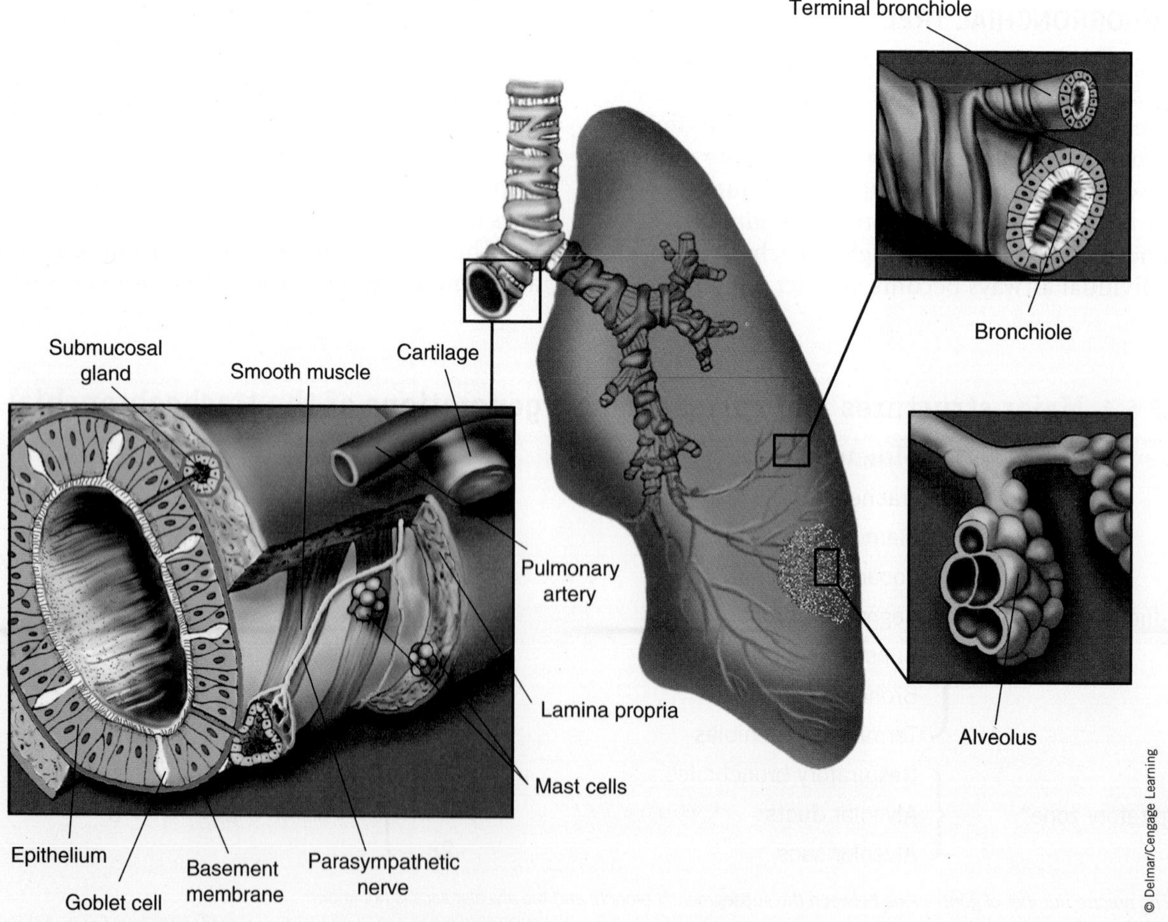

FIGURE 6-10 Histology of the tracheobronchial tree.

mostly water; the balance consists of glycoproteins, lipids, DNA, cellular debris, and foreign particles. Mucus is produced by goblet cells and submucosal glands. Goblet cells, which are interspersed between the ciliated cells, are present down to and within the terminal bronchioles. The submucosal, or bronchial, glands, which produce most of the mucus (100 mL per day), are located in the lamina propria. They are innervated by vagal parasympathetic nerve fibers (tenth cranial nerve). Increased parasympathetic activity increases mucus production; increased sympathetic activity and dehydration both decrease mucus production. The submucosal glands are present to the terminal bronchiole level.

The mucus blanket has two distinct layers: (1) the sol layer, which is closest to the ciliated cells, and (2) the more viscous gel layer, which is located nearest to the surface of the lumen. The gel layer traps foreign particles for removal from the airway. The cilia beat approximately 1300–1500 times per second through the sol layer, projecting the mucus blanket toward the head at a rate of 21.5 mm per minute.[1] At the larynx, the mucus and entrapments are coughed into the oropharynx for expectoration or swallowing. This process, called the mucociliary transport mechanism, or **mucociliary escalator**, is a valuable cleansing function for the tracheobronchial tree. Several factors slow the rate of mucociliary transport: cigarette smoke, dehydration, positive pressure ventilation, endotracheal suctioning, high F_IO_2 delivery, hypoxia, air pollutants, general anesthetics, parasympatholytic drugs, and certain disease states.

The lamina propria is the submucosal layer containing fibrous tissue that contains blood and lymphatic vessels, branches of the vagus nerve, and two sets of smooth muscle that wrap clockwise and counterclockwise around the tracheobronchial tree down into the alveolar ducts. The peribronchial sheath covers the outer lamina propria.

Mast cells are found in the lamina propria, in smooth muscles, intra-alveolar septa, and the submucosal glands. Mast cells are important in the two major immune response mechanisms: cellular immunity and humoral immunity. The *cellular immune response* (type IV, or delayed) is a hypersensitivity response responsible for tissue rejection in transplants. The *humoral immune response* involves circulating antibodies, which are immunoglobulins that defend against invading environmental antigens (e.g., pollen, animal dander). The IgE antibody is basic to the allergic response. The IgE antibody-antigen reaction mechanism is shown in Figure 6-12. When a susceptible person is exposed to an

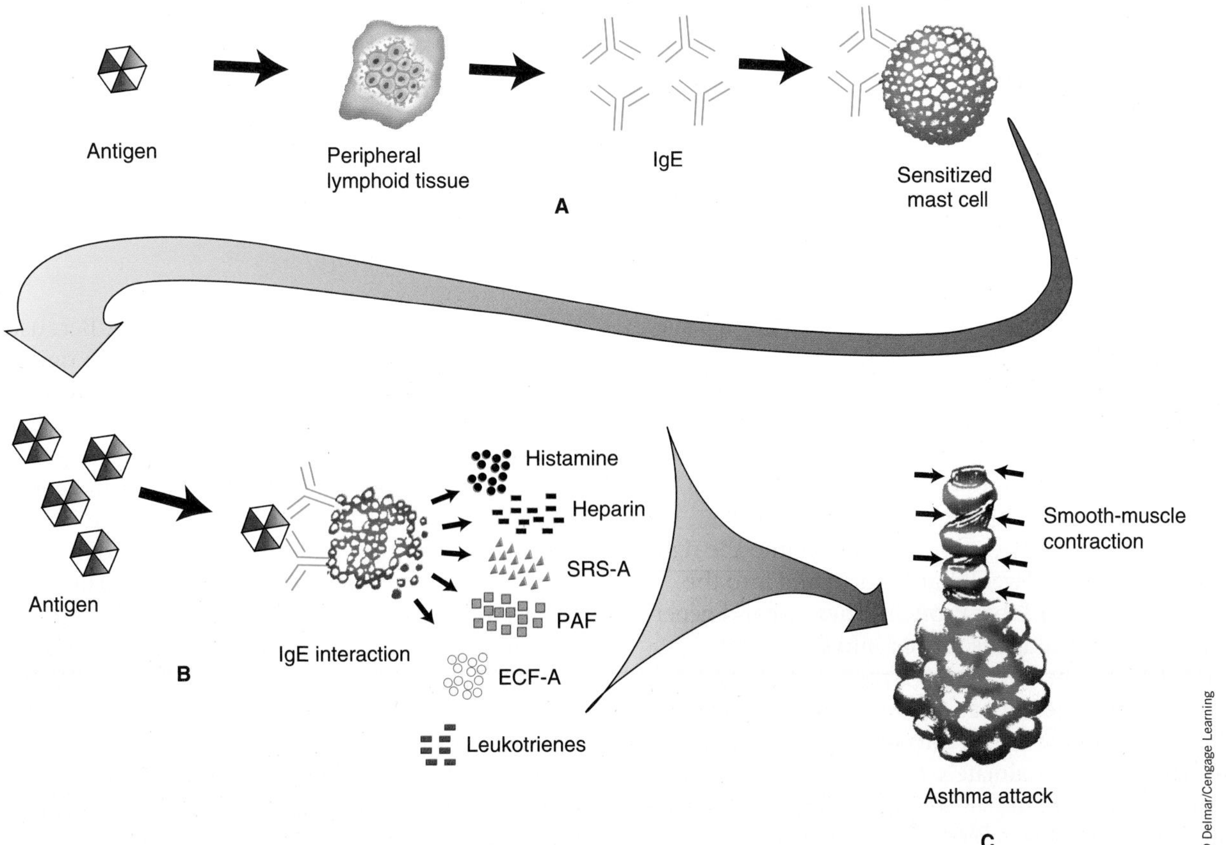

FIGURE 6-12 Immunological mechanisms.

antigen, lymphatic tissues release specific IgE antibodies that travel via the blood supply and attach to mast cell receptors. Once the antibodies have attached, the person is sensitive to that specific antigen, and continued re-exposure causes the antigen to be destroyed by chemical mediators of inflammation located on the mast cell surface. However, this process also causes the mast cell to break down, releasing chemicals [histamine, heparin, slow-reacting substance of anaphylaxis (SRS-A), and eosinophil chemotactic factor of anaphylaxis (ECF-A)] into the blood. These chemical mediators cause increased vascular permeability, smooth muscle contraction, increased mucus secretion, and vasodilation with edema. This reaction can be very dangerous and is found in allergic asthma, where the IgE levels can be greatly elevated. During an asthma attack, the person has airway narrowing due to bronchial edema, bronchospasm, and increased mucus production with plugging. The result is lung hyperinflation due to the trapping of air (air trapping). Together these effects can dramatically increase the work of breathing.

The cartilaginous layer is the outer layer of the tracheobronchial tree. It progressively diminishes decreases in thickness as the airways branch and become smaller. The cartilage is absent in bronchioles.

CARTILAGINOUS AIRWAYS

The *cartilaginous airways*, part of the conducting zone, conduct air. They consist of the trachea, main stem bronchi, lobar bronchi, segmental bronchi, and subsegmental bronchi (Figure 6-13). The adult trachea is 11–13 cm long and 1.5–2.5 cm in diameter.[2] The trachea extends from the cricoid cartilage of the larynx to the second costal cartilage, where it divides, or bifurcates, at the carina into the right and left main stem bronchi. The trachea gains support from 15–20 C-shaped cartilages that posteriorly share a fibroelastic membrane wall with the esophagus.

The main stem bronchi are the tracheobronchial tree's first generation. At birth, they form at relatively equal angles with the trachea. During development, the right becomes wider, more vertical, and shorter than the left, with the angle of the left diverging at a greater angle.[3] The two main stem bronchi divide into the right upper, middle, and lower lobar bronchi and into the left upper and lower lobar bronchi. These second-generation lobar bronchi divide further into segmental bronchi (third generation) that serve specific lung locations, 10 on the right and 8 on left. The subsegmental bronchi form the fourth through the ninth generations. They are approximately 1–4 mm in diameter and have a connective tissue sheath and contain nerves, lymphatics, and bronchial arteries. The connective tissue disappears in airways less than 1 mm in diameter.

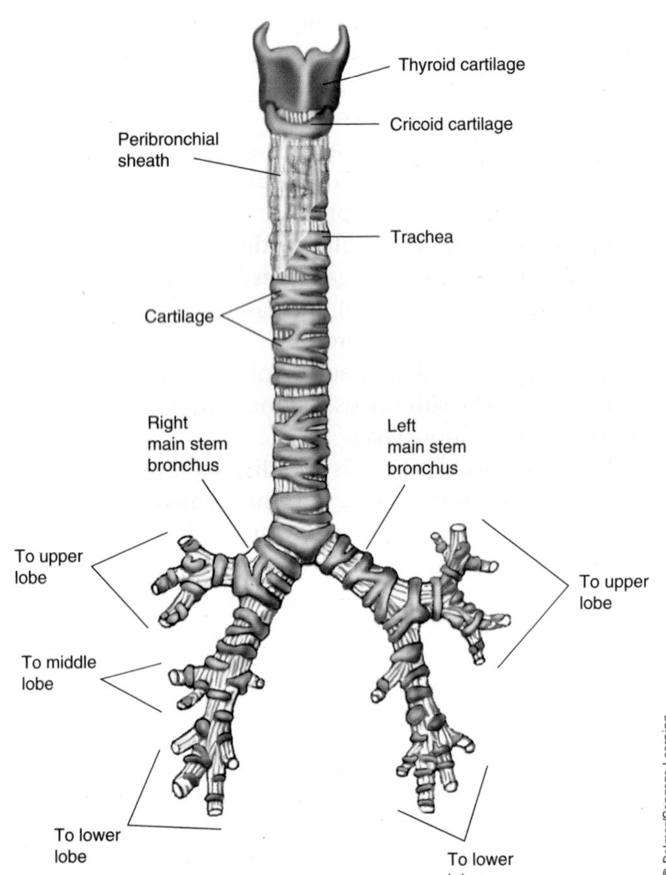

FIGURE 6-13 The cartilaginous airways.

NONCARTILAGINOUS AIRWAYS

The *noncartilaginous airways*, the bronchioles and terminal bronchioles, complete the conducting zone. The bronchioles are less than 1 mm in diameter and form generations 10 through 15. Because they lack cartilage for support, they are less rigid than the cartilaginous airways and more susceptible to alterations due to pressure differences or respiratory disease. Both conditions result in decreased airway patency. Terminal bronchioles form generations 16 through 19 and are about 0.5 mm in diameter. The epithelium flattens into a cuboidal shape, with the cilia and mucus glands disappearing. Terminal bronchioles have Clara cells with secretory functions. Also, collateral **ventilation** occurs at this level and is important in lung disease. Two types of collateral ventilation are *canals of Lambert*, small channels connecting a terminal bronchiole with an adjacent alveolus, and *pores of Kohn*, small channels connecting adjacent alveoli. The terminal bronchioles connect the conducting zone to the respiratory zone.

Bronchial Cross-Sectional Area and Bronchial Blood Supply

The total cross-sectional area inside the tracheobronchial tree increases from the trachea to the terminal bronchioles (conducting zone) and significantly increases beyond the terminal bronchioles owing to the increased number of branches of the respiratory zone (Figure 6-14). Ventilation (the mechanical movement of air into and out of the lungs) occurs down to the terminal bronchioles and requires the expenditure of energy (work of breathing). Molecular movement (diffusion) becomes the gas distribution mechanism in the respiratory zone.

The bronchial blood supply consists of the bronchial arteries (systemic circulation) that arise from the aorta. This bronchial supply is about 1% of the **cardiac output (CO)** and nourishes the tracheobronchial tree as far as the terminal bronchioles. About one-third of the bronchial venous blood returns to the right atrium (azygos, hemiazygos, intercostal veins), with the remaining two-thirds draining into the pulmonary circulation via bronchopulmonary anastomoses (bronchial, pleural, and Thebesian veins) and returning to the left atrium. This latter blood, being low in oxygen, mixes with the newly oxygenated pulmonary blood from the alveolar-capillary interface, creating what is termed *venous admixture.*

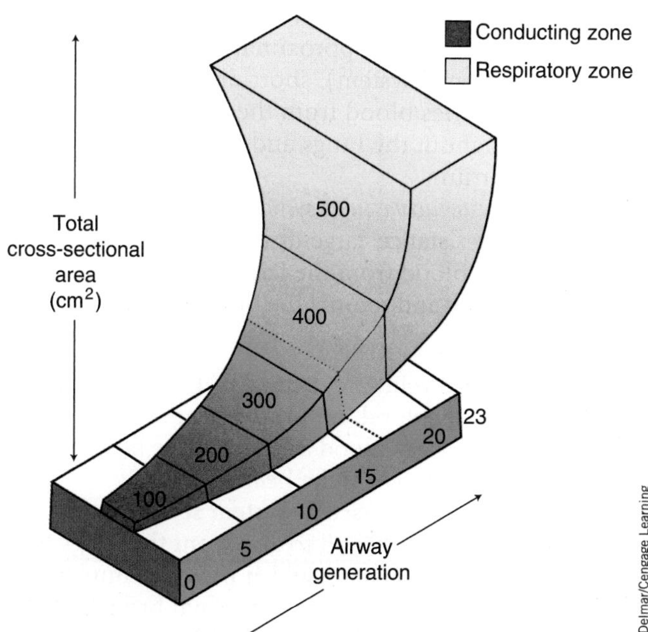

FIGURE 6-14 The cross-sectional area of the bronchial area. Note the major increase in total cross-sectional area of the respiratory zone.

SITES OF GAS EXCHANGE AND THE ALVEOLAR EPITHELIUM

The functional units of gas exchange, which are distal to the terminal bronchioles (Figure 6-15A), include generations 20 through 28. There are three generations of respiratory bronchioles with alveoli budding from their walls and three generations of alveolar ducts. The alveolar ducts are composed of alveoli separated by septal walls containing smooth muscle fibers and ending in 15–20 alveolar sacs that look like clusters of grapes. Most gas exchange takes place at the **alveolar-capillary membrane** (Figure 6-15B).

The adult male has approximately 300 million alveoli, each between 75 and 300 μm in diameter, with 85–95% of these alveoli covered by small pulmonary capillaries. This interface provides a huge surface area for gas exchange of from 50 to 100 m^2; 75 m^2 is the average area.[4] The *primary lobule* contains the respiratory bronchioles, alveolar ducts, and alveolar clusters. It is also called the acinus, terminal respiratory unit, lung parenchyma, and functional units.

There are three types of alveolar cell: I, II, and III. The alveolar epithelium comprises two principal cell types: type I (squamous pneumocyte) and type II (granular pneumocyte) (Figure 6-16). The type I cells are broad and thin (0.1–0.5 μm thick); they form 95% of the alveolar surface and are the major gas exchange sites. The type II cells are cuboidal; they have microvilli. These cells produce **pulmonary surfactant**, which, spread thinly on the alveolar type I cell's surface, decreases surface tension and promotes alveolar integrity. Pores of Kohn, which are small openings in the interalveolar septa, allow air to move between adjacent alveoli. They increase in number with lung parenchyma diseases, and their size increases with aging (Figure 6-15B). Alveolar macrophages, or type III pneumocytes (alveolar cells), protect the lung by removing bacteria and other foreign materials from the primary lobule.

INTERSTITIUM

Alveolar-capillary clusters are supported and shaped by the *interstitium*, which is a gel-like substance held together by a network of collagen fibers (connective tissue). Collagen limits alveolar distensibility, and, when overdistension occurs, pulmonary capillaries can be occluded, leading to collagen formation and alveolar damage. The interstitium is a tight space between the alveolar epithelium and the capillary endothelium (gas exchange area) and a loose space that surrounds the bronchioles and acinus area, which contain lymph vessels and nerve fibers.

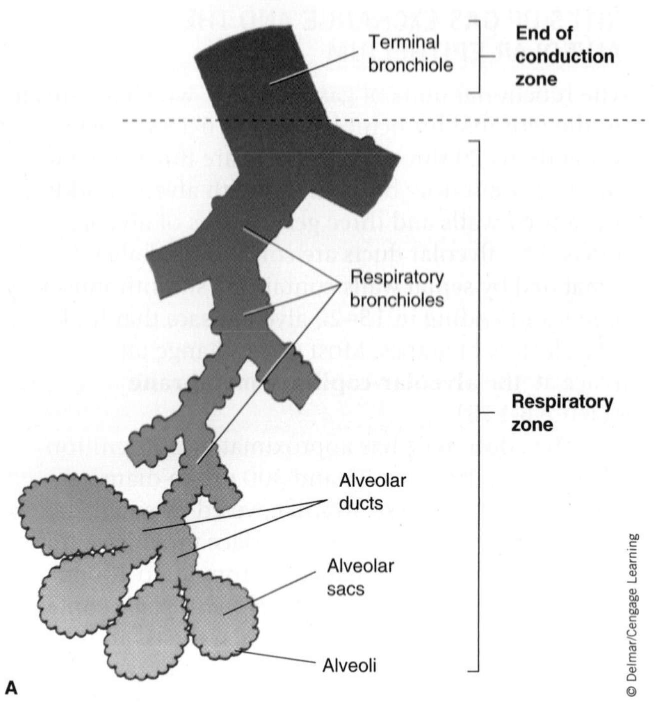

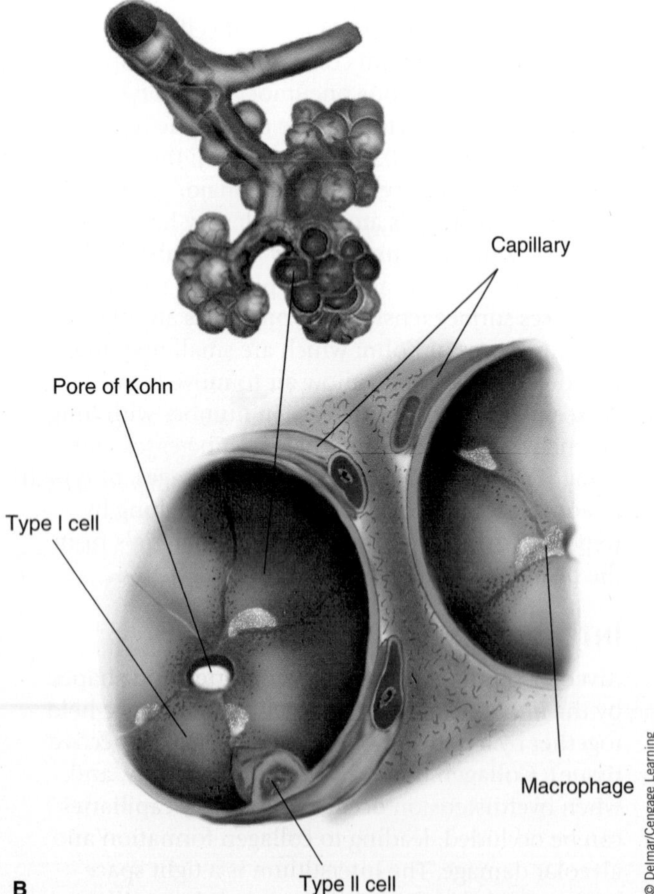

FIGURE 6-15 (A) Anatomical structures distal to the terminal bronchioles, called the primary lobule, or acinus. (B) The alveolar-capillary network.

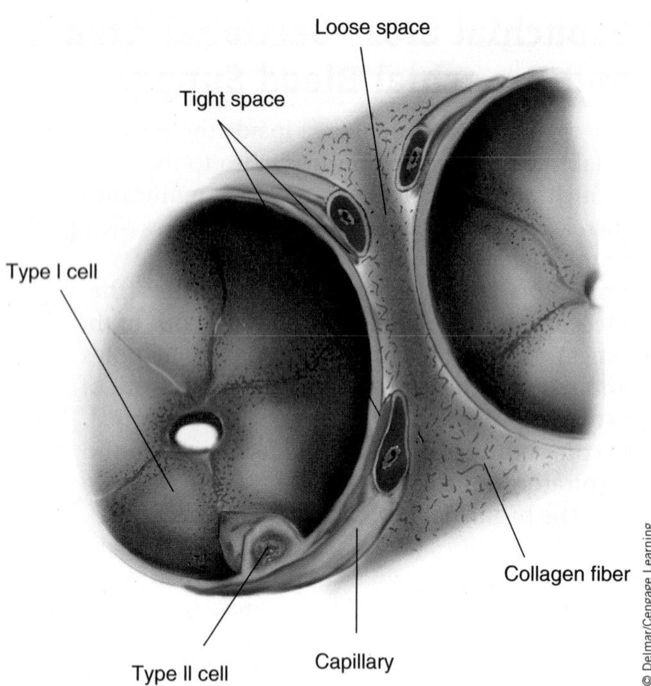

FIGURE 6-16 Alveolar structures and the interstitium.

PULMONARY AND SYSTEMIC CIRCULATORY SYSTEMS

The body has two distinct circulation, or vascular, systems: pulmonary and systemic.

- The *pulmonary vascular system* is a low-pressure, low-resistance (approximately one-tenth of systemic system), short-distance system that carries blood from the right ventricle throughout the lungs and returns it to the left atrium.
- The *systemic vascular system* is a high-pressure, high-resistance, large-distance system that carries blood from the left ventricle throughout the body and returns the blood to the right atrium.

Arteries and veins are defined by the direction in which they carry blood, not by the contents of the blood. Arteries carry blood away from the heart, and veins carry blood toward the heart.

The pulmonary vascular system serves two functions: It carries blood to and from the lungs for gas exchange with alveoli, and it provides nutrition for the structures distal to the terminal bronchiole level (acinus). The pulmonary vasculature contains arteries, arterioles, capillaries, venules, and veins—the same structures as found in the systemic vascular system.

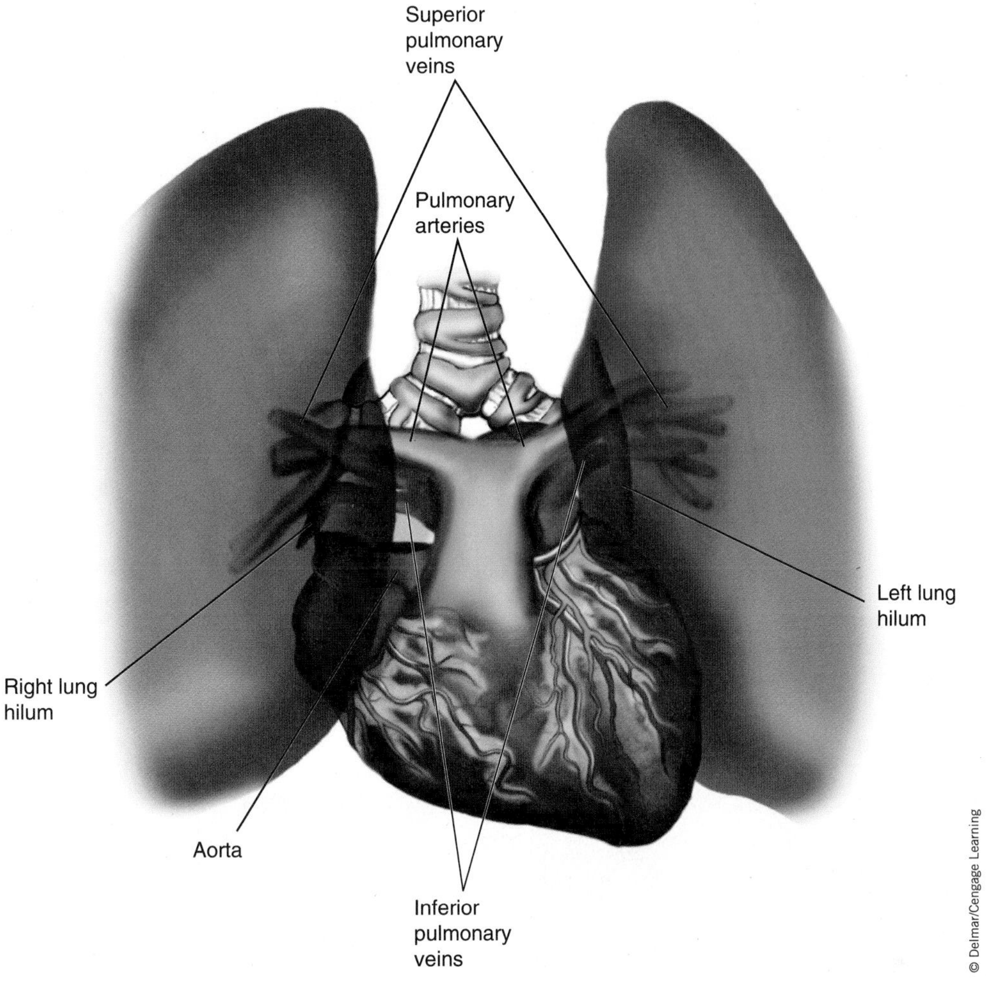

FIGURE 6-17 The major pulmonary vessels.

Pulmonary arteries (*PAs*) receive deoxygenated blood from the right atrium and divide into right and left branches (Figure 6-17). These branches pass through the hilum, where the main stem bronchi, vessels, and nerves also enter the lung. The pulmonary artery divides along the branchings of the tracheobronchial tree. Arterial walls have three layers (tunica intima, tunica media, tunica adventitia), making them relatively stiff; stiffness is necessary for carrying blood under high pressure, as in the systemic vascular system (Figure 6-18). The middle layer is the thickest and contains primarily connective tissue in large arteries and smooth muscle in medium and small arteries. The outer layer is connective tissue with blood vessels that serve all three layers.

Arterioles supply the acinus region, and their walls also have three layers (endothelial, elastic, smooth muscle). Arterioles, called *resistance vessels*, use their smooth muscle fibers for the distribution and regulation of blood.

Capillaries are an extension of the arteriole endothelial lining and form a network of vessels around the alveoli. They are very thin (less than 0.1 μm), have an external vessel diameter of about 10 μm, and are the site for gas exchange with their adjacent alveoli. The pulmonary capillary endothelium is selectively permeable to water, electrolytes, and sugars and is involved in the distribution of biologically active substances.

Venules are very small veins that collect blood from capillaries and empty into veins, which carry the blood back to the heart. Veins have three layers, like arteries, but they differ by having thinner walls and less smooth muscle. In the systemic system, veins in the lower extremities have one-way valves to assist blood flow back to the heart. Veins are called *capacitance vessels* because they can collect large amounts of blood with small pressure changes. The pulmonary veins merge into two large veins exiting the lungs at the hilum.

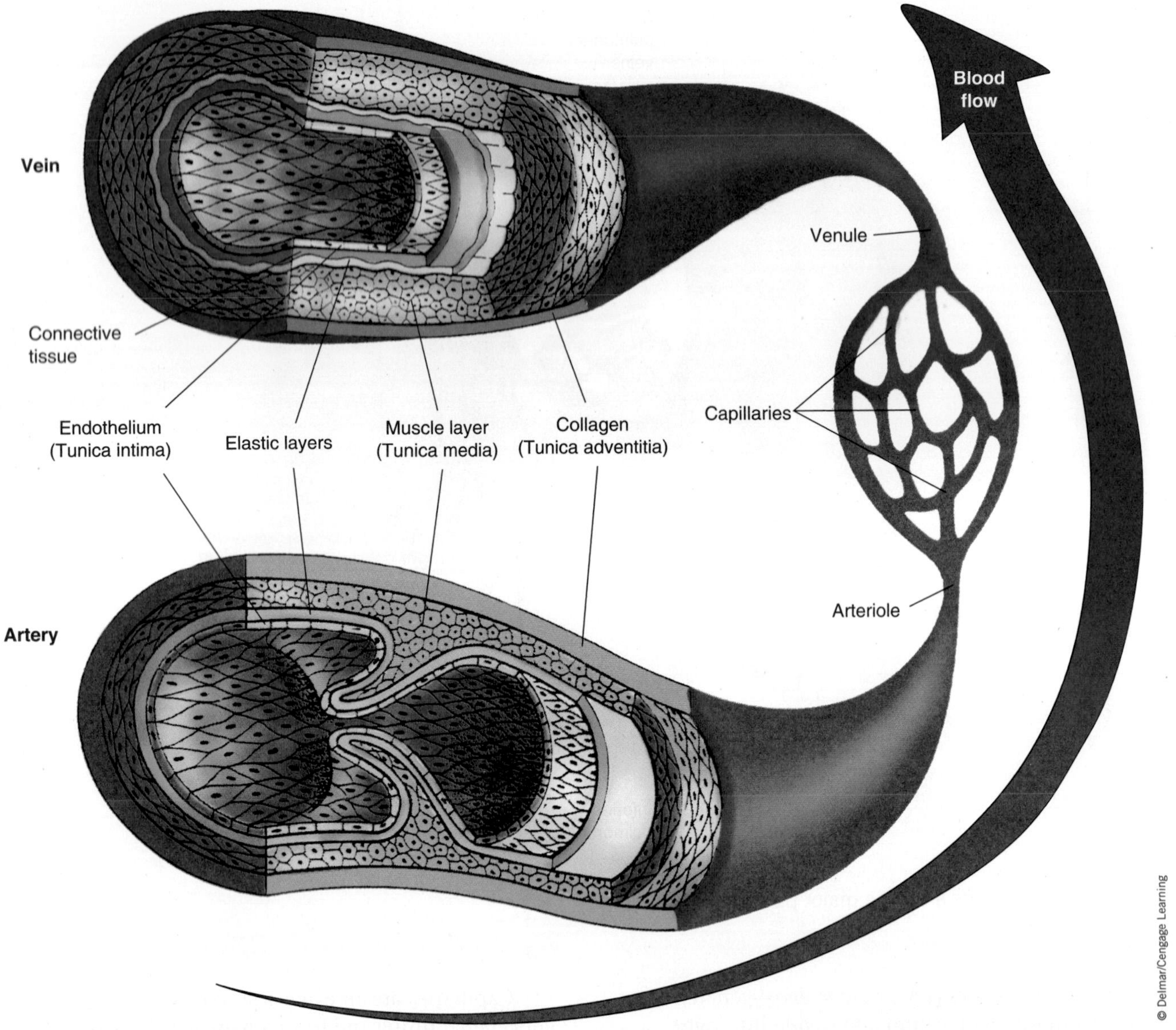

FIGURE 6-18 The components of the major blood vessels.

LYMPHATIC SYSTEM

Lymphatic vessels are found throughout the lungs and branch along with the airways and blood vessels. They remove excess fluid and protein molecules that leak from the capillaries. Lymph vessels end in *lymph nodes*, which are collections of lymphatic tissue. The nodes act as filters to keep particles from entering the bloodstream, and they produce lymphocytes and monocytes (Figure 6-19). There are more lymph vessels in the lower lung lobes, with more on the right lower lobe than on the left lower lobe.

NEURAL CONTROL OF THE LUNGS

The **autonomic nervous system (ANS)** regulates involuntary vital functions and controls the bronchial and arteriolar smooth muscle tone of the lungs, cardiac muscle, and glands (Table 6-2). The ANS has two divisions:

- The *sympathetic nervous system* relaxes bronchial smooth muscle (bronchodilation), speeds up the heart rate, and raises blood pressure.
- The *parasympathetic nervous system* constricts bronchial smooth muscle (bronchospasm), slows the heart rate, and increases intestinal peristalsis and glandular activity.

Smooth muscle tone is a reflection of the relative balance between the sympathetic and parasympathetic nervous systems. When the sympathetic nervous system is activated, the neural transmitters release

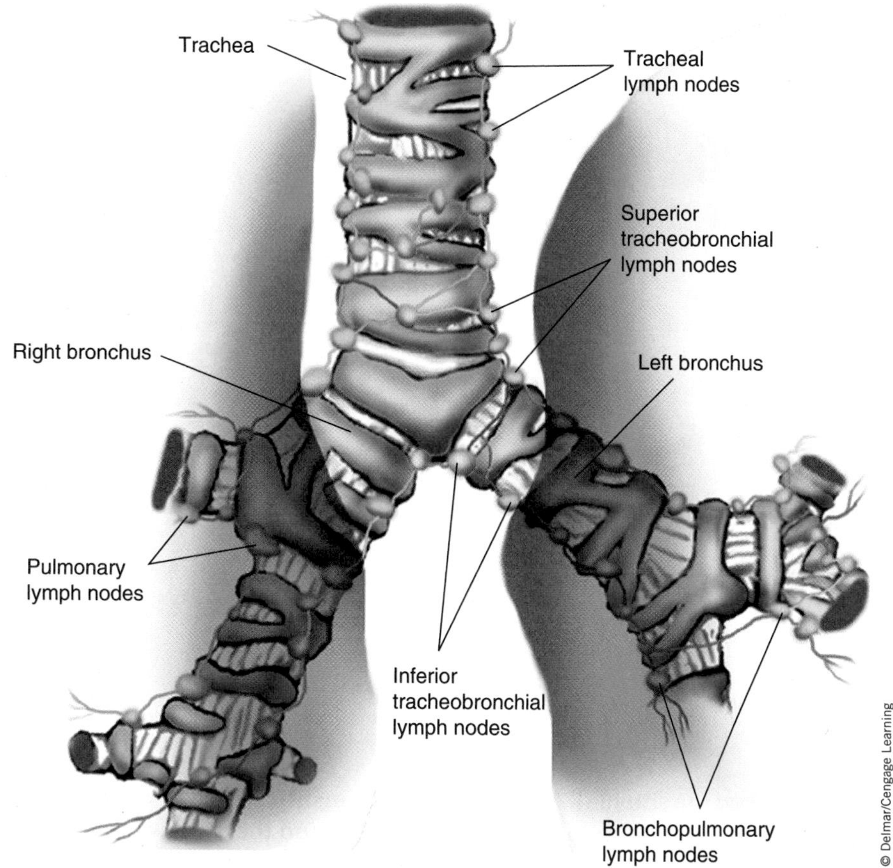

FIGURE 6-19 Lymph nodes of the trachea and the right and left mainstem bronchi.

epinephrine. They stimulate the beta 2 receptors in bronchial smooth muscle, causing bronchodilation. The alpha receptors in the arterioles' smooth muscle cause the pulmonary vascular system to constrict (vasoconstriction) and elevate blood pressure. When the parasympathetic nervous system is activated, the neural transmitter acetylcholine is released, causing constriction of the bronchial smooth muscle and increasing mucus production (secretions). Refer to Chapter 9 for a detailed description.

The Lungs

The *lungs* extend from the level of the first rib at the apex (top) and are continuous to the base anteriorly at the sixth rib (xiphoid process level) and posteriorly

TABLE 6-2 **Effects of autonomic nervous system activity**

Effector site	Sympathetic Nervous System	Parasympathetic Nervous System
Heart	Increases rate	Decreases rate
	Increases strength of contraction	Decreases strength of contraction
Bronchial smooth muscle	Relaxes muscle	Constricts muscle
Bronchial glands	Decreases secretions	Increases secretions
Salivary glands	Decreases secretions	Increases secretions
Stomach	Decreases motility	Increases motility
Intestines	Decreases motility	Increases motility
Eye	Widens pupils	Constricts pupils

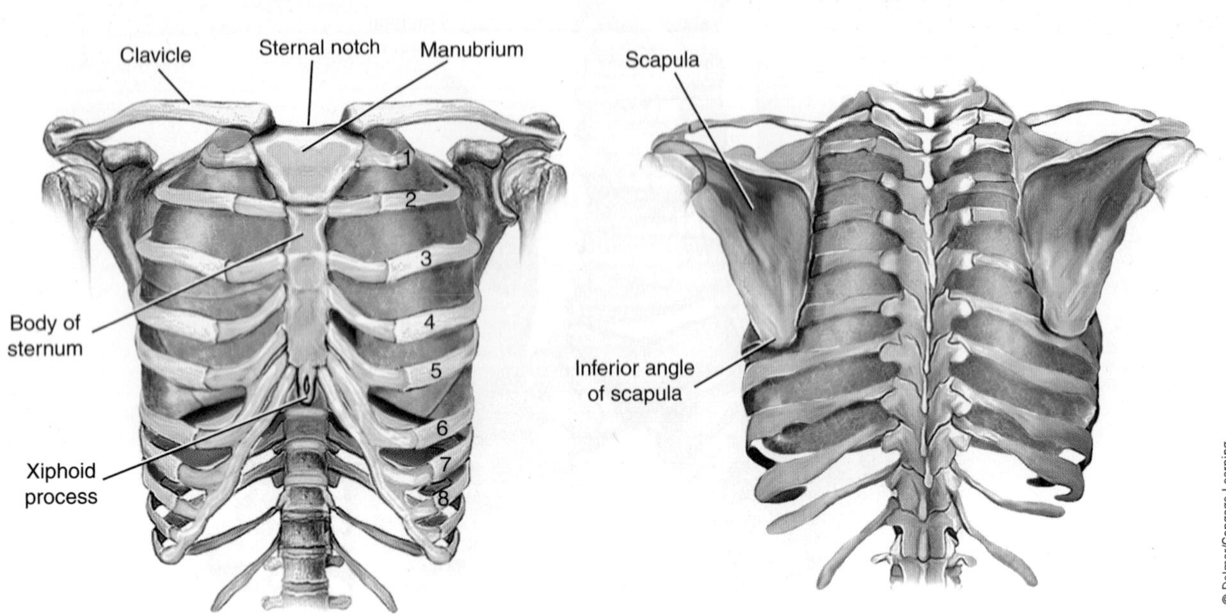

FIGURE 6-20 Anatomical relationship of the lungs and thorax.

to the eleventh rib (two ribs below the scapula) (Figure 6-20). The lungs are shaped to fit into the chest (thorax) along with the heart and mediastinal structures and to accommodate the convex diaphragm (Figure 6-21A). At the mediastinal border is the *hilum*, which allows the right and left main stem bronchi, blood and lymph vessels, and nerves to enter and exit the lungs (Figure 6-21B).

The right lung is larger, heavier, and shorter than the left lung and has three lobes (upper, middle, lower), which are divided by the oblique fissure (between the upper and middle lobes) and the horizontal fissure (middle and lower lobes). The left lung has two lobes, upper and lower, which are divided by the oblique fissure. All of the lobes are subdivided into bronchopulmonary segments (Figure 6-22).

MEDIASTINUM AND PLEURAL MEMBRANES

The *mediastinum* is the cavity between the lungs, sternum (anteriorly), and the thoracic vertebrae (posteriorly). It contains the trachea, heart, major blood vessels (great vessels), nerves, esophagus, thymus gland, and lymph nodes (Figure 6-23).

There are two pleural surfaces. The *visceral pleura* covers the lungs, and the *parietal pleura* covers the inside of the chest wall, the diaphragm, and the mediastinal surfaces (Figure 6-23). The space between the two pleural surfaces, called the *pleural cavity*, contains a small amount of serous fluid that allows smooth movement during breathing. The **lung-thorax relationship** describes the lungs' natural tendency to collapse and the chest wall's natural tendency to expand, which creates a subatmospheric (negative gauge) pressure in the pleural cavity.

THORAX

The *thorax* contains and protects the organs of the cardiopulmonary system. The sternum forms the anterior chest border and is composed of the manubrium, body, and xiphoid process. Twelve pairs of ribs are directly attached posteriorly to the thoracic vertebrae and attached indirectly by costal cartilage anteriorly to the sternum. Ribs 1 through 7 are true ribs, directly attached to the sternum by their cartilage. Ribs 8 through 10 are false ribs, and ribs 11 and 12 are floating ribs (Figure 6-24). Between the ribs are 11 *intercostal spaces*, containing nerves, arteries, and veins located below the lower rib border (Figure 6-25).

DIAPHRAGM AND ACCESSORY MUSCLES OF VENTILATION

Breathing has two primary phases:

- *Inspiration*, which has active muscle use and energy expenditure.
- *Expiration*, which in quiet breathing is a passive recoil of structures with minimal energy expenditure. During increased activity levels, expiration becomes active with the use of accessory muscles.

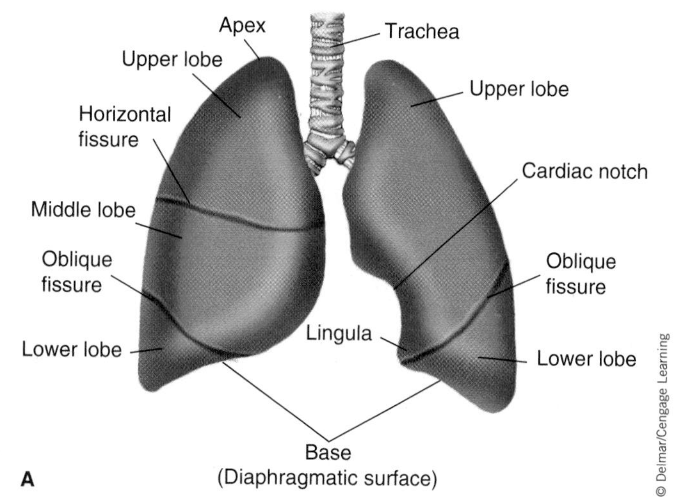

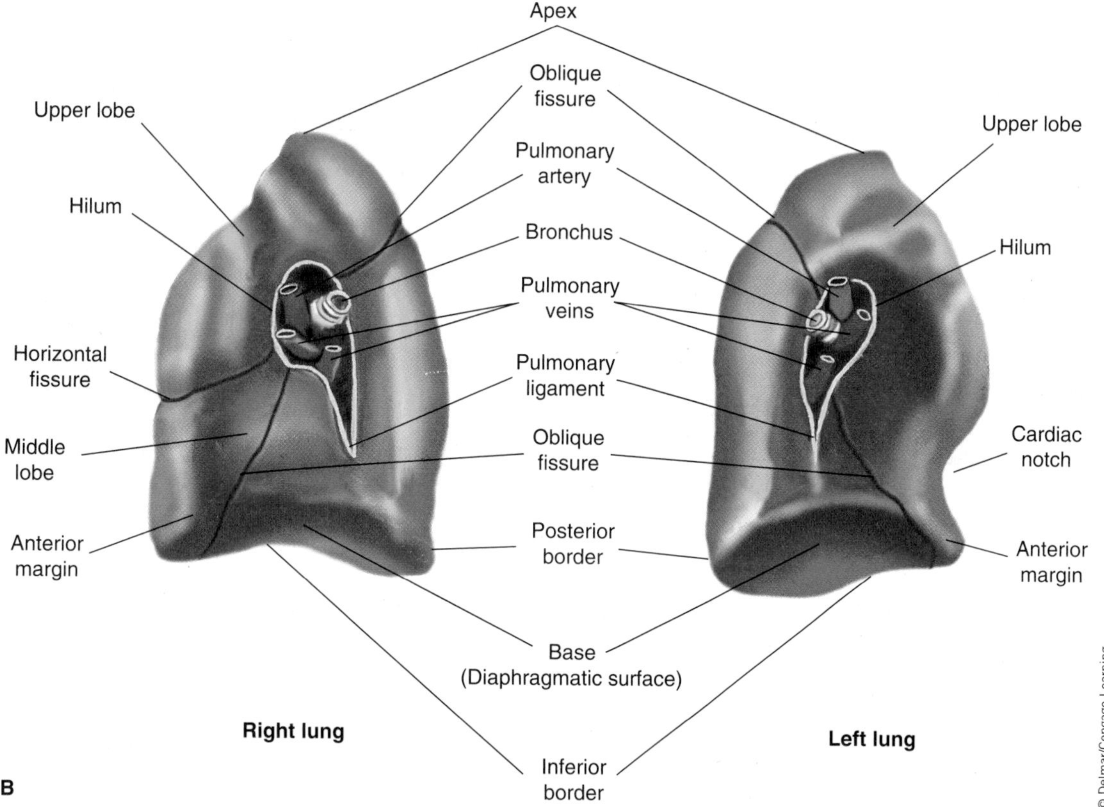

FIGURE 6-21 (A) Anterior view of the lungs. (B) Medial view of the lungs.

The *diaphragm* is the major muscle of respiration. It is made up of two dome-shaped muscles, the right and left hemidiaphragms, that merge into a central tendon. The right hemidiaphragm is slightly higher in the thoracic cavity than the left to allow room for the liver. The diaphragm separates the thoracic and abdominal cavities and is attached from the lumbar vertebrae, the costal margin, and the xiphoid process. Passing through the diaphragm are the esophagus, aorta, nerves, and inferior vena cava. The primary motor innervation of the diaphragm is from the phrenic nerves, which arise from cervical segments 3 through 5

Right lung		Left lung	
Upper lobe		Upper lobe	
Apical	1	Upper division	
Posterior	2	Apical/Posterior	1 & 2
Anterior	3	Anterior	3
Middle lobe		Lower division (lingular)	
Lateral	4	Superior lingula	4
Medial	5	Inferior lingula	5
Lower lobe		Lower lobe	
Superior	6	Superior	6
Medial basal	7	Anterior medial basal	7 & 8
Anterior basal	8	Lateral basal	9
Lateral basal	9	Posterior basal	10
Posterior basal	10		

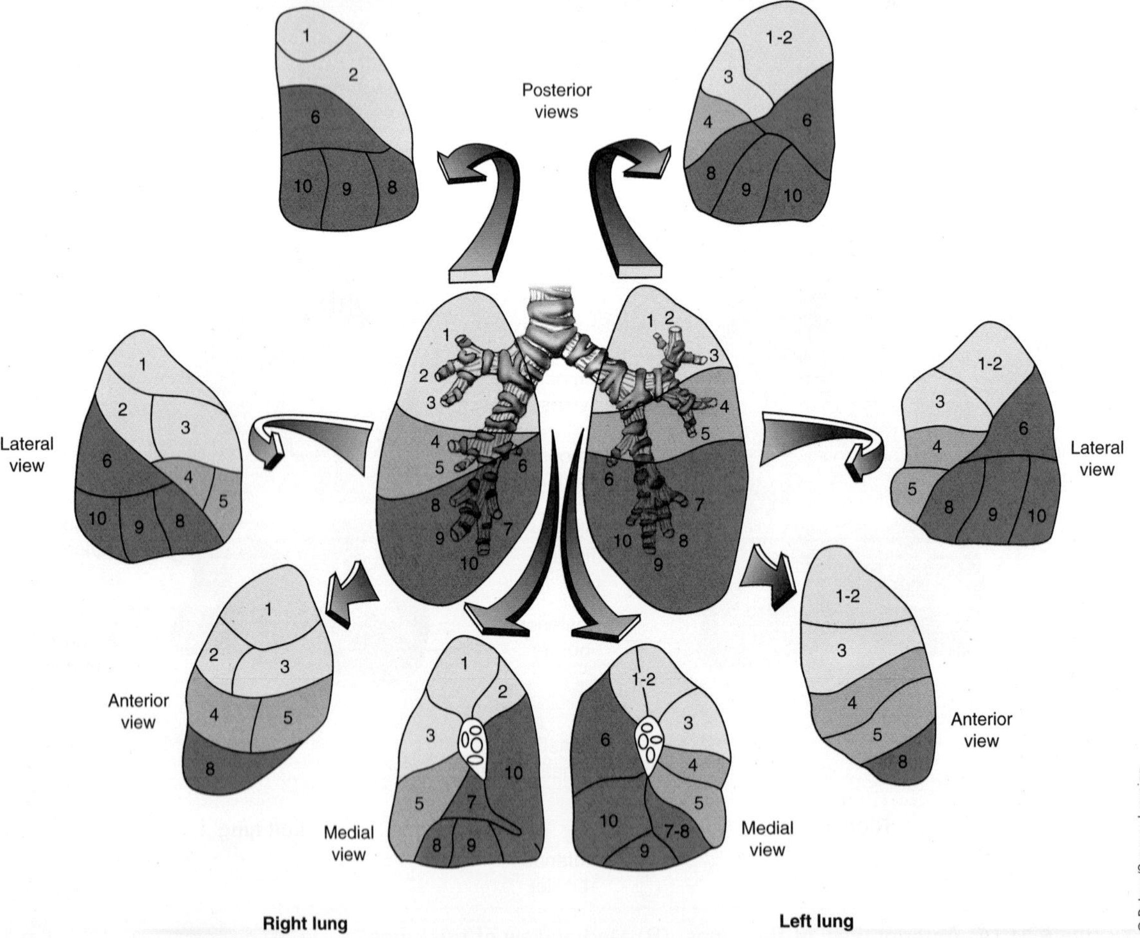

FIGURE 6-22 Lung segments.

(C 3–5), with the lower thoracic nerves also contributing to motor innervation.

When the diaphragm is stimulated, it contracts. The contraction moves the diaphragm downward and the lower ribs outward. This movement increases the thoracic volume, decreases the intrapleural and intra-alveolar pressures in the thorax, and, with a patent (open) airway, allows gas to flow into the lungs. Expiration results when the diaphragm relaxes and returns to its dome shape, thereby increasing pulmonary pressures and causing gas to flow from the lungs.

For normal ventilation, a healthy person can manage ventilation using the diaphragm alone. The accessory muscles of inspiration and expiration are activated to assist the diaphragm when increased

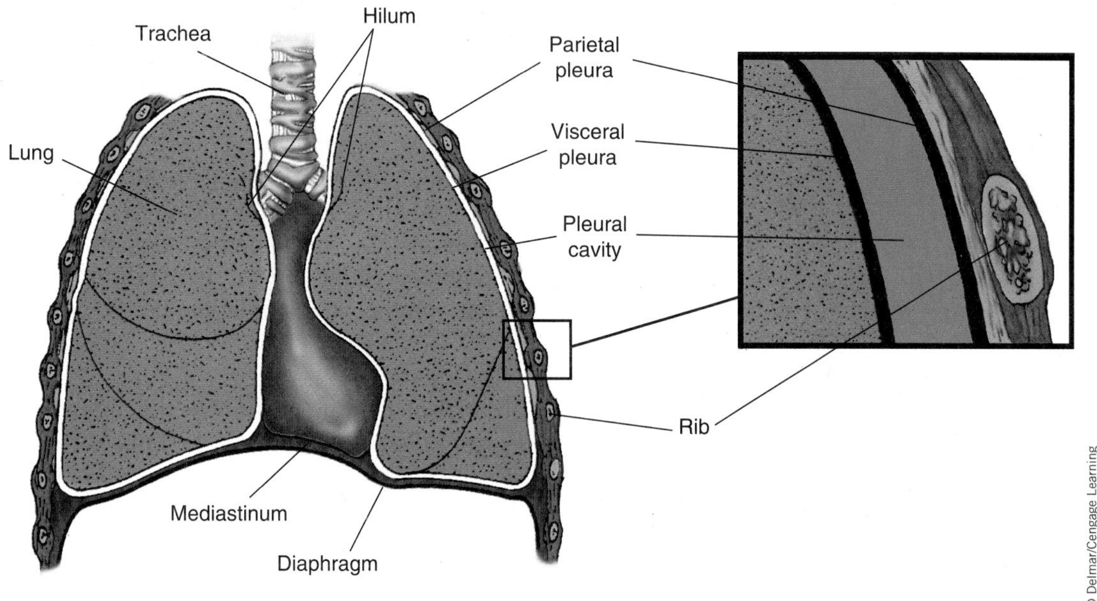

FIGURE 6-23 Major structures around the lungs.

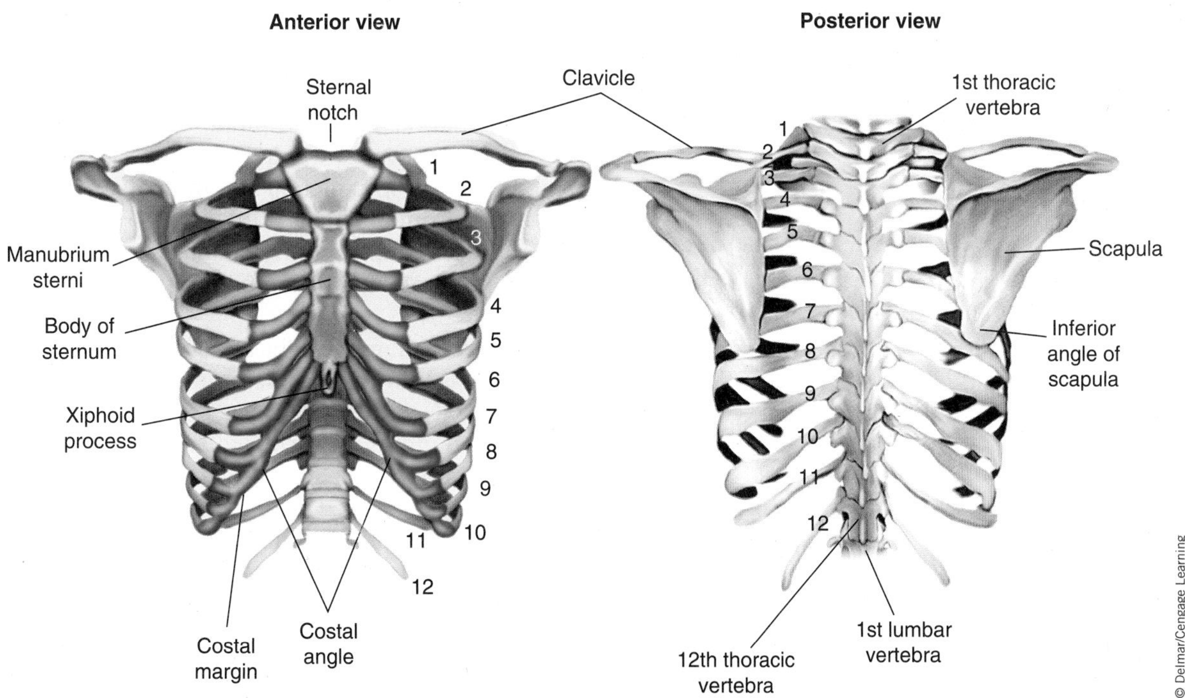

FIGURE 6-24 The thorax.

ventilation is needed, such as during exercise and in chronic obstructive pulmonary disease (COPD) and other disease states. The *accessory muscles of inspiration* generally work to expand the thorax. They include:

- The scalenes (elevate the first and second ribs).
- Sternocleidomastoids (increase the anterioposterior diameter of the chest).
- Pectoralis major muscles (increase the anterioposterior diameter of the chest).
- Trapezius muscles (elevate the thoracic cage).
- External intercostals (increase both lateral and anterioposterior diameters of the thorax).

The *accessory muscles of expiration* generally work to contract the thorax and help to overcome increased airway resistance. They include the:

- Rectus abdominis.
- External abdominis oblique.
- Internal abdominis oblique.

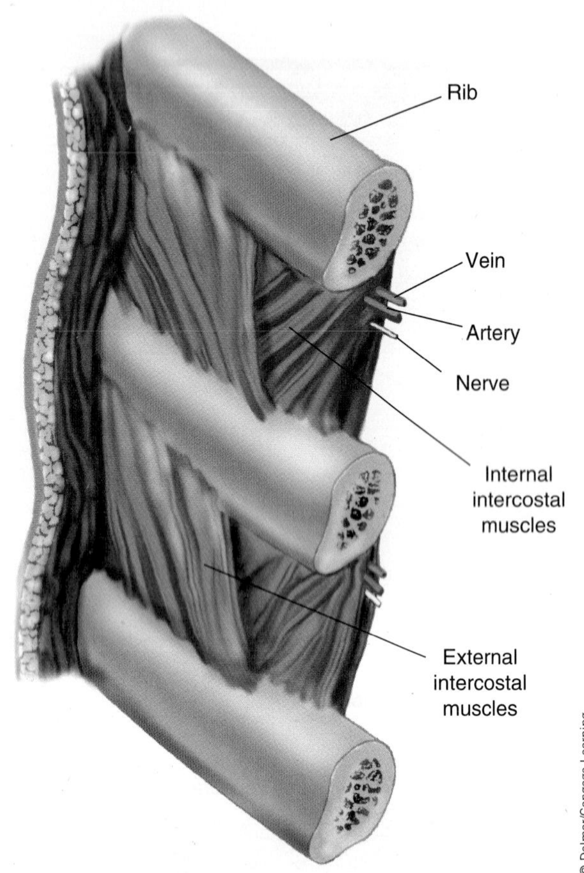

FIGURE 6-25 The intercostal space.

- Transversus abdominis (all four act to push the diaphragm into the thoracic cage).
- Internal intercostals (decrease lateral and anterio-posterior diameters and decrease lung volume).

Ventilation

Ventilation is the bulk movement of air into and out of the lungs. It is responsible for the exchange of oxygen and carbon dioxide between the alveoli and pulmonary capillary blood. The four characteristics describing ventilation are pressure differences, static lung characteristics, dynamic lung characteristics, and ventilatory patterns.

PRESSURE DIFFERENCES ACROSS THE LUNGS

Driving pressure is the difference between two points in a tube and is responsible for fluid movement through a tube. Fluids consist of gases and liquids. Barometric pressure (P_B) is the atmospheric pressure at the mouth and is normally 760 mm Hg at sea level. Transairway pressure (P_{ta}) is the pressure difference between the mouth (P_m), or airway pressure, and the alveolar pressure (P_{alv}). Transpulmonary pressure (P_{tp}), or alveolar distending pressure, is the difference between P_{alv} and pleural pressure (P_{pl}). Transthoracic pressure (P_{tt}) is the difference between P_{alv} and body surface pressure (P_{bs}). Gas flows through the airways because of these pressure differences.

Boyle's Law

Normal breathing is an application of Boyle's law, which states that volume is inversely related to pressure. The body plethysmograph, used to test pulmonary function and to measure total thoracic gas volume, is an application of Boyle's law.

Role of the Diaphragm in Ventilation. The contraction of the diaphragm moves it downward, increasing the thoracic volume and decreasing the intrapleural and intra-alveolar pressures. Gas flows through the tracheobronchial tree to the alveoli, from the higher P_B to the lower P_{alv} until these pressures equalize at end-inspiration. During expiration, the diaphragm relaxes and moves upward, decreasing thoracic volume and increasing intrapleural and intra-alveolar pressures. Gas flows from the lungs until the pressures equalize at end-expiration. The intrapleural pressure is always less than barometric pressure in normal breathing (Figure 6-26).

The normal movement of the diaphragm is about 1.5 cm at rest, with a normal intrapleural pressure drop of −3 to −6 cm H_2O. During a deep inspiration, the diaphragm moves 6–10 cm, with intrapleural pressures dropping as low as −50 cm H_2O (subatmospheric, or negative). For a forced expiration, intrapleural pressure can reach +70 to +100 cm H_2O above (positive) atmospheric pressure.

STATIC CHARACTERISTICS OF THE LUNGS

Static refers to matter at rest and to forces in equilibrium. After a normal expiration, the amount of air in the lungs, the *functional residual capacity* (*FRC*), reflects lung-thorax equilibrium. The two static forces causing an expanded lung to inwardly recoil are the lungs' elastic properties and the surface tension of the alveolar fluid lining layer.

Elastic Properties of the Lungs. Compliance is the volume (in liters, L) change per unit of pressure (cm H_2O) change. Compliance of the lung (C_L) is expressed as liters per centimeter H_2O change and provides the amount of volume attained for each pressure unit

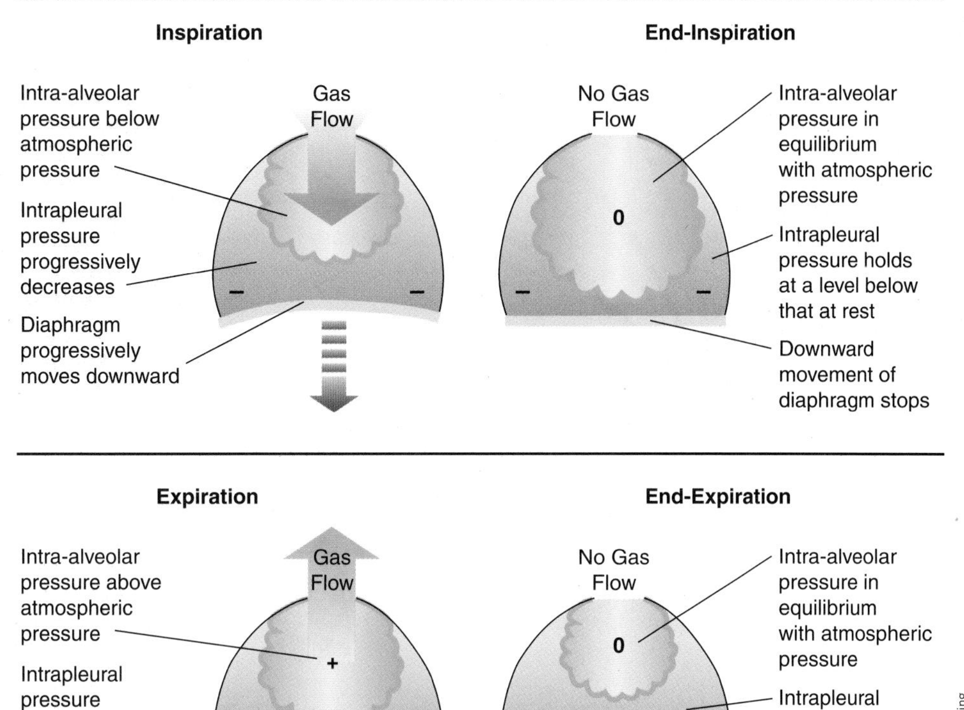

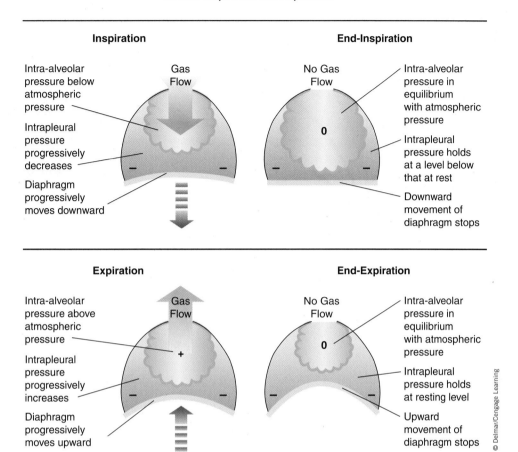

FIGURE 6-26 Diaphragm movement and pressure changes in the lungs during inspiration and expiration.

applied, either negative or positive. Normal lung compliance is 500 mL/5 cm H_2O = 100 mL/cm H_2O, or 0.1 L/cm H_2O.[5] The chest wall normally exerts a small static effect (chest wall compliance, or C_{CW}) that is increased in some diseases affecting the thorax.

Elastance is the lung's attempting to return to its original size and shape when force (pressure) is not being applied. Elastance is the reciprocal of compliance, and the two characteristics are inversely related. When a rubber band is stretched and then allowed to relax, it returns to its original dimensions, as does the lung during quiet expiration. When the lungs collapse, elastance is increased.

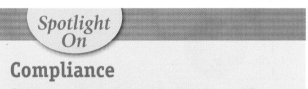

Compliance

Static compliance is measured without airflow. Dynamic compliance is measured using peak inspiratory pressure, which includes the effects of airflow through the tracheobronchial tree (airway resistance). See Figure 6-27 for an illustration of lung volume-pressure changes due to differences in compliance.

Surface Tension, Pulmonary Surfactant, and Effects on Lung Expansion. *Surface tension* is the molecular, cohesive force at the liquid-gas interface in the alveoli, which, if left unchecked, would cause the alveoli to collapse.

LaPlace's law describes the effect of distending pressure on a liquid bubble and is modified for use with alveoli that have one liquid-gas interface.

- The *distending pressure* of a liquid sphere (alveoli) is directly proportional to the liquid's surface tension and inversely proportional to the sphere's radius. Distending pressure varies inversely with the radius of the alveoli (Figure 6-28).
- *Critical opening pressure* is the high pressure needed to initially open a bubble by overcoming its cohesive force, such as blowing up a balloon.

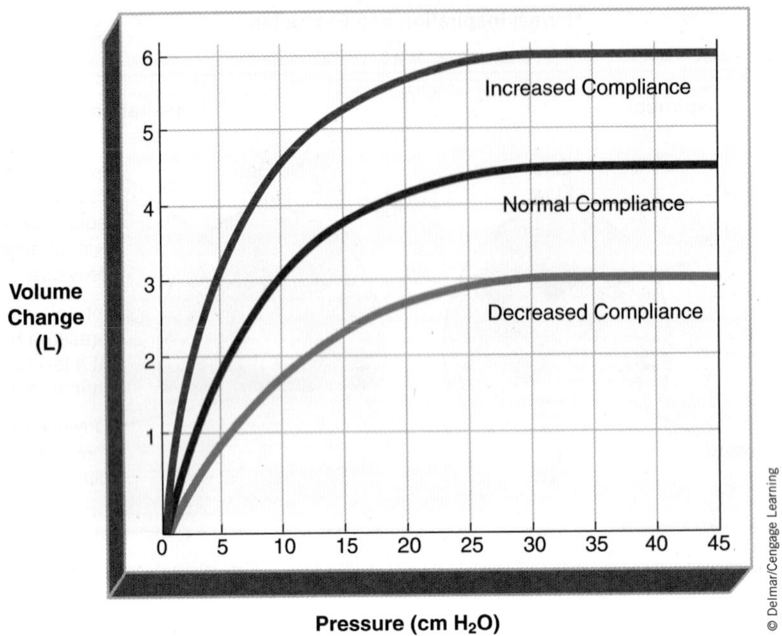

FIGURE 6-27 Lung compliance and volume-pressure curves.

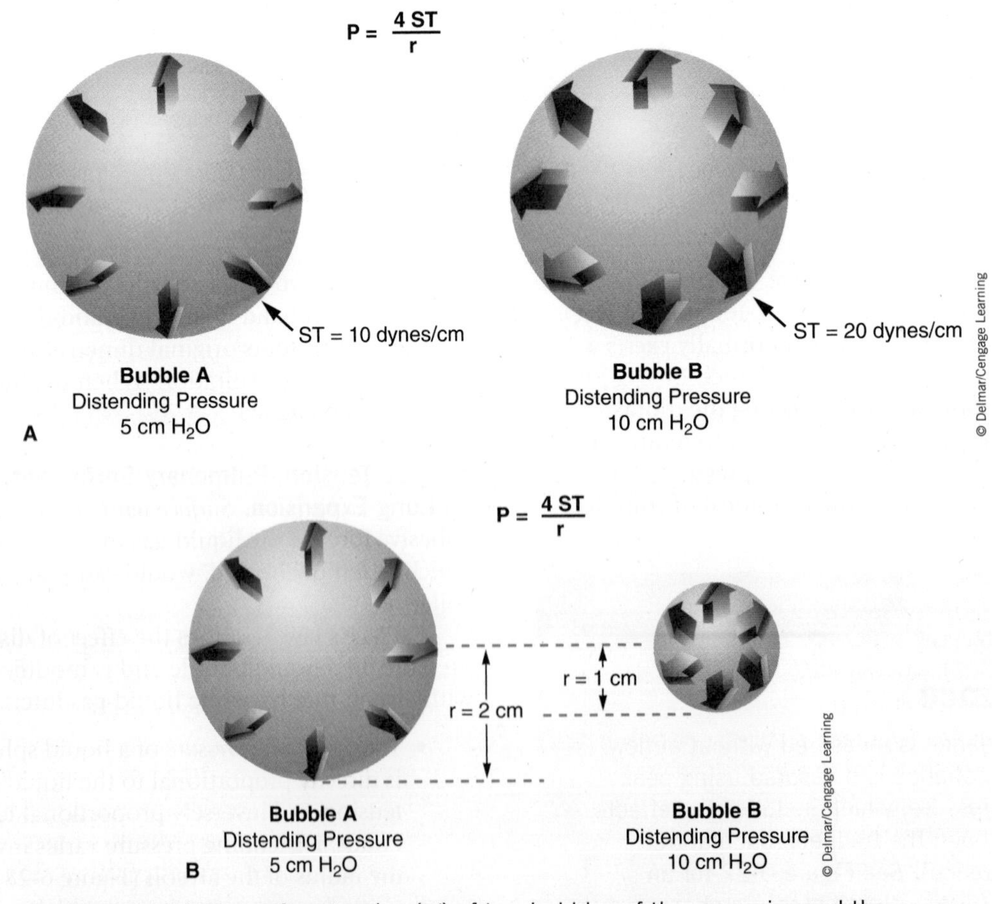

FIGURE 6-28 (A) The surface tension (*st*) of two bubbles of the same size and the distending pressures (*P*) needed to maintain their size. (B) The distending pressure needed to maintain the size of two bubbles of different sizes (r = radius).

When this pressure is reached, the volume rapidly increases with small, incremental pressure increases.
- *Critical closing pressure* is the point at which the liquid cohesive forces exceed the distending pressure and the sphere collapses.

Fortunately, in the healthy lung the natural tendency of the smaller alveoli to collapse is prevented by an extraordinary substance, pulmonary surfactant. *Pulmonary surfactant* is a phospholipid, with a major component being dipalmitoyl phosphatidyl choline. It is produced by the alveolar type II cells and functions to decrease alveolar surface tension in proportion to the ratio of surfactant to alveolar surface area. In alveolar size (volume) changes, surfactant is inversely related to surface area.

- When alveolar volume *increases*, the proportion of surfactant to surface area *decreases* and surface tension increases.
- When alveolar volume *decreases*, the proportion *increases*, decreasing surface tension and maintaining alveolar integrity.

Alveolar surface tension varies from 5 to 50 dynes per centimeter. **Atelectasis** is the collapse of small alveoli. Once collapsed, the alveolar walls with their liquid lining form a strong bond that resists re-expansion. Pulmonary surfactant deficiency results from clinical conditions that cause acidosis, hypoxia, hyperoxia, atelectasis, and pulmonary vascular congestion and from prematurity of the lung.

DYNAMIC CHARACTERISTICS OF THE LUNGS

Dynamic refers to the movement of gas into and out of the lungs and to the related pressure changes. These dynamic factors are Poiseuille's law for flow and pressure and airway resistance. Poiseuille's law describes the relationship between gas flow and pressure through tubes and, when applied to the lung, gas flow through nonrigid airways. During a normal inspiration, the intrapleural pressure decreases by -3 to -6 cm H_2O, causing passive dilation of the airways (increased length, increased diameter, and increased volume). During expiration, passive constriction occurs (decreased length, decreased diameter, and decreased volume). The application of this law shows that gas flow varies to the fourth power of the radius (r^4). If the airway radius is decreased by one-half, the airway pressure must be increased 16-fold to keep the flow constant. In normal breathing, this relation is not a problem. In respiratory disease states, however, bronchial narrowing results in decreased flows and increased pressures, resulting in an increased energy cost of breathing (work of breathing).

Airway Resistance. *Airway resistance* (R_{aw}) is the pressure difference between the mouth and the alveoli (transairway), divided by the flow rate (L/s). The difference is derived from Poiseuille's law. Resistance to airflow (friction) is created as gas molecules come into contact with the inner surface of the airways. Normal R_{aw} is 0.5–2.5 cm H_2O per liter per second.[6] Gas movement through airways can be laminar (streamlined and smooth, found with low flow rates and low pressure differences), turbulent (random and rough, found with high flows and high pressure differences), or transitional (tracheobronchial), a mixed condition found near airway branching.

Time Constants. A *time constant* is the time necessary to inflate an alveolus to 60% of its potential filling capacity and is a product of R_{aw} and C_L (Figure 6-29). Long time constants are found in lung regions with increased R_{aw} or increased C_L. Short time constants are found in regions with decreased R_{aw} or decreased C_L. Filling and emptying of lung regions are important components for normal breathing, and they become more important in respiratory disease, its treatment, and its management. If time constants vary significantly between alveoli and lung regions, so does ventilation.

Dynamic Compliance. *Dynamic compliance* is the change in lung volume divided by the change in transpulmonary pressure as measured by esophageal balloon. Dynamic compliance is measured during gas flow and includes R_{aw}, whereas static compliance is measured without gas flow. Normally the two types of compliance are equal, but with obstructed airways the ratio of dynamic to static compliance falls as the breathing frequency rises. This fall in the ratio occurs because the alveoli distal to the obstruction lack the time to fill because of the increased breathing rate (frequency dependent).

VENTILATORY PATTERNS

The ventilatory pattern consists of the tidal volume (V_T), ventilatory rate (f), and the ratio of inspiratory time (I) to expiratory time (E) (I/E ratio). *Tidal volume* is the volume of air inspired and expired in one normal breath and is equal to 3–4 mL/lb (7–9 mL/kg) of ideal body weight. The normal ventilatory rate (f) for an adult is about 12–20 breaths per minute.[6] The normal I/E ratio is 1:2, with inspiration being active and shorter and expiration passive and longer, including a brief pause before the next inspiration. At a ventilation rate of 20, which is 3 seconds per respiratory cycle, a normal 1:2 I/E ratio equals 1 second for inspiration and 2 seconds for expiration.

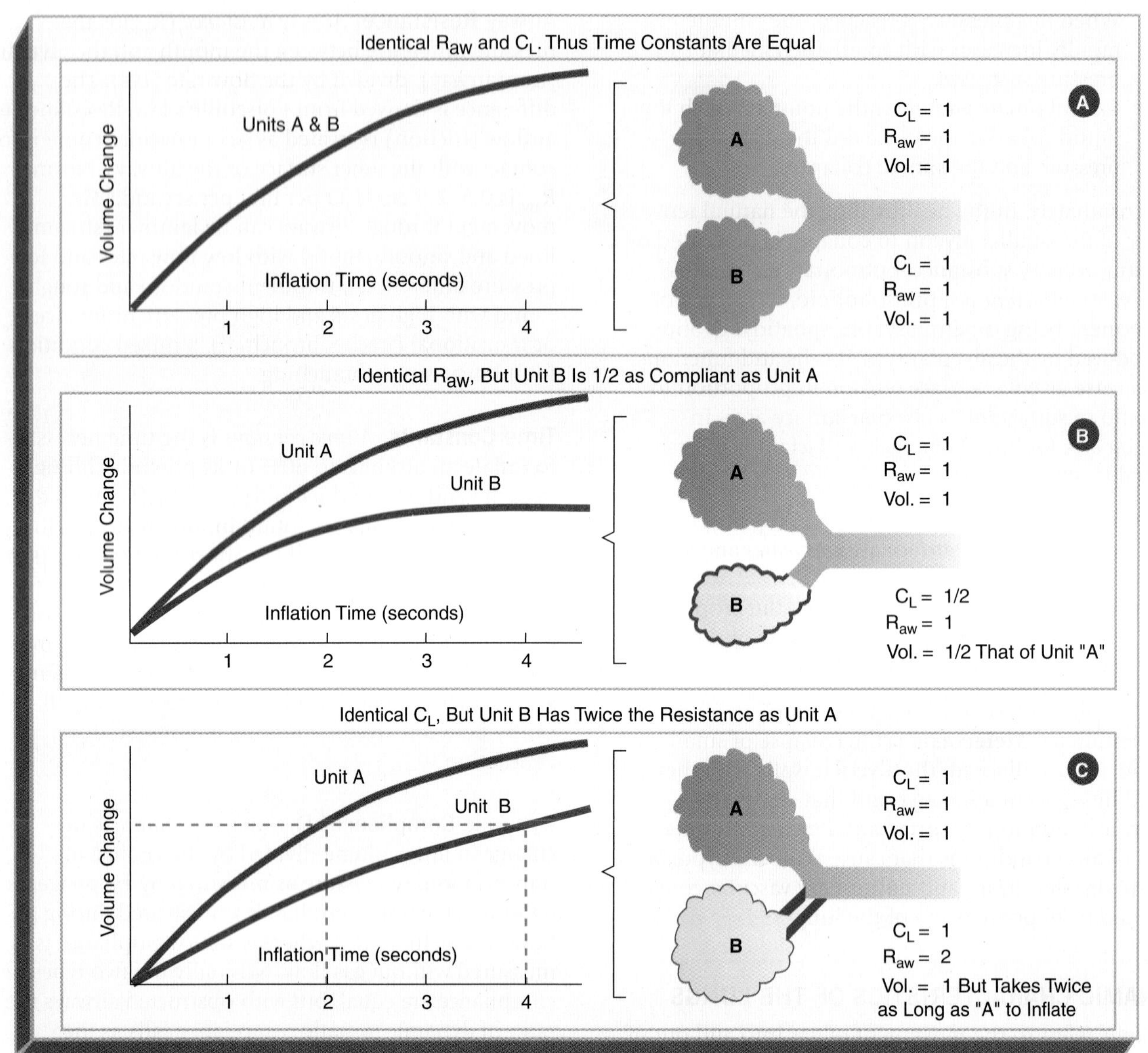

FIGURE 6-29 Time constants.

Minute Ventilation. Minute ventilation, $\dot{V}_E$, is the total volume of gas exhaled (or inhaled) per minute and is computed as $\dot{V}_T \times f$. A normal adult value is 500 mL × 12 f = 6000 mL (6.0 L).

Alveolar Ventilation. Alveolar ventilation ($\dot{V}_A$) is the volume of inspired gas that reaches the alveoli and that is available for gas exchange with pulmonary capillary blood. Minute alveolar ventilation, $\dot{V}_A$, is the volume of fresh gas entering the alveoli each minute and is computed as tidal volume minus dead space ($\dot{V}_D$) × f:

$$\dot{V}_A = (V_T - V_D) \times f$$
$$= (500 \text{ mL} - 150 \text{ mL}) \times 12$$
$$= 350 \text{ mL} \times 12 = 4200 \text{ mL } (4.2\text{L})$$

Dead Space. Dead space ventilation ($\dot{V}_D$) is the volume of gas in the lungs that does not participate in gas exchange. The three types of dead space are anatomic, alveolar, and physiologic.

- *Anatomic dead space* (V_{Danat}) is the volume of gas in the conducting airways and normally equals 1 mL/lb of ideal body weight. For example, a 150-lb person has 150 mL of V_{Danat}. The gas that enters the alveoli is a combination of V_{Danat} and atmospheric (fresh) gas. The fresh gas has to pass through the V_{Danat} to reach the alveoli (Figure 6-30).
- *Alveolar dead space* is the dead space that occurs when an alveolus is ventilated but not perfused with pulmonary capillary blood and therefore is not involved in gas exchange (as in pulmonary emboli).

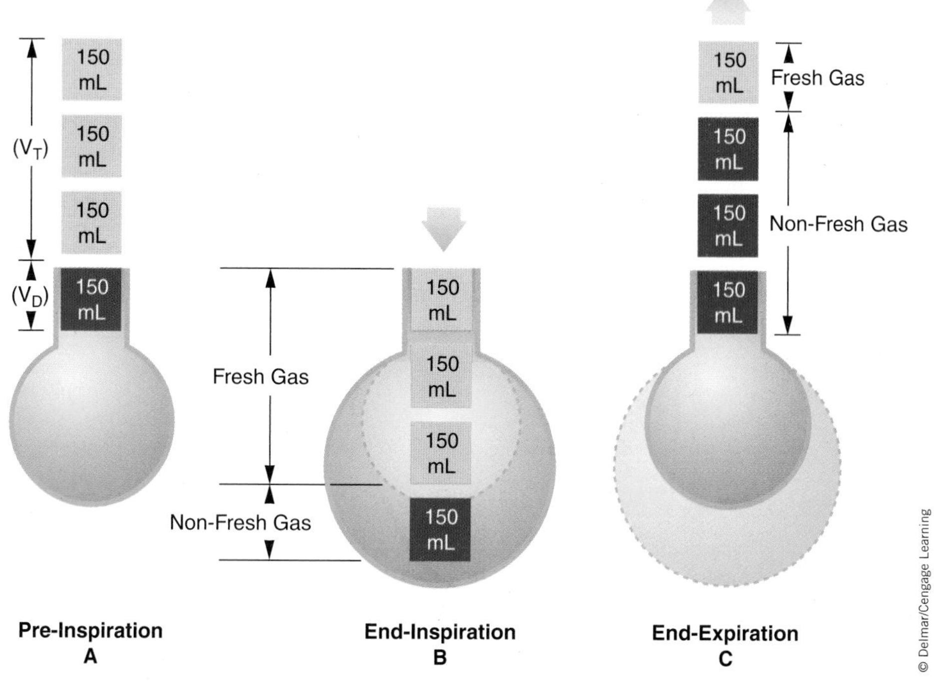

FIGURE 6-30 Relationship of alveolar ventilation and dead space.

- *Physiologic dead space* is the total dead space and is the sum of anatomic plus alveolar dead space.

Regional Differences in Normal Lung Ventilation. For the normal individual, there is an intrapleural pressure difference (gradient) from the lung apex (top) to the lung base (bottom). The lungs are suspended from the hilum and are gravity dependent. The lung bases weigh more than the apexes because of gravity and greater perfusion. This difference results in negative intrapleural pressures of −7 to −10 cm H_2O at the apex and −2 to −3 at the base (Figure 6-31). Alveoli respond to these intrapleural pressure differences and are larger at the apex. The alveoli at the base are smaller but more compliant. In the upright lung, ventilation is favored at the lung bases, where the alveoli have a greater potential to expand and have an increased ratio of surfactant to surface area. This relation is important when ventilation/perfusion matching is considered.

Effect of Airway Resistance and Lung Compliance on Ventilatory Patterns. The ventilatory pattern adopted by an individual is based on minimum work requirements rather than on efficiency. Normally, about 5% of an individual's total energy expenditure (5% of the oxygen uptake) is used for breathing. When lung compliance decreases, the ventilatory rate increases, and the tidal volume decreases, producing a rapid, shallow breathing pattern. When airway resistance increases, ventilatory rate usually decreases and tidal volume increases, producing a slower and deeper pattern that allows more time for exhalation.

Recognition of ventilatory patterns is important for respiratory care practice.

- *Eupnea* is normal, spontaneous breathing.
- *Apnea* is the complete lack of spontaneous breathing.
- *Hyperpnea* is an increased volume of breathing, with or without an increased ventilatory rate.
- *Hyperventilation* is any breathing pattern that results in a decreased arterial blood partial pressure of carbon dioxide (P_aCO_2).
- *Hypoventilation* is any breathing pattern that results in an increased arterial blood P_aCO_2.
- *Tachypnea* is a rapid rate of breathing.
- *Dyspnea* is difficulty in breathing, of which the individual is aware (subjective).

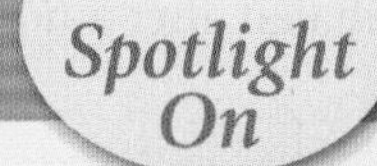

Breathing Pattern

Breathing pattern can dramatically affect alveolar ventilation (Table 6-3). An increased depth of breathing is far more effective in increasing total alveolar ventilation than an equivalent increase in breathing rate.

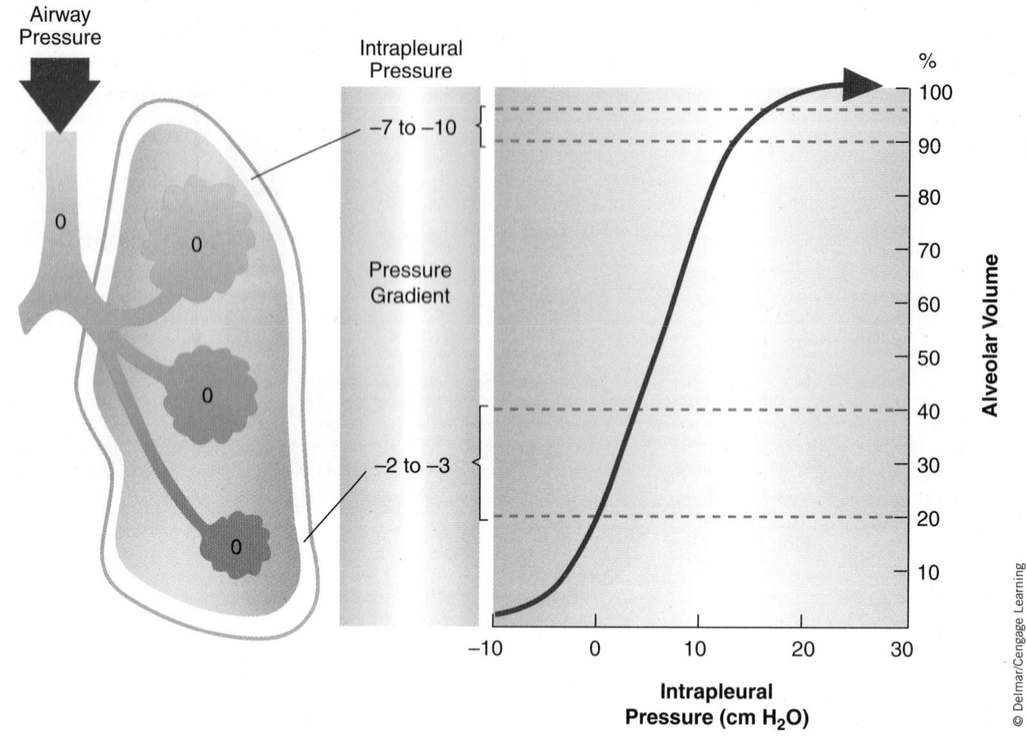

FIGURE 6-31 The intrapleural pressure gradient in the upright position.

Pulmonary Function Measurements

Pulmonary function measurements are an important application of assessing respiratory physiology. These include testing for lung volumes and capacities, flow rates, oxygen diffusion capacity, pulmonary mechanics, arterial blood gases and pH, and more specialized measurements, such as distribution of ventilation and blood flow.

LUNG VOLUMES

The total amount of air the lungs can hold is divided into four distinct lung volumes (Figure 6-32).

- *Tidal volume* (V_T) is the amount of air that moves into and out of the lungs in one normal breath.
- *Inspiratory reserve volume* (IRV) is the maximum amount of air that can be inhaled after a normal tidal volume inspiration.
- *Expiratory reserve volume* (ERV) is the maximum volume of air that can be exhaled after normal tidal volume expiration.
- *Residual volume* (RV) is the amount of air remaining in the lungs after a maximal expiration.

LUNG CAPACITIES

Lung capacities are combinations of two or more lung volumes or capacities (Figure 6-32).

- *Vital capacity* (*VC*) is the volume of air that can be exhaled after a maximal inspiration (*IRV* + V_T + *ERV*), or the amount of air that can be inhaled after a maximum exhalation.
- *Inspiratory capacity* (*IC*) is the volume of air that can be inhaled after a normal expiration (V_T + *IRV*).
- *Functional residual capacity* (*FRC*) is the volume of air remaining in the lungs after a normal expiration (*ERV* + *RV*) and is called the *resting level*.

TABLE 6-3 **Effect of breathing depth and frequency on alveolar ventilation**

Subject	Breathing Depth ($\dot{V}_T$) (mL)	Breathing Frequency (breaths/min)	Total Minute Ventilation (mL/min)	Total Dead Space Ventilation (mL/min)	Alveolar Ventilation (mL/min)
A	150	40	6000	150 × 40 = 6000	0
B	500	12	6000	150 × 12 = 1800	4200
C	1000	6	6000	150 × 6 = 9000	5100

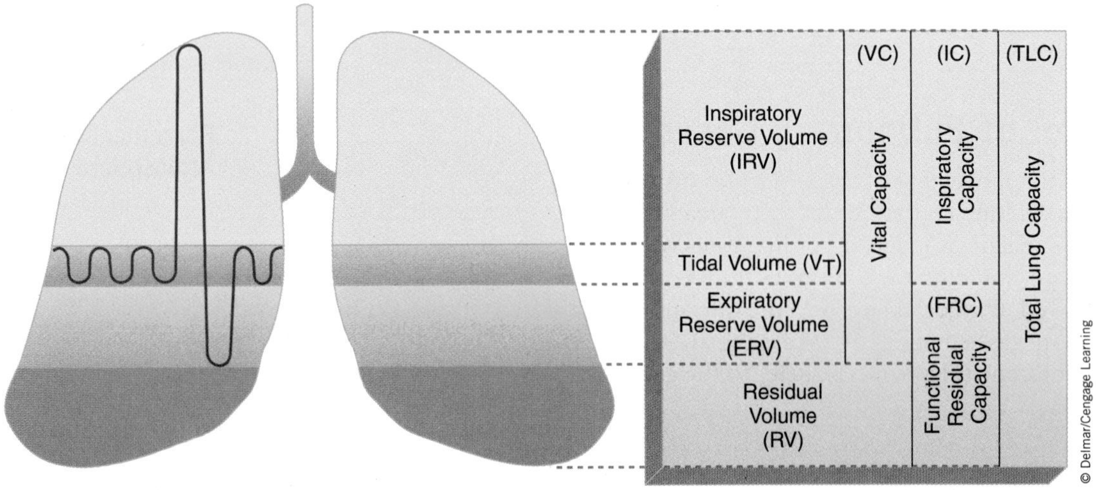

FIGURE 6-32 Normal lung volumes and capacities.

- *Total lung capacity* (*TLC*) is the maximum amount of air that the lungs can hold (*IC* + *FRC*).
- The ratio of residual volume to total lung capacity (*RV*/*TLC* × 100) is the percentage of the *TLC* occupied by the *RV*.

Normal lung volumes and capacities are listed in Table 6-4.

Measurements of pulmonary function, lung volumes, and lung capacities are important for patient assessment and treatment. Pulmonary function testing (see Chapter 17) is an important assessment and is used to identify the two primary types of lung disorder: obstructive (decreased expiratory flow rates) and restrictive (decreased volumes). In an *obstructive lung disorder*, *RV*, *FRC*, and *RV*/*TLC* are increased, and the *VC*, *IC*, *IRV*, and *ERV* are decreased. In a *restrictive lung disorder*, the *VC*, *IC*, *RV*, *FRC*, V_T, and *TLC* are all

Patient Assessment

Patient assessment is based on observing signs and symptoms, interviewing the patient for detail and clarity, and performing a physical assessment. The physical assessment includes chest examination, palpation, percussion, auscultation of the lungs, and review of pulmonary function study results. Comparison of the clinical findings with normal functions and values allows setting initial patient care plans and the trending of information for long-range patient management.

TABLE 6-4 **Approximate lung volumes and capacities in the average normal subject between 20 and 30 years of age**

	Male		Female	
Measurement	mL	Approximate Percentage of TLC	mL	Approximate Percentage of TLC
Tidal volume (V_T)	500	8–10	400–500	8–10
Inspiratory reserve volume (*IRV*)	3100	50	1900	30
Expiratory reserve volume (*ERV*)	1200	20	800	20
Residual volume (*RV*)	1200	20	1000	25
Vital capacity (*VC*)	4800	80	3200	75
Inspiratory capacity (*IC*)	3600	60	2400	60
Functional residual capacity (*FRC*)	2400	40	1800	40
Total lung capacity (*TLC*)	6000		4200	
Residual volume total lung capacity ratio (*RV*/*TLC* × 100)	6000	20	4200	25

decreased. Individuals may also have both types of disorder (*mixed disorder*).

Diffusion of Pulmonary Gases

Diffusion is the movement of gas molecules from an area of relatively high concentration to an area of low concentration. Each gas moves according to its own partial pressure gradients and continues until equilibrium is achieved. Oxygen and carbon dioxide are the two pulmonary gases that diffuse across the alveolar-capillary membrane (Figure 6-33). Refer to the gas laws in Chapter 3.

PARTIAL PRESSURES OF OXYGEN, CARBON DIOXIDE, AND WATER VAPOR

The weight of the atmospheric gases on the earth's surface is the barometric pressure (P_B), or atmospheric pressure. The normal value at sea level is 760 mm Hg. Barometric pressure decreases as elevation increases (when you are, say, climbing a mountain) and increases below the water's surface (diving). The percentage concentration of the atmospheric gases remains constant at high and low elevations (Table 6-5).

The partial pressures (P) of gases in an atmosphere are defined by Dalton's law of partial pressures. Table 6-6 displays the partial pressures of gases in the air, alveoli, and blood. Note that the partial pressures of oxygen (159 vs. 100) and of carbon dioxide (0.2 vs. 40) are quite different in the atmosphere and alveoli. As

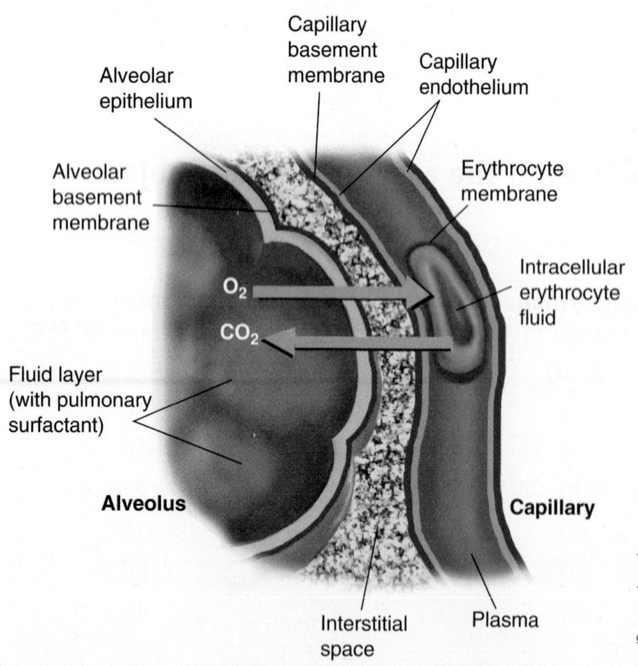

FIGURE 6-33 The alveolar-capillary membrane.

TABLE 6-5 Gases that compose the barometric pressure

Gas	Percentage of Atmosphere	Partial Pressure (mm Hg)
Nitrogen (N_2)	78.08	593
Oxygen (O_2)	20.95	159
Argon (Ar)	0.93	7
Carbon dioxide (CO_2)	0.03	0.2

oxygen diffuses into the alveoli, it is diluted with carbon dioxide (which diffuses from capillaries) and water vapor, both of which are higher than atmospheric pressure levels. Water existing as a gas (water vapor) exerts a partial pressure (pH_2O) of 47 mm Hg in the alveoli; that value represents 100% saturation at 37°C (body temperature). This water vapor weighs 44 mg/L. The balance of the atmosphere is composed of nitrogen (78%) and trace gases that are considered physiologically inactive.

IDEAL ALVEOLAR GAS EQUATION

The alveolar oxygen partial pressure, or tension, is computed for clinical use. The ideal alveolar gas equation for a normal individual breathing room air (room air has an oxygen concentration of 0.21, or 21%) is:

$$
\begin{aligned}
P_AO_2 &= F_IO_2 \times (P_B - PH_2O) - P_QCO_2 \times (1/R) \\
&= 0.21\ (760 - 47) - (40 \times 1.25) \\
&= (0.21 \times 713) - 50 \\
&= 150 - 50 \\
&= 100 \text{ mm Hg}
\end{aligned}
$$

where P_AO_2 is the partial pressure of oxygen in the alveoli, P_B is barometric pressure, PH_2O is water vapor pressure, F_IO_2 is the fractional concentration of inspired oxygen, and P_aCO_2 is the partial pressure of arterial carbon dioxide.[7] The factor 1.25 (R) represents variations in the F_IO_2 in the calculation of the respiratory exchange ratio (RR). The normal RR is 0.8 and is the comparison of 200 mL CO_2/minute diffusing into the alveoli divided by 250 mL O_2/minute diffusing into the capillaries (oxygen uptake). The detailed equation uses $1/R$, which equals $1 \div 0.8$, resulting in 1.25.

DIFFUSION OF OXYGEN AND CARBON DIOXIDE

Gas diffuses through the thin (0.36–2.5-μm) alveolar-capillary membrane, which has nine layers, as listed in Figure 6-33. In a healthy person, mixed venous

TABLE 6-6 **Partial pressure (mm Hg) of gases in the air, alveoli, and blood at standard pressure and temperature**

Gas	Dry Air	Alveolar Gas	Arterial Blood	Venous Blood
PO_2	159.0	100.0	95.0	40.0
PCO_2	0.2	40.0	40.0	46.0
PH_2O (water vapor)	0.0	47.0	47.0	47.0
PN_2 (and other gases in minute quantities)	600.8	573.0	573.0	573.0
Total	760.0	760.0	755.0	706.0

capillary blood (returned from the body) has a P_aCO_2 of 46 mm Hg and P_VO_2 of 40 mm Hg (P_VO_2 is venous oxygen). This mixed venous blood flows past alveoli and, within 0.25 second, via diffusion achieves values of 40 mm Hg and 100 mm Hg for carbon dioxide and oxygen, respectively (Figure 6-34). The pressure gradients are 6 mm Hg for PCO_2 (46 − 40) and 60 mm Hg for PO_2 (100 − 40).[1]

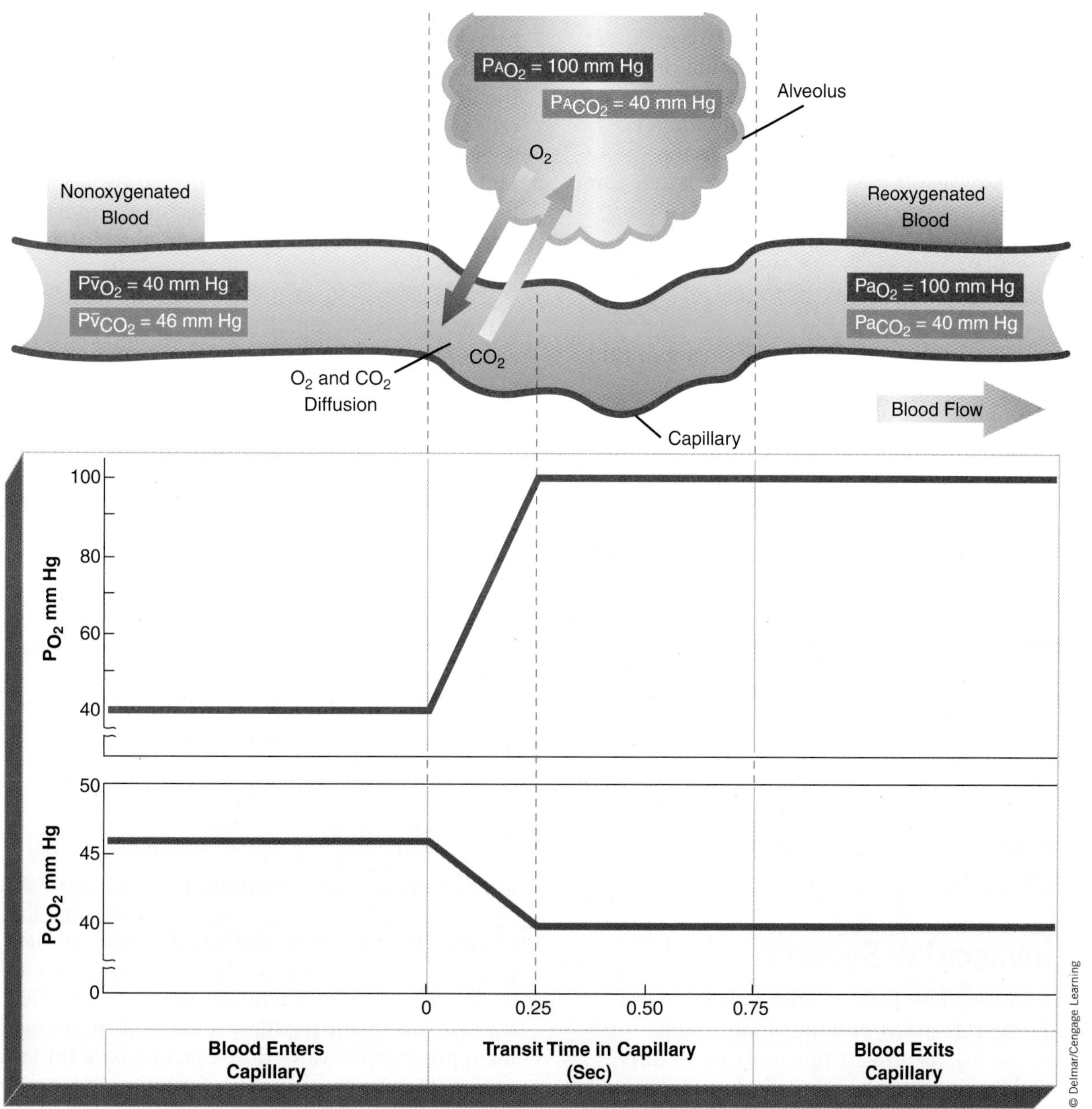

FIGURE 6-34 Alveolar-capillary gas exchange.

The average total time for blood to perfuse an alveolus is about 0.75 second, which leaves about a quarter of a second in reserve to meet increased gas exchange needs, such as during exercise or stress. With lung disease (fibrosis, pulmonary edema), the diffusion transit time may be lengthened, and gas equilibration may not be achieved (see Chapter 3). Basically, three situations decrease diffusion across the alveolar-capillary membrane: (1) decreased alveolar surface area, (2) decreased P_IO_2 or P_AO_2, and (3) increased alveolar-capillary thickness. The administration of increased amounts of inhaled oxygen can improve diffusion of oxygen by increasing the P_AO_2.

PERFUSION-LIMITED OR DIFFUSION-LIMITED OXYGEN

Perfusion-limited gas flow is the transfer of oxygen across the alveolar wall as a function of the amount of blood flow (perfusion) past the alveoli. Once equilibrium is reached, diffusion stops and resumes only when new perfusion occurs. *Diffusion-limited gas flow* is the movement of gas across the alveolar wall as a function of the alveolar-capillary membrane integrity (diffusion characteristics). Carbon monoxide (CO) is used to evaluate the lung's diffusing capacity (normal capacity is 25 mL/minute/mm Hg). As CO moves through the alveolar-capillary membrane and enters the red blood cell, it rapidly attaches chemically to hemoglobin (210 times faster than oxygen). Affinity is the natural attraction and measure of binding strength for oxygen and carbon monoxide to combine with hemoglobin. Once oxygen chemically combines with hemoglobin, the combined **oxyhemoglobin** no longer exerts a partial pressure.

When oxygen diffuses across the alveolar wall and dissolves in blood plasma as PO_2, it enters the red blood cell, combining chemically with hemoglobin. Hemoglobin quickly becomes saturated, oxygen stops entering the red blood cell, and the plasma PO_2 rises. Under normal circumstances, the diffusion of oxygen is perfusion limited. When an individual has a decreased cardiac output or anemia (decreased hemoglobin), the perfusion limitation may become significant. Under certain abnormal conditions, however, oxygen transfer may become diffusion limited (as in pulmonary edema).

Cardiovascular System

The *cardiovascular* (*circulatory*) *system* consists of the blood, the heart (cardio), and the blood vessels (vascular system). Its primary functions are to carry oxygen and nutrients to all body cells, to collect and remove metabolic waste products and carbon dioxide from the body, and to carry substances such as hormones from one part of the body to another.

BLOOD

Blood consists of 55% fluid (plasma) and 45% blood cells.[8] Serum is plasma without the factors involved with clotting. The blood contains specialized cells: erythrocytes (red blood cells, RBCs), leukocytes (white blood cells, WBCs), and thrombocytes (platelets).

The *erythrocytes* (RBCs) contain hemoglobin, which is a major carrier of oxygen and carbon dioxide. Red blood cells are made in the red bone marrow. The comparison of RBCs to total blood volume is called *hematocrit*, a viscosity measurement. Normal values are 45% for males and 42% for females.

Leukocytes (WBCs) function to protect the body from invaders, such as foreign bodies and bacteria, and include the polymorphonuclear granulocytes (neutrophils, eosinophils, basophils) and mononuclear cells (monocytes, lymphocytes). The *differential count* is the number of each type of WBC in 100 WBCs. Neutrophils and monocytes destroy bacteria; eosinophils become elevated in an allergic reaction; and lymphocytes produce antibodies that respond to antigens (invaders).

Platelets are cell fragments that cause blood clotting at trauma sites, stimulate smooth muscle contraction, and reduce blood flow (perfusion).

HEART

The heart is a muscular pump with four hollow chambers, valves, circulation, and an electrical conductive system (Figure 6-35). The two upper chambers, called *atria* (right, left), are separated by a muscular *interatrial septum*, or wall. The two lower chambers, or *ventricles* (right, left), are separated by the *interventricular septum*. The right atrium and right ventricle act as a single pump for sending underoxgenated blood to the lungs (pulmonary circulation); the left atrium and left ventricle work together circulating oxygenated blood to the body (systemic circulation).

Blood Flow Through the Heart. *Venous blood* (low oxygen, high carbon dioxide) returning from the body enters the right atrium from the superior vena cava and inferior vena cava and passes through the *tricuspid* (three-leaved) *valve* into the right ventricle (Figure 6-35). The tricuspid is a one-way valve stabilized by the chordae tendineae, which are attached to the ventricle by the papillary muscles. This arrangement prevents the valve from opening back into the atrium, thereby preventing regurgitation of blood back into the atrium. When the ventricles contract, the

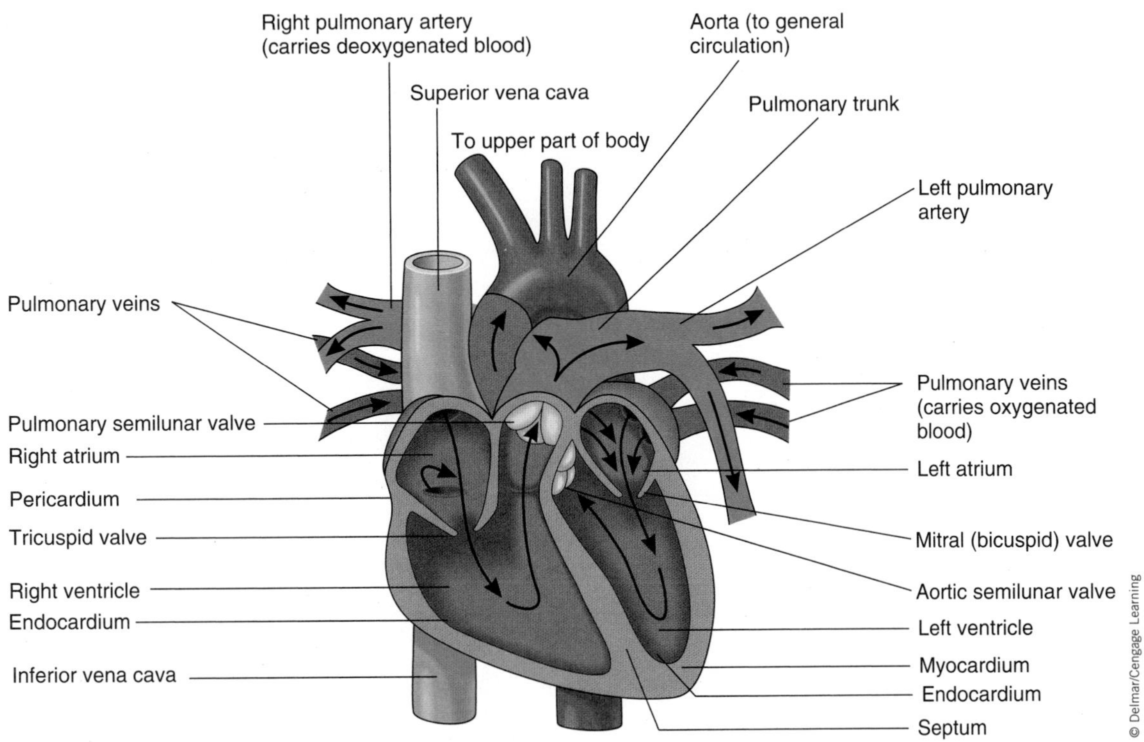

FIGURE 6-35 Blood flow through the heart.

tricuspid valve closes, and blood is sent through the *pulmonary valve* to the *pulmonary artery* and the lungs for oxygenation.

The blood returns from the lungs via the pulmonary veins and enters the left atrium before it goes through the mitral (bicuspid) valve to the left ventricle. The mitral valve is stabilized the same way as the tricuspid and prevents blood regurgitation back to the left atrium. When the left ventricle contracts, blood passes through the *aortic valve* and enters the *aorta*, the largest artery for distribution throughout the body. Both the pulmonary and aortic valves are one-way valves.

The atria contract slightly to increase emptying. However, when the ventricles contract (to eject blood) and then relax, they create a pressure drop inside the chamber that sucks most of the blood from the atria for efficient ventricular filling. The left ventricle's wall is thicker than the right ventricle's because it must pump against a higher resistance (aorta, arteries) and through the larger, whole body system.

The Heart Blood Supply. The heart receives systemic blood directly from the aorta through the left and right *coronary arteries*. These arteries are the first two branches off the aorta. The left coronary artery divides into the circumflex and anterior descending branches. About 5% of resting cardiac output passes through the coronary arteries to serve the heart. The coronary arteries cover the heart much as your fingers do when gripping a baseball.

The Heart Conducting System. The cardiac muscle has a special property, **automaticity**, or autorhythmicity, that enables it to initiate its own beat without outside stimulation. The heart's conducting system includes the sinoatrial (SA) node, atrioventricular (AV) node, bundle of His, right and left bundle branches, and Purkinje fibers (Figure 6-36). The *SA node* (pacemaker) in the right upper part of the right atrium sends an electrical impulse through the atrial muscles, resulting in simultaneous atrial contraction and blood flow to the ventricles. The *AV node*, located in the lower right atrium, receives the impulse and sends it to the ventricles via the bundle of His. The *bundle of His* then divides into the right and left bundle branches, and they further divide into the *Purkinje fibers*, which stimulate the ventricles to contract simultaneously. The autonomic nervous system also controls cardiac activity levels and contractions to meet always-changing bodily requirements. The cardiac centers of the medulla oblongata control cardiac acceleration (sympathetic) and inhibition (parasympathetic) to meet varying needs. Depolarization and repolarization of cardiac muscle can be recorded by chest electrodes. The resultant measurement is called an *electrocardiogram* (see Chapter 19).

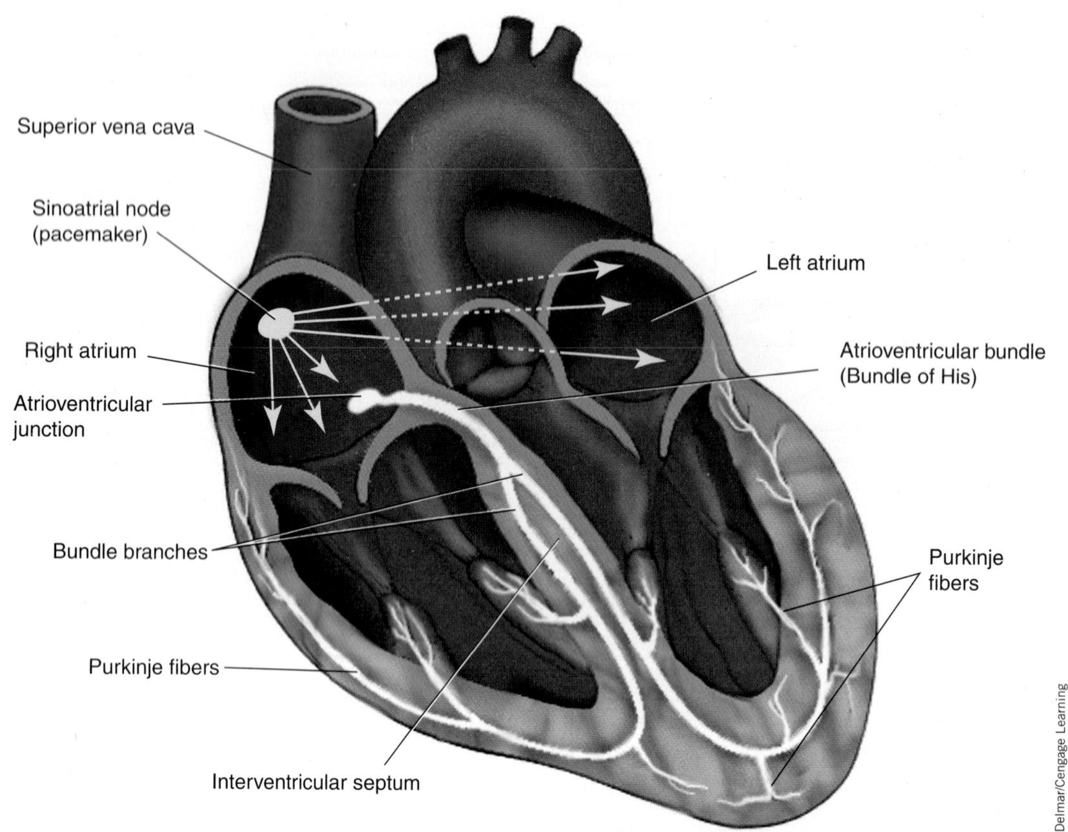

FIGURE 6-36 The conduction system of the heart.

PULMONARY AND SYSTEMIC VASCULAR SYSTEMS

The overall vascular system is divided into two subdivisions: the pulmonary vascular system (pulmonary artery to left atrium) and the systemic vascular system (aorta to right atrium).

Vascular structures become progressively smaller from arteries to arterioles to capillaries, and then increase in size from capillaries to venules to veins (Figure 6-37). Arteries carry blood away from the heart, can handle high systemic pressures, and divide into smaller arterioles that help regulate blood pressure. Small arterioles divide into thin-walled capillaries that allow gases, nutrients, and wastes to move through them. In the pulmonary capillaries, gases move between the air and the blood (external respiration); in the systemic capillaries, gases move between the blood and tissues (internal respiration). Venules collect the capillary blood and empty into veins. Veins carry blood toward the heart. They can hold large amounts of blood (about 60% of the body's blood volume) at small pressure changes (Figure 6-38).

Neural Control of the Vascular System. The blood vessels—primarily the arteries, arterioles, and, to a lesser extent, the veins—continuously receive sympathetic impulses from the vasomotor center in the medulla oblongata. These impulses result in a moderate contracted state called *vasomotor tone*. Blood flow through arteries is also affected by arterial baroreceptors (pressure receptors), by blood volume, and by the large veins through changes in intrathoracic and abdominal pressures.

> *Age-Specific Competency*
>
> **Normal Heart Rates**
>
> The normal heart rate is 60–100 beats per minute (bpm) for adults. It is affected by exercise, altitude, and disease states. The normal infant heart rate ranges from 100–190 bpm and averages 140 bpm.

The Baroreceptor Reflex. *Baroreceptors*, or *pressoreceptors*, located in the carotid arteries and aorta, contain nerve endings that sense the stretching of their walls. They respond by reflex action to maintain the most efficient and effective heart rate, force of cardiac contraction, arterial and venous constriction, and arterial blood pressure. When they sense decreased blood pressure, with a related decrease in stretch, the baroreceptors increase impulses to the medulla, which

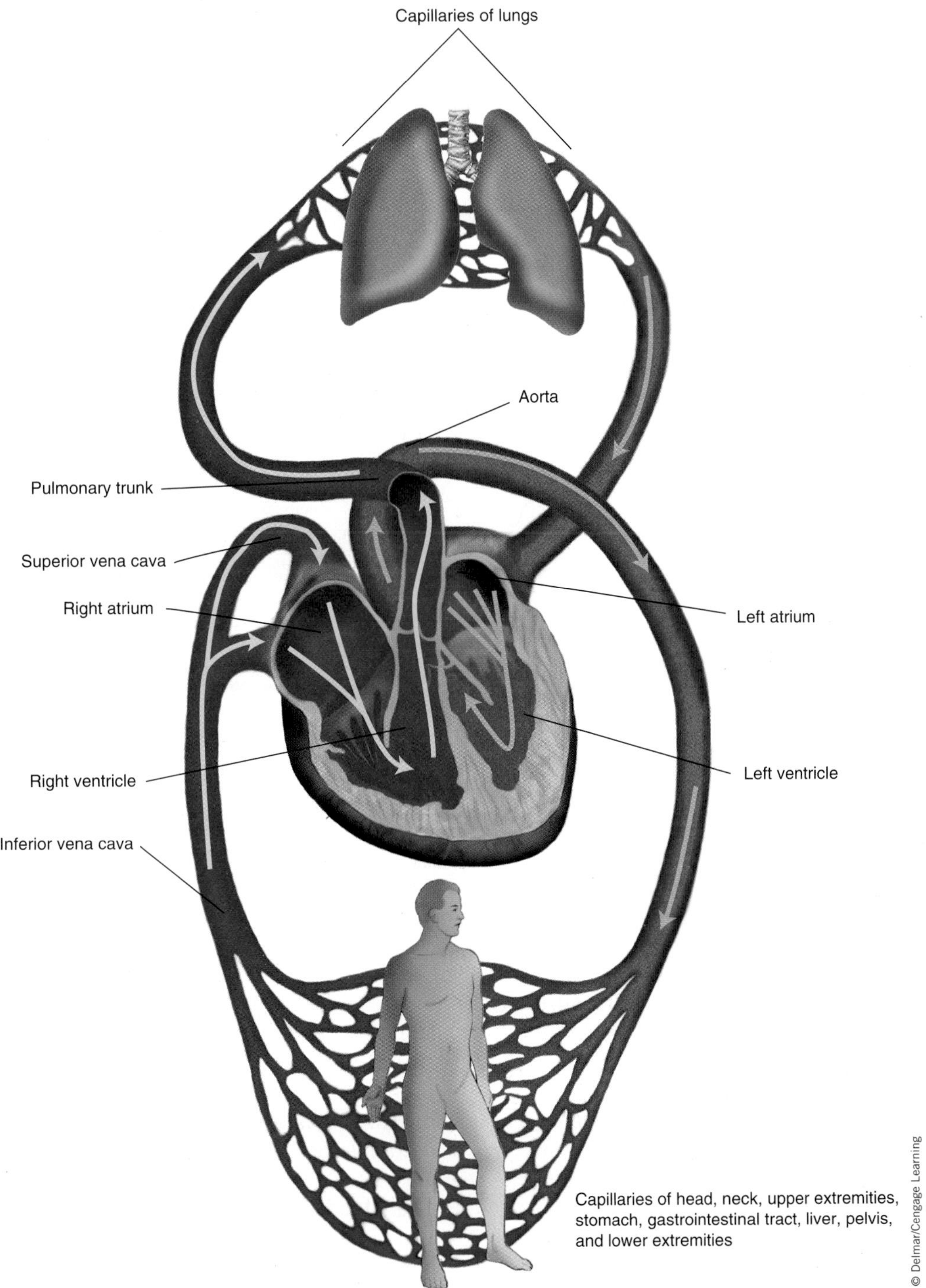

FIGURE 6-37 Vascular structures.

increases sympathetic impulses. The result is heightened arterial blood pressure. The opposite occurs when an increased arterial blood pressure is sensed.

BLOOD PRESSURES IN THE PULMONARY AND SYSTEMIC VASCULAR SYSTEMS

Three pressures are used for studying blood flow (perfusion):

- *Intravascular* (*intraluminal*), the actual pressure inside the vessel.
- *Transmural,* the difference between intravascular pressure and the pressure external to that vessel.
- *Driving pressure,* the difference in pressure at one point in a vessel and the pressure at any other point downstream in the same vessel.

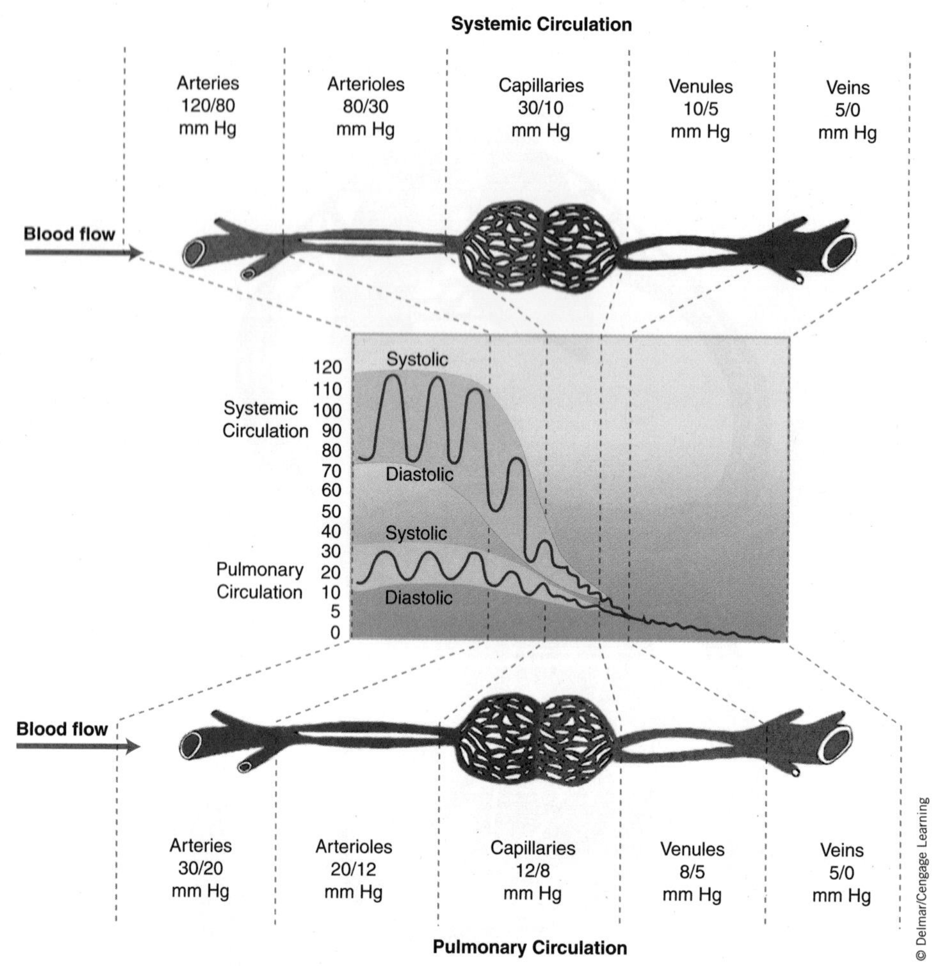

FIGURE 6-38 Blood pressures in the circulatory system.

The Cardiac Cycle and Effect on Blood Pressure. When the ventricles contract (*systole*) and eject blood to the arteries, the blood pressure in the arteries rises to its highest level; this point is called the *systolic pressure*. When the ventricles relax (*diastole*), the arterial blood pressure drops to its resting level; this point is called the *diastolic pressure* (Figure 6-38).

The systemic system is a high-pressure system, serving the body with a 120 mm Hg systolic pressure and an 80 mm Hg diastolic pressure (Figure 6-39). The pulmonary system is a low-pressure, large-volume, short-distance system with a blood pressure of 25 mm Hg systolic and 8 mm Hg diastolic. In general terms, the systemic system has a driving pressure about 10 times higher than that of the pulmonary system. The mean (average) pressures are 15 mm Hg in the pulmonary artery and 5 mm Hg in the left atrium; together, they equal a driving pressure of 10 mm Hg (15 − 5 = 10). For the systemic system, the mean aortic pressure is about 100 mm Hg and the mean pressure in the right atrium is 2 mm Hg; together, they equal a driving pressure of 98 mm Hg (100 − 2 = 98).

A surge of blood runs through the vessels as diastolic goes to systolic and then back again. This surge creates a waveform that is measured and used for monitoring a person's cardiovascular status. In addition, the surge of blood can be felt peripherally as the *pulse*, or *heart, rate*. See Figure 6-40 for sites to measure pulse rate.

The Blood Volume and Effect on Blood Pressure. The *cardiac output* (*CO*) is the amount of blood ejected by each ventricle each minute. It is measured by multiplying the heart rate (*HR*, beats per minute) by the **stroke volume** (*SV*, volume of blood ejected by each ventricular contraction).

$$CO = HR \times SV$$

The normal cardiac output is about 5040 mL/minute (pulse rate of 72 × stroke volume of 70 mL). Normally, cardiac output increases with an increase in either stroke volume or pulse rate, and it decreases with a decrease in stroke volume or pulse rate. The adult total blood volume is typically about 5 L, with 75% of the blood in the systemic system, 15% in the heart, and

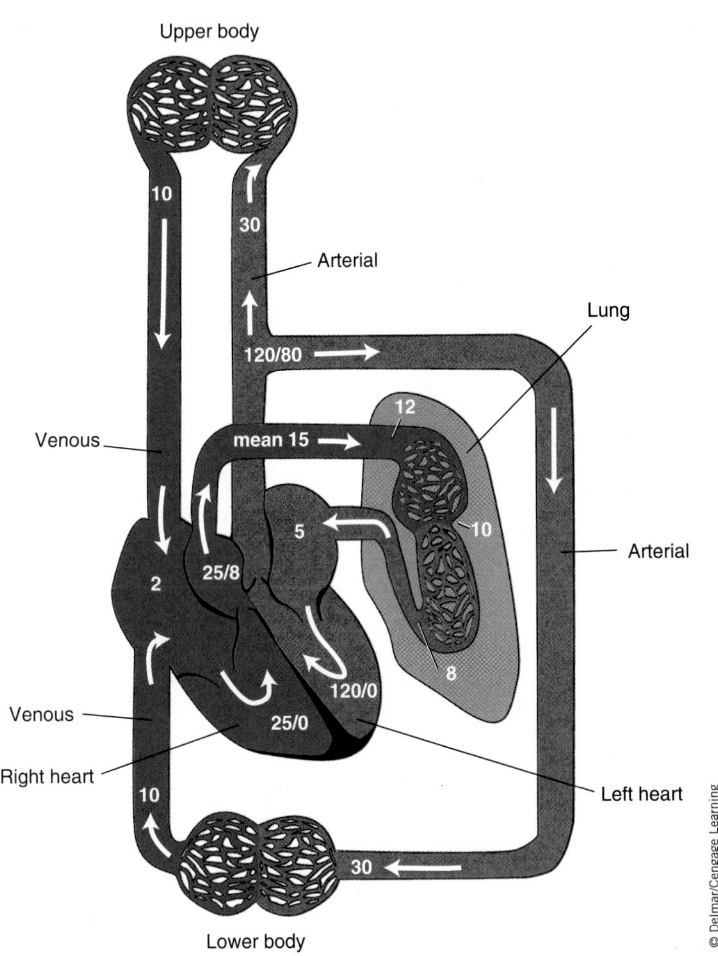

FIGURE 6-39 Mean intraluminal blood pressures (mm Hg).

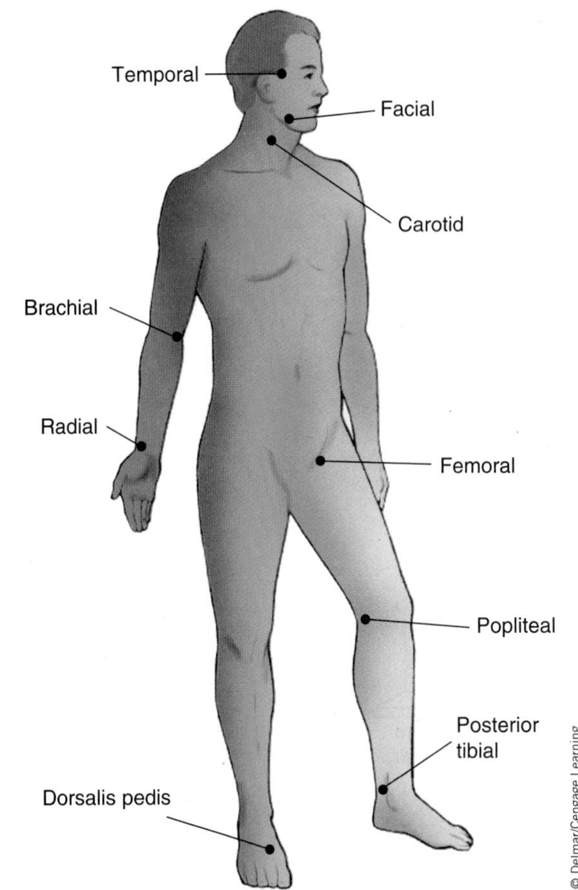

FIGURE 6-40 Major sites where an arterial pulse can be measured.

Best Practice

Clinical Use of Systemic Pulses

Systemic pulses are valuable for basic assessments during therapy, during cardiopulmonary resuscitation, and for drawing arterial blood for sampling. The sites are also easy to locate quickly. Practice finding the sites shown in Figure 6-40.

10% in the pulmonary system. The pulmonary capillary bed contains about 75 mL of blood but has a capacity of up to 200 mL for use in exercise.

DISTRIBUTION OF PULMONARY BLOOD FLOW

Blood flow progressively decreases from the lung base (bottom) to the lung apex (top). The factors affecting blood distribution are (1) gravity, (2) cardiac output, and (3) pulmonary vascular resistance.

Gravity. Gravity pulls most of the blood to the lower half of the lungs. The lungs are about 30 cm high; the pulmonary blood pressure must overcome this height to deliver blood to the lung apex. The effect of gravity is lessened when the person is supine (lying on the back) and the distance is shorter.

See Figure 6-41 for a description of the three-zone model of lung perfusion, showing the effects of gravity and alveolar pressures on the distribution of pulmonary blood flow.

Note:

- Zone 1 is nongravity dependent and has the least blood flow.
- Zone 2 has progressively increased blood flow moving down the lung toward zone 3.
- Zone 3 is gravity dependent and enjoys almost universal blood flow throughout.

Cardiac Output. Stroke volume is an important component of cardiac output. Three factors determine stoke volume: ventricular preload, myocardial contractility, and ventricular afterload.

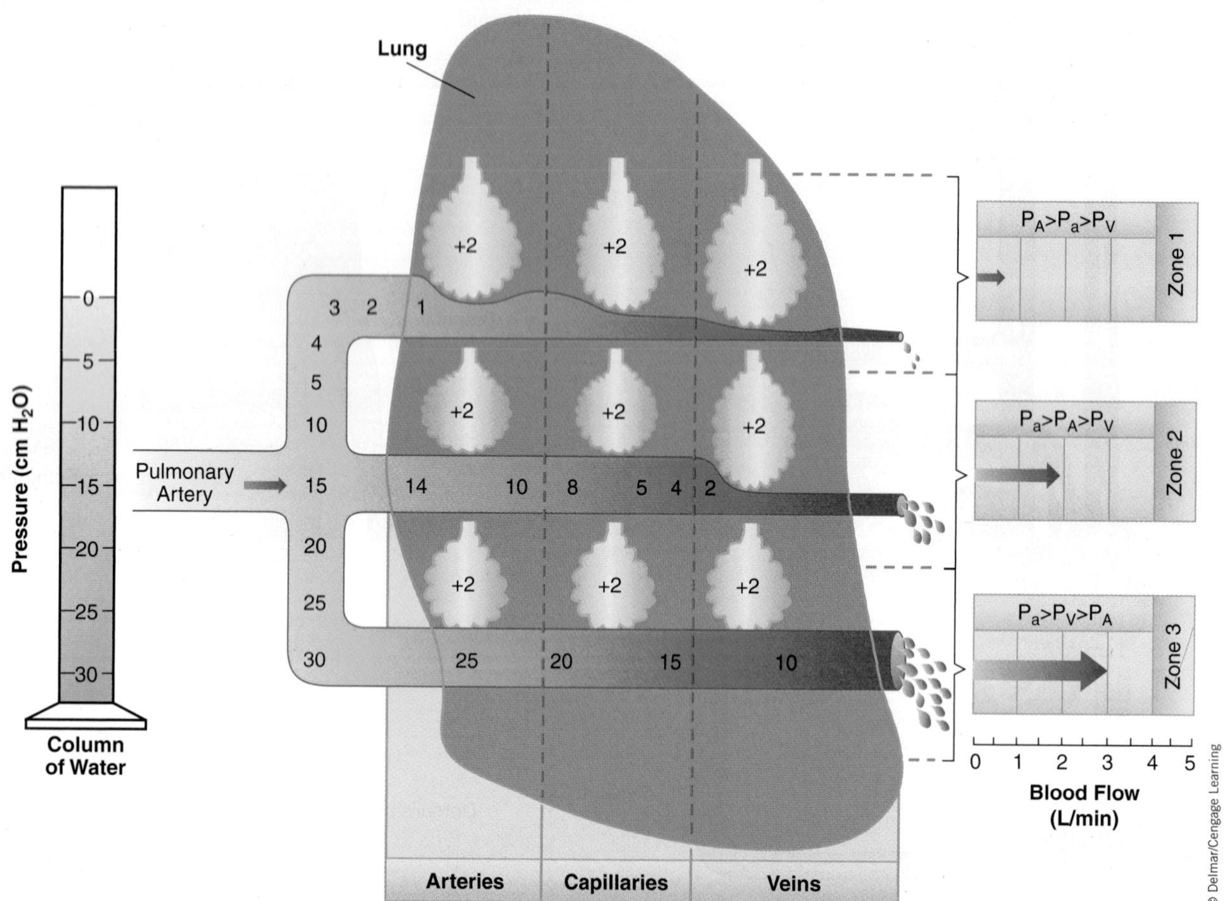

FIGURE 6-41 The three-zone model of lung perfusion. Pressures are expressed as cm H_2O.

- **Ventricular preload** is the amount the ventricle is stretched with blood (diastole) before the next contraction. In general, the more stretched the myocardial muscle fibers are (i.e., the higher the preload), the higher the stroke volume and cardiac output will be. This relationship between ventricular stretching and cardiac output is described by the **Frank-Starling principle**: more in, more out.
- **Myocardial contractility** is the force produced by the myocardial muscle fibers as they shorten. When contractility increases (called *positive inotropism*), cardiac output increases. When contractility decreases (called *negative inotropism*), cardiac output falls.
- **Ventricular afterload** is the force the ventricles must produce to eject blood. It is affected by blood volume and viscosity, peripheral vascular resistance, and the total vascular cross-sectional area being served (including the valve area). The arterial blood pressure is a very good measure of ventricular afterload because blood pressure equals cardiac output times vascular resistance.

See Chapter 19 for factors that affect preload, contractility, and afterload.

Vascular Resistance. *Vascular resistance* is found by dividing the mean blood pressure by the cardiac output. In general, when vascular resistance increases, blood pressure and afterload increase as a result. The opposite is also correct. Both active and passive mechanisms affect vascular resistance. Active mechanisms are:

- Decreased alveolar oxygen levels.
- Increased PCO_2.
- Lowered pH (more acidic blood).
- Pharmacologic stimulation.
- Pathologic conditions, such as pulmonary edema.

Passive mechanisms are:

- Pulmonary arterial pressure changes.
- Left atrial pressure changes.
- Lung volume changes.
- Alveolar pressure effects on vessel size (transmural pressure).
- Intrapleural pressure effects on large arteries and veins.

Vascular resistance is also affected by blood volume changes (increased blood volume, vascular resistance decreases) and by blood viscosity changes (viscosity increases are reflected by higher-than-normal hematocrit and vascular resistances).

Hemodynamic Measurements

Hemodynamic data can be obtained either directly or indirectly. Table 6-7 lists hemodynamic values directly obtained by pulmonary artery catheter. Table 6-8 lists computed hemodynamic values. (Refer to Chapters 12 and 19.)

Oxygen Transport

Oxygen transport is important in the study of pulmonary physiology, especially for the interpretation of arterial and mixed venous blood gas values. Oxygen is carried in the blood in two ways: dissolved and chemically bound to hemoglobin (Hb).

OXYGEN DISSOLVED IN BLOOD PLASMA

Oxygen that diffuses from the alveoli across the alveolar-capillary membrane dissolves in the blood plasma and is measured as PO_2 (partial pressure of oxygen). A PO_2 of 1 mm Hg equals 0.003 mL of dissolved oxygen.[4] For a normal person with a PO_2 of 100 mm Hg, the dissolved volume of oxygen is 0.3 mL per 100 mL of blood, or 0.3% volume ($100 \times 0.003 = 0.3$). This is a very small, but important, amount of the total oxygen content.

OXYGEN BOUND WITH HEMOGLOBIN

Most of the oxygen that enters the blood moves rapidly through the plasma as dissolved oxygen and enters the RBCs, where it chemically binds to hemoglobin (Hb). Hemoglobin is a specialized molecule made up of four heme (iron) groups and four protein chains (amino acids) that constitute the globin portion. At the center of the heme group, oxygen combines in a reversible reaction with the iron molecule, forming *oxyhemoglobin* (O_2Hb). Hemoglobin also transports carbon dioxide gas by combining chemically; the resulting compound is known as *reduced hemoglobin* (*Rhb, Hbr*, or *HbR*), or *deoxygenated hemoglobin*.

The normal hemoglobin value for males is 15 g/100 mL blood; the normal value for females is 14 g/dL blood. The average hemoglobin value for infants is 14–20 g/dL.

Hemoglobin makes up about 33% of the RBCs' total weight and carries the vast majority of oxygen. One gram of hemoglobin can carry 1.34 mL of oxygen. Therefore, the total oxygen that is chemically combined with hemoglobin is 20.1 mL O_2/dL blood: 15 g Hb × 1.34 mL oxygen × 100% (full) saturation. Normally about 3% of the hemoglobin is deoxygenated; so the true value is about 19.5 mL/dL ($20.1 \times 0.97 = 19.5$).

TOTAL OXYGEN CONTENT

Total **oxygen content** is calculated by adding the values for dissolved and combined oxygen ($0.3 + 19.5 = 19.8$ mL O_2/dL blood). Total oxygen content can be calculated for arterial blood (C_aO_2), mixed venous blood (C_vO_2), and pulmonary capillary blood (C_cO_2).

TABLE 6-7 **Hemodynamic values directly measured (pulmonary artery catheter)**

Hemodynamic Value	Abbreviation	Normal Range
Central venous pressure	*CVP*	0–8 mm Hg
Right atrial pressure	*RAP*	0–8 mm Hg
Mean pulmonary artery	*PA*	9–18 mm Hg
Pulmonary capillary wedge pressure (also called pulmonary artery wedge; pulmonary artery occlusion)	*PCWP* *PAW* *PAO*	4–12 mm Hg
Cardiac output	*CO*	4–8 Lpm

TABLE 6-8 **Computed hemodynamic values**

Hemodynamic Value	Abbreviation	Normal Range
Stroke volume	*SV*	60–130 mL
Stroke volume index	*SVI*	30–65 mL/beat/m^2
Cardiac index	*CI*	2.5–4.2 L/min/m^2
Right ventricular stroke work index	*RVSWI*	7–12 g-m/m^2
Left ventricular resistance	*LVSWI*	40–60 g-m/m^2
Pulmonary vascular resistance	*PVR*	20–120 dynes × s × cm^{-5}
Systemic vascular resistance	*SVR*	800–1500 dynes × s × cm^{-5}

Oxygen Dissociation Curve

On the steep part of the oxygen dissociation curve, small changes in P_aO_2 result in large changes in S_aO_2. The reverse is true on the flat upper part of the curve.

These calculations allow the objective study of pulmonary physiology and serve as a basis for patient care.

OXYGEN DISSOCIATION CURVE

The *oxygen dissociation curve* (also called the *oxyhemoglobin dissociation curve*) is S-shaped, reflecting the nonlinear relationship between dissolved oxygen and oxygen chemically bound to hemoglobin (% O_2Hb or SO_2). Figure 6-42 shows this relationship, with P_aO_2 on the horizontal and the SO_2 on the vertical. In addition, the corresponding oxygen content is listed on the right side of the figure. The part of the curve from a P_aO_2 of 10 to 60 mm Hg is vertically steep, reflecting the rapid uptake of oxygen by hemoglobin at the lung. Note that, at a P_aO_2 of 60 mm Hg, the hemoglobin is about 90% saturated. From a P_aO_2 of 60 to 100 mm Hg, the slope flattens, showing a small 7% gain in hemoglobin O_2 saturation. Increases above 100 mm Hg in P_aO_2 offer little increase in SO_2 because the hemoglobin is almost fully saturated.

FACTORS THAT SHIFT THE OXYGEN DISSOCIATION CURVE

The oxygen dissociation curve shows a rapid loading of oxygen at the lung and a rapid unloading of oxygen at the cellular level. In the presence of elevated carbon dioxide levels, hemoglobin tends to release oxygen; this phenomenon is called the **Bohr effect**. Changes in hemoglobin's affinity for binding oxygen—whether induced by carbon dioxide, pH, or temperature alterations—are rapid, resulting in enhanced oxygen uptake at the lung and its release at the systemic tissues.

Consider that venous blood returning to the right atrium has low oxygen and high carbon dioxide levels. At the *alveolar-capillary* (A-C) *surface,* carbon dioxide diffuses rapidly from the plasma into the alveoli. This drop in PCO_2 causes hemoglobin to release carbon dioxide into the plasma and drives carbon dioxide diffusion into the alveoli for equilibration. Also at the A-C level, oxygen diffuses from the alveoli into the plasma and dissolves as P_aO_2. The hemoglobin can then take up oxygen rapidly to replace the carbon dioxide that has vacated the hemoglobin chemical-bonding sites and raises the SO_2. The differences in arterial and

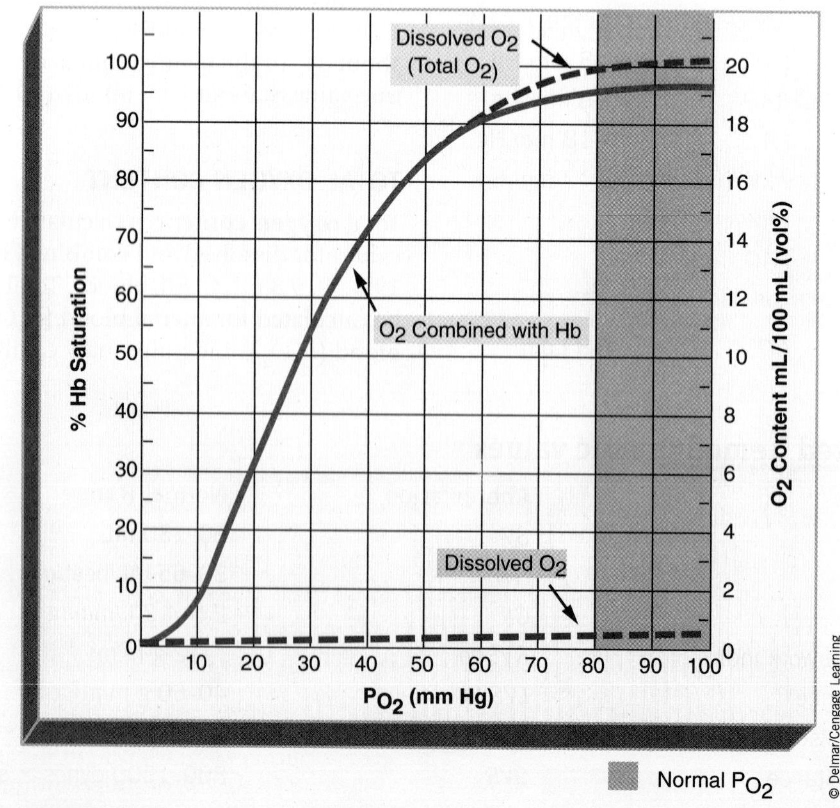

FIGURE 6-42 The oxygen dissociation curve.

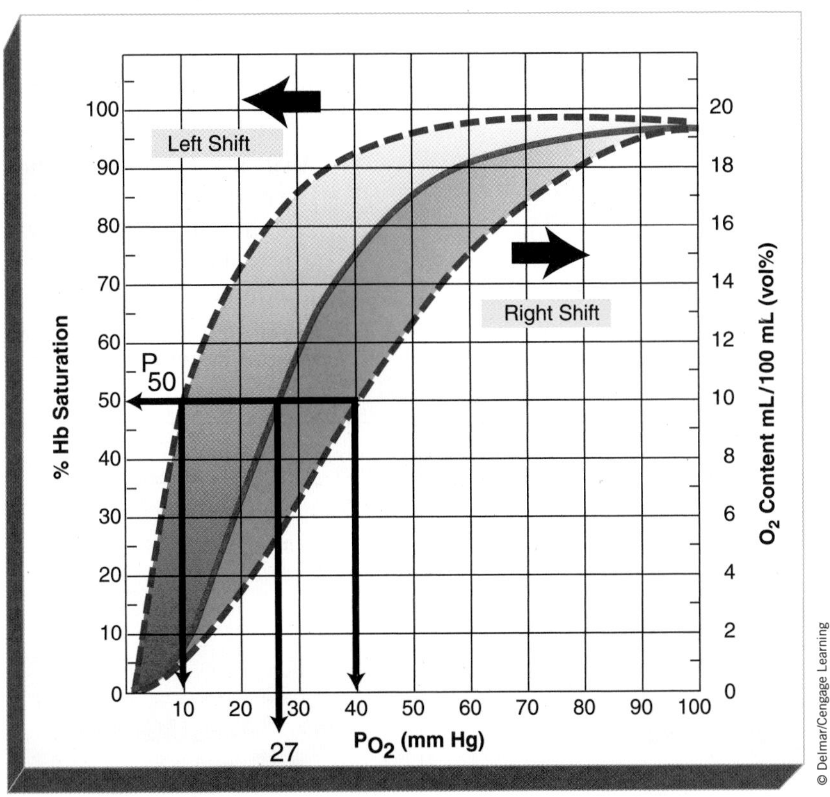

FIGURE 6-43 Factors that shift the oxygen dissociation curve to the right and left.

venous values are a reflection of tissue oxygen use and carbon dioxide production by the body.

Factors that affect the oxygen dissociation curve are pH, temperature, carbon dioxide, 2,3-diphosphoglycate (2,3 DPG), fetal hemoglobin (HbF), and carbon monoxide combined with Hb (carboxyhemoglobin, COHb). These factors affect hemoglobin in two ways: They either cause it to hold on to oxygen more tightly (shift the curve to the left) or release oxygen more easily (shift the curve to the right). A left shift has a higher %Hb saturation but oxygen available to unload at the cells because of increased affinity of the hemoglobin for oxygen. A right shift has a lower %Hb saturation and decreased affinity for oxygen and therefore less oxygen for release to the cells. Figure 6-43 summarizes these factors and their effects. Clinically, these must be considered in the interpretation of arterial blood gas and acid-base values.

OXYGEN TRANSPORT STUDIES

Arterial, mixed venous, and capillary oxygen contents are good indicators of cardiopulmonary function. The total oxygen content for delivery (DO_2) can be calculated by the equation

$$DO_2 = \dot{Q}_T \times (C_aO_2 \times 10)$$

Where Q_T is total cardiac output, C_aO_2 is arterial oxygen content, and the factor of 10 is needed to convert from C_aO_2 to milliliters of oxygen per liter. The difference between the arterial and venous oxygen contents ($C_{A\text{-}V}O_2$) is simply the arterial oxygen content minus the venous oxygen content (vol%). Oxygen consumption (oxygen uptake, VO_2) is the amount of oxygen extracted from the blood by the cells in 1 minute. It is calculated by the equation

$$\dot{V}O_2 = \dot{Q}_T \times (C_{A\text{-}V}O_2 \times 10)$$

The oxygen concentration ratio is the arterial-venous oxygen content difference divided by the arterial oxygen content:

$$O_2 \text{ extraction} = \frac{C_{(a\text{-}v)}O_2}{C_aO_2}$$

Mixed venous oxygen saturation is the measurement of blood from the pulmonary artery, sampled from an indwelling catheter. In addition, the volume of pulmonary blood flow (Q) is calculated by:

$$\dot{Q} = \frac{\dot{V}O_2}{C_aO_2 - C_vO_2}$$

where cardiac output through the lungs equals the volume of oxygen uptake per minute divided by the arterial-mixed venous oxygen content difference. The normal saturation of mixed venous blood is 75% with a $P_{\bar{v}}O_2$ of 40 mm Hg. Refer to Chapters 12 and 19.

Pulmonary Shunting and Venous Admixture

Pulmonary shunting is the part of cardiac output that enters the left side of the heart without having exchanged gases with alveoli (Figure 6-44). True shunting and shuntlike effect are two shunt mechanisms. In a *true shunt,* also called *absolute shunt,* no gas is exchanged, and the deoxygenated blood enters the left heart. Types of true shunt are anatomic and capillary.

- *Anatomic shunt* occurs when blood passes from the right side of the heart to the left without entering the pulmonary vasculature. Normally, this is about 2% to 5% of the blood; it is blood that drains via the bronchial, pleural, and Thebesian veins, emptying into the pulmonary venous system. Common pathologic causes of

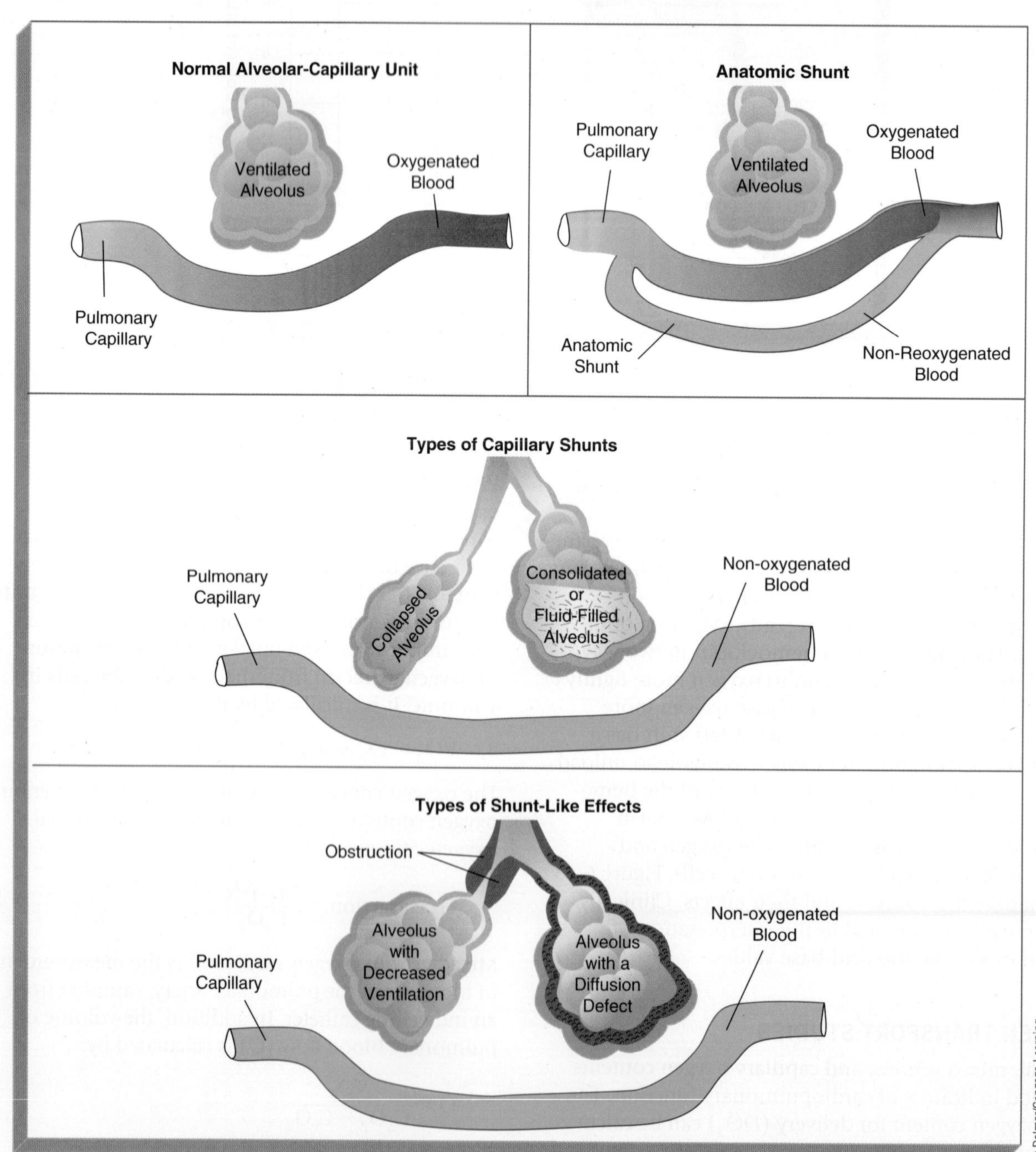

FIGURE 6-44 Pulmonary shunting.

anatomic shunting are congenital heart disease, intrapulmonary fistula, and vascular lung tumors.

- *Capillary shunting* is blood passing through the pulmonary capillaries without having exchanged gases with alveoli. The causes are atelectasis (alveolar collapse), liquid in the alveoli, and alveolar consolidation.

The physiological shunt is the total of anatomic and capillary shunts. These types of shunts do not respond to (i.e., they are refractory to) oxygen therapy.

Shuntlike effect occurs when pulmonary perfusion is more than alveolar ventilation. The causes are hypoventilation, uneven distribution of ventilation, and alveolar-capillary diffusion defects. Shuntlike effect responds positively to oxygen therapy.

Venous admixture (Figure 6-45) results when shunted deoxygenated blood mixes with freshly oxygenated blood distal to alveoli. This blood with differing oxygen levels mixes and equilibrates downstream, and it is measured via an arterial blood sample.

The amount of intrapulmonary shunting is calculated by the classic shunt equation:

$$\frac{\dot{Q}_s}{\dot{Q}_t} = \frac{C_cO_2 - C_aO_2}{C_cO_2 - C_vO_2}$$

where Q_S is the cardiac output that is shunt, Q_T is the total cardiac output, and C_cO_2, C_aO_2, and C_vO_2 are the oxygen contents of capillary, arterial, and mixed venous blood, respectively. The amount of pulmonary shunting is significant for patient care planning.

Tissue Hypoxia

Tissue hypoxia is a decreased amount of oxygen available in the tissues. The four main types of hypoxia are hypoxic hypoxia, anemic hypoxia, circulatory hypoxia, and histotoxic hypoxia.

- *Hypoxic hypoxia* is also called *hypoxemia* because of the low oxygen concentration in the blood (low P_aO_2). Hypoxemia results from (1) pulmonary shunting; (2) low alveolar PO_2 (P_AO_2) due to hypoventilation, ascent to altitude, or breathing gases lower than 21% oxygen; (3) diffusion impairment due to fibrosis or alveolar edema; and (4) ventilation/perfusion mismatches ($\dot{V}/\dot{Q}$ ratio).
- *Anemic hypoxia* is a low oxygen-carrying capacity due to either a low hemoglobin amount or abnormal hemoglobin, such as carbon monoxide poisoning. The PO_2 may be normal in this form of hypoxia.
- *Circulatory hypoxia* is characterized by a decreased amount of blood reaching the tissues, with the amount of oxygen available being inadequate for cellular needs.
- *Histotoxic hypoxia* occurs when the cells cannot use oxygen; the classic cause is cyanide poisoning.

Cyanosis and Polycythemia

Cyanosis is an observed discoloration, or blueness, of the lips, nailbeds, and mucus membranes. This is a variable sign and only a gross indicator of hypoxemia. Therefore, arterial blood gases should be used for a definitive diagnosis of low oxygen levels.

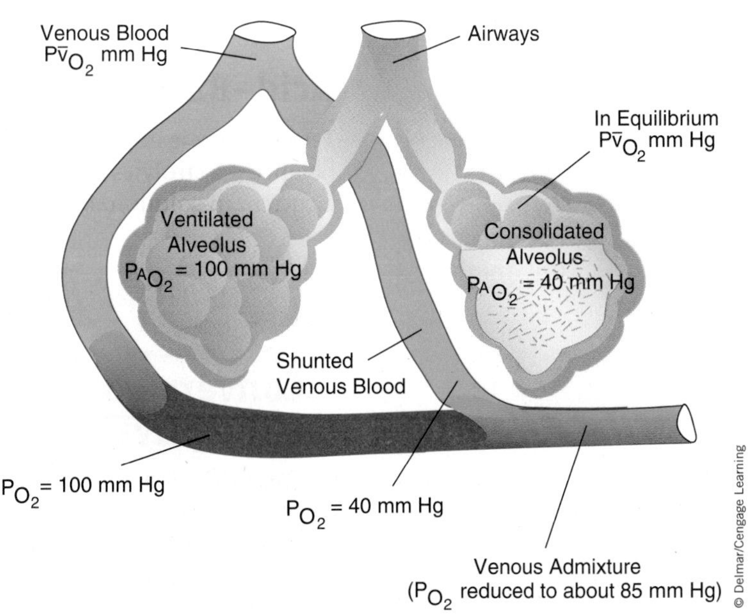

FIGURE 6-45 Venous admixture.

Polycythemia is an increased amount of circulating red blood cells (RBCs) (see Chapters 15 and 19). Secondary polycythemia occurs when the kidneys release erythropoietin owing to chronic hypoxemia, which stimulates an increase in RBC production. The resultant increase in hemoglobin and hematocrit (increased blood thickness) also increases oxygen-carrying ability. However, this increased hematocrit produces cor pulmonale, which is an increase in right ventricular size secondary to pulmonary disease.

Carbon Dioxide

Carbon dioxide must be transported from the tissues to the lungs for elimination.

CARBON DIOXIDE TRANSPORT

Carbon dioxide (CO_2) study is important for evaluating pulmonary physiology and acid-base balance and for interpreting arterial blood gas analyses. At rest, an adult produces 200 mL of carbon dioxide per minute and takes up 250 mL of oxygen per minute. The carbon dioxide is carried from the tissues, where it is a waste product of metabolism, to the lungs by six methods: three in the plasma and three in the RBCs (Table 6-9).

In plasma, carbon dioxide is transported as:

- Carbamino compound, bound to protein (about 1% of total).
- Bicarbonate (HCO_3^-), through slow but reversible hydrolysis (about 5% of total).
- Dissolved CO_2, measured as PCO_2 in arterial blood gas (about 5% of total).

TABLE 6-9 **Carbon dioxide transport mechanisms**

Carbon Dioxide Transport Mechanism	Approximate Percentage of Total CO_2 Transported to Lungs	Approximate Quantity of Total CO_2 Transported to Lungs (mL/min)
In plasma:		
Carbamino compound	1	2
Bicarbonate	5	10
Dissolved CO_2	5	10
In red blood cells:		
Dissolved CO_2	5	10
Carbamino-Hb	21	42
Bicarbonate	63	126
Total	100	200

In the red blood cells, carbon dioxide is transported as:

- Dissolved CO_2 (about 5% of total).
- Carbamino-Hb, combined with hemoglobin, which enhances oxygen release to the tissues (21% of total).
- Bicarbonate (approximately 63% of total).

The vast majority of carbon dioxide that enters the RBCs is converted to bicarbonate via hydrolysis. The reaction is speeded up by carbonic anhydrase (CA), an enzyme in the RBCs. Because of this rapid production, HCO_3^- diffuses from the RBCs into the plasma and, to maintain intracellular electrical neutrality, is replaced by chloride (Cl^-). This process is called the *chloride shift*, or *Hamburger phenomenon*.

CARBON DIOXIDE ELIMINATION AT THE LUNGS

When mixed venous blood enters the pulmonary capillaries, carbon dioxide is released to diffuse into the alveoli until equilibration is reached. This is the reverse of activities at the tissue level, where carbon dioxide diffuses into the plasma.

CARBON DIOXIDE DISSOCIATION CURVE

The carbon dioxide dissociation curve is linear, unlike the oxygen dissociation curve. For any PCO_2, there is a direct relationship between dissolved carbon dioxide and the total CO_2 in the blood. The effect of changes in oxyhemoglobin saturation on the relationship of carbon dioxide content to PCO_2 is called the **Haldane effect**. In the tissues, the unloading of oxygen from hemoglobin enhances its ability to take up carbon dioxide. The reverse occurs at the lung, where oxygen uptake enhances carbon dioxide unloading.

Acid–Base Balance

Terminology is important in the study of acid-base balance. Electrolytes are charged ions that conduct a current in solution. Buffers are substances that

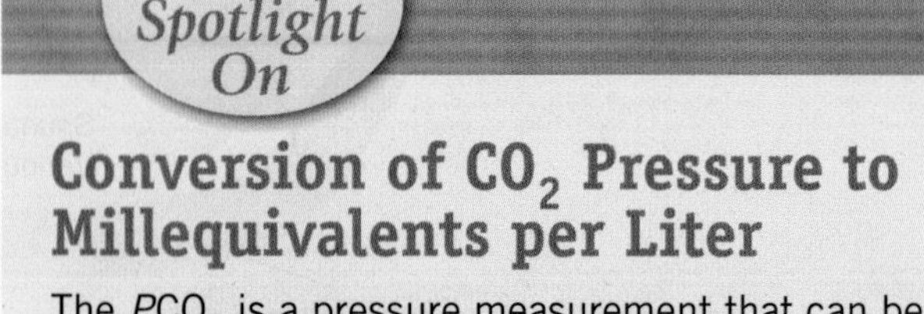

Conversion of CO_2 Pressure to Millequivalents per Liter

The PCO_2 is a pressure measurement that can be converted to millequivalents per liter by multiplying PCO_2 by 0.03. The normal value calculation for acid-base balance is:[4]

PCO_2 40 mmHg $\times$ 0.03 = 1.2 mEq/L H_2CO_3

neutralize acids and bases, preventing wide swings in pH. Acids dissociate (divide out) into hydrogen ions (H^+) in a solution. Bases react with water to form hydroxide ions (OH^-) in a solution. A dissociation constant is the equilibration between the molecular form and its ions, represented by the letter *k* in calculations of pH (see Chapter 4).

THE pH SCALE AND BUFFER SYSTEMS

The *pH* is defined as the negative logarithm (base 10) of the hydrogen ion concentration. A pH of 7.0 is neutral. The normal range for human arterial blood is 7.35–7.45. When there is an increase in acid, the pH number decreases (<7.40). Acids donate H^+ to solution, causing an increase in acidity and a drop in pH. When base increases, less acid is available, and the pH rises (>7.45). Bases accept H^+ and raise the pH value. The pH is maintained by means of the balance between buffer systems and the respiratory system's ability to eliminate carbon dioxide.

The Henderson-Hasselbalch (H-H) equation uses the bicarbonate–carbon dioxide relationship to arrive at the pH value:

$$\text{pH} = p_k + \log \frac{HCO_3^-}{CO_2}$$

Where p_k is the dissociation constant of the acid portion of the buffer combination.

Normally, the p_k is 6.1. With an HCO_3^- value of 24 mEq/L and a PCO_2 of 1.2 mEq/L (PCO_2 of 40 mm Hg × 0.03), the equation yields a pH value of 7.4:

$$\begin{aligned} \text{pH} &= 6.1 + \log \frac{24 \text{ mEq/L}}{1.2 \text{ mEq/L}} \\ &= 6.1 + \log 20{:}1 \\ &= 6.1 + 1.3 \\ \text{pH} &= 7.4 \end{aligned}$$

Spotlight On

Bicarbonate: Carbon Dioxide Ratio for pH

In the plasma, the ratio of HCO_3^- to PCO_2, in millequivalents per liter, is 24:1.2. This is reduced to a 20:1 ratio, with bicarbonate 20 times greater than carbonic acid (CO_2). This 20:1 ratio is a balance point for maintaining a normal pH (7.35–7.45). When the ratio is greater than 20:1, the blood is more alkaline (less acidic); when the ratio is less than 20:1, the blood is more acidic.

TABLE 6-10 **Normal blood gas value ranges**

Blood Gas Value	Arterial	Venous
pH	7.35–7.45	7.30–7.40
PCO_2	35–45 mm Hg (P_aCO_2)	42–48 mm Hg (P_vCO_2)
HCO_3^-	22–28 mEq/L	24–30 mEq/L
PO_2	80–100 mm Hg (P_aO_2)	35–45 mm Hg (P_vO_2)

Thus, the normal pH of 7.4 results from the 20:1 bicarbonate/PCO_2 ratio. See Table 6-10 for normal acid-base values.

RESPIRATORY ACID-BASE IMBALANCES

Respiratory changes brought on by acid-base imbalances are reflected in arterial blood gas sampling. For example, if ventilation slows or stops, PCO_2 rises in the plasma, increasing H^+ levels and lowering the pH. This condition is called *respiratory acidemia* (increased acid due to respiratory causes). If ventilation increases, a rapid decrease in PCO_2 causes a *respiratory alkalemia* (increased base). Respiratory system changes can bring on rapid changes in pH values (see Chapters 4 and 15).

METABOLIC ACID-BASE IMBALANCES

Disturbances due to metabolic conditions can lead to metabolic acidemia. Examples are:

- Lactic acidemia, resulting from inadequate tissue oxygenation, anaerobic metabolism, and the production of lactic acid that accumulates in the plasma.
- Ketoacidemia in the diabetic patient, caused by low insulin levels.
- Renal failure, in which H^+ accumulate in the plasma.

Metabolic alkalemia is caused by the elevation of other bases in the plasma. The causes are:

- Hypokalemia [decreased potassium (K^+)] resulting in the kidney's excreting increased amounts of H^+.
- Gastric suction, rapidly removing acidic stomach contents.
- Excessive administration of bicarbonate during cardiopulmonary resuscitation.

The body will compensate for disorders by attempting to bring acid-base imbalances back into balance. The buffer system controlled by the kidneys compensates for respiratory disorders. The respiratory system compensates for metabolic disorders (Table 6-11). In

TABLE 6-11 **Acid-base conditions and compensations**

	pH	PCO_2	HCO_3^-	Compensation*
Normal	7.40	40	24	Unchanged
Respiratory acidemia	Decreased	Increased	Unchanged	Primarily kidneys
Respiratory alkalemia	Increased	Decreased	Unchanged	Primarily kidneys
Metabolic acidemia	Decreased	Unchanged	Decreased	Respiratory system
Metabolic alkalemia	Increased	Unchanged	Increased	Respiratory system†

Compensation is always less than complete, with the pH moving toward normal without reaching a normal value.

†Respiratory compensation for metabolic alkalemia entails slowing breathing to increase PCO_2 levels. This mechanism is very limited because the respiratory control centers increase breathing to overcome this action.

addition, often mixed disturbances require in-depth analysis. See Chapter 15 for a detailed discussion.

BASE EXCESS OR DEFICIT

The *base excess* or *deficit* is reported in millequivalents per liter of base above or below the normal buffer base level. Use of a nomogram or software application reveals the amount of base excess or deficit and may lead to corrective treatment (see Chapter 15).

The Renal System and Its Effects on the Cardiopulmonary System

The kidneys are an important component of the body's acid-base regulatory system.

THE KIDNEYS

The kidneys are located against the posterior wall in the abdominal cavity. The blood composition is determined by the kidneys, through filtration and reabsorption of substances necessary to maintain normal body fluids. The *nephron* is the functional unit of the kidneys, with perfusion through blood vessels including arteries, capillaries, and veins.

URINE FORMATION

Urine is formed by glomerular filtration, tubular reabsorption, and tubular secretion.

- *Glomerular filtration* occurs because of hydrostatic pressure, which forces water and electrolytes out of the glomerular capillaries. Osmosis opposes hydrostatic pressure and attracts water into the blood vessel.
- Although *tubular reabsorption* occurs throughout all of the renal tubules, most of it occurs in the proximal convoluted tubule. Leaving the tubule are water, sodium, and glucose, with about 99% of glucose and amino acids reabsorbed. Approximately 50% of urea is reabsorbed, according to the body's needs.
- In *tubular secretion*, the opposite of tubular reabsorption, hydrogen ions and potassium enter the urine. Secretion regulates the blood levels of these substances, as well as the amount and composition of urine. The total normal volume of urine excreted daily is about 1500 mL per day.[9] This volume is reduced in hypotension (low blood pressure).

URINE CONCENTRATION AND VOLUME

The concentration and volume of urine are controlled to produce either a concentrated or a diluted urine. The countercurrent mechanism controls water reabsorption in the distal tubules and collecting ducts. Selective permeability of the collecting ducts is regulated by *antidiuretic hormone* (*ADH*). When blood volume and pressure increase, ADH production is inhibited, increasing urine volume and decreasing the concentration (dilute). When dehydration occurs, ADH production is stimulated and fluids are retained, urine volume decreases, and urine concentration increases. Normal blood volume is maintained at about 5 L.

REGULATION OF ELECTROLYTE CONCENTRATION

Important ions regulated by the kidney are sodium, potassium, calcium, magnesium, and phosphate. Sodium produces the majority of osmotic pressure and regulates the amount of water in the body. Potassium is essential for normal nerve and muscle function. Aldosterone stimulates potassium transport into the urine. The other electrolytes are regulated to maintain normal body function. The kidney also plays a major role in acid-base balance, primarily by regulating hydrogen ions through excretion and by the reabsorption of bicarbonate.

RENAL FAILURE

Renal failure is a life-threatening condition caused by congenital disorders, infections, obstructive disorders,

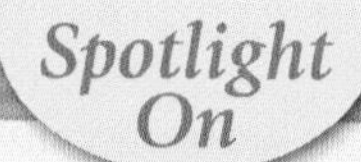

Mechanical Ventilation as a Cause of Renal Failure

The use of positive pressure ventilation (pressure above atmospheric) is a life-supportive therapy, but the higher pressures stimulate ADH production. The results are decreased urine formation and decreased urine elimination.

inflammation and immune responses, and neoplasms (new growths). Monitoring intake and output of fluids is a basic method to monitor renal function.

CARDIOPULMONARY PROBLEMS DUE TO RENAL FAILURE

Renal failure affects acid-base balance and the cardiopulmonary system. It can result in:

- Hypertension (increased blood pressure) and edema formation.
- Metabolic acidosis due to retention of hydrogen ions and potassium ions.
- Electrolyte imbalances.
- Anemia (decreased hemoglobin) due to reduced erythropoietin production.
- Bleeding and cardiovasculature disorders.

Ventilation/Perfusion Relationships

The interaction and effectiveness of the heart and lungs can be examined by determining the ventilation/perfusion ratio.

VENTILATION/PERFUSION RATIO

The matching of alveolar ventilation and pulmonary capillary perfusion is vital for life. Normally, alveolar ventilation is about 4 L/min, and pulmonary capillary blood flow (perfusion) is about 5 Lpm (Figure 6-46). The result is a ventilation/perfusion ratio of 4:5, or 0.8. Actually, this overall $\dot{V}/\dot{Q}$ reflects the sum of numerous regional $\dot{V}/\dot{Q}$ ratios.[5] For example, the alveoli in the lung apex receive moderate ventilation but little perfusion; they have a $\dot{V}/\dot{Q}$ ratio greater than 0.8. The opposite is true for the lung bases, where ventilation is increased but perfusion is greatly decreased. The result at the bases is a $\dot{V}/\dot{Q}$ of less than 0.8. The $\dot{V}/\dot{Q}$ ratio progressively decreases from the apex to the base of the upright lung (Figure 6-47).

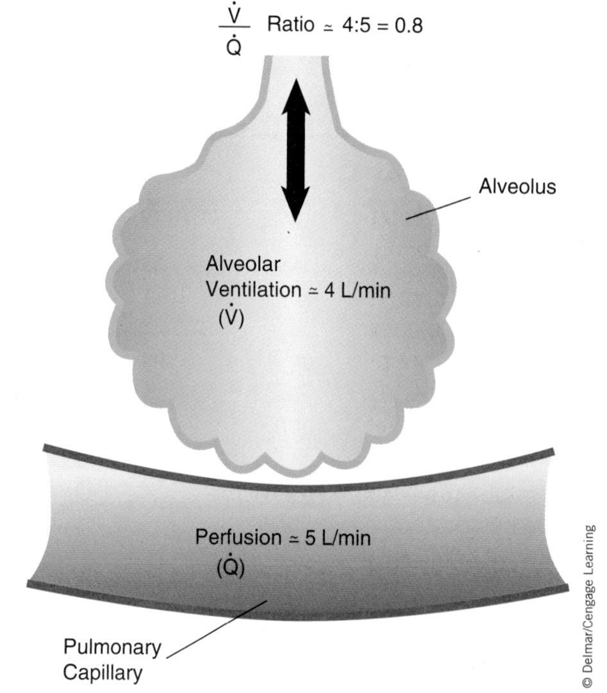

FIGURE 6-46 The ventilation/perfusion ratio.

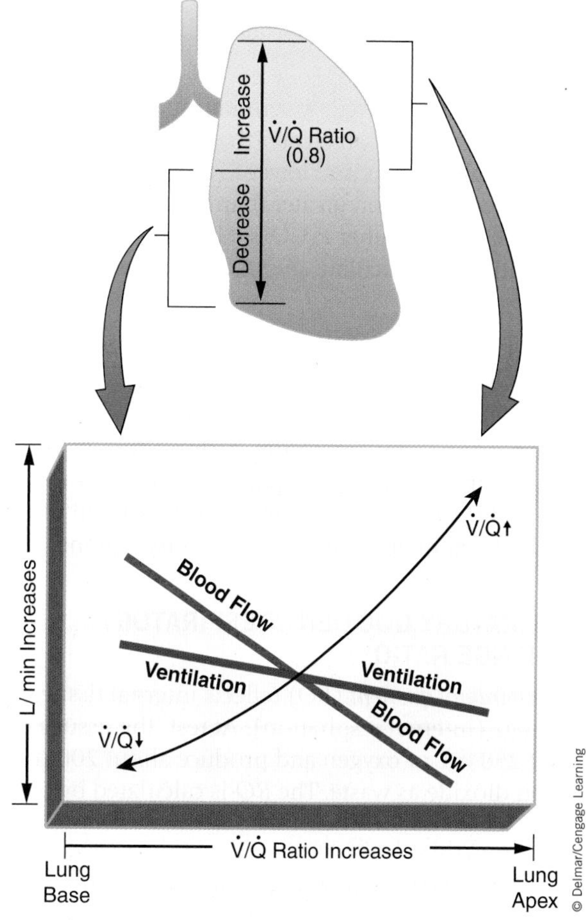

FIGURE 6-47 The ventilation/perfusion ratio in the upright lung.

Ventilation/Perfusion Considerations

The following relationships are for the normal, upright person:

- There is more ventilation in the lung bases than in the apexes.
- There is more perfusion in the bases than in the apexes.
- There is more ventilation than perfusion in the apexes.
- There is more perfusion than ventilation in the bases.

EFFECTS OF THE VENTILATION/PERFUSION RATIO ON ALVEOLAR GASES

Changing $\dot{V}/\dot{Q}$ ratios also alter alveolar gas composition for both P_AO_2 and P_ACO_2 and for arterial values as well. For P_AO_2, the value is determined by the amount of oxygen entering the alveoli and the oxygen removal by capillary perfusion. For P_ACO_2, the value depends on the amount of carbon dioxide entering the alveoli and on the amount removed by ventilation. Increased $\dot{V}/\dot{Q}$ ratios reflect ventilation greater than perfusion. This leads to higher P_AO_2s and lower P_ACO_2s. Decreased $\dot{V}/\dot{Q}$ ratios reflect perfusion greater than ventilation, with lower P_AO_2s and higher P_ACO_2s. Note that the alveolar air equation can calculate an estimate for use clinically.

EFFECTS OF THE VENTILATION/PERFUSION RATIO ON END-CAPILLARY GASES

As the $\dot{V}/\dot{Q}$ ratio progressively decreases from the apex to the base, the capillary values decrease for oxygen and increase for carbon dioxide, paralleling the changes in P_AO_2 and P_ACO_2. The pulmonary veins contain blood that has been mixed from all pulmonary regions.

RESPIRATORY QUOTIENT/RESPIRATORY EXCHANGE RATIO

The *respiratory quotient* (*RQ*) reflects internal tissue gas exchange (internal respiration). At rest, the tissues use about 250 mL of oxygen and produce about 200 mL of carbon dioxide as waste. The *RQ* is calculated by:

$$RQ = \frac{200 \text{ mL } CO_2/\text{min}}{250 \text{ mL } O_2/\text{min}}$$

The normal $RQ = 0.8$.

The *respiratory exchange ratio* (*REQ*) measures external pulmonary gas exchange between the alveoli and the atmosphere per minute. The normal value is also 0.8.

EFFECTS OF RESPIRATORY DISORDERS ON THE VENTILATION/PERFUSION RATIO

Increased $\dot{V}/\dot{Q}$ ratios result from disorders characterized by ventilation that is greater than perfusion (increased P_AO_2s, decreased P_ACO_2s). This condition is called *deadspace*, or *wasted, ventilation*. Disorders that cause increased deadspace are pulmonary emboli, obstructions of the pulmonary artery, increased pressure on the pulmonary blood vessels (pneumothorax, tumors), decreased cardiac output, and destruction of pulmonary vessels (emphysema).

Decreased $\dot{V}/\dot{Q}$ ratios reflect perfusion in excess of ventilation and an increased shunting of blood. These ratios result from obstructive lung diseases (asthma, bronchitis, emphysema), restrictive lung diseases (fibrosis, pneumonia, neuromuscular), and alveolar hypoventilation.

Control of Ventilation

Breathing is controlled automatically by neurons in the medulla oblongata and the pons of the brain and voluntarily, from the cerebral cortex, which allows specialized functions such as talking, coughing, and sniffing. Respiration is rhythmic and coordinated to meet changing ventilatory needs and to satisfy varying metabolic demands, ranging from sleep to extreme exercise.

RESPIRATORY COMPONENTS OF THE MEDULLA OBLONGATA

Two groups of respiratory neurons in the medulla oblongata are believed to coordinate the intrinsic rhythmicity of breathing. The dorsal (back, posterior) respiratory group and the ventral (belly, anterior) respiratory group.

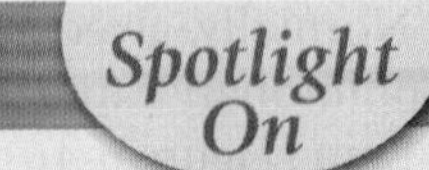

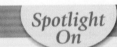

Sighing and Coughing

An effective and inexpensive method to help patients' breathing is to have them take a deep breath and cough. This action stretches the lungs and helps eliminate excess mucus. The deep breath is similar to a normal, periodic sigh, which also stimulates surfactant production.

Dorsal Respiratory Group. The *dorsal respiratory group* (*DRG*) contains primarily inspiratory neurons that are responsible for the basic rhythm of ventilation. The DRG receives input from the body, evaluates and prioritizes the signals, and responds via impulses (1–2 seconds each in duration) that stimulate the inspiratory respiratory muscles (diaphragm). During expiration, the lungs recoil naturally and without DRG input.

Ventral Respiratory Group. The *ventral respiratory group* (*VRG*) has both inspiratory and expiratory neurons, and, in quiet breathing, they are both inactive. During heavy exercise or stress, however, the expiratory neurons stimulate the expiratory muscles (abdominal) to become active. The inspiratory neurons also send impulses that stimulate the accessory muscles of inspiration (sternocleidomastoids).

PONTINE RESPIRATORY CENTERS

The pontine respiratory centers contain the apneustic and pneumotaxic centers, whose basic functions seem to modify the rhythmicity of breathing (Figure 6-48).

The *apneustic center*, in the middle to lower pons, sends signals continuously to promote a prolonged, unrestrained inspiration called *apneustic breathing*. Normally, the apneustic center receives suppressing signals that allow expiration.

- These signals are from the *pneumotaxic center* and the Hering-Breuer inflation reflex. The pneumotaxic center is in the upper third of the pons and functions to interrupt the apneustic center, promoting rhythmic breathing patterns. These impulses also stimulate shallower, more rapid breaths.

The medullary respiratory centers can be depressed by conditions such as decreased blood flow due to increased pressure, acute poliomyelitis, and drugs that depress the central nervous system (CNS).

MONITORING SYSTEMS THAT INFLUENCE THE MEDULLA OBLONGATA

The DRG and VRG of the medulla oblongata receive monitoring system input from the body, primarily from central chemoreceptors and peripheral chemoreceptors.

The *central chemoreceptors*, located bilaterally and ventrally, monitor the H^+ concentration in the *cerebral spinal fluid* (*CSF*). Hydrogen ions are the strongest stimulus to both the DRG and VRG neurons. The central chemoreceptors regulate breathing via the

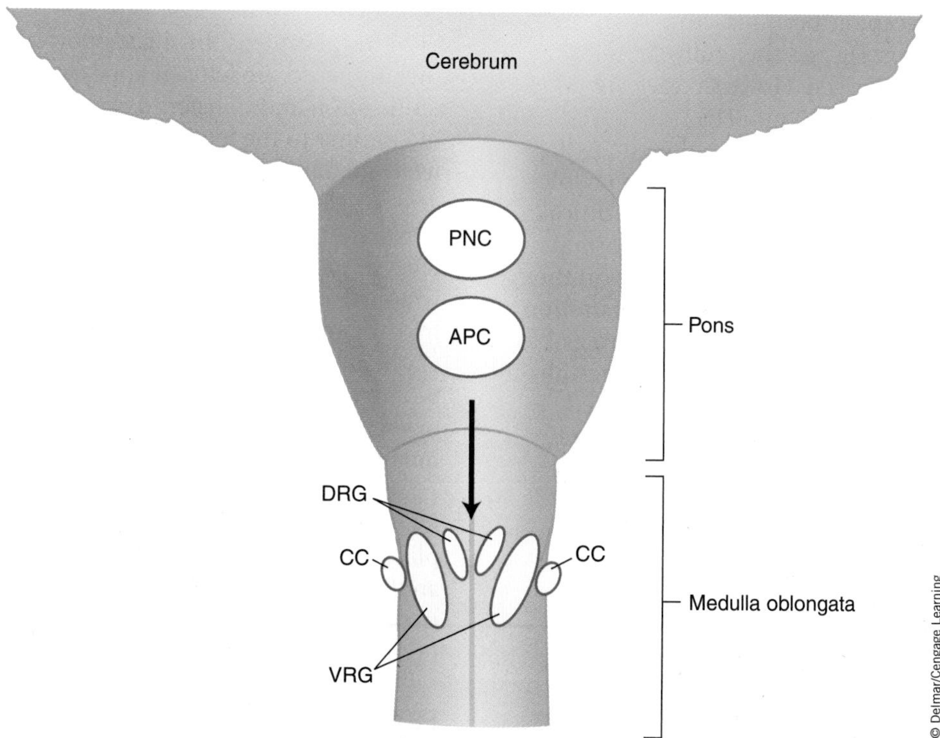

FIGURE 6-48 The respiratory centers in the brain stem: PNC, pneumotoxic center; APC, apneustic center; DRG, dorsal respiratory group; CC, central chemoreceptors; VRG, ventral respiratory group

indirect effects of carbon dioxide on the CSF pH level. The basic mechanism is:

1. CO_2 diffuses from the arterial blood through the semipermeable blood-brain barrier into the CSF.
2. CO_2 combines with water to form carbonic acid, which dissociates into hydrogen ion and bicarbonate.
3. Because the CSF has minimal buffering (low HCO_3^-, low protein levels), the pH rapidly decreases in the CSF.
4. The elevated H^+ stimulates the central chemoreceptors, which send signals to increase alveolar ventilation.
5. The increased ventilation reduces the arterial CO_2, reversing the stimulation process.

The result is decreased alveolar ventilation. The blood-brain barrier is basically impermeable to H^+ and HCO_3^- ions.

The *peripheral chemoreceptors* are specialized oxygen-sensitive cells in the carotid arteries (carotid bodies) and in the aortic arch (aortic bodies). The carotid bodies are in close contact with arterial blood and play a greater role in ventilation than do the aortic bodies. When a low P_aO_2 is sensed, afferent signals are sent via the ninth cranial nerve (glossopharyngeal) from the carotid bodies and via the tenth cranial nerve (vagus) from the aortic bodies. Efferent signals are sent to increase ventilation and elevate oxygen levels. The peripheral chemoreceptors become active at a P_aO_2 of approximately 60 mm Hg and then fully stimulated with further drops in oxygen. However, they are suppressed at P_aO_2s below 30 mm Hg.

In certain disease states (e.g., emphysema), the peripheral chemoreceptor drive to breathe may play a major role in ventilation. Patients with chronically high carbon dioxide levels may have their normal drive to breathe suppressed and have to rely on their peripheral drive mechanism. Careful administration and monitoring of oxygen therapy are encouraged to avoid oxygen-induced hypoventilation. The peripheral chemoreceptors are stimulated by decreased blood pH, hypoperfusion, increased temperature, nicotine (from smoking), and the direct influence of carbon dioxide. Peripheral chemoreceptors stimulate peripheral vasoconstriction, increased pulmonary vascular resistance, systemic arterial hypertension, tachycardia, and increased left ventricular performance.

REFLEXES THAT INFLUENCE VENTILATION

Reflexes also affect ventilation.

The Hering-Breuer reflex is a protective mechanism that prevents excessive lung inflation. Stretch receptors become excited when the bronchi and bronchioles are stretched during inhalation and then send inhibitory impulses to the medulla oblongata to stop inspiration.

- The deflation reflex becomes activated when the lungs are deflated.
- The irritant reflex, when stimulated by noxious gases, produces an increase in breathing rate, cough, and bronchoconstriction (spasm).
- Juxtapulmonary-capillary receptors (J-receptors) in the alveolar-capillary interstitium, when stimulated, cause a rapid-shallow breathing response.
- The dive reflex follows sudden immersion in cold water, resulting in apnea.
- Sudden pain results in apnea followed by tachypnea.
- Irritation to or pressure applied to the pharynx or larynx causes a brief apnea followed by coughing.

Cardiopulmonary Physiology of the Fetus and the Newborn

Adult anatomy and physiology differ markedly from those of the fetus and newborn. The development of the lungs is commonly divided into four periods (see Chapter 29): the embryonic period, the pseudoglandular period, the canalicular period, and the terminal sac. Sometimes a fifth period, the alveolar period, is considered to last from the 36th week of gestation onward.[10]

The placenta is the life support system from the mother to the fetus. It appears at the point of fertilization and transfers oxygen and nutrients from the mother to the fetus and eliminates wastes from fetal circulation. The placental segments, called *cotyledons*, provide the interface between maternal and fetal circulation. Deoxygenated blood is carried from the fetus to the placenta by two umbilical arteries, both wrapped around the umbilical vein. Oxygen transfers from maternal to fetal blood because of the pressure gradient, the higher hemoglobin concentration in fetal blood, and the greater affinity of fetal hemoglobin for oxygen. Carbon dioxide and wastes move from fetal to maternal blood at this time.

There are great differences between maternal and fetal blood values owing to maternal shunts and placental metabolism. Normal values for fetal blood are PO_2 20 mm Hg and PCO_2 55 mm Hg, whereas for maternal blood they are PO_2 80–100 mm Hg and PCO_2 33 mm Hg.

FETAL CIRCULATION, FETAL LUNG FLUIDS, AND ALVEOLI AT BIRTH

Fetal circulation is depicted in Figure 6-49.

- The umbilical vein carries oxygenated blood and nutrients from the placenta to the fetus.

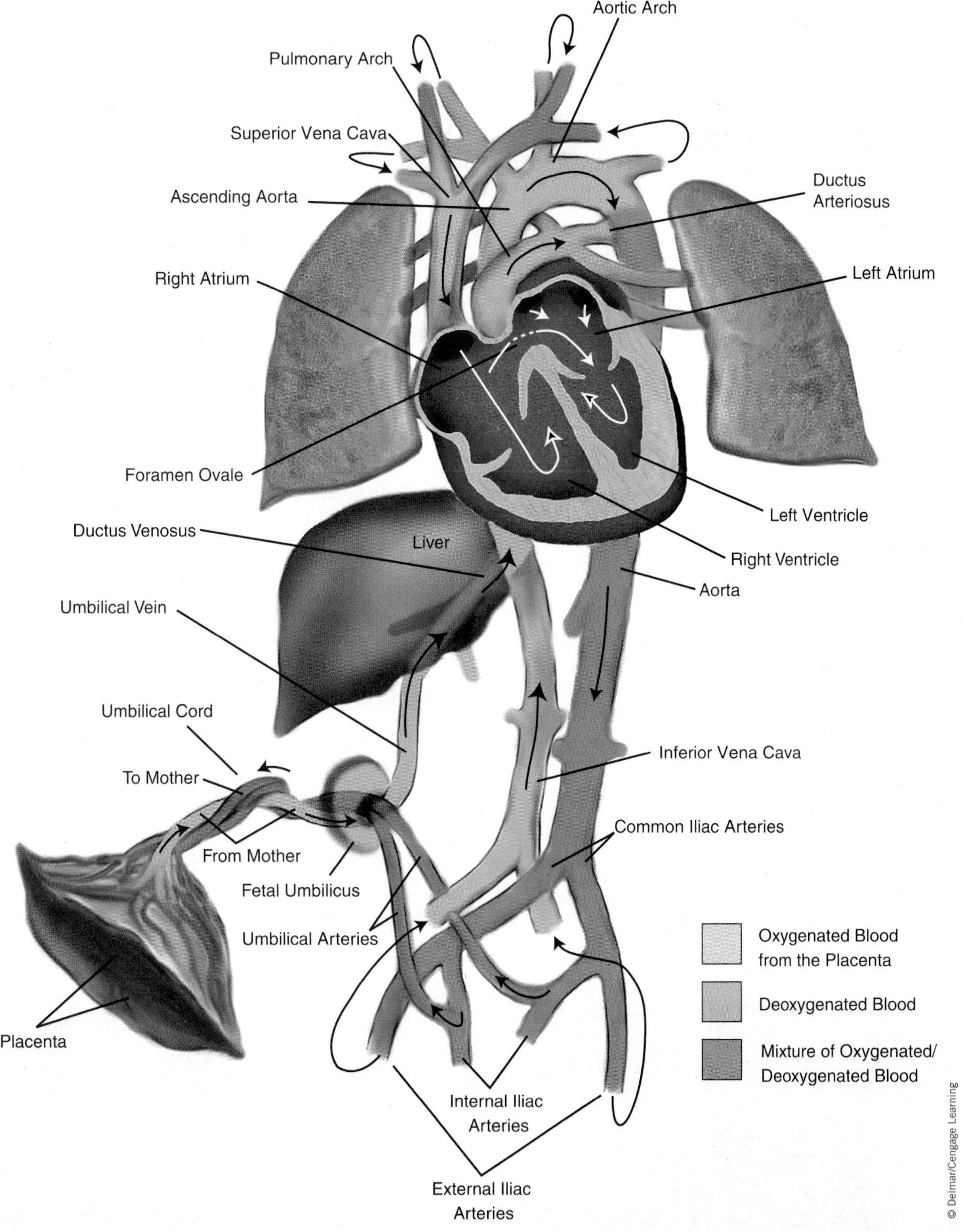

FIGURE 6-49 Fetal circulation.

- Half of this blood enters the liver, and the other half flows through the ductus venosus into the inferior vena cava (IVC), mixing with deoxygenated blood from the lower extremities.
- The blood travels via the IVC into the right atrium and mixes with deoxygenated blood from the superior vena cava (SVC).
- Most of the right atrial blood passes through the foramen ovale into the left atrium, where it mixes with deoxygenated blood from the pulmonary veins.
- The left atrial blood passes next into the left ventricle and is pumped to the heart and brain.

- The balance of blood in the right atrium flows into the right ventricle and is pumped into the pulmonary artery.
- About 85% of this blood bypasses the lungs and goes directly through the ductus arteriosis into the aorta. The balance (15%) passes through the lungs and returns to the left atrium via the pulmonary veins. The resultant PaO_2 in the descending aorta is about 20 mm Hg.
- Downstream, the blood passes into the internal illiac arteries and returns to the placenta.

After birth, the structures of fetal circulation become unnecessary and change to prepare for postuterine life.

At birth, the lungs are partially filled with liquid, roughly equal to the residual volume, produced by the alveolar cells during development. This fluid is removed from the lungs in the first 24 hours by three mechanisms:

- Squeezing of the chest during birth.
- Absorption by pulmonary capillaries.
- Absorption by the lymphatic system.

There are approximately 24 million alveoli at birth, increasing to more than 10 times that number in the normal adult. Alveoli continue to increase in number until 12 years of age; therefore, respiratory problems in childhood can significantly affect adult lungs.

BIRTH AND THE FIRST BREATH

After birth, rapid changes take place: The placenta stops functioning, the lungs open and begin breathing air, and features of adult circulation begin. The first breath marks the dramatic change from placental life support with liquid-filled lungs to newborn air breathing. Stimulation for taking the first breath is partly from placental failure, with decreasing PO_2s and increasing PCO_2s and pH, and from the sudden exposure to a noisy, bright, colder environment. In response to these stimuli, the newborn inhales.

CIRCULATORY CHANGES AT BIRTH

As the first breath is taken, *pulmonary vascular resistance* (*PVR*) decreases dramatically for two reasons: the rapid increase in alveolar PO_2, offsetting the fetal circulation's hypoxic vasoconstriction, and the mechanical increase in size of the pulmonary vessels, reducing resistance to perfusion. As the PVR drops, more blood passes from the right atrium to the right ventricle and more is returned to the left atrium. The volume and pressure in the left atrium increase, and the flap of the foramen ovale closes functionally. In addition, the fall in right atrial pressure assists closure of the foramen ovale. In the next few minutes, the elevated PO_2 causes the ductus arteriosus to constrict. Failure of alveolar expansion and increased oxygen levels keeps the ductus open,[11] contributing to the production of persistent pulmonary hypertension of the newborn (PPHN). The major cause of PPHN is continuing pulmonary hypertension.

Age-Specific Competency

The First Breath

The first air breath requires the infant to generate negative intrapleural pressures of from 40–80 cm H_2O. These large pressures are needed to overcome lung resistance, primarily due to viscous fluid in the lungs. This is similar to the effort needed to inflate an empty balloon. On the first and subsequent breaths, the residual volume and functional residual capacity are established. The average values for newborn lung compliance and airway resistance are 0.005 L/cm H_2O and 30 cm H_2O, respectively.

CONTROL OF VENTILATION IN THE NEWBORN

The central and peripheral chemoreceptors are active in stimulating the first breath. The peripheral chemoreceptors respond to hypoxemia by stimulating a transient increase, followed by a decrease in ventilation, which is stronger in the full-term newborn. The central chemoreceptors respond to elevated carbon dioxide levels similarly to the adult response.

INFANT REFLEXES

Several reflexes assist the newborn's breathing.

- In the trigeminal reflex, the cooling of the face results in a decrease in heart and respiratory rates.
- The irritant reflex causes slowing of respiration in the preterm infant but hyperventilation in the full-term infant.
- The head paradoxical reflex, which is a deep inspiration (sigh), results in increased lung volume, improved lung compliance, and the prevention of atelectasis.

NORMAL NEWBORN CLINICAL VALUES

The normal values for lung volumes and capacities and vital signs of newborns are listed in Table 6-12. The normal values for newborns' blood gas values are shown in Figure 6-50.

Age-Specific Competency

Lung Prematurity

Infants born before the 28th week of gestation are at risk because of their immature lungs. Surfactant production is necessary in large enough amounts to maintain alveolar stability for air breathing. Treatments for lung prematurity include continuous positive airway pressure (CPAP) and surfactant administration. Supporting the infant until the lungs grow and mature has been successful.

TABLE 6-12 **Approximate lung volume and capacity and vital sign values of the normal full-term newborn**

Lung Volumes	
Tidal volume (V_T)	15 mL
Residual volume (V_R)	40 mL
Expiratory reserve volume (V_{ER})	40 mL
Inspiratory reserve volume (V_{IR})	60 mL
Lung Capacities	
Vital capacity (*VC*)	115 mL
Functional residual capacity (*FRC*)	80 mL
Inspiratory capacity (*IC*)	75 mL
Total lung capacity (*TLC*)	155 mL
Vital Signs	
Respiratory rate (*RR*)	35–50 breaths/min
Heart rate (*HR*)	130–150 bpm

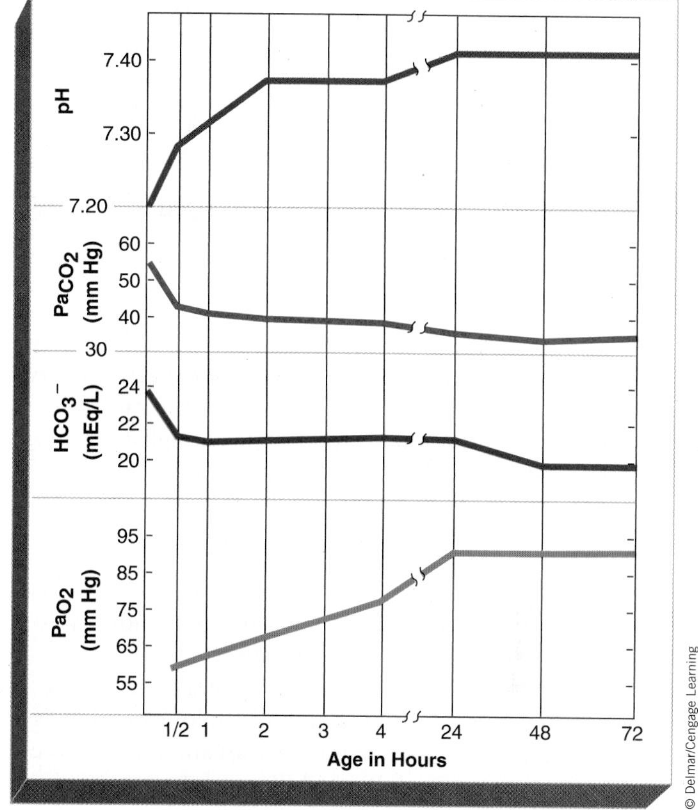

FIGURE 6-50 Average infant blood gas values during the first 72 hours after birth.

- Exercise tolerance is reduced, owing to decreased cardiac output.
- Diffusing capacity is decreased. Alveolar dead space is increased.
- Pressure differences between alveolar and arterial oxygen become greater.
- Hemoglobin is decreased (anemia).
- Ventilatory responses to carbon dioxide and oxygen are decreased.

In addition, environmental factors (occupation, smoking, trauma) and chronic pulmonary disease result in further decreases in function.

Effects of Aging on the Cardiopulmonary System

Like changes associated with aging from newborn to adult, other changes accompany aging during adulthood and into senior years.

INFLUENCE OF AGING ON THE RESPIRATORY SYSTEM

Aging is a normal process, and with it comes numerous normal changes.

- The chest wall becomes stiffer, and the respiratory rate slightly increases.
- The residual volume rises slightly. The forced vital capacity drops 21–25 mL per year after the 30th year.

INFLUENCE OF AGING ON THE CARDIOVASCULAR SYSTEM

Normal aging results in the following changes in the cardiovascular system.

- Cardiac output decreases, primarily because of decreased stroke volume.
- The maximal heart rate decreases.
- Fatty deposits and fibrosis form in the heart chambers.
- Fatty deposits (plaques) form on the arterial walls, leading to atherosclerosis and increased blood pressure.
- Peripheral vascular resistance increases.

Effects of Exercise and of High-Altitude and High-Pressure Environments on the Cardiopulmonary System

The cardiopulmonary system is challenged to respond and adapt to various stressors.

EXERCISE

During exercise, the cardiopulmonary system is stressed to meet the body's increased needs for oxygen delivery and carbon dioxide elimination. When the cardiopulmonary system is unable to provide enough oxygen for the working muscles, the body changes from aerobic (with oxygen) to anaerobic (without oxygen) metabolism. This point is called the *anaerobic threshold.*

Ventilation. Alveolar ventilation is increased in exercise to maintain normal oxygen and carbon dioxide levels in the body. The increased ventilation is probably a result of impulses sent from the cerebral cortex to the exercising muscles and the medulla oblongata, signals from proprioreceptors in the muscles and joints to the respiratory centers of the medulla, and the increase in body temperature. At rest, minute volume is about 6 L, but it can increase to about 120 L during heavy exercise.[4] The increase in alveolar ventilation is due primarily to an increased depth (tidal volume). Alveolar ventilation increases at the start of exercise, followed by a gradual increase and stabilization.

When exercise ends, alveolar ventilation drops (Figure 6-51). Cardiac output, not alveolar ventilation, is the major factor limiting aerobic performance. Oxygen consumption has a linear relationship with alveolar ventilation. At rest, oxygen consumption is 250 mL per minute. During exercise, this value rises to about 3500 mL per minute for an untrained person and to over 5000 mL per minute for the trained athlete.

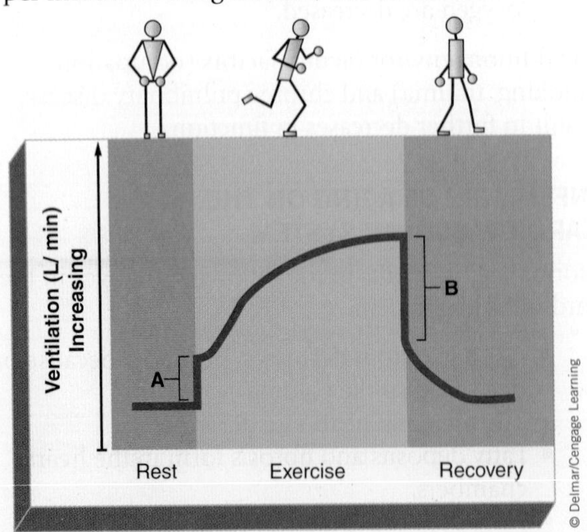

FIGURE 6-51 Relationship of exercise and ventilation: (A) onset of exercise warm up. (B) end of exercise cool down.

During exercise, P_AO_2 remains constant. The same is true for P_ACO_2 and pH, until they increase during heavy exercise. Oxygen diffusion capacity increases linearly during exercise because of increased alveolar-capillary surface area and increased cardiac output. The alveolar-arterial oxygen difference remains constant up to about 40% of maximal levels, and then widens to a value close to 33 mm Hg for distance runners.

Circulation. The circulatory system and muscles are equally important for determining exercise limits. Muscles are supplied with:

- Appropriate blood flow by increased sympathetic impulses, which stimulate the heart to increase its rate and contractile strength and to dilate the working muscles to increase perfusion.
- Increased cardiac output via heightened stroke volume (Frank-Starling mechanism) and increased heart rate.
- Increased arterial blood pressure, with the systolic pressure rising 20–80 mm Hg.

The maximal heart rate is calculated as

$$220 - \text{age (in years)}$$

This calculation is used for setting exercise and rehabilitation limits.

As oxygen consumption and cardiac output increase, the systolic and diastolic blood pressures also rise in the pulmonary vasculature. Oxygen uptake is increased because of distension of the pulmonary capillaries and the recruitment and opening of closed pulmonary vessels, allowing perfusion.

Muscle Work, Oxygen Consumption, and Cardiac Output Interrelationships. Increased muscle work results in increased oxygen consumption, increased perfusion in working muscles, greater venous return, and heightened cardiac output. Maximal cardiac outputs range from about 25 to 40 L/min.

The Training Influence. The trained athlete develops an increased heart chamber size and increased pumping action. At rest, the cardiac outputs of athletes and nonathletes are similar, but the athlete achieves it by having a higher stroke volume and lower heart rate. After exercise, the time the body needs to rest before continuing exercise is called the *recovery period.*

Body Temperature–Cutaneous Blood Flow Relationship. Heat is produced during exercise, and the body temperature may rise above normal. Sweating allows heat to dissipate, and as much as 5–10 lb of fluid may be lost. When liquid levels are inadequate before exercise or are not replaced after it, the body may experience heat stroke. This is a serious condition; symptoms include copious sweating, followed by no sweating, cramps, weakness, dizziness, confusion, and circulatory collapse. Before exercising, drink liquids (water), and then drink periodically during exercise. After exercise, take some time to cool down, stretch, and drink water to replace lost fluids.

HIGH ALTITUDE

Atmospheric pressure decreases with ascent to altitude. At 18,000 feet, the P_B is one-half of that at sea level (380 mm Hg). When an individual from a low altitude spends time at a high altitude, the body develops compensations, known collectively as *acclimatization*. Major cardiopulmonary acclimatization responses include:

- Increased alveolar ventilation via peripheral chemoreceptor stimulation.
- Secondary polycythemia, increased RBC production due to low oxygen levels.
- Development of respiratory alkalemia, due to the increased alveolar ventilation and carbon dioxide elimination.
- Increased oxygen diffusion capacity in native high dwellers, due to increased lung size.
- Increased alveolar-arterial oxygen difference.
- Improved ventilation/perfusion ratio.
- Increased cardiac output for nonacclimatized individuals.
- Increased pulmonary hypertension as a result of hypoxic vasoconstriction.

Other changes found at high altitude are poor sleep, increased myoglobin in skeletal muscles, acute mountain sickness, high-altitude pulmonary edema, high-altitude cerebral edema, and chronic mountain sickness. Seeking medical advice before ascending to high elevations is recommended.

HIGH-PRESSURE ENVIRONMENT

Breathing in gases at higher-than-atmospheric pressures affects the cardiopulmonary system. Scuba diving is the most commonly experienced high-pressure activity. Water is not compressible, and pressure increases directly with depth. For every 33 feet of descent below the water's surface, an additional atmosphere of pressure (760 cm H_2O) is added. At a depth of 33 feet, the total pressure exerted on the body is 2 atmospheres; at 66 feet, 3 atmospheres; and so forth. Subjected to these pressure increases, the lungs are compressed in size. The length of the dive is determined by the diver's metabolic rate and gas transport (oxygen and carbon dioxide). The feeling of breathlessness (dyspnea) signals the need for ascent. Interestingly, swallowing resets this feeling briefly.

The carbon dioxide–oxygen paradox occurs at depth. As the diver goes deeper, at some point alveolar carbon dioxide is greater than capillary carbon dioxide. At this point, carbon dioxide diffuses from alveoli into capillaries (the reverse directional movement of carbon dioxide). At the point during descent at which capillary oxygen is greater than alveolar oxygen, oxygen reverses its movement, going from capillaries to alveoli.

During a deep dive, gases in the blood move into the tissues. When the diver ascends back toward the surface, the pressure around the body is reduced (decompression). When ascent is done slowly, gases gradually move back into the blood for transport. At a rapid rate of ascent, however, the gases are released as bubbles; the bubbles then become trapped in the tissues causing *decompression sickness*, or *the bends*. These bubbles become trapped in tissues producing the signs and symptoms of the bends that include joint pain, chest pain, paralysis and circulatory failure that can result in death. Treatment for this life-threatening disorder is hyperbaric medicine (see Chapter 20), which reduces bubble size and resolution and increases tissue oxygenation.

Summary

The cardiopulmonary system brings atmospheric gas into the lungs, through successively smaller airways, to the alveoli. In the alveoli, these gases are brought into close contact with pulmonary capillary blood from the pulmonary vascular system, and oxygen rapidly moves into the blood and carbon dioxide out of it.

Breathing and circulation are controlled efficiently, balancing benefit and energy expenditure to meet the body's always-changing needs. General science principles clarify lung ventilation, gas diffusion, the perfusion of blood, gas transportation, and cellular-delivery mechanisms.

The fetus and newborn have different lung function and circulatory patterns than adults. Aging, exercise, and high-altitude and high-pressure environments all affect respiratory function.

Study Questions

REVIEW QUESTIONS

1. What are the lung structures (airway generations) from the trachea to the gas exchange area?
2. Name the tracheobronchial tree's lining layer and its functions.
3. Name the four characteristics that describe ventilation.
4. What are the static and dynamic characteristics of the lungs?
5. Trace one drop of blood as it flows through the adult heart, starting in the right atrium.
6. Name the components of the heart's conducting system.

7. Describe the lung-thorax relationship.
8. Discuss the two ways that oxygen is carried in the blood.
9. Name the six ways carbon dioxide is carried in the blood.
10. Discuss exercise and at least three effects on breathing.

MULTIPLE-CHOICE QUESTIONS

1. What is the minute ventilation, in milliliters, for a person with these values: respiratory rate (*f*) of 12, tidal volume of 600 mL, and dead space of 200 mL?
   a. 4800
   b. 6000
   c. 7200
   d. 9600
2. What is the average normal alveolar-capillary surface area, in square meters, for gas exchange?
   a. 50
   b. 75
   c. 100
   d. 125
3. Which blood cells contain hemoglobin?
   a. erythrocytes
   b. thrombocytes
   c. leukocytes
   d. platelets
4. What is the minute alveolar ventilation, in milliliters, for a person with these values: respiratory rate (*f*) of 12, tidal volume of 600 mL, and dead space of 200 mL?
   a. 4800
   b. 6000
   c. 7200
   d. 9600
5. The nephron is the functional unit of what organ?
   a. lung
   b. heart
   c. placenta
   d. kidney
6. Which of these is/are part of a true shunt?
   I. physiological shunt
   II. capillary shunt
   III. anatomic shunt
   a. I only
   b. II only
   c. I, II
   d. I, II, III
7. What is the oxygen content (volume percentage) for these values: P_aO_2 = 90 mm Hg, Hb = 14 g, O_2Sat = 95%?
   a. 0.27
   b. 17.8
   c. 18.1
   d. 19.0
8. How do the central chemoreceptors regulate breathing?
   a. by monitoring oxygen levels in the carotid arteries
   b. by the indirect effects of carbon dioxide on the cerebral spinal fluid
   c. directly from monitoring the medulla oblongata
   d. via input from the aortic bodies

CRITICAL-THINKING QUESTIONS

1. Using the four lung volumes and four lung capacities, list three different combinations that can describe vital capacity (VC).
2. A newborn infant with a P_aO_2 that remains below normal will have what circulatory effects?
3. When a person who lives at sea level travels to a mountainous area for a 2-week vacation, what changes occur?

References

1. Murray JF. *The Normal Lung*. 2nd ed. Philadelphia: WB Saunders Co; 1986.
2. Gorback MS. Chapter 29. In: Dantzker DR, MacIntyre NR, Bakow ED. *Comprehensive Respiratory Care*. Philadelphia: WB Saunders Co; 1995.
3. Slonim NB, Hamilton LH. *Respiratory Physiology*. 2nd ed. St. Louis: CV Mosby Co; 1971.
4. West J. *Respiratory Physiology: The Essentials*. 8th ed. Baltimore: Lippincott Williams & Wilkins; 2008.
5. Levitzsky MG. *Pulmonary Physiology*. 7th ed. New York: McGraw-Hill; 2007.
6. Oaks DF. *Clinical Practitioners Pocket Guide to Respiratory Care*. 7th ed. Old Town, ME: Health Educator Publications; 2008.
7. Ruppel GE. *Manual of Pulmonary Function Testing*. 9th ed. St. Louis: Mosby-Yearbook; 2008.
8. Anthony C, Thibodeau G. *Anthony's Textbook of Anatomy and Physiology*. 19th ed. St. Louis: CV Mosby Co; 2009.
9. *Mosby's Medical, Nursing, and Allied Health Dictionary*. 6th ed. St. Louis: Mosby-Yearbook; 2005.
10. Volpe M. Control of morphologic development of the lung. *Neonatal Respir Dis*. 1999;9:2.
11. Dantzker DR, MacIntyre NR, Bakow ED. *Comprehensive Respiratory Care*. Philadelphia: WB Saunders Co; 1995.

Suggested Reading

Des Jardins T. *Cardiopulmonary Anatomy and Physiology—Essentials for Respiratory Care*. 5th ed. Clifton Park, NY: Delmar Cengage Learning; 2008.

CHAPTER 7

Cardiopulmonary Pharmacology

Kenneth A. Wyka

OBJECTIVES

Upon completion of this chapter, the reader should be able to:

- Differentiate between the three phases of pharmacology: pharmaceutical, pharmacokinetic, and pharmacodynamic.
- Differentiate between tolerance and tachyphylaxis.
- Define the terms "additive effect," "cumulative effect," and "synergy," and explain the differences among these actions.
- Describe the types of drugs commonly administered by aerosol route and their mechanism of action.
- Describe the indications for, contraindications for, side effects of, and adverse reactions of aerosol drugs.
- Identify brand names and dosages of aerosol drugs.
- Determine the dosage of drug to be administered by either weight or volume.
- Describe drugs used in the management of asthma and COPD.
- List indications for and dosages of drugs used in advanced cardiac life support.
- Determine appropriate therapeutic actions when given a patient case scenario.

CHAPTER OUTLINE

(continues)

(continued)

KEY TERMS

adrenergic
additive effect
antagonism
anticholinergic
cumulative effect
mediator antagonists
mucolytics
pharmaceutical phase
pharmacodynamic phase
pharmacokinetic phase
potentiation
synergy
tachyphylaxis
therapeutic index (TI)
tolerance

Pharmacology is the study of drugs: their origin, nature, properties, and effects on living organisms. Respiratory therapists administer drugs by aerosol and instillation. They also routinely participate in the care of patients with complex metabolic and cardiovascular disorders, including those requiring resuscitation. This chapter introduces the general concepts of pharmacology as they are related to the care and support of patients with cardiopulmonary disorders. Specific information is provided regarding the selection and administration of bronchoactive drugs and selected cardiovascular agents used during advanced cardiac life support. This chapter is intended to be not a comprehensive pharmacology source but rather an overview and introduction to essential principles required for the practice of respiratory care.

Principles of Pharmacology

Drug action can be divided into three distinct phases: pharmaceutical, pharmacokinetic, and pharmacodynamic.

PHARMACEUTICAL PHASE

The term **pharmaceutical phase** refers to the method by which a drug is delivered to the body (i.e., the route of administration and drug form). Respiratory therapists commonly administer drugs in *aerosol* form by inhalation. The aerosol may consist of droplets of a liquid solution or a dry powder. Liquid solutions are typically administered by *small-volume nebulizer* (*SVN*) or *metered-dose inhaler* (*MDI*). Few medications are currently administered by *dry powder inhaler* (*DPI*); the ones that are designed for use with specific devices are marketed by the drug manufacturers.

The administration of a drug by the aerosol route offers several advantages:

- Immediate onset of action at the desired site
- Reduced side effects from systemic absorption
- Ability to administer smaller doses of potent drugs
- Ability of patients to self-administer medications

To administer a drug by *instillation*, a bolus of drug is injected directly into the tracheobronchial tree via tube or catheter. This route is typically used for the administration of wetting agents, mucolytics, surface-active agents (such as surfactant replacement), and advanced cardiac life support (ACLS) drugs during cardiac resuscitation.

Other common routes of administration include intravenous (IV), intra-arterial (IA), intramuscular (IM), oral (PO), and various routes of absorption (subcutaneous, sublingual, transdermal, rectal). The onset of drug action is directly related to its route of administration, as shown in Table 7-1.

TABLE 7-1 **Common routes of drug administration, their onset of action, clinical indications, and examples**

Route of Administration	Onset of Action	Clinical Indicators	Examples of Clinical Uses
Intra-arterial (IA)	< 1 minute	Drug delivery to specific target organ	Anticancer drugs
Intravenous (IV)	Within 1 minute	Emergencies; long-term infusion	ACLS, nutrient solutions, hydration, antibiotics, general anesthesia
Aerosol	Within 1 minute	Localized effect in respiratory tract; good systemic absorption of appropriate agents; self administration	Bronchoactive drugs in respiratory care; convenient noninvasive method for drugs such as insulin
Instillation	1–2 minutes	Useful when rapid onset is required and no IV is available; direct pulmonary activity desired	Instilled ACLS drugs; mucolytics or wetting agents for transtracheal oxygen therapy (TTOT) or during bronchosopy; surfactant replacement
Sublingual	Within minutes	Rapid systemic absorption required without IV access	Nitroglycerin for angina pectoris
Transdermal (topical)	15–30 minutes	Continuous low dosage, usually self-administered	Nitroglycerin patches, hormone patches, nicotine patches, analgesic ointments
Intramuscular (IM)	15–30 minutes	Drugs that have poor oral absorption; when higher serum levels are needed more rapidly than by oral route	Narcotics
Rectal	30 minutes	When patient is unable to take oral medication or does not tolerate PO route	Antinausea medications
Subcutaneous	30–45 minutes	Drugs that have poor oral absorption; when higher serum levels are needed more rapidly than by oral route but more slowly than by IM	Insulin, local anesthetic by hypodermic injection
Oral (PO)	30–60 minutes	Self-administered, convenient, immediate onset not required	Most medications, particularly over-the-counter preparations

PHARMACOKINETIC PHASE

The **pharmacokinetic phase** is the time required for drug absorption, drug action, drug distribution in the body, and the metabolization and excretion of the drug. Drugs must pass through cell membranes to reach the target tissue to exert their intended therapeutic effects. A *fully ionized drug* is not readily absorbed across lipid membranes. A *nonionized drug* is generally lipid soluble and will diffuse across cell membranes and into the bloodstream. For example, ipratropium bromide is a bronchodilator administered by aerosol that has few systemic effects because it is a fully ionized compound. Lipid-soluble nonionized drugs such as general anesthetics are readily absorbed into the central nervous system, where they alter neurological activity.

The distribution of a drug administered by the aerosol route depends on factors such as the person's breathing pattern (tidal volume and respiratory rate) and the aerosol's particle size. Although the intended site of action of inhaled bronchoactive drugs is the lung, some medication is inevitably deposited in the pharynx and will be swallowed. The portion of the drug that is deposited in the lung has therapeutic effects. Systemic effects are due to the absorption of the drug into the bloodstream through the gastrointestinal tract or the pulmonary mucosa.

PHARMACODYNAMIC PHASE

The term **pharmacodynamic phase** refers to the mechanism of action by which a drug causes its therapeutic effect. In the following sections, drugs administered by aerosol are described according to their mechanism of action. For example, both adrenergic and anticholinergic bronchodilators are used to enhance bronchodilation, but their mechanisms of action are different.

Drug Actions and Interactions

When a drug is administered repeatedly or when combinations of drugs are administered, the patient may experience a number of drug actions or effects. Some of these may be beneficial, and others may result in detrimental or harmful side effects. The major drug actions and interactions are:

- **Tolerance** is the effect when increased amounts of a drug are needed to produce the desired effect, possibly due in part to increased enzyme levels related to enzymatic activity that develops over a period of time. (The higher enzyme levels produced metabolize the drug faster and so a higher dose is needed to produce the effect. In other words, the individual is becoming tolerant to the drug.)
- **Tachyphylaxis** is the rapid development of drug tolerance.
- **Cumulative effect**, an exaggerated response and possibly toxic situation, occurs when doses of the same drug are administered before previous doses are inactivated and removed/eliminated from the body. The effect is especially likely if the drug has a long *half-life*, that is, the time required to metabolize 50% of the administered drug.
- **Additive effect**, an exaggerated response, occurs when two or more drugs are administered with the same effect on the body.
- **Synergy** is the result when two or more drugs produce an effect or response that neither could produce alone.
- **Potentiation** is the result either when two drugs produce an effect that is greater than what they usually produce when given alone or when one drug enhances the effect of another drug.
- **Antagonism** occurs when two drugs have opposite effects.
- **Therapeutic index (TI)** is the ratio of the lethal dose (LD_{50}) to the effective dose (ED_{50}). The LD_{50} is the dose that would be lethal to 50% of the test population, and the ED_{50} is the dose that would be effective for 50% of the test population.

Drug Calculations

Respiratory therapists must develop problem-solving skills when administering medications to their patients. *Drug calculations* follow basic mathematical principles. They include concentration calculations involving volume-to-weight and weight-to-volume problems or dilution calculations using volumes and concentrations.

CONCENTRATION CALCULATIONS

The *concentration* of any drug is the percentage solution of the active ingredient. This percentage is commonly found on the label or in the product information brochure. Respiratory therapists should be familiar with the following common drug calculations.

In the terminology of drug solutions, a *1% strength solution*, by definition, means that 1 g of the drug (the solute) is dissolved in 100 cc (or 100 mL) of a solvent. Most drugs, however, are expressed in milligrams (mg), not in grams. Therefore, in the setup of a drug problem, it is more appropriate to express the concentration as milligrams per milliliter (mg/mL). Then, for example, a 1% solution has 1000 mg/100 mL (1 g = 1000 mg). Simplified, the 1% strength solution contains 10 mg/mL. The following expression is used in solving many drug problems.

$$\text{mg} = \text{mL } x\% \times 10$$

Here is a sample problem: How many milligrams of drug are in 0.5 mL of a 2% strength solution? This problem may be set up and solved as follows: If a 1% solution contains 10 mg/mL, a 2% solution will contain 20 mg/mL. A simple mathematical calculation provides the answer:

$$\frac{20 \text{ mg}}{1 \text{ mL}} = \frac{x \text{ mg}}{0.5 \text{ mL}}$$

$$x \text{ mg} = 20 \times 0.5$$

$$x = 10 \text{ mg}$$

This problem can also be solved logically: A 2% solution containing 20 mg/mL has 10 mg/0.5 mL (half of the given amount).

RATIO CALCULATIONS

A drug solution may be expressed as a ratio instead of as a percentage. For instance, 1:100, 1:200, and 1:1000 are drug ratios often encountered; they all describe a strength of solution. Mathematically:

- A 1:100 solution is a 1% solution (1/100 × 100 = 1%).
- A 1:200 solution is 0.5% strength.
- A 1:1000 solution is 0.1% strength.

With this knowledge, respiratory therapists can convert ratio and percentage strengths and solve most drug problems.

Here is a sample problem: How many milligrams of drug are in 0.1 mL of a 1:100 strength solution? A 1:100 ratio solution is really a 1% strength solution containing 10 mg/mL. Therefore:

$$\frac{10 \text{ mg}}{1 \text{ mL}} = \frac{x \text{ mg}}{0.1 \text{ mL}}$$

$$x \text{ mg} = 10 \times 0.1$$

$$x = 1.0 \text{ mg}$$

Here is another sample problem: How many milliliters of a 0.5% strength solution should be used to administer 0.5 mg of a drug to a patient? A 0.5% solution contains 5 mg/mL. Therefore:

$$\frac{5 \text{ mg}}{1 \text{ mL}} = \frac{0.5 \text{ mg}}{x \text{ mL}}$$

$$0.5 = 5x$$

$$x = 0.1 \text{ mL}$$

DILUTION CALCULATIONS

At times, an available drug is too strong for the patient and must be diluted before it is administered. In these situations, a volume times concentration expression is set up to determine the appropriate amount of dilution. In most cases, normal saline is used as the diluent. A *dilution expression* is as follows:

$$\text{volume 1} \times \text{concentration 1} = \text{volume 2} \times \text{concentration 2}$$

where 1 represents the normal volume or concentration, and 2 represents the volume or concentration needed.

For example, a respiratory therapist (RT) has a 10% strength solution but needs to administer 2.0 mL of a 2.5% strength solution. How much drug should be used, and what dilution is needed? The problem should be set up in the following manner:

$$\text{volume 1} \times \text{concentration 1} = \text{volume 2} \times \text{concentration 2}$$

$$x \text{ mL} \times 10\% = 2 \text{ mL} \times 2.5\%$$

$$10x = 5$$

$$x = 0.5 \text{ mL}$$

To make 2.0 mL of a 2.5% strength solution, the RT has to dilute 0.5 mL of the drug with 1.5 mL of normal saline.

Here is another sample problem: How many milliliters of a drug with a 3% strength solution should be used to administer 0.75 mL of a 1% strength solution? To solve, set up the problem as follows:

$$\text{volume 1} \times \text{concentration 1} = \text{volume 2} \times \text{concentration 2}$$

$$x \text{ mL} \times 3\% = 0.75 \text{ mL} \times 1\%$$

$$3x = 0.75$$

$$x = 0.25 \text{ mL}$$

Age-Specific Competency

When drugs are to be administered to infants or children, smaller amounts (in milligrams or milliliters) are given on the basis of patient age or weight. Five basic rules or formulas are generally used:

1. Fried's rule (for patients younger than 1 year of age):

$$\text{pediatric dose} = \frac{\text{age in months}}{150} \times \text{adult dose}$$

2. Clark's rule (for patients older than 2 years of age):

$$\text{pediatric dose} = \frac{\text{weight in pounds}}{150} \times \text{adult dose}$$

3. Young's rule (for patients older than 2 years of age):

$$\text{pediatric dose} = \frac{\text{age in years}}{\text{age in years} + 12} \times \text{adult dose}$$

4. Cowling's rule (for patients older than 2 years of age):

$$\text{pediatric dose} = \frac{\text{age next birthday}}{24} \times \text{adult dose}$$

5. Body surface area (BSA) formula:

$$\text{pediatric dose} = \frac{\text{surface area of child (in mm}^2\text{)}}{1.7} \times \text{adult dose}$$

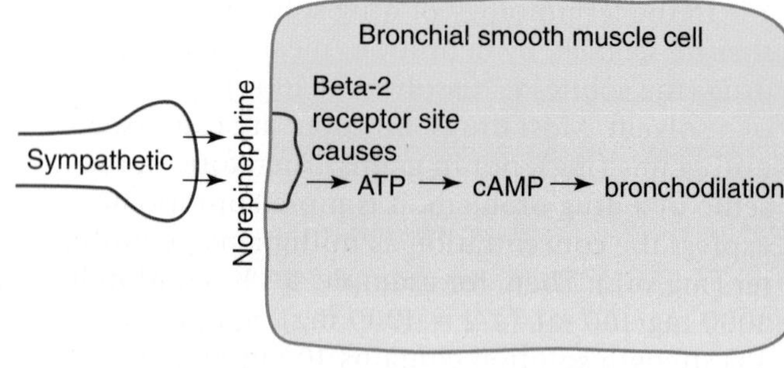

FIGURE 7-1 Sympathomimetic drugs stimulate cAMP.

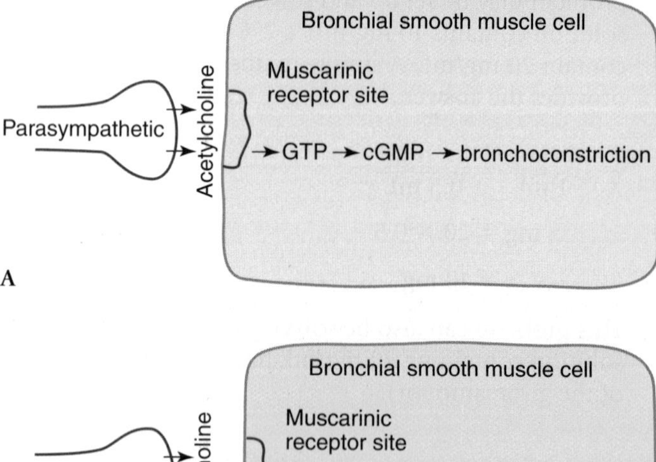

FIGURE 7-2 (A) Effect of parasympathetic stimulation in bronchial cells. (B) Anticholinergic drugs block parasympathetic stimulation.

To produce the prescribed 0.75 mL of the 1% strength solution, the RT dilutes 0.25 mL of the 3% strength drug with 0.5 mL of normal saline.

Bronchodilators

There are three commonly recognized mechanisms for inducing bronchodilation.

- Beta-adrenergic, or sympathomimetic, drugs directly stimulate the conversion of ATP to cyclic 3′5′-AMP via the enzyme adenyl cyclase (Figure 7-1).
- **Anticholinergic** drugs block the bronchoconstricting effects of the parasympathetic or cholinergic system (Figure 7-2).
- Xanthines inhibit phosphodiesterase to prevent the conversion of cyclic 3′-5′-AMP into GMP (Figure 7-3).

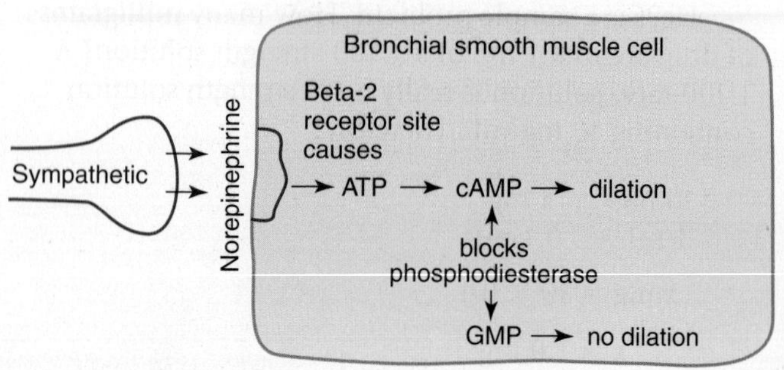

FIGURE 7-3 Xanthines inhibit phosphodiesterase.

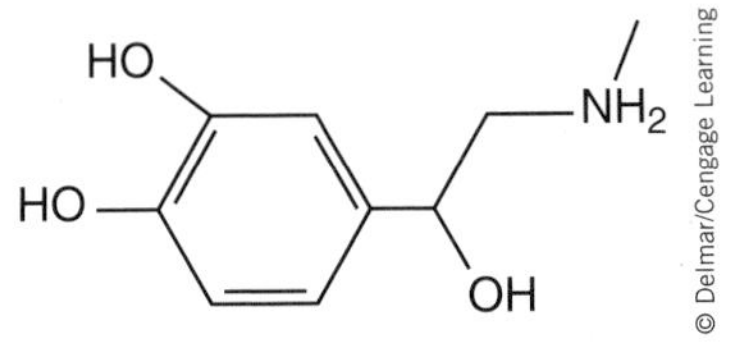

FIGURE 7-4 Catecholamine bronchodilator chemical structure: benzene ring (catechol nucleus) with placement of hydroxyl (OH) groups on the 3rd and 4th carbon sites of the ring, carbon side chain and terminal amino (NH_2) group.

SYMPATHOMIMETIC BRONCHODILATORS

Sympathomimetic bronchodilators promote the relaxation of bronchial smooth muscle by stimulating the intracellular production of cyclic 3′5′-AMP. They are also referred to as **adrenergic** because they promote bronchodilation via the neurotransmitter norepinephrine, which is similar to epinephrine (adrenalinelike, thus the term "adrenergic").

The first sympathomimetic bronchodilators were classified as catecholamines because they had a chemical structure that included a benzene ring (catechol nucleus) and a carbon side chain with a terminal amino (NH_2) group (Figure 7-4). The length of this carbon chain can vary and can impact the duration of action of some bronchodilators, many of which are noncatecholamine in chemical structure.[1] Bronchodilators with long carbon chains have longer durations of action.

Enzyme breakdown or deactivation can also affect the duration of catecholamine bronchodilation action. Catechol-O-methyl transferase (COMT) is the enzyme responsible for the rapid breakdown of the ultrashort-acting bronchodilators such as isoproterenol, resulting in a very short duration of action. On the other hand, the enzyme monoamine oxidase (MAO) works more slowly but also has an effect on deactivating catecholamine bronchodilators. For example, isoetharine is affected more by MAO and less by COMT, and therefore it has a longer duration of action (up to 3 hours) than isoproterenol.

Sympathetic system receptor sites include alpha, beta-1, and beta 2.

- *Alpha receptor* stimulation results in vasoconstriction.
- *Beta-1* receptors are located only in the heart, and stimulation results in increased heart rate.
- *Beta 2* receptors are located in the smooth muscle of the bronchi and uterus, and stimulation results in muscle dilation (relaxation).

Aerosol delivery of alpha agents is recommended for conditions associated with mucosal edema (e.g., croup, laryngeal trauma, postextubation laryngeal edema). Adrenergics are categorized as either catecholamine (having mixed beta-1 and beta 2 effects or alpha, beta-1, and beta 2 effects) or noncatecholamine (having strong beta 2 specificity). All newer beta agonists are noncatecholamine in nature, but both isoproterenol and racemic epinephrine (catecholamines) are still in use today.[1]

Some of the noncatecholamine bronchodilators are further classified as either resorcinols or saligenins on the basis of their chemical structure and drug action specificity.

- Resorcinols (metaproterenol and terbutaline) have a shift in the hydroxyl (OH) group from the 4th carbon site on the catechol nucleus to the 5th carbon site. This shift produces the resorcinol nucleus. COMT does not affect this nucleus, resulting in a drug duration of action of up to 6 hours.
- Saligenins, on the other hand, have a modification (OH group to CH_2OH group) at the 3rd carbon site. This produces the saligenin nucleus that is also not affected by COMT and MAO. Albuterol is classified as a saligenin bronchodilator with a duration of action up to 6 hours. An isomer of albuterol (levalbuterol, or Xopenex) has a long duration of action with reportedly fewer side effects. Another drug, Pirbuterol or Maxair, is very similar to albuterol except it has a pyridine ring structure (N at the 2nd carbon site) instead of the traditional benzene ring structure.

Another classification of bronchodilator is the prodrug variety. Bitolterol mesylate (Tornalate) is converted in the body, via esterase hydrolysis, to the active catecholamine, colterol. This agent also has a prolonged bronchodilator effect of up to 8 hours. However, Tornalate is no longer available in the United States.

The most common long-acting beta-agonist (LABA) bronchodilators are formoterol (Foradil) and salmeterol (Serevent). Formoterol is an analogue of catecholamine with very selective beta 2 activity. It has a duration of action of up to 12 hours, due in part to a lipid-soluble group on its structure that increases lipid solubility, resulting in greater beta 2 receptor binding. Salmeterol has enhanced beta 2 activity because of its chemical structure, which includes a very long carbon side chain. Its duration of action is also up to 12 hours.[1]

ANTICHOLINERGIC BRONCHODILATORS

Anticholinergic bronchodilators, also referred to as *parasympatholytics,* promote bronchodilation by blocking bronchoconstriction. Parasympathetic stimulation via the neurotransmitter acetylcholine induces bronchoconstriction; thus anticholinergic drugs block cholinergic-induced bronchoconstriction. This category currently includes four agents: atropine, ipratropium bromide (Atrovent), tiotropium bromide

(Spiriva), and glycopyrrolate. Of the four, atropine is not commonly delivered by aerosol.

Generally, anticholinergics have a longer onset than that of most beta-agonists but also have an extended duration of effectiveness. Anticholinergics are useful in managing chronic airflow obstruction associated with COPD but have limited usefulness in reversible airway diseases such as asthma.[2]

XANTHINES

Xanthines include caffeine, theobromine, and theophylline. Theophylline and its derivatives (aminophylline) are delivered by IV and oral routes in the management of chronic bronchospasm. Although xanthines are rarely administered by aerosol, some COPD patients receive oral xanthines as part of their overall pharmacologic management. Within bronchial smooth muscle cells, cyclic 3′5′-AMP is constantly degraded by the enzyme phosphodiesterase; one of the bronchodilating mechanisms of xanthines is their inhibition of phosphodiesterase.

Xanthines have numerous other effects, including pulmonary vasodilation, cardiac stimulation, skeletal muscle stimulation (including enhanced diaphragmatic contractility), central nervous system stimulation, and diuresis. Xanthines also have serious neurological and gastrointestinal side effects and must be kept within a narrow therapeutic range (10–15 μ/mL).

Xanthines also interact with a wide variety of drugs, most notably many of the cardiovascular drugs concurrently used in the complex management of many pulmonary patients. Beta-blockers (e.g., Inderal, Tenormin, Lopressor), calcium channel blockers (e.g., Procardia, Cardizem, Isoptin), corticosteroids, and many antibiotics tend to increase serum theophylline levels.[3]

INDICATIONS AND CONTRAINDICATIONS FOR BRONCHODILATORS

The general clinical indication for the administration of a bronchodilator is the presence of reversible airway obstruction, usually manifested by the presence of wheezing. Selection of the appropriate medication to treat wheezing depends on the cause of the airway obstruction. Wheezing is a symptom of bronchoconstriction, which may be due to bronchospasm, mucosal edema, or the presence of mucus. Bronchospasm is best reversed by the use of adrenergic or anticholinergic agents. Other conditions respond better therapeutically to the use of an adrenergic agent with alpha properties such as racemic epinephrine. An example is croup, manifested by laryngeal edema and bronchiolitis with associated mucosal edema.

Selection of an Adrenergic or Anticholinergic Bronchodilator. Adrenergic bronchodilators generally have a more rapid onset of action than anticholinergics because they directly stimulate the relaxation of bronchial smooth muscle cells. Anticholinergic agents have little application in the treatment of acute bronchospasm, such as asthma or exercise-induced bronchospasm, but they have been shown to be useful in the management of chronic bronchospasm associated with COPD. Concurrent use of an anticholinergic drug with a beta-agonist has also been shown to improve the effectiveness of each drug. Combivent is such a combination (MDI formulation of albuterol and ipratropium bromide); DuoNeb is a similar liquid formulation for aerosolization via a small-volume or hand-held nebulizer. Assessing the response to bronchodilator therapy at the point of care in terms of airflow, desired outcomes, patient monitoring, and presence of any side effects is thoroughly reviewed in an American Association for Respiratory Care (AARC) clinical practice guideline (CPG) published in 1995.[4]

Contraindications for Bronchodilators. All bronchodilators, regardless of their mechanism of action or beta 2 specificity, have some cardiovascular side effects. Respiratory therapists should always exercise caution when administering bronchodilators to patients who have a history of cardiac disease or arrhythmias.

SIDE EFFECTS OF AND ADVERSE REACTIONS TO BRONCHODILATORS

The most common side effects associated with inhaled bronchodilators are tachycardia, headache, nervousness, and nausea. Many patients experience tremors, which usually diminish with continued use. Although the newer drugs are formulated for more targeted beta 2 specificity, most patients still experience some degree of increased heart rate and nervousness. Headache is a commonly reported side effect, but it occurs almost as often in patients receiving a placebo. Table 7-2 summarizes the side effects associated with currently used aerosol bronchodilators.

BRONCHODILATOR DOSAGE GUIDELINES

The standard dosages for aerosolized bronchodilators are provided in Table 7-3. Recent clinical use of high-dose and continuous nebulization of bronchodilators has been shown to be useful in the management of intractable bronchospasm and status asthmaticus.

High-Dose Bronchodilator Protocol. When a patient presents in acute respiratory distress with diffuse wheezing, tachypnea, and a peak expiratory flow rate

TABLE 7-2 **Classification, receptors, and common side effects of aerosol bronchodilators**

Drug (Trade name)	Type	Receptors	Side Effects
Albuterol (Proventil, Ventolin)	Sympathomimetic	Primarily beta 2	Mild tremors, headache, insomnia, nervousness, nausea
Albuterol and ipratropium (Combivent)	Adrenergic, anticholinergic	Adrenergic, primarily beta 2; anticholinergic blocks muscarine receptors	Mild tremors, headache, insomnia, nervousness, nausea, dry mouth, cough
Bitolterol (Tornalate)	Sympathomimetic	Primarily beta 2	Mild tremors, headache, insomnia, nervousness, nausea
Epinephrine (Asthmahaler Bronitin Mist, Bronkaid Mist, Medihaler-Epi, Primatene Mist)	Catecholamine sympathomimetic	Strong alpha, beta-1, and beta 2	Profound tachycardia, hypertension, palpitations, vasoconstriction
Glycopyrrolate (Robinul)	Anticholinergic; parasympatholytic	Blocks muscarinic; receptors	Few, mild: dry mouth, cough
Ipratropium bromide (Atrovent)	Anticholinergic, parasympatholytic	Blocks muscarinic receptors	Few, mild: dry mouth, cough
Isoetharine (Bronkosol)	Catecholamine, sympathomimetic	Mild beta-1, primarily beta 2	Tachycardia, palpitations, nausea, headache
Isoproterenol (Isuprel)	Catecholamine, sympathomimetic	Strong beta-1 and beta 2	Profound tachycardia, palpitations, nervousness
Metaproterenol (Alupent, Metaprel, Pirbuterol (Tomalate)	Sympathomimetic	Primarily beta 2	Mild tremors, headache, insomnia, nervousness, nausea
Racemic epinephrine (Micronefrin, Vaponefrin, Racepinephrine)	Catecholamine, sympathomimetic	Alpha, beta-1, and beta 2	Mild tachycardia, shakiness, nausea, headache
Salmeterol (Serevent)	Sympathomimetic	Primarily beta 2	Mild tremors, headache, insomnia, nervousness, nausea
Terbutaline (Brethair, Brethine, Bricanyl)	Sympathomimetic	Primarily beta 2	Mild tremors, headache, insomnia, nervousness, nausea

(PEF) less than 50% predicted, it may be appropriate to administer a series of high-dose aerosol bronchodilator treatments with less than the usual time between treatments. A typical approach could include administering up to three aerosol treatments at 20-minute intervals with 1.0 mL albuterol (5.0 mg) and 1.0 mL normal saline.

Continuous Bronchodilator Aerosol. Situations such as status asthmaticus, refractory bronchospasm, or cystic fibrosis may indicate continuous aerosol by face mask or endotracheal tube. This dosage typically delivers a solution that provides 2.0 mL/hour (10 mg), which is administered until the patient's clinical condition improves.

Ultrashort-, Short, and Long-Acting Adrenergic Bronchodilators. As noted in Table 7-3, certain bronchodilators have an ultrashort duration of effectiveness or action (1–2 hours). These drugs include isoproterenol (Isuprel) and racemic epinephrine (Micronefrin). Others are short-acting beta-agonists (SABA) with 4–6 hours of pharmacologic action: albuterol (Proventil or Ventolin), levalbuterol (Xopenex), and metaproterenol (Alupent or Metaprel). Long-acting beta agonists (LABA), with up to 12 hours of action, are salmeterol (Serevent), formoterol (Foradil), and arformoterol (Brovana).

Isoproterenol is rarely used today because of its profound cardiovascular side effects and ultrashort duration of action. However, it may be useful in

TABLE 7-3 **Aerosol bronchodilator strengths, dosages, onsets, and durations of effectiveness**

Drug	Strength	Dosage	Frequency	Onset (minutes)	Peak	Duration
Albuterol	0.50% solution	0.50 mL	tid, qid	1–5	30–60 minutes	3–6 hours
Albuterol	MDI 90 μg/puff	2 puffs	tid, qid	1–5	30–60 minutes	3–6 hours
Albuterol and ipratropium	MDI 18 μg/puff Ipratropium and 90 μg/puff albuterol	2 puffs	qid	15	1–2 hours	4–6 hours
Bitolterol	0.20% solution	1.25 mL	tid	3–4	30–60 minutes	5–8 hours
Bitolterol	MDI 0.37 mg/puff	2 puffs	q 8 hours	3–4	30–60 minutes	5–8 hours
Epinephrine	1:100 (1.0%)	0.25–0.50 mL	q 2–4 hours	1–3	15 minutes	60 minutes
Glycopyrrolate	0.20 mg/mL	2.50–5.0 mL	tid, qid	15–30	1–2 hours	4–6 hours
Ipratropium	0.025% solution	1.0–2.0 mL	q 4–6 hours	15	1–2 hours	4–6 hours
Ipratropium	MDI 18 μg/puff	1–2 puffs	qid	15	1–2 hours	4–6 hours
Isoetharine	1.0% solution	0.25–0.50 mL	qid	1–3	15–60 minutes	1–3 hours
Isoproterenol	1:200 (0.50%)	0.25–0.50 mL	qid	1–3	5–30 minutes	30–120 minutes
Metaproterenol	5.0% solution	0.50 mL	tid, qid	1–5	30–60 minutes	3–4 hours
Metaproterenol	MDI 0.65 mg/puff	2–3 puffs	q 4 hours	1–5	30–60 minutes	3–4 hours
Pirbuterol	MDI 0.20 mg/puff	2 puffs	q 4–6 hours	3–4	30–60 minutes	5 hours
Racemic epinephrine	2.25% solution	0.25–0.50 mL	q 1–2 hours	1–3	15 minutes	30–60 minutes
Salmeterol	MDI 25 μg/puff	1–2 puffs	bid (morning and evening)	20	3–5 hours	12 hours
Terbutaline	MDI 0.20 mg/puff	2 puffs	q 4–6 hours	5	30–60 minutes	3–6 hours

selected clinical situations. Isoproterenol should not be given more often than every 4 hours, regardless of its very short therapeutic effects.

Racemic epinephrine, however, may safely be administered within 60 minutes of an initial treatment because it rapidly degrades and has few serious side effects.

Salmeterol is intended for the long-term maintenance and control of the chronic asthmatic. It does not have a rapid onset (as compared with other beta-agonists) and should not be used during an acute asthma attack. Asthmatics who use salmeterol should be instructed to carry a fast-acting beta-agonist (such as albuterol or levalbuterol) for use when an acute attack occurs.

BRONCHODILATOR ADMINISTRATION IN MECHANICALLY VENTILATED PATIENTS

Bronchodilators are routinely administered to patients on ventilators. The American Association for Respiratory Care (AARC) has published a clinical practice guideline (CPG) that recommends the selection of a device to administer the bronchodilator, how to administer it, and how to evaluate the response to therapy.[5] The CPG recommends use of metered dose inhalers (MDIs), small-volume nebulizers (SVNs), large-volume nebulizers (LVNs), and ultrasonic nebulizers for delivery of bronchodilators to mechanically ventilated patients. However, it states that dry-powder inhalers (DPIs) are not be suitable for use, suggesting that clinical trials are necessary to validate their use. Central to the CPG recommendations is that the tidal volume of an adult patient should be large enough to ensure that the drug will reach the small airways. The guideline suggests that the tidal volume be greater than 500 mL for adults and recommends the use of lower inspiratory flows or an inspiratory pause to improve the disposition of the aerosol. Either method should be used only if it does not compromise the patient and ensures that the patient's inspiratory needs are met.

Humidifiers and metered-dose drugs can pose extra problems for drug delivery to mechanically ventilated patients. Humidified gas can lower aerosol delivery, but the hazards of ventilating a patient with dry gas are greater. The guideline recommends that the humidifier remain inline, although an increase in aerosol dose may be necessary. The respiratory therapist may find it difficult to accurately time the activation of the metered-dose device with the onset of inspiration. The guideline recommends that the metered-dose device be fitted with a chamber that will hold the aerosol for the next inspiration.

Last, the CPG recommends that an inline nebulizer should be placed no farther than 30 cm from the proximal end of the endotracheal tube. The practitioner should also place a filter on the expiratory limb of the ventilator circuit to prevent aerosolized drug from entering any flow-sensing device in the ventilator. The nebulizer should never be left inline after the treatment is over.[5] The details of aerosol and humidity therapy are covered in Chapter 21.

Anti-Asthmatic and Anti-Inflammatory Drugs

Asthma affects an estimated 20 million Americans, and asthma mortality continues at a rate of 5000 deaths per year in the United States.[6] The primary clinical features of asthma are profound dyspnea and wheezing; thus, traditional therapy has long concentrated on controlling the bronchospasm, typically with inhaled or oral beta-agonists. Current asthma management addresses clinical manifestations of the disease: bronchospasm, inflammation with mucosal edema, and excessive airway secretions. Although asthma may be triggered by intrinsic or extrinsic causes, its primary manifestation is an acute inflammatory response, which is initiated by the complement cascade. Asthmatics exhibit airway inflammation with infiltration of the mucosa by activated T cells, mast cells, and eosinophils. T cells and mast cells release cytokines, which promote the production of IgE antibodies and the consequent increase in capillary permeability and mucosal edema.

The management of patients with asthma now focuses on the inflammatory elements of the disease. Treatment includes anti-inflammatory drugs such as corticosteroids and other controller drugs (e.g., mast cell inhibitors along with leukotriene inhibitors and antagonists).

INDICATIONS AND CONTRAINDICATIONS FOR ANTI-INFLAMMATORY DRUGS

Inflammation is associated with increased capillary permeability, which leads to mucosal edema. Administration of an alpha-adrenergic, such as racemic epinephrine, is indicated if the mucosal edema is associated with an inhalational injury (e.g., inhalation of smoke, fumes, or steam), trauma (e.g., intubation or extubation), or infectious process (e.g., croup, epiglottitis, bronchiolitis). In these situations, the mucosal edema is not secondary to an allergic response; therefore, the vasoconstricting action of an alpha-adrenergic drug is very effective. The dosage of racemic epinephrine is noted in Table 7-3.

Inflammation associated with a chronic inflammatory response such as asthma is controlled by corticosteroids. Inhaled corticosteroids (ICS) provide the advantage of reducing systemic side effects associated with long-term corticosteroid use. The primary indication for the use of ICS is to control the inflammation associated with mild to moderate persistent asthma.[7,8] Current drugs and drug administration guidelines for ICS are presented in Table 7-4.

The presence of a systemic fungal infection, renal failure, or severe diabetes mellitus contraindicates the use of corticosteroids.

SIDE EFFECTS OF AND ADVERSE REACTIONS TO CORTICOSTEROIDS

The systemic side effects of ICS have been documented and are similar to those of the oral variety (prednisone). The general side effects associated with inhaled steroids include hoarseness, dry mouth, dysphonia, and cough. Inhaled steroids may suppress the normal bacterial flora in the oropharynx and lead to fungal infections such as oral candidiasis or aspergillosis if the patient does not routinely rinse the mouth after inhalation of the steroid.[8]

Many asthmatics use multiple metered-dose inhalers (MDIs) and/or dry powder inhalers (DPIs) for symptom control. In such cases, the patients have to be

TABLE 7-4 **Aerosol corticosteroid dosages and onset of action**

Drug	Strength (μg/puff)	Dosage	Onset
Beclomethasone (Beclovent, Vanceril)	42	Adults: 2 puffs, tid, qid; children: 1-2 puffs, tid, qid	Usually within 24 hours
Budesonide (Rhinocort, Pulmicort)	200	Adults: 1–2 puffs, bid; children: (>5 years old): 1 puff bid	Usually within 24 hours
Dexamethasone(Decadron Respihaler)	84	Adults: 3 puffs, tid, qid; children: 2 puffs, tid, qid	Usually within 24 hours
Flunisolide (Aerobid)	250	Adults and children: 2 puffs, bid	2–3 days
Fluticasone diproprionate (Flovent)*	44	>12 years old, 2 puffs bid	2–3 days
Fluticasone diproprionate (Flovent)*	110	>12 years old, 1–2 puffs bid	2–3 days
Fluticasone diproprionate (Flovent)*	220	>12 years old, 1–2 puffs bid; maximum 880 μg/day	2–3 days
Triamcinilone (Azmacort)	100	Adults: 2 puffs, tid, qid; children:1–2 puffs, tid, qid	1–3 days

**Fluticasone dosages vary according to concurrent dosages of bronchodilators and oral corticosteroids; adrenal suppression occurs in 10%–16% of patients receiving 440 μg/day or more of fluticasone.*

instructed in the proper sequence of medication administration to both optimize the therapeutic effects and minimize adverse reactions. If multiple MDIs are used, the general sequence should be:

1. Bronchodilator (e.g., albuterol).
2. Mast cell inhibitor (e.g., Intal or Tilade).
3. Corticosteroid (e.g., Azmacort, Flovent, Pulmicort).

Regardless of the number of MDIs used, the corticosteroid should be taken last and the mouth thoroughly rinsed after inhalation. The most common DPI used in the management of asthma is Advair, a combination of the long-acting beta-agonist salmeterol and the corticosteroid fluticasone. Patients simply use this DPI, followed by any other prescribed MDI or DPI. Mouth rinsing after DPI use is also recommended.

Patient noncompliance is a possible cause of adverse effects or lack of effective asthma management. Corticosteroids have no bronchodilating properties but must be continued in the absence of symptoms. Many asthmatics do not understand or do not comply with treatment, which is intended to reduce the need for fast-acting beta-agonists. Corticosteroid MDIs are very expensive (some are two or three times as expensive as a bronchodilator); therefore, patients may "save" their steroids or, if money is an issue, discontinue them because they can rely on symptomatic treatment with beta-agonists. This practice is particularly troubling because corticosteroid use, even by aerosol, should be gradually tapered until finally discontinued by the physician. Patient education is a key component to the effective management of asthma.

MECHANISM OF ACTION OF ANTI-ASTHMATIC DRUGS

Mediator antagonists are drugs that compete for a receptor site and prevent a subsequent response to a stimulus. Two types of mediator antagonists are used in the management of asthma: mast cell inhibitors and leukotriene inhibitors. *Mast cells* are a component of the immune system that contain large quantities of histamine. These cells degranulate when exposed to an allergic or a nonallergic stimulus, releasing histamine and other mediators of inflammation [leukotrienes, formerly known as slow-reacting substance of anaphylaxis (SRS-A), prostaglandins, bradykinin, and platelet-activating factor].

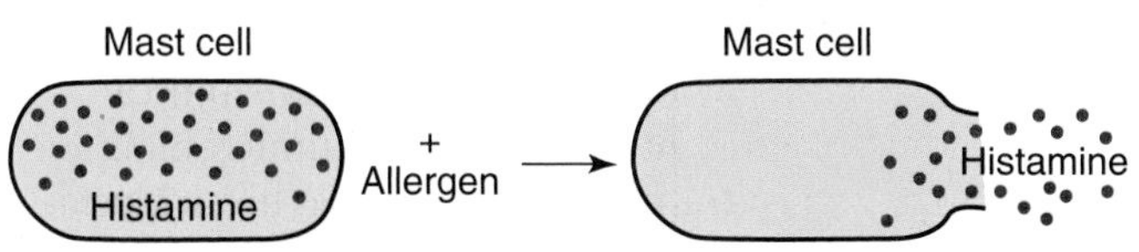

FIGURE 7-5 In the normal allergic response, ruptured mast cells release histamine.

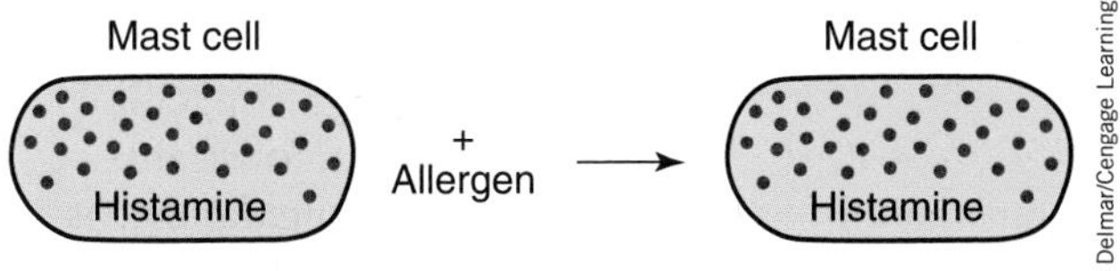

FIGURE 7-6 Cromolyn sodium and nedocromil stabilize mast cells to prevent histamine release.

These mediators cause bronchospasm and lead to the cascade of other mediators and the inflammatory response in the airway. Mast cell inhibitors (cromolyn sodium and nedocromil) prevent the degranulation of these cells and thus prevent the cascade of inflammatory events. Nedocromil has both mast cell inhibition and anti-inflammatory properties. Figure 7-5 illustrates the normal allergic response, and Figure 7-6 illustrates the mast cell inhibition by cromolyn sodium and nedocromil.

Leukotriene inhibitors either compete for leukotriene receptors (e.g., zafirlukast and montelukast) or inhibit the formation of leukotriene (e.g., zileuton). Leukotrienes stimulate leukotriene receptors and cause bronchoconstriction, mucus secretion, and chemotaxis of other inflammatory mediators. This family of drugs therefore prevents the leukotriene-stimulated inflammatory response.[9]

INDICATIONS FOR ANTI ASTHMATIC DRUGS

Several anti-asthmatic drugs are indicated for the prophylactic management of asthma. The leukotriene inhibitors are taken orally (they are not available by inhalation) and in tablet form two to four times a day. Cromolyn sodium and nedocromil are not available in oral forms and must be administered by aerosol (small-volume nebulizer, dry powder inhaler, or metered-dose inhaler). Patient compliance is also a concern with this group of drugs because their action is completely preventive and requires consistent dosing to maintain appropriate serum levels for therapeutic effect. Dosage guidelines for anti asthmatic drugs are provided in Table 7-5.

ASTHMA RELIEVERS AND CONTROLLERS

The National Asthma Education and Prevention Program (NAEPP) of the National Institutes of Health has established current guidelines distinguishing asthma medications as either relievers or controllers.[6] Short-acting beta agonist and anticholinergic bronchodilators are categorized as relievers; other bronchodilators (long-acting beta agonists and xanthines) are categorized as controllers. Respiratory therapists must understand the significance of this distinction when evaluating

TABLE 7-5 **Anti-asthmatic drugs and dosages**

Drug	Classification	Route of Administration	Strength	Dosage	Frequency
Cromolyn sodium (Intal)	Mast cell inhibitor	Aerosol metered-dose inhaler (MDI)	0.80 mg/puff	2 puffs	qid
Cromolyn sodium (Intal)	Mast cell inhibitor	Aerosol dry powder inhaler	20 mg/capsule	20 mg (1 capsule)	qid
Cromolyn sodium (Intal)	Mast cell inhibitor	Aerosol small-volume nebulizer	20 mg/2 mL	20 mg	qid
Montelukast (Singulaire)	Leukotriene inhibitor	Oral	5- and 10-mg tablets	1 tablet	qid
Nedocromil (Tilade)	Mast cell inhibitor	Aerosol MDI	1.75 mg/puff	2 puffs	qid
Zafirlukast (Assolate)	Leukotriene inhibitor	Oral	20-mg tablet	1 tablet	bid
Zileuton (Zyflo)	Leukotriene inhibitor	Oral	600-mg tablet	1 tablet	qid

TABLE 7-6 **Asthma relievers and controllers**

Quick-Relief Asthma Agents	Long-Term Asthma Controllers
Short-acting inhaled beta 2 agonists (albuterol, metaproterenol, bitolterol, pirbuterol, terbutaline)	Inhaled corticosteroids Mast cell inhibitors
Inhaled anticholinergic (ipratropium)	Leukotriene antagonists and inhibitors
Systemic corticosteroids	Long-acting beta 2 agonists (e.g., salmeterol and oral sustained–release tablets such as terbutaline and albuterol) Xanthines (theophylline, aminophylline) Oral corticosteroids

patient care and assessing its effectiveness, and they should explain the distinction to the patients. A summary of the NAEPP categories is provided in Table 7-6.

Drugs Used in the Management of COPD

As with asthma, the most important inhaled medications are the adrenergic bronchodilators, anti cholinergic bronchodilators (tiotropium bromide in particular), the selective use of xanthines, and inhaled corticosteroids. Both Advair (a combination of serevent and fluticasone) and Symbicort (foradil and budesonide) have been approved for pharmacologic management of the COPD patient.

Steroids, both oral and inhaled, are particularly beneficial in the management of COPD because of their anti-inflammatory effect in reducing mucosal edema in the bronchi and thereby decreasing airway resistance and work of breathing. Steroids may also potentiate the action of beta-agonist bronchodilators, increasing airway dilation. However, patients must be aware of potential side effects from long-term steroid use, and measures must be taken to avoid or manage associated problems such as osteoporosis, hypertension, steroid-induced diabetes, muscular atrophy, and/or increased gastric acidity.

In addition, mucolytics such as acetylcysteine (Mucomyst) may be used in COPD patients who have considerable mucus production secondary to chronic bronchitis and difficulty in expectorating the secretions. Antibiotics administered orally are also used in managing these patients when bronchial infection and/or pneumonia are present. Aerosolized antimicrobials are generally reserved for patients with either bronchiectasis or cystic fibrosis.

Finally, mention must be made about COPD patients with *alpha-1 antitrypsin* (*AAT*) *deficiency* and the use of Prolastin, or alpha-1 proteinase inhibitor (human). AAT deficiency is also known as *genetic emphysema* because it is triggered by defective family genes, resulting in individuals' having a congenital deficiency of alpha$_1$-PI in clinically demonstrable panacinar emphysema. This type of lung damage is similar to that caused by emphysema, but the clinical symptoms occur earlier in life (usually between 35 and 40 years of age).

For patients with this deficiency, Prolastin is indicated for chronic replacement therapy. It is administered once weekly intravenously. The usual adult dosage is 60 mg/kg, and it takes approximately 30 minutes to infuse the prescribed dose. It is recommended for adult use only because effectiveness in the pediatric population has not yet been established. Prolastin is contraindicated in individuals with selective IgA deficiency who are known to have an antibody against IgA (anti-IgA antibody). Side effects and adverse reactions may include flulike symptoms, allergiclike reactions, chills, dyspnea, rash, tachycardia and, rarely, hypotension, hypertension, and chest pain.[10]

Wetting Agents and Mucolytics

Bland aerosols and mucolytic agents are used in respiratory care to humidify the respiratory tract and to loosen, thin, and remove pulmonary secretions. Bland aerosols (e.g., normal saline, hypotonic or hypertonic saline, and sterile distilled water) do not actually disrupt the mucus molecule. **Mucolytics** (e.g., n-acetylcysteine, dornase alfa, and sodium bicarbonate) actually disrupt (or lyse) the mucus molecule (the long mucopolysaccharide chains) to facilitate secretion removal.

BLAND AEROSOLS

Bland aerosols are used primarily to humidify inspired air and irritate the airway to promote a cough. Sterile water, hypotonic saline, and hypertonic saline usually cause airway irritation (hypertonic saline may actually "draw" additional fluid into the lung to dilute the solution). They thus increase mucus production, which stimulates a cough reflex.[11] These solutions are not considered mucolytics, but they may be categorized as expectorants.

CASE STUDY 7-1

Michael Smith is a 58-year-old white male who was recently diagnosed with COPD and asthma. His physician has prescribed aerosolized albuterol qid via compressor/nebulizer followed by 2 puffs of Flovent bid via MDI. During the first week of therapy, the patient appeared to respond favorably.

During the next few weeks, however, Mr. Smith experienced a disrupted sleeping pattern along with persistent pharyngitis and the presence of white patches on his throat. He notified his physician, who modified his therapy accordingly with improved results.

Questions

1. What change, if any, do you think the physician made regarding the administration of aerosolized bronchodilator?
2. What was the likely cause of the patient's pharyngitis, and what could have been done to prevent it?

The AARC has published a CPG on the use of bland aerosols in respiratory care. Specifically, the CPG suggests that cool bland aerosols (water or saline) used for upper airway administration have a mass median aerodynamic diameter (MMAD) $\geq 5\ \mu m$. This size ensures that the aerosol is deposited in the upper airway. Hypo- and hypertonic saline solutions used for inducing sputum should have a MMAD between 1 and 5 μm. Finally, heated bland aerosols to correct humidity deficits when the upper airway is bypassed, as in patients with a tracheostomy, requires a MMAD of 2–10 μm.[12]

MECHANISM OF ACTION OF MUCOLYTICS

The mucus molecule is a mucopolysaccharide chain composed of strands of alternating amino sugars and amino acids that are connected by disulfide bonds (Figure 7-7). The three mucolytics in use disrupt the mucus molecule in three ways:

- N-acetylcysteine disrupts the disulfide bonds (Figure 7-8).
- Sodium bicarbonate disrupts the stability of the amino acid chains (Figure 7-9).
- Dornase alfa lyses mucus proteins or the proteinaceous secretions associated with infected sputum in cystic fibrosis patients.

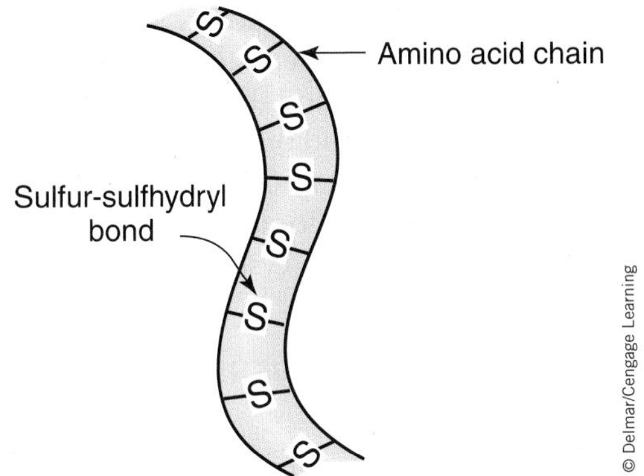

FIGURE 7-7 The structure of the mucus molecule.

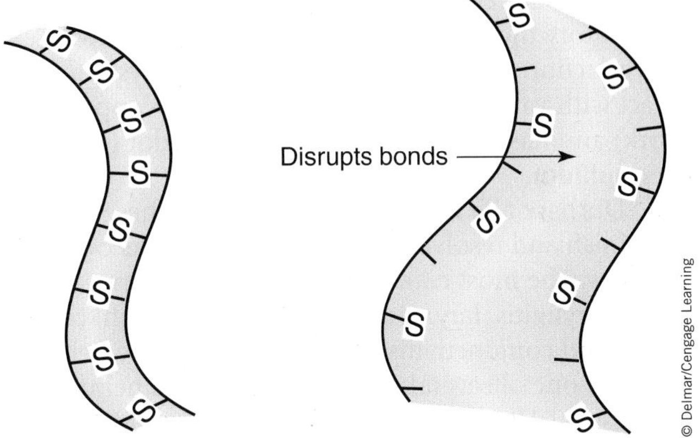

FIGURE 7-8 Mucolytic action of n-acetylcysteine.

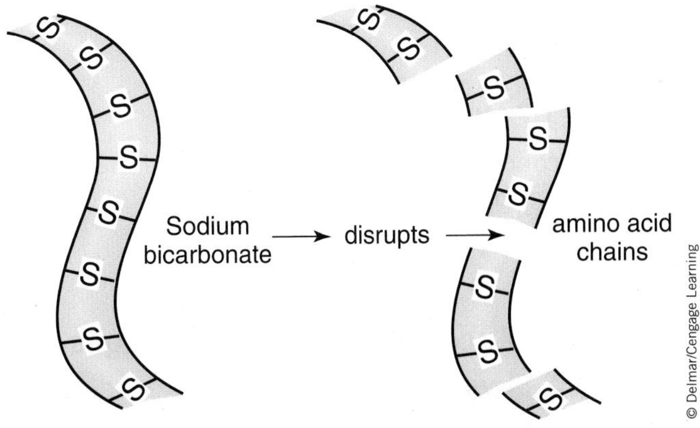

FIGURE 7-9 Mucolytic action of sodium bicarbonate.

INDICATIONS AND CONTRAINDICATIONS FOR MUCOLYTICS

Mucolytics may be administered by aerosol or by direct instillation into the airway (e.g., during bronchoscopy or lavage). A mucolytic should be considered for patients with thickened secretions who are capable of protecting their airway and generating a good spontaneous cough. Mucolytic therapy should be considered only after adequate systemic hydration (through oral or IV fluids), and the patient still exhibits persistent coarse rhonchi and difficulty in expectorating secretions. Both sodium bicarbonate and n-acetylcysteine may be used for mucolysis; dornase alfa is FDA-approved only for treating patients with cystic fibrosis.

SIDE EFFECTS OF AND ADVERSE REACTIONS TO MUCOLYTICS

N-acetylcysteine stimulates bronchospasm, especially in patients with bronchial asthma, and should always be given with a bronchodilator. When administering a mucolytic to any patient whose airway may be compromised by sudden mucolysis and airway obstruction, the respiratory therapist should exercise care and always have suction equipment available. N-acetylcysteine may react with various substances (e.g., rubber, copper, iron, cork) and has a characteristic rotten-egg odor (hydrogen sulfide).

Dornase alfa has few side effects, and these usually diminish and resolve in the first several weeks of therapy. The most common side effects of dornase alfa are pharyngitis, laryngitis, voice alteration, rash, chest pain, and conjunctivitis. Dornase alfa must be nebulized in one of several specifically approved nebulizers [Hudson T Up-draft II disposable nebulizer, Marquest Acorn II disposable nebulizer, and PARI LC (reusable) nebulizer with PARI PRONEB compressor]. Other aerosol medications (e.g., beta-agonists, anticholinergics) should never be mixed in the same nebulizer with dornase alfa.

DOSAGE OF MUCOLYTICS

Dosages, concentrations, and trade names of mucolytics are provided in Table 7-7.

CASE STUDY 7-2

Rose Johnson, a 62-year-old black female with chronic bronchitis, was prescribed acetylcysteine via nebulizer to help control her bronchial secretions and to assist with expectoration of mucus. Soon after the initiation of therapy, she experienced dyspnea with audible wheezing. She notified her physician after the first episode and was advised to reduce the dose of acetylcysteine. After subsequent treatments, she still experienced the shortness of breath and wheezing. Her physician decided to discontinue the mucolytic therapy.

Questions

1. What caused the patient's dyspnea and wheezing?
2. Besides discontinuing the acetylcysteine, what else could the physician have prescribed?

Aerosol Antimicrobial Therapy

Systemic administration of antimicrobial agents is the first-line approach in most cases of infection. Certain clinical situations and specific antimicrobial agents have been shown to be appropriate for aerosol administration. In particular, aerosolized antimicrobial agents in the prevention and treatment of ventilator-associated pneumonia (VAP) are being considered and investigated because of the emergence of multiple-drug-resistant gram-negative organisms that are resistant to systemic antimicrobial therapy.[13] Currently used aerosolized antimicrobials include antibiotics, antifungal drugs, antiprotozoal drugs, and antiviral drugs.

TABLE 7-7 **Mucolytic drugs and dosages**

Drug (Trade Name)	Action	Concentration	Dosage	Comments
Dornase alfa (Pulmozyme)	Proteolytic	Ampules contain 1.0 mg in 2.50 mL	1 ampule,* once or twice daily	Approved only for CF patients 5 years old and older
N-acetylcysteine (Mucomyst, Mucosol)	Disrupts disulfide bonds	10% and 20% solutions	3–5 mL, qid	Should be used with or after bronchodilator; 10% solution causes fewer side effects
Sodium bicarbonate	Disrupts stability of amino acid chains	4.2%	3–5 mL as needed	Few side effects, mild mucolytic

**Dornase alfa must be nebulized only with approved nebulizers and should never be mixed with other drugs for nebulization; administration by mouthpiece is recommended to avoid deposition in sinuses.*

INDICATIONS FOR AEROSOLIZED ANTIMICROBIAL DRUGS

There are several generally accepted indications for administering antimicrobial agents by aerosol:

- As an adjunct to systemic antimicrobial therapy that has been unsuccessful
- For direct topical deposition of an antimicrobial that is not appropriate for systemic administration (e.g., nystatin)
- For topical deposition in a pulmonary infectious process in which perfusion is limited and systemic therapy has failed (e.g., aspergillosis)
- For topical deposition of an antimicrobial that may be more effective, or better tolerated, by this route (e.g., pentamidine, which is used in the management of AIDS patients with HIV infections)
- To eliminate an organism that is colonizing the respiratory tract (e.g., infected sputum in cystic fibrosis and bronchiectasis patients)
- To help prevent and/or treat ventilator-associated pneumonia (VAP)
- To reduce the severity of systemic side effects (when an antimicrobial is selected that is poorly absorbed through the lungs)

Table 7-8 summarizes drugs, dosages, side effects, and clinical indications for currently utilized aerosol antimicrobials.

TABLE 7-8 **Selected aerosol antimicrobials**

Drug	Classification	Indication	Dosage	Side Effects/Comments
Amphotericin B	Antifungal	Pulmonary aspergillosis, coccidiomycosis, candidiasis	5–10 mg, nebulized 2–4 times/day	Fever, headache, anorexia, nausea, vomiting, malaise, muscle and joint pain
Colistin	Antibiotic	Colonized pseudomonas in CF patients	100 mg, nebulized 2–4 times/day	Parasthesia, numbness and tingling of tongue and extremities, itching and urticaria, GI upset, vertigo, slurring of speech
Nystatin	Antifungal	Pulmonary aspergillosis, Candida albicans	25,000 units, nebulized 2–4 times/day or instilled in ET tube	Nausea, vomiting, diarrhea
Pentamidine (Pentam, Pneumopent)	Antiprotozoal	Pneumocystis carinii pneumonia	600 mg in 6 mL SDW, nebulized* for 20–30 minutes, once/day	Fatigue is most common side effect; bronchospasm, cough, burning sensation in back of throat. Bronchodilator should be given if patient has history of asthma or smoking.
Ribavirin (Virazole)	Antiviral	Confirmed respiratory syncytial virus (RSV) pneumonia	300 mL of 2% solution, nebulized for 12–18 hours/day for 3–7 days	Deterioration of respiratory function, bacterial pneumonia, pneumothorax, apnea, ventilator dependence, rash, conjunctivitis. Drug is teratogenic and is a risk to visitors and health care providers; scavenger systems should be used. Drug may also precipitate in exhalation valve of ventilator circuits, inline particle filter is recommended.

**Pentamidine should be nebulized only in an approved micronebulizer.*

DISADVANTAGES OF AEROSOL ANTIMICROBIAL THERAPY

Because the effectiveness of most aerosol therapy is patient dependent, the aerosol delivery of antimicrobials is limited and may not achieve its therapeutic goal. Limitations and disadvantages of aerosolized antimicrobials are as follows:

- Bronchospasm is a common adverse reaction.
- Systemic side effects may occur.
- The drug may be inactivated by sputum proteins.
- Dosages for the aerosol delivery of antimicrobials have not been established.
- Optimal delivery and equipment techniques have not been determined.
- The drug may not be deposited at the desired (infected) site.
- Ambient air may be contaminated by the drug (exposing personnel, other patients, and visitors to the antimicrobial).
- The hospital's population of specific antimicrobial targets may develop a tolerance (see the previous list entry) and hospital-acquired infections may increase.

Surface Active Aerosols

Surface tension is the physical property that creates tension at a fluid-air interface. It is the result of the attraction (cohesion) of like molecules at the surface of a liquid. Molecules on the surface are attracted inward, making the liquid contract to minimize surface area. Detergents (e.g., surfactant) reduce surface tension. The presence of pulmonary surfactant reduces surface tension to ease the inspiratory work of breathing; the absence of surfactant (e.g., in infant and adult respiratory distress syndromes) increases the surface tension in alveoli, and the increased surface tension, in turn, opposes inflation and contributes to alveolar collapse. The concept of surface tension is applied in two very different clinical situations: infant respiratory distress syndrome (IRDS) and fulminating alveolar pulmonary edema.

SURFACTANT REPLACEMENT THERAPY

Premature or low-birth-weight infants often develop *infant respiratory distress syndrome* (*IRDS*). This syndrome is associated with difficulty breathing, poor ventilation and oxygenation, and excessive work of breathing, which leads to fatigue, cardiac dysrhythmias, and deteriorating blood gases. The primary clinical feature of the syndrome is a lack of surfactant at birth, and it may require up to 72 hours for adequate endogenous surfactant to be produced.[14] Surfactant-replacement drugs are generally administered by inhalation (nebulization) or by instillation into an endotracheal tube. The instillation is followed by vigorous manual ventilation and positional changes of the infant to enhance distribution. Currently available exogenous surfactant-replacement drugs fall into three categories based on the source and on the presence or absence of proteins in their chemical composition. These three categories and their corresponding surfactant preparations are as follows:[15]

- Nonprotein surfactants:

  Adsurf (pumactant, which is an artificial lung-expanding compound [ALEC])
  Exosurf (colfosceril palmitate)

- Protein-containing surfactants:

  HL-10
  Curosurf (poractant α)
  Alveofact (SF-Rl 1)
  BLES (bovine lipid extract surfactant)
  Infasurf (Calfactant CLSE)
  Newfacten
  Surfacten (surfactant-TA)
  Survanta (beractant)

- Peptide-containing synthetic surfactants:

  Venticute (rSP-C surfactant)
  Surfaxin (lucinactant)

Indications for Surfactant-Replacement Drugs. Surfactant-replacement drugs have both prevention and rescue protocols.

- The *prevention protocols* recommend the initial dosage of surfactant drug as soon as possible after birth (within 15 minutes) for infants born with a birth weight of 1250–1350 g or who exhibit signs of lung immaturity (e.g., an abnormal lecithin:sphingomyelin ratio).
- The *rescue protocol* is indicated for infants who develop IRDS, as manifested by radiographic findings and the need for mechanical ventilation.

Side Effects of and Adverse Reactions to Surfactant-Replacement Drugs. Bradycardia and oxygen desaturation occur in 10–20% of infants during the dosing procedure. If these occur, the dosing procedure should be interrupted and the infant resuscitated (but not suctioned). Less common adverse effects include bronchospasm, vasoconstriction, pulmonary hemorrhage, hypotension, hypocarbia, and apnea.[15]

Dosage Guidelines for Surfactant Replacement Drugs. Trade names and dosages of surfactant-replacement drugs are summarized in Table 7-9.

TABLE 7-9 **Surfactant replacement drugs**

Drug (Trade Name)	Prevention Protocol	Rescue Protocol	Supplied/Comments
Beractant (Survanta)	Initial dose within 15 minutes of birth for infants weighing less than 1250 g 100 mg/kg birth weight, divided into four equal quarter-doses and instilled into ET tube* Maximum of four doses given no more frequently than every 6 hours	Initial dose with 8 hours of onset of symptoms of IRDS 100 mg/kg birthweight, divided into four equal quarter-doses and instilled into ET tube* Maximum of four doses given no more frequently than every 6 hours	Single-dose 8 mL vials contain 25 mg/mL (200 mg/vial). Usual color is off-white to light-brown. Drug is refrigerated and should be warmed by standing at room temperature for 20 minutes or hand-warming for 8 minutes before administration; artificial warming methods should not be used; unused drug may be refrigerated only once.
Colfosceril palmitate, cetyl alcohol, tyloxapol (Exosurf Neonatal)	Initial dose as soon as possible after birth for infants weighing less than 1350 g 5.0 mL/kg birthweight, divided into two equal half-doses and instilled into ET tube* Usually three doses are but there is no maximum dosage	Initial does as soon as possible after onset of symptoms of IRDS 5.0 mL/kg birthweight, divided into two equal half-doses and instilled into ET tube* Usually two doses are adequate but there is no maximum dosage	Sterile lyophilized powder in 10 mL vials to which 8 mL sterile water is added. Reconstituted suspension is milky-white and contains 13.5 mg/mL. If suspension separates, it should be swirled before use; if large flakes or particles persist it should not be used.

**Both manufacturers have specific dosing guidelines, which are provided with illustrations and videotapes.*

In 1994, the AARC published a clinical practice guideline for surfactant replacement therapy. The guideline indicates that repeat doses of surfactant should be considered contingent on the continued diagnosis of IRDS. The clinical status of the patient dictates the frequency of repeat doses. The recommendation is that additional doses of surfactant should be given at 6- to 24-hour intervals for infants who experience increased ventilator requirements or who fail to improve after the initial dose.[16]

DRYING AGENT (ETHYL ALCOHOL)

Fulminant alveolar pulmonary edema is a rapidly occurring accumulation of fluid within the alveolar sacs (fulminant means "coming in lightninglike flashes"). This type of edema may be associated with life-threatening acute congestive heart failure or with traumatic causes such as head injuries (neurogenic), acute mountain (high-altitude) sickness, heroin overdose, burns, or acute inhalational injuries (e.g., poisonous fumes).

The use of ethyl alcohol as a surface active agent in fulminant alveolar pulmonary edema is based on the quick reduction in the alveolar-capillary diffusion barrier created by the frothy, foamy secretions associated with the edema. Ethyl alcohol alters the surface tension of the edema bubbles and causes them to burst. Bursting can be achieved by aerosolizing ethyl alcohol or by passing oxygen through a bubble diffuser filled with ethyl alcohol.[17]

Indications and Contraindications for Ethyl Alcohol. Ethyl alcohol, administered via nebulizer or humidifier, is indicated as an adjunct in the treatment of acute alveolar pulmonary edema. Treatment of the underlying cause of the edema should be ongoing, and traditional medical treatments (such as rotating tourniquets, diuretics, and digitalis) should continue. Patients with a history of alcohol abuse or those receiving Antabuse therapy for alcoholism should not receive aerosolized ethyl alcohol.

Side Effects of Ethyl Alcohol. Aerosolized quantities of ethyl alcohol rarely cause any adverse reactions, but the drying effects may irritate lung mucosa or cause bronchospasm. Mild intoxication may occur.

Dosage of Ethyl Alcohol. A short course of therapy (two to four treatments) is generally sufficient. The recommended dosage is 5–15 mL of 30–50% ethyl alcohol administered by small-volume nebulizer or intermittent positive pressure breathing (IPPB) with oxygen as the source gas. Treatments may be repeated every 30 minutes.

Note: Isopropyl or denatured alcohol must not be used for this purpose.

Assessing the Effectiveness of Aerosol Medications

The assessment of a patient before, during, and after receiving aerosol therapy is an integral part of the therapy and care plan. Before administering any aerosolized drug, the respiratory therapist should assess basic vital signs, breath sounds, and patient status. Except in the case of status asthmaticus, tachycardia in excess of 120 bpm is a general contraindication to the administration of beta-agonists. In status asthmaticus, the patient is in profound respiratory distress and is almost certain to be experiencing anxiety, fatigue, hypoxemia, and acid-base imbalance. In this case, the administration of effective fast-acting beta 2-selective drugs may actually result in a reduced heart rate when respiratory distress and hypoxemia are relieved.

The clinical decision regarding whether to proceed with a beta-agonist when a patient is experiencing tachycardia is a medical decision based on all factors in the case. When assessing the response to an administered bronchodilator, to the RT must consider airflow (both inspiratory and forced expiratory maneuvers), along with the presence or absence of an immediate response with regard to proper dose, the frequency of administration, and overall response to long-term therapy. The clinician must have complete knowledge of the main effects, mode of action, time course, side effects, and dosage constraints of any medications administered. This assessment is critical to documenting the desired patient outcomes and the need for continuing prescribed therapy.[18]

If a patient is unable to perform a reasonable inspiratory maneuver (because of muscle weakness, confusion, or inability or unwillingness to follow directions), then aerosol therapy may not produce the desired outcome. Administering the aerosol via IPPB may be appropriate for some patients; alternative delivery methods (e.g., oral, intramuscular, or suppository) may be required for others (e.g., oral, intramuscular, or suppository).

During an aerosol treatment, the therapist should continually monitor the patient's ventilatory pattern, posture, and general appearance. Many institutions require a midtreatment assessment of respiratory rate and heart rate for all therapy (not just adrenergic drugs).

After an aerosolized medication treatment, the patient should be assessed for a reasonable therapeutic response to the drugs and the presence of any adverse reactions. The assessment of the therapeutic response must be correlated with the goal of the therapy (e.g., a patient receiving a fast-acting bronchodilator should exhibit some improvement in breath sounds and, if appropriate, peak flow measurement). Patients receiving mucolytic therapy should be closely monitored for up to 20 minutes after a treatment. The mucolysis will likely continue beyond the treatment period, and the patient may require assistance in coughing or clearing the airway. The respiratory therapist can use the immediate post-treatment period for patient education as well as for clinical assessment.

Conscious Sedation

Sedation and *analgesia* imply a physical state in which a patient is able to tolerate an unpleasant or uncomfortable situation while maintaining adequate cardiopulmonary function. The patient should also maintain the ability to respond to verbal commands and tactile stimulation. The patient's ability to respond is important when respiratory therapists assist physicians during certain diagnostic and therapeutic procedures. Respiratory therapists can minimize associated risks by administering prescribed medications and closely monitoring patients during these types of procedures.

Recognizing the fact that respiratory therapists assist physicians with the administration of sedative and analgesic drugs during certain diagnostic and therapeutic procedures, the AARC published a position statement in December 1997 addressing this issue. This statement was revised in March 2000. The position statement notes that the American Society of Anesthesiologists (ASA) guidelines call on respiratory therapists to provide conscious sedation and that therapists complete formal training and competency assessment programs in order to provide this service under medical direction. The AARC's statement fully supports this formal training, resulting in competency certification, as well as respiratory therapists being permitted to provide the service in accordance with the ASA guidelines, any institutional policies and service operations, the requirements of the Joint Commission [formerly the Joint Commission on Accreditation of Healthcare Organizations (JCAHO)], and specific state requirements.[19]

Anesthesia Drugs

General anesthesia involves drugs that induce the absence of all sensation. Probably several types of mechanisms are at work to produce anesthesia. However, the current theory is that general anesthetics stabilize the membranes of excitable tissue by influencing synaptic transmission and consequently depressing the central nervous system (CNS). There are four stages of anesthesia:

- Stage I: State of analgesia (affects midbrain medullary centers and certain spinal cord areas)
- Stage II: State of excitation (affects subcortical inhibition centers causing excitation, delirium, and amnesia)
- Stage III: State of surgical anesthesia (affects midbrain and spinal cord in four distinct planes)
- Stage IV: State of medullary suppression (affects respiratory and cardiovascular centers, causing apnea, coma, and death)

There is no one ideal general anesthetic. Anesthesiologists use a combination of agents to produce safe and effective anesthesia, which include:

- Gases (nitrous oxide and cyclopropane).
- Volatile liquids (diethyl ether, halothane, methoxyflurane, isoflurane, and enflurane).
- Intravenous agents (droperidol or diazepam, fentanyl, ketamine, and propofol).

Before surgery, patients are usually given a preanesthetic agent such as morphine, triazolam, a barbiturate, or atropine to create sedation, reduce apprehension, or decrease salivary and bronchial secretions, depending on the type of agent used. Finally, some types of surgery necessitate complete paralysis. In this case, peripheral-acting muscle relaxants are used. These agents are classified as follows:

- Nondepolarizing neuromuscular blockers that compete with acetylcholine for the nicotinic-2 receptor site at the neuromuscular junction (e.g., d-tubocurarine, known as *curarin* or *curare*)
- Depolarizing neuromuscular blockers that cause a persistent depolarization at the motor end plate so that receptors cannot react with acetylcholine (e.g., succinylcholine or Anectine)
- Direct-acting neuromuscular blockers that interfere with the biochemical pathways and prevent the interaction of actin and mysosin in the muscle (e.g., dantrolene or Dantrium)

Ventilatory support must always be provided whenever these peripheral-acting muscle relaxants are used.

Advanced Cardiac Life Support Pharmacology

Respiratory therapists participate in cardiac resuscitation and may be directed to administer selected cardiovascular agents during a cardiac arrest. The American Heart Association (AHA) publishes standards regarding appropriate drugs, dosages, and sequences of interventions during cardiopulmonary resuscitation (CPR).[20] These standards are routinely reviewed, periodically updated, and published through the AHA. Resuscitation drugs primarily include agents that control cardiac rhythm and rate and agents that control cardiac output and blood pressure. Other advanced cardiac life support (ACLS) drugs include narcotic analgesics, volume expanders, and thrombolytics.

INTRAOSSEOUS (IO) ADMINISTRATION OF ACLS DRUGS

Narcan, atropine, valium, epinephrine, and lidocaine (NAVEL) may be administered via intraosseous (IO) access when an IV line cannot be established. This alternate method is preferred over instillation through an endotracheal tube because how much drug is actually delivered via the ET route is uncertain. Standard IV doses are used for IO administration. The delivery technique for IO access during CPR[20–24] is:

1. Insert needle directly through the bone's hard cortex and into the periosteum. Remove stylet and insert catheter.
2. The proximal tibia is often used, but the distal femur and iliac spine are alternate administration sites.
3. Administer drug via IO catheter.
4. Continue cardiac compressions.

DRUGS FOR CONTROL OF CARDIAC RHYTHM AND RATE

Drugs for the control of cardiac rhythm and rate include antiarrhythmics, beta-adrenergic blockers, calcium channel blockers, atropine, isoproterenol, adenosine, and magnesium. Specific clinical indications, contraindications, mechanisms of action, and dosages are provided in Table 7-10.

DRUGS TO IMPROVE CARDIAC OUTPUT AND BLOOD PRESSURE

Drugs to improve cardiac output and blood pressure include beta-adrenergic agents, inotropic agents, vasopressors, selective vasodilators, and nitrites. Specific clinical indications, contraindications, mechanisms of action, and dosages are provided in Table 7-11.

TABLE 7-10 **ACLS drugs that affect cardiac rhythm and rate**

Drug	Mechanism of Action	Clinical Indications	Contraindications/ Comments	Dosage/Route
Adenosine	Slows conduction through AV node	SVT (supraventricular tachycardia); narrow-complex PSVT (pulseless SVT)	Less effective in patients taking theophylline	6.0 mg (3mg/mL vial) by rapid IV push over 1–2 seconds
Atenolol	Beta blocker	Reduces incidence of ventricular fibrillation (VF) in post-MI patients not receiving thrombolytics	Concurrent administration with calcium channel blockers may cause hypotension; avoid in asthmatics	5.0 mg (0.50 mg/mL in 10 mL vial) by slow IV infusion (over 5 minutes)
Atropine	Inotropic and chronotropic	Symptomatic bradycardia; second drug (after epinephrine) for asytole or bradycardic pulseless electrical activity (PEA)	Use with caution in presence of myocardial ischemia and hypoxia; increases myocardial O_2 demand	0.50–1.0 mg IV repeated every 3–5 minutes up to maximum of 0.03–0.04 mg/kg (usually 3.0 maximum)
Bretylium	Anti-arrhythmic, elevates ventricular threshold	Persistent ventricular tachycardia (VT), VF, multifocal premature ventricular contractions(PVCs) when lidocaine and procainamide have failed	Contraindicated in heart block, asystole, PEA	5.0 mg/kg IV bolus for cardiac arrest from VF or VT; 5–10 mg/kg over 8–10 minutes for stable VT
Diltiazem	Slows conduction through SA node	Controls ventricular rate in atrial fibrillation and atrial flutter	Do not use concurrently with beta-blockers or calcium channel blockers	15–20 mg IV over 2 minutes for acute PSVT; 5–15 mg/hour titrated by heart rate for maintenance
Isoproterenol	Inotropic and chronotropic	Refractory torsades de pointes; temporary control of bradycardia in heart transplant patients	Increases myocardial O_2 demand; do not give with epinephrine	IV infusion 2–10 μg/minute, titrate to heart rate
Lidocaine	Anti-arrhythmic, elevates ventricular threshold	Drug of choice for ventricular ectopy, VT, multifocal PVCs, and VF	Contraindicated in heart block, asystole, PEA	IV bolus 1.0–1.5 mg/kg, may repeat every 5–10 minutes up to total of 3.0 mg/kg
Magnesium	Magnesium supplement	Cardiac arrest associated with torsades de pointes or hypomagnesemia; prophylactic after acute myocardial infarction (MI)	Renal failure	1.0–2.0 g mixed in 10 mL of D_5W IV push in cardiac arrest; 1.0–2.0 g in 50–100 mL of D_5 IV infusion
Procainamide	Anti-arrhythmic, elevates ventricular threshold	Persistent ventricular tachycardia (VT), VF, multifocal PVCs not controlled by lidocaine	Contraindicated in heart block, asystole, PEA	30 mg/min IV infusion up to17 mg/kg for cardiac arrest; 2–8 mg/kg/hour infusion to control dysrhythmias
Verapimil	Slows conduction and increases refractoriness in AV node	Drug of second choice after adenosine to terminate PSVT with narrow QRS and normal blood pressure	Do not use concurrently with beta-blockers or calcium channel blockers	2.50–5.0 mg IV bolus over 1–2 minutes; additional 5.0 mg bolus every 15 minutes as needed (up to 30 mg total dose)

TABLE 7-11 **ACLS drugs that affect blood pressure and cardiac output**

Drug	Mechanism of Action	Clinical Indications	Contraindications/ Comments	Dosage/Route
Amrinone	Inotropic; induces reflex peripheral vasodilation	Severe congestive heart failure (CHF) refractory to diuretics, vasodilators, and conventional inotropic agents	May exacerbate myocardial ischemia or worsen ventricular ectopy; do not mix with dextrose solutions or other drugs	Initial IV loading dose of 0.75 mg/kg over 2–3 minutes; maintenance infusion of 5.0–15.0 μg/kg/min
Calcium salts	Electrolyte	Known or suspected hyperkalemia or hypocalcemia; antidote for toxic effects of calcium channel blocker overdose	Do not routinely use in cardiac arrest: do not mix with other drugs	Initial IV dose, 10% calcium chloride solution, 2.0–4.0 mg/kg; calcium gluceptate 5.0–7.0 ml; calcium gluconate 5.0–8.0 mL
Digoxin	Slows ventricular response in fibrillation or atrial flutter	Third-line choice for PSVT (after adenosine, diltiazem, verapimil)	Avoid electrical cardio version if patient is receiving digoxin (if life-threatening, use lower current settings, i.e., 10–20 J)	IV loading dose of 10–15 μg/kg lean body weight; maintenance dose affected by body size and renal function
Dobutamine	Inotropic: may induce reflex peripheral vasodilation	Congestive heart failure or pulmonary congestion with systolic pressures of 70–100 mm Hg and no clinical signs of shock	Hypotension (systolic pressure <100 mm Hg) with signs of shock; may cause tachyarrhythmias, fluctuations in BP, headache, and nausea	2-20 μg/kg/minute IV infusion, titrate so heart rate does not increase more than10% of baseline; hemodynamic monitoring recommended
Dopamine	Dose-related: low doses cause renal and mesenteric vasodilation, higher doses cause peripheral vasoconstriction	Second drug (after atropine) for symptomatic bradycardia; hypotension when systolic BP is 70–100 mm Hg with signs of shock	Use in patients with hypovolemia only after volume replacement; caution in patients with cardiogenic shock and CHF; do not mix with sodium bicarbonate	Low dose: IV 1–5 μg/kg/minute; moderate dose: IV 5–10 μg/kg/min; high dose (vasopressor dose): IV 10–20 μg/kg/min
Epinephrine	Increases heart rate, force of contractions, and coronary perfusing pressures: vasoconstriction	Cardiac standstill; ventricular fibrillation; pulseless ventricular tachycardia, pulseless electrical activity (PEA); drug of choice in anaphylaxis	Increased blood pressure and heart rate may increase myocardial ischemia	1.0 mg IV push in cardiac arrest; may repeat every 3–5 minutes
Nitroglycerin	Selective coronary vasodilator	Acute angina pectoris; adjunct in unstable angina and CHF associated with acute MI	Do not mix with other drugs; patient should sit or lie down when taking this drug; with acute MI, limit systolic BP drop to10% in normotensive and 30% in hypertensive patients (do not allow systolic BP to drop below 90 mm Hg)	Sublingual: 0.3–0.4 mg repeated every 5 minutes IV; 10–20 μg/min, titrate to effect; hemodynamic monitoring recommended

(continues)

TABLE 7-11 **ACLS drugs that affect blood pressure and cardiac output *(continued)***

Drug	Mechanism of Action	Clinical Indications	Contraindications/ Comments	Dosage/Route
Nitroprusside	Potent peripheral vasodilation	Useful in heart failure with hypertension; may be useful in patients with low cardiac output and high systemic vascular resistance refractory to dopamine	Hypovolemia	Initial IV dose of 0.1–5.0 μg/kg/minute
Norepinephrine	Potent vasoconstrictor; inotropic	Severe cardiogenic shock and hemodynamically significant hypotension	Ischemic heart disease, hypovolemia	IV: 0.5–1.0 μg/min titrated improve BP

OTHER ACLS DRUGS

Advanced cardiac life support drugs with less direct myocardial or vasopressor effects may be critical during or after cardiac resuscitation. These drugs include analgesics, diuretics, and thrombolytics. Although sodium bicarbonate has been included in ACLS protocols, its use has become controversial. Current standards emphasize maintaining oxygenation and hyperventilation to ameliorate acid-base disturbances. Sodium bicarbonate may be useful in patients with a preexisting metabolic acidosis (i.e., diabetic ketoacidosis or lactic acidosis), hyperkalemia, or tricyclic or phenobarbitol overdose. In these cases, an initial dosage of 1.0 mEq/kg should be administered once the need has been established by arterial blood gas analysis. Specific clinical indications, contraindications, mechanisms of action, and dosages for the miscellaneous ACLS drugs are provided in Table 7-12.

TABLE 7-12 **Miscellaneous ACLS drugs**

Drug (Trade Name)	Mechanism of Action	Clinical Indications	Contraindications/ Comments	Dosage/Route
Flumazenil	Reverses sedative and respiratory depression effects of benzodiazepines	Benzodiazepine overdose or toxicity	Do not use suspected tricyclic overdose or in unknown drug OD; do not use in seizure-prone patients	0.20 mg IV over 15 seconds; if inadequate response administer 0.30 mg IV over 30 seconds; administer additional 0.50 mg over 30 seconds once every minute until adequate response or total of 3.0 mg is given
Furosemide (Lasix)	Loop diuretic	Adjuvant therapy of acute pulmonary edema in patients with systolic pressure >90 mm Hg; hypertensive emergencies; increased intracranial pressure	Do not use in hypovolemic or dehydrated patients	0.50–1.0 mg/kg IV infusion over 1–2 minutes
Mannitol	Osmotic diuretic	Increased intracranial pressure in management of neurological emergencies	Monitor fluid status and osmolarity; caution in renal failure because fluid overload may result	0.50–1.0 mg/kg IV over 5–10 minutes; additional doses of 0.25–2.0 g/kg every 4–6 hours as needed; use in conjunction with mild hyperventilation

TABLE 7-12 ***(continued)***

Drug (Trade Name)	Mechanism of Action	Clinical Indications	Contraindications/ Comments	Dosage/Route
Morphine	Narcotic analgesic	Chest pain and anxiety associated with acute myocardial infarction (MI) or cardiac ischemia	Administer slowly and titrate to effect, may compromise respiration; causes hypotension in volume-depleted patients	1.0–3.0 mg IV (over 1–5 minutes) every 5–30 minutes
Naloxone	Narcotic antagonist	Respiratory and neurological depression due to narcotic intoxication or OD	May cause narcotic withdrawal	0.4–2.0 mg every 2 minutes (use higher doses for complete narcotic reversal); may administer up to 10 mg over short period (<30 minutes)
Sodium bicarbonate	Alkalinizing agent	Preexisting hyperkalemia or metabolic acidosis (i.e., lactic acidosis, ketoacidosis)	Not recommended for routine use in cardiac arrest patients; adequate ventilation and CPR are major "buffer agents" in cardiac arrest	1.0 mEq/kg IV bolus, repeat half dose every 10 minutes; if ABGs available, manage by base deficit (BE) according to formula-HCO_3^- dosage = (–BE) (weight in kg) (0.3) = mEq HCO_3^-
Thrombolytic agents (e.g., Alteplase TPA tissue plasminogen activator. Streptokinase urokinase)	Thrombolytic activity	Acute MI with ST elevation 1 mm or more in at least two continguous leads, given <12 hours from onset of symptoms; acute ischemic stroke, given <3 hours from onset of symptoms	Do not use with active internal bleeding within 21 days, history of major surgery or trauma within 14 days, aortic dissection, severe uncontrolled hypertension, known bleeding disorders, lumbar puncture within 7 days, recent arterial puncture at noncompressible site, or history of cerebrovascular, intracranial, or intraspinal event within 3 months	*Alteplase: for AMI, 15 mg bolus, then 0.75 kg/mg over 30 minutes, then 0.50 mg/kg over 60 minutes not exceeding 100 mg total; for acute ischemic stroke: 60 mg IV first hour, then 20 mg/ hour for 2 hours; streptokinase: 1.5 million IU in a 1-hour infusion

**Dosing guidelines and procedures vary for thrombolytic agents; refer to current information for specific agent being used.*

Summary

A working knowledge of key pharmacological terms and concepts, as well as the dosages, actions, contraindications, and side effects of the major pharmaceutical agents, is critical to the practicing respiratory therapist in any area of patient care. Whether the practitioner is administering medicated aerosol treatments, providing conscious sedation during certain diagnostic and therapeutic procedures under medical supervision, or reviewing medications with a patient, this knowledge makes the respiratory therapist more clinically competent. Table 7-13 reviews and summarizes all of the medications that can be

TABLE 7-13 **Chart reviewing aerosolized medications used in the delivery of respiratory care (courtesy of Mohawk Valley Community College, Utica, NY)**

Generic Name	All Brand Names	% Solution	General Category	Chemical Structure	Receptors Stimulated or Action	Administration & Dosage	Adverse Effects	Special Considerations
Albuterol	Proventil Ventolin	0.5%	Sympathomimetic Bronchodilator	Saligenin	Beta 2	SVN: 2.5 mg MDI: 90 μg/puff	Muscle tremors	Used commonly as a rescue inhaler drug (MDI).
Levalbuterol HCL	Xopenex	Unit dose only	Sympathomimetic Bronchodilator	Saligenin R-isomer of albuterol	Beta 2	SVN: 0.63 mg & 1.25 mg Q6 to Q8 MDI:	Muscle tremors	Expensive when compared to cost of Albuterol.
Salmetrol xinafoate	Serevent	DPI only	Long-acting Sympathomimetic Bronchodilator	Saligenin	Beta 2	Diskus DPI: 1 capsule 50 mcg Q12H	Increases in heart rate & cardiac arrhythmias if overused.	Do not use in emergency situations!! Slow onset of action
Formoterol fumarate	Foradil	DPI only	Long-acting Sympathomimetic Bronchodilator	Saligenin	Beta 2	Aerolizer DPI: 1 capsule 12 mcg Q12H	Increased risk of toxicity with overuse of long acting drugs due to accumulation of drug in body.	Do not use in emergency situations!! Onset of action 3 to 4 minutes Peak action 30–60 minutes
Ipatropium bromide	Atrovent	Unit dose only	Parasympatholytic bronchodilator	quaternary ammonium compound	Blocks ACH at cholinergic receptor	SVN: 0.5 mg in unit dose MDI: 42 mcg/ puff (2p Qid)	Very few side effects	Used for people with problems associated with taking sympathomimetics. Commonly given with albuterol.
Tiotropium bromide	Spiriva	DPI only	Long-acting Parasympatholytic bronchodilator	quaternary ammonium compound	Blocks ACH at cholinergic receptor	HandiHaler DPI: 1 capsule 18 mcg/day	Very few side effects	Do not use as a rescue drug in an emergency.
Pirbuterol	Maxair	MDI only	Sympathomimetic Bronchodilator	Saligenin	Beta 2	Autohaler MDI: 2 puffs Q4H to Q6H 200 mcg/puff	Muscle tremors	Breath-actuated inhaler
Racemic epinephrine	Vaponephrine Micronephrine	2.25%	Sympathomimetic Bronchodilator	Catecholamine	a, B1, and B2	SVN: 0.25 to 0.5 mls/ 3 to 5 mis ns	Increases in: HR,BP	Duration of action is short 25 to 30 minutes for maximum effect.
Terbutaline	Bricanyl Brethaire Brethine	0.1% solution or MDI	Sympathomimetic Bronchodilator	Resorcinol	B2 > B1	SVN: I to 2 mg. MDI: 2 puffs	Tremors, increases in HR	
Acetylcysteine	Mucomyst	10% 20% solutions	Mucolytic	NA	Breaks the disulfide bond in mucus	SVN: 3 to 5mls TID or QID	Breaks the disulfide bond in mucus.	Bronchospasm due to acidity of solution. Nausea due to the smell. Give with a Beta 2 agonist
Dornase alfa	Pulmozyme		Proteolytic	enzyme	Breakdown of DNA in mucus chain	VN: 2.5 mg in 2.5 mls ns QD	Voice alteration, sore throat, etc.	Maintenance therapy drug must be taken everyday. Uses a special SVN.
Cromolyn sodium	Intal Arane	SVN solution + MDI	Anti-asthmatic	NA	Blocks Mast-cell degranulation	SVN: 20 mgs. tid or qid	Coughing and hoarsness	Propholactic type drug, it must be taken everyday. It may take up to 2 weeks for maximal effect.
Flunisolide	Aerobid	MDI	Anti-inflammatory	Corticosteroid	NA	250 μg/puff Bid	Possible immune & HPA suppression with higher doses	Thrush, if mouth is not rinsed out after use.

Budesonide	Pulmicort Respules Pulmicort Flexhaler	Liquid and DPI	Anti-inflammatory	Corticosteroid	NA	SVN: Respules UD 0.25 and 0.5 mg QD DPI: 90 & 180 mcg/ inhal. BID	Possible immune & HPA suppression with higher doses	Thrush, if mouth is not rinsed out after use.
Triamcinolone acetonide	Azmacort	MDI	Anti-inflammatory	Corticosteroid	NA	MDI: 2 puffs TID.QID 100 mcg/puff	Possible immune & HPA suppression with higher doses	Thrush, if mouth is not rinsed out after use.
Fluticasone propionate	Flovent HFA Flovent Diskus	MDI & DPI	Anti-inflammatory	Corticosteroid	NA	MDI: 2 puffs Bid DPI: Bid 44 mcg 50 μg HO mcg 100 μg 220 mcg 250 μg	Possible immune & HPA suppression with higher doses	Thrush, if mouth is not rinsed out after use.
Beclomethasone dipropionate	Qvar HFA	MDI	Anti-inflammatory	Corticosteroid	NA	MDI: 2 puffs 40 mc/ puff Bid 80 meg/puff Bid	Possible immune & HPA suppression with higher doses	Thrush, if mouth is not rinsed out after use.
Pentamidine	Pentam Nebupent	via Respigard II neb.	Anti-Protozoal Anti-Fungal	an aeromatic diamidine; it Interferes with cell wall metabolism	NA	SVN: 300 mg of powder in 6 ml sterile H_2O Q 4 weeks	Possible bronchospasm and increased risk of contracting TB from HIV patients	Must take precautions to protect the caregiver and environment. Respigard II neb,.neg pressure rooms HEPA filters etc.
Bitolterol mesylate	Tornalate	0.2%	Sympathomimetic Bronchodilator	PRO-drug/ catecholamine	Beta 2	MDI: 2 puffs BID-QID		No longer available in the USA
Salmelrol Xinafoate + Fluticasone Propionate	Advair	DPI & MDI HFA	Long-acting Sympathomimetic Bronchodilator + Anti-inflammatory	Saligenin + Corticosteroid	Beta 2	DPI MDI 100/50 45/21 250/50 115/21 500/50 230/21	Increases in heart rate & cardiac arrhythmias if overused.	Thrush, if mouth is not rinsed out after use.
Albuterol + ipratropium bromide	Duoneb	SVN unit dose	Sympathomimetic Bronchodilator + Parasympatholytic bronchodilator	Saligenin + Corticosteroid	Beta 2	SVN: 3 mg albuterol + 0.5 mg ipratropium bromide	Muscle tremors, same as other sympathomimetics	
albuterol + ipratropium bromide	Combivent	MDI				MPI:103 mcg albuteroH-18 mcg ipratropium bromide		
arformoterol tartrate	Brovana	Unit dose only	Long-acting Sympathomimetic Bronchodilator	Saligenin	Beta 2	SVN: 15 mcg/2 mls Q12H	Increases in heart rate & cardiac arrhythmias if overused.	Comes in a foil pack. Protect from light and excessive heat. Store in a refrigerator.
formoterol fumarate + budesonide	Symbicort	MDI with HFA	Long-acting Sympathomimetic Bronchodilator + Anti-inflammatory	Saligenin + Corticosteroid	Beta 2	2 strengths of MDI: 80/4. 5 mcg or 160/4.5 mcg	Increases in heart rate & cardiac arrhythmias if overused.	Thrush, if mouth is not rinsed out after use.

administered to the patient in aerosol form, through either an MDI, a DPI or a nebulizer, in terms of brand/generic name, category, chemical structure, receptor site activity, administration and dosage, adverse effects, and special considerations.

Study Questions

REVIEW QUESTIONS

1. What are the three phases of pharmacology?
2. What are the mechanisms of action of three types of drugs administered by inhalation?
3. What are some common indications for, contraindications for, and side effects of, and adverse reactions to aerosol drugs?
4. Name three aerosol drugs and their appropriate dosages.
5. How many milliliters are needed to administer 5 mg of a drug using a 2% strength solution?
6. What drugs are used in the management of asthma, and why are they used?
7. What are three drugs, including indications and dosages, used in advanced cardiac life support?
8. What is the appropriate action in a case involving a 22-year-old female asthmatic seen in the emergency room in respiratory distress? She is presently taking 16 puffs per day of her albuterol MDI with diminished response. She has been on this medication for 4 years.

MULTIPLE-CHOICE QUESTIONS

1. Delivering a drug via the inhalation route describes which phase of pharmacology?
   a. pharmaceutical
   b. pharmacokinetic
   c. pharmacodynamic
   d. pharmacologic
2. Sympathomimetic bronchodilators promote the relaxation of bronchial smooth muscle by stimulating the intracellular production of
   a. 5-AMP
   b. ADP
   c. ATP
   d. cyclic 39,59 AMP
3. Xanthines, such as aminophylline, produce bronchodilation by inhibiting which enzyme?
   a. monoamine oxidase
   b. catechol-O-methyl transferase
   c. phosphodiestarase
   d. adenyl cyclase
4. Epinephrine has which of the following receptor-site activities?
   a. alpha only
   b. alpha and beta-1
   c. beta-1 and beta 2
   d. alpha, beta-1, and beta 2
5. A 1.5% strength solution of a drug contains how many milligrams per milliliter?
   a. 0.15
   b. 1.5
   c. 15
   d. 150
6. How many milliliters of a drug are needed to administer 0.75 mg using a 0.5% strength solution?
   a. 0.15
   b. 1.5
   c. 0.3
   d. 3.0
7. A patient is receiving an aerosolized bronchodilator treatment when the respiratory therapist monitoring the patient notes a heart rate of 140. The baseline rate was 84. What action should the therapist take?
   a. Tell the patient to breathe more slowly and deeply.
   b. Ask the nurse what should be done.
   c. Stop the treatment, notify the patient's physician, and document the response in the patient's medical record.
   d. Add more saline to the nebulizer cup and continue with the treatment.
8. According to the American Heart Association, which of the following groups of drugs may be administered by endotracheal instillation as an adjunct or when an IV line cannot be established?
   a. epinephrine, atropine, and lidocaine
   b. norepinephrine, epinephrine, and sodium bicarbonate
   c. sodium bicarbonate, adenosine, and lidocaine
   d. adenosine, atropine, and verapamil
9. Which of the following agents produces a mucolytic effect by disrupting disulfide bonds?
   a. nedocromil sodium
   b. n-acetylcysteine
   c. sodium bicarbonate
   d. fluticasone propionate
10. Which of these antimicrobials can be nebulized for the treatment of *Pneumocystis carinii* pneumonia commonly associated with AIDS patients?
    a. amoxicillin
    b. pentamidine
    c. ribavirin
    d. amphotericin B

CRITICAL-THINKING QUESTIONS

1. Is it ever possible or permissible for a respiratory therapist who is administering aerosolized medications to patients to alter or change a physician's order in the patient's best interest? Identify a specific instance when a respiratory therapist might take such an action.
2. A physician orders a medication for a patient who the respiratory therapist knows is contraindicated and will result in harm to the patient. What actions should the therapist take? Explain your answer.
3. Why is it essential for respiratory therapists to be well versed in all areas of pharmacology when it seems as if the only medications they administer are aerosolized bronchodilators and mucolytics?

References

1. Op't Holt TB. Inhaled beta agonists. *Respir Care.* 2007;52,7:820–832.
2. Restrepo RD. Use of inhaled anticholinergic agents in obstructive airway disease. *Respir Care.* 2007;52,7:833–851.
3. Bills GW, Soderberg RL. *Principles of Pharmacology for Respiratory Care.* 2nd ed. Clifton Park, NY: Delmar Cengage Learning; 1998.
4. American Association for Respiratory Care. Assessing response to bronchodilator therapy at point of care. *Respir Care.* 1995;40,12:1300–1307.
5. American Association for Respiratory Care. Selection of device, administration of bronchodilator, and evaluation of response to therapy in mechanically ventilated patients. *Respir Care.* 1999;44:105–113.
6. National Heart, Lung and Blood Institute. Expert panel report 3: guidelines for the diagnosis and management of asthma: full report 2007. NIH publication 08-4051.
7. Baraniuk JN. Molecular actions of glucocorticoids: an introduction. *J Allergy Clin Immunol.* 1996; 97:141–142.
8. Phua G-C, MacIntyre NR. Inhaled corticosteroids in obstructive airway disease. *Respir Care.* 2007; 52,7:852–858.
9. Holgate ST, Bradding P, Sampson AP. Leukotriene antagonists and synthesis inhibitors. *J Allergy Clin Immunol.* 1996;98:1–13.
10. American Thoracic Society/European Respiratory Society Statement. Standards for the diagnosis and management of individuals with alpha-1 antitrypsin deficiency. *Am J Respir Crit Care Med.* 2003;168:818–900.
11. Robinson M, et al. Effect of hypertonic saline, amiloride, and cough on mucociliary clearance in patients with cystic fibrosis. *Am J Respir Crit Care Med.* 1996;153:1503–1509.
12. American Association for Respiratory Care. Bland aerosol administration. *Respir Care.* 2003;48,5:529–533.
13. Dhand R. The role of aerosolized antimicrobials in the treatment of ventilator- associated pneumonia. *Respir Care.* 2007;52,7:866–884.
14. Whitaker KC. *Neonatal and Pediatric Respiratory Care.* Clifton Park, NY: Delmar Cengage Learning; 1996.
15. Sinha S, Moya F, Donn SM. Surfactant for respiratory distress syndrome: are there important clinical differences among preparations? *Curr Opin Pediatr.* 2007;19:150–154.
16. American Association for Respiratory Care. Surfactant replacement therapy. *Respir Care.* 1994;39:824–829.
17. Ziment I. *Respiratory Pharmacology and Therapeutics.* Philadelphia: WB Saunders Co; 1978.
18. American Association for Respiratory Care. Assessing response to bronchodilator therapy at point of care. *Respir Care.* 1995;40,12: 1300–1307.
19. American Association for Respiratory Care. *Position Statement on Administration of Sedative and Analgesic Medications by Respiratory Care Practitioners.* Dallas: AARC; March 2000.
20. American Heart Association. 2005 American Heart Association (AHA) guidelines for cardiopulmonary resuscitation (CPR) and emergency cardiovascular care (ECC) of pediatric and neonatal patients: pediatric advanced life support. *Pediatrics.* May 2006;117,5:e1005–e1028.
21. Banerjee S, Singhi SC, Singh S, Singh M. The intraosseous route is a suitable alternative to intravenous route for fluid resuscitation in severely dehydrated children. *Indian Pediatrics.* 1994; 31,12:1511–1520.
22. Brickman KR, Krupp K, Rega P, Alexander J, Guinness M. Typing and screening of blood from intraosseous access. *Annals of Emergency Medicine.* 1992;21,4:414–417.
23. Frascone RJ, Jensen JP, Kaye K, Salzman JG. Consecutive field trials using two different intraosseous devices. *Prehospital Emergency Care.* 2007;11,2:164–171.
24. Davidoff J, Fowler R, Gordon D, et al. Clinical evaluation of a novel intraosseous device for adults: prospective, 250-patient, multi-center trial. *JEMS.* Supp. 2005;30,10:20–23.

Suggested Readings

Guntur VP, Dhand R. Inhaled insulin: extending the horizons of inhalation therapy. *Respir Care*. 2007;52,7:911–922.

Noonan M, Rosenwasser LJ, Martin P, O'Brien CD, O'Dowd L. Efficacy and safety of budesonide and formoterol in one pressurized metered-dose inhaler in adults and adolescents with moderate to severe asthma. *Drugs*. 2006;66,17:2235–2254.

Rau JL. *Respiratory Care Pharmacology*. 4th ed. St. Louis: Mosby-Yearbook; 1994.

Rubin BK. Mucolytics, expectorants, and mucokinetic medications. *Respir Care*. 2007;52,7:859–865.

Siobal, MS. Pulmonary vasodilators. *Respir Care*. 2007;52,7:885–899.

Szafranski W, Cukier A, Ramirez A, Menga G, Sansores R, Nahabedian S, Peterson S, Olsson H. Efficacy and safety of budesonide/formoterol in the management of chronic obstructive pulmonary disease. *Eur Respir J*. 2003;21:74–81.

CHAPTER 8

Pulmonary Infections

Barbara Ludwig

OBJECTIVES

Upon completion of this chapter, the reader should be able to:

- Describe the difference between bacterial and viral pneumonias.
- Discuss the effect of immunological disorders on the occurrence, clinical signs and symptoms, and treatment of pulmonary infections.
- Discuss the diagnosis and medical treatment of pulmonary infections.
- Describe the difference between a tuberculosis exposure and a tuberculosis infection.
- Explain the relationship between tuberculosis and HIV.
- Compare the differences between a tuberculosis infection and MAC infection.
- Discuss the geographic locations of common fungal infections.
- Compare the clinical appearance of a fungal infection in the patient with an intact immune system and the patient who is immunosuppressed.

CHAPTER OUTLINE

(continues)

(continued)

KEY TERMS

anergic
antibody titer
antigenic drift
antigenic shift
bullae
caseous necrosis
community-acquired pneumonia
coagulopathy
delayed hypersensitivity reaction
doubling time
empirical
Ghon complex
gray hepatization stage
hospital-acquired pneumonia
inflammatory stage
miliary tuberculosis
mycelium
nephrotoxicity
polymicrobial
primary infection tuberculosis
Ranke complex
reactivation tuberculosis
red hepatization stage
resolution stage

On the list of the 10 leading causes of death in 2005 in the United States [according to the National Center on Health Statistics (NCHS)], influenza/pneumonia is the eighth. In 2005, mortality rate increased significantly in several diseases; influenza/pneumonia was one of them. Of the deaths due to influenza/pneumonia, approximately 88% occurred in people 65 years or older. The age group with the highest death rate was in the oldest sector of the U.S. population, the 85 years and older group.[1] Although the mortality rate is very high in some vulnerable groups who contract influenza and pneumonia, complications of pulmonary infection can be serious in other age groups, and not all of the infections are viral or bacterial. This chapter covers many types of infections, both common and not so common. The respiratory therapist needs to know about all of them.

Pulmonary Infections

Viruses, bacteria, fungi, and parasites are microorganisms that cause infections of the respiratory system. Some of these infections are contagious and may cause serious respiratory disease with significant mortality in high-risk groups such as the chronically ill, the elderly, and persons with impaired immunity. Besides a significant cause of morbidity, a 1997 study reported the costs of medically treating respiratory infections and the effect on the workplace. The authors concluded that the cost to the employer for employees with respiratory infections was $112 billion and that included medical costs and time lost from work.[2] A comparison of the per-capita expenditures for people ill with lower respiratory tract infections to those for the average person reveals that the employee costs were almost three times more for that employee than for the average employee.[3]

Community-Acquired Bacterial and Viral Infections

Infections of the respiratory tract are among the most common afflictions of the human race. In the United States, respiratory tract infections are responsible for more visits to physicians than any other disease and for more time lost from work or school. In 1995, the National Health Interview Survey (NHIS) estimated that that there were 174 acute respiratory conditions per 100 persons per year. The NHIS indicated that, on average, everyone is afflicted with a respiratory condition or infection at least once a year.[2] The most common bacterial causes of respiratory infection are *Streptococcus pneumoniae, Haemophilus influenzae, Mycoplasma pneumoniae,* and *C. pneumoniae,* and the most common viral causes are adenovirus, influenza, metapneumovirus, and parainfluenza virus.

Community-acquired respiratory fungal infection is less frequent than bacterial or viral infection, but the common organisms in the United States are *Histoplasmosis capsulatum* and *Coccidiodes immitis.*[6]

VIRAL INFECTIONS AND PNEUMONIA

Respiratory viral infections cause everything from the common cold to severe viral pneumonia. A large majority of all respiratory infections are viral in origin. They cause considerable illness but few deaths, except in persons who are immunocompromised.

The most common viral pathogens that cause viral pneumonia in otherwise healthy adults, infants, and children are influenza A and B viruses (50% of cases). The elderly are susceptible to more viruses than healthy young adults because of diminishing immunity. Other common viruses that cause viral pneumonia in children are respiratory syncytial virus and parainfluenza virus.[6,7]

Influenza viruses A and B frequently cause annual epidemics and endemics. As the virus passes through the human population, it undergoes frequent antigenic mutation owing to viral RNA amino acid recombinations occurring on the viral surface proteins. These changes, called the **antigenic drift**, are sufficient to make the general population's current immune defenses inadequate against this new antigen mutation. The antigenic drifts are commonly associated with limited epidemics in the community.

Dramatic changes in viral subtypes can occur when RNA segments are exchanged between coinfecting viruses. This mutation significantly alters viruses' genetic makeup by means of new gene formation. This major change is an **antigenic shift**, and a serious epidemic or pandemic is possible. The population no longer has immunity against the changed virus.[7,9]

Severe influenza outbreaks generally occur every 10 to 30 years. The populations with the highest mortality in these influenza outbreaks are children, the elderly, and those with comorbid conditions such as chronic obstructive pulmonary disease, diabetes mellitus, cancer, heart disease, or renal disease. The worst influenza pandemic in history occurred in the closing years of World War I. An estimated 40 million people died during the flupandemic of 1918–1919.[7,9] The high death rates occurred in the vulnerable populations: children under the age of five and adults over the age of 70. Surprisingly, a group that is usually less affected, adults between the ages of 20 and 40, had devastating death rates that destroyed families and even entire communities.[10] Avian influenza A has recently taken a prominent position among the new viral infections that could develop into a flu pandemic. The avian virus usually does not infect humans, but since November 2003, nearly 400 cases have appeared in more than a dozen countries. The World Health Organization is keeping records of human cases, and public health officials are closely monitoring outbreaks because the virus has the potential to change and become infectious. The potential for an avian flu pandemic has resulted in medical communities preparing disaster plans for situations such as a viral pandemic that may be even more severe than the Great Influenza Pandemic of 1918.[11]

Viruses are transmitted from person to person by one of two mechanisms.

- The inhalation of virus-contaminated aerosolized secretions expelled into the air during a cough or sneeze by the person infected with the virus
- Direct upper airway contact, as would occur by getting the virus on your hand and touching your mouth, eye, or other mucus membrane surface[9]

With the invasion of the virus through the respiratory tract, the patient may develop a primary viral pneumonia or bronchitis. *Viral pneumonia* is a spread of the virus to the bronchi, bronchioles, alveoli, and alveolar interstitium. The virus damages the bronchi and bronchioles' epithelial layer, and the epithelial tissue sloughs to the basement membrane. This loss of the airway epithelium interferes with normal bronchial clearance. The affected areas of the parenchyma become edematous and hemorrhagic. The lungs' intense inflammatory response causes alveolar necrosis and the formation of hyaline membrane.[12]

Viral infections affecting the lower respiratory tract occur in three general situations:

- Infections confined to the lung alone, called *primary pneumonia,* such as respiratory syncytial virus, influenza, parainfluenza, and adenovirus
- Systemic infections involving the lung, which can result from measles, chicken pox, and adenovirus
- Viral infections that occur in the immunosuppressed,[12] who are vulnerable to pneumonia from cytomegalovirus, herpes zoster, chicken pox, and adenovirus.[12]

Most viral pneumonias are not fatal. In patients who die from their viral illness, the pathologic changes are mainly due to a secondary bacterial infection called a *secondary pneumonia,* or superinfection. Injury to the respiratory epithelium with a viral infection allows the bacteria attachment resulting in a bacterial pneumonia.[12] The most common bacteria causing postinfluenza pneumonia are *Streptococcus pneumoniae, Staphylococcus aureus,* and *Haemophilusinfluenzae.*[7]

The patient with an uncomplicated viral infection initially presents with classic features of influenza (fever, chills, malaise, headache, and body aches) with recovery after a few days. A worsening of respiratory symptoms suggests pneumonia. Primary influenzal pneumonia is rare, and its presence has a high mortality rate. The disease can rapid progress, leading to death within hours of onset.[12] If the viral illness is complicated by a secondary bacterial pneumonia, the morbidity and mortality also increase sharply.

The laboratory findings for a person with viral pneumonia are very different from those for a person with a bacterial infection. In primary viral pneumonia, the leukocyte count is normal. If the white count is elevated, the patient may have a superimposed bacterial infection. Although not often necessary, a specific diagnosis may be made by isolating the virus by demonstrating an elevated **antibody titer** of the person's serum (the reciprocal of the highest dilution of the serum in which the antibody is detectable). This test can identify the presence of viral proteins or assay the individual's respiratory secretions or nasopharyngeal washings for the presence of elevated antibody.[6,7]

Prevention. Antiviral vaccines (flu shots) play an important role in preventing influenza infections and decreasing the severity of the influenza illness. High-risk groups such as people with comorbid diseases, the elderly, or health care workers, are encouraged to be vaccinated yearly for influenza prevention.[9] The Centers for Disease Control and Prevention evaluates each year the appropriateness of administering the available antiviral drugs for prophylaxis and treatment of influenza A and B infections. Their recommendations are based on the circulating influenza A viruses, including two subtypes (H2N2 and H3N2) and influenza B viruses. These viruses circulate worldwide, but their prevalence within communities varies. Since 2006, the neuraminidase inhibitors (oseltamivir and zanamivir) have been the only antiviral drugs recommended because of resistance to the admantanes (amantadine, rimantadine). Local health department surveillance data and laboratory testing should help area physicians identify which antiviral drugs to use in preventing or reducing the severity of illness with the current viral strains.[13]

Other preventive antiviral drugs are the human monoclonal antibody palivizumab (Synagis) and respiratory syncytial virus immune globulin RSV-IVIG (RespiGam). These two medications effectively prevent the occurrence of respiratory syncytial virus in high-risk pediatric patients. Palivizumab is preferred because it does not interfere with vaccinations (measles-mumps-rubella, varicella), is an IM formulation, and has fewer complications than RSV-IVIG. However, RSV-IVIG provides additional protection against other viral infections and may be helpful in high-risk pediatric patients with an underlying immune deficiency or HIV infection. Neither drug is recommended for use for pediatric patients with congenital heart disease.[14]

Treatment

- *Acyclovir* is effective against herpes simplex virus, herpes zoster, or varicella (chickenpox).
- *Ganciclovir* and *immune globulin* are beneficial in the treatment of cytomegalovirus (CMV).[4] Patients with CMV pneumonia either are immunosuppressed by infection with HIV or are receiving immunosuppressive drugs (e.g., organ transplant recipients).
- *Aerosolized ribavirin* is no longer a recommended treatment for children with respiratory syncytial virus. However, ribavirin is effective for treating hepatitis C, and it has been administered by intravenous in immunocompromised children and neonates with adenovirus infection with local and disseminated involvement. The drug is given orally to adults. It is thought to reduce fever and viral shedding.[9]
- Two antiviral drugs—*zanamivir* and *oseltamivir*—are effective against both influenza A and B. Zanamavir is administered by inhaler or nasal route and should not be given to patients with reactive airways because of possible bronchospasm. Oseltamivir is administered orally. The drugs must be taken early in the onset of influenza symptoms and must be taken for 5 days.[7] Each drug is thought to reduce the viral symptoms by 1 day.[15]

Classifications of Pneumonia

In the past, there were only two major classifications of pneumonia: **community-acquired pneumonia** and **hospital-acquired** (*nosocomial*) **pneumonia**. Today, health care changes have caused less clear boundaries between the community and the hospital. More hospitalized patients have not totally recovered from their respiratory infections at the time of discharge from the hospital. Additionally, many patients are receiving medical care from outpatient facilities. In 2005, the American Thoracic Society and Infectious Diseases Society of America proposed a new category of pneumonia called *health-care-associated pneumonia*. This classification includes pneumonia cases of patients who recently had been hospitalized, had received hemodialysis or intravenous chemotherapy, or had been residents of a nursing home or long-term care facility. These patients either have serious health care issues or are living in institutions designed for senior citizens. Many are chronically ill. Although these patients previously were categorized as having community-acquired pneumonia, they are more ill than the typical case. Their need for hospitalization is different, as is their need for different and more potent antibiotics.

The current classifications of pneumonia are:

- Community-acquired pneumonia.
- Health-care-associated pneumonia.
- Hospital-acquired pneumonia.
- Ventilator-associated pneumonia.

The last three categories are associated with relatively serious pneumonias, longer hospital stays, and higher mortality rates.[4,5]

Community-Acquired Pneumonia

According to the National Center for Health, in 1997, 86,649 people died of influenza/pneumonia. It was the sixth leading cause of death by any means in the United States, and it was the leading cause of death due to infectious disease.[2,11] Most people with community-acquired pneumonia (CAP) are managed by their personal physician and are not admitted to the hospital. The most common bacterium found in people with CAP is *Streptococcus pneumoniae*. Other common organisms causing CAP are *Myocoplasma pneumoniae, Haemophilus influenzae,* viruses, and *Legionella species.* Often, the organism is never identified.[7]

RISK FACTORS OF COMMUNITY-ACQUIRED PNEUMONIA

Specific risk factors are common among people who develop community-acquired pneumonia (CAP): age, alcoholism, poor nutrition, smoking, comorbid conditions, and institutionalization.[7] These risks include senior citizens and the chronically ill living at home, military service personnel who are living in barracks or other communal facilities, and college students living in dormitories or in fraternity or sorority houses.

Each year a person lives after the age of 65 increases the risk for developing CAP. Research studies have identified this age group as the one at the highest risk of developing pneumonia from *Streptococcus pneumoniae*, the greatest risk of being hospitalized, and the greatest risk of death from pneumonia. This patient population also has the greatest incidence of underlying chronic conditions such as cardiovascular disease, chronic obstructive pulmonary disease (COPD), and diabetes. An additional problem is that the immune function of the elderly is less effective in the presence of infection than that of younger populations.[7]

A major mechanism of pneumonia is microaspiration of upper airway secretions. During sleep, 45% of normal subjects aspirate. People with impaired swallowing reflexes (e.g., stroke, amyotrophic lateral sclerosis (ALS), muscular dystrophy, postpolio syndrome) frequently microaspirate when compared to normal people. Therefore, their risk for pneumonia is higher.

Chronic excessive alcohol use has many negative effects that predispose alcoholics to pneumonia. Alcoholics routinely are undernourished or malnourished, and nutritional deficiencies compromise immune function. The oropharynx of alcoholics can be colonized with gram-negative bacteria, and, during intoxication, the glottic reflexes are obtunded. This can lead to microaspiration of upper airway secretions. Lastly, during sleep, alcohol impairs pulmonary clearance mechanisms (e.g., cough reflex, ciliary clearance). All of these factors combine to make the alcoholic more susceptible to pneumonia.[6,7]

Poor nutritional intake does not give the body adequate calories and protein to produce adequate numbers of immune cells. Therefore, individuals who are malnourished have impaired cell-mediated and humoral immunity. Malnourished people frequently have an underlying chronic condition, such as alcoholism, chronic lung disease, heart disease, or cancer, which may be the basis of their malnutrition.[6,7] These compounding risk factors put them at a greater risk of pneumonia and a fatal outcome.

Smoking also impairs pulmonary defense mechanisms, such as the mucociliary clearance, goblet cell function, and secretory IgA function. With lowered lung defenses secondary to smoking, these individuals are more susceptible to pulmonary infections.[7]

People with chronic diseases are susceptible to bacterial infections. Chronic lung disease patients have a greater incidence of CAP than do people with normal lungs. This patient population has a greater incidence of infections with *Streptococcus pneumoniae, Haemophilus influenza,* and *Moraxella catarrhalis.*[8] People with diabetes mellitus, neurological diseases, heart disease, or cancer also have a greater incidence of CAP, and they are at a greater risk of developing gram-negative infections. Research studies comparing the characteristics of patients dying of pneumonia with those of patients surviving it have shown that more of the deceased patients had comorbid conditions than did the surviving group.

PATHOGENESIS

The major mechanisms by which microorganisms invade the lower respiratory tract are by inhalation, by aspiration, or through the circulation. Community-acquired pneumonia primarily arises from aspirated bacterial invasion of the lower respiratory tract, not from inhalation or blood-borne bacteria.

The main reservoir of microaspiration is the oropharynx. The oropharynx usually harbors bacteria in the range of 10^7–10^8 organisms per milliliter of saliva, and it contains many anaerobes and gram-positive bacterial pathogens.[16] *Streptococcus pneumoniae* is a common pathogen of the oropharynx. Gram-negative bacilli are not present as commonly in the oropharynx, and only a small percentage of the general population harbor gram-negative bacteria in their oropharynx.

People normally aspirate oropharyngeal secretions during sleep, when the upper airway glottic reflexes are diminished. Usually, our lower airway defense mechanisms cope with this nightly onslaught of bacteria. The occurrence of pneumonia is determined by the interactions among the bacterial growth rate, the virulence of the organism, and the lower airway defense mechanisms. The first line of defense is ciliary clearance. If the organism reaches the lower airway and the host defenses are unable to control the proliferation of the bacteria, colonization swiftly changes to frank infection.[6,7]

PATHOLOGIC CHANGES

Bacterial CAP is classically described as a *lobar pneumonia*. It has four distinct pathologic stages:

- In the first 12–24 hours following infection, the lung is in the acute **inflammatory stage**. There is marked inflammatory pulmonary edema with engorgement of capillaries and exudation of acellular serous fluid into the alveolar spaces.
- The next stage of pneumonia progression is the **red hepatization stage**. These changes occur between 24 and 72 hours postinfection. The lung has a deep red, liverlike appearance. The alveolar spaces are full of coagulated exudate containing fibrin, red blood cells, polymorphonuclear leukocytes, and the causative bacteria.
- The pneumonic process changes to the **gray hepatization stage** 4–5 days postinfection. The lung is yellow-gray, and the alveoli contain many polymorphonuclear leukocytes and very few red blood cells.
- The **resolution stage** is the final (healing) phase of the pneumonic process. The enzymes released from the leukocytes liquefy the alveolar fibrinous exudate. The phagocytes reabsorb the liquid, and the atelectatic lung starts to reinflate. Necrosis of the lung is uncommon, but a transudative pleural effusion (neighborhood reaction) or an exudative pleural effusion or empyema may occur.[17]

These pneumonic stages are the effects of the bacteria on the tissues, the body's immune response to the infection, and the healing process. Not all parts of the lung are in uniform stages of consolidation. Some parts of the lung are infected initially, and the infection may spread. Therefore, one segment of the lung may be in the gray hepatization stage while another is in the resolution stage.[17]

BRONCHOPNEUMONIA

Bronchopneumonia has the same evolution of consolidation, but the infection is not confined to a lobe or lobes. The infection usually affects the alveoli contiguous to the bronchi. The consolidative changes are patchy and follow the pathway of the tracheobronchial tree. *Streptococcus pneumoniae, Staphylococcus aureus, Pseudomonas aeruginosa*, and *Escherichia coli* are some organisms that may cause this distribution pattern of pneumonia.[17]

DIAGNOSIS OF COMMUNITY-ACQUIRED PNEUMONIA

In trying to diagnose CAP, one must look at the individual's presenting symptoms (see Table 8-1). The classic constellation of fever, chills, body aches, cough productive of purulent sputum, chest pain, dyspnea, crackles, and bronchial breath sounds heard on auscultation, and dullness to percussion may not be present in many patients. Findings vary widely in people with CAP. For example, pneumonia in the elderly is frequently atypical in the clinical presentation. The elderly patient may be afebrile or even hypothermic. Mental confusion or obtundation is a common sign. In many cases, the patient may not exhibit abnormal breath sounds on auscultation or show evidence of consolidation on the chest radiograph.[6,7] In recent years, health care practices have changed considerably regarding the standard techniques used to diagnose CAP pneumonia. The routine tests of the past, such as chest X-ray, blood chemistry, and sputum culture, are not performed unless the patient is showing evidence of complications or has risk factors for unusual microorganisms or for a more severe disease.[7]

Infections with Specific Microorganisms. Some bacterial organisms cause a clinical picture that can help physicians identify them.

Mycoplasma pneumonia, an intermediate organism between a bacterium and a virus, causes a pneumonia process called *atypical pneumonia*.[15] Mycoplasma pneumonia accounts for 18% of all community-acquired pneumonia requiring hospitalization. This is

TABLE 8-1 **Pneumonia syndromes**

	Community-Acquired Bacterial	Viral	Immunocompromised Host
Signs	Abrupt onset Productive cough Crackles and rhonchi on auscultation, dullness to percussion over affected lung areas Purulent sputum, ± hemoptysis,	Acute onset of cough, sore throat, nasal discharge, dry cough, wheezing on auscultation Mucoid, non-purulent	Classic signs may be absent New development of worsening cough, increased respiratory rate May show new development of purulent secretions, or change in character or volume of secretions or increased suctioning requirements Crackles or bronchial breath sounds
Symptoms	Dyspnea, pleuritic chest pain	Dyspnea, pleuritic chest pain	Classic symptoms may be absent, ↑ dyspnea
Systemic manifestations	Toxic chills and high fever, body aches Altered mental state Metastatic infection may occur	Fever, body aches, headache, malaise	Fever, typical systemic features absent ≥ 70 years/old, altered mental status with no recognized cause
Suggested microbiology studies	Attempts to identify a pathogen not usually indicated. Exceptions for critically ill patients	Diagnostic tests of respiratory secretions: + Antigen-detection, + ELISA, Culture of secretions or tissue	BAL, protected brush or targeted bronchoscopy recommended
Chest radiograph	Localized infiltrates (lobar or segmental) Multilobar suggests *Streptococcal pneumoniae* or *Legionella pneumophilia* infection Interstitial infiltrates suggests *Mycoplasma pneumoniae* infection	Diffuse interstitial infiltrates or patchy infiltrates. RSV may also show atelectasis and/or hyperinflation.	New or progressive and persistent infiltrate OR Consolidation OR Cavitation OR Pneumatoceles (infants < 1 year)
Laboratory	Leukocytosis, Drop in SaO_2, Electrolytes and BUN and creatinine testing to identify hydration status	Normal WBC, Drop SaO_2,	Leukopenia or leukocytosis Positive blood culture not related to other source Drop in SaO_2, Increased oxygen requirements and/or increased ventilatory demands
Predisposing Factors	Age, smoking history, alcohol, comorbid disease, post-influenza, immunosuppressive drugs	Elderly, children, comorbid disease, communal living (dorms, military barricks)	Organ transplantation, malignancy, immunosuppression, comorbid diseases, HIV infection

(continues)

TABLE 8-1 **Pneumonia syndromes *(continued)***

	Community-Acquired Bacterial	Viral	Immunocompromised Host
Common microorganisms	*Streptococcal pneumoniae, Mycoplasma pneumoniae Chlamydia pneumonia Haemophilus influenzae, Staphylococcus aureus (methicillin/oxacillin sensitive), K. pneumonae*	Influenza, Parainfluenza, Respiratory Syncytial Virus, Adenovirus	**Early onset pneumonia** (<96 hrs) Bacterial: *Streptococcal pneumonae, Staphylococcus aureus, Haemophilus influenza, Moraxella catarrhalis,* enteric gram-negatives, *Serratia marcescens, Escherichia coli* *Viruses:* *Influenzae A and B* *Respiratory Syncytial Virus* **LATE onset pneumonia** (>96 hrs) Gram negative bacilli *(P. aeruginosa, Proteus* spp. *Acinetobacter* spp.) *S. aureus (MRSA/ORSA)* *VRE,* *L. pneumophila,* Viral: Influenza A and B Respiratory Syncytial Virus, Adenovirus Fungal: Yeasts, fungi, *P. jirovecii*

a frequency second only to pneumococcal pneumonia. The outstanding characteristic of this infection is that it is a disease of young people. It infects young adults or teens in the winter or summer months with a higher incidence in small communities such as schools, colleges, and military barracks. Infected individuals usually present with influenzalike signs and symptoms, which worsen over several days. Sufferers may also complain of headache and may have severe sore throat, earache, laryngitis, and conjunctivitis. The chest X-ray usually shows hilar infiltrates that may be bilateral. The mortality rate is low, and the chest X-ray changes usually resolve during convalescence.[6,7,12]

Staphylococcus aureus is a gram-positive coccus that usually appears on microscopic examination in clusters. This microorganism is seen as a cause of pneumonia in three major settings:[13]

- Secondary complication of a preceding viral respiratory tract infection
- Hospitalized patients who have host defense impairment and whose oropharynx is colonized with *Staphylococcus aureus*
- Complication of staphylococcus bacteremia or sepsis

The severity of the infection is determined by the degree with which the organism is resistant to common antimicrobials.

Methicillin-resistant *Staphylococcus aureus* (MRSA) is a serious staphylococcal infection that is very difficult to treat with common antimicrobials. Resistance to methicillin implies resistance to all beta-lactam antimicrobials such as penicillins, cephalosporins, carbapenems, and beta-lactamase inhibitor–beta-lactam combinations. Hospitalized patients with MRSA infection are placed in barrier isolation to prevent the spread of infection to others. The patient can be isolated in a private room or cohorted (roomed with other patients with the same infection). Personnel should wear gloves and gowns for direct contact and should wash their hands after removing their gloves. A mask should be worn if aerosolization or secretion splashing possible.

MRSA is transmitted commonly through the transiently contaminated hands of health care workers who have direct contact with an infected patient or with a contaminated surface and do not wash their hands properly. Airborne transmission can also occur. MRSA may also be transmitted by persons who carry MRSA in their nasopharynx. People who are nasal carriers of MRSA (patients or health care workers) can transmit the infection to other hospitalized patients; this mode of transmission, however, is uncommon.

The topical antibiotic Mupirocin has excellent antibacterial activity against staphylococcal infections and MRSA. Intranasal administration has been successfully used in patients and health care workers during MRSA outbreaks to reduce nasal carriage of the organism. Mupirocin use has reduced the number of MRSA outbreaks in a variety of clinical areas (e.g., neonatal nurseries, hemodialysis units, cardiothoracic surgery). At home, nasal carriers have not been identified as a source of infection to other healthy family members.[18]

In severe cases, staphylococcal pneumonia is known to cause formation of **bullae** (enlarged alveoli) and pneumothorax, as well as microabscesses, pleural effusion, and empyema. After recovery from pneumonia, the patient may have residual pulmonary lung damage such as fibrosis bronchiectasis and pulmonary cavities.[7,17]

Legionella pneumophila is an aerobic, gram-negative intracellular bacillus. This bacillus differs from others in that it fails to grow on standard media and requires a different culture technique. The organism thrives in warm, moist conditions such as soil or stagnant water reservoirs (e.g., faulty air-conditioning cooling towers, hospital showerheads, and faucets). Bacteria usually spread by air, and outbreaks commonly occur in the summer or autumn. Legionella pneumonia is most common in the elderly and cigarette smokers, as well as in people with chronic lung, heart, or kidney disease, diabetes, or suppressed immunosystems.[19] It is suggested that *Legionella* be tested for only if the patient is not responding to beta-lactam antibiotics or is immunosuppressed or if the suspicion of *Legionella* infection is high. *Legionella* organisms are known to affect multiple body organ systems in addition to the lung; they may cause liver dysfunction, kidney failure, or muscle necrosis.[6,7]

Chlamydia psittaci is the cause of psittacosis, which can be spread to humans by infected birds (e.g., parakeets, canaries, parrots). The more common clinical cause of chlamydia infection is the *Chlamydia pneumoniae*, or TWAR, organism. It was named TWAR because of its similarity to a conjunctival isolate from Taiwan (TW-183) and a pharyngeal isolate from the United States (AR-39).[15] TWAR is a very common organism that is known to cause pneumonia in the elderly and young adults, but its exact incidence is not known. Young adults have a clinical presentation similar to *Mycoplasma* pneumonia. By age 20, approximately 50% of the population has had the infection and reinfection appears to be common.[20] Research studies have shown a connection between *C. pneumoniae* and severe chronic adult asthma. It has been reported that 8.9% of patients presenting with acute asthma had serological evidence of *C. pneumoniae* infection.[21] In elderly people with a comorbid disease, it may have a lethal clinical course. This organism has been known to cause hospital-acquired pneumonia.[20]

Haemophilus influenzae is a small coccobacillary gram-negative organism that is found in two forms: the unencapsulated strain and the capsulated strain. It is often found in the nasopharynx of normal healthy individuals and in the lower airways of people with chronic obstructive lung disease.[19] The infected are often elderly or predisposed to pneumonia by alcoholism or chronic bronchitis. The person with chronic obstructive lung disease frequently develops an exacerbation of the lung disease secondary to infection with the unencapsulated strain, which may cause pneumonia or acute bronchitis.[13]

The pneumonia may take the form of either lobar pneumonia or bronchopneumonia. Factors that predispose the individual to oropharyngeal colonization by gram-negative bacteria and subsequent pneumonia are current or recent hospitalization, underlying disease or compromised host defenses, and recent antimicrobial therapy. Gram-negative pneumonia is frequently associated with abscess and empyema, and, after recovery, the person may be left with pulmonary fibrosis.[3,4]

TREATMENT OF COMMUNITY-ACQUIRED PNEUMONIA

The definitive treatment for CAP is antimicrobial therapy (Table 8-2). The treatment varies according to the microorganism and the sensitivity of the organism to specific drugs. The initial antimicrobial chosen for the person with CAP is **empirically** chosen (based on experience). Frequently, the organism is never isolated. Despite this lack of ability to isolate the causative organism, knowledge of a patient's health history and risk factors, a physical examination, and simple testing (SpO_2, chest X-ray) enable the physician to diagnose CAP and to identify a possible causative organism. An infiltrate on a chest X-ray has predictive values for specific clinical signs that, when present, increase the likelihood that the infiltrate is due to pneumonia. Increasing the probability that the patient has pneumonia are the presence of fever greater than 37.8°C, heart rate greater than 100 beats/minute, crackles on auscultation, and decreased breath sounds in a nonasthmatic.[6] For the person hospitalized for CAP, additional diagnostic procedures (see Table 8-1) may be necessary so that the appropriate antimicrobial therapy can be

TABLE 8-2 **Antibiotic therapy in bacterial pneumonia**

Microorganism	1st Line Antibiotic	Alternative Antibiotics	Treatment for Resistant Strains
Streptococcal pneumoniae	Semi-Synthetic Penicillins e.g. Penicillin G or V	Newer Fluoroquinolones e.g. Sparfloxacin, Gatifloxacin; 1st generation Cephalosporins e.g. Cephalexin, Cefazolin; Macrolides e.g. Erythromycin; Clindamycin	**Intermediately resistant** 3rd generation Cephalosporin Cefotaxime; Ceftriaxone **Highly resistant** Vancomycin + 3rd generation Cephalosporin Ceftriaxone, Cefotaxime; OR Fluoroquinolone e.g. Levofloxacin
Staphylococcal aureus	Strains sensitive to penicillinase–resistant penicillins (Oxacillin, Cloxacillin, Nafcillin)	1st or 2nd generation Cephalosporin e.g. Cefazolin, Cefuroxime; Clindamycin Carbapenenems e.g. Imipenem, Merepenem; Macrolides e.g. Erythromycin; Clindamycin; Gentamycin Vancomycin	**Methicillin/Oxacillin resistant *staphylococcus aureus* (MRSA/ORSA)** Vancomycin
Chlamydia pneumoniae (TWAR strain)	Tetracycline e.g. Doxocycline	Sulfonamide e.g. Trimethaprim-Sulfamethoxazole; Macrolides e.g. Erythromycin; Fluoroquinolone e.g. Ciprofloxacin	Treatment based on susceptability testing.
Mycoplasma pneumoniae	Tetracycline e.g. Tetracycline; Macrolides e.g. Erythromycin	Macrolides e.g. Clarithromycin, Azithromycin; Fluoroquinolone e.g. Levofloxacin	Treatment based on susceptability testing.
Hemophilus influenzae	Bronchitis: Sulfonamides e.g. Trimethaprim-Sulfamethoxazole; Serious infections: 3rd generation Cephalosporin e.g. Cefotaxime	Bronchitis: 2nd or 3rd generation Cephalosporin e.g. cefuroxime, cefotaxime; Fluoroquinolones e.g. Ciprofloxacin; Macrolides e.g. Azithromycin; Serious infections: 2nd generation Cephalosporin e.g. Cefuroxime; Chloramphenicol; Carbapenems e.g. Meropenem	Treatment based on susceptability testing.
Legionella pneumophilia	Macrolides e.g. Azithromycin, Erythromycin ± Rifampin Fluoroquinolone e.g. Levofloxacin ± Rifampin;	Tetracycline e.g. Doxycycline ± Rifampin; Sulfonamide e.g. Trimethaprim-Sulfamethoxazole	Treatment based on susceptability testing.
Klebsiella pneumoniae	3rd or 4th generation Cephalosporin e.g. Cefotaxime, Cefepime	Carbapenems e.g. Imipenim; Aminoglycoside e.g. Gentamicin; Extended spectrum penicillin e.g Pipercillin/Tazobactam (Zosyn) Sulfonamide e.g. Trimethaprim-Sulfamethoxazole	Treatment based on susceptability testing.
Stenotrophomonas Maltophilia	Sulfonamide e.g. Trimethaprime-Sulfamethoxazole	Tetracycline e.g. Minocycline; 3rd generation Cephalosporin e.g. Ceftaxidime; Fluoroquinolone e.g. Ciprofloxacin	Treatment based on susceptability testing.

(continues)

TABLE 8-2 **Antibiotic therapy in bacterial pneumonia *(continued)***

Microorganism	1st Line Antibiotic	Alternative Antibiotics	Treatment for Resistant Strains
Pseudomonas aeruginosa	Aminoglycoside e.g. Tobramycin, Gentamicin PLUS Extended Spectrum Penicillin e.g. Ticarcillin, Pipercillin	Carbapenems e.g. Imipenem, Meropenem PLUS Aminoglycoside e.g. Gentamicin	Treatment based on susceptability testing.
Escherichia coli	3rd or 4th generation Cephalosporin e.g. Cefotaxime, Cefepime; In severe illness: Add Aminoglycoside e.g. Gentamicin,	Penicillin e.g. Ampicillin ± Aminoglycoside e.g. Gentamicin; Extended Spectrum Penicillin e.g. Pipercillin, Aminoglycoside alone e.g. Tobramycin	Treatment based on susceptability testing.

administered. The decision regarding the need to hospitalize the patient is based on several indicators:

- Severe leukocytosis or leukopenia
- Significant hypoxemia (P_aO_2 less than 60 mm Hg and S_aO_2 less than 90%) or hypercarbia (P_AO_2 less than 50 mm Hg), acidosis (pH less than 7.30)
- Signs of multiple organ dysfunction
- Severe clinical manifestations (tachypnea, tachycardia, chest pain, high fever, cyanosis, hypotension)[6,7]

If the patient is hospitalized, in addition to intravenous (IV) antimicrobials, the following supportive therapies are frequently necessary: hydration with IV fluids, oxygen therapy, and bronchodilator therapy. If the patient's oxygenation or ventilatory defect is not reversed or controlled with intensive bronchial hygiene, invasive or noninvasive mechanical ventilation may be necessary until lung mechanics and oxygenation improve.

Hospital-Acquired Pneumonia

Hospital-acquired pneumonia (*HAP*) is defined as a pulmonary infection not present or incubating at the time of the patient's admission to the hospital.[20] HAP accounts for only about 15% of hospital-acquired infections, but it significantly affects patient morbidity, mortality, and hospitalization costs. The excess duration of length of stay attributed to hospital-acquired pneumonia has been estimated to be 6.8–30 days.[3]

The microorganisms causing HAP reflect the number of days after admission that the patients develop pneumonia.

- Patients with *early-onset HAP* develop symptoms in fewer than 5 days after admission to the hospital, and the organisms are closer to the causative agents of CAP. The common microorganisms causing early-onset HAP are *S. pneumonia, S. aureus, H. influenzae, Enterobacteriaceae, S. marcescens,* and *E. coli.*[12]
- In *late-onset HAP,* the infection occurs after day 5 of admission. The causative agents are different from early-onset HAP and reflect the patients' susceptibility to infection. Common organisms causing late-onset HAP are gram-negative bacilli (*H. influenza, P. aeruginosa*), *S. aureus* (*MRSA*), *Acinetobacter* spp., *K. pneumoniae,* and viruses.

PATIENTS AT RISK FOR HOSPITAL-ACQUIRED PNEUMONIA

The following is a list of the findings from numerous research studies examining which hospitalized patient groups are at the greatest risk for developing hospital-acquired bacterial pneumonia.[21]

- Older than 60 years of age
- Chronic lung disease or systemic disease
- Intubation (including surgery)
- Recent antibiotic history
- Large volume aspiration
- Depressed level of consciousness

Other clinical situations not listed put the patient at risk but to a lesser degree. Also increasing the specific patient's risk for hospital-acquired pneumonia is a host of factors (extremes of age, immune status, comorbid conditions, ICU admission) and clinical conditions. Patients for whom the ventilator circuit is changed every 24 hours have an increased risk of airway contamination. Patients receiving stress ulcer bleeding prophylaxis with H_2 blockers are at risk because H_2 blockers suppress gastric acidity and permit bacterial survival in the stomach. Patients who are in the supine position have a greater risk of aspiration.[21,22]

ETIOLOGIC MECHANISM

The mechanisms for development of HAP have similarities to those for CAP, but there are important differences. A highly significant shared etiology between CAP and hospital-acquired pneumonia is that of microaspiration of upper airway secretions, which is still by far the most frequent cause of pneumonia. CAP and hospital-acquired pneumonia are frequently caused by self-infection.[21] Other shared mechanisms are:

- Inhalation of contaminated aerosols (common).
- Blood-borne spread from a distant site (uncommon).
- Translocation of organisms from the gastrointestinal tract into the systemic circulation (increases the risk for bacterial overgrowth).
- Mucosal disruption of the bowel and impaired lymphatic clearance of organisms from the bowel.
- Cross-contamination from the hands of health care workers or contaminated gloves or devices (an important shared mechanism).
- Contaminated water supplies (showers, hospital cooling towers).[21]

Significant differences between the etiological mechanisms of CAP and hospital-acquired pneumonia are the additional sources of infection that the hospitalized patient is exposed to in the hospital environment and the organism pool of that specific hospital. With good handwashing among the hospital staff, bacterial monitoring, and infection control, these sources of infection can be reduced.

DIAGNOSIS

The clinical criteria for the diagnosis of hospital-acquired pneumonia are very general and may not be very helpful.[12,21] There are problems with using common criteria in diagnosing HAP pneumonia, especially in the ventilator patient. The chest X-ray is an insensitive tool, and it may show no changes even in the presence of infection. If an infiltrate is present, its pattern is not pathogen specific, and organism recovery and culture are needed. In addition, the presence of sputum or a change in its quantity or quality is also deceiving. Purulent sputum may be present with or without pneumonia. The upper airway sinusitis may be the source of the secretions. Other criteria, such as fever, leukocytosis, and immunoglobulin elevation, may also not be present in the patient with HAP. Many patients who are at risk for hospital-acquired pneumonia are immunosuppressed, and the immune system may not respond appropriately to the presence of infection.[12,21]

Bronchoalveolar lavage is the recommended way to obtain respiratory specimens and identify potential pathogens and to provide a guide to therapy. Fiberoptic bronchoscopy is a common diagnostic device that provides access to distal airways. Using a protected brush-sampling catheter or performing a bronchoalveolar lavage (BAL) or mini-BAL to obtain lung washings can recover uncontaminated specimens for culture. Uncontaminated specimens are necessary for proof of pneumonia and for determining which antimicrobial will be the most effective for treatment.

These distal airway–sampling techniques have limitations when used in the patient with a suspected hospital-acquired infection. The *protected specimen brush (PBS) catheter* has eliminated the problem of upper airway contamination of the sample, but the patient's current antimicrobial therapy reduces the diagnostic yield of organisms. False negatives are a big problem using this technique. *Bronchoalveolar lavage* is a diagnostic bronchoscopic procedure involving infusion of diluent or washing a lung segment and then aspirating and recovering the fluid for culture. A protected BAL catheter device is available. Normally, this technique involves lavaging the lung with approximately 20 mL of diluent, but a smaller lavage sample may be used with as little as 10 mL of diluent. The smaller lavage technique is termed a *mini-BAL*. When comparing the BAL and PSB in diagnosing pneumonia, researchers found that BAL was more accurate in diagnosing hospital-acquired pneumonia but that PSB was the more specific in diagnosing pneumonia.[5,22] "A positive BAL culture has a relatively low sensitivity (66%) but high specificity (90%) for a diagnosis of pneumonia. This means that a negative PSB culture does not exclude the presence of pneumonia, but a positive PSB culture confirms its presence with 90% accuracy."[23]

Treatment. When treating a newly admitted patient with community-acquired pneumonia, the physician should start an empirically determined antimicrobial immediately, with or without the organism identified. The antibiotic regimen should include agents that are in a different antibiotic class than what the patient had received previously.[5] Starting antimicrobial therapy very early reduces the likelihood that the infection will be fatal, providing the therapy is adequate. The treatment associated with the greatest patient survival is starting very early with the correct empiric antimicrobial therapy—possibly with a simple Gram stain coupled with patient signs and symptoms and knowledge of patient history and clinical course.[24]

- If the Gram stain indicates a great number of gram-negative bacilli with a likely *Pseudomonas* pneumonia, the patient is treated with combination therapy to cover the pseudomonas.
- If the infection is thought to be gram-positive cocci, the assumption is an infection with *Streptococcus pneumoniae* or *Staphylococcus aureus*.[23] Since there is a greater risk for MRSA infection or penicillin-resistant streptococci, vancomycin is preferred.
- The presence of mixed flora with no predominance on the Gram stain may indicate an anaerobic infection or a **polymicrobial** aerobic infection (by more than one species). This must be treated by a carbapenem such as imipenim, with a possible addition of an antipseudomonal antibiotic.[16]

Many patients with hospital-acquired pneumonia, ventilator-associated pneumonia, or health-care-associated pneumonia are infected with multi-drug-resistant microorganisms.[5] The American Thoracic Society has identified four principles of antibiotic management:

- Avoid untreated or inadequately treated HAP, VAP, or HCAP, because the failure to initiate prompt appropriate and adequate therapy has been a consistent factor associated with increased mortality.
- Recognize the variability of bacteriology from one hospital to another, specific sites within the hospital, and from one time period to another, and use this information to alter the selection of an appropriate antibiotic treatment regimen for any specific clinical setting.
- Avoid the overuse of antibiotics by focusing on accurate diagnosis, tailoring therapy to the results of lower respiratory tract cultures, and shortening duration of therapy to the minimal effective period.
- Apply preventative strategies aimed at modifiable risk factors.[5]

CASE STUDY 8-1

Hans Shultz is a 68-year-old male who lives in an assisted living facility and who has multiple hospital admissions for exacerbation of COPD. Prior to admission, he experienced two days of increasing dyspnea and cough. He complained of chills, fever, and body aches, and he was coughing grayish mucus. Mr. Shultz was admitted to the hospital and was taken to the pulmonary ICU.

The following laboratory studies and admitting clinical findings were obtained in the hospital's emergency department during initial evaluation and treatment.

Physical Exam:
Mr. Shultz is a cachetic (physical wasting with loss of weight and muscle mass due to disease), white male in obvious respiratory distress. He is using his accessory muscles to breathe and cannot lie flat.

Vital Signs: HR 116 beats/min, RR 23, BP—130/86 mm Hg, Temperature 38.3°C, SpO_2 85% on 2 liters nasal cannula. The oxygen liter flow rate was increased to 4 L/min.

Sensorium: Lethargic but arousable

Respiratory System: He states that he needs two pillows to sleep (he cannot lie flat). He has distant breath sounds with inspiratory and expiratory wheezing and crackles present in the right chest, especially in the middle lobe. He has slight end-expiratory wheeze in both bases.

Extremities: 2+ pitting edema

HEENT: Jugular venous distention

Laboratory Results:
CXR: Hyperlucent lung fields with infiltrates present in right middle and upper lobes, flat diaphragm with blunting of the costophrenic angle on the right, increased bronchial markings. Chest film from 3 months previously also had a lateral chest film available for review. The lateral chest film showed increased AP diameter and a large retrosternal airspace. Prominent pulmonary arteries were present.

ABG pH 7.28, $PaCO_2$ 66 mm Hg, PaO_2 58 on 4 L/min. nasal cannula

Hb. 13 g., Hct. 42%, WBC 13,000 mm^3

Questions

1. What information in this case is consistent with health-care-associated bacterial pneumonia?
2. What risk factor does this patient have for bacterial pneumonia?
3. What complications of COPD and bacterial pneumonia is this patient manifesting?

CASE STUDY 8-2

Mary Beth Allen is a 35-year-old Caucasian female with a history of multiple sclerosis and immune deficiency who presents to the hospital emergency department with worsening cough and increasing shortness of breath. The patient was hospitalized 4 weeks ago with *H. influenza* pneumonia, and she has been hospitalized 3 times in the last 12 months for health-care-associated pneumonia (HCAP) (MRSA × 1). Patient states she has experienced increased dyspnea over last 24 hours with cough production of brown "nasty" nonbloody sputum. She is still working as a nurse and "everyone has been sick" at home.

Social History:
Patient smokes a half a pack/day of cigarettes. She works as a nurse at a local hospital, and she has been taking care of patients with worsening pneumonia.

Vital Signs:
RR 16/min, HR 63, BP 147/80
Height 172 cm, Weight 83.1 kg
Chest X-ray results: Bilateral lower lobe pneumonia
Auscultation: Right upper, middle, and lower lobe have diminished breath sounds
Left upper lobe and left lower lobe show crackles
ABG
pH 7.55, $PaCO_2$ 20 mm Hg, PaO_2 68 mm Hg BE 3.5, HCO_3 17.2 mmol/dL on 2 L/min nasal cannula

Lab Chemistry:ds
Hb 11.2 gm/dL, Hct. 33.4%, RBC 4.0 m/uL, WBC 10.4 k/uL, Platelets 283 k/uL
Na^+ 132 mmol/dL, K^+ 2.7 mmol/dL Cl^- 106 mmol/dL BUN 6 mg/dL Creatinine 0.9 mg/dL, Lactic acid 2.4 mmol/L

3/11/11: Patient was admitted through the emergency department and transferred to the general medicine floors. The next morning she developed respiratory distress. The rapid response team was activated, they stablilized her, and a blood gas was drawn. It revealed a pH 7.35, $PaCO_2$ 39 mm Hg, PaO_2 36 mm Hg BE 4.1, HCO_3 21.1 mmol/dL on a nonrebreathing mask. She was then transferred to the Medicine ICU where they performed a bronchoscopy and a bronchial alveolar lavage (BAL). The BAL was negative for malignant cells. The Grocott stain was negative for pneumocystis and other fungal organisms. Bronchial wash fluid revealed the majority of cells were T cells with low CD4:CD8 ratio, which can be seen in a variety of lung diseases. The CXR showed bilateral subhilar infiltrates extending toward the lung bases consistent with pneumonia.

Medications:
Respiratory medications: Fluticasone/Salmeterol inhaler (500/50) and an Albuterol MDI
Nonrespiratory medications: Levofloxacin, Pipercillin/Tazobactam, Vancomycin, Enoxaparin injection, Fluoxetine, Interferon B-1A, Oxycodone/ Acetaminophen, Modafinil

Critical Thinking Questions

1. What risk factors does this patient have for health-care-associated pneumonia?
2. Why were ER staffers checking for malignancy and fungal infections?
3. What bacterial organisms are possible causes for her pneumonia?

Mycobacterium Infections

Several diseases are caused by organisms in the *Mycobacterium* genus, but the most common is tuberculosis (TB). Tuberculosis is a significant health problem throughout the world. Nontuberculous mycobacterial infections are more prevalent in immunocompromised patients, such as people who have HIV infections, although they may appear in patients with normal immune function. "HIV infection is the greatest single medical risk factor because cell-mediated immunity, which is impaired by HIV, is essential for defense against TB."[25]

MYCOBACTERIUM TUBERCULOSIS INFECTION AND DISEASE

In the year 2000, the World Health Organization estimated that nearly 2 billion people, or about a third of the world's population, had latent TB infection. This huge number of people could develop an active disease in their lifetime. Tuberculosis kills more adolescents and adults than any other infectious disease. The greatest proportions of people infected with tuberculosis are in developing countries, and the spread of tuberculosis is increasing. Many key determinants of health are outside the control of health

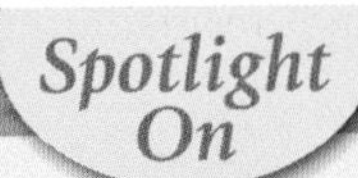

Tuberculosis and HIV Infection

The role that HIV infection has in tuberculosis is considerable. In 2006, there were an estimated 710,000 HIV-positive TB patients globally. Approximately 85% of them live in sub-Saharan Africa. The World Health Organization estimated that about 10.9 million people were coinfected with HIV and *M. tuberculosis* and have up to 15% risk of developing TB every year. The largest population infected with both organisms lives in sub-Saharan Africa, but South-east Asia also has a high incidence of this double infection. *Mycobacterium tuberculosis* is the leading killer in the HIV-positive population and is responsible for more than 50% of AIDS-related deaths.

From World Health Organization, "Tuberculosis," Fact Sheet 104 (November 2010). http://www.who.int/mediacentre/factsheets/fs104/en/index.html

officials and physicians (e.g., sanitation and water supply, education, trade, and environmental and climate change). The governments of many developing countries lack the resources to significantly change these risk factors.[26]

ETIOLOGY AND PATHOGENESIS

Mycobacterium tuberculosis is a nonmotile, non-spore-forming, aerobic, acid-fast bacillus. Unlike infections by the other mycobacterial organisms, *M. tuberculosis* infection is transmissible from person to person by way of inhalation of organisms suspended in aerosolized drops of saliva, respiratory secretions, or other body fluids. The infected person's coughing, sneezing, or talking suspends the organism in the air. There are other means of transmission:

- Ingestion of nonpasteurized milk from infected cattle
- Lab accidents causing direct inoculation through the skin
- Inhalation through contaminated fluids or materials (urine, feces, and sinus drainage).

However, touching inanimate objects such as eating utensils or clothing cannot transmit tuberculosis.[27]

Once the organism is inhaled, it is preferentially transmitted to the bases of the lungs, usually in only one site. When the infectious particle reaches the alveoli, it may be ingested by a macrophage. Its survival depends on the virulence of the organism and the killing ability of the macrophage. If it survives inside the macrophage, the organism may multiply slowly and eventually kill the macrophage. Inflammatory cells are attracted to the area and cause a tubercle and sometimes pneumonitis.

The organisms, now in greater numbers, spread in the lung and to distant body organs by way of the lymph system and the bloodstream. When the organisms reach areas of high oxygen partial pressures (the apices of lungs, kidneys, brain, long bones, vertebral bodies), further multiplication occurs. It takes 8 to 12 weeks for the immune system to process the organism and "recognize" it as foreign and nonself before the body's *cell-mediated immune* (*CMI*) *system* focuses on the organism.[25,27]

The activation of the CMI system activates macrophages to ingest and kill the organisms and directs T lymphocytes (killer T cells) to the bacillis, where they release lymphokines and other chemical killers. The CMI system contains the organisms and controls the spread of infection by walling off the organisms with a granuloma. A *granuloma* is the result of directed immunological cellular activity characterized by the presence of organized white blood cells (e.g., lymphocytes, macrophages) and capillaries that surround the organisms. In some of the granulomas, tissue necrosis occurs, producing a cheese-like material, in a process called **caseous necrosis**. The necrotic core of the granuloma contains latent live tuberculous bacteria. The initial pulmonary lesion of tuberculosis consists of a caseating granuloma and the adjacent enlarged hilar lymph node. The granuloma will calcify in time. Fibrosis and calcification of the layers of the granuloma frequently occur, seen as an isolated calcified density, called a **Ghon complex**, on the chest radiograph in the middle or lower lung zones. The term **Ranke complex** describes the lesion that includes the Ghon complex and the patient's calcified hilar lymph nodes.[25,27]

The other change secondary to activation of the CMI system is that the infected individual's TB skin test will convert from negative to positive.[25,27] The skin test conversion indicates that the immune system has an immunological memory of a previous infection with the *M. tuberculosis* organism. When re-exposed to the tuberculin protein in a TB skin test, the immune system shows a tissue reaction on the skin. The entire process of initial infection with the organism and the body's response is called **primary infection tuberculosis.** Many people with primary infection tuberculosis are asymptomatic and are unaware of the infection. If the initial primary infection occurs in someone who is immunosuppressed, the CMI system does not respond appropriately, and the infection progresses. Granuloma do not form, and *M. tuberculosis* spreads throughout the lungs and to other areas of the body.[25,27]

Three to five percent of people with a history of *M. tuberculosis* infection develop the disease tuberculosis within 1 year of initial infection. The occurrence represents poor immunological control of the infection. Other at-risk populations for progression from primary infection to tuberculosis disease are diabetics, cancer patients, and people who are HIV positive or poorly nourished or who have other causes of immunosuppression. Any decrease in immune function allows granulomata to break down, and *M. tuberculosis* organisms escape, causing disease activation. This condition is called postprimary tuberculosis, or **reactivation tuberculosis**. The lung areas frequently affected in postprimary tuberculosis are the apical and posterior segments of the upper lobe. Fifteen percent of the patients also have extrapulmonary disease. In this form of tuberculosis, active granulomata form, but, because immune function is reduced, it breaks down and continues to allow organisms to escape.[25,27]

Tuberculosis disease, if not controlled with drug therapy, causes lung necrosis, cavity formation, lung distortion, and fibrosis. Another form of tuberculosis is disseminated tuberculosis, known as **miliary tuberculosis**. It occurs when a tuberculous lesion erodes into a blood vessel and a large innoculum of organisms is disseminated throughout the body. It creates millions of metastatic tuberculous lesions 2–3 mm in diameter. The condition was named miliary because the lesions resemble millet seeds on an X-ray. The classic chest radiograph of miliary tuberculosis shows seeding of the lung with soft nodules approximately 2 mm in diameter. Other body organs are also seeded with infection and develop small abscess pockets. This fulminant spread of infection throughout the body can be rapidly fatal. The most vulnerable population groups to this type of infection are the elderly, newborns, children, and people with AIDS.[27]

PATHOPHYSIOLOGY

The changes in pulmonary function in people with active tuberculosis show a restrictive pattern (i.e., decreased lung volume) late in the disease. Because tuberculosis is equally unsparing of both the alveoli and the pulmonary blood vessels, the person's ventilation/perfusion relationship remains balanced, and hypoxemia and hypercarbia are infrequent.[27]

HISTORY AND CLINICAL MANIFESTATIONS

Health history is important in providing diagnostic clues, possibly giving the physician vital information necessary to make an accurate diagnosis.[28] The risk factors for infection are:

- Age.
- Prior TB or a positive TB skin test.
- Country or region of birth and residence.
- Exposure history.
- Recent travel.
- Socioeconomic status.

The risk factors for postprimary TB are:

- HIV-positive status.
- Silicosis.
- Immunosuppression secondary to disease.
- Drugs.
- Medical therapy.
- Lifestyle.

The clinical signs and symptoms that suggest pulmonary tuberculosis are:

- Respiratory symptoms (cough for longer than 3 weeks, hemoptysis, chest pain, and dyspnea).
- Constitutional symptoms (fever of unknown origin, fatigue, night sweats, and weight loss).[25,27]

DIAGNOSIS

Various tests can be performed to help in the diagnosis of tuberculosis. The *chest X-ray* and the *tuberculin skin test* are the initial screening tests and are good preliminary indicators of individuals who actually have the disease. If the results from these tests create a high index of suspicion that the patient has tuberculosis, then the procedures for organism recovery and sputum smear cultures are performed. With the help of these radiological and laboratory tests, a diagnosis of tuberculosis infection and disease can be made.[25,27]

Chest Radiograph. The *chest radiograph* is one of the most common diagnostic procedures used in the initial medical screening of a patient with suspected tuberculosis infection. If the patient has chest X-ray changes consistent with tuberculosis, then additional confirmatory testing is indicated. Computed tomography (CT) offers better imaging of possible cavities and is more accurate in locating lung involvement than is a regular chest X-ray.

In primary TB, the chest X-ray shows the mid- and lower lung zone, with or without nodular infiltrates, in the hilar adenopathy. The chest X-ray of an immunocompetent patient with postprimary tuberculosis shows upper lobe infiltrates (apical and posterior segments) with or without cavity formation. That of an HIV-positive or immunosuppressed patient shows hilar adenopathy, pleural effusion, and infiltrates in either the upper or lower lung zone.

Skin Testing. *Skin testing* (*Mantoux test*) is an important diagnostic tool to identify people with prior primary tuberculosis or asymptomatic active infection. A person infected with *M. tuberculosis* shows a characteristic reddened induration when tuberculin protein (PPD) is intradermally injected. This skin reaction is a **delayed hypersensitivity reaction** that is the result of the individual's T cells having been sensitized to the tuberculosis organism in a previous exposure. Five tuberculin units (TU), or 0.1, mL is injected intradermally. The diameter of the induration is read at 48–72 hours.[28]

- ≥20-mm induration indicates infection.
- 15-mm induration is positive if the patient is from a geographic area where nontuberculous mycobacterial infections are common.
- ≥10-mm induration is a positive test in U.S. regions where nontuberculous mycobacterial infections are uncommon.
- ≥5-mm induration is suspicious in HIV-positive or immunosuppressed individuals or in those in close contact with a person who has active TB.

False negative rates may be as high as 25%, and false positives are also common.

Sputum Testing. The actual percentage of people in the United States with active tuberculosis is small. However, patients with an unknown history of tuberculosis exposure who have a positive skin test must have their sputum tested for the presence of infection. Consequently, the steps involved in testing the sputum for mycobacterium are important for physicians, nurses, and respiratory therapists to know.[25,27]

Mycobacterial Culture. Does a sputum specimen that stains positive for the presence of acid-fast bacilli (AFB) represent active tuberculosis or colonization by nontuberculous mycobacterium? To diagnose the patient correctly, the clinician must culture the sputum smear. An egg- or agar-based medium could be used. Culturing is a slow process, taking from 3 to 8 weeks. A recently introduced automated culture system using carbon-14 as a liquid culture medium has reduced this time to 1–3 weeks.[26]

> *Best Practice*
>
> **Sputum Testing**
>
> - Morning sputum samples are taken or sputum is induced with warm saline for 3 consecutive days.
> - If sputum samples are negative or sputum could not be obtained, fiberoptic bronchoscopy (protected brush, BAL, or transbronchial biopsy specimens) is employed.
> - For children who cannot cooperate with sputum induction, an early morning gastric aspirate can be successful.

Direct Recognition of *Mycobacterium* Species. Rapid direct tests that detect *M. tuberculosis* nucleic acid are more desirable than the slow, expensive, and sometimes insensitive sputum cultures. For the patient who has a positive sputum smear, the *DNA probe* and the *polymerase chain reaction* (*PCR*) are direct tests of the sputum that give a faster confirmation than the traditional sputum culture and are very sensitive and specific.[29]

Under evaluation and not clinically available for rapid detection of TB are monoclonal antibodies, ELISA, radioimmunoassay, and dot-blot immunoassays.[28,30]

RESPIRATORY ISOLATION REQUIREMENTS

In the patient with unconfirmed suspected TB, all the risk factors for infection and disease progression are identified. The patient's clinical presentation, the chest radiograph findings, and the risk factors are carefully examined. If the patient information is suggestive of active tuberculosis, then respiratory isolation should be initiated pending the sputum smear results. The respiratory isolation recommendation can be communicated to the Public Health Services' TB control office, and the patient can be managed on an outpatient basis. Hospitalization is recommended only if the patient is acutely ill, if noncompliance is likely (due to alcoholism or past history of noncompliance), or if the home environment or social situation is unstable.[25,28]

TUBERCULOSIS RESISTANCE

Multi-drug-resistant tuberculosis (*MDR TB*) is defined as resistance to more than one antituberculosis drug. This label mainly refers to the two most common TB drugs—isoniazid and rifampin. *Extensively drug-resistant tuberculosis* (*XDR TB*) is defined as "resistance to at least isoniazid and rifampin among first line anti-tubercular drugs, resistance to any fluoroquinolone, and resistance to at least one second-line injectable drug (amikacin, capreomycin, or kanamycin)."[31] In 2006, the U.S. National TB Surveillance System (NTSS) published that 49 TB cases reported between 1993 and 2004 were XDR-TB. The NTSS found that the cases from the years 2000–2006 were likely to be foreign born and less likely to be persons with HIV infection. Drug resistance in the United States varies demographically and geographically. *Mycobacterium tuberculosis* resistance is common in dense population centers with large concentrations of people with HIV-positive disease or foreign-born Hispanic, Asian-Pacific Islanders, or

CASE STUDY 8-3

Ronald Carlyle recently discovered that he was HIV positive. His physician was performing a complete battery of tests, including chest radiograph, blood chemistry, urinalysis, and skin tests. One of the tests included a TB skin test. Ronald came back to the physician's office to have the skin test site examined. His tuberculin skin reaction was consistent with a positive skin test.

Clinical Manifestations: Fatigue, cough, weight loss of 10 pounds in the last 3 months, and night sweats.

Laboratory Workup:
Chest radiograph: Infiltrates in the upper posterior and apical segments of both upper lobes. The hilar lymph nodes are enlarged.

Laboratory findings: Normal fluid and electrolytes, Helper T cells (CD_4) 660 mm^3, other skin tests normal.

Questions

1. Does this patient have tuberculosis infection or tuberculosis disease? Explain your answer.
2. What is the definition of positive PPD test for an HIV-positive patient?
3. Describe two possible mechanisms that would cause TB disease in Mr. Carlyle.
4. Is a positive sputum test for acid-fast organisms necessary for an initiation of drug therapy for active tuberculosis?

African Americans. There is overlap among the individuals in ethnic groups with the HIV disease group.[25]

TREATMENT

Chemoprophylaxis is a term used to describe the drug treatment for an individual who is asymptomatic, is not shedding organisms in the sputum, and has a positive skin test. This person has a primary tuberculosis infection but not tuberculosis disease. If the person never received antituberculosis drug treatment, then he or she still has live organisms in lung granulomata, but the organisms are in the resting state. The small focus of infection that could potentially reactivate is treated by administration of a single drug to kill the still present occult infection. The drug needs to be taken over several months because of the slow **doubling time** (the time it takes to double in number) of the organisms in the resting state.[25]

Drug treatment (see Table 8-3) should be initiated as soon as an adequate sputum specimen is obtained and saved for culture.[25] With a negative smear and a high likelihood of infection, empiric therapy should be considered pending culture results. However, the presence of a negative smear may indicate that the patient is not highly infectious.

There are specific indications for antitubercular drug treatment in the patient with intact immune function who has a positive skin test. Individuals in this category include persons who:

- Recently developed a positive skin test.
- Have an unknown exposure history.
- Have known exposure to someone who has isoniazid-sensitive tuberculosis.
- Have known exposure to someone who has isoniazid-resistant tuberculosis.
- Have known exposure to MDR-TB.[28]

There are specific indications for antitubercular drug treatment in the patient who is HIV-positive. Individuals in this category are persons who:

- Currently have a positive skin test or a documented history of a positive skin test without known exposure to drug-resistant organisms.
- Are **anergic** (have diminished hypersensitivity) and a known exposure to drug-sensitive TB.
- Have a positive skin test and a known exposure to someone with isoniazid-resistant tuberculosis.
- Have a known exposure to MDR-TB and a high likelihood of infection (recent skin test converter or anergic to skin tests).[28]

The drug treatment for tuberculosis disease has varying schedules based on the individual's drug sensitivity, immune state, social and economic circumstances, and treatment compliance history. Antituberculosis drugs can be toxic, and some patients may not be able to tolerate certain medications. These patients will require drug substitutions and possibly longer treatment schedules.[28]

Nontuberculous *Mycobacterium* Infections

These organisms can be referred to in several ways: nontuberculous mycobacteria (NTM), atypical mycobacteria, and mycobacteria other than tuberculosis (MOTT).[25,31] This chapter will refer to infections with these organisms as NTM.

TABLE 8-3 **Treatment for acid-fast bacilli infection**

Acid-Fast Microorganism	Never Treated Give First Line Drugs	Multi-Drug Resistant	Specialized Treatment
Mycobacterium tuberculosis	**First 2 months** Isoniazid (INH) Rifampin (RMP) Pyrazinamide (PZA) Ethambutol (EMB) Stop EMB and PZA after 2 mos. **Additional 4 mos of INH + RMP** Neg. sputum, cultures and CXR **OR** Pos. sputum, cultures and neg. CXR **Additional 7 mos of INH + RMP** Pos. sputum, cultures and pulmonary cavities on CXR	**Treat 18–24 mos** Use remaining first line drugs (PZA, Streptomycin) **PLUS** Fluoroquinolone antibiotics **AND** Other Aminoglycoside antibiotics if resistant to streptomycin **Alternative Drugs** Levofloxacin/Ofloxacin/ Ciprofloxacin; Cycloserine; Capreomycin or Ethionamide; Clofazamine; Aminosalicylic Acid	**Extensively Drug Resistant** 3 drugs in order of preference: Capreomycin, PZA, Ethionamide, Cycloserine, Clofazimine, Fluoroquinolone e.g. Ofloxacin/ Levafloxacin; Aminoglycoside e.g. Kanamycin, Amikacin **INH resistant** RMP + EMB + PZA **HIV+** – same as conventional drug treatment but administer 3 mos. longer **Pregnant women** – same as conventional drug treatment but exclude PZA and Streptomycin
Mycobacterium kansasii	**Pos sputum and cultures and CXR** INH + RMP ± EMB or Aminoglycoside antibiotic Streptomycin	**Not common**	**Drug resistant** Not specified. Treatment based on susceptability testing.
Mycobacterium avium complex	**Treat 12–18 mos. or cultures neg for 12 mos.** Macrolide antibiotics Clarithromycin/Azithromycin PLUS ≥ 1 of the following: EMB, Fluoroquinolone antibiotic Ciprofloxacin, and/ or Rifabutin	**Common** Add RMP; Aminoglycoside antibiotic Amikacin	**Prophylaxis Therapy (1 or more)** Macrolide antibiotics: Azithromycin, Clarithromycin; Rifabutin **Disseminated disease in advanced AIDS** Combinations of 4 to 6 drugs that include: Rifabutin, Fluoroquinolone antibiotic Ciprofloxacin, Clofazimine, Aminoglycoside antibiotic Amikacin

These organisms are commonly occurring and have been recovered in many parts of the world and in varied environmental areas (soil, water, dairy products, house dust, animals).[32] The following is a noninclusive list of nontuberculous mycobacterial infections, with some general information about the infection, where exposure to the organisms could occur, and the population usually affected.

- *M. avium* complex: Common in AIDS patients, frequently disseminated throughout the body
- *M. kansasii*: Common in midwestern states; second most common NTM in AIDS patients
- *M. marinum*: Swimming pool granuloma, crustacean bites
- *M. scrofulaceum*: Granulomatous lymph nodes; found more in children than in adults
- *M. fortuitum*: Penetrating skin wounds and foreign body infections (porcine heart valves, breast implants)
- *M. xenopi*: Causes pulmonary disease in humans; water contaminant

In past years some geographic areas had a high incidence of NTM but little reported NTM disease, suggesting an environmental reservoir of infection.

In the United States, scientists report that the appearance of NTM disease appears to be increasing. In recent years, the number of isolates and the diagnosis of clinical disease are increasing. These results are mirrored elsewhere in the world. For example, in France, the incidence of NTM in HIV-negative persons was at one time estimated to be about 0.73 cases per 100,000 population with MAC (*Mycobacterium avium*-complex), *M. xenopi, M. kansasii*, and rapidly growing mycobacteria commonly seen in the isolates (*M. abscessus, M. chelonae, M. fortuitum*). Other than better laboratory diagnostic techniques, additional reasons for this increase in the number of NTM infections are a greater:

- Understanding of the disease.
- Availability of chest CT scanning.
- Number of people who are at risk for NTM (people with compromised immune systems and older adults).

Despite the fact that the organism is common, the medical community does not know the mode of transmission of NTM to humans. However, it is known that the transmission of disease, either from person to person or from animals to people, is not significant. Therefore, people with active NTM do not require respiratory isolation unless the patient also has a transmissible coinfection, such as *M. tuberculosis*.

There are three common presentations of pulmonary NTM in people with normal immunity.

- The first presentation is a tuberculosislike pattern with upper lobe involvement that appears in older men with a history of smoking and COPD.
- The second common presentation is in thin, nonsmoking women with skeletal abnormalities who complain of cough and have nodular bronchiectasis.
- The last occurs in people who develop a hypersensitivity pneumonitis after using a hot tub or a spa.

M. kansasii, M. xenopi, M. malmoense, and rapidly growing mycobacteria are commonly associated with the first two presentations, and MAC is associated with all of them.[32]

People with AIDS have an increased incidence for all of the NTM mycobacterial infections, but MAC is particularly worthy of mention. MAC is one of the AIDS-defining diseases.[27,31,33] It is the third most common opportunistic disease of AIDS patients in the United States, causing lung infection or bacterial colonization and frequently disseminating throughout the body. Up to 50% of HIV-positive individuals will develop disseminated MAC before their death.[33] It is now suggested that prophylaxis drug treatment for MAC be given to all AIDS patients with a CD4 count of $<75/mm^3$ and who have had prior opportunistic infections (see Table 8-3).[31]

Mycobacterium kansasii is the second most common NTM infection in AIDS patients. As is seen in people with MAC disease, it appears in people who are HIV positive late in the clinical course of the disease when the CD4 count is $<100/mm^3$. The disease remains confined to the lung in most cases but can disseminate to the bone marrow, lymph nodes, and skin.[33]

Other diseases—such as COPD, cystic fibrosis, gastroesophageal reflux disease, and chest wall disorders—are all associated with NTM. The exact relationship of these problems with NTM is unknown. However, the conditions could facilitate the development of NTM infection, and the organism's presence could certainly worsen these existing diseases. NTM infection is also a complicating condition in people with bronchiectasis and aspergillus lung disease. Apparently, NTM infection in people with bronchiectasis increases the risk for developing pulmonary aspergillosis. including the invasive form and aspergilloma (fungus balls).[32]

CLINICAL MANIFESTATIONS OF NTM DISEASE

NTM has nonspecific signs and symptoms. It can be a pulmonary infection or a disseminated infection, and the clinical manifestations reflect its origin. In pulmonary NTM, chronic cough with sputum production and fatigue are common but fever and night sweats appear in only 50% or fewer of cases.[32] The chest radiograph may be variable: with or without cavities, bronchiectasis, patchy infiltrates and nodules in the upper lobes, or isolated nodules without infiltrates.[25]

In AIDS patients with MAC infection, since the initial site of infection is thought to be the gastrointestinal (GI) tract, this patient population has GI symptoms (nausea, vomiting, diarrhea, enlarged liver or spleen, weight loss, and anorexia).[32] The infection disseminates to the bone marrow, liver, spleen, and lymph nodes. Since the lung is not directly infected, the lung may have colonies of organisms but not MAC lung disease. If the AIDS patient also has MAC lung disease, the chest radiograph is often normal but may show nodular or non-nodular infiltrates but no cavities.[31–33]

DIAGNOSIS OF NTM DISEASE

Unlike that of tuberculosis, the diagnosis of NTM is not made from simply culturing the organism from the lung. Using the high-resolution CT results with the microbiologic studies is essential for diagnosis.

The presence of organisms could represent colonization but not infection. Diagnosing NTM infection is made according to the following criteria:

- Clinical criteria: Clinical manifestations consistent with NTM, with the exclusion of other possible conditions, such as tuberculosis or cancer
- Imaging: Chest X-ray with infiltrates, nodules, or cavities OR HRCT showing multiple small noncalcified nodules and multiple locations of bronchiectasis with variable presence of cavities
- Bacteriology (any met within 1 year): >2 positive cultures from expectorated sputum; >1 positive culture from BAL or wash; transbronchial or other biopsy showing acid-fast bacillus or granulomatous inflammation[32]

TREATMENT OF NTM

The treatment of NTM in the immunocompetent population is very challenging. Unlike people with tuberculosis, most people with NTM are often resistant to many antimycobacterial drugs (e.g., isoniazid, pyrazinamide). They must be given a regimen of three or four antituberculous drugs (see Table 8-3).[32] For progressive disease, even other drugs might have to be added to this regimen. Consequently, there may be drug interactions or drug toxicity with complications.

Treating MAC pulmonary disease or disseminated MAC in people with AIDS poses even more challenges to the physician than the immunocompetent group. These patients are also receiving medications for their HIV disease, as well as possible prophylactic or definitive treatment for other opportunistic diseases (e.g., *Pneumocystis carinii*). Adding three more drugs to the treatment regimen may be difficult for the patient to tolerate.[19] Drug interactions, toxicity, and patient compliance are issues that must be carefully watched. Unlike MAC, *M. kansasii* responds well to the usual antimycobacterial antibiotics.[31]

Fungal Pulmonary Infections

Fungal pulmonary infections are uncommon in the immunocompetent host. Many fungal infections are classified as opportunistic infections that cause disease in people with depressed immune function (e.g., AIDS, chronic diseases, steroid therapy, cancer drugs). These diseases are in fact so pervasive in the immunosuppressed that the presence of specific fungal infections places the HIV-positive patient in the AIDS category of disease severity.[33]

In immunocompetent people who develop fungal infections, the disease occurs as an acute, benign, self-limiting respiratory infection. Patient history helps reveal the diagnosis with information on recent travels, geographic residence, and immunological function. Several fungal infections cause lung disease that predominate in certain areas of the United States: coccidioidomycosis, histoplasmosis, blastomyocosis.[34] The fungal organism is a normal inhabitant of soil in the specific location, existing in the **mycelium** form (as a mat of long, branching filamentous tubes). The spore breaks off from the fungus and becomes airborne. It is inhaled and deposits in the airways and alveoli. In the warm moist environment of the lung, it undergoes complex biochemical reactions and changes into the yeast form. The pulmonary scavenger macrophages ingest the yeast. The yeast survives and multiplies inside the macrophages. It then spreads throughout the lung and possibly throughout the body by way of the lymphatic and the bloodstream.

The immune response to the infection is in the form of a delayed hypersensitivity reaction mediated by the lymphocytes. This reaction promotes granuloma formation that is similar to the body's response to the mycobacterial organisms.[34] In the immunocompetent host, the organisms disseminate infrequently. If dissemination occurs, the skin and organs, such as the liver, spleen, kidney, bones, brain, and meanings of the brain, could become involved. When the infection is confined to the lung, the disease is usually self-limiting, and the host may be unaware of the infection. If the organism disseminates, the disease becomes chronic and slowly progressive. The person's symptoms are similar to those of tuberculosis (night sweats, fever, anorexia, weight loss) and, once diagnosed, can be treated with antifungal agents.[34]

In the immunosuppressed, the infection is usually subacute or chronic. The person has complaints that are subtle and vague, such as fatigue, weakness, and malaise. In the person with HIV disease, the symptoms manifest as an unexplained worsening. With progression and dissemination, the person could develop acute pneumonia, respiratory failure, and other signs of systemic involvement, such as hypotension and **coagulopathy** (a disorder in the blood's clotting system).[33,34]

COCCIDIOIDOMYCOSIS

Coccidioidomycosis is a fungal disease caused by the organism *Coccidioides immitis*. The organism is found in the soil in the southwestern United States, including the Central Valley of California, Arizona, and parts of New Mexico and western Texas. The area extends into northern Mexico, with some disease cases appearing in Central America and South America.[34,35] Because of its geographic predominance, this disease is also known as San Joaquin Valley Fever or Valley Fever.[35] If the infection disseminates, it affects many body organs and may penetrate into the cerebrospinal fluid and cause meningitis. Untreated disseminated coccidioidomycosis with meningitis is always fatal. Even when treated, fungal meningitis in HIV-positive patients has a very high mortality rate.[34,35]

HISTOPLASMOSIS

Histoplasmosis is a fungal disease caused by the organism *Histoplasma capsulatum*. This infection occurs throughout the world, but in the United States the organism is endemic to the Ohio and Mississippi river valleys, extending into Maryland, southern Pennsylvania, New York, and Texas. The organism is present in soil contaminated by avian droppings (e.g., chickens) and bat droppings. Inhalation of the airborne spores causes acute infection.

The infected individual may be asymptomatic or complain of a flulike illness. If the person inhaled a heavy concentration of spores, the infection could be severe and lead to severe hypoxemia and respiratory failure.[34,36] Chronic lung disease is a complication of chronic histoplasmosis. HIV-positive individuals with disseminated histoplasmosis have a 10% mortality rate.[33]

NORTH AMERICAN BLASTOMYCOSIS

The organism *Blastomyces dermatitidis* causes *North American blastomycosis.* Its geographic distribution is similar to that of *H. capsulatum* but extends farther north into the north-central Midwest, mid-Atlantic states, upstate New York, southern Canada, and the southeastern United States. The organism is contained in soil contaminated with animal excrement and decaying organic material. *Blastomyces dermatitidis* exists in the mycelium form until inhaled into the airway and alveoli, where it converts into yeast.[34,37]

The immunological response is a delayed hypersensitivity reaction that is monocyte derived. Macrophages phagocytize the yeast, and monocytes and giant cells infiltrate the infection site. They cause an inflammatory tissue reaction with granuloma formation and tissue necrosis with subsequent pulmonary fibrosis. Like other fungi, the organism can disseminate and cause bodywide infection and granuloma formation.[34,37] This fungal disease is known for causing skin lesions that abscess and scar. Other frequently affected areas are the bone, thyroid, prostate, epididymis, testes, and kidneys. The disease course is usually slowly progressive, but in some cases it can have a fulminant course. Untreated blastomycosis is fatal. Antifungal drugs are usually effective.[37]

DIAGNOSIS OF PULMONARY FUNGAL INFECTIONS

Serological tests of the patient's immune response may be helpful in diagnosing the fungal infection. Some of the organisms (e.g., *Histoplasma capsulatum* and *Cryptococcus neoformans*) have specific antigenic products that can be detected on blood sera studies. Diagnosis is usually confirmed by isolating the causative organism. Helpful in diagnosing the specific fungal organism are biopsy of skin lesions, cultures of sputum, urine, and blood, and bone marrow samples. Sputum culture alone is insufficient to diagnose actual fungal disease; the patient may have fungal colonization of the lung without infection. The invasiveness of the infection is the true diagnostic determination. To confirm the diagnosis of systemic fungal infection, cultures or biopsy findings from sites other than the lung, clinical evidence of infection, and the other clinical and laboratory findings are necessary.[34]

TREATMENT OF FUNGAL INFECTION AND FUNGAL PNEUMONIA

Drugs used to treat systemic fungal infections include flucytocine, amphotericin B, and others in the azole chemical family (see Table 8-4).[34] Amphotericin B is very nephrotoxic; patients receiving this drug must be monitored for **nephrotoxicity** (a kidney disorder resulting from ingestion of a toxic substance). If patients with normal kidney function at the beginning of therapy have a significant elevation in serum creatinine (3–4.5 mg/dL) or if the blood urea nitrogen (BUN) increases to >50 mg/dL, the dose of amphotericin B should be reduced. Permanent damage to the kidneys could occur. Aerosolized amphotericin B has been used to treat patients with colonization of fungal organisms in the lung. In addition to antifungal drugs, surgery to remove sites of localized infection may be effective in a limited number of cases.[34]

Summary

Infections of the respiratory tract are among the most common infections of the human race. In the United States, respiratory tract infections are responsible for more visits to physicians than any other diseases and for more time lost from work or school.

Viruses, bacteria, fungi, and parasites are organisms that cause infections of the respiratory system. Some of these infections are contagious and may cause serious respiratory disease. Pneumonia, an infection of one or both lungs, is extremely contagious and is the result of breathing in small droplets that get into the air when an infected person coughs or sneezes. Pneumonia can

TABLE 8-4 **Fungal lung disease treatment**

Microorganisms	Drug of First Choice	Alternative Drug Treatment	Specialized Treatment
Aspergillus spp.	**Invasive infections:** IV Amphotericin B ± Flucytosine	Oral Itraconazole	**Unresponsive Infection:** Lipid-associated formulations of Amphotericin B
Blastomyces dermatitidis	Itraconazole	**Mild disease in Itraconazole-intolerant** Fluconazole or Amphotericin B	**Life-threatening infections** Amphotericin B
Candida albicans	**Esophageal candidiasis** Fluconazole **Unresponsive esophageal candidiasis** Voriconazole	Itraconazole Caspofungin	**Invasive infection** Amphotericin B **Disseminated Disease** Voniconzole
Coccidiodes immitis	**Mild/moderate non-meningeal extrapumonary infection** Fluconazole **Severe illness** Amphotericin B	Itraconazole	**AIDS-associated severe disseminated infection:** Amphotericin B initially; maintenance with Itraconazole OR Fluconazole **Unresponsive Infection:** Lipid-associated formulations of Amphotericin B
Cryptococcus neoformans	**Systemic disease without meningitis** Fluconazole **More severe cases** IV Amphotericin B by Fluconazole maintenance in HIV+ patients	Fluconazole, Itraconazole; alternative maintenance (HIV+) Amphotericin B	**AIDS patients** Fluconazole and Flucytosine **AIDS–associated meningits:** Amphotericin B and Flucytosine **HIV$^+$ maintenance** Fluconazole or Itraconazole
Histoplasma capsulatum	Itraconazole	Amphotericin B	**AIDS-associated severe disseminated infection:** Amphotericin B initially; maintenance with Itraconazole

also result when bacteria or viruses from the mouth, throat, or nose inadvertently enter the lungs.

Antibiotics are used to treat pneumonia caused by bacteria, the most common cause of the condition. Pneumonia can also be caused by viruses, such as those that cause influenza (flu) and chickenpox (varicella). Varicella pneumonia, which is rare, can be treated with antiviral medicine.

In most cases pneumonia is a short-term, treatable illness. But frequent bouts of pneumonia can be a serious complication of a long-term (chronic) illness, such as chronic obstructive pulmonary disease (COPD).

M. tuberculosis infection is transmissible from person to person by way of inhalation of organisms suspended in aerosolized drops of saliva, respiratory tract secretions, or other body fluids. If the organisms are able to multiply in the lung, they can spread there and into other organs. Any patient with an evaluation suggestive of active tuberculosis should be placed in respiratory isolation.

Study Questions

REVIEW QUESTIONS

1. Name the common microorganisms that cause community-acquired bacterial pneumonia.
2. Patients in the hospital are at risk for developing hospital-acquired pneumonia due to the fact that most suffer from immunological disorders. Which group of patients is at the most risk for developing hospital-acquired pneumonia?

3. Tuberculosis is a pulmonary disease that is becoming more problematic because of the drug-resistant nature of some of the *mycobacterium.* What are the procedures for a diagnosis of tuberculosis?
4. Name common fungal diseases of the lung and the procedures for the diagnosis of this type of disease.

MULTIPLE-CHOICE QUESTIONS

1. Which of the following organisms is a virus?
   a. Influenza
   b. *Haemophilus influenzae*
   c. *Klebsiella pneumoniae*
   d. *Legionella pneumophila*
2. How long after the Mantoux test must you wait before checking for a tissue reaction?
   a. 8–16 hours
   b. 24–36 hours
   c. 48–72 hours
   d. 96–120 hours
3. What is the drug of choice for *mycobacterium tuberculosis* chemoprophylaxis?
   a. isoniazid
   b. rifampin
   c. pyrazinamide
   d. gentamycin
4. Which of the following nontuberculous mycobacterial organisms causes a common opportunistic infection in AIDS patients?
   a. *Mycobacterium chelonae*
   b. *Mycobacterium kansasii*
   c. *Mycobacterium fortuitum*
   d. *Mycobacterium avium-intracellulare*
5. What fungal infection is endemic to the Ohio and Mississippi river valleys?
   a. coccidioidomycosis
   b. histoplasmosis
   c. cryptococcus
   d. North American blastomycosis
6. What is the recommended antibiotic for MRSA infections?
   a. oxacillin
   b. erythromycin
   c. amikacin
   d. vancomycin
7. What changes in the virus is responsible for causing major epidemics or pandemics?
   a. protein mutation
   b. antigenic drift
   c. antigenic shift
   d. beta-lactamase mutation
8. What community-acquired pneumonia is associated with a high incidence in small communities such as schools, colleges, and military barracks?
   a. *Klebsiella pneumonia*
   b. *Staphylococcus pneumonia*
   c. *Chlamydia pneumonia*
   d. *Mycoplasma pneumonia*
9. What are clinical manifestations of community-acquired pneumonia?
   a. afebrile but acutely ill
   b. change in sputum color
   c. chills, high fever, body aches
   d. diffuse infiltrates on chest X-ray with normal breath sounds
10. What patient is *not* at risk for health-care-associated pneumonia?
    a. a 68-year-old woman living with her daughter
    b. a 10-year-old receiving outpatient chemotherapy for a brain tumor
    c. a 75-year-old man residing in an assisted living facility
    d. a 50-year-old woman going to an outpatient dialysis center 3 times a week

CRITICAL-THINKING QUESTIONS

1. During the acute inflammatory or consolidative stage of pneumonia, appropriate therapy selection would include antibiotics, bed rest, fluids and supplemental oxygen. Why might the use of other modalities be needed during the resolution stage? What other modalities might you include? What would be the rationale for each of the modalities you would add?
2. Why are the Occupational Safety and Health Administration guidelines for care of patients with active tuberculosis more complex than for patients with most other pulmonary infections?
3. Why might the various fungal diseases that impact the pulmonary system have geographical associations?
4. With all of the drug-resistant strains of bacteria being discovered, what could the health care community do to decrease the incidence of this problem?

References

1. Centers for Disease Control and Prevention. FastStats (A to Z). National Center for Health Statistics. "Deaths and Mortality." Cited October 15, 2008. http://www.cdc.gov/nchs/fastats/deaths.htm.

2. Birnbaum HG, Morley M, Greenberg PE, Colice GL. Economic burden of respiratory infections in an employed population. *Chest.* 2002;122(2): 603–611.
3. Birnbaum HG, Morley M, Leong S, Greenberg P, Colice GL. Lower respiratory tract infections: impact on the workplace. *PharmacoEconomics.* 2003;21:749.
4. Venditti M, Falcone M, Corrao S, Licata G, Serra P, Study Group of the Italian Society of Internal Medicine. Outcomes of patients hospitalized with community-acquired, health-care-associated, and hospital-acquired pneumonia. *Ann Intern Med.* 2009;150,1:19–26.
5. Guidelines for the management of adults with hospital-acquired, ventilator-associated, and healthcare-associated pneumonia. *Am. J. Respir. Crit. Care Med.* 2005;171,4:388–416.
6. Bartlett JG. Pneumonia. In: Beers M, et al, eds. *The Merck Manual of Diagnosis and Therapy.* Whitehouse Station, NJ: Merck Research Laboratories; 2006:423–437.
7. Huchon G, Roche N. Infectious diseases. In: Albert R, Spiro S, Jett J, eds. *Comprehensive Respiratory Medicine.* St. Louis: Mosby: 1999:20. 1–10, 21, 1–4, 22. 1–4, 23, 1–8.
8. Soto FJ, Varkey B. (2003) Evidence-based approach to acute exacerbations of COPD. *Curr Opin Pulm Med.* 2003;9:117–124.
9. Centers for Disease Control and Prevention. *Prevention and Control of Influenza: Recommendations of the Advisory Committee on Immunization Practices (ACIP).* MMWR: 2008;1–60.
10. Kolata G. The plague year. In: *"Flu" The Story of the Great Influenza Pandemic of 1918 and the Search for the Virus That Caused It.* New York: Simon & Schuster; 2001:2.
11. Centers for Disease Control and Prevention. *Avian Influenza: A Virus Infection in Humans.* Atlanta: CDC, 2008.
12. Corrin B. Viral, mycoplasmal and rickettsial infections. In: Corrin B, ed. *Pathology of the Lungs.* London: Harcourt Publishers Limited; 2000: 137–158.
13. Centers for Disease Control and Prevention. Interim antiviral guidance for 2008–2009. *Seasonal Flu 2008–2009.* February 11, 2009.
14. Rubin FH. Immunizations. In: Beers M, et al, eds. *The Merck Manual of Diagnosis and Therapy.* Whitehouse Station, NJ: Merck Research Laboratories, 2006:1399–1406.
15. Turner RB. Respiratory viruses. In: Beers M, et al, eds. *The Merck Manual of Diagnosis and Therapy.* Whitehouse Station, NJ: Merck Research Laboratories, 2006:1593–1603.
16. Marino PL. Nosocomial pneumonia. In: *The ICU Book.* Baltimore: Williams & Wilkins; 1998: 516–530.
17. Corrin B. Acute bacterial pneumonia. In: *Pathology of the Lung.* London: Churchill Livingstone; 2000:157–175.
18. Wessolossky MA, Daly J. Clinical considerations in gram-positive infections. In: Gates, RH, ed. *Infectious Disease Secrets.* Philadelphia: Hanley and Belfus, 1998:117–124.
19. Zacher LL. Community-acquired pneumonia: public enemy no.1. In: Gates, RH, ed. *Infectious Disease Secrets.* Philadelphia: Hanley and Belfus, 1998:268–272.
20. Centers for Disease Control and Prevention. *"Chlamydia pneumoniae."* Available from: http://www.cdc.gov/ncidod/dbmd/diseaseinfo/chlamydiapneumonia_t.htm.
21. Douglass J, O'Hehir RE. What determines asthma phenotype? Respiratory infections and asthma. *Am. J. Respir. Crit. Care Med.* 2000;161,3:S211–S214.
22. Torres A, El-Ebiary M. Bronchoscopic BAL in the diagnosis of ventilator-associated pneumonia. *Chest.* 2000;117(4 suppl 2): 198S–202S.
23. Marino PL. *Pneumonia in the ICU,* in *The ICU Book.* Philadelphia: Lippincott Williams & Wilkins; 2007:749–767.
24. Luna CM, Vujacich P, Niederman MS, Vay C, Gherardi G, Matera J, et al. Impact of BAL data on the therapy and outcome of ventilator-associated pneumonia. *Chest.* 1997;111,3:676–685.
25. Nardell EA. Mycobacteria. In: Beers M, et al, eds. *The Merck Manual of Diagnosis and Therapy.* Whitehouse Station, NJ: Merck Research Laboratories, 2006:1508–1522.
26. World Health Organization. "Tuberculosis." Fact sheet N 104 (November 2010). http://www.who.int/mediacentre/factsheets/fs104/en/index.html.
27. Broughton W, Bass J. Infectious disease: tuberculosis and diseases caused by atypical mycobacteria. In: Albert RK, Spiro SG, Jett JR, eds. *Comprehensive Respiratory Medicine.* St. Louis: Mosby; 1999:5.29. 1–5. 16.
28. Hammer J, Cohn D. The white plague revisited. In: Gates, RH, ed. *Infectious Disease Secrets.* Philadelphia: Hanley and Belfus, 1998:129–136.
29. Forbes B, Sahm D, Weissfeld A. Molecular methods for microbial identification and characteristics. In: *Bailey and Scott's Diagnostic Microbiology.* St. Louis: Mosby; 1998:188–207.
30. Gomez-Pastrana D, Torronteras R, Caro P, Anguita ML, López Barrio AM, Andrés A, et al. Diagnosis of tuberculosis in children using a polymerase chain reaction. *Pediatric Pulmonology.* 1999;28,5:344–351.

31. Karlin, N., *Mycobacteria other than tuberculosis*. In: Gates, RH, ed. *Infectious Disease Secrets*. Philadelphia: Hanley and Belfus, 1998:137–140.
32. Glassroth J. Pulmonary disease due to nontuberculous mycobacteria. *Chest.* 2008;133,1:243–251.
33. Miller RF, Lipman MCI. AIDS and the lung: pulmonary infections. In: Albert RK, Spiro SG, Jett JR, eds. *Comprehensive Respiratory Medicine*. St. Louis: Mosby; 1999:32, 1–32, 22.
34. Edwards, J.E., *Fungi*. In: Beers M, et al, eds. *The Merck Manual of Diagnosis and Therapy*. Whitehouse Station, NJ: Merck Research Laboratories, 2006:1523–1537.
35. Dooley D. Coccidioidomycosis. In: Gates, RH, ed. *Infectious Disease Secrets*. Philadelphia: Hanley and Belfus, 1998:146–152.
36. Dommaraju C, Everett E. Histoplasmosis. In: Gates, RH, ed. *Infectious Disease Secrets*. Philadelphia: Hanley and Belfus, 1998:156–158.
37. Dommaraju C, Everett E. North American blastomyocosis. In: Gates, RH, ed. *Infectious Disease Secrets*. Philadelphia: Hanley and Belfus, 1998:156–158.

CHAPTER 9

Airflow Limitation Diseases

Barbara Ludwig

OBJECTIVES

Upon completion of this chapter, the reader should be able to:

- Describe the difference between chronic bronchitis and emphysema.
- Describe the pharmacologic treatment of airflow limitation and compare the recommended drug therapy treatment of asthma to that of COPD.
- Describe the differences between COPD and asthma.
- Describe the clinical categories of asthma.
- Compare the clinical presentation of a patient with emphysema to that of a patient with asthma.
- Describe the different causes of bronchiectasis.
- Identify the bacteria commonly found in patients with chronic bronchitis and bronchiectasis.

CHAPTER OUTLINE

KEY TERMS

asthma
atopy
centriacinar emphysema
direct costs
indirect costs
panacinar emphysema
paraseptal emphysema
vagal tone

The primary airflow limitation diseases discussed in this chapter are asthma, bronchiectasis, chronic bronchitis, and emphysema.[1] *Asthma* is in a separate category of airflow limitation because it is a reversible disease that responds to bronchodilator therapy. Bronchiectasis, chronic bronchitis, and emphysema are known by the acronym *COPD* (*chronic obstructive pulmonary disease*). The airway obstruction in these diseases is not reversed by bronchodilators, and the diseases result in permanent and progressive changes. See Table 9-1 for the differences among these four disease states.

Asthma

Asthma is a chronic inflammatory disorder of the airways in which many immunological cells play a role. The predominant cellular elements are mast cells, T lymphocytes, eosinophils, macrophages, and neutrophils. In people who are susceptible to this disease, the inflammation causes recurrent episodes of wheezing, dyspnea, chest tightness, and coughing. The airflow obstruction may reverse spontaneously, or it may require treatment for reversal.

Asthma has several key characteristics. When these characteristics are committed to memory, the asthmatic patient's signs, symptoms, and treatment are easier to understand:[2]

- Chronic inflammatory disorder
- Recurrent episodes of breathing difficulties
- Characterized by airflow limitation
- Reversible

DEMOGRAPHICS AND STATISTICS

Asthma is the most common chronic childhood disease. It affects 22 million people, including approximately 6.5 million children.[2,3] The most recent statistics (2007) from the Centers for Disease Control and Prevention estimated that people with asthma account for approximately 444,000 hospitalizations annually with an average length of stay of 3.2 days. The inpatient hospital services are the largest single direct cost of asthma, at an estimated $1 billion per year. The indirect costs of asthma are related to a loss of school days, workdays, productivity, and productive years secondary to premature death. In 1998, the indirect cost of asthma was projected at $5.33 billion per year.[4] This includes family loss of income and productivity when parents stay home to take care of their asthmatic child. In 1999, over 5000 deaths were attributed to asthma, with most of the deaths in the 65-year-and-over age bracket.[3,4]

ATOPIC AND NONATOPIC ASTHMA

Asthma is classified as a chronic inflammatory disease. The inflammation is a consequence of the effects of activated inflammatory cells. This immune system response is classified as a *type 1 hypersensitivity reaction*, which is characterized by an IgE antibody–mediated inflammatory response. The immune reaction is initiated by exposure to an antigen protein to which that individual is sensitive; this sensitivity is called **atopy**. After birth, the mature immune system develops immunological tolerance. Atopic people's immune systems are intolerant of certain antigens, and they respond excessively to exposure to those antigens.[2,5] It is thought that atopy is a familial tendency, and it is considered the strongest predisposing factor for developing asthma.[6,7]

An individual with atopy has elevated IgE in the serum that has formed against specific antigens (allergens). The patient also has a positive skin test against the offending allergens. Many environmental substances are potential allergens or triggers (e.g., house dust mites, cats, pollen, and fungi), and each atopic person has a distinct allergic profile. The individual's immune system determines the strength of the inflammatory response to the allergen stimulus. Atopic asthmatics have an exaggerated or hypersensitive response to a trigger that would not elicit a response in a nonallergic individual.[5]

A *type IV hypersensitivity reaction* may also cause asthma in susceptible individuals. It is an IgG-mediated immune response. This immunological reaction may be secondary to exposure to environmental allergens, but it can also be secondary to triggers such as viral infections or aspirin. Some antigens are unknown.[8]

TABLE 9-1 **Airflow limitation diseases**

	Chronic Bronchitis	Emphysema	Bronchiectasis	Asthma
Etiology	Cigarette smoking, environmental pollution	Cigarette smoking, homozygotic α_1-antitrypsin deficiency, some connective tissue disorders, IV drug abuse,	**Infants and children** Congenital cause from a developmental arrest of the bronchial tree **Adults** Infectious insult Airway drainage impairment Airway obstruction Defect in host defense	Non-specific bronchial hyperreactivity to a variety of stimulants: airborn allergens, infection, pollution, drugs, emotion, exercise, gastroesophageal reflux
Pathologic changes	Bronchial mucus gland hyperplasia, basement membrane thickening, hyperplasia of mucus gland and goblet cells, narrowing of small airways	Air space enlargement of respiratory bronchioles and/or alveolar ducts, alveoli (Centriacinar and/or Panacinar)	Abnormal bronchial dilation with bronchial wall destruction and transmural inflammation Airway dilation is cylindrical, cystic, or varicose	Smooth muscle hypertrophy, hyperplasia of mucus glands and goblet cells, mucosal and submucosal edema, ↑ number of inflammatory cells, subepithelial fibrosis with collagen deposition
Clinical Features	Chronic productive cough (copious, purulent in acute exacerbations), ± hemoptysis, wheezing and rhonchi on auscultation, systemic evidence of cor pulmonale	Dyspnea, barrel chest, cachetic, pursed lip breathing, accessory muscles use, diminished breath sounds	**General Findings:** Digital clubbing, weight loss, nasal polyps, and chronic sinusitis **Respiratory Findings:** Cough, daily mucopurulent sputum production, hemoptysis, pleuritic chest pain related to coughing Aucultation: crackles, rhonchi, wheezing, +/− dyspnea, Multiple episodes of infection with increased sputum production over baseline, increased sputum viscosity, and foul odor of sputum	**During asthma attack** Tachypnea, dyspnea, accessory muscles use, pursed lip breathing, wheezing on auscultation
Precipitating Factors	Infection, atmospheric pollutants, temperature	Infection, atmospheric pollutants, temperature	Infection, other conditions related to the causes of bronchiectasis	Increased exposure to asthma triggers, infection

(continues)

TABLE 9-1 **Airflow limitation diseases *(continued)***

	Chronic Bronchitis	Emphysema	Bronchiectasis	Asthma
Chest radiograph	↑ bronchial markings, prominent pulmonary arteries	Hyperradiolucency, wide intercostal spaces, flattened diaphragm, long, narrow heart, ↑ retrosternal airspace (lateral)	**General Findings:** Increased pulmonary markings, honeycombing, atelectasis, pleural changes Specific Findings: Cylindrical form: Linear lucencies, and parallel markings radiating from the hila Varicose form: dilated bronchi Cystic: clustered cysts	**During asthma attack** Hyperradiolucency, wide intercostal spaces, flattened diaphragm, long, narrow heart, ↑ retrosternal airspace (lateral)
Pulmonary Function Changes	↓ Expiratory flows mild ↑ FRC, normal or ↑ RV, normal DL_{CO}	↓ Expiratory flows ↑ RV, FRC ↓ DL_{CO}	+/− Normal If abnormal, ↓ Expiratory flows, ↑ RV, FRC	↓ Expiratory flows, ↑ RV, FRC (in severe asthmatics) normal DL_{CO}
Arterial Blood Gas	↓ PaO_2, ± ↑ $PaCO_2$ (worsening in acute exacerbations)	↓ PaO_2 (worsening in acute exacerbations) Hypercapnia in acute exacerbations	↓ PaO_2 during acute exacerbations	**During asthma attack** ↓ PaO_2, variable $PaCO_2$
Complications	Frequent pulmonary infections, respiratory failure, cor pulmonale	Frequent pulmonary infections, respiratory failure, cor pulmonale	Recurrent pneumonia requiring hospitalization, empyema, lung abscess, hemoptysis, progressive respiratory failure, cor pulmonale	Bronchopulmonary Aspergillosis, Respiratory failure

ASTHMA TRIGGERS

Exposure to environmental triggers elicits an immunoglobulin-mediated hypersensitivity reaction in the bronchial epithelium of allergic patients. Patients who have inadequate control of their asthma or who have been exposed to a high concentration of allergens experience a rapid worsening in respiratory function secondary to asthma exacerbation (an asthma attack).

Allergic Triggers. Re-exposure to allergens in an atopic individual who is sensitized (who has elevated IgE in the serum) to that allergen has a worsening of asthmatic symptoms. Common allergic triggers are house dust and dust mites, pets, especially cats, pollens (tree, grass), roaches, and feathers.

- House dust contains organisms that may initiate an allergic reaction. Molds are a common cause.
- Dust mites are microscopic arachnids that eat the scales of human skin. They are present in cushioned furniture, carpet, and bedding.
- Cockroach proteins are a known allergic trigger. Roach-infested areas are a source of allergens for asthmatics.
- Animal dander from pets is in the house environment, permeates the house, and can even be carried on clothing.[5]

Infections. Infection by respiratory tract virus is a common cause of disease exacerbation in both children and adults. Viral infections elicit an immune response with similarities to the allergic mechanism. Infections also modulate the immune system and may enhance the allergic response. Viral infections increase the airways' responsiveness to triggers; this abnormality increases the response to activated inflammatory mediators and results in a severe worsening of symptoms.[6]

Exercise. Exercise in an individual with hyperresponsive airways triggers a worsening of asthmatic symptoms. The reaction is more severe in cold environments than in warm, moist environments (e.g., exercising outdoors versus exercising indoors). It is thought that the reaction is secondary to airway cooling resulting from water evaporation from airway mucosa. In addition, the evaporation of water results in hyperosmolarity of the sol layer on the mucosal surface and induces chemical mediator release. These effects are exaggerated in exercise because of increased minute ventilation. The cooling and increased mediator concentration in the hyper-reactive airway triggers asthma symptoms: wheezing, cough, chest tightness, and dyspnea.[7]

Medications and Preservatives. Certain drugs are known to trigger asthma symptoms. Sensitivity to aspirin and other nonsteroidal anti-inflammatory drugs (NSAIDs) is a known problem in some people with asthma. Other drugs that may worsen asthma symptoms are beta-blockers, both in oral tablets and topical forms.[5] Sulfite is a common preservative used in food and beverages such as processed potatoes, shrimp, dried fruit, beer, and wine. If people develop asthma symptoms after eating these items, asthma experts advise them to avoid those foods. Following exposure, they are at a greater risk for developing a severe asthma exacerbation or perhaps even status asthmaticus.[2]

Environmental Pollution. Asthmatics are extremely sensitive to environmental irritants, including cigarette smoke. If the concentration is significant, indoor and outdoor irritants trigger an asthmatic response.

- Indoor pollutants, such as chemical fumes given off by synthetic materials like rugs, furniture, aerosol sprays, particle board, wall coverings, and recent painting, may all cause symptoms in the asthmatic.
- Outdoor pollutants from motorized vehicles, manufacturing plants, and ozone can act as a trigger for asthma or add to the individual's existing breathing difficulties.
- Local meteorologists frequently broadcast air quality alerts, especially in the summer months, and the asthmatic should try to limit the time spent outdoors and, when outside, should wear a protective mask.

Exposure to pollutants may increase airway inflammation and increase the risk of allergic sensitization with exposure to multiple environmental allergens.[2,5]

Pathophysiology of Asthma. The cellular pathologic changes that occur in chronic inflammation are significant. The airway epithelium is damaged through its layers to the basement membrane. Collagen is deposited in the airway basement membrane. The airway is swollen. The mast cells are activated and release their intracellular mediators, and there is inflammatory cellular infiltration of the airway with eosinophils, neutrophils, and lymphocytes.[9]

Airway inflammation contributes to airway hyper-responsiveness, airflow limitation, symptoms, and chronicity. Three phases of airway inflammation are secondary to the activation of the inflammatory cells produced when the individual is exposed to an allergen (an acute asthma attack or exacerbation):

- The initial tissue changes in the acute inflammatory reaction are called the *acute phase response.* This is the initial cellular airway response to chemical mediator release from the mast cells of the airways and the basophils. The primary mediator in this response (histamine), along with many other mediators, creates inflammatory changes. This response is classically seen in the initial hours after an asthma exacerbation. The patient has bronchospasm, an outpouring of secretions, and mucosal edema with significant airflow limitation.
- In the *subacute phase,* the asthmatic patient's initial symptoms are being treated and controlled with appropriate medication, but a continuous inflammatory pattern is present. The patient's airflow limitation is still significant, and the patient's pulmonary function shows reduced expiratory flows. This phase continues for days to weeks after an asthma exacerbation.
- The *chronic inflammation* phase is present in asthmatics between asthma exacerbations. This is the inflammation that maintenance therapy is attempting to control.[2,10] Drug therapy with corticosteroids or drugs that control specific chemical inflammatory mediators, such as mast cell or leukotriene modifiers, are the primary means for control.

AIRWAY INFLAMMATION AND AIRFLOW LIMITATION

Airway inflammation causes *airway hyper-responsiveness,* that is, an exaggerated bronchospasm response to a stimulus (allergen, exercise, cold air, or infection). The individual has postexposure wheezing and breathlessness. The degree of airway hyper-responsiveness is correlated with asthma severity. Pulmonary function testing using methacholine/histamine inhalation challenge or nondrug stimuli inhalation such as cold, dry air can measure airway hyper-responsiveness. The testing includes the measurement of pre-exposure and postexposure expiratory flow rates. The patient who has a significant reduction in postexposure expiratory flows is diagnosed with hyper-responsive/hyper-reactive airways.[2,5]

Airway inflammation also causes bronchospasm. Bronchospasm is caused by many factors: IgE mediator release, aspirin or NSAIDs ingestion, non-IgE response, stress, or airway edema. Bronchospasm causes airflow limitation with wheezing and dyspnea.[2,10]

Chronic inflammation increases the rigidity of the airways, resulting from the chronic leakage of fluid from the blood vessels in the airway caused by chronic mediator release, mucosal thickening, and airway swelling. Acute airway rigidity is a type of airflow limitation in acute asthma that does not respond to bronchodilators. Rigidity can be reduced and controlled with anti-inflammatory medications.

However, if the chronic inflammation is not controlled with maintenance therapy, this aspect of airflow limitation becomes permanent because of airway structural changes. This end point of chronic inflammation is called *airway wall remodeling*. When the patient's airflow limitation is predominately secondary to airway wall remodeling, bronchodilators have no effect and the airflow limitation is fixed.[2,9] Mucus plugging also causes airflow limitation. The outpouring of secretions in the acute inflammatory phase can form plugs that obstruct the airway. Plugging usually occurs in the smaller airways and can seriously reduce airflow.[2,10]

DIAGNOSIS OF ASTHMA

The key elements of characterizing asthma mentioned earlier are very consistent with the cardinal diagnostic findings.[2,5] These clinical findings support the diagnosis of asthma:

- The presence of episodic symptoms of airflow limitation
- Airflow obstruction that is partially reversible
- The ruling out of alternative diagnoses

The techniques used to establish the diagnosis of asthma are:

- Patient history.
- Physical exam (respiratory tract, skin, and chest).
- Pulmonary function spirometry (demonstrate reversibility).
- Other studies.

Additional studies:

- Evaluate alternative diagnoses.
- Identify precipitating factors.
- Assess asthma severity.
- Identify potential complications (pneumothorax, atelectasis, and cor pulmonale).[10]

The signs and symptoms of someone presenting with undiagnosed asthma are very helpful in arriving at a diagnosis of asthma. In the asthmatic individual who is not having an asthma exacerbation, the clinical signs are less severe than those during an acute asthma attack. The asthmatic complains of wheezing and postexercise shortness of breath. Chest tightness and cough are frequent problems. The patient's symptoms are worsened with exposure to allergens or irritants. The typical signs and symptoms of an adult asthmatic in an asthma exacerbation are listed in Table 9-1.

Usually asthma attacks begin acutely. The patient has wheezing and chest tightness with intermittent coughing episodes. The cough is usually tight, nonproductive, and common at night. The wheezing worsens, is heard during inspiration, and is audible without a stethoscope. As airflow limitation increases, the ventilation/perfusion relationship becomes abnormal, and hypoxemia results. Dyspnea increases in severity, and the use of accessory muscles to breathe is obvious. Tachycardia and increased blood pressure are responses to stress and anxiety, as well as to hypoxemia. In severe asthma, which does not respond to beta-adrenergic drugs and other treatment modalities (status asthmaticus), hypoventilation occurs secondary to fatigue and severe ventilation/perfusion mismatching. In this scenario, the patient needs to be hospitalized and admitted to the intensive care unit. A critical element of an asthma attack is that a silent chest is a serious finding. If the airflow limitation is so severe that a wheeze cannot be heard, then this patient is critical and needs maximal therapy to avoid ventilatory failure and possible cardiopulmonary arrest.[2,5,10]

Age-Specific Competency

Asthmatic Children

Asthmatic children who are not in an asthmatic attack may show clinical manifestations that are not typically seen in the adult:

- Frequent headaches
- Irritability and depression
- Dark circles under the eyes (allergic "shiners")
- Rhinorrhea with yellow or green mucus or congestion with cough
- Sleeping difficulty, awakening with nightmares

TABLE 9-2 **Asthma classifications published by Asthma Expert Panel Report 2007**

	Symptoms		Lung Function		
Asthma Severity	**Daily**	**Night**	**Activity Limitation**	**Expiratory Flows**	**PF Variability**
Intermittent Asthma	<2 days/wk	≤2 nights/ mos	No limitations except during infrequent exacerbations	>80% of predicted	<20%
Mild Persistent	>2/wk but <1/day	>2/mos	Exacerbations may affect activity	>80% of predicted	20%–30%
Moderate Persistent	Daily	>1/wk	≥2/wk; may last days; exacerbations affect predicted activity	>60% – <80% of predicted	>30%
Severe Persistent	Continual	Frequent	Frequent exacerbations	<60% of predicted	>30%

ASTHMA CLASSIFICATIONS

Asthma has four severity classifications, and the intensiveness of the treatment varies directly with the asthma severity. With increasing asthma severity, the symptoms are more frequent, the airflow limitation is more severe, and the disease has a greater impact on the quality of life. The four asthma classifications (Table 9-2) are:

- Intermittent asthma
- Mild persistent asthma
- Moderate persistent asthma
- Severe persistent asthma

The patient's asthma severity is determined by assessing:

- Symptom frequency per week and at night, as well as activity restriction.
- Expiratory flow measures (e.g., peak expiratory flow (PEF) or forced expiratory flow in the first second of exhalation (FEV_1) and the flow rate variability during the day).[2,5,10]

ASTHMA MANAGEMENT

Asthma management takes two main directions. First, reduce the individual's exposure to environmental allergens. If allergen exposures can be significantly reduced, then the individual's asthma classification can be reassessed and the need for drug therapy reduced. The second main element of asthma management is drug therapy. The principles of asthma control are based on how the prescribed medications and reduction of environmental exposure improves the quality of life, reduces disease impairment, and lowers the risk of asthma exacerbations.[3] Table 9-3 summarizes the goals of asthma therapy.

Reduction of Exposure. Exposure reduction is an important part of asthma management. Controlling the environment of the asthmatic patient is one method of reducing exposure to the allergen. In fact, minimizing the contact with allergens cannot be stressed enough. If successful, exposure control reduces

TABLE 9-3 **Goals of asthma therapy published by the Asthma Expert Panel Report 2007**

Reducing Impairment	Reducing Risk
Prevent chronic and troublesome symptoms	Prevent recurrent exacerbations of asthma and minimize need for ED visits and hospitalizations
Require infrequent use (<2/wk) of Short Acting Beta 2 Agonist (SABA) for quick relief	Prevent progressive loss of lung function; for youths ≥ 12 years of age prevent reduced lung growth
Maintain (near) normal pulmonary function	
Maintain normal activity levels	Provide optimal pharmacotherapy with minimal or no adverse effects
Meet patients' and families' goals of asthma care	

asthma severity and improves the patient's quality of life.[2]

- Control animal dander.
  - Remove the pet from home or keep it out of the bedroom.
  - Close off the bedroom from free air circulation and place filters over air outlets.
- Control dust mites.
  - Essential: Encase mattress and pillows with allergen-impermeable covering; wash bedding weekly in hot water.
  - Desirable: Remove the carpet from the bedroom; minimize stuffed toys and wash them weekly; keep the home humidity less than 50%; avoid sleeping on upholstered furniture; remove carpets laid on concrete.
- Control cockroach allergen by the chemical control of cockroach infestation.
- Control indoor fungi by controlling dampness (dehumidifier); control fungi growth.
- Control exposure to outdoor allergens by staying in air conditioning with doors and windows closed (not so realistic a measure for children). If going out, try to schedule activities in the early morning.

Pharmacological Treatment. The drugs used to treat asthma are divided into two main categories: quick-relief and long-term control medications (Figure 9-1). Two drug groups are used as quick-relief medications:

- Short-acting beta 2 bronchodilators (SABA) and anticholinergic bronchodilators.
- Long-term control medications, such as the following drugs or drug groups: corticosteroids (inhaled, oral, or IV), long-acting beta 2 agonists, leukotriene receptor antagonists, cromolyn sodium and nedocromil sodium, and methylxanthines (see Table 9-4).

Quick-Relief Medications The *short-acting beta 2 bronchodilators* are used to provide the asthmatic quick relief of acute symptoms or to prevent exercise-induced bronchospasm. This drug group is the most effective treatment available for acute bronchospasm. The beta 2 agonists are taken by the inhaled route and give faster peak action with minimal side effects. These drugs should be taken only on an as-needed basis. If more than one canister of drug a month is used, then maintenance drug therapy should be changed. The regular use of short-acting beta 2 bronchodilators indicates a lack of pharmacological control of asthma and may result in frequent exacerbations requiring hospital treatment. Beta 2 medications have no effect on acute or chronic inflammation and are used to relieve patient symptoms arising from airway hyper-reactivity secondary to an acute worsening of inflammation.[2]

Anticholinergic bronchodilators make up the second medication group used for the quick-relief treatment of asthma. Ipratropium bromide may provide additional bronchodilation when used in conjunction with beta 2 agonists. Ipratropium helps patients with bronchospasm secondary to increased **vagal tone** (hyperexcitability of the parasympathetic nervous system). The drug may also serve as a primary bronchodilator for people who do not respond to beta 2 agonists. The lack of response indicates that either beta 2 bronchodilator has met with resistance secondary to overuse or that a larger element of increased parasympathetic tone is the cause of bronchospasm. The lack of response to the short-acting beta 2 drugs is more likely to occur in severe asthma exacerbations. One study reported that when pediatric asthma patients in an emergency department were given a maximum of three doses of ipratropium, they had 13% shorter duration of treatment and they received fewer beta 2 drug doses before discharge. However, the hospital admission rates did not change.[11] Another research study reported a significant reduction in hospitalization rates for children in a severe asthma exacerbation who were given ipratropium in the emergency department.[12] In another study, adult asthmatics admitted to the emergency department in an acute exacerbation of

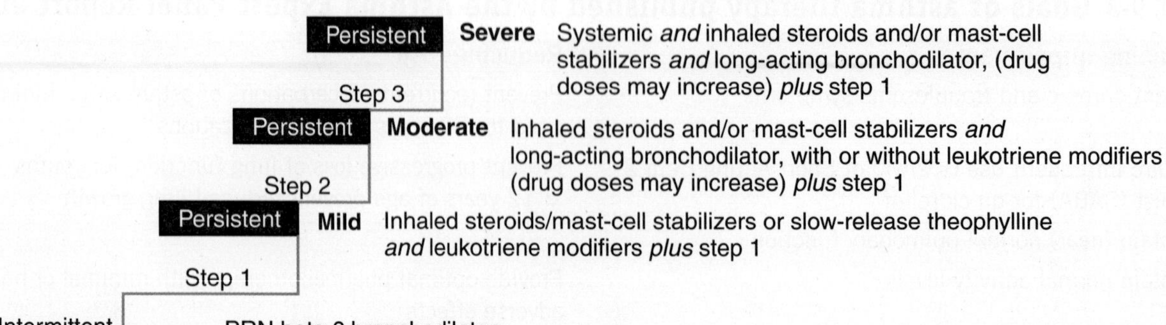

FIGURE 9-1 Steps in the pharmacological control of asthma.

TABLE 9-4 **Long-term asthma control published by Asthma Expert Panel Report 2007**

Step Phase	Preferred Treatment	Alternative Not Preferred Treatment
Intermittent Asthma		
Step 1	No Daily Medications PRN SABA Asthma Exacerbations • SABA Q4–6 hrs • Short course of oral steroids	None
Persistent Asthma		
Step 2	Low-dose Inhaled Steroids AND SABA (PRN)	Cromolyn OR Leukotriene Receptor Antagonists (Nedocromil) OR Sustained-Release Theophylline
Step 3	Low-dose Inhaled Steroids AND SABA (PRN) AND Inhaled Long-acting Beta$_2$ agonists	Medium-dose Inhaled Steroids OR Low-dose Inhaled Steroids AND Leukotriene Receptor Antagonists (Nedocromil) OR Sustained-Release Theophylline OR Zileuton
Step 4	Medium-dose Inhaled Steroids AND SABA (PRN) AND Inhaled Long-acting Beta$_2$ agonists	Medium-dose Inhaled Steroids AND Leukotriene Antagonists OR Sustained Release Theophylline OR Zileuton
Step 5	High-dose Inhaled Steroids AND SABA (PRN) AND Inhaled Long-acting Beta$_2$ agonists Consider adding Omalizumab Consult with asthma specialist	No alternatives identified
Step 6	High-dose Inhaled Steroids AND SABA (PRN) AND Inhaled Long-acting Beta$_2$ agonists AND Oral Steroids Consult with asthma specialist	No alternatives identified

asthma were given ipratropium in addition to beta 2 bronchodilators, and there was a distinct improvement in the patients' FEV_1 or PEF. In this study, the addition of ipratropium resulted in fewer hospital admissions.[13] Therefore, it is suggested that combination ipratropium–beta agonist therapy can be given to both children and adults in an acute asthma exacerbation.

Long-Term Control Medications. The asthmatic takes the long-term medications daily to control the disease. Minimizing asthma symptoms, decreasing the number of exacerbations, and increasing the person's quality of life are the goals of long-term asthma control. Because asthma is classified as a chronic inflammatory airway disease, the primary direction of asthma management is to reduce airway inflammation. Corticosteroids, leukotriene receptor antagonists, and cromolyn sodium or nedocromil reduce inflammation through different mechanisms. The patient takes one or more of these drugs.[2,10]

Corticosteroids (steroids) globally suppress the inflammatory response by suppressing the migration of polymorphonuclear leukocytes and fibroblasts. Inhaled steroids are the preferred therapy and are started when persistent asthma is diagnosed. Initiating inhaled steroids early in the disease course results in a heightened objective improvement in lung function. Steroids do not cure asthma, but research studies suggest that their early use, in conjunction with beta agonists, can reduce airway wall remodeling.[2,14] Steroids control airway inflammation in a dose-dependent fashion. Using the lowest possible dose of inhaled steroids is recommended. The inhaled form is employed the most frequently in long-term asthma control because of lower systemic effects. Since systemic or even inhaled steroids can inhibit growth and development in children, children's growth should be monitored for any abnormal slowing while they are taking steroids.[2]

Oral steroids also have a role in asthma therapy and are used in addition to inhaled steroids the asthmatic is taking. Oral steroids are indicated for asthmatics experiencing an acute exacerbation of symptoms but either not responding to or resistant to short-acting beta 2 bronchodilators.[2] Steroid administration can reverse or partially reverse the beta receptors' desensitization to sustained beta-adrenergic stimulation. A short course of systemic corticosteroids is recommended after an acute exacerbation of asthma. The temporary use of steroids reduces the number of asthma relapses and decreases use of the quick-relief beta 2 bronchodilator that the asthmatic usually needs in the postexacerbation period.[15]

Cromolyn sodium and nedocromil are not preferred anti-inflammatory drugs but can be used as an alternative medication. The individual properties of these two drugs are different from each other, but they both affect airway inflammation. Both drugs block chloride channels, which are thought to be the mechanism by which mast cell inflammatory mediator release is controlled. As a second-generation anti-asthmatic drug, nedocromil has a modulating effect not just on the mast cell but also on the airway epithelial cells, eosinophils, and sensory neurons. Both drugs are used in the treatment of asthma and may be used in place of or in addition to steroids. Their anti-inflammatory activity may be sufficient to control asthma in some people and may be preferred in the treatment of childhood asthma because they do not inhibit growth and development. Cromolyn and nedocromil are used to prevent asthma exacerbations and exercise-induced asthma. These drugs are not effective in the treatment of an asthma exacerbation.[2]

The duration of action of the long-acting beta 2 adrenergic agent salbutamol is approximately 12 hours. In providing long-term bronchodilation, salbutamol prevents nocturnal symptoms and helps provide attenuated control of exercise-induced bronchospasm. This drug has a prolonged duration of action because it is lipid soluble and has a delayed peak effect. Therefore, salbutamol should *not* be used for quick relief of symptoms or to treat an acute exacerbation of asthma. The short-acting beta 2 drugs are indicated for those emergency situations.

Methylxanthines have long been used in the treatment of asthma. Their role in asthma treatment has been open to question, but it is now accepted that theophylline is an alternative therapy for suppressing nocturnal asthma symptoms. Sustained-release preparations of the methylxanthine theophylline are an acceptable substitute for the long-acting beta 2 bronchodilator salbutamol. Issues such as cost may require the use of the less expensive methylxanthine. The drug is still not well understood and has been reported to have effects that may contribute to the overall reason for its effectiveness in asthma. Theophylline is a modest bronchodilator that is reported to have a slight anti-inflammatory effect and to strengthen diaphragmatic contraction. Since the difference between the therapeutic blood level and theophylline toxicity is

Best Practice

Salbutamol

Asthmatics using salbutamol should be carefully instructed that this drug should not be used in acute breathing problems and that to rely on this drug for relief is dangerous.

small, the drug blood levels must be regularly monitored for drug toxicity. People with theophylline toxicity complain of nausea, vomiting, and cardiac arrhythmias.[4]

Other types of anti-inflammatory drugs used in long-term control of asthma are the leukotriene modifiers. Leukotrienes are eicosanoids derived from arachidonic acid, a cell membrane phospholipid. The leukotriene molecules—LTC_4, LTD_4, LTE_4—were formerly known as the *slow-reacting substance of anaphylaxis* (SRSA). These chemicals are important mediators in asthmatic bronchoconstriction and airway inflammation. Bronchoconstriction persists in acute asthma exacerbations well beyond the acute phase because of the presence of these and other chemical mediators. Researchers have found that leukotrienes are acutely increased in the urine of atopic asthmatics exposed to an allergen to which they are sensitive. Also the urine of asthmatics with aspirin sensitivity contains chronically elevated levels when compared with the urine levels in non-aspirin-sensitive asthmatics.[6–9]

Treatment with leukotriene modifiers inhibits the production of leukotrienes, which control bronchoconstriction in people with atopic asthma, exercise-induced asthma, and aspirin-sensitivity-induced asthma. In addition, inhibiting leukotrienes reduces the airway hyper-responsiveness associated with airway inflammation.

The FDA approved the medications zafirlukast and zileuton for use in mild to moderate persistent asthma. They should not be used in patients with severe persistent asthma. The leukotriene receptor antagonists are approved for use in the pediatric patient. Zileuton is listed as an alternative leukotriene modifier in the adult and youths over the age of 12, but it is not a preferred drug because liver function monitoring is required.

THE ACUTE ASTHMA ATTACK

The classification system of asthma severity is helpful in determining the maintenance treatment of the asthmatic. However, any asthmatic with intermittent or persistent asthma who has an acute worsening of asthma symptoms—an asthma attack—can develop severe symptoms and need emergency department care and even hospitalization before the asthma can be controlled. There are three stages of an acute attack.[4] Treatment failure results in a seriously ill asthmatic at risk of respiratory arrest (see Table 9-5).

Stage 1 is considered a mild attack. In this severity of asthma exacerbation, the asthmatic's respiratory rate is increased, and end expiratory wheezing is heard on auscultation. But the attack does not limit the ability to lie flat, and the patient can talk in complete sentences without having to stop to breathe. If blood gases were measured, they'd be normal. The P_AO_2 and S_AO_2 are maintained within normal range because of the patient's hyperventilation. The heart rate and the blood pressure are still in the normal range.

Stage 2 is a moderately severe asthma attack. The asthmatic's respiratory rate is more elevated than in the previous stage, with obvious use of accessory muscles and audible inspiratory and expiratory wheezing. The asthmatic does not like to lie flat, and, because of dyspnea, talking is restricted to simple phrases. The arterial blood gases reveal two abnormalities: respiratory alkalosis and mild hypoxemia with an oxygen saturation greater than 90%. A moderately severe asthma attack is stressful, creating anxiety, ventilatory work, and mild to moderate hypoxemia, which causes an elevated blood pressure and tachycardia (100 and 120 bpm).

Stage 3 is a severe asthmatic attack. The asthmatic has a very rapid respiratory rate and must sit upright to breathe. He or she refuses to lie supine and is too short

TABLE 9-5 **Asthma attack severity stages**

Signs and Symptoms	Mild Attack	Moderate Attack	Severe Attack
RR	Increased over baseline	Tachypnea	Tachypnea
Dyspnea	+ Walking, Can lie flat	+ Talking, Prefers sitting to lying down	+ At rest, tripod position to breathe
Speaking	Full sentences	Partial sentences	Words
Wheezes (auscultation)	End expiratory	Inspiratory and expiratory	Decreased or Inaudible
Alertness	Normal	Agitated	Agitated or Drowsy
Pulsus Paradoxus	Normal <10 mm Hg	>10 mm Hg	>10 mm Hg
SpO_2	>95%	90–95%	<90%
PaO_2 (mm H)	Normal (ABG not necessary)	>60	<60 (possible cyanosis)
PCO_2 (mm Hg)	<35	35–45	>45
PEFR % personal best	>70–90%	50–70%	<50%

of breath to talk except in single words. Accessory muscle use is prominent during breathing, and wheezing may still be audible or it may decrease or even disappear. The heart rate is over 120 bpm, with accompanying hypertension. The extremely hyperinflated patient shows a paradoxical pulse (decreased pulse or blood pressure during inspiration). The arterial blood gas shows an elevated P_ACO_2 with hypoxemia, and oxygen saturation is less than 90%. Findings that herald respiratory arrest are:

- Paradoxical chest or abdominal movement during breathing.
- Minimal wheezing in a patient in severe respiratory distress.
- Exhaustion in presence of respiratory acidosis.
- Decreased level of consciousness.
- Bradycardia.
- Cyanosis.

In general, many asthmatics experiencing an acute exacerbation of asthma have a preliminary period of increased asthma symptoms that results in a visit or phone call to the physician's office. Drug treatment at home is intensified without alleviation of symptoms. The most critical element of asthma care for the asthmatic or the family is recognition of when to go to the emergency department. Asthma deaths occur with failure to come to the hospital or with delay in coming to the hospital until after deterioration into a treatment-refractory state.[5]

When to Come to the Emergency Department. If, after the patient has consulted the family physician or asthma specialist, the intensive home therapy is unsuccessful in controlling asthma symptoms (peak expiratory flow rate (PEFR) less than 60% of predicted or personal best), the patient should go to the hospital emergency department. Before starting for the hospital, the primary instructions for the patient are to:

- Continue taking the short-acting beta 2 bronchodilator.
- Take steroid tablets before leaving.
- Use oxygen if available.
- Call 911 if unable to drive.[15,17]

The management of the patient in the emergency department is very intense and complete. Emergency department treatment of the asthmatic includes oxygen, high-dose bronchodilators by nebulization, and steroids. The treatment regimen is determined by assessing asthma exacerbation severity and the response to that therapy; it follows the National Heart, Lung, and Blood Institute's Expert Panel guidelines on asthma management.[2]

The goals of treatment are to relieve acute symptoms and to prevent hospitalization. The asthmatic patient who is responding may receive treatment in the emergency department for up to 5 hours before being discharged from the hospital. The patient who shows a partial response to emergency department treatment may be admitted to the hospital or may be discharged. The decision is based on the patient's individual situation. The patient who shows poor response to treatment is admitted to the hospital. A good standard for discharge is pulmonary function performance. It is suggested that the PEFR should be greater than 70% of predicted or personal best unless otherwise directed by the attending physician.[2,5] Additionally, before discharge, the respiratory therapist should check the patient's inhaler technique and reinstruct the patient on its use.

Discharge medications commonly include systemic and inhaled steroids and quick-relief and long-acting beta 2 bronchodilators. The systemic steroids are gradually tapered off under the guidance of the physician and with careful monitoring of asthma symptoms. The patient's long-term pharmacological control regimen should be reassessed. An exacerbation of asthma is considered treatment failure and indicates reexamination and adjustment of home medications to prevent future exacerbations.[2,5]

Chronic Bronchitis (COPD) and Emphysema

In 2006 in the United States, 8.9 million noninstitutionalized adults were diagnosed with chronic bronchitis, and 3.8 million were diagnosed with emphysema. Chronic lower respiratory tract disease was the fourth greatest cause of death with 121,987. Most of the respiratory deaths were secondary to chronic obstructive pulmonary disease (COPD), and the majority of them were over the age of 55. This disease is one of senior citizens.[16]

The economic burden of a disease is reported as direct costs and indirect costs.

- **Direct costs** are the value of health care resources devoted to the diagnosis and management of a disease, including hospitalization, drug therapy, rehabilitation. These costs are generally reimbursed by health insurance.
- **Indirect costs** are the monetary consequences of disability, missed work, premature death, and the caregiver or family costs resulting from the illness. These costs reflect the shortened contribution of the afflicted individual to society and the burden on the family.

In developed countries, COPD exacerbations account for the greatest burden on the health care system. For example, the total direct costs of respiratory

CASE STUDY 9-1

This is one of numerous emergency department visits for Latonya Brewster, a 20-year-old female, for acute asthma exacerbation. She had been attending a family picnic when she started to feel chest tightness that was not relieved by using her albuterol inhaler. She became progressively more short of breath (SOB) despite taking her albuterol every 20 minutes. Her parents called the family physician. He told them to take her to the emergency department, and he would meet them at the hospital. The following were noted at the emergency department.

Physical examination: This 20-year-old female is in obvious respiratory distress. She is using her accessory muscles to breathe and can talk only in short phrases.

Vital signs: Heart rate 110, blood pressure 130/90, respiratory rate 25 breaths per minute, temperature 36.8°C, SpO_2 92%, peak expiratory flow rate ~60 Lpm.

Chest examination: Breath sounds revealed inspiratory and expiratory wheezing throughout the chest. Expiratory wheezing audible without a stethoscope.

HEENT (head, eyes, ears, nose, throat): Atraumatic normocephalic; she was using neck muscles during breathing.

Cardiovascular: Regular rhythm with sinus tachycardia

Medications taken for asthma: MDIs fluticasone, albuterol, salbutamol; montelukast. Her parents stated that her personal best PEFR is 70% of predicted, and it varies ~30%–35% throughout the day.

Oxygen therapy was started at 2 Lpm by nasal cannula. The respiratory therapist gave Latonya albuterol and Atrovent (ipratropium) administered by small-volume nebulizer every 20 minutes. An IV was started, and she was given the IV corticosteroid methylprednisolone.

Questions

1. In which stage of asthma exacerbation severity would you categorize Latonya Brewster's asthma attack?
2. On the basis of information supplied by her parents, in which asthma classification would you place Latonya? Explain your reasoning.
3. Would replacing Latonya's albuterol with a long-acting bronchodilator be a better treatment while she is in the emergency department?
4. Methylprednisolone was added to Latonya's emergency care. What is the benefit of methylprednisolone in the asthmatic?

disease in the European Union is about 6% of the total health care budget, with COPD responsible for approximately 56% of respiratory disease costs. In 2002, the direct and indirect costs of COPD to the United States' health care system were $18 billion and $14.1 billion, respectively.[1] Despite the higher direct costs, indirect costs have the largest impact on countries, reflecting the loss of human capital, which is the most important asset of any country.

DEFINITIONS

COPD is characterized by the presence of chronic bronchitis, emphysema, or both. The COPD patient has progressive airflow limitation that may be partially reversible in those with hyper-reactive airways. Although asthma is sometimes included in the label of COPD, asthma is a very different disease from bronchitis or emphysema. For many people with chronic bronchitis or emphysema, smoking is the underlying cause of their disease, and they respond differently to bronchodilator therapy and steroids.[17]

Emphysema is defined in pathological terms. Emphysema is present when there is abnormal permanent dilation and destruction of lung units distal to the terminal bronchioles, which include the respiratory bronchioles, alveolar ducts, and alveoli. Distribution in the lung is variable, but the involved areas exhibit abnormal lung architecture and abnormal exchange of oxygen and carbon dioxide. There are three main types of emphysema: panacinar, centriacinar, and paraseptal emphysema.

- **Panacinar emphysema**, also known as *panlobar emphysema,* has the same definition as emphysema. The entire lung unit—including the respiratory bronchioles, alveolar ducts, and alveolar sacs—is involved, hence the prefix "pan-," indicating "all." Panacinar emphysema usually occurs in the lower lobes of the lung. It can be caused by smoking and occurs in people with a genetic disease, alpha-1 antitrypsin deficiency.

- **Centriacinar emphysema** is the enlargement of the central part of the acinus and spares the distal lung units. It commonly occurs in the upper lobes of the lung and is strongly associated with smoking.
- **Paraseptal emphysema** preferentially involves the distal airway structures, such as the alveolar ducts and sacs. while sparing the respiratory bronchioles. This type of emphysema occurs in subpleural areas or along interlobular septa. It commonly occurs in the apices of the lung and is associated with bullae formation and subsequently is a cause of secondary pneumothorax in people with lung disease.

In most patients with COPD secondary to emphysema, these different forms of emphysema coexist.[18]

Chronic bronchitis is the predominant cause of COPD and accounts for approximately 90% of the COPD population. Chronic bronchitis is defined not pathologically but functionally. An individual with a chronically productive cough lasting 3 or more consecutive months for 2 successive years is diagnosed with chronic bronchitis. Before this diagnosis can be made, other diseases that cause similar symptoms—such as tuberculosis, lung cancer, and congestive heart failure—must be excluded from consideration.[17,19]

The classic relationship of asthma, emphysema, and chronic bronchitis is illustrated in Figure 9-2, which shows the variability of the COPD population.

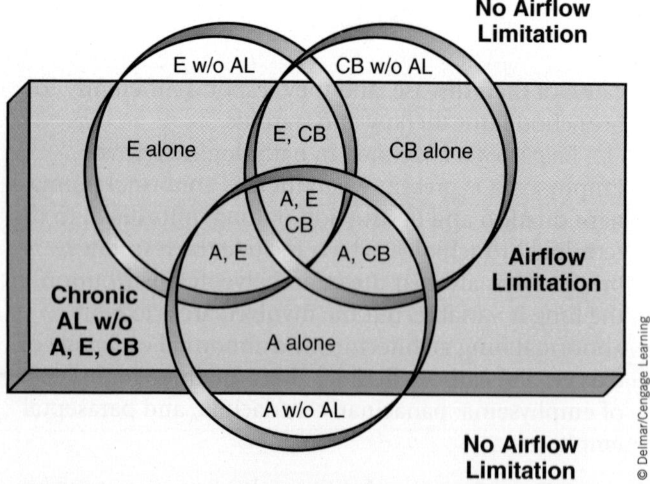

FIGURE 9-2 The combinations of disease overlap in populations diagnosed as having COPD. The rectangle represents airflow limitation as identified by a clinically significant decrease in FEV_1 or PEF. All patients with one or more of the three diseases in the rectangle can be classified as having COPD. CB = chronic bronchitis; E = emphysema; A = asthma; AL = airflow limitation.

Cookbook drug treatment does not work in treating patients with this disease. The figure helps to explain why medications are used in short-term trials. If the drug is beneficial, the medication is added to that patient's maintenance or emergency treatment regimen. If the drug does not improve the patient's clinical condition, the drug is stopped. Physicians attempt to discover the best treatment regimen for each person.

Asthma overlapping with chronic bronchitis is a patient group that needs special mention. This group is also described as having chronic asthmatic bronchitis. Some asthmatics have less than expected reversibility of their airflow limitation in response to beta 2 bronchodilators. In addition, they have chronic bronchitis. But this mix of asthma and bronchitis can also be examined when studying the chronic bronchitis patient population. Some patients with chronic bronchitis have significant partial reversibility of their airflow limitation that is not a characteristic of chronic bronchitis. These bronchitics have airway hyper-reactivity that is significantly responsive to beta 2 bronchodilators. Therefore, a diagnosis of chronic asthmatic bronchitis can describe these patients.[17,19]

RISK FACTORS

Specific risk factors are common among people who develop chronic bronchitis and emphysema: cigarette smoking, environmental pollution, and genetics. Knowledge gained from the Human Genome Project may show that genetic predisposition to lung disease is more important as a risk factor than was previously thought.

Cigarette Smoking. Cigarette smoking is the primary risk factor for COPD. Cigarette smokers have both a greater prevalence of COPD and a greater severity of clinical symptoms. The smoking variables that have the greatest effect on COPD morbidity and mortality are the age at which the COPD patient started smoking, the total pack-years, and the current smoking status.[17,19]

Despite the greater risk for COPD, only 20% of smokers actually develop COPD. Intensive research has been devoted to identifying why this population of cigarette smokers is predisposed to lung disease.[1,20]

Environmental Tobacco Smoke and Air Pollution. Environmental tobacco smoke, which has also been called *secondhand smoke,* is known to produce respiratory irritation such as cough, eye irritation, and increased respiratory infections. It is a known risk factor for lung cancer, and it may be an allergen trigger in asthmatics. Its role in COPD pathogenesis, however, is unknown.[21,22]

Air pollution is a respiratory irritant. Its role in precipitating sickness in people with cardiopulmonary disease is well documented. Officials who monitor air quality in urban and suburban areas announce alerts during the summer because of dangerously high levels of pollutants. High pollutant levels are a risk factor for exacerbation of COPD, but their role as a cause of COPD is small in comparison with cigarette smoking. High levels of pollution, dust, or chemical fumes irritate the respiratory tract and increase the patient's underlying airflow limitation.[19]

Alpha-1 Antitrypsin Deficiency. *Alpha-1 antitrypsin deficiency* is a genetic disease in which there is a decreased ability to produce the glycoprotein antitrypsin. Antitrypsin is necessary to block the activity of inflammatory proteases (proteolytic enzymes). Alpha-1 antitrypsin is a protein circulating in body fluids such as respiratory secretions, GI secretions, and saliva. A deficiency in this enzyme causes unopposed proteolysis of elastin in the lung and liver. The chronically increased breakdown of elastin, which is an important protein in the lung parenchyma structures, causes widespread lung destruction and panacinar emphysema. Liver disease or liver cirrhosis may also develop secondary to protease destruction of hepatocytes. Liver failure occurs in all ages, but this condition is especially severe in newborns. People who are born with this disorder and who smoke cigarettes develop early-onset panacinar emphysema in their twenties and thirties. Approximately 100,000 people in the United States have the severe form of the deficiency, and lung and liver transplantation are the only cure after the damage has occurred.[17,19]

PATHOGENESIS AND PATHOPHYSIOLOGY

Cigarette smoking is a cause of both pulmonary emphysema and chronic bronchitis. Why only 20% of smokers develop COPD is not understood. Research scientists have discussed the possibility of individual, genetic, familial, or environmental factors that provide protection. This question is being closely studied in COPD research.[21]

Pulmonary emphysema results from the proteolytic destruction of elastin, which is a large component of the structural matrix of the lung acinus. People with normal levels of alpha-1 antitrypsin can develop emphysema when the normal antiprotease-protease balance is disturbed by the addition of proteases such as neutrophil elastase, which is a product of cigarette smoke–induced inflammation. Smoking over an extended period of time produces a state of chronic inflammation. The pulmonary cells involved in the inflammatory reaction release chemical mediators that attract neutrophils to the lung. Neutrophil-derived elastase lyses lung tissue elastin. The injury is cumulative and becomes clinically evident when the patient has extensive destruction to the lung.

In some cases, chronic bronchitis occurs in nonsmokers. Research studies of the smoking and nonsmoking populations with chronic bronchitis support the hypothesis that the molecular and cellular characteristics of chronic inflammation that occur in the two different groups are different. Thus, the pathogenesis of chronic bronchitis in the smoker is different from that in the nonsmoker, although the end state is the same.[20,23] Table 9-6 lists the different presentations of smokers and nonsmokers with chronic bronchitis. This distinction indicates that the inflammatory process is different and that the initiating stimulus or trigger is different.[23] During acute exacerbations, the inflammatory cells are present in the airway wall epithelial tissue and mucus, and, during these episodes, bronchial injury is more severe. Chronic injury is thought to take place because of a disruption in the antiprotease-protease balance secondary to smoking irritants. The major proteases are neutrophil derived.

Chronic bronchitis causes tissue changes that are apparent both on gross examination and by microscope. The epithelial layer is red and edematous, with increased secretions pouring from the enlarged mucus glands. The affected bronchial epithelial layer has undergone permanent structural changes from the

TABLE 9-6 **Differences between smokers and non-smokers with chronic bronchitis**

Smokers	Non-Smokers
Increased macrophages	Increased mast cells
Increased neutrophils*	Increased non-activated eosinophils
Increased nonactivated eosinophils	Increased activated CD4+ T-lymphocytes
Increased activated $CD8^+$ T-lymphocytes	Increased Interleukin-5
Increased tumor necrosis factor alpha	Increased granulocyte-macrophage colony-stimulating factor genes
Increased interleukin-2 genes	Increased proteins
Increased proteins	

normal pseudostratified ciliated columnar epithelium to squamous, with a loss of the normal cilia. The smooth muscle may also hypertrophy. All of these changes decrease the bronchial lumen, especially in the smaller airways (the terminal bronchioles and respiratory bronchioles). As the disease progresses, the larger bronchi become more involved and the disease becomes apparent clinically.[19]

DIAGNOSIS OF COPD

The history and physical examination are helpful in establishing a diagnosis. Looking closely at risk factors for COPD, asking questions regarding the incidence of emphysema in the family (alpha-1 antitrypsin deficiency), asking about morning cough, sputum production, and shortness of breath provide the clinician valuable clues about the likelihood of COPD.[17] After identifying that a diagnosis of COPD is possible, the patient undergoes additional testing.

Chest Radiograph. The chest radiograph can identify X-ray changes consistent with chronic bronchitis or emphysema. People with emphysema show all the X-ray hallmarks of hyperinflation: low flat hemidiaphragm (on lateral), wide intercostal spaces, hypovascular lung showing excessive air, retrosternal air space (lateral), and long narrow heart. The chest X-ray changes classically seen in people with chronic bronchitis are less dramatic. Increases in lung markings indicate thickened airways containing mucus. These markings show as radiopaque linear densities on chest X-ray, and the pulmonary arteries are prominent in the hilar area. COPD patients with both disorders show a varying combination of these changes.[17,19]

Pulmonary Function Changes. Basic *spirometry testing* is the gold standard in diagnosing airflow limitation. Forced expiratory maneuvers identify airflow limitation and its severity. Testing the improvement of the FEV_1 after administering a short-acting beta 2 bronchodilator identifies the degree of reversibility of the airflow obstruction.

- The presence of a postbronchodilator FEV_1/FVC <70% and an FEV_1 <80% of predicted is diagnostic for airflow limitation that is not fully reversible.[1]
- An increase of 12% or more in the FEV_1 or FVC is the minimal improvement required for maintenance bronchodilator therapy.
- If the expiratory volumes improve more than 20%, the patient is diagnosed with an additional asthmatic condition; this degree of increase indicates partial reversibility.[24]

A *diffusion study* is a pulmonary function test that differentiates between emphysema and the other COPD diseases. Pulmonary emphysema is the only disease under the COPD triad (pulmonary emphysema, chronic bronchitis, and bronchiectasis) and asthma that shows a reduced single-breath carbon monoxide–diffusing capacity. Emphysema causes a loss of a large percentage of the alveolar capillary bed, and the reduced alveolar surface area decreases the diffusion capacity of the lung.[17]

Arterial blood gas measurement is used as supporting documentation in diagnosing COPD. Hypoxemia is present in both chronic bronchitis and late-stage emphysema. Hypercarbia is characteristic of a subpopulation of patients with chronic bronchitis and is seen in people with end-stage emphysema (FEV_1 <1 L).[17]

CLINICAL MANIFESTATIONS

Normally, patients do not have pure emphysema or pure chronic bronchitis. The signs and symptoms of COPD are a composite of the signs and symptoms of patients with varying combinations of asthma, emphysema, and chronic bronchitis. Patients with elements of more than one disease show combined symptoms:

- Dyspnea on exertion or at rest (emphysema)
- Productive cough of mucoid sputum (chronic bronchitis)
- Wheezing (chronic bronchitis)
- Distant breath sounds and use of accessory muscles (emphysema)
- Barrel chest (emphysema)
- Hypoxemia (chronic bronchitis, end-stage emphysema)
- Hypercarbia in end-stage disease (chronic bronchitis, end-stage emphysema)
- Slightly reversible airflow limitation in response to bronchodilators (chronic bronchitis)
- Systemic signs of cor pulmonale (early in chronic bronchitis, late in emphysema)[17,19]

The COPD patient with hyper-reactive airways (asthmatic component) demonstrates partial reversibility of airflow limitation in response to beta 2 bronchodilators. Emphysema patients may show no or little improvement in expiratory flows after bronchodilator therapy, and chronic bronchitics may be somewhere between the two extremes.[17,19]

STAGES OF COPD

The Global Initiative for Chronic Obstructive Lung Disease (GOLD) identified four stages of COPD: mild, moderate, severe, and very severe. These classifications are defined by postbronchodilator spirometry results (Table 9-7). The most general criterion for COPD is the

TABLE 9-7 **GOLD classifications of COPD**

Stages of COPD	Pulmonary Function Criteria	Clinical Manifestations
Stage I Mild COPD	FEV_1/FVC <70% FEV_1 ≥80% of predicted	Unaware of limitations ± Cough, sputum production
Stage II Moderate COPD	FEV_1/FVC <70% FEV_1 ≥50% to < 80% of predicted	Seeks medical attention because of symptoms or exacerbation episode Dyspnea on exertion ± Cough, sputum production
Stage III Severe COPD	FEV_1/FVC <70% FEV_1 ≥30 – <50% of predicted	↑ Dyspnea, reduced exercise tolerance, fatigue ± Cough, sputum production ↑ number of exacerbations
Stage IV Very Severe COPD	FEV_1/FVC <70% FEV_1 <30% of predicted OR FEV_1 <50% plus chronic respiratory failure (PaO_2 <60 mm Hg, ±$PaCO_2$ >60 mm Hg)	Evidence of cor pulmonale (pitting ankle edema, jugular venous distention) Dyspnea at rest, fatigue ± Cough, sputum production Life-threatening exacerbations

presence of airflow obstruction as indicated by FEV_1/FVC <0.70. Severity is determined by the FEV_1 in relation to its predicted value based on age, height, sex, and race.

COMPLICATIONS

The major complications of COPD are frequent infections, cor pulmonale, respiratory failure, sleeping disorders, and pneumothorax. These complications can cause deterioration in the patient's quality and length of life.[17,19]

Infections. An acute exacerbation is the cause of considerable morbidity and mortality in patients with COPD. Most of the exacerbations are secondary to lower respiratory tract infections. The most common microorganism strains cultured from the sputum are *Haemophilus influenzae*, *Streptococcus pneumoniae*, and *Moraxella catarrhalis*.[17,19] COPD patients in an acute exacerbation show a worsening of respiratory symptoms. They may have fever; the sputum changes from mucoid to purulent; the dyspnea worsens; and pulmonary function measurements deteriorate, with a drop in the P_AO_2, possible hypercarbia, and a decrease in FEV_1 or PEFR. They may also have a worsening of cor pulmonale in conjunction with the acute exacerbation. As the disease worsens, the acute exacerbation episodes occur more frequently and may cause acute respiratory failure.[17,19]

Cor Pulmonale. Cor pulmonale is defined as right heart failure secondary to lung disease. Cor pulmonale results from the effects of chronic hypoxemia on the pulmonary vasculature. Hypoxemia causes pulmonary vasoconstriction that increases the right ventricle's afterload. Pumping against the chronically high pulmonary vascular pressures increases right heart muscle work, which eventually causes right-sided heart failure. The treatment of cor pulmonale is to treat the underlying cause: lung disease. Maximizing the COPD patient's lung function and gas exchange is the best way to definitively treat cor pulmonale. Continuous oxygen therapy may be necessary to raise the P_AO_2 and to eliminate the stimulus for vasoconstriction. If pulmonary hypertension persists, long-term alpha-adrenergic antagonist therapy may be helpful in treating pulmonary hypertension and thus in improving heart function.[17,19]

Sleep Quality. Sleep quality is significantly affected in patients with COPD.[25] Insomnia, sleep-disordered breathing, and obstructive sleep apnea affect COPD patients, many of which have multiple health problems. Insomnia is common among people with COPD. Factors that could contribute to the inability to remain asleep at night are cough, dyspnea, and arousals associated with increasing P_ACO_2, oxygen desaturation, and medications that help breathing function but promote wakefulness.[26] During sleep, alveolar ventilation and P_AO_2 decrease and CO_2 increases in normal subjects. However, in the COPD population, their oxygen baseline values are lower than normal and their hypoventilation during sleep results in more severe drops in oxygen saturation, especially in REM (rapid eye movement) sleep. The acute episodes of hypoxemia during sleep lead to pulmonary vasoconstriction and put the person with COPD at a greater risk for developing persistent pulmonary hypertension and cor pulmonale. Obstructive sleep apnea (OSA) can occur in the COPD population. If they complain of disrupted sleep, daytime sleepiness, it may not be just insomnia. OSA should be considered by the physician as a possible problem in a patient who is complaining of insomnia.[26]

Acute respiratory failure is defined by a deterioration in the patient's arterial blood gas secondary to a worsening in lung function brought about by an acute infection, pneumothorax, or exacerbation of cor pulmonale. *Respiratory failure* is described as a state of alveolar hypoventilation in which the pH is less than 7.25, the P_ACO_2 is more than 60 mm Hg, and the P_AO_2 is less than 50 mm Hg. Intensive bronchial hygiene may help to avert intubation and mechanical ventilation. For the patient who is chronically hypercarbic, the arterial pH and P_AO_2 are used as the primary guidelines to determine respiratory failure.[19]

Pneumothorax. Pneumothorax is a possible complication of COPD. People with bullae are very vulnerable to rupture and subsequent pneumothorax. Other causes of pneumothorax are mechanical ventilation or other medical procedures that may lacerate the lung (e.g., a central IV line placement, thoracentesis).[19]

TREATMENT

Maintenance therapy in patients with COPD is very important in decreasing life-crippling symptoms, in decreasing the number of exacerbations, in improving quality of life, and possibly in extending life. The treatment regimen depends on disease severity (based on FEV_1) and on whether the patient has asthma as a component of the airflow limitation.

The first step in the treatment for COPD is to encourage the patient to stop smoking. This step is critical in mild to moderate COPD because smoking cessation slows disease progression. In severe COPD, smoking cessation reduces symptoms and exacerbation frequency. Many smoking cessation programs, quitting strategies, and behavior modification techniques may help the long-term smoker quit. When attempting to quit, the smoker is prone to relapses and may attempt to quit many times before being successful.[17,19]

Drug Therapy. The drugs used to treat COPD have many similarities to those used for asthma. An important difference is that the airflow limitation in COPD without an asthmatic component does not respond well to bronchodilator therapy. In COPD, the improvement is mild (about 12–15%), but the alleviation of symptoms may be appreciable. The goals of drug therapy in the treatment of COPD are to:

- Increase the positive effects of smoking cessation or reduction.
- Relieve dyspnea using bronchodilator therapy.
- Treat the episodic exacerbations of COPD.
- Preserve lung function and reduce its rate of decline.[17,19]

Bronchodilator medications are central to the management of people with COPD. They are given as rescue drugs for relief of persistent or worsening COPD and as maintenance drugs. The principle bronchodilators are beta 2 agonists, anticholinergics, and methlyxanthines. These medicines can be used alone or in combination.[1]

Beta 2 bronchodilators, used for many people with COPD, reduce airway obstruction secondary to bronchoconstriction. People with COPD have an irreversible or slightly reversible airflow limitation. If a patient does not initially respond to short-acting beta 2 agonists, a lengthy maintenance trial of this drug frequently results in symptomatic or pulmonary function improvement sometime after the bronchodilator trial. The relief of dyspnea without an accompanying increase in FEV_1 is sufficient cause for continuing to prescribe bronchodilator therapy to the patient with chronic lung disease. Improving quality of life is an important determinant of treatment efficacy.

Beta 2 agonists are available for inhalation as dry powder for self-actuation, in an MDI (metered-dose inhaler), and as liquids for nebulizing. The choice of the inhaler device depends on the physician, availability, costs, and individual coordination skills. People who have difficulty with the system can have an MDI space chamber added or use a breath-activated device.[1]

The anticholinergic drugs (ipratropium, oxitropium, and tiotropium bromide) have a greater role for relief of bronchospasm in COPD than in asthma. This drug group causes bronchodilation by blocking acetylcholine's effect on the M3 (muscarinic 3) receptors. They may also inhibit airway hyper-reactivity to nonspecific agents such as smoke or strong scents in cosmetics. This drug group has a longer duration of action than the short-acting beta 2 bronchodilators. Tiotropium, the longest acting of all the anticholinergic drugs, has a duration of action of 24 hours. It is suggested that ipratropium be used in mild to severe COPD. Combination therapy with a beta 2 drug should be added in moderate COPD. Anticholinergic drugs are available in an MDI or as a liquid for nebulization.[1,19]

Theophylline-based medications have been used in chronic lung disease for decades. The mechanism of bronchodilation is not well understood. Theophylline is known to have many beneficial effects for some people with COPD. Improvement in diaphragmatic contraction has been reported as well as an anti-inflammatory effect. One study of the therapeutic effects of theophylline reported the anti-inflammatory effect that theophylline demonstrated in a study on asthmatics.[27] The report indicated that, in the treatment of COPD, theophylline, when used in conjunction with other bronchodilator drugs, adds to the other drugs' bronchodilator effects. However, because of the potential for drug toxicity, inhaled bronchodilators are preferred.[1]

The routine use of antimicrobials in COPD is not indicated. Antimicrobial therapy is suggested as treatment for patients in an acute exacerbation secondary to a lower respiratory tract bacterial infection. The choice of antimicrobial therapy is based on the susceptibility of the likely pathogens. Drug-resistant strains are becoming a problem in treating pneumonia.[1,17,19]

Unlike their effect in asthma cases, oral and inhaled corticosteroids do not modify the progressive deterioration in lung function. However, the regular use of inhaled steroids in symptomatic Stage III and Stage IV COPD patients reduces the frequency of exacerbations and improves quality of life. Currently, maintenance treatment with inhaled steroids, especially the inhaled steroid combined with the long-acting beta 2 agonist, is recommended for a patient with more advanced COPD who is demonstrating repeated exacerbations.[1]

In the recent past, a trial of oral steroids was suggested for patients who are receiving optimal therapy and are still symptomatic. Discouraging steroid trials is the lack of clinical evidence that a short course of steroids can be used to predict the long-term response to inhaled steroids in COPD. Steroids cause too many serious side effects—such as diabetes, hypertension, and increased infections—in exchange for simply a greater sense of well-being.[1,17]

The use of oral steroids in COPD has changed in recent years. Short-term therapeutic trials of oral steroids are not recommended. Evidence suggests that a short-term trial of steroids does not predict the success of inhaled steroids in patients not responding to bronchodilator therapy. Additionally, evidence-based research does not support long-term treatment with systemic steroids. The systemic side effects are too severe to use these drugs without solid proof of their effectiveness.[1]

Other Treatment. Other directions for treating the patient with COPD are lung transplantation, lung volume reduction therapy, the replacement of alpha-1 antitrypsin, and pulmonary rehabilitation. These treatments are widely different in their impact on the patient's life. Their effects range from curative, as in the case of a lung transplant, to improving the quality of life for patients with a terminal illness, as in pulmonary rehabilitation.

Most COPD patients on the waiting list for *lung transplantation* have emphysema. The types of lung transplants are single-lung, double-lung, and living-related lung. Not all emphysema patients qualify for lung transplantation. They must meet stringent criteria before they are put on the transplant waiting list.[28] The criteria for lung transplantation are:

- Limited life expectancy.
- No alternative effective medical or surgical therapy.
- Being currently ambulatory.
- Having adequate nutritional status and acceptable left ventricular function without significant coronary artery disease.
- Age (single lung, younger than 65; double lung, younger than 60; heart-lung, younger than 55).

The exclusionary criteria are followed closely because of the desire to give the organ to people with the greatest chance of a successful outcome. The situations that disqualify a person for a lung transplant are:

- Recurring or active drug-resistant infections.
- Noncompliance with medical regimens.
- Being HIV-positive, hepatitis B–positive, or hepatitis C–positive status.
- Ventilator dependency.
- Receiving prednisone therapy of more than 20 mg/day.
- Mental instability.
- Current substance abuse.
- Malignancy within past 2 years.
- Dysfunction of other major organs.[28]

The most common type of lung transplant in the COPD patient is the single-lung transplant. This procedure is simpler than the others, does not require cardiopulmonary bypass, and has lower surgical and postoperative morbidity and mortality rates. Patients will need to be on immunosuppressive therapy for the rest of their lives.

Successful *lung volume reduction surgery* (*LVRS*) helps to reduce the number of COPD patients on the waiting list for lung transplantation. The surgery has reemerged as a treatment for end-stage COPD. Nonfunctioning areas of the emphysematous lung are removed to reduce hyperinflation and to improve lung mechanics and gas exchange. The National Emphysema Treatment Trial identified four subgroups of patients who had different surgical risks and different benefits from the surgery:

- Group 1 patients have mostly upper lobe emphysema and low exercise capacity.

- Group 2 patients have mostly upper lobe emphysema and high exercise capacity.
- Group 3 patients have diffuse emphysema and low exercise capacity.
- Group 4 patients have diffuse emphysema and high exercise capacity.

Groups 1 and 2 consist of the types of the patients who would benefit the most from lung volume reduction. They have localized disease, and removing the diseased lung decreases the areas of hyperinflation and improves lung mechanics, exercise tolerance, and quality of life. Groups 1 and 2 would benefit the most from lung volume reduction. Groups III and IV have disease that affect the entire lung so that, despite removing hyperinflated lung areas, the remaining lung would be still very diseased. These patients do not demonstrate significant improvement after surgery and are not candidates for LVRS. Their only possible avenue is lung transplant surgery.[28,29]

Small numbers of patients with COPD have premature emphysema secondary to alpha-1 antitrypsin deficiency (AAT). To qualify for alpha-1 proteinase inhibitor replacement therapy, patient must:

- Be a nonsmoker.
- Be over the age of 18.
- Have low serum concentration of A1-A <50 mg/dL or < 11μM/L or < 0.8g/L (35% of normal).
- Have progressive emphysema with a documented rate of decline in FEV_1.
- Be vaccinated with the hepatitis B vaccine series before administration.

The API drug is given by IV once per week or every 2–4 weeks, and the usual dose is 60 gm/kg/week. Patients must remain on this drug for the rest of their lives. There is a national registry for people who qualify for replacement therapy.[17]

Bronchiectasis

It is estimated that approximately 100,000 people in the United States have non–cystic fibrosis bronchiectasis. Most of the people with this type of bronchiectasis are over the age of 75. In recent years, the disease appeared to be more of historical interest. However, with the advent of more advanced imaging such as the high-resolution CT, the disease has been found to be more prevalent than previously thought.[30] Certain demographic groups have an increased risk for developing bronchiectasis, such as people with decreased access to health care, those with high rates of childhood pulmonary infections (cystic fibrosis is a prominent risk), and those with chronic airway disease such as chronic bronchitis.

"*Bronchiectasis* is an anatomic distortion of the conducting airways that results in chronic cough, sputum production and recurrent cough."[30] It was first described by Laennec in 1819 as abnormally dilated bronchi and bronchioles due to recurring episodes of infection and inflammation.[30,31] The airway dilation is chronic and irreversible and usually affects the medium-sized bronchi (4th–9th generations). The chronic airway inflammation and pooling of infected secretions sets up a cycle of repeated serious pulmonary infections with damage that is progressive and causes deteriorating lung function.

DIAGNOSIS

Someone with suspected bronchiectasis presents to the physician with a chronic cough productive of mucopurulent secretions. Although the physical findings are generic for many types of lung problems, the clinical findings are less common: hemoptysis, digital clubbing, and excessive sputum production with position change. Pulmonary function findings are unrevealing, with airway limitation ranging from mild to severe. The imaging study that definitively diagnoses bronchiectasis is the high-resolution CT (HRCT) scan. It has replaced the bronchogram as the gold standard for radiologic diagnosis of bronchiectasis.[30] HRCT findings reveal bronchial dilation with the appearance of the classic signet ring sign (the internal bronchial diameter is greater than the diameter of the accompanying bronchial artery) and the lack of bronchial tapering of the affected bronchial segmental generations. The three classic patterns of airway distortion in bronchiectasis are cylindrical, varicose, and saccular/cystic. Many people with bronchiectasis have all three abnormal changes to their bronchi. Those with a predominance of the saccular/cystic bronchiectasis have a higher incidence of *Pseudomonas aeruginosa* cultures and a poorer prognosis.[30,31]

ETIOLOGIES

The causes of bronchiectasis are organized as idiopathic, postinfection, or underlying disease. These categories overlap.

In the *idiopathic* category is a long list of diseases or conditions that frequently are unknown at the time the person is identified as having bronchiectasis but that are diagnosed at a later time. The idiopathic cause has subtypes such as:

- Secondary genetic immunologic dysfunction or autoimmune abnormalities.
- Genetic causes, such as cystic fibrosis, primary immotile cilia syndrome, and alpha-1 antitrypsin deficiency.

- IgG immune deficiency and immune-related dysfunction, such as allergic bronchopulmonary aspergillosis collagen vascular diseases and inflammatory bowel diseases.
- Chronic gastric aspiration, foreign body aspiration, and endobronchial tumors.

Nontuberculous mycobacteria (NTM) infections are associated with bronchiectasis, but it is not clear whether NTM actually causes or bronchiectasis or if bronchiectasis increases the patient's susceptibility to NTM.

Another group with a significant incidence of coexisting bronchiectasis is the COPD population. A study using HRCT revealed that 50% of a cohort of patients with stable COPD who had a mean FEV_1 <0.96 L had bronchiectasis. Additionally, COPD patients with bronchiectasis had more severe exacerbations, more colonization of their lower airway with bacteria, and more inflammatory markers in their sputum. Although asthmatics have a much lower reported incidence of bronchiectasis, a research study revealed a 3% incidence of bronchiectasis in a group of patients with severe persistent asthma.[30,32]

TREATMENT

Treatment of bronchiectasis is directed toward reducing the frequency of exacerbations and improving quality of life. The organisms commonly cultured from the diseased bronchi are nonenteric gram-negative bacteria, *Staphylococcus aureus*, and NTM. Cystic fibrosis (CF) should be ruled out in those with chronic cultures of *Staphylococcus aureus*. Approximately one-third of bronchiectasis patients are colonized with *Pseudomonas aeruginosa;* these patients have a greater number of exacerbations and greater deterioration in lung function.[30]

Oral or IV antibiotics are used only in acute exacerbations. However, studies on the benefit of inhaled maintenance antibiotics indicate that it may be beneficial to use a regimen of inhaled tobramycin or colistin in patients with frequent exacerbations. However, the concern is that the patient may develop antibiotic resistance.

Using the same respiratory medications and mechanical mobilization of secretions for CF-bronchiectasis and non-CF bronchiectasis is not recommended.

- Short-acting or long-acting beta adrenergic bronchodilators and anticholinergic bronchodilators are commonly used as maintenance therapy, but their effectiveness is not clear.
- The mucolytic agent, recombinant human dornase alfa, a standard of care in CF-bronchiectasis, causes adverse side effects in patients with non-CF bronchiectasis.
- Nebulized hypertonic saline (7%), a new form of therapy in CF-bronchiectasis, may be beneficial in non-CF bronchiectasis, but more evidence-based research should be performed before it is routinely used.
- Mechanical aids to augment sputum mobilization are effective in CF-bronchiectasis, but little research in the non-CF type of bronchiectasis is available. These treatments may still be used in both types of bronchiectasis, but their effectiveness is unproven.

Summary

The airflow limitation diseases discussed in this chapter are asthma, chronic bronchitis bronchiectasis, and emphysema. Asthma is in a separate category of airflow limitation because it is a reversible disease that responds to bronchodilator therapy. Chronic bronchitis, bronchiectasis, and emphysema are known by the acronym COPD. The airway obstruction in these diseases is not reversed by bronchodilators, and the disease results in permanent and progressive changes. In people who are asthmatic, the inflammation causes recurrent episodes of wheezing, dyspnea, chest tightness, and coughing. The airflow obstruction may reverse spontaneously, or it may require treatment for reversal. Exposure to environmental triggers elicits a hypersensitivity reaction in the bronchial epithelium of allergic patients, which may result in a rapid worsening in respiratory function. Other causes of exacerbation are viral infection, exercise, and inhalation of irritants.

COPD is characterized by the presence of chronic bronchitis, emphysema, or both. The COPD patient has progressive airflow limitation that may be partially reversible in those patients with hyper-reactive airways. Emphysema is present when there are permanent dilation and destruction of lung units distal to the terminal bronchioles.

Chronic bronchitis is the predominant cause of COPD. Chronic bronchitis is defined functionally as an individual having a chronically productive cough lasting 3 or more consecutive months for 2 successive years. Bronchiectasis is an anatomic distortion of the conducting airways that results in chronic cough, sputum production, and recurrent cough. The airway dilation is chronic and irreversible, usually affecting medium-sized airways. It is the result of recurring episodes of infection and inflammation.

A deficiency of alph-1 antitrypsin is a genetic disease involving a decreased ability to block the activity of proteolytic enzymes. A deficiency in the enzyme results in the unopposed proteolysis of elastin in the lung and the liver. The increased breakdown of elastin leads to the development of panacinar emphysema.

Basic spirometry is the gold standard for diagnosing airflow limitation. Forced expiratory maneuvers identify airflow limitation and its severity. The differentiation between emphysema and other diseases that limit airflow is based on the measurement of carbon monoxide diffusing capacity. Because emphysema results in the loss of alveolar surface area, the carbon monoxide diffusing capacity of the lung is decreased.

The major complications of COPD are frequent infections, cor pulmonale, respiratory failure, sleeping disorders, and pneumothorax. These complications can cause deterioration of the patient's quality and length of life.

Study Questions

REVIEW QUESTIONS

1. What are the differences between asthma, chronic bronchitis, and emphysema?
2. List and define the clinical categories of asthma.
3. Compare the clinical presentation of a patient with emphysema to that of a patient with asthma.
4. Differentiate between atopic and nonatopic asthma.
5. What are the three main types of emphysema? What are the differences among them?

MULTIPLE-CHOICE QUESTIONS

1. What postbronchodilator change in FEV_1 or FVC is considered a minimally acceptable improvement for prescribing bronchodilator therapy?
   a. 6%
   b. 12%
   c. 18%
   d. 20%
2. Which of the following diseases is not classified as an airflow limitation disease?
   a. pneumothorax
   b. asthma
   c. bronchiectasis
   d. chronic bronchitis
3. Which of following is *not* an etiology of bronchiectasis?
   a. cystic fibrosis
   b. immunologic dysfunction
   c. inflammatory bowel disease
   d. allergy to tree pollen
4. What is a common bacterial organism cultured from the sputum of patients with chronic bronchitis?
   a. *Pseudomonas aeruginosa*
   b. *Haemophilus influenzae*
   c. *Staphylococcus aureus*
   d. *Mycoplasma pneumonia*
5. What medication is preferred in patients receiving step 5 asthma maintenance therapy?
   a. low-dose inhaled steroids and a long-acting beta 2 bronchodilator
   b. medium-dose inhaled steroids and sustained-release theophylline
   c. high-dose inhaled steroids and inhaled long-acting beta 2 bronchodilator
   d. high-dose leukotriene antagonist and low-dose inhaled steroids
6. This asthma patient has an FEV_1 of 72% and complains of awakening at night about 1–2 times a week because of difficulty breathing, and his peak flow rates varies about 35% during the day. What is this patient's severity of asthma?
   a. mild intermittent asthma
   b. mild persistent asthma
   c. moderate persistent asthma
   d. severe persistent asthma
7. What is the recommended rescue medication for the patient with asthma?
   a. high-dose inhaled steroid
   b. inhaled cromolyn sodium
   c. leukotriene receptor antagonist
   d. short-acting beta 2 bronchodilator
8. This COPD patient has an FEV_1/FVC of 65%, FEV_1 of 62%. Using the GOLD classification, what is the severity of his COPD?
   a. Stage I
   b. Stage II
   c. Stage III
   d. Stage IV
9. What radiographic changes are consistent with pulmonary emphysema?
   a. air bronchogram extending to the peripheral lung fields
   b. increased radiodensity of the lung in the lower lobes
   c. increased bronchial markings
   d. low flat diaphragm
10. What clinical manifestation is commonly observed in patients with pulmonary emphysema?
    a. pronounced expiratory wheezing
    b. dyspnea on exertion
    c. digital clubbing
    d. cyanosis

CRITICAL-THINKING QUESTIONS

1. How are COPD with emphysema and emphysema caused by alpha-1 antitrypsin deficiency different? Briefly describe the typical course of therapy for each.
2. Define the two main elements of an asthma management program.
3. What are the three stages of an asthma attack? What are the differences between them? How would the treatment plan differ between stages?

References

1. Ishikawa N, Ohlmeier S, Salmenkivi K, Myllärniemi M, Rahman I, Mazur W, Kinnula VL. Hemoglobin α and β are ubiquitous in the human lung, decline in idiopathic pulmonary fibrosis but not in COPD. *Respir Res.* 2010;11,1:123.
2. *National Asthma Education and Prevention Program, Expert Panel Report 3: Guidelines for the diagnosis and management of asthma.* 2007.
3. Akinbami L. Asthma prevalence, health care use and mortality; United States, 2003–2005. In: *National Center for Health E-Stat.* Office of Analysis and Epidemiology. October 15, 2008. http://www.cdc.gov/nchs/products/pubs/pubd/hestats/ashtma03-05/asthma03-05.htm
4. Weiss KB, Sullivan SD. The health economics of asthma and rhinitis. I. Assessing the economic impact. *J Allergy Clin Immunol.* 2001;107,1:3–8.
5. Partridge M. Airway diseases:asthma:clinical features, diagnosis, and treatment. In: Albert R, Spiro S, Jet J, eds. *Comprehensive Respiratory Medicine.* St. Louis: Mosby: St. Louis; 1999:41, 1–41, 18.
6. Douglass J, O'Hehir RE. What determines asthma phenotype? Respiratory infections and asthma. *Am J Resp Crit Care Med.* 2000;161,3:S211–214.
7. Sandford AJ, Pare PD. The genetics of asthma. the important questions. *Am. J. Respir. Crit. Care Med.* 2000;161,3:S202–S206.
8. Rossenwasser LJ. Allergic and other hypersensitivity disorders. In: Beers M, et al, eds. *The Merck Manual of Diagnosis and Therapy.* Whitehouse Station, NJ: Merck Research Laboratories; 2006:1348–1364.
9. Elias JA. Airway remodeling in asthma, unanswered questions. *Am. J. Respir. Crit. Care Med.* 2000;161,3:S168–S171.
10. Martin RJ. Asthma. In: Beers M, et al, eds. *The Merck Manual of Diagnosis and Therapy.* Whitehouse Station, NJ: Merck Research Laboratories; 2006:381–399.
11. Zorc JJ, Pusic MV, Ogborn CJ, Lebet R, Duggan AK. Ipratropium bromide added to asthma treatment in the pediatric emergency department. *Pediatrics.* 1999;103,4:748–752.
12. Qureshi F, Pestian J, Davis P, Zaritsky A. Effect of nebulized ipratropium on the hospitalization rates of children with asthma. *N Engl J Med.* 1998;339,15:1030–1035.
13. Rodrigo GJ, Rodrigo C, Burschtin O. A meta analysis of the effects of ipratropium bromide in adults with acute asthma. *Am J Med.* 1999; 107,363–370.
14. Pedersen S. Why does airway inflammation persist? Is it failure to treat early? *Am J Resp Crit Care Med.* 2000;161,S182–S185.
15. Anderson GP. Interactions between corticosteroids and beta-adrenergic agonists in asthma disease induction, progression, and exacerbation. *Am. J. Respir. Crit. Care Med.* 2000;161,3:S188–S196.
16. Centers for Disease Control, *National Center for Health Statistics. 2006. Health, United States, with Chartbook on Trends in the Health of Americans. U.S. Department of Health and Human Services*: Hyattsville, MD: National Center for Health Statistics:1–559.
17. Celli B, Benditt J, Albert R. Airway diseases: chronic airflow limitation: chronic obstructive pulmonary disease. In: Albert R, Spiro S, Jett J, eds. *Comprehensive Respiratory Medicine.* St. Louis: Mosby: 1999:7.37.1–7.37.24.
18. Corrin B. *Diseases* Characterized by airflow limitation. In: *Pathology of the Lung.* Churchill Livingstone: London; 2000:79–120.
19. Wise RA. Chronic obstructive pulmonary disease. In: Beers M, et al, eds. *The Merck Manual of Diagnosis and Therapy.* Whitehouse Station, NJ: Merck Research Laboratories, 2006:400–412.
20. Saetta M. Airway inflammation in chronic obstructive pulmonary disease. *Am J Resp Crit Care Med.* 1990;160:S17–S20.
21. American Thoracic Society statement. Cigarette smoking and health. *Am J Resp Crit Care Med.* 1996;153:861–865.
22. Leonard C, Sach D. Environmental tobacco smoke and lung cancer incidence. *Curr Opin Pulm Med.* 1999;5:189–193.
23. Sun G, Stacey M, Vittori E, Marini M, Bellini A, Kieimberg J, et al. Cellular and molecular characteristics of inflammation in chronic bronchitis. *Eur J Clin Invest.* 1998;28:346–372.
24. American Thoracic Society. Standardization of spirometry. *Am J Resp Crit Care Med.* 1995;152:1107–1136.
25. Stege G, Vos P, van den Elshout F, Dekhuijzen R, van de Ven M, Heijdra Y. Sleep, hypnotics and chronic obstructive pulmonary disease. *Respir Med.* 2008;102,6:801–814.

26. Neubauer DN. *Insomnia and comorbid chronic obstructive pulmonary disease: a case study*. Medscape LLC. December 18, 2008.
27. Peleman R, Kips J, Pauwels R. Therapeutic activities of theophylline in chronic obstructive pulmonary disease. *Clin Exp Allergy.* 1998;28:53–56.
28. Dauber J, Corns P. Lung transplantation. In: Albert RK, Spiro SG, Jett JR, eds. *Comprehensive Respiratory Medicine*. St. Louis: Mosby; 1999:78.1–78.16.
29. Martinez F, de Oca M, Whyte R, Stetz J, Gay S, Celli B. Lung-volume reduction improves dyspnea, dynamic hyperinflation, and respiratory muscle function. *American Journal of Respiratory and Critical Care Medicine*. 1997;155,6:1984–1990.
30. O'Donnell AE. Bronchiectasis. *Chest.* 2008;134, 4:815–823.
31. Spencer H. Diseases of the bronchial tree In: *Pathology of the Lung*. New York: Pergamon Press; 1985:147–165.
32. Patel IS, Vlahos I, Wilkinson TMA, Lloyd-Owen SJ, Donaldson GC, Wilks M, et al. Bronchiectasis, exacerbation indices, and inflammation in chronic obstructive pulmonary disease. *Am. J. Respir. Crit. Care Med.* 2004;170,4:400–407.

CHAPTER 10

Diffuse Parenchymal Lung Diseases

Barbara Ludwig

OBJECTIVES

Upon completion of this chapter, the reader should be able to:

- Describe the difference categories of diffuse parenchymal lung diseases (DPLDs).
- Identify the four types of idiopathic interstitial pneumonias.
- Discuss the diagnosis and medical treatment of DPLDs.
- Describe an organization of different types of DPLDs.
- Identify the proposed mechanism of inflammation and fibrosis in diffuse lung disease.
- Describe the general X-ray changes in patients with DPLD.

CHAPTER OUTLINE

Diffuse Parenchymal Lung Diseases
- Incidence and Prevalence in the Population
- Mortality Rates
- Etiology
- Pathogenesis
- Phase 1: Antigen Trigger
- Phase 2: Chronic Inflammation
- General Clinical Appearance
- Diagnosis
- Complications
- Treatment

KEY TERMS

basement membrane
etiology
extracellular matrix
honeycomb lung
idiopathic
pathogenesis
video-assisted thoracoscopic surgery (VATS)

The terminology used to talk about diffuse parenchymal lung diseases is inconsistent. In various sources, these diseases may be referred to as restrictive lung diseases, interstitial lung diseases (ILDs), or pulmonary fibrosis. The American Thoracic Society/European Respiratory Society International Multidisciplinary Consensus Group refers to this disease group as *diffuse parenchymal lung diseases* (*DPLDs*). That organization also changed the classification of **idiopathic** (of uncertain or unknown origin) interstitial pneumonias. (See Table 10-1 for the new terminology.)[1]

Diffuse parenchymal lung diseases encompass all of the pulmonary and systemic diseases that cause infiltration into the alveolar airspace and the interstitium of the lung. The infiltration results in the thickening of the alveolar capillary membrane with an associated decrease in lung compliance and gas exchange. The wide variety of diseases that cause diffuse parenchymal and interstitial damage range, among many others, from idiopathic lung diseases, environmental lung diseases, drug toxicity, and collagen vascular diseases to hemorrhagic diseases of the lung.[1,2]

Approximately 190 disorders can cause diffuse parenchymal lung disease. The individual diseases or disorders are complex and are not specifically discussed in this chapter. Rather, employing a general perspective, the aim is to impart a broad understanding of the pathology, pathophysiology, clinical features, diagnosis, and treatment of diffuse parenchymal lung disease.

TABLE 10-1 **Classification of diffuse parenchymal lung diseases**

Categories	Specific Diseases	
DPLD of Known Cause	**Collagen vascular diseases**	
	Rheumatoid arthritis, Scleroderma, Systemic Lupus Erythematosus, Ankylosing spondylitis, Sjogren Syndrome, Mixed Connective Tissue Disease	
	Drug-induced interstitial disease	
	Cytotoxic agents, Certain antibiotics, Certain antiarrhythmics, Illicit drugs, Anti-inflammatory drugs	
	Radiation Exposure	
	Pulmonary Alveolar Proteinosis	
	Environmental Lung Diseases	
	Hypersensitivity Pneumonitis: *Farmers Lung, Baggassosis, Bird Breeder's Lung*	
	Pneumoconiosis: *Asbestosis, Berylliosis, Silicosis, Anthracosilicosis, Coal worker's lung*	
	Inherited DPLD	
	Familial IPF or Sarcoidosis, Tuberous sclerosis, Neurofibromatosis, Niemann-Pick disease, Gaucher disease, Hermansky-Pudlak syndrome	
Idiopathic Interstitial Pneumonias	**Idiopathic interstitial fibrosis** Formerly known as *Usual interstitial pneumonia* (UIP) or *end-stage lung*	**Other interstitial pneumonias:** *Desquamative interstitial pneumonia (DIP), Acute interstitial pneumonia (AIP) or Hamman-Rich syndrome,* *Non-specific interstitial pneumonia (NSIP),* *Respiratory bronchiolitis ILD, Cryptogenic organizing pneumonia (COP) formerly idiopathic BOOP* *Lymphocytic interstitial pneumonia (LIP)*
Granulomatous DPLD	Sarcoidosis	
Other DPLD	**Lymphangioleiomyomatosis (LAM)**	
	Langerhans' cell Histiocytosis/Histiocystosis X	
	Pulmonary/Renal vasculitis: *Wegener's Granulomatosis, Goodpasture's Syndrome*	
	Pulmonary Eosinophilic Syndromes	
	Loeffler's Syndrome (eosinophilic pneumonia), Churg-Strauss Syndrome	

Diffuse Parenchymal Lung Diseases

The DPLDs are a heterogeneous group of disorders that damage the pulmonary parenchyma secondary to various disease-causing processes. The type of inflammatory cells activated and the inflammatory pathway leading to lung injury depends on the etiologic trigger or antigen stimulus. Despite these differences, the end results are the same: widespread inflammation and fibrosis.[3] However, even though their effects are the same, their treatments, their responses to treatment, and their prognoses all vary.

INCIDENCE AND PREVALENCE IN THE POPULATION

Studies of people with intrinsic lung diseases revealed an overall prevalence (i.e., people already diagnosed) of 3 to 6 cases per 100,000 persons and a prevalence of idiopathic pulmonary fibrosis of 27 to 29 cases per 100,000 persons. When examining people over the age of 75, the prevalence exceeded 175 cases per 100,000 persons.[4–6] The prevalence of sarcoidosis in the United States is 10 to 40 cases per 100,000 persons. The incidence (i.e., people just diagnosed) of DPLD in people with collagen vascular disease is increasing for most of the diseases in this category.[4]

MORTALITY RATES

The morbidity and mortality rates of people with DPLD vary with the disease. Factors that directly increase the mortality rate of the patient with DPLD are:

- Increased age.
- Male sex.
- Smoking history.
- Severe dyspnea.
- Severe loss of pulmonary function.
- Severe X-ray changes.
- Poor response to therapy.
- Prominent fibroblasts on pathology report are all.

The following mean mortality rates of people diagnosed with idiopathic interstitial pneumonias have widely disparate time measures because they are from different research reports:[7]

- Idiopathic pulmonary fibrosis mean mortality rate: 68% (5–6 years)
- Acute interstitial pneumonia mean mortality: 62% (1–2 months)
- Desquamative interstitial pneumonia mean mortality rate: 27% (12 years)
- Nonspecific interstitial pneumonia mean mortality: 11% (17 months)

ETIOLOGY

Many of the DPLDs have an unknown **etiology** (the cause of a disease). However, of the diseases having known etiologies, a large group of diseases consists of the environmental (occupational) lung diseases. Environmental lung diseases are the most common disease classification of all the DPLDs. These diseases are distributed geographically according to the industry and occupational concentrations in specific areas of the country.[8]

Environmental lung disease (Tables 10-2 and 10-3) is secondary to the inhalation of allergens, chemical gases, and environmental pollutants that elicit an immunological reaction in the lung, causing deposition of fibroblasts in the airways or alveolar tissue.[9–12] Whether disease occurs in any one individual depends on several variables:

- Pollutant particle density.
- Duration of exposure.
- Chemical properties of the pollutant.
- The individual's susceptibility to that environmental material.[8]

Duration of Exposure. The particle size for optimal deposition in the respiratory bronchioles and alveoli is in the range of 0.5–5 μm. The density of environmental pollutants of this size determines the dose (quantity of an agent administered). If fewer than 10 particles per milliliter of air are inhaled, then all the pollutant particles are eliminated from the lung by its defense mechanisms. If 1000 particles per milliliter are inhaled, then 90% of the particles are eliminated. However, if the particle density is 1 million particles per milliliter, then a high percentage of these pollutants will be retained in the lung. This type of pollutant density overwhelms the lung's normal defenses, and the particles cannot be removed by the normal mechanisms (e.g., cough, mucociliary escalator). For example, if dust exposure occurs over months to years, then the dust may cause a low-level inflammatory response that causes progressive lung injury.

Chemical Nature of the Pollutant. The chemistry of a pollutant's impact on the individual should be answered by the following questions:

- Does the pollutant easily elicit an immunological reaction from the individual?
- Is the pollutant a known agent that causes fibrosis formation (e.g., silicosis, asbestosis)? If the pollutant is fibrinogenic, then the damage is progressive and continues even if the individual is removed from possible exposure. In this situation, disease may appear years after the exposure has ceased.

TABLE 10-2 **Environmental lung diseases**

Pneumoconiosis (inorganic dusts)		Extrinsic Allergic Alveolitis or Hypersensitivity Pneumonitis (organic dusts)	
Silicosis	Silicone Dioxide **Occupations:** rock mining, rock quarrying, tunneling, foundry work, manufacturing (pottery, porcelain, abrasives), sandblasting, stonecutting	**Malt workers Lung**	Moldy Malt Antigen: *Aspergillus clavatus* or *Aspergillus fumigatus*
		Farmers Lung	Moldy hay, bedding, compost Antigen: *Micropolyspora faeni*
Asbestosis	**Fibrous silicate** **Occupations:** insulation, shipyard and construction workers, auto repair workers exposed to brake linings	**Toxic chemicals (see Table 10-3)**	Acid fumes, aldehydes, ammonia, anhydrides, cadmium fumes
		Bird Breeders Lung	Parrots, parakeets, pigeons, chickens, etc. Antigen: Bird serum proteins in droppings
Coal Workers	Silica **Occupation:** coal mining		
Berylliosis	Beryllium **Occupations:** workers in aerospace, nuclear weapons and electronic industries	**Bagassosis**	Moldy sugar cane Antigen: *Thermoactinomyces saccharii, candidus, or viridus*

Susceptibility of the Individual. The third factor that determines disease occurrence with environmental exposure is the susceptibility of the individual to the pollutant. The individual's atopy or immune function affects the person's susceptibility or tolerance to any exposure to environmental pollution.[2,8]

PATHOGENESIS

With the existence of approximately 190 disorders causing DPLD, the **pathogenesis** (origination and development of a disease), or evolution, of disease will not be uniform. The pathogenesis of DPLD is described only in general terms so that the details of specific diseases do not cause confusion. Numerous pathways can lead to pulmonary fibrosis, and this description may not include all the ways in which inflammation, lung and interstitial injury, and fibrosis develop.

PHASE 1: ANTIGEN TRIGGER

The first phase in the pathogenesis of diffuse lung disease is the antigen trigger. It is the initial underlying cause of lung and/or vascular inflammation and subsequent parenchymal injury. How the initial stimulus or antigen begins the fibrotic process varies with the disease. The antigen trigger could be a virus or toxin, an inhaled organic or inorganic agent, an antibody released from the immune system, or an unknown trigger. Fibrosis is the result of chronic inflammation due to persistent or recurrent exposure to a stimulant, irritant, or antigen causing parenchymal injury.[1,13]

PHASE 2: CHRONIC INFLAMMATION

The release of inflammatory cell activation and mediator from the injured lung's epithelial cells and vascular endothelial cells is the second phase of pulmonary fibrosis development. The types of immune cells released and chemical mediators produced vary with the antigen trigger and determine the pathway of inflammation and subsequent fibrosis. Specifically activated inflammatory cells could include eosinophils, mast cells, macrophages, neutrophils, lymphocytes, and multiple types of cytokines. Activated inflammatory cells are attracted to the area of injury, where they release chemicals that damage and fibrose the alveolar capillary membrane (ACM).

TABLE 10-3 **Toxic gas inhalation injury**

Inhalant	Information	General Injury
High Water Solubility		
Ammonia	***Industries***: Fertilizer production and use; refrigeration; manufacturing of dyes and plastics Household cleaners Besides inhalation it can be ingested and injure the GI tract or injure by direct contact with skin, or eyes On airway tissue forms ammonium hydroxide in an exothermic reaction causing significant thermal injury Alkaline burn causes liquefaction necrosis and deeply penetrates tissue Mild exposures: Conjunctival and UA inflammation, pain Moderate exposures: exaggerated mild symptoms Severe exposures: respiratory distress, productive cough, pulmonary edema, dysphagia	Primarily upper respiratory tract: drooling, mucosal edema, cough, stridor, eye irritation, skin irritation Serious cases pulmonary edema and ARDS
Chloramine	***Industries***: Disinfectant in muncipile water systems, Risk for hemodialysis patients and fish (denature Hb. and causes hemolytic anemia)	
Methyl isocyanate	***Industries***: Carbamate pesticides, adhesives, and rubber production Involved in Bhopal disaster ~3800 deaths immediately and thousands experienced morbidity and premature death Respiratory tract, skin, and mucus membrane irritation Eye exposure causes: burning, photophobia, blepharospams, tearing, lid edema, corneal ulceration with reversible blindness ***Prolonged exposure***: vomiting, diarrhea, dyspnea, cough progressing to pulmonary edema and possible ARDS	
Sulfur dioxide	***Industries***: winemaking, winery sanitation, refrigerant, reagent or solvent in laboratories, combustion of fossil fuels, smelting of sulfide ores, volcanic emissions On airway tissues forms sulfuric acid and sulfurous acids Contributes to formation of acid rain Causes Bronchoconstriction in asthmatics Besides inhalation it can injure by direct contact with skin, or eyes Exposure: intensely irritating to the eye and respiratory tract • UA irritation, nosebleeds, dysphagia, coughing • In 5–15 minutes – bronchospasm • Continued exposure – high pitched crackles, chest pain, tracheitis, laryngeal edema, chemical bronchopneumonia, pulmonary edema, cyanosis, asphyxia, death Most common form of death is asphyxiation from glottic spasms	
Intermediate Water Solubility		
Chlorine	***Industries***: Chemical, paper, textiles; sewage treatment; Household and swimming pool accidents; Largest single cause of major toxic On airway tissue forms hypochlorous and hydrochloric acids Hallmark: Non-cardiogenic pulmonary edema Residual effects: non-specific airway hyper responsiveness, some people develop fibrosis or bronchiolitis obliterans release incidents	Affects all airways, potential for delayed symptoms. Combination of high and low water soluble symptoms

(continues)

TABLE 10-3 **Toxic Gas Inhalation Injury *(continued)***

Inhalant	Information	General Injury
Hydrogen Sulfide	***Industries***: petroleum, viscose rayon, rubber, and mining ***Other***: volcanic eruptions, exposure to sewers, liquid manure pits, ships' holds, sulfur springs Also called "acid rain" Forms sulfuric acid and sulfurous acids Inhalation, direct contact, possible histotoxic hypoxia resulting in asphyxiation • Low levels – irritation to mucus membranes and respiratory system • High levels – neurologic and pulmonary symptoms • Very high levels – cardiopulmonary arrest due to brainstem toxicity	
Nitrogen oxides	***Industries***: arc welders, firefighters, military and aerospace personnel, explosives, farmers NO_2 converted to NO, HNO_3 (nitric acid) and HNO_2 in distal airways • Toxic to alveolar Type I cells and ciliated airways • Alters macrophage and immune function, causing impaired resistance to infection • Methhemoglobinemia • ARDS 2–6 weeks post exposure patients can develop Bronchiolitis obliterans or diffuse alveolar damage	Terminal airway epithelial injury
Low Water Solubility		
Phosgene	***Industries***: Production of aniline dyes, polycarbonate resins, coal tar, pesticides, isocyanates, polyurethane, pharmaceuticals ***Found in***: household solvents, dry cleaning fluid Produced in the combustion of methylene chloride in paint remover or trichloroethylene in degreasing agents A chemical warfare agent Known as: carbonic dichoride, carbon oxychloride, carbonyl dichloride, chloroformyl chloride, d-stoff, and green cross Mechanisms of injury: • Hydrolysis: Forms CO_2 and hydrochloric acid in distal airways • Acylation: Denatures protein, disrupts enzymes activates inflammatory cascade	Lower airway injury with inflammation and necrosis Causes non-cardiogenic pulmonary edema (ARDS)

Acute ACM injury results in the destruction of Type I alveolar epithelial cells and the complementary pulmonary capillary endothelial cells. Chronic inflammation causes permanent loss of the ACM extracellular matrix, including the basement membrane, obliteration and fibrosis of the alveoli with fusion of adjacent basement membrane tissue remnants.

- The **extracellular matrix** consists of all the connective tissues and fibers that are not part of a cell but that provide support. It includes the interstitial matrix and the basement membrane. The interstitial matrix is present between cells in the interstitial space and acts as a protective buffer against stresses placed on the ECM. In diffuse parenchymal lung diseases, the damaged extracellular matrix does not allow the reestablishment of normal lung structure.
- The **basement membrane** is the anchor for organ cells. It is a thin membrane made up of proteins held together by type-IV collagen that is a vital component of the extracellular matrix. It forms an integrated structure that controls cell

position, cell motility, the permeability barrier, extracellular signal transmission to cells, and regulation of growth factors important to survival of alveolar epithelial and vascular endothelial cells. The epithelial cells of each body organ are anchored to this membrane and resemble a layer of tiles.

The focal areas of fibrosis are fused by connective tissue. It is thought that the focal organizing fibrotic areas represent permanent loss of alveolar structure to a respiratory lobule of the lung (terminal bronchioles to the alveoli). If the fibrotic process goes on unchecked, it ultimately destroys the entire lung lobule. This describes the idiopathic pulmonary fibrosis (usual interstitial pneumonia) found in end-stage lung in people with asbestosis (persistent exposure to the irritant), hypersensitivity pneumonitis (recurrent exposure to the antigen), collagen vascular disease (scleroderma, rheumatoid arthritis), or idiopathic (e.g., idiopathic pulmonary fibrosis [IPF]).[13]

Phase 3: Granuloma Formation. Depending on the type of DPLD, the third phase in pathogenesis may include the intermediate step of granuloma formation in addition to fibrosis development. Granulomatous pulmonary fibrosis is present in the lungs of people with hypersensitivity pneumonitis, eosinophilic pneumonia, and sarcoidosis. The inflammatory pathways that promote the granuloma formation in sarcoidosis are postulated to be mediated by activated T lymphocytes (CD4 cells) and activated macrophages. Idiopathic interstitial pneumonias have a different pathway for fibrosis development than does sarcoidosis.[14]

GENERAL CLINICAL APPEARANCE

The major clinical manifestation of people with interstitial lung disease is dyspnea. It is usually gradual in onset, with the patient believing that he or she is just "out of shape" until the dyspnea progresses ultimately to dyspnea at rest. In the very early stage of DPLD, dyspnea may be absent. The classic patient with DPLD is a 50- to 55-year-old male. His dyspnea worsens with exertion; he has bibasilar inspiratory crackles, a cough that is perhaps paroxysmal but nonproductive, and clubbing of his fingers and toes.[2,14]

DIAGNOSIS

For a diagnosis of DPLD (Table 10-4), the physician takes an extensive history of the patient's external risk factors and blood chemistry changes. During the evaluation of risk factors, the physician questions the patient about occupational and domestic environments—especially about asbestos, silica, and farm and animal dust exposures. The patient is also questioned about travel history and drug history, especially medications implicated in the genesis of DPLD, such as cytotoxic agents, amiodarone, gold, and some antimicrobials. Additionally, the physician's pursues the family history related to connective tissue diseases, sarcoidosis, and other genetically caused diffuse lung disease.[2,14]

Pulmonary Function Testing. All forms of DPLD decrease lung volumes but preserve expiratory flow rates unless the patient has airway involvement, is a smoker, or has an airflow limitation lung disease. The patients have a reduced total lung capacity, vital capacity, functional residual capacity, and FEV_1, along with a normal or increased FEV_1/FVC ratio. Studies of gas transfer typically show a reduction of carbon monoxide–diffusing capacity. The primary reason for the reduced diffusion is the destruction of alveoli and their capillaries, decreasing available surface area for gas exchange. This loss of surface area is the basis of the patient's hypoxemia. The patient's PaO_2 may be adequate at rest and drop with mild exertion, such as walking. Carbon dioxide is elevated only in end-stage pulmonary fibrosis.[2,14]

Chest Radiograph and Other Radiographic Studies. DPLD characteristically affects both lungs, and in some diseases it tends to dominate a particular lung zone. Sarcoidosis, silicosis, and hypersensitivity pneumonitis have upper lobe predominance; idiopathic interstitial pneumonias and asbestosis have lower lung zone predominance. Enlargement of the mediastinal lymph nodes is often associated with sarcoidosis or silicosis.

A common term used to describe severe pulmonary fibrosis on the chest radiograph is **honeycomb lung**, as seen in Langerhans histiocytosis X or late phase pulmonary fibrosis. The fibrotic lung zones of honeycomb lung are composed of cystic fibrotic air spaces, and the normal alveolar architecture is replaced with dense acellular collagen.[2,14]

High-resolution computed tomography (HRCT) brings much more definition to the usual CT scan. It samples 1- to 2-mm samples of lung tissue at 1-cm intervals and uses a high-resolution computer software algorithm. HRCT can bring into focus more detail than was possible with conventional CT scans (e.g., ground-glass opacification, diffuse or local involvement, airway structures). HRCT is valuable in detecting fine fibrotic, inflammatory changes, making it very helpful in identifying disease activity. Therefore, HRCT not only helps physician diagnose early fibrotic disease, but it also allows

TABLE 10-4 Diagnosis of interstitial lung disease

Diagnostic Clues

Diseases	History	Clinical signs and symptoms	Chest X-ray Findings	Laboratory Findings	Pulmonary Function Test Findings	Other Diagnostic Test Findings
Idiopathic Interstitial Pneumonias	Progressive DOE R/O occupational or drug related	Dyspnea at rest or exertion, digital clubbing, bibasilar crackles,	Diffuse basilar predominance (± nml. in early disease)	Hypoxemia at rest or during activity	Restrictive pattern with ↓ DL_{CO}	VTLB findings – areas of nml. lung, interstitial fibrosis & honeycombing > periphery HRCT – intralobular intersititial thickening, bronchiolar distortion with traction bronchiectasis peripheral honeycomb changes
Hypersensitivity Pneumonitis	Environmental exposure Diagnosis from history Variable illness depending on dose, exposure frequency, individual susceptibility	<u>Acute exposure:</u> Flu-like illness, respiratory distress, fever, cough, headache, diffuse fine bibasilar crackles <u>Chronic disease:</u> Progressive DOE, bibasilar inspiratory crackles, fatigue, weight loss, ± clubbing Cor Pulmonale in end-stage lung	Nml or ↑ lung markings between attacks <u>Acute exposure:</u> diffuse alveolitis, ground glass appearance <u>Chronic exposure:</u> Diffuse fibrosis with honeycombing	<u>Acute exposure:</u> Hypoxemia & hypocarbia IgG serum precipitins to inducing organic agent (↓'s in disease progression)	<u>Acute or Subacute</u> Restrictive pattern ↓ DL_{CO} for all forms of HP Many are hypoxemic at rest and desaturate with exercise <u>Chronic disease</u> Severe restrictive OR mixed obstructive & restrictive pattern	BAL – ↑ T-lymphocytes (≥60% of total lymphocytes) in acute exposure ↑ neutrophils, ↑ mast cells. TTB of lung, lymph nodes diagnosing patients with inadequate history. <u>Chronic HP disease</u> May mimic idiopathic pulmonary fibrosis or nonspecific interstitial pneumonia.
Langerhans Cell Histiocytosis (LCH) 3 syndromes: *Eosinophlic granuloma* *Hand-Schuller-Christian disease* *Letterer-Siwe disease*	Smoking may play a role > common in infants and young children; also affects adults Affects ≥1 organs	**Mild disease:** Asymptomatic or mild symptoms **Systemic disease:** Dyspnea, wheezing, hemoptysis, chest pain, fatigue, weight loss, fever Bone lesions, diabetes insipidus, ±digital clubbing	Reticular-nodular infiltrates predominance in UL, ML, clear costophrenic angles Advanced disease: bullae, cystic changes, pneumothorax	± hypoxemia at rest. ± desaturation with exercise	May have obstructive and restrictive disorder. Obstruction may be 2° to LCH &/or smoking ↓ DL_{CO} Abnml. exercise test	HRCT – Thin-walled irregular-shaped cysts, nodules ± cavitation, reticular densities & ground glass appearance. BAL or TTB – presence of Langerhans' positive cells in lung fluid or presence of Langerhans' cells in tissue sample VTLB or bone lesion biopsy

Sarcoidosis	2:1 male to female US – southeast > incidence in African-Americans	5% asymptomatic DOE, cough, chest pain, crackles on auscultation fever, anorexia, muscle aches,	Bilateral hilar lymphadenopathy, diffuse infiltrates ML, UL, End-stage: honeycomb lung	Hypoxemia or during exertion in moderate- to-severe sarcoidosis, Abnml lab tests specific to organ involvement (skin, eyes, heart, lungs, neurological)	Restrictive pattern some show obstruction Common- An isolated ↓ DL_{CO} Exercise testing indicates lung, heart involvement	HRCT may be helpful for staging and help locating site for biopsy TBB of lymph nodes & discrete, non-caseating granulomas. Epithieliod cell is dominant
Asbestosis	Environmental exposure Appropriate latent period High cancer risk with smoking	Progressive DOE, dry cough (± paroxsymal), bibasilar end-expiratory crackles, digital clubbing ~40% **Advanced:** Cor Pulmonale in end-stage lung	Lower lobe predominance with an irregular reticular pattern in periphery.	Earliest change is exertional hypoxemia	**Early:** ↓ $FEF_{25-75\%}$ ↓ FEV_1 with normal ratio **Late:** Restrictive pattern with ↓ DL_{CO}	HRCT Pleural or pleural-based abnormalities and cancer changes. Better definition of infiltrates. Early asbestos changes Peripheral septal thickening, honeycombing, areas of pleural thickening (placque), and bronchiolar thickening.
Cryptogenic Organizing Pneumonia (COP)	Flu-like onset, predromal URI Not described in children	Expiratory wheezing, no clubbing	Bilateral, patchy, migratory alveolar infiltrates		Restrictive pattern with ↓ DL_{CO} Airflow limitation may be present	HRCT – patchy consolidation and/or ground glass appearance Transbronchial biopsy or VTLB lung biopsy – intraluminal plugs of fibrobastic tissue in the conducting airways and alveolar ducts
Goodpastures Syndrome	Predromal viral upper respiratory infection	Severe dyspnea, hemoptysis, progressive renal failure	Progressive, migratory, asymmetric infiltrates found bilaterally	Presence of anti-basement membrane antibody in the blood + blood and protein in urine	Not necessary for diagnosis. If performed, the patient shows a restrictive pattern	Open lung biopsy – intraalveolar hemorrhage, macrophages containing hemosiderin Immunofluorescent staining of lung and kidney tissue showing deposition of anti-basement membrane antibody in the alveolar and glomerular basement membranes

close monitoring of the effects of drug treatment on active disease. In addition, information from this radiological technique can be used to identify potential locations to biopsy lung tissue for histopathologic diagnosis.[2,14] In some cases, HRCT is used to diagnose a patient with DPLD using information gained from patient history, bronchoalveolar lavage results, and pulmonary function testing. If more specific information is necessary (e.g., pathology results), then surgical lung biopsy is necessary. Common changes seen on HRCT performed on patients with DPLC are diffuse, patchy, reticular opacities with irregularly thickened interlobular fissures and honeycomb changes, especially in the bases.[14]

Clinical Laboratory Studies. Laboratory testing information is suggestive of some DPLD, but it is nondiagnostic. However, specific abnormalities can support a diagnosis of DPLD. For example:

- Abnormal erythrocyte sedimentation rate indicates autoimmune disease.
- The presence of serum precipitins is supportive of hypersensitivity pneumonitis.
- Antinuclear antibody and rheumatoid factors are supportive of collagen connective tissue diseases.
- Available blood tests, provide good supportive evidence of diffuse parenchymal lung disease.
- When used with clinical manifestations, pulmonary function test results, chest radiographs, and HRCT may be sufficiently specific to allow for a diagnosis without the need for a surgical lung biopsy or a transthoracic lung biopsy.[2,14]

Surgical Lung Biopsy. In most patients, surgical lung biopsy is not necessary to diagnose DPLD. A thorough history and physical exam, including appropriate blood chemistry studies, chest X-ray, and a HRCT imaging test, are performed before a surgical lung biopsy is considered. If the HRCT is not conclusive or more information is necessary, then the tissue biopsy may be needed.

Open lung biopsy (*OLB*) used to be the gold standard for the diagnosis of DPLD. Now many physicians use the less invasive **video-assisted thoracoscopic surgery (VATS)** in the place of OLB. Risks are associated with doing any surgical biopsy procedure. Patients with relatively severe cardiovascular-pulmonary impairment appear to be at the greatest risk for possibly fatal complications, such as acute exacerbation of idiopathic pulmonary fibrosis or unexplained acute lung injury. It is unclear whether the cause of the accelerated decline in lung function is the rapid disease progression in this population or a response to the anesthetic, to the surgical procedure, or to positive pressure ventilation. Before this procedure is performed, careful screening of patients for the presence of pulmonary hypertension, preoperative oxygen use, and lower total lung capacity (TLC) helps to identify poor candidates for surgical biopsy.[15]

The advantage of surgical lung biopsy is that it provides a histopathological diagnosis. The biopsy sample allows the pathologist to identify the type of inflammatory cells present in the lung sample, categorize the pulmonary changes and the extensiveness of the fibrosis, and arrive at a diagnosis. The pathologist can also help the physician ascertain whether the disease is at the end stage or whether the physician can give the patient some hope that the disease might respond to treatment. Recognition of ongoing inflammatory changes indicates that treatment with anti-inflammatory drugs may delay the progression to end-stage lung.[2,14]

Another technique of obtaining a lung sample for biopsy is through the fiberoptic bronchoscope. A *transbronchial needle biopsy* (*TBB*) permits sampling in the central, peribronchial areas. This technique is acceptable in testing for the presence of a DPLD associated with central lung involvement. Hilar lymph node sampling may provide sufficient tissue to permit a histopathological diagnosis for sarcoidosis or hypersensitivity pneumonitis. If the suspected DPLD involves primarily the peripheral lung, as would idiopathic pulmonary fibrosis, then OLB or VATS is necessary to obtain a large enough sample.[2,14]

Bronchoalveolar Lavage. *Bronchoalveolar lavage* (*BAL*) is a diagnostic procedure promoted as a possible technique to diagnose DPLD and eliminate the need for surgical lung biopsy. However, BAL has not proven to be an adequate substitute for surgical biopsy. Performing a pulmonary lavage and collecting the washing sample theoretically produce a representative sampling of the inflammatory cells responsible for the lung injury. However, BAL does not provide enough information for a diagnosis or determinations about the current state of the patient's lung disease.[2,14]

COMPLICATIONS

The major complications of DPLD are cor pulmonale, exacerbation of idiopathic pulmonary fibrosis, and progressive oxygenation failure. These complications can cause a significant decrease in quality and length of life.

Cor Pulmonale. *Cor pulmonale* is defined as an alteration in the structure and function of the right ventricle secondary to lung disease. The chronic effects of hypoxemia on the pulmonary vasculature cause cor pulmonale in patients with DPLD disease.

Doppler echocardiography is the most reliable noninvasive technique to estimate pulmonary artery pressure. Two-dimensional echocardiography identifies

CASE STUDY 10-1

Diffuse Parenchymal Lung Disease

Sean O'Connor, a 55-year-old male, went to his personal physician complaining of increased shortness of breath during exertion that had become worse over the last several months. He also complained of a dry nonproductive cough that interfered with sleep. His doctor performed a physical exam and general blood chemistry workup.

Physical Examination:

Vital Signs: HR 90, BP 145/85, RR 18, Temperature 36.8°C, SpO_2 94%

Respiratory: Inspiratory crackles heard bilaterally in the bases.

PFT: Simple spironmetry in the doctor's office: ↓ FEV_1 and ↓ VC, FEV_1/FVC 85%

Chest-radiograph showed ground-glass haziness in the bases, some streaky opaque shadows at the diaphragms, elevation of both diaphragms.

Cardiovascular: RRR without murmurs

ECG: 12 lead – no obvious problems visible

Extremities: No pitting edema in the legs, digital-clubbing present

Blood chemistry sent to Laboratory Services for analysis.

The patient was then intensively questioned regarding occupational exposure history. Mr. O'Connor denied exposure to any dusts or contaminants and denied any drug use. The doctor made arrangements for him to receive a full workup at the Pulmonary Function Lab that would include a diffusion study.

A week later, Mr. O'Connor came back to the doctor for discussion of his test results. The PFT revealed a restrictive ventilatory defect with a reduced total gas volume, normal expiratory flows, and a moderately reduced CO transfer. His walk test showed desaturation while walking to a nadir of 89%. His doctor told him that he had some type of diffuse interstitial pulmonary problem and that he would need to perform more diagnostic testing to see what type of diffuse disorder he had. Mr. O'Connor was given the facts that this may be a progressive disease and that the available treatment options may help.

Critical-Thinking Questions

1. What additional tests may be helpful in diagnosing Mr. O'Connor's lung disease?
2. What type of DPLD is Mr. O'Connor likely to have? Discuss the reasons for your choice.
3. Discuss why interstitial lung disease causes this pattern of pulmonary function abnormalities.

the signs of chronic right ventricular overload and its effect on cardiac function. If more precise measurements are necessary, right heart catheterization is the most accurate invasive test to confirm the diagnosis of cor pulmonale and to quantify the degree of pulmonary hypertension.[16] It can also give information about the patient's underlying lung disease that may aid in therapy.

The treatment of cor pulmonale is directed toward treating the underlying cause: lung disease. Maximizing the DPLD patient's lung function and gas exchange is the best way to definitively treat the condition. Continuous oxygen therapy may be necessary to raise the P_aO_2 and relieve hypoxic vasoconstriction. If pulmonary hypertension persists or is disproportionately high, a trial use of one or more drugs in primary pulmonary hypertension may improve exercise capacity and hemodynamics, as well as slow the rate of clinical deterioration in patients with secondary pulmonary artery hypertension. Sustained-release calcium channel blockers (nifedipine or diltiazem), intravenous or inhaled prostacyclin analog therapy, endothelin-receptor antagonists (bosentan), and sildenafil are all possible treatments that may reduce pulmonary pressure and improve right heart function.[16]

Exacerbation of Idiopathic Pulmonary Fibrosis. The causes of acute exacerbations of IPF are in many cases unknown. The effect may be the result of an acute direct stress on the lung, accelerating the speed of the fibrotic process or secondary to an occult viral infection or aspiration. Patients have no obvious infection, pulmonary embolism, or decompensated heart failure, but they demonstrate an acute pulmonary deterioration with worsening symptoms, gas exchange, and lung function. It is common for patients to present with severe hypoxemia, requiring mechanical ventilation.[17]

Although the definition of acute exacerbation of IPF is not standardized, an international group of pulmonary experts recommend the following diagnostic criteria to identify the patient in such a state:

- A diagnosis of IPF previously or on this admission
- Unexplained appearance or worsening of dyspnea within 30 days

- HRCT showing new bilateral ground glass abnormality and/or reticular or honeycomb pattern with superimposed consolidation consistent with UIP
- No bronchoscopic or tracheal aspirate evidence of infection
- Exclusion of new acute lung injury
- Left heart failure or pulmonary embolism.[17]

Cough, fever, and flulike symptoms can also be present, and many patients are admitted to the hospital with severe respiratory failure. The causes of acute respiratory failure in patients with DPLD are deterioration in the patient's P_aO_2 secondary to a worsening in lung function brought about by an acute infection, disease progression, or exacerbation of cor pulmonale. Intensive bronchial hygiene and increased F_IO_2 may help improve the patient's clinical status. Patients with end-stage pulmonary fibrosis have refractory hypoxemia and do not benefit from higher oxygen concentrations or continuous mechanical ventilation. These patients should be considered for organ transplantation.[4]

TREATMENT

Treatment of DPLD varies with the underlying disease, but the general treatment has not changed in some years. The initial direction in treatment is to control exposure to the precipitating antigens. Since many diseases causing DPLD do not have a known etiology, this measure is effective only in cases of environmental exposure.

The drug treatment used for people with DPLD is to prevent disease progression by suppressing the inflammatory process in the lung. This goal is accomplished by administering high-dose corticosteroids and monitoring disease activity by chest radiograph, HRCT, or other techniques. If steroids effectively reduce inflammation, the patient's dose is tapered to a level where inflammation suppression is sustained; this daily dose is maintained for long-term administration. Other drugs that may be used are cytotoxic drugs such as cyclophosphamide or azathioprine.

Patients' responses to steroids or cytotoxic drugs are variable, and the positive effects may not be sustained. For example, patients with idiopathic pulmonary fibrosis may initially respond to treatment early in the inflammatory phase of the disease with some stabilization of lung function, but, with disease progression, therapy becomes ineffective. In general, patients in end-stage pulmonary fibrosis do not respond to steroid therapy because the fibrotic process is well established at the time of diagnosis with little inflammation.[4,14] The median survival time for patients with interstitial pulmonary fibrosis is fewer than 3 years. Factors that affect survival are smoking history, pulmonary function deterioration, X-ray changes, response to therapy, and lung biopsy findings indicating loss of functional lung units.[4]

Continuous oxygen therapy is another treatment option that is predominately supportive. Continuous oxygen therapy may support the patient's oxygenation temporarily, but disease progression causes hypoxemia that is increasingly unresponsive to oxygen. Without a lung transplant, the patient will die when the disease process is so extensive that oxygenation cannot be maintained with supplemental oxygen.[4]

Lung transplantation is a definitive treatment for the patient with DPLD. Ideally, there should be early referral for lung transplantation. Waiting until the patient has end-stage pulmonary fibrosis may be too late. Many patients won't survive long enough to receive a new lung.[18]

Research is ongoing on identifying new agents that may be more effective in treating people with DPLD. The current treatment is minimally effective. Other forms of therapy must be developed to attack the disease process at the cellular level. Some treatment options under investigation are:[18]

- Antifibrotic therapy.
- Anti-inflammatory agents that directly control specific inflammatory cells (e.g., macrophage or T cell).
- Agents affecting the interaction of the fibroblast with lung parenchyma cells in the alveolar epithelium and capillary endothelium.
- Molecular therapy to promote lung repair (e.g., growth factors).

The number of diffuse parenchymal lung diseases makes the task of developing new effective therapies for this group of diseases all but insurmountable. Currently, scientists are spending considerable research dollars and time in investigating new treatments for the diseases with the poorest prognosis and for the greatest number of people. Idiopathic pulmonary fibrosis has no known cause and no effective treatment. If scientists are successful in developing therapies for this devastating disease, the diagnosis does not have to mean a terminal illness.

Summary

Diffuse parenchymal diseases encompass all of the pulmonary and systemic diseases that cause infiltration into the alveolar airspace and interstitium of the lung. The infiltration results in the thickening of the alveolar capillary membrane with an associated decrease in lung compliance and gas exchange. The wide variety of diseases that cause diffuse parenchymal and interstitial damage range, among many others, from idiopathic lung diseases, environmental lung diseases, drug toxicity, and collagen vascular diseases to hemorrhagic diseases of the lung.

Many of the DPLDs have an unknown etiology. However, of the diseases having known etiologies, a large group of diseases consists of the environmental (occupational) lung diseases. Environmental lung diseases are the most common disease classification of all the DPLDs. These diseases are distributed geographically according to the industry and occupational concentrations in specific areas of the country.

Fibrosis is the result of chronic inflammation due to persistent or recurrent exposure to a stimulant, irritant, or antigen causing parenchymal injury.

The major clinical manifestation of people with interstitial lung disease is dyspnea. It is usually gradual in onset, with the patient believing that he or she is just "out of shape" until the dyspnea progresses ultimately to dyspnea at rest.

All forms of DPLD decrease lung volumes but preserve expiratory flow rates unless the patient has airway involvement, is a smoker, or has an airflow limitation lung disease. The patients have a reduced total lung capacity, vital capacity, functional residual capacity, and FEV_1, along with a normal or increased FEV_1/FVC ratio. Studies of gas transfer typically show a reduction of carbon monoxide–diffusing capacity. The primary reason for the reduced diffusion is the destruction of alveoli and their capillaries, decreasing available surface area for gas exchange.

The major complications of DPLD are cor pulmonale, exacerbation of idiopathic pulmonary fibrosis, and progressive oxygenation failure. These complications can cause a significant decrease in quality and length of life.

Treatment of DPLD varies with the underlying disease, but the general treatment has not changed in years. The initial direction in treatment is to control exposure to the precipitating antigens. Because many diseases causing DPLD do not have a known etiology, this measure is effective only in cases of environmental exposure.

The drug treatment used for people with DPLD is to prevent disease progression by suppressing the inflammatory process in the lung. This goal is accomplished by administering high-dose corticosteroids and monitoring disease activity by chest radiograph, HRCT, or other techniques. If steroids effectively reduce inflammation, the patient's dose is tapered to a level where inflammation suppression is sustained; this daily dose is maintained for long-term administration. Other drugs that may be used are cytotoxic drugs such as cyclophosphamide or azathioprine.

Continuous oxygen therapy is another treatment option that is predominately supportive. Continuous oxygen therapy may support the patient's oxygenation temporarily, but disease progression causes hypoxemia that is increasingly unresponsive to oxygen. Without a lung transplant, the patient will die when the disease process is so extensive that oxygenation cannot be maintained with supplemental oxygen.[4] Lung transplantation is a definitive treatment for the patient with DPLD. Ideally, there should be early referral for lung transplantation.

Study Questions

REVIEW QUESTIONS

1. Briefly define the three phases of the pathogenesis of DPLD.
2. Describe the typical pattern of changes that might be seen on the pulmonary function tests performed on a patient with DPLD.
3. What is cor pulmonale?
4. Define hypersensitivity pneumonia.
5. Describe the general appearance of an individual with interstitial lung disease.

MULTIPLE-CHOICE QUESTIONS

1. Which of the following would cause hypersensitivity pneumonitis?
   a. bird breeder's lung
   b. rheumatoid arthritis
   c. asbestosis
   d. silicosis
2. Which of the following diffuse parenchymal lung diseases is caused by exposure to inorganic dusts?
   a. systemic scleroderma
   b. farmer's lung
   c. anthracosilicosis
   d. Niemann-Pick disease
3. Which of the following diseases do/does not have a known cause?
   a. environmental lung diseases
   b. pulmonary eosinophilic syndromes
   c. idiopathic interstitial pneumonias
   d. Wegener's granulomatosis
4. What occupations are associated with causing asbestosis?
   a. coal mining
   b. aerospace industry
   c. harvesting sugar cane
   d. shipyard and construction
5. What pulmonary function changes are seen in patients with idiopathic interstitial pneumonias?
   a. restrictive pattern with reduced DL_{CO}
   b. obstructive pattern that is refractory to bronchodilator therapy
   c. mixed obstructive and restrictive pattern
   d. cardiac limitation on exercise stress test

6. What clinical signs and symptoms are present in patients with chronic hypersensitivity pneumonitis?
   a. asymptomatic except during acute exacerbations
   b. hemoptysis, chest pain, fatigue, and weight loss
   c. progressive DOE, bibasilar inspiratory crackles, fatigue
   d. rhonchi, wheezing, and pleural friction rub on auscultation
7. Which of the following is *not* definitive but very important in helping to diagnose hypersensitivity pneumonitis?
   a. history of environmental exposure
   b. pulmonary function tests and reduced DL_{CO}
   c. chronic respiratory acidosis with hypoxemia
   d. transbronchial needle biopsy
8. What is a common cardiovascular complication of patients with severe DPLD?
   a. left ventricular failure and chronic pulmonary edema
   b. cor pulmonale and secondary pulmonary hypertension
   c. hypertensive heart disease secondary to systemic hypertension
   d. noncardiogenic pulmonary edema
9. What medication(s) is/are commonly used in the treatment of patients with DPLD?
   a. bronchodilators and inhaled steroids
   b. vasodilators and anticoagulants
   c. systemic anti-inflammatory drugs
   d. inotropic medications and vasodilators
10. What granulomatous DPLD is commonly associated with multiple organ involvement?
    a. systemic lupus erythematosis
    b. systemic scleroderma
    c. Goodpasture's syndrome
    d. sarcoidosis
11. What is a common problem with patients with DPLD during exertion?
    a. oxygen desaturation with exercise
    b. bradycardia with exercise
    c. leg pain and peripheral cyanosis
    d. syncope and hypotension during exercise
12. What DPLD is known to cause lung and kidney disease?
    a. sarcoidosis
    b. Langerhans cell histiocytosis
    c. Goodpasture's syndrome
    d. Wegener's granulomatosis

CRITICAL-THINKING QUESTIONS

1. Why are high-dose corticosteroids used in the treatment of DPLDs? What are the limitations of high-dose corticosteroids in treating DPLDs?
2. Describe the role of lung transplantation in the treatment of DPLDs.
3. What is the difference between hypersensitivity and allergic reaction?

References

1. American Thoracic Society/European Respiratory Society International Multidisciplinary Consensus Classification of the Idiopathic Interstitial Pneumonias. This Joint Statement of the American Thoracic Society (ATS) and the European Respiratory Society (ERS) was adopted by the ATS Board of Directors, June 2001 and by The ERS Executive Committee, June 2001. *Am. J. Respir. Crit. Care Med.* 2002;165,2:277–304.
2. Britton J, Evans A. Diffuse lung diseases: approach to diagnosis. In: Albert R, Spiro S, Jett J, eds. *Comprehensive Respiratory Medicine*. St. Louis: Mosby: 1999:44.1–44.8.
3. Mason RJ, Schwarz MI, Hunninghake GW, Musson RA. Pharmacological therapy for idiopathic pulmonary fibrosis. Past, present, and future. *Am. J. Respir. Crit. Care Med.* 1999;160,5:1771–1777.
4. Sharma S. (June 5, 2006) Restrictive lung disease. eMedicine Specialties: Pulmonology; Interstitial Lung Diseases.
5. Coultas D, Zumwalt R, Black W, Sobonya R. The epidemiology of interstitial lung diseases. *Am. J. Respir. Crit. Care Med.* 1994;150,4:967–972.
6. Raghu G, Weycker D, Edelsberg J, Bradford WZ, Oster G. Incidence and prevalence of idiopathic pulmonary fibrosis. *Am. J. Respir. Crit. Care Med.* 2006;174,7:810–816.
7. Katzenstein AA, Myers JL. Idiopathic Pulmonary Fibrosis: clinical relevance of pathologic classification. *Am. J. Respir. Crit. Care Med.* 1998:157,4:1301–1315.
8. Newman LS. Environmental pulmonary diseases. In: Beers M, et al, eds. *The Merck Manual of Diagnosis and Therapy*. Whitehouse Station, NJ: Merck Research Laboratories; 2006:469–480.
9. Peterson JS, Miller SM, Cairns CB. (June 10, 2008) Toxicity, Nitrous Dioxide. eMedicine Specialties: Emergency Medicine: Toxicology.
10. Mandavia S. (March 24, 2009) Toxicity, Hydrogen Sulfide. eMedicine Specialties: Emergency Medicine: Toxicology.

11. Noltkamper D, Burgher SW. (July 10, 2008) Toxicity, Phosgene. eMedicine Specialties: Emergency Medicine: Toxicology.
12. Issley S, Lang E. (March 14, 2007) Toxicity, Ammonia. eMedicine Specialties: Emergency Medicine: Toxicology.
13. Strieter RM. What differentiates normal lung repair and fibrosis? Inflammation, resolution of repair, and fibrosis. *Proc Am Thorac Soc.* 2008;5,3:305–310.
14. King Jr TE, Kline J. Interstitial lung diseases. In: Beers M, et al, eds. *The Merck Manual of Diagnosis and Therapy*. Whitehouse Station, NJ: Merck Research Laboratories; 2006:443–461.
15. Kreider ME, Hansen-Flaschen J, Ahmad NN, Rossman MD, Kaiser LR, Kucharczuk JC, et al. Complications of video-assisted thoracoscopic lung biopsy in patients with interstitial lung disease. *Ann Thorac Surg.* 2007;83,3:1140–1144.
16. Sovari AA, Dave RH. (September 3, 2008) Cor Pulmonale. eMedicine Specialties: Cardiology; Myocardial Disease and Cardiomyopathies.
17. Collard HR, Moore BB, Flaherty KR, Brown KK, Kaner RJ, King Jr TE, et al. Acute exacerbations of idiopathic pulmonary fibrosis. *Am. J. Respir. Crit. Care Med.* 2007;176,7:636–643.
18. Wells AU, Hogaboam CM. Update in diffuse parenchymal lung disease 2006. *Am. J. Respir. Crit. Care Med.* 2007;175,7:655–660.

CHAPTER 11

Atelectasis, Pleural Disorders, and Lung Cancer

Barbara Ludwig

OBJECTIVES

Upon completion of this chapter, the reader should be able to:

- Identify the four main cell types of malignant lung cancer.
- Discuss the diagnosis and the clinical manifestations of lung cancer.
- Describe the treatment for small-cell and non-small-cell lung cancer.
- Explain the different types of pneumothorax and their causes.
- Describe the clinical signs and symptoms a person shows with a tension and a nontension pneumothorax.
- Discuss the four mechanisms of pleural fluid formation in people with a pleural effusion.
- Identify the radiologic appearance of the various pleural disorders (effusion, empyema, pneumothorax).
- Explain the treatment for pleural disorders.
- Compare and contrast the types of atelectasis.
- Identify the radiologic changes seen in patients with atelectasis.

CHAPTER OUTLINE

KEY TERMS

adjuvant therapy
atelectasis
benign tumor
brachytherapy
carcinogen
carcinoma in situ
chemotherapy
cytology
decortication
empyema
exudates
malignant tumor
metastasis
open pneumothorax
palliative
paraneoplastic syndrome
pleural effusion
pneumothorax
radiation therapy
secondary spontaneous pneumothorax
thoracentesis
transudate

Atelectasis

Atelectasis means the incomplete expansion of the lung. It may be secondary to incomplete expansion at birth, called *primary atelectasis*, or secondary to a condition or disease that causes diminished volume for all or part of a lung. The different types of atelectasis can be categorized in several ways, but the simplest is dividing it into obstructive, nonobstructive, and special types of lung collapse.

OBSTRUCTIVE ATELECTASIS

Obstructive atelectasis, the most common type, results from the reabsorption of gas from the lung distal to the obstruction. The obstruction can occur at the level of the mainstem bronchi, or at lower-division bronchus. The most important of the many causes of a localized obstruction are tumors, aspirated foreign bodies, mucus plugs, or compression of the airway due to the enlargement of an adjacent structure.

The speed of lung collapse depends on two factors. First, if the person is breathing room air, atelectasis takes longer. The gas in the lung distal to the obstruction contains approximately 80% nitrogen, which absorbs into tissue spaces very slowly and slows the rate of lung deflation. The higher the F_IO_2 is, the faster gas resorption occurs.

Second, collateral air drifts through:

- Small holes between adjacent alveoli (pores of Kohn).
- Small channels between terminal and respiratory bronchioles and adjacent alveoli (canals of Lambert).
- Intersegmental respiratory bronchiole-to-bronchiole connections (Martin's channels).

The collateral air drift affects the pattern of atelectasis despite the presence of an obstruction interfering with normal airflow distribution.[1–3] Segmental and subsegmental lung collapse is less common because of collateral air drift through the alveolar and bronchiole communication channels. However, these communication channels do not occur across lung fissures; so the complete obstruction of the lobar bronchus results in the collapse of the entire lobe because collateral air drift cannot occur between lobes.[4]

Bronchial Neoplasms. Primary bronchogenic carcinoma is the most frequently encountered cause of localized bronchial obstruction. Squamous cell carcinoma and small cell carcinoma occur more in the central airways, and patients may initially come to their doctor because of respiratory problems.[1,5,6]

Foreign Bodies. Especially in children, inhaling foreign bodies is a common problem. Adults can also aspirate foreign bodies when they lose control of their airway protective mechanisms, such as in automobile crashes, during seizures, or after an overdose of depressant drugs. If a foreign body is aspirated because of vomiting, the presence of highly acidic gastric contents in the vomitus can produce acute lung injury and possible acute respiratory distress syndrome (ARDS).

The diagnosis of an endobronchial foreign body may not be identified immediately or seen on X-ray. If delayed, the signs and symptoms are consistent with a localized respiratory infection such as lobar pneumonia, or a lung abscess.[5]

Mucus Plugging. A mucus plug may become impacted in a bronchus and remain indefinitely. If infection develops, it can produce a classical clinical presentation identical to lung cancer. Diseases that can cause this type of problem are cystic fibrosis, asthma, and bronchopulmonary aspergillosis.[5]

External Compression of a Bronchus. Possible causes of external compression of the airway are:

- Enlarged lymph nodes infiltrated with cancer cells from bronchogenic carcinoma of the lung or lymphoma, which can compress, invade, and obstruct the bronchial lumen.
- **Malignant** or **benign tumors** of the mediastinum, which can compress the airway to the point of occlusion.

- Tuberculosis, which compress the airway by means of an infected lymph node putting pressure on the bronchus.[5]

NONOBSTRUCTIVE ATELECTASIS

Nonobstructive types of atelectasis are caused by an abnormal relationship between the visceral and parietal pleura, a loss of surfactant, or the replacement of normal lung parenchyma with scar tissue or cellular infiltrates.[1,5]

Pleural effusion, hemothorax, and pneumothorax are common causes of localized atelectasis secondary to a disruption of the normal lung-pleura relationship. The presence of fluid or air in the pleural space creates a positive intrapleural pressure, which is transmitted to the adjacent alveoli. The positive pressure in that part of the lung causes an appreciable decrease in ventilation to it. Consequently, underventilation and atelectasis occur in the lung areas directly adjacent to the affected pleura. Large accumulations of fluid or air can cause significant lung collapse and a decrease in lung compliance.

Adhesive atelectasis occurs because of increased surface tension secondary to surfactant loss. This problem can occur as the result of blunt chest trauma with significant lung contusion, radiation injury, and the many causes of acute lung injury and ARDS. The loss of surfactant makes the alveoli unstable, resulting in alveolar collapse. The atelectasis can be diffuse or localized.

Diseases that cause scarring (fibrosis) of the lung, along with the replacement of the normal alveolar epithelium with collagen, also cause diffuse atelectasis. The scar tissue distorts the normal architectural structure of the lung, causing the scarred areas to collapse and other areas to overdistend. Diseases associated with this type of atelectasis are interstitial pulmonary fibrosis, chronic tuberculosis, or severe fungal infections. This type of atelectasis is known as *cicatrization atelectasis*.[1]

SPECIAL TYPES OF ATELECTASIS

This third category of atelectasis consists of several types of special cases.

Postoperative Atelectasis. Acute atelectasis after surgery, especially procedures involving the thorax or upper abdomen, has long been associated with the loss of lung volume, causing complete or partial alveolar collapse. Pain, medications, increased secretions, and the inability to cough and to take deep breaths are common causes of postoperative atelectasis.[5] Postoperative atelectasis commonly affects areas of the lung in a segmental or subsegmental distribution.[1]

Plate or Discoid Atelectasis. Classic chest X-ray signs diagnose this type of atelectasis. Segmental and subsegmental atelectasis in the lung bases manifests on X-ray as narrow, straight bands or lines that run parallel to the diaphragm. Since the atelectasis does not follow known anatomical subdivisions of the lung, it is not obstructive. Because of its location in the peripheral bases of the lungs, it is likely the result of small areas of atelectasis secondary to hypoventilation, pulmonary embolism, pain associated with breathing (pleuritis or surgical pain), or poor diaphragmatic movement observed in obesity.[1,5]

DIAGNOSIS

Physical examination and laboratory studies assist in the diagnosis of atelectasis. However, chest X-rays and CT scans confirm the diagnosis. Other problems that show a similar clinical picture to atelectasis, such as pneumonia, pneumothorax, lung cancer, and other pulmonary diseases, need to be eliminated as the possible cause.[1,5]

Clinical Findings. The seriousness of the patient's clinical manifestations is related to the size of the affected lung area and to any other complicating problems, such as pneumonia. Patients will have dyspnea, tachypnea, fever, low S_pO_2 secondary to ventilation/perfusion mismatching, and possible cyanosis if the hypoxemia is severe. On physical exam, the patient will show dullness to percussion and diminished or absent breath sounds in the affected area, and the trachea will deviate to the atelectatic side.[1]

Radiographic Findings. The chest X-ray and CT scans show direct and compensatory changes that occur following alveolar collapse. The direct X-ray changes are:

- Increased radio-opacity of the affected lung.
- With nonobstructive atelectasis, the presence of an air bronchogram beyond the hilum appearing over the collapsed lung tissue.
- A fissure line with lobar lung collapse.

The compensatory changes reflect the loss of lung volume:

- The chest structures move to fill the vacated space left when the lung collapsed.
- The mediastinal structures (heart and trachea) move to the affected side.
- The hemidiaphragm is elevated on the affected side.
- The unaffected lung shows increased radiolucency because of overinflation.

The direct and compensatory changes are more pronounced with large areas of atelectasis.[1,5]

TREATMENT

The treatment of atelectasis depends on the underlying cause. The goal of treatment is lung reinflation by removing the cause of the lung collapse. If the problem is obstructive, the treatment is to remove the obstruction by flexible fiberoptic bronchoscopy or treat the cause of the obstruction, such as lung cancer or tuberculosis. If the patient has fluid in the pleural space, drainage (thoracentesis or chest tube) is the only way to improve ventilation and reinflate the atelectatic areas of the lung.

In patients with postoperative atelectasis, prevention is really the optimal approach.

- Limiting pain and sedative medications when practical.
- Early ambulation.
- Hyperinflation maneuvers (see Chapter 22).
- Antibiotic therapy if indicated.
- Oxygen therapy (if needed).
- Suctioning if the patient's cough is ineffective.[1,5]

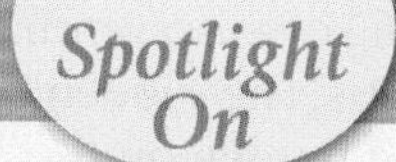

Spontaneous Pneumothorax

Primary spontaneous pneumothorax is most predominant among male smokers between the ages of 20 and 40. They are classically described as ectomorphs, having a tall, lean body frame. Cigarette smoking is the predominant risk factor. Smoking increases the risk for pneumothorax in females by a factor of 9 and in males by a factor of 22, with a direct relationship between the occurrence of spontaneous pneumothorax and the number of cigarettes smoked each day.

Pleural Disorders

Pleural disorders are pleural abnormalities that develop because of another primary disease or disorder. The pleural surface may become inflamed or irritated, or the pleural space may be filled with air, gas, or fluid. For the pleura to regain its normal function, the underlying cause of the pleural abnormality must be corrected or controlled. The pleural disorders discussed here are pneumothorax, hemothorax, and pleural effusion.

PNEUMOTHORAX

Pneumothorax is the presence of free air in the pleural space that causes partial or complete collapse of the affected lung. The classification of pneumothorax are primary spontaneous pneumothorax, secondary spontaneous pneumothorax, traumatic pneumothorax, catamenial pneumothorax, and iatrogenic pneumothorax.[7,8]

Primary Spontaneous Pneumothorax. This type of pneumothorax occurs in people without underlying lung disease. Typically, the person is an apparently healthy, young adult male in his teens or early twenties. The pneumothorax is thought to occur because of the rupture of subpleural apical blebs or bullae that may be present at birth or that may develop in those that smoke.[8] Ninety percent of primary spontaneous pneumothoraces occur at rest or during quiet activities. However, sometimes they occur during activities in which there may be an unequal transmission of pressure in the lung, such as skiing, sky- or underwater diving, or just flying in an airplane.[8]

The classical clinical appearance of people with a primary pneumothorax is pleuritic chest pain and dyspnea. Frequently, the pneumothorax is small, and symptoms may subside within 24 hours even if the condition goes untreated. If the pneumothorax is large, the person will come to the emergency department for treatment.[7] In a person with recurrent pneumothorax, chemical pleurodesis or surgical intervention is indicated.[5]

Secondary Spontaneous Pneumothorax. A **secondary spontaneous pneumothorax** occurs in people with chronic or acute lung disease. Commonly, it occurs because of rupture of a bleb or bullae in people with severe COPD or other lung diseases that cause injury to the lung parenchyma, such as interstitial lung diseases, infectious diseases, malignancies, connective tissue diseases, and many more. The clinical sequelae are more severe because these patients have a poor cardiopulmonary reserve as a result of their pulmonary disease. They have severe dyspnea, worsening hypoxemia, and possible hypotension. In people with chronic lung disease, the pneumothorax is more difficult to diagnose because its signs and symptoms are similar to those of an acute exacerbation of these patients' lung disease.[7]

A subtype of secondary spontaneous pneumothorax is *AIDS-associated pneumothorax*. This subtype is associated with infection with pneumocystis carinii pneumonia (PCP), caused by the organism *Pneumocystis jiroveci*. PCP causes cystic changes in the lung, and these cysts can rupture and cause a pneumothorax.[7]

Because of the underlying lung disease, ventilatory and oxygenation defects are present. The sudden onset of pneumothorax places an added burden on the patient's breathing, with sometimes life-threatening consequences. The individual's acute or chronic symptoms suddenly worsen significantly, with marked dyspnea, cyanosis, tachycardia, subcutaneous emphysema, and possible circulatory shock. These patients require emergency decompression of the pneumothorax with needle aspiration and chest tube placement for continuous air drainage. With recurrent pneumothorax, chemical pleurodesis is a treatment option. Because of the underlying severe lung dysfunction, surgery may be contraindicated, but chemical pleurodesis may prevent further episodes.[9]

Traumatic Pneumothorax. *Traumatic pneumothorax* is the result of direct or indirect trauma to the chest. It may be a complication of a medical diagnostic or therapeutic procedure, or it may be caused by penetrating or blunt chest trauma.[8,10,11]

Penetrating injury to the chest directly damages the chest wall, pleura, and lung. The injury to the lung and chest wall creates an **open pneumothorax**. The opening in the chest wall allows open communication between the atmosphere and the pleural space, and consequently air moves freely between the two areas during breathing. The pressure changes in the pleural space during breathing cause air to move from the atmosphere into the pleural space during inspiration. As a result, free lung movement is inhibited, causing air to retreat out of the pleural space during expiration. The results are large changes in pleural pressure and significantly reduced ventilation. The large changes in intrathoracic pressure may also affect venous return to the heart and cardiac output. The situation can be controlled quickly by placing a bandage over the open chest wound. The accumulating pleural air must also be removed with a chest tube.[8]

Blunt trauma to the chest can also cause pneumothorax. Rib fractures that lacerate the lung tissue or alveolar rupture from sudden chest compression (by a steering wheel or explosive energy). The person frequently has subcutaneous air from the air leak and experiences respiratory distress.[2]

Catamenial Pneumothorax. This type of pneumothorax represents 3–6% of all people with pneumothorax. It typically occurs within 48 hours of the onset of menstruation in premenopausal women or in postmenopausal women receiving estrogen. The cause is intrathoracic endometriosis. It is thought that endometrial tissue migrates through diaphragmatic openings, or it is released into the pelvic veins, travels to the lungs, and forms a pulmonary embolism. It usually affects the right lung (90–95%) and is a recurring problem in many women.

Iatrogenic Pneumothorax. This type of pneumothorax is secondary to medical procedures that could damage the pleura or lung tissue. Thoracentesis, transthoracic or transbronchial needle aspiration, central venous line placement, cardiopulmonary resuscitation, and mechanical ventilation are well documented procedural causes of pneumothorax.[7,8]. CPR is considered an iatrogenic, or hospital-induced, type of blunt chest trauma. After any medical procedure that has a risk of pneumothorax, the patient should have a chest radiograph as a precautionary measure.[9]

Tension Pneumothorax. Tension pneumothorax can develop in any category of pneumothorax. This condition occurs when the pleural pressure exceeds atmospheric pressure during the entire expiratory phase. This condition arises when a "one-way valve" condition is present in the patient's injured lung. Simply explained, the air can enter the pleural space through the ruptured alveoli, but it cannot exit. The air accumulates until the pressure of the trapped gas in the pleural space exceeds atmospheric pressure. This type of pneumothorax is frequently seen in patients receiving positive pressure ventilation.[9]

Tension pneumothorax is a life-threatening situation and a medical emergency. The high pleural pressure compresses the affected lung and may completely collapse it. The pressure also compresses the mediastinum and causes it to shift into the space occupied by the opposite lung. The shift distorts the structures inside the mediastinum (trachea, aorta, vena cava, and heart) and causes cardiovascular instability. The patient with tension pneumothorax shows all the signs of acute respiratory failure and circulatory shock:[8,9,11]

- Sudden deterioration in the clinical condition
- Rapid labored breathing, cyanosis
- Tachycardia, hypotension
- Physical exam of the chest: marked hyperexpansion of the affected lung and tracheal deviation to unaffected side
- Arterial blood gas: severe hypoxemia, with or without hypercarbia and respiratory acidosis

Immediate decompression of the tension is necessary using a 50-mL syringe. The needle should be inserted into the second anterior intercostal space at the midclavicular line. Large volumes of gas can be aspirated quickly. Then a chest tube is inserted once the patient is stabilized.[8,9,11]

Clinical Manifestations. The severity of symptoms varies widely from person to person. The scale ranges from the person who is asymptomatic to the person who is near death with respiratory failure and shock.[8] The identified manifestations include common signs and symptoms in addition to those the patient manifests with severe respiratory compromise.[9–11]

- Respiratory distress: dyspnea; chest pain, usually localized to side of pneumothorax; decreased S_pO_2
- Subcutaneous emphysema (may be expanding)
- Chest exam: reduced or absent breath sounds on affected side; ipsilateral expansion of the chest, with or without tracheal deviation to unaffected side; hyper-resonance to percussion on affected side
- Circulatory signs: tachycardia, with or without hypotension and shock

Diagnosis. The chest radiograph or the computerized tomography (CT) confirms the diagnosis of pneumothorax. To be detectable on a routine chest radiograph, the free pleural air must occupy approximately 20% of the thoracic volume. If a small pneumothorax is suspected, an expiratory chest film or a lateral decubitus chest radiograph may make the pleural air more visible.

The chest radiograph findings in the patient with pneumothorax identify the presence of pleural air with its attendant changes and indicate whether the air is under tension and is affecting the cardiovascular system.[9–11]

- Displacement of the mediastinum toward the normal or unaffected side
- Visible visceral pleural line on the side of the pneumothorax
- Absence of lung markings distal to the visceral pleural line
- Depressed hemidiaphragm on the side of the pneumothorax

Visible subcutaneous air in the soft tissue spaces or mediastinal air surrounding the heart. In addition, the diagnosis of pneumothorax should be considered if a patient who is being mechanically ventilated suddenly becomes agitated or begins "fighting the ventilator."[9]

Chest CT is increasingly used to predict the risk of pneumothorax recurrence. It is able to detect people with large or numerous blebs who are at high risk for recurring pneumothorax.[7]

General Treatment. The type of pneumothorax, the size of the pneumothorax, and the severity of the individual's symptoms determine the intervention. Any patient with a pneumothorax who is receiving positive pressure ventilation should have a chest tube inserted to prevent a tension pneumothorax. To treat the symptomatic patient, possible interventions that may be used include:

- Rest.
- Observation.
- Supplemental oxygen.
- Needle aspiration.
- Chest tube insertion and drainage of air.
- Chemical pleurodesis.
- Video-assisted surgery (VATS) with chemical pleurodesis (a procedure that causes the membranes around the lung to adhere and prevents the build-up of fluid in the pleural space), surgical clamping of bullae, or laser eradication of bullae.[11]

Chemical pleurodesis is a treatment for people with recurrent pneumothorax. Instilling talc slurry or 3 g of tetracycline into the pleural space through a chest intercostal tube scleroses the pleural space. This procedure is painful, so lidocaine can be added to the sclerosing mixture and a sedative drug be given before the procedure.[5]

Classification. Certain groups of patients are vulnerable to specific types of pneumothorax. If a patient is particularly susceptible to pneumothorax, the therapist must incorporate a routine assessment for this complication into the patient's care so that rapid treatment can be initiated to ensure a good outcome.

PLEURAL EFFUSION AND EMPYEMA

Pleural effusions are an accumulation of fluid in the pleural space. The estimated incidence of pleural effusion is 1 million cases per year.[12] They are a complication of a primary illness, with most effusions caused by infections, congestive heart failure, cancer, collagen diseases, pulmonary emboli, or cirrhosis of the liver. The most common cause of pleural effusion is congestive heart failure (30–40% of cases). The remaining 60–70% of the cases of pleural effusion are divided among nine primary diseases, with pneumonia as the second most common cause and malignancy as the third.[13] Of all the diseases that produce pleural effusion, four underlying physiological mechanisms can explain the reason for the effusion:

- Increased hydrostatic pressure (congestive heart failure)
- Increased capillary permeability (inflammatory and malignant effusions)
- Decreased plasma oncotic pressure (cirrhosis secondary to low serum protein)
- Impaired lymphatic drainage (malignancy, parasitic infections)

TABLE 11-1 Clinical signs of pleural effusion

Volume of Pleural Effusion	Lung Expansion	Tactile Fremitus	Percussion	Breath Sounds	Mediastinal Shift
<300 mL	Normal	High	Normal	Vesicular	None
300–1000 mL	Decreased	Medium	Dull	Decreased vesicular	None
1000–2000 mL	Decreased	Low	Dull	Decreased broncho-vesicular	Present
>2000 mL	Decreased	None	Dull	Decreased bronchovesicular	Present

There are two types of pleural fluid: transudate and exudate.

- A **transudate** is an ultrafiltrate of plasma, with a low concentration of protein. Transudate fluids form as the result of elevated hydrostatic pressure and decreased plasma oncotic pressure in the pulmonary circulation.
- An **exudate** is similar to plasma in that it has a high protein concentration. Increased capillary permeability and disturbed lymphatic drainage cause exudative fluid to form.

In some diseases, the pleural fluid can be a transudate or an exudate.[13]

Diagnosis. Pleural effusion is diagnosed with the help of physical signs and symptoms (see Table 11-1), imaging techniques, and **thoracentesis** (the extraction of fluid by inserting a needle into the pleural space). Common complaints that accompany a pleural effusion are dyspnea (particularly if the patient has chronic lung disease or if the effusion is large) and chest discomfort or pain. More than 300 mL of effusion fluid is necessary for abnormal chest percussion, but only 200–300 mL must be present to be visible on the chest radiograph. For smaller effusions, a lateral decubitus chest radiograph or ultrasound may be necessary to identify its presence. The actual presence of effusion fluid can be confirmed only by thoracentesis.[8,11]

An additional vocal sound heard in pleural effusion is *egophony*. "Egophony is a change in timbre (E to A) but not pitch or volume. It is due to a decrease in amplitude and increase in the intensity of the second formant, produced by solid (including compressed lung) interposed between the resonator and the stethoscope head."[14] When auscultating a patient with an effusion, the clinician asks the patient to say the letter "E" and listens to the chest in the area of the effusion. The sound of the patient saying "E" is heard as an "A" through the stethoscope. The high-frequency sounds are heard in compressed areas of the lung, and the low frequencies are filtered out. The bleating "A" sound is called egophony.

When removing pleural fluid during a thoracentesis, inspecting the aspirated effusion fluid for odor and appearance provides important diagnostic information and may even confirm the cause. For example, the color reveals considerable clues:

- Blood-tinged fluid may be due to the thoracentesis.
- Red fluid is blood secondary to trauma or bleeding.
- Black fluid indicates an aspergillus infection.
- Yellow-green fluid may be a rheumatoid pleuritis or pancreatic effusion.

If more specific information is necessary, the pleural fluid is analyzed. The minimum tests performed in the laboratory analysis of the pleural fluid are total protein and cytology. *Total protein* of the fluid identifies the fluid as a transudate or an exudate. **Cytology** examines the white count for the presence of infection and checks for the presence of bacteria and malignant cells. Additional clinical laboratory analysis may check glucose content, lactate dehydrogenase (LDH), cholesterol, amylase, hematocrit, and tumor markers. The information from these tests is the basis for a diagnosis and also indicates whether further diagnostic tests are needed.[8,13]

Empyema exists when pus is present in the pleural space. A complication of pneumonia, empyema is most likely to appear in the person with an underlying chronic condition such as COPD, diabetes, or renal failure. It should be suspected in the person who is still febrile despite receiving appropriate antimicrobial therapy or in the person who may be afebrile but still sick. A chest radiograph or CT scan identifies the presence of effusion. A thoracentesis confirms the presence of pus.[13]

Treatment. The treatment of pleural effusion is to treat the underlying cause and to relieve the patient's symptoms (i.e., give **palliative** care). Removing the fluid by either thoracentesis or chest tube drainage allows the lung to reexpand and may relieve dyspnea. If hypoxemia is present, oxygen therapy is indicated.

In a patient with an empyema, immediate and complete drainage by chest tube system is necessary. If tube drainage is unsuccessful, rib resection and surgical drainage of loculated pus pockets by blunt dissection or **decortication** (the removal of part or all of the outer surface of an organ) of the pleura may be necessary. Because an empyema usually indicates the presence of an anaerobic infection, antimicrobial therapy should be modified; additional antimicrobial changes may be necessary when culture results are known. The sequellae of inadequately treated empyema include fibrothorax, or "trapped lung."[8,13]

Lung Cancer

The American Cancer Society (ACS) identified cancer as the number two cause of death in the United States. Cancer accounted for nearly one-quarter of yearly deaths (559,312), exceeded only by heart disease (652,091). Lung cancer is the most common fatal cancer in both men (31%) and women (26%). Since 1990, the age-adjusted lung cancer death rate of men has decreased by 40%. In contrast, the lung cancer death rate for women more than doubled in the past 27 years, and in 1987, lung cancer mortality exceeded breast cancer, becoming the primary cause of cancer deaths in women.[15]

These statistical changes are reflected in cigarette smoking statistics. More women are smoking than are men, and fewer women are quitting.[16,17] The death rates are higher in men than in women in every racial and ethnic group. African American men and women have the highest cancer mortality, followed by whites, then American Indian/Alaskan natives, Hispanics, and finally Asian/Pacific Islander. Asian American and Pacific Islander men and women have the lowest cancer death rates, about half of the rate of African American men and women, respectively.[17]

The productivity costs to the U.S. economy secondary to cancer deaths—loss of paid employment, caregiving, and housekeeping activities—are significant. The estimated productivity losses in 2000 were approximately $116 billion. If the current survival rate does not improve, the costs will increase to $147.6 billion in 2020. The economic impact of death from lung cancer has been the most costly. Lung cancer alone was responsible for more than one-quarter of the total costs ($39 billion in 2010). Death from colon and rectum cancer was the second most costly ($12.8 billion in 2010), and death from female breast cancer was the third ($10.9 billion in 2010)."[18]

The following Surveillance and Epidemiology and End Results (SEER) statistics were released from the National Cancer Institute on the stage of lung and bronchus cancer at the time of diagnosis:[19]

- 16%—diagnosed while the cancer is still confined to the primary site (localized stage)
- 25%—diagnosed after the cancer has spread to regional lymph nodes or directly beyond the primary site (regional stage)
- 51%—diagnosed after cancer has metastasized (distant stage)
- 8%—staging information unknown

Diagnosis of advanced lung cancer in more than 75% of the cases explains why the 5-year survival rate for lung cancer is low and why the associated productivity costs are the highest.

The highest recorded 5-year survival rates are in the United States with 12.5% for men and 15.6% for women.[15,19] These values reflect the survival for *all* cell types of primary lung cancer. The developing world's 5-year survival is approximately 8%.

RISK FACTORS

Risk factors are the extrinsic or intrinsic elements in the environment that predispose an individual to a disease. Examples of factors are genetic predisposition to a disease, an antigen the individual is allergic to, social habits, and the state of the individual's immune function.

Cigarette Smoking. Lung cancer results from a combination of continued exposure of the bronchial mucosa to carcinogens and genetic susceptibilities.[20] Cigarette smoking is by far the most important risk factor for lung cancer and thought to be the primary risk factor for approximately 80% of all lung cancers.[21] About 15% of all people who smoke develop lung cancer, with the risk varying depending on the age at which smoking started and the number of cigarettes smoked.[22] Lung cancer risk increases by approximately the fourth power of smoking duration and by the square of the number of cigarettes smoked every day.[23] Tobacco smoke contains many **carcinogens** that are known to cause molecular abnormalities in bronchial epithelia. Respiratory epithelial chromosome damage is found in all chronic smokers.

People exposed to environmental tobacco smoke, including spouses and children of smokers, have an increased risk of about 17% for lung cancer.[24] In one study, people who had been exposed to tobacco smoke as children but not as adults did not appear to have any increased risk. Exposure to the smoking of family members and friends seems to be associated with the initiation of adolescent smoking.[23]

There are conflicting data regarding the relative risks of developing lung cancer from smoking for men and women. Two examples of conflicting reports are from the American Cancer Society and the Nurses Health Study of Women and Health Professional Follow-up Study of Men. The ACS performed two cancer prevention studies and identified that men who smoke had an increased risk of lung cancer compared to women who smoke.[15] Another large study studying cancer data from former and current smokers in both sexes found that women do not appear to have greater susceptibility to lung cancer than men.[25]

These conflicting results indicate the complexity of the subject and the need for further study. Reported differences in the histological subtypes are also not well understood.

- Women smokers appear to be at a higher risk of small-cell lung cancer than men smokers are.
- Men smokers seem to have an equal risk for squamous-cell and small-cell cancers.
- Women smokers have a greater incidence of adenocarcinoma than men smokers do, with a possible influence by estrogen.[26,27]
- Up to 15% of lung cancers in never-smokers are thought to be caused by second-hand smoke. (Cigarette smoke contains many carcinogens, such as aromatic polycyclic hydrocarbons and N-nitrosamines.) Urinary levels of tobacco-specific carcinogens were elevated in nonsmoking women exposed to environmental tobacco smoke. A nonsmoking woman has a 24% greater risk of developing lung cancer, if living with a smoker.[28]

Quitting smoking is the primary way to prevent lung cancer. However, it might be 15–20 years before the risk assumes a rate *almost* as low as nonsmokers' risk of lung cancer. Research has shown that the difference in risk between people who continue smoking and those who quit is explained by the differences between the two groups in the duration of smoking—the length of the exposure, not its intensity.[16,29]

Air Pollution. The pollutants emitted from motor vehicles, manufacturing, and the burning of coal contain carcinogens. The risk of lung cancer attributed to environmental pollution is thought to be small, but its real effect on cancer rates is not yet established.[16]

Occupations Linked to Lung Cancer. Uranium and asbestos workers have a much greater risk of lung cancer than any other occupational groups. A uranium worker who does not smoke has a seven-fold increase in cancer risk when compared with other nonsmokers. A uranium worker who smokes increases the risk of lung cancer to 38-fold compared to other nonsmokers. Asbestos workers' statistics are even more abysmal. An asbestos worker who does not smoke has a five-fold increased risk of lung cancer compared to other nonsmokers. But the asbestos worker who smokes has a 92-fold increased risk of lung cancer compared to nonsmokers. This risk is much greater than that of someone who smokes over two packs of cigarettes a day (64-fold risk increase).[16,30]

Radon Gas. *Radon gas* is a breakdown product of uranium and an environmental risk factor for lung cancer. Approximately 2–3% of lung cancer is thought to be caused by radon.[29] Because it is ubiquitous in the environment, it can seep into any dwelling. Many people are unaware that they are exposed to this pollutant in their own homes. A fact that is not appreciated is that radon and cigarette smoking *may* have a synergistic effect on lung cancer rates. Smokers, and possibly nonsmoking residents of smokers' households, may be at increased risk of lung cancer even when radon levels are relatively low. Kits are available to test the home for radon, and methods exist to remove it.

Family History. Genetics is under intense scrutiny as a possible lung cancer risk factor. One area of research is investigating the possibility of genetic susceptibility to environmental tobacco smoke. One study reported that individuals with a family history of lung cancer had a two-fold greater risk of developing lung cancer and that this risk was more pronounced in women.[15] The study found that women tend to carry more gene mutations that can increase their susceptibility to developing lung cancer.

Another direction of cancer research is in the area of familial tendencies to develop certain cell types of cancer, cancer at certain organ sites, and so on.[31] For example, current research suggests that a family history of cervical, ovarian, or uterine cancer may increase the risk of lung cancer in postmenopausal women. One study reported that a family history of ovarian cancer increases the risk by two-fold for adenocarcinoma of the lung, and a history of uterine and cervical cancer in a first-degree relative increases the risk slightly for squamous-cell and small-cell lung cancers. The higher risk occurred in both smokers and nonsmokers.[32] Studies also have indicated that women may have a greater genetic susceptibility to specific types of lung cancer due to female, X-linked inheritance (the inheritance of genes located on the X chromosome).[15]

Hormonal Influences. Hormones could present an increased risk for lung cancer. Researchers are looking at hormone replacement therapy, the age onset of a woman's first period, and the length of her menstrual cycle as possible risk factors for lung cancer. Estrogen is known to have a role at many levels in tumor production, and researchers are studying how estrogen affects abnormal cell growth as well as its role in cellular damage. Research in this area is one of the new directions in lung cancer studies.[15]

HISTOLOGICAL CELL TYPES OF LUNG CANCER

The two major classifications of lung cancer are non-small-cell lung cancer (NSCLC) and small-cell lung cancer (SCLC). NSCLC accounts for approximately 75% of all lung cancers, and it is a heterogeneous collection of three histological cell types: adenocarcinoma, squamous-cell carcinoma, and large-cell carcinoma. These histologies are classified together because the approaches to diagnosis, staging/prognosis, and treatment are similar. Small-cell lung cancer is very different from the other cancer classification with a different staging process, treatment approach, and prognosis (Table 11-2).

Non-Small-Cell Cancers. Adenocarcinoma accounts for about 35–40% of all lung cancers, and it is the most common type of NSCLC lung cancer in the United States. It occurs in smokers, but it is also the most common lung cancer found in nonsmokers. It is the usual cell type of 60–80% of cancers in nonsmokers.[6]

Adenocarcinoma may arise from a previous scar, and it usually does not cavitate. The tumor usually arises in the lung periphery and metastasizes early to other body organs through the circulatory and lymphatic systems. It usually metastasizes to the lymph nodes, pleura, adrenal glands, central nervous system, and bone. Adenocarcinoma tends to have a worse prognosis than squamous-cell cancer in all stages.[6]

Bronchoalveolar cell carcinoma is a subtype of adenocarcinoma that usually accounts for about 5% of all bronchogenic carcinomas. This type of cancer occurs in people with underlying interstitial lung disease and parenchymal scarring. It appears to arise from type II pneumocytes and may appear as a solitary peripheral nodule, multifocal disease, or a pneumonic form. The cancer may spread to other parts of the lung or to the other lung by transbronchial spread or by growing along the pulmonary interstitium. Spreading by these mechanisms is associated with a poor prognosis.[6]

Squamous-cell accounts for 20–25% of all lung cancers. It is strongly associated with cigarette smoking. The tumor commonly arises from large bronchi and spreads by direct invasion of neighboring tissues or lymph node **metastasis**. Squamous-cell cancers are frequently slow growing and can take several years to progress from a localized tumor to an invasive cancer.[6] On initial presentation, the patient frequently has significant airway obstruction secondary to the tumor and may be diagnosed with lung cancer after coming to the doctor for treatment of pneumonia.[16,29,30]

Large-cell cancer accounts for 10–15% of all lung cancers, and it is strongly associated with smoking. It is described as an undifferentiated cell type because it lacks glandular (adeno characteristics) and squamous characteristics. These tumors are often diagnosed by default when all other cell types have been excluded. They appear in the middle to peripheral lung areas and may extend to involve segmental and subsegmental bronchi. The large cell tumors are big, bulky, well-defined masses with extensive hemorrhage and necrosis. They grow rapidly and metastasize early through the lymphatics and bloodstream.

Giant-cell, a variant of large cell, is extremely aggressive and carries a very poor prognosis. The people with these tumors usually present with a large peripheral mass. The tumors do not involve the large airways unless they are spreading directly.[16,29,30]

Small-Cell Cancer. Small-cell lung cancer (SCLC) is a major classification as well as a cell type. SCLC has the highest association with cigarette smoking. Approximately 98% of patients with SCLC have a smoking history.[33] The disease originates in lung tissue next to central airways and major blood vessels. Because it grows so rapidly, SCLC is characterized by early metastasis to distant sites such as the mediastinal lymph nodes, liver, bones, adrenal glands, and brain; therefore, most patients already have detectable metastasis by the time it is first diagnosed. This cell type is also known for causing paraneoplastic syndromes, of which the most common are syndrome of inappropriate antidiuretic hormone (SIADH) and syndrome of ectopic adrenocorticotrophic hormone (ACTH) production. Neurologic syndromes may also occur such as Eaton-Lambert syndrome and sensory disturbances.[16,30,33]

CLINICAL MANIFESTATIONS

Fifteen percent of the people with lung cancer do not have symptoms at the time of diagnosis. Seventy percent of lung cancer patients have signs and symptoms of intrathoracic or distant metastasis at the time of diagnosis. Clinical manifestations in individuals with lung cancer include:

- Dyspnea (possible airway obstruction).
- Stridor and fever (possible atelectasis and infection).
- Hoarseness (involvement of the recurrent laryngeal nerve).
- Chest pain (pleural involvement).

Other clinical manifestations are listed in Table 11-2.[16,30]

TABLE 11-2 **Lung cancer**

		Non-Small Cell Lung Cancer			Other
	Small Cell	**Adenocarcinoma**	**Large Cell**	**Squamous Cell**	**Many Cell Types**
Distribution of cell types (%)	13	35–40	10–15	25–30	5
Specific Information	Highest correlation with smoking Central airways and blood vessels Highest occurrence of distant metastasis ↑ occurrence of paraneoplastic syndromes No Cavitation	Most frequent cause of lung cancer in non-smokers Peripheral lung Bronchoalveolar carcinoma is subtype Cavitary lesion	Smokers Undifferentiated Large peripheral mass with necrosis Metastasizes early Cavitary lesion	Smokers Central lesion in a proximal bronchus Cells shed and can be detected from cytology studies May be present for years before diagnosis	**Carcinoid:** slow growing malignant tumor ~2% of all primary lung tumors **Lymphoma:** primarily non-Hodgkin's <1% **Mucoepidermoid:** Derived from salivary gland tissue **Hamartoma:** Commonest benign tumor **Metastatic:** All cell types; result of spread from primary tumors (breast, head, neck)
Local Manifestations	*Asymptomatic*: ~25% of patients *Symptomatic*: Cough, new cough onset in smoker, hemoptysis, chest heaviness, dyspnea, digital clubbing, obstructive atelectasis or pneumonia *Local metastasis:* pleural involvement (pain, effusion), regional lymph node enlargement, superior vena cava syndrome (dilated neck veins, prominent veins on chest, facial edema, red coloring), superior sulcus tumor (Horner's syndrome, bony destruction, hand muscle atrophy)				
Metastasis	65–70% have disseminated or extensive disease at diagnosis *Common:* bone, liver, adrenal glands, pleura, CNS Symptoms give clues of metastasis	The more differentiated the cells, the slower the tumor growth and spread. Every body tissue could be the site of distant metastasis. Clinical manifestations give clues of metastasis			
Paraneoplastic Syndromes	*Associated systems:* muscloskeletal, cutaneous, neurologic, endocrine, hematologic/vascular *Musculoskeletal*: hypertrophic osteoarthopathy, myopathy *Cutaneous:* clubbing, pruritis, scleroderma *Endocrine:* Cushing's syndrome, syndrome of inappropriate antidiuretic hormone secretion (SIADH), hypercalcemia, carcinoid syndrome, thyroid-stimulating hormone, ACTH syndrome *Neurologic:* Lambert Eaton syndrome, neuropathy, psychosis, dementia *Vascular/hematologic:* anemia, polycythemia, arterial thrombosis, eosinophilia, hypercoagulability *Other:* wasting syndrome				

TABLE 11-2 **Lung cancer (*continued*)**

		Non-Small Cell Lung Cancer			Other
	Small Cell	**Adenocarcinoma**	**Large Cell**	**Squamous Cell**	**Many Cell Types**
Laboratory	Hypercalcemia: bony metastasis or secondary to parathyroid-like hormone from tumor cells Anemia: nutrition-related, bone marrow involvement, chemotherapy Decreased clotting time: not understood Hyponatremia and low serum osmolality: SIADH				
Diagnosis	*Initial screen*: patient symptoms, chest x-ray (incidental or first step in diagnosis) *Cell type diagnosis*: Bronchoscopy, needle aspiration, bronchial brushings, and washings, transbronchial biopsy, sputum cytology, or CT guided biopsy *Staging*: bronchoscopy with bronchial biopsy and lymph node biopsy, HRCT, pleural fluid cytology, mediastinoscopy and biopsy of mediastinal nodes, PET scan				
Treatment	*Solitary pulmonary nodule* Limited disease: surgical resection, chemotherapy, radiotherapy *Other cases*: Chemotherapy, radiotherapy, palliative tumor reduction, stent placement	*Varies with stage:* Surgery: Lobectomy; pneumonectomy; or segmental, wedge, or sleeve resection as appropriate if pulmonary function is adequate Systemic chemotherapy in combination with thoracic radiotherapy OR combined chemoradiotherapy Palliative tumor reduction Experimental – Biologic testing (various stages of testing)			
Prognosis (2005 data)	*Untreated:* <u>Limited disease</u> - median survival 12 wks <u>Extensive disease</u> - median survival 6 wks *Treated:* All stages: 5.9% Localized (at diagnosis confined to primary site) – 19.5% Regional (limited disease) – 12.5% Distant (extensive disease) – 2.2% Unstaged (stage not known) – 6.4%	All stages: 16.8% Localized – 51.2% (at diagnosis confined to primary site) Regional – 21.8% (spread to regional lymph nodes or directly beyond the primary site) Distant – 2.9% (diagnosed after metastasis to distant sites) Unstaged – 8.5% (unknown stage) Compared with people with squamous cell cancer, more patients with adenocarcinoma had cerebral metastasis within 5 years IIB disease – surgery and weight loss are significant independent predictors of 5-year survival			<u>All lung cancers</u> Localized – 49.5% Regional – 20.6% Distant – 2.8% Unstaged – 8.3%

PARANEOPLASTIC SYNDROMES

Paraneoplastic syndromes are nonpulmonary disorders that are caused by lung cancer. Many types are secondary to hormonelike chemicals or other substances released from the tumor that have metabolic or neurological effects. For example, digital clubbing, a common manifestation of lung cancer, involves the fingers and toes, with selective enlargement of the connective tissue to the distal phalanges. It is diagnosed by the loss of the angle between the cuticle and the base of the nailbed. The most common paraneoplastic problems (5–10%) are syndrome of inappropriate antidiuretic hormone (SIADH) and syndrome of ectopic adrenocorticotrophic hormone (ACTH) production. Neurologic syndromes may also occur, such as Eaton-Lambert syndrome and sensory disturbances.[16,30]

DIAGNOSIS AND STAGING

Diagnosing the cancer and staging the invasiveness of the involvement are intricately intertwined. The chest radiograph is a screening tool. Abnormalities on the chest radiograph, coupled with the patient's clinical manifestations, indicate whether further diagnostic tests are necessary. Cytology or histology aids in the diagnosis of lung cancer. The following tests are used in the initial diagnosis and staging of disease severity:[16,30]

- History and physical exam
- Laboratory studies: complete blood count, blood chemistry, including liver function tests
- High-resolution computer tomography (HRCT) of chest as well as CT of the liver, brain, and adrenal glands to identify distant metastasis.
- Bone scintigraphy if bone metastasis is suspected
- Positron emission tomography (PET scan)

The PET scan is more sensitive and accurate in staging mediastinal spread of the cancer. It can detect abnormalities not visible on CT scans.

Techniques Used in Cancer Diagnosis. The *fiberoptic bronchoscope* is frequently used in both cancer diagnoses and staging, especially if the suspicious lesion is centrally located:

- Obtaining tissue samples by transbronchial biopsy enables the clinician to determine cell type.
- It permits biopsy of regional lymph nodes for tumor staging.
- If the tumor is endobronchial, the bronchoscope also allows direct visualization of the tumor as help in later surgical resection.

Sputum samples for cytology testing can also be obtained when the tumor is too peripheral to be directly biopsied using the bronchoscope.

Mediastinoscopy is usually performed to visualize directly the mediastinal lymph nodes. It allows mediastinal node biopsy, which aids in cancer staging. The CT-guided biopsy is helpful when the lesion is located in the periphery of the lung. The CT identifies where the physicians should insert the biopsy needle to obtain a good tissue sample for determining malignancy.

If the patient has a pleural effusion, the fluid can be aspirated by thoracentesis and tested for cancer cells. This technique can be used to determine cell type and cancer stage. Other organs, such as the liver and adrenal glands, can be directly biopsied with needle aspiration to aid in cancer staging.

Video-assisted surgery has proved useful in cancer diagnosis of indeterminate isolated pulmonary nodules. This visual technique has also been used in surgical removal of the lung in high-risk or elderly patients. Its current use in the management of patients with malignancy is being studied.[34,35]

Lung Cancer Staging. Cancer staging criteria help the clinician identify the extent and prognosis of tumors. Lung cancer staging criteria are different for the two main cell types. The cell type of the lung tumor and the degree of invasiveness determine treatment options and patient prognosis.

Cancer *clinical staging*, which describes the extent of disease, is determined following completion of the diagnostic work-up. The work-up includes the:

- Pathology report from tissue obtained during bronchoscopy, needle (or other technique) biopsy.
- Blood tests.
- Imaging tests (e.g., abdominal ultrasound of the liver, radionuclide bone scans, HRCT, MRI scan of brain, chest and abdomen) that were indicated by a high index of suspicion based on patient clinical manifestations.[6,30,33]

The purpose of staging is to determine resectability and operability because surgical resection is the only cure for lung cancer. Pulmonary function tests should be performed in people with resectable cancer to decide operability. If the estimated postoperative lung function ($<$40% FEV_1 and $<$40% DL_{CO}) indicates that the patient is inoperable, then exercise testing is performed to confirm this estimation. If surgery is not indicated, the patient receives other definitive care.[4]

Staging of Non-Small-Cell Lung Cancer. The *TNM staging system* was implemented in 1997 after revisions of the stage groupings: *T* is the primary tumor, *N* is for the regional lymph nodes, and *M* is for distant metastasis. The system is used for all lung carcinomas *except* small cell.

- *T* describes tumor size and its location in relation to bronchi, carina, major blood vessels, pleura, and chest wall (TX, T0, Tis, T1, T2, T3, T4).
- *N* describes lymph node involvement and whether the involvement is on the ipsilateral side or contralateral side of the primary tumor (NX, N0, N1, N2, N3).
- *M* is either present or absent (MX, M0, M1).

The *X* designation in each category indicates that the subset was unable to be assessed, and the *Tis* indicates carcinoma *in situ*.

Carcinoma in situ is a premalignant neoplasm in which the tumor cells are confined to the epithelium of origin and have not invaded the basement membrane. A diagnosis of carcinoma in situ is associated with a high incidence of progression to invasive cancer. Neoplastic changes in squamous or glandular epithelium can occur in the body wherever these cells are common, such as in the cervix, anus, bronchi, esophagus, uterine endometrium, or vagina.

There are four stages for NSCLC, with further subdivisions of stages I–III into A and B designations. The severity of the disease worsens with the increased numerical designation. The A and B designations in stages I, II, and III are expansions of the classification system to indicate gradations of severity within the stage. There are many possible combinations of tumor size, tumor invasiveness, and lymph node metastasis in stages IIB, IIIA, and IIIB.[6,16,30]

- Stage 0 (carcinoma in situ)
- Stage IA (T1N0M0), Stage IB (T2N0M0)
- Stage IIA (T1N1M0), Stage IIB (T2N1M0 or T3N1M0)
- Stage IIIA (T3N1M0, T1N2M0 or T2N2M0 or N3N2M0)
- Stage IIIB (T4N0M0, T4N1M0 or T4N2M0 or T1N3M0, T2N3M0 or T3N2M0, T4N3M0)
- Stage IV (any T, any N, M1)

Staging is the primary method used to determine whether surgery will benefit the patient. In stages I, II, and IIIA, the tumors are operable if the patient has no complicating medical problems.[16] Additionally, the oncology team needs to know the individual's cancer severity stage to design the treatment plan.[6]

Staging of Small-Cell Lung Cancer. The TNM system is primarily used to stage NSCLC. In very few patients with small-cell lung cancer (<5%), a very detailed staging is helpful. However, in most cases, the TNM staging system is of limited use in determining a prognosis for patients with SCLC because most of the patients are in stage III/IV at the time of diagnosis. An older system, developed by the Veterans Administration group, is still used today to stage patients with SCLC. This system consists of two stages: limited disease and extensive disease.

- *Limited disease* is disease that is confined to one hemithorax and its ipsilateral mediastinal and supraclavicular lymph nodes. Malignant pleural effusion is excluded. Thirty-five to forty percent of patients are in this stage when diagnosed. This circumscribed anatomical area is based on the fact that it falls within 1 radiation field, using radiation therapy settings as the limitation.[29] [**Radiation therapy** is treatment with high-energy rays (such as X-rays) to kill or shrink cancer cells. The radiation may come from outside the body (external radiation) or from radioactive materials placed directly in the tumor (brachytherapy or internal radiation). This therapy may be used to shrink the cancer before surgery, to destroy any remaining cancer cells after surgery, or as the main treatment. It may also be used as palliative treatment for advanced cancer.]
- *Extensive disease* is disease that has spread beyond the limited-stage anatomical area and cannot be encompassed in 1 radiation field. Any tumor cells found in contralateral lymph nodes, tumor-laden lymph nodes above the clavicle, malignant pleural effusion, or distant organ metastasis is classified as extensive disease.[29]

TREATMENT

The treatment of lung cancer depends on the cell type: non-small-cell lung cancer or small-cell lung cancer. The sensitivity of the tumors to radiation, chemotherapy, and the ability to surgically remove the tumor all vary in these two cancer classifications.

Non-Small-Cell Lung Cancer. The 5-year survival rate of lung cancer is reported to be approximately 16%. Approximately 50% of all patients with NSCLC have distant metastasis at the time of diagnosis (stage IV). There is no cure for these people, but oncologists are developing treatment regimens that may in the future prolong life. Currently, treatment focuses on the palliation of symptoms and disease control.[16,29,30]

The primary treatments for non-small-cell lung cancer are surgery and radiation therapy. Stages I, II, and in some cases IIIA are considered operable. Stage IIIA may be surgically curable, but the risk is high and the benefit is marginal. Surgery provides the best 5-year survival rates in the treatment of NSCLC: stage 1A, about 70%; stage IB, 50–60%; stage IIA, 40–55%; stage IIB, 40%; and stage IIIA about 25%.[16]

Radiation therapy is sometimes indicated before surgery to shrink the tumor, after surgery to kill remaining cancer cells, or at both times. But, even with the surgical removal of the lung, the recurrence rates are high.

Chemotherapy (or *chemo*) is an **adjuvant therapy** (an auxiliary treatment) to kill any cancer cells present in the body. In cases of recurrence, radiation and chemotherapy are used to relieve patient symptoms such as coughing and shortness of breath. Tumor reduction is one of the goals of adjuvant therapy. It relieves airway obstruction secondary to the endobronchial tumor, enabling the patient to breathe more comfortably. Other adjuvant therapies are:[16,30,36]

- Stent implantation (maintains airway patency in the presence of external compression of the trachea from tumor).
- Laser therapy (palliative reduction of endobronchial tumor mass).
- Photodynamic therapy (causes tumor light sensitivity and induces tumor cell death when the tumor is exposed to a concentrated laser beam).
- **Brachytherapy** (intraluminal application of radiation to patients with tumor-caused airway obstruction).

Small-Cell Lung Cancer. Surgery has a very limited place in the treatment of SCLC. It is suggested that patients with a solitary pulmonary nodule have lung resection followed by chemotherapy and thoracic radiotherapy. Other presentations of SCLC do not show improved survival with surgical resection.

Limited-stage SCLC is treated with multiple-drug chemotherapy usually containing a platinum-containing regimen and concurrent thoracic radiotherapy (see Table 12-1). The patient who goes into complete remission should be offered prophylactic cranial radiation therapy. Approximately 50% of patients achieve complete remission, but they relapse within 2 years.

Approximately two-thirds of SCLC patients have extensive-stage disease when initially diagnosed. Patients with extensive-stage SCLC respond to combination chemotherapy using a platinum-containing regimen, but the relapse rate is very rapid. Prophylactic cranial irradiation should be offered to all patients with extensive-stage disease who are responding to chemotherapy. It reduces brain metastasis, improves disease-free time, and prolongs life.[33] The adjuvant therapy available to patients with SCLC is the same as in NSCLC. New chemotherapy agents for SCLC have not appeared, but some experimental treatment strategies in the area of angiogenesis blocking agents have been are tested. Researchers hope that these drugs can stop blood flow to the tumors and starve them of the nutrients necessary for growth.[16,30,33]

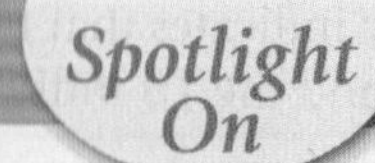

Racial Disparities in Lung Cancer

Lung cancer death and survival rates differ between African Americans and non-African Americans. According to statistics released from the American Cancer Society, African Americans have the highest death rate and the shortest survival rate of any racial and ethnic group in the United States. The reasons are complex and include social and economic differences. "These include inequalities in work, wealth, income, education, housing and overall standard of living, barriers to high-quality health care, and racial discrimination." Although, this disparity is decreasing, as of 2010, the overall cancer death rate was still 33% higher in African American men and 16% higher in African American women.

Source: *Statistics for 2009: Cancer Facts and Figures for African Americans 2009–2010*, American Cancer Society Inc. http://www.cancer.org/docroot/STT/STT_0.asp.

Summary

Atelectasis is the incomplete expansion of the lung. It can be categorized in several ways, but the simplest is dividing it into obstructive, nonobstructive, and special types of lung collapse. *Obstructive atelectasis*, the most common type, results from the reabsorption of gas from the lung distal to the obstruction. *Nonobstructive* types of atelectasis are caused by an abnormal relationship between the visceral and parietal pleura, a loss of surfactant, or the replacement of normal lung parenchyma with scar tissue or cellular infiltrates. One of the common *special* types of atelectasis is acute atelectasis after surgery, especially procedures involving the thorax or upper abdomen, has long been associated with the loss of lung volume, causing complete or partial alveolar collapse. Pain, medications, increased secretions, and the inability to cough and to take deep breaths are common causes of postoperative atelectasis. The treatment of atelectasis depends on the underlying cause. The goal of treatment is lung reinflation by removing the cause of the lung collapse.

Pleural disorders are pleural abnormalities that develop because of another primary disease or disorder. The pleural surface may become inflamed or irritated, or the pleural space may be filled with air, gas, or fluid. Pneumothorax is the presence of free air in the pleural space that causes partial or complete collapse of the affected lung. Pleural effusions are an accumulation of fluid in the pleural space. The most common cause of pleural effusion is congestive heart failure (30–40% of cases). The remaining 60–70% of the cases of pleural effusion are divided among nine primary diseases, with pneumonia as the second most common cause and malignancy as the third.

The two major classifications of lung cancer are non-small-cell lung cancer (NSCLC) and small-cell lung cancer (SCLC). NSCLC accounts for approximately 75% of all lung cancers, and it is a heterogeneous collection of three histological cell types: adenocarcinoma, squamous-cell carcinoma, and large-cell carcinoma. These histologies are classified together because the approaches to diagnosis, staging/prognosis, and treatment are similar. Small-cell lung cancer is very different from the other cancer classification with a different staging process, treatment approach, and prognosis.

The treatment of lung cancer depends on the cell type: non-small-cell lung cancer or small-cell lung cancer. The sensitivity of the tumors to radiation, chemotherapy, and the ability to surgically remove the tumor all vary in these two cancer classifications.

Study Questions

REVIEW QUESTIONS

1. Identify the four main cell types of malignant lung cancer.
2. Discuss the four mechanisms of pleural fluid formation leading to the development of a pleural effusion.
3. Compare and contrast the types of atelectasis.
4. Describe the clinical signs and symptoms of tension pneumothorax.
5. Describe the treatment for small-cell and non-small-cell lung cancer.

MULTIPLE-CHOICE QUESTIONS

1. Which lung cancer is most frequently found in nonsmokers?
   a. small cell
   b. adenocarcinoma
   c. large cell
   d. squamous cell
2. What is/are the cause(s) of collateral air drift in the lung?
   a. pores of Kohn
   b. canals of Lambert
   c. Martin's channels
   d. all of the above
3. What is a cause of obstructive atelectasis?
   a. pleural effusion
   b. bronchogenic carcinoma
   c. decreased lung surfactant
   d. lung fibrosis
4. What findings are present in a patient with a pleural effusion of 700 mL?
   a. increased bronchovesicular breath sounds
   b. hyper-resonance to percussion over the affected area
   c. mediastinal shift on chest X-ray
   d. decreased lung expansion in the effusion area
5. What cell type of lung cancer is associated with causing paraneoplastic syndromes?
   a. adenocarcinoma
   b. squamous cell
   c. large cell
   d. small cell
6. In which type of lung cancer is extensive disease present in 65–70% of patients at diagnosis?
   a. adenocarcinoma
   b. squamous cell
   c. large cell
   d. small cell
7. What is the curative treatment for the patient with non-small-cell cancer?
   a. surgery
   b. chemotherapy
   c. radiation therapy
   d. b and c
8. What are the radiographic findings in a patient with a tension pneumothorax?
   a. mediastinal shift to the affected side
   b. absence of pulmonary vascular markings on the affected side
   c. increased radio-opacity of the lung on the affected side
   d. blunting of the costophrenic angle on the affected side
9. What type of atelectasis is associated with lobar collapse?
   a. compression atelectasis
   b. nonobstructive atelectasis
   c. obstructive atelectasis
   d. adhesion atelectasis
10. What are the characteristics of a transudate?
    a. The fluid is an ultrafiltrate of plasma and contains less protein than plasma.
    b. The fluid is similar to plasma and has a higher level of protein.
    c. Transudates are usually present in pneumonia.
    d. b and c

CRITICAL-THINKING QUESTIONS

1. How might external compression of a bronchus result in atelectasis? Develop a treatment plan for the atelectasis caused by external compression of a bronchus.
2. How would decreased lung expansion after surgery lead to the development of atelectasis? What would you recommend to prevent the development of postoperative atelectasis?
3. In a patient with significant atelectasis, compensatory changes may be seen in the unaffected lung. Describe the compensatory changes and provide a rationale for their existence.

References

1. Sharma S. Atelectasis. eMedicine Specialties: Pulmonology: Aspiration and Atelectasis. June 14, 2006. http://emedicine.medscape.com/article/296468-overview.
2. Murray JF. Postnatal growth and development of the lung. In: *The Normal Lung*. Philadelphia: WB Saunders Co; 1976:51–53.
3. Martin HB., Respiratory bronchioles as the pathway for collateral ventilation. *J Apple Physiology*. 1966;21,5:1443–1447.
4. Miller WT. Acute alveolar opacities and atelectasis. In: *Diagnostic Thoracic Imaging*. New York: McGraw-Hill Professional; 2006:217–281.
5. Hingham H, Murray JF. Disorders of the airway. In: *Diseases of the Chest*. Philadelphia: WB Saunders Co; 1980:606–617.
6. Sharma S. Lung Cancer, non-small cell. eMedicine Specialties: Radiology: Chest. August 10, 2005.
7. Alhameed FM, Sharma S. Pneumothorax. eMedicine Specialties: Radiology of the Chest. December 11, 2008. http://emedicine.medscape.com/article/360796-overview.
8. Light R.W. Mediastinal and pleural disorders. In: Beers M, et al., eds. *The Merck Manual of Diagnosis and Therapy*. Whitehouse Station, NJ: Merck Research Laboratories; 2006:488–499.
9. Tammemagi CM, Freedman MT, Church TR, Oken MM, Hocking WG, Kvale PA, et al. Factors associated with human small aggressive non small cell lung cancer. *Cancer Epidemiol Biomarkers Prev.* 2007;16,10:2082–2089.
10. Vanderschueren R. Pleural diseases: pneumothorax. In: Albert R, Spiro S, Jett J, eds. *Comprehensive Respiratory Medicine*. St. Louis: Mosby: 1999: 65.1–65.4.
11. Hanley M. Pneumothorax. In: Parsons P, ed. *Critical Care Secrets*. St. Louis: Mosby-Yearbook: 1992:341–344.
12. Rubins J. Pleural effusion. eMedicine Specialties: Pulmonology. June 5, 2008. http://emedicine.medscape.com/article/299959-overview.
13. Loddenkemper R. Pleural diseases: pleural effusion. In: Albert R, Spiro S, Jett J, eds. *Comprehensive Respiratory Medicine*. St. Louis: Mosby: 1999: 66.1–66.10.
14. Sapira JD. About egophony. *Chest*. 1995;108,3: 865–867.
15. Novello S, Vavala T. Lung cancer and women. *Future Oncol*. 2008;4,5:705–716.
16. Midthun D, Jett J. Lung tumors. In: Albert R, Spiro S, Jett J, eds. *Comprehensive Respiratory Medicine*. St. Louis: Mosby: 1999:43.1–43.24.
17. Cancer Facts & Figures. American Cancer Society. 2008. http://www.cancer.org/docroot/STT/STT_0.asp.
18. Bradley CJ, Yarbrough KR, Adman B, Fewer EJ, Marriott A, Brown ML. Productivity costs of cancer mortality in the United States: 2000–2020. *J. Natl. Cancer Inst.* 2008;100,24:1763–1770.
19. Rise L, Elbert D, Rancho M, Stinchcomb D, Howlader N, Horner M, et al. *SEER Cancer Statistics Review, 1975–2005*. Bethesda, MD: National Cancer Institute; 2008. http://seer.cancer.gov/csr/1975_2007/index.html:, based on November 2007 SEER data submission, posted to SEER Web site, 2008.
20. Shields P. Molecular epidemiology of lung cancer. *Ann Oncol*. 1997;10:S7–S11.
21. Bach PB, Kattan MW, Thornquist MD, Kris MG, Tate RC, Barnett MJ, et al. Variations in lung cancer risk among smokers. *J. Natl. Cancer Inst.* 2003;95,6:470–478.
22. American Thoracic Society statement. Cigarette smoking and health. *Am J Respir Crit Care Med*. 1996;153:861–865.
23. Franceschi S, Bidoli E. The epidemiology of lung cancer. *Ann Oncology*. 1999. 10: p. S3–S6.
24. Leonard C, Sachs D. Environmental tobacco smoke and lung cancer incidence. *Curr Opin Pulm Med*. 1999;5:189–193.
25. Bain C, Feskanich D, Speizer FE, Thun M, Hertzmark E, Rosner BA, et al. Lung cancer rates in men and women with comparable histories of smoking. *J. Natl. Cancer Inst.*, 2004;96,11:826–834.
26. Bennett WP, Alavanja MCR, Blomeke B, Vahakangas KH, Castren K, Welsh JA, et al. Environmental tobacco smoke, genetic susceptibility, and risk of lung cancer in never-smoking women. *J. Natl. Cancer Inst.* 1999;91,23:2009–2014.
27. Yang P, Cerhan JR, Vierkant RA, Olson JE, Vachon CM, Limburg PJ, et al. Adenocarcinoma of the lung is strongly associated with cigarette smoking: further evidence from a prospective study of women. *Am. J. Epidemiol.* 2002;156,12:1114–1122.

28. Hackshaw A, Law M, Walkd N. The accumulated evidence on lung cancer and environmental tobacco smoke. *BMJ*, 1997;315:980–988.
29. Maghfoor I, Perry M. Lung cancer, non-small cell. EMedicine Specialties: Oncology: Carcinomas of the lung and other intrathoracic carcinomas. December 13, 2005. http://emedicine.medscape.com/article/279960-overview.
30. Hong WK, Tsao AS. Tumors of the lungs. In: Beers M, et al, eds. *The Merck Manual of Diagnosis and Therapy*. Whitehouse Station, NJ: Merck Research Laboratories; 2006:503–511.
31. Schwartz A, Rothrock M, Yang P, Swanson G. Increased cancer risk among relatives of non-smoking lung cancer cases. *Genet Epidemiol.* 1999;17:1–15.
32. Anderson K, Woo C, Olson J, Sellers T, Zheng W, Kushi L, et al., Association of family history of cervical, ovarian, and uterine cancer with histological categories of lung cancer: the Iowa Women's Health Study. *Cancer Epidemiol Biomarkers Prev,* 1997;6,6:401–405.
33. Maghfoor I, Perry M. Lung cancer, oat cell (small cell). eMedicine Specialties: Oncology: Carcinomas of the lung and other intrathoracic carcinomas. October 15, 2008. http://emedicine.medscape.com/article/280104-overview.
34. Brown W. Video assisted thoracic surgery: the Miami experience. *Semin Thorac Cardiovasc Surg.* 1998;10:305–312.
35. McCarthy J, Hurley J, Wood A. The diverse potential of thoracoscopic assisted surgery. *Int Surg.* 1997;82:29–31.
36. Stohr S, Bollinger C. Stents in the management of malignant airway obstruction. *Monaldi Arch Chest Dis.* 1999;54:264–268.

CHAPTER 12

Diseases That Affect the Pulmonary Vasculature

William Atkinson and Barbara A. Ludwig

OBJECTIVES

Upon completion of this chapter, the reader should be able to:

- Describe the pathophysiology of the various forms of pulmonary edema.
- List the differences between hemodynamic pulmonary edema and edema associated with acute lung injury.
- Explain the various ventilation/perfusion imbalances associated with acute pulmonary embolism and the mechanism of restoring balance as the clot dissipates and blood flow is restored.
- Name major causes of venous stasis in the lower extremities that are risk factors in the development of deep venous thrombosis.
- Explain cor pulmonale and discuss the various lung pathologies that are precursors to the condition.
- Name several mechanisms by which patients develop pulmonary hypertension.
- Discuss the hypoxemia that occurs by means of many different mechanisms in heart and lung disease.

CHAPTER OUTLINE

KEY TERMS

ACE inhibitors
acute respiratory distress syndrome (ARDS)
amyloidosis
angiotensin receptor blockers (ARBs)
aortic insufficiency (AI)
aortic stenosis (AS)
barotrauma
cardiac markers
cardiogenic shock
constrictive pericarditis
CT angiogram (CTA)
diaphoresis
diastolic dysfunction
diastolic gallop
fibrinolysis
granulomatous
hepatojugular reflux
Homan's sign
hydrostatic pressure
intrapulmonary shunting
J-type juxtapulmonary receptors
Kerley's lines
kyphoscoliosis
loop diuretics
lupus erythematosus
mitral regurgitation
mitral stenosis
oncotic pressure
palpitations
paroxysmal nocturnal dyspnea
perfusion pressure
pulmonary edema
pulsus alternans
sarcoidosis
systolic dysfunction
Westermark's sign

This chapter explains various syndromes so that the respiratory therapist is able to understand their pathophysiology and mechanisms. Diagnosing is discussed, and, in some cases, treatment strategies are outlined. Special emphasis is placed on respiratory therapy modalities as they apply to this group of illnesses.

Hemodynamic Pulmonary Edema

Hemodynamic pulmonary edema is the accumulation of hypotonic fluid in the interstitial space of the lung caused by an imbalance of the capillary **perfusion pressure** and the pulmonary venous pressure.

PHYSIOLOGIC CONSIDERATIONS

Fluid accumulates in the interstitial space of the lung if either the capillary perfusion pressure or the pulmonary venous pressure is too high. In the first instance, the capillary bed is stretched, and the spaces between the vascular endothelial cells allow for leakage of fluid into the interstitial space under the increased pressure. In the second instance, leakage is caused by increased **hydrostatic pressure** in the pulmonary venous system resulting from a number of cardiac causes.

If the changes in pressure are small, the increase in interstitial water can be cleared by the lymphatic system. This system can remove 18–20 mL of fluid per hour and direct it to the pleural space, ultimately clearing it through the thoracic duct. An acute rise in the capillary perfusion pressure can far exceed the **oncotic pressure** in the interstitium and flood the space. In that case, the lymphatic system cannot keep up with this rapid water accumulation even though, under these circumstances, it can increase its clearance capacity to up to 200 mL per hour.[1]

As a consequence of increased lung water, the lung stiffens, with decreased compliance requiring increased work of breathing and dyspnea, even though there may not be deterioration of oxygen transfer early in the process. As pulmonary venous pressures increase, interstitial water continues to accumulate. The accumulation of fluid in the interstitium can compromise the small airways and lead to mild hypoxemia. **J-type juxtapulmonary receptors** J-receptors, which modulate respiration, are stimulated and lead to tachypnea. With accumulations of more than 500 mL of interstitial fluid, the alveolar epithelium is violated, and alveolar flooding and frank **pulmonary edema** follow, with severe hypoxemia and respiratory failure.

Physiologic note: Even given high pulmonary venous pressures, the structure of the alveolar capillary relationship prevents leakage into and the flooding of the alveolar space until late in the process. On one side of the vascular space is wide interstitial space that is away from the alveolar membrane; this space allows fluid to accumulate in the interstitium without violating airspace. On the opposite side of the capillary wall, the alveolar membrane abuts the capillary endothelial membrane and protects the alveolar airspace with tight intercellular junctions between the alveolar lining cells. Only after these tight junctions break down can alveolar flooding occur.[2]

PATHOPHYSIOLOGY

The outflow of blood from the left atrium is the common denominator for most causes of cardiogenic pulmonary edema. The edema (fluid from inside blood vessels seeps outside the blood vessel into the surrounding tissues) may take the form of obstruction at the level of the mitral valve, as seen in the **mitral stenosis** or acute **mitral regurgitation** associated with papillary muscle dysfunction during acute myocardial infarction.

So-called **systolic dysfunction** occurs with syndromes that interfere with the cardiac output (CO) and stroke volume of the cardiac pump: acute infarction, left ventricular outflow obstruction and overload (the case with aortic valve disease), and septal hypertrophy and obstruction.

Diastolic dysfunction as a cause of cardiogenic pulmonary edema occurs when the left ventricle is incompletely filled during diastole, as seen in severe hypertensive disease associated with left ventricular hypertrophy. Infiltrative cardiac disease, such as seen in **amyloidosis**, produces the same picture. Pericardial effusion and **constrictive pericarditis** prohibit diastolic relaxation and filling of the left ventricle, leading to increases of left atrial pressure and cardiac failure.

The classification of systolic and diastolic heart failure may be a bit artificial because many of these conditions are associated with the features of both.

- Fluid overload and increased left ventricular end diastolic pressures are common to many of these conditions, especially when the left ventricle starts to dilate. Typically, these are the effects of **aortic insufficiency (AI)** and end-stage **aortic stenosis (AS)**.
- They are also a consequence of mitral regurgitation because the L ventricle is not protected as it is in mitral stenosis. Noncardiac conditions associated with fluid overload occur in *renal failure*, the hypoproteinemic state associated with nephritic syndrome and iatrogenic overinfusion of fluids and blood products.
- Often unrecognized causes of pulmonary edema occur in the elderly and chronically ill patients who have a number of comorbidities, including low serum albumin from poor nutrition, anemia, and modest levels of hypoxemia associated with unappreciated pulmonary disease. These patients develop interstitial fluid and edema at much lower L atrial pressures than normal because of low intravascular oncotic pressures. In addition, oxygen-carrying capacity and delivery in the presence of anemia, coupled with hypoxemia associated with primary pulmonary disease, further impair cardiac function. Even with only minimal impairment of cardiac function such as in a small myocardial infarction that would otherwise not cause edema, these comorbidities can lead to life-threatening pulmonary edema.[3]

DIAGNOSTIC FEATURES

Pulmonary edema is often caused by heart failure. As the heart fails, pressure in the pulmonary venous system starts to rise. As the pressure in these blood vessels increases, fluid is forced into the interstitial spaces and ultimately into the alveoli. This fluid reduces oxygen diffusion into the blood, resulting in hypoxemia.

Pulmonary edema may be caused by damage directly to the lung or severe infection. Lung damage with a build-up of body fluid is also seen in kidney failure. Pulmonary edema may also be a complication of a mechanical inefficiency due to heart attack, leaking or narrowed mitral or aortic valves, or weakening or stiffening of the heart muscle.

The health care provider will perform a history, physical exam, laboratory evaluation, measurement of blood oxygen levels, chest X-ray, electrocardiogram (ECG), and other tests.

History. The patient often has a history of previous heart disease or a heart murmur. At times, a family member has had premature heart disease or a congenital lesion that had to be corrected. Some types of arrhythmias and metabolic defects that run in families may be important, and one should ask about previous kidney and lung disease.

The usual symptoms are as follows:

- Air hunger and dyspnea are symptoms, but unassociated with cough and sputum production.
- When sputum is present, it is usually not thick or purulent, but thin, colorless, and foamy. It may be pink or blood tinged, but not bloody.
- Patients tend to want to sit and not lie down because the dyspnea increases as a consequence of gravity and redistribution of fluid from the lower extremities. Often, a patient is much more comfortable sleeping with several pillows (orthopnea). There may or may not be a history of ankle and leg edema.
- Because of the redistribution of fluid with gravity, some patients will waken from sleep with acute dyspnea and sit on the side of the bed or go to the window to catch their breath (**paroxysmal nocturnal dyspnea**).
- A patient with ischemic heart disease may complain of precordial pressure, jaw pain, or pain radiating to the L shoulder and medial portion of the L arm.
- **Diaphoresis** and **palpitations** are common, and the patient may be peripherally vasoconstricted and cyanotic, complaining of being cold.
- Patients are almost never febrile and do not complain of chills or rigor.

TABLE 12-1 **Comparison of pulmonary edema with pneumonia**

Characteristics	Pulmonary Edema	Pneumonia
Profound	Dyspnea	Variable
Non-productive and unusual	Cough	Productive
Thin and foamy occas. pink tinged	Sputum	Copious, thick, and colored gray, yellow, or green
Never unless associated pneumonia or sepsis	Fever	Usual often with chills and rigor
Diffuse	Distribution	Localized
Rare	Leukocytosis and left shift	Usual unless viral
Common	Cardiomegaly	Never unless associated cardiac disease
Common	Peripheral edema	Never
Usual	Tachycardia	Common
Usual	S3	Rare unless concomitant CHF

Table 12-1 distinguishes the presentation of pulmonary edema from pneumonia.

Physical Examination. The patient presents with varying degrees of respiratory distress. Unless the left heart failure has led to subsequent right-sided overload and right heart failure, or both sides are involved (as can be seen in pericardial tamponade, cardiomyopathy, and infiltrative myocardial disease), peripheral signs of right heart failure are absent. These include ankle and leg edema, liver engorgement and enlargement, **hepatojugular reflux**, and distended pulsatile neck veins at 45 degrees of head elevation.

The main physical findings of cardiogenic pulmonary edema are fine inspiratory rales at the posterior lung bases. As the edema becomes more severe and the alveolar space is flooded, coarse, bubbly rales can be heard throughout, in addition to harsh breath sounds and severe respiratory distress. Tachycardia is always present in the absence of heart block, and the primary auscultatory findings are a ventricular **diastolic gallop** (S3) and **pulsus alternans**. Patients are usually cyanotic. The hectic cardiac rhythm often precludes identifying other abnormalities or valvular lesions by auscultation.

Laboratory Evaluation. A blood count should determine whether the patient is anemic. Normally, the white blood cell count is minimally elevated, but there rarely is a left shift with immature neutrophils present, which should make infectious disease (pneumonia) less likely.

A metabolic panel assesses the degree of renal insufficiency. One may see modest elevations of the BUN with normal creatinine if renal perfusion is decreased or the patient is dehydrated. The blood chemistries should also reveal abnormalities of potassium and magnesium, which could be the result of excess diuresis. A low serum albumin suggests malnutrition and makes the treatment of the edema and diuresis all the more difficult.

Cardiac markers should be done to be sure that myocardial ischemia or myocardial cell death has not occurred. These include serial measurements of CPK-MB and Treponon levels. B-naturetic peptide levels add very little to the diagnosis, but they are useful as guides to the effectiveness of treatment and to follow the treatment over the long-term course of the disease.

Electrocardiography. The *electrocardiogram* has no specific findings caused by pulmonary edema and congestive heart failure. However, the presence of left ventricular hypertrophy or left bundle branch block may suggest aortic valve disease or a hypertensive heart. An electrocardiogram can also be very helpful when it shows evidence of ischemia or of current injury, suggesting acute myocardial damage as the cause of the pulmonary edema. Various arrhythmias may also provide clues to the reason the heart suddenly failed to pump efficiently. These patients should be put on continuous electrocardiographic monitoring as soon as they come to the hospital to detect any arrhythmias or heart block.

Arterial Blood Gasses and Pulse Oximetry. Initial arterial samples should be taken as part of the assessment. The *arterial blood gasses* (*ABG*) gives not only the level of oxygenation, but also the effectiveness of ventilation from the pCO_2 and the acid-base state to be sure there is no underlying acidosis as overventilation. Alkylosis should be present in uncomplicated cases.

Pulse oximetry should be used only to follow the patient's ability to oxygenate. It is not a measure of ventilation and often misleads caregivers toward wrong conclusions about the effectiveness of their therapy.

Imaging. Standard *posteroanterior* (*PA*) and *lateral chest X-rays* may not be possible if the patient is in respiratory distress. So some of the subtleties and classical features of cardiac failure and congestive heart failure cannot be appreciated. Portable PA chest films are then done to help establish the diagnosis. Classical findings include:

- Cephalization of the pulmonary vessels with fuzzy indistinct definition of their outlines.
- Cardiac enlargement.
- Blunting of the costophrenic angles and/or obvious pleural effusion.
- **Kerley's lines** leading to the pleura, indicating engorged lymphatics and a hazy ground glass appearance of the lung fields themselves (see Chapter 14).

Two-dimentional echocardiography can often be done at the bedside with portable machines. Valvular disease, as well as presence of pleural effusion, can be easily detected. Adynamic segments of L ventricular myocardium are ominous signs of ischemia or infracted segments of the ventricular wall. Diastolic volume of the left ventricle and ejection are good indications of cardiac output and efficiency. If the pulmonary edema is the consequence of an acute ischemic cardiac event, the patient should be stabilized and taken to the cardiac catheterization lab where the coronary arteries can be imaged and a revascularization procedure performed.

BEDSIDE MONITORING

The goals of treatment can be reached with monitoring as a guide to therapy. In addition to continuously monitoring vital signs, urinary output and oxygenation should be tracked.

By means of the following tools, pulmonary arterial pressure monitoring and periodic measurements of pulmonary capillary wedge pressure are used to track cardiac output.

- In mechanically ventilated patients, frequent arterial blood gas analysis is warranted.
- In patients with pump failure, overwhelming pulmonary edema, or **cardiogenic shock**, intra-arterial continuous blood pressure (BP) monitoring and right heart catheterization with a Swan-Ganz line are frequently employed.

Urinary output must be maintained even in hypotensive states. In addition to diuretics, a low-dose dopamine drip might be used to increase renal blood flow. The pulmonary capillary wedge pressure and the pulmonary artery diastolic pressure reflect L atrial pressure. As cardiac output improves with inotropic therapy, afterload reduction, diuresis, and oxygenation, the wedge pressure, and the pulmonary artery diastolic pressure should all increase, as well as the mixed venous O_2 content. Instances of cardiogenic shock with low cardiac output and low blood pressure call for adrenergic blood pressure support with dopamine and dobutamine. If that fails, intra-aortic balloon placement through the femoral artery and counterpulsation therapy may be warranted until cardiac function and blood pressure are restored.[4]

OXYGENATION AND MECHANICAL VENTILATION

Oxygen, one of the hallmarks of therapy, must be given to all patients in cardiac failure. If patients can maintain ventilation on their own, assisted ventilation may not be needed. In most instances with pulmonary edema and alveolar flooding, neither oxygenation nor ventilation can be sustained, and mechanical ventilation is required. In recent years, BiPAP (bidirectional airway pressure) therapy without intubation has become popular. BiPAP gives a ventilatory assist and maintains intratracheal expiratory pressure in an attempt to recruit alveoli and increase functional residual capacity.

Hypoxic patients are often confused and combative because of air hunger and are therefore intolerant of the BiPAP mask. In such instances, sedation and intubation are necessary before the patient deteriorates. With the newer, more sophisticated mechanical ventilators available today, many techniques can be employed. Often one starts with plain assisted ventilation, but often the patient overrides the ventilator because of air hunger and tachypnea. Ineffective ventilation and oxygenation are the result. A better tactic is to use volume-controlled ventilation with pressure limitation and autoflow. Another effective maneuver is to use positive end-expiratory pressure (PEEP). Both techniques tend to recruit new alveoli, increase lung compliance, and, within limits, enhance oxygenation and cardiac output. If PEEP is used in excess, the mean intrathoracic pressure is increased, and venous return impaired, thus decreasing cardiac output.[5]

DRUG THERAPY

In addition to oxygen and ventilation therapy, several drugs are useful in treating pulmonary edema.

Diuretics. **Loop diuretics**, especially furosamide, are central to the treatment of pulmonary edema. The patients have water excess and are often hypervolemic with decreased renal blood flow. Loop diuretics are the most effective agents to clear fluid from the intravascular space and ultimately improve cardiac function. The medication is usually given intravenously to patients in the acute state, either by direct injection or continuous infusion. The drug acts quite quickly, and diuresis is substantial as long as renal blood flow can be maintained and the patient is not hypovolemic.

Nitroglycerine and Nitroprusside. Nitroglycerine in its varying forms reduces preload rapidly and reduces afterload to some degree. Given intravenously in a drip, the dose can be titrated gradually up to as high as 100 μg/min.

Nitroprusside is a potent preload and afterload reducer that causes smooth muscle relaxation. Given in an intravenous drip, it rapidly increases cardiac output but can cause significant reduction in BP, which must be monitored. Prolonged use can cause thiocyanate toxicity.

ACE Inhibitors and Angiotensin Receptor Blocker. **ACE inhibitors** and **angiotensin receptor blockers (ARBs)** reduce afterload, increase cardiac output, and lower BP. They are given orally and are usually reserved for the outpatient setting and the general hospital setting. Better drugs can be used in the acute setting. However, after an acute episode, these drugs need to be given when the patient is discharged to the nonacute setting, either in the hospital or home.

Morphine Sulfate. Morphine sulfate has been used for many years in the treatment of acute pulmonary edema. It reduces preload to some degree, but its main effect is to reduce the anxiety and rapid shallow breathing associated with the syndrome. Its main problems are oversedation, decreased cardiac output, and respiratory depression, often leading to intubation and ICU admission.

Dopamine and Dobutamine. Dopamine and dobutamine are both useful adrenergic agents in the treatment of acute pulmonary edema and cardiac failure.

The effects of dopamine are dose dependant, and it is given by continuous intravenous infusion. In low doses, the drug increases renal blood flow and hence urinary output. Higher doses increase cardiac contractility and cardiac output. Very high doses have an alpha adrenergic effect, cause vasoconstriction, and increase blood pressure. Higher doses are arrhythmogenic and should be used with caution.

Dobutamine is a beta-1-receptor agonist and to some degree has beta 2 activity. It has significant inotropic activity and increases cardiac output. It produces significant vasodilatation; if the patient becomes hypotensive, the dose has to be reduced.

Norepinephrine. Norepinephrine is an alpha adrenergic agonist reserved for patients in profound shock whose BP cannot be supported by other means. It increases afterload and decreases cardiac output.

Newer Agents. Nesiritide is a recombinant BNP (B-Naturetic peptide) that decreases right-sided pressures, wedge pressure, and systemic vascular resistance, increasing cardiac output.

Phosphodiesterase inhibitors have a positive inotropic effect, decrease afterload, and decrease pulmonary vascular resistance. They work by increasing intracellular cyclic AMP by preventing its breakdown.

Pulmonary Heart Disease

Diseases of the lungs can cause right heart disease and subsequent right heart failure—a condition referred to as *cor pulmonale*. In 84% of cases, the hypertrophy of the right ventricle associated with this condition is caused by chronic obstructive lung disease (COLD). Other causes are:

- Interstitial lung disease.
- Thoracic cage deformity.
- Obstructive sleep apnea.
- Neuromuscular diseases.
- Obesity hypoventilation syndrome.
- Pulmonary fibrosis associated with a number of systemic diseases, the most common of which are the collagen vascular diseases.

Separate consideration should be reserved for the syndromes of idiopathic (primary) pulmonary hypertension and recurrent pulmonary embolism. Acute massive pulmonary embolism is often a lethal cause of acute cor pulmonale.

OBSTRUCTIVE LUNG DISEASES

The common denominator in the development of pulmonary hypertension in the obstructive lung diseases (emphysema, chronic bronchitis, and chronic asthma) is chronic hypoxemia. This leads to endothelial proliferation and vasoconstriction in the pulmonary arterial bed. The toxic effects of cigarette smoke (vasoconstriction and oxidation) are the primary, but not the only, causes of the pathological evolution of these changes.[6] Over time, the changes become permanent, leading to so-called *fixed pulmonary hypertension*. Ultimately, right heart failure follows.[7]

CASE STUDY 12-1

A 75-year-old man presented to the emergency room with the chief complaint of shortness of breath, which had become progressive over the past 4 days. He had additional complaints of cough and fever up to 102°F and was producing gray-green sputum. On the day of admission, he produced sputum mixed with blood. Upon questioning, he admitted to being short of breath for a considerable amount of time prior to this present illness. He had been able to walk to the light pole on the street without dyspnea. He also complained of sharp right supraclavicular pain, which was worse with respiration and associated with precordial chest heaviness. The patient had a known elevated right hemidiaphragm, which was presumed to be from a paralyzed phrenic nerve.

His past history included treatment for hypertension, left knee arthroplasty, and colonoscopy with removal of benign polyps. A prostatectomy was done 6 years prior to admission for adenocarcinoma. When he developed recurrence the year prior to admission, he underwent a course of radiation therapy. Following his knee surgery, he developed chest pain. Evaluation for ischemic cardiac disease proved negative, but he was later shown to have esophageal candidiasis and, when he was given antifungal agents, the chest pain resolved.

He never smoked.

System review was negative except for chronic constipation and anxiety.

Physical Examination:
He was in moderate respiratory distress on oxygen with a temperature of 102°F. His BP 137/76, pulse 102 and regular, respiratory rate of 20 and an O_2 saturation of 86% on room air, which increased to 92% on 2 LO_2 by nasal cannula. There were decreased breath sounds at both lung bases, greater on the right, with a right-sided pleural friction rub over the lateral chest. There were no cardiac abnormalities except the tachycardia, and the remainder of the physical examination was normal.

X-ray of the chest showed atelectasis of both lower lobes and bilateral apical pleural parenchymal scarring. He had no pleural effusion or pneumothorax. The sputum culture showed no pathogens and only normal oropharyngeal flora.

Laboratory data was normal except for mild elevation of the transaminases and bilirubin, an arterial PO_2 of 61 torr and a slightly low PCO_2. White blood cell count was normal without a left shift, and he was not anemic. Cardiac markers were normal.

Initial treatment consisted of oxygen, third-generation cephalosporins, and doxycycline.

After arriving to the floor, the nurse noted that he desaturated to 88% on 4 L nasal oxygen and improved to only 94% with 5 L nasal O_2 and deep breathing. He had persistent, blood-tinged sputum. A standard two-view PA and lateral chest showed only right-sided atelectasis and a small pleural effusion. Subsequent **CT angiogram (CTA)** of the chest showed multiple filling defects bilaterally in the pulmonary arterial system. He was subsequently anticoagulated with intravenous heparin, which was later switched to low-molecular-weight heparin subcutaneously. A 2-D echocardiogram showed elevated right-sided pressures (estimated) but no other abnormalities of significance.

On the second hospital day, the patient developed acute respiratory distress while moving from his bed to the chair. Oxygen saturation at that time was 93% on 4 L nasal O_2. Breath sounds were reduced in the lower lobes, and the episode resolved with bronchodilator inhalation. Electrocardiogram revealed a right bundle branch block. X-ray was unchanged.

Over the next few days, the patient showed progressive improvement, was switched to warfarin, and was discharged using oxygen at night to be followed as an outpatient.

Outpatient Follow-up Visit:
The patient was seen in the outpatient department 12 days after discharge and was found to be adequately anticoagulated. He continued to be desaturated at night and thus remained on nocturnal oxygen. His vital signs were normal, but he continued to be in mild respiratory distress, especially in the supine position. He had some airway sounds, but the rest of the physical exam was normal. He had no evidence of deep venous thrombosis. Repeat pulmonary CT angiogram showed persistent filling defects, which had only partially resolved and which appeared to be adherent to the vessel walls.

Assessment:
Since his dyspnea can be traced back to the prostate surgery and radiation, it is likely that at

(continues)

(continued)

least some of the emboli are old, especially since they failed to resolve after a considerable period of anticoagulation. The acute illness appeared clinically to be an infectious process that precipitated respiratory failure. Some of the clots could have been new, but there was no obvious source. This patient will likely need prolonged and even lifetime anticoagulation.

Discussion Questions

1. Describe the changes in ventilation and perfusion that occur acutely in pulmonary embolism.
2. What are the causes of hypoxemia in acute pulmonary embolism?
3. In this specific case, describe the possible sources of the emboli.
4. In this case, describe the features that favor embolism and those that favor pneumonia.
5. In pulmonary embolism, describe the changes that occur in ventilation and perfusion that compensate for the imbalance and restore effective oxygenation in the days after the acute event.

Cor pulmonale can often be suspected clinically in patients with chronic lung disease who are shown to be chronically hypoxemic. They often have a history of repeated episodes of respiratory failure and show clinical evidence of diminished air entry, hyperaeration, cardiac enlargement (by chest X-ray), and peripheral edema. These patients often have very loud pulmonic second heart tones with a widely split second sound, a right ventricular heave, and a tricuspid regurgitant murmur. Two-dimensional echocardiography is usually sufficient to establish right ventricular hypertrophy, but right heart catheterization and measurement of pulmonary artery pressures with and without oxygen prove the diagnosis. The wedge pressure must be normal to rule out left heart disease, and there must not be evidence of left to right shunting, overloading the right heart.[8]

OTHER CAUSES

Kyphoscoliosis and other severe deformities of the chest wall lead to underventilation of large portions of one or both lungs with overdistention of other portions, leading to a large imbalance between ventilation and pulmonary perfusion. Over time, as the abnormality progresses, chronic hypoxemia ensues, resulting in pulmonary hypertension, which ultimately becomes fixed and leads to cor pulmonale and right heart failure.

There is a long list of lung diseases (see Chapter 10), many of whose etiologies are not known, that cause diffuse infiltration of the lung parenchyma. In their chronic states, these processes, whatever their cause, result in lung fibrosis and interference with oxygen diffusion at the level of the alveolar-capillary membrane. An example is idiopathic interstitial fibrosis (IPF), often called usual interstitial pneumonia (UIP). This disease has a number of etiologies; some are inhalational, some infectious and inflammatory, and some immunogenic. The disease usually has a protracted course with fibrosis and ultimately the destruction of the architecture of the lung and so-called honeycombing, a characteristic radiographic finding. At end stage, severe irreversible pulmonary hypertension results in cor pulmonale and right heart failure. Sudden death often results from fatal cardiac arrhythmias or sudden cardiac collapse with low cardiac output state. An acute form of the disease has been described and referred to the as *Hamman-Riche syndrome*, which is rapidly progressive and fatal; its histopathology is indistinguishable from the more protracted form of the disease.

The chronic **granulomatous** diseases of the lung deserve special mention, primarily because the fibrosis is often patchy and the infiltrates nodular, not linear and diffuse. For example, **sarcoidosis** is a granulomatous inflammatory process in the lung; the immunologic reaction has gone wild, leading to fibrosis and the destruction of the lung architecture. The etiology is not known, but some cases respond to anti-inflammatory and immunosupressive therapy.

Berylliosis, a granulomatous disease with a known etiology (inhalation of beryllium dust from machined metal alloy) causes an immunologic reaction in the lung with progressive granuloma formation and fibrosis, leading to pulmonary hypertension.

Obstructive Sleep Apnea (OSA) and Obesity Hypoventilation Syndrome (OHS). Obstructive sleep apnea (OSA) and obesity hypoventilation syndrome (OHS) are considered together because they often occur together and because they both result from chronic hypoxemia. The entities are often accompanied by COLD, but not always. Although obesity is universal in OHS, it is not always in OSA. In obesity hypoventilation, chronic hypoventilation results in both hypoxemia and hypercarbia and eventual in pulmonary hypertension. In sleep apnea, the patients obstruct their upper airway during sleep and become apneic. They oxygen-desaturate during these episodes, develop pulmonary as well as systemic hypertension, and experience chronic sleep deprivation. Over a prolonged period of time, without intervention, the pulmonary hypertension in both diseases becomes fixed. In the case of OSA, treatment includes nocturnal continuous positive airway pressure breathing (CPAP); in OHS, it consists of weight reduction, assisted ventilation, and low-flow oxygen.

Neuromuscular Diseases. A number of neuromuscular diseases, such as muscular dystrophy of the Duchenne's variety and amyotrophic lateral sclerosis (Lou Gehrig's disease), cause progressive loss of skeletal muscle function including the muscles of respiration. Progressive ventilatory failure occurs, terminally leading to pulmonary hypertension. Additionally, the heart muscle itself may be affected further, adding to the cardiopulmonary insult. Progression of the pulmonary complications can be delayed by oxygen supplementation, but eventually assisted ventilation is needed to maintain life. Other diseases, including poliomyelitis, Guillain–Barré syndrome, and myasthenia gravis, have similar consequences in their terminal state.

IDIOPATHIC (PRIMARY) PULMONARY HYPERTENSION (IPH)

This term is reserved for a syndrome that occurs primarily in young women and that is rapidly fatal. The disease is thought to be immunologically mediated with a primary change in the pulmonary arterioles themselves. An endothelial proliferation of the vessels is the primary lesion with progressive onion skinning of the arteriole and ultimate obliteration of the vessels and progressive pulmonary hypertension.[9] IPH is often accompanied by a number of markers of collagen vascular diseases, such as antinuclear antibodies, without findings of the disease itself. Occasionally scleroderma or another collagen vascular disease becomes obvious after pulmonary hypertension is well established.[10] Because of this relationship and similar pathology, the collagen diseases and IPH are often lumped together.

PULMONARY VASCULITIS

Rapidly developing pulmonary hypertension occurs in vasculitis of the pulmonary vessels. This inflammatory process can be part of a connective tissue disease such as **lupus erythematosus** or rheumatoid arthritis. It can also be the primary lesion as in Churg-Strauss disease, which is associated with eosinophilia and usually presents as asthma. Pathologically, these diseases are accompanied by inflammatory cells seen in the pulmonary vessel walls as opposed to the pathologic changes in scleroderma. These forms of pulmonary hypertension are usually responsive and largely reversible with corticosteroid or immunosupressive therapy.

PULMONARY EMBOLISM

Embolization of the pulmonary vascular bed usually comes from clots formed in the deep veins of the femoralpopliteal system in the lower extremities. Stasis in these veins is the precursor to clot formation. The stasis may be associated with diseased veins, long periods of immobility such as occurs in prolonged bed rest or hospitalization, long bus or plane rides, underlying right-sided cardiac failure, or the immobility associated with restricting plaster casts applied for fractures of the lower extremity. In rare instances, circulating clotting factors, either hereditary or acquired as a result of a systemic disease, can predispose one to clot as part of a hypercoaguable state. Such is the case with lupus erythematosus, where proteins C and S are identified with clotting; in these cases, the clotting need not be restricted to the leg veins. These clots at times dislodge and travel to the pulmonary arterial bed. This event leads to wide discrepancies between ventilation and perfusion with dead space ventilation, **intrapulmonary shunting**, and overperfusion of the remaining lung, producing hypoxemia. Local hypoxemia in the lung may lead to bronchospasm and redistribution of the inspired air.[11] If the embolism is not large and occludes less than 50% of the pulmonary vascular bed, cardiac output can usually be maintained. If the obstruction is greater than 50%, circulatory collapse, low cardiac output, and a hypotensive state can lead to catastrophic consequences, including arrhythmia and sudden death. Normally, the percentage of intrapulmonary shunt is less than 10%. When the intrapulmonary shunt is greater than 30%, resultant hypoxemia does not improve with supplemental oxygenation because the shunted blood does not come in contact with the high oxygen content in the alveoli. P_AO_2 continues to fall proportionately as the shunt increases.

In the diagnosis of pulmonary embolism:

- The patient usually complains of a sharp pleuritic pain in the chest with the sudden onset of dyspnea.
- Hemoptysis (the coughing up of bloody sputum) may or may not occur.
- Patients often have a sense of impending doom and are very air hungry.
- A pleural rub is often not present.
- Wheezing is occasionally heard.
- Tachycardia is almost always present, along with varying degrees of hypoxemia.

Signs of right-sided cardiac overload and hypertension are common if a significant clot load has migrated to the pulmonary vascular bed. These signs include:

- Distended neck veins.
- Loud pulmonary component of the second sound.
- Increased split of S2 and an occasional right-sided third heart sound (gallop).

One must search diligently for signs of deep vein thrombosis of the lower extremities, including:

- Unilateral calf tenderness and edema.
- Varicosities and signs of stasis.
- A positive **Homan's sign** (pain in the ipsilateral calf when the calf is flexed passively).[12]

Laboratory tests are helpful but not diagnostic.

- Low arterial PO_2s are the rule. It has been said that, if the arterial PO_2 is above 90 torr, a pulmonary embolism is not present. This cutoff does not exclude many patients because most of them have depressed blood oxygen values anyway due to underlying cardiac or pulmonary disease.
- Elevated blood transaminases in the past have been used to help confirm pulmonary emboli, but they are rarely helpful.
- Elevated blood fibrin split products and other markers of clot formation and dissolution are not helpful.
- An electrocardiogram can be helpful if it shows a mean QRS axis that has shifted to the right and back to the left again. One may also see EKG evidence of right ventricular overload and strain, right bundle branch block, and various atrial tachyarrhythmias, none of which are diagnostic.
- Ventilatory function studies, including diffusion capacity, are not useful and should not be done in an acute situation.

The standard PA and lateral chest X-ray is usually normal. If abnormalities exist, they are often subtle. Occasionally one sees a small pleural effusion or an elevated diaphragm on the side of the pain. A unilateral segment of lung with no lung markings and a prominent proximal pulmonary artery on that side (**Westermark's sign**) or a wedge-shaped density with bowing of the fissures and pleural effusion (Hampton's hump) indicate not only pulmonary embolism, but frank infarction of a portion of lung. However, these are rarely seen.

In the past, ventilation/perfusion lung scans were used to confirm the diagnosis. Albumin tagged with iodine 131 was infused in the venous system, and radioactive xenon was inhaled, held in the lungs, and washed out in one sitting. The radio-labeled albumin was trapped in the pulmonary capillary bed, and the chest was subsequently scanned to determine the evenness of perfusion. One looked for wedge-shaped, pleural-based areas of nonperfusion. A second scan was done for xenon distribution, and the evenness of ventilation was determined. The two scans were matched, looking for areas of ventilation that are not perfused. It is largely accepted that a normal perfusion excludes a significant pulmonary embolism. However, the patient with underlying pulmonary disease already has an existing mismatch of ventilation and perfusion, such that the significance of perfusion defects is less certain.

Until recently, the pulmonary angiogram has been regarded as the gold standard test to confirm the presence of pulmonary embolism. The test required a pulmonary artery catheterization, rapid injection of iodinated dye, and a sophisticated vascular radiology suite. In the presence of pulmonary hypertension, arrhythmias often occur, leading to an occasional cardiac arrest. The dye loads were substantial, and transient renal insufficiency frequently occurred, especially if the patient had preexisting renal disease. Now, with the advent of advanced CT scanners and digital radiography, dye can be rapidly dripped in a peripheral vein, and the patient can be scanned shortly after the diagnosis is suspected. The images can be rapidly transmitted digitally by phone lines or by satellite to off-site reading stations, either to distant radiographic reading rooms or to the covering radiologist's home. CT angiography is now accepted as the standard of care.[13]

In both procedures, iodine hypersensitivity requires the pretreatment of the patient with corticosteroids, which does not absolutely eliminate the possibility of an allergic reaction.

The goals of treatment are to maintain oxygenation and to prevent further extension of the clot until **fibrinolysis** can occur.

- Oxygen is always given to maintain an O_2 saturation above 90%. In a few cases, ventilatory support is required.
- Heparin is the anticoagulant of choice to prevent further clotting while fibrinolysis occurs. The most common practice is to give an 8- to 10-thousand-unit bolus of heparin intravenously and follow that with a heparin drip of 1000 units an hour. The partial thromboplastin time (PTT) is usually checked every 4 hours until a stable and therapeutic value is achieved.
- Thrombolysis can be enhanced with thromboplastin activation (TPA), urokinase, or streptokinase intravenous thrombolytics. The preferred drug is TPA because it can be directly injected

into the pulmonary artery and has fewer idiosyncratic allergic reactions. If thrombolytics are to be used, the heparin needs to be stopped and the PTT normalized.

Initially, patients are kept in bed until they are hemodynamically stable and there is no residual evidence of deep venous thrombosis. They can then be ambulated and the anticoagulation changed to an oral agent (warfarin). Minimum treatment is 6 weeks, but persistent venous thrombosis or severe stasis may require longer anticoagulation.

Surgical intervention with thrombectomy is a last-resort measure reserved for patients with massive clotting and cardiovascular collapse in a low cardiac output state. In these instances, BP and adequate oxygenation cannot be maintained. This operation requires putting the patient on cardiac and pulmonary bypass therapy and manually extracting the clot from the pulmonary artery. Rarely successful, the procedure is statistically not as good as early use of thrombolytic.

Noncardiogenic Pulmonary Edema: Acute Lung Injury

Acute lung injury (ALI) was first described in the 1960s during the war in Vietnam, and it was then called *DaNang Lung*. Exsanguinated battlefield casualties facing delayed transfusion were often supported in the field with plasma to maintain blood pressure and transported rapidly by helicopter to hospitals where they were resuscitated and stabilized. After reperfusion, a progressive hypoxemia developed, requiring increasing inspired concentrations of oxygen. Ultimately many of these patients required mechanical ventilation to maintain oxygenation, and even then the oxygen requirements increased relentlessly. The clinical picture was one of hemorrhagic atelectasis with stiff, low-volume lungs that were difficult to ventilate. It was later learned that, in addition to the acute exsanguination/reperfusion injury, type 2 alveolar cell proliferation caused by the toxic effects of high inspired oxygen concentrations increased the barrier to oxygen diffusion at the alveolar capillary membrane. This created a vicious cycle of increasing respiratory failure and death.

In the intervening years, it has been learned that the primary injury is to the alveolar-capillary interface; alveolar leaks permit the exudation of blood and plasma and the flooding of the alveolar space. Further, there are many other predisposing conditions of this syndrome unrelated to exsanguination injury (see Table 12-2). These conditions all have in common acute injury to the alveolar-capillary interface with hemorrhagic atelectasis.

TABLE 12-2 **Clinical risk factors for the development of ARDS**

Sepsis syndrome
Aspiration of gastric contents
Drug overdose
Near drowning
Pulmonary contusion
Multiple transfusions
Multiple major fractures
Head trauma

Hudson LD, Millierg JA, Anardi D, et al. 1995. Clinical risks for the development of the acute respiratory distress syndrome. Am. J. Respir. Crit. Care Med. *151:298–301.*

RISK FACTORS

Many risk factors are commonly associated with ALI/ARDS. Hudson and coworkers, who studied 695 ICU patients with a predisposing risk for **ARDS (acute respiratory distress syndrome)**, reported that one out of four patients developed the syndrome.[14] Patients with sepsis syndrome and patients who had received multiple blood transfusions were the most common groups that developed ALI/ARDS. Garber and coworkers found in a retrospective study of multiple research publications that the risks for ALI/ARDS with the strongest supporting evidence for a cause-and-effect relationship were sepsis, aspiration, trauma, and multiple transfusions. The weakest connection of cause and effect for developing ALI/ARDS was disseminated intravascular coagulation.[15]

DIAGNOSIS OF ALI/ARDS

In 1994 an American-European Consensus Conference established clinical criteria for the diagnosis of ARDS. The criteria include five basic categories:

- Sudden clinical onset.
- A demonstrated risk factor for ALI/ARDS.
- Poor gas exchange measures (e.g., P_AO_2/F_IO_2 ratio of <200 regardless of PEEP level).
- Diffuse bilateral infiltrates on frontal chest X-ray.
- A pulmonary capillary wedge pressure of <18 mm Hg.

Conditions that mimic ALI/ARDS are pneumonia, acute pulmonary embolism, pulmonary edema secondary to cardiac disease, and acute exacerbation of chronic lung disease. These conditions must be ruled out before making the diagnosis of ALI.[16]

Although the routine chest X-ray is not reliable for telling whether the pulmonary edema is secondary to ALI/ARDS or to cardiac origin, the chest radiograph is

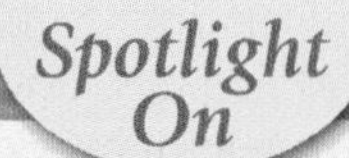

ARDS

A National Institute of Health (NIH) research study entitled ARDSnet Protocol vs. Open Lung Approach in ARDS is trying to determine whether the addition of a decremental PEEP trial after a recruitment maneuver improves patient outcomes during low tidal volume ventilation.

The recruitment maneuver involves:

- Sedating the patient,
- Preoxygenating the patient for 5–10 minutes and ventilating via pressure or volume ventilation with small V_T (4–6 mL/kg).
- Increasing the PEEP to 30 cm H_2O for 30–40 seconds.
- Lowering the PEEP by 2 cm H_2O every 5–20 minutes while oxygenation (S_PO_2) or compliance is monitored (S_PO_2 increases as PEEP decreases, and then decreases or plateaus as PEEP is further decreased). The optimal PEEP is the pressure associated with the best oxygenation or compliance during the decremental trial.
- Then performing the recruitment maneuver again and setting the PEEP 2 cm H_2O above the optimal PEEP identified in the decremental PEEP trial.
- Change F_IO_2 to the lowest level that maintains PO_2 in the target range.

The study started in January 2007 and is expected to conclude in March 2013. Visit the ARDSnet Web site (http://www.ardsnet.org/) for additional information and updates *(ARDSnet Protocol vs. Open Lung Approach in ARDS.* available at http://clinicaltrials.gov/ct2/show/NCT00431158).

Kacmarek RM, Kallet RH. Should recruitment maneuvers be used in the management of ALI and ARDS? Resp Care. *2007;52,5:622–635.*

one of the primary methods used to support the diagnosis of ARDS.[16] An additional complicating factor of using the chest X-ray as a diagnostic tool for ALI/ARDS is that the X-rays may vary with different mechanisms of injury (e.g., direct or indirect injury). The chest X-ray differences are described as diffuse, bilateral pulmonary infiltrates with greater density in the dependent areas of the lung. The infiltrates predominately involve the peripheral lung areas. An air-bronchogram may be visible, and the heart size is usually normal.

Hemodynamic changes using the pulmonary artery flow-directed catheter are helpful in differentiating the mechanism of pulmonary edema. The pulmonary capillary wedge pressure (PCWP) is less than 18 mm Hg in the patient with ALI/ARDS, except in patients with underlying cardiac disease. This type of pulmonary edema is known as noncardiogenic pulmonary edema or increased permeability edema (Table 12-3). In the patient with pulmonary edema secondary to cardiac disease, the PCWP is more than 18 mm Hg. This edema is called *cardiogenic pulmonary edema* or *hydrostatic pulmonary edema*.[16]

Laboratory analysis of edema fluid that is extracted from the respiratory tract and that reveals an edema/plasma ratio (protein levels) greater than 0.7 indicates

TABLE 12-3 **Clinical features of noncardiogenic pulmonary edema (ALI/ARDS) and cardiogenic pulmonary edema**

Feature	Noncardiogenic Pulmonary Edema	Cardiogenic Pulmonary Edema
Occurance of hypoxemia	Early	Late
Radiographic findings	Bilateral infiltrates on frontal x-ray, without Kerley B lines	Patchy, hilar and basilar, with Kerley B lines
Pulmonary capillary wedge pressure	$<$18 mm Hg or no clinical evidence of left atrial hypertension	$>$18 mm Hg
Ratio of total protein of edema fluid to total protein of plasma	$>$0.7	$<$ 0.5
Common clinical risk factors	Sepsis, trauma, multiple transfusions, pneumonia	Coronary artery disease, acute myocardial infarction, congestive heart failure

ARDS or noncardiogenic pulmonary edema. Protein levels less than 0.5 are indicative of hydrostatic or cardiogenic pulmonary edema. In ALI/ARDS, the protein concentration of the alveolar edema fluid is similar to that of plasma because the mechanism of pulmonary edema in ARDS is increased capillary permeability caused by capillary endothelial injury. The alveolar capillary membrane is severely injured and allows free seepage of inflammatory cells, capillary plasma, and red blood cells into the alveolar space.[16]

CLINICAL PRESENTATION OF ALI/ARDS

The clinical appearance of ALI/ARDS is time related. The early signs and symptoms occur within hours of the causative event. The inciting clinical cause may result in one or more of the following early clinical manifestations of ARDS.[16]

- Tachypnea out of proportion to the blood gas changes
- Progressive hypoxemia
- Few early radiological changes
- Decreasing vital capacity

In the ensuing 24–48 hours, the chest X-ray begins to reveal diffuse infiltrates, and the patient is increasingly dyspneic. Arterial oxygenation continues to decrease and is no longer responsive (is refractory) to increasing F_IO_2. A low ventilation/perfusion ratio (shunt effect) and atelectasis are the primary causes of oxygenation problems. The patient's deteriorating lung function results in acute oxygenation failure and eventual ventilatory failure, both of which require mechanical ventilation.

The earlier this syndrome can be recognized, the earlier treatment can be started and the better the outcome will be. The goal is to oxygenate the patient without causing further injury to the lung from oxygen toxicity and to allow the lung to heal. Early measures to more effectively ventilate a stiff low volume lung with loss of functional residual capacity (FRC) is to use positive airway pressure throughout the respiratory cycle (PEEP or CPAP), thus enhancing the recruitment of alveoli, decreasing compliance, and increasing FRC. As oxygenation improves, the F_IO_2 can be gradually lowered to 40% to preclude further injury. High inflation pressures and high PEEP pressures are associated with **barotrauma** to the lung, resulting in pneumothorax, pneumomediastinum, and increased sensitivity to the toxic effects of oxygen.

To determine the optimal—or "best"—PEEP, the clinician makes use of the fact that cardiac output is optimal at FRC and lower at extremes of lung volume. Most patients in this degree of respiratory failure have pulmonary artery catheters, so one can monitor the cardiac output directly or use variations in the mixed venous PO_2 to adjust the PEEP pressures up or down to achieve normal FRC and optimal oxygen delivery. Another way to determine optimal PEEP is to create a no-flow condition with the ventilator. Then, with the ratio of volume and pressure, determine "ventilator" static compliance. When resting lung volume is increased toward normal FRC, the compliance increases. When optimal ventilating lung volume is exceeded, compliance drops off, and the PEEP should be reduced.

Patients with acute lung injury are critically ill and need to be treated in an ICU setting. They are likely to be on ventilators and need extensive cardiac and respiratory monitoring. Fluid and blood products are given to maintain BP and intravascular volume, being mindful of the fact that overtransfusion or giving excess fluids can make pulmonary edema worse. Diuretics are often given if the patient is not hypotensive. Vasopressors to maintain blood pressure are often needed. The underlying cause of the illness must be determined and treated promptly, whether it is shock, an undrained abdominal abscess, or unrecognized ruptured viscus.

Note: The use of corticosteroids in this syndrome for their anti-inflammatory effect is controversial in recent years and has been largely discounted.

Summary

Pulmonary edema is a condition caused by excess fluid in the lungs. This fluid collects in the interstitial spaces and may enter the alveolar space, interfering with ventilation and gas exchange. In most cases, cardiac problems cause pulmonary edema. Fluid can accumulate for other reasons, including pneumonia, exposure to certain toxins and medications, exercising, or living at high elevations and malnutrition. Treatment for pulmonary edema varies depending on the cause but generally includes supplemental oxygen and medications.

Cardiogenic pulmonary edema—also known as congestive heart failure—occurs when the diseased or overworked left ventricle can not effectively pump out the blood it receives from your lungs. As a result, pressure increases inside the left atrium and then in the pulmonary veins and capillaries, causing fluid to be pushed through the capillary walls into the interstitial spaces and alveoli.

If not treated, pulmonary edema can raise pressure in the pulmonary artery, and eventually the right ventricle will begin to fail. The increased pressure backs up into the right atrium and then into various parts of your body. When not treated, acute pulmonary edema can be fatal. In some instances it may be fatal even if you receive treatment. Oxygen administration is the first step in the treatment for pulmonary edema. It may be necessary to assist ventilation mechanically.

Diseases of the lung can cause right heart disease and subsequently right heart failure (cor pulmonale). Although other conditions can cause hypertrophy of the right ventricle associated with cor pulmonale, very often it is caused by chronic obstructive pulmonary disease.

Embolization of the pulmonary vasculature is generally the result of blood clots (thrombi) in the lower extremities. When emboli form in the lungs, they block venous circulation to distal alveoli, resulting in dead space ventilation. Obstruction of the pulmonary vascular bed greater than 50% can be catastrophic. The goals of treatment for pulmonary embolism are to maintain oxygenation, and prevent new thrombus formation and further extension of the embolus until fibrinolysis can occur.

In ARDS, structural changes occur: alveolar and interstitial edema, alveolar consolidation, loss of pulmonary surfactant, and atelectasis. The general management of ARDS requires modalities such as oxygen therapy, mechanical ventilation using a lung protective strategy and techniques to reinflate collapsed alveoli.

Study Questions

REVIEW QUESTIONS

1. List the differences between hemodynamic pulmonary edema and edema associated with acute lung injury.
2. Name several mechanisms by which patients develop pulmonary hypertension.
3. Describe the pathophysiology of the various forms of pulmonary edema.
4. Explain the various ventilation/perfusion imbalances associated with acute pulmonary embolism and the mechanism of restoring balance as the clot dissipates and blood flow is restored.
5. Discuss the hypoxemia that occurs by means of many different mechanisms in heart and lung disease.

MULTIPLE-CHOICE QUESTIONS

1. Causes of deep venous thrombosis include all of the following except:
   a. a long bus ride across the United States from New York to San Francisco.
   b. pelvic malignancy with spreading to the posterior pelvic wall.
   c. prolonged use of excessive amounts of the drug Viagra.
   d. prolonged hospitalization with coma.
   e. fracture of the tibia with prolonged immobilization in a plaster cast.
2. What is the cause of hypoxemia in acute pulmonary embolism?
   a. alveolar-capillary block
   b. interstitial edema
   c. dead space ventilation
   d. L-sided heart failure
   e. lymphatic engorgement
3. Typical vital signs and lab values for a patient with acute pulmonary embolism are:
   a. T 102F, BP 150/95, P 120, RR 12, PO_2 95, PCO_2 34, and pH 7.50.
   b. T 99.2F, BP 105/70, P 120, RR 20, PO_2 72, PCO_2 34, and pH 7.50.
   c. T 102F, BP 150/95, P 78, RR 12, PO_2 95, PCO_2 55, and pH 7.34.
   d. T 99.2F, BP 105/70, P 78, RR 12, PO_2 95, PCO_2 40, and pH 7.40.
   e. T 98.6F, BP 120/80, P 78, RR 20, PO_2 105, PCO_2 55, and ph 7.50.
4. In acute pulmonary embolism, the most common finding on a chest X-ray is:
   a. normal chest X-ray
   b. Westermark's sign
   c. large pleural effusion
   d. Hampton's Hump
   e. enlarged heart
5. Findings in acute pulmonary embolism include all of the following except:
   a. hypoxemia.
   b. pleural friction rub.
   c. cough and sputum production.
   d. pleuritic chest pain and dyspnea.
   e. hemoptysis.
6. Direct causes of ARDS include:
   a. sepsis.
   b. hemorrhagic shock.
   c. pancreatitis.
   d. pulmonary contusion.
7. The primary mechanism of hypoxemia in the patient with ARDS is:
   a. hypoventilation.
   b. dead space ventilation.
   c. intrapulmonary shunting.
   d. histotoxic hypoxia.
8. The first recognition of ARDS appeared in patients with:
   a. hemorrhagic shock.
   b. overwhelming infection.
   c. viral pneumonia.
   d. chest trauma.

9. What are edema fluid differences between cardiogenic and noncardiogenic pulmonary edema?
   a. the presence of neutrophils in the cardiogenic edema fluid and eosinophils in the noncardiogenic edema
   b. the presence of more protein in the edema fluid from patients with noncardiogenic edema
   c. the presence of blood in the edema fluid from patients with cardiogenic pulmonary edema
   d. no difference in the fluid characteristics between the two types of pulmonary edema
10. What are primary causes of cor pulmonale?
   a. left heart failure
   b. primary pulmonary hypertension
   c. chronic lung diseases
   d. autoimmune diseases

CRITICAL-THINKING QUESTIONS

1. How does ARDS result in decreased lung compliance?
2. What is the mechanism for the development of pulmonary edema concomitant with malnutrition?
3. What is the mechanism for the pulmonary edema that might result from mitral valve stenosis?

References

1. Fishman A.P. Pulmonary edema. The water-exchanging function of the lung. *Circulation.* 1972;46,2:390–408.
2. Nunn JF, Aaron S. Nunn's Applied Respiratory Physiology (Fourth Edition). *Critical Care Med.* 1995;23,10:1794.
3. Parmley WW. Pathophysiology and current therapy of congestive heart failure. *J Am Coll Cardiol.* 1989. 13,4:771–785.
4. Connors Jr AF, Speroff T, Dawson NV, Thomas C, Harrell Jr FE, Wagner D, et al. The effectiveness of right heart catheterization in the initial care of critically ill patients. SUPPORT Investigators. *JAMA,* 1996;276,11:889–897.
5. Mehta S, Jay GD, Woolard RH, Hipona RA, Connolly EM, Cimini DM, et al. Randomized, prospective trial of bilevel versus continuous positive airway pressure in acute pulmonary edema. *Crit Care Med.* 1997;25,4:620–628.
6. Peinado VI, Pizarro S, Barbera JA. Pulmonary vascular involvement in COPD. *Chest.* 2008;134,4:808–814.
7. Vizza CD, Lynch JP, Ochoa LL, Richardson G, Trulock EP. Right and left ventricular dysfunction in patients with severe pulmonary disease. *Chest.* 1998;113,3:576–583.
8. Weitzenblum E. Chronic cor pulmonale. *Heart.* 2003;89,2:225–230.
9. McGoon M, Gutterman D, Steen V, Barst R, McCrory DC, Fortin TA, et al. Screening, early detection, and diagnosis of pulmonary arterial hypertension: ACCP evidence-based clinical practice guidelines. *Chest* Supp. 2004;126,1:14S–34S.
10. Kawut SM, Taichman DB, Archer-Chicko CL, Palevsky HI, Kimmel SE. Hemodynamics and survival in patients with pulmonary arterial hypertension related to systemic sclerosis. *Chest.* 2003;123,2:344–350.
11. Elliott CG, Pulmonary physiology during pulmonary embolism. *Chest.* Supp. 1992;101,4:163S–171S.
12. Fedullo PF, Tapson VF. Clinical practice. The evaluation of suspected pulmonary embolism. *N Engl J Med.* 2003;349,13:1247–1256.
13. Weiss CR, Scatarige JC, Diette GB, Haponik EF, Merriman B, Fishman EK. CT pulmonary angiography is the first-line imaging test for acute pulmonary embolism: a survey of US clinicians. *Acad Radial.* 2006;13,4:434–446.
14. Hudson L, Milberg J, Canard D, Maunder R. Clinical risks for development of the acute respiratory distress syndrome. *Am Review Respir Crit Care Med.* 1995;151:293–301.
15. Garber BG, Hebert PC, Yelled J.-D, Hotter RV. Adult respiratory distress syndrome: a systematic overview of incidence and risk factors. *Crit Care Med.* 1996;24,4:687–695.
16. Marino PL. Acute respiratory distress syndrome, 3rd edition. In: *The ICU Book.* Philadelphia: Lippincott Williams and Wilkins; 2007:419–435.

SECTION III

Essential Diagnostics

CHAPTER 13

Comprehensive History, Assessment, and Documentation

William F. Clark

OBJECTIVES

Upon completion of this chapter, the reader should be able to:

- Recognize the need for clear and complete understanding during a patient interview.
- Describe the general guidelines and techniques for interviewing a patient.
- Describe the basic structure and parts of a complete history of an adult patient.
- Recognize the differences between an adult history and a pediatric history.
- Perform a clinical evaluation of an adult patient.
- Perform inspection, palpation, percussion, and auscultation on an adult patient.
- Perform the collection of vital signs on an adult patient.
- Recognize the need for confidentiality when dealing with patient data.
- Document a history and physical of an adult patient using the problem-oriented medical record technique.

CHAPTER OUTLINE

KEY TERMS

active listening
adventitious breath sounds
auscultation
bradycardia
bradypnea
central cyanosis
fremitus
gallop rhythm
inspection
intimate space
kyphoscoliosis
kyphosis
lordosis
murmur
palpation
pectus carinatum
pectus excavatum
percussion
peripheral cyanosis
personal space
physical examination
problem-oriented medical record (POMR)
pulse pressure
scoliosis
SOAP
social space
source-oriented charting method
sphygmomanometer
tachycardia
tachypnea
voice sounds

For many years, respiratory therapists have been the acknowledged experts in cardiopulmonary care. They are taught to perform a thorough, focused pulmonary history and physical. Through the use of clinical simulations, the profession has increased its effectiveness in the area of focused cardiopulmonary care. Health care is changing, however, and the profession must change with it. Respiratory therapists of the future must be able to address the patient as a whole, not just the patient's pulmonary status.

As health care changes, the need for respiratory therapists to be multicompetent is more important than ever. One such competency is the ability to perform an extensive history and physical on a patient. The American Association for Respiratory Care (AARC) offers a course on physical assessment. As more and more practitioners start working in alternative sites and become case managers for health care organizations, the ability to perform a complete history and physical becomes even more vital to their success in alternate site positions.

Patient History: The Interview

A *complete patient history*, an extremely important but underused procedure, is as important as any lab test or diagnostic procedure in determining a patient's health status. Asking the correct questions in a manner designed to collect the appropriate information ensures that the subsequent laboratory tests and diagnostic procedures confirm a suspected diagnosis instead of uncovering a new condition.

The health care provider must be able to elicit enough information from a patient to understand the problem. Although gathering data efficiently is necessary, a good interview takes time and effort. The health care provider must also respond to the patient's emotions and develop rapport. Illness arouses different emotions in patients. How the health care provider responds to these emotions determines the type of rapport established with the patient and family. Without good rapport and trust, the health care provider cannot hope to elicit accurate information. Finally, the health care provider must also use this time to provide patient education and motivation. As the patient and the family understand the illness better, they have greater motivation to adhere to the medical plan developed for the patient.[1]

GENERAL GUIDELINES FOR INTERVIEWING

Many factors affect the interview process, some of which are impossible to control. Internal factors such as previous experiences, attitudes, values, cultural heritage, religious beliefs, self-concept, listening habits, preoccupations, and the feelings of both the interviewer and the patient are impossible to control. However, many factors are controllable. Thus, the interview environment is important.

The correct use of space helps establish rapport with the patient. Introduce yourself, making sure the patient can hear and see you. Move toward the patient until the patient recognizes you, usually when the distance between you is 4–12 feet, also known as **social space**. The social space is where initial rapport with the patient is established and where general, nonpersonal questions can be asked. Once the initial rapport has been established, the health care provider may enter the **personal space**, but only after receiving the patient's verbal or nonverbal consent. As shown in Figure 13-1, in the personal space ($1^1/_2$–4 feet), the health care provider is close enough to ask questions without being overheard by others in the room. The

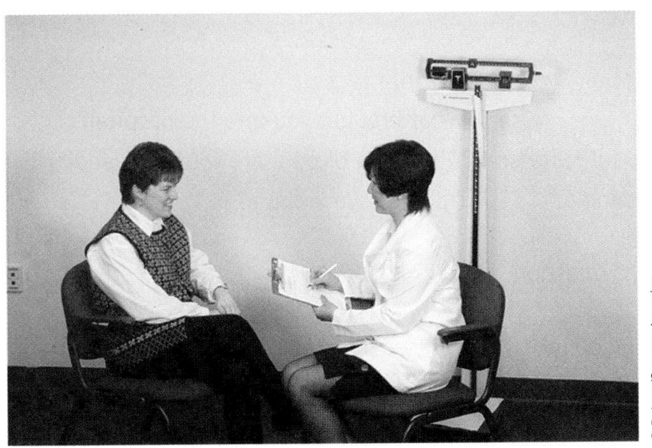

FIGURE 13-1 The patient interview.

final area, **intimate space** (less than $1^1/_2$ feet), is where the actual physical examination is performed.[2] It should be noted that personal and intimate space is greatly influenced by culture and ethnicity. The patient's privacy should be honored at all times.

In addition to space, other environmental factors influence the interview. Room lighting, noise, and temperature can be controlled to provide the best interview conditions. The room should be well lit so that the health care provider and the patient can see each another clearly. All extraneous noise should be kept to a minimum to allow for complete attention. Keep interruptions to a minimum to allow for the free flow of information and to prevent having to repeat information.

Another key factor is communication style. Verbal barriers, such as the use of jargon, should be kept to a minimum. The interviewer should also choose words and voice tone that minimizes patient anxiety, stress, and fear. Likewise, the interviewer should use appropriate nonverbal communication such as body movement, facial expressions, and dress to ease the communication pathway. Finally, the interviewer should always act professionally and show warmth and interest during the interview process.

BASIC INTERVIEWING TECHNIQUES

Interviewing is not a science but an art that must be practiced and developed over time. The bulk of the interview consists of asking questions to elicit information. The kinds of questions asked, how those questions are framed, and proper probing for information all make the interview a success. Just as vital as the questions asked are **active listening** skills, which are verbal and nonverbal techniques to indicate interest and comprehension. During the interview, the interviewer should observe the manner of the patient and how the patient reacts to different questions.

CASE STUDY 13-1

William Smith is a 35-year-old male who has come to the clinic and who has been waiting for over 2 hours. Mr. Smith is finally called into a treatment room, and the practitioner enters to start the history and physical. As the practitioner enters the room, she observes an anxious Caucasian male sitting on a chair. The patient looks up as the practitioner approaches. (*Note:* Mr. Smith will be the patient throughout most of the chapter. For simplicity and clarity, the patient in the text will be assumed to be male, the practitioner female.)

Questions

1. How far away should the practitioner be when she makes her initial introduction?
2. When can the practitioner move into the room and enter the personal space?
3. What should the practitioner do to make the environment more comfortable for the patient?

Questioning a patient can be stressful to both the practitioner and the patient. To put the patient at ease and to help reduce the stress felt during the interview, the practitioner should be careful how the questions are asked. The tone of voice can speak volumes, even for a simple response such as "oh." Practice asking all questions and making statements in a neutral tone so as not to offend, scare, or anger the patient. Volume is closely related to tone. Because volume can send subtle messages, the practitioner should practice speaking at a level that the patient can hear but that does not convey a personal judgment or opinion.[3]

Every interview should begin with *open-ended questions*, which need more than a yes or no or otherwise limited response. A typical open-ended question is, "What brought you into the hospital?" To be less threatening to the patient, open-ended questions can be reworded as indirect statements that elicit information but do not make the patient feel as if he or she is being questioned. *Direct questions* can be used to focus the patient; these guide the patient to give more information in the areas of interest to the interviewer. To pinpoint a specific item, the interviewer should use *closed questions*, that is, questions that can be answered with a simple yes or no. When asking probing closed questions always keep in mind the four Ws and the one H: what, when, where, why, and how. Table 13-1

TABLE 13-1 **Verbal interviewing techniques**

Skill	Reason for Use	Example
Open-ended questioning	Starts flow of information	What brought you into the hospital?
Direct questioning	Guides patient to area of interest to interviewer	What kind of pain are you experiencing?
Closed questioning	Usually a yes or no question addressing a specific area	Do you have asthma?
Indirect questioning	Between an open-ended and a direct question; usually less threatening to patient	Tell me about your problems.
Facilitating	Helps keep the patient talking during open-ended questioning	Phrases such as "Yes" or "Go on" or repeating the last words said by the patient.
Checking or restating	Checks the accuracy of information received	Let me see if I understand you correctly. You said . . .
Surveying	Ensures that there is nothing else wrong	What else is bothering you?
Clarifying	Checks your understanding of ambiguous words	What do you mean by the words *a cold?*
Summarizing	A short summary of what the practitioner heard	You said you have had a fever for 4 days and been coughing up yellow sputum.
Empathizing	Indicates you care about the patient's problems; can be used as a bridge to another type of question	"That must have been difficult for you," or, "I can only imagine how that must have felt."
Interpreting	Keeps the focus of the interview on the patient while elaborating on patient's statements (The practitioner should always give the patient a chance to either confirm or deny the interpretation, since the practitioner can only guess what the patient is feeling.)	Patient: "Before I was sick, I could help other people. Now I just sit around and do nothing." Practitioner: "I understand you to say that your illness has limited you. Is it possible that you are feeling lonely since you cannot help other people?" Patient: "You could be right. I miss being needed."
Reflecting	Communicates that the practitioner observes feeling or emotion from the patient	I can see that you're upset at the moment.
Legitimizing or validating	Communicates acceptance and validation of an emotional experience	I understand why you are so upset.
Supporting	Communicates that the practitioner can help the patient (must be honest)	Please let me know what I can do to help you.
Partnering	Communicates that the practitioner wants to promote a partnership in the treatment of the patient	After we have finished this interview, maybe we can discuss some solutions for your problems.
Respecting	Communicates that the professional has respect for the patient's problems (similar to empathy)	I am impressed by the way you have been able to cope with this problem.

illustrates the different types of verbal techniques that can be used in an interview to elicit information.

No one interviewing method is better than another; the practitioner should be familiar and comfortable with all techniques. Changing techniques in an interview can be a very effective method of keeping the patient at ease and maintaining rapport. Avoid any behavior that can block the flow of communications: showing anger, responding to emotions inappropriately, giving advice, giving false reassurance, moralizing, defending, arguing, or belittling. Finally, do not be afraid to use silence. Silence is counterproductive when it creates tension between the patient and the practitioner, but it can be used effectively to signal the patient to continue talking or to elaborate. It also eliminates the

TABLE 13-2 **Active listening techniques**

Nonverbal Techniques
Maintaining eye contact as much as possible
Using supportive gestures such as nodding your head to indicate understanding or leaning forward toward the patient
Taking notes (if the patient is comfortable with the note taking)
Listening with an open mind
Listening to the content rather than the delivery
Keeping facial expressions neutral or supportive
Verbal Techniques
Keeping the tone of your statements neutral
Using facilitating statements such as "Go on" or "And what else did you feel?"
Using checking statements such as "Is this what you are telling me, . . ."
Paraphrasing the basic message and giving the patient a chance to confirm or deny the message
Soliciting the patient's reactions to your interpretation
Clarifying any vague or incomplete ideas

possibility of sending the wrong signals about what the practitioner wants to hear.

Always end the interview by asking whether the patient wants to discuss or needs anything else. This final surveying of the patient allows for final reflections or further information.[1,3–6]

Just as important as interviewing techniques are the *listening skills* that an interviewer uses to indicate active listening. Table 13-2 lists nonverbal and verbal techniques that indicate that the practitioner is listening.

The practitioner needs to understand what is being said and to ascertain the accuracy and validity of the information. The listener must be open to all the information being given. Because of past experience, the listener might fail to hear, being "certain" of what is going to be said. This failure occurs because the interviewer's frame of mind distorts the meaning of the words to fit the personal ideas instead of being open to different interpretations. Active listening also requires the listener's undivided attention. If there are constant interruptions or if the senses become overloaded, active listening cannot take place. The interview must take place in an environment that limits interruptions or sensory overload. Finding such an environment in a hospital setting is difficult, but care should be taken to limit distractions.

The *powers of observation* are also an important aspect of an effective interview. During the introduction, the practitioner should be aware of any nonverbal messages the patient may be sending. When approached, does the patient look down dejectedly or look up expectantly? Watch for subtle messages sent by the patient that indicate whether rapport is being established. Watch for body movement, facial expressions, and the tone and manner of answering questions for indications of the patient's emotional status. The practitioner's ability to observe these messages can furnish further meaning to the words of the patient.

STRUCTURE OF THE INTERVIEW

The *structure of the interview* is the agenda the practitioner has in conducting it. Nothing is gained by a stream-of-consciousness, free-ranging discussion with no structure or reason; a free-for-all interview confuses the patient and usually wastes the practitioner's time. Each practitioner should form a structure for each interview and develop a checklist so that nothing is missed. However, the practitioner needs to remember not to force the patient to respond. The practitioner should also not be afraid to stray from the structure if a topic not on the list seems to need discussion.

The Opening. Every interview starts with the opening. The *opening* consists of the introduction, establishing the goals of the interview, obtaining consent for the interview, establishing the initial rapport, and ensuring of the patient's comfort.

Legally, all health care providers must *introduce* themselves to the patient, including their name and department. They should call the patient by name and identify the patient as the person to be interviewed. The introduction should be started when the practitioner is in the social space and continue as the practitioner moves into the personal space. Although a handshake is usually a good rapport builder, be aware that some cultures frown on touching in this manner. Next, the practitioner should give the patient a short explanation of the purpose of the visit, making clear the interview's purpose and the practitioner's expectations. Then the practitioner is legally bound to obtain the patient's consent for the interview. Most patients want to talk to you, but verbal consent is necessary for the interview to continue. Here is an opening that has all these elements:

> Good morning, my name is Jane Simons, and I am a Respiratory Therapist from the respiratory care department. You are Mr. William Smith? Dr. Agrwal has asked me to interview you and take your medical history. Would you be willing to talk to me for a few minutes?

CASE STUDY 13-2

It is 7:00 p.m., and the practitioner (Jane Simons) has entered the treatment room and introduced herself to William Smith. She then establishes initial rapport and moves toward the patient. She closes the curtain to give herself and Mr. Smith some privacy and sits down across from him. She begins the interview by explaining what she is going to do and asks permission to continue. Mr. Smith answers that he came here directly from work and is very upset that it took over 2 hours to get to see anyone. As Jane Simons prepares her papers and equipment, Mr. Smith sits in the chair fidgeting and muttering. When Ms. Simons begins to ask her first question, Mr. Smith stands up and starts to pace back and forth in the small room.

Questions

1. What active listening skills should Jane Simons use to help put Mr. Smith at ease?
2. What verbal interviewing techniques should she have used before starting to ask questions?
3. What patient mannerisms should have warned the practitioner not to begin immediately asking questions?
4. Does Jane Simons have the right to continue with the interview?

THE COMPREHENSIVE HISTORY

The items of a comprehensive history vary depending on the age, sex, and illness of a patient; however, the practitioner must have an exhaustive checklist available. Time and the goals of the interview dictate how many of the items are covered and in what detail. A comprehensive history includes essentially two parts.

- The first part is the patient history, described in Table 13-3.
- The second part (Table 13-4) is a comprehensive review of systems.

Pediatric histories are different and are discussed later in the chapter.

The *history of the present illness* and the *past health history* of the patient are documented before the review of the systems is conducted. The chief complaint should be directly quoted in the patient's words when possible. When documenting the present illness, the practitioner should be sure to make the information clear and put it in chronological order, but the information must come from the patient. The history of the present illness section should include all of the principal symptoms, described in detail as to location, duration, quality, and quantity or severity. It should also include any associated factors such as aggravating factors and alleviating factors. Also included should be

TABLE 13-3 **Patient history**

Date
Time
Identifying Data
Name
Address
Age
Gender
Marital status
Occupation
Source of history (patient, parent, child, friend, etc.)
Chief complaint(s) (presenting problem)
History of the Present Illness
Symptoms (location, duration, quality, quantity or severity, associated aggravating factors and alleviating factors)
Negative symptoms
Past Health History
Childhood illnesses and immunizations
Adult illnesses
Obstetric or gynecologic history (if relevant)
Psychiatric illnesses
Injuries
Blood transfusions
Surgical history
Hospitalizations
Current Health Status
Current medications
Allergies
Tobacco use (type, amount, and duration of use)
Alcohol use
Drug or related substance use
Diet
Screening tests (dates and results)
Immunization status (date of each vaccine)
Sleep habits
Exercise/leisure
Environmental hazards
Safety measures
Family History (note age and health of all living members and cause of death of all deceased members)
Social History
Educational level
Home environment
Significant others

TABLE 13-4 **Review of systems**

General
Patient's perception of general state of health at the present, difference from usual state, vitality and energy levels

Psychological
Irritability, nervousness, tension, increased stress, difficulty concentrating, mood changes, suicidal thoughts, depression

Integumentary System
Rashes, itching, changes in skin pigmentation, black and blue marks (ecchymoses), change in color or size of mole, sores, lumps, change in skin texture, odors, excessive sweating, acne, loss of hair (alopecia), excessive growth of hair or growth of hair in unusual locations (hirsutism), change in nails, amount of time spent in the sun

Eyes
Blurred vision, change in visual acuity, glasses, contacts, sensitivity to light (photophobia), excessive tearing, night blindness, double vision (diplopia), drainage, bloodshot eyes, pain, blind spots, flashing lights, halos around objects, glaucoma, cataracts

Ears
Hearing deficits, hearing aid, pain, discharge, lightheadedness (vertigo), ringing in the ears (tinnitus), earaches, infection

Nose and Sinuses
Frequent colds, discharge, itching, hay fever, postnasal drip, stuffiness, sinus pain, polyps, obstruction, nosebleed (epistaxis), change in sense of smell

Mouth
Toothache, tooth abscess, dentures, bleeding/swollen gums, difficulty chewing, sore tongue, change in taste, lesions, change in salivation, bad breath

Throat/Neck
Hoarseness, change in voice, frequent sore throats, difficulty swallowing, pain/stiffness, enlarged thyroid (goiter)

Respiratory System
Shortness of breath (dyspnea), shortness of breath on exertion, phlegm (sputum), cough, sneezing, wheezing, coughing up blood (hemoptysis), frequent upper respiratory tract infections, pneumonia, emphysema, asthma, tuberculosis

Cardiovascular System
Shortness of breath that wakes you up in the night (paroxysmal nocturnal dyspnea), chest pain, heart murmur, palpitations, fainting (syncope), sleep on pillows to breathe better (orthopnea; state number of pillows used), swelling (edema), cold hands/feet, leg cramps, myocardial infarction, hypertension, valvular disease, pain in calf when walking (intermittent claudication), varicose veins, inflammation of a vein (thrombophlebitis), blood clot in leg (deep vein thrombosis), anemia

Breasts
Pain, tenderness, discharge, lumps, change in size, dimpling

Gastrointestinal System
Change in appetite, nausea, vomiting, diarrhea, constipation, change in bowel habits, black tarry stools (melena), vomiting blood (hematemesis), change in stool color, excessive gas (flatulence), belching, regurgitation, heartburn, difficulty swallowing (dysphagia), abdominal pain, jaundice, hemorrhoids, hepatitis, peptic ulcers, gallstones

Urinary System
Change in urine color, change in voiding habits, painful urination (dysuria), hesitancy, urgency, frequency, excessive urination at night (nocturia), increased urine volume (polyuria), dribbling, loss in force of stream, bedwetting, change in urine volume, incontinence, pain in lower abdomen (suprapubic pain), kidney stones, urinary tract infections

Musculoskeletal System
Joint stiffness, muscle pain, back pain, limitation of movement, redness, swelling, weakness, bony deformity, broken bones, dislocations, sprains, gout, arthritis, osteoporosis, herniated disc

Neurological System
Headache, change in balance, incoordination, loss of movement, change in sensory perception/feeling in an extremity, change in speech, change in smell, fainting (syncope), loss of memory, tremors, involuntary movement, loss of consciousness, seizures, weakness, head injury

(continues)

TABLE 13-4 **Review of systems (*continued*)**

Female Reproductive System
Vaginal discharge; change in libido; infertility; pain during intercourse; menses: last menstrual period (LMP), age period started (menarche), regularity, duration, amount of bleeding, prementrual symptoms, intermenstrual bleeding, painful periods (dysmenorrhea); menopause: age of onset, duration, symptoms, bleeding; obstetric: number of pregnancies, number of miscarriages/abortions, number of children, type of delivery, complications, type of birth control, estrogen therapy
Male Reproductive System
Change in libido, infertility, sterility, impotence, pain during intercourse, age at onset of puberty, testicular pain, penile discharge, change in erectile function, emissions, hernias, enlarged prostate, type of birth control
Endocrine System
Bulging eyes; fatigue; change in size of head, hands, or feet; weight change; heat/cold intolerances; excessive sweating; increased thirst; increased hunger; change in body hair distribution; swelling in the anterior neck; diabetes mellitus

any negative symptoms (for example, "no urinary problems") that may help in differentiating the diagnosis.

The past health history should include any childhood and adult illnesses. Childhood illnesses should be listed as well as any immunizations for chickenpox, measles, mumps, and polio. Adult illnesses should include medical problems such as high blood pressure, diabetes, asthma, chronic bronchitis, emphysema, tuberculosis, and HIV disease. Any surgical and obstetric procedures or history should be documented as well as any accidents or injuries, especially if they resulted in transfusions. Hospitalizations and psychiatric illness should also be documented.

In *current health status*, the practitioner documents the patient's current lifestyle:

- Current medications being taken and any allergies
- Use of tobacco, drugs, alcohol, or related substances
- Diet along with any restrictions
- Current immunizations such as tetanus, influenza, or hepatitis B
- Recent screening tests such as mammograms, Pap smears, tuberculin tests, or cholesterol tests
- Lifestyle information such as sleep habits, exercise, environmental hazards, and safety issues

This information is especially vital if there is a possible exposure to harmful substances. If the patient is retired, ask about his or her occupation because some exposures such as asbestos can take many years to affect the body.[4]

In the *family history section*, the practitioner should document:

- Any health- or age-related problems of each immediate family member.
- The cause of death of any deceased immediate family member.

In the *social history section*, the patient's home environment and significant others are documented.

The *review of systems* (Table 13-4) should be done carefully, starting from the head and working down. The practitioner should follow the same method every time to develop a personalized system. When asking about general health, the practitioner should focus on general changes in the patient's health, either recently or in the past. For each system, the practitioner should try to use open-ended questions first and then direct questioning, clarifying, and surveying to ensure that all aspects of the system are reviewed. Finally, the practitioner should summarize to allow the patient to correct any misunderstandings. Refer to Table 13-4 for a list of some of the problems that a patient may experience in each of the systems. The list is by no means complete; it is provided to help the practitioner with areas that may need closed questions.

Most respiratory therapists do a focused *review of systems* that may not be as complete as the one in Table 13-4; however, as the practitioners move out of the hospital into alternative settings, they should be able to do a complete review of the systems if necessary. The practitioner should start each system with an

Best Practice

Pack-Years History

Cigarette smoking should be documented in *pack-years*, that is, the total number of years smoking times the highest number of packs ever smoked per day. For example, a patient who has smoked two packs a day for 30 years has a 60-pack-year history. If the patient has quit smoking, document how long ago the patient quit.

CASE STUDY 13-3

Mr. Smith becomes calmer and sits down in the chair in the treatment room. The practitioner (Jane Simons) pulls out the chart that has been started on Mr. Smith. She sees that the face sheet lists him as a 35-year-old male factory worker who is at the clinic because of occasional chest pain. She starts interviewing Mr. Smith, who gives her the following information when asked what has brought him to the clinic.

> There are times when I find it hard to breathe. I also sometimes have a pain in the center of my chest. It's not all the time, but it's been bothering me for about 2 to 3 weeks and more lately. I'm having trouble walking up stairs.

As the practitioner continues the interview, Mr. Smith relates that he had allergies when he was young. He takes only aspirin and cold medicine. He says that he had all the normal childhood diseases and had very few medical problems until 3 or 4 months ago. He has had no serious injuries and has had his tonsils removed. He smokes up to two packs of cigarettes a day, and he started smoking at age 15. He drinks socially two to three beers a night and denies any drug or substance abuse. He cannot remember any immunizations other than the usual childhood shots, but he had a tetanus shot 3 years ago when he cut himself with a knife at work. Mr. Smith also relates that he has had cold- and flulike symptoms for over 3 months, but the symptoms have been mild and he has not felt the need to seek medical attention until now.

Mr. Smith says that he lives at home with his wife and one child, age 7. The wife seems to be in good health, but the boy was diagnosed with asthma 3 years ago. Mr. Smith's father and mother are both living, and he has no brothers or sisters. His father has been diagnosed with coronary artery disease and had bypass surgery 2 years ago. His mother also has some heart problems and suffered a heart attack last year. He says that all other family members are deceased, but he cannot remember what they died from.

Mr. Smith says he works in a sheet metal factory and graduated from high school. His hobbies include working on classic cars and watching television.

Questions

1. Does the practitioner record the identifying data as written on the face sheet or as given by the patient?
2. How would the practitioner write the chief complaint?
3. What kind of interviewing technique would the practitioner use to clarify the type of chest pain and the shortness of breath?
4. What are the principal symptoms the practitioner would list for this patient?
5. How could the practitioner further clarify the symptoms to better understand what is happening?
6. What other questions would be appropriate to clarify the present illness, the past health history, the current health status, and the social history?
7. How should the practitioner use the information about the flulike symptoms for over 3 months other than recording them in the chart?

open-ended question such as, "Please describe to me any respiratory problems you may have had." This is now a open-ended inquiry. Once the flow of information from this type of question starts to slow down, however, the practitioner should also ask about other specific ailments to find out whether there is a negative response or if the patient just forgot to mention them.

PATIENT BEHAVIOR DURING THE INTERVIEW

The practitioner must frequently employ *checking*, as described in Table 13-1, to ensure that the information is correct. While surveying a list of problems, the practitioner often has to *probe* to ensure completeness. The problem with checking and probing is that they can be stressful to the patient. Likewise, the practitioner must understand that an ill patient may not be able to communicate well and may feel threatened. The practitioner must understand the possible perceived threats (Table 13-5), which can cause stress to a patient, because even normal responses may be clouded by them.

A patient's normal reaction to stress is to lapse into denial, regression, suppression, repression, anxiety, anger, and sadness. These emotions color patients' responses to questions and even affect their ability to answer. The practitioner should keep the influence of stress in mind when conducting an interview.

CASE STUDY 13-4

The practitioner (Jane Simons) continues interviewing Mr. Smith with the review of systems. When asked how he usually feels, Mr. Smith states that he usually feels fine but that he has felt as if he had the flu for over 3 months. He denies any weight changes, fatigue except when climbing stairs, and fever. He admits that he has had some weakness in the legs and arms lately. He admits to getting headaches at work but denies any other problems with his head. He states that his eyes and ears are normal but admits that he has a runny nose quite often and sometimes blows his nose so forcefully that it bleeds. The patient states that his mouth and neck are normal. He states that his chest is normal but admits to coughing up small amounts of thick white sputum, especially in the morning. He relates that he feels short of breath when he exercises but not at rest. He says that he sometimes has shortness of breath after eating, but that it is not bad. He does not know if he wheezes but denies that he has any respiratory problems. The chest pain he feels is a pressing type of pain that is near the center of his chest. It does not radiate out to the arm or jaw. He denies any other cardiac problems. No gastrointestinal or urinary problems are elicited. He says he eats normally and has been watching his diet since his mother's heart attack. He admits that he has some coolness in the fingers at times and weakness of the legs and arms. All other systems are normal according to the patient's responses.

Questions

1. What aspects of the review of systems are important and should be noted in the chart?
2. Would it be appropriate to list the negative responses in the chart?
3. Which system areas need to be emphasized when doing a physical examination?
4. On the basis of the patient's answers, should the practitioner suspect the problem is respiratory or cardiac in nature? Why?

TABLE 13-5 **Stress of illness**

Threats	Patient Manifestation of the Threat
Threat to efficiency	Illness saps a person's ability to deal with normal events. Patient must cope with loss of ability to cope with normal aspects of life and the accompanying loss of esteem.
Threat of separation	Hospitalization induces the fear of being separated from family or loved ones. Even the most independent person has a basic fear of separation.
Threat of loss of love	Many patients fear that illness will make them unattractive or unloved by people around them.
Threat of loss of bodily function	Especially for hospitalized patients, this fear is the greatest. Incontinence makes a person feel helpless to control even the simplest bodily functions.
Threat of loss of bodily parts	This can be either a physical or a psychological reality. Some illnesses result in physical loss, and some patients fear they will lose use of some of their body parts.
Threat of loss of rationality or cognitive function	Some patients dread the possibility of losing control or the ability to communicate.
Threat of pain	Most patients do not want to feel pain or to suffer.
Threat of loss of privacy	Most of the usual privacy people enjoy at home is lost in the hospital.
Threat of loss of home	Many people find it difficult to sleep or relax in a strange environment. The hospitalized patient is forced to live in a strange and unnatural environment.
Threat of loss of independence	This is the hardest for many patients. Hospitals force patients to do things by the hospital's schedule.

Compiled from Cohen-Cole SA. The Medical Interview: The Three-Function Approach. *St. Louis: Mosby-Yearbook; 1991:101–103; and Purtilo R, Haddad A.* Health Professional and Patient Interaction. *5th ed. Philadelphia: W.B. Saunders Co; 1996:119–128.*

Age-Specific Competency

Patient History of a Child

In addition to the information obtained in an adult history, the following must be ascertained for a child.

- Identifying data
  - Date and place of birth
  - Nickname
  - First name of parents (and last names, if different)
  - Parents' occupations and where they can be reached during work hours
- Chief complaint(s) (making clear whether it is a patient concern, a parent concern, or both)
- History of the present illness (include thoughts of family members concerning symptoms)
- Past health history
  - Birth history (important in first 2 years of life)
  - Prenatal history (maternal health and substance abuse during pregnancy)
  - Natal history (nature of labor and delivery)
  - Neonatal history (any problems at birth and gestational age)
  - Illnesses (any recent exposures to childhood illnesses)
- Feeding history (important in first 2 years of life)
  - Infancy (method of feeding and problems with or parental concerns about growth)
  - Childhood (eating habits, amount, and types of food eaten)
- Growth and development history
  - Physical growth (actual or approximate weight and length at birth and beyond; any slow or fast gains or losses)
  - Developmental milestones
    - Age patient held up head in prone position
    - Age rolled over from front to back and back to front
    - Age sat with support and then alone
    - Age said first words, combinations of words, and sentences
    - Age tied own shoes
    - Age dressed without help
    - Age of tooth growth and loss pattern
    - Growth according to growth chart
  - Social development
    - Sleep
    - Toileting
    - Speech
    - Personality
    - Discipline
    - Schooling
    - Sexuality
- Family history (age and health of individuals who live in the child's home)

Source: Adapted from Bickley LS, Hoekelman RA. Bates' Guide to Physical Examination and History Taking. *7th ed. Philadelphia: JB Lippincott Co; 1999:39–42.*

Not every patient behaves normally during an interview. The practitioner's ability to understand abnormal responses and employing effective coping strategies can mean the difference between a successful interview and a trying experience for both the practitioner and the patient.

- One type of maladaptive patient is the *persistently angry* patient. These patients lash out with every response. Sometimes it is helpful to allow angry patients to vent their feelings and then to try to continue. Another coping mechanism is to legitimize the feeling (Table 13-1). If the anger persists, continuing the interview is not advisable; instead, have another person try or seek psychiatric help for the patient.
- A second type of maladaptive patient is the one who is in a *major depression*. Empathizing and legitimizing can usually break the mood enough for the patient to answer questions. If the depression is too deep to penetrate, the patient requires psychiatric help.
- A third type of maladaptive patient suffers from *severe anxiety*. This patient is liable to suddenly become anxious that he or she has the diseases you are listing during a review of systems. He or she can also become severely agitated when questioned. If the practitioner can maintain a calm and controlled demeanor during an interview with this patient, he or she may respond. However, if his or her mood is intractable, psychiatric evaluation should be encouraged.

Other types of patients that a practitioner may encounter are those who are compulsive, dependent, histrionic, masochistic, narcissistic, psychotic, delirious, or demented. Practitioners should be aware of these patients and be prepared to deal with them.[1]

Barriers to Communication. In addition to emotions and personality disorders, cultural and language differences may act as major barriers to communication. Every culture has its own customs and traditions that affect how the patient responds to questions and touching by the practitioner. Although learning all the different cultural influences is impossible, the practitioner should be well aware of varying traditions and watch for verbal and nonverbal clues as to how the patient is tolerating the interview and subsequent physical examination. In this area, the family may be able to help the respiratory therapist understand their cultural practices and their expectations of the health care experience. In some cases, an interpreter may be needed to ensure that the information gathered is accurate and complete.

Interviewing a Child. A pediatric history is more challenging because it may be coming from the parent or guardian rather than from the patient. Whenever possible, engage the patient in the process unless the child is too young to be able to respond.

Assessment

A **physical examination** is a thorough assessment of a patient for all positive and negative medical conditions. The physical examination requires keen observational and analytical skills. The practitioner must be able to interact with a patient in such a way that he or she trusts the practitioner. Because the physical usually follows the history, the rapport built during the history can be used as a vehicle for the physical examination. Along with the history, a complete and comprehensive physical often leads a practitioner to a diagnosis without the use of expensive and often invasive clinical tests. The clinical tests can then be ordered to confirm the suspected diagnosis.

PHYSICAL EXAMINATION TECHNIQUES

A practitioner should follow some general guidelines to make the physical examination as easy and as nontraumatic as possible. The physical examination environment should ensure the patient's privacy at all times. In the hospital, privacy curtains should always be drawn. At other sites, a private, quiet room should be used. The room should be well lit, and the temperature should be comfortable for the patient. The practitioner should schedule enough time to be able to complete the exam without interruption. A complete physical does more than reassure a healthy person; it can provide important opportunities for health education, baseline data for future encounters, and opportunities to find minor problems before they become major.

The physical examination techniques are inspection, palpation, percussion, and auscultation. Seeing, feeling, and hearing still form the backbone of the complete physical examination. The practitioner can use the sense of smell. Odors sometimes help the practitioner make clinical judgments, because distinctive odors provide clues to the diagnosis of certain conditions.

Inspection. **Inspection** is the process of observing a patient's outward appearance for positive and negative signs and symptoms. The practitioner must observe as much as possible. Inspection as part of the physical examination starts even before the history is taken. The patient's demeanor, which can reveal emotional and mental status, can be observed at the beginning of the interview during the introduction. The patient should also be observed during the interview for any changes in demeanor or mental status. Likewise, the practitioner should watch for changes during the interview, such as shortness of breath, patient posture, and whether the patient must stop talking after a few words or sentences. The practitioner should inspect each part of the body under direct light to reveal any changes, discoloration, or textures. Tangential or indirect light can also be useful for seeing any lumps, bumps, or distortions of the skin.[4,7,8]

Palpation. **Palpation** is using touch to perform a physical examination. There are two types of palpation:

- *Shallow, light, or superficial palpation* is pressure to about 1 cm deep, which is done to feel surface abnormalities (see Figure 13-2).
- *Deep palpation* is pressure to about 4 cm deep, which is done to feel abnormalities deep beneath the surface and to detect tenderness or guarding (see Figure 13-3).

As shown in Figure 13-4, different parts of the hand are used for palpation. To palpate abnormalities, whether superficial or deep, the practitioner should use fingerpads. Therefore, fingernails should be cut short so as not to injure the patient. To palpate **fremitus** (vibrations transmitted through the skin), the practitioner can use the fingerpads or the ulnar (front) surface of the hands. To palpate temperature, the practitioner should use the dorsal (back) surface of the hand.

Vocal fremitus is performed to detect changes in the transmission of vibrations through the tracheobronchial tree. Have the patient repeat the number 99 while systematically palpating the chest with the ball

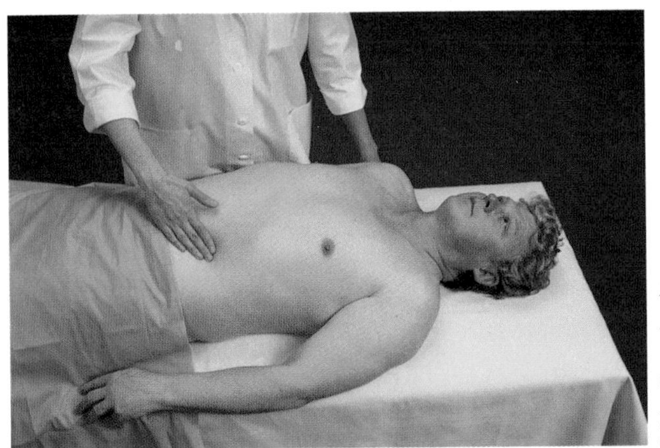

FIGURE 13-2 Light palpation.

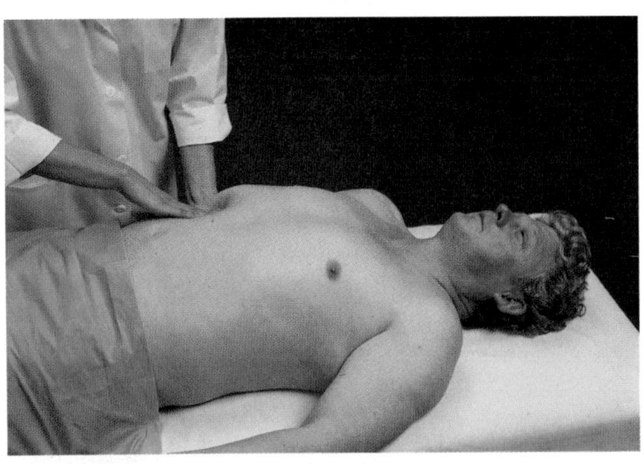

FIGURE 13-3 Deep palpation.

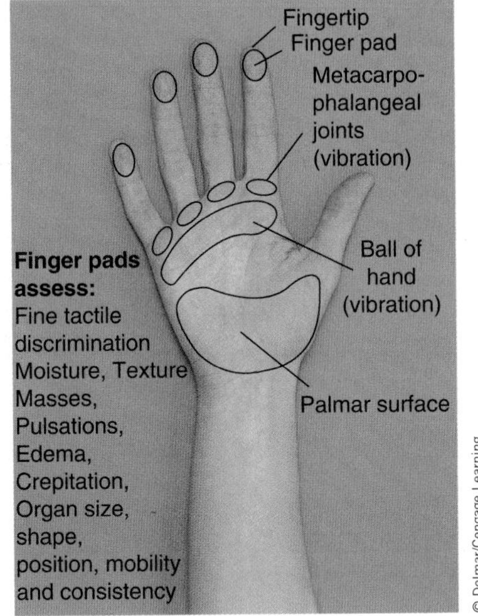

Palmar surface

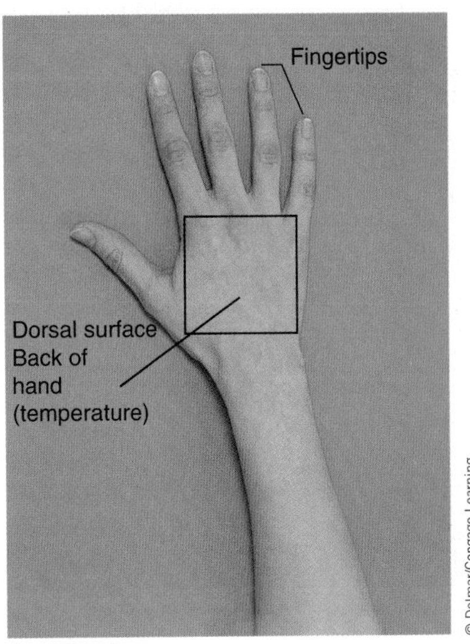

Dorsal surface

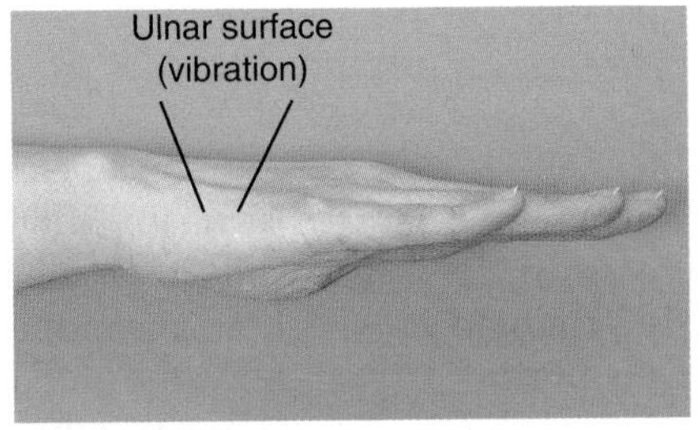

Ulnar surface

FIGURE 13-4 Parts of the hand used in palpation.

or the ulnar surface of the hand and comparing areas of the chest bilaterally. Vocal fremitus can indicate areas of pulmonary complications. Decreased vocal fremitus, or the lack of vibration transmission, can be caused by fluid or air in the pleural space, complete obstruction of the airways, or changes in residual capacity as with emphysema. Increased vocal fremitus, or increased vibration transmission, can be caused by pneumonia, atelectasis, consolidation, pulmonary edema, and lung masses. Figure 13-5 indicates the pathways to be used to palpate tactile or vocal fremitus of the chest.

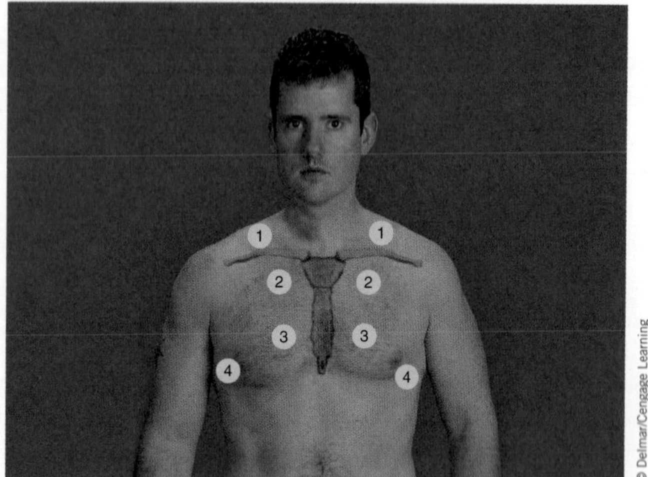

A. Anterior thorax

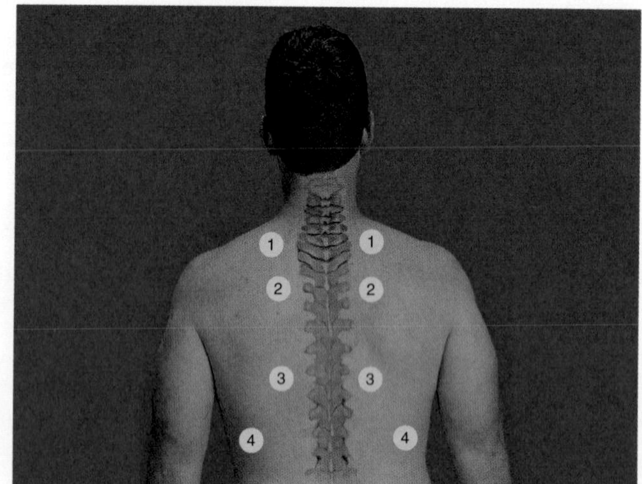

B. Posterior thorax

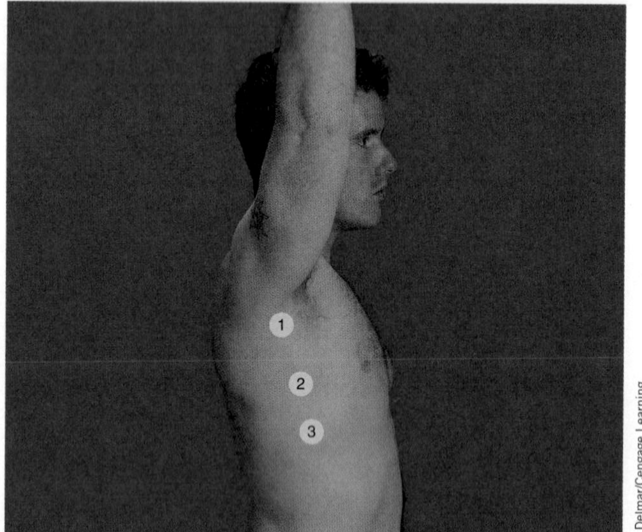

C. Right lateral thorax

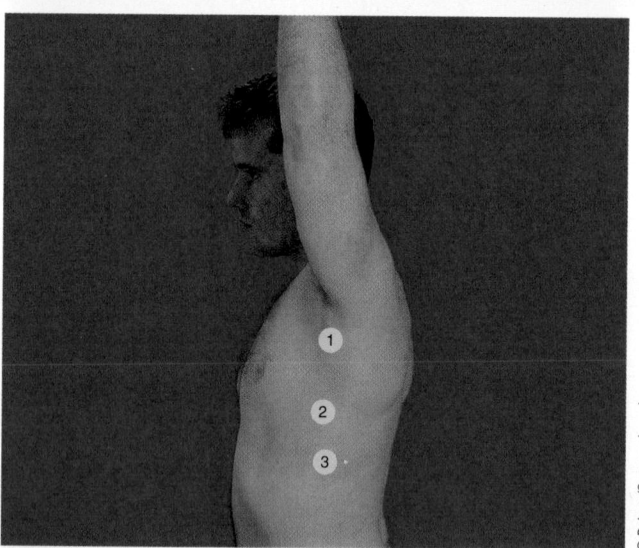

D. Left lateral thorax

FIGURE 13-5 Patterns for vocal or tactile fremitus.

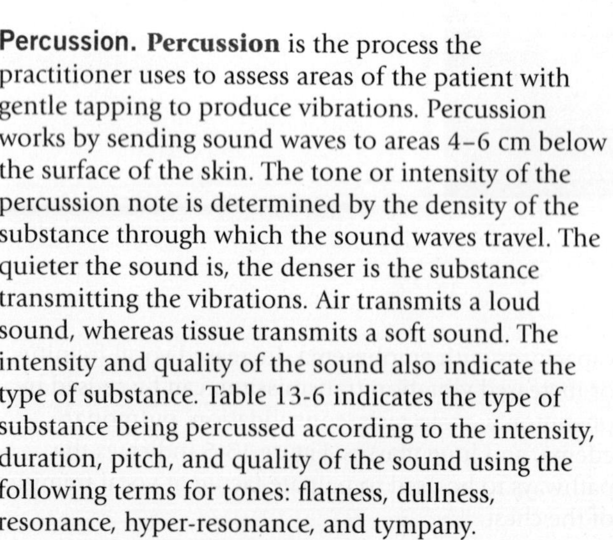

Percussion. **Percussion** is the process the practitioner uses to assess areas of the patient with gentle tapping to produce vibrations. Percussion works by sending sound waves to areas 4–6 cm below the surface of the skin. The tone or intensity of the percussion note is determined by the density of the substance through which the sound waves travel. The quieter the sound is, the denser is the substance transmitting the vibrations. Air transmits a loud sound, whereas tissue transmits a soft sound. The intensity and quality of the sound also indicate the type of substance. Table 13-6 indicates the type of substance being percussed according to the intensity, duration, pitch, and quality of the sound using the following terms for tones: flatness, dullness, resonance, hyper-resonance, and tympany.

Proper percussion technique is essential. Perform the percussion indirectly by tapping the finger of one hand while it is resting against the patient's skin. Figure 13-6 shows the proper percussion technique, and Figure 13-7 shows the proper positioning of the hands for percussion. Be sure that the passive hand (the one being tapped) is placed firmly on the surface to be percussed. Separate the fingers of the passive hand so that the vibrations are transmitted to the patient and not dampened by the adjoining fingers. Do not move your entire hand when percussing. Instead, tap by moving only the finger that is percussing. Use the tip of your finger when percussing, not the pad. Perform percussion systematically and bilaterally to ascertain any differences from right to left. Figure 13-8 shows a recommended path for percussion of the chest to determine bilateral differences.

TABLE 13-6 **Characteristics of percussion sounds**

Sound	Intensity	Duration	Pitch	Quality	Normal Location	Abnormal Location	Density
Flatness	Soft	Short	High	Flat	Muscle (thigh) or bone	Lungs (severe pneumonia)	Most dense
Dullness	Moderate	Moderate	High	Thud	Organs (liver)	Lungs (atelectasis)	
Resonance	Loud	Moderate to long	Low	Hollow	Normal lungs	No abnormal location	
Hyperresonance	Very loud	Long	Very low	Boom	No normal location	Lungs (emphysema)	
Tympany	Loud	Long	High	Drum	Gastric air bubble	Lungs (large pneumothorax)	Least dense

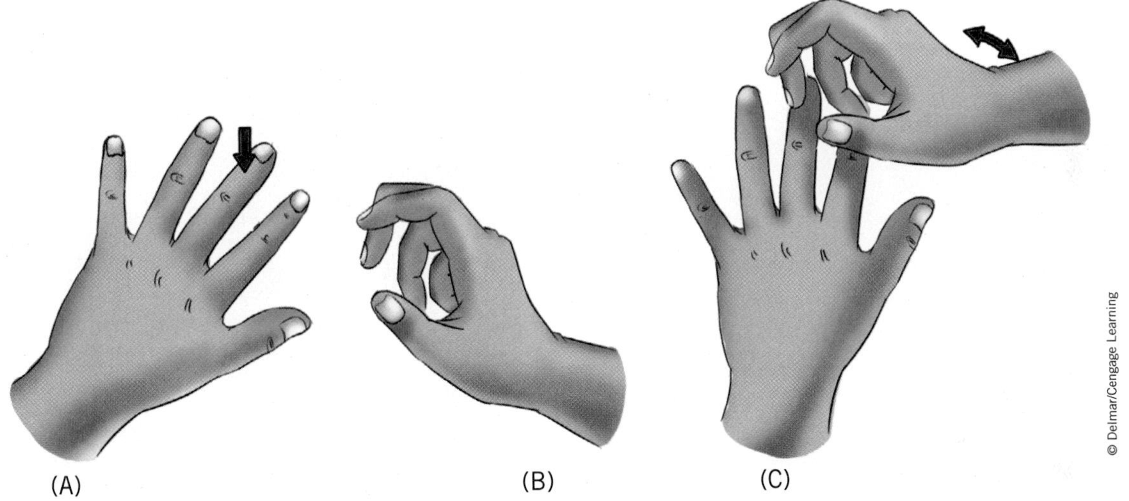

FIGURE 13-6 Percussion technique: (A) Hyperextend the middle finger of the nondominant hand and press the distal phalanx and joint firmly on the surface to be percussed. (B) Cock the hand upward, with the middle finger partially flexed and poised to strike. (C) Strike the middle finger of the nondominant hand with the tip of the middle finger of the dominant hand.

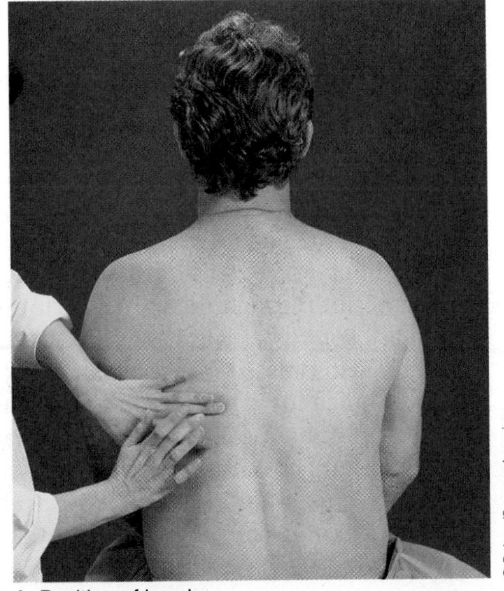

A. Position of hands

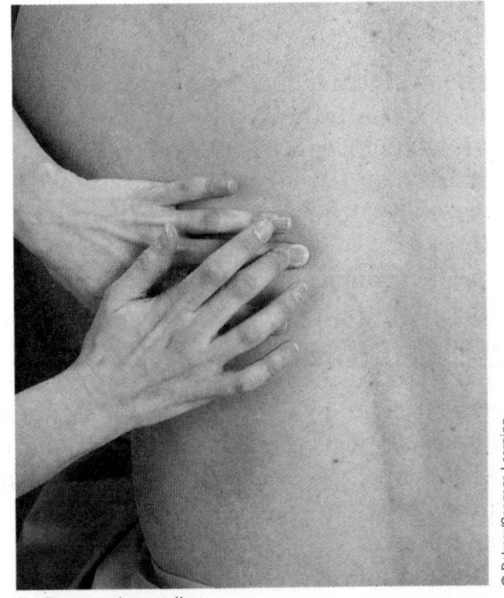

B. Percussion strike

FIGURE 13-7 Posterior thorax percussion.

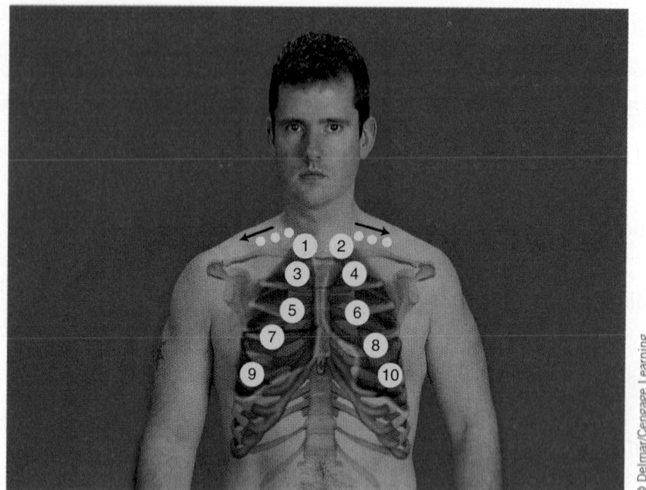

A. Anterior thorax

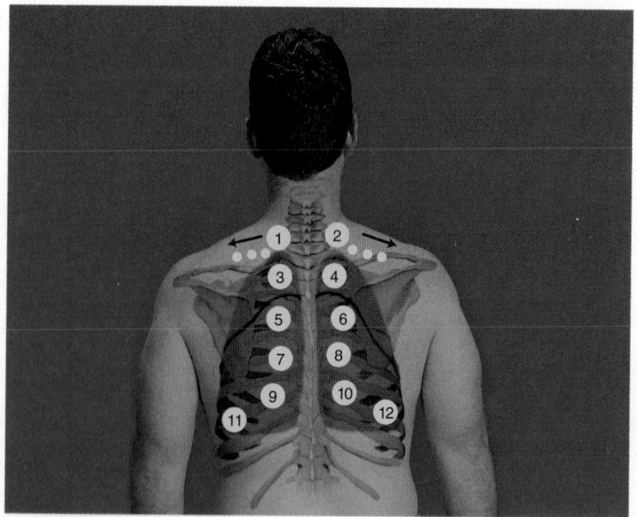

B. Posterior thorax

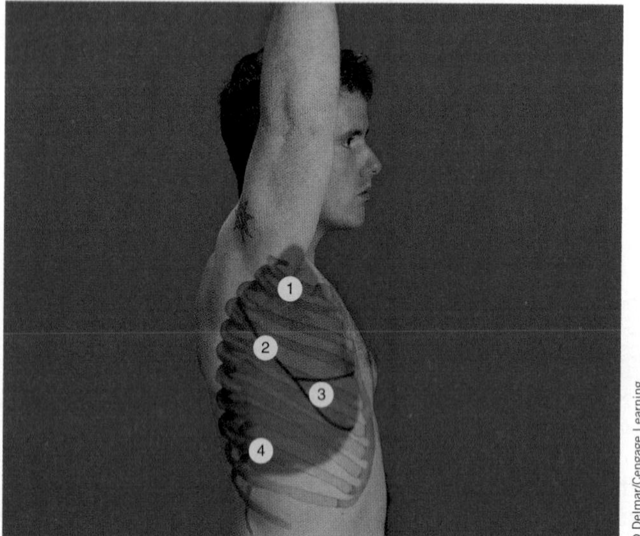

C. Right lateral thorax

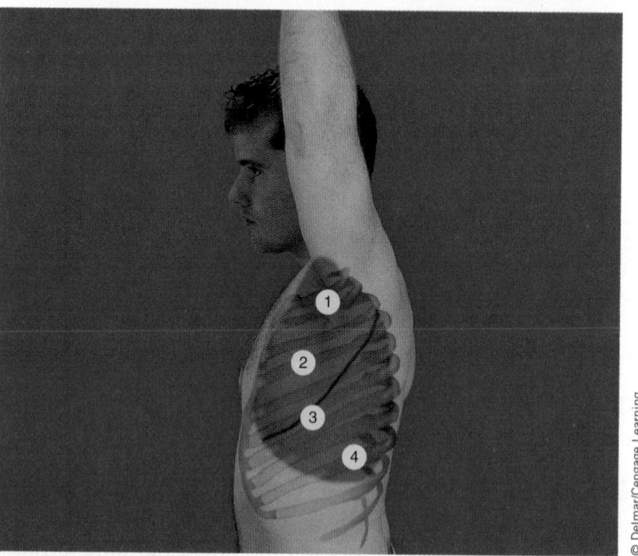

D. Left lateral thorax

FIGURE 13-8 Percussion patterns.

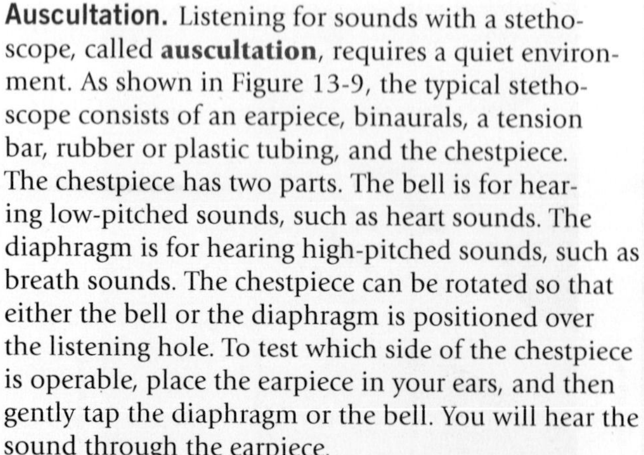

Auscultation. Listening for sounds with a stethoscope, called **auscultation**, requires a quiet environment. As shown in Figure 13-9, the typical stethoscope consists of an earpiece, binaurals, a tension bar, rubber or plastic tubing, and the chestpiece. The chestpiece has two parts. The bell is for hearing low-pitched sounds, such as heart sounds. The diaphragm is for hearing high-pitched sounds, such as breath sounds. The chestpiece can be rotated so that either the bell or the diaphragm is positioned over the listening hole. To test which side of the chestpiece is operable, place the earpiece in your ears, and then gently tap the diaphragm or the bell. You will hear the sound through the earpiece.

When using the stethoscope to listen to breath sounds, be careful to stabilize it firmly against the patient's chest by positioning the chestpiece of the stethoscope between your index and middle finger and using your hand to stabilize the chestpiece against the skin (Figure 13-10). Disinfect the chestpiece with alcohol and warm it before placing it against the patient's chest. Be sure, especially when listening for breath sounds, to auscultate over bare skin, not through the patient's clothing. Cloth can mask sounds or vibrate against the chestpiece. Chest hair also causes noise that can mask breath sounds; minimize these effects by dampening the hair. When auscultating the chest, use a systematic bilateral technique, following the same pattern for auscultation as for percussion (see Figure 13-8); however, with auscultation, start the pattern at the bases and work upward.[4,8]

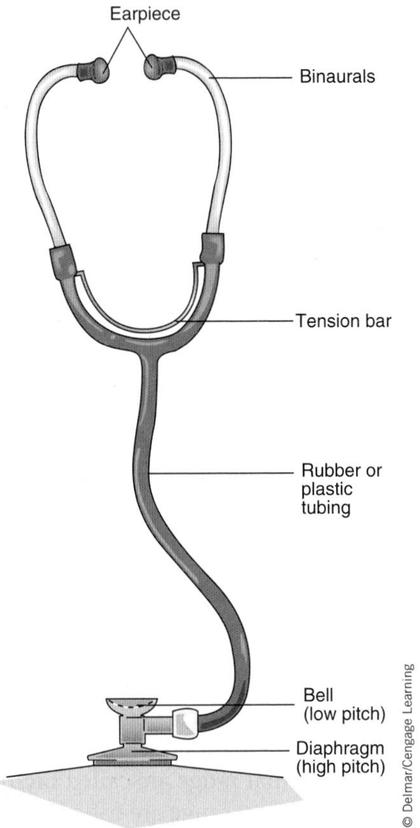

FIGURE 13-9 Acoustic stethoscope.

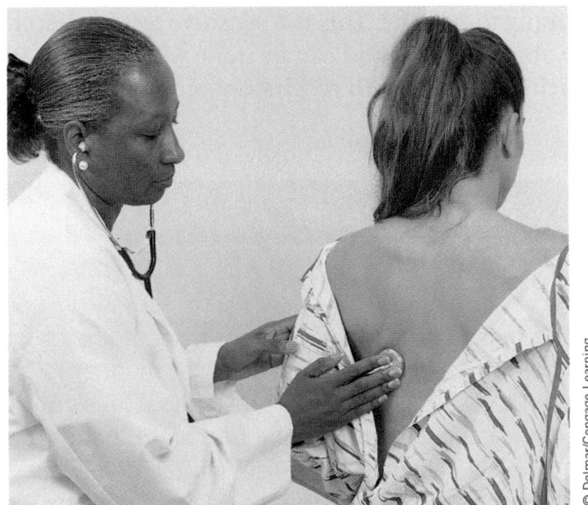

FIGURE 13-10 Correct way to hold a stethoscope.

PHYSICAL EXAMINATION OF THE ADULT

Presenting a total physical examination of the adult patient is not possible in this chapter because the process is complex and each finding leads to another. The combination of all the findings can help in determining a diagnosis. Therefore, an overview of the entire process is presented here, with a focus on the chest and cardiovascular system.

Mental Status. Upon approaching the patient and engaging him in conversation, the practitioner starts checking the patient's mental status and continues to observe his appearance and behavior during the interview.

- Assess the level of consciousness. Is the patient alert and responsive to verbal stimuli, or is he lethargic, obtunded, stuporous, or comatose?
- Assess the patient's posture and motor behavior, observing the range, characteristics, and appropriateness of the patient's movements. Are these normal, or is the patient restless, agitated, or immobile? The patient may also exhibit bizarre postures or involuntary movements.
- While the patient is answering questions, assess his speech and language patterns, noting the clarity, loudness, quantity, and rate of speech. These observations can indicate conditions such as aphasia, dysphonia, or dysarthria.
- Finally, assess the patient's mood, noting, for example, elation, depression, anxiety, anger, or indifference.[4]

Another part of evaluating mental status is assessing the patient's thought processes and perceptions. By listening to the patient's answers, the practitioner can assess coherence.

- Carefully probe any unusual or unpleasant thoughts introduced by the patient, being careful not to agitate him.
- Ask about any unusual perceptions the patient might have, such as illusions or hallucinations.

Finally, establish the patient's orientation, attention, and memory.

A patient *oriented* to time, place, and person is said to be "oriented times three" (written × 3). If not oriented times three, the patient is said to be "disoriented." The Glasgow Coma Scale is the gold standard for assessing a patient's level of *consciousness*, especially if the patient is recovering from a coma or lapsing into a comatose state, has suffered head trauma, or has been sedated or received anesthesia.[9] Table 13-7 shows the Glasgow Coma Scale.

Attention is established by assessing digit span, serial sevens, or spelling backward.

- *Digit span* is tested by having the patient repeat forward and backward a seven-digit phone number spoken by the practitioner.
- *Serial sevens* tests the patient's ability to subtract seven repeatedly from a starting number of 100.
- *Spelling backward* a five-letter word such as *world* is another test of attention.

TABLE 13-7 **Glasgow Coma Scale**

Eye-opening response	Spontaneous opening	4
	To verbal response	3
	To pain	2
	None	1
Most appropriate verbal response*	Oriented	5
	Confused	4
	Inappropriate words	3
	Incoherent	2
	None	1
Most integrated motor response	Obeys commands	5
	Localizes pain	4
	Flexion to pain	3
	Extension to pain	2
	None	1
Normal consciousness is a score of 14, and coma is a score of 3.		

Intubated patients cannot speak, so their scores are modified as 3 through 10, with 10 as normal consciousness.

- *Memory* is tested by asking the patient to answer questions such as the current date, his or her birth date, the name of the president, or his or her high school. Questions such as these test short-term and long-term memory.
- Recent *memory* can be tested by asking the person about his or her activities for the past 24 hours.

Poor performance on any of those tests is common in a delirious or demented patient; however, it can also be a result of language or educational barriers or of learning disorders.

General Appearance. After observing the patient's mental status:

- Observe the patient's general state of health, height, weight, build, and sexual development.
- Generally inspect the patient for odors, grooming, and personal hygiene, especially in home care or nonhospital settings.
- Assess motor activity, facial expressions, and reactions.
- Observe and note skin color, signs of distress, and posture.[10]

Vital Signs. Typically, four vital signs are recorded as part of the comprehensive physical examination: pulse, respiratory rate, blood pressure, and temperature.

Pulse is measured by placing the fingers on a pulse point and counting the pulse for at least 30 seconds. Common pulse points are the radial artery, the brachial artery, and the carotid artery. If using the carotid, make sure that pressure does not impede the flow of blood to the brain and that the carotid sinus is not stimulated (stimulating the carotid sinus can result in bradycardia). Evaluate the pulse for strength, rhythm, and rate.

- The *strength* of the pulse is the **pulse pressure**, the difference between the systolic and diastolic blood pressures. A weak pulse can be an early indication of the compromise of systemic blood pressure.
- The *rhythm* should be regular (see Figure 13-11 for common abnormal pulse patterns).
- The *rate* should fall within the normal range for the patient's age. A heart rate above the normal range is called **tachycardia**, and one below it is called **bradycardia**. Table 13-8 gives the normal ranges for vital signs by age.

The *respiratory rate* should be counted for at least 30 seconds as well. Because a patient can become self-conscious when someone is directly watching his or her chest, observe the respiratory rate, rhythm or pattern, and depth indirectly. Once the pulse has been taken, the practitioner should keep her fingers on the pulse point but, out of the corner of her eye, observe the rise and fall of the patient's chest. Respiratory rates above the normal range are called **tachypnea**. Rates below the normal range are called **bradypnea**. The pattern of breathing should also be observed. Table 13-9 describes some common abnormal breathing patterns. Additionally, during the interview process, count the number of words a patient can say before stopping to breathe. This is a sensitive test for respiratory abnormalities and can be done without the patient noticing. Patients with respiratory problems tend to

Best Practice

Pulse

The pulse rate can be different from the heart rate. If an electrocardiogram (ECG) monitor is used to establish the heart rate, the vital sign should be documented as a heart rate, not as a pulse. By designating "pulse" on the chart, the practitioner indicates that she actually felt for a pulse and counted it for at least 30 seconds. Because of some cardiac anomalies, not every heartbeat on the ECG results in a pulse. Also, pulse oximeters are not as accurate as the practitioner's own fingers in establishing what is a pulse and what could be artifact. So the practitioner must take an actual pulse when performing vital signs and not rely solely on electronic devices.

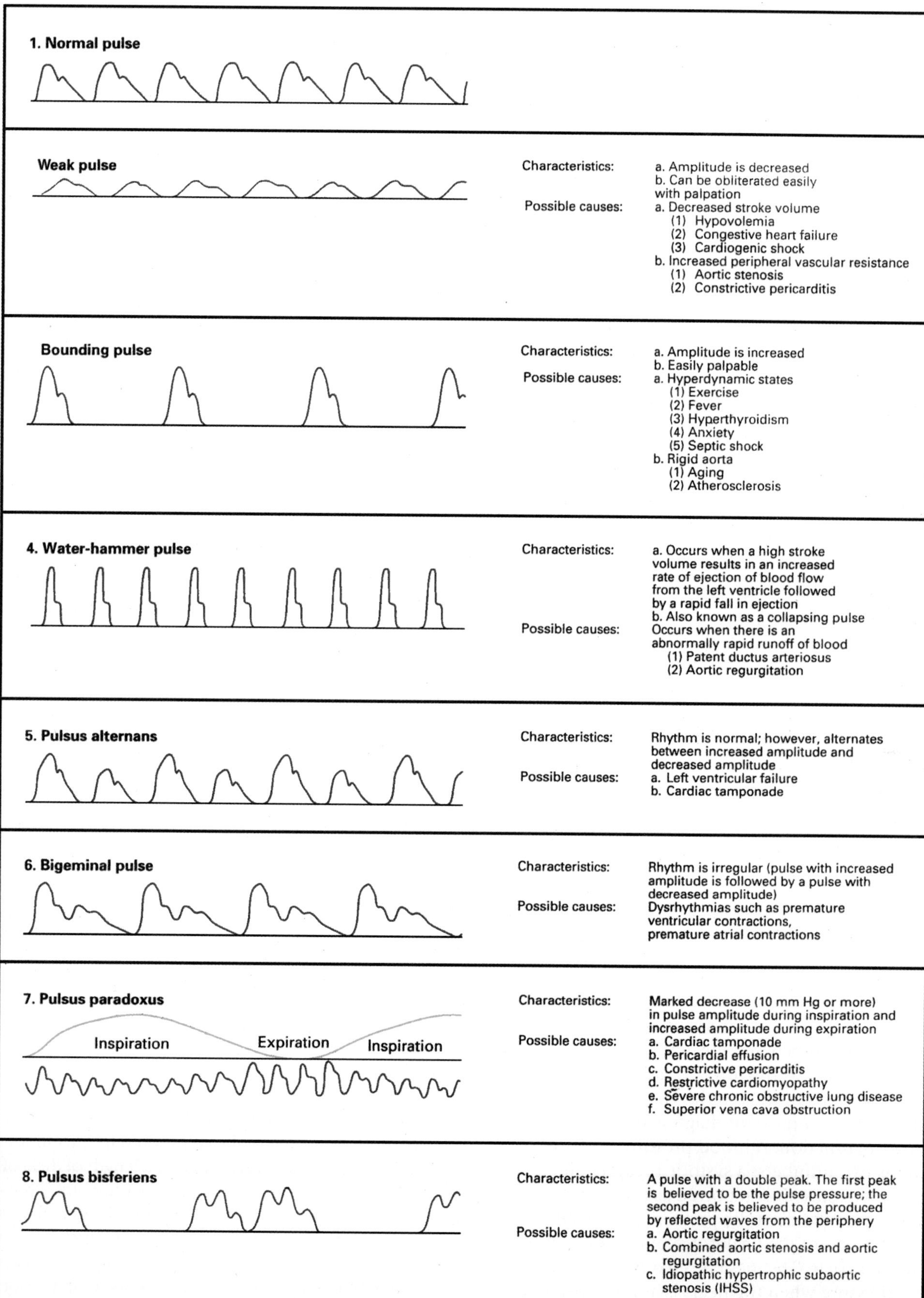

1. Normal pulse
Weak pulse
Characteristics: a. Amplitude is decreased
b. Can be obliterated easily with palpation
Possible causes: a. Decreased stroke volume
(1) Hypovolemia
(2) Congestive heart failure
(3) Cardiogenic shock
b. Increased peripheral vascular resistance
(1) Aortic stenosis
(2) Constrictive pericarditis
Bounding pulse
Characteristics: a. Amplitude is increased
b. Easily palpable
Possible causes: a. Hyperdynamic states
(1) Exercise
(2) Fever
(3) Hyperthyroidism
(4) Anxiety
(5) Septic shock
b. Rigid aorta
(1) Aging
(2) Atherosclerosis
4. Water-hammer pulse
Characteristics: a. Occurs when a high stroke volume results in an increased rate of ejection of blood flow from the left ventricle followed by a rapid fall in ejection
b. Also known as a collapsing pulse
Possible causes: Occurs when there is an abnormally rapid runoff of blood
(1) Patent ductus arteriosus
(2) Aortic regurgitation
5. Pulsus alternans
Characteristics: Rhythm is normal; however, alternates between increased amplitude and decreased amplitude
Possible causes: a. Left ventricular failure
b. Cardiac tamponade
6. Bigeminal pulse
Characteristics: Rhythm is irregular (pulse with increased amplitude is followed by a pulse with decreased amplitude)
Possible causes: Dysrhythmias such as premature ventricular contractions, premature atrial contractions
7. Pulsus paradoxus
Inspiration
Expiration
Inspiration
Characteristics: Marked decrease (10 mm Hg or more) in pulse amplitude during inspiration and increased amplitude during expiration
Possible causes: a. Cardiac tamponade
b. Pericardial effusion
c. Constrictive pericarditis
d. Restrictive cardiomyopathy
e. Severe chronic obstructive lung disease
f. Superior vena cava obstruction
8. Pulsus bisferiens
Characteristics: A pulse with a double peak. The first peak is believed to be the pulse pressure; the second peak is believed to be produced by reflected waves from the periphery
Possible causes: a. Aortic regurgitation
b. Combined aortic stenosis and aortic regurgitation
c. Idiopathic hypertrophic subaortic stenosis (IHSS)

FIGURE 13-11 Normal and abnormal pulse patterns.

TABLE 13-8 **Normal vital sign ranges by age**

Age	Pulse (beats/min)	Respiration (breaths/min)	Blood Pressure
Newborn	130–160	30–60	50–52/25–30 mm Hg
Child	80–120	18–30	95–118/62–75 mm Hg
Adult	60–80	12–20	<140/<89 mm Hg

TABLE 13-9 **Abnormal breathing patterns**

Abnormality	Description	Pathology
Kussmaul	Rapid deep breathing	Metabolic acidosis, anxiety
Cheyne-Stokes*	Periods of deep breathing with periods of apnea	Heart failure, cerebral damage
Ataxia	Unpredictable irregularity; breathing may be deep or shallow with apnea	Respiratory depression, medullary brain damage
Biots	Irregular breathing with long periods of apnea	Increased intracranial pressure
Obstructive pattern	Prolonged exhalation	Asthma, emphysema
Retractions and bulging	Skin at apices and in intercostal areas retracts inward during inhalation or bulges outward on exhalation	Severe airflow obstruction and large swings in pleural pressures
Abdominal paradox	Abdomen sinks inward during inhalation	Diaphragmatic fatigue or paralysis
Respiratory alternans	Periods of only diaphragmatic breathing alternating with only chest wall breathing	Diaphragmatic fatigue or significant inspiratory muscle fatigue
Orthopnea	Shortness of breath that starts or increases as patient lies flat	Suggestive of left ventricular failure or mitral stenosis but may accompany obstructive lung disease
Platypnea	Shortness of breath increases in the upright position	Suggestive of right to left intracardiac shunt
Paroxysmal nocturnal dyspnea	Sudden onset of shortness of breath and orthopnea that awakens patient after a period of sleep	Suggestive of left ventricular failure or mitral stenosis and may be mimicked by nocturnal asthma attacks

Compiled from Bickley LS, Hoekelman RA. Bates' Guide to Physical Examination and History Taking. *7th ed, Philadelphia: J.B. Lippincott Co; 1999:269; and Wilkins RL.* Physical Examination of the Patient with Cardiopulmonary Disease. *In: Wilkins RL, Krider SJ, Sheldon RL, eds.* Clinical Assessment in Respiratory Care. *3rd ed. St. Louis: Mosby-Yearbook; 1995:38.*

**This pattern can be normal in young children or in aging people during sleep.*

breathe more often when expending energy by speaking: the more serious the problem, the fewer the number of words between breaths.

Blood pressure is the force of the blood exerted against the walls of the arteries as it moves through them and is an important diagnostic measure of circulatory function. A blood pressure measurement contains two numbers: a systolic pressure and a diastolic pressure. It is reported as the systolic pressure over the diastolic pressure. The *systolic pressure* measures the peak force of contraction of the left ventricle. The *diastolic pressure* measures the blood pressure when the heart is at rest. The *pulse pressure* is the difference between these two measurements.

A **sphygmomanometer** is a device used to measure blood pressures. Using the correct cuff size when measuring blood pressure is important. A cuff that is too wide gives erroneously low values, and too small a cuff gives erroneously high values. A small cuff often causes erroneously high readings in obese and very muscular patients. The bladder of the cuff should be a width of 40% of the arm circumference and a length of 80% of the arm circumference.[4] To accurately measure blood pressure, center the bladder of the cuff over the brachial artery, with the lower border of the cuff at least 1 inch above the antecubital crease. The cuff should be snug enough on the arm to stay in place but not too snug. A cuff that is too loose does not exert sufficient pressure when inflated. Too snug a cuff can mask the diastolic pressure sounds.

The most effective sequence for accurately measuring blood pressure is as follows:

First, establish the *palpable systolic blood pressure.* Place the fingers of one hand over the brachial or radial artery.

1. Rapidly inflate the cuff until the pulse is no longer felt.
2. Then inflate 20–30 mm Hg above that point.
3. Deflate the cuff slowly at a rate of 2–3 mm Hg per second until you feel at least two beats of the brachial pulse. This is the palpable systolic blood pressure. Deflate the cuff immediately.

Next, establish the *diastolic and systolic pressures.*

1. Place the bell of the stethoscope over the brachial artery.
2. Pause for 30 seconds.
3. Then inflate the cuff until it is 20–30 mm Hg above the palpable systolic pressure.
4. Deflate the cuff slowly, while listening for the following sounds:
    - Two consecutive beats indicate the systolic pressure and the beginning of the Korotkoff sounds.
    - In some cases, the Korotkoff sounds are heard, then disappear, and reappear when the cuff pressure has decreased 10–15 mm Hg. This is the ausculatory gap, which can occur in patients with systolic hypertension or severe aortic regurgitation. Not being aware of the possibility of this gap can cause misreading.
    - The Korotkoff sounds change from crisp to muffled. This is the first diastolic sound, believed to be the closest to the actual diastolic arterial pressure. This sound signals the imminent disappearance of Korotkoff sounds (not to be confused with ausculatory gap).
    - Note the point at which sounds disappear completely. This is the second diastolic sound.

The American Heart Association recommends recording systolic and both diastolic readings (for example, 110/80/72). If only two values are recorded, they should be the systolic and the second diastolic.[7]

Normal values for blood pressure change with age; however, the Seventh Report of the Joint National Committee on Detection, Evaluation, and Treatment of High Blood Pressure established the following guidelines in 2004.

- For adults over age 18, optimal blood pressure is a systolic of less than 120 mm Hg and a diastolic of less than 80 mm Hg.
- The high normal range is a systolic of 120–129 mm Hg and a diastolic of 80–84 mm Hg. Although a high normal alone is not a problem, if combined with other risk factors such as smoking, overweight, and high cholesterol values, high normal blood pressure can indicate pending cardiovascular problems.
- Hypertension is rated as Stage One (mild, 140–159/90–99 mm Hg), Stage Two (moderate, 160–179/100–109), and Stage Three (severe, 180 or above/110 or above).

Finally, critically ill patients often suffer from shock, which produces very low blood pressures. Hearing systolic and diastolic sounds may be impossible, especially if the pulse pressure is lower than 30 mm Hg. In these cases, only a palpable blood pressure is reported. *Palpable blood pressure* is reported as the systolic number only, with the word "palpable" after it to designate how the pressure was obtained.

Temperature is the fourth vital sign usually reported. A patient's temperature can be taken in four ways: oral, rectal, axillary, and aural. Each method has its restrictions and usefulness; however, with the newer, more accurate tympanic thermometers, the aural route has become the avenue of choice. The aural method usually registers almost one degree higher than the oral method and is very close to the reading of the rectal method, which is considered the closest to the patient's core temperature. Normal adult oral and rectal temperatures are between 37° and 38°C or 98.6° and 100.5°F. Temperature fluctuates during the day; it is lower in the morning upon awakening and slowly rises throughout the day until late afternoon. Hypothermia, or low temperature, is relatively common and usually results in the hypothalamus initiating shivering to generate energy and vasoconstriction to conserve body heat.[9]

Face and Skin. The next segment of the physical examination consists of examining the patient's face and skin. With the patient sitting on the edge of the bed or on an examining table, stand in front of the patient to examine the face for any discoloration, lesions, or injuries, noting their location, size, type, color, and number. Study the patient's head, scalp, and

> *Best Practice*
>
> **Temperature**
>
> Hyperthermia, or fever, in a patient is vital to assess, especially for respiratory patients, because oxygen consumption and carbon dioxide production increase approximately 10% for each 1°C rise in body temperature above normal.

hair for any problems. Examine the patient's hands and nails for any discoloration, pallor, or temperature difference, all of which can indicate inadequate peripheral circulation.

Also note the presence of any cyanosis or clubbing, and assess capillary refill. *Cyanosis*, a bluish discoloration of the skin, exists when the hemoglobin is reduced by 1.5 volume percent or more.[8] Two types of cyanosis can be discovered:

- **Peripheral cyanosis** is the blueing of the fingers or nailbeds. It indicates peripheral venous obstruction or a decreased blood flow because of circulation problems.
- **Central cyanosis** is the blueing of the lips and mucus membranes. It indicates advanced lung disease, congenital heart problems, or abnormal hemoglobin.[4] In most cases, central cyanosis indicates a lack of oxygenation.

Clubbing is a condition in which the ends of the fingers enlarge and the fingernail loses its angle. In advanced stages, the ends of the fingers begin to look like clubs, with the ends larger than the fingers themselves. Figure 13-12 illustrates early clubbing compared with a normal finger. Clubbing takes years to develop, but it can be determined in the early stages by palpating the base of the nails, which take on a spongy feeling. Clubbing is found in patients with chronic pulmonary disease such as emphysema and cystic fibrosis, bronchogenic carcinoma, and chronic cardiovascular disease.[8]

Capillary refill is the time it takes for capillary blood flow to return to an area and indicates the adequacy or inadequacy of peripheral circulation. To assess capillary refill, gently press and release a place on one of the patient's extremities, such as a fingernail or a toenail, or on the back of the hand or top of the foot. Observe how long it takes for the nail or skin to return to its normal or original color. With normal refill, the color returns within 3 seconds. A refill time of greater than 3 seconds can indicate a lack of adequate peripheral circulation.

Eyes, Ears, Nose, and Throat. After inspecting the hair, scalp, skull, face, and skin, the practitioner examines the patient's eyes, ears, nose, and throat.

Examine the *eyes* for acuity and for position, alignment, and the ability to follow a moving object (accommodation). Inspect the eyelids, sclera, and conjunctiva of each eye. Compare the pupils, and test their reaction to light. The abbreviation *PERRLA* is used to indicate "pupils equal, round, and reactive to light and accommodation."

Next, inspect the *ears*, including the auricles, canals, and eardrums, noting any structural irregularities, inflammation, discharge, or presence of wax or foreign objects. Then examine the outside of the nose, and, with a light, inspect the inside: nasal mucosa, septum, and the turbinates. Palpate the nose and the frontal and maxillary sinuses for tenderness.

Next, examine the *mouth and throat* with a light. Inspect the lips, oral mucosa, gums, teeth, tongue, palate, tonsils, and pharynx for swelling, ulceration, discoloration, or irritation. The tongue should also be inspected for texture, color, and any nodules.

Neck. The neck should be inspected and palpated for any masses, swollen lymph nodes, or unusual pulsations. Gently tracing the trachea with the index and middle finger on either side from the chin down to the sternal angle allows a practitioner to assess whether the trachea is midline or has shifted.

Because jugular venous pressure (JVP) reflects right atrial pressure, assess the jugular veins for distention. As shown in Figure 13-13, raise the head of the bed or examination table to higher than 45 degrees above horizontal. At 60 degrees the top of the visible jugular veins should not be more than 3–4 cm above the sternal angle. If the top is above 4 cm, jugular venous distention (JVD) is present. This most likely indicates right-side heart failure, which can be caused by chronic hypoxemia or pulmonary hypertension; it can also be secondary to left-side heart failure.

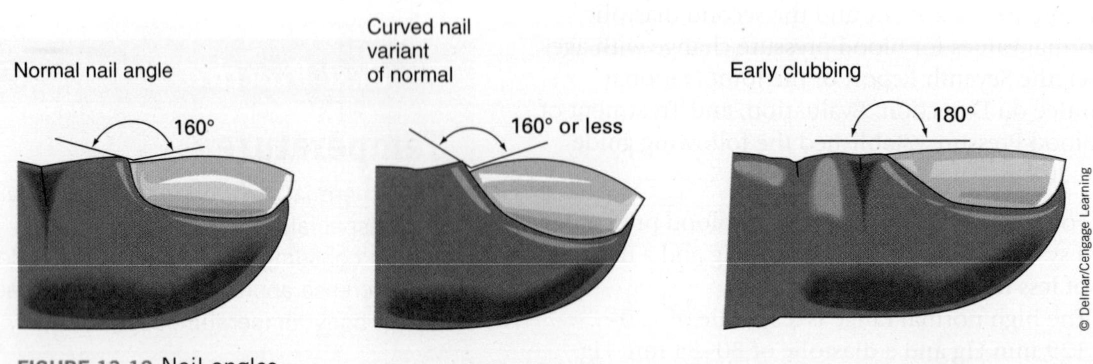

FIGURE 13-12 Nail angles.

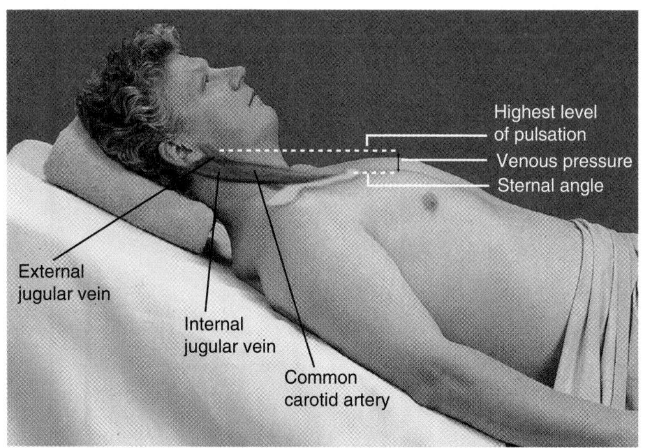

FIGURE 13-13 Inspection of jugular venous pressure.

Respiration/Thorax. After examining the neck, examine the thorax. Knowing the basic anatomy of the chest is essential for accurately assessing the respiratory system. Figure 13-14 shows the pathway of the respiratory tract. When examining the chest and documenting the results, use as reference points the standard surface landmarks, as shown in Figure 13-15. Also remember the surface landmarks that mark the various internal organs to be examined. Figure 13-14 shows the location of the tracheal bifurcation, and Figure 13-16 shows the lobes of the lung. Figure 13-17 shows the location of lung fissures.

Inspect the anterior and posterior chest for any deformities or asymmetry. Observe any abnormal retractions of the supraclavicular area or intercostal spaces, note chest symmetry, and compare the chest anterior-posterior (A-P) diameter with the lateral diameter. A normal chest has a larger lateral than A-P diameter (see Figure 13-18). A person with an A-P diameter equal to the lateral diameter is classified as having a "barrel chest." Other thoracic abnormalities are **pectus carinatum** (sternal protrusion) and **pectus excavatum** (sternal depression). While examining the posterior view of the thorax, observe for spinal deformities such as (see Figure 13-19):

- **Kyphosis**—abnormal anteroposterior curvature.
- **Scoliosis**—abnormal lateral curvature.
- **Kyphoscoliosis**—combination of kyphosis and scoliosis.
- **Lordosis**—abnormal posteroanterior curvature.

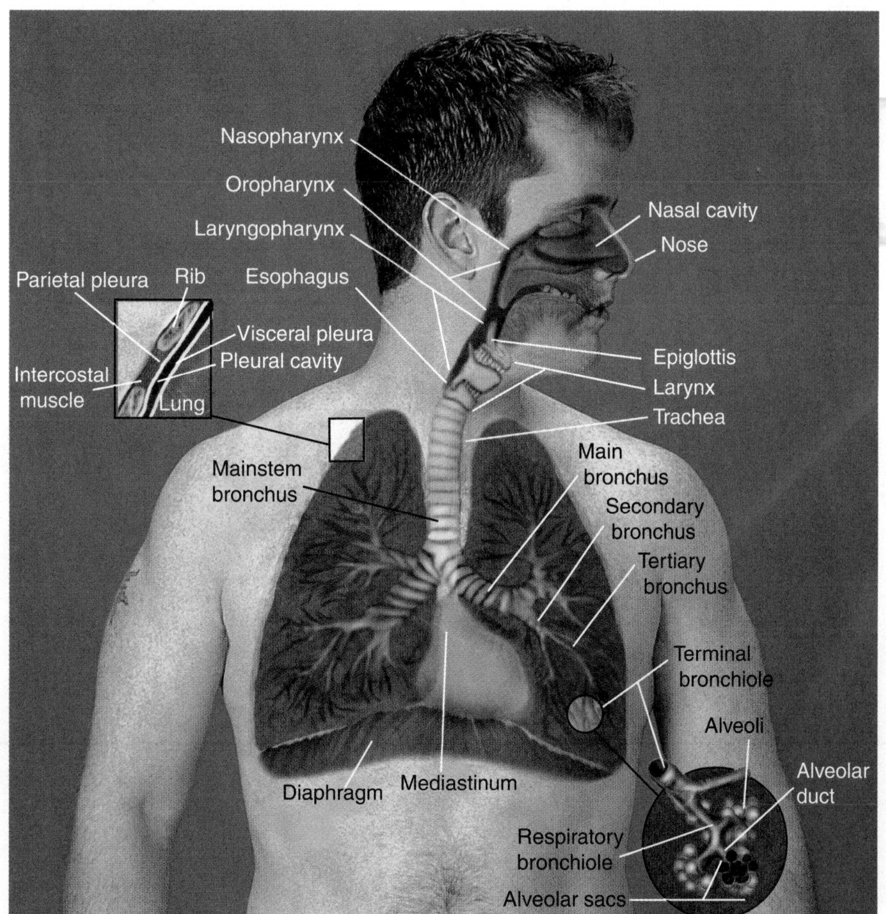

FIGURE 13-14 Pathway of the respiratory tract.

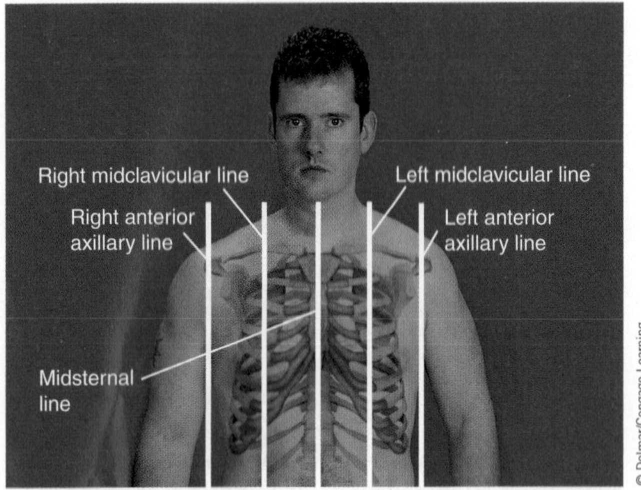

A. Anterior view

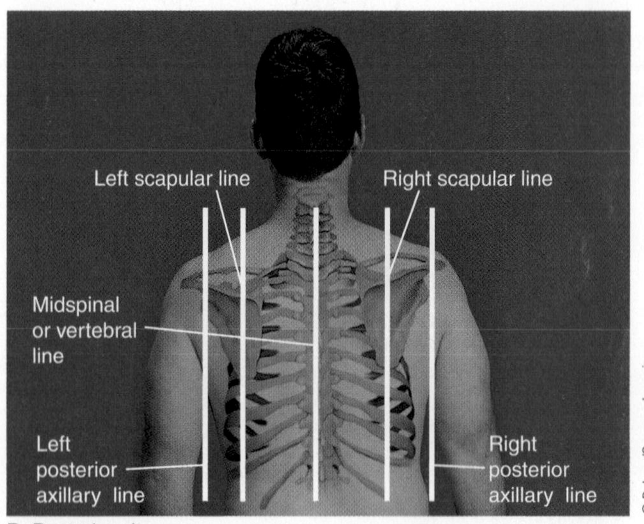

B. Posterior view

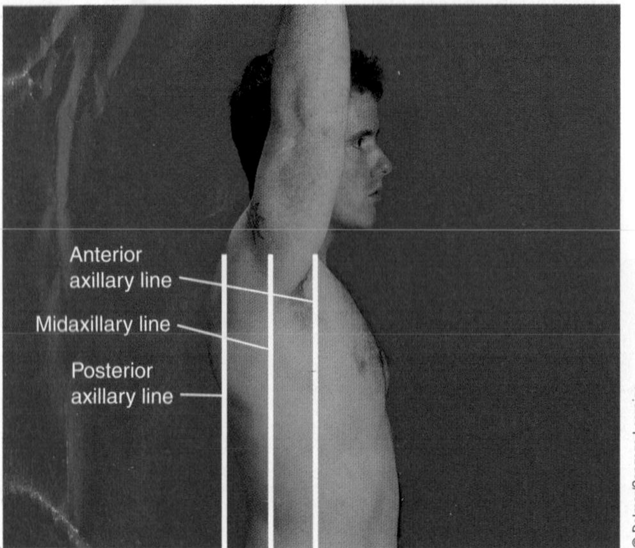

C. Right lateral view

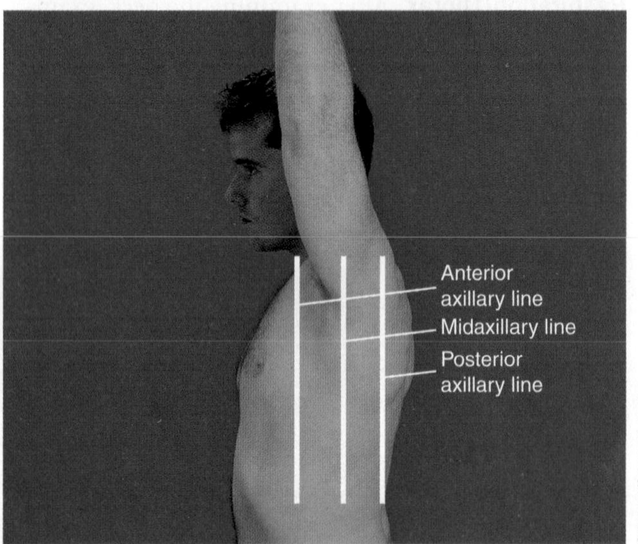

D. Left lateral view

FIGURE 13-15 Thoracic surface landmarks.

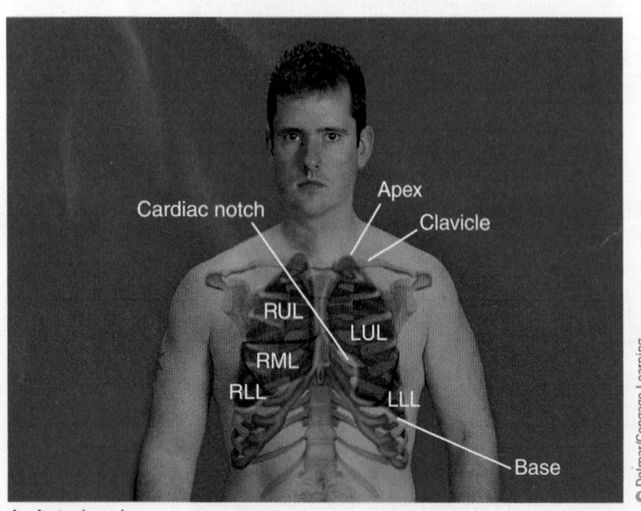

A. Anterior view

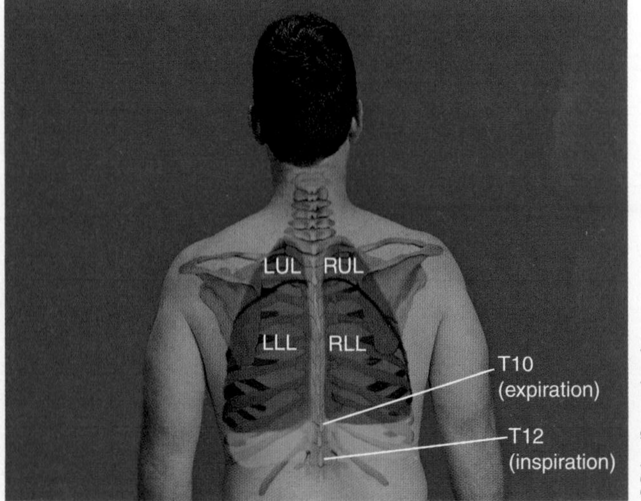

B. Posterior view

FIGURE 13-16 Lobes of the lungs. RUL = right upper lobe; RML = right middle lobe; RLL = right lower lobe; LUL = left upper lobe; LLL = left lower lobe.

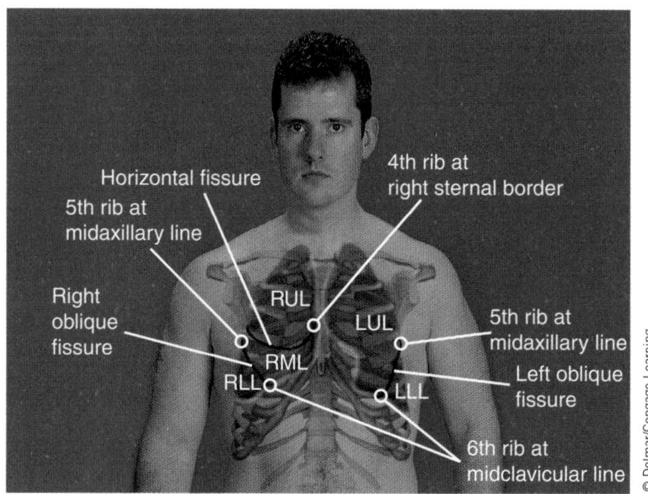

A. Anterior view

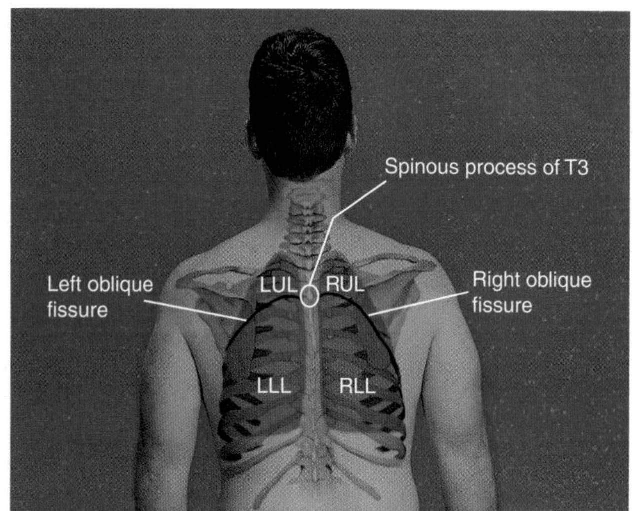

B. Posterior view

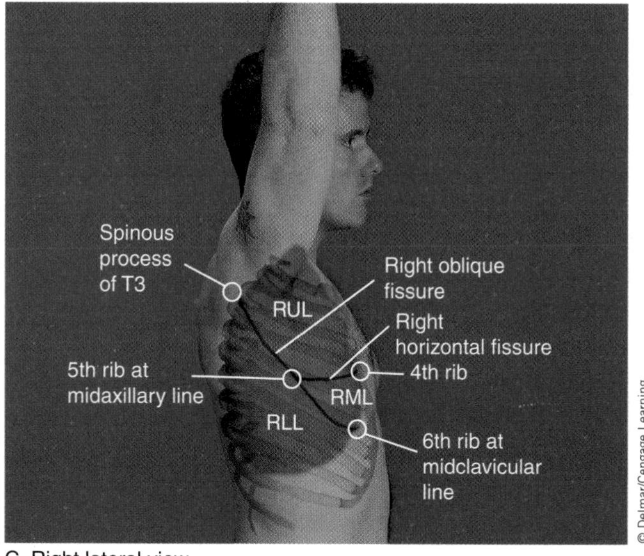

C. Right lateral view

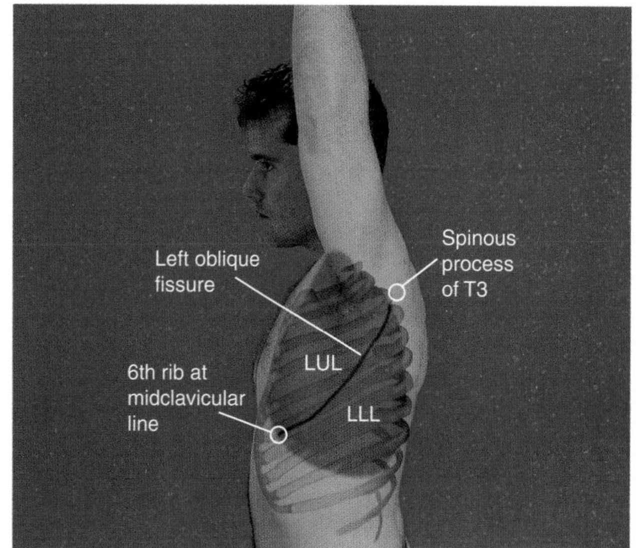

D. Left lateral view

FIGURE 13-17 Fissures of the lungs. RUL = right upper lobe; RML = right middle lobe; RLL = right lower lobe; LUL = left upper lobe; LLL = left lower lobe.

After examining and observing the exterior of the thorax, assess the interior structures. Using superficial palpation, the examiner palpates the anterior and posterior chest for any tenderness or abnormalities in the skin and chest wall, such as subcutaneous emphysema or lesions. To palpate the patient's chest wall expansion, the practitioner places her thumbs posteriorly at approximately the eighth thoracic vertebra with her fingers extended toward the midaxillary lines. Anteriorly, she places her thumbs at the xyphoid process and extends her fingers laterally along the ribs toward the midaxillary lines. Figure 13-20 shows anterior and posterior hand placement. At full exhalation, she places the thumbs so that they are together, and then asks the patient to take a deep breath. Each thumb should move from the midspinal line equally about 3–5 cm. *Bilateral reduction of chest expansion* can be caused by such problems as neuromuscular diseases and respiratory diseases that result in severe hyperinflation or air trapping (for example, emphysema or a severe asthma attack). *Unilateral reduction in chest wall expansion* suggests lobar consolidation, atelectasis, pleural effusion, pneumothorax, or unilateral diaphragmatic paralysis. During this part of the examination, the practitioner should also palpate anteriorly and posteriorly for changes in vocal fremitus.[4,8]

After chest palpation, percussion should be performed on both the anterior and posterior chest. Because percussing over bone is not diagnostic, it should be done on the intercostal spaces and away

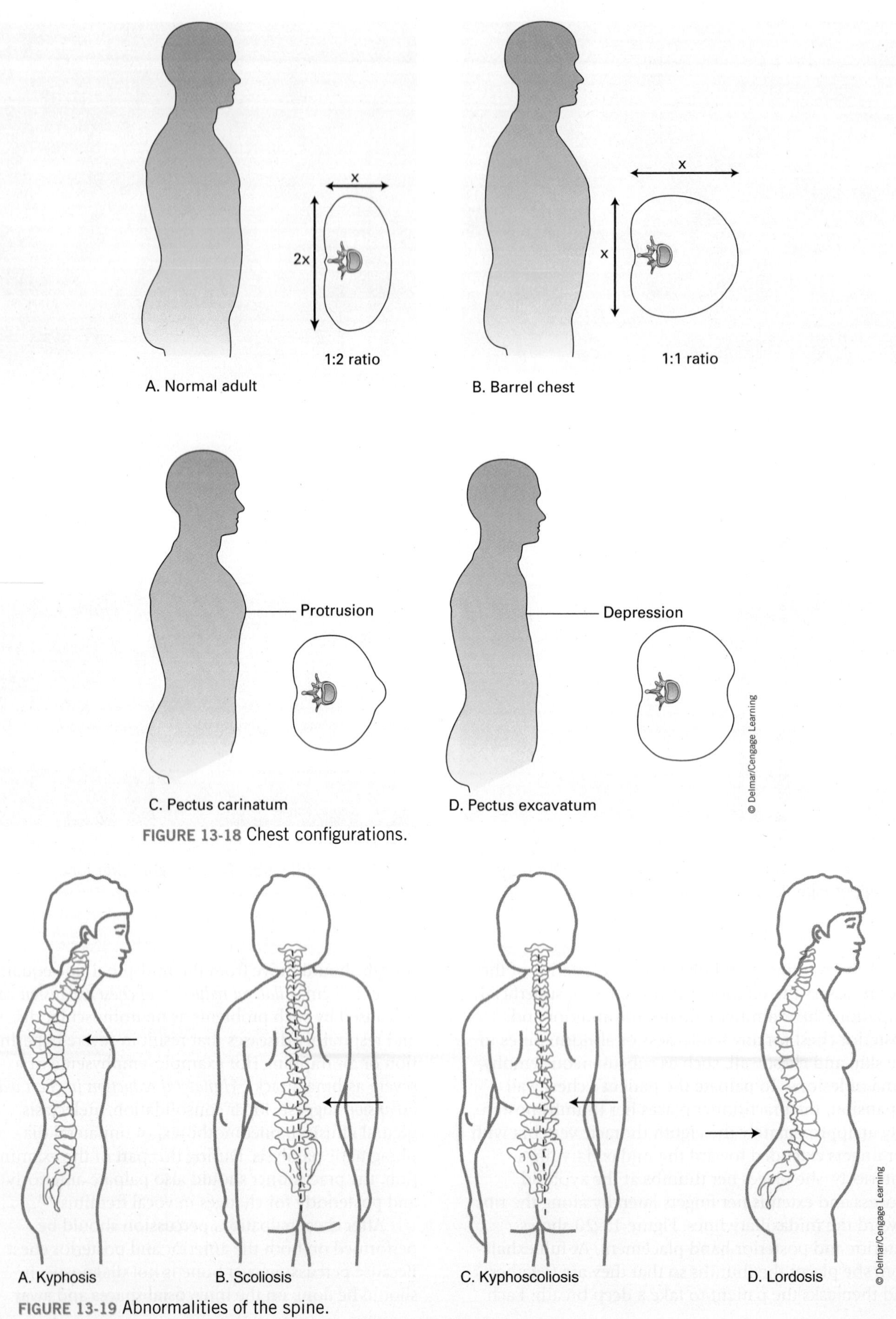

FIGURE 13-18 Chest configurations.

FIGURE 13-19 Abnormalities of the spine.

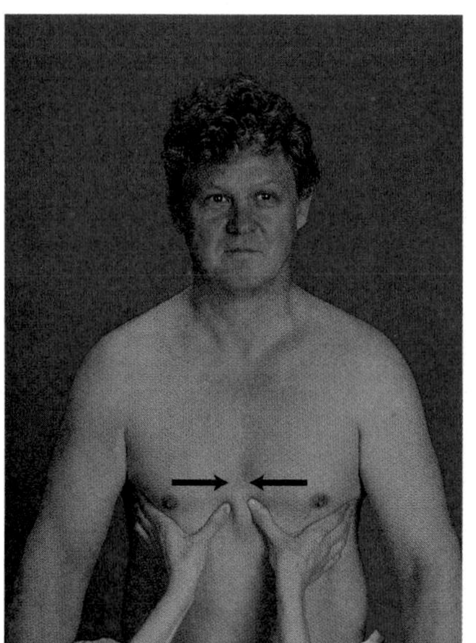

A. Anterior

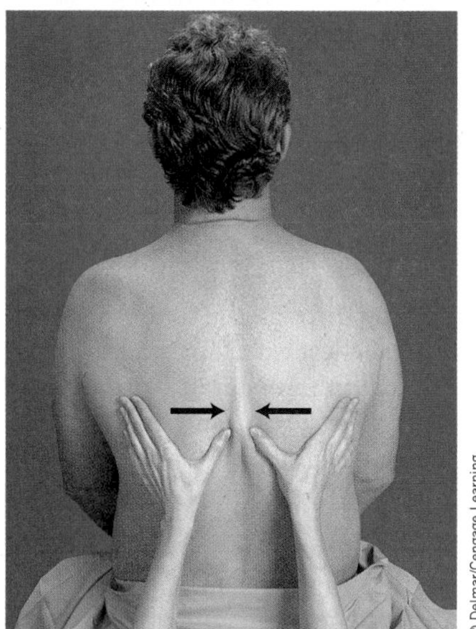

B. Posterior

FIGURE 13-20 Hand placement for palpating chest wall expansion.

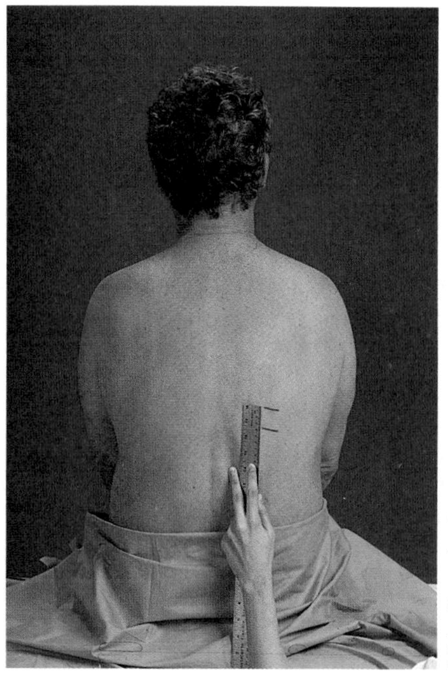

FIGURE 13-21 Assessment of diaphragmatic position.

from the scapulae. Percussion may have limited diagnostic value in patients who are obese or overly muscular. However, the practitioner can assess many abnormalities with percussion. For example, it is useful for assessing diaphragmatic excursion. As the patient fully exhales, the practitioner percusses the posterior chest downward until a dull note is heard. This is the level of the diaphragm, and a line is drawn on the patient's skin at this point. The patient takes a deep breath and holds it. The practitioner then percusses from the line down until the dull note is heard again and draws another line. The process is repeated on the other side of the posterior chest. (The practitioner should work quickly so that the patient does not become short of breath.) Normal diaphragmatic movement is approximately 5–7 cm during a deep breath. Although percussion can give only an approximate position of the diaphragm and its movement, any decrease in movement bilaterally or unilaterally can help in the diagnosis of respiratory problems. Figure 13-21 shows the assessment of diaphragmatic position.

After palpation and percussion, the next step is assessing respiration through auscultation. Using auscultation to distinguish between normal and abnormal breath sounds is one of the most important aspects of the physical examination of the chest. Auscultation must be performed in a quiet environment with care being taken to auscultate all areas of the lung.

To understand abnormal and **adventitious breath sounds** (sounds not usually heard in the lungs, such as wheezing and crackles), a practitioner must be able to identify normal breath sounds. The three types of normal breath sounds are tracheal or bronchial breath sounds, vesicular or normal breath sounds, and bronchovesicular breath sounds.

- *Tracheal or bronchial breath sounds*, normally heard over the trachea, are high-pitched, loud sounds, with the expiratory component equal to the inspiratory component.
- *Vesicular or normal breath sounds*, heard over the peripheral areas of the lungs, are low-pitched, soft sounds, with only a minimal expiratory

component. Bronchial breath sounds have been described as the sound of air passing through a tunnel, and vesicular breath sounds have been described as the rustling of leaves in a gentle breeze.

- *Bronchovesicular breath sounds,* normally heard over the main bronchi, have characteristics of both bronchial and vesicular breath sounds and occur when auscultating in a location, such as near the scapulae, where both sounds can be heard.

In addition to these normal breath sounds, abnormal sounds may be heard.

- Abnormal breath sounds include normal breath sounds heard in abnormal areas of the chest. For example, bronchial or bronchovesicular breath sounds heard in the peripheral areas of the chest can indicate consolidation or atelectasis that is in communication with the large airways and transmitting the harsher sounds to the periphery of the lung.
- Other abnormal breath sounds are those that are either diminished in one area or diminished throughout the chest. *Unilateral diminished breath sounds* suggest either a blocked bronchial tube, such as a large mucus plug, or a space-occupying mass in the pleural space, such as a pleural effusion or pneumothorax. *Bilateral diminished breath sounds* indicate hyperinflation or severe air trapping such as in a patient who has emphysema or is having a severe asthma attack.
- The final adventitious sound is a *pleural friction rub,* which occurs if the pleural surface becomes inflamed or loses its lubricating fluid. The sound is continuous throughout inhalation and exhalation, resembling the sound of Velcro being pulled apart.

Adventitious breath sounds also indicate abnormal lung process. The American Thoracic Society and the American College of Chest Physicians recommend standardized descriptions and terminology for adventitious breath sounds, described in Table 13-10. Adventitious sounds are characterized as *discontinuous* (fine or course crackles) or *continuous* (wheeze or rhonchi).

Voice sounds, or vibrations of spoken letters or words heard via auscultation, are useful if other examination techniques suggest a respiratory abnormality. These sounds are egophony, bronchophony, and whispered pectoriloquy.

- *Egophony* exists when the patient says the letter "e" and the practitioner hears the letter "a" over the peripheral chest wall. This difference suggests compressed lung tissue, usually identified only above a pleural effusion.
- *Bronchophony* is when spoken sounds increase in clarity and intensity, indicating increased lung tissue density. Bronchophony is usually easier to detect if it is unilateral and suggests consolidation of lobar pneumonia.
- *Whispered pectoriloquy* describes the selective transmission of high-pitched sounds. When a patient whispers "one, two, three," normal lung tissue filters out most of the high-pitched sounds. The practitioner hears a very faint, low-pitched whispering through the stethoscope on the peripheral chest wall. Areas of selective lung consolidation transmit the sounds clearly to the peripheral chest wall, and the practitioner hears the sounds clearly over the affected lung area.[8]

The total examination of the thorax can suggest many pulmonary disorders. Table 13-11 describes some of these disorders as well as the corresponding inspection, palpation, percussion, and auscultation results.

TABLE 13-10 **Lung sounds**

Type	Sound	Name	Pathology
Discontinuous	High-pitched, low amplitude, short duration at end of inspiration	Fine crackles	Atelectatic alveoli opening; does not clear with cough
	Low-pitched, high amplitude, long duration during inspiration	Coarse crackles	Sudden opening of proximal bronchi as in chronic bronchitis; unaffected by cough
Continuous	High-pitched, musical; heard only or loudest during exhalation	Wheeze	Polyphonic—small airway obstruction; monophonic—large airway obstruction
	Low-pitched, coarse sound; heard most often continuously during both inhalation and exhalation	Rhonchi	Thick mucus in trachea and large airway; usually clears with cough

Adapted from Seidel HM, Ball JW, Dains JE, Benedict GW. Mosby's Guide to Physical Examination. *4th ed. St. Louis: Mosby-Yearbook; 1999:381–382.*

TABLE 13-11 **Possible physical findings associated with common respiratory conditions**

Condition	Inspection	Palpation	Percussion	Auscultation
Asthma	Tachypnea, dyspnea	Tachycardia, diminished fremitus	Occasional hyperresonance, occasional diaphragm at lower level and limited movement	Prolonged exhalation, wheezes, diminished lung sounds
Atelectasis	Diminished chest wall movement, respiratory lag, narrowed intercostal spaces on affected side, tachypnea	Diminished fremitus, apical cardiac impulse, and trachea shifted toward affected side	Dullness over affected lung	Wheezes, rhonchi, and crackles in varying amounts, depending on extent of collapse
Bronchiectasis	Tachypnea, respiratory distress, hyperinflation	Few, if any, consistent findings	No unusual findings if no other pulmonary problems	A variety of crackles, usually coarse, rhonchi, sometimes disappearing with cough
Chronic obstructive lung disease	Respiratory distress, audible wheezing, cyanosis, neck vein distention, peripheral edema in presence of right-sided heart failure	Limited diaphragm mobility, diminished vocal fremitus	Occasional hyperresonance	Diminished breath sounds, rhonchi, wheezing, and fine crackles
Emphysema	Tachypnea, prolonged exhalation, pursed-lip breathing, barrel chest, thin, underweight	Apical impulse may not be felt, liver edge displaced downward, diminished fremitus	Hyperresonance, limited diaphragmatic movement, dullness, liver pushed downward	Diminished breath and voice sounds, diminished heart sounds, occasional adventitious sounds
Pleural effusion and/or thickening	Diminished chest wall movement and respiratory lag on affected side	Unilateral diminished chest wall movement or lag, cardiac apical pulse and trachea shifted away from affected side, diminished fremitus over affected area, tachycardia	Dull note over affected area	Diminished to absent breath sounds over affected area, bronchophony, whispered pectoriloquy, and egophony in area superior to effusion, occasional pleural rub
Pneumonia	Tachypnea, shallow breathing, occasional cyanosis, splinting and limited motion on affected side	Increased fremitus in presence of consolidation, decreased fremitus in presence of concomitant empysema or pleural effusion, tachycardia	Dullness if consolidation is large enough	A variety of crackles and occasional rhonchi, bronchial breath sounds, egophony, bronchophony, and whispered pectoriloquy
Pneumothorax	Tachypnea, cyanosis, respiratory distress, bulging intercostal spaces (if tension pneumothorax), respiratory lag on affected side, tracheal deviation away from affected side	Cardiac apical pulse, mediastinal and tracheal shift away from affected side, diminished to absent tactile fremitus over affected area, tachycardia	Hyperresonance	Diminished to absent breath sounds, succussion splash audible if air and fluid mix, sternal and precordial clicks and crackling if air underlies sternal area, diminished to absent voice sounds

Courtesy of Seidel HM, Ball JW, Dains JE, Benedict GW. Mosby's Guide to Physical Examination. *4th ed. St. Louis: Mosby-Yearbook; 1999:392–393.*

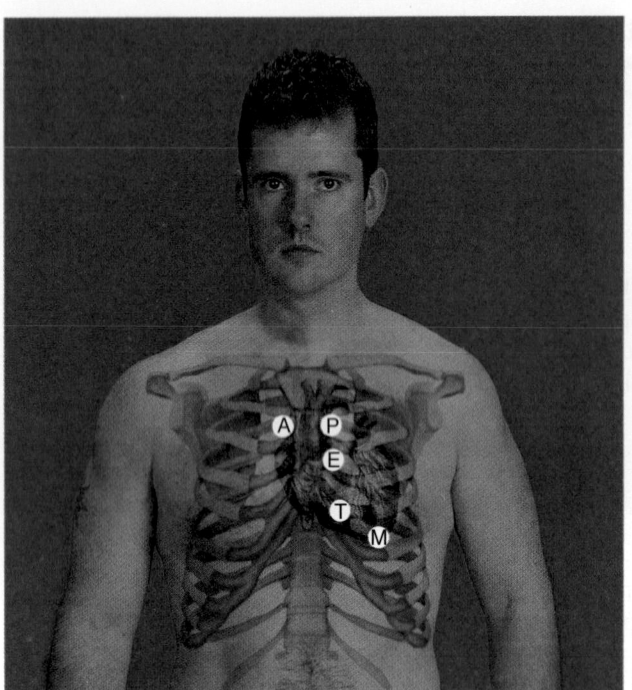

FIGURE 13-22 Cardiac landmarks: A = aortic area; P = pulmonic area; E = Erb's point; T = tricuspid area; M = mitral area.

Cardiovascular System. As with the respiratory system, the practitioner must know the underlying anatomy of the cardiovascular system before performing an examination. The heart lies between the lungs slightly on its side, with the right atrium inferior to the left atrium and the right ventricle anterior to the left ventricle. The apex of the heart consists of the ventricles and extends slightly downward and into the left chest almost to the midclavicular line. The base of the heart consists of both atria and lies beneath the body of the sternum. Figure 13-22 shows the anatomical position of the heart as well as the positions for auscultating the valves.

While inspecting and palpating the chest, the practitioner should also inspect and palpate the area around the heart. While inspecting the anterior chest, the practitioner, in some cases, is able to visualize the apical impulse in the left intercostal space between the fifth and sixth ribs near the midclavicular line. The *apical pulse*, the pulsation of the ventricles when they contract, can usually be palpated and is called the *point of maximal impulse (PMI)*. The PMI is difficult to assess on patients with emphysema because the increase in A-P diameter moves the apex of the heart away from the chest wall or, if it is felt at all, the PMI may shift inferiorly owing to the diaphragm's having a lower resting point. Shift of the PMI also occurs when the mediastinum is shifted because of some pulmonary problem. The closure of the pulmonic valve usually cannot be palpated; vibrations felt at the left sternal border between the second and third ribs suggest pulmonary hypertension.

After inspection and palpation of the chest, auscultation is performed. Auscultation of the heart requires that the practitioner understand and be able to identify normal heart sounds: S_1, E_j, and S_2.

- S_1, the first heart sound, is the closure of the mitral valve during systole and ventricular contraction. As the left ventricular pressure rises, it exceeds the afterload pressure in the aorta, and the aortic valve opens, accompanied by the early systolic ejection sound, or E_j.
- The second heart sound, S_2, is the sound of the aortic valve closing (also referred to as A_2), when the ventricles have finished contracting and the ventricular pressure drops below the aortic pressure. Normally, there is a long pause between S_2 and the next S_1, reflecting the diastole of the heart. During S_2, the pulmonic valve also closes, but this sound, referred to as P_2, is usually masked by the louder aortic valve sound. If right heart enlargement and pulmonary hypertension exist, the pressure closing the pulmonic valve may be enough to make it as loud as the aortic valve sound. This is referred to as a loud P_2 and is a common finding in cor pulmonale.

During inhalation, these two sounds sometimes separate slightly and become audible; this separation is called *splitting of the heart sounds*. The mitral valve opening is usually a silent event unless there is mitral stenosis or prolapse, in which case the practitioner might hear a snap right after S_2.

Two other sounds may be heard:

- A thrill-like sound that occurs after the opening of the mitral valve is the rapid filling of the ventricles. This sound, normal in children and young adults, is called the S_3 sound.
- The final sound, not usually heard in adults, is S_4, or atrial contraction.

Abnormal heart sounds, such as diastolic and systolic murmurs and gallop rhythms, can also be auscultated.

A **murmur** is caused by rapid blood flow across a normal valve, the backflow of blood through an unclosed valve, or blood flow through a stenotic valve. A murmur should be described by the practitioner according to its location, timing, shape, pitch, and intensity. Where the murmur is heard can indicate the *location* of the affected valve. For example, a mitral valve murmur is most likely to be heard at the fifth intercostal space at the left midclavicular line. *Timing* is the next part of a murmur to assess.

- If the murmur occurs between S_1 and S_2, it is a systolic murmur.
- If it occurs between S_2 and the next S_1, it is a diastolic murmur.

These types of murmurs can be further classified:

- A systolic murmur that is loudest in the middle of the S_1 and S_2, with breaks between the S sounds and the murmur, is referred to as a *midsystolic murmur*.
- If there are no gaps and the sound is constant, the murmur is referred to as a *pansystolic murmur*.
- A *late systolic murmur* occurs after the midpoint between S_1 and S_2 and persists up to S_2.
- *Diastolic murmurs* are either early, midway, or late depending on when they occur during S_2 and the next S_1.

The *shape* refers to the pattern of sound over time and can be:

- Crescendo (goes from soft to loud).
- Decrescendo (goes from loud to soft).
- Crescendo-decrescendo (louder in the middle).
- Plateau (has the same pattern throughout).

Pitch is whether the sound can be classified as high, medium, or low. It can be reported descriptively as blowing, harsh, rumbling, and musical.

Murmurs are also graded by *intensity*, with six grades of loudness from very faint to very loud. Table 13-12 gives the grades of murmur intensities.

A **gallop rhythm** is an abnormal heart sound with S_3, S_4, or both present. The sequence of sounds suggests the gallop of a horse. A gallop rhythm suggests ventricular distention during diastole as would occur after a myocardial infarction, ventricular disease, a left-to-right shunt, or ventricular failure.[8]

TABLE 13-12 **Grading heart murmurs**

Grade	Characteristics
I	Very faint; heard only after a period of concentration
II	Faint; heard immediately
III	Moderate intensity
IV	Loud; may be associated with a trill
V	Loud; stethoscope must remain in contact with the chest wall in order to hear; trill palpable
VI	Very loud; heard with stethoscope off of chest wall; trill palpable

Abdomen and Legs. The next segment of the physical examination is the abdomen and legs. With the patient in the supine position, the practitioner should inspect, palpate, and auscultate the abdomen for most of the abdominal examination.

- First inspect the abdomen for any scars, rashes, or lesions. Examine the contour of the abdomen for any distention, protrusions, or bulges. Observe the abdomen for normal aortic pulsations at the epigastrium.
- Next, palpate superficially for any tenderness, muscular resistance, and palpable masses. Perform deep palpation to delineate any masses and to assess tenderness.
- Finally, auscultate the abdomen, listening for active bowel sounds (clicks or gurgles occurring approximately 5–34 times per minute). If a patient has high blood pressure, *bruits*—vascular sounds that resemble a murmur—may be heard. Bruits in the upper quadrant and epigastrium may indicate renal artery stenosis.

Examine the legs, assessing the peripheral vascular system, the musculoskeletal system, and the neurological system.

- Note any swelling, discoloration, or ulcers.
- Palpate for edema, noting whether it is pitting or nonpitting edema. With *pitting edema*, when the practitioner gently pushes in on the skin, the indentation remains. In *nonpitting edema*, the skin returns to its previous shape, with no indentation.
- Palpate and evaluate the dorsalis pedis, posterior tibial, and femoral pulses.
- When examining the musculoskeletal system, note any joint enlargement or deformity, and check the range of motion if indicated.

Finally, examine the neurological system of the legs to ascertain any abnormal movements or neurological deficit. This examination has three components.

- Test the patellar and Achilles reflexes with a rubber hammer and note whether the reflexes are normal or deficient.
- Ascertain movement and the patient's ability to follow commands. Ask the patient to flex the foot up and down and wiggle the toes.
- Assess sensation by asking the patient to close his eyes. Then, touching the end of the rubber hammer to various points on the legs, have the patient indicate when he can feel touch. Assessing sensation also includes determining whether the patient can distinguish between a sharp and a dull stimulus. Most hammers have a tool on the end to perform this assessment. Do not use a safety pin or other object that can pierce the skin.

CASE STUDY 13-5

Mr. Smith consents to a physical examination. The practitioner (Jane Simons) asks him to remove his shirt and put on a gown. She leaves and comes back in a few minutes to find Mr. Smith still pacing about the room. He appears to be in generally good health, weighs 220 pounds, and is 6 feet 2 inches tall, with a generally stocky build. Mr. Smith exhibits good grooming and personal hygiene. He is frowning and looks a little anxious. His arms are crossed across his chest, and he is watching Ms. Simons closely.

The practitioner approaches Mr. Smith and explains that she wants to take his vital signs. Mr. Smith consents and sits down, but on the edge of his seat. The practitioner records the following vital signs:

Pulse	110
Respirations	25
Blood pressure	150/95
Temperature	37°C (aurally)

While taking Mr. Smith's vital signs, the practitioner notices the following. His pulse is strong but exhibits some pulsus paradoxus. Respirations are shallow, and there seems to be some obstruction to flow. Owing to the muscular chest wall, retractions are not observed.

A general examination of the face, extremities, and skin reveals no lesions, discoloration, clubbing, or injuries. There is some peripheral cyanosis, and capillary refill is about 5 seconds. There seems to be some bilateral weakness in his arms and grip.

Eyes, ears, nose, and throat are unremarkable.

Neck is supple, and the lymph nodes are of normal size. The trachea is midline, and there is no jugular venous distention.

The patient's chest is of normal configuration, and there are no spinal abnormalities. Chest expansion is bilaterally equal but seems less than normal. Vocal fremitus seems equal bilaterally. Percussion reveals slightly hyper-resonant tone bilaterally, and the posterior diaphragmatic excursion is less than 5 cm. Upon auscultation, the practitioner hears bilateral diminished breath sounds, as well as faint polyphonic wheezes during exhalation. Voice sounds are diminished but otherwise normal.

While inspecting and palpating the chest, the practitioner notices nothing remarkable about the cardiac system. Upon auscultation, the practitioner notes a grade II, medium-pitched, late-systolic plateau murmur. There are no other abnormal heart sounds.

The abdomen shows no rashes or lesions, and it seems normal to palpation, with no tenderness or guarding. Bowel sounds are normal, and there are no abnormal findings.

Examination of the legs reveals no swelling, discoloration, edema, or ulcers. The pedal pulses seem a little weak, and there is some peripheral cyanosis and temperature deficit of the feet. The legs seem to show a little bilateral neurological deficit.

Questions

1. Should the practitioner do anything before starting the physical examination after returning to the room?
2. How would the practitioner classify the vital signs?
3. What does the examination of the patient's extremities indicate to the practitioner?
4. What should the practitioner suspect after the examination of the chest and abdomen?
5. Why is this patient experiencing shortness of breath and chest pain?
6. Should any other questions be asked to help distinguish the diagnosis?

Documentation and the Medical Record

Whenever the practitioner comes into contact with a patient professionally, the results of the encounter must be documented. Documentation chronicles the patient's medical history from birth through death. Over the patient's lifetime, distinct episodes focus on the illness of that moment, such as an acute illness or injury; other episodes are less critical, such as routine physical examinations. Many practitioners contribute to this overall medical record, and each practitioner must recognize the importance of each record and make sure to document every encounter with the patient accurately and clearly. Each institution has its own method for recording medical documentation; however, the formal medical record must be documented accurately and kept confidential.

Age-Specific Competency

Physical Examination of the Child or Infant

Most of the techniques used to perform the adult examination are applicable to both infants and children. However, when performing a physical examination of a child or an infant, the practitioner should be aware of the need to alter the examination to meet the patient's special needs. Infants are the most difficult to examine because of their inability to follow directions or to keep still. The parent can be helpful in holding the infant and keeping his attention while the practitioner performs the examination. A unique approach to examining a child or an infant is to perform painful or distressing maneuvers out of sequence, at the end of the physical examination. Auscultating the lungs and heart should be done early, whereas examining the ears and mouth and palpating the abdomen should be done last. There may be some resistance to the examination, and the child may be crying or screaming during the exam. The practitioner should understand and not show anger or frustration but allow time for the child to adapt to the surroundings and the situation. Flexibility in the exam process and in the order of the physical exam is necessary to focus on what is important, particularly if the time for the examination is limited.

CONFIDENTIALITY

The patient's medical record, whether written or entered into a computer system, is a legal document indicating exactly what was done to the patient and what happened as a result. Patients expect this document to be kept confidential, and anyone not directly involved in their care should refrain from violating this confidence. Likewise, practitioners directly involved with the patient should ensure at all costs that the patient's right to privacy is respected. As stated in the Hippocratic Oath, "What I may see or hear in the course of treatment or even outside of treatment in regard to the life of men, which on no account must be noised abroad, I will keep to myself holding such things shameful to be spoken about." All health care practitioners are subject to the same ethical code. Table 13-13 details the fundamental elements of confidentiality. Failure to maintain confidentially violates the Health Insurance Portability and Accountability Act (HIPAA) of 1995 and may carry significant legal penalties. See Chapter 2.

TABLE 13-13 **Confidentiality**

1. Keep all client records secure.
2. Consider carefully the content to be entered into the record.
3. Release information only with the patient's written consent and full discussion of the information to be shared, except when release is required by law.
4. Use professional judgment deliberately regarding confidentiality when the client is a danger to self or others.
5. Use professional judgment deliberately when deciding how to maintain the confidentiality of a minor. The rights of the parent or guardian must also be considered.
6. Disguise clinical material when used professionally for teaching and writing.

LEGIBILITY

Everyone knows the jokes about physicians' handwriting. The problem is that illegible handwriting can result in medical errors and confusion concerning treatment. Likewise, if the medical record is used as a document in a legal matter, illegible handwriting can put the writer in jeopardy. When documenting anything in the medical record, take time to write the entry clearly to prevent any misunderstandings among practitioners.

Although abbreviations allow the practitioner to chart quickly, they can also lead to confusion. For the most part, avoid abbreviations if possible, or use only those approved by the institution (the list is usually maintained by the medical records department). Consult with medical records before writing any abbreviations in the patient's chart.

COMPUTERIZED MEDICAL RECORDS

To decrease the incidences of illegible handwriting and to facilitate access to medical records, many institutions have converted to a computerized system. Computerized medical records have many advantages.

- The record is always available wherever a computer terminal is available. Even if the patient is in one department for care, the medical record is available simultaneously to the practitioner treating the patient, to the doctor who is responsible for the patient, and to other practitioners who may need to see the patient at a later time, even if they are in different departments or even outside the institutional walls.

- The computerized medical record is legible and current because what is entered is immediately available and in printable form.
- Computer systems act as checklists for practitioners by providing a preplanned charting system that includes all the elements to be included in the record.
- Results of tests can be attached directly to the computerized patient record at the point of practice rather than being printed out and then placed on the paper chart later.
- Departments can list commonly used terms and then preprogram them into the computer. The terms can be accessed by a single key code, bar code, or touch screen.
- Finally, the record is complete, and no page is missing, as can happen with a paper chart.

Some of these advantages are also disadvantages.

- Because of instant access, people who understand computer systems could get unauthorized access to the patient record without too much trouble. Each institution tries to minimize this possibility by establishing security barriers. The most elementary barrier is the practitioner's password. However, in most institutions the number of people who need and who are legally authorized to access patient records is staggering. These people must remember and keep confidential their personal passwords. And, unless passwords are changed frequently, the possibility of someone else getting a practitioner's password increases, making the system vulnerable to breakins.
- Preprogramming commonly used terms increases charting compliance, but the quality of the charted notes may be less comprehensive than if the practitioners compose the notes themselves.
- Even though computer records work well, many institutions do not plan well enough for when the computer system malfunctions. Inevitably, systems fail. The practitioner should be thoroughly familiar with the paper back-up system to be used until the electronic system is restored. As computer systems become more complex and more comprehensive, the need to periodically review the back-up procedures becomes more acute. Also, at times, the system may not be available because of routine maintenance. At these times, the paper back-up system must be used for any of the tasks that the computer usually performs.

PROBLEM-ORIENTED MEDICAL RECORD

In the past, hospitals and other medical institutions organized the patient chart according to the **source-oriented charting method**. Each department or practitioner (source) had a separate section of the patient chart in which to record information. This method hindered communication among disciplines because each discipline had to read the entire chart to get a complete picture of the patient. Everything in the chart was organized in chronological order or, in some institutions, in reverse chronological order (i.e., the most recent note was first in each section). The source-oriented method made it difficult to treat the patient in the new multidisciplinary environment, and no two institutions used the same organizational structure.

Because of the need to standardize medical records, most institutions have adopted the **problem-oriented medical record (POMR)**. As medicine becomes more dependent on teamwork and a multidisciplinary approach to treating patients, the POMR system helps ensure accurate documentation. The POMR consists of the database, the problem list, the problem-related plans, flowcharts, and the progress notes.

Database. The practitioner should list all aspects of the health history and record the patient's answers to the questions as well as the practitioner's observations. All negatives should also be recorded to indicate that they are negatives and that they were not overlooked. If the practitioner who takes the first history does a complete job, it does not have to be redone each time the patient is seen. The next practitioner just has to confirm aspects of the history and then "fill in" the time since the last history. The physical examination also should be recorded accurately by the practitioner performing it. With an accurate and complete history and physical, the practitioner can construct a complete problem list on the patient.

Problem List. The problem list is the fundamental part of the POMR. After taking the history and performing the physical exam, the practitioner should list all the problems that were uncovered. This initial master problem list is placed in the front of the chart. As another problem is discovered or a problem is solved, it is either added to or deleted from the list. Each problem is listed in order of importance or acuity, with the date it was entered on the list, not the date the patient first discovered it. In time, the problem list is divided into two categories: *active problems*, which require action, and *inactive problems*, which do not require action but may be important for other practitioners to know. The problems can be established diagnoses, physical signs and symptoms, laboratory tests, areas uncovered during the history, or special risk factors.

Next to the problem list, a differential diagnosis list should be established. As each problem is investigated and the diagnosis is refined, the list includes monitor or treatment lists to indicate how the problem is being handled.

CASE STUDY 13-6

The following documentation includes information gathered from follow-ups suggested by questions in preceding case studies.

Patient History:

Date: 12/17/11 1900 hours
William Smith, 35-year-old male, married
Address: 1 Main St., Morris Plains, NJ
DOB: 10/2/76
Sheet metal factory worker
Source of history: Patient
Chief complaints: (1) Shortness of breath, (2) chest pain, (3) weakness of extremities

History of the Present Illness:

1. Shortness of breath: Started 2–3 weeks ago and is getting worse. Now has trouble walking up stairs. Shortness of breath worse at end of workweek, better by end of weekend. Also can occur after eating.
2. Chest pain: Noticed for the last 3 weeks. Nonradiating pressure to center of the chest getting worse over the 3-week period. Pressing-type pain. Associated with the shortness of breath.
3. Weakness of the extremities: Noticed by patient for the last 3 days. Associated with weakness of grip and in legs.

Patient had episode today that brought him to the clinic. Episode involved not being able to walk up one flight of stairs without resting. Shortness of breath, chest pain, and weakness seemed worse at time, getting better since leaving work area.

Past Health History:

Patient feels he is in general good health, with some recent problems with breathing, chest pain, and weakness.

Childhood illnesses: Patient remembers having chickenpox, measles, and mumps as a child. No history of diphtheria, whooping cough.

Childhood immunizations: Remembers having "the usual shots." Salk vaccine for polio. No adverse reactions.

Adult illnesses: No past history of adult illnesses. *Flulike symptoms* for 3 months subsided about 2 weeks ago.

Psychiatric illnesses: No history of psychiatric problems

Injuries: Small cut to hand by knife 3 years ago

Blood transfusions: No transfusions

Surgical history: Tonsillectomy, 1981

Hospitalizations: No other hospitalizations

Current Health Status:

Current medications: Aspirin and cold medicines

Allergies: Allergy to mold, pollen, dust, and grass as child; treated with desensitizing shots until age of 12; shots discontinued because symptoms stopped

Tobacco use: 40-pack-year history—*still smoking*

Alcohol/drug use: 2–3 beers per day, no other substance abuse

Diet: No restrictions. Diet is high fat and patient does not restrict intake of salt.

Screening tests: None remembered

Immunization status: Tetanus 3 years ago

Sleep habits: Normal with no nocturnal dyspnea

Exercise/leisure: Relatively sedentary lifestyle with no regular exercise program; never traveled abroad

Environmental hazards: Work hazards of *fumes and metal dust*; at home, some paint fumes

Safety measures: Patient uses seatbelt.

Family History:

Father: 60, alive (bypass surgery 2005)

Mother: 58, alive (MI, 2006)

Wife: 35, alive and well

Son: 7, alive (asthma)

No brothers or sisters. Grandparents deceased, causes unknown

No family history of TB

Social History:

A 35-year-old sheet metal factory worker who recently moved to a smaller work area where metal is being cut with torches. Exposed to fumes and metal dust in poorly ventilated room. Married to housewife who also works at home as a freelance sign painter. Father of one 7-year-old boy who was diagnosed 3 years ago as having asthma. Live together in house in suburbs with large lawn. One dog, which is usually kept outside.

(continues)

Educational History:

The patient has a high school diploma and 1 year of community college. Mother has 2 years of college. Father dropped out of high school after grade 11 but plans to complete GED and start community college part time.

Systems Review:

General: No weight change, appetite normal, flulike symptoms for over 3 months

Psychological: No indication of illness

Integumentary system: No rashes or lesions, no varicose veins, no edema or swelling, some *peripheral cyanosis*

Eyes: Normal vision

Ears: Hearing good with no tinnitus, vertigo, or infections

Runny nose sometimes yellow mucus; some nosebleeds with blowing of nose. Some *postnasal drip* noticed.

Mouth: Normal; last dentist visit over 3 years ago

Throat/Neck: No lumps, goiter, or pain

Respiratory system: Progressively worsening *shortness of breath. Morning cough* with small amounts of thick white sputum. No hemoptysis. *Exertional dyspnea* and some shortness of breath after eating.

Cardiovascular system: Nonradiating *chest pain* associated with shortness of breath; no orthopnea, palpations, edema, or nocturnal dyspnea; some exertional dyspnea

Breasts: No dimplings on inspection; no pain, tenderness, or lumps on palpation

Gastrointestinal system: Good appetite; no nausea, vomiting, indigestion; bowel movements normal about once daily; no diarrhea or bleeding; no pain, jaundice, gallbladder, or liver trouble

Urinary system: No dysuria, hematuria, or nocturia

Musculoskeletal system: No back pain or joint pain

Neurological system: Some *poor balance* and *weakness of grip*; no fainting, seizures, or trouble swallowing; memory good; *headaches* associated with workplace; no head injuries

Endocrine system: No known thyroid problems, temperature intolerance; sweating average; no symptoms or history of diabetes

Physical Examination:

General appearance: Mr. Smith is a tall, stocky male who walks and moves easily. He responds to questions quickly but seems agitated and anxious. His appearance is well groomed and neat. His color is good, and he sits and lies without discomfort. When answering questions, shows some trouble breathing, with some use of accessory muscles. Breathlessness seems to increase agitation.

Vital signs: Pulse: 110 regular with some *paradoxical pulse*

Respirations: 25/min and shallow

BP: 150/95 right arm lying down; no appreciable difference in left arm

Temperature: 37°C (aurally)

Skin: Palms cool and dry; normal color and texture; no visible lesions; some peripheral cyanosis and prolonged capillary refill; no clubbing; some temperature deficit in fingers; some cyanosis with no edema or varicose veins; no calf tenderness; feet cool to touch; scattered superficial burn scars on hands and lower arms

Head: Hair, scalp, skull, and face appear normal.

Eyes: Vision 20/20 in each eye; no contact lenses or eyeglasses; field of vision full by confrontation; PERRLA; extraocular movement intact

Ears: Ear canals clear, and drums intact; acuity good to whispered voice

Nose: Nose intact, mucosa slightly inflamed, septum midline; some sinus tenderness

Mouth: Lips and mucosa pink, some irritation noted in back of throat; teeth in good repair; tongue midline; tonsils absent

Neck: Supple, with no lymphadenopathy; trachea midline; no JVD

Chest: Normal configuration, and no spinal abnormalities; no masses palpated; decreased bilateral chest expansion; hyper-resonant percussion note bilaterally, with decreased diaphragmatic excursion; diminished breath sounds bilaterally, with faint bilateral polyphonic wheezes on exhalation; diminished bilateral voice sounds

Cardiovascular system: Good carotid pulses; no S_3 or S_4; grade II/VI medium-pitched late systolic plateau *murmur* at 2nd right interspace—does not radiate to the neck; diastole clear; apical impulse absent due to muscular chest.

Abdomen: No rashes or lesions; slightly enlarged but normal to palpations and percussion; normal bowel sounds; liver normal span but displaced inferiorly; no bruits noted

Pulses:

	Radial	Femoral	Popliteal	Dorsalis Pedis	Posterior Tibial
RT	N(paradoxical)	N	↓	↓	↓
LT	N(paradoxical)	N	↓	↓	↓

Musculoskeletal system: No deformities, no swollen or tender joints; good range of motion in hands, wrist, elbows, shoulders, spine

Neurological system: Mental status: tense, agitated, alert, and anxious but cooperative; thought coherent; oriented ×3; cognitive testing not done; cranial nerves intact.

Motor: Some flaccidity noted in extremities; muscle strength rated 4/5; some weakness of grip; gait normal with some hesitation and unsteadiness

Sensory: Intact; reflexes: 2+, no ptosis

Problem List

Date Problem Entered	No.	Active Problem	Inactive Problem
12/17/11	1	Shortness of breath	
12/17/11	2	Chest pain	
12/17/11	3	Weakness of extremities	
12/17/11	4	Exertional dyspnea	
12/17/11	5	Grade II murmur	
12/17/11	6	Morning cough	
12/17/11	7	Headaches	
12/17/11	8	Runny nose	
12/17/11	9	Peripheral cyanosis	
12/17/11	10	Flulike symptoms	
12/17/11	11	Paradoxical pulses	
12/17/11	12	Allergies	
12/17/11	13	Smoking	
12/17/11	14	Possible high blood pressure	
12/17/11	15	Environmental hazards	
12/17/11	16	Diet high in calories, fat, and salt	
12/17/11	17	Sedentary lifestyle	

(continues)

Patient Record Note [in part]:

Diagnosis: Asthma

Assessment: Supporting this diagnosis are tachypnea, shallow respirations, paradoxical pulses, hyper-resonant lung percussion note bilaterally, bilateral inferior diaphragm placement, and decreased diaphragmatic exertion, polyphonic wheezes bilaterally, childhood history of allergies, nonradiating pressing pressure in middle of chest, use of accessory muscles, and bilateral diminished breath and voice sounds. Possible occupational asthma evidenced by timing of incidents.

Plan: Diagnostic: Pre- and postbedside spirometry if possible, pre- and postpeak flow measurement. Eosinophil count. Chest X-ray. Schedule for full pulmonary workup with pulmonary function testing and possible bronchial challenge testing and/or allergy testing. *Therapeutic:* Inhaled bronchodilator treatment now and continue until peak flows improve. *Education:* Discuss nature of asthma, need for avoidance of environmental hazards, need for smoking cessation.

Questions

1. Does any aspect of the documentation need to be expanded?
2. Write an assessment and plan for the problems in the problem list that were not covered in the asthma notes.
3. In your opinion, can this patient be sent home, or should he be admitted? Explain your reasoning.

Initial Problem-Related Plan. As each initial problem is listed, a problem-related plan is developed. The plan includes any diagnostic tests needed, any monitoring tests needed, what treatments are being prescribed, and what education is necessary for the patient and family. Each problem must have a plan, even if it is a simple plan such as "monitor patient until other signs or symptoms occur." The plan is updated with each updated problem list. Once a disease or condition has been resolved and moved to the inactive list, an arrow is used to indicate the observations showing that the disease or condition has been resolved and what follow-up may be needed.

Flowcharts. The POMR lends itself naturally to flowcharts to show the patient's progress. Clinical, diagnostic, and monitoring tests and observations are often done and repeated during the course of an illness. A flow sheet is a convenient way to keep a record of these tests, and the flowchart makes it easy for the practitioner to determine trends in the values of the various tests. A perfect example is the vital signs flowchart that most hospitals use for each patient. As the practitioner takes the vital signs, the numbers are recorded on a sheet, accompanied in most cases with a graphic display. At a glance, every practitioner who comes into contact with the patient can assess quickly the latest vital signs and whether the patient is stable, getting better, or getting worse.

Progress Notes. The progress notes record the day-to-day progress of the patient. Each practitioner should make a progress note every time she interacts with the patient. The note should be brief and succinct, and it should focus on what was performed or on the change being documented. The progress note should follow the **SOAP** method of documentation: subjective, objective, assessment, and plan.

- The *subjective* part of the progress notes should indicate (in the patient's own words when possible) what the patient is feeling or the problem the patient is expressing.
- The *objective* part of the note records any physical signs, diagnostic or clinical tests, and physical findings that may result from a treatment or changes that may affect the problem list and plan for the patient.
- The *assessment* should include whether the practitioner feels that the subjective and objective data confirm the plan or alter it according to assessment of the data.
- Finally, the *plan* indicates what the practitioner will do after making the assessment. Any modification to the problem list and plan for the patient should be documented here and on the problem list as well.

PATHWAYS

Medicine, particularly the large health maintenance organization (HMO), has embraced the use of clinical or critical pathways as a way to standardize treatment across the United States. *Pathways* are interdisciplinary flowcharts that show what tests, treatments, counseling, and interventions should be done to a typical patient with a certain diagnosis. They are "plans of care that outline the optimal sequencing and timing of interventions for patients with a particular diagnosis, procedure, or symptoms."[11] All pathways should contain four aspects: patient outcomes, a timeline for the pathway, collaboration among disciplines, and comprehensive care of the patient. Pathways sequence naturally into case management of diseases because of a standardized plan for the disease management.

CARE PLANS OR PROTOCOLS

Care plans are the disciplinary part of the pathways. Based on an accepted standard of care, care plans sequence the patient's treatment, based on the problem list. Every problem listed in the active part of the problem list usually has an initial care plan to address the problem. Most care plans or protocols are patient driven in that the patient's signs and symptoms generate the sequencing of the care plan.

LEGAL REQUIREMENTS

No discussion of medical records would be complete without a discussion of the legal issues involving the records. Medical records are legal documents and frequently requested by attorneys representing patients or their survivors to serve as evidence in malpractice cases, real or perceived. What is in the record or not in the record is often a key element in the legal processes during medical malpractice, workers' compensation, and personal injury cases. RTs must record completely their actions and patient outcomes to all therapy interventions. Recording vital signs before and after therapy, recording ventilator settings before and after making adjustments, and noting patent conditions before and after treatments are all important parts of patient care. The medical-legal axiom is, "If it isn't recorded, it wasn't done." The corollary is, "If it was done, it should be recorded."

Experience tells us that respiratory therapists are increasingly being named in lawsuits as defendants in medical malpractice cases. These cases include hospital, long-term care sites, and home care practice. Therapists are being held responsible for their actions, their misactions, and their inactions. The importance of a complete and accurate medical record cannot be overstated. RTs may be asked to remember that patient they took care of three years ago on Wednesday the twenty-third at 6:50 p.m. Odds are they will not be able to cite the activities and actions they took with any degree of clarity, unless the medical record is complete and accurate. Therapists may not assume that someone else will record their activity.

Summary

A health care professional must act like a detective to determine what is wrong with a patient. Thorough questioning and an in-depth examination of the patient should reveal any medical problems. In most cases, an extensive history and physical exam decreases the need for invasive testing and accurately indicates what tests are necessary. Also, as respiratory therapists are called on to do more and more, the ability to perform a complete history and physical may help the practitioner perform in alternative sites.

Once information has been gathered, the ability to share it with other health care providers is essential for a seamless continuum of care. Documentation must be done in a way that facilitates the dissemination of information. Clear, concise, complete documentation is the key to multidisciplinary care of the patient.

Study Questions

REVIEW QUESTIONS

1. Why is clear and complete understanding needed during a patient interview?
2. What are the general guidelines and techniques for interviewing a patient?
3. What are the basic areas covered in the patient history of an adult patient?
4. What are the areas covered in the review of systems of an adult patient?
5. Why is it necessary to perform inspection, palpation, percussion, and auscultation on a patient?
6. What are the vital signs collected on an adult?
7. Why is confidentiality necessary when dealing with patient data?
8. What is the basic structure of a problem-oriented medical record?

MULTIPLE-CHOICE QUESTIONS

1. Recognition is usually established in which of the following?
   a. general space
   b. social space
   c. personal space
   d. intimate space
2. The interview is usually performed in which of the following?
   a. general space
   b. social space
   c. personal space
   d. intimate space
3. Most of the physical examination must be performed in which of the following?
   a. general space
   b. social space
   c. personal space
   d. intimate space

4. To elicit a free flow of information, the interviewer should use which of the following?
   a. open-ended questions
   b. direct questions
   c. closed questions
   d. surveying
5. To focus the patient on specific information, the interviewer should use which of the following?
   a. open-ended questions
   b. direct questions
   c. closed questions
   d. surveying
6. To pinpoint a specific piece of information, the interviewer should use which of the following?
   a. open-ended questions
   b. direct questions
   c. closed questions
   d. surveying
7. To ensure that all information has been collected, the interviewer should use which of the following at the end of each set of questions?
   a. open-ended questions
   b. direct questions
   c. closed questions
   d. surveying
8. Which of the following are nonverbal active listening techniques?
   I. taking notes
   II. maintaining eye contact
   III. listening to how the patient is speaking rather than to what is being said
   IV. using supportive gestures to indicate understanding and support
   a. I, II, III, and IV
   b. I, III, and IV only
   c. I, II, and III only
   d. I, II, and IV only
9. Which of the following are verbal active listening techniques?
   I. keeping your voice tones neutral
   II. accepting vague and incomplete statements
   III. using checking statements to summarize what is being said
   IV. using facilitating statements such as "Go on"
   a. I, II, III, and IV
   b. I, III, and IV only
   c. I, II, and III only
   d. I, II, and IV only
10. Which of the following is *not* part of the history of the present illness?
   a. location
   b. quality
   c. age
   d. timing
11. When the practitioner is checking the past health history, which of the following is *not* included?
   a. tobacco use
   b. medical problems
   c. accidents or injuries
   d. childhood illnesses
12. When performing a review of the systems, the practitioner should begin with:
   a. questions concerning the head.
   b. questions concerning the eyes, ears, nose, and throat.
   c. questions concerning the skin.
   d. questions concerning general health.
13. Some of the barriers to communication include which of the following?
   I. emotions
   II. language problems
   III. cultural differences
   IV. personality disorders
   a. I, II, III, and IV
   b. I, III, and IV only
   c. I, II, and III only
   d. I, II, and IV only
14. Which of the following are required to perform a physical exam?
   I. privacy
   II. soft dim lighting
   III. comfortable temperature
   IV. no interruptions
   a. I, II, III, and IV
   b. I, III, and IV only
   c. I, II, and III only
   d. I, II, and IV only
15. According to the Glasgow Coma Scale, a score of 3 is considered
   a. obtunded.
   b. confused.
   c. coma.
   d. normal.
16. Which of the following pulse patterns are associated with decreased compliance of the aortic wall?
   a. weak pulse
   b. bounding pulse
   c. pulses alternans
   d. paradoxical pulse
17. Which of the following pulse patterns are associated with obstructive lung disease?
   a. weak pulse
   b. bounding pulse
   c. pulses alternans
   d. paradoxical pulse

18. Which of the following pulse patterns are associated with left ventricular failure?
    a. weak pulse
    b. bounding pulse
    c. pulses alternans
    d. paradoxical pulse
19. Which of the following is the range for child's a normal pulse rate?
    a. 130–160
    b. 80–120
    c. 60–80
    d. 40–60
20. Which of the following is considered bradycardia for an adult?
    a. 130–160
    b. 80–120
    c. 60–80
    d. 40–60
21. Which range of respiratory rates is considered normal for a newborn?
    a. 30–60
    b. 18–30
    c. 12–20
    d. 80–120
22. With age, the blood pressure normally
    a. decreases.
    b. increases.
    c. stays the same.
    d. decreases and then increases.
23. Which of the following breathing patterns is associated with asthma?
    a. Kussmaul
    b. ataxia
    c. biots
    d. obstructive
24. Which of the following breathing patterns is associated with increased intracranial pressure?
    a. Kussmaul
    b. ataxia
    c. biots
    d. obstructive
25. Which of the following breathing patterns is associated with diaphragmatic fatigue?
    a. retractions
    b. abdominal paradox
    c. ataxia
    d. orthopnea
26. Which of the following breathing patterns is associated with respiratory depression?
    a. retractions
    b. abdominal paradox
    c. ataxia
    d. orthopnea
27. Which grade of murmur is considered quiet but can be heard immediately after placing the stethoscope on the chest?
    a. grade II
    b. grade III
    c. grade IV
    d. grade VI
28. Which of the following are considered part of confidentiality?
    I. All records should be kept secure.
    II. Information can be released with verbal consent.
    III. A practitioner should consider carefully what is to be entered into the record.
    IV. Material should be disguised if used for teaching and writing.
    a. I, II, III, and IV
    b. I, III, and IV only
    c. I, II, and III only
    d. I, II, and IV only
29. Which of the following is *not* an aspect of problem-oriented medical record keeping?
    a. the problem list of all past and present patient problems
    b. the database of all findings, both positive and negative, of the history and physical exam
    c. a subjective statement of the patient's illness in the patient's own words
    d. flowcharts that show the progress of the patient

CRITICAL-THINKING QUESTIONS

1. What could hinder a practitioner from gathering adequate information from a patient?
2. Why is it necessary for a respiratory therapist to understand the entire history and physical exam rather than concentrating only on the respiratory history and physical exam?
3. Where in the entire process of dealing with the patient could confidentiality be compromised? How would you go about preventing the loss of confidentiality?

References

1. Cohen-Cole SA. *The Medical Interview: The Three-Function Approach*. 2nd ed. St. Louis, MO: Mosby-Yearbook; 2000.
2. Wilkins RL. Preparing for the patient encounter. In: Wilkins RL, Krider SJ, Sheldon RL, eds. *Clinical Assessment in Respiratory Care*. 6th ed. St. Louis, MO: Mosby-Yearbook; 2009.

3. Purtilo R, Haddad A. *Health Professional and Patient Interaction*. 7th ed. Philadelphia: WB Saunders Co; 2007.
4. Bickley LS. *Bates' Pocket Guide to Physical Examination and History Taking*. 6th ed. Philadelphia: JB Lippincott Co; 2009.
5. Tamparo CD, Lindh WQ. *Therapeutic Communications for Health Professionals*. 3rd. ed. Clifton Park, NY: Delmar Cengage Learning; 2007.
6. Wilkins RL, Hodgkin JE. History and physical examination of the respiratory patient. In: Burton GG, Hodgkin JE, Ward JJ, eds. *Respiratory Care: A Guide to Clinical Practice*. 4th ed. Philadelphia: JB Lippincott Co; 1997.
7. Seidel HM, Ball JW, Dains JE, Benedict GW. *Mosby's Guide to Physical Examination*. 7th ed. St. Louis, MO: Mosby-Yearbook; 2010.
8. Wilkins RL. Physical examination of the patient with cardiopulmonary disease. In: Wilkins RL, Krider SJ, Sheldon RL, eds. *Clinical Assessment in Respiratory Care*. 6th ed. St. Louis, MO: Mosby-Yearbook; 2009.
9. Krider SJ. Vital signs. In: Wilkins RL, Krider SJ, Sheldon RL, eds. *Clinical Assessment in Respiratory Care*. 6th ed. St. Louis, MO: Mosby-Yearbook; 2009.
10. Estes MEZ. *Health Assessment & Physical Examination*. 3rd ed. Clifton Park; NY: Delmar Cengage Learning; 2006.
11. Ignatavicus DD, Hausman KA. *Clinical Pathways for Collaborative Practice*. Philadelphia: WB Saunders Co; 1995:10.

Suggested Reading

Chan PD, Winkle PJ. *History and Physical Examination in Medicine*. 10th ed. Laguna Hills, CA: Current Clinical Strategies Publishing; 2002.

Edge RS, Groves JR. *Ethics of Health Care: A Guide for Clinical Practice*. 3rd. ed. Clifton Park, NY: Delmar Cengage Learning; 2005.

Epstein O, Perkin GD, de Bono DP, Cookson J. *Clinical Examination*. 4th ed. London: Mosby-Yearbook Europe; 2008.

Lindh WQ, Pooler MS, Tamparo CD, Cerrato JU, eds. *Clinical Medical Assisting*. 4th ed. Clifton Park, NY: Delmar Cengage Learning; 2010.

Swartz MH. *Pocket Companion to Textbook of Physical Diagnosis*. 3rd. ed. Philadelphia: WB Saunders Co; 1998.

CHAPTER 14

Radiology for the Respiratory Therapist

Glendon G. Cox and Paul J. Mathews

OBJECTIVES

Upon completion of this chapter, the reader should be able to:

- Discuss why a respiratory therapist should be able to identify major abnormalities on chest radiographs.
- List the various types of radiological studies.
- Discuss the rationale for ordering specific radiological studies.
- Explain the principles of various radiological studies.
- Differentiate between a regular and a portable chest X-ray.
- Describe a sequence for systematically reviewing a chest radiograph.
- Discuss the diagnostic values of various types of radiographic studies.
- Given a list of conditions, select the appropriate studies for their evaluation and justify the choices.
- Identify common abnormalities on a chest film.

CHAPTER OUTLINE

(continues)

(continued)

Alveolar (Air-Space) Infiltrates and Air Bronchograms
Lobar Atelectasis
Lung Cancer
Tuberculosis
Congestive Heart Failure, Pulmonary Edema, and Pleural Effusion
Pneumothorax
Tension Pneumothorax
Pneumoperitoneum
Aortic Aneurysm, Aortic Dissection, and Traumatic Aortic Injuries
Pulmonary Thromboembolism
Adult Respiratory Distress Syndrome

Device Positioning
Endotracheal Tubes
Swan-Ganz Catheters
Nasogastric Tubes and Feeding Tubes
Chest Tubes
Aortic Balloon Pumps

Internal Cardiac Pacemakers and Defibrillators

Chest Trauma
Flail Chest
Subcutaneous Emphysema
Penetrating Chest Wounds
Foreign Body

KEY TERMS

air bronchogram
angiogram
arteriography
atelectasis
barotrauma
bullae
computerized (axial) tomography
contrast
Doppler sonography
echocardiography
flail chest
fluoroscopy
hemothorax
hot-lighting
lateral decubitus
magnetic resonance imaging (MRI)
positron emission tomography (PET)
radiodensity
radiograph
radiology
radiopaque
subcutaneous emphysema
Swan-Ganz catheter
transducer
ultrasound
ventilation/perfusion ($\dot{V}/\dot{Q}$) scan

Respiratory therapists can enhance their contribution to the care of their patients and their value to the clinical care team if they have a basic knowledge of chest radiology. **Radiology** is the use of X-rays and other forms of energy to generate images of the internal structures of the chest in the diagnosis and treatment of disease). Almost all hospital patients requiring an evaluation of their pulmonary function or treatment for pulmonary disease or whose care involves services by respiratory therapy undergo diagnostic imaging studies. Such studies are ordered because they allow the treating physician or the respiratory therapist to learn things about patients' internal structure and function that are not readily available through observation, physical examination, history taking, or laboratory testing. Even a tool as important as breath sounds has significant limitations in diagnosing the cause of a patient's cardiopulmonary complaints. In many cases, lungs really are simply better seen than heard.

Why Should a Respiratory Therapist Learn Radiology?

A respiratory therapist should learn some basic radiology to develop the ability to:

- Get information not available by physical examination.
- Identify conditions that require respiratory care or emergent treatment.
- Assess a patient's response to respiratory care.
- Identify complications of respiratory care.

- Conduct a preliminary assessment of radiographs when radiologists and physicians are not available.
- Confirm proper positioning of devices, tubes, and monitor leads.

Radiological studies of the chest, typically chest **radiographs**, are often the primary means by which physicians and therapists identify the diseases or processes that are responsible for a patient's shortness of breath or chest pain. These diseases range from conditions that are relatively easy to manage, such as atelectasis, to more severe, sometimes life-threatening conditions, such as pneumonia, adult respiratory distress, or tension pneumothorax. Radiographs can be used in judging the response to a variety of medical and surgical treatments, including responses to antibiotics, diuretics, therapeutic bronchoscopy, and chest tube or artificial airway placement. Chest radiographs are used to screen for complications of respiratory care procedures including **barotrauma** (damage caused by excessive pressure during mechanical ventilation), misplaced lines and tubes, or volume loss (**atelectasis**, or airlessness of a pulmonary segment, a lobe, or an entire lung).

A respiratory therapist (RT) should have some basic skills in analyzing radiographs because many studies are done and available for review only when the radiologist or treating physician is at another hospital, at home, or otherwise unavailable. A respiratory therapist who can identify a pneumothorax or a misplaced endotracheal tube before the physician makes rounds or the radiologist interprets a study can, by notifying appropriate personnel, prevent complications and in some cases save a life.

Today's "X-rays" are more likely to be viewed and stored in a digital format or as digitalized images rather than as films. In fact, the images in this chapter are mostly from digital sources. However, the term "film" is still used because it is a useful cognitive aid for learners and because films still exist and are still frequently encountered when comparisons to older imaging studies are required. With increased use of digital radiography, physicians with appropriately designed computer systems have access to the results of radiographic studies in their offices or at their homes 24 hours a day. As *teleradiology*, the interpretation of medical imaging studies at sites remote from the hospital or imaging facility, evolves and expands, remote reading and analysis of radiographic images, especially images that require subspecialty expertise, will become commonplace. Respiratory therapists who are trained to insert or maintain artificial airways or to manage pulmonary artery or umbilical catheters can help prevent complications of these therapeutic interventions by learning how to verify the proper placement of these devices using chest radiographs.

How Can This Knowledge Be Gained?

Reading this chapter is the first step toward becoming comfortable viewing and doing basic analysis of chest radiographs. The key to becoming proficient, however, is practice. The more radiographic studies respiratory therapists look at and analyze, the better they become at distinguishing what is normal from what is not and the more conditions they learn to recognize. Respiratory therapists should make a habit of examining as many radiographic studies as possible. Examining radiographs is easy to do in intensive care areas, which often have display systems or digital access to the complete image files of all of the patients in the unit. Increasingly, the review of radiographs of any inpatient and most outpatients can also be accomplished either at specialized display consoles or on appropriately configured personal computers. Also, a number of Web-based resources that are dedicated to chest radiology and imaging can be accessed by a simple Internet search. These sites are invaluable as learning tools for even the most seasoned respiratory therapist.

In addition to viewing and studying radiographs, the RT should take advantage of every opportunity to draw information from others who have more experience and knowledge and who can explain and point out findings. A respiratory therapist who works in a teaching hospital should try to attend the daily X-ray rounds with the attending physicians or radiologists. Asking the attending or covering physician to discuss a film is an excellent way to build rapport with the physician and simultaneously to build expertise in this important skill. In a short time, quite a bit of proficiency can be gained in this way. Respiratory therapists who work in non-teaching hospitals should approach staff physicians, the medical director, the emergency room doctors, and on-call radiologist about teaching them the fundamental skills. Remember that physicians learn by teaching other physicians and medical students. They are often happy to pass on their knowledge.

Body Planes and Directional Terminology

To ensure accurate communications and the reproducibility of imaging studies, clinicians must use common frames of reference with regard to anatomic positions and projections. Locations of structures are often referred to in relation to the body surface. For example:

- A structure close to the surface is said to be *superficial* to structures or organs lying farther from the skin surface. Obviously, structures lying farther from the body surface are referred to as *deep*. Using this convention, the muscles of the chest wall are deep to the skin and subcutaneous fat layers.
- The front of the body is referred to as *anterior* or *ventral*, and the back of the body is *posterior* or *dorsal*.
- The right and left sides of the patient's body are *right lateral* and *left lateral*, respectively.
- Locations of structures or body parts can also be referred to in terms of their relationships to the body's *center of mass*. Structures located farther away from the central mass than an arbitrary reference point or landmark are said to be *distal* to that landmark, and structures that are nearer the center of mass are *proximal*. For example, the wrist is distal to the elbow, and the hip is proximal to the knee.
- Another frame of reference identifies the relative position of two structures in relation to the midline of the body. A structure located farther from the midline than an arbitrary landmark is said to be *lateral* to the landmark, and a second structure located closer to the midline is said to be *medial*. In the standard anatomic projection, with the palms facing forward, the thumbs are lateral to the little fingers, and the little fingers are medial to the thumbs.
- Finally, the relative locations of landmarks may be specified in terms of their relationships to the head or tail (in Latin, *cauda* is the word for "tail") or feet (in the case of tail-less humans). If you were to draw a line starting from the top of the sternum to the pubis, the direction that you would move your pen would be *craniocaudal*—from the head, toward the tail or feet.

Many modern imaging systems produce cross-sectional images of the body. The *planes of section* are described in relation to three primary, orthogonal (mutually perpendicular) planes:

- The *sagittal plane* lies in the midline of the body and divides its right and left sides. The sagittal suture of the skull takes its name from the sagittal plane.
- The *coronal plane* is perpendicular to the sagittal plane and divides the body into anterior and posterior portions. The coronal suture that separates the frontal and parietal bones of the skill lies in the coronal plane.

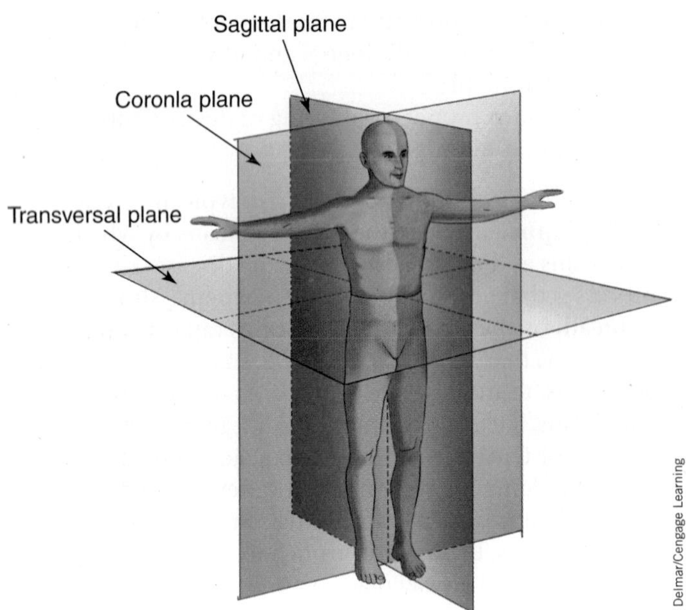

FIGURE 14-1 The three primary planes of the body.

- The *transverse* (or *axial*) plane divides the body into cranial and caudal portions. In a standing human, the transverse plane is parallel to the ground.

Figure 14-1 illustrates these three primary planes of reference. Each primary anatomic plane defines an infinite set of parallel planes along which the body can be imaged. More generally, the transverse, or axial, plane is perpendicular to the longitudinal, craniocaudal axis. Any sectional set of images is described based on the primary anatomic plane to which the planes of section of the images are parallel. For example, many of the computerized tomography (CT) images generated by examinations of the chest and abdomen are in planes perpendicular to the longitudinal axis of the body, parallel to the primary transverse plane; they are referred to as *axial images*. In fact, early CT scanners could generate only images in transverse, hence an obsolete term for CT scanning was *computerized axial tomography*, or CAT.

The use of standard terminology is essential in describing the exact position or direction of the organs and anatomic structures, medical instrumentation and implants, or foreign objects that may be found in the body. The terminology is also necessary to ensure accurate communication between physicians and radiologic technologists in prescribing examinations and positioning patients.

In radiology, as in many areas of life, the need for the rapid and accurate transmission of data has led to the adoption of specialized terms, abbreviations, and nicknames for procedures. For example, a chest

Best Practice

Use of Abbreviations

The use of abbreviations may confuse communications because many abbreviations have several meanings. For example, PA can refer either to a posterior-anterior radiographic projection (the direction of the X-ray beam as it passes through the body) or to the pulmonary artery. Abbreviations are often specific to a discipline, with the same abbreviation having different meanings in different fields of practice. Even when used in context, these phrases and others like them can be confusing. Consequently, current best practices and accreditation criteria require that the use of abbreviations in communications be restricted or eliminated.

radiograph may be referred to as a CXR, a chest film, a picture, a radiograph, or a "X-ray." A computed tomographic study may be referred to as a CT (or, archaically, as a CAT scan). Magnetic resonance studies are often referred to as MRs or MRIs.

Types of Radiological Studies

Many types of radiological studies are encountered in clinical practice, and more are added as the science advances. Respiratory therapists should be familiar with the types of studies available at the institution where they work.

CHEST RADIOGRAPHY

Chest radiographs, often referred to as *chest films* in a nod to the passing era when chest radiographs were produced and stored on 14×17-inch films, are among the most commonly performed imaging studies. They are the type of X-rays most people are familiar with. The patient's chest is placed between an X-ray detector, historically a sheet of X-ray film, and a source of X-ray energy. The "shadows" cast on the film after a short exposure to the X-rays are recorded. The "colors" white, black, and grays on the film are determined by the relative ability of various tissues, devices, and substances to block the X-rays from reaching the film. By convention, the images are viewed in a white-on-black format. Black areas represent low-density substances, such as air, that do not block X-rays very effectively. White areas represent high-density substances, such as metal or bone, that are more efficient in blocking the X-rays. Materials that have densities lying between these two extremes appear as various shades of gray.

Best Practice

Radiograph Formats

In some countries and for certain specialized clinical applications, the images are viewed in a black-on-white format in which low-density areas are white instead of black.

Radiographs are the most simple, inexpensive, and available studies. They are most useful when the tissues being studied have density differences sufficient to show the details needed for the purpose intended. Radiographs of the chest rely on the different densities of aerated and nonaerated lung tissue, bones, the heart, and other mediastinal structures, as well as the many artificial devices such as endotracheal or chest tubes or venous catheters.

Figure 14-2A is a normal chest radiograph showing the four basic densities in plain film radiography: bone, soft tissue, fat, and air. Figure 14-2B is the corresponding normal left lateral view of the chest in which the patient's left side of the chest is placed against the X-ray detector or film cassette. Lateral views are helpful in identifying fluid accumulations, such as pleural effusions. Alternatively, **lateral decubitus** views can be used to detect small amounts of pleural fluid. To obtain a lateral decubitus view, the patient is placed on a table or cart, lying with the affected side down. This allows any fluid present in the pleural space to layer along the dependent (lowest) portion of the parietal pleural. The image is obtained by shooting the X-ray beam parallel to the table top.

Correct Orientation for Viewing Chest Radiographs. By convention, all chest X-rays, whether PA or anterior-posterior (AP, from front to back), are displayed as if the observer (reader) were facing the patient; the patient's left is to the observer's right. Normal chest images in the PA view should show the heart, specifically the cardiac apex, on the patient's left, or your right when viewing the image. The right diaphragm is normally slightly higher than the left by about 1–2 cm (about ½–1 inch). Gas in the upper portion of the stomach—the *gastric bubble*—is usually readily apparent under the left diaphragm.

When the PA radiograph is obtained, the patient's arms should be raised or the shoulders rotated upward and forward toward the cassette, thereby elevating the clavicles (collar bones) and moving the scapulae forward and laterally so that they are projected as much as possible away from the lungs. The lengths of the collar bones should appear to be equal and their

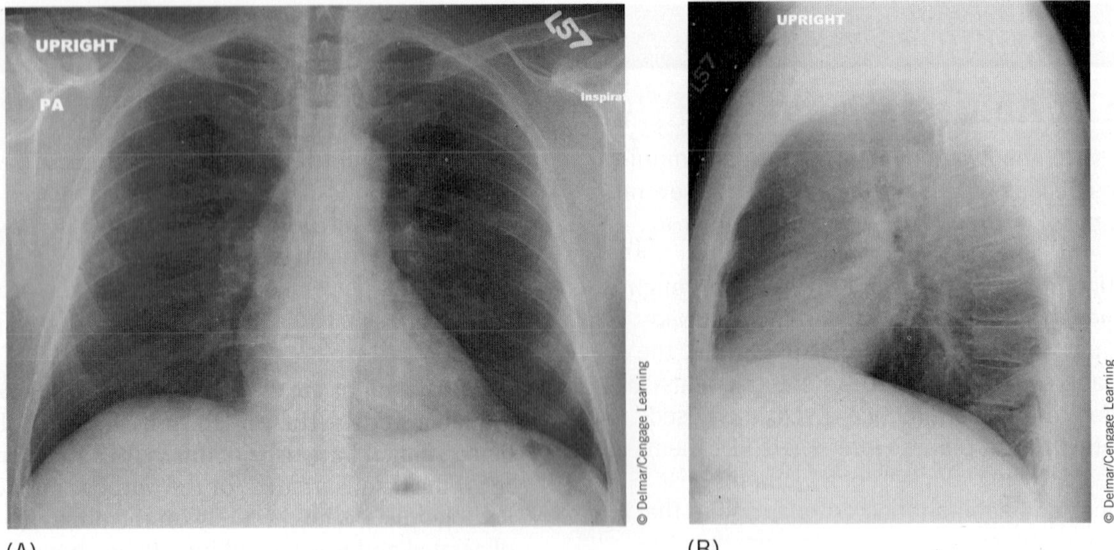

(A) (B)

FIGURE 14-2 (A) Normal inspiratory PA view: This illustrates the relative radiodensities of bone, soft tissues, fat, and air. Note the wide intercostal spaces (ICS), long thin heart, and relatively flat diaphragms bilaterally. Also note the presence of a gastric air bubble below the left diaphragm. (B) A normal inspiratory left lateral view with the left side of the patient's chest near the X-ray detector.

proximal ends should lie equidistant from the posterior spinal processes of the upper thoracic vertebra, which are used as marker of the midline on the PA or AP radiograph. The trachea and mediastinum should also lie near the midline under the sternum; otherwise the patient may be rotated into an oblique position or there may be a disease process resulting in tracheal or mediastinal shift.

Inspiratory versus Expiratory Studies. The reader of chest X-rays has to be able to distinguish between inspiratory and expiratory radiographs. Ideally, chest radiographs are taken at full inspiration. ("Take in a deep breath and hold it.") Occasionally, expiratory views are taken in special situations, such as attempting to demonstrate small pneumothoraces or to look for evidence of bronchial obstruction or air trapping. With practice, RTs can recognize the differences between inspiratory and expiratory chest radiographs based on their different characteristics—some subtle, some obvious.

- Inspiratory films (Figure 14-3) show wide intercostal spaces (ICS) with increased transverse (side-to-side) and AP diameters, and a flattened diaphragm. The heart appears relatively vertical and narrow in the standard upright inspiratory chest film.
- Expiratory films (Figure 14-4), on the other hand, have narrow intercostal spaces and the diaphragm is upwardly domed. The AP and transverse diameters of the chest are shorter, and the heart appears somewhat broader and more horizontally oriented. In a comparison of inspiratory and expiratory films on the same patient, the lower lung zones appear more dense and the vessels in the lower lobes are crowded together.

Portable Versus Nonportable Studies. Chest radiographs can be made using either fixed equipment in the radiology department or portable equipment in intensive care units, emergency departments, or other settings. Portable studies are most frequently used when patients are difficult or impossible to move

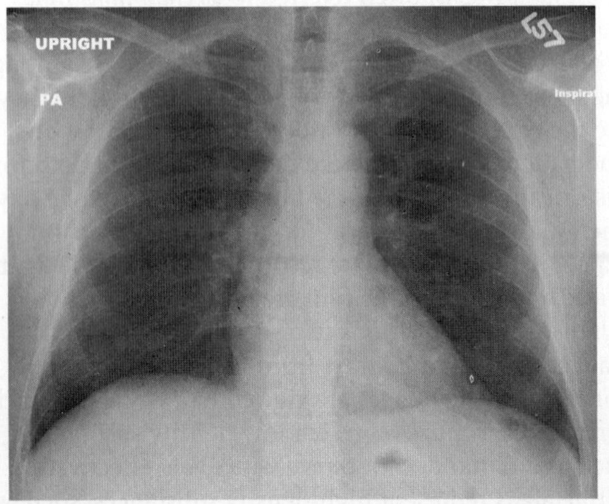

FIGURE 14-3 Normal inspiratory PA view: Note the wide ICS, increased side to side and front to back diameters. Note the flattened diaphragms and elongated narrow heart.

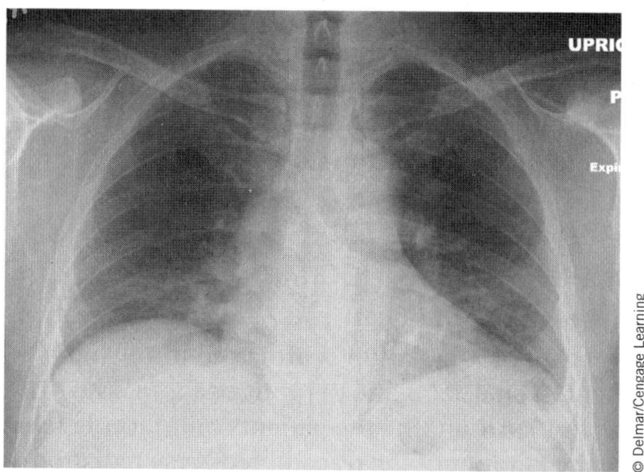

FIGURE 14-4 Normal expiratory film: Note the narrow ICS, domed diaphragm, thickened lower lobes, and decreased AP and transverse diameters with a relatively wider and shortened heart image.

because of either their condition or equipment (ventilators, chest tubes, and so on). The quality of portable studies is frequently limited, however, owing to nonstandard positioning, nonstandard distance, and other factors. Chest radiographs done in the radiology department are almost always of better quality than those done with portable techniques. The portable studies can be useful, however, provided the interpreter is aware that (1) the study was obtained using a portable unit and (2) portable techniques have certain limitations.

In standard chest radiography obtained in a PA projection (Figure 14-5), the patient stands upright with the anterior chest wall against the imaging detector or film cassette. The X-ray tube is positioned 6 feet behind the patient. The PA designation indicates the direction of the X-ray beam as it traverses the body from back (posterior) to front (anterior). The patient's arms are either raised or the shoulders are rolled forward toward the detector or cassette, stretching the thoracic cage while spreading and raising the scapulae.

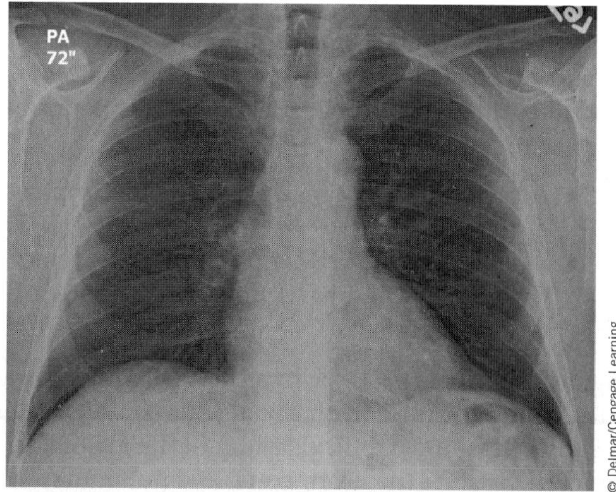

FIGURE 14-5 Posterior-anterior (PA) view, sometimes called a *standard view:* These films are taken in an X-ray or radiology lab. The patient's front chest wall is positioned against the image detector. The patient is normally standing (erect). Note the raised arms.

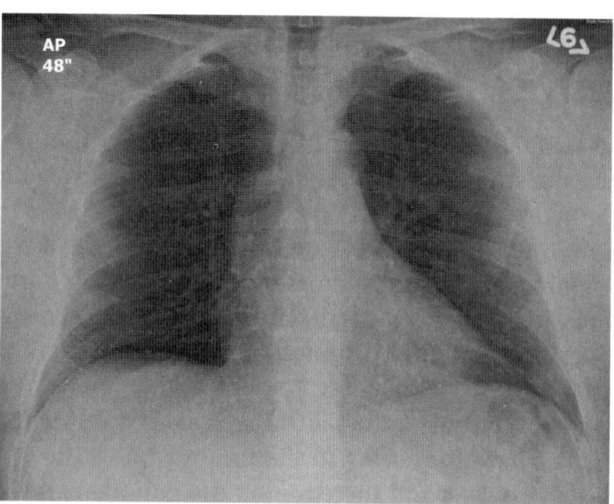

FIGURE 14-6 A portable radiograph, usually an AP view: The patient is normally on his or her back or sometimes propped up in bed in a seated or semirecumbent position. Note the magnification effect caused by the shorter focal length of the X-rays and the increased distance from the chest wall to the heart.

Portable radiographs are usually taken with the patient in a semirecumbent or recumbent position (Figure 14-6). In these positions, the arms are not raised over the head and the chest wall is not elevated and elongated. These films are commonly shot from front to back, hence the AP designation. Unlike PA radiographs where the tube-to-receptor distance is standardized at 72 inches, the tube-to-receptor distance for portable AP chest radiographs is generally no more than 48 inches, and it is often as short as 36 inches. Due to the combined effect of the shorter tube-to-receptor distance and the fact that the heart is farther away from the receptor in the AP projection, the shadow of the heart (the *cardiac silhouette*) is magnified compared to its appearance in PA.

Best Practice

AP versus PA Radiographs

Observers who are unaware of this single difference between AP and PA radiographs find themselves erroneously diagnosing enlargement of the heart (cardiomegaly) in their patients.

Radiographic Studies Using Contrast Materials

Standard radiographic techniques are not very useful when the structures of interest are surrounded by other structures of the same or very similar density. For example, an X-ray of the chest does not show the aorta or esophagus as distinct structures in the mediastinum because they are both of soft tissue density, the same as the density of all the surrounding structures in the central portion of the chest. To demonstrate these structures, contrast materials must be used; **contrast** materials have the ability to significantly block the passage of X-rays and thereby alter the radiodensities of the structures into which they are introduced. For example, in *arteriography*, the technique used to visualize arteries on radiographs, a liquid contrast agent that contains atoms of iodine bound to organic ring molecules is injected into an artery while images are obtained. The contrast agent mixes with the arterial blood, making the blood **radiopaque** (i.e., capable of blocking a greater proportion of the X-ray beam). As a result, the artery is *opacified*, that is, its density is increased to show the interior of the vessel. Similarly, in performing a study of the esophagus and stomach, commonly referred to as an *esophogram and upper GI*, either a barium sulfate suspension or Gastrographin (another water-soluble, iodine-based liquid contrast agent) is ingested to fill the esophagus and stomach, allowing the internal features of these structures to be seen. Contrast agents, particularly intravascular contrast agents, are also useful in CT scanning to distinguish pathological abnormalities, such as tumors, abnormally enlarged lymph nodes, or blood clots from normal vascular structures.

FLUOROSCOPY

In **fluoroscopy** (or fluoro), an image intensifier attached to a video system is used to generate and record the X-ray images. Unlike radiography, in which a single image—a snapshot—is obtained, fluoroscopy generates a series of radiographic images, closely spaced in time, creating a kind of movie or video of internal organs such as the heart, blood vessels, esophagus, or stomach as they function. The resulting video files allow the reader to see moving pictures instead of still images.

Fluoroscopy is useful in guiding a catheter, needle, or biopsy forceps to a particular point inside a patient. It is also helpful in clarifying whether a nodule that projects over the lung on a plain film is within the lung parenchyma or attached to the chest wall. This distinction is made by rotating the patient under fluoroscopy as the nodule is viewed; the movement of the nodule can be compared with the movement of structures behind or in front of it to get a better appreciation of its location and shape. Fluoroscopy is frequently used during bronchoscopic procedures, such as transbronchial biopsies, to verify that the forceps got to the area of pathology and that it is not on the pleural surface (so as to prevent a pneumothorax).

COMPUTERIZED TOMOGRAPHY

In **computerized (axial) tomography (CT** or **CAT)**, a thin beam of X-radiation is projected through the patient in an axial plane to produce a *scan*. Rings of detectors surrounding the patient continuously measure the amount of the transmitted X-ray radiation. A computer processes these measurements to produce a two-dimensional image of the patient. Normal and pathological anatomy is displayed as if the patient were cut into cross sections (hence the term "tomography"—to create a picture of a cut surface or slice).

To assure that the region of interest is appropriately included on the scan, a *scout image*—a digital radiograph produced by the CT scanner—is used to create the CT exam prescription. The *exam prescription* specifies the locations, thicknesses, and spacing of the cross-sectional images as well as the amount of X-ray energy to be used. Figure 14-7A is an example of a CT scout image. The scout image is annotated with superimposed lines that identify the start and end positions of the scan and the locations of proposed so-called cuts; examining it ensures the completeness of the examination. Figure 14-7B shows the same scout image view annotated with slice location data.

The thickness of the slices used to create an image set can be varied depending on the degree of detail and the size of the structures of interest for a particular examination. A typical slice thickness ranges from 1.5 to 10 mm.

When studying CT images, the contrast and brightness are adjusted to best display the anatomic structures of interest. These adjustments are performed by changing the:

- *Window width*, or range of different gray values displayed.
- *Window center* (*level*), or position of the center value of the window width along the range of possible gray values.

Figure 14-8A is an example of a chest CT with intravascular contrast using a mediastinal window accentuating the differing radiographic densities of the major structures such as the heart, aorta, and pulmonary artery. By adjusting the window width and level, the same image can be modified to display the internal structures of the lungs (Figure 14-8B).

By obtaining thin CT slices and changing how the computer processes the data, radiologists can obtain very detailed, sharp images of small structures in the

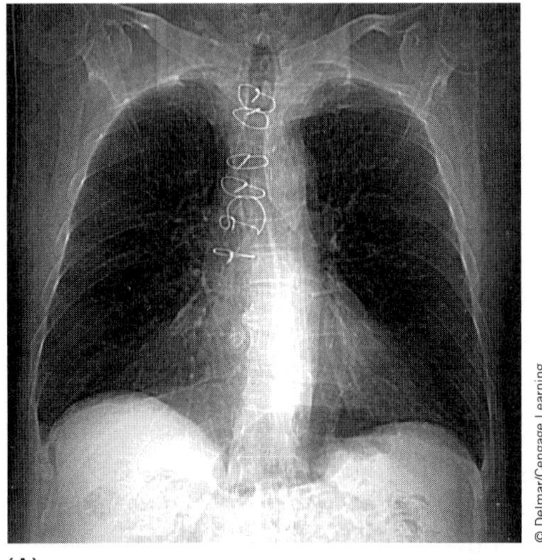

(A)

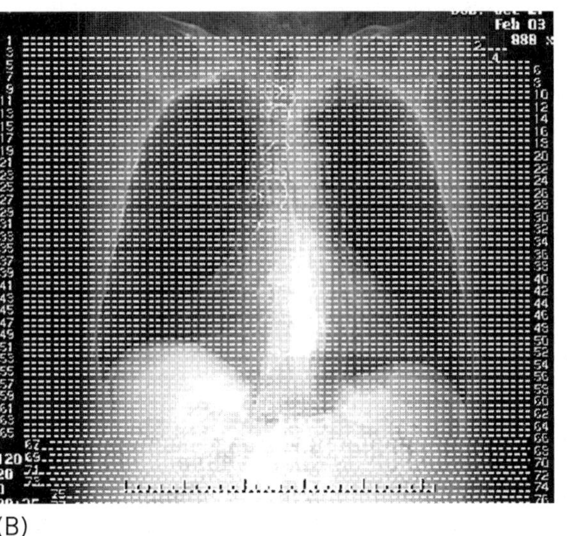

(B)

FIGURE 14-7 (A) A scout image of a computerized tomography (CT) scan: This is used to determine the slice locations for a full CT study. (B) The same scout image: The image now includes the cut location data.

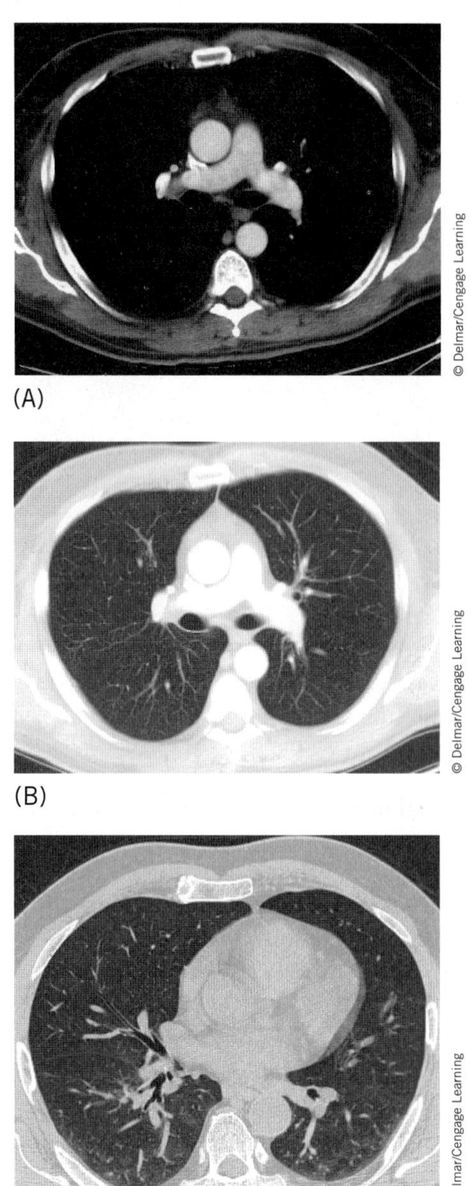

(A)

(B)

(C)

FIGURE 14-8 (A) A chest CT with intervascular contrast highlighting the mediastinal structures using a mediastinal window. (B) The same patient with the window expanded to study the internal lung structures. (C) A high-resolution CT: The HRCT enhances the small peripheral structure of the scanned area—in this case the lung. Note the superb detail.

parenchyma of the lung. This technique is commonly referred to as *high-resolution computed tomography* (*HRCT*). Figure 14-8C is an example of an image from an HRCT of the lung showing the exquisite detail of the small vascular and bronchiolar structures achievable using this technique.

Though the basic CT data set is used to generate a set of "stacked" axial images, the computer can reconstruct slices in any desired plane without having to rescan the patient. *Three-dimensional* (*3-D*) *images* of structures can also be generated. By combining basic CT techniques with the use of intravascular contrast and applying some

Best Practice

CT Settings

Because simultaneously displaying bone, mediastinal (soft tissue), and lung at their optimal window and level values is impossible, a complete review of a chest CT involves looking at each image using several different window and level settings.

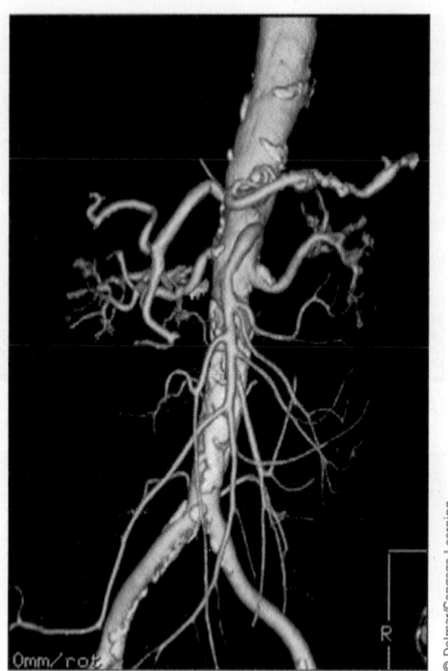

FIGURE 14-9 An image of a 3-D reconstruction of a CT angiogram of the abdominal aorta and its subdivisions.

of the special imaging-processing capabilities of modern CT systems, technicians can create 3-D images of many vascular structures. Figure14-9 is an example of a 3-D reconstruction of a CT **angiogram** of the abdominal aorta and its major branches.

For patients with pulmonary problems, CT scans are frequently used to determine the nature and location of various infiltrates or masses. Computerized tomography is the most sensitive means of detecting bronchectosis and is very sensitive for detecting and quantifying pleural fluid (effusion), pleural thickening (plaques), or pneumothorax. It can also be used to guide needle biopsies (i.e., a tissue sample usually obtained by an invasive method) and to allow for precise placement of catheters to drain abscesses or other localized fluid collections. The most advanced CT scanners currently in wide clinical use acquire up to 64 channels of attenuation data simultaneously as the table moves the patient continuously through the X-ray beam. This technique, commonly referred to as *spiral CT*, creates a data set with no gaps between adjacent slices, making it possible to create exquisitely detailed images of the human body. These systems make it possible to image structures as small as the coronary arteries or peripheral branches of the pulmonary artery and to diagnose coronary artery stenosis or pulmonary emboli with high specificity and sensitivity.

MAGNETIC RESONANCE IMAGING

Whereas CT creates images based on differences in the abilities of various tissues to block, or attenuate, an X-ray beam, **magnetic resonance imaging (MRI)** creates cross-sectional images based on the behavior of hydrogen nuclei (protons) in a magnetic field. To understand the basic physics of MRI, think of the single protons in the hydrogen nuclei as tiny bar magnets (magnetic dipoles), similar to the needle in a compass. A powerful magnet is used to cause the dipoles of the hydrogen nuclei to align with the external magnetic field. Radio frequency pulses are then used to excite, or tip, the dipoles out of alignment with the external field. Once the exciting radio frequency pulse is turned off, the protons relax back to the ground state in which they align again parallel to the external field. As the protons realign, the scanner "listens" for a radio frequency signal emitted from the body. The computer system of the MR scanner then processes the emitted signals to form the images. MRI, unlike CT and radiography, uses no ionizing (X-ray) radiation. As a result, numerous closely spaced images in several different planes can be generated with excellent detail and tissue differentiation without the risk of overexposure to radiation, which is a growing concern in CT imaging.

An MRI study involves putting the patient in a small tunnel, and some patients experience feelings of claustrophobia. Recently, open, or C-shaped, MRI scanners have allowed even claustrophobic patients to undergo MRI procedures. Because it can take several seconds to obtain the data for each standard MR data set, imaging moving objects, such as the heart, was difficult. However, specialized fast scanning techniques that allow imaging of the heart and great vessels are now widely available.

The appearance of an MR image depends on how the radiofrequency data are obtained. The amount of time between the radiofrequency pulses used to excite the protons is referred to as *TR*. The amount of time between an exciting pulse at the time at which the scanner is listening for the radiofrequency signal, or echo, is called the *TE*. By systematically varying TR and TE, one can accentuate the differences between tissues and translate these differences into differences in brightness, or contrast, in the MR images. Figure 14-10A is an axial (transverse) image of the brain using a short TR/short TE, or T_1-weighted pulse sequence. (By convention, axial images are oriented so that the patient is facing up and the patient's right is to your left.) On T_1-weighted images:

- Water and similar materials produce the lowest signal and appear dark, as illustrated by the cerebrospinal fluid (CSF) in the ventricular system.
- Solid materials, such as the gray-and-white structures of the cerebral hemispheres, show signals of intermediate intensity and show up as various shades of gray.

Best Practice

MRIs and Magnets

Because of the strength of the magnets used in MRI, patients with certain metallic implants or electronic devices, such as pacemakers or cochlear implants, cannot be imaged. In addition, patients with metallic foreign bodies, especially in the eye or orbit, should not be imaged because there is a danger of displacing magnetic metals. MRI can also erase computer disks or credit cards brought into the MRI suite. Because of these dangers, most mechanical ventilators and many monitors cannot be used near an MRI scanner. However, specially designed and fabricated systems are becoming available to allow scans of critically ill patients. Until these new devices become available, these patients may have to be manually ventilated while they are being scanned. Also, furniture, gas cylinders, medical devices, or other objects containing ferrous materials (iron compounds) or other magnetic metals are banned in MRI suites. Additionally, pagers, cell phones, PDAs, watches, jewelry (especially piercings), and medical/dental implants may contain ferrous compounds. These objects can be pulled into the bore of the magnet at high velocities, posing the risk of serious bodily injury to patients and staff, not to mention significant damage to the very expensive MRI equipment.

- Finally, fat in the subcutaneous tissues and in the marrow space between the inner and outer layers of the skull show the highest signal and appear as white.

Compare this image with Figure 14-10B, an image obtained using a long TR/long TE, or T_2-weighted pulse sequence.

- The highest signal is emitted from the CSF in the ventricular system, which appears as white.
- The gray-and-white matter of the cerebral hemispheres emit signals of lower intensity and appear as dark gray.
- The signal emitted by fat is of intermediate intensity between those of CSF and soft tissue.

A third commonly used pulse sequence is the long TR/short TE, which produces *spin density*: the signal is weighted in proportion to the number of protons per unit volume in a given area.

In addition to modifying the tissue contrast by changing how an MR signal is obtained and processed, coronal or sagittal images can be generated directly by changing how the radio frequency signal is detected. Figure 14-10C shows a T_2-weighted midline, sagittal image of the head and cervical spine. Here the convention is to display the image as if the patient were facing to the reader's left. Figure 14-10D is a coronal, T_1-weighted image of the brain.

MRI currently has relatively limited clinical applications with regard to the lungs, though a variety of possible uses are being actively investigated. Most patients who require MRI while under the care of a respiratory therapist are imaged for neurological conditions.

ULTRASOUND

Ultrasound, or sonography, uses high-frequency sound waves to generate cross-sectional images of the body. Various tissues differ in their abilities to transmit, absorb, or reflect high-frequency sound waves. To generate an ultrasound image, a **transducer** (a device that can convert one form of energy to another and back again) is placed against the surface of the body. The transducer converts an electronic signal into a pulse of high-frequency sound waves that is transmitted into the body. This acoustic pulse passes through some tissues (usually liquids) very well, but soft tissues absorb some of the acoustic energy. Some energy is scattered away from the transducer, and some is reflected back toward it from the interfaces where two tissues of slightly different acoustic properties touch one another. Once the transducer has generated and transmitted the initial pulse, it "listens" for the echo of sound reflected back from the patient's internal organs. In the listening mode, the transducer converts the acoustic energy of the reflected ultrasound pulse to a series of electronic signals. The computer of the ultrasound unit uses data about the strength and timing of the reflected sound waves to create an image. The frequency of the sound waves used for most medical imaging is 3.5–10 million cycles per second (MHz), far above the range of human hearing.

Ultrasound is a minimally invasive method that does not use either ionizing or nonionizing radiation. The sound transmission and reflection characteristics of a tissue are completely different from the properties that contribute to **radiodensity** or MR tissue contrast. Consequently, ultrasound differentiates tissues in ways completely unlike conventional radiography, computed tomography, or MRI.

Ultrasound images may be recorded as two-dimensional images, frozen at a particular point in time, or they can be stored and viewed as real-time video or movie files. Although most ultrasound imaging is rendered as two-dimensional cross sections,

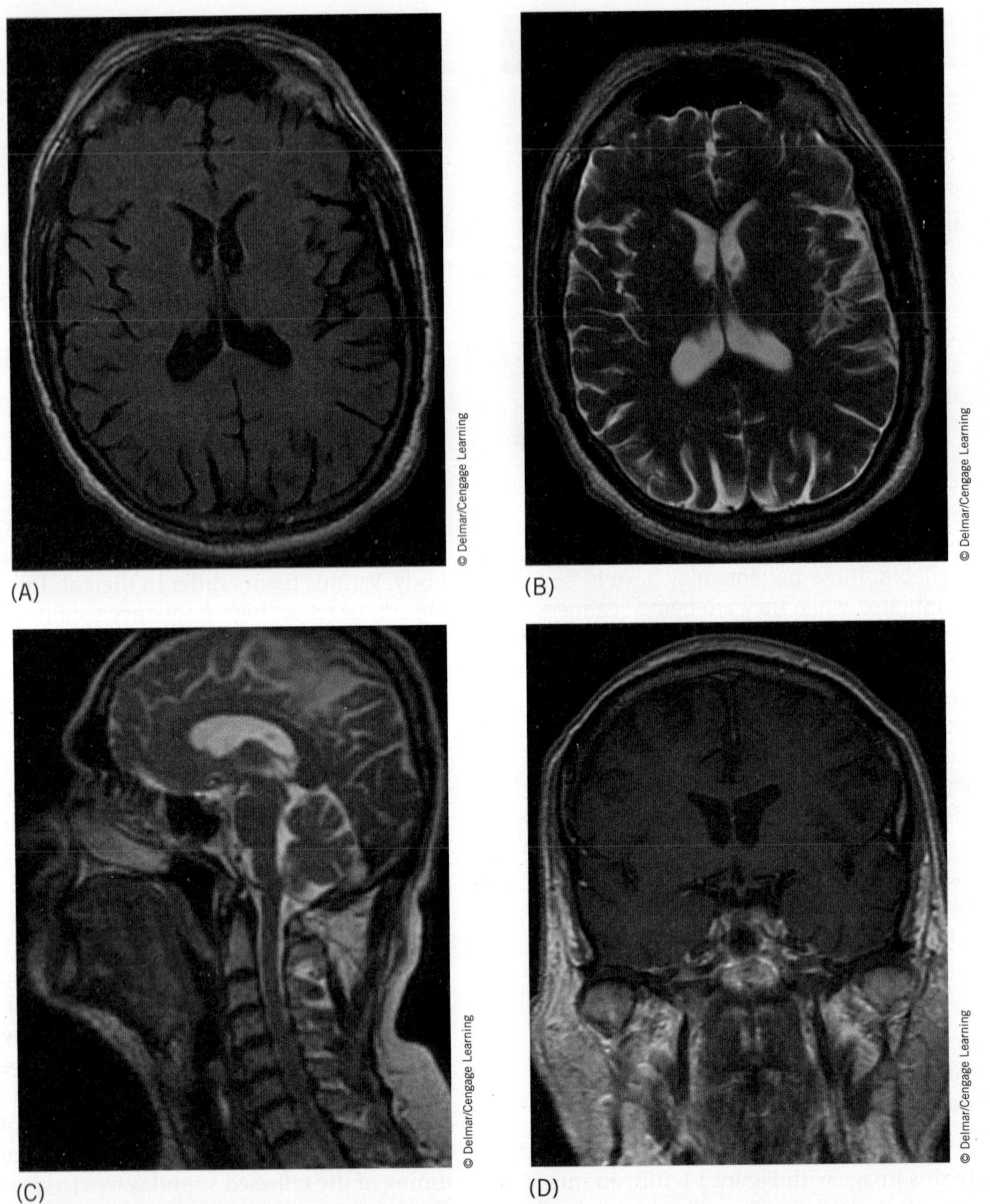

FIGURE 14-10 (A) an example of an axial (transverse) image of the brain using a short TR/short TE, or T_1-weighted pulse sequence. (B) An image obtained using a long TR/long TE, or T_2-weighted pulse sequence. (C) A T_2-weighted midline, sagittal image of the head and cervical spine (the image is displayed as if the patient were facing to the reader's left). (D) A coronal, T_1-weighted image of the brain.

a number of available systems can generate three-dimensional, real-time images.

When imaging the chest, several factors limit the use of ultrasound as compared to CT or MR. First, the ability of the sound waves to penetrate and therefore to image the human body decreases with their frequency. On the other hand, the ability of ultrasound to demonstrate small structures increases as the frequency of the beam increases. Consequently, ultrasound works best for imaging structures near the surface of the body. Furthermore, some substances, such as bone or air, block the transmission of ultrasound waves into the underlying tissues, making it impossible to image structures in the aerated lung or directly beneath the ribs or scapulae.

In imaging of the chest, ultrasound is commonly used to evaluate pleural effusions and to guide drainage of effusions (thoracentesis) or other pleural or

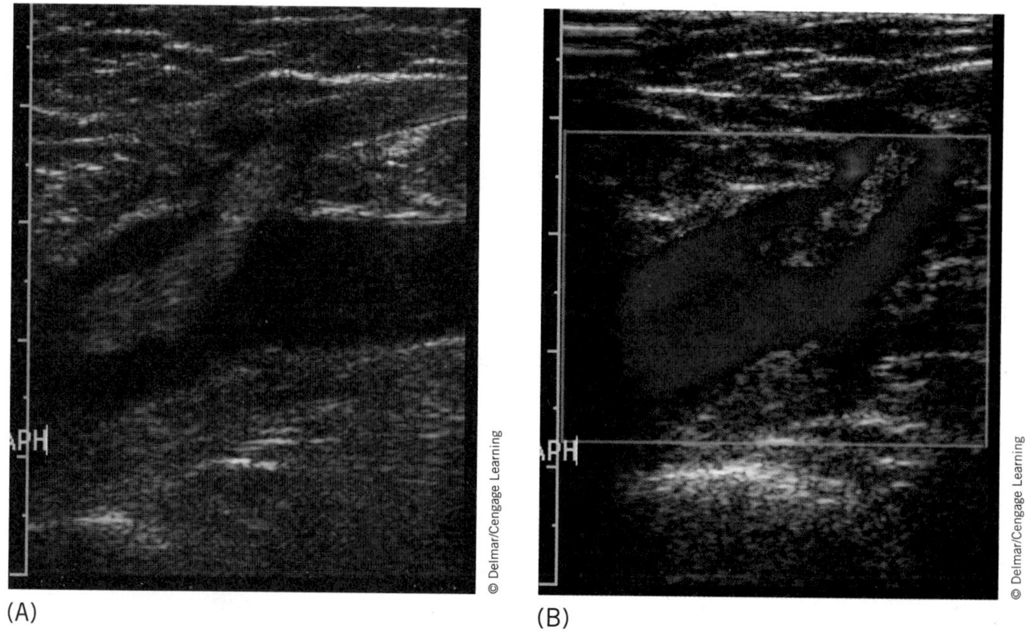

FIGURE 14-11 (A) A 2-D grayscale sonographic image of the right common femoral vein showing a nonocclusive clot (thrombus) against a black background due to the absence of reflected echoes from the blood flowing around the clot. (B) A color Doppler image of the same area: The ultrasound unit has been adjusted to detect signals reflected from the moving red cells in the vein and to translate them to a blue color. In this image, the clot is seen as a gray structure partially surrounded by the blue color representing nonclotted, flowing blood.

pericardial fluid collections. More common applications for ultrasound are:

- Imaging abdominal or pelvic organs, including the prenatal evaluation of fetal growth and development.
- Imaging the arteries and veins of the extremities and neck.
- **Echocardiography**, a specialized form of ultrasound used to image the heart in motion.

Doppler sonography is useful for documenting blood flow and measuring the degree of narrowing, or stenosis, in diseased vessels. In the intensive care unit, where patients are at increased risk of developing deep venous thrombosis and pulmonary embolism, Doppler sonography can detect clots in the deep veins of the lower extremities. Figure 14-11A is a 2-D grayscale sonographic image of the right common femoral vein showing a nonocclusive clot (thrombus) against a black background due to the absence of reflected echoes from the blood flowing around the clot. Figure 14-11B is the color Doppler image of the same area. The ultrasound unit has been adjusted to detect signals reflected from the moving red cells in the vein and to translate them to a blue color. In this image, the clot is seen as a gray structure partially surrounded by the blue color representing nonclotted, flowing blood. With the advent of smaller, lightweight, and more technologically advanced systems, ultrasound devices are being used in surgery, in emergency room ICUs, and sometimes on patient floors.

NUCLEAR MEDICINE STUDIES

Nuclear medicine studies involve administering a small amount of a radioactive material (called a *radiotracer, tracer, radioisotope,* or *isotope*) to the patient. Imaging is performed by placing the patient under a camera that detects the photons of energy emitted by the tracer as the isotope with which it is labeled decays. The radioisotope tracer is carried to and accumulated by the tissues and organs of interest by a number of different mechanisms in the areas of interest. For instance, in a perfusion lung scan, particles of a material called macro-aggregated albumin are tagged with a radioactive isotope of technetium and injected into the patient's vein. Due to the size of the albumin particles, they and the isotope they carry become trapped in pulmonary capillaries in the perfused parts of the lung. When the patient is placed under a camera, the image (Figure 14-12A) is a map of the perfused parts of the lungs. Similarly, ventilation can be mapped by having the patient breathe either a radioactive gas, usually an isotope of xenon (Figure 14-12B), or a radioactive aerosol. The two images make up a **ventilation/perfusion ($\dot{V}/\dot{Q}$) scan** for the patient. By comparing the images

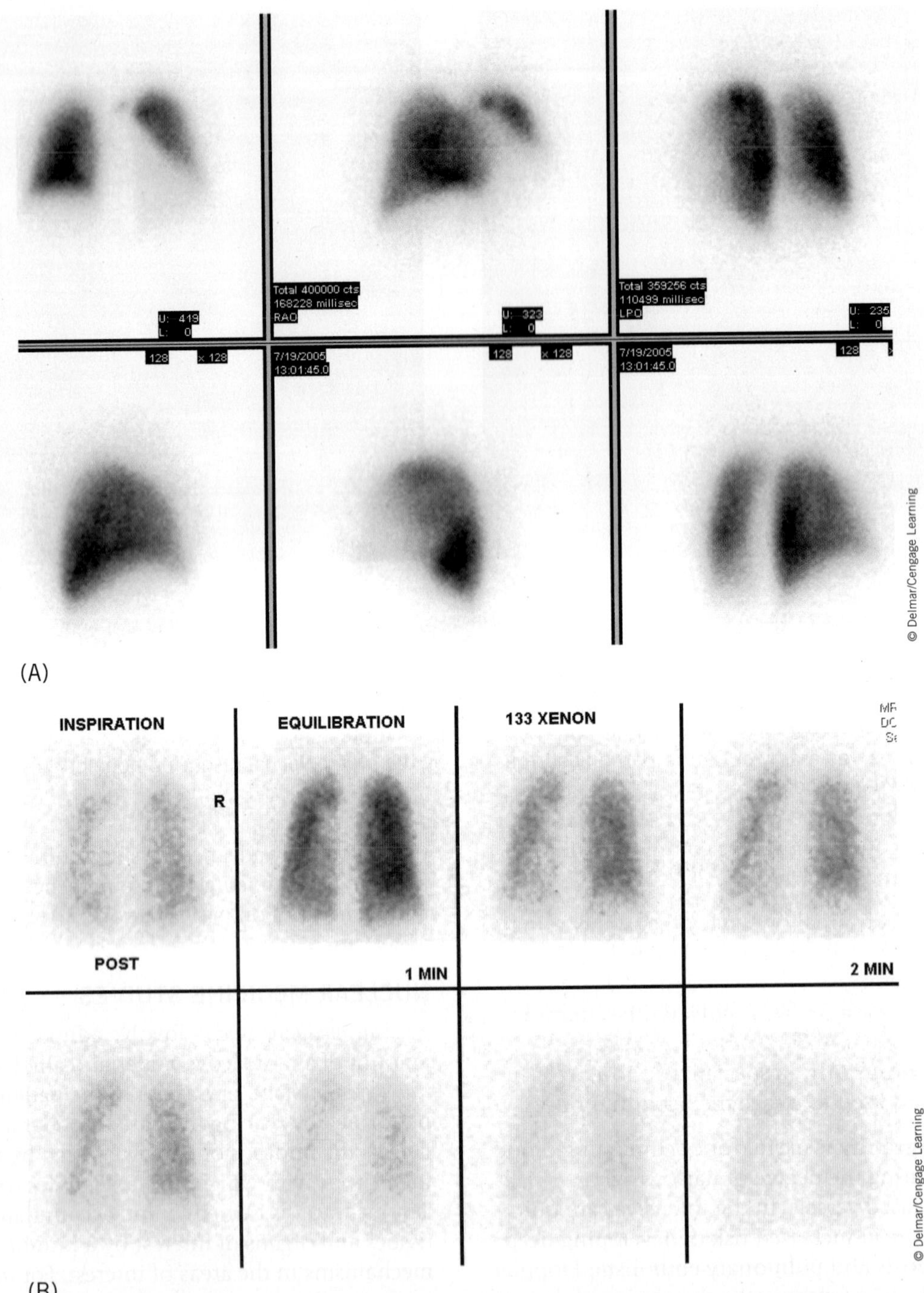

FIGURE 14-12 (A) A perfusion lung scan, showing the trapped isotopes in the pulmonary capillaries in the perfused parts of the lung. (B) Mapping of ventilation when the patient breathes a radioactive gas, usually an isotope of xenon.

and looking for areas of the lung that are ventilated but not perfused, to the reader can detect pulmonary emboli.

Another example of nuclear medicine imaging is the use of indium-labeled white blood cell scans to localize infectious or inflammatory processes. In this type of study, white blood cells (WBCs) labeled with radioactive indium^{111} are injected into the bloodstream. White blood cells are naturally attracted to areas of infection or inflammation. Consequently when radio-labeled WBCs are injected, they and the isotope are concentrated in any sites of active inflammation. Such scans are sometimes used to detect occult (hidden) abscesses or other inflammatory processes when other diagnostic tests have been unsuccessful.

Still another common type of nuclear medicine imaging is the use of the radioisotope thallium^{201} to evaluate the blood flow to the heart in patients suspected of having myocardial ischemia (angina pectoris).

Positron emission tomography (PET) is yet another application of nuclear medicine imaging. In this technique, chemical compounds, such as glucose or other sugars, are labeled with positron-emitting isotopes. These compounds are actively taken up by cells during their metabolism. A positron is a unique particle in that, when a single positron collides with an electron, both particles disappear in a phenomenon called *annihilation*. Positron annihilation results in the emission of two high-energy photons that travel in opposite directions along a straight line. The photons can be detected using a special scanner that can identify the "coincident" photon pairs and map their locations in the body with much greater accuracy than is achievable with a standard nuclear medicine camera. By assigning different colors, or grayscale values, to various levels of activity of tracer uptake, one can actually see the accumulation and concentration of the labeled materials. Because the radio-labeled compounds used for PET imaging are actively taken up by living cells during metabolism, groups of actively growing and dividing cells appear as foci of increased activity—so called *hot spots*—on PET images.

PET can be used to image infectious or inflammatory processes. However, it is most widely used for assessing the growth and spread (metastasis) of malignant tumors. For example, using a glucose derivative labeled with the positron-emitting isotope fluorine^{18} (F-18 fluorodeoxyglucose, or FDG), PET scanning can detect malignancies such as lung cancer because many cancers are metabolically active and tend to accumulate the modified glucose molecules to a greater degree than normal tissues. Figure 14-13 presents a typical coronal projection PET scan image in a patient with a history of cancer of the urinary bladder treated by cystectomy; the patient has developed metastases to the left hilar lymph nodes.

Often, PET images are combined with CT or MR images (a process sometimes referred to a *fusion imaging*) to allow physicians to localize lesions anatomically with greater confidence than is possible using PET images alone. Figure 14-14 is an example of a PET-CT fusion image in a patient with a left hilar lung cancer. The colored PET data are mapped over the grayscale CT data for an axial image at the level of the tumor.

The formal interpretation of imaging studies requires knowledge and skills that can be fully acquired only through years of medical education. In the hospital setting, the final interpretations of radiographic studies are usually performed by *diagnostic radiologists*, physicians who have completed at least four years of training after medical school. Although the formal interpretation of medical imaging studies is beyond the scope of this chapter and not a part of respiratory therapy practice, RTs need to understand the range of imaging techniques that can be brought to

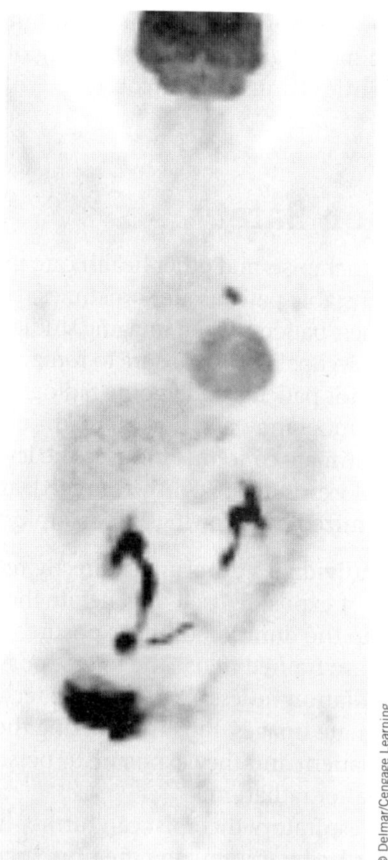

FIGURE 14-13 A typical coronal projection PET scan image in a patient who has a history of cancer of the urinary bladder treated by cystectomy and who has developed metastases to the left hilar lymph nodes.

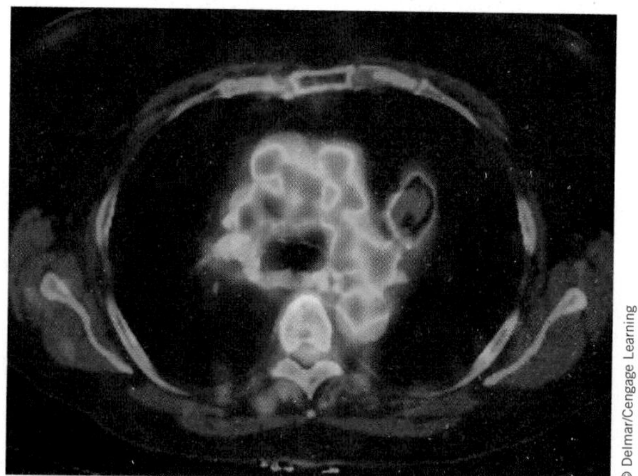

FIGURE 14-14 An example of a PET-CT fusion image in a patient with a left hilar lung cancer.

bear when evaluating lung structure and function, and they should have a general understanding of the types of abnormalities commonly encountered in clinical practice.

Radiation Safety

Respiratory therapists and other health care professionals managing unstable patients are sometimes required to tend to their patients when imaging studies are performed. Occupational exposure to ionizing radiation while caring for patients undergoing radiography, computed tomography, and nuclear medicine examinations is a legitimate concern. However, the levels of occupational exposure are tightly regulated, and the risks can be minimized by following a few simple rules.

- An individual's exposure is directly related to the level of exposure used to generate the images and to the duration of the exposure. Technologists are trained to use the lowest possible dose of radiation necessary to produce technically adequate images, thus minimizing the dose to the patient and they exposure to personnel due to scatter radiation.
- The respiratory therapist can further limit exposure by minimizing the time spent in a room while a study is being obtained.
- The RT who must be in the room during an exposure should ask the technologist for appropriate shielding equipment, such as lead aprons or screens.
- Radiation dose varies inversely with the square of the distance from the source (the inverse square law, Chapter 3). So increasing the distance from the source of exposure, typically the patient rather than the imaging device itself, significantly decreases exposure. Increasing the distance to the patient's bedside from 1 to 2 feet, reduces the scatter dose by a factor of 4.
- Finally, if the RT is in a position that requires regular attendance during imaging examinations, the facility's safety office should provide a personal dosimeter to monitor the cumulative exposure over time.

Ultrasound and MR examinations do not entail exposure hazards. However, MR does present significant physical hazards due to the effect of the powerful magnetic fields on certain metal objects such as chairs, gas canisters, and medical devices. Also, personnel and patients with medical devices such as pacemakers or cochlear implants should not enter the MR suite without first checking with the MR supervisory staff.

How to Interpret Studies

In interpreting (reading) radiology studies, the reader must fully understand the context in which the study was obtained. Before a study is interpreted and management decisions are made based on the findings, the images should be reviewed for technical adequacy in light of the following questions:

- Does the examination obtained match the examination that was ordered?
- Is the patient clearly identified by markings or annotations that are either a part of the images or permanently linked to the study in the electronic medical record (EMR)?
- Are the date and time of the image also included on the images or linked to the study in the EMR?
- Is the position of the patient clearly indicated (upright, supine, decubitus, or oblique)?
- Is the view or projection (PA, AP) clearly indicated on the images?
- Is the region of interest completely included on the images?
- Are the exposure factors adequate?
- Was the X-ray beam of sufficient energy, and was the length of exposure sufficiently long to produce an image of diagnostic quality?
- Was a sufficient amount of X-ray attenuation data collected to generate CT images that are of diagnostic quality?
- Were an adequate number of photons counted to generate nuclear medicine images that can be confidently interpreted?
- Did the way in which the image was acquired either create artifacts or degrade the image?
- Were all garments, jewelry, overlying devices (lines, tubes, etc.), surgical instruments, and other foreign bodies removed? If not, does their presence compromise or limit the diagnostic quality of the examination?
- Are the images degraded by patient movement (breathing, cardiac motion, changes in position)?

PREANALYSIS

In addition to knowing the type of study being read, the reader must know how the patients were prepared and positioned for examinations. For example, one needs to know whether a chest radiograph was obtained in the upright or supine position. Depending on the position, a suspected pleural effusion shows up either as a blunting of the costophrenic angle in the upright position or as generalized increase in the density of the involved lung (hemithorax) due to the fluid lying behind the lung in the supine position.

Best Practice

Exposure of the Chest Radiograph

As a general rule, in a radiograph of the chest, the penetration and exposure should be such that the intervertebral spaces in the thoracic spine are just visible.

One must also be certain that the region of interest is completely and appropriately imaged. For example, if the concern is for a pneumothorax, a radiograph performed in a supine position or one that *clips* (does not include) the lung apices, is inadequate.

The overall quality of the film must also be assessed. When a chest radiograph is too dark (overexposed), a pneumothorax, which is also dark on a plain film, is difficult to detect. Using intense back lighting (called hot-lighting or spot lighting) details can be enhanced in overexposed (dark) films. If the radiograph is too light (underexposed), important mediastinal landmarks or the tips of devices, such as endotracheal tubes, central venous lines, or a Swan-Ganz catheter, may not be visible.

Cardiac or respiratory motion can blur the images of medical devices, particularly those in or near the heart and great vessels, such as Swan-Ganz catheters or internal cardiac pacemakers. Artifacts or foreign objects on an image may confuse the reader. For example, consider a portable chest X-ray obtained while a patient is in the operating room that shows a surgical clamp overlying the left lung. Without additional information or additional lateral or oblique views, the reader cannot determine absolutely whether the clamp is inside the patient's chest or lying on the surgical drapes covering the chest wall. Finally, at some point during the review of every examination, the reader should locate and identify all foreign objects and devices and compare them with previous examinations to determine whether there are any new devices or lines or any of the previously noted devices and lines have changed significantly in their positions. As an exercise, take a look at the two images in Figure 14-15, which were obtained immediately before (A) and after (B) a trip to the operating room. Even a relatively cursory comparison of the two images shows an endotracheal tube (ET), a Swan-Ganz (pulmonary arterial) catheter, a left thoracostomy tube, and several additional sternal wires that were placed as a part of the patient's coronary artery bypass surgery. Although it is easy to become lackadaisical in the checking routine postsurgical tubes, drains, and lines, attention to these details can prevent adverse events such as the retention of surgical drains, sponges or instruments—events that are considered completely avoidable and inexcusable by patients and their families.

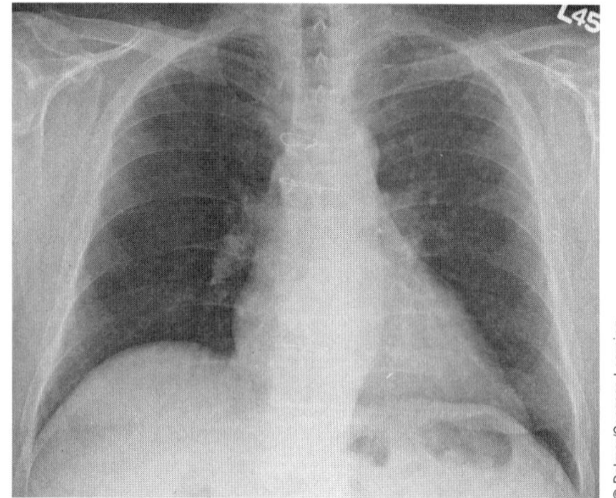

(A)

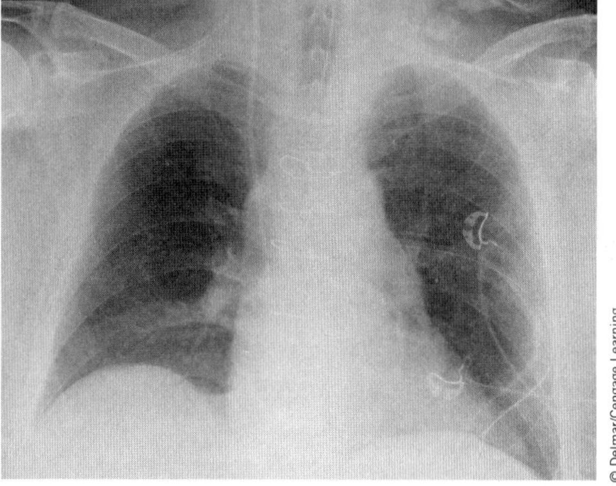

(B)

FIGURE 14-15 Two radiographs taken before (A) and after (B) surgery: Note the endotracheal tube (ET), a Swan-Ganz (pulmonary arterial) catheter, a left thoracostomy tube, and several additional sternal wires that were placed as a part of the patient's coronary artery bypass surgery.

REVIEW OF THE STUDY

Be systematic! Always look at images and examinations in a consistent and systematic way. The order in which an image is reviewed is not critical, as long as the method or sequence used is logical to the reader. The method should ensure that the entire image, including all edges, corners, and image annotations, are examined. Consider a commonly used sequence for evaluating a chest radiograph by reviewing Figure 14-16:

1. Check the identity of the patient.
2. Check the date and time of the study.

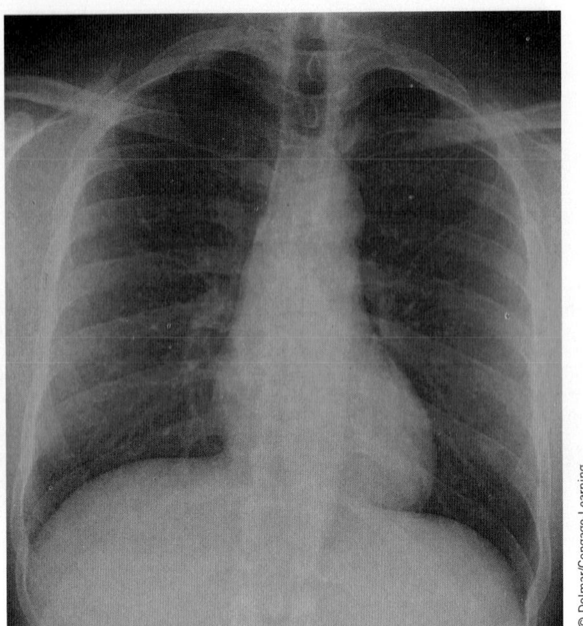

FIGURE 14-16 Review of the chest radiograph.

For purposes of publication, the patient identifying information and date and time of the study are suppressed. This information is generally recorded or displayed as image annotations at the corners of the image.

3. Identify the type of study (know what was ordered, what was done, position, view).
4. Evaluate the technical quality of the image.
5. Identify any and all artifacts.
6. Identify all foreign objects (e.g., tubes, lines, devices).
7. Evaluate extrathoracic soft tissues (e.g., subcutaneous emphysema, foreign material).
8. Evaluate bony structures and joints (e.g., fractures, dislocations, normal variations, abnormal densities).
9. Evaluate the pleura, including the apices and costophrenic angles (e.g., a pneumothorax, pleural effusion).
10. Evaluate the upper, middle, and lower zones of the lungs, using the corresponding regions of the opposite lung to improve your sensitivity to focal abnormalities (e.g., masses, nodules, infiltrates, cavities). Pay particular attention to the areas beneath the clavicles and first ribs, behind the heart, and beneath the domes of the diaphragm.
11. Evaluate the right and left hilum, again using the opposite hilum for comparison (e.g., enlargement of one as compared to the other).
12. Assess the size and configuration of the heart (e.g., cardiomegaly, abnormal shape).
13. Evaluate the aorta, main pulmonary artery, and other mediastinal soft tissue landmarks, including the superior mediastinum (e.g., a shift of the mediastinum, mass, aneurysm, abnormal calcification).
14. Evaluate the trachea and central bronchi (e.g., masses, foreign bodies).

Be careful to review the entire image. A radiograph of the chest can reveal a critical abnormality in the abdomen, or an abdominal film might identify something critical in the chest. In many cases, an additional study may be required to completely evaluate the incidentally identified abnormality. However, do not make the mistake of ignoring free gas in the abdomen beneath the diaphragm or similar "incidental findings" on an otherwise normal chest radiograph just because a chest X-ray rather than an abdominal study was obtained.

The image used for this exercise (Figure 14-16) is essentially normal. Nevertheless, the patient's first ribs are asymmetric and small, particularly on the patient's left. This happens to be an incidental finding or normal variant, but it is still a good test of an RT's observational skills.

COMPARISON WITH PREVIOUS STUDIES

Always compare the current study with the most recent studies of the same anatomic region to detect new abnormalities and to reduce the tendency to mistake

Best Practice

Systematic Review

Having a systematic process of reviewing films is helpful. RTs should follow the same sequence every time they review a film to prevent missing important facts. Sometimes changing your perspective by moving around the film - go to the left - to the right - go forward and go backwards. Changing your point of view can help you "find" variations in the film.

Age-Specific Competency

Minimizing Patient Movement

Infants, small children, patients who are confused or combative, and patients with Parkinson's disease, seizure disorders, or tremor-producing disorders may be very difficult to X-ray or perform scans on. If X-rays or scans are critically important, either such patients must be physically or chemically restrained, or the practitioner has to settle for a poorer-quality film and analysis.

Best Practice

Image Verification

The reader must verify that the image set is of the correct patient and was taken at the correct time. An image or study that is not properly labeled should be interpreted with caution, if at all. Critical errors in patient management can be made if someone accidentally reads a study of a wrong patient or from last year while assuming that the image represents the patient in question today.

stable lesions or normal variants as pathological findings. The comparison is also helpful in the assessment of the rate of change of new lesions or of lesions appropriate for radiographic follow-up rather than biopsy or surgical removal. A single study is only a snapshot in time; without comparing it to older studies, the reader cannot tell whether a process is improving, worsening, stable, or chronic. As a general rule, a lesion, such as a lung nodule, can be considered benign if it shows no change in size or border contour over a two-year period. However, even relatively minor changes in the size or border features of a nodule are cause for concern because certain lung cancers, particularly those arising in regions where the parenchyma is scarred, can evolve relatively slowly.

CORRELATION OF FINDINGS WITH CLINICAL SITUATION

Accuracy in interpreting a radiograph improves greatly when the radiographic findings are compared with what is known about the patient's clinical presentation and clinical course. The reader is not only more likely to look for information that is pertinent to the patient's situation, but also more likely to correctly identify the pathology. For example, a diffuse infiltrate in an ICU patient could represent pulmonary edema, acute respiratory distress, pneumonia, or pulmonary hemorrhage, among many other conditions. The clinician is much more likely to correctly identify pulmonary hemorrhage as the underlying cause of the infiltrates if he or she is aware that the nurse has reported significant hemoptysis and that the morning laboratory findings show a significant drop in the patient's hemoglobin or a marked prolongation of the patient's bleeding time.

FINAL INTERPRETATION

The final interpretation of a radiological study should describe all observations that are believed to be important and mention any so-called *pertinent negatives*. For example, in a patient with a resolving pneumonia, the final interpretation might be, "The lobar consolidation noted on the previous study has now resolved, and there are no new areas of consolidation."

The reader then reports an impression that, as concisely as possible, explains possible reasons for the observations. Consider, for example, a chest radiograph obtained following drainage of a moderate left pleural effusion. The image shows a patchy, air-space infiltrate in the left lower lobe (the description of your major finding), a small residual left pleural effusion, and no evidence of a pneumothorax (a pertinent negative in a patient who has just undergone a procedure that may be complicated by the development of a pneumothorax). The patient's morning examination indicates that she has a productive cough, a fever, and an elevated white blood cell count. The explanation of the radiographic findings could be that the patient has a left lower lobe pneumonia associated with a parapneumonic effusion.

Note: The impression should reflect and can be influenced by all of the information known about the patient (e.g., a productive cough, fever, and elevated white count). However, the observation and description of findings should reflect only the findings revealed by the images and should not be influenced (biased) by other available clinical information.

Example Cases

The cases and commentaries in this section illustrate how a variety of clinical conditions and disease processes manifest themselves radiographically. A number of technical and clinical factors related to the radiographic findings are also discussed.

NORMAL CHEST

The normal PA chest radiograph (Figure 14-17) may show many features that reflect anatomic variations among individuals.

- Common variations are in the thickness of the soft tissues of the chest wall, the shape of the heart, and the heights of the domes of the diaphragm.
- In Figure 14-17, note the symmetric soft tissue densities overlying the lower lungs due to the normal breast shadows in this female patient.
- Another common normal finding related to both the male and the female breast is the presence of unilateral or bilateral solitary soft tissue "nodules" over the lower lobes. On careful review, though sometimes only after a repeated examination with radiopaque markers placed on

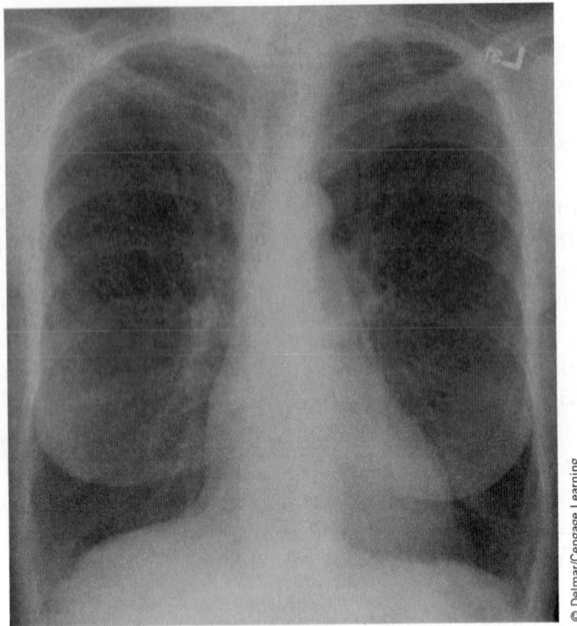

FIGURE 14-17 The normal chest.

the nipples, these are shown to be false nodules due to the soft tissue of the nipples.

- Other normal variants are the presence of additional ribs associated with the lowest cervical vertebra, the absence or hypoplasia of the last thoracic ribs, and deformities of the sternum and anterior ribs such as pectus excavatum (sunken chest) or pectus carinatum (pigeon breast).

Only through practice and experience does one become proficient in recognizing normal variations and distinguishing normal and normal variant anatomy from pathological findings.

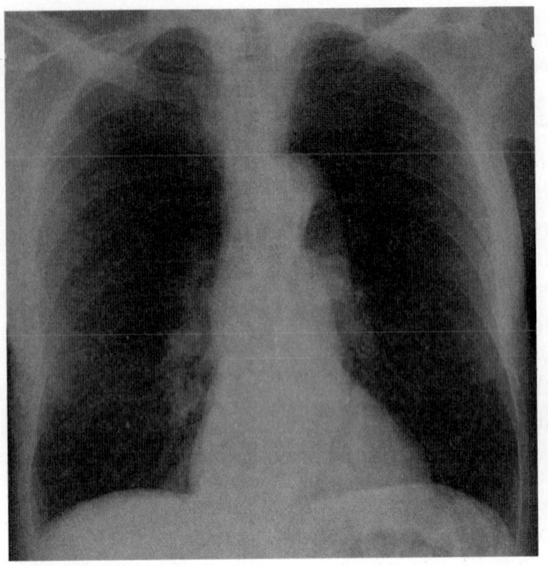

(A)

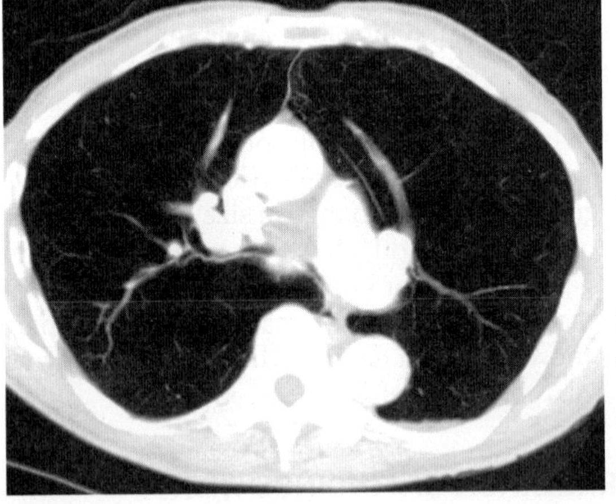

(B)

FIGURE 14-18 Emphysema and bulbous lung disease: (A) Radiograph. (B) CT.

EMPHYSEMA AND BULBOUS LUNG DISEASE

Emphysema is an irreversible enlargement of the airspaces (alveoli) in the lung with destruction of the alveolar walls. The resulting cystic airspaces may become large enough to see with the naked eye and are called **bullae**. Because air does not move efficiently out of these abnormal air cysts, over time the size of the bullae and of the lungs themselves tend to increase, resulting in increased diameters of the chest and a flattening of the diaphragm. The vessels in the most involved regions tend to be reduced in number, smaller in caliber, and stretched lengthwise due to the increased volume of the diseased pulmonary parenchyma.

In extreme cases, the structural elements of the lung, including the blood vessels, are very diminished in number. It is difficult to tell whether a collection of air in the chest cavity is a pneumothorax in the pleural space or an air-filled bulla in the substance (parenchyma) of the lung itself. The radiograph in Figure 14-18A and the CT scan in Figure 14-18B are from a patient with marked changes of emphysema with bulbous disease. Note the increased lucency of the lungs and the flattening of the diaphragm illustrated by the chest X-ray. The CT also shows the loss of normal lung markings, the hyperlucency, and the formation of innumerable bulla that displace and stretch the remaining vascular and septal structures. Making the distinction between a bulla and a pneumothorax is critical. Placing a chest tube into a bulla on the mistaken impression that it is a large pneumothorax can lead to severe complications, such as a persistent air leak and chronic pneumothorax. Occasionally, bullae may become infected or filled with fluid, in which case air-fluid levels may be seen on upright chest radiographs or on CT.

LOBAR PNEUMONIA

Infection in the lung is called *pneumonia*. Infections can involve the air spaces (alveoli), the conducting airways (bronchi and bronchioles), the walls and supporting elements of the lung (interstitium), or any combination of these. *Interstitial pneumonias*, often caused by viruses, produce an increase in the linear markings in the lung and a thickening of the interlobular septa, similar to the pattern seen in interstitial pulmonary edema (discussed in Congestive Heart Failure, Pulmonary Edema, and Pleural Effusion on page 368). Infections of the alveoli or conducting airways produce a focal area of increased density in the lung parenchyma that can be identified on chest X-ray, but their appearance differs in ways that can suggest one causative bacterium over another.

Pneumonia developing at the level of the alveolus often presents as a *lobar process*—a condition that involves much or all of one or more of the anatomic lobes of the lung. To identify lobar diseases, the reader must have a knowledge of the basic lobar anatomy of the lung. The right lung normally has three lobes (upper, middle, and lower), and the left lung has only two (upper and lower). The lobes are separated from one another by the interlobar fissures: two on the right (the major and minor fissures) and one on the left (the major fissure). The fissures separating lobes are not especially prominent on a chest radiograph, but they can become much more evident should fluid accumulate in the fissure or should a lobar infiltrate develop in the adjacent lung.

Lobar processes tend to produce a relatively uniform, often quite dense, opacification of the involved portions of the lung. Figure 14-19 is an example of a lobar pneumonia involving portions of the right upper lobe. On the PA projection (Figure 14-19A), the right minor fissure sharply defines the inferior border of the infiltrate, indicating involvement of the anterior segment of the right upper lobe. However, the lateral view (Figure 14-19B) is somewhat confusing because the area of consolidation is also partially delineated by the cephalad portion of the right major fissure, which normally defines one border of the posterior segment of the right upper lobe. This unusual appearance is due to the involvement of portions of both the anterior and posterior segments of the right upper lobe while sparing the apical segment. This pattern of involvement is sometimes referred to as pneumonia of the *axillary segment*, based on reports of a normal variant *axillary bronchus* supplying these regions of the lung. Classically, lobar pneumonia is caused by *Streptococcus pneumoniae*, though many other bacteria can produce this pattern of disease.

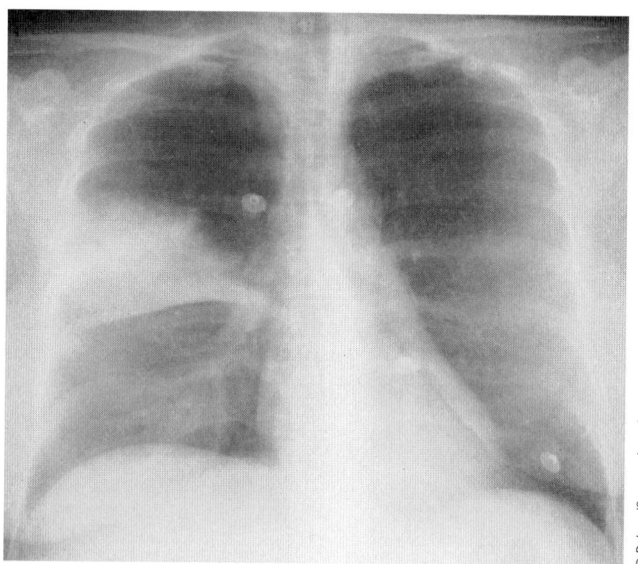

(A)

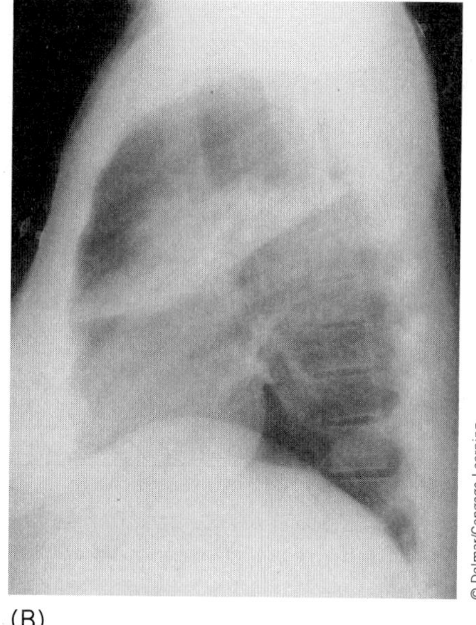

(B)

FIGURE 14-19 Lobar pneumonia: (A) PA projection showing the right minor fissure sharply defining the inferior border of the infiltrate, indicating involvement of the anterior segment of the right upper lobe. (B) Lateral view showing an area of consolidation partially delineated by the cephalad portion of the right major fissure, which normally defines one border of the posterior segment of the right upper lobe.

BRONCHOPNEUMONIA

Bronchopneumonia is a second common pattern of pneumonia produced by bacterial and, less commonly, viral or mycoplasmal (fungal) infections of the lung. The classic agent is *Staphylococcus aureus*. In this case,

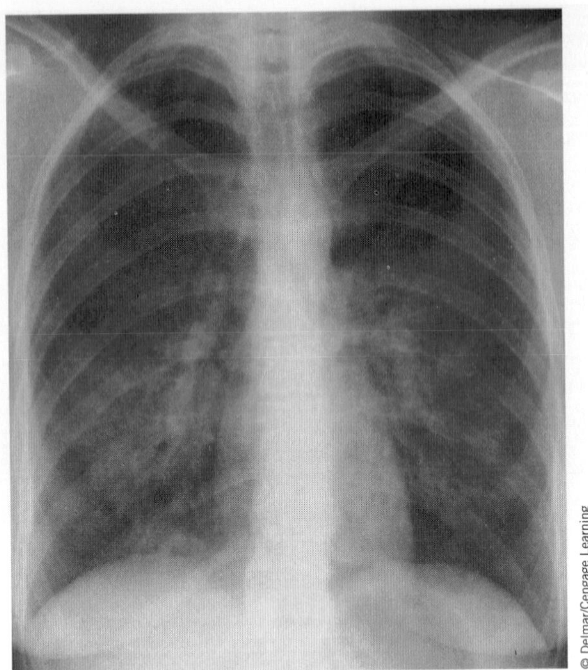

FIGURE 14-20 The typical, patchy, inhomogeneous appearance of the infiltrates of a bronchopneumonia involving all lobes in a patient infected with *Mycoplasma pneumoniae*.

the initial focus of infection is in the airways, and the infectious agent can be passed relatively freely from one area to another as secretions are transported centrally and the patient coughs. The infection starts with the bronchioles and bronchi, and then the alveoli supplied by the affected airways become involved. Unlike lobar pneumonias, no anatomic barriers, such as the fissures, act as barriers to the spread of the process. Consequently a bronchopneumonia often involves more than one lobe, and in many cases both lungs are affected. Figure 14-20 illustrates the typical, patchy, inhomogeneous appearance of the infiltrates of a bronchopneumonia involving all lobes in a patient infected with *Mycoplasma pneumoniae*.

ALVEOLAR (AIR-SPACE) INFILTRATES AND AIR BRONCHOGRAMS

Lobar pneumonia is one example of a whole range of conditions that result in alveolar, or air-space. consolidation (infiltrates). Air-space disease starts peripherally and progresses centripetally (toward the center), displacing the air from the lung parenchyma. Because the central airways have more effective ways of clearing mucus and debris than do the peripheral air-spaces, they tend to remain filled with air. As the lung surrounding the air-filled bronchus becomes more radio-dense due to the accumulation of fluid, cells, bacteria, pus, or blood in the airspaces, the bronchus

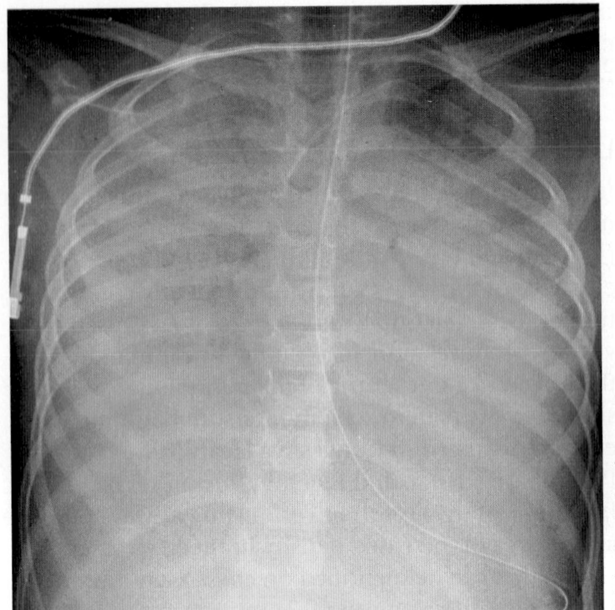

(A)

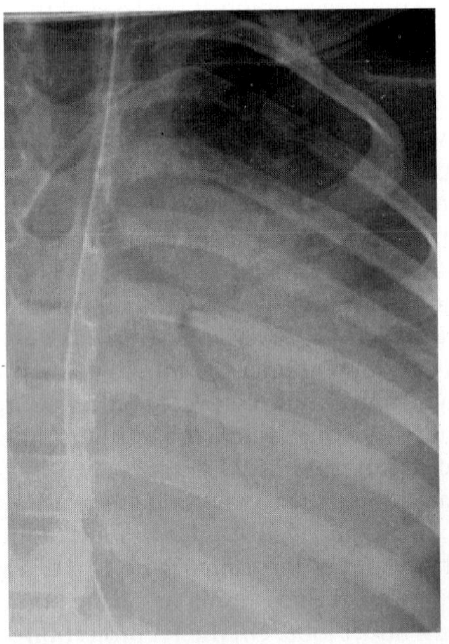

(B)

FIGURE 14-21 (A) Air bronchograms against a background of extensive alveolar consolidation in a patient with overwhelming sepsis and diffuse alveolar damage. (B) A number of branching lucencies radiating from the left hilum and extending well into the periphery of the left lung.

becomes clearly defined as a *linear* or *cylindrical lucency* in the area of consolidation. These lucencies are referred to as **air bronchograms.** Figure 14-21 illustrates air bronchograms against a background of extensive alveolar consolidation (Figure 14-21A) in a patient with overwhelming sepsis and diffuse alveolar damage. This radiograph (Figure 14-21B), on careful examination, shows a number of branching lucencies radiating from the left hilum and extending well into the periphery of the left lung. This is an extreme example of air bronchograms. An air bronchogram is said to be present if airways can be followed to their segmental or subsegmental branches in a lobe (roughly three or four generations of branching from the carina). The clinical settings in which alveolar infiltrates are common include lobar pneumonia, the adult respiratory distress syndrome, neonatal hyaline membrane disease (infantile respiratory distress syndrome), and pulmonary edema or pulmonary hemorrhage (see Chapter 8).

LOBAR ATELECTASIS

Atelectasis is the technical term for volume loss or the collapse of a portion of the lung. If the air is removed from the lung parenchyma, the volume of the remaining soft tissue is quite small. *Lobar atelectasis*, or airlessness and volume loss of an entire lobe, typically occurs when a central airway is blocked and the air distal to the blockage is absorbed into the bloodstream. As a result, the lobe supplied by the obstructed bronchus becomes smaller and more radio-dense. Atelectasis results in the displacement or bowing of adjacent fissures toward the involved lobe, and it may also result in the displacement of the hilum and the elevation of the diaphragm on the involved side. Because an airless lobe can be very small, changes of complete lobar atelectasis can be easily overlooked, particularly on a single view of the chest. Figure 14-22 illustrates the radiographic appearance of complete atelectasis of the right middle lobe. Figure 14-22A is a PA radiograph of a patient with complete atelectasis of the right middle lobe, showing only subtle loss of the definition of the right heart border. The corresponding lateral view (Figure 14-22B) shows the atelectatic right middle lobe as the thin band of soft tissue projected obliquely over the cardiac silhouette.

Figure 14-23 is a second example of complete lobar atelectasis.

- Figure 14-23A shows a radiograph of some soft tissue fullness overlying the area between the aortic arch and the main pulmonary artery (the aorticopulmonary window), hyperlucency of the upper portion of the left hemithorax, and stretching and splaying of the vessels in the upper portion of the left lung.
- The lateral view (Figure 14-23B) shows a thin band of soft tissue density against the anterior wall of the hemithorax, increasing the density of the normally radiolucent retrosternal clear space.

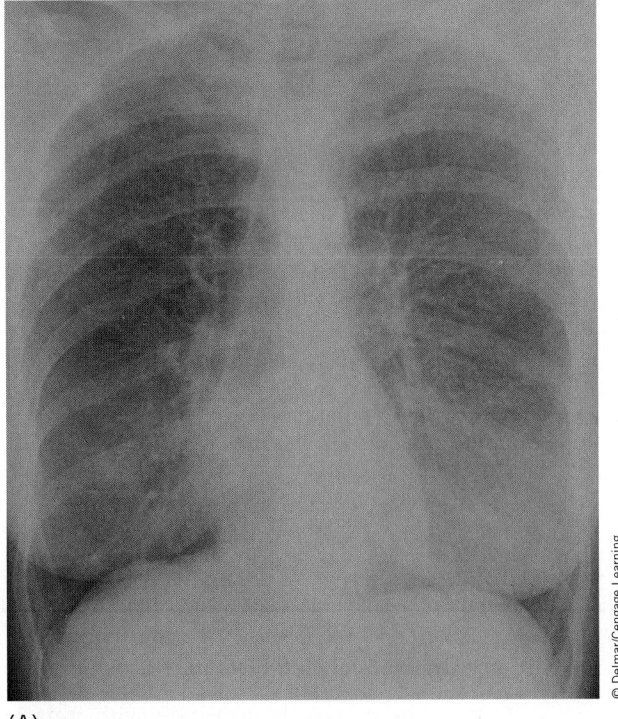

(A)

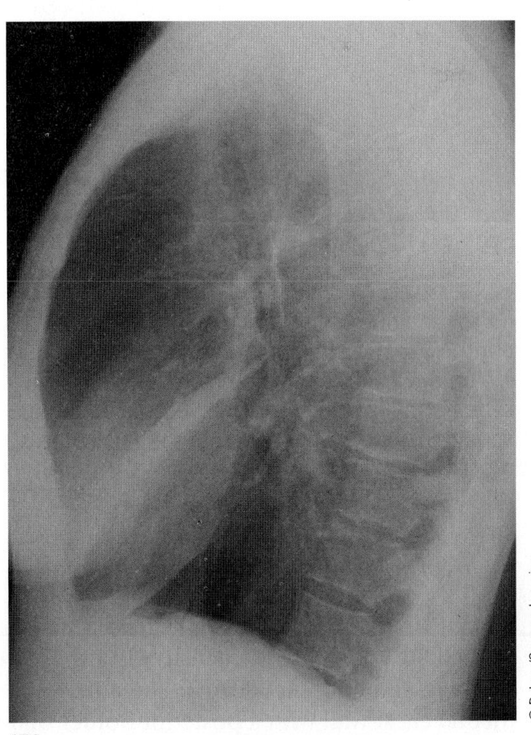

(B)

FIGURE 14-22 (A) A PA radiograph of a patient with complete atelectasis of the right middle lobe showing only subtle loss of the definition of the right heart border. (B) The corresponding lateral view shows the atelectatic right middle lobe as the thin band of soft tissue projected obliquely over the cardiac silhouette.

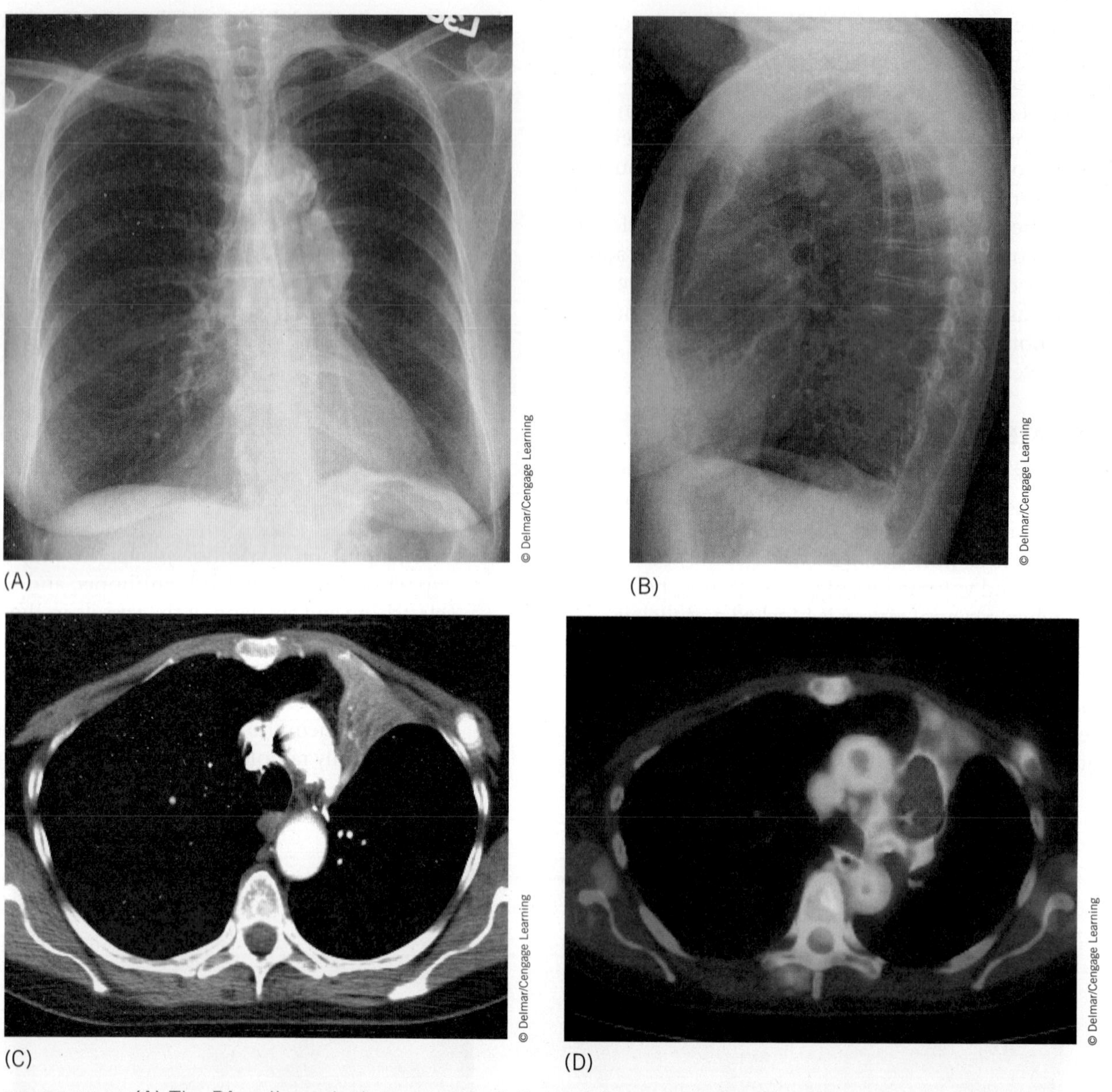

FIGURE 14-23 (A) The PA radiograph shows some soft tissue fullness overlying the area between the aortic arch and the main pulmonary artery (the aorticopulmonary window), hyperlucency of the upper portion of the left hemithorax, and stretching and splaying of the vessels in the upper portion of the left lung. (B) The lateral view shows a thin band of soft tissue density against the anterior wall of the hemithorax, increasing the density of the normally radiolucent retrosternal clear space. (C) The CT image shows a wedge-shaped area of soft tissue density closely applied to the left anterior mediastinal and anterior-medial chest wall with a posterior border that is bowed inward, toward the density. (D) A representative image from the patient's PET/CT, showing intense focal uptake of the F-18 labeled FDG in red.

- The CT image (Figure 14-23C) shows a wedge-shaped area of soft tissue density closely applied to the left anterior mediastinal and anterior-medial chest wall with a posterior border that is bowed inward, toward the density. This patient had a complete obstruction of the left upper lobe bronchus due to lung cancer, resulting in complete atelectasis of the left upper lobe.
- Figure 14-23D is a representative image from the patient's PET/CT, showing intense focal uptake of the F-18 labeled FDG in red.

Both of these cases demonstrate, with atelectasis, that there is always a loss of volume in the affected area and that other structures—other segments or lobes, fissures, the heart, and/or mediastinum—are pulled

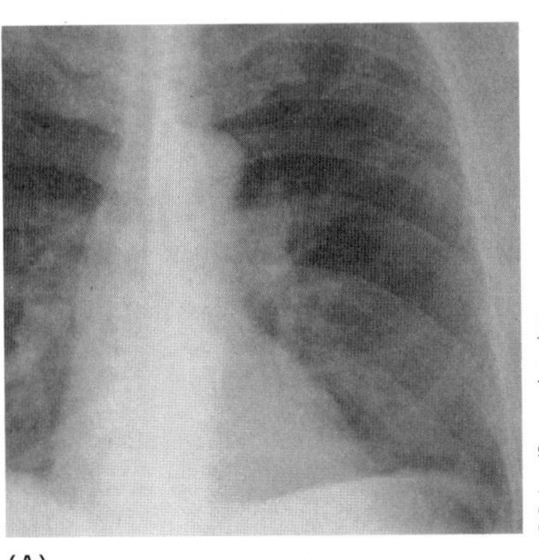

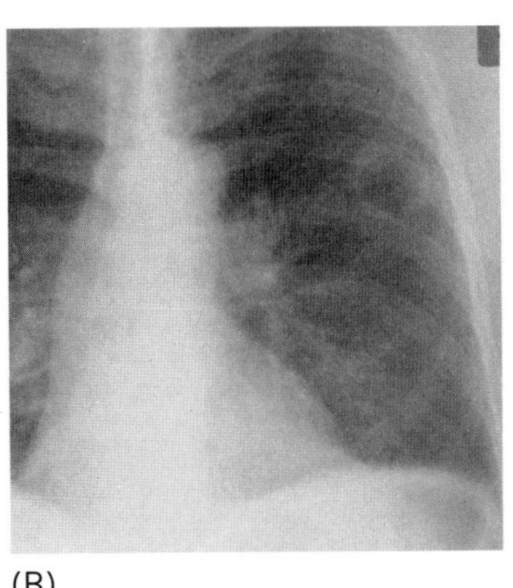

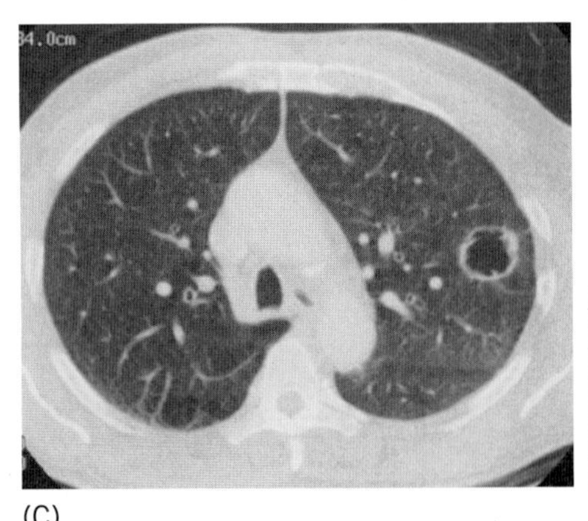

(A) (B) (C)

FIGURE 14-24 (A) A thin-walled cavitary lesion that was initially thought to be infectious or inflammatory in origin. (B) The follow-up study showing a significant increase in the thickness and irregularity of the wall of the cavity—changes highly suggestive of malignancy. (C) A CT scan, acquired on a lung window setting, that confirmed the aggressive, irregular, nodular wall of the lesion, one of the common presentations of the squamous cell type of bronchogenic carcinoma.

toward the area of atelectasis. In the most extreme cases, when the right or left main bronchus is obstructed—for instance, by tumor—the entire lung on the involved side collapses, and the heart and mediastinum shift toward the involved side, resulting in complete opacification (white-out) on the side of the lesion and hyperexpansion of the uninvolved lung on the opposite side.

LUNG CANCER

Respiratory therapists frequently are called on to evaluate and help manage patients with lung cancer, or bronchogenic carcinoma. The radiographic appearance of primary malignancies of the lung is highly variable, ranging from solitary pulmonary nodules or masses with more or less well-defined margins, through irregularly marginated masses and cavities, to ill-defined masses and infiltrates or diffuse infiltrates resembling lobar or bronchopneumonia. Other patients present with no abnormalities in the lungs but have mediastinal or hilar masses due to disease spreading to the lymph nodes. Still others, like the patient in Figure 14-23, present primarily with atelectasis. Finally, unfortunately, for many patients, their tumors produce no detectable radiographic abnormalities; their cancers are radiographically occult.

When a lung cancer presents as a mass or nodule, the lesion shows growth over time. Typically, lung cancers double in volume within 6 weeks to 6 months. (For spheres, only a 25% increase in diameter produces a two-fold increase in volume.) Lesions with volume doubling times longer than 6 months tend to be benign, such as granulomas or hamartomas (benign tumors containing several different types of tissue); lesions that double in less than 6 weeks tend to be inflammatory or infectious in origin. The patient in Figure 14-24 presented for an annual physical examination with a new, thin-walled cavitary lesion (Figure 14-24A) that was initially thought to be infectious or inflammatory in origin. However, a slight irregularity of the wall was noted; so the patient had a follow-up chest X-ray to see whether the cavity resolved or progressed. The follow-up study (Figure 14-24B) showed a significant increase in the thickness and irregularity of the wall of the cavity—changes highly suggestive of malignancy. The CT scan in Figure 14-24C was acquired on a lung window setting and obtained to evaluate the patient's hilar and mediastinal nodes before removal of the lung. It confirmed the aggressive, irregular, nodular wall of the lesion, one of the common presentations of the squamous cell type of bronchogenic carcinoma.

TUBERCULOSIS

Tuberculosis (TB), an infection caused by *Mycobacterium tuberculosis*, was once relatively well controlled in the United States, but it has experienced a resurgence due to the prevalence of HIV/AIDS and to the expanding use of immunosuppressive therapies for a variety of malignant and nonmalignant conditions. Two forms of tuberculosis are generally described: primary and postprimary (reactivation).

Primary tuberculosis occurs on an individual's first exposure to the bacillus and often goes undetected clinically or radiologically. If a patient happens to have a chest X-ray during the initial infection, the appearance is one of a nondescript focal infiltrate and/or hilar adenopathy, especially in children. In most individuals, the infection is contained, and the X-ray shows little or no detectable residual abnormality. In some patients,

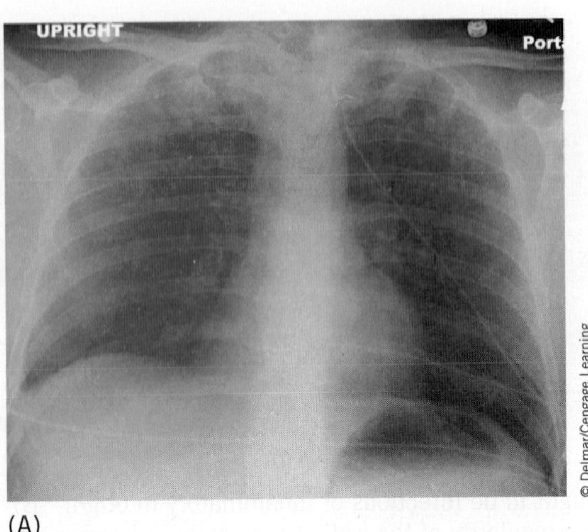

(A)

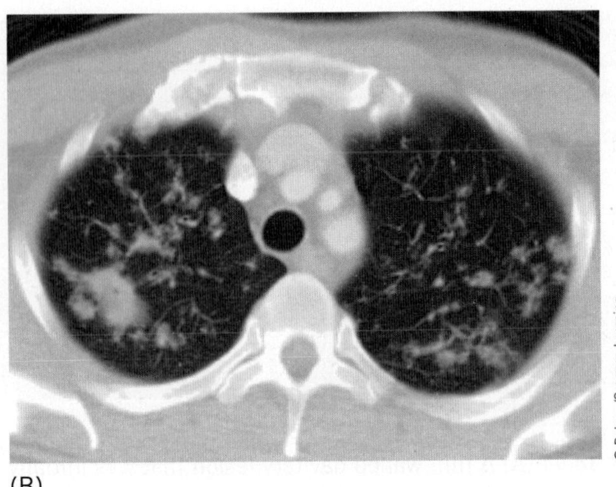

(B)

FIGURE 14-25 (A) A chest X-ray illustrates bilateral patchy apical inflitrates with nodules typical of early reactivation TB. (B) The CT scan shows the same patient's pathology depicting patchy areas of alveolar consolidation in the apices of both lungs.

the healed focus of infection can be seen as a soft tissue nodule, called a *granuloma*, which may calcify over time. Some patients with healed primary tuberculosis also show calcifications in hilar or mediastinal lymph nodes.

Postprimary, or *reactivation, tuberculosis* occurs in patients with a previously contained primary infection. In such patients, alterations in the ability to fight infection due to the weakening of the immune system allow the bacillus to reemerge. The radiographic changes are those of patchy consolidation (broncho-pneumonia), often involving the apical segment of the upper lobe or superior segment of the lower lobe in one or both lungs. Figure 14-25A is a chest X-ray of a patient with early reactivation TB showing patchy, nodular infiltrates in the apices of the lungs. Figure 14-25B is the patient's CT scan showing patchy areas of alveolar consolidation in the apical segments of both upper lobes. The early changes of postprimary disease often progress to *cavitation*, the radiographic hallmark of reactivation TB. In many patients, the infection is ultimately contained by host responses or by treatment with specific drugs. However, even in patients who recover from reactivation TB, the involved areas often become fibrotic and scarred, resulting in bronchial dilatation and volume loss in the affected lobes.

In severely immunocompromised patients, TB is less likely to have the characteristic apical distribution or cavitation. Instead, the disease demonstrates a pneumonialike pattern similar to that seen in primary tuberculosis. In some patients, the tuberculosis bacillus spreads through the bloodstream, seeding the interstitial spaces of the lungs and producing a pattern of fine nodularity throughout the lungs—a pattern called *miliary TB* because the nodules are generally 1–3 mm in size, comparable in size to millet seeds.

CONGESTIVE HEART FAILURE, PULMONARY EDEMA, AND PLEURAL EFFUSION

Patients with congestive heart failure due to chronic coronary artery insufficiency, previous myocardial infarctions, or chronic cardiomyopathy frequently have cardiomegaly. The cardiothoracic ratio cannot be used to assess cardiomegaly on AP or supine radiographs because the heart is magnified to a greater degree than on the PA projection.

In congestive heart failure, the progression of changes in the pulmonary vascular anatomy, interstitium, and airspaces is relatively predictable based on the severity of the left ventricular dysfunction and the resulting elevation in left atrial, pulmonary venous, and pulmonary capillary pressure.

- Early in the course of progression, the pulmonary venous pressure increases, resulting in an equalization of the sizes of the upper and lower

Best Practice

The Cardiothoracic Ratio

On upright PA chest radiography, the ratio of the width of the cardiac silhouette to the widest diameter of the thorax between the inner cortical margins of the ribs (the cardiothoracic ratio) is normally less than 0.5.

lobe pulmonary veins. (Remember that, in the normal upright patient, the upper lobe veins are smaller in caliber due to the hydrostatic pressure gradient between the upper and lower lung zones.)

- With further deterioration in left ventricular function and the resulting increases in left atrial and pulmonary venous pressures, fluid begins to leak from the intravascular space into the pulmonary interstitium. This results in the thickening of the septal structures in the lung, particularly the interlobular septa.
- The thickening of the interlobular septae results in an increase in the linear markings in the lungs, which is easily appreciated in the peripheries of the lower lobes. A pattern of short, 1- to 2-cm-long lines perpendicular to the visceral pleura (Kerly B lines) may be seen.
- The accumulation of interstitial fluid may also appear as a thickening of the fissures and of the peribronchial soft tissues (peribronchial cuffing).
- Finally, with the most marked elevations of left atrial pressure, fluid begins to fill the airspaces, resulting in alveolar consolidation, often in a perihilar (batwing or butterfly) distribution.

Figure 14-26 illustrates the increased prominence of the upper lobe veins, increased linear (interstitial) markings in the central (perihilar) zones, and numerous Kerley B lines in a patient with congestive heart failure and interstitial pulmonary edema. If the patient's congestive heart failure can be effectively treated, these findings may resolve relatively rapidly. Patients with congestive heart failure also often develop pleural effusions, indicated by a rounding off or blunting of the costophrenic angles laterally or posteriorly (see Chapter 13).

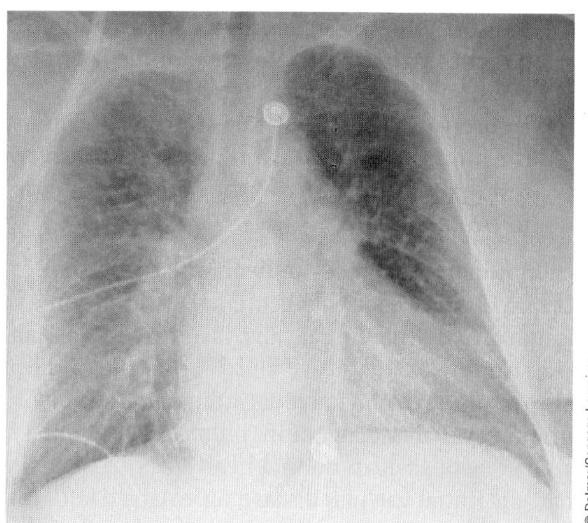

FIGURE 14-26 This patient demonstrates radiographic evidence of congestive heart failure (CHF) and interstitial pulmonary edema: increased upper lobe vascular markings, increased interstitial markings in the perihilar area, and many Kerly B lines.

Figure 14-27 illustrates a common sequence of radiographic changes in a patient with an acute myocardial infarction (a heart attack).

- Figure 14-27A was taken at the time of the patient's admission to the emergency department and shows bilateral air-space infiltrates due to acute, alveolar pulmonary edema.
- Figure 14-27B shows partial clearing of the edema but development of bilateral blunting of

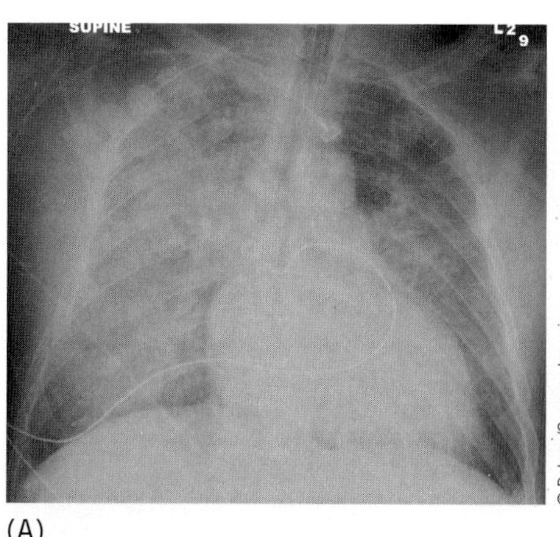

(A)

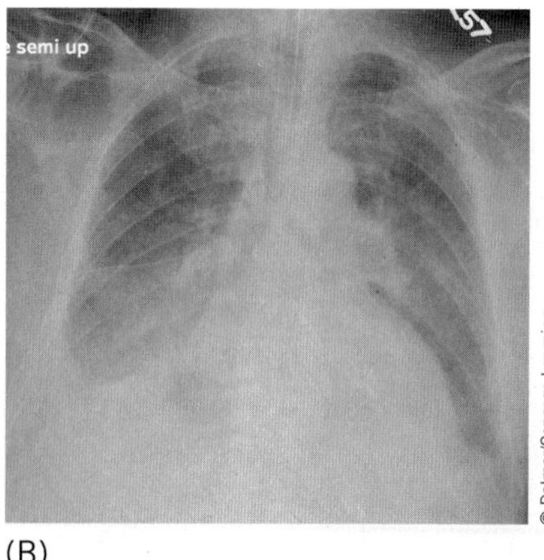

(B)

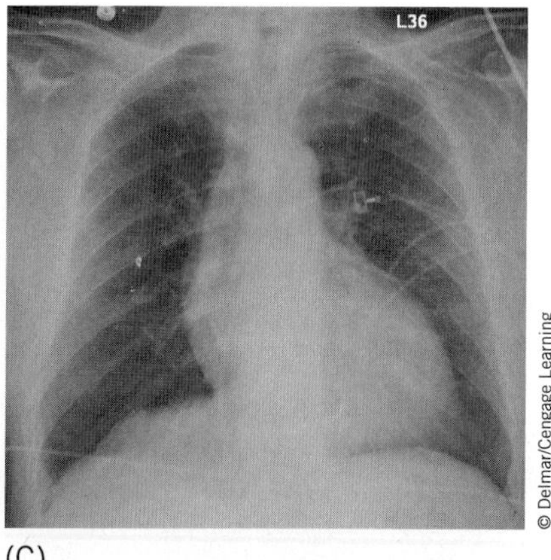

(C)

FIGURE 14-27 (A) The first of three films documenting the sequence of radiographic changes in a patient admitted to the ER with a heart attack (myocardial infarction, MI): This first film shows bilateral air-space infiltrates due to acute alevolar pulmonary edema. (B) The partial clearing of the acute pulmonary edema, but development of bilateral blunting of the costophrenic angle, which is most apparent on the right due to development of pleural effusion. (C) The clearing of the pulmonary edema and pleural effusions in response to treatment: However, there is a residual cardiomegaly (increased size of the heart).

the costophrenic angles, more apparent on the patient's right, due to the development of pleural effusions.
- Figure 14-27C demonstrates the resolution of the pulmonary edema and pleural effusions with residual cardiomegaly as the patient responded to treatment.

Pulmonary edema due to heart disease is usually associated with cardiac enlargement. However, some conditions, such as acute mitral valve insufficiency (as can be seen in rupture of a papillary muscle) or acute cardiomyopathy resulting from viral myocarditis can result in pulmonary vascular congestion, pulmonary edema, and pleural effusions with a normal heart size on chest X-ray. In chronic mitral valvular disease, an enlarged left atrium is frequently seen in association with the changes of vascular congestion and pulmonary edema.

PNEUMOTHORAX

A *pneumothorax* occurs when air enters the pleural space, allowing the lung on the affected side to collapse. Pneumothoraces, particularly small ones, are easy to miss on a chest X-ray if the study is not carefully reviewed. The signs of a pneumothorax are the presence of a radio-dense visceral pleural line that separates the lung, with its normal vascular and interstitial marking from the air-containing pleural space. Obviously, the air in the pleural space lacks the vascular and interstitial markings and soft tissue components of a normal lung. So it appears more radiolucent than the adjacent lung, as illustrated by Figure 14-28, which shows a moderate left pneumothorax. The detection of a pneumothorax may be difficult due to its size or the presence of other conditions, particularly the presence of air in the chest wall, a condition called **subcutaneous emphysema**. Careful examination of Figure 14-29 reveals that, in addition to the moderate right pneumothorax, there is a striped, or striated, pattern of alternating bands of density and lucency, best seen over the right costophrenic angle. This striated appearance is one of the radiographic signs of subcutaneous emphysema.

The identification of pneumothoraces on supine radiographs is also problematic unless the reader searches for specific features. A classic indicator in a supine image is the *deep sulcus sign*—the extension of the pneumothorax into the nondependent portions of the costophrenic sulcus, resulting in a deep and more radiolucent costophrenic angle on the involved side. Figure 14-30 illustrates a deep sulcus sign in the left costophrenic angle in a patient who suffered a small-caliber gunshot wound to the left chest. Another, often very subtle, finding is increased lucency either in the region of the diaphragm on the involved side or along the heart border or adjacent to the mediastinum.

It is easy to underestimate the size of a pneumothorax if the reader considers only the distance between the edge of the lung and the chest wall. Significant portions of the pneumothorax may be located anterior or posterior to the lung, and they may not be well appreciated on a single AP or PA view. The lateral view of a chest radiograph, if available, should also be used

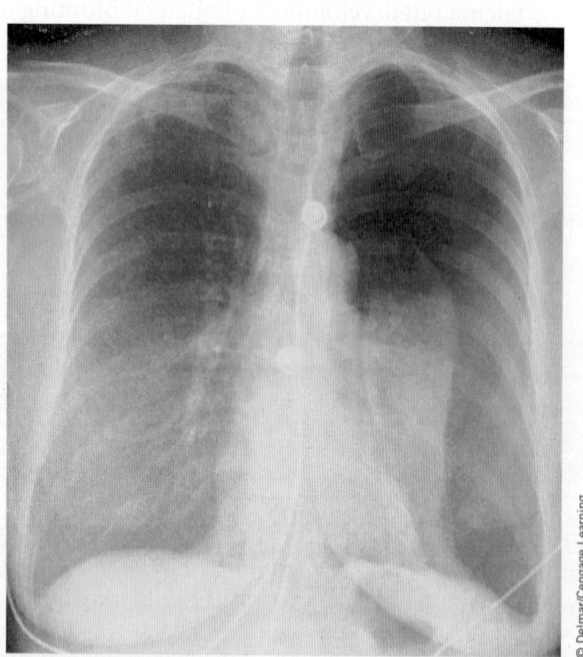

FIGURE 14-28 A moderate left pneumothorax.

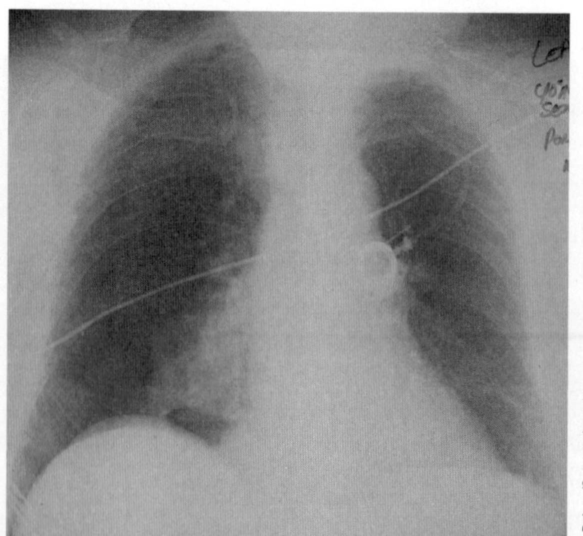

FIGURE 14-29 A right pneumothorax of moderate size and what appears to be subcutaneous emphysema over the right costophrenic angle (appearing as a striped light and dark pattern).

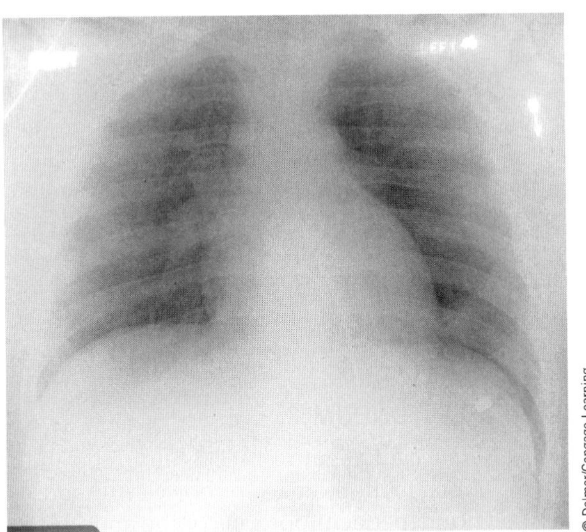

FIGURE 14-30 A supine view of a patient who was shot in the left chest with a small-caliber gun. Note the prominent costophrenic angle on the left side as compared to the right side, illustrating a pneumothorax.

in estimating the size and location of a pneumothorax. CT scanning is much more sensitive at identifying and estimating the volume of a pneumothorax than is a radiograph. CT should be used in questionable cases and when the severity of the patient's clinical condition is disproportionate to the apparent size of the pneumothorax on the radiograph.

TENSION PNEUMOTHORAX

In a *tension pneumothorax* (see Chapter 11), the air in the pleural space results in an increase in enough intrapleural and/or intrathoracic pressure to affect the function of other organs, particularly the heart. They can occur from a variety of injuries to the lung or chest wall, but they are particularly common in penetrating trauma, such as stab wounds. Wounds of this type often result in a one-way, or flap, valve at the tissue defect. During inspiration, air is pulled into the pleural space by the negative intrathoracic pressure, but on expiration, the tissues surrounding the wound draw together, closing the defect and preventing air from leaving the pleural space. Over multiple respiratory cycles, air progressively accumulates, intrapleural and intrathoracic pressures progressively increase, and a tension pneumothorax evolves.

Another common setting for tension pneumothorax is in ventilated patients who require significant positive pressures to maintain oxygenation. Tension pneumothoraces tend to result in the kinking and/or compression of the superior and inferior vena cava, leading to decreased venous return to the heart, decreased cardiac output, shock, and, in untreated cases, death.

Whenever pneumothorax is identified on imaging, the interpretation should include a comment on whether there is evidence of tension. Signs of a tension pneumothorax (Figure 14-31A) include flattening or

Best Practice

Pneumothorax

A pneumothorax should be assumed to exist until proved otherwise in any patient in whom subcutaneous emphysema (air under the skin) is seen or in whom abnormal lucencies (clear areas) are seen overlying the lung or mediastinum.

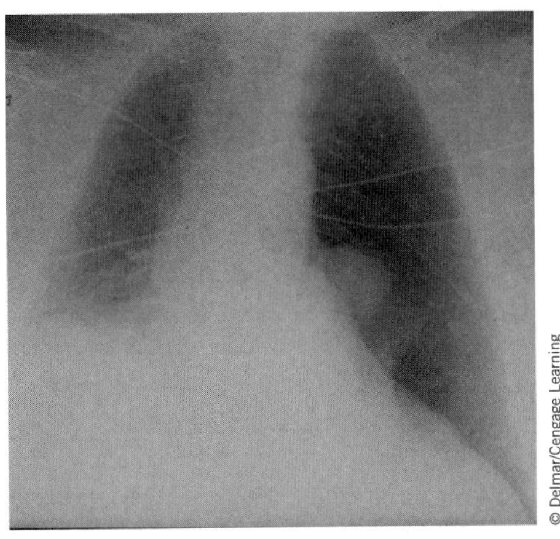

(A)

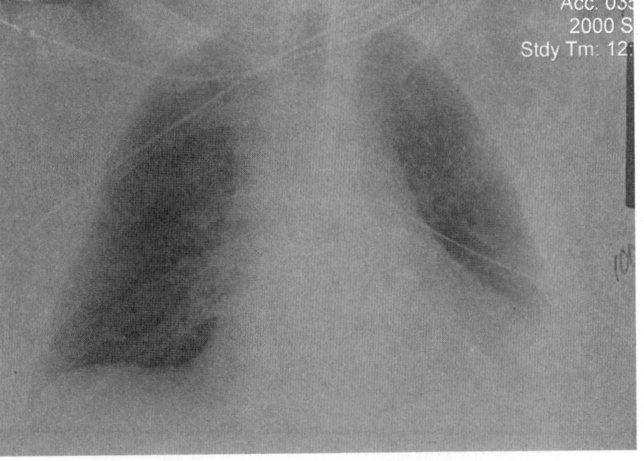

(B)

FIGURE 14-31 (A) A patient with a tension pneumothorax: The film exhibits a tracheal, cardiac, and mediastinal shift toward the unaffected (contralateral) lung. (B) The treatment of a pneumothorax with the insertion of a chest tube: This film shows the almost complete reexpansion of the lung.

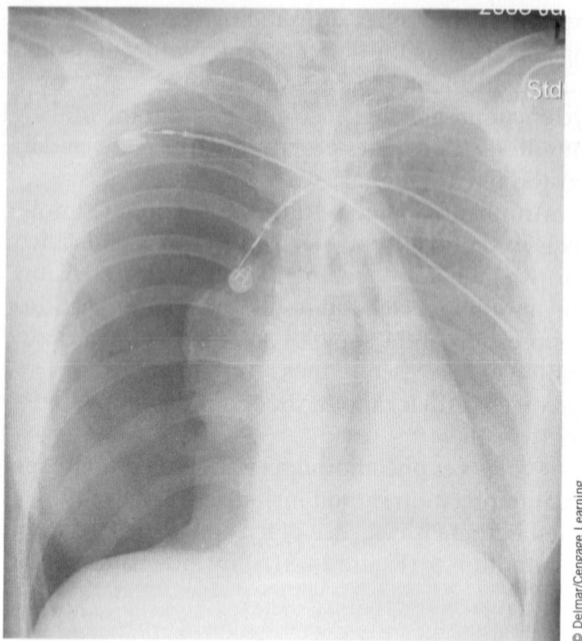

FIGURE 14-32 A right tension pneumothorax with marked widening of the ICSs and bulging of the parital pleura between the ribs: Note the shift of the heart, mediastinal structures, and the trachea to the right.

even inversion of the diaphragm on the side of the pneumothorax and a shift of the trachea, mediastinum, and heart away from the side of the pneumothorax. Other findings of a tension pneumothorax are illustrated in Figure 14-32, the radiograph of a patient with a right pneumothorax. Note the marked widening of the intercostal spaces and bulging of the parietal pleura between the ribs in addition to the shift of the trachea, mediastinum, and heart from right to left.

A tension pneumothorax is treated by the prompt placement of a chest tube (thoracostomy) (Figure 14-31B), which generally results in rapid resolution of the hemodynamic instability attributable to increased intrathoracic pressure. In Figure 14-31B, note the marked decrease in the size of the pneumothorax and the nearly complete reexpansion of the collapsed left lung.

Two final notes about tension pneumothoraces:

- Be aware that the degree of collapse of the lung on the involved side has no reliable correlation to the degree of elevation of the intrapleural pressure, especially in ventilated patients or those with underlying lung disease. Pulmonary edema, fibrosis, and other conditions decrease the tendency of the lung to collapse completely, and the positive ventilatory pressure tends to keep the lung inflated, leading to the paradoxical situation of a tension pneumothorax with relatively limited collapse of the lung. In patients with underlying lung disease, even small pneumothoraces can lead to a life-threatening elevation in intrathoracic pressure.
- In those uncommon cases of bilateral tension pneumothoraces, the heart tends to be small and the diaphragm is pushed down far below its normal position. However, the mediastinum may or may not be shifted, depending on the relative pressures in the two pleura.

PNEUMOPERITONEUM

A *pneumoperitoneum* (Figure 14-33) is air in the abdominal cavity outside the stomach or bowel. Air tends to rise to the nondependent portions of the abdomen; so this condition is typically diagnosed on an upright abdominal or chest radiograph, appearing as increased radiolucency due to gas between the diaphragm and liver or other upper abdominal organs. In these cases, the diaphragm appears as a thin, soft tissue density arc separated from the liver and other organs by a lucent crescent representing the free gas. As with pneumothoraces, the identification of a pneumoperitoneum on a supine radiograph is problematic. Consequently, in patients who cannot stand or sit upright, it may be necessary to resort to lateral decubitus views, with the patient lying on the side and the X-ray beam parallel to the exam table, to evaluate for the presence or absence of free gas.

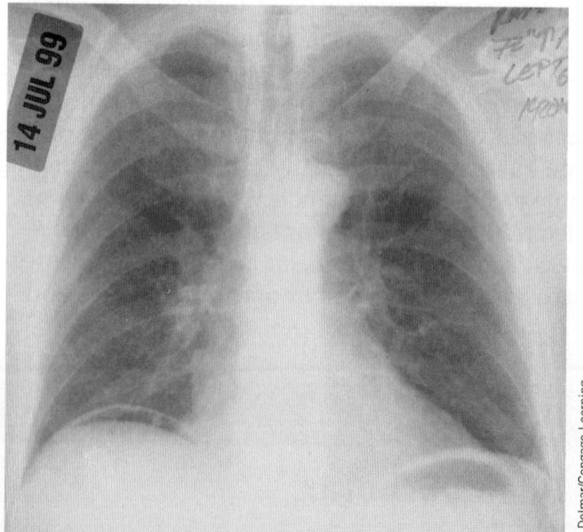

FIGURE 14-33 An upright abdominal pneumoperitoneum caused by free gas or air in the abdominal cavity: The preferred technique for these pictures are either an upright abdominal or chest X-ray. Note the increased lucency of the film due to the presence of gas.

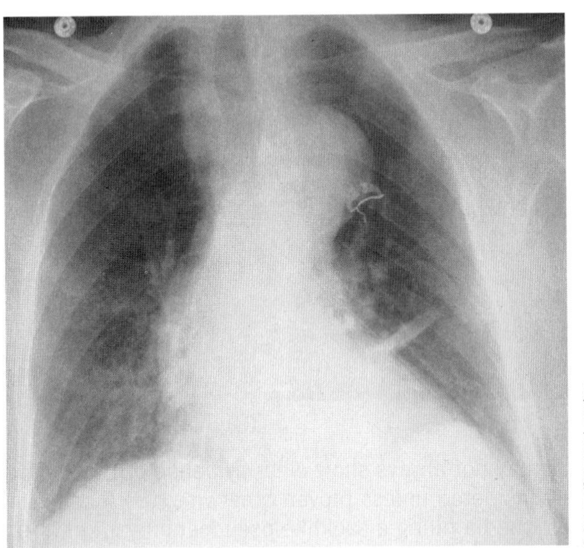

FIGURE 14-34 Enlargement of the thoracic aortic arch indicating a thoracic aortic aneurysm.

AORTIC ANEURYSM, AORTIC DISSECTION, AND TRAUMATIC AORTIC INJURIES

An *aortic aneurysm* is an abnormal dilatation, or ballooning, of the aorta. The wall of the aneurysm includes all three histological layers—tunica intima, tunica media, and tunica adventitia—that normally make up the wall of the aorta. Figure 14-34 is a chest radiograph on a patient with a thoracic aortic aneurysm showing the abnormal enlargement of the aortic arch.

An *aortic dissection* is a separation of the inner layer of the aortic wall (the intima) from the other two layers (media and adventitia) by a false channel of flowing or clotted blood. Figure 14-35 is an image from a CT scan on a patient with a dissection of the ascending thoracic aorta showing the thin, soft-tissue lucency of the so-called intimal flap outlined by the opacified blood in the true and false lumens of the dissection.

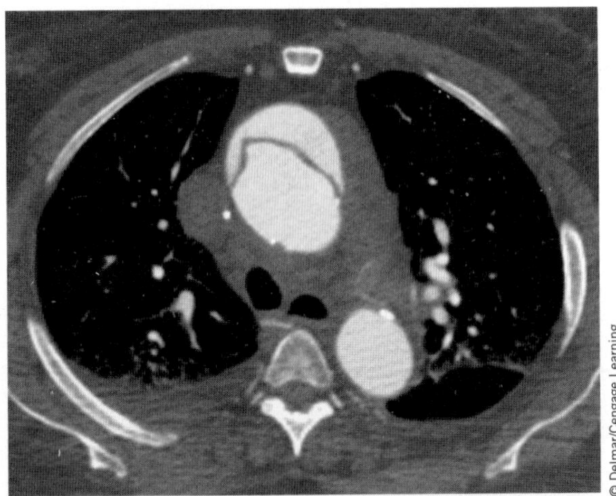

FIGURE 14-35 A CT scan of a patient with a dissecting ascending thoracic aorta aneurysm. These conditions can rapidly become life-threatening.

Aneurysms and dissections are two distinct pathologic entities, but they frequently coexist. Both are often related to underlying atherosclerosis. Clinically, aortic aneurysms are often silent and discovered in the course of a workup for other conditions, particularly coronary artery disease. In contrast, aortic dissections often present as severe, acute chest pain. The radiographic findings in both conditions are often relatively unimpressive, particularly in the case of aortic dissection where aortic dilatation may not be a feature. Although large aneurysms may appear as a dilatation of the involved segment of the thoracic aorta, many small, though clinically significant, aneurysms may produce no apparent radiographic changes.

High-speed trauma or crush injuries of the chest may produce a range of *traumatic aortic injuries*, including intimal laceration, traumatic dissections, transmural lacerations (tears), and posttraumatic aortic pseudoaneurysms.

- *Intimal lacerations* are focal defects in the inner lining of the aorta that are usually radiographically occult, though they can be symptomatic particularly if they are associated with local thrombosis and arterial occlusion.
- *Traumatic dissections* are simply separations of the intima from the media by a false lumen in the setting of trauma.
- *Transmural lacerations* are tears of the wall of the aorta that involve all three layers.
- *Aortic pseudoaneurysms* are formed when a traumatic laceration or other through-and-through injury of the aortic wall is contained by the surrounding mediastinal soft tissues and hematoma (Figure 14-36).

Chest radiographs in patients with traumatic aortic injuries are usually unimpressive, but some show a widening of the superior mediastinum and the loss of definition of the aortic arch (Figure 14-36A). CT scanning has now become the gold standard for the initial diagnosis of traumatic aortic injuries. It is capable of demonstrating the full range of findings from relatively subtle, isolated intimal injuries to obvious complete lacerations of the aorta with their associated hematomas and pseudoaneurysms. Figure 14-36B is an image from the CT scan obtained on the patient with the widened mediastinum illustrated in Figure 14-36A, showing contrast filling a saccular pseudoaneurysm anterior to the proximal descending aorta surrounded by the soft-tissue density of the associated hematoma. Many thoracic surgeons

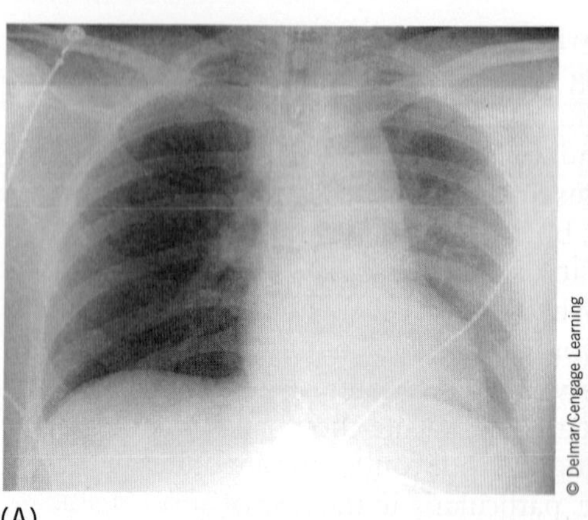
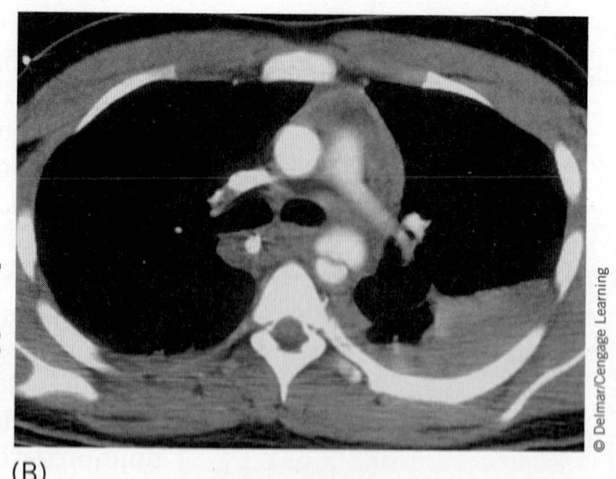
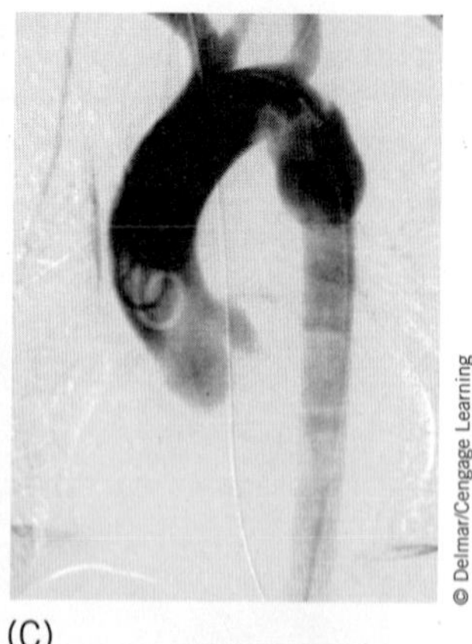

(A) (B) (C)

FIGURE 14-36 (A) Chest X-rays of patients with traumatic aortic injury may not always show clear evidence of those injuries. But in all cases of high-velocity or crush trauma, they must be considered unless proven otherwise. (B) A contrast CT of the patient shown in the previous figure: The CT shows contrast media filling a sacklike pseudoaneurysm in front of the proximal descending thoracic aorta. The hazy area around the sack is a hematoma for the aortic leak. (C) A single frame of the associated thoracic aortogram: The aneurysm shown in "C" (right upper darkness at the top of the long tube-like structure is the pseudoaneurysm. In "B" it shows as the white projection in the right side of the chest – note the light gray chicken leg shaped object.

have become accustomed to taking patients directly to surgery based on the CT diagnosis of a traumatic aortic injury. However, aortography, which can show the detail of intimal injuries, dissections, and pseudoaneurysms, still has a role, particularly in patients who are candidates for endovascular stent grafting—a relatively new technique that involves placing tubular grafts in the lumen of the aorta via a catheter placed in the femoral artery and advanced to the site of the injury. Figure 14-36C is a single frame from a thoracic aortogram that demonstrates the pseudoaneurysm initially diagnosed on the CT image (Figure 14-36B).

Best Practice

Thoracic Trauma

Traumatic aortic injuries, particularly aortic tears and pseudoaneurysms, are life-threatening conditions with exceptionally high mortality rates if they are undiagnosed. The vast majority of patients who are undiagnosed and/or untreated are dead within 7–10 days of their trauma. Occasionally, patients beat these odds and survive for extended periods, as illustrated by the patient whose CT (Figure 14-37A) and aortogram (Figure 14-37B) shows a chronic pseudoaneurysm nearly 5 years after his chest injury. Traumatic aortic injuries should be suspected in all cases of significant chest trauma, especially in moderate- to high-speed motor vehicle collisions.

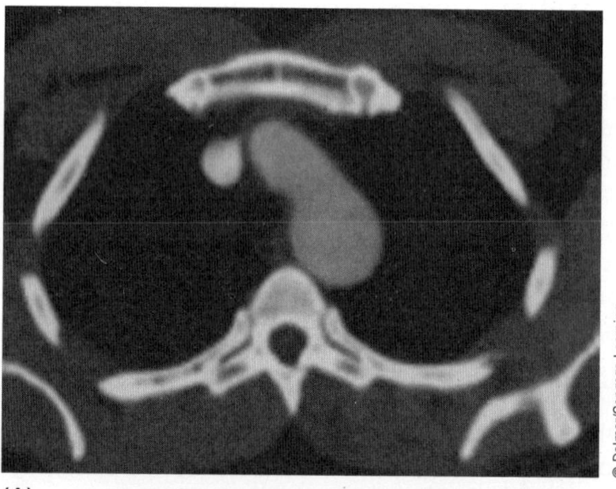

(A)

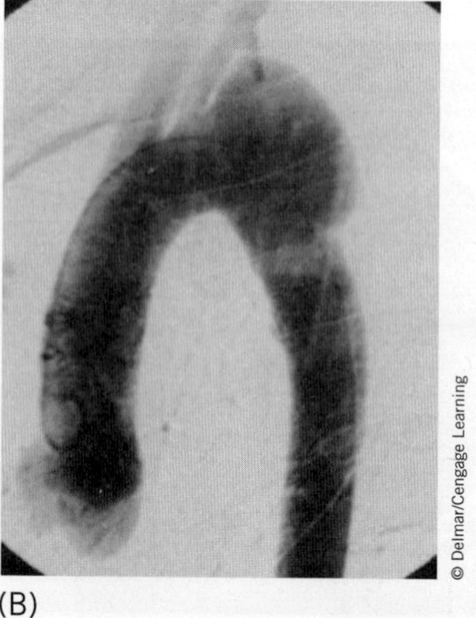

(B)

FIGURE 14-37 A 5-year follow-up of the patient from Figures 14-36A–C. (A) The follow-up CT. (B) The 5-year post–chest trauma single frame of his aortogram.

PULMONARY THROMBOEMBOLISM

In *pulmonary thromboembolism*, or more simply *pulmonary embolism* (*PE*), blood clots that have formed in a peripheral vein break free and migrate through the right atrium and right ventricle to lodge in one or more branches of the pulmonary artery. Risk factors for the development of pulmonary emboli include prolonged bed rest and immobilization. Patients with acute pulmonary emboli often present with chest pain, shortness of breath, and rapid breathing. Pulse oximetry or arterial blood gas analysis generally shows significantly decreased levels of arterial oxygen (hypoxemia).

The most common site of origin of pulmonary emboli is in the deep veins of the legs. Although preventive measures, such as early mobilization after surgery, the use of compression stockings or pneumatic compression devices, and/or the use of anticoagulants such as heparin, are widely used in high-risk patients, pulmonary embolism is a significant, often preventable, cause of increased morbidity and mortality among hospitalized patients.

The most common radiographic presentation of an acute pulmonary embolism is a normal chest X-ray. However, other types of medical imaging play a central role in the diagnosis of this condition. Until recently, the primary diagnostic imaging technique was ventilation/perfusion lung scanning. In patients with pulmonary emboli, the ventilation portion of the study remains relatively normal while the perfusion images show one or more areas of decreased activity in the pulmonary segments that are deprived of blood flow by the blockages in their arterial supply. Figure 14-38A is the ventilation study from a patient with proven acute pulmonary emboli showing the preservation of normal distribution of the inhaled xenon gas. Figure 14-38B is the perfusion study from the same patient showing numerous areas of little or no activity in the portions of the lungs where blood flow has been cut off by clots that occlude branches of the pulmonary arteries.

The development of multidetector, helical, or spiral CT scanning has significantly altered the radiologic workup of patients with suspected pulmonary emboli. So-called *CT angiograms* can now be prepared that are of sufficient quality to detect emboli directly. In addition, the CT study for pulmonary embolism takes significantly less time than that required for preparing and administering the radioisotopes in $\dot{V}/\dot{Q}$ scanning. A CT pulmonary angiogram is obtained by scanning the patient while a bolus of intravenous contrast is injected. The scan is timed in such a way as to obtain images during peak opacification of the pulmonary arteries. On CT angiography, pulmonary emboli appear as low-attenuation (darker) filling defects outlined by the more attenuating (lighter) contrast containing blood in the pulmonary arterial bed. Figure 14-38C is an axial CT image in a patient with a large, acute

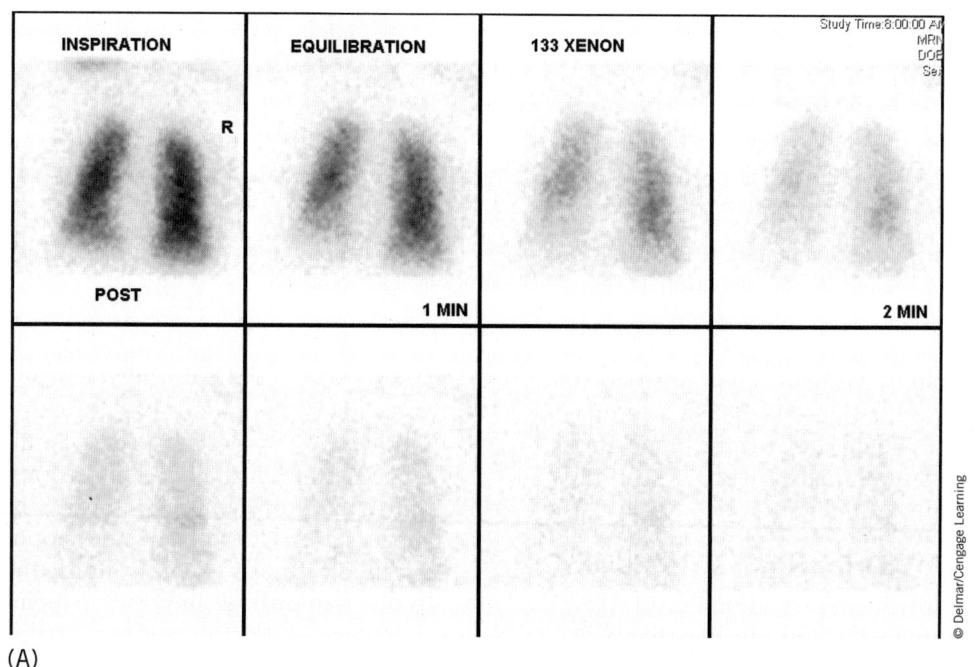

(A)

FIGURE 14-38 (A) The ventilation scan of a patient with a known history of pulmonary emboli: The radioactive gas distribution appears normal. (*continues*)

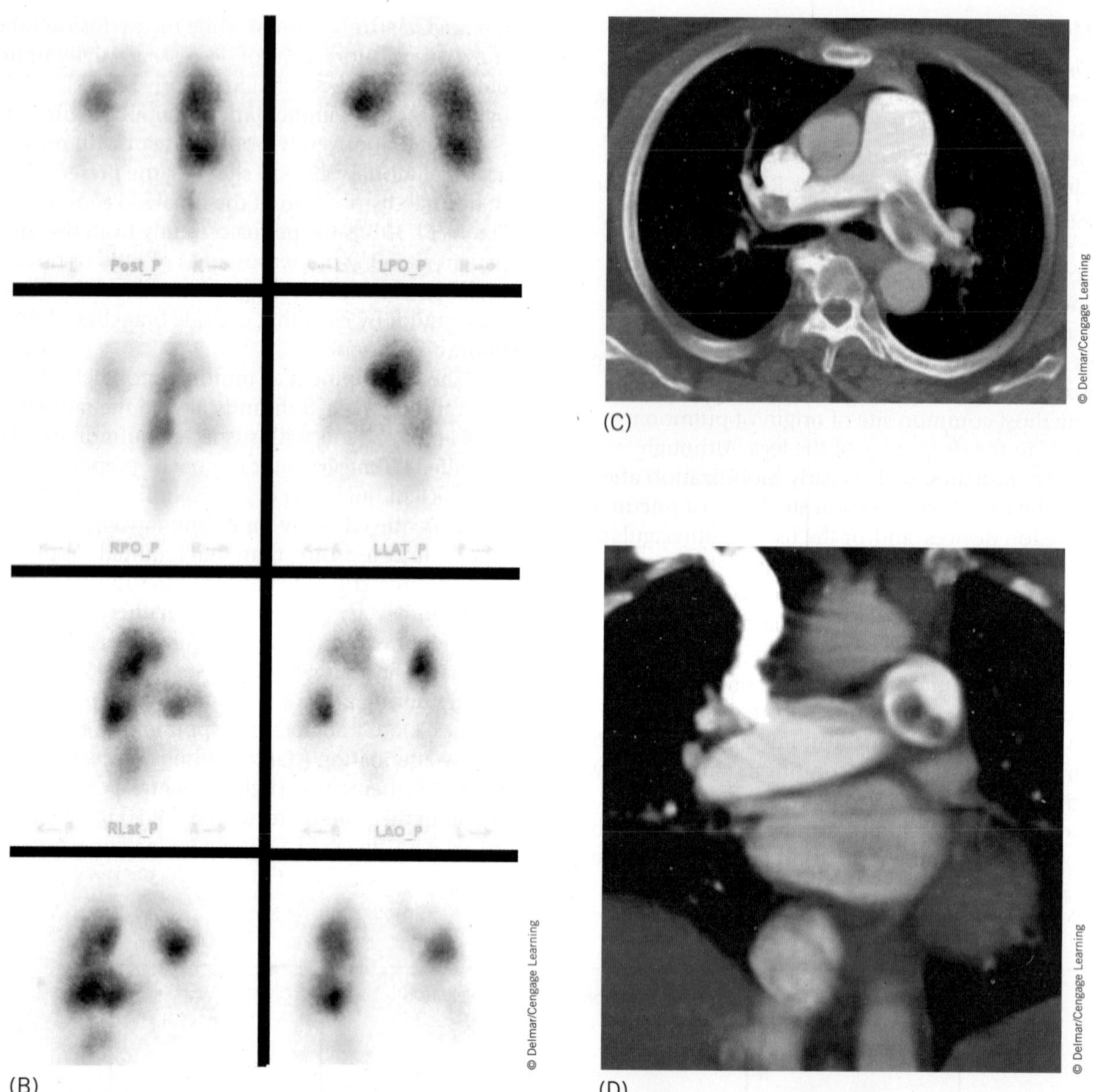

FIGURE 14-38 (B) The perfusion study of the same patient: Areas of the lung show very poor perfusion secondary to the emboli blocking branches of the pulmonary circulation. A comparison of the two images reveals areas of $\dot{V}/\dot{Q}$ mismatch. (C) An axial CT image of a bilateral pulmonary artery emboli. (D) A coronal CT image of the left pulmonary artery portion of the emboli described in C.

pulmonary embolus that involves both the right and left pulmonary arteries. Figure 14-38D is a coronal CT image of the same patient showing the branching embolus in the left pulmonary artery.

ADULT RESPIRATORY DISTRESS SYNDROME

The adult respiratory distress syndrome (ARDS) is commonly encountered in critically ill patients. Virtually any systemic insult can result in the development of ARDS, common ones being trauma, shock, sepsis, aspiration, or pneumonia. The clinical features are severe shortness of breath, tachypnea, refractory hypoxemia, and more-or-less diffuse pulmonary infiltrates on the chest X-ray. ARDS inflicts diffuse damage at the alveolar level in the lung parenchyma. As a result of the damage to the alveolar wall, the airspaces in the early stage of development are flooded with fluid (alveolar edema). Shortly thereafter, areas of alveolar hemorrhage and hyaline membrane formation can be seen on microscopic examination.

Should the patient survive the initial period of respiratory failure, the lung attempts to heal itself. However, for reasons that are not clearly understood,

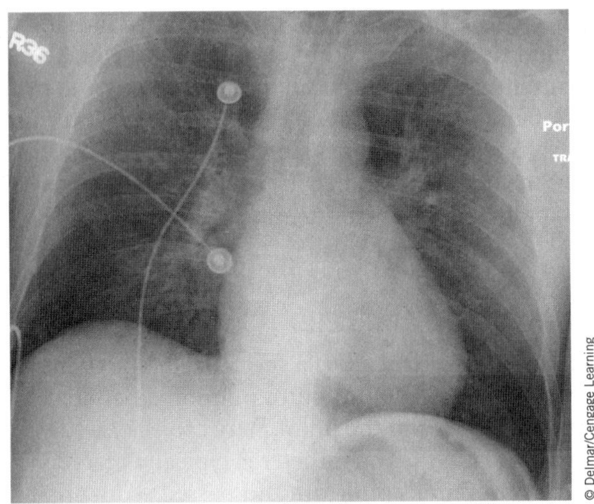

FIGURE 14-39 The ground glass appearance of a patient with early stage acute respiratory distress syndrome (ARDS) 48 hours after the initial symptoms were noted.

the reparative process is unchecked and the involved portions of the lung develop fibrosis and scarring. The fibrotic stage of the disease can be severe enough to result in permanent impairment lung function. Figure 14-39 shows the diffuse, so-called ground-glass infiltrates of the earliest stage of ARDS in a trauma patient that, over the course of the first 48 hours in the intensive care unit, developed progressive and refractory hypoxemia, ultimately requiring intubation.

Device Positioning

The chest radiographs and CT scans in this section demonstrate the positions of thoracic tubes, lines, catheters, and medical or surgical appliances or devices. Some of these illustrate correct positioning and placement; others show misplaced or dislodged devices.

ENDOTRACHEAL TUBES

Radiographs are two-dimensional representations of three-dimensional structures. Do not assume that an endotracheal tube overlying the trachea is actually in the trachea. Normally, the esophagus lies just behind the trachea, and an esophageal intubation can be missed on an AP radiograph. A lateral view is diagnostic because it shows an appropriately positioned endotracheal tube overlying the air filled cervical segment of the airway, whereas a tube in the esophagus lies posterior to the trachea. Frequently, the initial placement of an endotracheal tube is too deep, resulting in intubation of one of the main bronchi. In these cases, the tube tends to be directed into the right rather

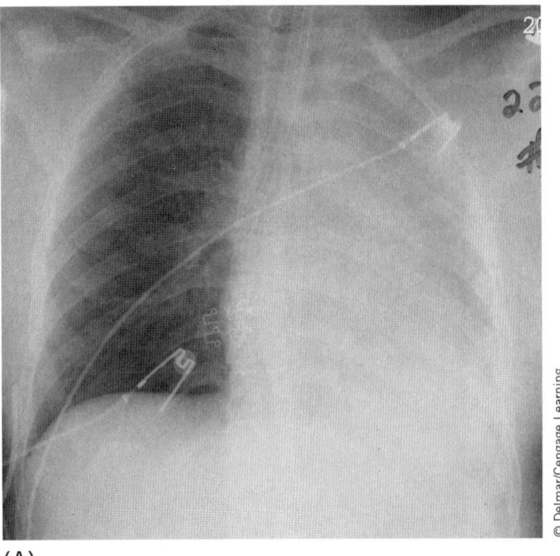

(A)

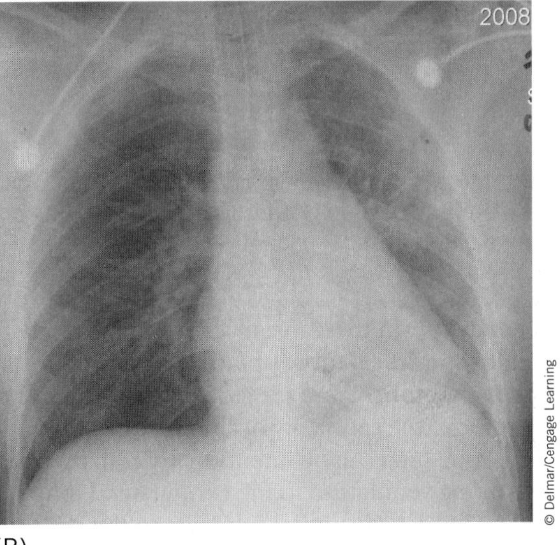

(B)

FIGURE 14-40 (A) A misplaced endotracheal tube: This is a right mainstem bronchus. The left lung is not being ventilated. (B) The same patient after the endotracheal tube has been repositioned to the correct position.

than the left bronchus due to its more vertical course from the carina. Figure 14-40A shows misplacement of an endotracheal (ET) tube with intubation of the right bronchus, resulting in atelectasis of the unventilated left lung. Figure 14-40B shows the same patient after repositioning of the ET tube so that its tip is at an appropriate level in the trachea with nearly complete resolution of the atelectasis on the left. These images were obtained 15 minutes apart, illustrating the transitory nature of atelectasis when the cause of the volume loss is identified and treated.

In some patients, usually those undergoing cardiac or pulmonary surgery, the lungs need to be ventilated

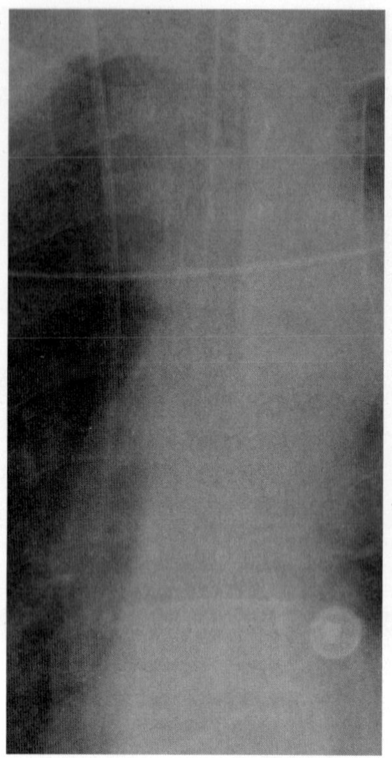

FIGURE 14-41 A double lumen endotracheal tube, which is used when it is desirable to either isolate one lung or to ventilate one lung independently from the other.

independently. In these instances, a special, dual-lumen endotracheal tube is placed with its tip in one of the main bronchi and the side port of the second lumen above the carina. By occluding one of the lumens, one lung can be intentionally collapsed while maintaining ventilation to the contralateral lung, allowing improved surgical exposure to the structures on the side of the collapsed lung. Figure 14-41 shows a double-lumen endotracheal tube with its tip in the left main bronchus.

When using cuffed endotracheal tubes, pay attention to the tube cuff. If cuff inflation is maintained with too great a pressure, erosion or necrosis of the tracheal wall can occur. A sign that suggests overinflation or necrosis is the bulging of the contour of the cuff beyond the margins of the tracheal air-shadow. The occurrence of this complication has been reduced by the use of endotracheal tubes designed with low-pressure cuffs. In patients with a history of prolonged intubation, tracheal stenosis may be apparent as a narrowing or tapering of the subglottic tracheal air-shadow.

Best Practice

Endotracheal Tube Placement

Ideally, the distal tip of an endotracheal tube should be at least 1–2 cm above the carina. If the carina cannot be visualized, the top of the aortic arch or between the fourth and sixth thoracic vertebra are good landmarks for placement of the tip in adults.

SWAN-GANZ CATHETERS

A **Swan-Ganz catheter** is a specialized type of intravascular catheter used to monitor pulmonary arterial pressure (PAP) and the pulmonary capillary wedge pressure (PCWP). The catheter is typically placed via a subclavian venous puncture and passed sequentially through the innominate vein, superior vena cava, right atrium, right ventricle, pulmonary outflow tract, and pulmonary artery. The unwedged catheter may be left in place for several hours or days as a means of assessing how much the pulmonary edema is due to cardiac failure (elevated pulmonary capillary wedge pressure) or to noncardiac factors (normal wedge pressure).

When the wedge pressure is measured, the tip of the catheter is advanced, often with the assistance of a floatation balloon incorporated into the distal portion of the catheter, until the tip of the catheter occludes a small pulmonary artery branch and a relatively flat, nonpulsatile pressure tracing, characteristic of the capillary wedge pressure, is obtained. Once the capillary pressure is obtained, the catheter is withdrawn so that its tip is in the more proximal pulmonary artery. In the parked position, the tip of the catheter should be no more than 2–4 cm beyond the margin of the hilum. Figure 14-42 shows a Swan-Ganz catheter placed, via the right jugular vein, passing:

- Caudally to the level of the right atrium.
- Across the tricuspid valve and out the pulmonary outflow tract.
- Through the pulmonic valve and main pulmonary artery into the right pulmonary artery.
- Parked with its tip projected over the right hilum.

NASOGASTRIC TUBES AND FEEDING TUBES

Nasogastric (NG) tubes should be positioned so that their tips and all side holes are below the gastroesophageal junction. A nasogastric tube with its tip or one or more of its side holes in the esophagus does nothing to alleviate symptoms related to gastroesophageal reflux or to lessen the risk of aspiration. Feeding tubes are positioned with their tips either in the stomach or duodenum, depending on the particular medications or feeding solutions.

Best Practice

Placement of the Swan-Ganz Catheter

Failure to park the catheter in a more proximal position can result in thrombosis of a branch artery to a portion of the lung and pulmonary infarction. Figure 14-43 demonstrates a Swan-Ganz catheter with its tip parked in too peripheral a location. Note also the unusual course of the catheter due to the patient having a left-sided superior vena cava. If the catheter is inserted too far or if the balloon is inflated while the catheter is in its wedged position, pulmonary artery perforations, pulmonary hemorrhage, or a pulmonary artery aneurysm can occur. Figure 14-44 is a CT image from a patient with acute hemoptysis following removal of a peripherally inflated Swan-Ganz catheter; it shows opacification of a pulmonary artery pseudoaneurysm in the medial right lower lobe, surrounded by an area of consolidation due to pulmonary hemorrhage. On the other hand, pulling the catheter so far back that its tip is in the right ventricle may cause arrhythmias, injury, or even perforation of the right ventricular wall.

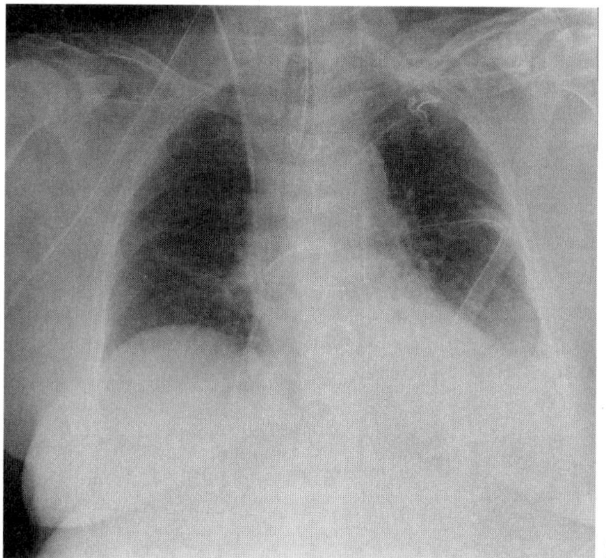

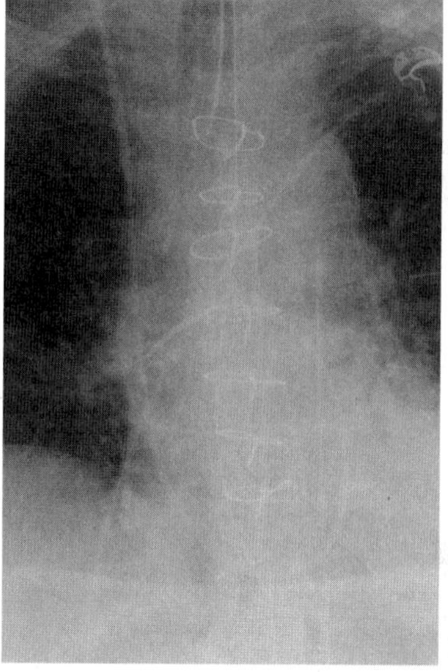

FIGURE 14-42 A Swan-Ganz catheter placed in the right jugular vein and threaded through the heart into the right pulmonary artery.

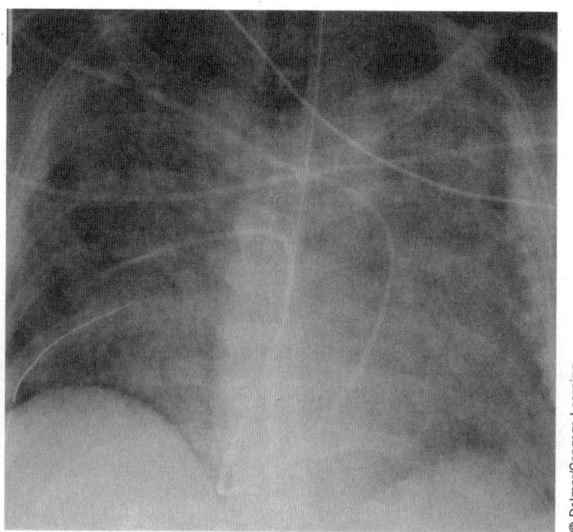

FIGURE 14-43 A Swan-Ganz catheter that was advanced too far: Note the abnormal position of the superior vena cava, which is on the left rather than on the right.

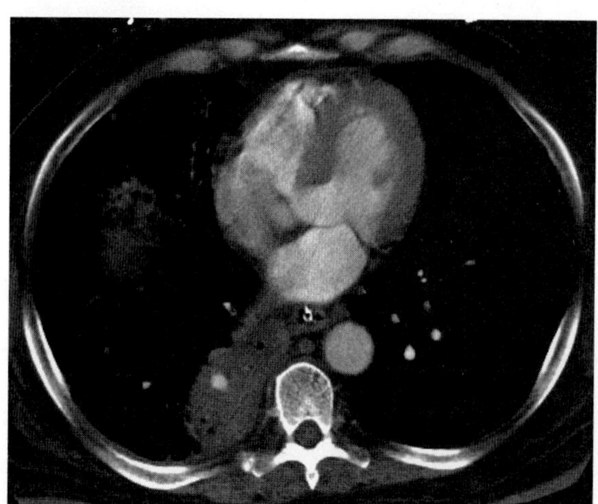

FIGURE 14-44 A CT of a pulmonary artery pseudo aneurysm following a Swan-Ganz catheter being placed too far into the pulmonary artery.

Best Practice

Placement of a Nasogastric Tube

Radiographic confirmation of appropriate NG or feeding tube placement is important because occasionally the tube is inadvertently placed in the trachea or advanced into a more peripheral bronchus.

Misplacements are generally easy to identify by chest radiography. Failure to confirm appropriate placement, especially of tubes being used for feeding or medication, can result in *iatrogenic* (resulting from medical care) aspiration pneumonia. Figure 14-45 is a radiograph that demonstrates both appropriate positioning of a nasogastric tube, which loops in the gastric fundus, and inappropriate positioning of a feeding tube, which is directed into the right lower lobe bronchus.

CHEST TUBES

Chest (*thoracostomy*) *tubes* are inserted to drain and remove fluids and gases from the pleural space. During their placement, an attempt may be made to direct the

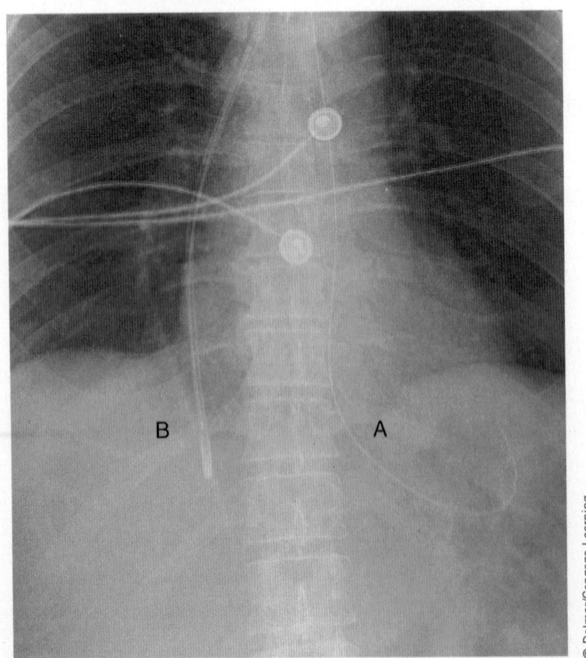

FIGURE 14-45 A: A correctly positioned nasogastric (NG) tube. B: An incorrectly placed feeding tube. Note the feeding tube is in the right lower lobe bronchus.

Best Practice

Placement of a Chest Tube

The placement of a chest tube should always be checked by chest X-ray. Figure 14-46 shows a left chest tube in a patient treated for a left tension pneumothorax. Note the extensive subcutaneous emphysema.

position of the tube tip since a final location in the upper portion (apex) of the pleural space is advantageous for the evacuation of a pneumothorax. On the other hand, a position in the posterior, lower pleural space or costophrenic angle aids in the drainage of fluid.

AORTIC BALLOON PUMPS

Intra-aortic balloon pumps are specialized balloon catheters that are placed from a femoral artery approach and positioned in the descending thoracic aorta. The inflation of the balloon is timed to occur during diastole, when the aortic valve is closed, to decrease the amount of pressure that the left ventricle must work against while improving diastolic perfusion of the coronary arteries. A radiopaque, metallic marker is embedded in the tip of the catheter and should be positioned in the proximal descending aorta, just below the aortic notch. On chest X-rays obtained during diastole, the inflated balloon can be seen as a cylindrical lucency within the descending aorta (Figure 14-47).

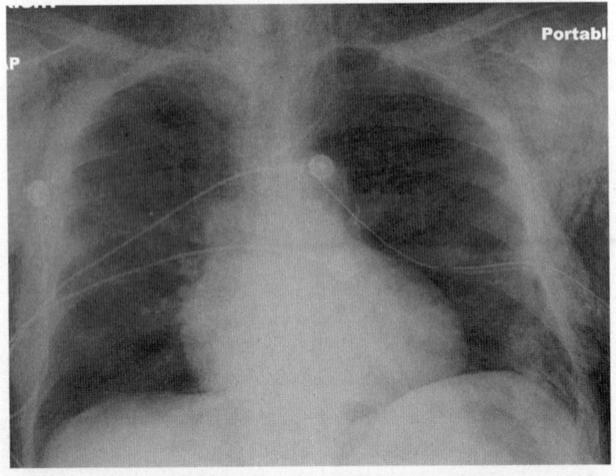

FIGURE 14-46 A chest drainage tube in the left chest: The patient is being treated for a left tension pneumothorax. Note the position of the tube relative to the patient's anatomy and the large area of subcutaneous emphysema.

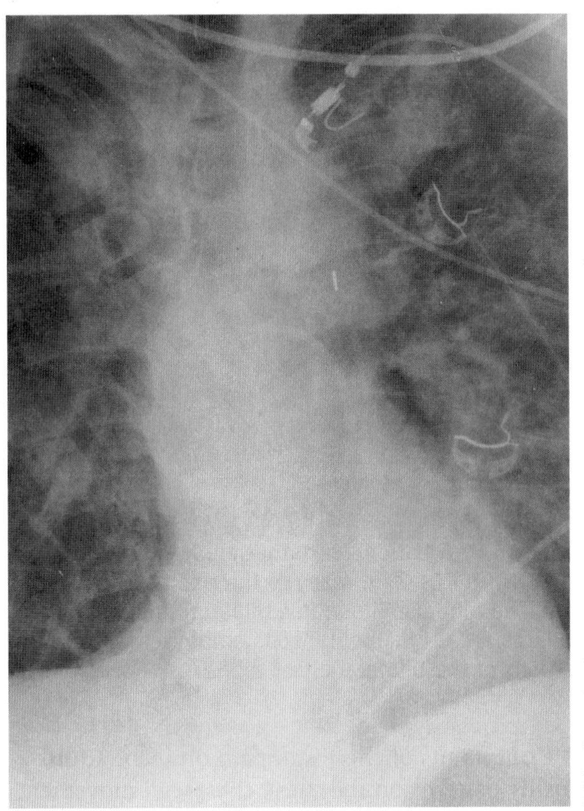

FIGURE 14-47 An aortic balloon pump catheter with its tip properly placed distal to the aortic notch: These devices are also known as *ventricular assist devices.*

INTERNAL CARDIAC PACEMAKERS AND DEFIBRILLATORS

Internally placed cardiac pacemakers and defibrillators are among the most common implanted devices encountered in the outpatient setting. *Pacemakers* are used to control the rhythm of the heart. Internal *defibrillators* are programmed to shock the heart back into a regular rhythm when the normal electrical signals controlling the heartbeat become disorganized, as in ventricular fibrillation. The leads for these devices are generally threaded from the subclavian vein, through the superior vena cava and into the right atrium. Depending on the condition being treated, the tips of one or more electrodes may be placed in the right atrium, right ventricle, and/or coronary sinus (for left ventricular pacing). Internal defibrillators generally have two leads that are distinguished from simple pacemaker leads by additional coils along segments of the atrial and ventricular leads. These units are powered and controlled by a battery and microchip contained in a battery pack that is implanted in the subcutaneous tissues of the chest wall. Today, many of these devices combine the functions of a pacemaker and a defibrillator.

Chest radiographs are routinely used to confirm the placement of the electrodes and to evaluate for broken leads in patients who experience implant failures. One of the possible pitfalls in the interpretation of chest films of patients with pacemakers or defibrillators is that portions of the lung are obscured by their battery packs. Consequently, the reader could miss subtle or slowly developing lesions in the lung beneath the battery packs. Such a case is shown in Figure 14-48. The initial chest X-ray (Figure 14-48A) shows four electrodes: one defibrillator electrode each in the right atrium and the right ventricle, an additional right ventricular pacemaker electrode, and a pacemaker electrode in the coronary sinus. The battery pack is overlying the left upper lobe. The study otherwise looks essentially normal, but several coarse bands of soft-tissue density extend toward the area of the lung obscured by the battery pack. However, due to his

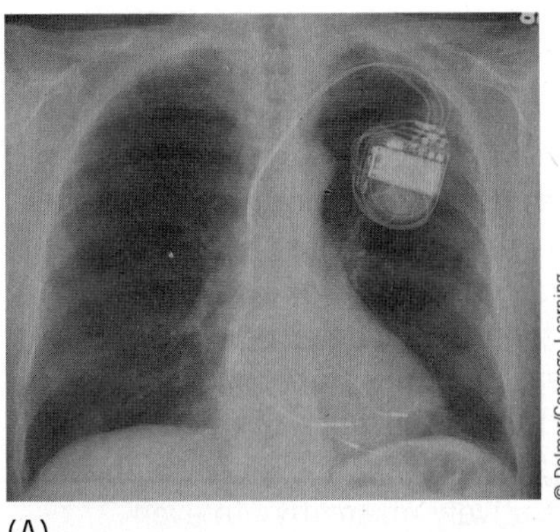

(A)

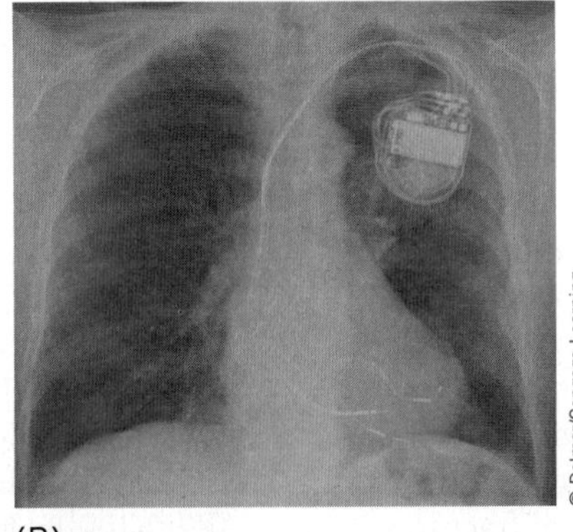

(B)

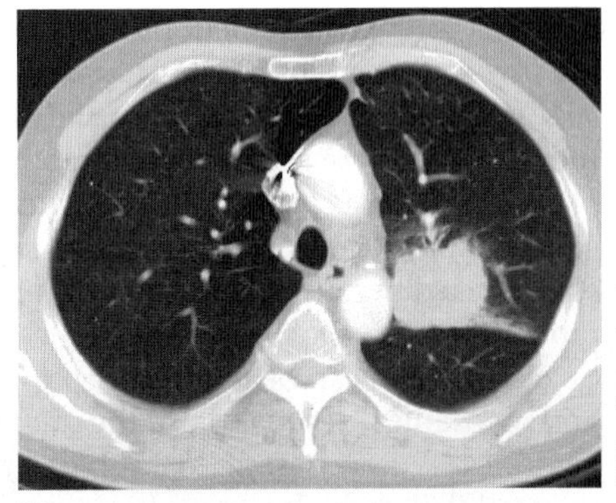

(C)

FIGURE 14-48 (A) The chest X-ray shows 4 electrodes: 2 defibrillator electrodes in the right atrium and right ventricle, 1 pacemaker electrode in the right ventricle, and another pacemaker electrode in the coronary sinus. The pacemaker's battery pack is also imaged on this view. The film was assessed as being essentially normal. (B) A repeat chest X-ray, done 6 months later: Note the large soft tissue mass that was obscured by the battery pack in the previous study. (C) A CT scan performed still later, confirming the findings of a left upper lobe bronchiogenic carcinoma hidden by the power pack in the first study.

persistent cough, the patient returned to see his physician 6 months later and had a repeat chest X-ray. The study in Figure 14-48B showed a large, soft-tissue mass extending from the hidden portion of the lung toward the left hilum. The CT (Figure 14-48C), obtained after the second chest radiograph, confirmed the presence of a left upper lobe bronchogenic carcinoma that had been obscured on the initial radiograph.

Chest Trauma

Radiology is extremely important in the assessment and diagnosis of damage done by various forms of chest trauma. Common injuries range from fractures of the ribs, sternum, spine, or clavicles to injuries of the lung, bronchi, pulmonary vessels, or pleura. The resulting conditions can be pulmonary contusion, pulmonary hemorrhage, pneumothorax, pneumomediastinum, pneumopericardium, or **hemothorax** (blood in the pleural space). Other possible injuries are to the heart or great vessels, resulting in hemopericardium, atrial or ventricular perforation, traumatic aortic injuries, or mediastinal hematomas. Knowledge of the mechanism of injury provides important diagnostic clues to the potential injuries.

FLAIL CHEST

A **flail chest** results from multiple fractures of adjacent ribs. The precise number of ribs involved to qualify as a flail chest varies based on the experts questioned. Some say as few as two adjacent ribs with two or more fractures each is a sufficient criterion. In practice, the diagnosis of flail chest is based largely on the clinical observation of paradoxical motion of any portion of the chest wall as the patient breathes. In other words, the involved segment moves *inward* on inspiration and *outward* on expiration—the opposite of the normal movements. These asynchronous motions affect pressure gradients in the thorax, reducing the efficiency of ventilation. The depth and rate of respiration are also affected because pain responses result in shallow, rapid breathing. Obviously, the observation of paradoxical motion can be made only prior to intubation and mechanical ventilation of the trauma victim. Figure 14-49 is a chest radiograph of a patient with a bilateral flail chest due to multiple segmental fractures of the right and left second–ninth ribs, bilateral pneumothoraces, and extensive subcutaneous emphysema. The right chest tube is appropriately positioned, but the left chest tube is kinked and does not enter the pleural space.

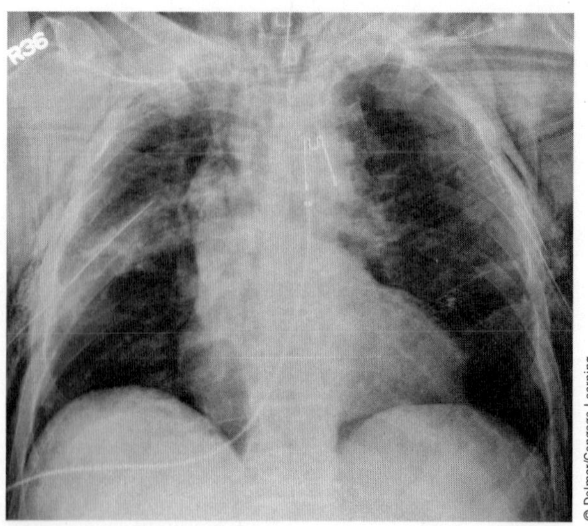

FIGURE 14-49 A patient with multiple fracture of the ribs bilaterally in ribs 2–9; many of the ribs have several fractures: The film also illustrates bilateral pneumothoraces and large areas of subcutaneous emphysema. Note the positions of the bilateral chest tubes.

Complaints of chest wall pain on inspiration, bruising patterns on the chest, chest wall movement that lags on one side, or paradoxical movements of the chest are all indicative of the need to look for fractured ribs or sternum. The presence of downward diagonal bruising on the chest wall indicates seat belt injuries: left to right for driver-side occupants, right to left for passenger-side occupants. These bruising patterns are often clues to rib fractures and chest wall muscular injuries.

Best Practice

Rib Fractures

Chest radiography is a relatively insensitive method for identifying fractures, especially non-displaced fractures. Nearly 50% of rib fractures may be missing on the initial chest radiographs obtained in the trauma suite. In the care of trauma patients, therefore, a good practice is to closely examine each rib, the sternum, the spine, and the clavicles for the presence of fractures. Also keep in mind the fact that single-view chest radiographs are relatively insensitive to even major injuries of the chest wall, great vessels, or heart. Consequently, CT examinations are routinely used in the evaluation of individuals presenting with chest injuries.

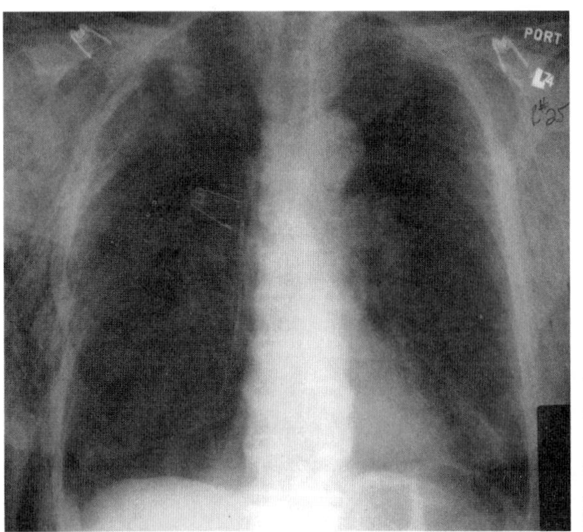

FIGURE 14-50 A trauma victim with subcutaneous emphysema: Findings of subcutaneous emphysema in trauma patients are commonly associated with injury to the chest, heart, and trachea.

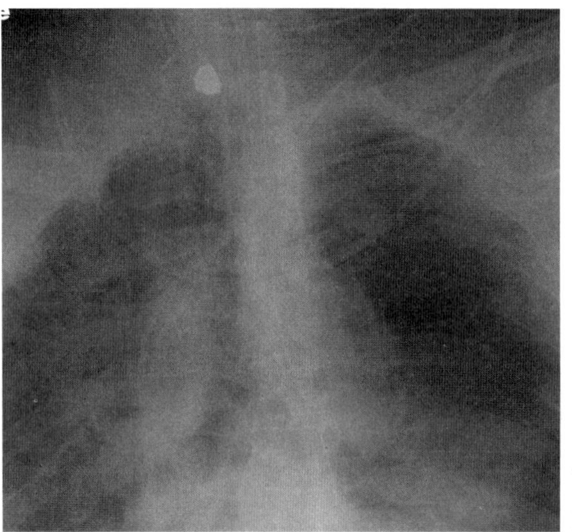

FIGURE 14-51 A dental cap that was loosened and aspirated during an endotracheal intubation: The dental cap can be seen beside the ET tube in the trachea.

SUBCUTANEOUS EMPHYSEMA

Subcutaneous emphysema presents as palpable bubbles of air under the skin. These bubbles have a classic feel referred to as *crepitus*; the feeling has been described as resembling the feeling of popping Rice Krispies® or bubble wrap. In a trauma patient, subcutaneous emphysema (Figure 14-50) almost always indicates a pulmonary, tracheal, or bronchial injury and is almost always associated with a pneumothorax injury or a pneumothorax. Intubated, tracheostomized, and ventilated patients are at increased risk of subcutaneous emphysema due to tracheal wall puncture, false passage intubation, and the increased pressure gradients that result from positive pressure ventilation, either mechanical or manual. These injuries often cut through other tissues in the head, neck, and chest, leaving subcutaneous air in these locations. The build-up of gas pressure can lead to vascular resistance and deceased perfusion to the affected areas.

PENETRATING CHEST WOUNDS

Penetrating wounds from knives, especially stab wounds (as opposed to slash injuries), are more likely to lead to a tension pneumothorax than a gunshot wound. A knife entrance wound allows air to leak into the pleural space from a punctured lung but does not provide a way for air to leave the pleural space as would a gunshot wound. Penetrating trauma frequently leads to a *hemothorax* (which looks like a pleural effusion). Blunt trauma with fractured ribs can also lead to injury to the lung or abdominal contents, leading to pneumothorax, hemothorax, or a lacerated liver or spleen.

FOREIGN BODIES

Inspect all chest X-rays, particularly those of trauma patients, for evidence of foreign bodies in the chest wall, lungs, mediastinum, or airway. Frequently, teeth or dental appliances are dislodged during a traumatic event or, less often, during the intubation of an unstable patient. Figure 14-51 demonstrates a metallic dental cap that was inadvertently dislodged during intubation and aspirated into the trachea, where it now lies alongside the endotracheal tube.

CASE STUDY 14-1

Figure 14-52 shows the chest film of a man who had unsuccessfully attempted suicide by hanging. The chest X-ray was taken at the same time as a cervical spine film that showed only soft tissue injury—no neck fracture (fx).

Questions

1. What could account for this rather startling chest film?
2. What is the probable cause of the pulmonary edema?

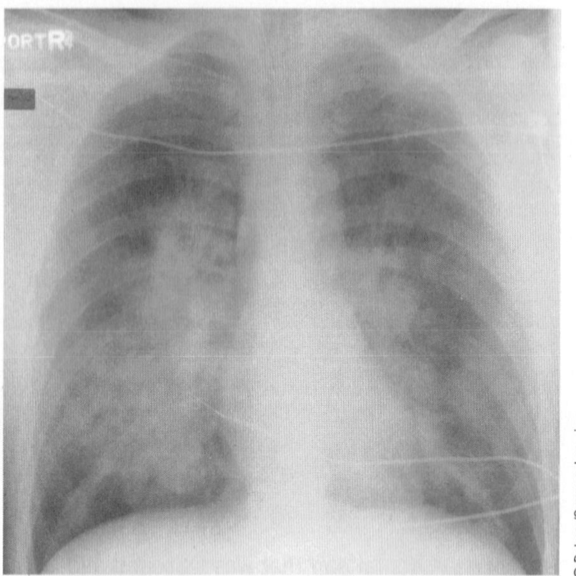

© Delmar/Cengage Learning

FIGURE 14-52 Supine portable chest indicating diffuse pulmonary edema: This film was taken contemporaneously with a C-spine film of a patient who attempted suicide by hanging. The neck was not fractured, but the associated soft tissue swelling and airway narrowing of the trachea indicate mechanical asphyxiation by strangulation. (Courtesy of Glendon Cox, M.D., University of Kansas Medical Center)

Best Practice

Safety Practices

Respiratory therapists are often involved in supporting ventilation during the application of ionizing radiation, for either diagnostic or treatment purposes. They are typically given lead aprons and lead shields to protect the gonads and thymus while in the procedure room. If RT is supporting the patient's head or neck, wearing lead-lined gloves is appropriate.

It is far less common for respiratory therapists to wear radiation dose meters (dosimeters), which provide an ongoing and cumulative record of radiation exposure over time. RTs who are stationed in the ICU or ER or who frequent transport and support procedures in the radiology department should wear a dosimeter. If they are not provided with a dosimeter, they should request one.

Summary

A respiratory therapist should be able to effectively review and analyze radiographic studies, should know how various imaging modalities can contribute to a patient's diagnosis and treatment, and should be able to use the information obtained from medical imaging to improve patient care. Such a knowledgeable RT is an asset to patients, to other health care workers, and to the health care facilities at which they work. To properly use medical imaging information, a respiratory therapist must understand the basic principles of how the study is created and how to systematically evaluate studies for their technical quality and meaning. Proficiency can be obtained and maintained only through frequent practice and learning from mentors and teachers.

Study Questions

REVIEW QUESTIONS

1. Why should a respiratory therapist be able to read and interpret chest radiographs?
2. What are the major types of radiological studies?
3. What factors influence the ordering of specific radiology studies?
4. Explain the principles of various radiological studies.
5. Differentiate between a regular and a portable chest X-ray.
6. List a sequence for systematically reviewing a chest radiograph.
7. Identify common abnormalities on a chest film.

MULTIPLE-CHOICE QUESTIONS

1. Which of the following is characteristic of a portable chest film?
   a. high quality
   b. low visibility of spine
   c. prominent spinal column
   d. erect position
2. Your patient, Mrs. J, is having difficulty breathing and diminished breath sounds in the right base and is complaining of "pain in my lower right chest when I inhale." Which of the following radiographic examinations would be most sensitive to rule out a small (<50 mL) right pleural effusion?
   a. a right lateral oblique
   b. a left lateral decubitus
   c. an AP lateral
   d. a bronchogram with contrast

3. Mr. P's PA chest radiograph shows that his right clavicle and ribs appear larger than do those on his left. Which of the following is a probable cause of this effect?
   a. Mr. Plump is rotated so that his left anterior chest wall is closer to the imaging cassette.
   b. Mr. Plump has a growth disorder, causing the right side to develop more than the left.
   c. The X-ray machine was partially set on the magnify setting.
   d. The film was a left lateral radiograph, and this result is normal for that view.
4. A patient is suspected of having an obstructive lesion, and the lesion's size, shape, and location have to be precisely delineated. Which of the following radiological tests would you suggest?
   I. plain chest film
   II. a lateral decubitus chest film
   III. MRI scan
   IV. CT scan
   V. $\dot{V}/\dot{Q}$ scan
   a. I only
   b. II and IV
   c. I and V
   d. III and VI
5. Which of the following radiographic features would be expected in a CT scan of an untreated tension pneumothorax?
   I. mediastinal shift away from the pneumothorax
   II. mediastinal shift toward the pneumothorax
   III. extra pulmonary air in the contralateral chest cavity
   IV. air-fluid level
   V. foreign object in the chest cavity
   a. I, II, and V
   b. I only
   c. II, IV, and V
   d. III and IV only
6. In a thoracic CT scan of an acute hemopneumothorax that is not under tension, which of the following is likely?
   I. mediastinal shift toward the lesion
   II. mediastinal shift away from the lesion
   III. foreign object in the chest cavity
   IV. air in the contralateral chest cavity
   V. air-fluid level in the ipsilateral (affected-side) pleural space
   a. II and V
   b. I only
   c. II, IV, and V
   d. III and IV only
7. Which of the following is indicative of an expiratory portable CXR?
   a. wide intercostal space
   b. depressed sternum
   c. AP view
   d. domed diaphragm
8. Which of the following techniques should be employed to reduce heart magnification in chest X-rays (CXRs)?
   I. Have CXR shot during expiration.
   II. Have CXR done in radiology department.
   III. Have CXR done as a portable study.
   IV. Use the PA view.
   a. I, II, and III
   b. I and II only
   c. II and IV
   d. IV only
9. Which of the following is not an appropriate safety precaution for reducing the respiratory therapist's occupational exposure to radiation?
   I. Wear a dosimeter and be enrolled in a monitoring program.
   II. Avoid caring for persons likely to need radiological procedures.
   III. Wear a lead apron and shield when exposure is necessary.
   IV. Limit exposure as appropriate.
   a. I, III, and IV
   b. II and IV only
   c. II, III, and IV
   d. I only
10. Which of the following statements is true regarding radiological procedures in chest trauma?
   a. Owing to their complexity, CT scans are often inappropriate for use in trauma.
   b. Prone and lateral positions are the most valuable when assessing chest trauma.
   c. Upright, PA films are seldom the view of choice in severe chest trauma.
   d. Supine AP and lateral films are likely to be useful for initial diagnosis in chest trauma.

CRITICAL-THINKING QUESTIONS

1. What variations should a reader expect to see a standard, plain chest radiograph were compared with a portable one taken a few minutes apart on the same patient?
2. What are the limitations of X-rays when it comes to making a diagnosis of pulmonary diseases?
3. Is it necessary that just about every patient who comes into the hospital have a chest X-ray? Explain your answer.
4. Mr. K is a 2-day postcode patient who remains on a ventilator with increasingly high pressures. Observation of the patient reveals that his face and neck appear to be bloated. What are the possible reasons for this observation?

Suggested Readings and Web Resources

Fraser RS, Colman N, Muller NL, Pare PD. *Synopsis of Diseases of the Chest*. 3rd ed. Philadelphia: Saunders/Elsevier; 2005.

Goodman L. *Felson's Principles of Chest Roentgenology: A Programmed Text*. 3rd ed. Philadelphia: Saunders/Elsevier; 2007.

Muller NL, Silva IS. *Imaging of the Chest, Vols. I and II*. Philadelphia: Saunders/Elsevier; 2008.

Society of Thoracic Radiology Pulmonary Resources, http://education.thoracicrad.org/pulmonary_imaging.htm.

Society of Thoracic Radiology Cardiac Resources, http://education.thoracicrad.org/cardiac_imaging.htm.

University of Virginia ICU Chest Radiology, http://www.med-ed.virginia.edu/courses/rad/chest/

University of Miami Interactive Chest Radiology, http://www.med.miami.edu/articulate/Rad_INTERACCXR/CXR0413.html.

Webb WR, Higgins CB. *Thoracic Imaging: Pulmonary and Cardiovascular Radiology*. Philadelphia: Lippincott Williams & Wilkins; 2005.

CHAPTER 15

Clinical Laboratory Studies

Ingo S. Kampa

OBJECTIVES

Upon completion of this chapter, the reader should be able to:

- Explain the functions of electrolytes and the causes and consequences of alterations in their concentration.
- Be able to describe the chemical concepts of analyzing electrolytes.
- Describe the causes of various acid-base disturbances and typical laboratory findings.
- Understand the importance of ionized magnesium and calcium ions.
- Identify the current biochemical markers for acute myocardial infarction.
- Outline the statistical methods used to validate analytical assay runs.

CHAPTER OUTLINE

KEY TERMS

coefficient of variance (CV)
coulometric-amperometric titration method
electrolyte
ionized calcium
ionized magnesium
ion-specific electrode (ISE)
Leland Clark electrode
osmolality
standard deviation (SD)

Electrolytes consist of *anions* (negatively charged particles) and *cations* (positively charged particles). The major cations in a physiological system are sodium (Na^+), potassium (K^+), calcium (Ca^{2+}), and magnesium (Mg^{2+}). The major anions are chloride (Cl^-), bicarbonate (HCO_3^-), HPO_4^-, dibasic phosphate (HPO_4^{2-}), and sulfur dioxide (SO_4^{2-}).[1] Electrolytes have numerous functions in the body. Essentially all metabolic reactions are controlled or influenced by electrolytes. In addition, electrolytes regulate water movement, osmotic pressure, pH, and numerous other factors. As a result, the accurate determination of electrolytes is important in the diagnosis and treatment of many disorders.

Body fluids contain large quantities of inorganic electrolytes. The large concentrations of sodium (largely confined to the extracellular space) and potassium (found in the intracellular space) have a major influence on both the distribution and retention of body fluids. Because water is freely diffusible, changes are influenced to a large extent by sodium and potassium concentrations in the various compartments. Both electrolytes have a significant effect on **osmolality**, which in turn determines the flow of water between extra- and intracellular compartments. Increased electrolyte dehydration can occur during periods of water restriction or when the rate of water loss exceeds the rate of electrolyte loss. This difference in loss rates can result in intracellular dehydration because the compensatory mechanism shifts water from the cells to the extracellular space. Typical symptoms of this condition include severe thirst and possibly nausea and vomiting. Excess ingestion of electrolyte-free water as a response to the depletion of both water and electrolytes results in an extracellular electrolyte dilution or deficit. The result is intracellular edema because water passes into the cells from the extracellular compartment.

Monitoring body water disturbances and their effects on acid-base and metabolic disturbances requires accurate measurement of electrolytes. However, several factors should be kept in mind in the evaluation of fluid and electrolyte status. Laboratory measurements are made on plasma or serum and urine samples, which represent a small compartment, or portion, of body fluids, and interpretation must be related to the total body fluid compartments. Therefore, the disease status must be considered along with the clinical status of the patient. Also, laboratory electrolytes are reported in concentration units and may not represent the total amount of electrolytes in the plasma.

Body Fluids and Electrolytes

Body fluid is distributed in three separate compartments: the *plasma*, the *interstitial fluid (ISF)*, and the *extracellular fluid (ECF)*. The fluids in these compartments are not homogeneous but consist of subcompartments containing varying concentrations of electrolytes.[2]

The electrolytes consist of cations (positive charge) and anions (negative charge).[1] The important cations are sodium (Na^+), potassium (K^+), calcium (Ca^{2+}), inorganic phosphorus, and magnesium (Mg^{2+}). Important anions discussed in this chapter are chloride (Cl^-) and bicarbonate (HCO_3^-) (Figure 15-1).

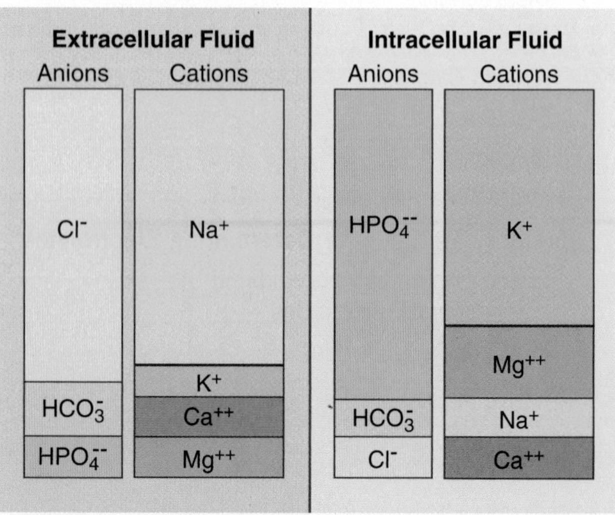

FIGURE 15-1 Anions and cations in body fluid.

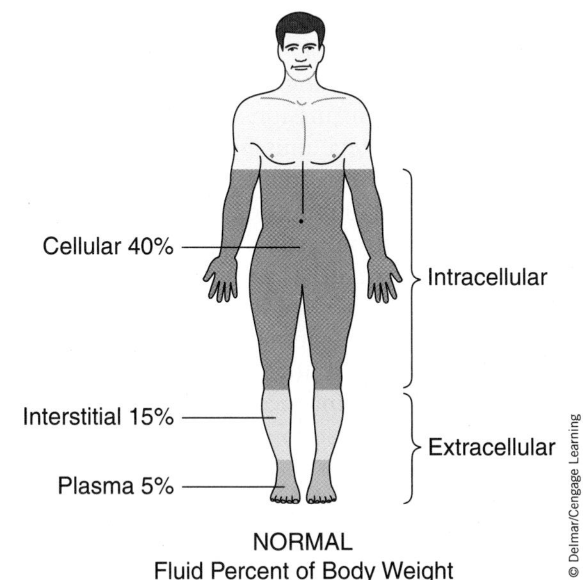

FIGURE 15-2 Body fluid compartments.

WATER

The most abundant compound in a human living body is water, representing 65–90% of the total weight of an individual (Figure 15-2). Water is contained in individual cellular compartments, usually referred to as *intracellular fluid* (*ICF*), and outside of cells; water outside cells is collectively referred to as *extracellular fluid* (*ECF*). The fluid within individual cells is relatively constant; thus, cellular fluid in the numerous separate cells can be referred to as a single compartment. Extracellular fluid is a more heterogeneous mixture that consists mainly of plasma, interstitial fluid, and transcellular fluids.

Water is constantly lost from the body through water vapor from lungs, perspiration through the skin, urine via the kidney, and feces via the intestine (Figure 15-3). Water loss by urine can be measured easily and is called *sensible water loss*. The water loss that cannot be measured (exhaled, in feces, and through perspiration) is called *insensible water loss*. The amount of insensible water loss is substantial, ranging between 1500 and 2000 mL daily by an adult.

SODIUM

Sodium, the most plentiful electrolyte, is found in high concentration in extracellular fluid and in low concentration in intracellular fluid (Figure 15-1). (The normal plasma sodium value is 135–145 mmol/L.) Sodium is involved in the maintenance of intracellular and total body fluid volumes, the maintenance of osmolality, neuromuscular excitation processes, and hydrogen ion metabolism. Potassium concentration is the opposite of sodium concentration; that is, it is high in the intracellular compartment and low in the extracellular compartment. Cell membranes maintain these

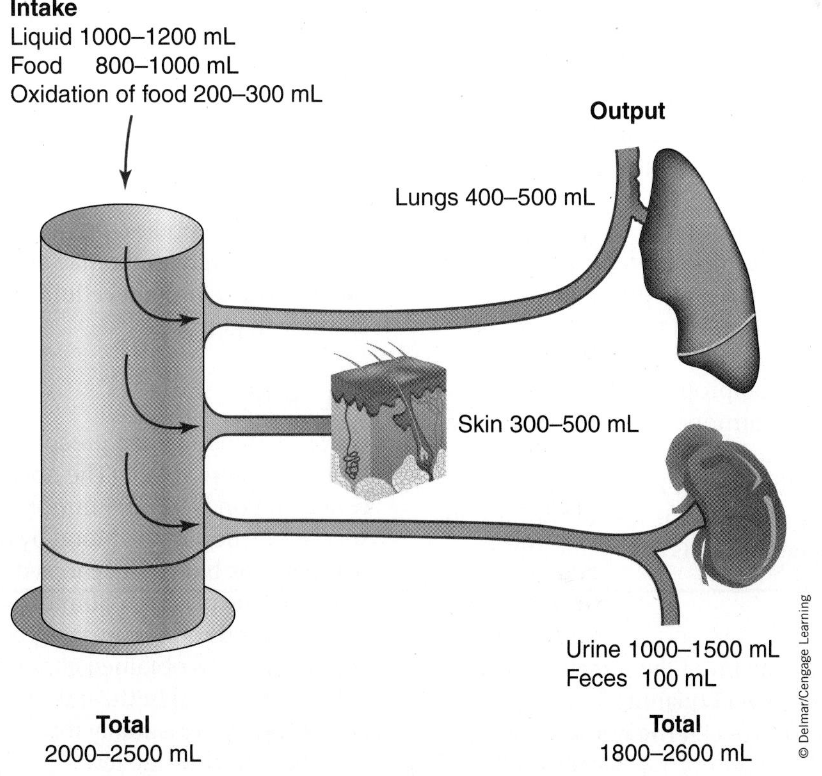

FIGURE 15-3 Normal pattern of water intake and loss.

concentration differences. Maintaining these differences in concentration requires the movement of sodium from the intracellular compartment to the extracellular compartment.

The cell must continuously expend energy to preserve these ionic conditions against the concentration gradient. These conditions are preserved by the Na^+, K^+-ATPase system, which is activated by the high-energy compound adenosine 59-triphosphate (ATP). Because sodium has a high concentration in the blood, it is the source of over half of the inorganic ions that produce the plasma osmolality. The average daily sodium consumption of 8–15 g is almost entirely absorbed by the gut. Daily sodium requirements are only 1–2 mmol/day. The kidneys excrete the vast excess of sodium.

Elevated plasma sodium concentrations (*hypernatremia*) may result if the body's water storage is depleted. Other causes may be:

- Increased mineralocorticoid production.
- Decreased antidiuretic hormone (ADH) production.
- Decreased renal tubular sensitivity to the antidiuretic hormone.
- Inappropriate administration of saline as a result of parenteral therapy.

The kidney's ability to concentrate urine in the presence of depleted water stores is limited. Insensible water losses through the lungs, skin, and stool aggravate the condition. In chronic water starvation, the kidney's compensatory ability to increase sodium excretion proportionally may be overwhelmed. Adrenal tumors are a common cause of increased mineralocorticoids, resulting in increased tubular reabsorption of sodium. A decrease in or an absence of antidiuretic hormone, or diabetes insipidus, results in the decreased ability of retaining body water.

Decreased plasma serum sodium levels (*hyponatremia*) are often caused by decreased intake of sodium and is exaggerated by vomiting and prolonged diarrhea. Extracellular fluid expansion without a concomitant increase in sodium, as seen in edema, is another cause of hyponatremia. Inappropriate increased secretion of antidiuretic hormone can result in plasma expansion without an increase in sodium levels. Metabolic acidosis, as observed in ketoacidosis in uncontrolled diabetes, results in the loss of sodium due to coexcretion with large amounts of organic anions.

POTASSIUM

Potassium, the most abundant of the intracellular cations, is found in only small quantities in the extracellular fluid (Figure 15-1). (The normal plasma potassium value is 3.5–5.0 mmol/L.) The intracellular concentration is maintained by actively transporting potassium into the cells against the concentration gradient. This task requires energy and is accomplished by the action of the Na^+, K^+-ATPase pump. Potassium is important in maintaining ionic gradients required for nerve impulse transmission and contractility of both cardiac and skeletal muscles.

The daily dietary requirement of potassium is approximately 50–150 mmol/day. Potassium is rapidly absorbed in the gastrointestinal tract. The cellular uptake is relatively small. As a result, nearly all of the dietary potassium is excreted in the urine, and the urine output generally reflects the dietary intake of potassium. Other factors affecting or regulating potassium secretion are plasma levels of aldosterone and acid-base balance. Aldosterone enhances potassium secretion, whereas acidosis affects renal regulation of potassium secretion. High levels of potassium result in weakness and numbness. Cardiac arrest and death may be the consequences as potassium concentrations exceed 7.0 mmol/L.

Excessive plasma potassium levels (*hyperkalemia*) are often the result of later stages of renal disease, as a result of damage to cells, hemolytic anemia, and the excessive use of dietary supplements containing potassium. Addison's disease increases potassium levels by causing sodium depletion. Symptoms of hyperkalemia are cardiac and central nervous system depression. Bradycardia, peripheral vascular collapse, and ultimately cardiac arrest are the consequences of severe hyperkalemia.

Potassium levels of less than 3.0 mmol/L (hypokalemia) are associated with neuromuscular abnormalities and indicate severe critical intracellular depletion. Low levels of plasma potassium are often the result of prolonged gastrointestinal loss through vomiting and diarrhea, prolonged administration of laxatives, diuretic therapy, and metabolic acidosis. The excretion of potassium is also increased by excessive quantities of corticosteroids and corticotrophin; such an increase may result in a potassium deficit. Insulin therapy in diabetic hyperglycemia may also result in hypokalemia owing to concomitant cellular uptake of potassium along with glucose.

CHLORIDE

Chloride is maintained predominately in the extracellular fluid (Figure 15-1). (The normal plasma chloride concentration is 97–108 mmol/L.) Chloride plays a special function in the blood by maintaining electrical neutrality. As bicarbonate ions diffuse out of the erythrocytes into the plasma, equimolar quantities of chloride enter the erythrocytes, in a process known as the *chloride shift*. Chloride is obtained almost entirely as sodium chloride absorbed in the intestinal tract, and its intake and output are essentially inseparable from sodium.

Elevated chloride levels (*hyperchloremia*) are associated with metabolic acidosis, kidney dysfunction, Cushing's disease, hyperventilation, dehydration, and salicylate intoxication. Decreased chloride levels (*hypochloremia*) are observed in diabetic ketoacidosis and excessive gastrointestinal losses through prolonged vomiting or diarrhea. Hypoventilation, heat exhaustion, and Addison's disease also promote excessive chloride excretion.

BICARBONATE

Carbon dioxide is a component of the most important buffer in plasma, referred to as bicarbonate (HCO_3^-) (Figure 15-1). (The normal plasma bicarbonate value is 22–32 mmol/L.) It serves as the primary mechanism for eliminating acids because lungs can readily dispose of carbon dioxide. Laboratory methods for measuring carbon dioxide or bicarbonate usually consist of measuring the bicarbonate ion (HCO_3^-) carbon dioxide bound loosely to the amine group of proteins and carbonic acid.

Lung disease and impaired carbon dioxide excretion (*respiratory acidosis*) result in decreased blood pH. The loss of stomach content through prolonged vomiting (*metabolic alkalosis*) results in decreased stomach acid content with an elevation of carbon dioxide. Overmedication with sodium bicarbonate or diuretics also results in an increase in carbon dioxide.

During hyperventilation, carbon dioxide concentrations commonly decrease and pH increases. Hyperventilation can result from overstimulation of the portion of the brain that controls breathing, often caused by anxiety or intake of toxic substances. In diabetic metabolic acidosis, both carbon dioxide and pH are decreased.

CALCIUM

Calcium is present in the body in larger amounts than any other mineral element. About 99% of body calcium is found in the skeleton and teeth; only about 1% circulates in the bloodstream. (The normal plasma calcium value is 8.5–10.0 mg/dL.) The unbound, or ionized fraction, constituting approximately 40% of the total, is thought to be more important physiologically. Approximately 45% of the body's calcium is bound to proteins, and the remainder of the calcium complexes with bicarbonate, citrate, lactate, and phosphate. Calcium is important in the transmission of nerve impulses, in the normal contractility of muscles, as a cofactor in certain enzyme reactions, and in the coagulation of blood.

Calcium ions are absorbed in an active transport process in the upper small intestine. Calcium uptake in the intestine is regulated by a metabolite (1,25-dihydroxycholecalciferol) of vitamin D. Its synthesis in the kidney is in response to low plasma concentrations of **ionized calcium** (calcium that is not bound to proteins or diffusible ligands). The body eliminates calcium through excretion in urine and feces.[3]

Parathyroid hormone (*PTH*) regulates plasma calcium concentrations, operating as a typical feedback regulation. A hyperactive or adenomatous parathyroid gland results in a large accumulation of plasma calcium (12–22 mg/dL). In many cases of hyperparathyroidism, the total calcium is not elevated, but increases in ionized calcium levels are diagnostic of hyperparathyroidism. A low concentration of ionized calcium stimulates the synthesis of PTH, which mobilizes calcium from bone, increasing the renal reabsorption and the intestinal absorption of calcium.

> *Best Practice*
>
> **Carbon Dioxide Concentration**
>
> Changes in carbon dioxide concentration are early signs of dysfunction of the acid-base status. However, because the acid-base balance must be maintained in a narrow range to sustain life, changes in plasma carbon dioxide concentration may occur only after substantial damage has already been incurred. Also, the nature of the acid-base imbalance cannot be determined from the carbon dioxide changes alone.

IONIZED CALCIUM

Many published studies attest to the importance of monitoring ionized calcium. It has been known for some time that ionized (free) calcium determinations are more useful than total calcium in critically ill patients. (The expected reference intervals for ionized calcium levels are 1.15–1.35 mmol/L, or 4.6–5.4 mg/dL.) Critically ill patients undergoing major surgery, such as cardiopulmonary bypass procedures, and receiving citrated blood or platelets, heparin, and bicarbonates have high total calcium and often critically low ionized calcium. These patients are likely to have abnormal protein levels, along with alterations in blood pH and temperature. Measurements of free calcium levels in patients receiving citrated blood platelets, intravenous solution of bicarbonate, calcium, or heparin are found to be more accurate than measurements of total calcium and provide better maintenance of cardiac function than does measurement of total calcium. Monitoring free calcium levels, along with potassium levels and blood gases, has benefited patients undergoing cardiopulmonary bypass. Ionized calcium determinations have been important, also, in the diagnosis of hypercalcemia.

A problem encountered with free calcium levels is the instability of free calcium in blood samples.

Best Practice

Ionized Calcium

Patient preparation for the measurement of ionized calcium is important. The patient must be relaxed, and the tourniquet application procedure must be as brief as possible. Bed rest is also important because it may elevate ionized calcium levels into the abnormal range. The practice of calculating ionized calcium from nomograms using total calcium and albumin or proteins has been shown to produce erroneous results.

Source: From National Committee for Laboratory Standards, Standardization of Sodium and Potassium Ion-Selective Electrode Systems to the Flame Photometric Reference Method; Approved Standard C-29A. *Wayne, PA: National Committee for Laboratory Standards; 1995.*

Samples must be sealed completely after centrifugation to prevent the loss of carbon dioxide from them. New instrumentation and new studies have resulted in increased interest in ionized calcium levels. Highly accurate instrumentation for measuring ionized calcium levels has become routinely available. It can measure the pH of aerobically collected blood samples and adjust the ionized calcium to a level at a pH of 7.4.

PHOSPHORUS

Phosphorus (inorganic or organic phosphate) is distributed throughout the body. (The plasma reference interval for phosphorus in a normal individual is approximately 2.5–4.5 mg/dL.) The largest amount is combined with calcium in bones and is a major component of hydroxyapatite. Phosphorus is also a constituent in carbohydrates, lipids, and proteins. It is an essential energy compound owing to the formation of the high-energy phosphate bond in adenosine triphosphate (ATP). As a result, phosphorus is involved in the regulation of carbohydrate, lipid, and protein metabolic pathways. This element is available in nearly all foods and is readily absorbed in the intestine and excreted in urine.

Plasma phosphorus concentrations are normally inversely related to the calcium levels. Thus, phosphorus levels are usually elevated in conditions causing hypocalcemia and decreased in hypercalcemia. Increased plasma phosphorus levels (*hyperphosphatemia*) are commonly seen in renal disease and can be a prominent cause of acidosis in severe renal disease. Low plasma phosphate levels (*hypophosphatemia*) are seen in certain malabsorption syndromes as well as in hyperparathyroidism and celiac disease. In most cases of malabsorption, both plasma calcium and plasma phosphorus levels are reduced.

MAGNESIUM

Magnesium is one of the most important cations in the body. (The plasma reference intervals for magnesium in a normal individual are approximately 0.6–1.1 mmol/L.) Next to potassium, it is the most prevalent intracellular ion, involved in activating or catalyzing many enzymes. It acts by binding to enzyme active sites, by binding to ligands in enzymes that require ATP, and by promoting aggregation in multienzyme complexes.

Very high levels of magnesium (*hypermagnesemia*) may result in the loss of sensations of touch, temperature, and pain and even in cardiac arrest. Increased magnesium levels can be expected in diabetic acidosis and Addison's disease. Low plasma magnesium levels (*hypomagnesemia*) produce impaired neuromuscular function, which, if not corrected, may result in prolonged involuntary muscle spasm. Hypertension and atherosclerosis have also been linked to low magnesium levels. Magnesium is absorbed in the gastrointestinal tract. The kidneys control plasma concentrations by regulating the excretion of magnesium.[4]

IONIZED MAGNESIUM

Magnesium exists in three forms in plasma. **Ionized magnesium** (iMg) is the physiologically active form and represents approximately 55% of the total plasma magnesium. (The whole blood reference intervals for ionized magnesium in a normal individual range from approximately 0.45 to 0.60 mmol/L.) The other two forms—protein-bound and ligand-complex—are unavailable for biological processes. The iMg is believed to be in equilibrium with the intracellular compartment and represents the biologically active form. Ionized magnesium levels could change significantly in critically ill patients without accompanying changes in the total plasma calcium.[5]

Changes in pH, acid-base status, and ligands can alter the iMg concentration. The bicarbonate ion, sometimes administered during hypoxia (associated with increased lactate levels), binds with iMg, reducing its concentration. A decrease in iMg in critically ill patients may have serious consequences because iMg is essential for maintaining electrical integrity across cell membranes.[6] The Na^+, K^+-ATPase pump is iMg dependent. This pump maintains high potassium and low sodium cellular concentrations by pumping potassium into the cell and removing sodium from it. A disruption of this process can disrupt electrolyte gradients and have fatal consequences in a critically ill patient. In addition, high intracellular sodium concentrations cause sodium-calcium exchange, resulting in an increase of intracellular calcium concentrations.

The functions of anions and cations in the body are summarized in Table 15-1.

TABLE 15-1 **Electrolytes and their functions**

	Sodium	Chloride	Potassium	Bicarbonate	Calcium	Phosphorus	Magnesium
Neuromuscular	• Transmission and conduction of nerve impulses		• Transmission and conduction of nerve impulses • Contraction of skeletal and smooth muscle		• Transmission of nerve impulses • Contraction of skeletal muscles	• Normal nerve and muscle activity	• Transmits neuromuscular activity • Mediator of neural transmissions in CNS
Body fluids	• Osmolality of vascular fluids • Regulation of body fluid	• Osmolality of vascular fluids • Regulation of body water balance	• Regulates osmolality of intracellular fluids				
Cellular	• Sodium pump • Enzyme activity		• Enzyme activity for cellular energy production • Deposits glycogen in liver cells		• Maintenance of cellular permeability • Coagulation of blood	• Forms high-energy compounds • Formation of red blood cell enzymes • Utilization of B vitamins • Transmits hereditary traits • Metabolizes carbohydrates, fats, and proteins	• Carbohydrate and protein metabolism • Transports sodium and calcium across cell membrane • Influences utilization of potassium, calcium, and protein
Acid-base levels	• Regulation of balance	• Regulation of balance • Acidity of gastric juices		• Elimination of acids		• Maintains acid-base balance in body fluids	
Cardiac			• Nerve conduction and contraction of the myocardium		• Contraction of heart muscle		• Contraction of heart muscle
Bones and teeth					• Formation of bones and teeth	• Formation, strength, durability	

Laboratory Methods for Determining Electrolytes

A variety of specimen types can be used to measure electrolytes. In the clinical laboratory, serum is still the most common type of specimen. However, the use of heparinized plasma samples and whole blood is gaining popularity quickly because they eliminate the time required for clotting and serum separation.

Measuring Electrolytes

Analytical electrolyte (Na, K, Cl, and CO_2) values differ among serum, plasma, and whole blood. With the exception of potassium, these differences are small and not clinically significant. The potassium concentration in plasma is approximately 0.3 mmol/L less than that in serum. Potassium concentrations in whole blood are approximately 0.2 mmol/L greater than in serum.

Source: National Committee for Laboratory Standards, *Standardization of Sodium and Potassium Ion-Selective Electrode Systems to the Flame Photometric Reference Method; Approved Standard C-29A. Wayne, Pa: National Committee for Laboratory Standards; 1995.*

FLAME PHOTOMETRY AND INDIRECT ION-SPECIFIC ELECTRODES

For many decades, flame emission photometry was the most common procedure to quantitatively measure sodium and potassium in body fluids. However, since the mid-1990s flame emission photometry has rapidly disappeared from the clinical laboratory and is no longer used. These results are then compared to the original results from flame photometry, which is still considered the reference method.[7]

The basis for flame photometry is that many metallic elements, when supplied with sufficient energy, emit this energy at a wavelength that is characteristic for the specific element. When energy is supplied to a solution of serum in the form of a hot flame, the absorbed energy is released by both sodium and potassium in a characteristic spectrum for each element. Sodium emits a visible yellow light, and potassium emits a violet light. Specific wavelengths in the sodium and potassium spectra that emit the largest amount of energy are selected and compared with the energy emitted from a standard solution of sodium and potassium. The light intensity produced at a specific wavelength is directly proportional to the concentration of atoms in the solution. The mathematical comparison of the emitted spectra of the unknown sample with those of the standard reveals the actual concentration of either sodium or potassium.[7,8] Figure 15-4 shows a typical schematic of a flame photometer.

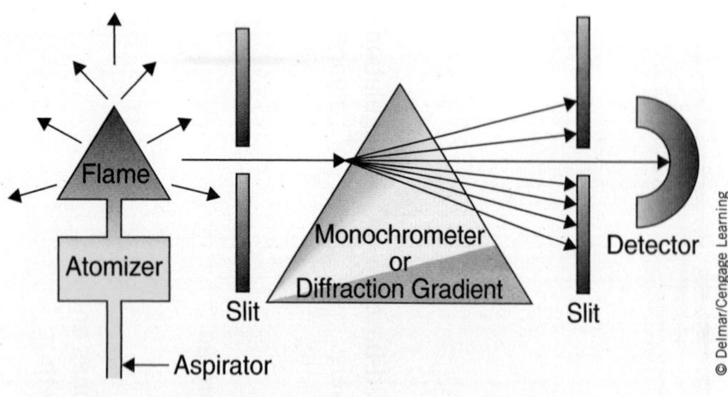

FIGURE 15-4 Schematic of a flame photometer.

Flame photometry had always been plagued with problems. It was difficult to maintain a constant and controlled supply of energy to the solution that contained the analytes. Other problems were:

- The danger of using gases to produce the flame.
- The continuous emissions caused by the burning of nonionic products.
- Signal enhancement (mutual excitation) caused by high sodium concentrations in the sample.

ION-SPECIFIC ELECTRODES

Today, sodium and potassium are measured with **ion-specific electrodes (ISEs)**, which consist of sodium electrodes with glass membranes and an electrode with a liquid ion-exchange membrane. Measuring the electron potential on a selective membrane requires a complete electrical circuit. There are two electrodes: a reference and an ion-specific electrode. The potential of the reference electrode is maintained constant and that of the ISE electrode varies. As sodium ions penetrate the ion-exchange membrane, a change in the membrane potential is detected and then related to sodium concentration.

Potassium measurements are accomplished similarly. The potassium ISE contains a valinomycin membrane that excludes the large sodium ion while allowing the smaller potassium ion to penetrate.

Electrodes measuring total carbon dioxide consist of a carbon dioxide–permeable membrane and a pH electrode. The bicarbonate ion and protein-bound carbon dioxide are converted to carbon dioxide gas, which can diffuse through the membrane to dissolve in a bicarbonate buffer solution. The diffused carbon dioxide causes a change in the pH, which is measured with the pH electrode.

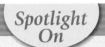

Ion-Specific Electrodes

Ion-specific electrode methods can be divided into two types: the direct method and the indirect method. In the *indirect method*, the sample is diluted with a diluent of high ionic strength before being presented to the electrode. In the *direct method*, undiluted serum, plasma, or whole blood is introduced directly into the ion-specific electrode. The latter approach allows the use of whole blood and thus is compatible with the simultaneous determination of blood gases.

BIOSENSOR TECHNOLOGY

Biosensors are devices that combine ion-specific electrodes, enzymatic methodology, and solid-phase technology to selectively recognize an element with a transducer. Thus, biosensors can be defined as devices in which an immobilized biochemical component reacts with an analyte, such as an ion, to produce a signal. The signal is proportional to the quantity of the analyte.[8–10] (Although the potassium electrode uses a biocomponent, valinomycin membrane, it is not considered a biosensor because the electrode does not incorporate biorecognition in its measuring process.)

Biosensors

The major manufacturers' blood gas analyzers use direct ISE methods. Earlier ISEs using the indirect method consisted of a rather large electrode surface, requiring a large volume to cover the electrode. With the development of smaller electrodes, smaller sample volumes have eliminated the need for sample dilution.

Workable biosensors have been used for such analytes as creatinine, glucose, lactate, and urea nitrogen. Biosensors have also been developed for blood gases, heparin, homocysteine, and protein.

Some technical hurdles related to sensitivity and specificity have to be overcome before biosensors are used commonly as routine measuring devices.

Laboratory Methods for Determining Arterial Blood pH, Carbon Dioxide Pressure, and Oxygen Pressure

The pH electrode consists of an Ag/AgCl electrode and a calomel electrode. The calomel electrode (the reference) consists of mercury covered by a thin layer of $HgCl_2$. The Ag/AgCl (indicator) electrode is surrounded by a glass membrane immersed in a reference solution. Hydrogen ions in the test solution penetrate the glass membrane of the indicator electrode, effecting a change in the reference solution. The potential charge difference between the test solution and the reference solution is calibrated into pH units. Figure 15-5 illustrates the components of a pH electrode.

The PCO_2 (Stow-Seringham) electrode consists of a glass pH electrode separated from the blood or plasma to be measured by a thin, gas-permeable membrane consisting of Teflon, silicon rubber, or other material that allows gas but not liquid to permeate. Blood, plasma, or gas is introduced into a temperature-controlled chamber that is separated from a compartment containing bicarbonate buffer by a thin (0.001-in.) gas-permeable membrane. The membrane allows uncharged particles such as carbon dioxide to permeate but prevents charged particles (nongaseous substances) from penetrating. The diffused gas reacts with the bicarbonate solution, resulting in the following reaction:

$$CO_2 + H_2O \leftrightarrow H_2CO_3 \leftrightarrow H^+ + HCO_3^-$$

The hydrogen ions produced penetrate the gas electrode, and the Ag/AgCl internal electrode detects the change in potential. Figure 15-6 illustrates the components of a PCO_2 electrode.

The PO_2 electrode, also known as the **Leland Clark electrode**, consists of a platinum cathode and an Ag/AgCl anode in a phosphate buffer. The platinum electrode is separated from the test solution by a gas-permeable membrane. When the cathode is set at −0.65 V in the absence of oxygen, the current is zero. When oxygen diffuses across the membrane, it is reduced at the cathode, resulting in a current flow between the two electrodes. The current flow is

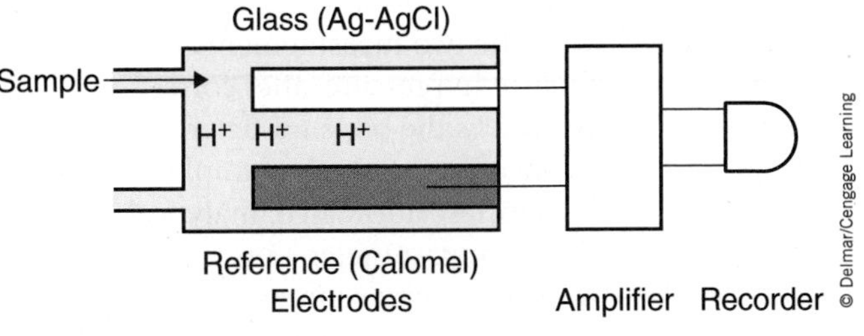

FIGURE 15-5 Components of a pH electrode.

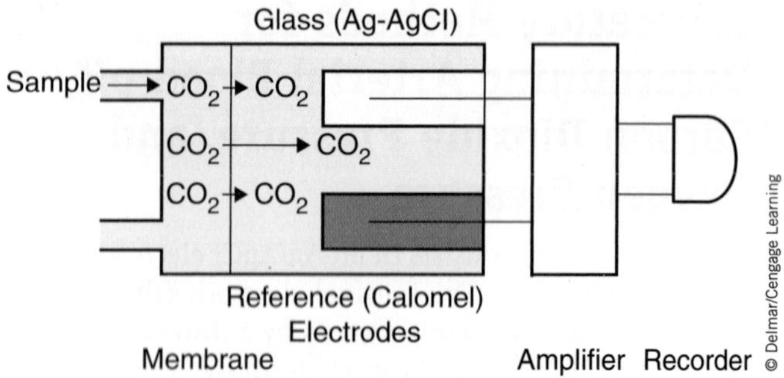

FIGURE 15-6 Components of a PCO_2 electrode.

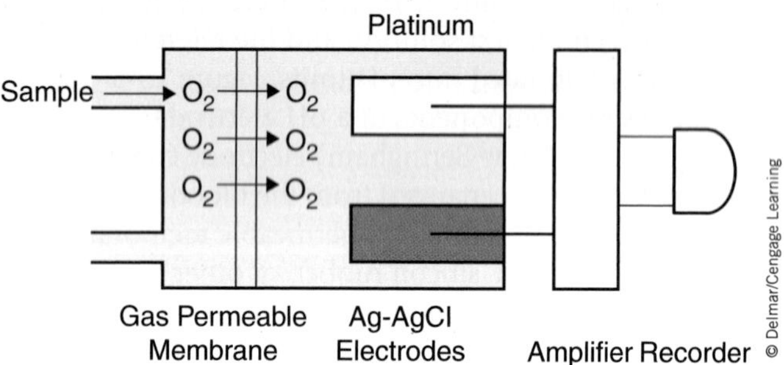

FIGURE 15-7 Components of a PO_2 electrode.

calibrated to the oxygen concentration in the test sample. A typical PO_2 electrode is shown in Figure 15-7. Chapter 16 provides additional details on acid-base and blood gas analysis.

Laboratory Methods for Analyzing Carbon Dioxide and Chloride

Historically, numerous methods have been used to measure carbon dioxide.[1] One of the earlier and more reliable assays is the manometric method popularized by Samuel Natelson, known as the *Natelson microgasometer*. This method is based on the pressure resulting from the carbon dioxide released when acid is added to a solution in an enclosed system. After the barometric pressure in the solution has been measured, the mixture is treated with alkali, and the dissolved carbon dioxide is absorbed into the solution. The barometric pressure of the resulting solution is measured, and the difference between the two measurements is established. The difference in pressure, after correction for atmospheric pressure, is the basis for determining the carbon dioxide concentration in the sample.

In most laboratories, automated analytical assays have replaced the microgasometer. One of the more successful methods is an *enzymatic assay*. It requires the conversion of all forms of carbon dioxide to the bicarbonate ion. The resulting solution, containing the bicarbonate ion, is reacted with the substrate phosphoenolpyruvate and the enzyme phosphoenolpyruvate carboxylase to form oxaloacetate. That is, in turn, reacted with nicotinamide adenine dinucleotide hydrogen (NADH) and malate dehydrogenase to form malate and reduced nicotinamide adenine dinucleotide (NAD^+). The decrease in absorbance is measured at a wavelength of 340 nm and is used to quantitate the carbon dioxide concentration.

Nearly all other methods in use today use a *carbon dioxide electrode*. The carbon dioxide electrode consists of a carbon dioxide gas–permeable membrane and a pH electrode. The sample is acidified to convert all bicarbonate, both free and protein bound, into carbon dioxide gas. The liberated carbon dioxide diffuses through a permeable membrane and dissolves in the internal filling solution. The dissolved carbon dioxide in the internal filling solution causes a pH change in the solution, which is measured by the pH electrode. The magnitude of the pH change is a function of the total carbon dioxide content of the sample and is converted to carbon dioxide concentration units.

Traditional methods for plasma chloride determinations included photometric (use of a spectrophotometer) and **coulometric-amperometric titration methods**.[11]

- *Coulometry* is an electrochemical titration in which the titrant is electrochemically generated and the end point is detected by amperometry.
- *Amperometry* is the measurement of the current through an electrolyte solution.

A typical spectrophotometric analysis reacts mercuric thiocyanide with chloride ions in plasma or serum to form mercuric chloride and free thiocyanate ions. The free thiocyanate ions are reacted with Fe^{3+} to form ferric thiocyanate, which is spectrophotometrically quantitated at a wavelength of 480 nm.

Coulometric-amperometric titration methods for quantitating chloride levels are based on the generation of silver ions at a constant rate from a silver electrode. The generated silver ions react with chloride ions to form insoluble silver chloride. When all of the chloride ions have been used in the formation of silver chloride, the generation of silver from the silver electrode is terminated. The time interval between the beginning and end of the reaction is directly related to the amount of chloride ion in the sample. Comparing the time of analysis of a known standard against the time of analysis of the unknown sample allows the quantitation of chloride in the sample.

Ion-specific electrodes (ISEs) have become the new methodology in measuring chloride concentration in plasma, serum, and whole blood.[12] Typically, a reference electrode and an ion-specific electrode are used. The potential of the reference electrode remains constant; that of the ISE varies depending on the activity of the chloride ion across the membrane. The change in potential is predicted by the Nernst equation and allows for the quantitation of the unknown chloride sample.[7] The ISE electrode used for chloride measurements is a silver chloride membrane electrode, one of whose drawbacks is that therapeutic levels of bromide and iodide in blood can cause significant errors in chloride levels. The silver chloride electrode selectively recognizes these halogens as compared with chloride. Thus, small therapeutic levels of bromide and iodide could result in falsely elevated chloride results.

Laboratory Findings in Acid-Base Disturbance

As described in Chapter 4, acid-base disturbance due to changes in the bicarbonate levels in blood is of metabolic origin. Low blood bicarbonate levels without a change in H_2CO_3 are defined as *acidosis*, and excess bicarbonate levels as *alkalosis*. Changes in CO_2 as a result of altered ventilation are *respiratory acidosis* (increased CO_2) or *respiratory alkalosis* (decreased CO_2).[13]

LABORATORY FINDINGS IN METABOLIC ACIDOSIS

Metabolic acidosis is based on the loss of extracellular buffers, the accumulation of fixed acids, or both. Common conditions causing metabolic acidosis include diabetic ketoacidosis, excess production of lactic acids, uremia and chronic renal disease, diarrhea, and the administration of drugs.

Diabetic ketoacidosis occurs in insulin-dependent diabetes mellitus (IDDM, type I) and in advanced stages of non-insulin-dependent diabetes (NIDDM, type II). In both cases, the severely abnormal carbohydrate and lipid metabolism results in large increases in the production of keto-acids such as hydroxybutyric acid and acetoacetic acid.[14] In this condition, an increased anion gap is found [anion gap = $Na^+ - (Cl^- + HCO_3^-)$]. Common laboratory findings are large increases in blood glucose, increased chloride concentrations, and significant reductions in bicarbonate levels. An increase in urine ketone bodies and positive plasma acetone levels is also expected. Blood gas findings include increases in hydrogen ion concentrations, as indicated by lower blood pH, and decreases in PCO_2 levels. The administration of insulin results in significant improvements.

Renal tubular acidosis is characterized by the inappropriate reabsorption of bicarbonate ions by the proximal tubules.[15] The deficiency in the reabsorption of bicarbonate ion results in the increased reabsorption of chloride ion. Laboratory data show decreased PCO_2 levels, along with decreased blood pH, and increased plasma chloride concentrations. Differential laboratory tests require renal function tests.

Metabolic acidosis caused by increased lactic acid can have a variety of causes, including anaerobic metabolism. Other causes are:

- Alcohol consumption.
- Diabetes mellitus.
- Glycogen storage diseases.
- Tumors.
- Idiopathic causes.
- Vomiting and diarrhea, which can cause a significant loss of bicarbonate ion and other conjugate bases.
- Inappropriate administration of hydrochloric acid and administration of ammonium chloride during treatment procedures in medical settings.

The compensatory response to metabolic acidosis is primarily neuromuscular and secondarily renal. Increased alveolar ventilation results in rapidly decreasing PCO_2 levels. Renal compensation also involves increasing the elimination of hydrogen ions by increasing the ammonium ion loss.

LABORATORY FINDINGS IN METABOLIC ALKALOSIS

Common causes of metabolic alkalosis include excessive losses of noncarbonic acids from the upper gastrointestinal tract, diuretic therapies, and increases in corticosteroids.

- Prolonged and excessive vomiting and gastric suction in medical settings are the most common causes. The greater chloride concentration in the gastrointestinal fluid results in chloride depletion and excessive retention of the bicarbonate ion; these effects result in increases of plasma bicarbonate and decreases in plasma chloride levels.
- Diuretic therapy and laxatives cause impairment in the reabsorption of potassium ion and increased excretion of hydrogen ions by the kidney.
- Hyperaldosteronism and steroid therapy are less common causes of metabolic alkalosis. Both of these steroids cause increased secretion of potassium and hydrogen ions.

Laboratory findings in metabolic alkalosis show increases of both dissolved carbon dioxide and bicarbonate ion, resulting in an increase of PCO_2. A decreased concentration of plasma chloride and potassium is common, and an elevation in plasma sodium is possible. Patients with potassium deficiency show general weakness, decreases in tendon reflexes, and, in more severe cases, tachycardia and cardiac arrhythmia. Compensatory mechanisms are not clearly understood and usually include decreased alveolar ventilation.

LABORATORY FINDINGS IN RESPIRATORY ACIDOSIS

Respiratory acidosis demonstrates an elevation of PCO_2 (*hypercapnia*) and is caused by defects in the excretion of bicarbonate ion. Defects in respiration include obstructive lung disease and trauma to the respiratory center, resulting in CNS depression. Chronic obstructive lung disease and the overuse of respiratory depressant drugs are probably the most common causes of respiratory acidosis. Chronic bronchitis, emphysema, pulmonary edema, and fibrosis are common conditions resulting in chronic obstructive lung disease. CNS depression has multiple causes: inappropriately prescribed antidepression and narcotic drugs, self-administered narcotics, and overdoses of prescription drugs.

Laboratory findings before compensation show high PCO_2, decreases in PO_2, and low pH levels.

Renal compensation is the primary response to respiratory acidosis. A decrease in arterial pH (increased hydrogen ion concentration) and an increased PCO_2 level are powerful stimuli for bicarbonate ion reabsorption by the kidneys. The kidneys' response is not immediate, however; it takes 2–5 days to fully develop. Laboratory findings after compensation show increases in the bicarbonate ion and total carbon dioxide levels. The ratio of bicarbonate ion to dissolved carbon dioxide is decreased, causing a further decrease in blood pH level.

LABORATORY FINDINGS IN RESPIRATORY ALKALOSIS

Respiratory alkalosis is the result of excessive alveolar ventilation, which leads to an excessive loss of carbon dioxide, thereby lowering PCO_2 levels. Alveolar hyperventilation that occurs repeatedly without apparent reason is known as *hyperventilation syndrome*. Emotional states such as excitement, hysteria, and anxiety increase alveolar hyperventilation. Metabolic acidosis, pulmonary emboli, and mild restrictive lung diseases are other causes of respiratory alkalosis. Subnormal levels of PO_2 stimulate the respiratory center, resulting in increased breathing. A variety of drugs are also known to cause alveolar hyperventilation.

Normal and relatively rapid responses to respiratory alkalosis consist of buffering and intra- and extracellular ion shifts. Compensatory mechanisms in acute and prolonged respiratory alkalosis consist of a decrease in the urine's secretion of hydrogen ion and decreased retention (increased excretion) of bicarbonate ion in an effort to lower blood pH.

The primary laboratory findings in respiratory alkalosis are reductions in PCO_2 and dissolved carbon dioxide, resulting in increased blood pH. Table 15-2 summarizes the lab values found relative to acid-base disturbances.

CURRENT BIOCHEMICAL MARKERS IN ACUTE MYOCARDIAL INFARCTION

Biochemical markers to diagnose acute myocardial infarction have been in use since the mid-1950s with the initial use of *aspartate aminotransferase* (*AST*). Since

TABLE 15-2 **Lab Values of Acid-Base Disturbances**

Acid-Base Disturbance	Common Lab Values
Metabolic acidosis	• Large increases in blood glucose • Increased chloride concentrations • Significant reductions in bicarbonate levels • Increase in urine ketone bodies • Positive plasma acetone levels • Increase in hydrogen ion concentrations • Lower blood pH • Decreases in PCO_2 levels
Metabolic alkalosis	• Increases of both dissolved carbon dioxide and bicarbonate ion • Increase of PCO_2 • Decreased concentration of plasma chloride and potassium (common) • Elevation in plasma sodium (possible)
Respiratory acidosis	Before compensation: • High PCO_2 • Decreases in PO_2 • Low pH levels After compensation: • Increases in the bicarbonate ion and total carbon dioxide levels • Decreased ratio of bicarbonate ion to dissolved carbon dioxide • Decrease in blood pH level
Respiratory alkalosis	• Reductions in PCO_2 • Dissolved carbon dioxide • Increased blood pH

then, other markers for acute myocardial infarction (AMI) that have been used are:

- Lactic dehydrogenase isoenzymes.
- Total creatine kinase (CK).
- Creatine kinase isoenzymes by electrophoresis.
- Creatine MB determinations by immunoassay techniques (CK-MB).
- Creatine kinase isoforms.

The difficulties with these markers included the lack of specificity and, in some cases, the length of the assay procedure. Since 1992, *troponin T* (*cTnT*) and soon thereafter *troponin I* (*cTnI*) have become the predominant AMI markers. These later markers are:

- Highly specific for cardiac muscle injury.
- Have a high assay sensitivity.
- Appear very early after myocardial infarction.
- Display prolonged elevation after myocardial injury.[16,17]

The striated muscle in the cardiac tissue contains a protein complex consisting of three polypeptides that are involved in calcium regulation. Two of these, troponin I and troponin T, are considered highly specific for cardiac muscle injury because they have not been demonstrated in other types of skeletal muscle.[18] Troponin is elevated in 4–8 hours after an acute myocardial infarction and thus is similar to CK-MB. Unlike CK-MB, however, troponin T and troponin I are highly specific for striated muscle tissue and remain elevated for several days.

In addition to the troponins and CK-MB, *myoglobin* determinations are frequently used because of their early increases in patients' blood.[19] Myoglobin becomes abnormal within 2 hours after an acute myocardial infarction and peaks within 6–9 hours. The early elevations are of particular importance because thrombolytic therapy for AMI patients is most effective when used within the first 6 hours of an AMI. Because myoglobin is an acute-phase reactant, however, its elevation alone is not a confirmation of AMI. It must be used along with electrocardiogram and clinical evaluation.

Best Practice

Drug Overdoses

Salicylate overdose and excessive doses of anabolic drugs, epinephrine, and progesterone are known to result in alveolar hyperventilation. Increased alveolar ventilation is a normal response to metabolic acidosis.

Statistical Quality Control

Good laboratory practice and the enactment of the Clinical Laboratory Improvement Amendments of 1988 (CLIA-88) require that all laboratory testing processes be monitored using quality control specimens and the appropriate use of statistical quality control (QC) procedures.[20]

ESTABLISHING PRECISION GOALS

The analytical performance of an analyte needs to be monitored in order to assess the performance of an analytical test method.[21,22] Precision is a measure of reproducibility and is determined by analyzing the same material repeatedly over time. If the observed concentration of the control is plotted against the frequency of the occurrence of observed concentrations, a normal, or Gaussian, distribution is obtained (Figure 15-8). The same distribution curve of data can also be obtained by calculating the mean and standard deviation of the data.

The *mean* is simply the average value of the data points and is calculated as follows:

$$\bar{x} = \frac{\Sigma x_1 + x_2 + x_3 + \ldots x_n}{n}$$

where $\bar{x}$ = mean; Σ = sum of all values; n = the number of determinations.

Standard deviation (SD) is a measure of dispersion (the spread of the data around the mean). It is the square root of the sum of the squares of the observed data minus the mean value of the observed data

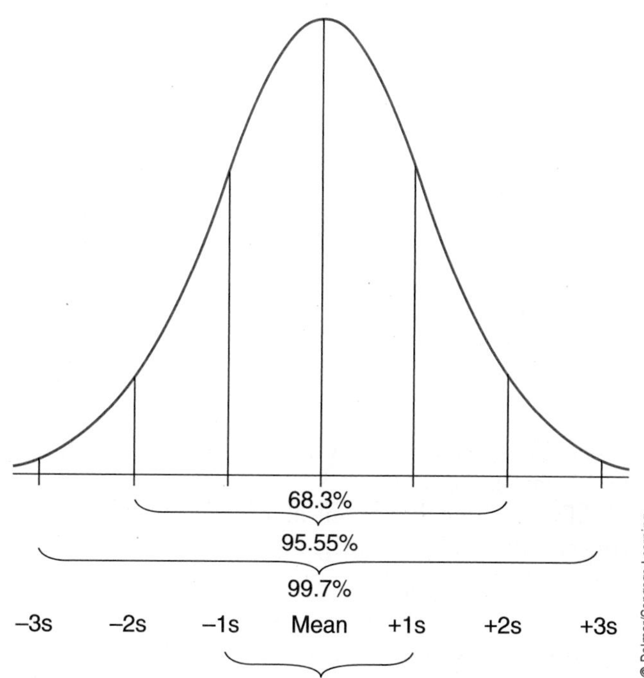

FIGURE 15-8 Gaussian distribution of data.

Best Practice

Analyte Performance

Analyzing control materials of various concentrations can monitor the performance of an analyte. Control materials are usually commercially produced lyophilized serum products that contain analyte concentrations below, within, and above reference intervals. The observed values are then compared with acceptable upper and lower limits for the specific analyte. An analytical assay run is then evaluated as successful or unsuccessful according to certain established criteria.

divided by the number of observations. It is calculated as follows:

$$SD = \sqrt{\frac{\Sigma(x_i - \bar{x})^2}{n}}$$

where SD = standard deviation; x_i = value of observed data points; $\bar{x}$ = mean value of observed data; and n = number of determinations.

As shown in Figure 15-8, the normal distribution of data can be divided into areas corresponding to ±1 SD, ±2 SD, and ±3 SD. The percentages of values in these distinct areas are 68.3, 95.55, and 99.7, respectively.

This range, however, may be too narrow for analytes, which have excellent precision and thus a very narrow acceptable, perhaps unrealistic, range for controls. Also, by statistical design, nearly 5% of the control assays fall outside the acceptable range. Using plus and minus 3 SD enlarges the range for acceptable controls to 99.7% of the control samples. Observations (data) which falls outside the 3rd SD are also known as *"outliers"*.

Another approach to create reference intervals for control values is to use a **coefficient of variance (CV)**, which is the standard deviation expressed as a percentage of the mean. A CV of 5% is considered an acceptable analytical performance. This requires that a theoretical standard deviation be calculated using the mean and a CV of 5%. This is calculated as follows:

$$CV = \frac{100 \times SD}{\bar{x}}$$

where CV = coefficient of variation, $\bar{x}$ = mean, and SD = standard deviation.

If we assume that a control for PCO_2 has a mean concentration of 55 mm Hg, then:

$$5 = \frac{100 \times SD}{55}$$

$$100\ SD = 275$$

$$SD = 2.75$$

Thus, the reference interval for an acceptable control value is the mean ±2 SD, or 49.5–60.5 mm Hg.

Best Practice

Standard Deviations

Standard deviations can be used to establish the upper and lower limits of a control material. Plus and minus 2 standard deviations (2 SD) from the mean are traditionally used as control limits.

The coefficient of variation (CV) is more meaningful than standard deviation because it expresses the standard deviation as a percentage of the mean. Assume that two PCO_2 controls have means of 55 and 110 mm Hg and standard deviations of 6 and 8 mm Hg. The CV of the lower control is 10.91, and that of the higher control is 7.27. The value obtained with the higher control is more precise even though it has a higher standard deviation.

MONITORING THE ANALYTICAL PRECISION OF A TEST

The two types of errors a laboratory needs to monitor are random and systematic errors.

- *Random errors* are an indication of the precision of a test method. They are observed by the scatter of control data points around the mean of the control value. The scatter of control values should be randomly distributed above and below the mean.
- On the other hand, *systematic errors* are reflections of the accuracy of the method. *Accuracy* has been defined as the agreement between the best estimate of a quantity and its true value. These can be detected by the comparison of laboratory data with those obtained from other laboratories using the same methodology.

Once a control material, along with the upper and lower control limits, has been established, the performance of the assay needs to be monitored. Control results are ideally distributed randomly around the mean value of the control. The number of control values outside control limits (i.e., out of control) in a properly performing assay depends on the method used to determine the control limits. If ±2 standard deviations is used to establish the control limits, then 5%, or 1 out of 20, control values will be outside the control limits. At 3 SD, only 3 out of 1000 will fall outside control limits. If a CV of 5%, is the basis for setting control limits, then failure will depend on the precision of the particular assay. If the precision of the assay is at or near 5%, then a larger number of control results will fall outside the limits. When an analytical run is performed, a judgment needs to be made whether a run is in control or out of control. If the run is in control, then the patient results are acceptable for clinical interpretation. If the run is considered out of control, patient values cannot be used, and corrective actions need to be initiated.

Various criteria can be used to judge whether a run is in or out of control. A common procedure used in laboratories is the *multirule procedure* developed by Westgard and coworkers.[23] The multirule method is often incorporated into instrument computer quality control modules, into laboratory information systems (LIS), and into hospital information systems (HIS). It entails a simple approach to interpreting control values and determining the rejection or acceptance of an analytical run. Table 15-3 outlines the rules. Clinical laboratories extensively use the first three rules to evaluate the performance of their assays.

Other approaches include the use of *Levey-Jennings charts,* as depicted in Figure 15-9.[24] These charts are simple and convenient to use because laboratory and hospital computer information systems can produce them automatically. The Levey-Jennings charts can be used to monitor internal quality control by the Westgard multirule method and by trend analysis.[25]

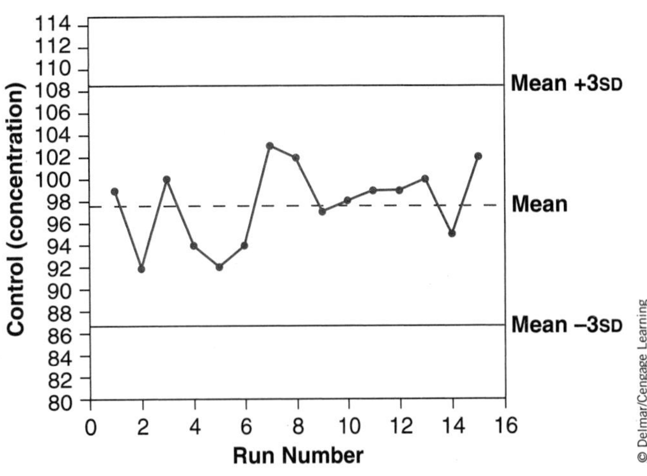

FIGURE 15-9 Levey-Jennings control chart: Control limits are set at the mean ±3 SD.

CONDUCTING INTERLABORATORY COMPARISONS

Various manufacturers of quality control material conduct external laboratory quality assurance (QA) programs. Laboratories using the same lot number of control samples submit their monthly quality control

> **Best Practice**
>
> **Trend Analysis**
>
> Trend analysis can be useful in monitoring the deterioration of either the quality control material or the calibration curve. Deviations of control values from the mean over a period of time are indications of trends, whereas sudden changes of control values involving a shift in either direction often require immediate attention. A good laboratory uses a variety of these methods to monitor quality control.

TABLE 15-3 **Westgard's rules**

$1_{2\,SD}$	The value of one control exceeds the mean by +/–2 SD.	Warning rule: further evaluation required Evaluate rules $1_{3\,SD}$, $2_{2\,SD}$, $R_{4\,SD}$, 10_x. Accept the run if it passes these rules. Reject the run if it fails any of these rules.
$1_{3\,SD}$	The value of one control exceeds the mean by +/–3 SD.	Reject the run.
$2_{2\,SD}$	The values of two consecutive controls exceed the mean by +/–2 SD.	Reject the run.
$R_{4\,SD}$	The value of one control exceeds the mean by +2 SD; another exceeds the mean by –2 SD.	Reject the run.
$4_{1\,SD}$	Four consecutive control values exceed the mean by +1 SD or –1 SD.	Reject the run.
10_x	Ten consecutive control values fall above the mean, or 10 consecutive control values fall below the mean.	Reject the run.

Source: From Westgard OJ, Klee GG. Quality management. In: Burtis CA, Ashwood ER, eds. Tietz Textbook of Clinical Chemistry. *3rd ed. Philadelphia: WB Saunders Co; 1999; 384–418.*

results, which consist of the mean and standard deviation for each analyte tested. The submitted data are statistically compared with the data submitted by other laboratories. A common statistical comparison is the *standard deviation interval* (*SDI*), calculated as follows:

$$\text{SDI} = \frac{\text{laboratory mean} - \text{group mean}}{\text{group standard deviation}}$$

The group mean is the mean of values in analyses of an analyte obtained from all participant laboratories using an identical method. The group standard deviation is a calculated standard deviation of the mean values from all laboratories submitting data.

The laboratory SDI value can then be used to evaluate the analyte performance of an individual laboratory in the group. An SDI of less than +2 SD or −2 SD is an indication that the laboratory result is in good agreement with data submitted by other laboratories using identical methods. A value that exceeds ±2 SD is an indication of a lack of agreement.

SDI units can also be presented in a Youden plot (Figure 15-10). This plot requires two control materials of different concentrations to be used. The SDI value of control 1 is plotted on the *y*-axis, and the SDI value of control 2 is plotted on the *x*-axis. Under ideal conditions, the point of intersection should fall at 0.0. Data points drifting to the right are indications of proportional errors. Displacement of the point downward or upward is an indication of a constant error or constant errors. The difficulties are the number of participating laboratories and the fact that a laboratory with bad data can affect the group mean and the group standard deviation.

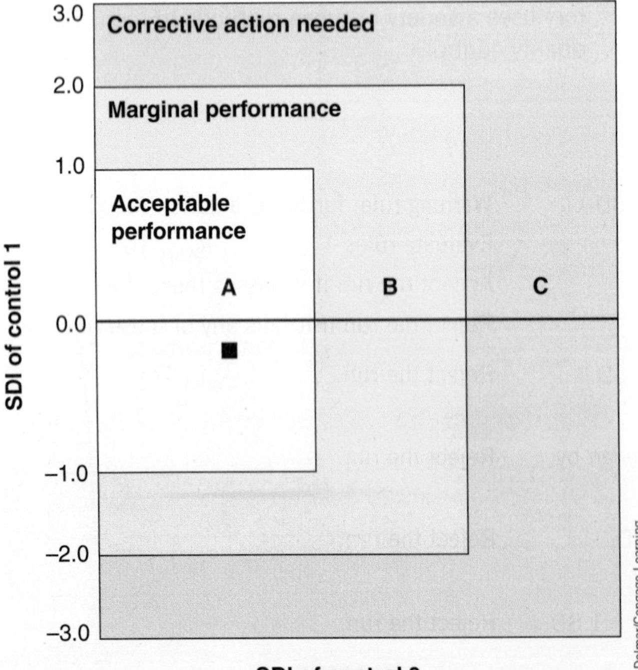

FIGURE 15-10 Representation of the Youden plot: Comparing the standard deviation interval (SDI) values of two control materials. All values on the *x*-axis are 0.0 SD. Coordinate for the observed mean of control 1 versus the observed mean of control 2.

> *Best Practice*
>
> **Interlaboratory Comparisons**
>
> Interlaboratory comparison data are available to participants of group data comparison studies. Such studies are conducted by companies that sell quality-control material and organizations that provide quality control surveys, such as the College of American Pathology (CAP).

DETERMINING THE ACCURACY OF AN ANALYTICAL ASSAY

Accuracy is a measure of truth or adherence to consensus for an analytical test method. Ideally, a test method in a clinical laboratory should be traceable to a reference material. The accuracy of a test method can be ascertained by analyzing the recovery of a reference material. Often, the unavailability or cost of obtaining reference material makes this approach impractical. Manufacturers of reagents use reference material as their calibrators or have their calibrators traceable to reference materials. Thus, the laboratory is relying on manufacturers for the accuracy of the laboratory method.

In addition, laboratories rely on regional quality control programs and on government-mandated or accrediting agency–mandated proficiency testing for acceptable accuracy performance of their analytical methods. In interlaboratory comparisons, the laboratory results are evaluated against results obtained by other laboratories using the same reagents and instrumentation. In mandatory proficiency testing for analyses monitored by the Centers for Medicare & Medicaid Services (CMS, formerly the Health Care Financing Administration (HCFA)I, the laboratory results are compared with the results obtained by other laboratories or with methodologies considered to be accurate. Several professional organizations and many individual states provide these surveys for a fee. The laboratory survey results are monitored by CMS, and an acceptable passing score must be obtained.

CASE STUDY 15-1

After completing the normal morning maintenance on the blood gas analyzer, the laboratory technician analyzed three control samples and obtained the following results (acceptable values ±2 SD; the variations in the normal ranges given in parentheses are attributable to the lot number, the manufacturer, and other factors):

Control 1:

pH = 7.320 (7.28–7.36)
PO_2 = 98 mm Hg (95–105 mm Hg)
PCO_2 = 60 mm Hg (57–64 mm Hg)

Control 2:

pH = 7.128 (7.132–7.184)
PO_2 = 45 mm Hg (46–51 mm Hg)
PCO_2 = 35 mm Hg (35–41 mm Hg)

Control 3:

pH = 7.456 (7.436–7.510)
PO_2 = 68 mm Hg (65–74 mm Hg)
PCO_2 = 75 mm Hg (71–79 mm Hg)

Questions

1. After evaluating the quality control run, which of the following should the technician do?
   a. Report the results to the physician.
   b. Recalibrate the analyzer and repeat the controls.
   c. Rerun the quality control material.
   d. Follow the troubleshooting procedure for the test on the analyzer.
2. Why are controls essential to the operation and maintenance of a blood gas analyzer?

CASE STUDY 15-2

A 10x alert comes up on a sodium assay during a daily quality control assay. The sodium quality-control results show that the sodium values of the normal and high controls are 121 and 149 mmol/L, respectively. The control ranges (±2 SD) for these controls are 120–128 and 148–154 mmol/L, respectively. A review of the quality-control values for the past month reveals that the control values for both sodium controls have been slowly drifting downward. All of the other analytes produce acceptable results without error flags. The sodium methodology on the analyzer is an ion-specific electrode, placed on the analyzer 6 months ago.

Questions

1. Determine which of the following actions to take:
   a. No actions are required, both quality-control values are within acceptable limits.
   b. Perform maintenance and reanalyze quality-control samples.
   c. Replace the sodium ISE electrode, perform maintenance, and repeat quality-control samples.
   d. Replace the reagents; they are probably deteriorating.
2. Why are quality controls essential to electrolyte analysis?

Summary

The respiratory therapist must have a basic understanding of chemistry and the various properties of atoms, bonds, and the atomic structure of biological molecules. This knowledge is necessary to understand how electrolytes influence and control metabolic reactions. Both sodium in the intracellular space and potassium in the extracellular space have a major influence on the distribution and retention of body fluids and on osmolality. Thus, electrolytes and body fluids affect changes in HCO_3^-, PCO_2, and pH.

Also helpful is an understanding of the various factors that control the concentration of both anions and cations in the body. Ionized calcium and ionized magnesium have been shown to be better indicators of cardiac function after cardiopulmonary bypass than the total levels of calcium and magnesium, consisting of both bound and free forms.

Respiratory therapists must be familiar with the various cardiac markers and their release into the blood.

The understanding of basic quality control, along with basic concepts of measuring various analytes, allows the respiratory therapist to monitor the accuracy of analytical results. Thus, proper and accurate information is provided to the physician or health care provider.

Study Questions

REVIEW QUESTIONS

1. Describe how element 11 (Na) differs from element 19 (K), and describe how the two elements are similar.

2. Biological molecules are usually classified into four groups: carbohydrates, lipids, proteins, and nucleic acids. Which group is the most important source of energy?
3. Identify some functions of electrolytes in the human body.
4. List three methods of analyzing for electrolytes, and indicate why one of these methods is now used almost exclusively.
5. Diabetes mellitus is a common cause of metabolic acidosis. Detail the typical laboratory results seen in this condition.
6. Explain the significance of measuring ionized magnesium levels in critically ill patients.
7. Explain why the measurement of myoglobin alone is not a reliable indicator for the diagnosis of myocardial infarction.
8. What are the statistical requirements to validate and monitor an analytical assay?

MULTIPLE-CHOICE QUESTIONS

1. Which of the following plasma analyses is the least affected by hemolysis?
   a. potassium
   b. chloride
   c. lithium
   d. sodium
2. A principal cause of metabolic acidosis is the formation of organic acids at a rate exceeding their breakdown. In diabetic patients with uncontrolled diabetes mellitus, there is an overproduction of organic acids such as acetoacetic acid and beta-hydroxybutyric acid, which leads to metabolic acidosis. Another common cause of metabolic acidosis is:
   a. late stages of salicylate poisoning.
   b. fat loss due to vigorous exercising.
   c. severe hypothermia.
   d. moderate consumption of ethanol.
3. The following laboratory findings were obtained
   pH = 7.24
   PCO_2 = 24 mm Hg
   Total carbon dioxide = 18 mmol/L
   These values are consistent with:
   a. respiratory alkalosis.
   b. respiratory acidosis.
   c. metabolic alkalosis.
   d. metabolic acidosis.
4. Bicarbonate diffuses from the red blood cells into the plasma through an exchange mechanism with:
   a. sulfate.
   b. lipids.
   c. chloride.
   d. phosphate.
5. When you are calibrating pH, PCO_2, and PO_2 in a blood gas analyzer, it is not necessary to
   a. control electrical drift.
   b. maintain the temperature at 37°C.
   c. determine the barometric pressure and make necessary adjustments.
   d. prime the instrument using a whole blood sample.
6. Ion-specific electrodes (ISEs) are based on the principle of:
   a. oxidation-reduction reactions.
   b. electrochemical reactions.
   c. potentiation.
   d. coulometric-amperometric analysis.
7. A number without units used to show deviation regardless of the concentration of a control is:
   a. standard deviation.
   b. coefficient of variation.
   c. mean.
   d. trend.
8. *Accuracy* refers to the:
   a. true value of an analyte.
   b. precision of an analyte.
   c. standard deviation of a control value.
   d. reliability of the assay result.
9. The coefficient of variation is equal to:
   a. standard deviation × 100%.
   b. (mean/standard deviation) × 100%.
   c. (standard deviation × 100%)/mean.
   d. standard deviation × mean × 100%.
10. Which of the following statements about the PCO_2 electrode is not true?
    a. It measures the rate of change of the oxygen concentration.
    b. Oxygen diffuses across an O_2-permeable membrane.
    c. Silver is oxidized at the anode; oxygen is reduced at the platinum electrode.
    d. The CO_2 gas diffuses through the membrane, altering the pH of the bicarbonate solution.
11. The potassium electrode is different from the sodium electrode in that it:
    a. contains a valinomycin membrane.
    b. contains a silver electrode.
    c. consists of a double glass system.
    d. allows for a change in pH.
12. "Chloride shift" refers to:
    a. the shift of plasma chloride to the red blood cells.
    b. an abnormally high concentration of plasma chloride.
    c. an abnormally low concentration of plasma chloride.
    d. the irreversible binding of chloride ions to plasma proteins.

13. The Teflon membrane on the PCO_2 electrode prevents the transition (diffusion) of:
    a. oxygen.
    b. hydrogen ion.
    c. dissolved CO_2.
    d. ionized magnesium ions.
14. A state of elevated carbon dioxide in blood is called:
    a. hypercalcemia.
    b. hypocapnia.
    c. hypernatremia.
    d. hypercapnia.
15. The most specific marker for myocardial infarction (MI) is:
    a. myoglobin.
    b. troponin T or troponin I.
    c. creatine kinase MB.
    d. lactic dehydrogenase (LD).
16. The extent to which the true value of an analyte agrees with the analytical measurement is known as:
    a. reproducibility.
    b. accuracy.
    c. precision.
    d. reliability.

CRITICAL-THINKING QUESTIONS

1. A whole blood sample was analyzed for electrolytes (Na, K, Cl, CO_2), iCa, and iMg. The following results were obtained (the normal reference interval is given in parentheses):

   Na = 209 mmol/L (135–145)

   K = 5.5 mmol/L (3.5–5.0)

   Cl = 104 mmol/L (97–108)

   CO_2 = 29 mmol/L (22–32)

   iCa = 1.4 mmol/L (1.15–1.35)

   iMg = 0.7 mmol/L (0.45–0.60)

   The very high Na level required further investigation before the results could be reported. An examination of the whole blood specimen revealed slight hemolysis. A nonheparinized sample was obtained and allowed to clot. The resulting serum specimen was analyzed in the main laboratory with the following results:

   Na = 149 mmol/L

   K = 5.2 mmol/L

   Cl = 103 mmol/L

   CO_2 = 26 mmol/L

   iCa = 1.4 mmol/L

   iMg = 0.55 mmol/L

   The serum results were reported to the physician. Because the Na level was now closer to the normal range (135–145 mmol/L), slight hemolysis was considered the most likely cause of the elevated Na. Determine the most likely cause for the elevated sodium. Was it indeed a critical value, or was hemolysis or sample contamination the most likely cause?
2. A severely ill patient admitted in the emergency room had the following laboratory results (the normal reference interval is given in parentheses):

   Na = 158 mmol/L (135–145)

   K = 5.9 mmol/L (3.5–5.0)

   Cl = 124 mmol/L (97–108)

   CO_2 = 33 mmol/L (22–32)

   Glucose = 340 mg/dL (70–110)

   Osmolality = 271 mOsm/kg (280–300)

   iCa = 1.6 mmol/L (1.15–1.35)

   iMg = 0.85 mmol/L (0.45–0.60)

   Detect inconsistencies with respect to the values. Provide the reasons for these.
3. Two blood gas analyzers are being considered for possible purchase for the department. The goal is to select the instrumentation with the better precision. The evaluation is conducted by two respiratory therapists, each using a control material over a period of 14 days. The following results of this evaluation are to be used to make a purchase decision:

		Data from Instrument 1	Data from Instrument 2
pH	Mean	7.124	7.591
	SD	0.094	0.102
	CV	1.26	1.34
	n	14	14
PCO_2	Mean	55 mm Hg	99 mm Hg
	SD	4.02	5.03
	CV	7.31	5.08
	n	14	14
PO_2	Mean	55 mm Hg	99 mm Hg
	SD	0.094	0.102
	CV	1.26	1.34
	n	14	14

   Select an instrument, and provide reasons for your selection.
4. An arterial blood gas analysis is performed on a patient with the following results:

   pH = 7.38

   PO_2 = 75 mm Hg

   PCO_2 = 49 mm Hg

   HCO_3^- = 25 mmol/L

The specimen has been recapped and refrigerated. Two hours later, the physician questions the result and asks for a repeat analysis on the same sample. The following results are obtained:

pH = 7.39

PO_2 = 75 mm Hg

PCO_2 = 38 mm Hg

HCO_3^- = 41 mmol/L

How would you explain the changes to the physician?

5. A blood gas analysis is performed on an arterial specimen, and the following results are obtained:

pH = 7.35

PO_2 = 98 mm Hg

PCO_2 = 35 mm Hg

HCO_3^- = 32 mmol/L

Moderate hemolysis was also observed, which was noted on the report.

The physician requested some additional chemistry tests on this specimen. The results were as follows (normal reference intervals are given in parentheses):

Na = 144 mmol/L (135–145)

K = 7.1 mmol/L (3.5–5.0)

Cl = 109 mmol/L (97–108)

CO_2 = 31 mmol/L (22–32)

Glucose = 85 mg/dL (70–110)

iCa = 1.33 mmol/L (1.15–1.35)

Evaluate the validity of these results.

References

1. Scott MG, Heusel JW, LeGrys VA, Siggaard-Anderson O. Electrolytes and blood gases. In: Burtis CA, Ashwood ER, eds. *Tietz Textbook of Clinical Chemistry*. 3rd ed, Philadelphia: WB Saunders Co; 1999:1056–1092.
2. Brueckner PJ. Water, electrolyte and/hydrogen ion disorders. In: Gornall AG, ed. *Applied Biochemistry of Clinical Disorders*. 2nd ed. Philadelphia: JB Lippincott Co; 1986:99–128.
3. Ladenson JH, Lewis JW, McDonald JM, Slatopolsky E, Boyd JC. Relationship of free and total calcium in hypercalcemic conditions. *J Clin Edocrinol Metab.* 1978;48:393.
4. Polancic JE. Magnesium: metabolism, clinical importance, and analysis. *Clin Lab Sci.* 1991;4:195.
5. Shiry TL. Critical care profiling for informed treatment of severely ill patients. *Am J Clin Pathol.* 1995;104:579–587.
6. Aglio LS, Stanford GG, Maddi R, Boyd III JL, Nussbaum S, Chernow B. Hypomagnesemia is common following cardiac surgery. *J Cardiothorac Vasc Anesth.* 1991;5:201–208.
7. D'Orazio P, Miller WG, Myers GL, et al. Standardization of sodium and potassium ion-selective electrode system to the flame photometric reference method. Approved standard. 2nd ed. *CLSI.* 2000; 20:1–22.
8. Durst RA, Siggaard-Anderson O. Electrochemistry. In: Burtis CA, Ashwood ER, eds. *Tietz Textbook of Clinical Chemistry*. 3rd ed. Philadelphia: WB Saunders Co; 1999:133–149.
9. Freitag R. *Biosensors in Analytical Biotechnology* Austin, TX: RG Landis Co; 1995.
10. Wang J. Electro analysis and biosensors. *Anal Chem.* 1995;67:487R–492R.
11. Wrotnowski C. Biosensor technology advances. *Genet Eng News.* 1998:18:132.
12. Karselis TC. *The Pocket Guide to Clinical Laboratory Instrumentation.* Philadelphia: FA Davis Co; 1994.
13. Oech U, Ammann D, Simon W. Ion-selective membrane electrodes for clinical use. *Clin Chem.* 1986;32:1448–1459.
14. Heusel JW, Siggaard-Anderson O, Scott MG. Physiology and disorders of water, electrolyte, and acid-base metabolism. In: Burtis CA, Ashwood ER, eds. *Tietz Textbook of Clinical Chemistry*. 3rd ed. Philadelphia: WB Saunders Co; 1999:1095–1124.
15. Sacks DB. Carbohydrates. In: Burtis CA, Ashwood ER, eds. *Tietz Textbook of Clinical Chemistry*. 3rd ed. Philadelphia: WB Saunders Co; 1999;750–808.
16. Lash JP, Arruda JAL. Laboratory evaluation of renal tubular acidosis. *Clin Lab Med.* 1993;13:117–129.
17. Apple F, Henderson R. Cardiac injury. In: Burtis CA, Ashwood ER, eds. *Tietz Textbook of Clinical Chemistry*. 3rd ed. Philadelphia: WB Saunders Co; 1999:1178–1203.
18. Wu ABH. Introduction to coronary artery disease (CAD) and biochemical markers. In: Wu AHB, ed. *Pathology and Laboratory Medicine: Cardiac Markers.* Totowa, NJ: Humana Press; 1998:3–20.
19. Greaser ML, Gergely J. Reconstitution of troponin activity from three different components. *J Biol Chem.* 1971;246:4226–4233.
20. Vaidya HC, Vaananen HK. Myoglobin and carbonic anhydrase III. In: Wu AHB, ed. *Pathology and Laboratory Medicine: Cardiac Markers.* Totowa, NJ: Humana Press; 1998:103–112.
21. U.S. Department of Health and Human Services. Medicare, Medicaid, and CLIA programs: regulations implementing the clinical laboratory improvement amendments of 1988 (CLIA). Final rule. *Fed. Regist.* 1992;57:7002–7186.
22. Kringle RO, Bogovich M. Statistical procedures. In: Burtis CA, Ashwood ER, eds. *Tietz Textbook of Clinical Chemistry*. 3rd ed. Philadelphia: WB Saunders Co; 1999:365–409.

23. Westgard JO, Klee GG. Quality management. In: Burtis CA, Ashwood ER, eds. *Tietz Textbook of Clinical Chemistry*. 3rd ed. Philadelphia: WB Saunders Co; 1999:384–418.
24. Westgard JO. *OPSpecs Manual—Expanded Edition: Operating Specifications for Imprecision, Accuracy, and Quality Control*. Oggunquit, ME: Westgard QC; 1996.
25. Levey S, Jennings ER. The use of charts in the clinical laboratory. *Am J Clin Pathol*. 1950;20: 1059–1066.

Suggested Readings

Clark LC. A family of polarographic enzyme electrodes and the measurement of alcohol. *Biotechnol Bioeng*. 1972;3:377.

Ebbing DD, Gammon SD. *General Chemistry*. 9th ed. Belmont, CA: Brooks Cole; 2010.

Elion-Gerritzen WE. Quality control in clinical chemistry—two-sample plot and improvement in laboratory performance. *Am J Clin Pathol*. 1977;67:91–96.

Mercer DW. Role of cardiac markers in evaluation of suspected myocardial infarction: selecting the most clinically useful indicators. *Postgrad Med*. 1997;102:113–117,

National Committee for Laboratory Standards. *Standardization of Sodium and Potassium Ion-Selective Electrode Systems to the Flame Photometric Reference Method; Approved Standard C-29A*. Wayne, PA: National Committee for Laboratory Standards; 1995.

Seager SL, Slabauch MR. *Chemistry for Today: General, Organic, and Biochemistry*. 6th ed. Minneapolis, MN: West Publishing Co; 2007.

Steel RGD, Torrie JH. *Principles and Procedures of Statistics*. 3rd ed. New York: McGraw-Hill Book Co; 1996.

CHAPTER 16

Arterial Blood Gases and Noninvasive Monitoring of Oxygen and Carbon Dioxide

Paul J. Mathews and Larry Conway

OBJECTIVES

Upon completion of this chapter, the reader should be able to:

- List the normal measured and calculated values for arterial blood gases.
- Given examples, select blood gases that indicate abnormal conditions, such as respiratory acidosis, respiratory alkalosis, metabolic acidosis, metabolic alkalosis, and mixed metabolic and respiratory conditions.
- Calculate and explain the significance of anion gap variations.
- Given a clinical scenario, choose the correct acid-base status of the patient.
- Supplied with adequate information, calculate projected blood gas values.
- Determine the oxygen-carrying capacity and content of blood.
- Differentiate between S_aO_2, S_PO_2, and O_2 content.
- Determine whether the available information is sufficient to perform blood gas prediction equations.
- Define oxygen saturation, oxygen content, oxygen combining capacity, oxygen dissociation curve, pulse oximetry, and buffer.
- Select and order the steps in blood gas sampling by arterial puncture, arterial line aspiration, and capillary-sampling techniques.
- Discuss the principles of operation for transcutaneous and gas-sampling techniques.
- Identify the strengths and weaknesses of various types of invasive and noninvasive analysis techniques.
- Identify the indications and contraindications associated with various blood gas analysis and monitoring techniques.

CHAPTER OUTLINE

(continues)

(continued)

KEY TERMS

Allen's test (modified)
analyte
anion gap (AG)
arterial blood gases (ABG)
capnogram
capnometer
conjugate pairs
co-oximetry
dyshemoglobins
glycolysis
metabolism
plethysmography
respiration
spectrophotometry
S_PO_2
tricarboxylic acid (TCA) cycle
ventilation

The goals of this chapter are to provide an understanding of the principles of acid-base balance and the arterial blood gases as they apply to the body's quest for homeostasis. Also discussed are the methods used to sample arterial blood gases and pH. The factors that affect the normal blood gases and those that can adversely affect the results of the analysis are examined.

Arterial blood gases (ABGs) are the diagnostic tests that best define the function of the lungs in their task of supplying oxygen to and removing carbon dioxide from the body. Arterial blood gases provide a window through which we can examine ventilation, respiration, metabolism, and acid-base balance during health and disease. Arterial blood gas analysis is perhaps the single most important diagnostic tool in the treatment and diagnosis of respiratory and respiratory-related disease.

This chapter details the normal values of the measured and calculated ABGs and the variations in these measures that signal disease states. Factors that influence the arterial blood gases and acid-base balance and the methods of estimating and measuring these values are discussed. The role of hemoglobin and its structural and biochemical variations in oxygen transport and ABG analysis are explained. The concept and importance of anion gap are detailed. Sampling, analysis, quality control, and possible error-causing factors are covered. In addition, some new and emerging technologies to assess the blood gases are discussed. Through the use of several case studies, the information provided in this chapter is applied.

Blood Gases

The study of blood gases entails the study of gases carried in the blood, in most cases, in the arterial circulation.

WHAT ARE THE BLOOD GASES?

Blood gases are physiological indicators of the efficiency and effectiveness of internal and external respiration and of ventilation. **Respiration** is the movement of gases across biological membranes by diffusion. **Ventilation** is the gross movement of gas into and out of the lungs. In other words, ventilation is an external process, and respiration is an internal process. More precisely, ventilation is composed of at least three internal functions: pulmonary respiration, tissue respiration, and cellular respiration.

Once the oxygen reaches the cell or tissue level, it is drawn into the cells. There, it undergoes a chemical bonding with other substances in a process called *oxidative phosphorylation*, which is part of a complex series of biochemical reactions that utilize oxygen to produce energy. Carbon dioxide, water, other chemical substances, and heat are by-products of this process. The total process is called **metabolism**. The major pathway of metabolism is called the Krebs cycle. Figure 16-1 illustrates the major components of the TCA cycle.

THE TCA CYCLE

The **tricarboxylic acid (TCA) cycle** is one of three subpaths of metabolism (Figure 16-1). In the first, **glycolysis**, two molecules of adenosine triphosphate (ATP) and heat are produced by the reaction of pyruvic acid and glucose ($C_6H_{12}O_6$). Enzymes in the body break the glucose down into 2 units of pyruvic acid [CH_3, 4 hydrogen ions, and energy expressed as heat (Δ)]. Chemical shorthand expresses this reaction in the following formula:

$$C_6H_{12}O_6 \rightarrow 2\ CH_3 = O = COOH + 4H^+$$
$$+ \text{ glucose} \rightarrow \text{pyruvic acid}$$

$$CH_3 = CHOH = COOH + \Delta$$
$$\rightarrow \text{lactic acid}$$

Because no oxygen is used, this reaction is known as an *oxidative* or *anaerobic* (without oxygen) form of metabolism. Note in the formula that the original 6 oxygen molecules from the glucose are still present in the 2 molecules of pyruvic acid that resulted from the reaction. At this point, the TCA cycle is activated in aerobic situations, producing acetyl coenzyme A, 2 hydrogen, and 2 carbon dioxide molecules, producing

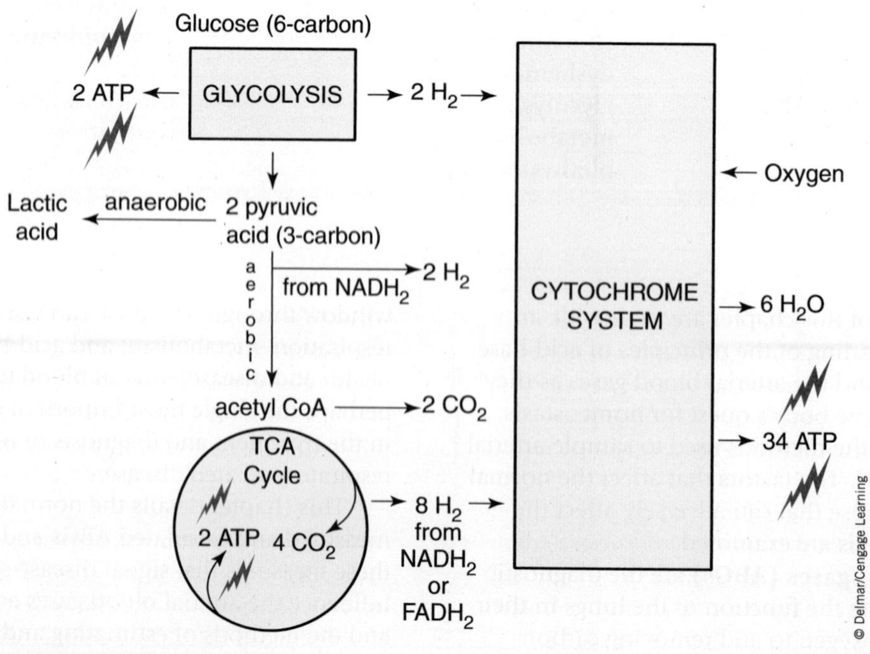

FIGURE 16-1 The TCA cycle.

2 more ATP molecules, 8 H_2 molecules, and 4 CO_2 molecules:

$$2\,CH_3 = C = COOH + O_2 \rightarrow 2\,H_2 + 2\,CO_2 + \text{acetyl CoA}$$

pyruvic acid

If sufficient oxygen is available, the reaction proceeds to the third, or aerobic, subpathway—more formally called the *cytochrome* or *oxidative phosphorylation system*. In this subsystem, oxygen and 10 H_2 molecules enter the system and produce 6 H_2O molecules and 34 ATP molecules.[1,2]

Figure 16-1 illustrates these three oxygen- and glucose-consuming, energy-producing, and carbon dioxide–producing systems. Note the glycogen and glucose reaction is dynamic and reversible, indicating that glycogen stores are conserved. Clearly, the body's ability to acquire and use oxygen and to eliminate carbon dioxide is a critical function.

The chapters on applied physics (Chapter 3) and pulmonary anatomy and physiology (Chapter 6) discussed how the body provides for the bulk movement of gases into and out of the lungs. In this chapter is a discussion of how these respiratory gases, mainly oxygen and carbon dioxide, are transported throughout the body. The first area of discussion is how the circulatory system carries these gases to the tissues and organs of the body.

GAS TRANSPORT IN THE BLOOD

The respiratory gases are carried in the blood in one of three ways. They may be:

- Dissolved in the liquid (plasma) portion of the blood.
- Chemically bound to other substances.
- Attached to hemoglobin.

Each of these methods has different characteristics and affects gases in a different way.

Gases that are dissolved in the plasma exert a partial pressure in response to Dalton's law (see Chapter 3). The partial pressure exerted is proportional to the fractional (percentage) concentration of the gas in the inhaled gas volume. For example, room air is composed of 20.93% oxygen, 0.03% carbon dioxide, 78% nitrogen, and small percentages of trace gases.

For this example, assume a sea level normal barometric pressure (P_B) of 760 mm Hg and an ambient temperature in a range suitable for human life. Also assume that the well hydrated human body is normally capable of warming (or cooling) the inhaled gas to a temperature of about 37°C and humidifying it to 100% saturation by the time it reaches the carina.

As a result of this warming and addition of water vapor, the volume of gas now has a water vapor pressure (PH_2O) of 47 mm Hg and a water vapor content of 43.9 mg/L³. Take the barometric pressure, deduct the water vapor pressure, and then calculate the partial pressure of each inspired gas by multiplying the adjusted barometric pressure by its fractional concentration (F). The result is the partial pressure (P) of each gas in the mixture. For example, room air (RA) has the following partial gas pressures under the assumed conditions:

$$P_B = 760 \text{ mm Hg}$$
$$PH_2O = 47 \text{ mm Hg}$$
$$P_{B(adj)} = 713 \text{ mm Hg}$$

$$P_{B(adj)} \times F_IO_2 = P_aO_2$$
$$P_{B(adj)} \times 0.2093 = P_aO_2$$
$$713 \text{ mm} \times 0.2093 = 149.2309 \text{ mm Hg } P_aO_2$$
$$713 \text{ mm} \times 0.003 = 2.139 \text{ mm Hg } P_aCO_2$$
$$713 \text{ mm} \times 0.78 = 556.14 \text{ mm Hg } P_aN$$
$$713 \text{ mm Hg} \times 0.0077 = 5.4901 \text{ mm Hg } P_{trace}$$
$$713.00 \text{ mm Hg} = P_{total}$$

After compensation for the water vapor pressure, the partial pressures of the other gases equal 713 mm Hg, with each gas having a pressure proportional to its fractional concentration (its percentage in the inspired gas) in the atmosphere. This fact holds true for all altitudes to which an unaided human might travel. The PH_2O changes only with changes in temperature. The pressure exerted by water in the gas is called its *water vapor pressure*.

Acid-Base Balance

In addition to blood gases, other factors govern the acidity (pH) of the blood. *Acid-base balance* is the dynamic equilibrium between the substances in the body that are proton donors and those that are proton acceptors (Chapter 4). This balance in the normal individual is such that the pH, or balance of alkalinity and acidity, in the body remains stable within a very fine but slightly alkaline range of 7.35–7.45 pH.

To restate this concept, acid-base balance is that part of the homeostatic function of the body that maintains the fluids in the body in the correct acidity range to promote optimum biological and chemical function. Not all body fluids are in that pH range, but, on average, the normal human adult body is in that range. Infants have slight differences in the acid-base homeostasis (Chapter 29).

The major systems that maintain optimal pH are the respiratory system (by controlling carbon dioxide levels) and the renal or urinary system [by controlling bicarbonate (HCO_3^-)]. The balance between the production and excretion of the two substances results in a buffer system (Chapter 4). The buffer systems referred to in this chapter, in general, result from the reactions of weak acids and weak bases. The particular weak acid and weak base pair of interest is the weak acid carbonic acid (H_2CO_3) and the weak base bicarbonate (HCO_3^-). The reversible reaction formed by these substances is shown in the formula:

$$\underset{\text{Weak acid}}{H_2CO_3} \quad \leftrightarrow \quad \underset{\text{Weak base}}{H^+ + HCO_3^-}$$

Such pairs of acids and bases, and others like them, are called **conjugate pairs** (i.e., a weak base and its conjugate acid or a weak acid and its conjugate base). The body has four types of H^+ buffering: ventilatory, renal, intracellular, and extracellular buffering.

VENTILATORY BUFFERING

Carbon dioxide regulation (hyper- or hypoventilation) is the most rapid method the body has to alter and control acid-base status. It is also very fatiguing and produces metabolic acids, primarily lactic acid, as a result of the energy expenditure required.

RENAL BUFFERING

The kidneys regulate H^+ through blood filtering and urine production. Renal buffering is energy sparing but slow in effect. In addition, it puts a strain on the kidney and at times on the heart and circulatory system.

INTRACELLULAR BUFFERS

Intracellular buffers include protein, phosphates, and hemoglobin (Hb). Carbon dioxide buffering by the red blood cells (RBCs) triggers a response that results in the following transformation:

$$H^+ + Hb^- \leftrightarrow HHb$$

The RBC buffering also assists the movement of HCO_3^- out of the cell and the movement of chloride ions (Cl^-) into the cell to balance cellular electrical charges. This is known as the *chloride shift*.

Excess H^+ moving into the cell causes the movement of both Na^+ (sodium ions) and K^+ (potassium ions) out of the cells and into the circulating plasma in order to retain the cell's electrical neutrality. The increase in circulating sodium generally has little effect owing to the already high concentration of plasma sodium. The addition of small amounts of potassium may have little effect because of its initial low concentration, but it can have dramatic and sometimes lethal effects if hyperkalemia ensues.

EXTRACELLULAR BUFFERS

Bicarbonate and blood proteins have small but important effects on acid-base balance. They stabilize and maintain the acid-base balance in homeostatic ranges as the plasma and blood proteins circulate in the body.

Measurement of ABG and Acid-Base Results

Arterial blood gases and acid-base balance are generally measured simultaneously because they are interrelated and interdependent. Additionally, they can be measured using the same blood sample; the patient does not have to undergo another arterial needlestick and the associated discomfort. The P_aCO_2 level is integral to the acid-base balance represented by the measured pH value and the calculated bicarbonate (HCO_3^-). An acute change in the P_aCO_2 produces relatively immediate changes in the pH through the relationships of the major buffering systems described by the Henderson-Hasselbalch (H-H) equation.

Best Practice

Henderson-Hasselbalch Equation

The relationship of the weak acid H_2CO_3 and the weak base HCO_3^- is defined in the Henderson-Hasselbalch equation:

$$\text{pH} = \text{pK} + \log \frac{[HCO_3^-]}{[H_2CO_3]}$$

In this equation, HCO_3^- represents the metabolic (kidney) component, and the H_2CO_3 represents the respiratory (lung) component. H_2CO_3 can be calculated from measured P_aCO_2 using the constant factor 0.03. For a person with textbook normal ventilation ($P_aCO_2 = 40$) and bicarbonate ($HCO_3^- = 24$), the equation transforms to:

$$\begin{aligned} \text{pH} &= pK + \log \frac{[24]}{[40 \times 0.03]} \\ &= pK + \log \frac{[24]}{[1.2]} \\ &= pK + \log [20] \end{aligned}$$

Since pK is a constant with a value of 6.1, and the log of 20 is 1.3, the equation further resolves to:

$$\begin{aligned} \text{pH} &= 6.1 + 1.3 \\ &= 7.4 \end{aligned}$$

Thus, pH for a person with normal ventilation (indicated by a normal concentration of CO_2) and bicarbonate levels is 7.40. The two primary components in this buffering system are the lungs and the kidneys.

Alternatively, the body's most immediate response to pH changes caused by other buffering systems is to modify breathing patterns. The response is to alter the P_aCO_2:

- Either by increasing the minute volume of gas reaching the alveoli (alveolar hyperventilating) for increased P_aCO_2 or decreased pH.
- Or by reducing gas volumes per minute delivered to the alveoli (alveolar hypoventilation) for decreased P_aCO_2 or increased pH.

The minute volume change can be changed by changing either the frequency (rate) of ventilations, the tidal volume of each breath, or both rate and volume. The general relationship between pH, P_aCO_2, and HCO_3^- can be described with the illustration in Figure 16-2.

First, consider the illustration to be a seesaw, with the HCO_3^- as the unmoving pivot point. (Figure 16-2A). When the P_aCO_2 falls, as in simple hyperventilation, the pH rises. This rise produces simple, uncompensated respiratory alkalemia. Alternatively, if the P_aCO_2 rises, as in simple hypoventilation, the pH falls. This fall produces uncompensated respiratory acidemia.

Next, consider that the P_aCO_2 is the unchanging pivot point of the line (Figure 16-2B). If the HCO^{3-} falls, as in diabetic crisis, the pH is "pulled down" as the center of the lever is lowered. This fall in pH produces uncompensated metabolic acidemia. If the HCO_3^- rises, the lever is "pushed up," and the pH rises, resulting in metabolic alkalemia.

In addition to these interactions, the pH affects the placement and shape of the oxyhemoglobin dissociation curve (Figure 16-3). The shape and shift of this curve directly affect the loading, unloading, and transport of oxygen in the lungs and at the tissues. Given the dramatic and direct relationships, ABGs and acid-base balance have to be addressed together.

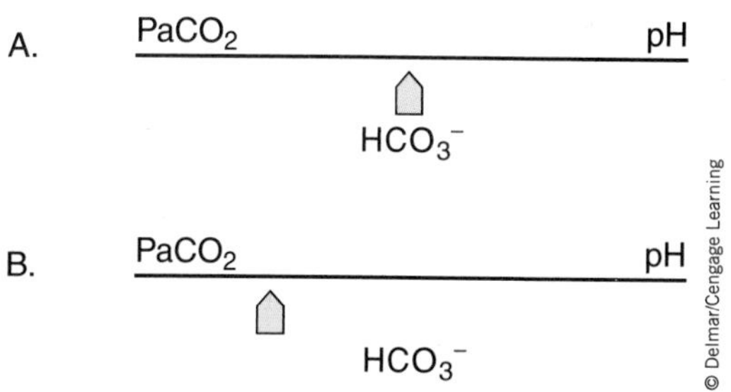

FIGURE 16-2 Simple acid-base balance model: (A) The pivot point is at the HCO_3^-. Therefore, if HCO_3^- is stable, as P_aCO_2 rises, pH falls. If P_aCO_2 falls, pH rises. This is a respiratory-based change. (B) The pivot point is located at the P_aCO_2, indicating that P_aCO_2 is the stable component: As HCO_3^- rises, pH also rises. If HCO_3^- falls, pH also falls. This is a metabolic-based change. Actual clinical scenarios often include combinations in which, for example, HCO_3^- has changed a lot and P_aCO_2 has changed a little, causing a combined change on the pH.

Oxygen Saturation

Oxygen saturation (SO_2) can be determined in several ways, leading to some confusion and misunderstandings about this variable. The most common method of expressing the oxygen saturation (SO_2) is as the S_pO_2,

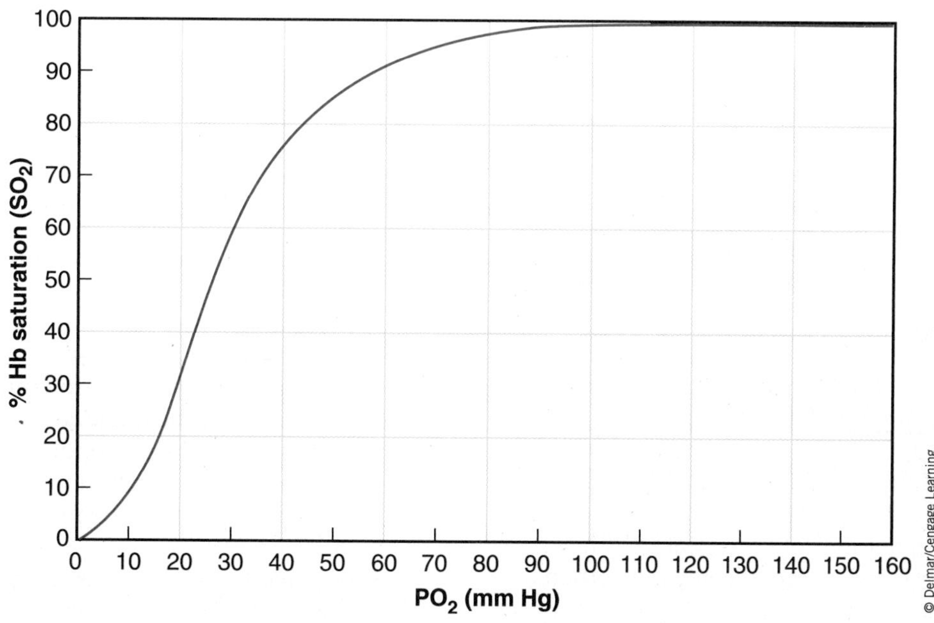

FIGURE 16-3 The oxyhemoglobin dissociation curve.

where the subscripted "P" indicates that this value is determined by pulse oximetry (discussed in detail later in this chapter). The S_PO_2 value is an expression of the ratio of the hemoglobin with oxygen attached to the total amount of hemoglobin present in the circulation that passed the pulse oximeter's sensor during the sampling period. The hemoglobin with oxygen attached is called *saturated hemoglobin* or *oxyhemoglobin* (HbO_2). Hemoglobin without oxygen attached is known as *unsaturated*, or reduced, *hemoglobin* (Hbr, RHb, or HbR). Recall that hemoglobin carries about 97% of the O_2 circulating in the blood.

The other 3% of the circulating O_2 is dissolved in the blood plasma and is readily available to the tissues and their cells. This volume of O_2 also has a saturation, called the *saturation of arterial oxygen* (S_aO_2) or *venous oxygen saturation* (S_VO_2) depending on where the sample was obtained. For the most part, the arterial value is reported as part of an arterial blood gas report. The S_aO_2 and S_VO_2 values represent the percentages of the actual, as opposed to the potential, partial pressures of oxygen in the plasma. This concept is the same as that for expressing relative humidity, where the actual is compared to the potential water vapor pressure. Be aware that the S_aO_2 oxygen value is calculated, not measured. and that it represents only 3% of the circulating O_2 mass. Also, S_aO_2 and S_PO_2 do not represent the same data and should not be taken to be interchangeable even though their values may at times be similar.

From the definition, clearly at least three factors influence oxygen saturation: the amount of oxygen available, the amount of hemoglobin available, and the ability of the hemoglobin to carry oxygen. When the partial pressure of oxygen in the arterial blood is plotted against the %Hb saturation (SO_2), the plot assumes a characteristic S-shaped, or sinusoidal, curve (Figure 16-3). For more information on the factors that affect the oxygen saturation curve, see Chapter 6.

Best Practice

Oxygen Saturation

Oxygen saturation (SO_2) is expressed as a percentage of saturation, that is, the percentage of the available hemoglobin (Hb) that is combined with oxygen. Common abbreviations for this value are S_aO_2, % SO_2, SO_2%, O_2 Sat, and Sat. This ratio does not indicate the total oxygen content of the blood. It reports only the portion of the oxygen bound to hemoglobin.

Nomenclature

There is widespread misapplication of certain terms related to blood gases and acid-base balance. In general:

- Terms ending in "-ia" refer to conditions at the tissue level (e.g., anoxia).
- Terms ending in "-emia" refer to conditions in the blood (e.g., hypoxemia).

Scientific and medical accuracy, both in communications and in application, demands that all personnel use correct and appropriate terminology in patient care, research, and oral or print communications. To do otherwise invites error and chaos. Here are some confused or confusing terms and their correct meanings:

- *Acidemia*—Blood pH less than 7.35
- *Acidotic*—Having a lower than normal pH (less than 7.35)
- *Alkalemia*—Blood pH greater than 7.45
- *Alkalotic*—A higher than normal pH (greater than 7.45)
- *Anoxemia*—The total lack or absence of oxygen in the blood
- *Anoxia*—The total lack or absence of oxygen in the tissues
- *Hypercapnea*—A higher than normal P_aCO_2 (greater than 45 mm Hg), caused by hypoventilation
- *Hyperoxia*—A higher than normal level of oxygen at the tissues
- *Hyperventilation*—Alveolar ventilation sufficient to lower P_aCO_2 to below normal (less than 35 mm Hg)
- *Hypocapnea*—A lower than normal P_aCO_2 (less than 35 mm Hg)
- *Hypoventilation*—Alveolar ventilation decreased sufficiently to cause a P_aCO_2 above normal (greater than 45 mm Hg)

Note: Hyper- and hypoventilation address changes in minute alveolar ventilation by changes in respiratory rate, in volume, or in both. Breath-by-breath changes may not result in hypo- or hyperventilation.

- *Hypoxemia*—A lower than normal level of oxygen in the blood
- *Hypoxia*—A lower than normal (but adequate) level of oxygen at the tissues
- *Metabolic*—In blood gas interpretation, a condition driven by the kidneys
- *Mixed*—An acid-base condition in which the respiratory and metabolic systems (lungs and kidneys) are driving the pH variance in the same direction
- *Respiratory*—In blood gas interpretation, a condition driven by the respiratory system (e.g., changes in P_aCO_2 of the lungs)

Homeostasis

The role of a buffer is to resist or diminish the level of pH change in a system. A buffer system is a combination of a weak acid and a weak base that, together, absorb the introduction of a strong acid or base, resulting in a smaller change in acid-base balance. Therefore, the effect of a buffer system is to moderate changes in pH and to maintain homeostasis.

The purpose of buffering is to maintain a relatively narrow balance of pH (normal 7.35–7.45). This dynamic balance, or equilibrium—called *homeostasis*—represents the optimum pH for bodily functions. That is the pH range where metabolic functions are most efficient and most effective. By far the most important buffering system in controlling pH is the *bicarbonate (bicarbonate–carbonic acid) system*. Although this is a very poor chemical buffer system, it is an effective physiological buffer. This system is all the more powerful because it is an open system; that is, one of its constituent parts (CO_2) can be added or removed quickly.

Other, lesser buffering systems are nonbicarbonate systems and closed; that is, the constituent parts remain in the system. These are hemoglobin itself, proteins, and phosphate.

- Hemoglobin is quantitatively the most important so-called chemical buffer in the red blood cell.
- Protein buffers (Pr^-/HPr) are the most important chemical buffers in the plasma, but they are quantitatively less important than hemoglobin.
- The phosphate buffer system ($HPO_4^-/H_2PO_4^-$) is relatively unimportant as a body-buffering system.

LUNGS

The lungs, through the adjustment of the P_aCO_2, are a primary means of maintaining pH homeostasis in the body. The placement of the H_2CO_3 in the Henderson-Hasselbalch equation indicates that P_aCO_2 and pH are inversely related. In general, every 20-mm-Hg rise in P_aCO_2 results in a decrease of 0.1 pH units; conversely a 10-mm-Hg fall in P_aCO_2 causes an increase of 0.1 pH units. The impact of the lungs on pH can be rapid, almost instantaneous. A patient's maximal hyperventilation to lower the P_aCO_2 to offset the falling pH of diabetic ketoacidosis (DKA) dramatically demonstrates the power of the lungs in this regard and the extent to which the body goes to maintain pH homeostasis.

To a lesser extent, the body uses the lungs to compensate for elevated pH. Decreasing ventilation and allowing the P_aCO_2 to rise lowers the pH somewhat. In general, in the absence of other factors, such as sedation, the body limits the level to which the P_aCO_2 rises to accomplish compensation for alkalosis.

KIDNEYS

The kidneys are an effective but much slower means to compensate for acid-base imbalances. Their response can take 24 hours or more to produce significant impact. By retaining or excreting more HCO_3^-, the kidneys can offset an acidemia or an alkalemia, effects that are commonly seen in chronic lung disease patients. Many of these patients live day to day with relatively elevated P_aCO_2 levels, which cause lower pH (acidemia). Over time, the kidneys retain more HCO_3^- that "pushes up" on the center of the lever described in Figure 16-2, raising the pH to a more normal level. Likewise, the kidneys can compensate for acid-base disturbances caused by other buffering systems by adjusting the level of HCO_3^- maintained in the body.

Arterial Blood Gas

The most accurate and complete assessment of acid-base and gas status is the arterial blood gas. Analysis of arterial blood not only gives direct measurement of pH, P_aCO_2, and P_aO_2 but also derives values for HCO_3^-, S_aO_2, and base excess (BE). Oxygen saturation (S_aO_2) can also be measured directly by **co-oximetry**, which is also used to measure total hemoglobin and to recognize and quantify **dyshemoglobins**. Dyshemoglobins are types or species of hemoglobin that do not readily attract, carry, or release oxygen (discussed later in the chapter). Both the arterial blood gas and co-oximetry require an invasive puncture. Although arterial blood gas analysis is more accurate than noninvasive means, it is an isolated and static measurement. It cannot reflect continuous changes in oxygenation status.

COLLECTING THE ABG SAMPLE

ABG sampling requires a physician's order or a patient care protocol that is established and approved by the institution. The first step of any analysis is collecting an acceptable specimen. In the case of ABG/acid-base analysis, the sample is arterial blood. It must be collected under aseptic conditions and maintained and transported in a way to avoid ambient air contamination. Care must also be taken to prevent or diminish the ongoing metabolism of the blood cells from significantly altering the values in the sample before analysis. Therefore, the sample must be obtained with a minimum of air bubbles in the sample, and the sample must be either iced or analyzed within a very short time. The AARC clinical practice guidelines for arterial blood gases state that the "sample should be immediately chilled or analyzed within 10–15 minutes if left at room temperature."[3] It is not always possible or desirable to ice the sample because icing can produce errors if other **analytes** (substances being analyzed), such as electrolytes, are to be measured from the sample.

Historically, acquiring samples for ABG/acid-base analysis has been done in three ways:

- Single, separate arterial punctures at one of several common sites
- Capillary sampling
- Drawing blood from indwelling arterial lines.

Arterial Punctures. Standard arterial punctures (*arteriotomies*) to obtain arterial samples are relatively easy to perform once the technique is perfected. However, they carry significantly higher risks than venipuncture.

A number of sites are available for arterial puncture, as is shown in Figure 16-4. The most commonly used is the radial artery at the wrist. It is relatively easy to access, it is relatively shallow in the tissue, and the bone structure makes it fairly easy to limit movement of the artery. Generally, the collateral blood supply is adequate should some arterial interruption occur, and the site is generally easy to compress and to monitor after the puncture. There remains controversy over which site, if any, has a clear advantage regarding the risk of adverse outcomes.

> *Age-Specific Competency*
>
> **Sites for Arterial Puncture**
>
> The femoral artery is used in situations in which the radial and the brachial arteries are not accessible. The dorsalis pedis and the temporal or superficial cranial arteries are sometimes used in neonates and children or in adults whose primary preferred sites are unavailable.

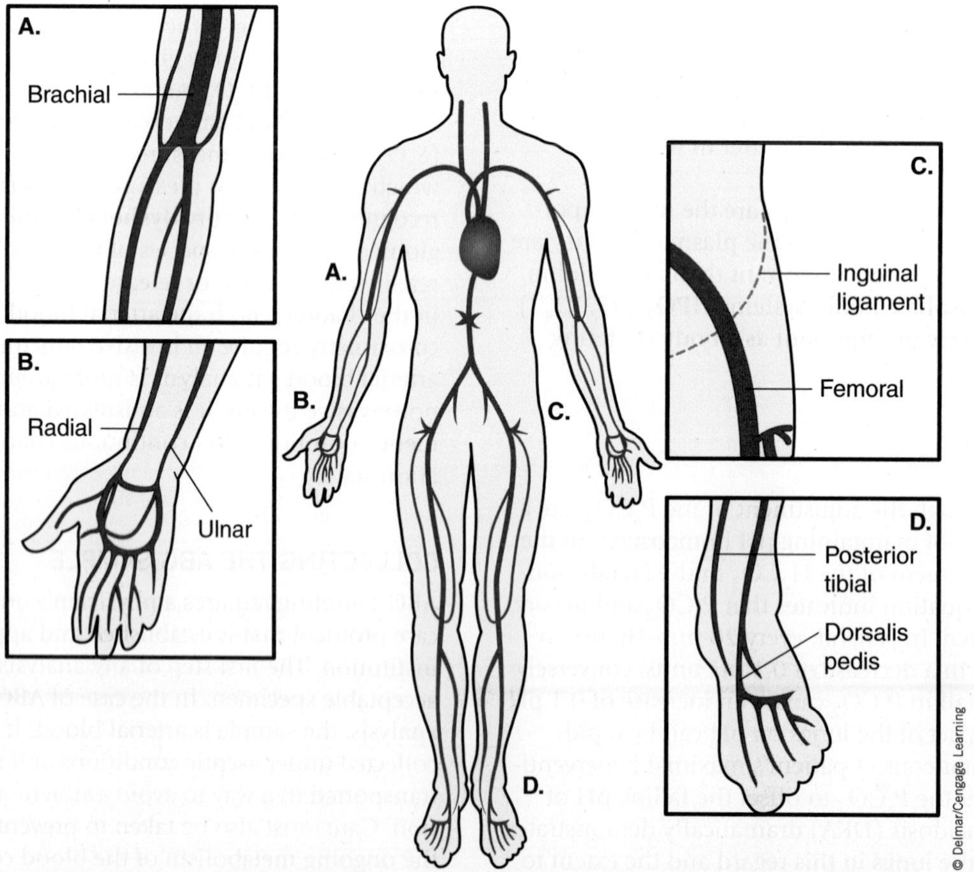

FIGURE 16-4 The four most common sites for arterial puncture: (A) The brachial artery. (B) The radial artery. (C) The femoral artery. (D) The dorsalis pedis artery. Collateral circulation for the radial artery is generally the greatest and most reliable, whereas collateral circulation for the femoral artery is the least reliable, making the femoral the least attractive site for puncture.

Best Practice

Dangers of Arterial Punctures

Greatest among the risks of arterial punctures is the possible interruption of blood flow distal to the puncture site. In worst-case situations, fingers or hands have been rendered useless or lost. Patients must be assessed before puncture for conditions or medications that increase the risk of prolonged bleeding, hematoma, and subsequent blood-flow interruption. It is also critical that the puncture be assessed shortly after the procedure to ensure that blood flow has returned to normal.

Best Practice

The Allen's Test (modified)

The **Allen's test** (Figure 16-5) is a clinical test during which both the radial and ulna arteries in the wrist of the sample site arm are occluded by manual pressure by the person doing the arterial puncture. The patient is instructed to hold the sampling arm above heart level and to "pump" the hand for 30 seconds to a minute. The palm of the hand should blanch from the lack of arterial blood flow. At this point, the caregiver releases pressure on only the ulnar site and observes for a return of color to the hand. Color should return within 20 seconds of relieving the pressure. Failure to recolor is indicative of reduced or absent collateral blood flow to that hand. The respiratory therapist should then select another puncture site.

A sample procedure for arterial punctures is outlined in Procedure 16-1. Specifics regarding site selection, modified Allen's, the test use of ice, the size of sample, the use of adhesive bandages on puncture sites, and the required label information can vary from facility to facility or depend on equipment requirements.

Capillary Sampling. Capillary sampling is a common procedure in the care of neonatal patients. Capillary sampling of blood is a fairly common technique that involves heating the patient's extremities to dilate the underlying vessels. This dilation promotes increased blood flow to the warmed part. In capillary sampling for estimation of arterial values, the site is first warmed in an attempt to *arterialize* the capillary bed beneath the site by increasing arterial flow to the area. The increased blood flow carries with it the increased arterial oxygen content and hence has higher oxygen

Best Practice

Use of Bandages

The use of adhesive bandages and other dressings that visually obscure the puncture site should be avoided because they may prevent the timely notice of hematoma formation or continuous bleeding from the site.

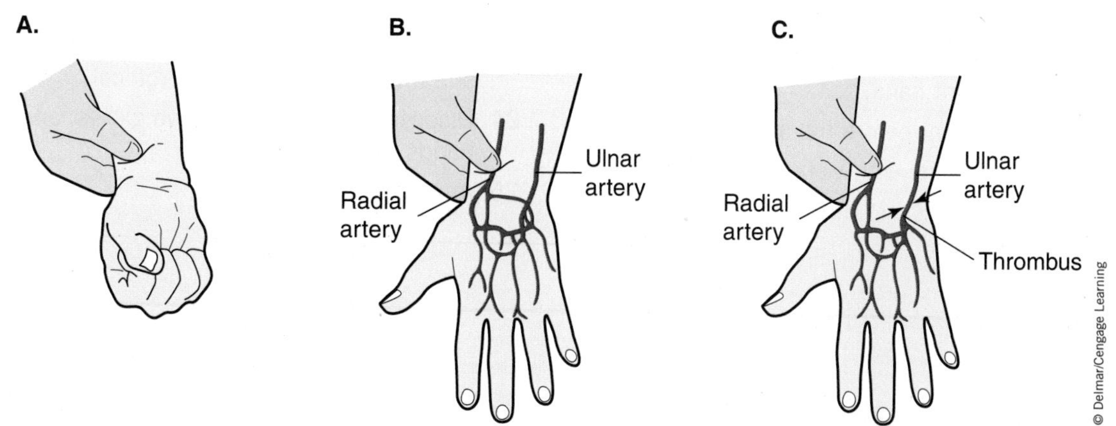

FIGURE 16-5 Modified Allen's test: (A) Pallor is initiated by compressing the radial artery with the fist clenched. (B) A patent ulnar artery reveals the return of palm perfusion despite radial artery compression. (C) An occluded ulnar artery results in continued pallor of the hand while the radial artery is still compressed.

PROCEDURE 16-1

Sample ABG Puncture Procedure

Equipment required (Figure 16-6):

- Arterial blood gas kit
- Biohazard plastic bag for sample
- Gloves (nonsterile)
- Equipment to anesthetize site (optional)
- Ice
- Disinfectant swab (e.g., Betadine) and alcohol
- Face shield, mask, or goggles

Procedure:

1. Assemble disposable blood gas kit according to manufacturer's specifications.
2. Obtain ice for the sample (if hospital policy).
3. Verify physician's order.
4. Review chart for anticoagulant or bleeding disorder status.
5. Verify patient's identity.
6. Maintain standard precautions.
7. Explain the procedure to the patient.
8. Wash hands.
9. Don gloves.
10. Select the site for the puncture. If it is the radial artery, perform a modified Allen's test to verify good collateral circulation. If adequate collateral circulation not present, follow hospital policy to select an alternate site.
11. Maintain aseptic technique.
12. If hospital policy, swab the site with a hospital-approved cleanser or disinfectant, such as Betadine. Follow the manufacturer's instructions for use.
13. If hospital policy, anesthetize the site.
14. Localize the target artery using the fingers of the nondominant hand.
15. Inform the patient before the actual puncture.
16. Swab puncture site with Betadine. Wipe clean with alcohol.
17. Perform the puncture (Figure 16-7).
    a. Insert the needle with the bevel up.
    b. Insert at approximately 45-degree angle.
    c. Point syringe "upstream" relative to blood flow.
    d. Use smooth, consistent advancement of the needle. If any redirection of the needle is required, withdraw to just under the skin and then readvance. Avoid deep side-to-side movement of the needle.
    e. Watch for flash of blood in the hub of the needle.
    f. Consistent with the type of syringe kit used, allow blood to fill to an adequate sample size (often 2.5–3 cc for adults 0.5–1.0 cc for infants and children) under arterial pressure.
18. Remove the needle and apply pressure for 3–5 minutes or until the site has stopped bleeding.
19. Expel all air from the sample, remove the needle, and cap the syringe. (Dispose of the needle in an appropriate biohazard container.)
20. Mix the blood thoroughly.
21. Label the sample (Figure 16-8): Name and room number (required on all samples); ventilation parameters; F_IO_2; time; patient temperature; puncture site; doctor.
22. Place sample in ice and transport to the blood gas lab. (If the sample will be run within a few minutes of drawing, it is not necessary to use ice to transport it.)
23. Assess the patient's puncture site. Ensure that all bleeding has stopped. Check for distal pulse. Place adhesive bandage securely over puncture site if required by facility protocol.
24. Dispose of all waste, remove gloves, and wash hands.
25. Analyze the blood.

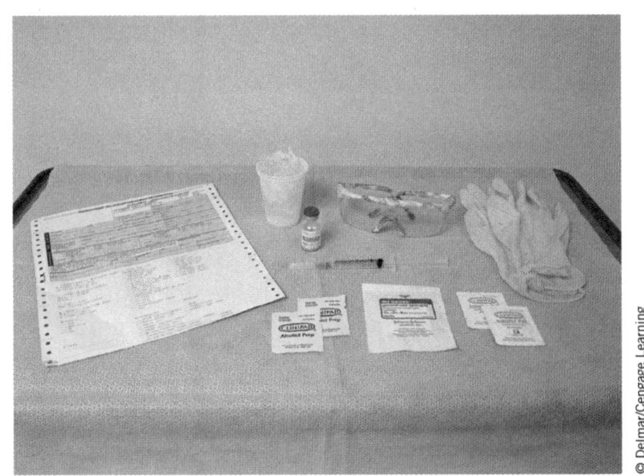

FIGURE 16-6 Equipment needed for arterial puncture: alcohol, syringes, gauze, heparinized solution, and a cup of ice.

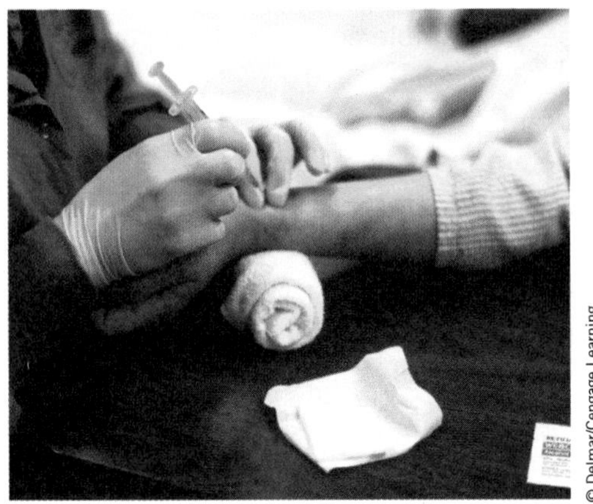

FIGURE 16-7 Insert the needle with the bevel up at a 45-degree angle.

Name____________________________

Date__________Time________________

Room No.__________Temp.________

F_IO_2 _____ V_T_____Puncture site____

Doctor____________________________

FIGURE 16-8 Sample ABG label.

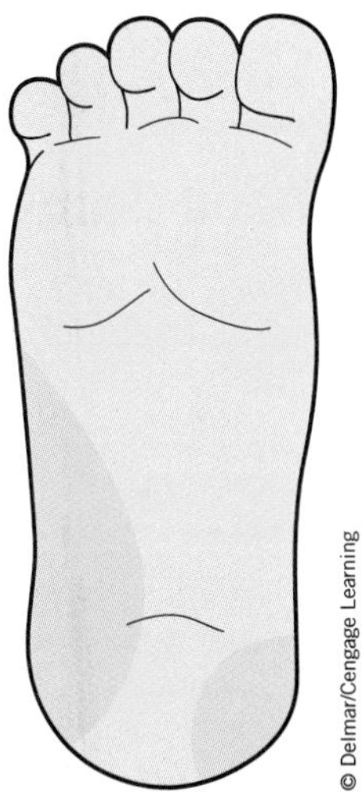

FIGURE 16-9 Sites for capillary refill in an infant (shaded area).

content than does venous blood; that is, the blood is arterialized.

Capillary samples are typically obtained from infants and neonates. Great care must be used in the warming process to avoid burning the skin and underlying tissue, especially in neonates. Common sites for capillary sampling are the heels of the feet or digits, either fingers or toes.

Capillary gas values, especially the P_aO_2, should not be taken as absolute equivalents of arterial values. Capillary values should instead be considered approximations, assuming optimal site preparation and quick collection free of room air contamination. Figure 16-9 shows capillary-sampling sites. Procedure 16-2 provides a sample procedure for capillary sampling.

Arterial Lines. For patients who are expected to require numerous ABG/acid-base analyses, indwelling arterial

Age-Specific Competency

Capillary Sampling

Capillary sampling is not true arterial blood sampling. It is an alternative for patients or in situations in which a traditional arterial puncture is not appropriate. Capillary sampling is used most often in the pediatric and neonatal settings, partly to avoid the risk of injury to very small and fragile arteries.

PROCEDURE 16-2

Capillary Blood Sampling

Equipment required:

Heel warmer (lab) or appropriate warming device
Lancet/Accu-Jet
Betadine and alcohol wipes
Sterile gauze
Gloves
Heparinized capillary tube
Capillary tube caps
Ice
ID label
Metal mixing "fleas" (optional)
Magnet (optional)

Procedure:

1. Gather equipment and ice.
2. Verify physician's orders.
3. Observe standard precautions.
4. Identify yourself to patient (or family). Verify the patient's identity.
5. Explain procedure and purpose.
6. Wash hands.
7. Select the puncture site area, and use a heel warmer or other appropriate device to establish increased regional circulation.
8. Swab site with Betadine and blot dry with sterile gauze.
9. Don gloves.
10. Firmly puncture area so that it forms drops of blood rapidly. Do not squeeze, or "milk," the site to increase blood flow! If flow is inadequate, another, more aggressive, puncture is required.
11. Fill the tube from the middle of the drop. Avoid admission of air. Keep the tip of the tube that is in the blood drop slightly lower than the other end to avoid air entry in the sample stream.
12. (Optional) If it is departmental policy, insert mixing "flea" in sample.
13. Cap the capillary tube with the cap provided.
14. (Optional) If it is departmental policy, use the magnet to move the "flea" throughout the sample to mix the heparin and blood.
15. Label the sample according to departmental policy.
16. Ice sample. (If the sample will be used to determine electrolytes, icing may be inappropriate.)
17. Tend to the puncture according to departmental policy.
18. Transport the sample and analyze it according to departmental policy.

catheters (arterial lines) are generally placed to avoid subjecting the patient to multiple punctures. The lines also offer the advantage of providing a continuous display of arterial blood pressure and heart rate. Clotting of the blood in the line is prevented by flushing the line with heparin (an anticlotting medication) after each sampling.

Both heparin and a permanent line in the arterial system carry risks.

- Indwelling lines carry an increased risk of infection for the patient.
- The arterial line (A-line) could become disconnected and allow for significant blood loss by the patient. Because the catheter is in the arterial (high pressure) part of the circulatory system, blood loss can occur rapidly and in large volumes. Careful attention is warranted when dealing with these indwelling lines, especially in patients receiving anticoagulants such as heparin. Their blood is slow or unable to clot, compounding the bleeding problem.
- Clots can form around the line and then break away to float in the circulation.

Best Practice

Squeezing the Sample Site

Avoid "milking," or squeezing, the capillary sampling site to increase the blood flow. Squeezing increases the venous component of the sample and causes decreased accuracy in reflecting the true values. Therefore, an aggressive puncture technique must be developed to avoid repeated discomfort from multiple ineffective attempts.

In some facilities, respiratory therapists are authorized to place arterial lines once a prescribed course of training and competence demonstrations have been completed. In other facilities, placement of arterial lines remains the domain of physicians.

The collection of a sample involves allowing the heparin solution that fills the catheter between samplings to empty so that a true unadulterated arterial sample is collected. Procedure 16-3 presents a sample procedure for arterial line collection.

Indwelling Blood Gas Analyzer Electrodes

There has long been hope for indwelling electrodes or sensors that continually measure and display ABG values, making these parameters dynamic rather than snapshots of the clinical status of the patient. Numerous designs for these sensors have been proposed and actually produced and utilized. In some designs, the sensor actually is placed in the artery and transfers values to a display. In other designs, blood is

PROCEDURE 16-3

Arterial Line Sample Collection

Equipment required:

- Arterial blood gas sample kit
- One 15-mL syringe (if drawing blood for labs)
- Face shield or mask and goggles
- One 6- to 8-mL syringe
- Sterile gloves
- Betadine swab

Procedure:

1. Assemble the necessary equipment.
2. Verify the orders.
3. Explain the procedure to the patient (if the patient is alert).
4. Wash hands.
5. Don gloves and goggles.
6. Swab the access port on the stopcock with Betadine swab and wait 3–4 minutes for the antimicrobial effect.
7. Note the patient's temperature. If the patient is on an E_TCO_2 or S_aO_2 monitor, note the values and record.
8. Change to sterile gloves. Use the wrapper to form a sterile field under the access port.
9. Ensure adequate pressure on the IV pressure bag.
10. Using aseptic technique and, with stopcock in the off position to the access port, remove the deadhead cap and replace with a 6-mL sterile syringe. Turn the stopcock off to the transducer line. For adults, draw 3 mL of blood from the catheter and discard it. For babies and neonates, institutional policy usually limits the amount of blood withdrawn. Policy may also require reinfusion of "presample" blood to minimize overall blood loss and the need for transfusion.
11. Turn the stopcock halfway toward the sideport. (Caution: If stopcock is turned off to the sideport, blood is diluted with flush solution.)
12. Attach the sterile 15-mL syringe. (ABG syringe if only obtaining ABGs; if blood is drawn for ABGs only, skip steps 12–15.)
13. Turn the stopcock off to the transducer line.
14. Draw 12 mL of blood for the lab.
15. Return the stopcock halfway toward the side port.
16. Remove the syringe and attach the ABG syringe.
17. Turn the stopcock off to the transducer line.
18. Draw 2.5–3 mL of blood.
19. Turn the stopcock off to the patient.
20. Flush the side port of the stopcock with flush solution. Be careful not to contaminate the system by touching the port while clearing it.
21. Replace the deadhead cap.
22. Turn the stopcock off to the side port; flush the line thoroughly; remove all blood from the catheter.
23. Remove all waste material from the patient's bed.
24. Discard the blood in an appropriate container.
25. Remove the gloves and wash hands.
26. Transport the blood to the lab and analyze it according to procedure.

periodically withdrawn from the artery, analyzed, and returned to the patient, eliminating blood loss. Unfortunately, most designs and sensor types have failed to demonstrate benefits that outweigh the risks and costs. Several companies have introduced and marketed versions of this technology but have failed to be financially successful. As a result, these units are not in widespread use today.

Noninvasive Methods Used to Measure Oxygenation Status

Although noninvasive methods of monitoring oxygenation status may not be as accurate as arterial blood gas analysis, they have certain advantages. The most obvious is patient comfort. Also, the risk of complications is minimal with noninvasive monitoring. Noninvasive monitoring can provide the practitioner with a continuous display of the patient's oxygenation status, rather than isolated, static measurements. These continuous measurements allow for the detection of trends in real time and promote early interventions in developing patient conditions. Reliable noninvasive methods of assessing ABGs are an ultimate goal.

Noninvasive procedures are often considered less expensive than invasive alternatives. However, no single noninvasive method has been developed that can provide all the parameters of an ABG. When the cost of all the current noninvasive procedures that are required to provide information comparable to the ABG is considered, it may actually be greater. Of course, not every patient requires all the information that an ABG provides, so clinical judgment and risk-benefit analysis are vital.

PULSE OXIMETRY

Pulse oximetry is the most commonly used noninvasive method of assessing a portion of the ABG data: oxygen saturation. *Pulse oximetry* uses the pulsate nature of arterial flow to focus on arterial rather than on venous blood. It analyzes the absorption of certain light wavelengths and compares the absorption with the known absorption of specific light wavelengths by hemoglobin (Figure 16-10). Oxygen saturation determined by pulse oximetry is referred to as S_PO_2. This technique provides information on the oxygen saturation obtained by pulse oximetry (S_PO_2), not the arterial oxygen saturation (S_aO_2). The two values may not always be the same. (The principles of operation of pulse oximetry are discussed elsewhere in the chapter.)

Pulse oximetry has three shortcomings.

- It is able to provide only an indirect measure of a single analyte available from ABGs; it does not determine either pH or P_aO_2.

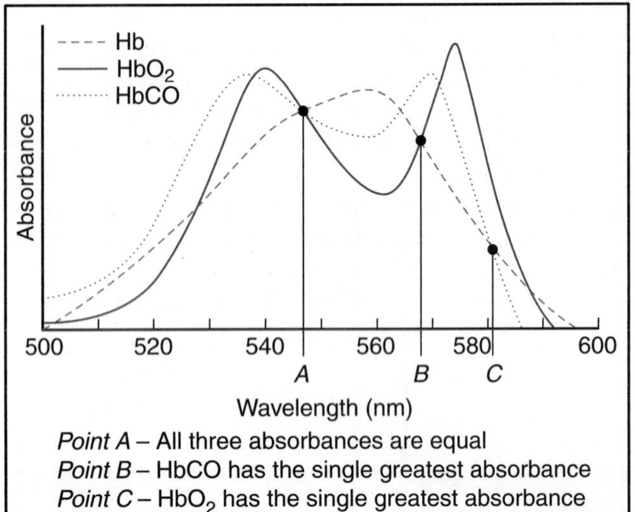

FIGURE 16-10 Principle of spectrophotometric oximetry: Various forms of hemoglobin absorb light differently at different wavelengths. The relative proportion of each can be measured by comparing points of equal absorbance (isobestic points) between different pairs of hemoglobin species.

- The S_PO_2 cannot be directly related to the P_aO_2. The shape and shift of the oxyhemoglobin dissociation curve are not constant and are not assessed by pulse oximetry.
- The oxyhemoglobin curve is relatively flat at P_aO_2s above 60 mm Hg. Therefore, S_PO_2 is inaccurate in determining saturations below 80 mm Hg. S_PO_2 is a poor indicator of ventilation status, so its use alone for patients with suspected ventilator compromise is not sufficient.

Clinical applications of pulse oximetry include the following:

- Continuous monitoring of oxygenation during anesthesia
- Adjusting F_IO_2 or titrating oxygen liter flow during oxygen therapy
- Documenting S_PO_2 during long-term oxygen therapy for purposes of Medicare requirements for reimbursement for disability
- Continuous monitoring of oxygenation during weaning from mechanical ventilation
- Prevention of retinopathy of prematurity (ROP) in neonates (although transcutaneous monitoring is more sensitive)
- Monitoring oxygenation during diagnostic procedures such as bronchoscopy, sleep studies, and exercise testing
- With appropriate remote auditory alarms, serving as an alarm system in non-ICU situations such as long-term care or ventilator-weaning facilities.

TISSUE OXYGEN SATURATION (S_TO_2)

Tissue oxygen saturation (S_TO_2) is a new technology that uses photo spectrometry to determine peripheral tissue oxygenation.

TRANSCUTANEOUS MONITORING

Transcutaneous monitoring is a measurement of the partial pressures of the gases that diffuse through the skin. The transcutaneous probe heats the skin to increase the rate of diffusion, thus increasing the gas pressures at the transcutaneous sensor to more closely mirror arterial levels. The transcutaneous partial pressures of both oxygen (T_CO_2) and carbon dioxide (T_CCO_2) can be measured simultaneously by incorporating into the same probe a Clark electrode for measuring PO_2 and a Severinghaus electrode for measuring P_aCO_2. The probe is secured to the skin by an adhesive and connected to a monitor for continuous readings. A heater and a thermistor inside the probe are connected to an external heat source to control skin temperature.

Transcutaneous oxygen monitors are typically used to monitor oxygenation status and oxygen therapy in neonates and newborns. Transcutaneous monitoring is much more sensitive than pulse oximetry in these patients, and it is not affected by ambient light or movement of the patient. It can also serve to reflect cardiopulmonary compromise.

Transcutaneous oximetry has great potential but has not fulfilled its promise. It is used mostly in pediatric and neonatal patients. The two greatest problems with this technique are the requirement of heating the site and the variability of the T_CO_2 relationship with the P_aO_2. In neonates, and even pediatric and adult patients, the monitoring site must be moved frequently to avoid injury to the skin and underlying tissues. Also, it can be difficult to ensure correlation between true arterial values and the transcutaneous values.

Additional types of transcutaneous monitors are currently in development, in clinical testing, and available for patient care. Among these are monitors that use technology similar to T_CO_2 monitors or to the pulse oximetry. These devices can measure muscle O_2 and tissue O_2 and some work has been done using these techniques to measure blood glucose and other electrolytes.

GAS SAMPLING

At its simplest, *gas sampling* is merely the collection and analysis of exhaled gases. The complex part of this process is the technology that allows the collection and analysis to occur rapidly and without significantly impeding ventilation. There are two major clinical reasons for gas sampling:

- Analysis of exhaled carbon dioxide and oxygen for purposes of metabolic assessment (not within the scope of this chapter and not discussed here)
- Analysis of exhaled carbon dioxide through capnometry

A **capnometer** simply provides digital readings of the carbon dioxide in respiratory gases during the respiratory cycle. A **capnogram**, or capnograph, may or may not display the values but provides a graphic waveform of the partial pressure of the exhaled carbon dioxide throughout the breathing cycle. Through analyses of these waveforms, much complex information can be derived.

Age-Specific Competency

Infant Transcutaneous Monitoring

Transcutaneous monitoring is the preferred method of monitoring oxygenation status in infants younger than 2 weeks of age. The skin composition is such that the correlation of T_CO_2 and P_aO_2 is excellent. Transcutaneous monitoring is more sensitive than pulse oximetry. There is a much wider range in P_aO_2 relative to S_aO_2. Pulse oximetry is unable to reflect hyperoxia, because a large increase in P_aO_2 presents as only a small increase in S_aO_2 above a P_aO_2 of 80 mm Hg. Transcutaneous monitoring is a great benefit in preventing conditions such as retinopathy of prematurity (ROP), in which oxygenation should be monitored continuously.

Best Practice

Transcutaneous Monitoring

Whenever the T_CO_2 is decreased, an arterial blood gas should be drawn. If the P_aO_2 is normal, a perfusion or circulatory impairment should be suspected. The heating requirements for the probe to alter the T_CO_2 toward P_aO_2 levels should be used to verify altered perfusion. Higher-power (heat) requirements suggest lower blood flow. Decreases in both the T_CO_2 and the P_aO_2 reflect pulmonary impairment.

By assessing the carbon dioxide levels, various *deflection points* (places where there is a change in the direction of the waveform), and *slopes* (steepness) on the capnogram, one can determine:

- Deadspace ventilation volume.
- The severity of pulmonary disease.
- The response to therapy.
- The integrity of the ventilator circuit.
- The effects of esophageal versus tracheal intubation.

Various studies have evaluated the usefulness of the capnogram in assessing bronchospasm. You and coworkers found a strong correlation between spirometry and the angle between the ascending and alveolar phases.[4] Yaron et al. reported that the plateau phase of the capnogram is a rapid, effort-independent, noninvasive measure that indicates significant bronchospasm in adult emergency room patients.[5] They found that this method is correlated well with the peak expiratory flow rate (PEFR).

The potential for the use of a capnogram to assess bronchospasm in children is especially exciting because the measurements from the capnogram are noninvasive and effort independent, as opposed to traditional pulmonary function studies. This benefit is of particular interest to persons studying lung function and asthma in children, especially children who are too young to understand and follow complex directions.

Age-Specific Competency

Testing in Children

Because children, especially those of a young age, either cannot or do not cooperate and give voluntary best-effort spirometric attempts, tests that are highly cooperation- and effort-dependent are not suited for testing in this age group. Testing methods that do not require a high level of effort or cooperation should be encouraged and used to provide high-quality and repeatable results.

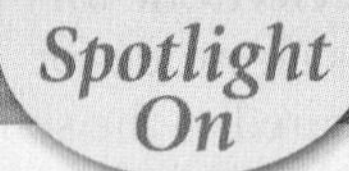

Capnograms in ARDS

Capnograms are also being evaluated for their value in predicting cardiac output changes and monitoring ventilatory disturbances in ARDS patients. Capnography also may be a strong predictor of post resuscitation survival.

Normal Values

Normal values are generally cited as a numerical value and an index of variability, usually the standard deviation (SD). Normal blood gas data are shown in Table 16-1. These data are shown as the mean (average), data, and the first and second standard deviation (SD) ranges of the means. The first SD ranges encompass nearly 68% of the population; the second SD ranges include about 95% of the population. Most texts show second standard deviation ranges as the normal range. Table 16-1 shows both ranges on the assumption that, if the first SD range is accepted, the health care provider becomes proactive at recognizing and responding to alteration of the ABGs.

When analyzing, interpreting, and reporting ABGs and pH, remember that some of the values are directly measured, whereas others are calculated from the measured values. The values generally measured for arterial blood gas analysis are:

- pH
- PO_2
- P_aCO_2

TABLE 16-1 **Normal blood gas values with 1-SD and 2-SD ranges**

		Arterial			Venous		
Value	Units	Mean	1-SD Range	2-SD Range	Mean	1-SD Range	2-SD Range
PH		7.40	7.38–7.42	7.35–7.45	7.36	7.35–7.38	7.31–7.41
P_aCO_2	mm Hg	40	38–42	36–44	46	44–48	41–51
P_aO_2	mm Hg	97	94–99	80–104	33	35–38	25–40
HCO_3^-	mEq/L	24	22–26	20–28	23	21–22	21–25
S_aO_2	%	97	95–98	93–99	75	65–85	70–80
BE/D	mEq/L	0	−2.4–2.3	+/− 3.0	Same	Same	Same
Lactate	mg/dL	9.45	4.5–14.4	NA	12.15	4.5–19.8	NA

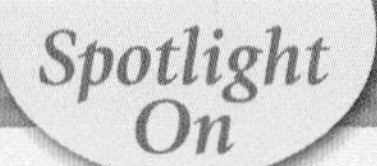

Normal Physiological Data

Normal values for physiological data have been determined through the efforts and talents of many clinical and basic scientists. Many of the so-called "normal values" are the results of data collected in the U.S. Army's World War I and World War II Selective Service physical examinations. The values may not be normal for all individuals or, for that matter, for all groups. In fact, at this time, most normal values are biased toward white males. The addition of studies and data from other ethnic and racial groups and from females is reducing this bias.

Hemoglobin (Hgb) is measured in some ABG analyzers, as are serum electrolytes and lactate (a derivative of lactic acid).

The values generally calculated for arterial blood gas analysis are:

- HCO_3^-
- Base excess/base deficit
- O_2 saturation

MEASURED ACID-BASE VALUES

The sole routinely measured acid-base value is pH. Note that the pH is dimensionless. The technique uses an electrode based on pH-sensitive glass. The operation of the pH electrode is detailed elsewhere in this chapter.

The measured blood gas values are generally the P_aO_2 and the P_aCO_2. These are measured using the Clark and Severinghaus electrodes, respectively. The operation of these electrodes is discussed elsewhere in this chapter.

CALCULATED VALUES

The calculated values are derived from the measured values by means of a series of mathematical equations called *regression equations* or by means of algorithms within the microprocessors in the blood gas analyzer.

Acid-Base Balance. The most common calculated acid-base values are HCO_3^- and base excess (or base deficit). The relationship between pH, P_aCO_2 (measured), and HCO_3^- (calculated) is defined in the Henderson-Hasselbalch (H-H) equation. This equation essentially calculates pH by determining the ratio of H_2CO_3 to CO_2, taking the logarithm of that ratio, and adding it to a constant value for human blood (the dissociation constant, 6.3).

The value of the concentration of carbon dioxide (CO_2) can be calculated using a constant value and the measured P_aCO_2. The HCO_3^- value is calculated using algorithms in the analyzer based on this equation. An HCO_3^- value developed in this way cannot be used as a test of the validity of the pH or P_aCO_2 measurement because the HCO_3^- is derived from the suspect data.

Base excess (sometimes called *base deficit* when its value is negative) is a calculation intended to quantify the nonrespiratory acid-base status. It is sometimes loosely defined as the excessive amount of base if the pH were instantaneously corrected to 7.40.

Blood Gases. The most often reported calculated blood gas value is oxygen saturation. It is calculated on the basis of the predicted slope of the oxyhemoglobin dissociation curve, given a known measured pH, temperature, P_aCO_2, and P_aO_2. However, not all labs report calculated oxygen saturations. With the advent of more blood gas analyzers with built-in co-oximetry, actual measured oxygen saturation values, rather than calculated ones, are becoming more common. Co-oximeters are devices that measure the actual percentage of hemoglobin that is carrying (i.e., is saturated with) oxygen (discussed later in this chapter).

Best Practice

Analyzers

The measured and calculated values may vary from analyzer to analyzer. Each year, more tests are being added both to the overall range of tests performed on the arterial blood sample and to the list of calculated and measured tests. Respiratory therapists should know the capabilities of the analyzers used in their institutions.

Best Practice

Calculated Values

Respiratory therapists must know that calculated values are not always the same as measured values. The discrepancies may be small, but they may be nonetheless important in some cases. When in doubt, get measured values to confirm the results.

Deviations from Normal

Because arterial blood gas analysis includes both the determination of acid-base status and the analysis of the functions of gas diffusion and transport, several variations from normal are possible. In addition, several of the quantities measured are not only interdependent but may also change simultaneously. The usual method of interpreting arterial blood gas results is to begin with the acid-base status and then to evaluate the gas exchange condition.

ACID-BASE VARIANCES

The four primary types of acid-base variances, or disturbances, are named according to their pH abnormality and the primary system causing the variance:

- Respiratory alkalemia
- Respiratory acidemia
- Metabolic alkalemia
- Metabolic acidemia

The names are modified by stating whether the values are compensated or uncompensated. *Compensated* means that the body is responding to a change in the pH and has brought it back to normal (fully compensated) or toward normal (partially compensated). Thus:

- Respiratory alkalemia is an uncorrected, uncompensated alkalemia (high blood pH) caused by a decrease in the P_aCO_2 (respiratory).
- Respiratory acidemia is an uncorrected, uncompensated acidemia (low blood pH) caused by an increase in the P_aCO_2.
- Metabolic alkalemia is an uncorrected, uncompensated alkalemia caused by an increase in the HCO_3^- (metabolic system).
- Metabolic acidemia is an uncorrected, uncompensated acidemia caused by an decrease in the HCO_3^-.

> **Best Practice**
>
> **Terminology**
>
> In most clinical references, acidemia and alkalemia are referred to as acidosis (acidotic) and alkalosis (alkalotic), instead of by their more proper names of acidemia or alkalemia.

The changes characteristic of these primary variances are displayed in Table 16-2.

Not all variances are simply one of these primary types. There are also cases of mixed alkalemia and acidemia. In a mixed variance, both the metabolic and respiratory systems are contributing to the pH displacement, as displayed in Table 16-3.

Once a variance has been going on long enough for the body to attempt to return to homeostasis, the result is always a mixed variance, referred to as *compensated*. The compensating system shifts in the direction necessary to correct the pH toward normal. The compensation is generally not complete, so a slight pH shift remains in the direction of the primary variance, as detailed in Table 16-4.

Metabolic Acidosis. In cases of *metabolic acidosis*, nonrespiratory acid levels increase relative to the respiratory and metabolic bases and the respiratory acid. The P_aCO_2 represents respiratory acid. Metabolic acids are difficult to measure and are detected by decreased (more acid) pH, while P_aCO_2 remains within its normal range; that is, they are detected by exclusion. Various metabolic conditions can result in metabolic acidosis, including anaerobic metabolic states, diabetes, and the ingestion of alkalinizing substances.

TABLE 16-2 **Primary acid-base variances**

Imbalance	pH	HCO_3^-	P_aCO_2	Base Excess
Respiratory alkalemia	Increase	No change	Decrease	Increase
Respiratory acidemia	Decrease	No change	Increase	Decrease
Metabolic alkalemia	Increase	Increase	No change	Increase
Metabolic acidemia	Decrease	Decrease	No change	Decrease

TABLE 16-3 **Mixed acid-base variances (respiratory and metabolic)**

Imbalance	pH	HCO_3^-	P_aCO_2	Base Excess
Alkalemia	Increase	Increase	Decrease	Increase
Acidemia	Decrease	Decrease	Increase	Decrease

TABLE 16-4 **Compensated variances**

Imbalance	pH	HCO_3^-	P_aCO_2	Base Excess
Respiratory alkalemia	No change (slight alkalemia)	Decrease	Decrease (primary)	No change
Respiratory acidemia	No change (slight acidemia)	Increase	Increase (primary)	No change
Metabolic alkalemia	No change (slight alkalemia)	Increase (primary)	Decrease	No change
Metabolic acidemia	No change (slight acidemia)	Decrease (primary)	Increase	No change

Respiratory Alkalosis. *Respiratory alkalosis* occurs when arterial CO_2 levels are abnormally low, causing pH to rise above 7.45. Respiratory alkalosis results when the patient is exhaling too much carbon dioxide. This condition often occurs when people are undergoing manual or mechanical ventilation with faster than normal rates or volumes or a combination of both.

Hyperventilation or, more properly, alveolar hyperventilation can rapidly decrease P_aCO_2. Fear, exercise, mechanical ventilation, hypoxia, and even the discomfort and anxiety associated with the drawing of the ABG are reasons for hyperventilating. Trauma, certain drugs, and various psychological states can also lead to hyperventilation.

One of the most important results of hyperventilation is to reduce—some would say "blow off"—CO_2, decreasing the P_aCO_2. The effect of the reduced P_aCO_2 in the absence of corrective factors is to swing the pH to a physiologic alkalotic state. Recall that the body is normally slightly alkalotic (pH 7.35 to 7.45), although, from a chemical point of view, acidotic states begin below pH 7.00, and alkalotic states begin above pH 7.00.

CASE STUDY 16-1

A. H. is a 34-year-old female who is confused and lethargic. She has had "flu" for 3 days and has not eaten in that time. She is an insulin-dependent type I diabetic who missed her injections while ill. On 40% face mask, her ABGs are as follows (all normal values are 2 SD normal ranges):

pH 7.29 (normal 7.35–7.45)

P_aCO_2 34 mm Hg (normal 35–45 mm Hg)

HCO_3^- 12 mEq/L (normal 22–26 mEq/L)

P_aO_2 198 mm Hg (normal 95–100 mm Hg on 21% O_2, >200 on 40%)

S_aO_2 94% (normal 96–99%)

Serum glucose 690 mg/dL (normal <100 mg/dL; diabetic normal <150 mg/dL)

ABG interpretation. pH is acidotic; P_aCO_2 is just below normal; HCO_3^- is very low (acidotic); P_aO_2 is high; S_aO_2 is low; and glucose is extremely high.

Diagnosis: Acute metabolic acidosis (diabetic ketoacidosis) with partial compensation and hyperoxia. Probable Kushmaul's respirations if not corrected.

Question

1. Why is Ms. H.'s HCO_3^- so low? What result of diabetes caused the decline in bicarbonate being delivered?

CASE STUDY 16-2

J. L. was seen in the postoperative recovery room after relatively minor surgery under general anesthesia. He was having difficulty coming out of anesthesia and was being mechanically ventilated at high volumes and rates. His F_IO_2 was 0.30. Arterial blood gases were obtained, with the following results:

pH 7.52

P_aCO_2 23 mm Hg

P_aO_2 145 mm Hg

HCO_3^- 26 mm Hg

S_aO_2 99%

Respiratory rate 35, respiratory volume = 1.5 × normal

The P_aO_2 and pH are high; HCO_3^- and P_aCO_2 are low.

Questions

1. With the low P_aCO_2 and HCO_3^- normal, and in light of the pH, is this a metabolic or a respiratory disorder?
2. What actions do you recommend to stabilize Mr. L.?
3. What is Mr. L.'s oxygenation status?

Respiratory Acidosis. *Respiratory acidosis* occurs when the P_aCO_2 increases. The increased P_aCO_2 causes the pH to decrease and become more acidic. In the absence of compensatory measures, the pH remains in a physiological acidotic range, and the blood becomes acidemic. P_aCO_2 increases because of alveolar hypoventilation, that is, a reduction in the gas entering the alveoli via the respiratory system. Causes of reduced alveolar ventilation include obstruction and neuromuscular and restrictive conditions.

For example, in an automobile accident victim, chest wall and lung surface injuries may cause restriction of inspiratory movement because of pain. The restriction results in lower lung volumes. The patient tries to accommodate this condition by increasing respiratory rate but is unable to compensate for the reduced alveolar ventilation. This is a classic differentiation of hypoventilation versus tachypnea. Do not confuse hypoventilation (low alveolar ventilation) with bradypnea (low respiratory rate) or hyperventilation (excessive alveolar ventilation) with tachypnea (rapid respiratory rate).

Respiratory acidosis occurs when the lungs are unable to excrete carbon dioxide owing to one or more of three mechanisms:

- Diffusion problems at the alveolar capillary (a–c) membrane
- The failure of the ventilatory pump to bring sufficient gas flow to and from the alveoli and other respiratory structures in the lungs
- Failure of the circulation to reach the a–c membrane

Often combinations of these mechanisms affect a patient's status.

Best Practice

Organ Control

P_aCO_2 can change rapidly, whereas HCO_3^- changes slowly. The reason is that the principle organ controlling P_aCO_2 level is the lung, while HCO_3^- depends on the slower-acting kidney for its control.

Mixed Metabolic and Respiratory Acidosis. On occasion, both metabolic and respiratory conditions occur, each of which would result in an acidotic condition. When they occur simultaneously, a mixed acidosis is evident. These mixed conditions are characterized by HCO_3^- and P_aCO_2 values that would individually result in a pH in the acidotic range. A factor that may be involved is the anion gap.

The **anion gap** (AG) is the difference between the serum anions and the serum cations. It represents the fixed or volatile acids generated as metabolic end products. (The anion gap is discussed more fully later in the chapter.) Anions are negatively charged ions, and cations are positively charged ions. Anions can be produced from the breakdown of acids, and cations can be formed by the breakdown of alkaline, or base, substances. For instance, the substance H_2SO_4 (sulfuric acid) breaks down to 2 H^+ (hydrogen) + SO_4^- (sulfide) in a dynamic equilibrium reaction

$$H_2SO_4 \leftrightarrow 2H^+ + SO_4^-$$

CASE STUDY 16-3

M. J., a 16-year-old male automobile accident victim, was admitted to the emergency room with an ETT (endotracheal) tube in place, and he was on 100% O_2. He had a fractured pelvis and possibly internal bleeding and lung contusions. PE – P = 130, BP = 90/50, RR = 36 – IVs × 2. ABGs were ordered, obtained, and reported as follows:

pH 7.25
P_aCO_2 65 mm Hg
HCO_3^- 23 mEq/L
P_aO_2 55 mm Hg
S_aO_2 85%

ABG interpretation: pH is in the acidic range, <7.35; the P_aCO_2 is increased; the HCO_3^- is in the low normal range; P_aO_2 and O_2 Sat are both markedly decreased.

Diagnosis: Respiratory acidosis secondary to reduced tidal volume (V_T), question of pleural effusions, question of early acute respiratory distress syndrome (ARDS), decreased compliance and increased WOB (work of breathing) secondary to abdominal injury. Probable stage II shock.

Questions

1. What are the likely causes of the changes from normal in the blood gases reported?
2. What features of this blood gas indicate whether it is a chronic or an acute condition?
3. How can we use the answer to the previous question to treat the pH abnormality?

From this breakdown, we derive an end product acid (H^+) and its conjugate base (SO_4^-).

Metabolic end products are substances that are created as the body performs its functions but that are not utilized. These include lactic and pyruvic acids, as well as more complex organic acids. To get a more accurate picture of the total acid-base state, calculate the difference between the acid and base influences on serum pH. The normal anion gap range is between 12 and 14 mmol/dL.

Metabolic Alkalosis. *Metabolic alkalosis* occurs when HCO_3^- (the base) rises in relation to P_aCO_2. The cause may be a chronic condition, in which case the kidneys reserve bicarbonate—a slow process. Or the cause may be acute, such as the ingestion of a solution or substance high in bicarbonate that can cause metabolic changes in a short period of time. Finally, rapid loss of systemic acids can be reflected in an acid-base imbalance. Prolonged vomiting and diarrhea are often associated with metabolic alkalosis.

CASE STUDY 16-4

I. S., a 69-year-old, 110 pack-year smoker was readmitted to the intensive care unit on 2 Lpm of oxygen by nasal cannula. Her chief complaint (CC) on admission was, "I can't breathe. Can I have a smoke?" Her admission ABGs were:

pH 7.36
P_aCO_2 53 mm Hg
HCO_3^- 32 mEq/L
P_aO_2 68 mm Hg
S_aO_2 82%

ABG interpretation: pH is low normal; P_aCO_2 is very high (respiratory acidosis); HCO_3^- is very high (metabolic alkalosis), indicating renal compensation; S_aO_2 is low even on 2 Lpm O_2 by nasal cannula.

Diagnosis: Compensated respiratory acidosis and hypoxemia secondary to COPD and long-term tobacco addiction.

Questions

1. What if any effect does Ms. S.'s pH have on her oxygenation status?
2. Why is her pH within "normal limits"?

CASE STUDY 16-5

L. T. is a 24-year-old power company lineperson who was electrocuted 45 minutes ago. She arrived in the emergency room in full arrest. She was being manually ventilated via ET tube with 90+% O_2. Three ampoules of sodium bicarbonate had been given in the field, along with chest compression. CPR was started 1 minute postarrest. Arterial blood gases were drawn and analyzed, with the following results:

pH 7.12
P_aCO_2 56 mm Hg
HCO_3^- 26 mEq/L
P_aO_2 320 mm Hg
S_aO_2 99+%
Anion gap* 25 mmol/dL

ABG interpretation: pH is acidotic; P_aCO_2 is very acidotic; HCO_3^- is slightly alkalotic; PO_2 and the anion gap are very high.

Diagnosis: Mixed acidosis secondary to high P_aCO_2 and unmeasured organic acids (lactic, pyruvic, etc.); hyperoxygenation.

The resuscitation efforts resulted in increased bicarbonate. It was not enough to offset the acidosis that occurred secondary to the hypoxia during the arrest and the production of lactic and other organic acids that led to the anion gap (AG) while the patient was using anaerobic metabolism to provide energy. The P_aCO_2, although high and in the acidosis-producing range, is not high enough to produce a pH of the level shown. Additional acids must be causing this effect. These acids must come from the metabolic processes. This effect is called the *anion gap.*

Questions

1. What metabolic acid is the most likely cause of acidosis in the hypoxic individual, and why is your answer correct?
2. What is the compensation mechanism for respiratory acidosis in patients with chronic lung disease?

Best Practice

Antacid Use

The overuse of antacids can also result in shifts of the pH into the alkalotic ranges. In cases of chronic metabolic alkalosis, dietary habits and history should always be investigated during the history and physical, as well as use of home remedies.

During protracted vomiting and diarrhea, gastrointestinal acids are purged from the body. This lowering of total body acid results in a downward shift of hydrogen (H^+) ion concentration, resulting in a disturbance of the acid-base balance. The treatment of the diarrhea and vomiting, as well as reducing or ceasing antacid intake, should resolve the cases of metabolic alkalosis for these causes.

Compensated Metabolic Alkalosis. Compensation occurs when the body takes action in an attempt to return the acid-base status to a normal or homeostatic condition. The body's goal is to maintain the pH at its physiological optimum range of 7.35–7.45. To compensate for metabolic alkalosis the body must conserve respiratory acid (P_aCO_2). It can do this either by breathing more slowly, by breathing less deeply, or doing some combination of the two.

Some cases of metabolic alkalosis occur secondary to the use of folk remedies, such as eating clay to treat the complications of the early stages of pregnancy such as nausea. These cases illustrate not only a cause of metabolic alkalosis but also that the use of folk remedies, herbs, and other self-prescribed practices can have marked effects even on patients presenting for standard scientific medical evaluation and treatment.

Best Practice

Treatments and Drug Use

Always question patients about all their drugs and treatments, whether prescribed, over-the-counter (OTC), or folk cures.

CASE STUDY 16-6

M. C. is a 67-year-old female who presented to the emergency room complaining of "nausea and vomiting for 3 days." She was diaphoretic and her vital signs were RR = 16; pulse = 124; BP = 135/88. Arterial blood gas (ABG) analysis revealed the following values:

pH 7.51
P_aCO_2 40 mm Hg
HCO_3^- 33 mEq/L
P_aO_2 92 mm Hg
S_aO_2 96%

ABG interpretation: pH is alkalotic (normal, 7.35–7.45); P_aCO_2 is normal (35–45); HCO_3^- is high (22–6).

Diagnosis: Acute metabolic alkalosis; "acid dumping" secondary to vomiting and possible antacid overuse.

Questions

1. Will slowing this patient's respirations and reducing alveolar hyperventilation, with no other treatment, reduce or increase the alkalosis? Explain your answer.
2. What would be the effect of increasing respiratory rate and increasing alveolar hyperventilation in this case with no other treatment? Explain your answer.

CASE STUDY 16-7

J. M. is a 72-year-old, long-term congestive heart failure patient who was admitted to the critical care unit for "decompensation." He was on the usual cardiac drugs, including Lasix and Attenalol. He was on 2 Lpm O_2 by nasal cannula. His ABGs revealed the following:

pH 7.45
P_aCO_2 50 mm Hg
HCO_3^- 33 mEq/L
P_aO_2 74 mm Hg
S_aO_2 94%
RR 8 breaths per minute

Tidal volume 380 mL/breath (normal for Mr. M. would be 480–500 mL)

ABG interpretation: pH is high normal; P_aCO_2 is high; HCO_3^- is high; P_aO_2 is within normal limits for his age.

Diagnosis: Compensated metabolic alkalosis secondary to long-term use of diuretics. Oxygenation is normal.

Questions

1. Why is it necessary to correct this condition if Mr. M. is able to compensate so well?
2. Why is age a requirement for compensation of the P_aO_2 but not of the P_aCO_2?

Best Practice

Calculating Normal P_aO_2

Increased age brings a reduced normal range. The expected or normal P_aO_2 can be adjusted for age in patients over 60 years old by subtracting 60 from the patient's age and then subtracting the remainder from 80 mm Hg. For example, the expected, or age-adjusted, P_aO_2 for a 72-year-old patient is 68 mm Hg:

$$80 - (72 - 60) = 68$$

Respiratory Alkalosis. *Respiratory alkalosis* results when the P_aCO_2 (the acid) decreases in relation to the HCO_3^-. This situation can occur from alveolar hyperventilation or tachypnea or both. Some toxic substances such as methyl alcohol bind CO_2 and can essentially strip away dissolved CO_2, reducing the CO_2 levels to extremely low values. Even in the short run, the CO_2-to-H_2CO_3 discrepancy in these cases can result in a profound respiratory alkalosis.

Table 16-5 indicates the acid-base status for nonmixed and uncompensated acid-base disorders, the problem, examples of their causes, and the usual treatments.

Mixed Respiratory and Metabolic Alkalosis. Sometimes treatments and the body's compensatory mechanisms overlap, producing mixed states in which both respiratory and metabolic processes are occurring simultaneously.

Mixed or combined alkalotic conditions are found when HCO_3^- increases and P_aCO_2 decreases simultaneously but not necessarily proportionally. In a patient on ventilation or undergoing resuscitation, a combination of too much HCO_3^- administered over a short period of time and overventilation (hyperventilation) may set this condition into action. The HCO_3^- cannot be processed and removed by the kidney quickly enough, so it remains in the circulation. Overly enthusiastic manual or mechanical ventilation can blow off carbon dioxide. The result is two approaches to alkalemia: The low CO_2 works to increase alkalinity while the high increased HCO_3^- raises the base portion of the blood serum acid-base balance, resulting in a mixed respiratory and metabolic alkalosis.

Nonproportional changes in HCO_3^- and P_aCO_2 lead to partial compensation; proportional changes lead to full compensation. This fact bears repeating; the speed of change depends on whether P_aCO_2 or HCO_3^- is changing.

CASE STUDY 16-8

L. T., the 24-year-old power company lineperson from Case Study 16-6, is given 2 more amps of bicarbonate and placed on a ventilator via an endotracheal tube. Her fraction of inhaled oxygen (F_IO_2) is 80+%, and her tidal volume (V_T) is 600 mL. Her respiratory rate is 20 breaths per minute, and she is on positive end-expiratory pressure (PEEP) of 5 cm H_2O. Her estimated weight is 120 pounds. Gases are drawn 20 minutes after the bicarbonate infusion with the following values reported:

pH 7.56
P_aCO_2 28 mm Hg
HCO_3^- 34 mEq/L
P_aO_2 240 mm Hg
S_aO_2 99+%
AG 18 mmol/dL

ABG interpretation: pH is very alkalotic; P_aCO_2 is very low; HCO_3^- is very high. The P_aO_2 is also very high; AG is stabilizing toward normal. These blood gases can be interpreted as indicating a metabolic and a respiratory alkalosis occurring at the same time. The diagnosis is mixed alkalosis secondary to overaggressive ventilation and resuscitation drugs.

Questions

1. Another scenario in which this condition is likely to occur is that of the patient in kidney failure. What events might lead to such a situation?
2. Because the patient is in acute mixed alkalosis, what treatment strategies would be appropriate?

BLOOD GAS VARIANCES

Gas variances, as the term suggests, are changes not of the acid-base components of the blood gases but rather of the measured gas values. They are related to the P_aO_2 (oxyemia) and the P_aCO_2 (carbia).

Oxyemia. *Oxyemias* are conditions or states affected by the amount of oxygen in the blood. The phrase generally refers to the relative amount of oxygen that is dissolved in the plasma and that exerts a partial pressure. Therefore, to refer to a person as having an altered oxyemia by virtue of oxygen saturation, as is commonly done, is incorrect. The measurement of P_aO_2 is the proper analysis technique to determine a patient's oxyemia status.

TABLE 16-5 **Characteristics of the four, basic acid-base states**

Condition	Problem	Causes	Treatment
Metabolic acidosis	Loss of bicarbonate Increased fixed acids	Kidney failure, diabetic ketoacidosis, ingestion of toxic substances such as antifreeze, aspirin overdose Diarrhea Sepsis Lactic acidosis	Sodium bicarbonate
Metabolic Alkalosis	Potassium depletion, diuretics, high bicarbonate	Chloride-responsive alkalosis (urine chloride <20 mEq/L) Vomiting NG suction Thiazides and loop diuretics (after discontinuation) Post hypercapnia Cystic fibrosis Chloride-resistant alkalosis (urine chloride >20 mEq/L) Hypertension Adrenal adenoma or cancer Primary hyperaldosteronism Use of diuretics in hypertension Cushing syndrome Mineralocortocoids or glucocorticoids Renal hypertension Severe potassium depletion Current use of thiazides and loop diuretics, reduced magnesium *Other causes:* Alkali administration Antacids $NaHCO_3$ therapy renal failure Metabolism of lactic or keto acids IV penicillin Massive blood transfusion Hypercalcemia	Hydrochloric acid Potassium replacement Ammonium chloride Acetazolamide (Diamox)
Respiratory acidosis	Ventilation deficit	Drug depression of respiratory center (by opiates, sedatives, and/or anesthetics) CNS trauma Infarct, hemorrhage or tumor Hypoventilation of obesity (Pickwickian syndrome) C-spinal cord trauma/lesions at or above C4 level High central neural blockade Tetanus Poliomyelitis Cardiac arrest with cerebral hypoxia	Increase ventilation Intubation Reduced sedation
Respiratory alkalosis	Hyperventilation	Anxiety, pain, fever, sepsis, shock Pulmonary emboli	Sedation Pain relief Relaxation techniques Increased ventilation

Source: Adapted from Shoulders-Odom B. Using an algorithm to interpret arterial blood gases. Dimensions in Critical Care Nursing. *January/February 2000;19,1:36–41.*

Age-Specific Competency

Infant Hyperoxyemia

Be sure that the P_aO_2 of infants is not too high. Infants are at increased risk for retinopathy of prematurity (ROP), oxygen toxicity, and bronchopulmonary dysplasia (BPD).

Hyperoxyemia The prefix "hyper-" indicates high. Therefore, hyperoxyemia is an abnormally high P_aO_2. In general, high P_aO_2 is not a critical problem in short-term exposures. However, exposure to high oxygen concentrations can lead to complications, including oxygen toxicity and ARDS, so avoid clinically unnecessary exposure to significant elevations of F_IO_2.

Best Practice

Factors That Affect P_aCO_2

Some patient-associated variables, such as pain, emotional stress, fear, agitation, or crying, may result in hyperventilation or tachypnea. These states can result in abnormal P_aCO_2 findings. To prevent misinterpretation, note the presence of these conditions on the blood gas request and report forms.

Hypoxemia The more problematic oxyemia is *hypoxemia,* which means a low P_aO_2. In general, this is understood to mean a P_aO_2 of less than 80 mm Hg when a patient is breathing room air (F_IO_2 0.21). Hypoxemia is problematic because it has the greater risk of causing harm to the patient and because, depending on its cause, it may be very difficult to overcome.

- P_aO_2 values between 60 and 80 mm Hg represent mild hypoxemia.
- Those in the 40–60-mm-Hg range are moderate.
- P_aO_2 values below 40 mm Hg represent severe hypoxemia.

When treating patients for hypoxia by administering supplemental oxygen and monitoring the effects of the treatment by ABGs and/pulse oximetry, note in the patient record that seemingly "good" or "normal" oxygenation values are "assisted" by the supplemental oxygen.

In cases involving blunt force chest trauma, do serial chest X-rays (CXR) and closely monitor oxygenation and CO_2 elimination status. Oxygenation status should be monitored both by continuous pulse oximetry and by periodic blood gas analysis to correlate the oxygenation findings with the F_IO_2 and PEEP levels.

Carbia. *Carbia* is the root form for words that refer to conditions affecting or affected by carbon dioxide levels in the blood or gases in the lung. Many sources use the root form "capnea" instead of "carbia."

CASE STUDY 16-9

J. J. is a 58-year-old post–open-heart patient. His postextubation blood gases on a 40% Venturi mask revealed the following results:

pH 7.43
P_aCO_2 36
P_aO_2 210
HCO_3^- 22
O_2 Sat 99+%

The patient's acid-base status was normal, with only mild hyperventilation, perhaps from the pain of the arterial puncture.

The oxygen status reveals a hyperoxyemia, since the P_aO_2 is greater than the normal 80–120 range. It is not unusual for open-heart patients to be maintained for a few hours at elevated oxygen levels, but this patient's P_aO_2 level is probably too high for that application. Unless there is another indication for maintaining a high P_aO_2, a 28% or 32% Venturi would probably provide a more appropriate P_aO_2.

Questions

1. On the basis of the assumption of a linear P_aO_2 response to increased F_IO_2, which Venturi mask (28% or 32%) would bring this patient's P_aO_2 closer to 150 mm Hg?
2. For at least the immediate postoperative period, open-heart patients require close monitoring of ventilation and ABGs. What conditions make this an important factor in their care?

CASE STUDY 16-10

R. M. is a 58-year-old Hispanic male with a smoking history of 80 pack-years. He is in the doctor's office for a routine visit. He has a barrel chest and is slightly tachypneic. His resting, room air arterial blood gases reveal the following:

pH 7.36

P_aCO_2 67 mm Hg

P_aO_2 65 mm Hg

HCO_3^- 35 mmol/dL

O_2 Sat 93%

The patient has a significant hypercarbia, but it has been compensated for by a rise in HCO_3^-. Since HCO_3^- is slow to change, the hypercarbia must have been present for some time (i.e., it is chronic). The patient also has borderline hypoxemia that he tolerates fairly well. Given the history, the patient probably has emphysema or chronic obstructive pulmonary disease (COPD), although other testing is required to clearly define the nature of his chronic lung disease.

Questions

1. What can Mr. M. expect to happen if he should contract the flu or pneumonia during the fall or winter? How would his blood gas values change?
2. As Mr. M. continues to age, his pulmonary function values will decline through the normal aging process. Given his smoking history and current condition, what steps are appropriate to reduce his risk of respiratory system failure?

CASE STUDY 16-11

E. W. is a 33-year-old asthmatic. She was brought to the emergency room in respiratory distress. She had pronounced wheezing in all lung fields throughout the respiratory cycle at a rate of 30 bpm. She was placed on 2 Lpm oxygen by nasal cannula. Blood gas analysis revealed:

pH 7.57

P_aCO_2 23 mm Hg

P_aO_2 105 mm Hg

HCO_3^- 23 mmol/dL

O_2 Sat 99%

The patient has a significant hypocarbia, driven by her struggle to breathe with the bronchospasm. At this point, a low P_aCO_2 is a good sign; it indicates that she has not tired to the point of failure. A rise in P_aCO_2 to or above normal before treatment may indicate impending respiratory failure.

Questions

1. The ability to drive the P_aCO_2 below normal indicates what physiologically?
2. What indicator means that this is an acute condition? Why?

Hypercarbia An elevated P_aCO_2 is termed *hypercarbia,* or *hypercapnea.* It generally indicates diminished alveolar ventilation or an increase in carbon dioxide production. In any case, the patient is unable to adequately remove the carbon dioxide produced by the body.

Hypocarbia The prefix "hypo-" indicates low. *Hypocarbias,* or *hypcapneas,* are blood gas variances with low P_aCO_2. They can be caused by a number of conditions and can be positive signs in some clinical settings and disturbing in others. Their correlation with the clinical scenario is a key factor in determining causality and diagnosis.

Best Practice

Monitoring Oxygenation Status

It is easy to see how P_aO_2 is reacting to PEEP and how F_IO_2 changes by keeping a trend line graph that plots PEEP, F_IO_2, and P_aO_2 on the *y*-axis and time on the *x*-axis. If the patient is improving, P_aO_2 should rise or remain constant relative to the PEEP and F_IO_2 lines. If the patient is not improving or is getting worse, the gaps between the PEEP and F_IO_2 lines widen.

Best Practice

S_PCO_2 Accuracy

Sometimes blood gas results do not seem to make sense. One example is a patient who presents with an extremely low to nonexistent P_aCO_2. The question is, "Why doesn't this patient have a P_aCO_2? Was he drinking methyl alcohol?" Organic compounds sometimes bind carbon dioxide so that you cannot measure P_aCO_2.

A patient who does not have a measurable P_aO_2 or who has an extremely low P_aO_2 could be metabolizing oxygen at a very rapid rate. Patients with hyperleukocytosis may have very rapid utilization of oxygen stores. Such issues must be raised in puzzling cases.

Analysis Techniques

Analysis of the blood gases and acid-base balance is of great importance in modern medicine. The techniques used to obtain blood gas values range from invasive and complex electrochemical analysis to simple noninvasive spectrophotometric devices. The accuracy and utility vary with the patient and with the environmental and medical conditions.

ARTERIAL BLOOD GAS ANALYZERS

Blood gas analyzers use three key electrodes:

- The Clark (O_2) electrode
- The Sanz (pH) electrode
- The Severinghaus (CO_2) electrode

Many also incorporate co-oximetry and other parameters, such as hemoglobin (Hgb) levels, hematacrit (crit), basic electrolytes, lactose, and glucose. The operational bases of the electrolyte and glucose electrodes are outside the scope of this chapter and are not specifically discussed here.

The *Clark* (O_2) *electrode* uses a half cell design with positive and negative electrodes. This device measures oxygen by assessing the varying electrical current generated by the reduction of oxygen. In a reduction reaction, a substance gains electrons. The higher the oxygen concentration is, the more rapid the reaction and the higher the electrical current will be. As current increases, more electrons are attracted to the positive pole of the Clark electrode. The Clark electrode is a miniaturized polarographic electrode (Figure 16-11) that is housed in a chamber that optimizes the conditions for measuring oxygen. As the current flows, a sensor measures the current and reads out the current flow as PO_2 based on a factor determined during the calibration procedure using a known PO_2.

The modern pH electrode uses pH-sensitive glass and is commonly referred to as the *Sanz electrode*. By

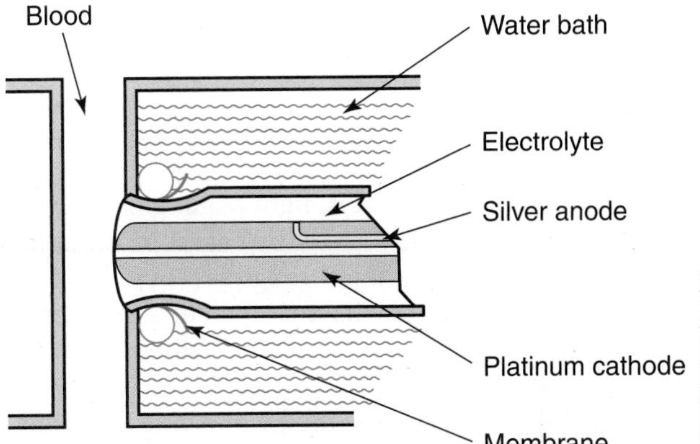

FIGURE 16-11 Schematic of a Clark electrode.

assessing electrical conduction through a blood specimen, the Sanz electrode assesses the concentration of hydrogen ions (H), which is the defining characteristic of pH.

The *Severinghaus* PCO_2 *electrode* builds on the simpler Sanz electrode. The introduction of carbon dioxide into an aqueous bicarbonate solution causes changes in the pH:

$$CO_2 = H_2O \leftrightarrow H_2CO_3 \leftrightarrow H^+ + HCO_3^-$$

The PCO_2 electrode actually measures changes in pH. However, the change in pH is directly related to the PCO_2 in an isolated environment; the pH change causes change in the electrical flow in the electrode. The electrical flow is calibrated to the corresponding pH levels, allowing the analyzer to display the P_aCO_2 of the sample.

PULSE OXIMETERS

Pulse oximetry provides a revolutionary and completely noninvasive method of measuring oxygen saturation: no need to puncture arteries or veins; no need to invade the body with tubes, needles, or catheters. Instead, a small lightweight device is fitted over the patient's finger, toe, or earlobe, or it is attached to the forehead. This device is painless and, best of all, provides continuous information.

The principles of operation for pulse oximetry are spectrophotometry and plethysmography.

- **Spectrophotometry** is the measurement of light intensity generated at a known wavelength and passed through a substance and the measurement of the intensity of that light as it leaves the solution. Because substances absorb or reflect different wavelengths of light, the analysis of the difference between the light entering and leaving a substance allows determination of the substance's constituent materials. The solution in this instance is the arterial blood.
- **Plethysmography** is the study of changes in the shape or size of an organ. It is used to distinguish static or unchanging factors from dynamic or variable components in the system being measured. In other words, plethysmography measures pulsate waves, felt as the difference in pressures noted when taking a pulse.

These two principles enable pulse oximeters to measure different wavelengths of light in pulsate waves, giving them the specific ability to focus on arterial, or pulsate, blood (Figure 16-12). Figure 16-13 illustrates the application of this principle.

Modern pulse oximeters use two wavelengths of light: one in the red wave band and the other in the infrared portion of the spectrum. The two wavelengths

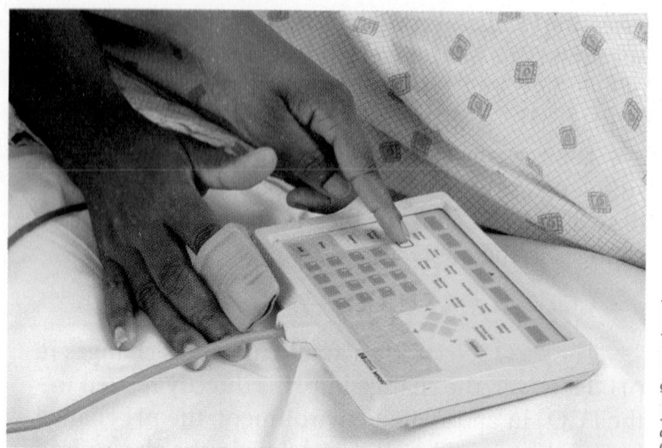

FIGURE 16-12 The pulse oximeter probe can be placed on any finger, though the index finger is most common. Consideration of circulation, skin pigmentation, and finger or fingernail discoloration should go into the decision of which finger to use.

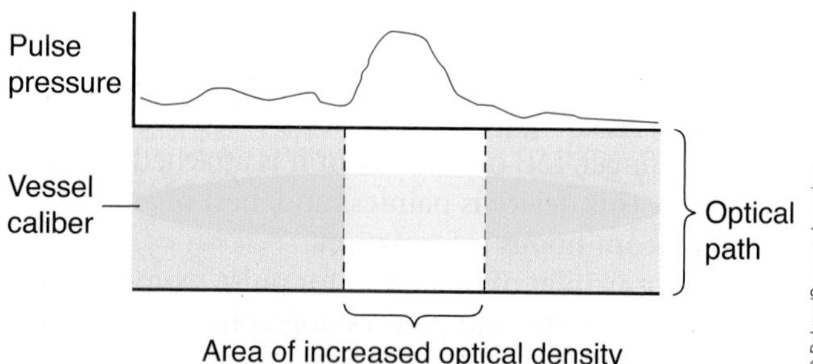

FIGURE 16-13 Pulsatile versus nonpulsatile blood flow and optical density: The tissue bed increases in density as the increased blood flow during pulsate flow expands the vessel, resulting in an increased extravascular tissue density due to the compression forces of the pulse pressure. Vessel caliber (diameter) increases as internal pressure increases.

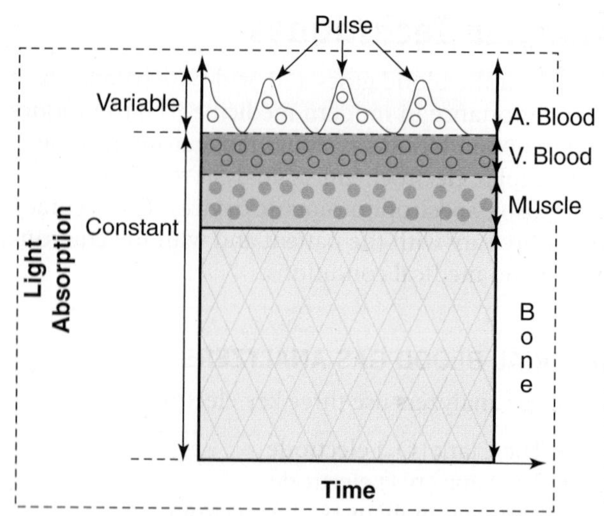

FIGURE 16-14 Light transmission across a tissue block: The light or optical path remains relatively stable over time, with the exception of the volume added during pulsate flow. With the relative inability of the bone, muscles, and extracellular fluid to change their size, added length to the optical path must be caused by the pulse pressure.

of light are transmitted from a light-emitting diode (LED) through the body part (the artery) to a photo detector. At the red wavelength of 660 nm, red light passes through oxyhemoglobin (HbO_2) and is absorbed by reduced hemoglobin, or deoxyhemoglobin (RHb). At the infrared wavelength of 940 nm, infrared light passes through reduced hemoglobin and is absorbed by oxyhemoglobin. Figure 16-14 demonstrates the concept behind the use of pulsate wave forms to coordinate sampling in pulse oximetry. The pulse oximeter reports samples obtained only during the period of pulsate flow.

Pulse oximeters compare oxyhemoglobin and reduced hemoglobin, using two wavelengths of light. The percentage of oxygen saturated with hemoglobin can be determined by applying the following formula:

$$\% \text{ HbO}_2 = [\text{HbO}_2/(\text{R Hb} + \text{HbO}_2)] \times 100$$

This is a measure of functional saturation. Pulse oximetry does not take into account the presence of dyshemoglobins. *Dyshemoglobin* is an abnormal type of hemoglobin such as carboxyhemoglobin (COHb), methemoglobin (MetHb), and sulfhemoglobin (SulfHb). These dyshemoglobins interfere with the binding of oxygen, greatly decreasing the oxygen-carrying capacity of hemoglobin and significantly lowering the C_aO_2. However, because the pulse oximeter differentiates only between bound and unbound hemoglobin, in the presence of dyshemoglobins, the pulse oximeter reading will be falsely high.

Pulse oximetry has technological and physiological limitations. The technological limitations are as follows:

- Motion artifact due to shivering, tapping the sensor on a bed rail, or continuous moving or twitching of the probe site
- Ambient light, such as bright sunlight, xenon lamps, fluorescent, and infrared lights, masking the spectrographic waves in the critical wavelengths
- *Optical shunting,* that is, light passing from the LED to the photodetector by passing around the body part rather than through it (For example, the LED probe may have slipped to a transverse position rather than being in an anterior-posterior alignment.)
- Vascular dyes, such as methylene blue or cardiogreen, blocking light passage at critical near-infrared wavelengths

TABLE 16-6 **Physiological factors affecting pulse oximetry**

Low Saturation	Low Perfusion	Dyshemoglobin
False high readings at S_aO_2 below 80%	Cardiac arrest Hypothermia	COHb MetHb
Inaccurate readings at S_aO_2 below 65%	Peripheral shunting Vasoconstriction Shock	SulfHb

- Deeply pigmented skin blocking light passage (The S_PCO_2 readings may be off because the accuracy of the sensors declines as light passes through dark skin.)
- Nail polish, such as black, blue, or green, hindering the effectiveness of probes applied to darkly colored nails
- Low perfusion

Physiological limitations of pulse oximetry are inaccuracies caused by very low saturations, low perfusion states, and the presence of dyshemoglobins. Table 16-6 summarizes these limitations.

The pulse oximeter does more than measure O_2 saturation. Because it measures only during pulsate flow, it also measures (or counts) pulse rate. Further, because it detects pulse, it also detects perfusion through the area being sampled (the pulse pressure drives perfusion).

Be aware that the pulse indicated on a pulse oximeter may not match the pulse rate shown on an ECG monitor. The ECG monitor counts electrical activity in the heart, whereas the pulse oximeter counts pulsate waves. Some abnormal heart diseases cause periods of pulseless electrical activity (PEA) and may result in incorrect pulse rates, while the pulse oximeter reports actual pulse episodes. Variances in these two rates should be noted in the patient's record and reported to the patient's nurse.

CO-OXIMETERS

Co-oximetry, like pulse oximetry, uses the principle of absorption of light by hemoglobin to analyze blood samples. However, co-oximetry utilizes four wavelengths of light rather than two and therefore measures all common dyshemoglobins. The result is a measure of fractional saturation, not the simpler functional saturation yielded by pulse oximetry. We therefore can determine the composition of the total hemoglobin by hemoglobin subtype or species.

Some dyshemoglobins are incapable of carrying or releasing oxygen. The hemoglobin molecule's ability or inability to carry oxygen is largely dependent on its geometry. Dyshemoglobins have structural abnormalities that alter the shape of the molecule, making the bind/release ability more difficult or impossible. These geometric changes are caused by chemicals such as carbon monoxide (CO) or by genetic agents as in the case of sickle cell disease.

The fractional concentration of hemoglobin is determined by comparing oxyhemoglobin with total hemoglobin, as shown in the following formula:

$$\%\ HbO_2 = HbO_2/(HbO_2 + RHb + COHb + MetHb) \times 100$$

Because an arterial blood sample must be obtained, this is an invasive procedure. Co-oximetry is usually performed in conjunction with arterial blood gas analysis. Most modern blood gas analyzers include or offer built-in co-oximetry modules that allow the use of a single sample. The newer co-oximeter may also be capable of measuring other hemoglobin characteristics such as Hb A1-C, a measure of average blood glucose over time; this is a good indicator of the stability of serum glucose in diabetic patients.

END-TIDAL CO_2 ANALYZERS

Two types of end-tidal CO_2-measuring devices are currently marketed. They are classified according to the basis of their method of providing output data.

- The *capnometer* provides digital readings of the percentage of end-tidal CO_2 (sometimes converted to a partial pressure).
- The *capnograph* provides a waveform displaying the percentage of CO_2 per unit of time for each breathing cycle. The capnograph produces this waveform, or capnogram, either on a breath-by-breath basis or as a trend chart illustrating a sequence of CO_2 production for a series of breaths.

A third type of end-tidal CO_2 monitor combines the features of both the capnometer and the capnograph.

End-tidal CO_2 ($E_{TC}O_2$) analyzers are fundamentally of two kinds: mainstream and sidestream.

- On a *mainstream* analyzer, the sensor is within the main flow of gas.
- On a *sidestream* analyzer, a sample is extracted to a sidestream sensor.

The principle of operation is basically the same for both types. Both mainstream and sidestream systems have advantages and disadvantages. Fortunately, newer technology has reduced the problems with both designs.

Best Practice

Calculation of Oxygen Content

Neither P_aO_2 nor S_aO_2 provides complete information about the capacity of the blood to deliver oxygen to the tissues, which, of course, is the key point. Hemoglobin levels and hemoglobin's oxygen-carrying capacity must be included in determining oxygen content. In addition, some oxygen is carried dissolved in the blood. Oxygen content is the total of all oxygen carried in 100 milliliters (mL) of blood, either bound to hemoglobin or dissolved.

Hemoglobin levels are expressed in grams percent (g%), that is, the grams of hemoglobin in 100 mL of blood. Oxygen content is expressed in volume percent (vol%), that is, the volume in milliliters of oxygen in 100 mL of blood. Research has indicated that 1 g of hemoglobin can carry (or bind with) 1.34 mL of oxygen if fully saturated. Some studies have indicated this number could be as high as 1.39 mL O_2/g Hgb, but we will use 1.34 mL O_2/g Hgb. Finally, the Bunsen solubility coefficient for oxygen in blood is 0.003 mL O_2/100 mL blood; that is, 0.003 mL of oxygen will dissolve in 100 mL of blood.

With these factors in place, the math is simple. Given a patient with Hg = 15 g%, P_aO_2 = 95 mm Hg, and S_aO_2 = 98%:

(a) O_2 attached to Hb $= \text{Hb (g\%)} \times 1.34 \times S_aO_2$
$= 15\text{ g\%} \times 1.34 \times 0.98$
$= 20.1 \times 0.98$
$= 19.70$ vol%

(b) Oxygen dissolved $= P_aO_2 \times 0.003$
$= 0.29$ vol%

(c) Total oxygen content = A + B = 19.99 vol%

Thus, for this patient scenario, each 100 mL of blood can carry 19.99 mL of oxygen to the tissues. Remember, however, that this is only part of the answer. If the heart fails, or if circulation is restricted, the oxygen content of the blood is of little use, no matter how great. No single component of patient assessment or laboratory testing is all-revealing.

Mainstream. As the name implies, a *mainstream end-tidal CO_2 monitor* places the CO_2 sensor within the main flow of patient gases. This positioning has the advantage of not requiring aspiration and transport of a sample via tubing. But the mainline sensors and adapters can be bulky, awkward, and affected by water vapor rainout and other contaminants.

Best Practice

Measurement Mismatches

The pulse oximetry reading is high and the ABG says low. What is happening? When S_pCO_2 and S_aO_2 do not match, think hemoglobin abnormality. Examples of such abnormal conditions include:

- COHb.
- Sickle cell disease.
- SulfHb.
- Thalesemia.
- MethHb.
- Cooley's anemia.
- Cyanide poisoning.
- Iron deficiency anemia.
- Organophosphate poisoning.
- Antirejection drugs.

Sidestream. A *sidestream system* requires that a sample of patient gas be aspirated from the main flow and transported to a sensor. This approach reduces the bulk and awkwardness at the patient's airway, but water or mucus often makes its way into the sampling tubing, blocking the narrow sampling tube and disrupting the sampling process.

A rapid-response CO_2 analyzer is the major component of any end-tidal CO_2 monitor. Rapid analysis may be performed using a variety of devices: carbon dioxide–specific infrared cells, Raman scattering, mass spectrometry, or photo-acoustic technology.

The most commonly used technology is *infrared absorption*. In this technique, infrared light is filtered to a specific frequency, and the resultant beam is split using mirrors. Each beam of light is then passed through one of two sampling chambers. One sample chamber is for reference, and the other contains the patient's exhaled respiratory gas sample. Carbon dioxide absorbs infrared light. The higher the partial pressure of carbon dioxide is in the sample, the lower will be the amount of infrared reaching the infrared sensitive detector cell (or sensor). The infrared sensor emits an electrical current that is proportional to the amount of infrared light reaching it.

The level of CO_2 in the patient sample can be determined by comparing the expiratory sample sensor's current with the reference sample current. This information is then displayed numerically, graphically, or both ways.

Although the end-tidal CO_2 is measured as a percentage of the total gas, some analyzers mathematically convert the percentage data into a partial pressure using an algorithm based on Dalton's law (Chapter 3). Alternatively, clinicians can do the conversion themselves by solving the equation for Dalton's law. The ET_CO_2 of most patients closely approximates the P_aCO_2 with results within 1–2 mm Hg of each other. This similarity is due to the high rate of diffusion of CO_2 across the alveolar capillary membrane.

TRANSCUTANEOUS GAS ANALYSIS

The principle of operation of transcutaneous monitoring (T_C) is the same for both oxygen (T_CO_2) and carbon dioxide (T_CCO_2). Modified Clark and Severinghaus electrodes are incorporated into a sensor that is attached to the skin. The skin is heated to 44°–45°C, to promote vasodilation of the capillary bed and increase perfusion to the area. The increased perfusion raises the diffusion of oxygen and carbon dioxide. The resulting T_CO_2 and T_CCO_2 measurements should correlate with P_aO_2 and P_aCO_2, assuming optimal conditions.

The most significant hazard of transcutaneous monitoring is burns caused by the sensor. The risk of burns increases greatly during conditions of low perfusion because the heat is not dissipated as well owing to the diminished blood flow in the area of the sensor.

Transcutaneous Oxygen Sensing. Various factors determine how well T_CO_2 correlates with P_aO_2.

Skin Thickness Thicker skin yields a longer diffusion pathway for oxygen. The correlation between blood gas values and T_C values are not strong; the T_CO_2 is lower than the actual P_aO_2.

Oxygen Consumption Regional oxygen consumption in the area of the sensor site affects correlation. The T_CO_2 is lower than the P_aO_2 as regional oxygen consumption increases.

Perfusion Status Adequate or even hyperperfusion must exist for an accurate correlation; this is the rationale behind heating the skin.

- In low-perfusion states, such as a decreased cardiac output resulting from vasoconstriction or hypothermia, the T_CO_2 is substantially lower than the P_aO_2.
- If adequate perfusion exists (that is, a cardiac index of 2 Lpm/m²), the T_CO_2/P_aO_2 ratio is 70%, plus or minus 12%. As a result, the T_CO_2 is 70% (±12%) of the P_aO_2.

Temperature

- If the skin temperature is too low, adequate peripheral perfusion is not present, and the T_CO_2 is lower than the P_aO_2. If the skin temperature is too high, the T_CO_2 is higher than the measured P_aO_2 (as temperature increases, the diffusion coefficient increases and observed pressure increases).

So the diffusion coefficient is directly related to patient temperature and T_CO_2.

Age Transcutaneous monitoring is used almost exclusively in neonates and newborns. Their skin is much thinner than that of adults, decreasing the length of the diffusion pathway. Under proper conditions, the correlation of T_CO_2 and P_aO_2 is excellent. T_CO_2 can actually equal P_aO_2 if the proper temperature is maintained, adequate perfusion exists, and the infant is younger than 2 weeks old. This positive correlation decreases with age as the skin thickens.

Transcutaneous CO_2 Sensing. Because carbon dioxide diffuses more rapidly and easily across the skin than does oxygen, T_CCO_2 generally is correlated with P_aCO_2 more reliably than T_CO_2 is with it. In addition, CO_2 is not consumed by surrounding tissue, thereby affecting the T_CCO_2 relationship to P_aCO_2. However, other factors that affect T_CO_2 can also affect the T_CCO_2.

Skin Thickness Although CO_2 crosses the skin more easily than O_2, skin thickness can still affect the T_CCO_2, though not to the degree it affects T_CO_2.

Perfusion Status Inadequate blood flow in the region causes the T_CCO_2 to be lower than the P_aO_2.

Temperature Temperature affects the T_CCO_2 just as it does the T_CO_2. A lower temperature causes lower

Best Practice

Preventing Burns

To prevent burns, rotate the sensor site for the transcutaneous probe every 2–4 hours and never place it over a bony area.

perfusion and thus lower than actual T_CCO_2. Higher temperatures increase the pressure, as higher temperatures do to all gases, including those dissolved in liquids, resulting in an artificially heightened T_CCO_2.

Age The direct impact of aging on T_CCO_2 is less evident than on T_CO_2, but the physiological changes associated with aging, such as thickening skin and decreased perfusion, can affect the T_CCO_2, generally causing it to read lower than actual. T_CCO_2 can be a valuable monitor in pediatric patients who are on high-frequency ventilation.

POINT OF CARE TESTING

Point of care (*POC*) *units,* such as i-STAT™, have many potential advantages over the traditional benchtop analyzer found in pulmonary or clinical laboratories. The term "point of care" refers to the fact that these units are small and simple to use; they can be used at the patient's bedside, potentially speeding the availability of results. The principle of operation of POC units is no different, essentially, from that of benchtop units. Variants of the Sanz, Clark, and Severinghaus electrodes are in place, though miniaturized and self-contained. The key difference is the short-term disposability of the electrodes and the reduced size of the units.

Although the design and operation of the various POC units vary, they generally eliminate the repeated use of a set of electrodes. Instead, they use a disposable cassette that contains both the electrodes and the electrolyte reagent in a sampling chamber. The performance of the electrodes is tested immediately before the analysis is done, and the electrodes are discarded after the analysis.

POC units have several advantages:

- Discarding the electrodes eliminates the need to plot the ongoing performance of the electrodes. Statistical analysis and charting of the electrodes' performance status are unnecessary because the same electrode is never used twice.
- Calibration and quality control materials are often part of the electrode pack, eliminating the need for inventories of separate supplies. In some cases, electronic calibrations eliminate the need for calibration materials entirely.
- Sampling-to-report time is reduced.
- Sample transport requirements are eliminated.
- The number of "bad" samples due to delay is reduced.
- Depending on the institution's staffing and policies, staff spend more "on location" when they do not have to transport the sample to another location.

Age-Specific Competency

POC Units

POC manufacturers claim that point of care units need a smaller sample size than other analyzers, reducing blood loss. Although the consideration of reduced blood loss is important in neonatal patients and small children, it is rarely relevant in the care of adolescents and adults. Even so, compared with modern benchtop analyzers, POC units offer virtually no advantage in sample size if the benchtop unit is being used optimally.

All of these advantages come at a price, however. The sample analysis packs can be expensive. Some POC analyzers have bulk calibration and electrode packs that are used over several analyses, but they also have expiration periods of 3–14 days from instillation and activation. If the number of procedures performed during the calendar life of the pack is not within the expiration range, the cost per analysis goes even higher. The number and frequency of blood gas analysis must be carefully evaluated to determine which unit is best for a facility or even whether POC makes sense in the facility.

Various studies have alternately validated and questioned the accuracy of POC units compared with analyzers. Many facilities have adopted POCs house-wide. Others have integrated POC and benchtop units. Still others have rejected POC units, opting instead for satellite laboratories that bring the benchtop analyzers closer to the bedside. The future of POC testing rests on many factors, including pricing of supplies and units, the ongoing accuracy of the units, the size and nature of health care facilities, and the makeup of the clinical staff.

Role of Hemoglobin and Its Variants in ABG Analysis

The hemoglobin (Hb) molecule is a complex structure with many variables. Its ability to combine with many different substances is at once valuable and hazardous. Closely related to the myoglobin found in cardiac muscle, hemoglobin consists of two distinct parts: *heme*—a cluster-like arrangement of molecules—and *globulin*—a polypeptide chain—form the functional hemoglobin molecule (Figure 16-15).

Adult hemoglobin (HbA) has a molecular weight of 64,500, and each red cell (erythrocyte) carries about 280 million Hb molecules. The body produces between

Spotlight On

New and Emerging Techniques

Several new technologies that are being discussed in research journals and at professional meetings may prove to be clinically valuable in the near future.

Ultrasound is being used in a wide variety of ever-growing applications in medicine. Recently, an ultrasound device for measuring blood sugar noninvasively has been tested very successfully in a small group of individuals. The ability to refine the use of ultrasound will make it an attractive technology for investigation for future noninvasive measurement of more substances, including ABGs.

The potential of *indwelling sensors* will continue to attract research efforts, and improved strategies for their use will emerge. As technology improves and methods are developed to reduce clot formation and motion artifact, the use of these sensors should become more widespread. The ability to obtain real-time, in vivo data on blood gases and acid-base balance will make these improved optic sensors valuable additions to critical care technology.

The use of newer applications of *light absorption, frequencies, wavelengths*, and better *filters* and *sensors* will refine the accuracy and specificity of light absorption technology, allowing for expanded use and greater accuracy.

2 million and 10 million red blood cells in the bone marrow each day. Each erythrocyte has a life of approximately 120 days. Normal hemoglobin levels of adults are 13.5–18.0 g/dL for males and 12.0–16.0 g/dL for females. One gram of hemoglobin can carry 1.34 g of oxygen.

The shape of the Hb molecule plays an important role in its ability to attract, carry, and release oxygen and carbon dioxide. Even slight alterations of this shape can prevent O_2 and CO_2 from binding with the molecule. If the receptor sites are not properly aligned, the O_2 and CO_2 cannot dock properly, and the ability of the hemoglobin to carry those molecules is reduced.

Think of the molecule of Hb as a lock; only certain keys allow the lock to function, and no other lock works. If the shape of the key changes, the lock does not open, or if the lock itself changes shape, the key does not fit. If the heme molecule and its four iron molecules, which are normally bound to oxygen, are reconfigured by replacement of the oxygen with carbon monoxide, sulfur, or a methyl group, instead of oxyhemoglobin (HbO_2), the species of hemoglobin

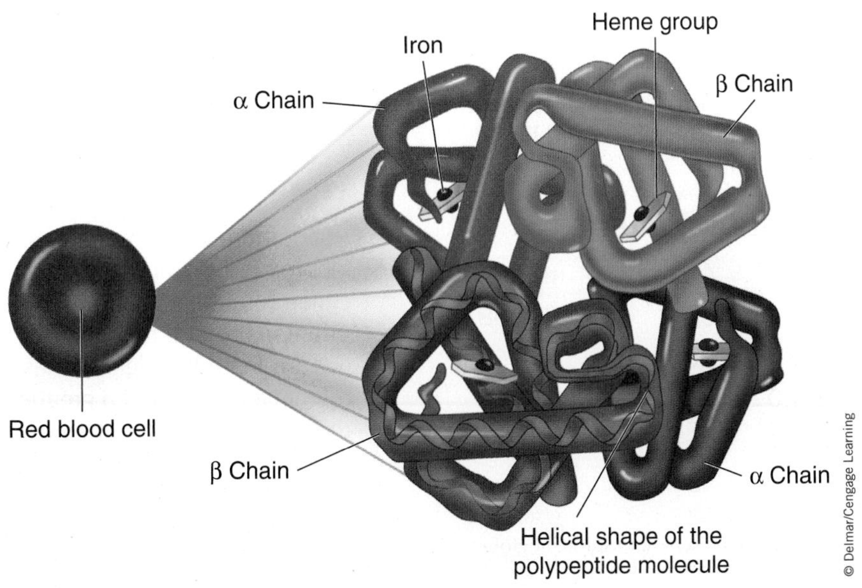

FIGURE 16-15 Hemoglobin molecule.

changes; it could be carboxyhemoglobin (HbCO), sulfhemoglobin (HbS),* or methhemoglobin (HbM). Each of these has different physical and chemical properties than oxyhemoglobin, and each has decreased ability to attract, transport, and release oxygen and carbon dioxide. This is an example of how the geometry of a compound can affect both its function and its limitations.

Normally, small quantities of these Hb species are in the blood. Methhemoglobin* levels of 1–2% are typical (Hbmet). Sulfhemoglobin (HbS) levels of <1% are normal, and, in persons living and working in rural areas with low levels of environmental hydrocarbon pollutants, levels of less than 1–2% are normal. Carboxyhemoglobin (HbCO) levels of 5–10% in city dwellers—especially smokers—are not uncommon. It is believed that normal metabolic processes may result in incomplete combustion of organic compounds, thus establishing a so-called normal level of CO in the body. HbSulf is far more common in blacks than in other racial groups and has been linked to sickle cell disease.

Other Factors That Affect ABG Results

Additional factors that affect the procurement or accuracy of ABGs and that are causes of potential error are the anion gap, sampling errors, and problems with the analysis itself.

ANION GAP

Physiological factors include the anion gap (AG), the difference between the anions (negatively charged electrolytes) and the cations (positively charged electrolytes) in the blood plasma. The cations are Na^+, K^+, Ca^{2+}, and Mg^{2+}, and the anions are Cl^-, HCO_3^-, and PO_4^{2-}. Table 16-7 presents the normal values for serum electrolytes. In normal subjects, the AG should be about 12 ±2 mEq/L. To determine the anion gap (AG), subtract the sum of the anions from the sum of the cations. For convenience sake, when performing anion gap calculations, ignore the ions with very low values (Ca^{2+}, Mg^{2+}, K^+, PO_4^{2-}); they have little effect on the AG. Thus the formula for anion gap (AG) is:

$$AG = Na^+ - (Cl^- + HCO_3^-)$$

Significance of the Anion Gap. The anion gap accounts for unmeasured anions such as ketones, sulfates, anionic proteins (proteins without an electrical charge), and lactic acid. The calculation indicates the effect of organic and volatile acids that are difficult to isolate and analyze. These effects can often explain otherwise puzzling results in the acid-base portion of ABG analysis. Coexisting conditions, such as diabetes, malnutrition, or kidney disease, or conditions causing increases in anaerobic metabolism cause most of the alterations in the AG.

Interpretation of the Anion Gap. Interpretation of anion gap data is tied to the overall acid-base status, for example, with metabolic acidosis:

- *High AG*—This can result from alkali (HCO_3^-) deficit secondary to increased unmeasured anions (e.g., ketones).
- *Normal AG*—Alkali deficit may occur secondary to direct loss of HCO_3^- and fluid (e.g., an inability to form or reabsorb HCO_3^- or an excess infusion of Cl^-).
- *Decreased AG*—This may be a sign of lab error of decreased unmeasured anions (e.g., hyperalbuminemia), or of increased unmeasured cations (e.g., lithium overdose).

TABLE 16-7 **Normal serum values**

Cations (+)	mEq/L	Anions (–)	mEq/L
Na^+	135–145	Cl,$^-$	95–108
K^+	3.5–5.0	HCO_3^-	22–26
Ca^{2+}	3.5–4.0	PO_4^{2-}	1.7–2.6
Mg^{2+}	1.3–2.1		

*The abbreviation "HbS" is used to represent both sulfhemoglobin and sickle cell disease. Be careful not to confuse the two. To avoid this issue in this chapter, the nonstandard abbreviation "HbSulf" is used.

Age-Specific Competency

Hemoglobin Variants

In addition to carboxyhemoglobin, sulfhemoglobin, and methhemoglobin, a normal variant called fetal hemoglobin (HbF) exists in fetuses, infants, and to a much lesser extent in adults (<2%). Fetal hemoglobin has different abilities than does HbO_2 and a greater affinity for oxygen than does HbA (adult hemoglobin), in order to enable the fetus to extract oxygen from the mother's blood. HbF concentration falls from 95% at 10 weeks gestation to about 50% at birth, and it should be at 5% at 6 months of age, reaching adult levels soon after.

SAMPLING ERRORS

Errors in sampling technique can substantially affect the results of blood gas analysis. Consider the following potential errors by sampling route or site.

Arterial Puncture. Since the vast majority of arterial blood gases are obtained by arterial puncture, consider the problems associated with that method first.

Room Air Contamination The presence of room air bubbles in a sample alters the values toward those of room air. P_aCO_2 moves toward zero, and PO_2 moves toward 150. Since the level of P_aCO_2 affects the pH through the hydration reaction, pH is shifted upward. The impact of a bubble increases with the size of the bubble and with the duration of the presence of the bubble in the sample.

Venipuncture Inadvertent puncture of the venous circulation is a fairly common error. Clearly, upon analysis, the blood gas values appear to be venous. Although venous pulse pressures are substantially lower than arterial pressures, some patients have high enough venous pressures to cause syringe filling. Lack of spontaneous filling of the syringe should be a signal that one of three conditions has occurred:

- A venous sample was obtained.
- There is a regional perfusion problem.
- The patient is extremely hypertensive.

Prolonged Puncture Prolonged and/or painful puncture can result in patient hyperventilation, altering the values significantly from their true resting state. Patients sometimes breathe rapidly or deeply in anticipation of pain during a needle insertion. Other patients may hold their breath as they anticipate the puncture and during the puncture procedure itself, resulting in a hypoventilation state.

Residual Heparin Although most ABG kits use preheparinized syringes, sometimes nonheparinized syringes may be used. Liquid heparin poses a special concern. Too much heparin remaining in the dead space of the sampling device can shift the sample's values toward those of the heparin. Also, dilution of the sample can cause errors in hemoglobin and co-oximetry measurements. Many institutions use preassembled and preheparinized ABG kits, which greatly reduce the chance of heparin-related problems.

Arterial Lines. Arterial lines (or A-lines) are the other major source of blood gas samples. They come with their own special types of potential sampling errors.

Inadequate Flushing of the Line Between samplings, arterial lines are flushed with a heparin solution to prevent blood clotting. If the solution is not adequately removed before sampling, the resulting sample is diluted with the flushing solution. This dilution alters all the results by moving gas values toward those of the flushing solution. The pH is shifted owing to the change in P_aCO_2, and any co-oximetry values from this sample are also affected.

Best Practice

Heparin Type

Some types of heparin can affect specific values. For example, sodium heparin is not best if your sample will be used to measure sodium in an electrolyte analysis. In these cases, use lithium heparin.

Sampling from the Wrong Line Care must be taken to avoid mistakenly withdrawing samples from venous, central venous, or intracardiac lines instead of arterial lines. The blood gas values normally range widely among these sampling sources. All lines should be color coded or identified with labels that indicate their purpose.

Capillary Sampling. In capillary sampling, the sampling site is usually an earlobe or, in children and infants, more commonly the heel. The chosen site is warmed with warm (not hot) wet gauze pads or with a specially designed chemical heating pack for 10–15 minutes. This part of the procedure is critical because warming dilates the blood vessels in the area, promotes perfusion, and thus arterializes the blood in the area of the sampling site.

After warming, the sample site is cleaned with Betadine and alcohol:

- Make a stab incision on the fatty part of the heel using a no. 11 scalpel blade, lancet, or other appropriate instrument. The incision needs to be deep enough to produce a free flow of blood but not so deep as to incise the muscle layer.
- When active bleeding is accomplished, introduce a capillary tube into the blood flow. At this point, blood should be drawn into the tube by capillary action.
- Seal the tube at both ends and ice it in preparation to be sent to the lab for analysis.
- Wipe away the remaining blood at the sample site.
- Apply firm, but not tight, manual pressure to the site with a gauze pad until the bleeding stops in about 2–5 minutes.

- Document the puncture site, holding time, and success of the capillary stick on the lab request form and in the patient's chart, along with the patient's oxygenation status, temperature, and toleration of the procedure, including excessive crying.

Capillary sampling is largely confined to infants and small children, but it poses some significant problems related to technique. The patient's sample volume-to-surface area sets the diffusion rate across the collection device's walls.

Room Air Contamination The impact of room air contamination on capillary samples is the same as it is for arterial punctures.

Aggressive Squeezing Ideally, a capillary sample is acquired with no squeezing of the site to prompt blood flow. Squeezing (milking) causes the forced introduction of venous capillary blood into the sample. Milking shifts the values toward venous values, generally causing a lower PO_2, a higher P_aCO_2, and a lower pH.

Poor Site Preparation Inadequate heating of the site results in a poorly arterialized sample, causing the sample to reflect more venous values.

ANALYSIS

The analysis itself can give rise to problems when analyzing ABGs, from several potential sources.

Out-of-Calibration Analyzer. The lab standard values (the normal range of values) should conform to national and regional norms.

- *Critical values* are those that fall outside the normal lab values.
- *Panic values* are analysis results that indicate a need for swift and decisive intervention by the caregivers.

These values should be justifiable by reference to current literature and cross-analysis with peer and reference labs. Membership in a reference group is highly desirable for any lab. In addition, ongoing recording and trending of calibration and quality assurance results provide added safeguards and reference points for improved lab practices.

An out-of-calibration analyzer compromises all the results since the last calibration. Whether all those results are accurate or, if not accurate, how they vary from correct results cannot be known. Performing analysis using an out-of-calibration analyzer places laboratory accreditation at risk. Calibrations should be scheduled on the basis of the analyzer's use pattern and the recommendations of the manufacturer, and the calibration schedule should be strictly enforced. Personnel performing the analysis should be rigorously trained in calibration and in verification rationales and techniques. Any question as to whether the ABG values obtained result from an instrument that is out of calibration should lead to immediate reanalysis of the sample on a second analyzer.

The issue of reporting the suspected out of calibration results along with the results of the second unit's analysis is a matter of debate. One group says that both sets of data should be reported along with the perceived out-of-calibration condition of the primary analyzer. Others contend that only the secondary results need reporting, either with or without the out-of-calibration statement.

Of course, the primary analyzer should be examined immediately to determine the cause of the out-of-calibration status and to resolve it as soon as possible. Until the situation is resolved, the analyzer must be taken out of service and have a "Out of Service" sign placed on it.

Out-of-Control Analyzer. As with results from an uncalibrated analyzer, any results from an out-of-control analyzer are of questionable accuracy and value. Reporting results from an out-of-control analyzer also jeopardizes the laboratory's accreditation.

Out-of-control, in this context, means that the analyzer gives an incorrect response to quality control (QC) samples at a frequency beyond that predicted by normal, random variation. In other words, the results of the analysis of quality control samples are outside the accuracy range of the known quality control samples. The QC range is usually 1–2 standard deviations (SD) from the known mean of the QC sample. A 2-SD QC range represents the range of values within which one would expect to find 95% of all sample values or 95% of the population from which the sample was selected. A 1-SD range is equivalent to the results found in 68% of the population samples.

Inasmuch as the standard deviation range is generally distributed equally on either side of the mean data value, in the case of 2 SD, 47.5% of the data is below the mean and 47.5% of the data is above the mean. In nonbiological data, this distribution of values, when viewed in terms of their frequency of occurrence, forms a bell-shaped or normal curve. Biological data often form a curve that is skewed or tipped slightly to the right. This type of curve, called a *Gaussian curve*, means that more data fall on the high side of the mean than on the left, or low, side of the curve. For QC purposes, assume a normal curve because the range of normal values used is very small and the population is very large.

Best Practice

Icing Samples

Icing a sample that will also be used for electrolyte analysis yields inaccurate results for some of the electrolytes. When the sample will be used for multiple types of analysis, the respiratory therapist walks a delicate line in deciding whether to ice it. One solution is to split the sample:

- Allow additional blood to enter the ABG syringe.
- Inject an appropriate amount of the ABG sample into the proper blood collection tube or tubes.
- Then ice the ABG sample but not the other tubes of blood.

Another method, which requires another pair of hands, is to:

- Insert a three-way stopcock between the needle and hub of the ABG syringe before inserting the needle into the patient.
- Make sure that the three-way valve is set to allow blood flow from the needle to the ABG syringe.
- Have another syringe ready to place on the free hub of the three-way stopcock as the blood flow to the ABG syringe is halted by turning the stopcock to the off position.
- Attach the other, needle-less, syringe on the empty hub and turn the stopcock so that blood flows into the new syringe.
- When this is getting full again, turn the stopcock off.
- Remove both the needle and the new syringe.
- Transfer the contents of the new syringe into the correct venopuncture tube.

Improperly Handled Samples. Allowing a sample to remain at room temperature for more than 15 minutes allows metabolism within the sample to lower the PO_2, raise the P_aCO_2, and lower the pH. The blood cells within the sample are still alive and are still metabolizing. Inside the sampling syringe, oxygen is still being used to create energy, and carbon dioxide continues to be produced. As metabolism continues, the amount of oxygen in the sample is decreasing, and the amount of carbon dioxide in the sample is increasing in the sample.

These changes in key values are affected by the *rate of metabolism*, which is a factor of the amount of metabolism per unit of time and the temperature of the metabolic system. These two facts mean that we can control the changes in P_aO_2 and P_aCO_2 by reducing the time from draw to analysis (decreasing the time effect) or by reducing the temperature of the sample. Or we can do both: Ice the sample, and then transport it quickly for analysis.

Inadequately Mixed Sample. Poor mixing of the sample before analysis can result in a nonhomogeneous sample. The separation of the formed elements and the plasma tends to alter the distribution of both electrolytes and dissolved gases. This alteration can cause unpredictable changes in the results for any measured ABG parameters.

To prevent separation, always agitate the sample by holding it upright (be absolutely sure that the transport cap is on correctly and tightly), and then move the wrist rhythmically from side to side for 1–2 minutes. This action adequately mixes the sample.

Note: Rolling the sample syringe between the palms does not provide adequate mixing.

Quality Control, Quality Assurance, and Performance Improvement

Anyone who is involved in health care, particularly in direct patient care, needs to be aware of the need for a well developed and defined system of quality control. Such systems include several components in which:

- Limits are set and defined (quality control, QC).
- Limits are measured and tested (quality assurance, QA).
- Remediation of errors is addressed (performance improvement, PI).

QUALITY CONTROL

A most important and, sadly, most misunderstood issue surrounding blood gas analysis is quality control. Too many therapists mistake quality control as a mechanism to get them into trouble or to provide busywork when clinical analysis requirements are slow. Nothing could be further from the truth. Precise and accurate performance and recording of successful and unsuccessful control samples are required to ensure

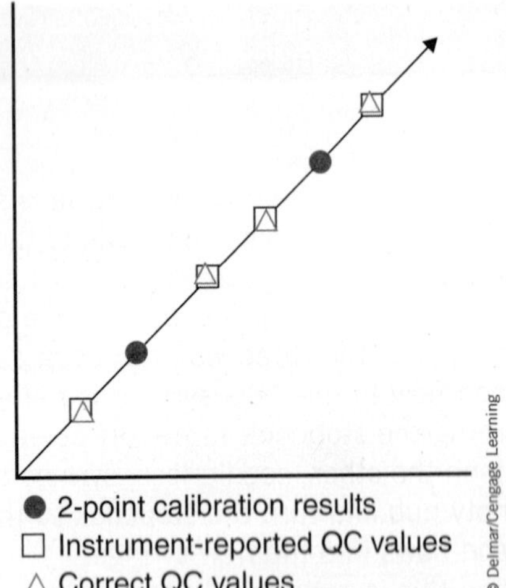

FIGURE 16-16 The ideal electrode performance documents fully linear relationships between the electrical signal and the displayed values. Not only the calibration points, but the reported values for the quality control sample, fall linearly.

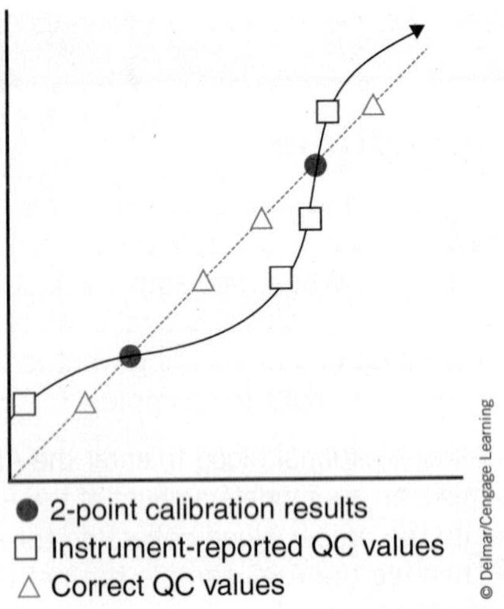

FIGURE 16-17 Out-of-control electrode performance: Although the calibration points fall linearly, the quality control points do not. This is the most problematic electrode performance because the calibrations alone indicate that the instrument is working properly. Only the QC samples reveal the nonlinear (and thus nonpredictable) nature of the electrode's readings.

accurate test results. The accurate control of sample procurement and analysis helps to avoid problems and trouble in the future and to protect the patient from being treated on the basis of faulty information and erroneous data.

The purpose of quality controls (QC) is to determine the measurement characteristics of the analyzer. Even though an instrument may be measuring properly at the points tested during calibration, proper measurement performance at other points along the measurement continuum has to be confirmed. Figure 16-16 shows the hoped-for ideal performance of an electrode. The response of the electrode to a given value in the sample is linear, passing through the calibration points and the sample points in a predictable and linear fashion. However, Figure 16-17 illustrates what the response of the electrode could be: nonlinear and unpredictable. Although the response passes through the calibration points for the electrode, away from the calibration points, the curve is far from linear. Notice that the sample points are far different from the values illustrated in Figure 16-16 because the response curve is distorted. In the scenario presented in Figure 16-17, running calibrations alone could lead the respiratory therapist to mistakenly assume that the analyzer is measuring properly.

Quality controls (*QCs*) are predefined samples placed at other points along the expected response curve; some are in the normal range, some are high, and some are low. Together, they check the performance across a clinically relevant range. If they are not measured and reported properly by the analyzer, it indicates a potential problem.

Sometimes the cause of an out-of-range measurement is normal, random variation. Sometimes it is a real machine problem. How does the operator tell the difference and avoid unnecessary troubleshooting and maintenance? That question bothered Dr. James Westgard, and in the late 1970s he applied statistics to the problem. What resulted were his so-called Westgard rules.[7] The so-called rules are based on 1, 2, and 3 standard deviations and the percentage of probability associated with data falling within each range.

Recall that a single standard deviation (1 SD) is equivalent to approximately a 68%-confidence interval; that is, 68% of all potential values should fall within that 1-SD range. Two standard deviations (2 SD) is a 95% confidence interval, meaning that 95% of all results should fall within the 2-SD range. Three standard deviations (3 SD) is a 99.7% confidence interval, meaning that 99.7% of all results should fall inside the 3 SD range. Beyond the 3rd SD are *outliers*, samples that may really belong to another population rather than the one being studied.

Now turn this notion around. In a 2-SD range, 5 of 100 results could or should fall outside the range; these results represent simple random variation within the system. Although 5 of 100 is not a large number, it is not all that unlikely that a single result will fall outside the range. However, a 3-SD range indicates that only 3 of 1000 results is normally expected to fall outside the range; this is a small enough expectation that a single value outside the range is truly suspect. That is how the Westgard rules approach QC values.

Suppose the respiratory therapist runs controls on the blood gas analyzer. The P_aO_2 value for the QC falls outside the 2-SD range but is within the 3-SD range. Is this a real problem? The solution is to repeat the QC. If the P_aO_2 falls within the 2-SD range on the repeat test, a safe assumption is that this was just one of those 5 of 100 that fall outside the range. However, if the repeat is also outside the 2-SD range, there must be a real problem; the probability that two consecutive results would be part of the 5 of 100 is quite low. The repeat result should be treated as a real problem, and troubleshooting and documentation should be done.

If the QC is outside the 3-SD range when the control is run the first time, this is a problem because a value outside the 3 SD is expected to occur only 3 times out of 1000. The probability is that data which is outside the 3 SD range represents samples that are "outliers" and likely are from a different or variant population. Troubleshooting and documentation should be done. The instrument should be out of service until the problem is resolved, and the measurement is reliably falling within the 2-SD range.

The question, however, is whether those out-of-range QC values should be recorded and kept in the database or be discarded. Many therapists choose to discard them, but discarding them creates problems in the long run. The first QC value that was out of range should be retained in the database. The repeat value, along with any repeat failures performed during the troubleshooting, should not be retained because they are defined as not-normal variations. Why is discarding the data an issue, and what problem will discarding it cause? Standard deviation is calculated on the basis of all values in the database. Figure 16-18 illustrates a Levy-Jennings plot (also known as a Levy-Jennings chart or graph), in which analysis results are plotted in terms of their standard deviation distribution from the mean control values. Throwing out all out-of-range values means throwing out the "normal" 5% that fall outside the 2-SD range through normal variation and that are thus valid. The SD range progressively shrinks, producing a QC target that the lab cannot hit.

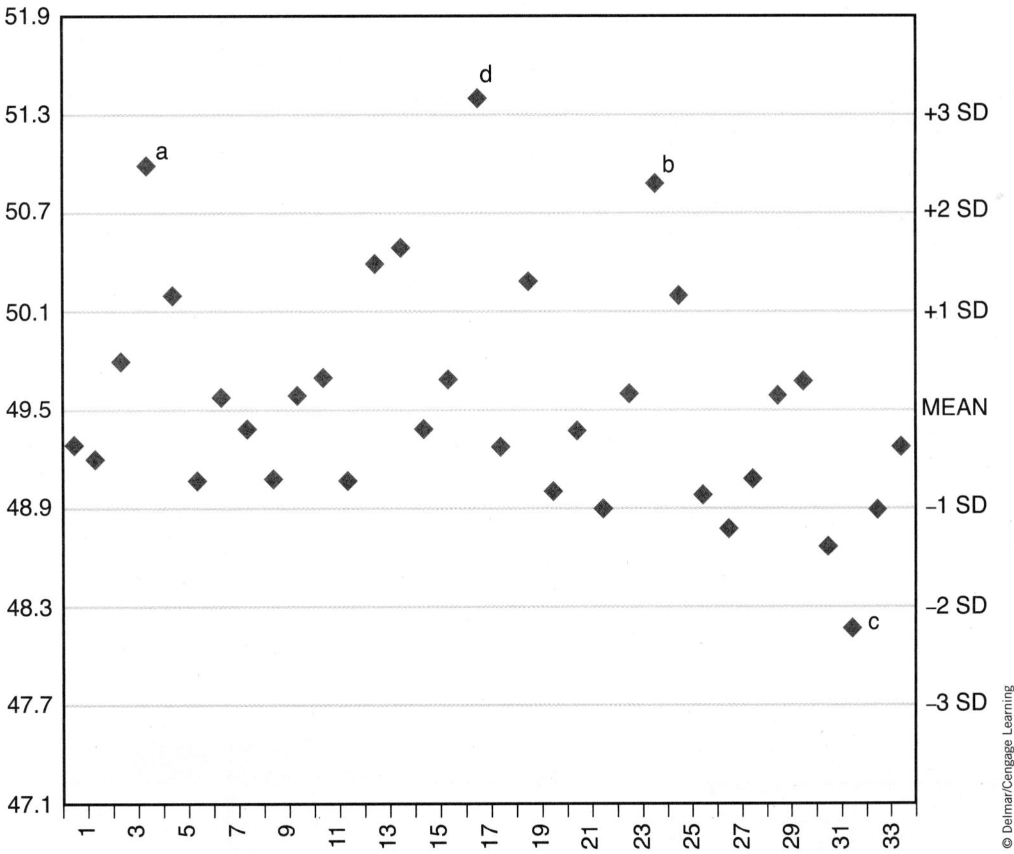

FIGURE 16-18 Levy-Jennings QC plot: Results of individual quality control runs are plotted in a graphic display to make trends more apparent. Individual points are plotted against the mean, ±1 standard deviation (SD), ±2 SD, and ±SD. Note that points a, b, and c fall beyond 2 SD from the mean and require repeat analyses. Because the repeat falls within 2 SD, no further action was carried out.

Numerous other Westgard rules help in determining whether a pattern of performance is likely to represent normal variation or a system problem. If they were all applied to a single lab, getting any results reported successfully would be difficult. So a few should be selected that best protect the validity of the data from the individual blood gas lab. By all means, all therapists must protect the validity and completeness of the QC database by properly retaining or discarding the data. Additionally, a detailed, comprehensive and contemporaneous QC/QA log should be rigorously maintained. A lab that consistently documents fewer than 5% 2 SD violations is suspect because random variation should be an expected outcome.

QUALITY ASSURANCE

Quality assurance and *quality control* are terms that are often used interchangeably. They are, however, very different. Quality assurance (QA) has recently become known as *performance improvement* (PI), but its focus remains to detect systemic problems and to use them to improve the system. The idea is to:

- Perform ongoing monitoring to ascertain the quality of the outcome.
- Determine where improvements should be made.
- Then devise and carry out a plan to make the improvements.

A key concept is that the QC/QA process must be treated as a system, not as independent parts and practices. The blood gas *system* is made up of more than just the machine. The system also consists of the order processing, the therapists, the sample collection and transport mechanisms, the sample-handling procedures, and the result-reporting mechanism. The system includes anything, including pre- and post-analysis processes, that can affect the quality of the results (Figure 16-19). If a respiratory therapist receives blood gas orders on the wrong patient, the mistake has nothing to do with the blood gas machine, but it is a blood gas system problem. If the

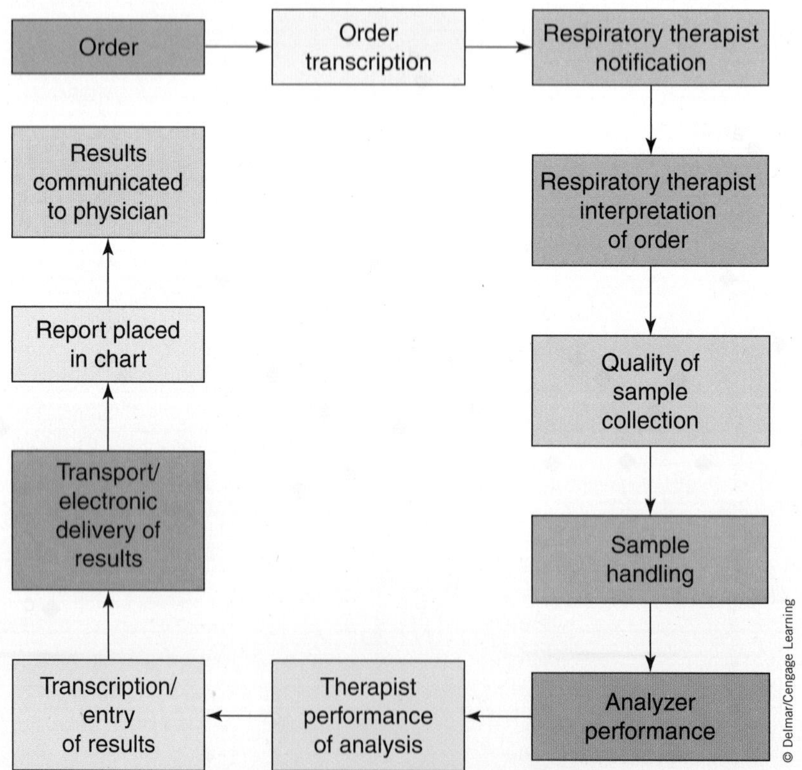

FIGURE 16-19 Blood gas quality control components: Potential sources of quality-control problems with blood gases range far beyond instrument performance. These other sources are often classified as preanalytical and postanalytical. Potential issues are the appropriateness and clarity of the order, misentry or misinterpretation of the order, collection errors, errors in transcription of results, and errors in report generation by computer systems.

computerized blood gas reporting system transposes numbers in results, that error is a blood gas system problem. If the ABG results do not fit the patient's clinical signs and symptoms picture, the reason may have to do with other ABG system failures unrelated to the results.

PERFORMANCE IMPROVEMENT

Performance improvement (*PI*) monitors (tests and processes to check the integrity of the system) should be designed to cover all aspects of the system, although not all at the same time. Trying to monitor everything all the time is a virtual guarantee of failure. The monitors should be selective and change periodically. Once or twice a year, a monitor should compare blood gas machine output with actual printed results at the patient unit. This practice checks the reporting system. Periodic monitoring of turnaround times for blood gases helps in the detection of problems in the ordering, handling, or processing of orders. Table 16-8 indicates some PI issues that have risen in the literature, along with their possible solutions.

Of course, monitoring technical performance should be a part of PI. For example, what is the rate of necessary repeated punctures? What is the rate of patient complaints about punctures? The Clinical Laboratory Improvement Act of 1988 (CLIA) requires the performance of proficiency testing (PT) throughout the year to determine a lab's proficiency at accurately running and reporting blood gases, and PT should be included in any PI program.

Even though regulators and accrediting organizations act as guardians of proficiency, a sound PI program is just plain good for your patients and your organization. All the many parts of the ABG system, other than the blood gas analyzer, may be a potential source of error. Juvenal, the Roman satirist, wrote, "*Quis custodiet ipsos custodes?*" (Who will guard the guardians?). In the case of ABG results, all the participants in the system must act as guardians if patient care is to be enhanced, safe, and effective.

TABLE 16-8 **Performance improvement issues**

Issue	Sample Indicator	Remediation
ABG punctures	Percentage failure	Manikin practice observed punctures
Air bubble	Number of contaminated samples	Reinstruct practice
Report speed	Number of complaints, mean response time	Electronic reports, time and motion study

Interpreting Blood Gas Analysis Results

Before interpreting the results of an ABG analysis, the respiratory therapist, lab technician, and physician should have all the information needed to understand the results. For example, they must know the patient's:

- Age.
- Temperature.
- Ventilator status.
- Diagnosis.
- Respiratory rate.
- F_IO_2.
- Tidal volume.

METHODS AND RULES

Of the many techniques for interpreting ABG results, the system offered here is one of the many commonly used methods. Practicing this skill will make the respiratory therapist an even better interpreter of blood gases.

ABG Interpretation Method Made Simple. First determine the acid-base status of the patient as indicated by the results of the blood gas analysis. Then interpret the patient's oxygenation and ventilation status. Recall that the ABG results indicated by the blood gases must be correlated with the patient's clinical status and treatment regime.

A simple yet accurate method of interpretation of ABG findings is called the *four-step acid-base analysis*.[6] These four easy steps enable the respiratory therapist to quickly master the art of blood gas interpretation. However, each step must be followed carefully and taken in order.

1. List the three values responsible for acid-base balance: pH, P_aCO_2, HCO_3^-.
2. Compare these with the normal values and determine whether they are acid (A), base (B), or normal (N). Write "A," "B," or "N" beside each value:
   pH 7.50—B
   P_aCO_2, 25—B
   HCO_3^- 24—N
3. Circle any letters that are the same, usually pH and either P_aCO_2 or HCO_3^-.
   pH 7.50—B
   P_aCO_2, 25—B
   HCO_3^- 24—N

Best Practice

Things to Know Before ABG Interpretation

Things the RT *must* know:

- F_IO_2
- Patient's temp (There is some controversy on this point.)
- Ventilator status
- PEEP
- Patient's age
- Comorbidity

Things the RT *should* know:

- Hgb/Hct
- Drugs given
- Fraction type specific Hgb
- Chief complaint
- Diagnosis
- Respiratory rate
- V_T or MV
- Intake and Output (fluid balance)

4. Determine whether the uncircled value has moved in the opposite direction of the circled ones. If it has, compensation is occurring; if it has not, compensation is absent.

In addition, the RT might wish to know whether the changes are acute (sudden) or chronic (old) changes. The following formula will help in making that determination.

Acute: pH and 1 factor change (e.g., pH and P_aCO_2 or HCO_3^- or AG)

Chronic: More than pH +1 factor changes (e.g., pH and P_aCO_2 and HCO_3^- change and/or AG)

PREDICTING AND ESTIMATING CHANGES IN BLOOD GAS VALUES

The ability to predict what blood gas levels should be under given conditions is helpful in the interpretation of ABG results. Tables 16-9 to 16-11 present prediction formulas that enable the respiratory therapist to determine the expected values for many variables under a number of conditions.

TABLE 16-9 **Blood gas prediction formulas**

Respiratory-Driven pH Changes
Acute acidosis/alkalosis
pH change = 0.008 units/1 mm Hg P_aCO_2 change
Chronic acidosis
pH change = 0.003 units/1 mm Hg P_aCO_2 change
Chronic alkalosis
pH change = 0.0017 units/1 mm Hg P_aCO_2 change
Metabolically Driven P_aCO_2 Changes
Metabolic acidosis
P_aCO_2 = 1.54 (HCO_3^-) +8 (±2)
Metabolic alkalosis
P_aCO_2 = 0.7 (HCO_3^-) +20 (±1.5)
If the P_aCO_2 predicted is greater than the observed, there is a superimposed respiratory alkalosis.
If the P_aCO_2 predicted is less than the observed, there is a superimposed respiratory acidosis.

TABLE 16-10 **Respiratory-driven pH or P_aCO_2 changes**

To predict pH or P_aCO_2 change:
Assume pH = 7.40, P_aCO_2 = 40 mm Hg
For each *acute* 10 mm Hg *rise* of P_aCO_2, pH will *decrease* by 0.05 unit.
For each *acute* 10 mm Hg *fall* of P_aCO_2, pH will *increase* by 0.1 unit.

New and Emerging Technologies

Although the understanding of blood gas physiology does not change radically in short periods of time, fine-tuning regularly occurs. The technologies certainly change, as does the understanding of how to measure associated physiologic variables. For example:

- An improved understanding of how to reduce interference in pulse oximetry sampling has led to pulse oximeters that dampen the effects of artificial environmental light and movement artifact. These devices have proved to be much more accurate and reliable.
- Other improvements over the last 5–10 years are waveform stabilization through signal processing to remove interfering patterns, filtering data, and ultrafast sampling techniques.
- Research on the near infrared (NIR) wavelength absorption by various hemoglobin species has lead to improvements in and the expansion of

TABLE 16-11 Miscellaneous prediction formulas

pH Changes
If $P_aCO_2 > 40$ mm Hg:
$7.40 - \frac{(\text{measured } P_aCO_2 - 40)/100}{2}$
If $P_aCO_2 < 40$ mm Hg:
$pH = 7.40 - \frac{(40 - \text{measured } P_aCO_2)}{100}$
HCO_3^- Changes
To predict HCO_3^- from P_aCO_2 change:
HCO_3^- decreases 2 mmol/L per 10 mm Hg decrease in P_aCO_2.
HCO_3^- increases 1 mmol/L per 10 mm Hg rise in P_aCO_2.
Age-Compensated P_aO_2
$P_aO_2 < 1$ mm Hg per year of age over 60 from a base of 80 mm Hg
$P_aO_2 = 80 - (\text{age} - 60)$

the ability to accurately determine the fractional concentration of these species.

- Pulse oximeters no longer are limited to using photospectometry to determine S_PCO_2.
- Hemoglobin of several species (HbO_2, MetHb, SulfHb, COHb) can now be measured by mimicking the co-oximeter.
- Several types of ABG analyzers include co-oximetry and Hb determination.
- Some ABG analyzers can provide information on electrolytes, thanks to ongoing research on microsampling technology.
- Blood glucose measurement by transcutaneous, photospectrometric methods is currently under study and will, if successful, be a welcome instrument for millions of diabetics worldwide.
- Without doubt, patient care will be improved by:

  The ability to measure and quantify physiologic variables, such as exhaled nitric oxide, gastric, and esophageal pH, via minimally invasive sensors.

  The use of ultrasound vascular location devices to minimize failed arterial and venous punctures.

  The use of pulse oximetry data to determine perfusion index, differential perfusion, and pulse waveform analysis.

- Measurement of tissue O_2 (S_TO_2) by transcutaneous photospectometric methods has recently become a reality.
- Microtechnology, including nearly nanorobots (nanobots) and cameras have opened new vistas (figuratively and in reality) for treatment and diagnosis.
- Enhanced data storage and display abilities through the microization of computers will clearly allow faster, more accurate trend analysis and response to changing physiology, drug delivery, and improved disease and injury survival rates.
- Advances in radiologic technology have already changed the face of medicine. Medical imaging has allowed us to see into the deep spaces of the body that were previously hidden from us.

Summary

Arterial blood gas values are a key diagnostic tool in many diseases and conditions. They allow the measurement and analysis of acid-base balance. This technique involves the examination and determination of pH, P_aCO_2, and HCO_3^-. By examining the ratios of acid (P_aCO_2) and base (HCO_3^-) in relation to the pH, respiratory therapists can, at least broadly, determine the source of acid-base disturbances. With knowledge of the anion gap, they can further define these alterations in acid-base homeostasis. Acid-base and blood gas physiology are among respiratory care's most important knowledge bases. Very often the respiratory therapists are the experts in this area, and their knowledge is critical for the survival of the patient.

ABGs can be measured directly by invasive sampling and direct analysis of blood and noninvasively and indirectly through the use of sophisticated devices such as photospectrometers and pulse oximeters. Some of the methods and devices used, such as blood gas analyzers, provide actual measured data; others, such as the capnograph, provide data that are more valuable when looking at trends over time. Remember that ABGs are like a static picture, giving a look at the respiratory physiology at a single second in time. Trend data are more like a video, enabling the RT to see how the physiology has acted over time. So the choice becomes the desirability of a static glimpse at the ABG values or a dynamic presentation of real-time physiology under current conditions.

Arterial blood gas procurement, analysis, and interpretation are skills that must be learned, practiced, and evaluated repeatedly over time. In addition to maintaining current skill levels, the respiratory therapist must be aware that blood gas analysis technology, techniques, and procedures are constantly being upgraded and improved. Such change only further emphasizes the need for continuous training in this area of respiratory therapist practice. An ongoing program of quality assurance, remediation, and review is a mandatory part of offering a blood gas service.

Study Questions

REVIEW QUESTIONS

1. Choose the correct acid-base status of this patient: pH 7.32; P_aCO_2 36 mm Hg; P_aO_2 97 mm Hg; HCO_3^- 17 mmol/dL; S_aO_2 98%.
   a. respiratory acidosis
   b. mixed metabolic and respiratory
   c. metabolic alkalosis
   d. metabolic acidosis
2. Choose the condition indicated by the following ABG values: pH 7.52; P_aCO_2 28 mm Hg; P_aO_2 97 mm Hg; HCO_3^- 24 mmol/dL; S_aO_2 98%.
   a. respiratory acidosis
   b. respiratory alkalosis
   c. metabolic acidosis
   d. metabolic alkalosis
   e. mixed metabolic and respiratory alkalosis
3. Choose the correct acid-base status of this patient: pH 7.32; P_aCO_2 36 mm Hg; P_aO_2 97 mm Hg; HCO_3^- 17 mmol/dL; S_aO_2 98%.
   a. respiratory acidosis
   b. mixed metabolic and respiratory
   c. metabolic alkalosis
   d. metabolic acidosis
4. Given the following information, calculate predicted blood gas values: pH 7.25; P_aCO_2 __ mm Hg; P_aO_2 __ mm Hg; HCO_3^- 17 mmol/dL; S_aO_2 98%. The patient is 69 years old and on room air.
   a. P_aCO_2 50 mm Hg, P_aO_2 93 mm Hg
   b. P_aCO_2 65 mm Hg, P_aO_2 85 mm Hg
   c. P_aCO_2 70 mm Hg, P_aO_2 73 mm Hg
   d. P_aCO_2 30 mm Hg, P_aO_2 103 mm Hg
5. What is the correct definition of each of the following terms?

a. oxygen saturation	____	a modifier of acid-base reactions
b. oxygen content	____	the proportion of HbO_2 to Hb_{total}
c. O_2 combining capacity	____	relationship between P_aO_2 and S_aO_2
d. O_2 dissociation curve	____	actual amount of O_2 present
e. pulse oximetry	____	ability of Hb to carry O_2
f. buffer	____	light absorption oxygen determination

6. Put the following steps in the proper order for blood gas sampling by arterial puncture.
   a. Assemble disposable blood gas kit according to manufacturer's specifications.
   b. Don gloves.
   c. Inform the patient before the actual puncture.
   d. Insert needle with the bevel up, at approximately a 45-degree angle.
   e. Introduce yourself and explain the procedure to the patient.
   f. Transport sample to lab and analyze.
   g. Wash hands.
   h. Expel all air from sample.
   i. Remove needle; cap syringe.
   j. Dispose of needle in appropriate biohazard container.
   k. Allow blood to fill to adequate sample size under arterial pressure.
   l. Select the site for the puncture.
   m. Establish collateral circulation, if possible, for site.
   n. Obtain needed supplies, including ice if hospital policy.
   o. Watch for flash of blood in the hub of the needle.
   p. Swab puncture site with Betadine; wipe it clean with alcohol.
   q. Use smooth, consistent advancement of the needle. If redirection is required, withdraw needle to just under the skin and advance it again.
   r. Dispose of all waste, remove gloves, and wash hands.
   s. Remove the needle, apply pressure for 3–5 minutes or until the bleeding stops.
   t. Review chart for physician order and anticoagulant or bleeding disorder status.
   u. Mix the blood thoroughly.
   v. Label the sample.
   w. Localize the target artery using the fingers of the nondominant hand.
   x. Place sample in ice if hospital policy.
   y. Assess puncture site. Ensure bleeding has stopped; check for distal pulse.
   z. Verify patient's identity.
7. Discuss the principles of operation for transcutaneous and gas-sampling techniques.
8. Identify the strengths and weaknesses of various types of invasive and noninvasive analysis techniques.
9. Identify the indications and contraindications associated with various blood gas analysis and monitoring techniques.

10. What are the normal values for arterial blood gases, both measured and calculated at sea level?

	pH	P_aCO_2 mm Hg	P_aO_2 mm Hg	HCO_3^- mmol/dL	S_aO_2 %	AG mmol/L
a.	7.35–7.50	25–32	80–105	8–15	88–96	22–34
b.	7.35–7.45	35–45	95–100	22–26	96–99	12–14
c.	7.45–7.55	40–50	106–115	18–32	85–92	10–15
d.	7.38–7.42	38–35	89–94	14–28	85–95	13–18

MULTIPLE-CHOICE QUESTIONS

1. Low hemoglobin levels has what effect on S_PCO_2 readings?
   a. S_PCO_2 reads higher than actual.
   b. S_PCO_2 readings are not affected.
   c. S_PCO_2 reads the same as S_aO_2 readings.
   d. S_PCO_2 reads lower than actual.
2. Which of the following does not adversely affect S_PCO_2 data?
   a. decreased peripheral perfusion
   b. Black Pearl nail polish
   c. increased methemoglobin level
   d. increased pulse pressure
3. Which of the following represents a 1-SD range of normal blood gas values?
   a. pH 7.42–7.45; P_aCO_2 35–37 mm Hg; P_aO_2 105–110 mm Hg
   b. pH 7.38–7.42; P_aCO_2 38–42 mm Hg; P_aO_2 95–98 mm Hg
   c. pH 7.35–7.45; P_aCO_2 35–45 mm Hg; P_aO_2 105–110 mm Hg
   d. pH 7.42–7.45; P_aCO_2 35–37 mm Hg; P_aO_2 105–110 mm Hg
4. A quality control tool that plots sample results as a function of standard deviation is the:
   a. Levy-Jennings plot.
   b. Westgard rules.
   c. May-Optely figure.
   d. Thomas–Quigley chart.
5. Correction of respiratory acidosis is ________ than that of metabolic acidosis because ________.
   a. slower ... the lungs have a larger surface area than the kidneys
   b. faster ... we can change pH by holding our breath
   c. faster ... it is easier to get rid of CO_2 than HCO_3^-
   d. slower ... the urine is more acidic than expired air
6. In "normal" individuals, the ratio of HCO_3^- to CO_2 is:
   a. 20:1.
   b. 1.5 mmol/L.
   c. 0.80.
   d. 18 g/dL.
7. The major energy-producing process in the body is known as *oxidative transphosphorylation* or:
   a. respiration
   b. ventilation
   c. cyclic AMP
   d. TCA cycle
8. Regarding "normal values," which of the following statements is correct?
   a. Normal values are universal for each physiological and biochemical value analyzed.
   b. Normal values tend to be specific to each major demographic, ethnic, or racial group.
   c. Most normal values are biased toward white males of European ancestry.
   d. Normal values are not variable within a culture.
9. The anion gap (AG):
   a. is the difference between the anions and the other chemicals in the body.
   b. accounts for the effects of unmeasured organic acids on the acid-base balance.
   c. roughly approximates the P_aCO_2 less the pH and is used to estimate HCO_3^-.
   d. determines the electrolyte difference between fluid intake and output.
10. The term "6.3" in the Henderson-Hasselbalch equation represents:
    a. the slope of the line comparing P_aCO_2 with P_aO_2.
    b. the relationship between gas saturation and partial pressure.
    c. the dissociation constant for human blood plasma.
    d. the intercept of the pH (x-axis) and P_aCO_2 (y-axis) on the O_2 dissociation curve.
11. Is the available information in Review Question 5 sufficient to perform blood gas prediction equations?
    a. Yes
    b. No
    c. No, the F_IO_2 is needed
    d. Yes, but not necessary

CRITICAL-THINKING QUESTIONS

1. What are the possible consequences of borderline hypoxemia due to the shape of the oxyhemoglobin curve?
2. Alterations of the anion gap (AG) can have profound effects on the patient's acid-base balance, yet these alterations can be difficult to resolve. What are some diseases that cause these alterations, and why are effective solutions so difficult to initiate?
3. The use of noninvasive technologies has, without doubt, enhanced our ability to monitor and care

for our patients. However, these gains have some drawbacks. What are some of the real and potential problems with noninvasive monitoring?

4. What is the significance of the Latin phrase "Quis custodiet ipsos custodes?" in relation to QA/QI systems?

References

1. Brooks SW. *Integrated Basic Science*. 3rd ed. St. Louis, MO: Mosby; 1970.
2. Wojciechowski WV. *Respiratory Care Sciences: An Integrated Approach*. 3rd ed. Clifton Park, NY: Delmar Cengage Learning; 2000.
3. American Association for Respiratory Care. Sampling for arterial blood gas analysis. *Respir Care*. 1992;37:913–917.
4. You B, Pesin R, Duvivier C, Dang Vu V, Grilliat JP. Expiratory capnography in asthma: evaluation of various shape indices. *Eur Respir J*. 1994;7:318–323.
5. Yaron M, Padyk P, Hutsinpiller M, Cairns CB. Utility of the expiratory capnogram in the assessment of bronchospasm. *Ann Emerg Med*. 1996;28:403–407.
6. Tasota FJ, Wesmiller SW. Balancing act. *Nursing 98*. 1998;28:35–41.
7. Westgard JO, Lott JA. Critical reviews in clinical laboratory sciences, 1549–781X, V13, N4, 1981: 283–330.

Suggested Reading

Davila F. A comparison of clinical and research oxygen-related physiologic equations. *Intens Care World*. 2000;15:182–188.

CHAPTER 17

Pulmonary Function Testing

Robert A. Whitman and Susan A. Holland

OBJECTIVES

Upon completion of this chapter, the reader should be able to:

- List the indications for spirometry and for postbronchodilator studies.
- Explain how to perform pre- and postbronchodilator spirometry and interpret the results.
- Explain the results of a cardiopulmonary stress test.
- List the indications for more testing after spirometry is done, specifically MVV, diffusing capacity, lung volumes, lung compliance, airway resistance, single-breath nitrogen washout, and bronchoprovocation.
- List the indications for cardiopulmonary stress testing.
- Explain how to perform the following tests and interpret the results: lung volumes, diffusing capacity, single-breath nitrogen washout, MVV, airway resistance, lung compliance, and a CO_2 response curve.
- Check equipment for proper function and explain infection control measures in pulmonary function testing.

CHAPTER OUTLINE

KEY TERMS

airway conductance (G_{aw})
airway resistance (R_{aw})
anaerobic threshold (*AT*)
body plethysmography
bronchoprovocation
calibration
differential pressure pneumotachometer
diffusing capacity
lung capacities
lung compliance
lung volumes
maximum voluntary ventilation (MVV)
obstructive lung disease
pneumotachometer
pressure transducer
restrictive lung disease
shutter
spirometry
thermal pneumotachometer
ultrasonic pneumotachometer

Pulmonary function testing consists of a group of tests designed to measure aspects of lung function. The most commonly performed test is spirometry, frequently referred to as a *forced vital capacity maneuver*. Spirometry measures the maximal flows that a patient can generate and is the most useful in determining whether airway obstruction is present. Spirometry also measures how much volume a patient can exhale; a reduced volume can indicate the presence of restrictive lung disease. Spirometry can be performed using portable equipment, allowing for on-site occupational screening, patient bedside testing, and even testing at health fairs and in shopping malls.

Other, more sophisticated tests allow for a more specific diagnosis of the type of lung disease (obstructive, restrictive, or a combination) and for further assessment of the severity of the disease. These tests require larger, more sophisticated, and more expensive equipment, so they are usually performed in a pulmonary function laboratory.

Indications for Pulmonary Function Testing

A pulmonary function test (*PFT*) is typically done to:

- Establish the presence or absence of lung disease and assess level of severity.
- Evaluate operative risks.
- Perform surveillance for occupational or environmental exposure.
- Evaluate disability or impairment.

More specialized tests provide additional information (obstructive, restrictive, or combined) about a lung disease. The severity and reversibility of the impairment can be assessed as well. The effect of exercise on breathing can be assessed using exercise testing.

Follow-up testing or monitoring is used to check periodically on the progression of lung impairment. It is also done to assess the effectiveness of medications and treatments prescribed. Follow-up exercise testing can assess the effectiveness of a rehabilitation or exercise program.

The purposes of pulmonary function testing are summarized in Table 17-1.

LUNG ASSESSMENT THROUGH PFT

Several pulmonary function tests measure the following aspects of lung function.

- The *condition of the airways* is assessed by measuring flows.
- *Lung volumes* are measured both directly (by physical measuring) and indirectly (through mathematical calculation).
- The *resistance of the airways* and the *compliance of the lung and thorax* are also measured.

TABLE 17-1 **Purposes of pulmonary function testing**

Screening
General population
Occupational risk
Disability determination
High-risk groups
Preoperative evaluation
Diagnosis
Type of disease
Severity of disease
Reversibility of disease
Follow-up
Progression of disease
Effectiveness of medications
Effectiveness of rehabilitation

TABLE 17-2 Parameters assessed in pulmonary function testing

Exhaled flows
Inhaled flows (with some equipment)
Airway resistance
Lung compliance
Gas distribution in the lungs
Exercise tolerance
Diffusing capacity
Reversibility of lung disease
Airway hyper-reactivity
Response to increased CO_2

- The *distribution* of air in the lungs can be assessed, as well as the *rate* at which oxygen is able to diffuse from the lungs into the blood.
- The *degree to which a medication reverses a lung disease* can be assessed by giving a subject a bronchodilator treatment after all other tests have been completed and then repeating some of the tests.
- The subject's *response or sensitivity to increased concentrations of CO_2* can also be measured.

Table 17-2 lists the parameters assessed in pulmonary function testing.

GENERAL DISEASE PATTERNS

Lung diseases are classified as restrictive, obstructive, or a combination of the two patterns.

Restrictive Lung Diseases. Restrictive lung diseases are characterized by an inability to inhale as much as normal. This condition is due to one of the following problems or a combination of them:

- The lung tissue itself is stiff (with scar tissue or fluid accumulation).
- The chest wall cannot expand normally (due to chest wall or spinal abnormalities).

Both cause a decrease in compliance, which restricts the expansion of the lungs. The defining characteristic of restrictive lung disease is a *reduced total lung capacity* (*TLC*). Examples of restrictive lung disease are pneumoconiosis, pulmonary fibrosis, pleural thickening, scoliosis, lordosis, and kyphoscoliosis.

Obstructive Lung Diseases. Obstructive lung diseases are characterized by an inability to exhale as quickly as normal. This limitation is shown in reduced maximal effort flow measurements and is defined by an increase in airway resistance. The conducting airways have become narrowed because of any one or a combination of the following:

- Inflammation
- Accumulation of secretions
- Bronchospasm (muscle spasms in the airways)
- Loss of the supporting tissue in the airways, causing them to partially collapse during exhalation

Examples of obstructive diseases are asthma, chronic bronchitis, bronchiectasis, and emphysema.

Normal or Predicted Values

The results of a subject's tests are compared with the normal or predicted values for that subject. Of the several sets of predicted values, some are more commonly used than others. All of these sets were developed by testing many people who did not have lung disease. Regression analysis (prediction equations) or nomograms were then developed for all parameters. These equations take into account the age, height, and sex of the subject. Some sets of predicted values also include race or body surface area as variables. Separate sets of predicted values have been developed for children, adolescents, and adults.

Computerized equipment has the predicted value sets installed. The subject's performance in each test is automatically compared with what is predicted. When noncomputerized equipment is used, predicted normal values can be determined by manual calculation of predictive equations or the use of nomograms (the graphical plots of predictive equations).

Normal or predicted values are described in terms of *BTPS* (*body temperature and pressure saturated*). Measurements made by pulmonary function equipment are actually taken at *ATPS* (*atmospheric pressure and temperature saturated*). According to Charles's law (Chapter 3), the volume of a gas at room temperature is less than the volume at body temperature; so a conversion to BTPS must be made. Computerized equipment makes that correction automatically, and results are reported in BTPS. When noncomputerized equipment is used, the adjustment must be made by multiplying the results by a factor that is determined by the room air temperature and the barometric pressure. Tables listing these correction factors are widely available from equipment manufacturers and in books on pulmonary function.

Lung Volumes

Lung volumes are the four segments into which the amount of air moving into and out of the lungs is divided. **Lung capacities** are combinations of two or more lung volumes. The respiratory therapist (RT) must be aware of the distinction between volume and capacity to understand the significance of the results of several pulmonary function tests.

Three of the lung volumes are measured directly using spirometry, and one can be measured indirectly. The four capacities are calculated from the measured volumes or, if possible, directly. The RT should learn the following definitions before continuing this chapter.

- *Tidal volume* (V_T), measured directly, is the amount of air moved into and out of the lungs in a normal (resting) breath. Tidal volume is important because several of the other volumes and capacities are defined by reference to it.
- *Inspiratory reserve volume (IRV)*, measured directly, is the maximum amount of air that can be inhaled after a resting tidal inhalation.
- *Expiratory reserve volume (ERV)*, measured directly, is the maximum amount of air that can be exhaled after a resting tidal exhalation.
- *Residual volume (RV)* is the amount of air that remains in the lungs after a maximal exhalation (i.e., after *ERV* has been exhaled). It cannot be measured directly, but tests have been developed to measure residual volume indirectly.
- *Inspiratory capacity (IC)* is the maximum amount of air that can be inhaled after a resting tidal exhalation. This is the sum of the tidal volume and the inspiratory reserve volume ($V_T + IRV$). It can be measured directly by spirometry.
- *Functional residual capacity (FRC)* is the amount of air that remains in the lungs after a resting tidal exhalation. This is the sum of the expiratory reserve volume and the residual volume ($ERV + RV$).
- *Vital capacity (VC)* is the maximum amount of air that can be forcibly exhaled after an inhalation. This capacity is the sum of the inspiratory reserve volume, the tidal volume, and the expiratory reserve volume ($IRV + V_T + ERV$). It can be measured directly by spirometry.
- *Total lung capacity (TLC)* is the maximum amount of air that the lungs can hold. This capacity is the sum of all the volumes ($IRV + V_T + ERV + RV$, or $IC + FRC$).

Figure 17-1 shows these lung volumes in terms of a volume-time spirometry tracing and two bar graphs. Normal lung volumes and capacities are shown in Table 6-4.

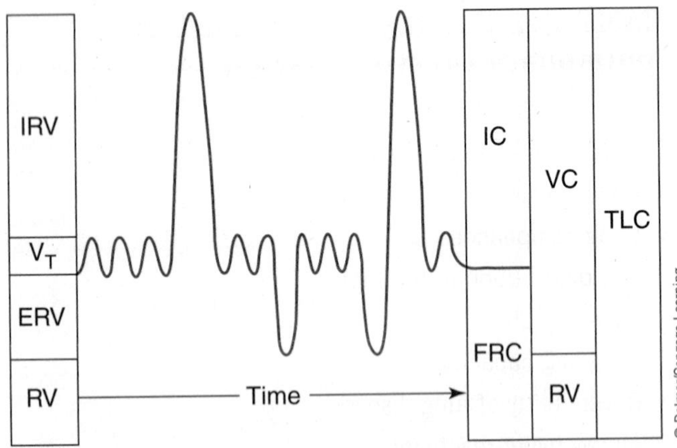

FIGURE 17-1 Lung volumes (left) and capacities (right).

Spirometry

Spirometry is a test to assess pulmonary mechanics under dynamic conditions. Spirometry is the most common test performed in assessing lung function and is frequently performed at the bedside, in the physician's office, at health fairs, as well as in the laboratory. Spirometry consists of a series of forced vital capacity maneuvers in which both volume and flow rates are measured.

FORCED VITAL CAPACITY

The *forced vital capacity* (*FVC*) *test* measures the *VC* of the subject and, with a V_T measurement, allows the calculation of the *IRV* and the *ERV*. Because the test is done with the subject exhaling as hard as possible from *TLC* (full) to *RV* (empty), flows during various portions and at specific times during the FVC can also be measured. Indications, contraindications, hazards, procedure, and so on are discussed in the American Association for Respiratory Care (AARC) clinical practice guideline for spirometry.[1]

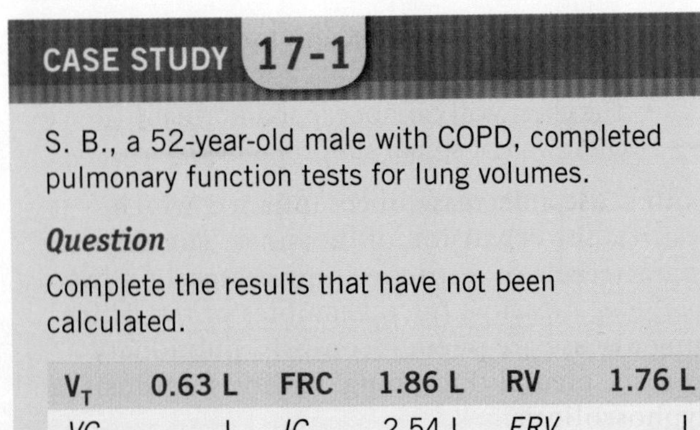

CASE STUDY 17-1

S. B., a 52-year-old male with COPD, completed pulmonary function tests for lung volumes.

Question

Complete the results that have not been calculated.

V_T	0.63 L	FRC	1.86 L	RV	1.76 L
VC	L	*IC*	2.54 L	*ERV*	L
TLC	L	*IRV*	L		

Best Practice

FVC Test

The subject should not perform a glottic closure (closing the glottis, as is done before a cough) during the inspiratory hold. To avoid glottic closure, instruct the subject to continue to try to inhale more air during the 2-second hold.

- Coaching is very important in this test because maximal effort must be obtained. The subject should be encouraged to blow hard until the recommended 6 seconds have passed or until the equipment has not sensed any flow for 1 second.
- There should be no coughing during the forceful exhalation. If the subject cannot refrain from coughing at the end of the forced exhalation, the results can be reported with the coughing noted on the report.
- The position of the subject (seated or standing) should be the same for all FVC maneuvers. Usually subjects are seated.

Patient Maneuver. The patient maneuver for the FVC test is as follows:

- The subject generally wears noseclips for the FVC test to ensure that all exhaled air is captured. The best way to make sure that the clips are tight enough to prevent any airflow through the nose is to ask the subject to try to sniff air through the nose with the mouth closed. If airflow occurs, tighter noseclips are needed.
- Have the subject place the teeth and lips tightly around the mouthpiece. If the subject wears dentures, they should be removed, and the subject should be instructed to place the gums and lips tightly around the mouthpiece.
- Instruct the subject to relax and breathe normally to establish normal tidal volume.
- At the end of a tidal exhalation, tell the subject to inhale as much air as possible and then immediately exhale as forcefully and for as long as possible. The exhalation should continue for at least 6 seconds, unless there is an obvious plateau with no flow occurring for 1 second. If the equipment used measures only exhalation, the test is completed at this time, and the subject can take his or her mouth off the mouthpiece.

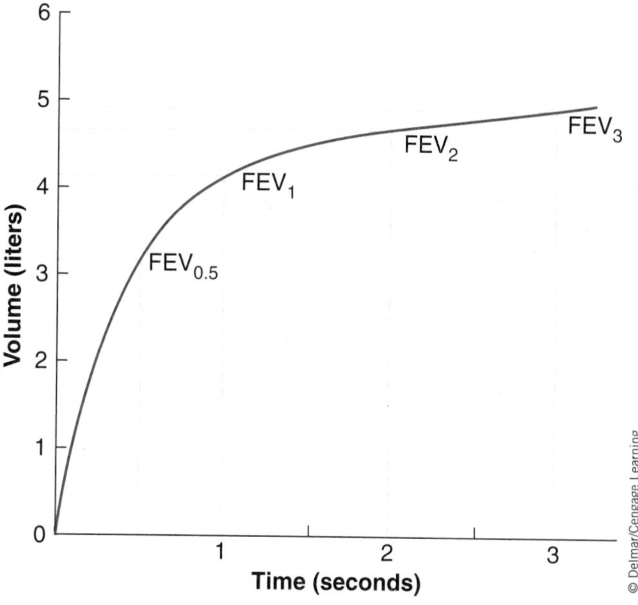

FIGURE 17-2 A volume-time curve for timed volumes.

- If the equipment also measures inhalation, the subject should then be instructed to inhale as quickly as possible up to *TLC* (full). Most computerized equipment has these criteria built in so that poor test performance is not accepted as valid.

Graphics. The results of the patient's forced vital capacity (FVC) maneuver can be displayed graphically in two ways.

One shows the FVC with time on the horizontal and volume on the vertical side of the graph. Depending on the equipment used, the time may be recorded from left to right or from right to left, and changes in volume may be recorded with exhalation going from top to bottom or from bottom to top. This graph is called a *volume-time curve*. Seven measurements can be made from a volume-time curve (Figures 17-2 and 17-3):

- FVC (forced vital capacity)—the maximum amount of air that can be forcefully exhaled after a maximal inhalation. This indicates the volume available for ventilation, which is decreased in restrictive disease and in advanced cases of obstructive disease.
- FEV_t [timed (forced) exhaled volume]—the amount of air exhaled in the first half second ($FEV_{0.5}$), first 1 second (FEV_1), or first 3 seconds (FEV_3) of a forced vital capacity maneuver. The FEV_1 is the most commonly reported value. The FEV_1 is decreased in both obstructive and restrictive lung disease.

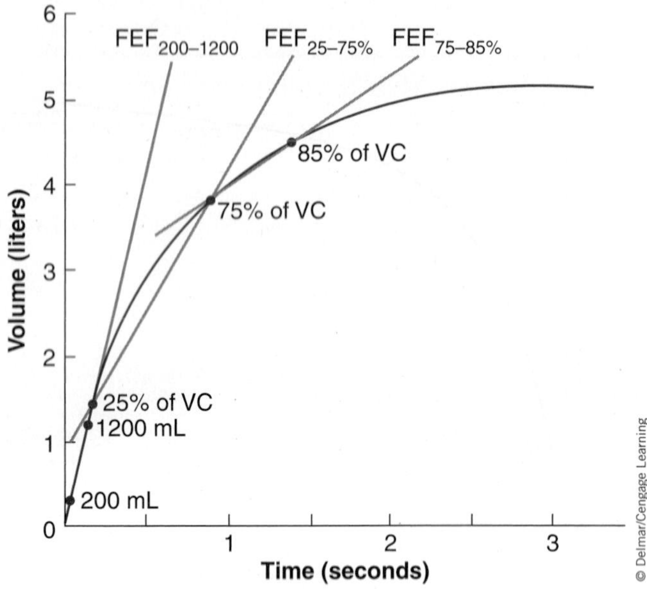

FIGURE 17-3 Volume-time curves for average flows.

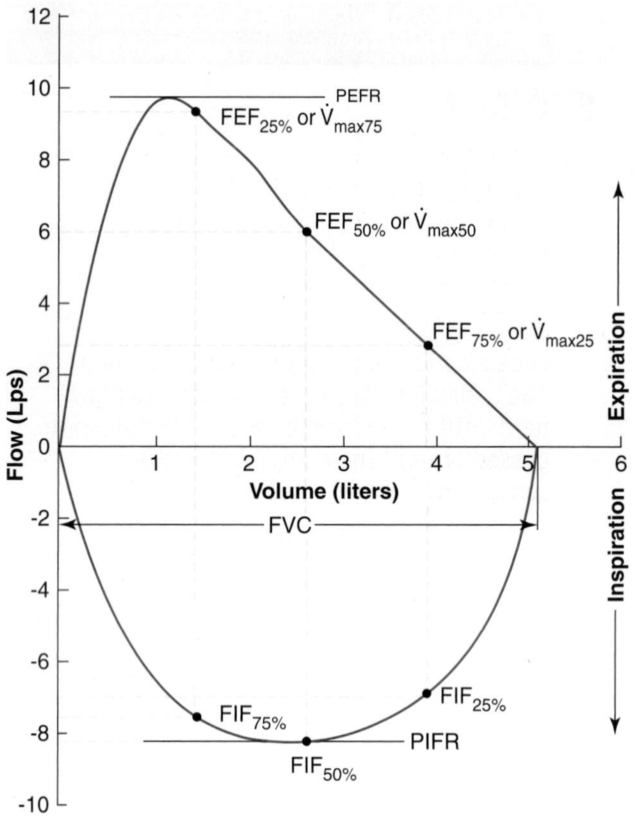

FIGURE 17-4 Flow-volume loop for flows and volumes.

- $FEV_{t\%}$ (ratio of the FEV_t to the FVC as a percentage)—FEV_1 is usually written as FEV_1/FVC. This value is decreased in obstructive lung disease and is normal or increased in restrictive disease.
- $FEF_{200-1200}$ (forced expiratory flow from 200 to 1200 mL)—the average flow produced in the forced vital capacity after the first 200 mL has been exhaled until 1200 mL has been exhaled. This measurement assesses the large airways.
- $FEF_{25-75\%}$ (forced expiratory flow from 25% to 75% of the FVC, sometimes called the *midflow*)—the average flow generated in the middle 50% of the FVC. This measurement assesses the small airways.
- $FEV_{75-85\%}$ (forced expiratory flow from 75% to 85% of the FVC)—the expiratory flow rate at the end of exhalation, after 75–85% of the volume (FVC) has been expired.
- PEFR or PEF (peak expiratory flow rate or peak expiratory flow during the FVC)—the highest flow rate generated during a forced vital capacity maneuver. It generally occurs at or near the beginning of the FVC maneuver and is sometimes used to assess patient effort in the FVC maneuver.

The other graphic for the FVC is the *flow-volume curve* or *loop* (Figure 17-4). This shows the FVC maneuver, with volume on the horizontal axis and flow on the vertical axis. The flow-volume curve shows exhalation only; the flow-volume loop shows both exhalation and inhalation. Both the curve and the loop show FVC and PEFR (the highest point on the curve or loop). In addition to the preceding seven measurements, the following measurements can be shown on a flow-volume curve or loop:

- $FEF_{25\%, 50\%, 75\%}$ (forced expiratory flow at 25%, 50%, and 75% of the FVC)—instantaneous flows, not average flows like the $FEF_{25-75\%}$. They are the flows generated by the subject at the exact instants when 25%, 50%, and 75% of the FVC have been exhaled. This flow can be shown on both a curve (the expiration portion of Figure 17-4) and a loop.
- PIFR or PIF (peak inspiratory flow rate or peak inspiratory flow)—the highest inspiratory flow generated during the FVC maneuver. This can be shown only on a flow-volume loop. It is the lowest point on the inspiratory curve.

Reporting Results. The American Thoracic Society (ATS) has made recommendations about performing spirometry to ensure that the results reported are valid (i.e., that any abnormalities reported are real, not the result of poor performance).[2] The ATS recommends that:

- At least three acceptable maneuvers be saved.
- Among these three, the largest FVC must not vary more than 0.150 L from the second largest

CASE STUDY 17-2

The following are the FVC and FEV_1 results from one subject:

	Trial 1	Trial 2	Trial 3
FVC	1.20 L	1.26 L	1.27 L
FEV_1	0.92 L	0.98 L	0.94 L

Questions

1. According to ATS standards, are the results of these three maneuvers acceptable?
2. What should be reported as the largest FVC?
3. What should be reported as the largest FEV_1?
4. According to the ATS standards, which trial should be reported as the best?
5. According to the ATS, from which trial should all other measurements be made?

FVC, and the largest FEV_1 must not vary more than 0.150 L from the second largest.

- Of a series of at least three maneuvers, the largest FVC and the largest FEV_1 should be reported.
- The test in which the sum of the FVC and the FEV_1 is the largest is to be chosen as the best test, and all reported flow rate measurements are to be made from this test.

Pre- and Postbronchodilator Studies. A patient who is already taking bronchodilating medications should stop using them before testing unless symptom control is not possible without them.

- Short-acting beta-adrenergic bronchodilators and anticholinergics should be stopped at least 4 hours before testing.
- Long-acting beta-adrenergic bronchodilators and methylxanthines should be stopped 12 hours before testing.
- Slow-release methylxanthines, cromolyn sodium, and necromodil sodium should be discontinued 24 hours before testing.
- Leukotriene inhibitors should be stopped 24 hours before testing.

Table 17-3 summarizes the withholding time schedules for these medications.

After all testing has been completed, the bronchodilator is administered. A fast-acting beta-adrenergic bronchodilator is usually given, unless another medication is specified.

TABLE 17-3 **Withholding medications before pulmonary function testing**

Medication Type	Withholding Time Before Testing (hours)
Short-acting beta-adrenergics	4
Anticholinergics	4
Long-acting beta-adrenergics	12
Methylxanthines	12
Slow-release methylxanthines	24
Cromolyn sodium, necromodil sodium	24
Leukotriene inhibitors	24

- If the medication is administered by a small-volume nebulizer, the subject should be instructed to take deep breaths with a 3-to 5-second breath-hold.
- If the medication is given by metered-dose inhaler (MDI), the subject should wait for 2 minutes between puffs.
- If a beta-adrenergic medication is administered, retesting should be done after a 10- to 15-minute wait.
- If an anticholinergic is administered, retesting should be done after 45–60 minutes.

Blood pressure and pulse should be monitored during and after the administration of the medication. The test that is usually repeated after the bronchodilator is the FVC maneuver, although airway resistance (see Other Specialized Tests on page 469), lung volume determination, and diffusing capacity (see Additional Laboratory Assessment on page 464) may also be done.

The amount of change in any parameter after bronchodilation is generally reported as the percentage change from the baseline value. A significant response to the bronchodilator, according to the ATS, is at least a 12% and 200-mL improvement in the FEV_1 or FVC. The response is also considered to be significant if the airway resistance is reduced by 30–40%. The ATS states that if the response is less than 12%, a bronchodilator can still be prescribed if it results in improved symptoms or exercise tolerance. A follow-up study is recommended in these cases because the response of some subjects can improve over time. Contraindications, hazards, assessment of outcome, monitoring, and other topics are covered in the AARC clinical practice guideline for assessing the response to bronchodilator therapy at the point of care.[3]

Interpretation of Results. Interpretation follows a few simple rules:

- If the measurement of a parameter is between 80% and 120% of the predicted value, it is considered to be normal.
- In general, any result value that is less than 80% of the normal value is considered decreased and therefore abnormal.
- The *TLC* is also considered to be abnormal if it is over 120% of the predicted value.
- One exception to these general rules is the $FEV_1\%$, for which any reduction from the normal percentage is abnormal.

The pattern of abnormalities allows the interpreter to distinguish between obstructive disease, restrictive disease, and a combination of the two.

Obstructive disease develops progressively, and the number of abnormal values slowly increases. Before obstructive disease can be diagnosed, the $FEF_{25-75\%}$ is decreased (i.e., the small airways are narrowed). Then the medium-sized airways become narrowed, resulting in a decreased FEV_1. This narrowing, in turn, results in a decrease in the $FEV_1\%$. As air trapping develops, as evidenced by an increase in *TLC* (>120%), the FVC decreases below 80% of predicted. Further tests, such as lung volumes and diffusing capacity, are indicated to assess the severity of the disease. Postbronchodilator retesting is indicated to assess the reversibility of the disease.

With *restrictive disease*, the FVC is decreased. The FEV_1 is normal at first, and then it decreases. (In severe cases, the predicted FEV_1 is greater than the subject's actual FVC.) Although both FVC and FEV_1 may be decreased, the $FEV_{1\%}$ remains within normal limits or increases relative to normal individuals. Because the presence of restrictive lung disease is defined by a decrease in *TLC*, lung volume tests are indicated. Also, a diffusing capacity test is indicated to assess the effect of the restrictive disease on the ability of oxygen to diffuse from the lungs to the blood. This are decreased in disease caused by lung tissue abnormalities and normal in disease caused by chest wall abnormalities.

Combined disease states show characteristics of both patterns.

See Table 17-4 for a summary of these patterns.

Interpretation of results should be approached methodically to avoid confusion and errors. To interpret FVC test results, three parameters need to be examined: the FVC, the FEV_1, and the FEV_1/FVC ($FEV_1\%$).

- The measured FVC and FEV_1 are abnormal or decreased if they are less than 80% of the predicted value.
- The $FEV_1\%$ is considered abnormal if it is less than the predicted value.

TABLE 17-4 **Abnormal spirometry values in restrictive and obstructive lung diseases**

	Restrictive	Obstructive
FVC	< 80% predicted	Normal or < 80% predicted
FEV_1	Normal or < 80% predicted	< 80% predicted
$FEV_1\%$	≥ predicted	< predicted

- If the FVC is normal (≥ 80% of the predicted value) and the FEV_1 is normal (equal to or greater than predicted), the test is normal.
- If the FVC is normal and the FEV_1 is less than 80% of its predicted value, obstructive disease is indicated. Postbronchodilator studies can reveal the reversibility of the disease.
- If the FVC is decreased and the $FEV_1\%$ is at or above the predicted value, restrictive disease is suggested. Further testing should be performed to confirm that the *TLC* is less than 80% of the predicted value.
- If the FVC is decreased and the $FEV_1\%$ is below its predicted value, obstructive disease is indicated. Again, postbronchodilator studies reveal the degree of reversibility of the disease.

The method described is summarized in the flowchart in Figure 17-5.

The shape of a flow-volume loop can provide valuable information for interpretation (Figure 17-6). When a subject has obstructive disease, the expiratory curve has a concave, or dishlike, shape because the flows that the subject can produce are limited by the decreased diameter of the medium-sized and small airways. If a normal flow-volume loop is available for comparison, the restrictive one is a miniature of the normal one because the *TLC* is reduced.

The flow-volume loop is particularly useful in diagnosing upper airway obstructions.

- A fixed obstruction causes flat expiratory and flat inspiratory curves because the obstruction limits flow on both inhalation and exhalation.

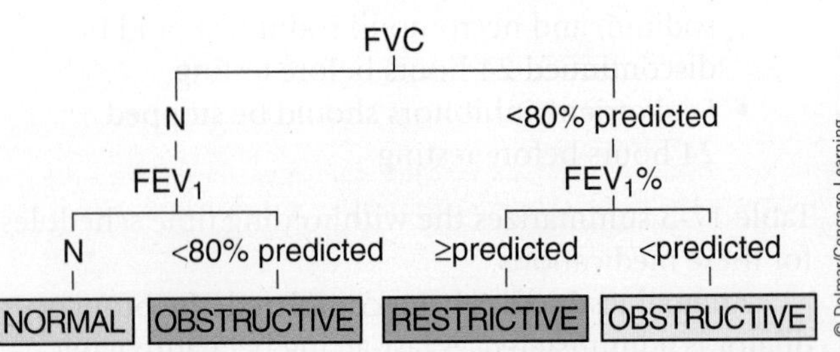

FIGURE 17-5 A flowchart for interpretation of spirometry.

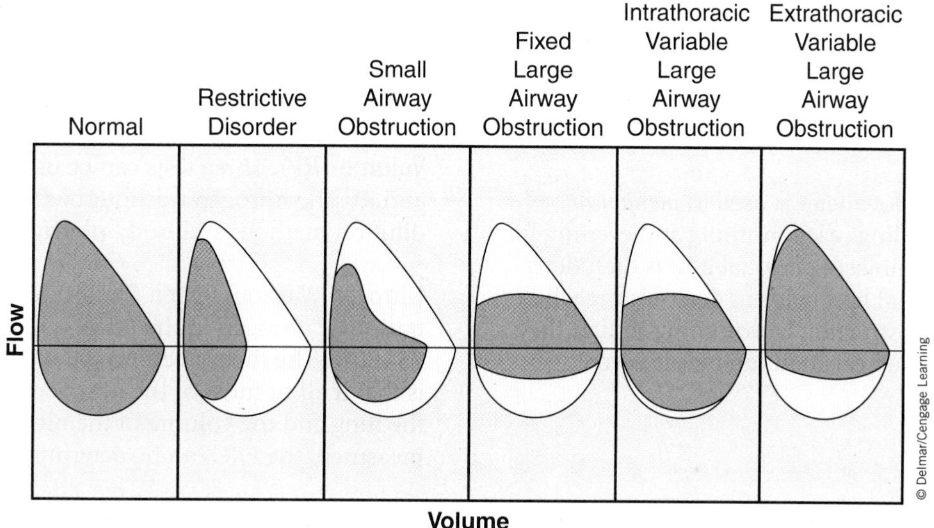

FIGURE 17-6 The shape of flow-volume loops for restrictive and obstructive lung disease and upper airway obstruction.

- A variable extrathoracic obstruction (airway exposed to atmospheric pressures) causes a flat inspiratory curve and a normal expiratory curve. The negative intrathoracic pressures (less than atmospheric) generated on inspiration cause the obstruction to narrow, while the positive pressures generated on exhalation cause the obstructed area to widen.
- A variable intrathoracic obstruction (airway exposed to intrathoracic pressures) causes a flat expiratory curve and a normal inspiratory curve. The positive intrathoracic pressures generated on exhalation cause the obstruction to narrow, while the negative intrathoracic pressures generated on inspiration cause the obstructed area to widen.

PEAK FLOW

Small portable devices, called *peak flowmeters*, are used to monitor peak flow for subjects who have asthma or hyper-reactive airways. They can be used in clinics, hospitals, or the home.

CASE STUDY 17-3

P. J. is a 52-year-old black male. He is 65 inches tall and weighs 222 pounds. The following are his spirometry results, pre- and postbronchodilator (BD):

	Predicted	Pre-BD	Percentage Predicted	Post-BD	Percentage Predicted
FVC	3.59 L	2.34 L	65	2.62	73
FEV_1	2.94 L	0.88 L	30	0.90	31
FEV_1/FVC	82%	38%	46	34%	41
$FEF_{25-75\%}$	189 Lpm	16 Lpm	8	15 Lpm	8
PEFR	462 Lpm	152 Lpm	33	170 Lpm	37

Questions

1. What is your interpretation of the prebronchodilator results?
2. Is P. J. response to bronchodilator significant? (*Hint:* Calculate the percentage change.)
3. Why is the postbronchodilator FEV_1/FVC less than the prebronchodilator FEV_1/FVC?

To detect *effort-induced bronchospasm*, first zero, or set, the peak flowmeter. Then the subject inhales maximally, places teeth and lips around the mouthpiece, and exhales as forcefully as possible. This performance should be repeated three times, with all results recorded.

When a peak flowmeter is used to *monitor an asthmatic*, take readings each morning and evening for a few weeks. The subject's personal best is then determined. The personal best helps in determining when subjects' airway obstruction is worsening so that they can seek further medical attention before severe obstruction occurs.

Additional Laboratory Assessment

If the spirometry results of a subject are normal, no further testing is needed. If the results are abnormal, a physician may order further tests to confirm the presence of restrictive lung disease or to assess the severity of either restrictive or obstructive lung disease. The equipment used to perform these further tests is not portable; therefore, they must be done in a pulmonary function laboratory.

The tests done in a pulmonary function laboratory can assess several aspects of lung function.

- Lung volumes and capacities can be measured and calculated.
- Diffusing capacity, airway resistance, lung compliance, and the evenness of the distribution of air in the lungs can be assessed.
- Specialized testing regimens (bronchoprovocation) can be performed to determine the presence or absence of airway hyper-reactivity and exercise-induced asthma.
- The ventilatory response of the subject to increasing CO_2 concentrations can be evaluated.

DETERMINING LUNG CAPACITIES AND VOLUMES

Spirometry can be used to measure the three lung volumes and two lung capacities: V_T, *IRV*, *ERV*, *IC*, and *VC* (which account for all usable lung volume). Procedures for determining slow vital capacity, functional residual capacity, and residual volume are discussed here.

Slow Vital Capacity (SVC or VC). The patient performs the same maneuver as for forced vital capacity (FVC), except that exhalation is slow rather than forceful. From this maneuver, *VC*, V_T, *IRV*, *IC*, and *ERV* are measured. If the *VC* is larger than the FVC, the difference indicates the amount of early airway closure (preventing further exhalation) that has occurred in the FVC.

Functional Residual Capacity (*FRC*) and Residual Volume (*RV*). Three tests can be used to determine *FRC* and *RV*: the nitrogen washout method, the helium dilution method, and **body plethysmography**.

Nitrogen Washout (Open Circuit) Method The concentration of nitrogen in the lungs is approximately 75–80%. The theory behind the *nitrogen washout test* is that if all or most of the nitrogen is removed from the lung and the volume of the nitrogen exhaled is measured, the *FRC* can be determined.

- Place noseclips on the subject's nose.
- The subject places lips tightly around the mouthpiece, breathes normally, and then is given time to relax.
- At the end of exhalation, the subject is switched to 100% oxygen.

The computerized system measures the volume exhaled in each breath and has an in-line nitrogen analyzer to determine the volume of nitrogen exhaled with each breath. Continue the test until the concentration of nitrogen in the exhaled gas is reduced to approximately 1%. For normal subjects, this concentration should be reached within 3–7 minutes. Subjects who have obstructive disease take longer because of the uneven distribution of gas in their lungs. Subjects with restrictive disease complete the test in the normal 3–7 minutes. See Figure 17-7 for an illustration of this test, along with the equation for determining results.

- The *FRC* can then be calculated, thereby enabling the calculation of *RV* and *TLC* as well.
- The *ERV*, already known from the SVC test, can be subtracted from the *FRC*, measured by the nitrogen washout, to calculate the *RV* ($FRC - ERV = RV$).
- The *TLC* is calculated by adding the *VC* (measured in the SVC) to the calculated *RV* ($VC + RV = TLC$).

The calculated results are for atmospheric conditions (ATPS), so a correction factor for BTPS must be applied before reporting results if this has not already been done by the computerized equipment.

Helium Dilution (Closed Circuit) Method The theory behind the *helium dilution test* is that if a known concentration of an inert gas is rebreathed by a subject until its concentration is the same on inhalation as it is on exhalation, the change in the concentration of the

GAS VOLUME AND N2 CONCENTRATION IN LUNGS BEFORE NITROGEN WASHOUT WITH OXYGEN

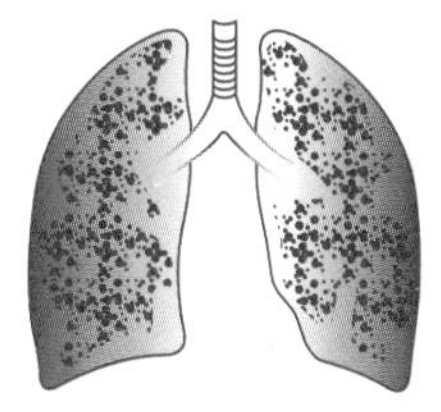

$C_1\ V_1$

$C_{Alv}N_2 = 0.75$

V_{FRC} = Unknown

COLLECTED EXHALED GAS VOLUME AND N2 CONCENTRATION AFTER NITROGEN WASHOUT WITH 100% OXYGEN

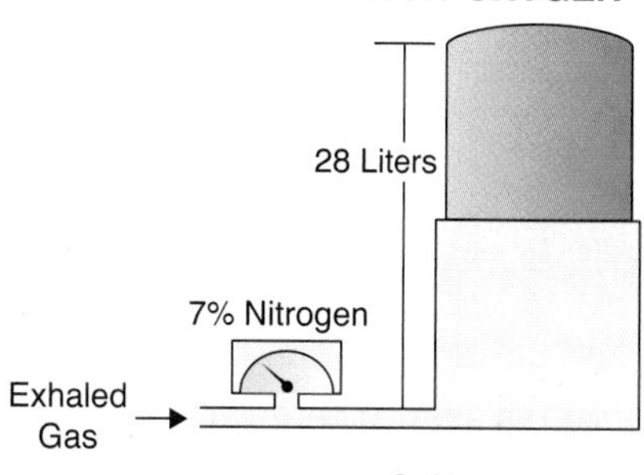

$C_2\ V_2$

$C_{Exh}N_2 = 0.07$

V_{Exh} = 28 liters

$$V_1 = \frac{C_2\,V_2}{C_1} \text{ or } V_{FRC} = \frac{(V_{Exh})\,(C_{Exh}N_2)}{C_{Alv}N_2}$$

$$V_{FRC} = \frac{(0.07)(28 \text{ liters})}{0.75}$$

$$V_{FRC} = 2.61 \text{ liters}$$

C = Concentration of gas (N_2)
V = Volume of exhaled gas

FIGURE 17-7 Equipment set-up and graphics for the nitrogen washout test.

Best Practice

Nitrogen Washout Method

1. A sudden increase in the nitrogen concentration indicates a leak in the system. Terminate the test at that time.
2. If the nitrogen concentration does not go down to 1%, the subject may have a punctured eardrum, which allows room air to enter the airways through the eustachian tube.
3. Retesting should be done after a 10-minute wait to allow nitrogen to build up to normal levels in the lungs.

inert gas is due to dilution of the gas by the subject's *FRC*.

- With noseclips in place, the subject first breathes normally through an open circuit.
- At end-exhalation, the patient is switched into a spirometer or reservoir containing a known volume of air with a known concentration of helium (usually 10–15%).
- An in-line CO_2 absorber on the exhalation side keeps the CO_2 from building up in the reservoir, and oxygen is added to keep the F_IO_2 at or above 21%.
- The patient continues normal breathing until equilibrium is reached (i.e., the concentration of helium exhaled is the same as the concentration of helium in the reservoir). The equilibration time is usually about 7 minutes in normal subjects. Subjects with obstructive disease take longer.
- The final concentration of helium in the reservoir is then measured after thorough mixing.

The *FRC* is then calculated, leading to the calculation of *RV* and *TLC* in the same way they are calculated when nitrogen washout is used. See Figure 17-8 for the equipment used and the process of equilibration.

Body Plethysmography *Body plethysmography* measures changes in volume and pressure in the thorax. The patient sits in an airtight booth and breathes through a

Best Practice

Helium Dilution Method

1. Helium concentration readings should decrease by less than 0.02% in 30 seconds or until 10 minutes have passed.
2. A sudden decrease in helium concentration indicates a leak in the system; the test should be terminated.

TESTS FOR PULMONARY VOLUMES AND VENTILATION

SPIROMETER SYSTEM BEFORE HELIUM DILUTION

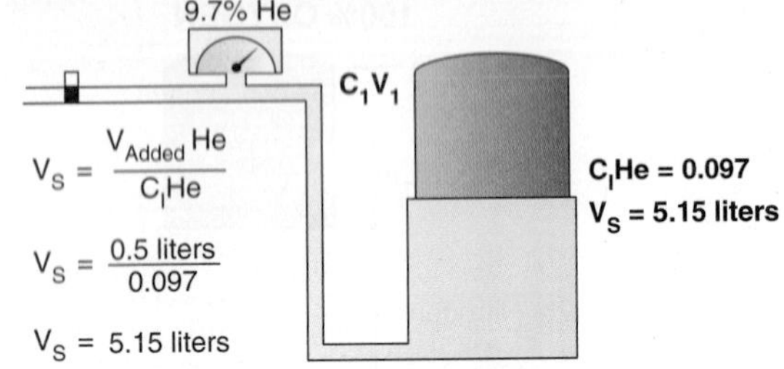

SUBJECT/SPIROMETER SYSTEM AFTER HELIUM DILUTION

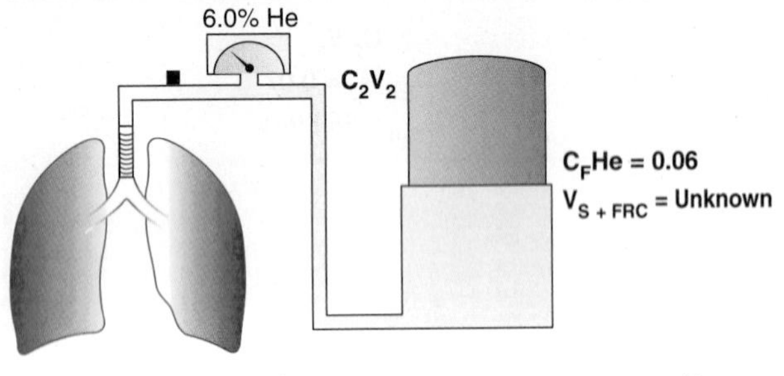

$$\frac{C_1 V_1}{C_2} = V_2 \text{ or } \frac{(V_S)(C_I He)}{C_F He} = V_{S + FRC}$$

$$\frac{(0.097)\ (5.15 \text{ liters})}{0.60} = V_{S + FRC}$$

$$8.33 \text{ liters} = V_{S + FRC}$$

$$V_{FRC} = V_{S + FRC} - V_S$$

$$V_{FRC} = 8.33 \text{ liters} - 5.15 \text{ liters}$$

$$V_{FRC} = 3.18 \text{ liters}$$

FIGURE 17-8 Equipment set-up and procedure for the helium dilution test.

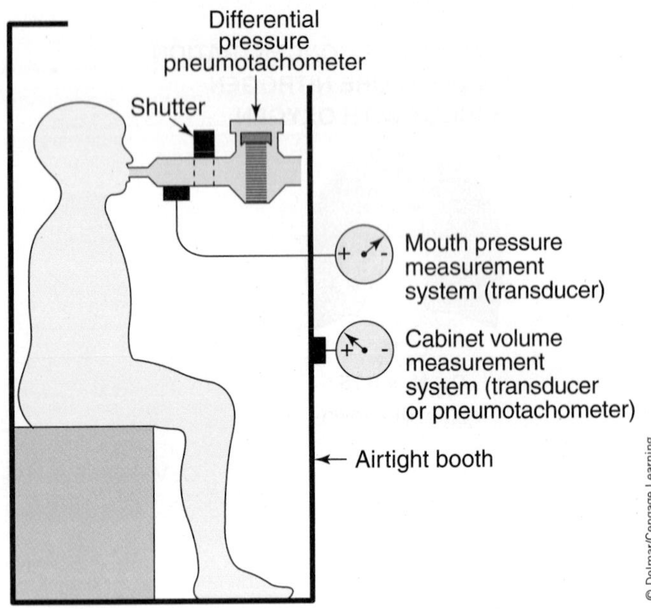

FIGURE 17-9 Components of the body plethysmograph system.

mouthpiece that is open to room air. In-line are a **pneumotachometer** (a flow sensor), a pressure manometer, and a **shutter** that cuts off airflow. The booth contains a flow sensor or pressure transducer (depending on the methodology used). See Figure 17-9 for the arrangement of these components.

Although several tests can be done with this device, only two tests require an airtight booth: airway resistance and volume of thoracic gas. The volume of air in the thoracic cavity at *FRC* is determined on the basis of Boyle's law ($P_1 \times V_1 = P_2 \times V_2$, when temperature is constant).

- The subject pants against the closed shutter, and mouth pressures and changes in the volume of air in the booth (displaced by the expansion of the thorax) are measured.
- The subject, with noseclips tightly in place and sitting in the booth with the door closed, breathes normally through the mouthpiece. The temperature in the booth rises because of the subject's body heat, so it takes several minutes for equilibration to be reached. Equilibration is indicated by the end-tidal level remaining stable on the computer screen.
- The subject then puts hands over the cheeks to prevent their expansion when panting against the closed shutter.
- Instruct the subject to pant (in small pants) through the mouthpiece one or two times per minute.
- At end-exhalation, close the shutter, and tell the subject to try to pant against the closed shutter.
- The shutter is then opened, and the test is complete.

It is recommended that the test be repeated three times. The AARC clinical practice guideline for body plethysmography covers contraindications, hazards, and equipment requirements.[4]

The volume of thoracic gas (V_{TG}) is determined using the principle of Boyle's law, where V_1 is the volume of thoracic gas (V_{TG}), V_2 is the change in alveolar volume, P_1 is atmospheric pressure, and P_2 is the change in alveolar pressure. An SVC test in the same session of testing is required to calculate all lung volumes.

An oscilloscope is used to show pressure and volume changes during panting, with volume on the horizontal axis and pressure on the vertical axis. The oscilloscope display allows the test giver to be sure that the pants are small enough to produce measurable loops (see Figure 17-10).

DIFFUSING CAPACITY (SINGLE-BREATH METHOD)

Of the several tests available to assess lung **diffusing capacity** (the rate at which oxygen diffuses from the alveoli to the capillaries), the single-breath method is the most common. Because oxygen is already in the

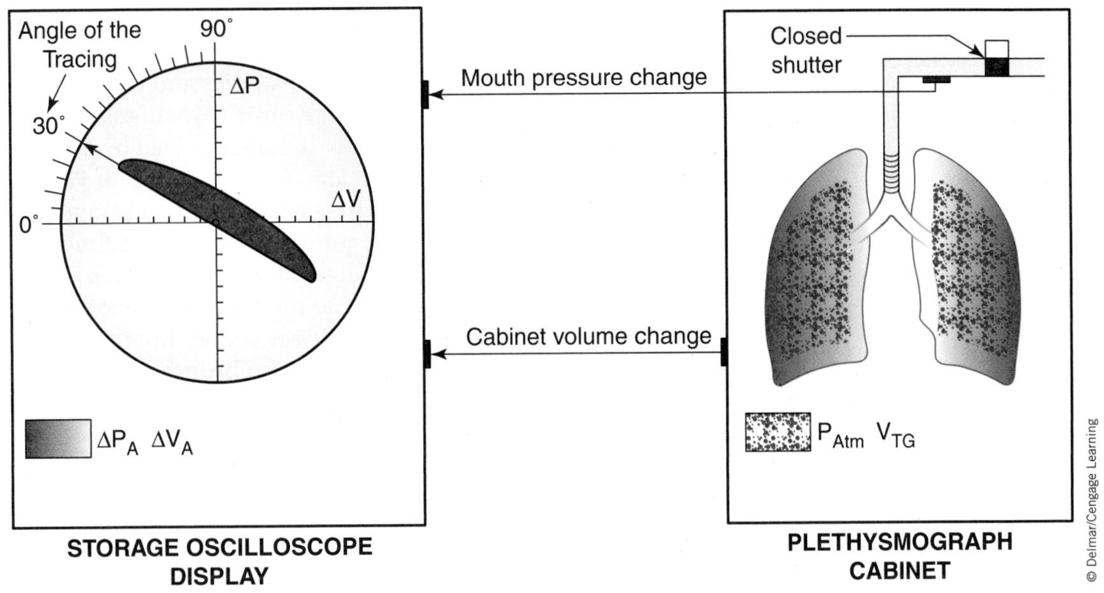

FIGURE 17-10 Oscilloscope display for body plethysmography.

lungs and in the blood, measuring how much diffuses from the lung into the blood in one breath is impossible because the partial pressure of oxygen in the capillary blood cannot be determined. Therefore, another gas (carbon monoxide, CO) is used in a very low concentration. Carbon monoxide has diffusing characteristics similar to those of oxygen and is carried in the blood in the same way as oxygen, and because CO is almost completely taken up by the hemoglobin, no back pressure exists in the capillary blood and is assumed to be zero. The amount of CO that diffuses from the lung into the blood (D_LCO) gives a direct indication of the rate at which O_2 diffuses from the lung into the blood. The relationship between the diffusion of carbon monoxide and oxygen can be expressed as:

$$D_LO_2 = D_LCO \times 1.23.$$

The change in CO concentration between inhalation and exhalation is not all due to diffusion out of the lungs. Some of the change is due to dilution by the gases that are still in the lungs when the test starts. Therefore, a known concentration of an inert gas (called a *tag gas*), such as helium (He) or neon (Ne), is added to the gas mixture inhaled by the subject. Because this gas does not diffuse or combine with anything in the lung, the change in its concentration gives a dilution factor. This dilution factor can be used to calculate the amount of CO that is actually diffused out of the lung.

- With noseclips in place, the subject makes a tight lip seal around the mouthpiece and breathes normally.
- Instruct the subject to exhale down to *RV* and then inhale up to *TLC* as quickly as possible. The gas inhaled is a special mixture containing 0.3% CO, 10% He, 21% O_2, and balance N_2.
- The subject holds his or her breath at *TLC* for approximately 10 seconds and then exhales as quickly as possible.

During the exhalation, the first 750–1000 mL is discarded because it is deadspace volume where no diffusion takes place. If the subject's *VC* is less than 2.0 L, the washout volume may be reduced to 500 mL. Then a small volume of exhaled gas is collected, usually 500 mL, and the sample is analyzed for He (or Ne) and CO concentrations.

Computerized equipment makes all calculations. The first step is to make the dilution correction to get the initial alveolar CO concentration using the changes in He or Ne concentration. The second step is to calculate alveolar volume. Then the D_LCO is calculated. Results are reported at STPD as milliliters of carbon monoxide per minute per millimeter of mercury (mm Hg is the partial pressure gradient across the alveolar-capillary membrane). The normal value is around 25 mL CO/min/mm Hg.

Factors other than abnormalities in the alveolar-capillary membrane can cause abnormal results in this test: reduced lung volume, anemia, the presence of carboxyhemoglobin in the blood, and altitude.[5] Correction factors are available to account for these conditions.

Best Practice

Diffusing Capacity: Single-Breath Method

1. The subject should be instructed not to smoke for 24 hours before testing.
2. The test should be repeated only after a 4-minute wait.
3. The inspiratory volume should be at least 90% of the previously measured *VC* or FVC.
4. Two or more tests should be averaged and should be within 10% of each other.
5. If the subject has a decreased hemoglobin (Hb) or an elevated carboxyhemoglobin (COHb), less CO diffuses out of the alveoli than if the subject had normal levels. Hemoglobin carries almost all the O_2 and CO that enters the blood from the alveoli. If the hemoglobin is less than normal, less CO than normal is able to diffuse into the blood. If the COHb is abnormally high, some of the hemoglobin already carries CO, so less CO diffuses out of the alveoli into the blood. Therefore, corrections should be made in the results to compensate for abnormal Hb and COHb. Both corrected and uncorrected values should be reported.

INTERPRETATION

Several sets of predicted values are available. Computerized equipment units have these values installed, and some manufacturers offer a choice of sets to install. In general, results are normal if they are between 80% and 120% of the predicted value for the subject. The predicted values for each measurement are determined by the subject's gender, height, and age.

Abnormal values typical of obstructive lung disease are the same as in the interpretation of FVC results. Postbronchodilator studies and D_LCO results help to further classify the obstructive disease.

Reversibility is demonstrated by a 12% and a 200-mL or greater increase in FVC or FEV_1 postbronchodilation. In general, asthma responds the most dramatically, sometimes returning abnormal values to the normal range. Chronic bronchitis improves to a lesser degree, and the increase may or may not be significant. Emphysema does not improve postbronchodilation because no bronchospasm is involved in this disease. In some cases, however, both emphysema and chronic bronchitis are present.

The D_LCO is decreased in emphysema because of the destruction of alveolar air space. Usually, the D_LCO is normal in asthma and chronic bronchitis, although it may become reduced in the presence of significant ventilation/perfusion mismatching.

In restrictive disease, spirometry results show a decrease in all lung volumes and capacities. The FEV_1 is normal or decreased, but the FEV_1% is normal or increased. Lung volumes reveal a decrease in *TLC*. There is no response to bronchodilators because no bronchospasm is involved in any of the restrictive lung diseases.

The D_LCO helps in identifying the cause of the restrictive lung disease. Diseases caused by chest wall abnormalities (kyphosis, scoliosis, neuromuscular diseases) have a normal D_LCO when adjusted for reduced lung volume. Parenchymal diseases (fibrosis, pneumoconiosis, some connective tissue disorders) have a decreased D_LCO.

Table 17-5 summarizes the abnormal laboratory values associated with obstructive and restrictive diseases. Figure 17-11 shows a flowchart that can be used to interpret a combination of spirometry, lung volume, and D_LCO tests. The tests are examined in the following order:

1. FVC (spirometry): FVC, FEV_1, FEV_1%
2. Lung volumes: *TLC*, *RV*, *VC*
3. D_LCO

TABLE 17-5 **Abnormal laboratory values in restrictive and obstructive and lung diseases**

	Restrictive	Obstructive
FVC	< 80% predicted	Normal or < 80% predicted
FEV_1	Normal or < 80% predicted	< 80% predicted
FEV_1%	≥ predicted	< predicted
VC	< 80% predicted	Normal or < 80% predicted
TLC	< 80% predicted	Normal or > 80% predicted
RV	< 80% predicted	Normal or < 80% predicted
Postbronchodilation	Not significant	Significant or not significant
D_LCO	Normal or < 80% predicted	Normal or < 80% predicted

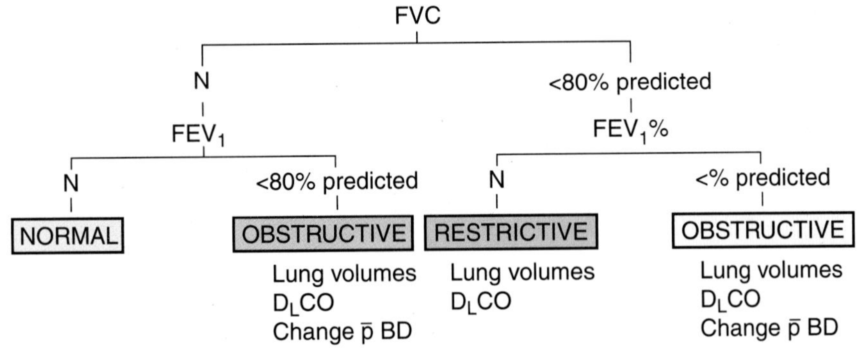

OBSTRUCTIVE

- Lung volumes: normal, progressing to increased RV and decreased VC, and then to increased TLC
- D$_L$CO: normal—asthma, chronic bronchitis (unless there is significant $\dot{V}/\dot{Q}$ mismatching)
  decreased—emphysema
- pBD (Postbronchodilator) change: significant—asthma, some chronic bronchitis
  not significant—emphysema and some chronic bronchitis

RESTRICTIVE

- Lung volumes: decreased TLC and all other volumes and capacities
- D$_L$CO: normal—chest wall diseases
  decreased—parenchymal diseases

FIGURE 17-11 Interpretation of pulmonary function tests.

OTHER SPECIALIZED TESTS

The following tests are used to measure very specific aspects of lung function and to assess the effect of lung disease or other diseases on the subject's activity level.

Maximum Voluntary Ventilation. The **maximum voluntary ventilation (MVV)** is the maximum amount of air a subject can move into and out of the lungs in 1 minute, measured in liters per minute (L/min). The patient is instructed to breath deeply and rapidly for a 12-second interval at an ideal respiratory rate of 90 breaths per minute. The volume moved in the 12-second interval is then extrapolated for a period of 1 minute. This test is extremely effort dependent, so much coaching and encouragement are required. The results are then compared with normal values based on gender, height, and age. This test is particularly valuable for subjects with very mild neuromuscular disease. These individuals may be able to perform spirometry well and achieve normal values. With the sustained effort required for this test, the subject may tire as the test proceeds. The test is also useful as an indicator of exercise tolerance in subjects with lung disease.

Airway Resistance. The airway resistance (R_{aw}) test can be performed only with body plethysmography.

- Place noseclips on the subject and instructed the subject to place the hands on the cheeks to stabilize them.

Best Practice

Maximum Voluntary Ventilation

1. To have the patient perform at personal best, give the instruction to pretend that a large bag has to be blown up as much as possible.
2. This test should be done at least twice; the largest MVV should be reported.
3. Subjects with airway hyper-reactivity may achieve lower than expected results owing to bronchospasm induced by hyperventilation.
4. Results are acceptable if the volume moved is 35 times the FEV$_1$.

CASE STUDY 17-4

J. T. is a 39-year-old Caucasian female. She is 62 inches tall and weighs 237 pounds. She is a nonsmoker who works as a department store salesclerk. Her test results are as follows:

Spirometry

	Predicted	Pre-BD	Percentage Predicted	Post-BD	Percentage Predicted	Percentage Change
FVC	3.12 L	2.65 L	85	2.89 L	93	9
FEV_1	2.65 L	2.03 L	78	2.36 L	89	16
$FEV_1\%$	86	77	—	82	—	6
$FEF_{25–75\%}$	186 Lpm	100 Lpm	54	145 Lpm	78	45

Lung Volumes

	Predicted	Actual	Percentage Predicted
VC	3.12 L	2.64 L	85
TLC	4.66 L	4.40 L	94
RV	1.49 L	1.76 L	118

Single-Breath Diffusion

	Predicted	Actual	Percentage Predicted
D_LCO	20.9	21.6	103

Questions

1. How would you interpret the spirometry, lung volumes, and D_LCO values?
2. Is there a significant response to bronchodilation?

- Seal the door to the plethysmograph.
- The subject breathes normally through the mouthpiece.
- The subject then pants through the mouthpiece, and pressure changes at the mouth and the flow through the mouthpiece are measured.
- Close the shutter.
- The subject continues to try to pant against the closed shutter.

Airway resistance is calculated by dividing the pressure change at the mouth by the flow measured at the mouth, using the following formula:

$$R_{aw} = \frac{\text{change in pressure}}{\text{flow at the mouth}} = \frac{\Delta P}{\dot{V}_{mouth}}$$

Normal values range from 0.6 to 2.4 cm H_2O/L/sec. Specific airway resistance (SR_{aw}) is also calculated by dividing the airway resistance by the V_{TG}, determined during the closed-shutter panting ($SR_{aw} = R_{aw}/V_{TG}$).

An airway resistance test reports two other parameters:

- **Airway conductance (G_{aw})**—a measure of the ease with which air passes through the conducting airways of the pulmonary system—and specific airway conductance (SG_{aw})
- **Airway resistance ($G_{aw} = 1/R_{aw}$)**—the difficulty with which air passes through the airways.

Airway conductance is the inverse, or the reciprocal, of airway resistance. The specific airway conductance (SG_{aw}) is calculated by dividing the airway conductance by the V_{TG} at which the closed-shutter panting was performed. If airway resistance (R_{aw}) is above normal, the airway conductance (G_{aw}) is below normal.

Obstructive diseases such as asthma, chronic bronchitis, emphysema, bronchiectasis, and airway hyper-reactivity increase airway resistance (R_{aw}).

Lung Compliance. To test **lung compliance** (a measure of the distensibility of the lung):

- Insert a catheter with a balloon near its end into the esophagus. The catheter is attached to a pressure transducer to get intrathoracic pressure readings.
- With noseclips in place, the subject inhales maximally to *TLC* and then holds the breath with an open glottis.
- The patient then exhales slowly and, at periodic intervals, holds the breath.
- Record the pressure and volume measurements.

The pressures required to achieve a change in volume are used to calculate *static compliance* (compliance measured without airflow):

$$\Delta V/\Delta P = C_L$$

Compliance is measured in liters or milliliters per centimeter H_2O. *Normal lung compliance* is 0.2 L/cm H_2O.

Restrictive diseases that affect the lung parenchyma (e.g., pulmonary fibrosis) reduce lung compliance. Emphysema typically results in an increase in lung compliance.

Single-Breath Nitrogen Gas Distribution Test (Closing Volume, Single-Breath Nitrogen Washout). This test is used to assess the distribution of ventilation in the subject's lungs, as well as the closing volume. *Closing volume* (*CV*) is the volume remaining in the vital capacity when the small airways start to close during a slow exhalation. *Closing capacity* (*CC*) is the volume of air remaining in the lungs when the small airways start to close (*CV* + *RV*). Results are often reported as a ratio between these two results: *CV*/*CC*.

- The subject first exhales maximally and then maximally inhales 100% O_2.
- Then the subject immediately exhales very slowly. As the subject exhales, an in-line nitrogen analyzer monitors the exhaled nitrogen concentration, and a flow sensor measures volume.
- The results are recorded on a graph, with the nitrogen concentration on the vertical axis and volume on the horizontal axis. As shown in Figure 17-12, the tracing is divided into four phases.

Phase I is the exhalation of deadspace gas.

Phase II is a mixture of deadspace gas and alveolar gas.

Phase III is all alveolar gas.

Phase IV is the closing volume (CV).

The start of phase IV is when the small airways start to close. The distribution of ventilation in the subject's lungs is assessed by the slope of phase III, reported as the change in nitrogen (ΔN_2). Subjects with an uneven distribution of ventilation have a steep phase III, and, in severe cases, it may be difficult to determine the onset of phase IV. A steep phase III is characteristic of moderate to severe obstructive lung diseases.

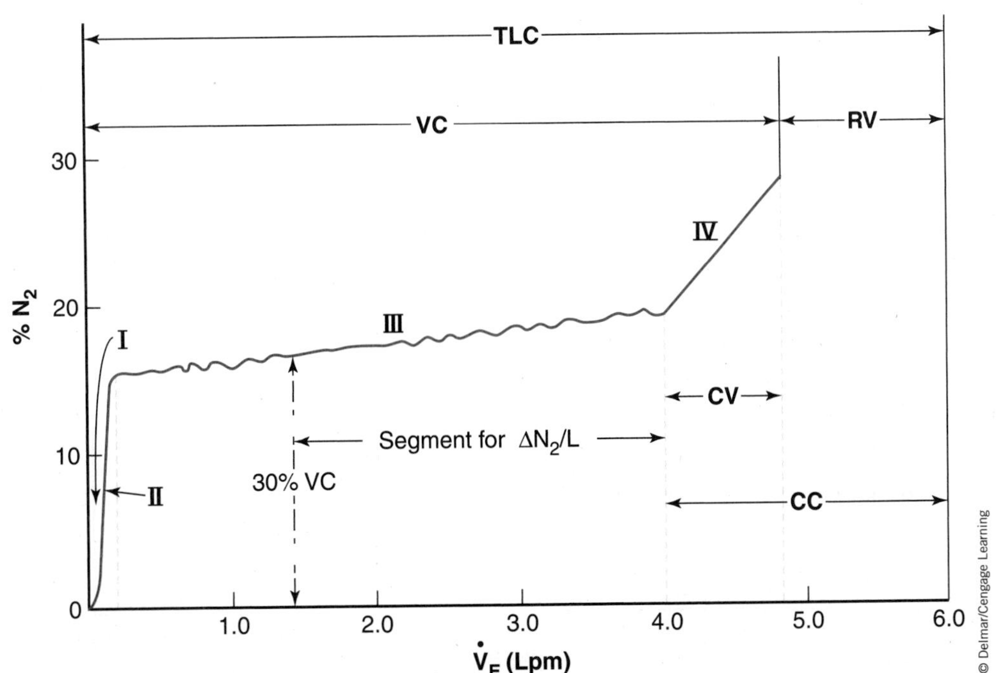

FIGURE 17-12 Phases of the nitrogen washout gas distribution test.

Cardiopulmonary Stress Testing. In *cardiopulmonary stress testing* (*CPX test*), subjects go through a series of increasing exercise levels. During the exercise, the responses of the pulmonary system, such as minute volume, CO_2 production, and O_2 consumption, are assessed. The responses of the cardiovascular system, such as blood pressure, stroke volume, cardiac output, and cardiac rate and rhythm, are also assessed.

Normal Exercise Physiology Exercise increases the metabolic need of the tissues for oxygen. Both the pulmonary system and the cardiovascular system must meet this increased demand. Diseases in either of these systems can result in exercise limitation.

The pulmonary system increases the amount of oxygen available at the alveolar-capillary membrane by increasing minute volume (V_E). This increase in alveolar ventilation is accomplished mostly by increasing tidal volume and, in more strenuous exercise, by increasing the respiratory rate (RR) as well. The minute volume can be increased in a normal fit subject as much as 20 times the resting minute volume. Figure 17-13 illustrates these changes as the exercise workload is increased.

The cardiovascular system increases the rate of oxygen delivery to the tissues by increasing the cardiac output (CO). This increase is accomplished first by an increase in stroke volume (SV, the volume of blood pumped with each ventricular contraction), and then by an increase in heart rate (HR). The CO can be increased as much as 6 times the resting CO in a normal fit subject. Figure 17-14 illustrates these cardiac responses to an increasing exercise workload.

If the workload is steadily increased, as it usually is in stress testing, oxygen consumption continues to rise until the maximum oxygen consumption level (VO_{2max}) is reached. The production of CO_2 (VCO_2) also continues to rise until the body cannot continue to metabolize aerobically. When the body switches over to anaerobic metabolism, the rate of production of CO_2 increases dramatically owing to the increase in lactic acid production, which is buffered by serum bicarbonate. This point is called the **anaerobic threshold (*AT*)**. Figure 17-15 illustrates the determination of the anaerobic threshold.

Arterial blood gas measurements during exercise show that the P_aO_2 remains stable throughout incremental exercise. The P_aCO_2 falls slightly until the anaerobic threshold (AT) is reached, and then decreases more rapidly, probably because of the chemoreceptor response to the increased lactic acid produced in anaerobic metabolism. Figure 17-16 shows these changes.

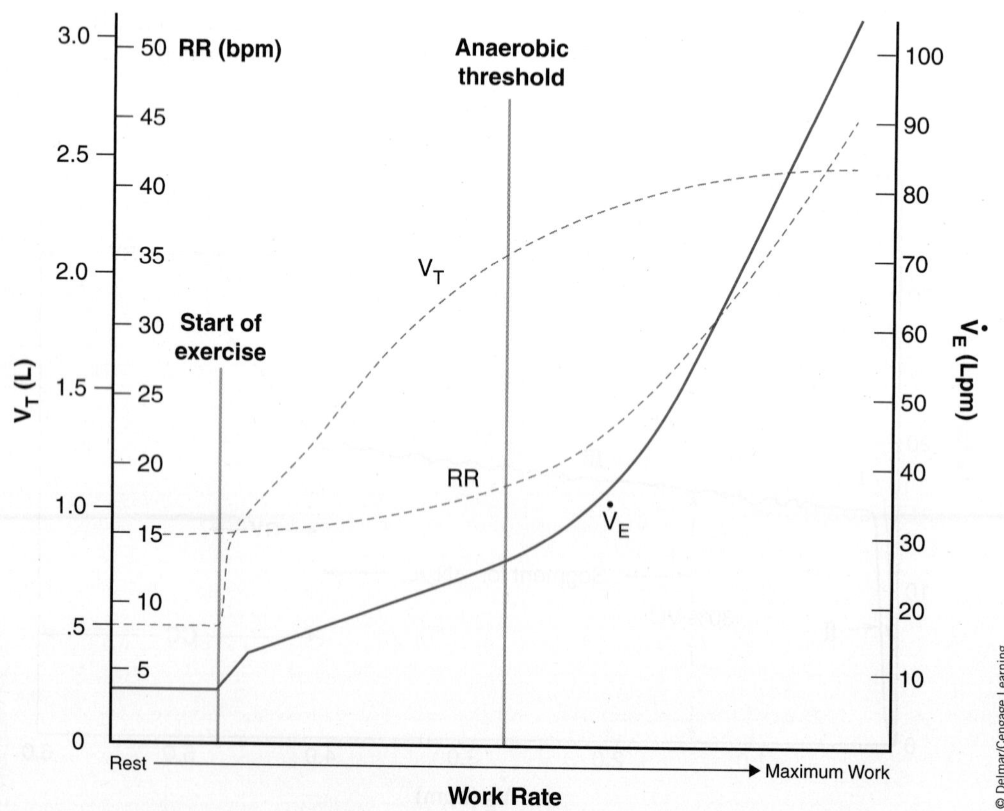

FIGURE 17-13 Response of the pulmonary system to increasing exercise workloads.

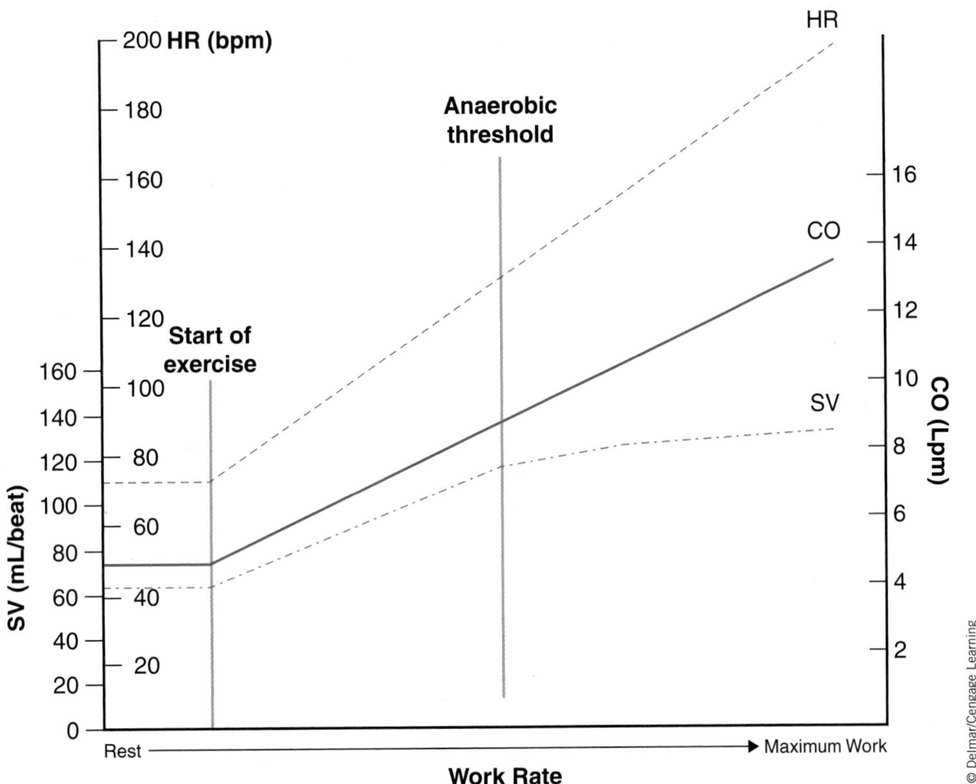

FIGURE 17-14 Response of the heart to increasing exercise workloads.

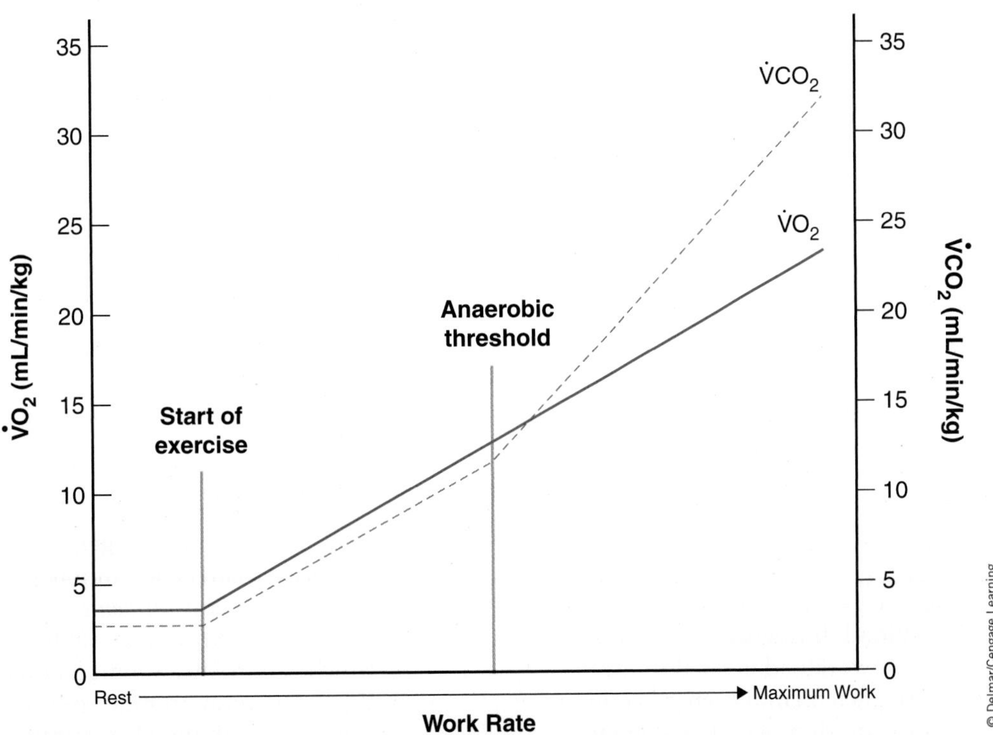

FIGURE 17-15 Oxygen consumption and carbon dioxide production in increasing exercise workload.

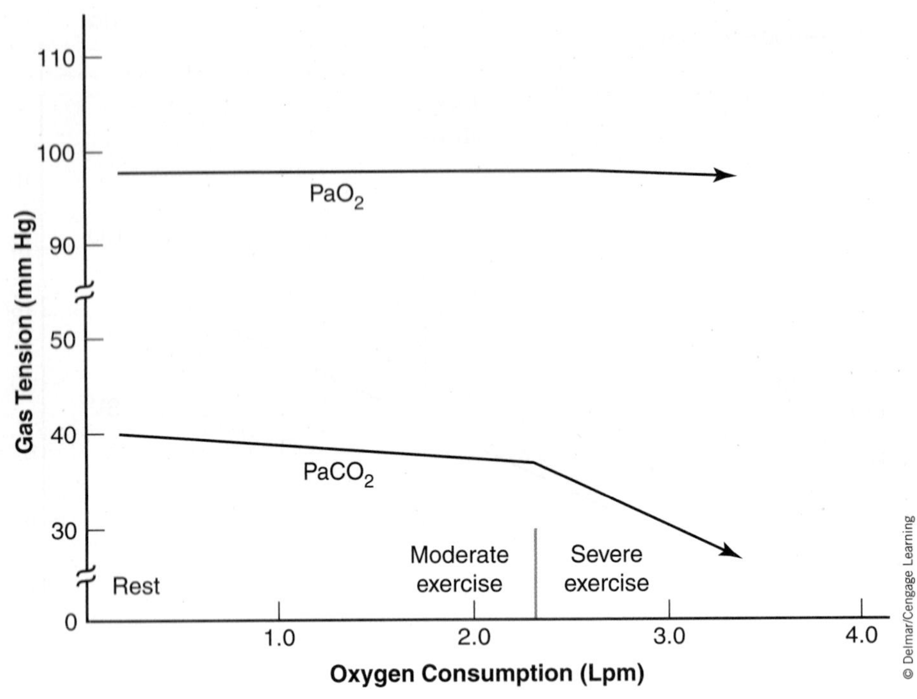

FIGURE 17-16 Changes in arterial blood gases in response to increasing exercise workloads.

Indications Cardiopulmonary stress testing is indicated for:

- Evaluating unexplained dyspnea upon exertion to determine whether the cause is a problem in the pulmonary or cardiovascular system.
- Monitoring the effect of previously diagnosed pulmonary, cardiovascular, or neuromuscular disease on exercise tolerance.
- Determining the magnitude of hypoxemia for oxygen prescription.
- Evaluating fitness or the patient's progress in a rehabilitation program.

Contraindications There are a number of absolute and relative contraindications to cardiopulmonary stress testing, mainly severe or potentially life-threatening cardiovascular conditions. For a more detailed discussion of contraindications and hazards, see the AARC clinical practice guideline for exercise testing.[6]

Testing Procedure The exercise used can be *steady state* (the same workload throughout the test) or *incremental* (increased workload at fixed intervals throughout the test). Incremental exercise is the more common. Either a treadmill or a cycle ergometer (exercise bicycle) can be used. The patient continues to exercise until he or she is unable to continue.

During the test, a number of parameters are monitored.

- A pneumotachometer (an electronic device used to measure flow) is used to measure minute volume, respiratory rate, and tidal volume.
- A pulse oximeter is used to monitor oxygen saturation (S_PO_2).
- Oxygen and carbon dioxide analyzers are used to monitor exhaled oxygen and carbon dioxide concentrations, respectively. Arterial blood gases should be performed before exercise to establish the correlation between the S_aO_2 and the S_PO_2 and may be repeated during and after testing.
- In addition, an electrocardiogram (ECG) is run continuously to monitor heart rate and rhythm.
- Blood pressure is taken periodically.

The following are some of the data collected and calculated during and after the test:

- $\dot{V}O_{2max}$ (maximum oxygen consumption) is expressed as liters per minute (L/min) or in units called *metabolic equivalents of energy expenditure* (METs). One MET is the subject's $\dot{V}O_2$ at rest, which is normally 3.5 mL/kg/min.
- $\dot{V}_{max}$ (maximum minute volume) is usually compared with the MVV acquired in another test and is expressed as $\dot{V}_{max}$/MVV.
- HR_{max} (maximal heart rate)

TABLE 17-6 Patterns of abnormalities at maximal exercise level in cardiopulmonary stress testing

	Pulmonary Disease*	Cardiovascular Disease*	Deconditioned*
$\dot{V}O_{2max}$	↓	↓	↓
$\dot{V}_{Emax}$	↑	↓	↓
S_pO_2	Often ↓	N	N
AT	Not achieved	Achieved at low $\dot{V}O_2$	Achieved at low $\dot{V}O_2$
HR_{max}	↓	↑	↑
ECG rhythm	N	Dysrhythmias	N

*↓, *less than predicted;* ↑, *greater than predicted; N, normal.*

- P_aO_2 and/or S_pO_2 (arterial partial pressure of oxygen and/or Hb saturation with O_2 measured by pulse oximeter)
- ECG (heart rate and rhythm)
- AT (anaerobic threshold) is the workload at which the subject changes from aerobic metabolism to anaerobic metabolism. This is indicated by a sharp increase in CO_2 production ($\dot{V}CO_2$).

Interpretation Abnormal results can be due to three causes: pulmonary disease, cardiovascular disease, and deconditioning or unfitness. Table 17-6 summarizes the results associated with each of these causes.

- Subjects with *pulmonary disease* are ventilation limited in exercise. They may not achieve the anaerobic threshold, and their maximal minute volume ($\dot{V}_{Emax}$) is greater than 70% of their MVV. The ECG is normal, and their maximal heart rate is less than 85% of the predicted rate.
- Subjects with *cardiovascular disease* are circulation limited in exercise. Their heart rate is greater than 85% of the predicted rate, and the ECG may show dysrhythmias, or S-T segment changes, or both. Their anaerobic threshold is reached sooner than predicted, and their maximal minute volume is typically less than 50% of their MVV.
- A *deconditioned subject* has the same abnormal results as a subject with mild cardiovascular disease.

Bronchoprovocation. The purpose of a **bronchoprovocation** test is to detect the presence of airway hyper-reactivity. It is indicated:

- When a subject has the symptoms of bronchospasm but normal pulmonary function tests.
- When there is occupational risk.
- As a baseline study before occupational exposure.

Follow-up testing is also indicated to check for changes in the hyper-reactivity or its severity. The AARC clinical practice guideline for bronchial provocation covers contraindications, hazards, and limitations.[7]

The most common inhaled agents used for bronchoprovocation are methacholine (a cholinergic agent) and histamine. Hyperventilation using cold air or room air may also be used. For suspected exercise-induced bronchospasm (EIB), testing is done after exercise.

Before any bronchoprovocation test, all bronchodilators should be withheld.

- Beta-adrenergics and anticholinergics should be withheld for 8 hours.
- Sustained-action theophylline, cromolyn sodium, necromodil sodium, and leukotriene inhibitors should be withheld for 48 hours.
- Caffeine, smoke, and smoking should be avoided for 6 hours before testing.
- Inhaled or oral steroids may be continued.

Table 17-7 summarizes the schedule for withholding medications.

TABLE 17-7 Prebronchoprovocation withholding schedule for bronchodilating agents

Agent	Hold Time (hours)
Beta-adrenergics	8
Anticholinergics	8
Sustained-action theophylline	48
Cromolyn sodium	48
Necromodil sodium	48
Leukotriene inhibitors	48
Caffeine	6
Smoke and smoking	6

Methacholine and Histamine Procedure. The procedure is as follows:

- Prebronchoprovocation spirometry is done. The FEV_1 should be > 60–70% of the predicted value.
- The subject is given nebulized normal saline, and the spirometry is repeated. If there is a 10% reduction in the FEV_1, the test is positive for airway hyper-reactivity. No further testing should be done. Continue if the reduction is equal to or greater than 10%.
- At fixed intervals, increasing doses of methacholine or histamine are given by nebulizer. A number of protocols for the dosing are widely available. Spirometry is done at 30–90 seconds after each dose, and the test procedure and results must meet the current ATS acceptability guidelines. A 20% decrease in FEV_1 is considered a positive test for airway hyper-reactivity, and at that time the testing is stopped. The dose after which this decrease occurs is the PD_{20} (the provocation dose resulting in a 20% or greater decrease in FEV_1).
- A bronchodilator is administered to reverse the bronchospasm. The reversal is documented by a return to prebronchoprovocation values.

Hyperventilation Procedure. The procedure is as follows:

- Prebronchoprovocation spirometry is performed. The FEV_1 should be either >80% of the predicted value or >80% of the highest previous value for that subject to continue the testing.
- The subject hyperventilates either room air or cold air (21–22°C or 69.8–71.6°F) for 4–6 minutes.
- Spirometry is then performed at fixed intervals of up to 20 minutes. Again, the results must be reproducible (per ATS acceptability guidelines). If the FEV_1 is reduced by 20% in that time, the test is positive for airway hyper-reactivity.

Exercise Challenge. The procedure is as follows:

- On a treadmill or ergometer, the subject exercises to 60–80% of the predicted heart rate for 6–8 minutes. The ECG and blood pressure are monitored during the exercise period.
- After exercise, spirometry is done 1–2 minutes postexercise and then every 5 minutes. In a positive test, the FEV_1 decreases by 10–20% (usually in 5–10 minutes) and then returns to baseline (usually in 20–40 minutes).

- Severe bronchospasm may require the administration of a bronchodilator, with documentation of reversal done with spirometry.

CO_2 Response Curve. The purpose of this test is to evaluate the subject's response to increased levels of CO_2 while P_aO_2 is maintained within normal limits. The results are reported in liters per minute per millimeter mercury (L/min/mm Hg).

Two methods can be used. One uses an open circuit and the other, a closed circuit.

- In the *open-circuit method*, the subject breathes varying percentages of CO_2 (usually 1–7%). For each percentage, the end-tidal CO_2 ($P_{et}CO_2$), the minute volume ($\dot{V}_E$), and the O_2 saturation (S_pO_2) are monitored and recorded.
- In the *closed-circuit method*, a gas mixture containing 7% CO_2 is placed in a reservoir. The subject rebreathes from this reservoir. An in-line analyzer measures $P_{et}CO_2$, a pneumotachometer measures $\dot{V}_E$, and a pulse oximeter monitors S_pO_2. The F_IO_2 is maintained at 0.21 by adding O_2, as an oxygen analyzer indicates the need. The subject continues to rebreathe from the reservoir until the $P_{et}CO_2$ is higher than 9%, or for 4 minutes, whichever occurs first.

The results are recorded on a graph, plotting minute volume on the vertical axis and $P_{et}CO_2$ on the horizontal axis. The response to increased concentrations of CO_2 is linear, as shown in Figure 17-17. The normal increase in $\dot{V}_E$ is 3 L/min/mm Hg, with a range of 1–6 L/min/mm Hg. Some subjects with obstructive disease have a reduced response to increases in CO_2 concentrations; others do not.

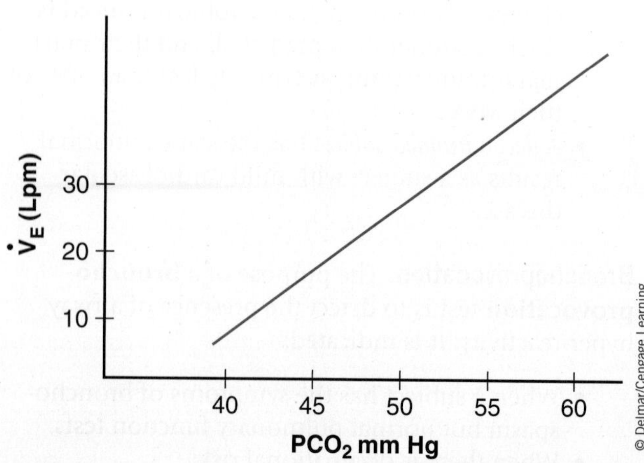

FIGURE 17-17 Normal response to the inhalation of increasing partial pressure of carbon dioxide.

Spirometers

There are two types of spirometer: volume displacement and flow-sensing.

VOLUME DISPLACEMENT DEVICES

Volume displacement devices measure volumes directly through changes in volume inside the device. The volume displacement is recorded on graph paper; either a pen is moving over the paper at a set speed, or the paper moves under the pen at a set speed. Flows and volumes can be measured from the volume-time curve. There are three types of volume displacement devices: water seal spirometers, rolling dry seal spirometers, and bellows spirometers.

Water Seal Spirometers. In these devices, water provides a leakproof seal to record changes in volume in the bell. A pen attached to the bell records changes in volume on a recorder that is moving at a set speed, producing a volume-time curve. This type of spirometer is shown in Figure 17-18.

Rolling Dry Seal Spirometers. In these devices, a flexible dry seal provides an airtight seal around a piston. A potentiometer senses the movement of the piston and electronically records the movement of the piston as the subject exhales into it. The electronic signals received are converted to a flow-volume loop and to numerical measurements of flow and volume. Figure 17-19 illustrates this type of device.

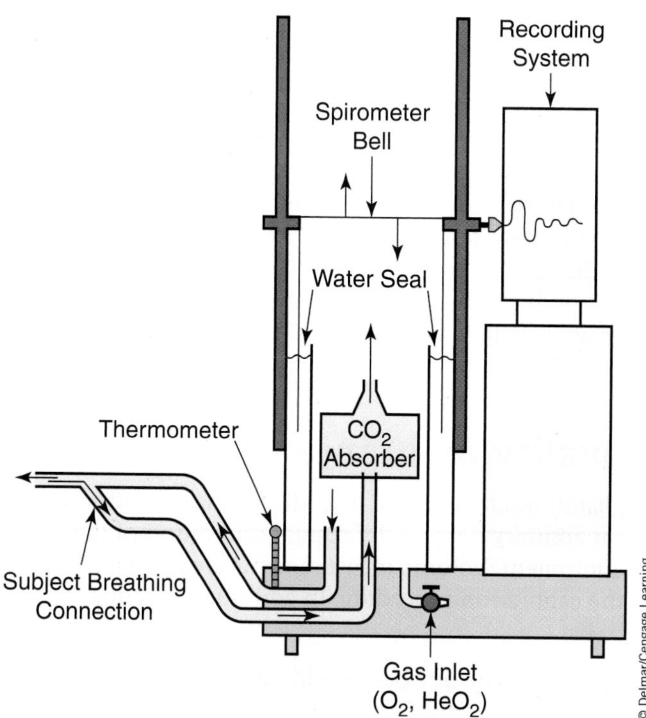

FIGURE 17-18 A water seal spirometer.

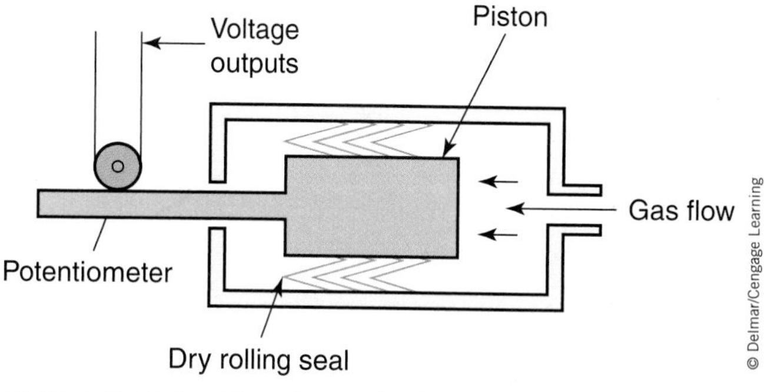

FIGURE 17-19 A rolling dry seal spirometer.

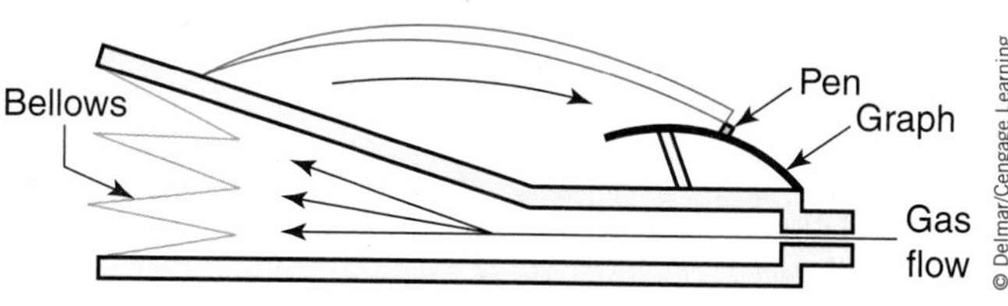

FIGURE 17-20 A bellows spirometer.

Bellows Spirometers. As the subject exhales into the opening of the bellows, the added gases are recorded by a pen, which records the change in volume either on graph paper moving at a set speed or by moving at a set speed across stationary graph paper. A volume-time curve is recorded, from which measurements are made. Figure 17-20 shows a bellows spirometer.

FLOW-SENSING DEVICES

Flow-sensing devices measure flows electronically and then convert the measurements to volumes. Flow-sensing devices are also called **pneumotachometers**, which are electronic devices that measure flows. For volume measurements, the computer converts the flow measurements over time to volume measurements.

Flow-sensing devices have largely replaced volume-displacement devices in modern computerized pulmonary function equipment. It is beyond the scope of this chapter to discuss each of the several types of pneumotachometer in detail.

- **Differential pressure pneumotachometers** (Figure 17-21) measure flow by the change in pressure that occurs as gases pass through a resistive device with a known resistance.
- **Thermal pneumotachometers** (Figure 17-22) measure flow through the change in temperature of a heated element as the gases pass over it.
- The **ultrasonic pneumotachometer** (Figure 17-23) uses the disturbance of ultrasonic waves as the gases pass through them to measure flow.

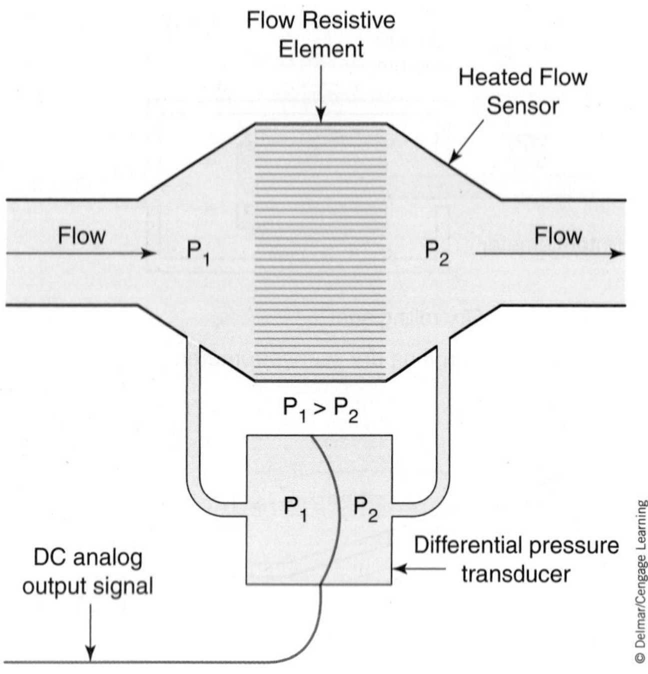

FIGURE 17-21 A differential pressure pneumotachometer.

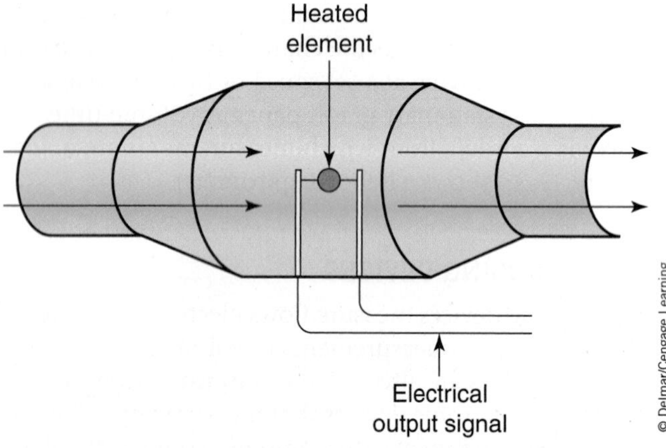

FIGURE 17-22 A thermal pneumotachometer.

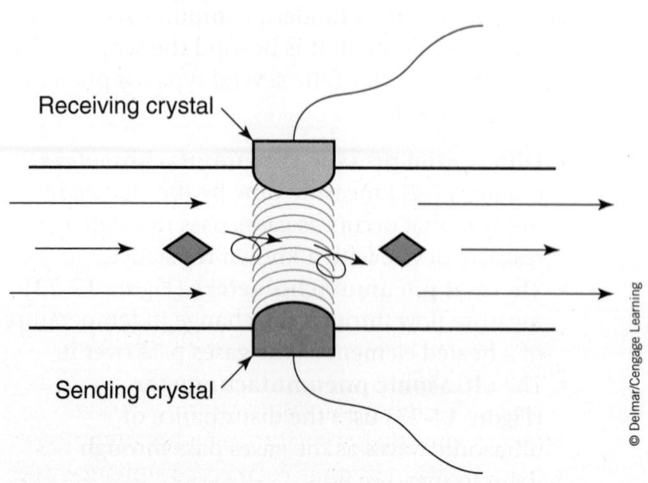

FIGURE 17-23 A ultrasonic pneumotachometer.

Body Plethysmograph

Although it is used to perform spirometry, MVV, and other tests, the body plethysmograph was developed to make two measurements: V_{TG} and R_{aw} (discussed earlier in the pages 466 and 469). There are five basic components in a body plethysmograph (Figure 17-9).

- A booth that can be sealed airtight is needed
- A differential pressure pneumotachometer to measure flows
- A **pressure transducer** to measure pressure changes at the mouth
- A **shutter** to stop airflow at the mouth
- Either a pressure transducer in the plethysmograph or a pneumotachometer in the wall of the booth to measure changes in pressure or in the volume of air in the booth that occur as a result of the subject's expanding the thorax in an attempt to pant against the closed shutter.

Calibration

Calibration is the testing and adjusting of equipment to make measurements more accurate. Calibration is usually done using a special calibrated 3-L syringe made for this purpose. The manufacturer prescribes the procedure and frequency of calibration. Computerized spirometers self-adjust after the calibration test using a correction factor.

Calibration should be performed at least once on any day the equipment is used. If the equipment is moved, it should be calibrated at each site. If a large number of tests are being performed, calibration should be done every 4 hours.

Check volume displacement devices daily for leaks before the calibration is performed. Leaks can be detected by applying a weight or constant pressure against the spirometer when it is full. If no change in volume is recorded over a period of time, there is no leak.

Body plethysmographs have automatic calibration systems. Follow the manufacturer's calibration procedure.

Quality Assurance

Quality assurance is the periodic testing of equipment for accuracy beyond the regular calibration of the equipment. Volume measurements are checked daily in the calibration procedure. In addition, on a quarterly basis:

- Volume devices should be checked with a wide variety of volumes.
- Flow-sensing devices should be checked with a wide variety of flows.

- Flow-measuring accuracy should also be checked quarterly. This check is not needed with flow-sensing devices because, if the unit is measuring volumes accurately, the flow measurements are accurate.
- Volume displacement devices should be checked with accurate flow-generating devices over a range of flows.
- Check the recorder of volume displacement devices. The recorder is started, and volume changes are introduced at fixed intervals that are timed with a stopwatch. The tracing is then checked to ensure that the recorder matches the actual time interval.

The American Thoracic Society has defined acceptable degrees of error in spirometers. In general, for diagnostic spirometers, accuracy must be within ±3% or ±50 mL, whichever is larger.[2]

Quality assurance can also be interpreted to mean that all tests are performed correctly by the subject and that the results reported are valid. This type of quality assurance requires technologists who are well trained not only in giving the subject instructions but also in judging whether the subject has followed them. The technologist must also be well versed in the recommendations for reporting results.

Infection Control

There is very little risk of cross-contamination among subjects or to technologists if certain commonsense precautions are taken. Transmission among subjects can be prevented by:

- The use of disposable mouthpieces and noseclips.
- The cleaning of nondisposable noseclips between uses.
- The disinfection or sterilization of nondisposable mouthpieces.
- Good handwashing techniques between patients and after handling contaminated equipment.
- Following the manufacturer's recommended method and frequency for cleaning other parts of the equipment.

Age-Related Considerations

The tests discussed in this chapter can be performed for adults, young children, and adolescents. For young children and for adolescents, there are different regression equations and nomograms, and these should be used to arrive at an accurate assessment. (Pulmonary function testing performed on infants requires special equipment and special techniques, which are beyond the scope of this chapter.)

No matter what the age of the subjects, the criteria for judging whether they can be tested are:

- Whether they can understand the instructions.
- Whether they are able to perform the required maneuvers.

Summary

In pulmonary function testing, spirometry or forced vital capacity measurements are used to find out whether the subject's lung function is normal or abnormal. Abnormal findings indicate a need for further testing to assess the type and degree of lung impairment. Such tests include lung volumes, diffusing capacity, postbronchodilator spirometry, maximum voluntary ventilation, airway resistance, lung compliance, the nitrogen washout gas distribution test, and the CO_2 response curve. Specialized test regimens, such as cardiopulmonary stress testing and bronchoprovocation, help assess the severity of lung disorders.

Equipment should be calibrated on a regular basis according to manufacturers' recommendations. Spirometers should have quality assurance assessments quarterly to ensure their accuracy. Infection control is easy to achieve by the use of disposable mouthpieces and noseclips and the sterilization of nondisposable items after each use. Handwashing is, of course, important after handling equipment and between subjects.

Study Questions

REVIEW QUESTIONS

1. What are the indications for spirometry?
2. When are postbronchodilator studies indicated?
3. How would you instruct a subject to do a forced vital capacity maneuver?
4. How are spirometry results interpreted?
5. In the results of cardiopulmonary stress tests, what are the patterns of abnormal values for cardiovascular disease, pulmonary disorders, and deconditioned subjects?
6. What are the indications for the following additional tests after spirometry: postbronchodilator MVV, diffusing capacity, lung volumes, compliance, airway resistance, single-breath nitrogen washout, and bronchoprovocation?
7. What are the indications for cardiopulmonary stress testing?
8. How are the following tests performed: lung volumes, diffusing capacity, single-breath nitrogen washout, MVV, airway resistance, compliance, and the CO_2 response curve?

9. What are typical results of the following tests in obstructive and restrictive diseases: lung volumes, diffusing capacity, single-breath nitrogen washout, MVV, airway resistance, compliance, and the CO_2 response curve?
10. How are spirometers calibrated and how often?
11. What quality-assurance tests should be performed quarterly on spirometers?
12. How is infection control achieved in using pulmonary function equipment?

MULTIPLE-CHOICE QUESTIONS

1. The amount of air a subject can forcefully exhale after a maximal inhalation is the:
   a. *ERV.*
   b. *FRC.*
   c. FVC.
   d. *RV.*
2. The amount of air remaining in the lungs after a maximal exhalation is the:
   a. *ERV.*
   b. *FRC.*
   c. *VC.*
   d. *RV.*
3. If a subject can still inhale air through the nose with the noseclip on while performing an FVC maneuver, the measured volumes will:
   a. be less than actual.
   b. be more than actual.
   c. be measured correctly.
   d. not be measurable.
4. The ATS recommends which of the following criteria for choosing the best FVC maneuver?
   a. the one with the largest FVC
   b. the one with the largest FEV_1
   c. the one with the highest peak flow
   d. the one with the largest sum of the FVC and the FEV_1
5. A sudden increase in the nitrogen concentration of exhaled air during a nitrogen washout test indicates:
   a. air trapping.
   b. therapist error.
   c. a leak in the system.
   d. patient fatigue.
6. The results of a nitrogen washout, a helium dilution, and a body plethysmograph are the same in subjects with:
   a. emphysema.
   b. pulmonary fibrosis.
   c. chronic bronchitis.
   d. cystic fibrosis.
7. In a single-breath nitrogen gas distribution test, the subject inhales a full vital capacity of 100% oxygen and is to maintain a breath-hold for:
   a. 0 seconds.
   b. 4–8 seconds.
   c. 5–10 seconds.
   d. 9–11 seconds.
8. When exhaled gas in a diffusing capacity test is being collected, the first 750 mL is discarded because:
   a. the subject is not exhaling as fast as possible at that time.
   b. these gases occupied alveolar deadspace.
   c. that volume was not involved in gas exchange.
   d. that volume is mostly helium.
9. In an airway resistance test, the subject first pants with the shutter open, and then with the shutter closed. The closed-shutter panting segment is used to determine:
   a. airway resistance.
   b. compliance.
   c. *FRC.*
   d. V_{TG}.
10. Which of the following is the formula for calculating lung compliance?
    a. $\Delta P/V$
    b. $V/\Delta P$
    c. $\Delta V/\Delta P$
    d. $\Delta P/\Delta V$
11. On the graph produced in a single-breath nitrogen gas distribution (or closing volume) test, phase III is analyzing:
    a. deadspace gas.
    b. a mixture of alveolar and deadspace gas.
    c. alveolar gas.
    d. closing volume.
12. In incremental exercise (the workload is increased at specific intervals), the shift to anaerobic metabolism is indicated by:
    a. a marked reduction in O_2 consumption.
    b. a marked increase in minute volume.
    c. a marked increase in CO_2 production.
    d. a marked drop in P_aO_2.
13. Which of the following is a cholinergic agent used in bronchoprovocation testing?
    a. acetylcholine
    b. histamine
    c. methacholine
    d. atrovent
14. Which of the following is considered to be a positive methacholine challenge test result?
    a. a 10% reduction in FEV_1
    b. a 20% reduction in FEV_1
    c. a 20% reduction in $FEF_{25-75\%}$
    d. a 20% reduction in $FEV_1\%$

15. If pulmonary function equipment is being moved to several different sites in one day, the equipment should be calibrated:
    a. before testing is started.
    b. every 4 hours.
    c. after arrival at each site.
    d. daily.

CRITICAL-THINKING QUESTIONS

1. Maximal subject effort in a forced vital capacity (FVC) maneuver is necessary for the results to be valid. How can a therapist tell whether the subject has made a maximal effort?
2. If a subject who has obstructive lung disease has a larger slow vital capacity than forced vital capacity, can the test results be valid?
3. A subject with obstructive lung disease has been in a pulmonary rehabilitation program for several months. Should pulmonary function tests or cardiopulmonary stress testing be used to assess the subject's progress? Explain your answer.
4. A subject who has moderate obstructive lung disease is doing the nitrogen washout test to determine *FRC*. The subject has been doing the washout for 12 minutes, and the exhaled nitrogen concentration is still 9%. There is no evidence of a leak in the system. Should the test be continued or terminated? Explain your answer.

References

1. American Association for Respiratory Care. AARC clinical practice guideline: Spirometry, 1996 update. *Respir Care*. 1996;41:629–636.
2. American Thoracic Society/European Respiratory Society Task Force. Standardization of spirometry. *Eur Respir J*. 2005;26:319–338.
3. American Association for Respiratory Care. AARC clinical practice guideline: Assessing response to bronchodilator therapy at point of care. *Respir Care*. 1995;40:1300–1307.
4. American Association for Respiratory Care. AARC clinical practice guideline: Body plethysmography: 2001 revision & update. *Respir Care*. 2001;46: 506–513.
5. American Association for Respiratory Care. AARC clinical practice guideline: Single-breath carbon monoxide diffusing capacity, 1999 update. *Respir Care*. 1999;44:91–97.
6. American Association for Respiratory Care. AARC clinical practice guideline: Exercise testing for evaluation of hypoxemia and/or desaturation: 2001 revision & update. *Respir Care*. 2001;46: 514–522.
7. American Association for Respiratory Care. AARC clinical practice guideline: Methacholine challenge testing: 2001 revision & update. *Respir Care*. 2001;46:523–530.

Suggested Readings

American Association for Respiratory Care. AARC clinical practice guideline: Static lung volumes: 2001 revision & update. *Respir Care*. 2001;46:531–539.

Chang DW. *Respiratory Care Calculations*. 2nd ed. Clifton Park, NY: Delmar Cengage Learning; 1999.

Des Jardins T. *Cardiopulmonary Anatomy and Physiology*. 5th ed. Clifton Park, NY: Delmar Cengage Learning; 2007.

Madama, VC. *Pulmonary Function Testing and Cardiopulmonary Stress Testing*. 2nd ed. Clifton Park, NY: Delmar Cengage Learning; 1998.

Ruppel GL. *Manual of Pulmonary Function Testing*. 9th ed. St. Louis: Mosby; 2009.

Wanger J. *Pulmonary Function Testing*. Philadelphia: Williams & Wilkins; 1996.

White GC. *Equipment Theory for Respiratory Care*. 4th ed. Clifton Park, NY: Delmar Cengage Learning; 2005.

Wilkins RL, Dexter JR, Heuer A. *Clinical Assessment in Respiratory Care*. 6th ed. St. Louis: Mosby; 2010.

CHAPTER 18

Polysomnography and Other Tests for Sleep Disorders

Robert A. Whitman

OBJECTIVES

Upon completion of this chapter, the reader should be able to:

- List the four stages of sleep and describe the cycling of sleep stages that characterizes normal sleep architecture.
- Discuss the EEG, EOG, and EMG criteria used to identify each sleep stage.
- Identify the cardiovascular and respiratory changes associated with each stage of sleep.
- Identify and discuss the four most common sleep disorders.
- Describe the electrode configuration used to monitor EEG activity during sleep.
- Describe the various technologies available to monitor breathing during sleep to include monitoring of airflow, respiratory effort, and arterial oxygen saturation.
- Discuss the technical and procedural aspects of performing polysomnography.
- Identify the scoring criteria for staging sleep, quantifying respiratory events, and quantifying limb movements.
- Explain the concept of CPAP and bilevel PAP therapy and describe the general protocols for titrating each.
- List the two tests used to assess daytime sleepiness and explain the rational for their use.

CHAPTER OUTLINE

(continues)

(continued)

KEY TERMS

apnea
apnea/hypopnea index (AHI)
artifact
autotitrating CPAP
bilevel positive airway pressure
cataplexy
central apnea
central sleep apnea
continuous positive airway pressure (CPAP)
electroencephalogram (EEG)
electromyogram (EMG)
electrooculogram (EOG)
epoch
excessive daytime sleepiness (EDS)
high-frequency filter
hypnagogic
hypnogogic
hypopnea
inductance plethysmography
low-frequency filter
mixed apnea
nonrapid eye movement (NREM)
obstructive apnea
obstructive sleep apnea (OSA)
obstructive sleep disordered breathing (OSDB)
patient calibration
periodic limb movements in sleep (PLMS)
polygraph
polysomnogram
polysomnography (PSG)
rapid eye movement (REM)
REM latency
respiratory disturbance index (RDI)
restless legs syndrome (RLS)
scoring
sleep apnea
sleep architecture
sleep deprivation
sleep disordered breathing (SDB)
sleep fragmentation
sleep histogram
sleep latency
sleep paralysis
slow-wave sleep

Polysomnography is the primary diagnostic tool used by sleep specialists to characterize abnormal physiological patterns associated with sleep disorders. Frequently referred to as a *sleep study*, **polysomnography (PSG)** is the monitoring and recording of physiological patterns during sleep; it is used in the clinical setting for the diagnosis of sleep disorders.

Sleep disorders and the technology used to diagnose them are specialized and complex. To become fully proficient, respiratory technologists need on-the-job training, usually teamed with an experienced therapist, as well as extensive education in data collection and interpretation. (Contact the Association of Polysomnographic Technologists and the Association of Sleep Technologists for credentialing requirements.)

The purpose of this chapter is to introduce respiratory technologists to the characteristics of normal sleep and to the most common sleep disorders, as well as to provide a basic review of polysomnography application and interpretation and the related tests.

Normal Sleep

Researchers began to study patients with sleep complaints in the 1960s. Their work subsequently evolved into an organized methodology for the study of sleep called *polysomnography*. In an effort to standardize sleep staging, in 1968 Rechtshaffen and Kales developed a manual for scoring normal adult sleep (commonly referred to as the *R&K manual*).[1] The rules described in the manual have been used to characterize sleep patterns in adults for nearly 40 years. The scoring rules were based on normal values from young adults and did not accurately cover sleep criteria for children and older adults. Adjustments have been since made to the rules to cover these patient populations in clinical practice.

In March 2007, the American Academy of Sleep Medicine (AASM) introduced a new manual for scoring sleep that incorporated recommended guidelines for scoring sleep and other parameters commonly monitored during polysomnography.[2] These guidelines are based on current scientific evidence and expertise in the advancing field of sleep medicine. Because the R&K sleep stage scoring rules have been used for many years and permeate the scientific literature, the therapist must be able to make the appropriate mental adjustments when reading prior literature. In this chapter, the rules for scoring sleep are based on the new AASM scoring guidelines. Significant differences between the current rules and the R&K rules are noted.

Distinct patterns of brain activity are associated with wakefulness and sleep. The characteristic patterns observed during normal sleep can be divided into distinct stages, and the typical distribution of these stages throughout the night is termed "sleep architecture." In addition, characteristic cardiovascular and respiratory changes are associated with sleep.

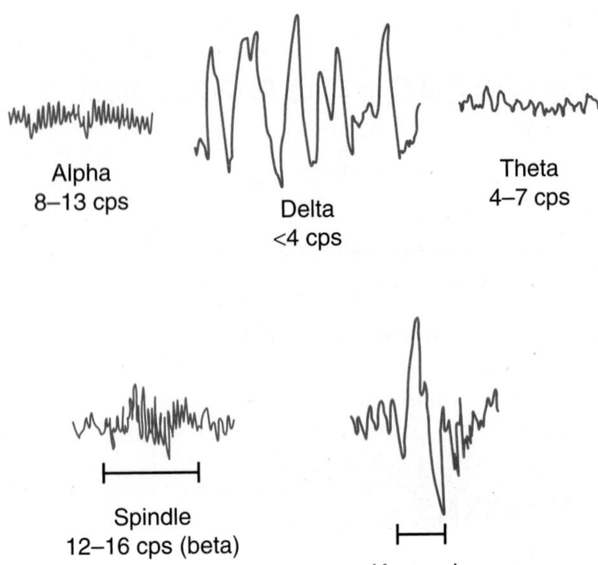

FIGURE 18-1 Examples of common waveforms found on the electroencephalogram (EEG) that are the basis for sleep staging: The values below each waveform represent the range of frequencies in cycles per second (cps) that define each type.

SLEEP TYPES AND STAGES

Sleep is typically divided into two distinct types: **nonrapid eye movement (NREM)** and **rapid eye movement (REM)**. As the names suggest, REM sleep is characterized by the occurrence of phasic rapid eye movements, which are absent in NREM sleep. Both respiratory and cardiac rhythms are regular during NREM sleep but fluctuate significantly during REM sleep.

NREM sleep is divided into three stages based on combined elements of:

- **Electroencephalogram (EEG)** patterns.
- Eye movements, or the **electrooculogram (EOG)**.
- Muscle activity from **electromyogram (EMG)** recordings, typically, the chin muscles (submental EMG).

Electroencephalographic activity is generally described by the frequency of the measured activity in cycles per second (cps). Frequencies are designated alpha, beta, delta, and theta (Figure 18-1). In addition to these signals, sleep spindles and K-complexes are also used to define sleep stages. *Sleep spindles* are waxing and waning bursts of 11- to 16-Hz (beta) activity lasting 0.5 or more seconds. *K-complexes* are characterized by a well-delineated negative sharp wave immediately followed by a positive component with a duration equal to or greater than 0.5 seconds. The stages of NREM sleep are labeled N1, N2, and N3, with N designating REM sleep.

- During resting wakefulness in the adult with eyes closed, the EEG is characterized by a dominant rhythm in the frequency range of 8 to 13 Hz, or *alpha activity*.
- With the transition to sleep, the rhythm changes to a mixed low-amplitude frequency (4- to 7-Hz *theta activity*), termed *Stage N1 sleep*, the first stage encountered, and is generally short in duration. Sharp vertex waves (sharply contoured waves with duration <0.5 seconds) may be seen. The EOG shows slow, rolling eye movements.
- *Stage N2 sleep* is characterized by the same low-voltage, mixed-frequency activity seen in Stage 1; in this stage, however, sleep spindles or K-complexes or both appear. Eye movements are generally absent.
- *Stage N3* is defined by the presence of delta waves comprising at least 20% of the record and often is referred to as **slow-wave sleep**, or *delta sleep*. Eye movements are absent. Slow-wave sleep is the deepest sleep; in this stage, arousing an individual is much more difficult than in the other stages of sleep. In the R&K manual, slow-wave sleep comprised Stages 3 and 4 sleep, in which Stage 4 sleep was defined as slow-wave activity accounting for 50% or more of the time.

- In *Stage REM* sleep, the EEG pattern is similar to Stage N1 sleep: a relatively low-voltage, mixed-frequency pattern. Unique to REM sleep, however, are phasic periods of rapid eye movements. Alpha activity may also be seen. Also characteristic of REM sleep is a low level of muscle tone compared with other sleep stages, seen as decreased amplitude of the chin EMG. In the REM stage of sleep, most dreaming occurs, and the loss of muscle tone protects against acting out the dreams.

SLEEP ARCHITECTURE

The distinct cycling of sleep stages throughout the night is referred to as the **sleep architecture**. The cycle begins with NREM sleep, progressing from Stage N1 through Stages N2 and N3 and followed by a REM sleep period. The duration of this cycle is approximately 90 minutes. The time from sleep onset to the end of the first REM period is the first sleep cycle. The second and subsequent sleep cycles are the sleep periods between the end of a preceding REM period and the end of the next REM period, including the intervening NREM sleep, which is usually devoid of Stage N1 sleep. An individual typically has four to six sleep cycles during a normal night's sleep.

Brief awakenings generally occur during the night, although the individual is usually unaware of them unless they are of sufficient duration. Figure 18-2 shows the typical normal progression of sleep stages, known as a **sleep histogram**, or hypnogram.

The time it takes for a sleep stage to first occur is termed the "latency" for that stage. Of interest are the sleep onset latency and the latency to the first REM period. The sleep onset latency, or **sleep latency**, is the time it takes from going to bed until Stage N1 sleep occurs. The time between the initial sleep onset and the first REM period is the **REM latency**. These two latencies are typically used to describe abnormal alterations in sleep architecture.

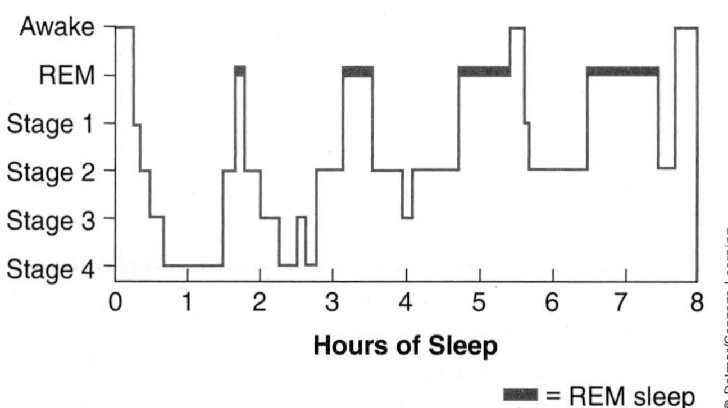

FIGURE 18-2 Hypnogram depicting the normal progression of sleep stages through the night for a normal adult: The solid bars represent the occurrence of REM sleep.

The microstructure of sleep changes significantly over the human lifespan (Figure 18-3). In general, these changes are:

- An increase in sleep latency with age.
- The percentage of Stage N1 increases with age.
- The percentage of Stage N3 decreases with age.
- The percentage of REM sleep decreases with age in adults.

Slow-wave sleep shows the greatest decrease over the lifespan, making up 40% of the total sleep time in early childhood and decreasing steadily until old age. There is also a significant and steady increase in *wake after sleep onset* (*WASO*) over the lifespan.

CARDIOVASCULAR AND RESPIRATORY CHANGES

In normal individuals, measurable changes occur in both respiratory and cardiovascular variables with sleep. Respiratory changes are as follows:

- During NREM sleep and when compared with wakefulness, minute ventilation falls by approximately 0.5–1.5 L/min, primarily owing to a reduction in tidal volume.
- Respiratory rate typically increases.
- Both tidal volume and respiratory rate become stable and rhythmic in slow-wave sleep.
- During REM sleep, the respiratory pattern varies, with most of the variation occurring during phasic REM when bursts of actual rapid eye movements are seen.
- Upper airway resistance increases during sleep as a result of *hypotonia* of the upper airway muscles that normally dilate the airway. During NREM sleep, there is hypotonia of the intercostal muscles with essentially normal function of the diaphragm.
- In contrast, REM sleep is characterized by *atonia* of the intercostal muscles and hypotonia of the diaphragm. The reduced respiratory muscle activity with sleep results in a decreased functional residual capacity.

Cardiovascular changes during sleep can be observed as changes in blood pressure and heart rate.

- Blood pressure falls by 5–14% during NREM sleep and fluctuates during REM sleep.
- Heart rate decreases during NREM sleep and remains stable. However, heart rate can be quite variable in REM sleep and periods of bradycardia may be seen.

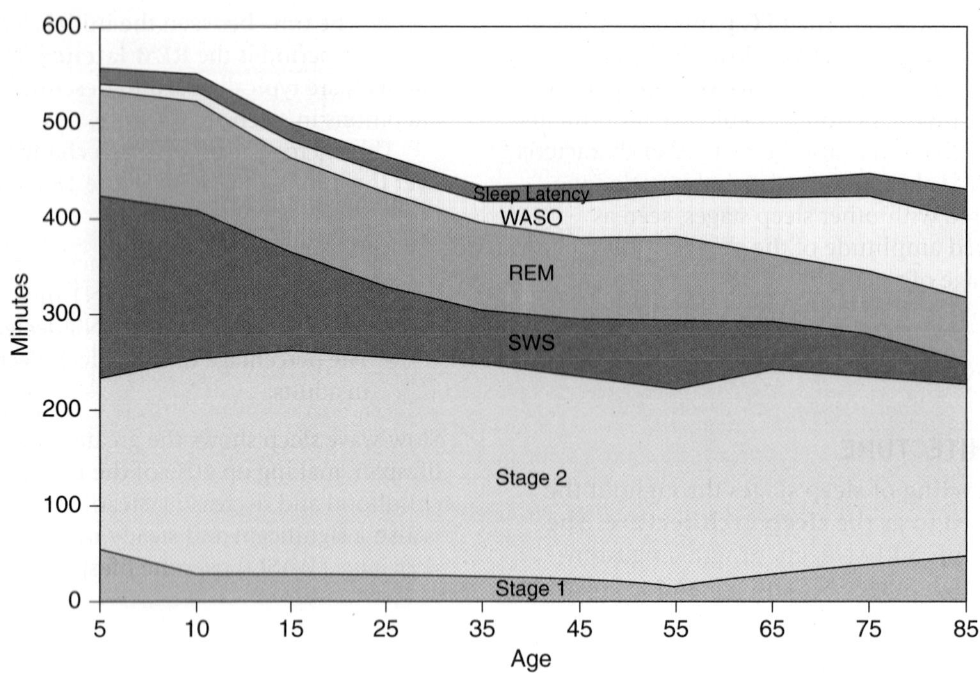

FIGURE 18-3 Age-related trends for Stage N1 sleep, Stage N2 sleep, Stage N3 (slow-wave) sleep, Stage REM sleep, wake after sleep onset (WASO), and sleep latency in minutes. (From Phayon MM, Carskadon MA, Guilleminault C, Vitiello MV, Meta-analysis of quantitative sleep parameters from childhood to old age in healthy individuals: developing normative sleep values across the human lifespan. *Sleep.* 2004;27:1255.)

Sleep Disorders

When sleep is not of sufficient duration (**sleep deprivation**) or when sleep is disturbed by frequent arousals (**sleep fragmentation**), an individual usually complains of **excessive daytime sleepiness (EDS)**, or *hypersomnolence*. Most normal individuals experience occasional EDS; chronic EDS, however, may indicate a pathologic abnormality. A complaint of EDS must be taken seriously because the condition can markedly affect psychosocial function, school performance, and work performance, and it can endanger the individual's and the public's safety.

There are over 84 known sleep disorders. The four most frequently encountered ones are insomnia, sleep disordered breathing, narcolepsy, and restless legs syndrome. For a more in-depth discussion of known sleep disorders, see the *International Classification of Sleep Disorders*.[3]

INSOMNIA

Insomnia is the most prevalent sleep-related complaint. Insomnia can be situational, lasting a few days to weeks, or chronic, lasting more than a month. Almost everyone occasionally suffers from short-term insomnia resulting from stress, jet lag, diet, or many other factors. It is estimated that chronic insomnia affects 9–12% of the population. The causes of insomnia are many and range from psychological to medical, and in some cases the condition is of a primary etiology.

Insomnia is defined as difficulty initiating or maintaining sleep. It can take the form of difficulty initiating sleep after going to bed, difficulty going back to sleep after an awakening, waking up frequently during the night, or waking up early in the morning and being unable to go back to sleep for the rest of the night. Many of the more than 84 known sleep disorders have insomnia as a symptom; in fact, insomnia is as much a symptom as it is a diagnosis. Patients with insomnia frequently report EDS.

SLEEP DISORDERED BREATHING

Sleep disordered breathing (SDB), or **sleep apnea** or hyponea syndrome, is by far the most common diagnosis in patients presenting to a sleep disorders clinic. Sleep disordered breathing is categorized as either central or obstructive, depending on the physiological mechanism involved. **Central sleep apnea** results from a transient failure of the central respiratory system to activate inspiratory effort.

Obstructive sleep apnea (OSA) is a continued effort to breathe against an occluded airway (apnea) or partially occluded airway (hypopnea). This obstruction can include:

- Soft tissue occlusion of the airway, as might be caused by an extremely elongated soft palate, large tonsils and adenoids, an edematous uvula, and occasionally macroglossia (large tongue).
- Craniofacial abnormalities that result in the narrowing of the oropharyngeal space.
- Nasal pharyngeal abnormalities, such as a deviated nasal septum, large or swollen turbinates, or allergic nasal polyps, which increase upper airway resistance, leading to more negative airway pressures and promoting the collapse of the airway.

OSA is by far the most common form of sleep apnea. The collapse of the upper airway leads to an increase in respiratory effort, which in turn leads to an arousal or an awakening. This cycle of apnea followed by arousal or awakening can occur hundreds of times each night, resulting in sleep fragmentation and presenting as EDS.

In addition to EDS, sleep apnea has other physiological consequences. With OSA, the repeated obstruction of the airway and associated large negative intrathoracic pressures lead to predictable hemodynamic changes. Additional effects may be seen in patients who have significant hypoxemia (Table 18-1).

- Many of these hemodynamic effects are magnified when chronic lung disease is also present.
- OSA has been linked to increased risk for cardiovascular disease, arrhythmias, and stroke.

TABLE 18-1 **Potential cardiovascular effects of obstructive sleep disordered breathing**

Systemic hypertension
Pulmonary hypertension
Ventricular hypertrophy
Serious arrhythmias
Sinus bradycardia
Asystoles
Second-degree antrioventricular block
Runs of ventricular tachycardia
Myocardial infarction
Aggravation of existing cardiac problems
Stroke
Increased release of atrial natriuretic peptide
Death

- Patients with OSA have 2 to 3 times greater odds of having systemic hypertension.
- The incidence of pulmonary hypertension is also increased, likely the result of the acute cyclic hemodynamic changes associated with the repeated obstructive events.
- There is a strong association of OSA with myocardial infarction.
- OSA has been shown to be an independent risk factor for atrial fibrillation.
- There is growing evidence for the involvement of OSA and sleep loss in general in the development of glucose intolerance and insulin resistance.

NARCOLEPSY

Narcolepsy is a disorder of the central nervous system of unknown origin (i.e., idiopathic), characterized primarily by severe EDS. Secondary symptoms, which may or may not be present, are cataplexy, sleep paralysis, and hypnagogic hallucinations.

- **Cataplexy** is a sudden loss of muscle tone, typically triggered by emotion, such as happiness, excitement, or anger. The loss of muscle tone may be extensive, causing the individual to fall down, or it may be very subtle and indiscernible, merely causing an eyelid to droop. Many experts feel that cataplexy must be present for a diagnosis of narcolepsy.
- **Sleep paralysis** is total-body paralysis, with the exception of respiration and eye movements. It can last from seconds to minutes and can initially be very frightening to the individual.
- **Hypnagogic** (occurring during the transition from wakefulness to sleep) hallucinations are characterized as extremely vivid, often frightening dreams that may be associated with sleep paralysis. Hallucinations may also occur upon awakening **(hypnogogic)**.

The sleep of patients with narcolepsy is typically fragmented. A classic finding with this disorder is the early occurrence of REM sleep—frequently within minutes—after sleep onset.

Narcolepsy usually begins to appear in adolescence or early adulthood, although the initial onset can occur in early childhood or later in adult life. A period of progressive onset is usually followed by a fairly stable course with rarely any remission in symptoms. There is a known genetic basis for narcolepsy, and the risk for narcolepsy is much higher for children of narcoleptics and first-degree relatives than for individuals without a family history of narcolepsy.

RESTLESS LEGS SYNDROME

Restless legs syndrome (RLS) is a neurological disorder that is characterized by four specific complaints.

- An urge to move, usually a result of uncomfortable sensations in the legs, described as creeping, burning, itching, pulling, or tugging.
- The most uncomfortable symptoms when the individual is at rest, only partially relieved by moving the affected extremity.
- The worse symptoms in the evening and early part of the night than during the day.
- Relief from the discomfort by moving, particularly walking.

A feature frequently associated with RLS is **periodic limb movements in sleep (PLMS)**. Periodic limb movements are stereotypical, repetitive movements that occur most frequently during the first half of the night. They are usually found during NREM sleep and are uncommon in REM sleep. Most patients with RLS exhibit PLMS, but patients with no RLS symptoms can also have PLMS. Although periodic limb movements in sleep may occur at any age, the frequency increases dramatically in the elderly.

The Polysomnogram

Polysomnography involves the use of equipment and techniques to produce a recording of sleep data, called the **polysomnogram**. The type of equipment used to collect physiological data varies considerably. However, certain approaches to collecting and processing data are common to all types of equipment:

- EEG, EOG, and EMG
- Respiratory airflow and effort
- Arterial oxygen saturation
- Electrocardiogram

Table 18-2 shows those parameters typically measured with a standard polysomnogram. (Refer to *The AASM Manual for the Scoring of Sleep and Associated Events* for additional information.) A clinical practice guideline (CPG) published by the American Association for Respiratory Care outlines the generally accepted standards of practice for polysomnography.[4]

EEG, EOG, AND EMG

EEG. The AASM guidelines recommend the monitoring of at least three EEG channels for staging sleep. EEG is monitored by placing electrodes on the scalp according to the international 10–20 system of electrode placement.[5] In this neurodiagnostic procedure, electrodes are placed at equally spaced locations on the scalp, using identifiable skull landmarks (Figure 18-4). The electrodes are labeled according to:

- Their location: for example, F for frontal, C for central, and O for occipital.
- The side of the scalp. Even numbers designate the right side, and odd numbers designate the left side. Numbers are larger farther from the midline.

So C_4 would designate the central electrode on the right side farther from the midline.

The electrodes are then referenced to a second electrode, either at the left mastoid process (designated M_1) or at the right mastoid process (designated M_2), but always on the opposite side. [This positioning

TABLE 18-2 **Parameters typically recorded on a standard polysomnogram**

Channel*	Parameter
1	EEG (central lead)
2	EEG (occipital lead)
3	EOG (right eye)
4	EOG (left eye)
5	EMG (chin)
6	EMG (right leg)
7	EMG (left leg)
8	ECG
9	Airflow
10	Thoracic effort
11	Abdominal effort
12	Arterial oxygen saturation

**Additional channels may include snoring, position, and CPAP pressure, as well as back-up EEG channels.*

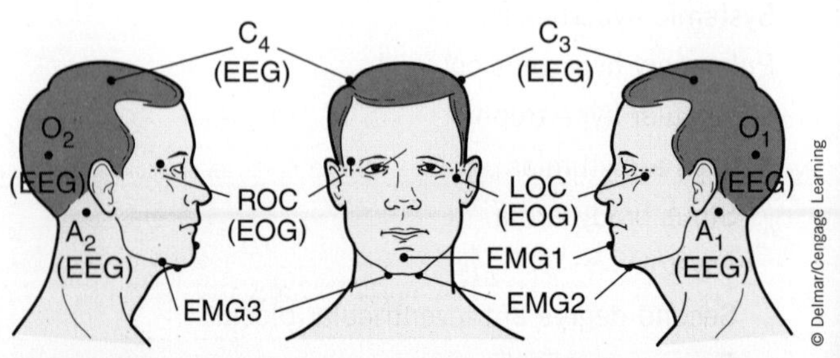

FIGURE 18-4 Standard placement of EEG, EOG, and EMG leads used in sleep studies: EEG electrodes are designated and placed according to the international 10–20 system. Note the placement of one eye electrode slightly above and one slightly below the horizontal center of the eyes. ROC = right outer canthus; LOC = left outer canthus.

creates a reference point—like longitude and latitude—and completes an electrical circuit to allow measurement of electrical potential across the distance (C4−M1).] Thus, C_4 would be reference to M_1 (designated C_4-M_1). The recommended derivations for scoring sleep are F_4-M_1, C_4-M_1, and O_2-M_1. Backup electrodes are usually applied with derivations of F_3-M_2, C_3-M_2, and O_1-M_2. The frontal electrode is preferred for detecting sleep-wave activity, and the occipital electrode is best for detecting awake alpha activity.

EOG Rapid eye movements characterize REM sleep, and slow eye movements generally accompany the transition from wakefulness to sleep as well as the transition back to Stage 1 during sleep. An electropotential exists from the front to the back of the eye; the front is positive with respect to the back. Eyeball movement produces spatial changes in this potential. The EOG electrodes are therefore typically applied to the outer canthus of each eye, one slightly above and one slightly below the horizontal plane (Figure 18-4). The two eye electrodes are typically referenced to the same reference electrode (either M_1 or M_2). With this configuration, both vertical and horizontal movements of the eyes are detected and appear opposite in polarity (out of phase) on the recording. This arrangement facilitates the differentiation of real eye movements from artifact because any EEG interference appears as in-phase potentials.

EMG. The chin EMG facilitates detection of REM sleep and helps distinguish the waking state from REM sleep. Typically three electrodes are placed: One electrode is placed in the midline 1 cm above the inferior edge of the mandible. The other two are placed 2 cm below the inferior edge of the mandible and 2 cm to the right and left of the midline. Either of the inferior electrodes is referenced to the midline electrode. The third electrode serves as a backup in case one fails during the study (Figure 18-4).

RESPIRATORY AIRFLOW AND EFFORT

Because sleep disordered breathing is a frequently diagnosed disorder in the sleep laboratory, a vital part of standard polysomnography is monitoring the breathing pattern, which is accomplished by measuring airflow and respiratory effort. Pneumotachometers provide a quantitative measure of airflow, but they are bulky and must be attached to a mask. They are not comfortable for the patient and can interfere with sleep quality. So, historically, airflow has been monitored using *temperature-detecting sensors*, either thermistors or thermocouples. These sensors detect the temperature difference between inspiration (room temperature) and expiration (body temperature) and produce a change in voltage proportional to temperature change. These types of devices do not provide a quantitative assessment of airflow but are preferred because of their small size for patient comfort and their simplicity of operation. These types of sensors are best at detecting the absence of airflow (apnea).

More recently, *nasal pressure monitoring* has been used to monitor airflow. The system used to measure nasal pressure consists of a nasal cannula connected to a pressure transducer. Nasal pressure is positive during expiration and negative during inspiration. Nasal pressure is directly proportional to airflow and thus is more sensitive to changes in airflow than thermistors or thermocouples. The AASM recommends nasal pressure monitoring for detecting hypopneas.

Although several techniques are available to monitor respiratory effort, the two most frequently used methods are piezoelectric transducers and inductance plethysmography. *Piezoelectric technology*, a fairly recent addition, uses crystals that produce an electrical current when squeezed. These crystals are attached to bands that go around the patient's chest and abdomen. When the band is stretched, the crystals are squeezed, producing a small current that is amplified by the polygraph. The amount of current produced is directly related to the circumference changes of the thorax and abdomen.

Inductance plethysmography uses a transducer composed of an insulated wire sewn in sinusoid shape onto an elastic band. One band is placed around the thorax and one around the abdomen. Changes in lung volume produce changes in the cross-sectional areas of the rib cage and abdomen, which translate into changes in the diameter of the bands. Changing the diameter of the bands directly affects their self-inductance properties, providing an output proportional to effort. This type of technology can quantify airflow at the mouth by summing the rib cage and abdominal signals using a unique calibration protocol. Inductance transducers are configured to deliver either calibrated or uncalibrated signals.

The AASM guidelines recommend using either esophageal manometry or inductance phethysmography for monitoring effort. *Esophageal manometry* (esophageal pressure monitoring) involves inserting a balloon-tipped catheter into the esophagus. The catheter is connected to a pressure transducer. Pressure changes in the esophagus reflect intrathoracic pressure changes, which represents effort. Esophageal manometry is considered the gold standard for measuring effort. However, most patients do not tolerate the technique well due to its invasive nature of this form of monitoring. The AASM recommends *inductance plethysmography* as the standard technique for monitoring

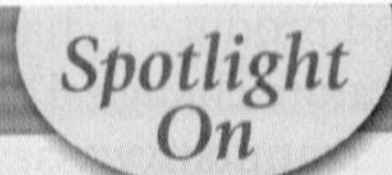

Airflow Monitoring

Since the 1970s, when polysomnography began to be used in the clinical detection of sleep apnea, thermistors and thermocouples were the primary sensors for monitoring airflow. Because these types of sensors monitor the temperature changes between inspiration and expiration, they provide only a qualitative indicator of airflow. It was later realized that these types of airflow sensors were poor at detecting hypopneas (reduced airflow). In the late 1990s and early 2000s, devices designed to measure nasal pressure changes during inspiration and expiration were developed. They began to replace thermistors and thermocouples as the primary airflow-measuring device in many sleep laboratories. These devices gave a more quantitative measure of airflow and were able to detect reductions in airflow similar to that provided by a pneumotachometer. However, for large reductions in airflow, the pressure change was difficult to detect, and many hypopneas were classified as apneas. As a result, in 2007, the AASM recommended both thermal detectors and nasal airflow transducers in the detection of respiratory conditions: thermistor/thermocouples for detecting apneas and nasal pressure devices for detecting hypopneas.

effort as piezo belts are not felt to give a satisfactory refection of respiratory effort.

ARTERIAL OXYGEN SATURATION

The measurement of arterial oxygen saturation is vital to determining the severity of obstructive sleep disordered breathing or the presence of alveolar hypoventilation. *Oximeters* (or more accurately pulse oximeters) measure the relative absorbance of two wavelengths of light: infrared and near infrared. This measurement allows the determination of total hemoglobin and oxygenated hemoglobin that is read out as a percentage saturation of arterial blood, commonly designated as S_PO_2. *Pulse oximetry* is the oximeter's ability to analyze the difference between light absorbed by the tissues and light absorbed by blood that is pulsing through the vascular bed with each heartbeat. The pulsing value represents oxygen saturation. To ensure accuracy, anyone using pulse oximetry to monitor oxygenation must be aware of the following issues:

- Oximeters are unable to distinguish between hemoglobin bound with oxygen and hemoglobin bound with carbon monoxide. As a result, the reading for oxygen saturation in patients with elevated carboxyhemoglobin levels, such as smokers, can be artificially high.
- Impaired systemic circulation may give false readings.
- Pigmented skin may affect the oximeter reading. Newer technology has greatly reduced this problem.
- There is a delay between the time blood passes through the lung and the time it reaches the oximeter probe, which is usually placed on the ear or finger. This delay results in a change in saturation 6–30 seconds after the decrease in ventilation is seen on the polysomnogram recording.

Pulse oximetry has become the standard for monitoring oxygenation in all types of patients in many situations. It is well suited for monitoring saturation during sleep, specifically for detecting arterial oxygen desaturation associated with apneas and hypopneas in sleep disordered breathing.

ELECTROCARDIOGRAM

A single-channel electrocardiogram (ECG) is typically included with polysomnography to monitor heart rate and rhythm. Typically, either ECG electrodes or standard cup electrodes (used for EEG, EOG, and EMG) are employed, with one electrode placed below the right clavicle and a second electrode placed on the left side at about the level of the seventh rib.

The Polysomnographic Recording

The individual physiological signals must be amplified and conditioned for display. Amplification and conditioning are typically accomplished with a multichannel recording system, referred to as a **polygraph**, configured to meet the requirements for sleep studies. The number of channels of information that can be processed varies and is usually dictated by the sleep laboratory requirements. Regardless of the specific type of instrumentation used, to produce a quality recording, technologists must understand several important capabilities of sleep recording equipment.

SENSITIVITY

Sensitivity is the ratio of signal voltage to the amount of deflection observed on the recording device. A standard sensitivity for bioelectrical signals (EEG, EOG, EMG) is 7 μV/mm; that is, every 7 μV of bioelectrical activity causes the displayed signal to move vertically 1 mm. Sensitivity is equal to input voltage (microvolts) divided by the output deflection on the display (millimeters). Because input activity can vary considerably, a number of increasing sensitivity settings are available to obtain the best display. As the microvolts per millimeter sensitivity values decrease, signal amplification increases. Thus, 1 μV/mm is highly sensitive, whereas 50 μV/mm represents a very low sensitivity. A sensitivity of mill volts per centimeter of display deflection can record stronger electrical potentials, such as those recorded on the electrocardiogram (ECG).

FREQUENCY FILTERS

Frequency filters eliminate or attenuate **artifact**, that is, activity from the bioelectrical signal that interferes with or distorts the desired signal. Three types of filters are typically employed.

- A **low-frequency filter** minimizes unwanted low-frequency artifact such as swaying of the EEG caused by respiration, perspiration, and motion. A typical setting is 0.3 Hz.
- **High-frequency filters** filter out any high-frequency artifact. A setting of 35–70 Hz is generally used. The specific filter setting chosen reduces the activity at that particular frequency by 20%. As the signal frequencies increase (as with high-frequency filters) or decrease (as with low-frequency filters), the signal is attenuated.
- The third type of filter is a *60-Hz notch filter*, which sharply attenuates frequencies between 58 and 62 Hz. This filter reduces the 60-Hz activity from AC electrical interference. Activity outside the 58–62 Hz range is barely affected. Sixty-hertz filters should not be routinely used. In most cases, 60-Hz artifact can be eliminated through proper electrode application and good amplifier operation. An exception is when recording in an electrically active environment, such as an intensive care unit.

CALIBRATION

Calibration checks the accuracy of a recording device. A calibration check should be performed both before and after the PSG recording. Typically, a device has a calibration button with a known voltage, such as 50 μV. When this known signal is used, the effect of the instrumentation on the bioelectrical signal can be evaluated. Pushing the calibration button introduces a positive signal and causes an upward deflection; releasing the button causes a downward deflection. Thus the polarity of the signal is checked. In addition, introducing a known calibration signal of 50 μV/mm with a sensitivity setting of 7 μV/mm should produce a display signal with an amplitude of 7 mm. The display amplitude should be plus or minus 5% of the expected amplitude.

Make sure that extreme filter settings are not set. Use high-frequency filters of 70 Hz or low-frequency filters of 1 Hz or less. At the end of the study, a calibration check is performed at the final sensitivity and filter settings used during the study.

Recording and Monitoring During the Night

After completion of the patient hookup, the patient should make preparations for bed, including such rituals as brushing teeth and using the restroom. When the patient is in bed and comfortable, all electrodes and other monitoring devices should be plugged into the polygraph interface box, commonly called a *jack box*. Inform the patient at this time that the patient:

- Should feel free to change position at any time during the night.
- Will be monitored throughout the recording period.
- Should use the intercom or other communication system (and should be instructed on how to use it).
- Should call whenever he or she needs to use the restroom or has any other problem or request.
- Should let the sleep technologist disconnect electrodes if he or she needs to get up.

Also at this time, perform any other required procedures: blood pressure and temperature measurements, presale questionnaire, and so on.

PATIENT CALIBRATION

The next step is **patient calibration**, or biological calibration, which:

- Identifies any problems with the recording system.
- Allows repair before the test begins.
- Provides qualitative signals that can be used later to facilitate accurate analysis of the record.

Patient calibration is performed immediately before lights-out. Ask the patient to lie quietly face up and listen for instructions, which vary depending on the types of biological signals being recorded. For a standard PSG, the instructions typically consist of the following:

- "With your eyes open, look straight ahead." Have the patient maintain this state for 30 seconds without moving.

- "Please close your eyes and lie very still." Have the patient hold this position for 30 seconds. This procedure allows a baseline reading of alpha activity when the patient is awake and relaxed with eyes closed, as may occur during the recording. The technologist must verify that the patient's eyes are closed during this period.
- "Open your eyes and, without moving your head, look to the right, look to the left, look up, look down, relax." This step ensures that the EOG signals are deflecting appropriately (out of phase). It also characterizes the pattern of slow, rolling eye movements that typically occur during the transition from wakefulness through Stage 1 sleep.
- "Holding your head still, blink your eyes slowly five times." This step allows recognition of blink artifact, to differentiate wakefulness from REM sleep.
- "Grit your teeth, and then relax." This step should produce an increase in the EMG activity and should note muscle artifact in both the EOG and EMG signals.
- "Inhale and hold your breath . . . . Now exhale and breathe normally." This step allows you to calibrate respiratory channels.
- "Flex your right ankle, relax. Now flex your left ankle, relax." This step calibrates the anterior tibialis EMG channels.

During each of these calibration procedures, record the type of activity performed.

Throughout the process of patient hook-up and calibration, the patient should not be allowed to fall asleep. Keeping a hypersomnolent patient awake may be difficult, and, on occasion, patient calibration may be impossible because of the patient's inability to maintain wakefulness.

After patient calibration, ask the patient to get comfortable and then turn out the lights.

RECORDING PROCEDURES

The sleep therapist's responsibility is to ensure that a quality polysomnographic recording is obtained. Constant vigilance is also needed to identify and correct problems with the recording equipment and electrodes, to document any observations that would affect later analysis and interpretation of the data, and to recognize any patient safety issues such as life-threatening arrhythmias or unsafe activities. The therapist accomplishes all this by monitoring the PSG recording and using other monitoring equipment such as video and sound equipment to observe the patient.

Sleep laboratories typically use some form of standardized documentation to record routine interval checks. For example, a half-hour check sheet may be used to record various physiological parameters observed, such as stage of sleep, heart rate, arterial oxygen saturation, the presence of respiratory events, arrhythmias, arousals, and so on.

In addition, the technologist should note on the recording whenever:

- The recording is altered in any way, for example, changes made in sensitivity, filter settings, and electrode configuration.
- Any patient activity is required to accurately analyze the data—for example, coughing, moving, position changes, talking while asleep.
- Anything else happens that may affect the evaluation of the data, such as external noises, a therapist entering the room to make repairs, or any other necessary intervention.

At the conclusion of the recording period, awaken the patient. Be sure to caution the patient before turning on the lights. Perform a post-test patient calibration at this time along, with any post-test measurements such as blood pressure. A posttest questionnaire assessing the patient's perceived quality of sleep and alertness, as well as any experiences the

Age-Specific Competency

Although the general procedures for performing polysomnography for children are similar to those for adults, children present with a wide range of physical, developmental, and behavioral challenges that must be considered during polysomnography. In addition, a child may be easily frightened by the unfamiliarity of the sleep laboratory and the attachment of numerous monitoring devices. Thus, personnel performing the study should be:

- Skilled in dealing with the specific needs of infants, children, and adolescents.
- Demonstrate knowledge of childhood behavior.
- Be able to deal with the emotional responses likely to be encountered.
- Understand the differences in procedural protocol between children and adults, such as timing of the study and techniques for placement and securing of monitoring devices.
- Be certified in pediatric cardiopulmonary resuscitation.

Best Practice

Technologist Responsibilities

Because polysomnography is a diagnostic test, the technologist is responsible for ensuring the quality of information and for documenting all observations that may be important in the interpretation of the results. Generally, each technologist monitors no more than two patients at a time. Monitoring more than two patients increases the chance of missing important observations or of failing to keep a complete record during the study. Monitoring should be limited to only one patient per technologist in situations in which frequent intervention is anticipated, such as with very ill patients, mentally disadvantaged patients, and small children.

patient had that may have interfered with sleep, is commonly completed. Highly recommended is the therapist's summary of the nighttime activity, including any unusual occurrences, recording difficulties, or other factors that may affect the interpretation of the results such as the use of a fan, open window, or elevation of the head of the bed.

A typical PSG record consists of 14 or more channels of data collected over 6–8 hours. The process of **scoring** reduces the recorded PSG data to a meaningful summary or, put another way, assigns values and meaning to a series of physiological waveforms. These values, used in combination with other observations of unusual events, are used to interpret the study. Thus, scoring:

- Identifies the stages of sleep.
- Quantifies respiratory events.
- Quantifies leg movements.
- Identifies any other abnormalities noted in the record.
- Establishes other indices of sleep quality such as the degree of sleep fragmentation, which can explain symptoms of daytime sleepiness.

STAGING SLEEP

Identifying the stages of sleep, or staging sleep, is based on the criteria initially described by Rechtschaffen and Kales and subsequently revised by the AASM. Sleep is broken down into consecutive 30-second periods called **epochs** to facilitate scoring. Each epoch is staged independently based on the following general rules:

- If criteria exists that meets the definition for more than one stage is present in an epoch, the stage that consumes the greatest portion of the epoch is recorded.
- Scoring Stage N1 requires a clear, discernible slowing of the EEG tracings and an evident onset of theta activity for more than 50% of the epoch. Slow rolling eye movements may or may not be present but, if present, aids in the scoring of N1.
- Score Stage N2 sleep if one or both of the following wave activities occur during the first half of the epoch or the last half of the preceding epoch:
  - One or more K complexes unassociated with arousals
  - One or more sleep spindles
- Score Stage N3 sleep when 20% or more of an epoch consists of slow-wave activity.
- Score Stage R sleep when the EEG is a low-amplitude, mixed-frequency with low chin EMG tone, and rapid eye movements are present

Becoming proficient at staging normal sleep takes time and practice, and accurately staging abnormal sleep takes even longer. Consult the AASM's scoring manual for a more in-depth description of the scoring rules.

IDENTIFYING AROUSALS

Many sleep disorders involve frequent, brief arousals that result in excessive daytime sleepiness. Arousals occur frequently in patients with sleep disordered breathing, periodic limb movement disorder, and many other sleep disorders. Assessing the frequency of arousals is important in establishing the cause of EDS. Arousal can occur in all stages of sleep.

An *arousal* can be defined as any clearly visible abrupt shift of EEG frequency, including alpha, theta, and/or frequencies greater than 16 Hz (that are not spindles) that last as least 3 seconds. There must be at least 10 seconds of stable sleep preceding the change. To score an arousal in REM sleep, there must be a concurrent increase in submental (chin) EMG lasting at least one second. Arousals are summed and reported as an arousal index (number of arousals per hour of sleep).

QUANTIFYING RESPIRATORY EVENTS

To establish a diagnosis of sleep disordered breathing, an abnormal respiratory pattern has to be demonstrated. The **respiratory disturbance index (RDI)**, commonly called the **apnea/hypopnea index (AHI)**, is the universal method used to establish a diagnosis of sleep disordered breathing. Respiratory events are generally categorized as either a hypopnea or an apnea on the basis of specific criteria.

Age-Specific Competency

The rules for scoring sleep stages and respiratory events for children may vary significantly from those for adults. Infants younger than 6 months have continuous developmental aspects with respect to their central nervous system. Scoring of sleep and wakefulness is based on both behavioral and polysomnographic characteristics. In general, the sleep of infants younger than 2 months is classified as either quiet sleep, active sleep, or indeterminate sleep. Behavioral observations are necessary in differentiating between wakefulness and sleep. The scoring of sleep in infants and children at 2 months of age and older is based on adult scoring rules with some modifications that account for the developmental aspects of the infant.

The scoring of sleep-related respiratory events is also affected because children differ from adults both physiologically and in the way sleep-related upper airway obstruction is manifested. Healthy children rarely have obstructive respiratory events during sleep, so all obstructive apneas, regardless of length, are regarded as significant. During scoring:

- Central apneas greater than 20 seconds that are not related to a sigh or to movement should be scored.
- Central apneas less than 20 seconds should be scored if the duration is at least two standard breaths and a decrease in saturation of 3% or greater.
- An obstructive apnea is scored when the apnea lasts at least two standard breaths and there is a drop in baseline flow of greater than 90%.
- Score respiratory hypopneas when there is a 50% or greater decrease in nasal or oral airflow amplitude and the duration is equal to or greater than 2 breaths.

Measurement of end-tidal PCO_2 may be helpful in assessing hypoventilation. If measured, record the peak end-tidal PCO_2 and the duration of the end-tidal PCO_2 that is greater than 50 mm Hg, expressed as a percentage of total sleep time.

Source: American Thoracic Society. Standards and indications for cardiopulmonary sleep studies in children. Am J Respir Crit Care Med. *1996;153:866–878.*

Hypopneas are defined as a reduction in airflow for at least 10 seconds. As mentioned earlier, the AASM rules require the use of nasal pressure monitoring to establish the presence of a hypopnea. The nasal pressure signal amplitude must drop by 30% or more of baseline and be associated with a 4% or greater decrease in saturation.

An **apnea** is the absence of airflow for a minimum of 10 seconds and is scored when the thermal airflow sensor signal has decreased 90% or more of the baseline value that existed prior to the event. Apneas are designated as either a central apnea, obstructive apnea, or mixed apnea (Figure 18-5).

- The apnea is scored as **central apnea** if no effort is detectable in either the chest or abdominal effort signal.
- The apnea is scored as an **obstructive apnea** when there is a paradoxical pattern between the chest and abdominal signals; that is, the signals are out of phase and frequently show increasing amplitude (increasing effort) as the event continues.
- In addition, events classified as **mixed apneas** are routinely reported. These events start off looking like a central apnea; however, recognizable respiratory effort begins to appear during the latter part of the event (Figure 18-5). Mixed apneas must last a minimum of 10 seconds to be scored. Many laboratories consider this type of event to be obstructive and do not report it as a separate type.

Figures 18-6 and 18-7 illustrate the characteristics of central and obstructive apneas and obstructive hypopneas, as would be observed on a standard polysomnogram.

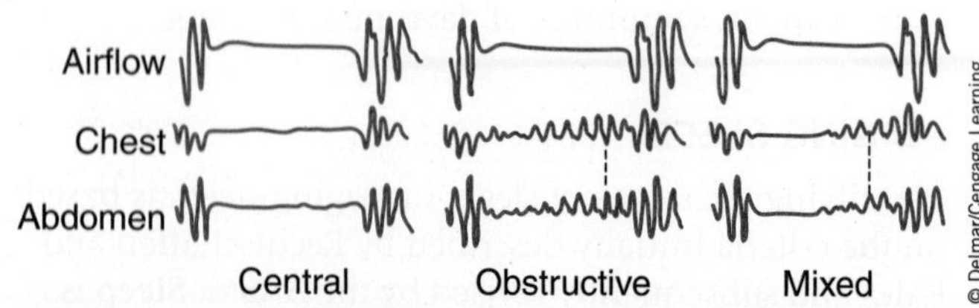

FIGURE 18-5 The three types of respiratory apnea found on a polysomnogram in patients with sleep disordered breathing: Flat lines represent absence of airflow or absence of respiratory effort or both. Vertical dashed lines show that the chest and abdomen are moving in a paradoxical manner.

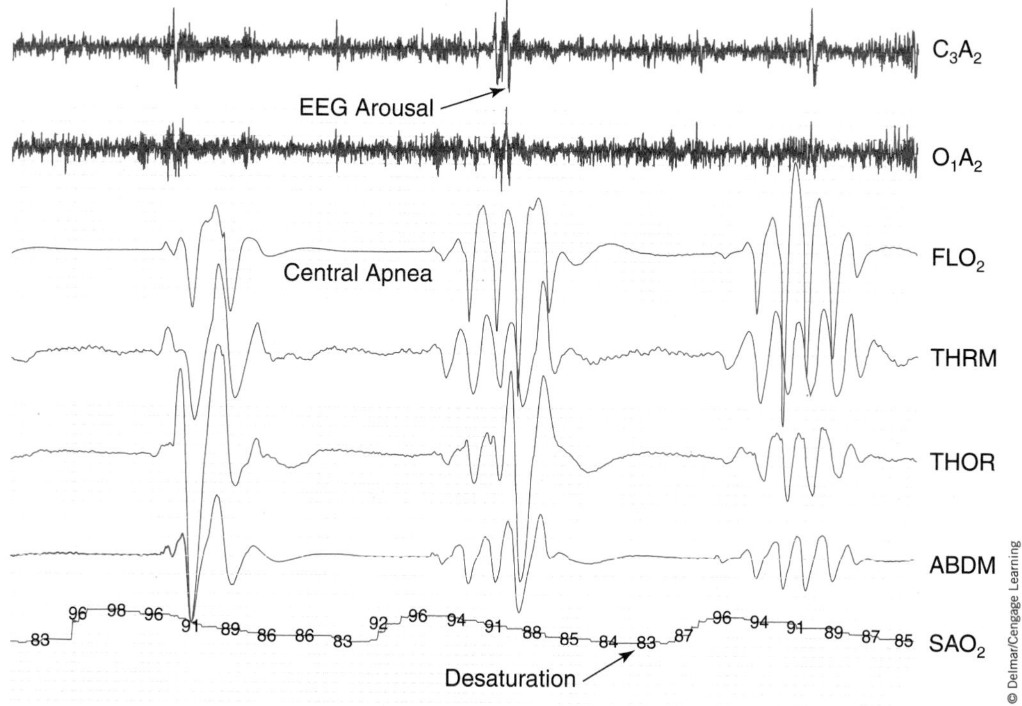

FIGURE 18-6 Example of a central apnea: Airflow is absent in both the nasal pressure (FLO_2) and thermo sensor (THRM). In addition, there is the absence of effort in the thoracic (THOR) and abdominal effort (ABDM) signals, indicating the absence of a neural drive to breath. An associated decrease in saturation is delayed due to the transit time from the lungs to the finger sensor. Central apneas may or may not be associated with an arousal, as indicated in the EEG signal (C_3–A_2).

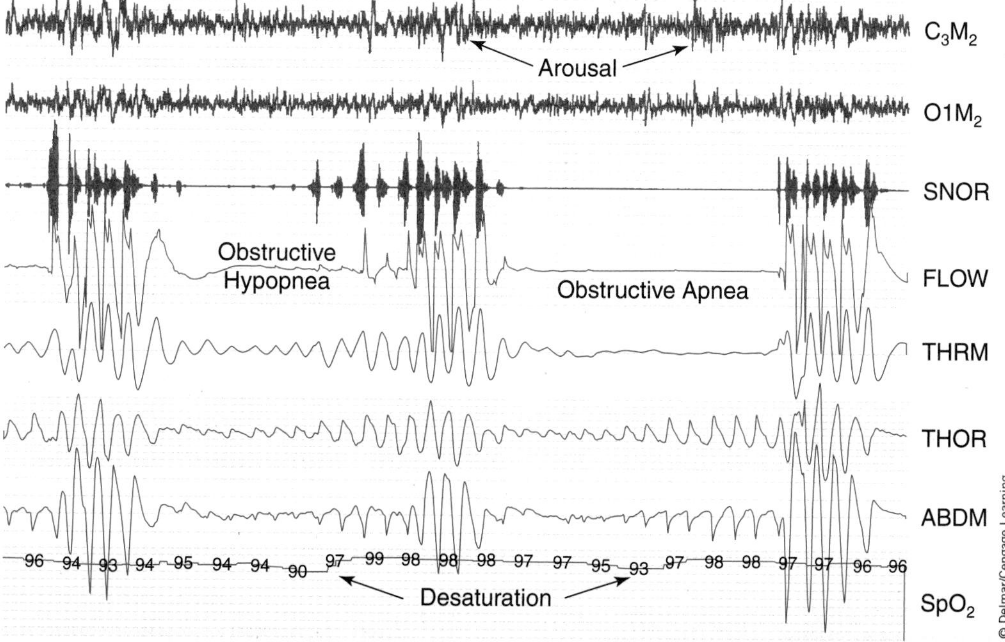

FIGURE 18-7 Example of an obstructive apnea and obstructive hypopnea from a polysomnogram: With an obstructive apnea (right side of figure), airflow is absent in both the nasal pressure and thermo sensor signals, but a continued effort to breathe, as indicated by the progressively increasing amplitude in the thoracic (THOR) and abdomen (ABDM) sensor signals with a typically paradoxical motion of the two effort sensors. An obstructive hypopnea (left side of figure) looks similar to an obstructive apnea except that there is evidence of airflow in the thermo sensor and nasal pressure sensor. Obstructive events are typically terminated with an arousal as evident in the EEG signal (C_3–M_2). An associated decrease in saturation is delayed due to the transit time from the lungs to the finger sensor.

Once the scoring of respiratory events is complete, the total number of each type of event is divided by the total hours of sleep to obtain a frequency index. For example, if 140 obstructive apneas were scored during a study that took a total sleep time of 7.0 hours, the obstructive apnea index would be 20 events per hour of sleep.

When all events are summed and divided by the total sleep time, the respiratory disturbance index (RDI), or apnea/hypopnea index (AHI), is obtained. The RDI is used to define the severity of the disorder.

- A respiratory disturbance index over 5 per hour is considered abnormal.
- An apnea index of 5 to 15 per hour is considered mild.
- An index of 15–30 is considered moderate.
- An index greater than 30 is considered severe.[6]

QUANTIFYING LEG MOVEMENTS

Leg movements or leg jerks are recorded using bioelectrical electrodes placed over the anterior tibialis muscle of both legs. A leg jerk or movement is identified when a burst of leg EMG activity lasts 0.5–10 seconds and has an increase in amplitude of at least 8 μV in EMG voltage above the resting EMG level. Movements occurring synchronously (within less than 5 seconds of each other) are considered one movement. Movements may occur simultaneously in both legs or appear in one leg only. Frequently, movements switch from one leg to the other or occur in both legs but out of phase; this type of movement is referred to as *alternating leg muscle activation* (*ALMA*).

To be used in the assessment of *periodic limb movements in sleep* (*PLMS*), a movement must occur as part of a series of rhythmic jerks with intermovement intervals of 5–90 seconds. There must be a series of at least four movements. PLMS are generally scored as being either associated with or not associated with an arousal or an awakening. An overall PLMS index (number of movements per hour of sleep) is typically reported, and an index of greater than 5 per hour of sleep is considered pathologic.

Best Practice

Reporting Data

There is generally a uniform approach to preparing a final report.

- Data are usually presented in either a tabulated or a narrative form or in a combination of the two formats. At minimum, presented data should show the time in bed, total sleep time, and the time spent in the various sleep stages.
- Other data—such as respiratory events (RDI, type and number of events, saturation levels), cardiovascular events (occurrence of arrhythmias), and limb movements—are included when relevant. The extent of data included in the report may vary considerably among sleep laboratories.
- Finally, the sleep disorders clinician renders a narrative conclusion, relating the findings from the polysomnogram to a final diagnosis.

CASE STUDY 18-1

J. G., a 43-year-old male with a complaint of excessive daytime sleepiness, was referred to the sleep disorders center for evaluation. His history and physical examination showed a morbidly obese male with disruptive snoring, a large neck, a large soft palate, and systemic hypertension. A nocturnal polysomnogram was performed with the following results:

Sleep latency	20 minutes
REM latency	294 minutes
Slow-wave sleep	2%
Sleep efficiency	88%
RDI	38/h
Mean arterial oxygen saturation	94%
Percentage time with saturation less than 85%	8.5%
Arousal index	52/h
PLMS index	2/h

Questions

1. On the basis of these data, what primary sleep disorder is present? Can the severity be classified?
2. Do the data suggest the presence of a second sleep disorder?
3. Is there significant sleep disturbance? On what data is the decision based?

Nasal Continuous Positive Pressure Therapy

Obstructive sleep disordered breathing is by far the most common sleep disorder encountered in the sleep disorders laboratory. Although a number of interventions exist to treat this disorder—such as weight loss, positional training, oral appliance, and surgical intervention—the most effective and accepted form of therapy is **continuous positive airway pressure (CPAP)**. With this form of therapy, first described in 1981, a positive pressure, established in the patient's airway, acts as a pneumatic splint to prevent the airway from collapsing.

A blower that establishes airflow is attached via a length of wide-bore tubing to the patient's airway. Interfaces such as masks or nasal prongs are used. A positive pressure is generated through changes in airflow and resistance within the system (Figure 18-8). Most CPAP systems can deliver pressures from 2 to 20 cm H_2O. Pressure is controlled either by adjusting the speed of the blower fan or by a valve in the blower housing that controls the amount of flow delivered to the patient's airway.

An important requirement of a CPAP system is venting to allow exhaled gas to be flushed from the patient interface, thus preventing rebreathing. Venting is typically accomplished by establishing a vent hole in the patient interface that provides a leak of at least 10–15 Lpm at low CPAP pressures. This amount is sufficient to flush the system of all exhaled carbon dioxide.

CPAP TITRATION

Obstructive sleep disordered breathing is a complex disorder. The nature of the obstruction varies among individuals and depends on structural and functional abnormalities, positional effects, sleep stage, weight, and behavioral factors such as alcohol consumption. As a result, the level of positive pressure required to eliminate upper airway obstruction also varies among individuals. The therapeutic or effective CPAP pressure is determined through titration.

Typically, CPAP titration is performed with full polysomnography (PSG) on a second night after the patient's initial diagnostic evaluation. Performing full PSG along with CPAP titration allows an objective assessment of the most effective pressure for eliminating all evidence of upper airway obstruction and for verifying the effect on sleep quality. Of equal importance is the presence of an experienced sleep technologist, who can influence how well a patient responds to CPAP therapy.

- Sleeping with a mask over the nose and the pressure sensation encountered during CPAP can lead to significant anxiety. An experienced technologist can explain CPAP, decrease anxiety, and increase cooperation.
- An experienced technologist is required to determine the best type of airway interface and to ensure an appropriate fit, both very important in the patient's acceptance of CPAP.
- The technologist manually titrates pressure upward when evidence of obstruction persists and validates that all evidence of flow limitation is absent at the optimal pressure.
- Technologist intervention may be required during titration to correct leaks, add humidification if needed, and address any concerns or side effects the patient may experience.

These topics are discussed in more detail in the following sections.

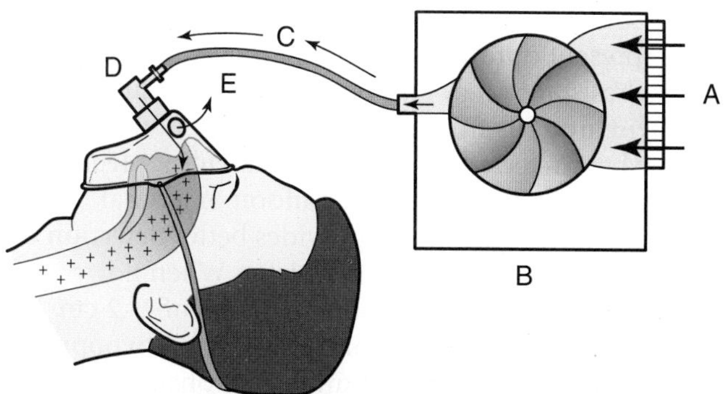

FIGURE 18-8 A nasal CPAP system and the mechanism by which airway obstruction is prevented: (A) Entrainment of room air through a filter. (B) Blower unit capable of delivering a high airflow that enables a constant positive pressure output during respiration. (C) Wide-bore tubing. (D) Nasal mask. (E) Vent allowing washout of deadspace in the mask to prevent rebreathing. + = positive pressure in airway produced by nasal CPAP.

Patient Education. Explaining CPAP, how it works, and its possible side effects—all before beginning the treatment—goes a long way in getting the patient to accept this form of therapy. Some patients want to touch or examine the equipment. The videos provided by equipment manufacturers are an excellent medium for educating the patient about obstructive sleep disordered breathing and CPAP therapy. The technologist should also be available to answer the patient's questions.

Choosing the Airway Interface. Once the patient becomes knowledgeable about CPAP, the next step is to determine the most suitable airway interface. Three general types of interface are available (Figure 18-9):

- A nasal mask that encircles and seals around the patient's nose.

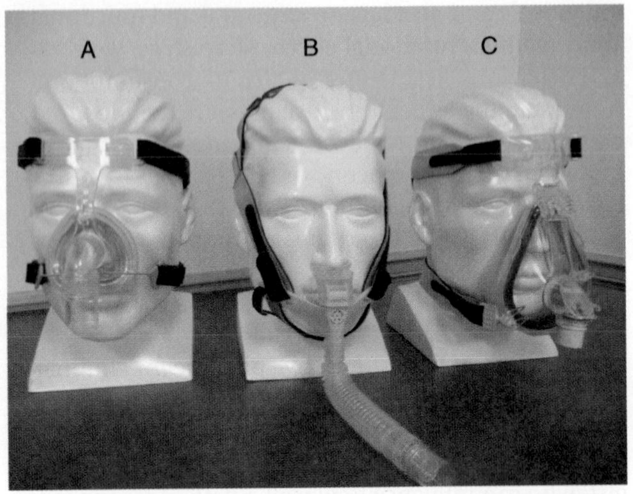

FIGURE 18-9 Three common styles of CPAP mask: (A) Nasal mask. (B) Nasal pillows or prongs. (C) Full face mask.

- Nasal prongs or bellows that form a seal at the opening to the nacres.
- An oral-nasal mask (full-face mask) that encircles both the nose and the mouth.

The nasal mask and nasal prongs are the most frequently used. Which one is selected as the interface usually depends on patient preference; however, the use of one type over the other may be based on its ability to provide a seal and thus effective therapy. In some circumstances, a patient may be intolerant of the nasal mask or nasal prongs, or the mask or nasal prongs may not provide an adequate seal. Or the patient may have a problem keeping the mouth closed while asleep, leading to an inadequate positive pharyngeal pressure or significant sleep disruption. In many cases, a chinstrap, available from some CPAP equipment manufacturers, may help keep the mouth closed. However, a chinstrap may not be effective, and, in some cases, an oral-nasal mask should be considered. Full-face masks are less likely to be accepted because they may induce claustrophobia.

Other considerations in choosing the type of interface are risk of aspiration if the patient should vomit and the theoretical concern of limited ability to breathe if the machine should fail. Safety valves should be present in the circuit close to the patient in the event of machine failure to allow the patient to breathe fresh air.

Both masks and prongs are available in different sizes to accommodate variations in facial contours, thereby reducing leaks. Nasal masks are also available in a variety of shapes; trying several shapes gives patients some freedom about choice and comfort. All varieties of interface are attached to the face by headgear that fits over the head. Headgear is designed specifically for a given mask, and interchanging headgear is not recommended.

Once an appropriate interface has been determined, have a practice session before starting the polysomnogram. In the practice session, the patient wears the CPAP mask and experiences both low and high pressures. This session can improve tolerance during the study.

CPAP TITRATION PROTOCOL

There is no universally agreed-on method for how CPAP titration should proceed. As a general rule, the initial CPAP pressure is set low and is titrated incrementally to higher pressures until the optimal pressure is determined. There are several reasons for this approach. First, starting at low pressures enhances patient tolerance and allows the subject to achieve sleep. Second, low pressures may be enough to be therapeutic in some patients. Third, higher pressures are generally associated with mask leaks and patient discomfort, and so they are to be avoided unless required therapeutically.

CPAP is typically initiated with a low pressure of 4 cm H_2O and increased in steps (at a minimum of 1 cm H_2O). CPAP pressure is usually increased rapidly when obstructive events are frequent and at a slower rate when respiratory events become less frequent. CPAP pressure is increased until:

- Either evidence of obstruction has been eliminated.
- Or a maximum pressure of 20 cm H_2O is reached.
- Or the patient is unable to tolerate the pressure.

This protocol results in optimal treatment at the lowest possible pressure.

The elimination of apneas and hypopneas may not represent optimal treatment. Elevated upper airway resistance may still be present and result in frequent arousals from sleep. Inspiratory flow limitation is best detected by the measurement of pleural pressure using an esophageal balloon or a nasal pressure transducer, which provides better detection of flow characteristics than a thermistor. When flow limitation is detected, pressure increases of 1–2 cm above that needed to eliminate apneas and hypopneas are generally sufficient to eliminate all obstruction and resulting arousals. The technologist must monitor the effects of CPAP in REM sleep and, if possible, in the supine position because higher CPAP pressures are typically required to resolve upper airway obstruction in these situations.

Dealing with Side Effects. CPAP is generally well tolerated, but it has some side effects or conditions that may lead to arousals and reduce CPAP tolerance or

TABLE 18-3 **Common side effects associated with CPAP use and possible remedies**

Side Effect	Possible Remedies
Mask-related:	
Pain or abrasion on bridge of nose	Loosen mask headgear if too tight
	Switch to nasal prongs
Leaks around mask	Check for proper mask size
	Switch to nasal prongs
Oral air leaks (mouth drops open)	Chinstrap
	Full-face mask
CPAP-related:	
Nasal dryness/ irritation	Saline spray/gel
	Humidification
	Chinstrap if air is escaping from mouth
Nasal congestion	Antihistamine
	Nasal steroids
	Full-face mask
Difficulty exhaling	Use ramp function
	Use bilevel PAP to lower expiratory pressure
Claustrophobia	Switch to nasal prongs
	Bilevel PAP
	Behavioral desensitization training
Air swallowing	Bilevel PAP to lower expiratory pressure
	Raise head of bed

effectiveness (Table 18-3).The technologist must address side effects during CPAP titration because they may affect how the patient receives the long-term therapy. Most side effects are related either to the patient interface (e.g., mask, nasal prongs) or to the sensation of high pressure or high airflow.

- Poor mask fit can lead to air leaks around the mask; those occurring around the eyes are the most disruptive.
- Frequently, the patient relaxes the lower jaw, producing an oral leak. This leak not only may produce arousals but also frequently reduces the effectiveness of CPAP. A chinstrap designed to hold the lower jaw closed may help.
- A full-face mask may also help but is generally less preferred by the patient.
- Pressure-related side effects include difficulty exhaling, nasal congestion, and nasal dryness. Adding humidification to the airflow may help and is now the standard of practice with CPAP.
- Some patients may feel claustrophobic on their first encounter with CPAP. Progressive desensitization and using nasal prongs rather than a mask may help.
- A few patients simply refuse CPAP.

Best Practice

Ensuring CPAP Compliance

Good therapeutic effectiveness on the CPAP titration night does not guarantee that the patient will be compliant with CPAP use at home. Factors that may lead to reduced use or to nonuse (noncompliance) are generally related to its side effects. Early follow-up can help identify and resolve problems that patients may have with CPAP. Follow-up at regular intervals thereafter is helpful in ensuring continuing compliance.

BILEVEL POSITIVE AIRWAY PRESSURE

Bilevel positive airway pressure (bilevel PAP) is a variation of CPAP that allows inspiratory and expiratory pressures to be adjusted independently. During the respiratory cycle, a critical level of pressure is needed to maintain a patent airway. With complete or nearly complete airway occlusion, the expiratory pressure required to prevent the collapse of the airway is the same as the inspiratory pressure required to prevent anemic events. Bilevel PAP takes advantage of the fact that if positive pressure is applied to inspiration, thus eliminating the anemic obstruction, then less pressure is required to maintain the airway during exhalation. Thus, with bilevel PAP, the inspiratory positive airway pressure (IPAP) is similar to the pressure titrated with standard CPAP. However, expiratory positive airway pressure (EPAP) is typically 4–6 cm H_2O lower than IPAP. A bilevel device cycles between the preset IPAP and EPAP pressures by monitoring changes in respiratory flow.

The titration of bilevel PAP is more complex than that of conventional CPAP because it involves establishing two separate pressures. IPAP and EPAP pressures are independently adjusted and thus generally require more time to establish therapeutic levels. A typical protocol for the titration of bilevel PAP is to:

- Begin with an IPAP of 8 cm H_2O and an EPAP of 4 cm H_2O.
- If obstructive apneas persist, EPAP is increased to equal IPAP.

- If obstructive apneas still continue, then increase IPAP and EPAP together until apneas are eliminated. EPAP is left at the pressure that eliminated apneas while IPAP is increased incrementally until all evidence of obstruction has been eliminated (e.g., snoring, desaturation, arousals).

Variations in the protocol can be found between laboratories.

Bilevel PAP devices are frequently used in noninvasive nasal ventilation of patients with respiratory failure, especially patients with neuromuscular or chest wall disease. These patients may be sent to the sleep disorders laboratory for a PSG and to establish ventilatory parameters using bilevel PAP. Bilevel PAP is also used in patients who have difficulty tolerating CPAP, especially at higher CPAP pressures (i.e., greater than 15 cm H_2O). These patients tolerate lower expiratory pressures better.

SPLIT-NIGHT POLYSOMNOGRAPHY

A full night of recording is generally needed to establish and assess the degree of obstructive sleep disordered breathing. For patients with severe obstruction, however, a diagnosis may be feasible after only a few hours of monitoring. In such cases, CPAP titration could be performed on the same night to detect and assess the disorder. Condensing the assessment and titration segments in this way is referred to as a *split-night polysomnogram*. The trend toward using split-night studies reflects an effort to reduce costs and to decrease waiting time for a sleep disorder assessment, which may be weeks or months.

However, making a split-night study the routine has its disadvantages. First, apneas may occur only during REM sleep or only when the patient is supine. REM sleep is the most plentiful during the second half of the night, and sufficient supine sleep, especially in conjunction with REM sleep, may not occur during the first half of the night. Therefore, the severity of the disorder may not be adequately assessed during the first half of the study. Second, confining CPAP titration to just half of the night may not allow sufficient time to titrate to the optimal pressure, especially in patients with severe obstructive sleep disordered breathing. This problem is compounded when bilevel PAP is used because it requires a more complex titration protocol.

The AASM recommends that an AHI of at least 40 events per hour be documented during a minimum of 2 hours of diagnostic PSG before considering a split-night study.[7] Split-night studies may sometimes be considered at an AHI of 20–40 events per hour, based on clinical judgment (e.g., if there are also repetitive long obstructions and major destructions). CPAP titration should be carried out for a minimum of 3 hours to ensure adequate PSG documentation that CPAP eliminates or nearly eliminates the respiratory events during REM and NREM sleep, including REM sleep with the patient in the supine position.

AUTOTITRATING CPAP

The level of CPAP pressure required to eliminate upper airway obstructions in sleep-disordered breathing varies with conditions. The optimal pressure may vary during the night with respect to position changes and sleep stage. It may also vary from night to night because of alcohol consumption, sedative medication, and previous sleep deprivation. The hypothesis that changing CPAP according to the patient's need at any given time could improve CPAP compliance has resulted in the development of **autotitrating CPAP** devices that automatically adjust pressure according to the patient's requirements. Autotitrating CPAP machines continuously adjust the positive pressure level depending on the presence of flow limitation. These machines use flow, pressure, sound, or vibration—or a combination of those variables—to establish whether flow limitation is present. They increase or decrease pressure in predetermined increments to maintain the lowest effective pressure. Autotitrating CPAP has been advocated for use in CPAP titration studies, both attended and unattended, and as a standard mode of therapy for patients.

Measuring Daytime Sleepiness

Daytime somnolence or sleepiness is a hallmark symptom of many sleep disorders. Assessing the degree of sleepiness may be useful in diagnosing certain sleep disorders and in monitoring the effects of treatment. Two tests are currently in use to objectively assess sleepiness: the multiple sleep latency test (MSLT) and the maintenance of wakefulness test (MWT). The MSLT was the first such test to be described and remains the most commonly used test. The AASM practice parameter for the clinical use of the MSLT and MWT describes the protocols for both tests.[8]

The *multiple sleep latency test* consists of a series of four or five nap opportunities given at 2-hour intervals throughout the day. The test is usually preceded by a nocturnal PSG to provide accurate documentation of the preceding night's sleep, which influences the accurate interpretation of MSLT results. The first nap is performed 1.5–3 hours after the nocturnal PSG ends.

During the monitoring of the naps, sleep onset is determined, and sleep stages are identified. The standard montage includes a C_3 or C_4 EEG lead, right and left EOG leads, and a chin EMG. A second occipital lead is frequently monitored to help in distinguishing wakefulness from sleep. Additional channels include ECG and airflow if snoring was noted in the nocturnal PSG.

The MSLT must be performed in an environment conducive to sleep. The sleeping area should be quiet and dark. Intermittent noises should be avoided. Maintaining quiet may necessitate being away from elevators, toilets, outside traffic, and heavily used hallways. Any audible noises that could interfere with sleep onset must be documented to facilitate accurate interpretation.

In addition, specific patient preparation routines need to be followed.

- The patient should change into street clothes sometime before preparing for the first nap.
- Keep the patient awake except during the actual nap time. Keeping the patient awake requires the attendance of laboratory staff throughout the day.
- Patients who smoke should stop smoking 30 minutes before nap time.
- Fifteen minutes before nap time, the patient should prepare for bed. This preparation includes using the restroom, removing shoes, and loosening restricting clothing.
- The patient should be in bed and relaxed 5 minutes before nap time. At this time, perform a biological calibration similar to one done during the nocturnal PSG.
- Immediately before lights-out, ask the subject to get into a comfortable position, and given a short set of instructions that encourage falling asleep, such as, "Close your eyes, lie still, and let yourself fall asleep." (Repeat the same set of instructions before each nap.)

There are also specific criteria for terminating the nap.

- Terminate the nap if, after 20 minutes, the patient has not fallen asleep.
- If the patient falls asleep within 20 minutes, continue the nap for 15 minutes after the first epoch of sleep to assess any occurrence of REM sleep, which is useful in establishing a diagnosis of narcolepsy. Sleep latency is calculated from data gathered from combined nap periods.

The *maintenance of wakefulness test* is similar to the MSLT in that a series of five nap opportunities is given at 2-hour intervals and a mean sleep latency is reported. In contrast to the MSLT, however, the patient remains upright in a dimly lit room and is instructed to try to stay awake for 40 minutes. The test is terminated if sleep is noted or after 40 minutes if the patient remains awake. This test is used less frequently than the MSLT and no clear standards exist for interpreting the results.

Summary

Normal sleep consists of alternating periods of rapid eye movement and nonrapid eye movement sleep. Sleep patterns and stages can be observed by using EEG, EOG, and EMG and by monitoring breathing and arterial oxygen saturation. The resulting data can be interpreted to detect the presence of sleep disorders, including sleep-disordered breathing, narcolepsy, and periodic limb movements in sleep.

The polysomnogram is used to report sleep data. The therapist sets filters and sensitivities for the equipment used and prepares the patient for the testing, including patient or biological calibration to ensure accurate data collection and minimal artifact. The therapist also monitors the test in progress. The data collected are scored or interpreted to determine whether any sleep disorders are present.

Effective forms of therapy for sleep-disordered breathing include continuous positive airway pressure, in which positive pressure established in the patient's airway acts as a pneumatic splint to keep the airway open. CPAP may be applied with a mask or other device, depending on the patient's needs and tolerance. The amount of pressure must be titrated to produce maximum therapeutic results while maintaining patient comfort. Bilevel positive airway pressure allows inspiratory and expiratory pressure levels to be adjusted independently, and autotitrating CPAP devices automatically adjusts pressure according to patient requirements.

Study Questions

REVIEW QUESTIONS

1. Identify the four stages of sleep, and discuss the relative percentages of each stage and the pattern of occurrence through the night.
2. Define excessive daytime sleepiness, and identify three common sleep disorders for which this is a prominent symptom.
3. Identify the physiological parameters typically measured on a standard polysomnogram, and discuss available technologies for monitoring each of them.
4. Define and discuss the importance of sensitivity, frequency filters, and impedance checking when performing a polysomnogram.
5. Discuss the importance of performing a patient calibration before starting a polysomnogram.
6. Identify four common side effects of CPAP therapy, and discuss methods to reduce or eliminate each.

MULTIPLE-CHOICE QUESTIONS

1. An EEG frequency ranging between 4 cps and 8 cps is classified as:
   a. delta rhythm.
   b. theta rhythm.
   c. alpha rhythm.
   d. beta rhythm.
2. A patient experiences 78 impaired respiratory events throughout the night. She has a total sleep time of 312 minutes during a recording period of 400 minutes. This patient's respiratory disturbance index is:
   a. 10 per hour.
   b. 15 per hour.
   c. 25 per hour.
   d. 40 per hour.
3. An epoch is an interval of time used when staging sleep, and in polysomnography it has a standard duration of:
   a. 15 seconds.
   b. 20 seconds.
   c. 30 seconds.
   d. 60 seconds.
4. Which of the following MSLT results is the most consistent with a diagnosis of narcolepsy?
   a. a mean sleep latency of 15 minutes and no sleep onset REM periods
   b. a mean sleep latency of 2.5 minutes and no sleep onset REM periods
   c. a mean sleep latency of 8 minutes and a sleep onset REM period in the first nap
   d. a mean sleep latency of 4.5 minutes and sleep onset REM periods in naps 1, 3, and 4
5. Which of the following controls on the polygraph can be used to reduce electrical supply line interference in the EEG channels?
   a. sensitivity
   b. high-frequency filter
   c. low-frequency filter
   d. 60-Hz notch filter
6. An impaired respiratory event that is characterized by the cessation of airflow for at least 10 seconds and is accompanied by continuous paradoxical motion between the thoracic and abdominal effort channels is defined as:
   a. a central apnea.
   b. an obstructive apnea.
   c. a mixed apnea.
   d. an obstructive hypopnea.
7. A relatively low-voltage, mixed-frequency EEG pattern with variable occurrences of K-complexes and sleep spindles is characteristic of which stage of sleep?
   a. REM
   b. Stage N1
   c. Stage N2
   d. Stage N3

CRITICAL-THINKING QUESTIONS

1. What approach might be taken to convince a patient to try CPAP therapy on the CPAP titration night after he has refused to wear the nasal mask because of feelings of claustrophobia?
2. During monitoring of a standard nocturnal polysomnogram, the onset of a cardiac arrhythmia is observed and identified as ventricular tachycardia. What action should be taken?

References

1. Rechtschaffen, A., and Kales, A., eds. *A Manual of Standardized Terminology, Techniques and Scoring System for Sleep Stages in Human Subjects*. Washington, DC: U.S. Government Printing Office; 1968.
2. Iber C, Ancoli-Israel S, Cheeson A, Quan SF. *The AASM Manual for the Scoring of Sleep and Associated Events: Rule, Terminology and Technical Specifications.* Westchester, IL: American Academy of Sleep Medicine; 2007.
3. American Academy of Sleep Medicine. *International Classification of Sleep Disorders, 2nd ed: Diagnostic and Coding Manual*. Westchester, IL: American Academy of Sleep Medicine; 2005.
4. American Association for Respiratory Care. Cardiopulmonary Diagnostic CPG Focus Group and the Association of Polysomnographic Technologists. AARC-APT clinical practice guidelines—polysomnography. *Respir Care*. 1995;40:1336–1343.
5. Harner PF, Sannit T. *A Review of the International Ten-Twenty System of Electrode Placement*. Quincy, MA: Grass Instrument Co; 1974.
6. The report of the American Academy of Sleep Medicine Task Force. Sleep-related breathing disorders in adults: recommendations for syndrome definition and measurement techniques in clinical research. *Sleep*. 1999;22:667–689.
7. Kushida CA, Littner MR, Morgenthaler T, et al. Practice parameters for the indications for polysomnography and related procedures: An update for 2005. *Sleep*. 2005;28:499–521.
8. Standards of Practice Committee of the American Academy of Sleep Medicine. Practice parameters for clinical use of the multiple sleep latency test and the maintenance of wakefulness test. *Sleep*. 2005;28:113–121.

Suggested Readings

Berry RB. *Sleep Medicine Pearls*. 2nd ed. Philadelphia: Mosby; 2003.

Butkov N, Lee-Chiong T. *Fundamentals of Sleep Technology.* Philadelphia: Lippincott Williams & Wilkins; 2007.

Chokroverty S. *Atlas of Sleep Medicine.* Boston: Butterworth-Heinemann; 2005.

Chokroverty S. *Sleep Disorders Medicine: Basic Science, Technical Considerations, and Clinical Aspects*. Philadelphia: WB Saunders; 2009.

Keenan SA. Polysomnography: technical aspects in adolescents and adults. *J Clin Neurophysiol.* 1992;9:21–31.

Kryger MH. *Atlas of Clinical Sleep Medicine*. Philadelphia: Elsevier Saunders; 2009.

Kryger MH, Roth T, Dement WC, eds. *Principles and Practice of Sleep Medicine*. 5th ed. Philadelphia: Elsevier Saunders; 2010.

Lee-Chiong TL. *Sleep: A Comprehensive Handbook.* Hoboken, NJ: Wiley; 2005.

Loube DI, Gay PC, Strohl KP, Pack AI, White DP, Collop NA. Indications for positive airway pressure treatment of adult obstructive sleep apnea patients—a consensus statement. *Chest*. 1999;115:863–866.

Niedermeyer E, Lopes da Solva FH. *Electroencephalography: Basic Principles, Clinical Applications, and Related Fields.* 4th ed. Philadelphia: Lippincott Williams & Wilkins; 2004.

Positive Airway Pressure Task Force of the American Academy of Sleep Medicine. Clinical guidelines for the manual titration of positive airway pressure in patients with obstructive sleep apnea. *J Clin Sleep Med.* 2008; 4(2):157–171.

Rechtschaffen A, Kales A, eds. *A Manual of Standardized Terminology, Techniques and Scoring System for Sleep Stages of Human Subjects*. NIH Publication #204, 1968. American Electroencephalographic Society. Polygraphic assessment of sleep-related disorders (polysomnography). *J Clin Neurophysiol.* 1994;11:116–124.

CHAPTER 19

Cardiac and Hemodynamic Monitoring

Barbara Ludwig and L. Micky Mathews

OBJECTIVES

Upon completion of this chapter, the reader should be able to:

- Describe the timing of electrical and mechanical events of the cardiac cycle.
- Identify the lead placement for the 12-lead ECG.
- Identify the steps involved in analyzing an ECG strip.
- Correctly identify various abnormal ECG patterns from a selection of examples.
- Identify and choose lethal arrhythmias from a sample of ECG tracings.
- Given a sample ECG tracing, calculate the heart rate.
- Identify the signs, symptoms, and causes of cardiac dysfunctions.
- List the factors that affect preload, afterload, and contractility, and discuss the impact of preload, afterload, and contractility on cardiac output.
- Given the appropriate data, calculate various hemodynamic variables.
- Discuss the significance of monitoring mixed venous oxygenation to evaluate hemodynamic status.
- Describe the thermodilution method of measuring cardiac output, and identify the thermodilution curve associated with poor injection technique and with normal, high, and low cardiac output.

CHAPTER OUTLINE

(continues)

(continued)

KEY TERMS

action potential
afterload
AV dissociation
bicycle ergometer
cardiac cycle
cardiac output (CO)
cardiac tamponade
catheter whip
compensatory pause
contractility
damped pressure curve
depolarization
diastasis
diastole
myocardial scintigraphy
overwedging
pericarditis
preload
pulmonary vascular resistance (PVR)
pulsus alternans
pulsus bisferiens
pulsus paradoxus
pulsus parvus
P-R segment
P-wave
QRS complex
refractory period
repolarization
S-T segment
systemic vascular resistance (SVR)
systole
T-wave
T-wave inversion

This chapter presents an explanation of basic cardiac function, the normal ECG waveform, the basics of electrocardiography, the analysis of the ECG tracing, and the collection and interpretation of hemodynamic data. Common cardiac abnormalities, both electrical and functional, are discussed. The effects of altered cardiac function, blood flow, and pressure in the cardiovascular system are illustrated, and the concepts of shock are detailed. The reader is advised to review the discussion in Chapter 6 of the structure and function of the circulatory system.

The Cardiac Cycle

The **cardiac cycle** (one complete heartbeat) consists of two phases: a period of relaxation called **diastole** followed by a period of contraction called **systole**. The diastolic phase has four components: isovolumetric relaxation, rapid ventricular filling, reduced ventricular filling and diastasis, and atrial systole.

- During the *isovolumetric relaxation* period, the myocardial cells are relaxed; all four of the cardiac valves are closed. Venous blood returning to the atria causes the pressure in the atria to increase.
- After the atrial pressure exceeds ventricular pressure, the atrioventricular valves open, allowing for *rapid ventricular filling*. During this period, venous blood returns to the atria quickly but passively, filling the ventricles. As the ventricles begin to fill with blood, the pressure within the ventricles rises and becomes equal with that of the atria.
- As the pressure equalizes, the rate at which blood flows from the atria into the ventricles begins to slow (*reduced filling*) and eventually

comes to a virtual standstill **(diastasis)**. At this point, the atria contract in response to an electrical impulse generated by the sinoatrial (SA) node.
- The contraction of the atrial muscle cells (systole) increases pressure in the atria and propels the remaining atrial blood into the ventricles. This propulsion is referred to as the *atrial kick*. After the atrial kick, pressure within the atria drops, and the atrioventricular valves close, thereby ending diastole.

Systole occurs in response to electrical activation of the ventricular myocardial cells. The systolic phase of the cardiac cycle has three components: isovolumetric contraction, rapid ejection, and reduced ejection.

- Once the ventricular myocardium has received a nerve impulse, the muscles contract; however, the semilunar valves remain closed initially. Because there is no change in the ventricular volume at this point, this component is referred to as *isovolumetric* (*iso-* means "same") *contraction*. Contraction of the ventricular myocardial cells increases the pressure in the ventricles. When the intraventricular pressure becomes greater than the pressure in the aorta and pulmonary artery, the semilunar valves are pushed open.
- With the opening of the semilunar valves, blood is *rapidly ejected* into the great vessels.
- The rapid ejection period is followed by the *reduced ejection* period. Although the ventricular muscle cells remain contracted during the reduced ejection period, the flow of blood out of the ventricles begins to slow as the volume of blood in the ventricles diminishes.

Secondary to the reduction in blood flowing out of the ventricles, pressure in the ventricles and the great vessels begins to drop. When the electrical stimulus is no longer present, the ventricular muscle fibers relax. During relaxation, pressure in the ventricles drops so dramatically that the pressure in the aorta and pulmonary artery is greater than that in the ventricles; the difference in pressure pushes the semilunar valves closed. Once the aorta and pulmonary valves are closed, isovolumetric relaxation begins, and the cardiac cycle repeats.[1]

The events of the cardiac cycle involve a series of complex electrical, chemical, and physical events in the cardiac cells. When cardiac cells are at rest, they are electrically polarized; specifically, the inside of the cell is negatively charged, and the outside of the cell is positively charged. (This difference in charge from inside to outside is called the *transmembrane potential*.) The resting cell remains polarized owing to the action of a membrane pump that maintains the proper balance of ions (potassium, sodium, chloride, and calcium).

- **Depolarization** (a change in transmembrane potential from negative toward positive) is referred to as the *fundamental electrical event* of the heart because it stimulates the cardiac cells to contract. Depolarization spreads from cell to cell, producing a wave of electrical current that spreads (is propagated) throughout the myocardium.
- **Repolarization** (a change in transmembrane potential from positive toward negative) occurs after depolarization is complete. With repolarization, the cardiac cells return to their resting potential (i.e., negative inside, positive outside).[1]

One electrical cycle of depolarization and repolarization within a single cell is an **action potential**, and it is the stimulus that initiates the contractile process. An action potential is generated (initiated) by a change in cardiac cell membrane permeability to specific ions (sodium and calcium). This change allows a sudden influx of positively charged ions into the cell, thus causing depolarization. Every time an action potential is generated, it stimulates adjacent cells to depolarize until the entire heart has been depolarized.[1,2]

There are three basic types of cardiac cells in the atria and ventricles: pacemaker cells, conducting cells, and myocardial cells.

- The *pacemaker cells* are the electrical generators of the heart. These cells spontaneously discharge an action potential at a "preset" rate. The primary pacemaker of the heart is the SA node, which generates action potentials at a rate of 60–100 times per minute. This rate can vary considerably depending on the activity of the autonomic nervous system and the demands of the body for more blood flow.[1,2]
- Each time the SA node fires an action potential, it propagates depolarization throughout the heart via the *conducting cells*. These cells, found in both the atria and the ventricles, carry the electrical current quickly from the pacemaker cells to the myocardial cells.
- As the electrical impulse spreads to the *myocardial cells*, muscle contraction occurs. The contraction is secondary to a process called *excitation-contraction coupling*, which is the response of the muscle fibers to the excitation signal with rapid depolarization followed by a mechanical response, in this case cardiac contraction. The myocardial cells contain the contractile proteins actin and myosin, which are necessary for the heart to contract. When the myocardial cells are depolarized, calcium is released into the cell. The calcium allows the

coupling of actin and myosin for contraction. After depolarization is complete, the cardiac cells repolarize, returning to their resting polarity, calcium is no longer available, the bond between actin and myosin molecules is broken, and the cell relaxes.[1,2]

The normal cardiac cycle begins with the stimulus originating from the SA node. The electrical impulse is conducted through the atrial muscle cells to the *atrioventricular (AV) node*. The transmission of the electrical impulse is momentarily delayed at this point to allow the atria to contract, ejecting the last bit of blood into the ventricles. From the AV node, the electrical impulse is conducted through the bundle of His to the ventricles via the left and right bundle branches. From the bundle branches the impulse is then carried through the Purkinje fibers to the ventricular muscle.[1,2]

The *electrocardiogram* (*ECG*) records the electrical impulse as it moves through the conducting system of the heart by means of electrodes placed on the body. The waveforms inscribed on the ECG reflect the waves of depolarization and repolarization.

- As the wave of depolarization spreads through the atria, the ECG records a positive deflection called the **P-wave**.
- After the atrial depolarization, the wave of depolarization is delayed at the AV node. This AV nodal delay is recorded as a straight line called the **P-R segment**.
- Depolarization of the ventricles is also recorded as a positive deflection, called the **QRS complex**.
- Because the atria repolarize during ventricular depolarization, atrial repolarization is not seen on the ECG.
- For a short time following ventricular depolarization, the ventricular muscle cells are refractory to further stimulation. This **refractory period**, called the **S-T segment**, is seen as a straight line on the ECG.
- Following the refractory period, the ventricles repolarize; the cardiac cell has recovered its normal resting membrane potential. On the ECG, ventricular repolarization is seen as another positive deflection, called the **T-wave**.

One complete cardiac cycle is represented by the P-wave, QRS complex, and T-wave.[1,2]

Cardiac Leads

The standard 12-lead ECG comprises bipolar and unipolar leads that record the electrical activity of the heart from 12 different views. Leads are placed on the patient's chest and limb skin surface. Each lead acts as an "eye" that looks at the heart from a unique perspective.

STANDARD 12-LEAD ECG

The three bipolar leads are the original leads selected by Einthoven to record the electrical impulses of the heart in the frontal plane. (Willem Einthoven was a Dutch physician who received the Nobel Prize for physiology and medicine in 1924 for the invention of the electrocardiograph.) Electrodes are applied to the body limbs: the right arm (RA), left arm (LA), and left leg (LL), as shown in Figure 19-1. The right leg (RL) electrode is the ground (G), or neutral, electrode. The RA electrode is always the electrically negative pole. The LA electrode is electrically positive in lead I and negative in lead III. The LL is always the electrically positive pole.[1,3,4]

- Lead I: Left arm positive (+) and right arm negative (−)
- Lead II: Left leg positive (+) and right arm negative (−)
- Lead III: Left leg positive (+) and left arm negative (−)

The relationship among the three leads is expressed mathematically by Einthoven's equation:

electrical potential of lead II = electrical potential of lead I + electrical potential of lead III

The limb electrodes have standard color designations to help the practitioner attach the correct ECG machine leads to the patient's surface limb electrodes:[1,3,4]

- Right arm (RA) is white.
- Left arm (LA) is black.
- Right leg (RL or G) is green.
- Left leg (LL) is red.

Unipolar leads are divided into different types: limb leads, precordial (V) leads, and intraesophageal leads. Of these three types, only the intraesophageal leads are not included in the 12-lead ECG. Unipolar limb leads resemble bipolar frontal leads in several ways. They measure the patient's cardiac activity in the frontal plane, and they have the same electrically positive pole. The unipolar limb leads differ from bipolar leads in that, instead of a negative electrode, the unipolar leads have a so-called *indifferent electrode*.[1,3,4]

The indifferent electrode is the average of the other two augmented leads acting as the negative electrode (RA, LA, LL). Therefore, when the electrodes are placed on the extremities (RA, LA, LL), the ECG deflections represent the difference in potential between the selected limb lead and the average potential of the remaining two unipolar limb leads.

The unipolar limb leads are termed aV_R, aV_L, and aV_F.

- The *a* before V_R, V_L, and V_F indicates that waveforms are amplified (1.5 times). The amplification is necessary to see ECG deflections.
- The *V* identifies that it is a unipolar lead.
- The letters *R* (right), *L* (left), and *F* (left leg) refer to the limb lead that acts as the positive electrode.[1,3,4]

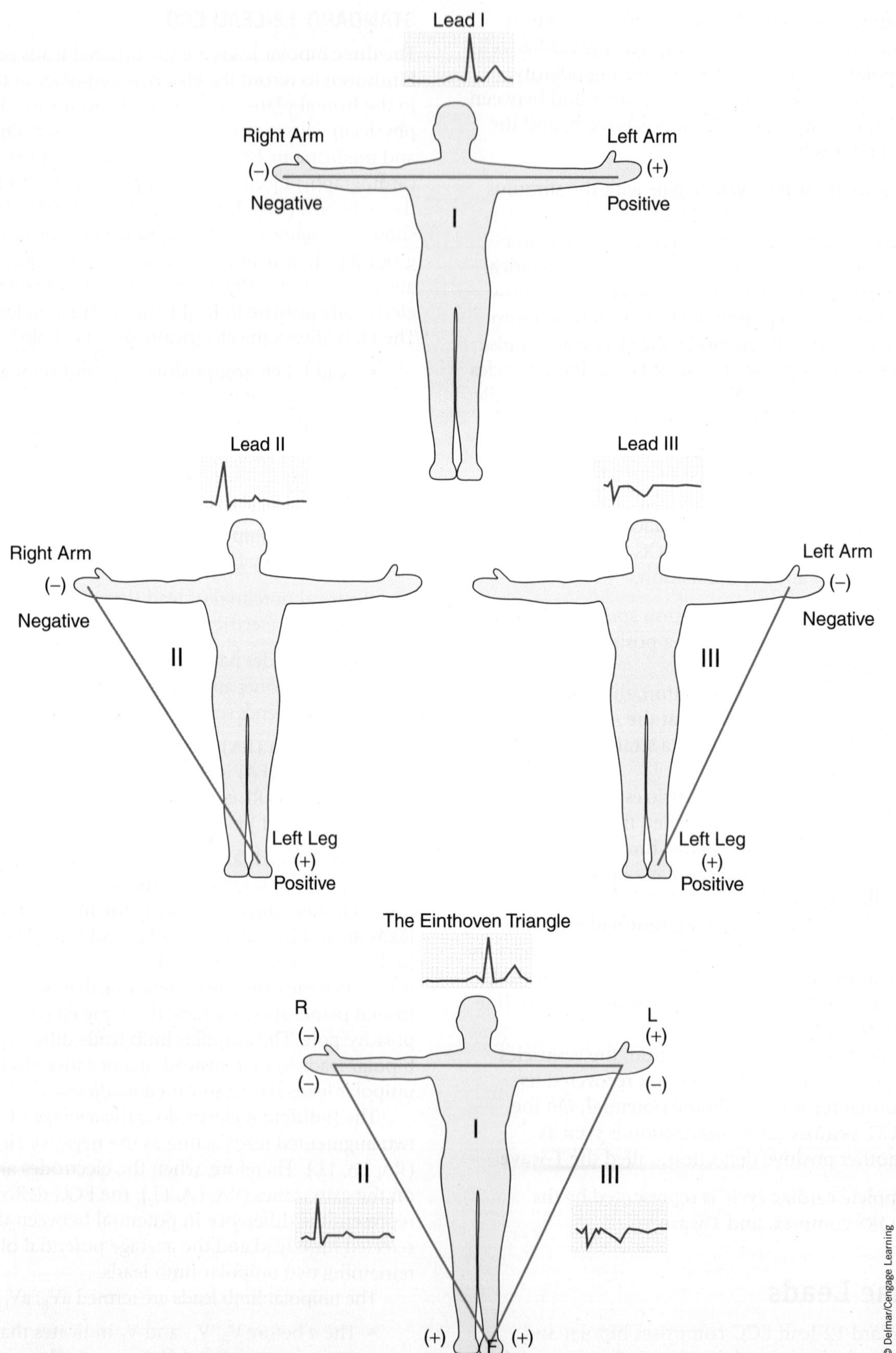

FIGURE 19-1 The six frontal plane leads consist of three bipolar leads (I, II, III) and three unipolar leads (aV_R, aV_L, aV_F). The electrode placements for the frontal leads are the right arm (RA), left arm (LA), and the left leg (LL), with the ground, or right leg, designated as G. The electrode polarity (+ or −) is identified for each lead electrode placement site.

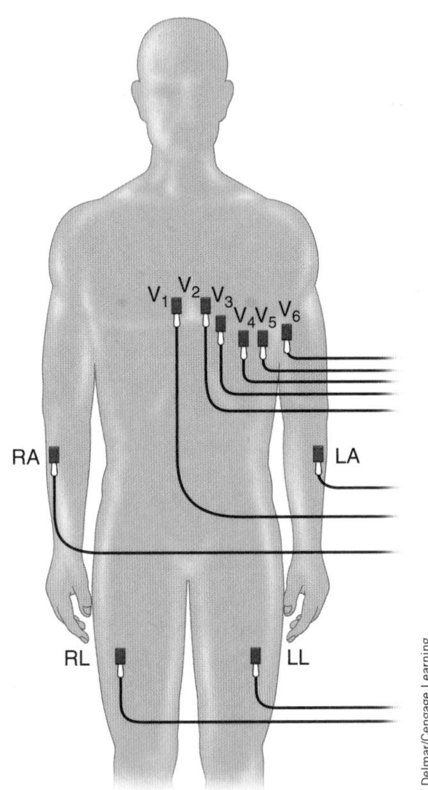

FIGURE 19-2 Six standard precordial leads: The *V* before the lead number identifies it as a unipolar lead.

Six unipolar precordial, or chest, leads (V_1–V_6) are placed on specific areas of the anterior chest wall (Figure 19-2). These leads measure the heart's electrical activity in the horizontal plane. The common chest positions of precordial leads are as follows:

- V_1: Fourth intercostal space, right sternal border
- V_2: Fourth intercostal space, left sternal border
- V_3: Fifth intercostal space midway between V_2 and V_4
- V_4: Fifth intercostal space, midclavicular line
- V_5: Fifth intercostal space, anterior axillary line
- V_6: Fifth intercostal space, midaxillary line

Bedside monitors can be used to obtain a 12-lead ECG. Software available on bedside monitors allows clinicians to intermittently obtain a 12-lead printout using the monitor leads.[1,3,4]

ALTERNATIVE LEADS

Any lead may be placed on any part of the body to obtain an ECG tracing. These alternative leads are standardized and used in clinical electrocardiography.

MCL System. An alternative bipolar lead system is the *MCL (modified chest left arm) system*, which is frequently used for continuous monitoring in intensive care units. A common lead of this system is MCL_1, which is a modification of the precordial lead V_1. The positive electrode (exploring electrode) is placed at the V_1 position (fourth intercostal space, to the right of the sternum). The left arm is the electrically negative pole, and the ground, or neutral, electrode is in the RA position (Figure 19-3).

The primary use of this lead in continuous ECG monitoring is to detect bundle branch conduction abnormalities. MCL_6 is also commonly used to identify bundle branch conduction abnormalities (Figure 19-4). The Lewis lead is a special bipolar chest lead that amplifies atrial waves and makes it easier to identify the presence and possible physiological mechanism of atrial dysrhythmias (Figure 19-5). The other precordial chest leads could also be used for monitoring and diagnostic purposes.[1,3,4]

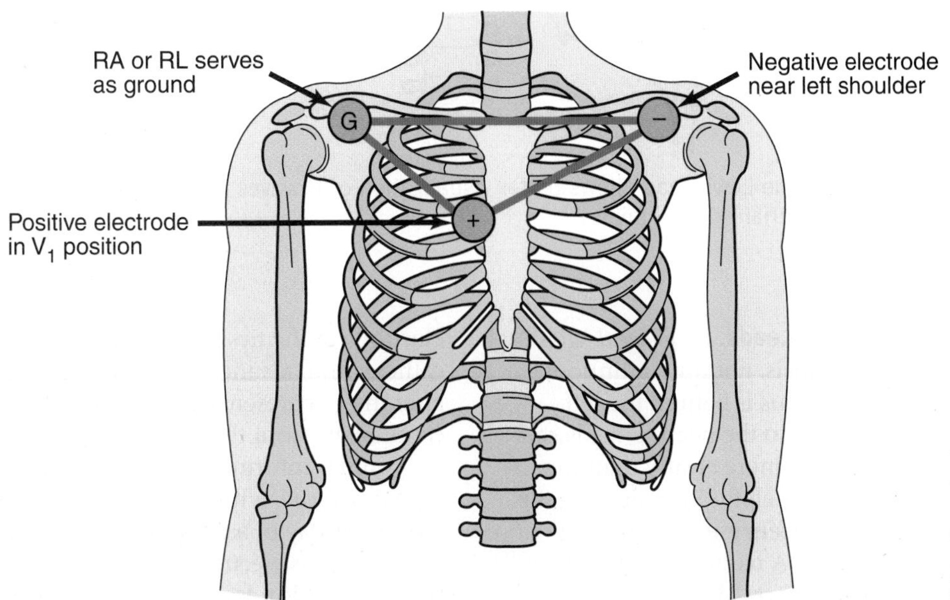

FIGURE 19-3 The MCL_1 lead helps in the differential diagnosis of a bundle branch block.

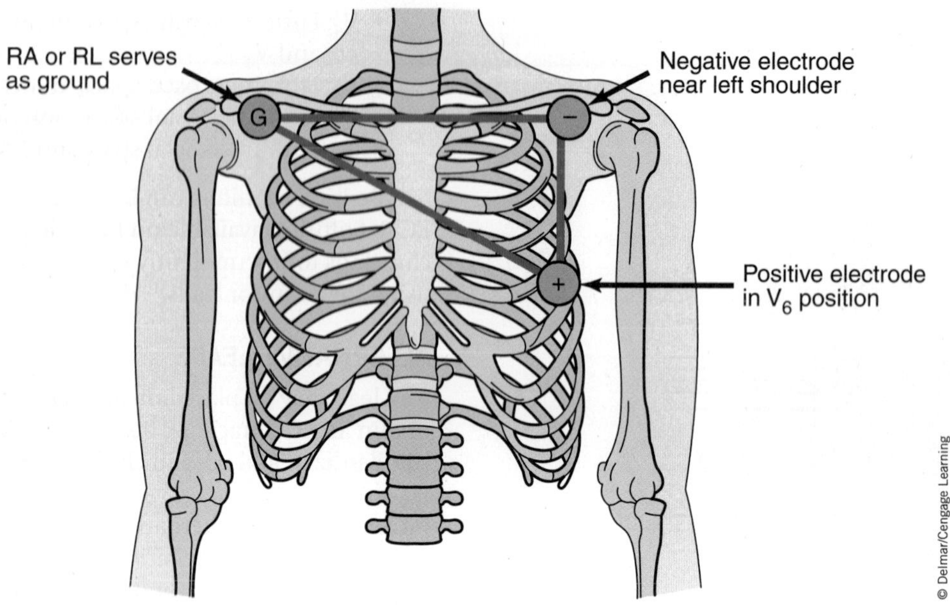

FIGURE 19-4 The MCL_6 lead helps in the differential diagnosis of a bundle branch block.

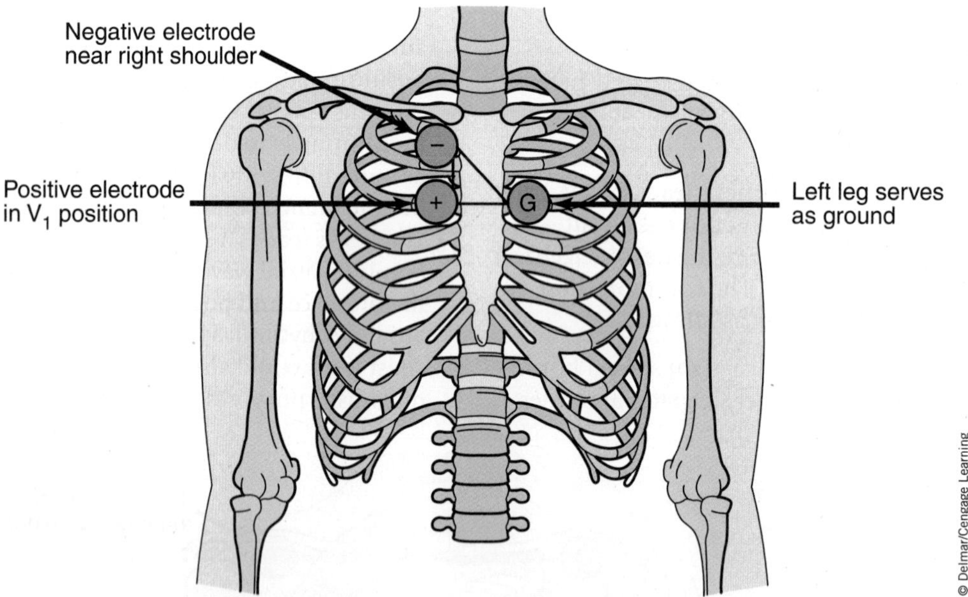

FIGURE 19-5 The Lewis lead allows better visualization of P-waves and aids in the diagnosis of atrial dysrhythmias.

Esophageal and Intra-Atrial Leads. *Esophageal leads*, or *E-leads*, are used for diagnosis, not for continuous monitoring. Since the esophagus is behind the left atrium and in close proximity to the heart, E-leads can be used to reveal atrial activity more clearly than the standard leads.[5] They are also helpful in evaluating the function of the conducting system and in revealing mechanisms of dysrhythmias. A nasal catheter is introduced into the patient's nares. A wire with the electrode at the tip is threaded through the nasal catheter and advanced into the esophagus. The number after the *E* represents the distance of that electrode in centimeters from the nares.[6,7]

Similar information can be obtained with *an intra-atrial lead*, which is inserted directly into the right atrium by way of a peripheral vein. The lead permits bundle of His electrical studies, which provide definitive information for diagnosing cardiac dysrhythmias.[7]

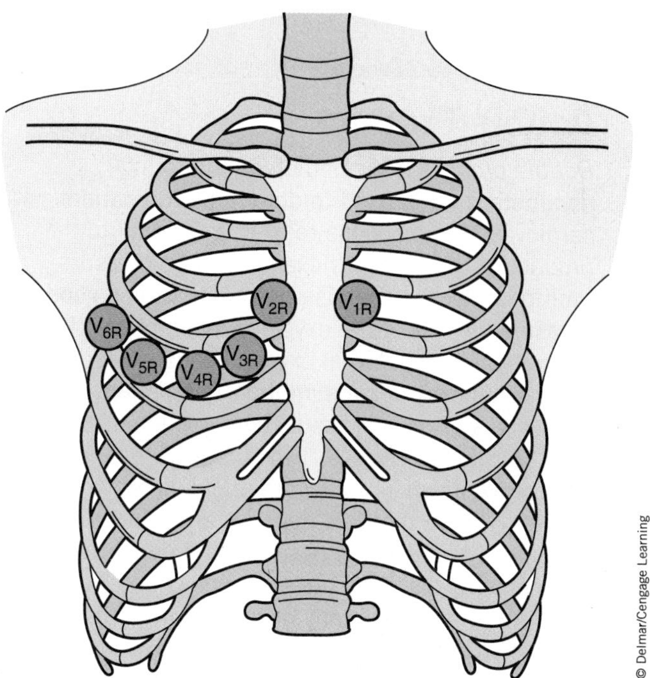

FIGURE 19-6 Alternative precordial lead placement: The ECG leads are placed on the right side of the chest in the same location as the left-sided leads; for example, V_{2R} is the same as V_1.

Other Unipolar Precordial Lead Systems. *Unipolar precordial leads* can be positioned in different locations on the anterior and posterior chest.

- They can be continued to the vertebral border on the left posterior chest and, if so, are designated V_1–V_9.
- They may be placed on the right side of the chest. The placement mirrors the left-sided electrode placement, and the leads are designated V_{1R}–V_{9R}.
- They can also be placed on the right side of the chest at one intercostal space higher than the traditional placement on the left chest and designated $3V_{3R}$–$3V_{6R}$ or $3V_{9R}$.

The positions of the special leads allow examination of the electrical activity of the posterior wall of the heart or of the right ventricle (Figure 19-6).[1,4]

Continuous ECG Monitoring

Continuous bedside ECG monitoring is often performed. Up to 12 leads can be monitored continuously from the patient's bedside.

A *three-lead monitoring system* uses one electrode designated as positive (+), a second designated as negative (−), and a third as a ground. Any two of the limbs (RA, LA, LL) may be identified as the positive electrode and negative electrode. The electrode positions determine the lead monitored—lead I, II, or III. MCL_1 may also be continuously monitored using the three-lead system. The positive electrode is placed in the V_1 position, and the negative electrode is placed under the left clavicle (LA). The ground is usually positioned on the RL, LL, or RA. Placing the positive electrode in the appropriate precordial chest position can also monitor other modified chest leads (MCL_{2-6}).

A *five-electrode monitoring system* uses four limb electrodes (RA, LA, RL, LL) in the traditional locations. The fifth electrode may be placed in the desired MCL_{1-6} position. This five-electrode system permits monitoring of one or more of all 12 leads at the patient's bedside.[1,4]

Special Diagnostic Monitoring

Holter monitoring is a type of continuous monitoring used to diagnose the occasional dysrhythmia. The *Holter monitor* is a portable ECG monitor with a memory. The patient wears the monitor for 24–48 hours. Since these patients' dysrhythmia occurs infrequently, it is more likely to occur within this extended time period than in a short office visit. The Holter equipment records two or three channels of the ECG onto a cassette tape or flash card for analysis by the cardiologist after the 48-hour period. The leads are usually modified chest leads that resemble V_1 and V_5 because they are more sensitive at detecting atrial dysrhythmias and bundle branch blocks. The patient's chest is wrapped in an elastic bandage to keep the leads in place. Patients are instructed to keep a diary and write down the precise times they experience symptoms. The diary is then compared with the downloaded ECG recordings to determine whether a dysrhythmia occurred at the time that the patient felt symptoms.[6]

For patients whose dysrhythmias occur too infrequently for the Holter monitor to record them, a *transtelephonic event monitor* may be necessary. Patients wear the unit and activate it only when they experience symptoms, such as palpitations or dizziness. The unit records the ECG for 3–5 minutes and stores it in memory. The patient then attaches the unit to a modem and transmits the ECG information for evaluation. This diagnostic technique allows monitoring for months, making the dysrhythmia diagnosed accurate.[6]

The *cardiac stress test*, or *exercise tolerance test*, is a diagnostic procedure that allows assessment of the individual's cardiovascular response to exercise. This noninvasive procedure is used as the initial screening test for the detection of coronary artery disease. An ECG monitor and a noninvasive blood pressure cuff

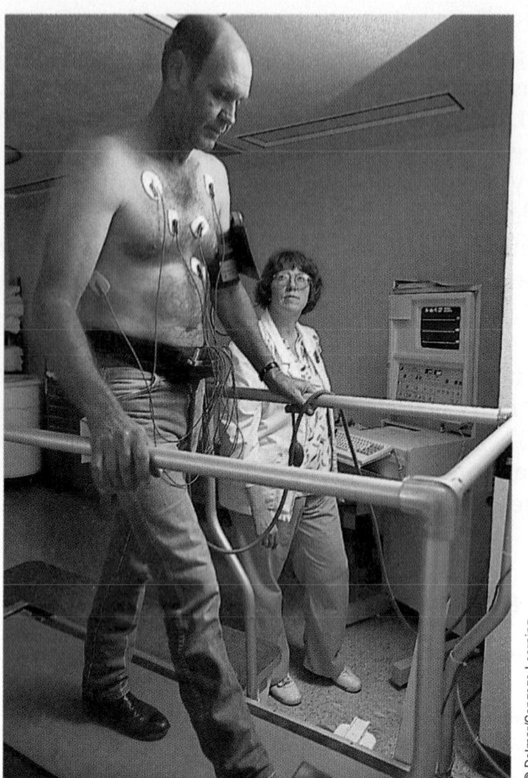

© Delmar/Cengage Learning

FIGURE 19-7 A stress test is performed to test cardiac function.

Best Practice

Double Product

Double product is a calculated monitoring parameter that is used to determine the patient's cardiovascular response to exercise. Equal to the product of the patient's exercise blood pressure multiplied by the exercise heart rate, it is a good measure of myocardial oxygen consumption. If the patient's myocardial oxygen needs exceed myocardial oxygen consumption, the patient will show signs of myocardial ischemia, such as chest pain, and ECG changes. Two such ECG changes are **T-wave inversion** (a symmetrical, sharply pointed T-wave that has negative amplitude in leads that are typically positive) and depressed ST segment (discussed later in this chapter). If the patient manifests any of these symptoms, the cardiac stress test must be terminated, and the patient must be closely monitored for continuing or worsening symptoms.

$$\text{Exercise BP} \times \text{Exercise Heart Rate} = \text{Double Product}$$

are attached to the patient, who then ambulates on a treadmill (a **bicycle ergometer** may also be used) at gradually increasing speeds and angles of incline (Figure 19-7). If a bicycle ergometer is used, the resistance is gradually increased. According to the American College of Cardiology/American Heart Association (ACC/AHA), it is an absolute indication to stop an exercise stress test when the patient:[8,9]

- Is unable to continue.
- Experiences moderate to severe angina.
- Reaches the maximum exercise heart rate {predicted maximum HR = [210 − (patient's age × 0.65)]}.
- Is manifesting cardiac symptoms such as ST segment elevation, poor tissue perfusion, or sustained ventricular tachycardia.

A cardiac stress test is by no means infallible. The results can be false positive or false negative. A positive test result indicates coronary artery disease (CAD), but this finding must be closely examined in light of the individual's risk factors, such as age, family history of CAD, smoking history, diabetes, hyperlipidemia, or hypertension. A positive stress test in an otherwise healthy young individual with minimal risk factors may lead the physician to recommend a **myocardial scintigraphy** study in conjunction with the exercise stress test. Injecting the patient with radioactive imaging agents during the stress test permits visualization of areas of poor coronary circulation. If no defects are observed, the patient does not have to go through cardiac catheterization, which is more invasive and associated with more complications.[8,9]

The ECG: Waveforms and Intervals

The ECG produces a printout that shows the electrical events in all the leads (Figure 19-8). The ECG waveforms represent the electrical activity of the cardiac chambers during systole and diastole. The intervals between waveforms are time measures that indicate the amount of time in fractions of a second that the heart requires to depolarize and repolarize the atria and ventricles (Figure 19-9 and Table 19-1).[1]

P-WAVE

The P-wave is the first waveform seen on the ECG and represents atrial depolarization. Normally, the atrial tissue does not initiate the electrical impulse. The P-wave reflects atrial depolarization after the SA node impulse reaches the atria.[1,10]

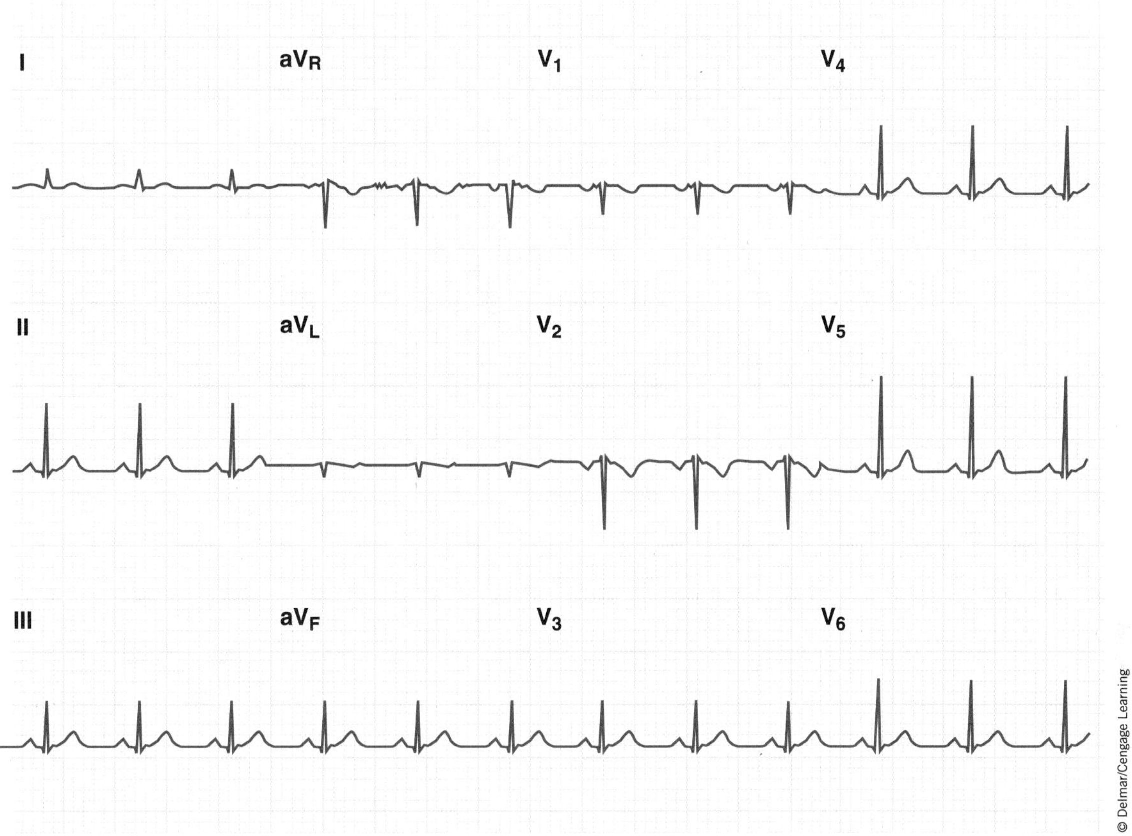

FIGURE 19-8 The 12-lead ECG consists of three standard leads and three augmented leads that view the heart in the frontal plane, and six precordial chest leads that view the heart in the horizontal plane.

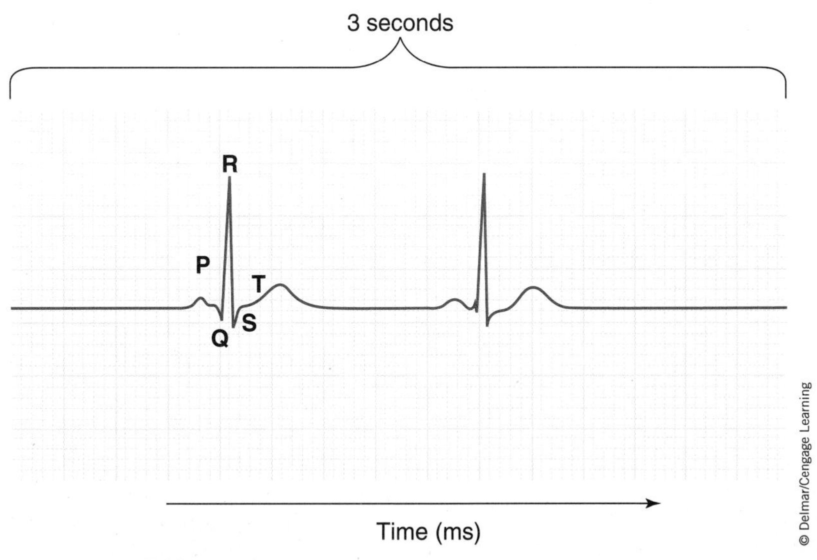

FIGURE 19-9 ECG waveforms.

P-R INTERVAL AND SEGMENT

The P-R interval (P-RI) and the P-R segment are time measures. The P-R interval lasts from the beginning of the P-wave to the beginning of the Q-wave. The P-R segment is a component of the P-R interval (Figure 19-10), lasting from the end of the P-wave to the beginning of the Q-wave. Any changes in the P-R segment alter the P-RI. Because the P-RI is easier to calculate, it is the more commonly used of the two time measures (Table 19-2). Although the P-RI is

TABLE 19-1 **ECG Waveforms**

Waveform Characteristic	P-Wave	QRS Complex	T-Wave	U-Wave
Shape	Symmetrical, gently rounded	Sharp and narrow; consists of ≥1 waves representing ventricular electrical activity (Q-, R-, and S-waves)	Variably shaped; usually asymmetrical and slightly rounded	Symmetrical and round
Amplitude	0.5–2.5 mm	Deflection height from baseline—positive or negative—varies from 2 to 15 mm	<5 mm	Usually flat; <2 mm
Duration	<0.11 s	<0.12 s	0.10–0.25 s	Not known
Direction	Positive in lead II; variable in other leads	Variable, depending on lead and patient's electrical axis; net amplitude may be positive, negative, or equally positive and negative	In lead II, positive; in other leads, variable	In lead II, positive; in other leads, direction parallels the preceding T-wave
Miscellaneous information	Normal P-wave indicates normal origin of electrical impulse with normal depolarization of right and left atria	Normal QRS indicates ventricular activation occurred through the normal conduction pathway	Abnormal T-wave indicates abnormal ventricular repolarization (premature ventricular contraction, bundle branch block, electrolyte disturbance, medication, myocardial infarction)	Abnormal U-wave information seen in hypokalemia, hyperthyroidism, left ventricular hypertrophy, certain cardiac drugs; not observed in most ECGs

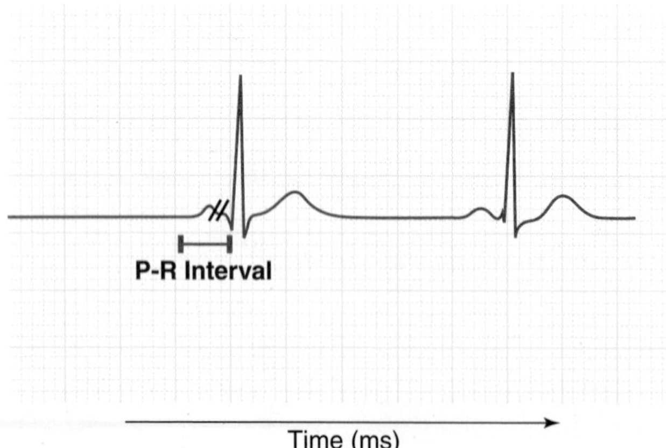

FIGURE 19-10 The P-R interval (bar between vertical lines) and the P-R segment (portion of wave between diagonal lines).

predominately used as an indicator of electrical conduction through the AV junction, remember that P-RI normally changes with heart rate. The primary causes of P-RI abnormalities are slowed or blocked conduction caused by parasympathetic nervous system stimulation, by severe heart disease and the effects of the disease process on conductivity, and by medications affecting the autonomic nervous system.[1,10]

QRS COMPLEX

The QRS complex represents ventricular depolarization. It is the waveform from the beginning of the Q-wave to the end of the S-wave. The time from Q to S is referred to as the *QRS time* or *QRS duration*. The complex consists of one or more of the following: a positive deflection called the *R-wave* and two negative deflections called the *Q-wave* and the *S-wave*. Each wave represents a different aspect of ventricular depolarization (Figure 19-9).[1,10]

Q-Wave. The *Q-wave* is the first negative deflection in the QRS complex that is not preceded by an R-wave. The Q-wave deflection represents ventricular septal depolarization.

R-Wave. The *R-wave* is the first positive deflection in the QRS complex. If the QRS complex has additional

TABLE 19-2 **ECG timing and intervals**

Characteristic	P-R Segment	P-R Interval	R-R Interval	S-T Segment	Q-T Interval
Significance	Detects changes in AV nodal conduction; short line seen in junctional dysrhythmias and sinus or atrial tachycardia; long line seen in first-, second-, and third-degree heart blocks	Same as P-R segment; lengthens in bradycardia	Detects changes in heart rate and rhythm regularity; short interval seen in tachydysrythmias; long intervals seen in bradydysrhythmias; variable intervals seen with premature beats, some heart blocks, atrial fibrillation or flutter	Deviation indicates abnormal ventricular repolarization; elevation indicates acute myocardial infarction; depression indicates myocardial ischemia	Deviation reflects changes in time required for ventricular repolarization; prolonged Q-T interval more common than shortened one: caused by some cardiac drugs, hypokalemia and calcemia, and acute myocardial infarction; patient is susceptible to lethal dysrhythmias
How calculated	Time from end of P-wave to start of QRS complex	Time from start of P-wave to start of QRS complex	Measured by number of large or small squares from beginning of one QRS complex to end of next QRS complex	Time from end of S-wave to beginning of T-wave; normal allowed baseline deviation: 2 mm above, 0.5 mm below	Time from the beginning of the QRS complex to the end of the T-wave
Normal duration	0.05–0.08 s	0.12–0.20 s	Consistent with rate 60–100 pbm	≤ 0.20 s	Heart rate dependent; less than half of preceding R-R interval
Miscellaneous Information	Less practical than P-RI	Varies with heart rates	Variation indicates rhythm irregularity	Duration is heart rate dependent	Trend changes more important than absolute values

positive deflections, the second positive wave is called *R′* (R prime), and the third positive wave is called *R″* (R double prime). The R-wave deflection represents early ventricular depolarization.

S-Wave. The *S-wave* is the first negative deflection after an R-wave. If the QRS complex has more than one negative deflection after the R-wave, then the second negative deflection is called *S′* (S prime), the third is called *S″* (S double prime), and so on. The S-wave deflection represents late ventricular depolarization.

QS-Wave. A *QS-wave* is a wave in the QRS complex with a single negative deflection and no positive deflection (i.e., no R-wave).[3,10]

S-T SEGMENT

The S-T segment is usually observed as an isoelectric (straight) line or as a sloping shape relative to the baseline on the ECG tracing. It represents the early part of ventricular repolarization, the time from the end of an S-wave to the beginning of the T-wave. During the S-T segment, the ventricles are absolutely refractory to additional electrical stimulation. The area on the ECG tracing where the QRS complex ends and the S-T segment begins is called the *junction*, or *J point*. The S-T segment extends to the point at which the T-wave begins (Figure 19-11).[1,3,10]

T-WAVE

The T-wave (Figure 19-9) represents ventricular repolarization. The T-wave always occurs after a QRS complex, even though it may be difficult to see because of low amplitude.[1,11]

U-WAVE

The *U-wave* is not observed in most ECG tracings. It is thought to represent the final stage of Purkinje fiber repolarization. It is a small deflection after the T-wave in a direction that usually parallels that of the T-wave.[1,11]

Q-T INTERVAL

The *Q-T interval* (Figure 19-12) is not normally used in ECG analysis, but it is something the respiratory therapist should understand. Measured from the beginning of the QRS complex to the end of the T-wave, the Q-T interval represents ventricular depolarization and repolarization. Normally it varies with gender, age, and heart rate. The term *QT(c)* is the Q-T interval that has been "corrected" or adjusted for the patient's heart rate.[3,4] For a heart rate of 70 bpm, the QT(c) is ≤0.40 s. It is calculated by Bazett's Formula:[12]

$$QT(c) = \frac{QT}{RRR \text{ (in seconds)}}$$

For every 10 bpm increase above 70, subtract 0.02 s, and for every 10 bpm decrease below 70, add 0.02 s. For example:

$QT \leq 0.38$ @ 80 bpm

$QT \leq 0.42$ @ 60 bpm

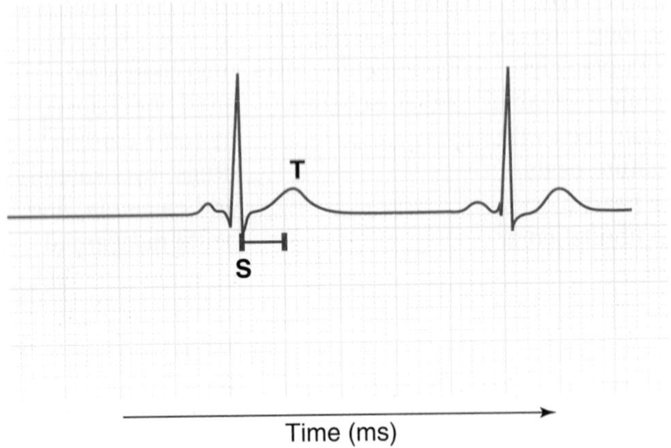

FIGURE 19-11 The S-T segment.

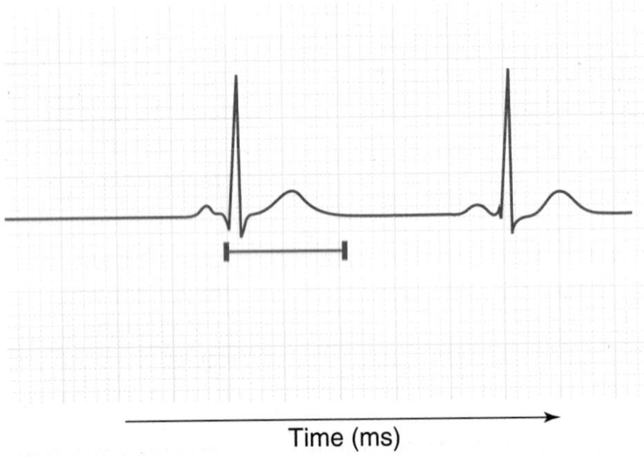

FIGURE 19-12 The Q-T interval.

Determination of Heart Rate

Two of the various techniques that can be used to determine the patient's heart rate using the ECG tracing are discussed here.

Timing is measured by the grid on the ECG paper. Time markers (1 second, 3 seconds, 6 seconds) appear on some ECG paper. If they do not, just remember that there are 30 large squares in 6 seconds, 15 large squares in 3 seconds, and 300 large squares in 1 minute (Figure 19-13).

SIX-SECOND TECHNIQUE (UNIVERSAL TECHNIQUE)

If the patient has an irregular rhythm, use a sampling procedure to determine heart rate (the most common is to count the heart rate for 6 seconds). To use this technique, count the number of R-waves (which is the same as the number of QRS complexes) in a 6-second sample of the ECG strip and then multiply that number by 10. The result is a close estimation of the actual

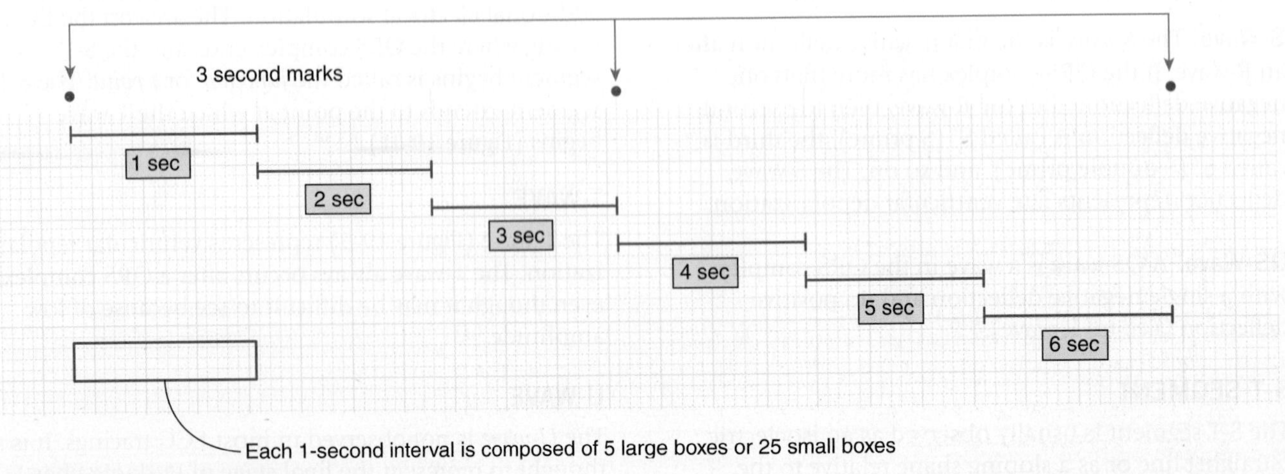

FIGURE 19-13 ECG intervals.

heart rate (beats per minute). (Also count the number of P-waves if the P-wave rate is needed to help with dysrhythmia interpretation.) Using a 3-second sample of R-waves and then multiplying by 20 is possible, but the resulting heart rate estimation is less accurate.

REGULAR RHYTHM RATE CALCULATION TECHNIQUE

When the patient has a regular rhythm, use the following heart rate calculation technique: Count the number of large squares between two QRS complexes and divide the count into 300. The quotient is the heart rate.

If the QRS complexes do not fall exactly on the large square lines, an alternative method is to count the number of small squares between two QRS complexes and divide that number into 1500 (there are 1500 small squares in 1 minute of ECG paper). The quotient is the heart rate.[1]

Steps in Dysrhythmia Recognition

When interpreting an ECG, the keys to accuracy are consistency and thoroughness. The key to interpreting an ECG is similar to that for performing any clinical procedure: Follow the same steps every time when analyzing each ECG. Using a systematic approach ensures that nothing is overlooked. Although no one set sequence is standard, analyzing the QRS complexes must always come first because it identifies life-threatening cardiac dysrhythmias that require emergency treatment. The following suggested sequence for interpreting an ECG enables the interpreter to eliminate possibilities at each step. Through this process, the reader can identify whatever dysrhythmia appears.

Step 1: Analyze the QRS complexes.

- Are there recognizable or normal QRS complexes? If not, consider ventricular fibrillation, asystole, or ventricular tachycardia—all pulseless rhythms.
- In the presence of normal QRS complexes, does the patient have a pulse? If not, consider pulseless electrical activity—a cardiac emergency.
- After determining that the patient does not have a life-threatening dysrhythmia, identify the shape and duration of each QRS complex. Do all the QRS complexes look the same? If not, identify normal and abnormal QRS durations. With a normal QRS duration, the rhythm is supraventricular; a wide QRS indicates a ventricular rhythm or a conduction disturbance in the ventricle.[5]

Step 2: Analyze the heart rate.

- Is the rate normal? The rate eliminates a large group of dysrhythmias from the possibilities. Tachycardia eliminates bradycardias and AV blocks. Bradycardia eliminates atrial tachycardia, sinus tachycardia, and ventricular tachycardia.

Step 3: Analyze the ventricular rhythm.

- Is the R-R interval regular or irregular?
- Is there a pattern to the irregularity, or does it occur unpredictably?
- If the rhythm is irregular, eliminate the problems that would show a regular rhythm, such as sinus bradycardia and tachycardia.

Step 4: Analyze the P-waves.

- Are P-waves present?
- Do all the P-waves look the same?
- Is the P-wave upright or inverted in lead II?
- Is the P-P interval regular or irregular? Are F- or f-waves present? (See Atrial Dysrhythmias on page 520.)

Step 5: Analyze the PQRST relationship to determine whether a heart block or ectopic beats are present.

- Is there one P-wave for each QRS complex?
- How long is the P-RI?
- If the relationship of the P-wave to the QRS complex is abnormal, does the abnormal pattern repeat in a constant time interval, or does the interval vary?

Step 6: Identify the site of the dysrhythmia.

- Is the dysrhythmia supraventricular or ventricular in origin?
- Are the P-waves upright in lead II (sinus), or are they inverted (junctional)?
- Is the QRS complex of normal duration (supraventricular)?
- If the QRS complex is wide, is it really a ventricular beat, or is a conduction delay in the ventricle causing the prolonged QRS duration?

Step 7: Now the dysrhythmia should be identifiable.[1]

Causes of Cardiac Dysrhythmias

There are many causes of cardiac dysrhythmias (abnormal cardiac rhythms): coronary artery disease, electrolyte imbalance, congestive heart failure, drug toxicity, and many more. But all these clinical problems cause just three abnormalities in cardiac electrophysiology: abnormal automaticity, abnormal conductivity, or a combination of the two.[1]

DISORDERS OF AUTOMATICITY

The heart rate is determined by the inherent rate of self-depolarization by specific cardiac cells (*automaticity*).

The SA node, AV junction, and ventricular conducting system have their own intrinsic levels of spontaneous depolarization that determine their pacemaker rates. The working cells of the myocardium do not normally possess the property of automaticity but can become more excitable in disease states such as coronary artery disease and congestive heart failure. Clinical situations that disturb the inherent excitability of the pacemaker tissue or the myocardial tissue of the atria and ventricles can cause the heart rate to speed up, slow down, or be irregular. A few examples of dysrhythmias that may be caused by a disturbance of automaticity are sinus bradycardia, premature ventricular contractions, and ventricular tachycardia.[1]

DISORDERS OF CONDUCTIVITY

Conductivity is determined by many variables, such as electrolyte balance, stimulus intensity, and repolarization disparity. If conduction is accelerated or slowed, then the wave or segment duration is shortened or prolonged. For example, if conduction is slowed through the AV junction, as one would see in a heart block, then the P-R interval is prolonged (more than 0.20 second).

Another common cause of a conductivity problem is the phenomenon known as *reentry*, which occurs when there are unequal refractory periods in the heart. This situation might occur with a premature (early) beat such as a premature atrial contraction. The P-wave occurs too early in the cardiac cycle, and part of the conducting system is still refractory to electrical stimulation. Consequently, the depolarization wave travels only through the part of the conducting system that has recovered. This abnormal depolarization pathway takes longer than the normal one. When the previously unresponsive part of the heart muscle has recovered, it depolarizes and creates a new depolarization wave that restimulates the heart. Essentially, the premature atrial complex has set up a circular wave of self-depolarization, and the resulting dysrhythmia is a very fast, self-perpetuating tachycardia. This dysrhythmia is called *paroxysmal supraventricular tachycardia (PSVT)*.

Other examples of conduction disturbance are first-degree heart block and second-degree type I heart block. In both of these dysrhythmias, conduction is slowed through the AV junction. This conduction problem is reflected by a prolonged P-R interval. In some cases, the conduction can be so delayed that the depolarization wave does not propagate through the AV junction to the ventricle.[1]

COMBINED DISORDERS OF AUTOMATICITY AND CONDUCTIVITY

A *combined disorder* involving both automaticity and conductivity occurs when an abnormal rate of spontaneous depolarization and a conduction disturbance exist together. These problems may be present in a variety of clinical situations. For example, ventricular tachycardia or sinus bradycardia might be combined with first-degree heart block. Or premature atrial contraction may coexist with a ventricular bundle branch block. These problems may be transient or permanent, and they may range from fairly benign to lethal.[1]

Types of Cardiac Dysrhythmia

Of the many categories of dysrhythmia, in this chapter dysrhythmias are categorized as sinus, atrial, junctional, AV block, and ventricular. The dysrhythmias discussed are those included in the Advanced Cardiac Life Support Course offered by the American Heart Association. They are common cardiac dysrhythmias seen in critically ill patients and may require maintenance or emergency treatment.

It is paramount during the analysis of a dysrhythmia that you keep in mind the *best monitor* of how the patient is handling the dysrhythmia is clinical observation of the patient. You are first and foremost treating the patient NOT the monitor.

SINUS DYSRHYTHMIAS

In sinus dysrhythmias, the electrical impulses originate in the sinus node. The electrical current follows the normal electrical path through the atria, the AV junction, and the ventricles. The ECG has normal waves in the normal sequence. The basic abnormality is the heart rate or the regularity of the waveforms. Table 19-3 lists the causes of sinus tachycardia and sinus bradycardia, and Table 19-4 lists their physiological mechanisms and their ECG characteristics.

Sinus Tachycardia. *Sinus tachycardia* is a common dysrhythmia in both healthy and critically ill individuals. It has the same characteristics as a normal sinus rhythm except for the heart rate.

Description Sinus tachycardia occurs when the baseline rate sinus node discharge is greater than 100. As the most common dysrhythmia in critically ill patients, it is the result of a physiological need for greater **cardiac output (CO)**, the amount of blood ejected by the left ventricle each minute. Because the causes are so diverse, the physician must identify the underlying cause before attempting to control the dysrhythmia. Figure 19-14 shows the ECG of a patient with sinus tachycardia.

Clinical Significance Sinus tachycardia is the most common dysrhythmia in the critically ill. Because it can be the result of any of myriad clinical problems, the

TABLE 19-3 **Causes of sinus dysrhythmias**

Causative Category	Sinus Tachycardia	Sinus Bradycardia
Autonomic nervous system	Sympathetic nervous system stimulation: exercise, emotion, fever, pain, hypoxemia, acidosis, hypercarbia, stimulants (coffee, tea, nicotine, chocolate)	Parasympathetic nervous system stimulation: carotid massage, vomiting, suctioning, increased intracranial pressure
Drugs or drug toxicity	CNS stimulants: norepinephrine, epinephrine, isoproterenol, dopamine, cocaine, amphetamines, methamphetamines; parasympathetic stimulants: anticholinergic drugs, tricyclic antidepressants	Beta-adrenergic blockade, calcium channel blockade, organophosphate poisoning, adenosine, cholinergic drug toxicity
Diseases or conditions	Acute myocardial infarction, congestive heart failure, acute pulmonary embolism, pulmonary edema, shock, hyperthyroidism, sepsis	Well-conditioned athlete, sick sinus syndrome, inferior wall, myocardial infarction

TABLE 19-4 **Sinus dysrhythmia: physiological mechanisms and ECG characteristics**

	Sinus Tachycardia	Sinus Bradycardia
Physiological mechanism	Increased automaticity of the SA node	Decreased automaticity of the SA node
Rate	100–150 bpm (may go up to 180 bpm)	40–60 bpm (may be lower)
Ventricular rhythm	Regular	Regular
P-wave	Regular sinus P-waves; P-wave rate is same as QRS rate; P-wave upright in lead II	Same as sinus tachycardia
PQRST relationship	Normal sequence: one P-wave for each QRS complex	Normal sequence
QRS complex	Usually normal ≥0.12 s if bundle branch block or anomalous ventricular conduction pathway is present	Same as sinus tachycardia
Waveform intervals	P-RI and Q-T interval may be shorter than normal	P-RI and Q-T interval may be longer than normal

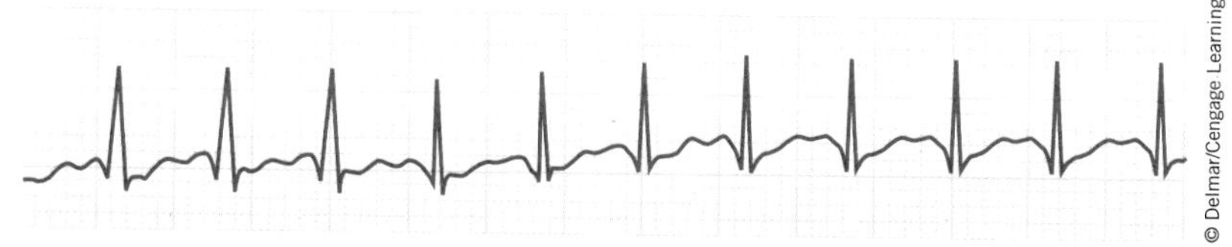

FIGURE 19-14 Sinus tachycardia: The rhythm is regular, and the rate is approximately 136 bpm. The P-wave is visible, and all the P-waves look the same.

best approach is to treat the underlying mechanism. For example:

- If fever is the cause, the treatment may be the administration of an antipyretic.
- If the cause is a bacterial pneumonia with hypoxemia, then antimicrobial and oxygen therapy may be sufficient to decrease the heart rate.
- If the sinus tachycardia is associated with heart failure, then improving heart function by administering cardiac drugs may decrease the heart rate.
- In the elderly or individuals with underlying cardiovascular disease, the reduced ventricular filling time associated with tachycardia may significantly reduce cardiac output. These patients may require additional treatment to stabilize their cardiovascular function.[1]

Sinus Bradycardia. Sinus bradycardia may occur in normal individuals with a healthy heart, such as well-conditioned athletes. Sinus bradycardia has the same characteristics as a normal sinus rhythm except for the slower-than-normal heart rate.

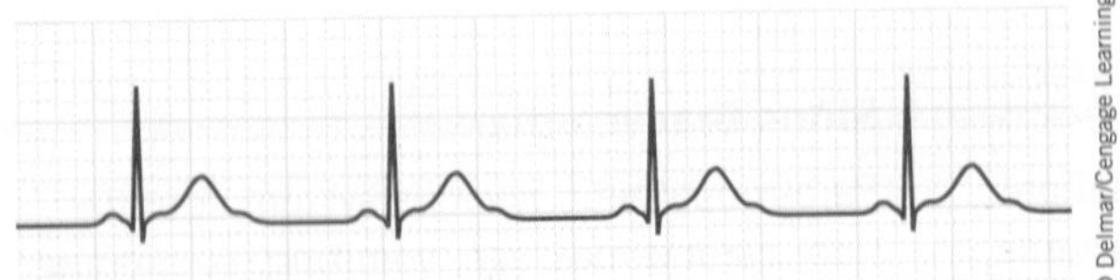

FIGURE 19-15 Sinus bradycardia: The rhythm is regular, but the rate is only about 33 bpm. The P-wave is visible, and all the P-waves look the same.

Description Sinus bradycardia occurs when the baseline rate of sinus node discharge is less than 60 bpm. Found in many situations, this dysrhythmia is most common in individuals with underlying heart disease. Many cardiac drugs may also cause sinus bradycardia. Mild sinus bradycardia is well tolerated, but for severe drops in heart rate (<50 bpm), medical treatment is necessary. Figure 19-15 shows the ECG of a patient with sinus bradycardia.

Clinical Significance The individual with sinus bradycardia is not usually symptomatic until the heart rate falls below 50 bpm. With the increasing numbers of people doing regular *physical workouts*, the incidences of otherwise healthy persons having bradycardia has risen. When manifesting symptoms, the person usually complains of dizziness, faintness, and lightheadedness. These symptoms appear because of decreased cardiac output and reduced perfusion of the brain.

For the individual who has suffered an *acute myocardial infarction*, a mild sinus bradycardia has some positive benefits. The slower heart rate decreases the work of the heart and thereby lessens the oxygen requirements of the heart muscle. If the heart rate is too slow, however, cardiac output decreases, reducing coronary blood flow and coronary perfusion of the heart muscle. When the heart muscle is not adequately perfused, it becomes oxygen deprived (ischemic), and systolic function deteriorates.

Another complication of sinus bradycardia is the increased incidence of *ventricular escape beats*. These premature beats help support the cardiac output by adding to the heart rate. However, they also increase the risk of precipitating serious ventricular dysrhythmias, such as ventricular tachycardia, ventricular fibrillation, or ventricular asystole. The ventricular premature beats are not specifically treated because they help support the patient's cardiac output. The basic direction of treatment is to increase the rate of the sinus node. This increase in rate may suppress the patient's premature ventricular contractions.[1,11]

ATRIAL DYSRHYTHMIAS

Atrial dysrhythmias originate not from the sinus node, but from the atrial tissue or atrial conducting structures. Consequently, the P-wave (atrial depolarization) may have a different shape, duration, and direction than on a normal ECG. The P-wave alterations depend on the ectopic (abnormal) beat's origin in the atria and on the ECG lead in which you are viewing the waveforms.

- If the ectopic beat arises from atrial tissue close to the sinus node, the P-wave is similar to the P-wave of a sinus rhythm.
- If the ectopic beat arises from tissue close to the AV junction, the P-wave may be negative (below baseline) because the electrical stimulus depolarizing the atria is traveling in an opposite direction from normal.

A disturbance in automaticity, conductivity, or a combination of the two may cause atrial dysrhythmias (Table 19-5). Table 19-6 describes the physiological mechanisms and ECG characteristics of atrial dysrhythmias.[1,13]

Premature Atrial Contraction. Premature atrial complexes or contractions (PACs) are also known as atrial premature contractions (APCs).

Description An early atrial beat is caused by an ectopic pacemaker in the atria. The ectopic atrial pacemaker spontaneously depolarizes before the next sinus node discharge and causes a premature P-wave. The early P-wave, called a *P'* (P prime), is different in morphology from the sinus-generated P-wave. Usually, the P'-wave is conducted and is followed by a normal or an abnormal QRS complex. If the P' wave is too premature, the AV junction or the bundle branches may still be refractory from the previous depolarization wave and does not propagate the impulse. Consequently, the PAC is not conducted to the ventricle. Figure 19-16 shows the ECG of a patient with premature atrial contractions.

Clinical Significance In the normal person, premature atrial contractions are usually benign and not significant. In individuals with underlying heart disease, PACs indicate increased automaticity of the atrial tissue or a conduction disturbance. The sudden appearance of frequent PACs warns of greater cardiac irritability and may indicate worsening of cardiac function. When symptomatic, the individual usually complains of dizziness, faintness, and lightheadedness. These symptoms appear because of decreased cardiac output and reduced perfusion of the brain.[1]

TABLE 19-5 **Causes of atrial dysrhythmias**

Causative Category	Premature Atrial Contraction (PAC)	Paroxysmal Atrial Tachycardia	Nonparoxysmal Atrial Tachycardia	Atrial Flutter	Atrial Fibrillation
Autonomic nervous system	Increased sympathetic tone, increased catecholamines, emotion, infection, hypoxemia, stimulants (coffee, tea, nicotine, chocolate)	Same as PAC	Increased sympathetic tone, increased catecholamines	Normal individuals, secondary to excessive stimulants (coffee, tea, nicotine, chocolate) or emotional distress	Normal individuals secondary to excessive stimulants (coffee, tea, nicotine, chocolate), or emotional distress
Drugs or drug toxicity	Sympathomimetic drugs, digitalis toxicity	Same as PAC	Digitalis toxicity	Digitalis toxicity (rare)	Digitalis toxicity (rare)
Diseases or conditions	Occurs in people with apparently healthy heart; heart diseases: myocardial ischemia, acute myocardial infarction, early congestive heart failure, mitral valve disease	Occurs in people with apparently healthy heart; heart diseases: coronary artery disease, rheumatic heart disease, acute myocardial infarction	Heart diseases: coronary artery disease or cor pulmonale	Small incidence in people with apparently healthy heart; heart diseases: rheumatic heart disease, hypertensive heart disease, coronary artery disease, congestive heart failure, thyrotoxicosis	Small incidence in people with apparently healthy heart; heart diseases; mitral valve disease, congestive heart failure, coronary artery disease, myocardial infarction, hypertensive heart disease

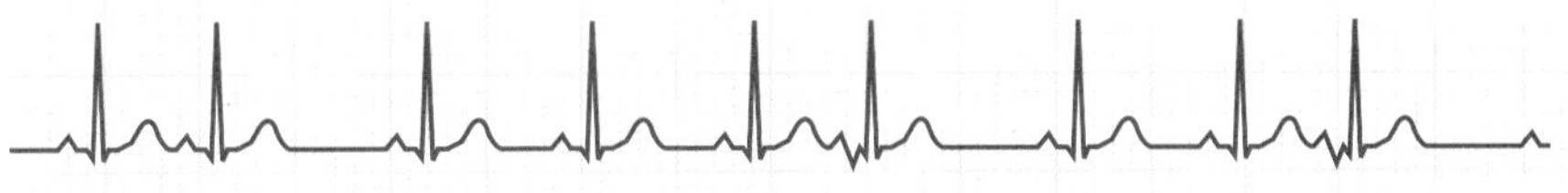

FIGURE 19-16 Premature atrial contractions: The sinus rhythm has three premature atrial contractions (beats 2, 6, and 9). These early beats have a positive P-wave before each early QRS. These premature P-waves differ in appearance from the normal sinus P-waves. The rhythm strip is irregular, and the total rate is 70 bpm, with an underlying sinus rate of 68 bpm.

Atrial Tachycardia. *Atrial tachycardia* applies to dysrhythmias that originate in the left or right atria and have identifiable, uniform P-waves preceding the QRS. This definition excludes atrial flutter, atrial fibrillation, and multifocal atrial tachycardia. Atrial tachycardia accounts for about 15% of cases of supraventricular tachycardias in adults and up to 23% in children. It may be secondary to reentry (*paroxysmal*) or to abnormal automaticity (*nonparoxysmal*). The reentry, or paroxysmal, form is a much more common mechanism of atrial tachycardia in adults. However, in children, reentry and automaticity occur approximately in the same proportion (11–12%). If this dysrhythmia becomes a chronic problem in children, the mechanism is usually secondary to automaticity.[14]

Best Practice

Leads for PAC

The best leads for assessing PACs are II, aV_F, and V_1 because the P-wave is more prominent in these leads.

TABLE 19-6 **Atrial dysrhythmia: physiological mechanisms and ECG characteristics**

	Premature Atrial Contraction (PAC)	Paroxysmal Atrial Tachycardia	Nonparoxysmal Atrial Tachycardia	Atrial Flutter	Atrial Fibrillation
Physiological mechanism	Increased automaticity of an ectopic arterial pacemaker or reentry circuit in the atria	Rapid reentry circuit in the atria	Increased automaticity of ectopic atrial pacemaker	Increased automaticity of ectopic atrial pacemaker or rapid reentry circuit in the atria	Increased automaticity of ectopic atrial pacemaker or multiple rapid reentry circuit in the atria
Rate	Adds to patient's baseline rate	160–240 bpm	160–240 bpm	Atrial rate 240–400 bpm; ventricular rate may be half or one third of atrial rate	Atrial rate 360–700 bpm; ventricular rate slower
Ventricular rhythm	Irregular, secondary to early beat	Regular	Regular, with constant AV conduction, or grossly irregular with variable AV conduction block (digitalis toxicity)	Usually regular, or irregular with variable conduction ratio	Irregular
P-wave	Early P-wave arises from atrial tissue; morphology different from sinus P-waves	Not visible in PSVT, but may be seen at lower atrial rates	Ectopic P-waves have different appearance from sinus P-waves	P-waves (called F-waves) with saw-toothed appearance	P-waves called F-waves; atrial rate not determinable; baseline may look wavy or flatline
PQRST relationship	Normal relationship, usually; in nonconducted PACS, early P-wave occurs during refractory period; noncompensatory pause present	Varies with origin of dysrhythmia (atria or AV junction)	Usually normal, except physiological AV block may exist at atrial rates > 200 bpm; in digitalis toxicity, AV block may exist, with more P-waves than QRS complexes	Conduction ratio usually constant but may vary	One-half to one-third of F-waves are randomly conducted; ventricular stimulation controlled by physiological AV block
QRS complex	Normal duration unless early-wave occurs when ventricle is variable refractory; then the QRS ≥0.12 s	Usually normal; ≥0.12 s if bundle branch or anomalous ventricular conduction pathway is present	Same as paroxysmal atrial tachycardia	Same as paroxysmal atrial tachycardia	Same as paroxysmal atrial tachycardia
Waveform intervals	R-R interval irregular	P-RI not determinable in PSVT because P-wave not seen; Q-T may be short	Normal P-RI and R-R intervals, except prolonged P-RI and/or irregular R-R interval in physiological AV block or secondary to digitalis toxicity	P-RI usually equal but may vary; R-R interval usually regular, except variable R-R intervals with varying AV block	R-R interval varies widely, except in atrial fib with superimposed third degree AV block

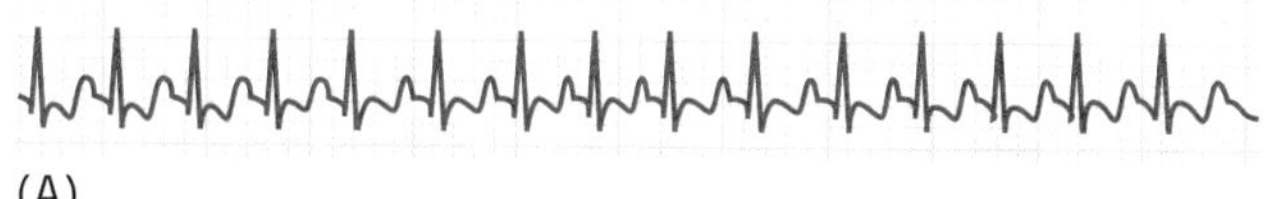

(A)

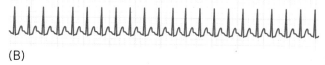

(B)

FIGURE 19-17 (A) Paroxysmal atrial tachycardia (supraventricular tachycardia): The rhythm is regular, with 1:1 conduction. The rate is approximately 188 bpm. (B) Paroxysmal supraventricular tachycardia: The rhythm is regular, and the P-wave is not seen. The rate is approximately 188 bpm.

Description Atrial tachycardia occurs when there are at least three successive ectopic atrial complexes. The atrial heart rate is very fast, and, in the paroxysmal form, the relationship is usually 1:1 between the ectopic atrial beat and a ventricular response.

Atrial tachycardia is thought to be the result of one of two mechanisms: enhanced automaticity of an area of the atrial tissue (nonparoxysmal atrial tachycardia) or, more commonly, a reentry conduction disturbance that is started by a PAC occurring when part of the heart is still refractory (paroxysmal atrial tachycardia). Figure 19-17 identifies important clinical differences between the two types of paroxysmal atrial tachycardia. By convention, when there is a single wave between the QRS complexes and no visible P′-wave, the atrial dysrhythmia is simply called a *supraventricular tachycardia*. If the onset is sudden, the dysrhythmia may be called *paroxysmal supraventricular tachycardia*.[1]

Clinical Significance The tolerance to atrial tachycardia depends on the heart rate and the presence of underlying heart disease. A common symptom of atrial tachycardia is palpitations. Other symptoms are the result of a rapid decrease in cardiac output and cerebral blood flow: dizziness, fainting, sweating, pallor, and dyspnea.

In the elderly or individuals with underlying cardiovascular disease, the rapid heart rate reduces ventricular filling, and the reduced ventricular filling may significantly reduce cardiac output. The reduction in cardiac output also decreases coronary blood flow (an estimated drop of 25%) and coronary perfusion of the myocardium. Consequently, individuals with coronary artery disease or congestive heart failure may quickly develop myocardial ischemia and have a catastrophic deterioration in ventricular function. This is a life-threatening emergency that requires immediate treatment.[1]

Atrial Flutter. *Atrial flutter* (Tables 19-5 and 19-6) is a supraventricular dysrhythmia that is sometimes difficult to distinguish from paroxysmal atrial tachycardia. A helpful clue is that the atrial flutter waves are continuous on the ECG, whereas the P-waves of atrial tachycardia are separated by a short isoelectric line (compare Figures 19-17 and 19-18).

Description Atrial flutter (Table 19-6) is a tachycardia in which the atrial rate is very rapid: between 240 and 400 bpm (average, 300 bpm). The electrophysiological mechanism of atrial flutter is the presence of an ectopic focus in the atria, with a rapid atrial rate that is maintained by either enhanced automaticity or reentry. The atrial wave, known as the *F-wave*, is characteristically described as having a saw-toothed or picket fence appearance. A classic feature of atrial flutter dysrhythmia is a 2:1 conduction ratio: very regular F-waves have a rate of 300 per minute with a ventricular rate of 150 bpm. The ventricular rate is commonly one half or less of the atrial rate; the conduction ratio is usually constant but it may vary.

Atrial flutter occurs rarely in people with a normal heart and infrequently in people with heart disease. It is more often seen in patients with diseases involving the right heart such as tetralogy of Fallot, cor pulmonale caused by severe lung disease, or pulmonary embolism. Frequently, atrial fibrillation may develop during atrial flutter, and the patient may fluctuate

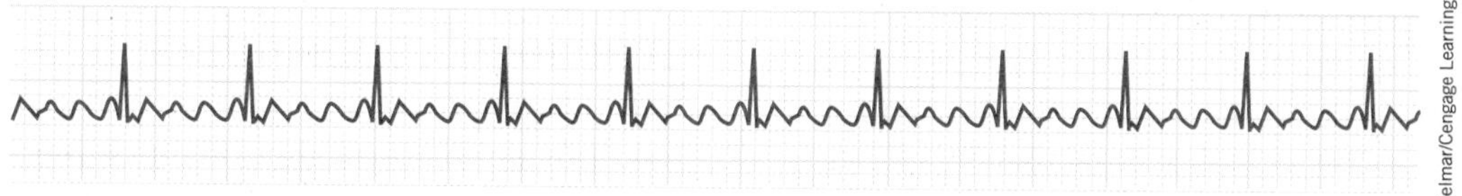

FIGURE 19-18 Atrial flutter: This rhythm is regular, but there is a 4:1 conduction ratio (four F-waves for each QRS complex). The flutter rate is approximately 273 bpm, and the ventricular rate is approximately 68.

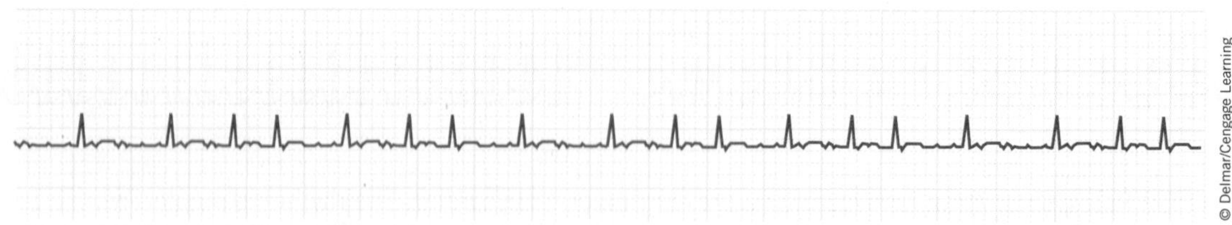

FIGURE 19-19 Atrial fibrillation: The rhythm is regular, with no recognizable P-waves. The f-wave rate is not determinable, but the ventricular rate is approximately 110 bpm. This dysrhythmia is called *uncontrolled* because the ventricular rate is greater than 100 bpm.

between the two rhythms. The term used to describe this phenomenon is *flutter-fibrillation*.[14]

Clinical Significance The problems associated with atrial flutter are similar to those of atrial tachycardia. Patient tolerance depends on the heart rate and on the presence of underlying heart disease. The usual symptoms are palpitations, dyspnea, and breathlessness, which are characteristic of all tachycardias. An additional problem with atrial flutter is the loss of effective atrial contraction during atrial systole. Therefore, this atrial dysrhythmia may decrease cardiac output by as much as 25% because of impaired ventricular filling, and it may increase the severity of symptoms.[1,14]

Atrial Fibrillation. *Atrial fibrillation* has the most rapid atrial rate of all the atrial dysrhythmias. A hazard of atrial fibrillation is the formation of blood clots in the atrium because of stagnant blood in the atrial chamber secondary to absent atrial muscle contraction during atrial systolic time. Heparin is indicated for patients with chronic atrial fibrillation to prevent clot formation and to lessen the risk of stroke or pulmonary embolism. The most important single factor encouraging the onset of atrial fibrillation in high-risk clinical problems is the advancing age of the patient. Most people with atrial fibrillation have structural heart disease such as a valve disease, coronary artery disease, hypertension, cardiomyopathy, and myocarditis.

The dysrhythmia can be short-lived or chronic.

- In the short-lived type, the rhythm either converts spontaneously or responds to cardioversion.
- In chronic atrial fibrillation, the rhythm is refractory to cardioversion, and therapy is directed to improving cardiac function. [14]

Description Atrial fibrillation (Tables 19-5 and 19-6) arises from multiple ectopic areas in the atria and causes a chaotic "twitching" of atrial tissue. The atrial rate can range from 360 to 700 depolarization stimuli per minute. The AV junction is bombarded with this outpouring of stimuli from twitching atrial tissue, and its depolarization timing in turn becomes chaotic. Consequently, the ventricular rate is rapid and very irregular. The electrophysiological mechanism that sustains atrial fibrillation is enhanced automaticity, or a reentry phenomenon, or a combination of the two.

The atrial waves in atrial fibrillation (Figure 19-19) are known as the *f-wave*. They are characteristically described as coarse or fine waves located between normal-appearing but very irregular supraventricular QRS complexes. Sometimes the net electrical amplitude of the 400+ atrial depolarization waves (f-waves) is so small that the sections between the QRS complexes are flat, or isoelectric. *Fine atrial fibrillation* has deflections of less than 1 mm; *coarse atrial fibrillation* has deflections of more than 1 mm. This deflection is equivalent to one small square on the ECG paper.

Clinical Significance The problems associated with atrial fibrillation are more serious than with atrial flutter. Usually atrial flutter has a regular ventricular rate, and the ventricular rate is usually lower than in patients with uncontrolled atrial fibrillation. Patients with atrial fibrillation have no atrial systole, but they also have an irregular cardiac rhythm and a rapid cardiac rate. Because ventricular filling time varies with the irregular tachycardic pattern, the blood pressure changes from one beat to the next, creating hemodynamic instability. A simple clinical test can detect this problem. If you listened to the apical pulse of a patient with atrial fibrillation and also feel the patient's peripheral pulse at the same time, many times the apical pulse is higher. This clinical sign, called a *pulse deficit*, occurs because stroke volume varies from beat to beat. Some cardiac contractions may have so little stroke volume that the pulse wave heard at the cardiac apex is imperceptible at the peripheral pulse points.[14]

JUNCTIONAL DYSRHYTHMIAS

Junctional dysrhythmias (Tables 19-7 and 19-8) are the result of automaticity abnormalities in pacemaker cells of the junctional tissue, or of conduction abnormalities in the AV junction, or of both. The AV node and the bundle of His make up the AV junction. The AV junction's primary role is to act as a conduction

CASE STUDY 19-1

This is the first admission for D, G., a 49-year-old white male, who was admitted for a cardiac catheterization. His chief complaint was that of a 4-month history of angina. At approximately 0800, he was taken to the cardiac lab, where the catheterization was performed. After the procedure was finished, Mr. G. complained of shortness of breath and lightheadedness. This was his ECG tracing:

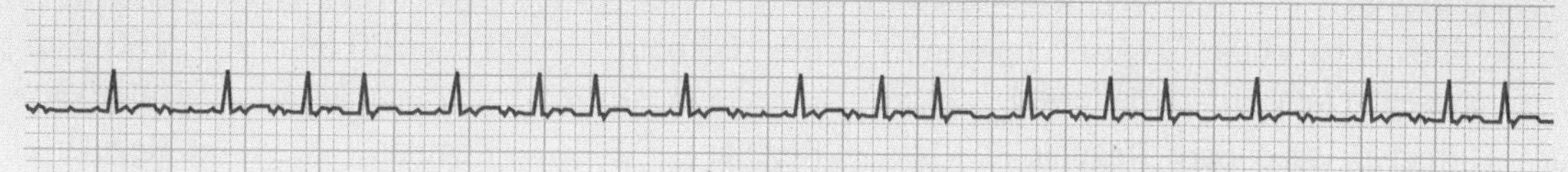

Questions

1. Discuss the patient's rhythm strip, and relate the strip to his symptoms.
2. What are possible causes for this patient's dysrhythmia?

TABLE 19-7 **Causes of junctional dysrhythmias**

Causative Category	Premature Junctional Contraction	Junctional Escape Rhythm	Nonparoxysmal Junctional Tachycardia: Accelerated Junctional Rhythm	Nonparoxysmal Junctional Tachycardia: Junctional Tachycardia	Paroxysmal Junctional Tachycardia (same as PSVT)
Autonomic nervous system	Sympathetic nervous system stimulation; stimulants (coffee, tea, nicotine, chocolate)	Excessive vagal depression of the SA node	Not a cause	Not a cause	Increased sympathetic tone; increased catecholamines, emotion, infection, hypoxemia, stimulants (coffee, tea, chocolate)
Drugs or drug toxicity	Digitalis toxicity	Digitalis toxicity	Digitalis toxicity	Digitalis toxicity	Sympathomimetic drugs, digitalis toxicity
Diseases or conditions	Normal finding, or congestive heart failure (CHF), myocardial ischemia, coronary artery disease (CAD), valvular heart disease, hypokalemia	Inferior wall myocardial infarction (MI), CHF, valvular heart disease, AV node ischemia	Inferior wall MI, acute rheumatic fever, CHF, valvular heart disease, AV node ischemia	Same as accelerated junctional rhythm	Occurs in persons with apparently healthy heart or heart disease (CAD, rheumatic heart disease, acute MI)

"bottleneck" so that the atria have sufficient time to adequately fill the ventricles with blood during atrial systole. The speed of AV nodal conduction is slowed or enhanced by changes in autonomic control.

A secondary but important role of the AV junction is to act as the back-up pacemaker for the heart. If the SA node fails to initiate an electrical stimulus because of either disease, drugs, or increased parasympathetic tone, the AV junction may initiate the stimulus and assume the pacemaker role. The pacemaker cells of the AV junction have an inherent excitability; therefore, if not suppressed by the normal functioning of the SA

TABLE 19-8 **Junctional dysrhythmia: physiological mechanisms and ECG characteristics**

			Nonparoxysmal Junctional Tachycardia		
	Premature Junctional Contraction	**Junctional Escape Rhythm**	**Accelerated Junctional Rhythm**	**Junctional Tachycardia**	**Paroxysmal Junctional Tachycardia (PSVT)**
Physiological mechanism	Increased automaticity of AV junction or reentry circuit involving the AV junction	Decreased automaticity of the SA node or decreased conductivity of the SA node impulse	Increased automaticity on the AV junction	Same as accelerated junctional rhythm	Reentry circuit in the AV junction or increased automaticity of AV junction
Rate	Adds to patient's baseline rate	40–60 bpm (may be lower)	60–100 bpm	100–150 bpm	160–240 bpm (may vary)
Ventricular rhythm	Irregular, secondary to early beat	Regular	Regular	Regular	Regular
P-wave	Early P-wave arises from junctional tissue; if present, the P-wave is inverted	May be absent or present; differs from sinus P in size, shape, and direction and is inverted in lead II	Same as junctional escape rhythm	Same as junctional escape rhythm	Usually absent, especially at the faster rates
PQRST relationship	Early P-wave may be before, during, or after, the QRS; if P-wave occurs simultaneously with QRS, P-wave is not visible	Early P-wave may be before, during, or after, the QRS; if P-wave occurs simultaneously with QRS, P-wave is not visible	Same as junctional escape rhythm; if P-wave is visible it may have no electrical relation to the QRS; this is AV dissociation	Same as junctional escape rhythm	If P-waves are not seen, it is called PSVT; cannot be differentiated from paroxysmal atrial tachycardia
QRS complex	Normal duration unless early P-wave occurs when ventricle is variable refractory; then the QRS $\geq$ 0.125 second	Normal duration unless preexisting bundle branch block is present	Same as junctional escape rhythm	Same as junctional escape rhythm	Same as junctional escape rhythm
Waveform intervals	If P-wave is before QRS, PR-I is $\leq$0.12 second R-R intervals equal	If P-wave is before QRS, PR-I is $\leq$0.12 second R-R intervals equal	Same as junctional escape rhythm	Same as junctional escape rhythm	Same as junctional escape rhythm

node, the cells self-depolarize at a rate of 40–60 times per minute.

Junctional dysrhythmias caused by automaticity or reentry disturbances are:

- Premature junctional contraction.
- Junctional escape.
- Nonparoxysmal junctional tachycardia.
- Paroxysmal supraventricular tachycardia.

Premature Junctional Contraction. *Premature junctional contractions (PJCs)* (Figure 19-20) are premature beats arising from the AV junction. Like all premature beats, they occur in normal hearts but occur less commonly than premature atrial or ventricular contractions. The electrophysiologic mechanism of premature junctional contractions is either increased automaticity or reentry.[1]

Description An ectopic stimulus in the AV junction is the primary cause of an early junctional beat. The ectopic junctional pacemaker spontaneously depolarizes before the next discharge of the sinus node and causes an early beat. Because the pacemaker stimulus occurs out of the normal sequence in the conduction

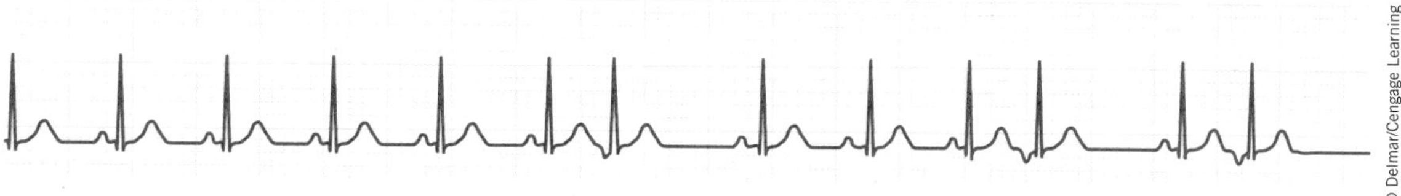

FIGURE 19-20 Premature junctional contraction: There are three premature junctional contractions (beats 7, 11, and 13). The P-wave is visible and inverted before each premature beat. Each QRS complex is <0.12 second, and each premature beat has an abnormally short P-RI. The rhythm is irregular, and the rate is 68 bpm.

network, the atrial depolarization is backward, or retrograde. In lead II, this retrograde conduction creates an inverted or negative P-wave. Conversely, the QRS complex remains normal because the conduction direction is unchanged in the ventricles.

The location of the ectopic pacemaker in the AV junction determines the placement of the P-wave in the ECG tracing. These are the possible variations of P-wave placement in the patient's ECG:

- If the ectopic stimulus arises from an area close to the atrial tissue, it depolarizes the atria before the ventricles, and the inverted P-wave occurs *before* the QRS complex. Because the stimulus originated from an area close to the atria, the P-RI is *abnormally fast* (<0.12 second).
- If the ectopic stimulus comes from the middle of the AV node, then the atria are depolarized *at the same time* as the ventricles, and the inverted P-wave is *hidden* in the QRS complex—not visible.
- If the ectopic stimulus arises from a site in the AV node that is closest to the ventricular tissue, then the ventricles are depolarized *first*, and the P-wave appears *after* the QRS complex.[1]

Clinical Significance In the normal person, premature junctional contractions are usually benign and not clinically significant. Some nonbenign causes of persistent PJCs are:

- Digitalis toxicity.
- Increased automaticity of the AV junction.
- Increased vagal tone on the SA node.
- Cardiac drugs.
- Hypoxia.
- Heart disease.

Since PJCs can occur in individuals with underlying heart disease, their presence indicates a situation of increased automaticity of the junctional tissue or a conduction disturbance. The sudden appearance of frequent PJCs suggests cardiac irritability and a worsening of cardiac function, requiring immediate treatment.[1]

Junctional Escape Rhythm. *Junctional escape rhythm* is the pacing of the heart by the AV junction. If the AV junction supports the heart rate for under 3 consecutive beats, then those beats are junctional escape beats, not junctional escape rhythm. Physiologically, the AV junction is a secondary or default pacemaker and does not normally pace the heart, a persistent junctional escape rhythm is too slow for long-term support.[1]

Description Two situations allow the AV junction to take over as the cardiac pacemaker.

- First, if the baseline discharge rate of the sinus node falls below the normal discharge rate of the AV junction, then the AV junction has escaped from the inhibitory control of the SA node and has become the cardiac pacemaker (Figure 19-21). The normal stimulus discharge rate of the AV junction is 40–60 bpm. If the SA node increases its rate of discharge to above that of the AV junction, the SA node again becomes the dominant pacemaker.
- Second, if the impulse from the sinus node does not reach the AV junction because of SA node disease or a conduction abnormality, then the AV junction takes over as the pacemaker.[1,14]

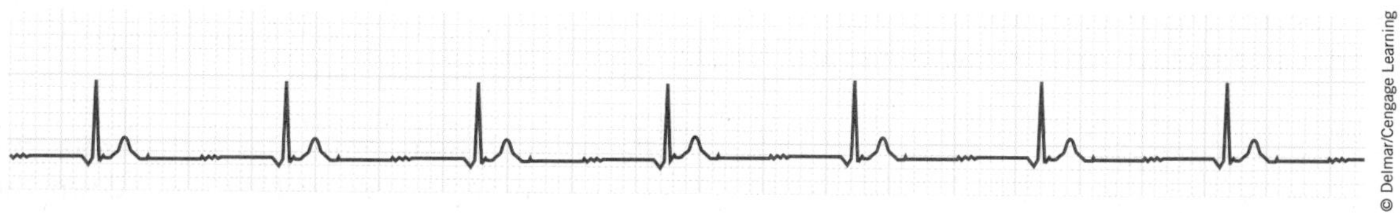

FIGURE 19-21 Junctional escape rhythm: The rhythm is regular with a rate of 40 bpm, and there is an inverted P-wave before each QRS complex. The QRS is <0.12 second, and the P-RI is abnormally short.

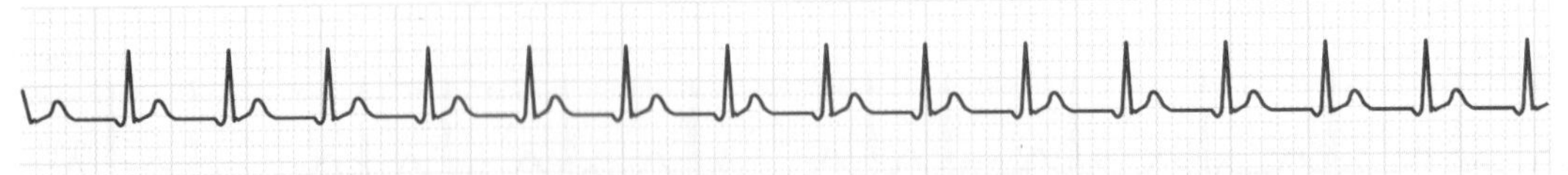

FIGURE 19-22 Accelerated junctional rhythm: The rhythm is regular, with a rate of 83 bpm, and an inverted P-wave precedes each QRS complex. The QRS complex is <0.12 second, and the P-RI is abnormally short.

Clinical Significance Individuals with junctional escape rhythm have the same clinical manifestations as those with sinus bradycardia. If the junctional escape rhythm is persistent and if attempts to reestablish the SA node as the pacemaker fail, then a permanent pacemaker is inserted. Back-up pacemakers such as the AV junction are not reliable, and there is a risk of AV node failure and deterioration into a very slow ventricular escape rhythm or ventricular asystole.[1,14]

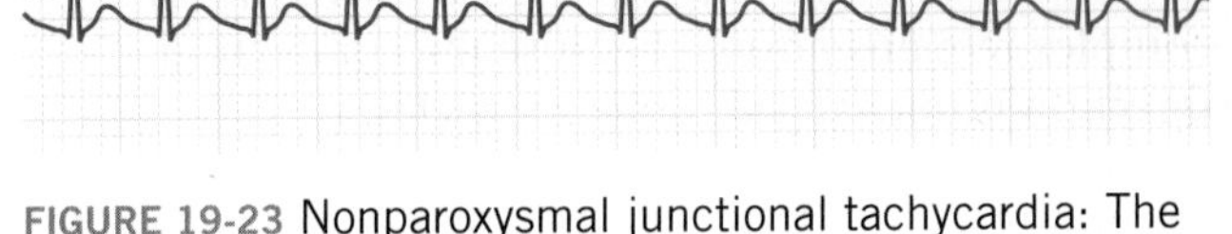

FIGURE 19-23 Nonparoxysmal junctional tachycardia: The rhythm is regular, and the rate is approximately 167 bpm. P-waves are inverted and precede the QRS complexes.

Nonparoxysmal Junctional Tachycardia (Accelerated Junctional Rhythm and Junctional Tachycardia). The mechanism of *nonparoxysmal junctional tachycardia* is increased automaticity. The ectopic focus in the AV junction takes over as the pacemaker because the rate is faster than the SA node. The rhythm is regular, with a rate that ranges from 60 to 150 beats/minute.[1]

Description Nonparoxysmal junctional tachycardia includes two distinct cardiac dysrhythmias:

- A junctional rhythm with a rate of 60–100 is *accelerated junctional rhythm*.
- With a rate greater than 100, it is *junctional tachycardia*.

The rhythm is regular, and, as with PJCs, the innervation of the ventricle is controlled by the ectopic pacemaker in the AV junction, not by transmission from the SA node. Therefore, the P-wave does not have the normal relationship to the QRS.

Nonparoxysmal junctional tachycardia is classically gradual in starting and stopping because it is due to enhanced automaticity of the AV junction. It takes time to develop this condition, and it takes time for treatment to suppress the cause.[1,14]

Both accelerated junctional rhythm and nonparoxysmal junctional tachycardia (Figures 19-22 and 19-23) can develop with digitalis toxicity. Other causes are:

- Drugs that increase automaticity (sympathomimetics).
- Hypoxemia.
- Electrolyte disturbances. (Low potassium can worsen the effects of digitalis.).
- Injury to the AV junction following a myocardial infarction.

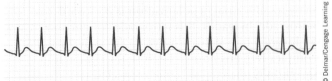

Any patient with this dysrhythmia is at risk for developing a more lethal rhythm, and treatment is necessary.[1]

A condition called **AV dissociation** occurs when the atria and ventricles beat independently. It appears for two reasons:

- Either the sinus rhythm is slightly less than the normal AV junctional rate. In this case, the rates of both pacemakers are very close, and the P-wave rate is slightly less than the ventricular rate.
- Or the AV junction has increased automaticity. With enhanced automaticity, the AV junction's rate is higher than normal, and the AV junction usurps pacemaker control from the sinus node. The atrial rate is also less than the ventricular rate, but the ventricular rate is greater than the usual AV pacemaker's rate, ranging from 60 to 240 beats/minute.[1]

Clinical Significance The presence of nonparoxysmal junctional tachycardia raises the red flag for digitalis toxicity. If digitalis is the likely cause, treatment must be started before the patient develops a life-threatening dysrhythmia. The clinical manifestations of rapid nonparoxysmal junctional tachycardia are the same as those for atrial tachycardia.[1]

Paroxysmal Supraventricular Tachycardia. *Paroxsymal supraventricular tachycardia* (*PSVT*) is a dysrhythmia arising as a result of an reentry circuit, or loop, within the AV node or between the AV node and an accessory pathway located between the atria and the ventricles. The rate is usually very fast, ranging from 160 to 240 beats/minute (rates may be lower or higher). P-waves are usually not visible. The rate is so high that the P-waves are hidden in the QRS complex or the P-waves merge with the T-wave, showing T/P-waves separating the QRS complexes.

The onset and termination of PSVT are sudden. A common event precipitating the rhythm is a premature atrial contraction, which occurs when part of the heart is still refractory. This creates a reentry pathway, allowing a sudden rapid tachycardia. Table 19-8 identifies important clinical differences between the two types of junctional tachycardia: nonparoxysmal and paroxysmal. By convention, a narrow-QRS tachycardia with no distinct P-wave, is supraventricular tachycardia (SVT) unless the onset is sudden, then the dysrhythmia is paroxysmal supraventricular tachycardia.[1]

Clinical Significance The clinical manifestations of PSVT are the same as those with atrial tachycardia. However, clinicians must be aware of an additional problem identified in patients with PSVT. When the rhythm suddenly terminates, the SA node does not immediately pace, and patients' experience dizziness or even lose consciousness during this asystolic period.[1]

DISTURBANCES OF ATRIOVENTRICULAR CONDUCTION

Atrioventricular (AV) block is a conduction disturbance occurring between the initiation of the sinus impulse and the ventricular response to that impulse (Tables 19-9 and 19-10). The primary method used to categorize the different types of AV block is by degree:

- First-degree AV block
- Mobitz type I second-degree AV block
- Mobitz type II second-degree AV block
- Third-degree AV block

Other terms, *complete* and *partial*, separate these conduction disturbances according to the extent of the block.

Partial AV Block. *Partial AV block* refers to the degree of conduction impairment through the AV junction. If some of the P-waves are conducted and activate the ventricular muscle, the block is partial.

First-Degree AV Block. First-degree heart block is the least serious of the heart blocks (Figure 19-24). This block is associated with digitalis toxicity and should be monitored for progression to more serious AV blocks.

Description First-degree AV block is a disorder of slowed conduction in the AV junction, characterized by a prolonged P-R interval (>0.20 second). The underlying ventricular rate may be normal. The ECG has the normal P-QRS-T-wave sequence, and the appearance and duration of the waves are normal.

Clinical Significance First-degree AV block is not common in young healthy adults. As people age, the PR interval lengthens beyond 0.20 to 0.24 seconds, even in those without heart disease. This abnormal conduction

TABLE 19-9 **Causes of AV block**

		Second-Degree (Partial)		
Causative Category	**First-Degree (Partial)**	**Type I Second-Degree**	**Type II Second-Degree**	**Third-Degree (Complete)**
Autonomic nervous system	Increase in vagal (parasympathetic) tone of the AV junction	Increase in vagal (parasympathetic) tone of the AV junction	Not applicable	Increase in vagal (parasympathetic) tone of the AV junction (transient third-degree block)
Drugs or drug toxicity	Digitalis toxicity	Digitalis toxicity (e.g., digitalis, beta-blocker, calcium channel blocker)	Not applicable	Drug toxicity (e.g., digitalis, beta-blocker, calcium channel blocker)
Diseases or conditions	Acute inferior myocardial infarction (MI), ischemia of the AV junction	Acute inferior MI; ischemia of the AV junction; infection causing rheumatic fever or myocarditis; electrolyte imbalance	Acute anteroseptal MI (necrosis of conduction network)	Acute inferior MI; ischemia of the AV junction; chronic degenerative aging changes in the conduction network; infection causing rheumatic fever or myocarditis; electrolyte imbalance

TABLE 19-10 **AV block: physiological mechanisms and ECG characteristics**

		Second-Degree (Partial)		
	First-Degree (Partial)	Type I Second-Degree	Type II Second-Degree	Third-Degree (Complete)
Physiological mechanism	Decreased conductivity of AV junction	Repetitive cycle of progressive decrease in conductivity through AV junction until conduction is completely blocked	Defective conduction through AV junction or ventricular bundle branches, with regular or unpredictable episodes of complete AV block and absent conduction	Absent conduction at the level of the AV node, bundle of His, or ventricular bundle branches; AV junctional pacemaker or ventricle pacemaker controls ventricular rate
Rate	Does not affect rate of underlying rhythm	Ventricular rate is less than atrial rate; rate is determined by the underlying primary rhythm	Same as type I	Rate controlled by pacemaker controlling the ventricle rate: AV junction: 40–60 bpm; ventricular pacemaker: <40 bpm
Ventricular rhythm	Does not affect underlying rhythm	Irregular; atrial rhythm is regular	Same as type I	Usually regular
P-wave	Regular sinus P-waves; P-wave rate same as QRS rate; P-wave upright in lead II	Regular sinus P-waves; P-wave rate greater than QRS rate; P-wave upright in lead II	Regular sinus P-waves; P-wave rate greater than QRS rate; P-wave upright in lead II; conduction ratio may be variable or constant	P-wave rate determined by underlying atrial rhythm
PQRST relationship	Normal sequence: one P-wave for each QRS complex	Abnormal relationship; nonconducted P-waves present	Same as type I	No electrical relationship between atria and ventricles; each beat independently (AV dissociation)
QRS complex	Usually normal; ≥0.12 second if bundle branch block or anomalous ventricular pathway is present	Same as first-degree	Usually abnormal (≥0.12 second) because AV block is below bundle of His	Usually abnormal (≥0.12 second): block is below bundle of His; normal duration if block is in AV junction or the bundle of His
Waveform intervals	P-RI is prolonged (>0.20 second) and does not vary	P-RI varies: progressively lengthens until P-wave is not conducted through AV junction; R-R intervals irregular, with interval decreasing during cycles of increasing P-RI	P-RI may be abnormal but is usually constant	P-RI varies (AV dissociation); R-R intervals regular and P-P intervals regular but do not have electrical relationship

does not typically cause any clinical signs and symptoms, and it therefore does not require treatment.[15] The conventional wisdom is that any P-RI greater than 0.45 sec does not conduct the P-wave through the AV junction. However, in rare cases, the P-RI conducting the P-wave has been as long as 1 second.[16]

Mobitz Type I Second-Degree AV Block. This category of heart block, also called the *Wenckebach phenomenon* (Figure 19-25), is one of the less clinically significant AV blocks. Most patients do not require definitive treatment, but in some cases they should be monitored for clinical deterioration.

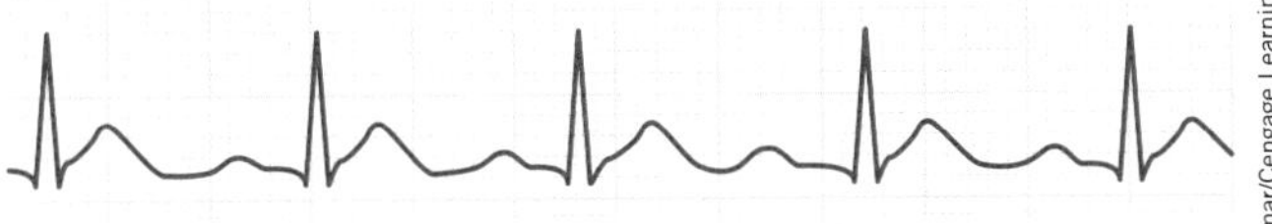

FIGURE 19-24 First-degree AV heart block with accompanying sinus bradycardia: The rhythm is regular, and the rate is approximately 55 bpm. The P-RI is very prolonged.

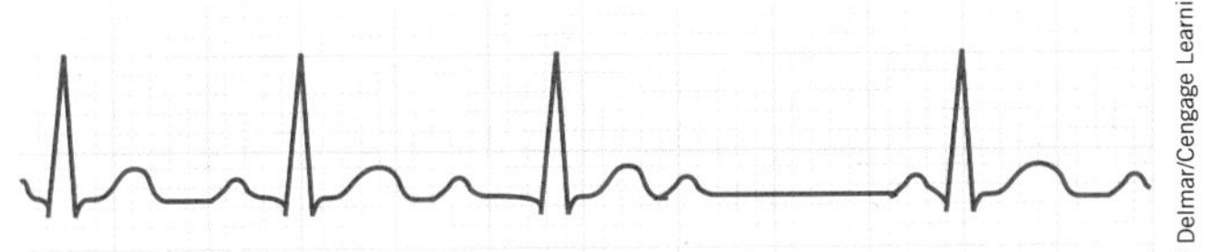

FIGURE 19-25 Type I second-degree AV block (Wenckebach phenomenon): The rhythm is irregular, and the rate is approximately 60 bpm. One nonconducted P-wave appears between the third and fourth ventricular beats. The P-RI increases in duration before the nonconducted P-wave.

Description This dysrhythmia represents a greater abnormality in AV conduction than first-degree heart block. Type I second-degree AV block, or Wenckebach phenomenon, is characterized by the progressive lengthening of AV conduction time for a series or group of electrical stimuli until the AV node becomes totally refractory and the last stimulus is blocked and does not activate the ventricle. The ECG of a patient with Wenckebach phenomenon shows a group of P-QRS-T-waves that are close to each other and are separated from the other groups by a pause. This configuration is called *grouped beating*. Within each group, the P-RI for each successive P-wave is longer than that of the preceding one, and the R-R interval becomes progressively shorter. This pattern continues until finally the last P-wave is not conducted. The pause between groups represents a failure of AV conduction. During this pause, the AV node recovers, and the process starts again. Marriott called this pattern "the footsteps of Wenckebach."[16]

Clinical Significance Type I second-degree AV block occasionally occurs in people with a normal heart. If present, it is usually transient or reverses with treatment. Most patients do not develop significant clinical problems with this dysrhythmia. In some patients, however, this partial AV block progresses to a complete block. Therefore, high-risk patients must be carefully monitored, and, if deterioration is detected, aggressive treatment should be given. Drug toxicity can also cause partial AV block, and medical treatment is always necessary.

> *Best Practice*
>
> **Wenckebach Phenomenon**
>
> Here is a memory jogger to help identify the Wenckebach phenomenon on an ECG.
>
> - First, there are more P-waves than there are QRS complexes with a varying R-to-R interval.
> - Second, the P-RI varies.
>
> Two variables, or "V's," put together, make the letter "W"—for Wenckebach. So the rule is "*v*ariable PR and *v*ariable RR is Wenckebach."

Mobitz Type II Second-Degree AV Block. This block, also known simply as *Type II AV block*, is always serious and requires close monitoring and treatment (Figure 19-26). In particular, patients suffering from an anterior wall myocardial infarction are at risk of developing a life-threatening dysrhythmia.[1,16]

Description The presence of a Type II second-degree AV block indicates that the patient has a serious abnormality in the conduction network. Its appearance indicates irreversible tissue necrosis. The conduction block typically occurs below the bundle of His, in the bundle branches, and involves a complete block of one bundle branch and intermittent block of the other bundle branch.[1] The ECG characteristics of Type II second-degree AV block show a constant PRI with episodes of AV conduction block and nonconducted P-waves. The AV block may show a repeating pattern or be unpredictable. The QRS complex is usually wider than normal (>0.12 second), indicating the bundle

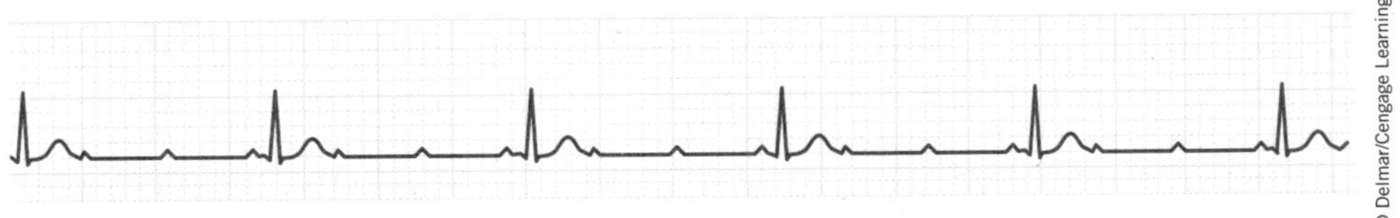

FIGURE 19-26 Type II second-degree AV block: The rhythm is regular with a ventricular rate of 34 bpm. There are three P-waves for each QRS complex with a constant P-R interval of 0.14 second. The QRS is <0.12 second; therefore the patient's block is in the AV junction.

branch block. More rarely, a normal QRS duration (0.10 sec) may indicate that the block is at the level of the bundle of His without an existing bundle branch block.[1,16]

Clinical Significance Mobitz Type II second-degree AV block does not appear in someone with a normal heart. When present, it is usually a permanent or recurrent dysrhythmia. Most people with this conduction disturbance are not hemodynamically stable and are symptomatic. Many have just suffered an anterior wall myocardial infarction, and they are manifesting signs and symptoms of circulatory insufficiency and need emergency care. The insertion of a permanent pacemaker is an emergency procedure, not elective. These patients are at high risk for deterioration, which may take the form of complete heart block or a pulseless rhythm, such as asystole.[1]

Second-Degree 2:1 and Advanced Heart Block. These types of heart block are not the classic Type I or Type II second-degree AV block. Patients with these rhythms have defective conduction in the AV junction and/or the bundle branches, and the pattern reveals a P-to-QRS ratio of 2:1 or greater, with or without a bundle branch block.

Description Closely associated with Type I AV block is a 2:1 AV block *with* a normal QRS duration. The ECG shows:

- Two P-waves for each QRS.
- Regular rhythm.
- Normal or prolonged P-RI.

Two-to-one heart block and advanced heart block *with* wide QRS complexes are associated with Type II AV block because the wide QRS indicates bundle branch conduction defects. Any conduction ratio of 3:1 or greater is a high-grade, or advanced, heart block. The ECG characteristics show:

- A constant P-RI that may be normal or prolonged.
- Regular or irregular rhythm, depending on whether the conduction ratio remains constant.
- Either a normal QRS time duration, indicating an AV node conduction delay, or a prolonged duration, indicating a bundle branch block.

Clinical Significance In patients with 2:1 heart block *with* wide QRS complexes and advanced heart block *with* wide QRS complexes, these rhythms are more serious and can deteriorate into complete heart block or asystole. If the heart rate is excessively slow, the signs and symptoms are the same as in clinically significant sinus bradycardia. The insertion of a cardiac pacemaker is necessary.[1]

Complete Heart Block or Third-Degree AV Block. In *complete AV block*, there is a total absence of conduction between the atria and the ventricles. The conduction defect could be anywhere from the AV junction through the bundle branches. The only block in this category is third-degree AV block. If the block is located below the bundle of His, this rhythm requires aggressive treatment because the patient is in danger of deteriorating into asystole without warning.

Description Third-degree AV block exists when there is a complete lack of electrical communication between the atria and the ventricles (Figure 19-27). Atria are controlled by a supraventricular pacemaker and the ventricles are paced by the AV node or ventricular pacemaker cells. In the absence of His-bundle recordings, the location of the block may be identified by the width of the QRS complex and the ventricular rate.

- If the QRS complex is *narrow*, the block is proximal to the bundle of His in the AV node, and the underlying rate is consistent with a junctional pacemaker (40–60 bpm).
- If the QRS complex is *wide* (>0.12 second), the block is distal to the bundle of His, and the underlying ventricular rate is slower (<40 bpm). This ventricular pattern is typically described as an *idioventricular rhythm*.[1]

The ECG characteristics of third-degree AV heart block are:

- Normal P-P intervals.
- Normal R-R intervals.
- Variable PR intervals.

The atrial rate is usually faster than the ventricular rate because of the difference in automaticity of the respective pacemakers.

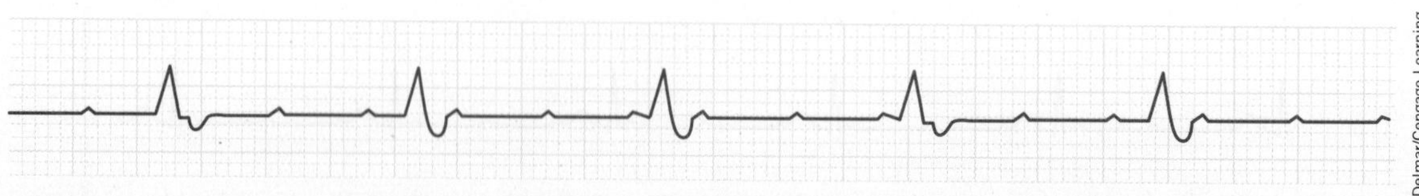

FIGURE 19-27 Third-degree AV block: The rhythm is regular with a rate of approximately 34 bpm. The R-R interval is constant, and the P-RI is variable. The QRS is 0.12 second, indicating a ventricular pacemaker.

Complete heart block has a varying duration. In the presence of acute myocardial infarction, a conduction defect in the intraventricular conduction system indicates significant irreversible disease, and the patient needs a permanent pacemaker.[1]

Clinical Significance The clinical presentation of a patient in third-degree AV block is the same as that of a patient with any symptomatic bradycardia. These patients complain of dizziness and syncope. Their blood pressure is low, secondary to reduced cardiac output.

If the conduction defect is in the AV node, the heart block is reversible and responsive to treatment. If the conduction defect is in the ventricle, as evidenced by a wide QRS complex, the prognosis is more serious because permanent damage to the ventricular conduction network has occurred. All patients in a third-degree block should be treated because of the possibility of backup pacemaker failure, with the sudden development of asystole.[1,16]

VENTRICULAR DYSRHYTHMIAS

Ventricular dysrhythmias (Tables 19-11 and 19-12) are the most serious of all cardiac dysrhythmias. None of these dysrhythmias can sustain life. Ventricular escape or ventricular tachycardia may initially support life, but they cannot create a stable blood pressure that can sustain life. Ventricular fibrillation and asystole are always pulseless rhythms. Patients with ventricular tachycardia may initially have a pulse and blood pressure, but continuation of the rhythm usually results in cardiovascular instability and deterioration into a pulseless state. Patients with these dysrhythmias need advanced life-support measures to convert the cardiac rhythm into one that supports life.

Premature Ventricular Contraction. *Premature ventricular contraction* (*PVC*) is a common dysrhythmia that is found in people with normal or abnormal hearts (Figure 19-28). The treatment varies according to the clinical situation.

Description An early ventricular beat is caused by an ectopic stimulus that arises in any part of the ventricular myocardium. The ectopic ventricular pacemaker spontaneously discharges before the next expected sinus beat. The premature ventricular contraction does not stimulate the SA node because the AV node is usually refractory to retrograde conduction; thus, the SA node timetable is not disturbed. Therefore, the interval between the sinus beats before and after the premature ventricular beat is two times the normal R-R interval. This **compensatory pause** is found for each PVC.[1]

PVCs indicate increased ventricular automaticity or reentry in the bundle of His–Purkinje network.

PVCs may be unifocal or multifocal and may have a repeating pattern. That is, they may occur in couplets, salvos (a number of events in regular succession), or regular coupling intervals.

Clinical Significance In people with a normal heart, premature supraventricular beats are more common than premature ventricular contractions. If present in the normal heart, PVCs are usually benign. More commonly, however, premature beats occur in people

TABLE 19-11 **Causes of ventricular dysrhythmias**

Causative Category	Idioventricular Rhythm or Ventricular Escape	Accelerated Idioventricular Rhythm	Ventricular Tachycardia	Ventricular Fibrillation	Ventricular Asystole
Autonomic nervous system	Decreased automaticity of the higher pacemakers	Increased automaticity of ectopic pacemaker in ventricular bundle branches	Increased automaticity of ventricular ectopic pacemaker in bundle branches, Purkinje network, or myocardium or reentry circuit in the ventricle	Increased automaticity of ventricular ectopic pacemaker in bundle branches, Purkinje network, or myocardium or reentry circuit in the ventricle	Absent automaticity of pacemakers
Drugs or drug toxicity	<40 bpm	40–100 bpm	>100 bpm	300–500 bpm with no effective cardiac output	0
Diseases or conditions	Usually regular	Usually regular	Usually regular	Chaotic, totally irregular	Absent

TABLE 19-12 **Ventricular dysrhythmia: physiological mechanisms and ECG characteristics**

	Premature Ventricular Contraction	Idioventricular Rhythm or Ventricular Escape	Accelerated Idioventricular Rhythm	Ventricular Tachycardia	Ventricular Fibrillation	Ventricular Asystole
Physiological mechanism	Increased automaticity of ectopic ventricular pacemaker or reentry circuit in the ventricle	Decreased automaticity of the higher pacemakers	Increased automaticity of ectopic pacemaker in ventricular bundle branches	Increased automaticity of ventricular ectopic pacemaker in bundle branches. Purkinje network, or myocardium or reentry circuit in the ventricle	Increased automaticity of ventricular ectopic pacemaker in bundle branches. Purkinje network, or myocardium or reentry circuit in the ventricle	Absent automaticity of pacemakers
Rate	Adds to patient's baseline rate	<40 bpm	40–100 bpm	>100 bpm	300–500 bpm with no effective cardiac output	0
Ventricular rhythm	Irregular, very early beat	Usually regular	Usually regular	Usually regular	Chaotic, totally irregular	Absent
P-wave	P-wave may be present	May be present or absent; if present, rate is different from ventricular rate	May be present or absent; if present, rate is different from ventricular rate	May be present or absent; if seen, the wave is usually inverted	Absent	P-waves may be present or absent
PQRST relationship	P-wave not related to QRS complex and occurs with normal sinus time; T-wave opposite in polarity to QRS; compensatory pause present	If present, P-waves have no set relationship to QRS; AV dissociation may be present	P-waves are electrically unrelated to QRS; AV dissociation is present	P-waves are electrically unrelated to QRS; AV dissociation is present	None	No relationship present
QRS complex	≥0.12 s increased amplitude	≥0.12 s	≥0.12 s	≥0.12 s	Absent	Absent
Waveform intervals	P-RI not present; Q-T interval prolonged; R-R interval irregular	P-RI usually absent; R-R intervals may be equal or vary	P-RI absent; R-R intervals may vary	P-RI usually absent; R-R intervals may be equal or vary	No intervals present; *fine v-fib:* amplitude <3 mm; *coarse v-fib:* amplitude >3 mm	No intervals present

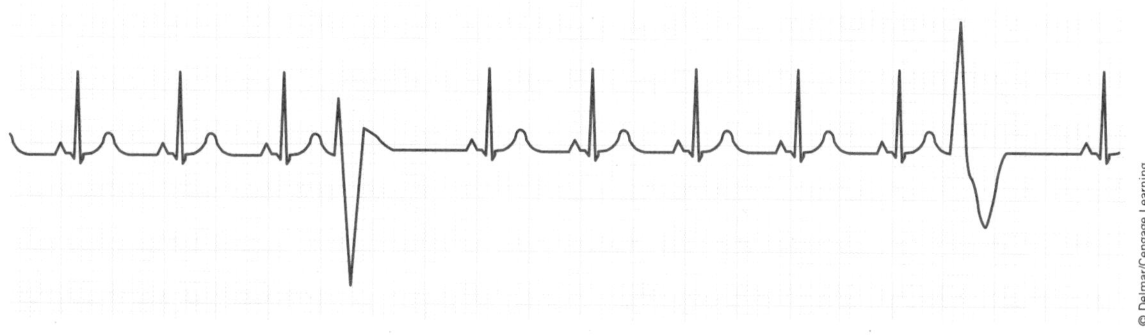

FIGURE 19-28 Premature ventricular contraction—multifocal: The rhythm is irregular with a ventricular rate of 70 bpm. The two premature ventricular contractions do not have the same direction and amplitude. The premature beats have a duration of >0.12 second, and the other sinus beats have a normal QRS duration.

with heart disease. The sudden appearance of frequent PVCs suggests cardiac irritability and a worsening of cardiac function, which requires immediate evaluation. Digitalis toxicity is a cause of many cardiac dysrhythmias, and PVCs is one of them.

A classification system for ranking the severity of the patient's ventricular ectopy is a helpful clinical guide.

- Currently, patients are not treated with an anti-arrhythmic medication unless they are at high risk of developing a life-threatening dysrhythmia. Examples of PVCs that place the patient at risk are runs of three or more PVCs in a row, couplets of PVCs, and R on T PVCs.
- Less serious categories of PVC, such as multifocal PVCs or frequent PVCs, are considered in conjunction with the patient's clinical condition before treatment decisions are made.
- Usually, anti-arrhythmics treatment is given for patients with a suspected myocardial infarction and for patients showing evidence of cardiac ischemia with accompanying ectopic ventricular irritability. These PVCs place the patient at a high-risk of a lethal dysrhythmia.

Anti-arrhythmic agents are not given to all heart disease patients with ventricular ectopy because sometimes the treatment is worse than the ailment. Anti-arrhythmic therapy is used sparingly because these drugs have side effects that may be serious, especially in elderly patients. Clinical drug studies have shown that anti-arrhythmics do not increase patient survival, and some drugs may actually increase the risk of death. Therefore, these drugs are limited to patients at risk for sudden death.

Ventricular Escape Rhythm (Idioventricular Rhythm) and Accelerated Idioventricular Rhythm. These two rhythms are very separate despite their being grouped together.

- *Idioventricular rhythm* (Figure 19-29) is a slow escape pacemaker rhythm that is incompatible with life.
- *Accelerated idioventricular rhythm* (Figure 19-30) is also known as "slow ventricular tachycardia."

Description Idioventricular rhythm occurs when the SA node and AV junction fail as cardiac pacemakers. Before its onset, there is a pause because of SA node failure. When the AV junction also fails to discharge, the tissue of the bundle of His–Purkinje network initiates the impulse and prevents asystole. If the pacemaker failure persists, the ventricle acts as the

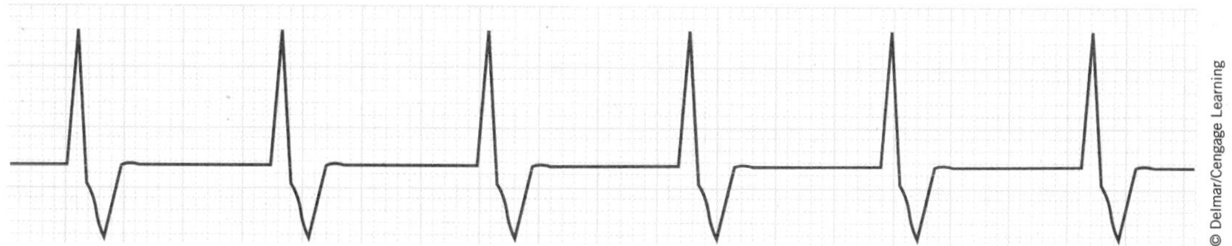

FIGURE 19-29 Idioventricular rhythm (ventricular escape): The rhythm is regular with a ventricular rate of 40 bpm. Each ventricular complex is wide with a QRS duration of >0.12 second and no visible P-waves.

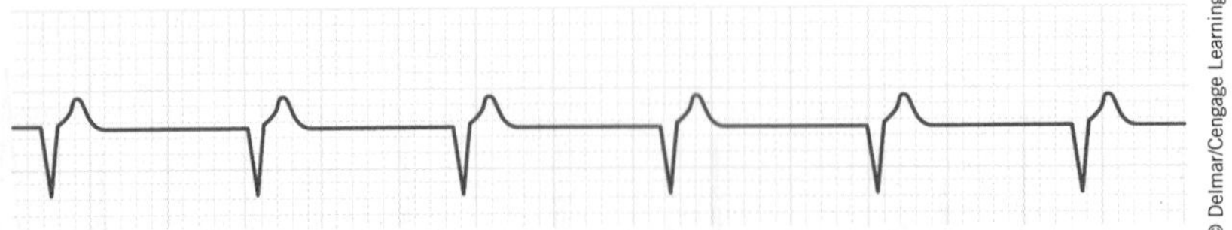

FIGURE 19-30 Accelerated idioventricular rhythm: The rhythm is regular with a ventricular rate of 44 bpm. Each ventricular complex is wide with a QRS duration of >0.12 second and no visible P-waves.

pacemaker, and the established rhythm is ventricular escape or idioventricular rhythm with AV dissociation. The rate is usually <40 bpm. A rate that is greater than 40 but less than 100 bpm is *accelerated idioventricular rhythm.*

Clinical Significance People in ventricular escape are symptomatic because of their very slow heart rate. They manifest all the signs and symptoms of low tissue perfusion, such as low blood pressure, dizziness, and fainting episodes. In more severe cases, they may deteriorate into cardiogenic shock. These people need emergency care to elevate the heart rate and reestablish a viable cardiac output.

People with an accelerated idioventricular rhythm are usually not symptomatic at the higher ventricular rates. This rhythm is usually transient and does not require treatment.

Ventricular Tachycardia. *Ventricular tachycardia* is a rapid heart rate that constitutes a cardiac emergency (Figure 19-31). If untreated, it rapidly deteriorates into ventricular fibrillation.

Description Either an increased automaticity of an ectopic area in the ventricle or a reentry disturbance in the bundle of His–Purkinje system causes ventricular tachycardia. Like supraventricular tachycardia, ventricular tachycardia usually starts with a premature beat. If increased automaticity is the mechanism, the ectopic ventricular pacemaker spontaneously discharges before the next expected sinus beat. The ventricular ectopic pacemaker discharges at a faster rate than the sinus node and usurps that pacemaker's function. If a reentry loop exists, the rhythm is self-sustaining, with a faster discharge rate than other pacemakers. Converting out of the rhythm requires interruption of the reentry loop.[1,17]

Three scenarios exist for the patient in ventricular tachycardia:

- The dysrhythmia is sustained and does not convert despite treatment.
- It is treated and converts into another rhythm.
- It spontaneously converts into another rhythm.

The newly established rhythm is either life-sustaining or incompatible with life. In the latter case, the patient needs immediate cardiac life support.

Clinical Significance The rate and duration of ventricular tachycardia and the individual's own cardiac function primarily determine tolerance to this dysrhythmia. A person in ventricular tachycardia who has severe heart disease is probably not able to maintain adequate heart function. Cardiac filling is severely hampered secondary to two major hemodynamic alterations that occur with ventricular tachycardia. First, the fast heart rate severely limits filling time. Second, in the presence of AV dissociation, there is no synchronous, coordinated atrial systole to aid in filling the ventricles. Therefore, ventricular tachycardia causes a significant decrease in the amount of blood pumped out of the heart. The individual may be hypotensive or experience a severe drop in arterial blood pressure that it is incompatible with life.[1,17]

Ventricular Fibrillation *Ventricular fibrillation* is a cardiac rhythm that does not provide circulation (Figure 19-32). The rhythm requires immediate conversion into a viable rhythm, or the patient will not survive.

Description Ventricular fibrillation is an extremely rapid, chaotic dysrhythmia, with unsynchronized twitching of the heart muscle. It is secondary to either enhanced automaticity or a reentry conduction disturbance with multiple conduction pathways that

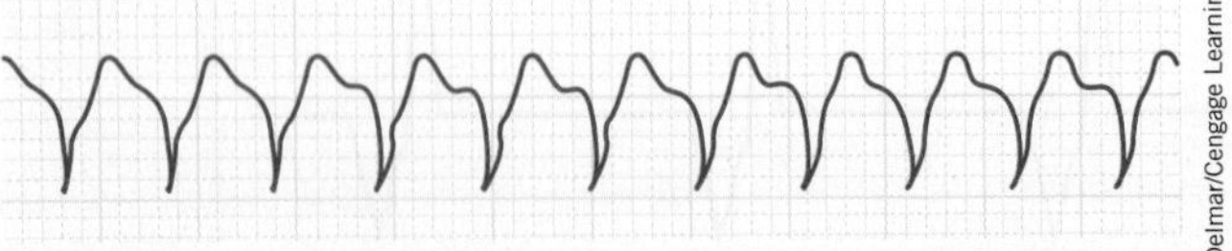

FIGURE 19-31 Ventricular tachycardia: The rhythm is regular, with a ventricular rate of approximately 136 bpm. No P-waves are present.

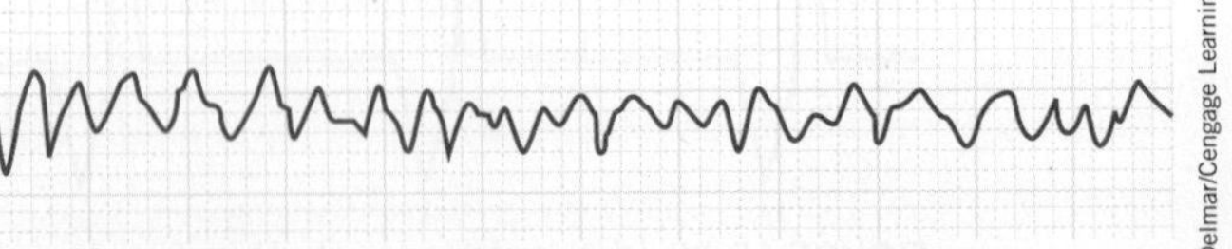

FIGURE 19-32 Ventricular fibrillation: The rhythm is chaotic with no ventricular rate.

vary in size and direction. In ventricular fibrillation, minute parts of the ventricular muscle are in various stages of depolarization and repolarization. Consequently, the ventricular muscle does not depolarize as a unit, and the muscle contraction is totally ineffective, with a twitching heart muscle that is unable to fill up with or eject blood. In effect, the heart is in a state of cardiac arrest. This dysrhythmia is fatal if left untreated.

The two classifications of ventricular fibrillation—coarse and fine—are distinguished from each other by wave amplitude.

- *Coarse* ventricular fibrillation exists when wave amplitude is more than 3 mm (3 small squares). Coarse ventricular fibrillation is of a more recent onset than fine and is likely to respond to defibrillation.
- When the amplitude is less than 3 mm, the rhythm is classified as *fine* ventricular fibrillation. Fine ventricular fibrillation is close to ventricular asystole, and someone with this rhythm is likely to need epinephrine and anti-arrhythmic medications in addition to defibrillation in order to convert the rhythm.[1]

Clinical Significance Ventricular fibrillation is a cardiac emergency that is incompatible with life. The patient must be treated immediately. The recommended treatment is CPR, electrical shock (defibrillation), and medications, if necessary.

- Chest compressions and artificial ventilation keep the individual alive until a life-sustaining heart rhythm is reestablished.
- The first definitive treatment is electrical shock. Defibrillation immediately depolarizes the entire heart in synchrony. This action stops the heart's chaotic electrical activity and allows the opportunity for the normal cardiac pacemakers to resume control of the heart's rate and rhythm.
- If defibrillation fails to convert the patient to a viable rhythm, then medications are administered to aid in rhythm conversion.

Ventricular Asystole. *Ventricular asystole*, or ventricular standstill, is a rhythm characterized by an absence of electrical activity (Figure 19-33). This rhythm is commonly known as *flatline*, although the baseline may not be completely isoelectric.

Best Practice

Use of an Automatic Implantable Cardiac Defibrillator

A large randomized study (MADIT II) of patients with a left ventricular ejection fraction of ≤30% and a history of a heart attack compared the effect of an automatic implantable cardiac defibrillator (AICD) to the that of conventional medical therapy. The study revealed that the AICD significantly reduced mortality. The reduction in sudden cardiac death was reduced by 68% in patients under 65 years, by 65% in patients between 65 and 74 years, and by 68% in patients aged 75 years. New guidelines released by the American College of Cardiology with the American Heart Association recommend the AICD with a class I indication for many types of patients with preexisting heart problems who are high risk for sudden death. Additionally, the AICD is now used to treat patients with congestive heart failure who need synchronization of the heart rhythm to improve cardiac function.

This needs several safety warnings:

- don't apply external defibrillation paddles over the AED or lead locations.
- do not defibrillate over medication patches
- do defibrillate between automatic shocks or pacemaker initiated beats.

Source: Aronow WS. Treatment of ventricular arrhythmias in the elderly. Geriatrics. *2007;63,8:20–28.*

Description Ventricular assystole exists when there is an absence of electrical activity and of contraction in the ventricles. If atrial electrical activity is still present and the dysrhythmia has only P-waves on the ECG, it is *ventricular standstill*. Death is imminent without immediate intervention.

When asystole occurs outside the hospital, it has likely developed from the deterioration of a ventricular

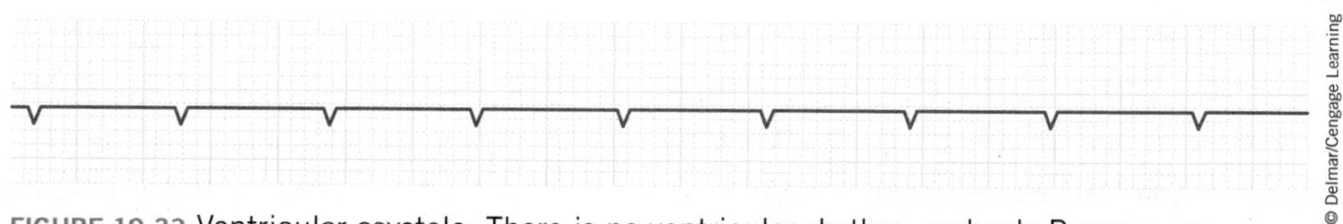

FIGURE 19-33 Ventricular asystole: There is no ventricular rhythm, and only P-waves are present. The ventricular rate is 0, and the atrial rate is approximately 55 bpm.

fibrillation and indicates prolonged cardiac arrest. The prognosis is better when asystole occurs when the person is in the hospital. Besides the obvious benefit of rapid discovery and treatment by trained professionals, another explanation of improved survival is that patients with specific causes of asystole respond well to resuscitation measures. If the mechanism is massive parasympathetic discharge resulting in excessive vagal tone, or heart block, atropine administration suppresses the vagus nerve and improves AV conduction so that a heart rate and rhythm may return. When asystole develops because of severe heart disease, the possibility of survival is poor.

Clinical Significance Ventricular asystole is a cardiac emergency that is incompatible with life. The patient must be treated immediately.

Pulseless Electrical Activity

One can never interpret an ECG strip as pulseless electrical activity (PEA) unless a patient is attached to the monitor and the patient's pulse can be obtained at the same time that the ECG is being observed.

DESCRIPTION

Pulseless electrical activity (*PEA*) is not a dysrhythmia; it is a clinical condition that exists when there is no detectable pulse or blood pressure but there is a viable rhythm on the ECG. The heart is showing electrical activity, but there is no effective mechanical contraction, and the patient has no cardiac output. The types of cardiac dysrhythmias seen on the ECGs for patients with PEA are:

- Supraventricular rhythms.
- Wide QRS rhythms such as accelerated idioventricular rhythm or ventricular escape.
- Very slow bradycardia.

There are different degrees of PEA. The most severe form occurs when the heart has no ventricular contraction; it is totally motionless. A less severe form of PEA is the presence of ventricular contractions that are too weak to produce a pulse or blood pressure.

Treatment is always attempted because the underlying cause may be reversible. In addition to the standard treatment of cardiac arrest—CPR and drug therapy—attempting to determine the cause of PEA and reversing the problem are necessary to resuscitate the patient.

CLINICAL SIGNIFICANCE

PEA is a cardiac emergency that is incompatible with life. The patient must be treated immediately.

Hemodynamic Evaluation

The goal of hemodynamic monitoring is to ensure adequate delivery of oxygen to the tissues, primarily through the manipulation of cardiac output. Because it is the product of heart rate times stroke volume, cardiac output can be altered by altering either of those two factors.

Heart rate is primarily controlled by the central nervous system. Sympathetic stimulation increases heart rate, and parasympathetic stimulation decreases heart rate (Table 19-13). The parasympathetic nervous system predominantly keeps the heart rate within normal limits (60–100 bpm). In general, increases in heart rate raises cardiac output up to a point. When the heart rate becomes too rapid, however, diastolic filling time is greatly reduced; thus, cardiac output may drop. Decreases in heart rate usually do not significantly reduce cardiac output because slower heart rates allow for improved ventricular filling, thereby increasing stroke volume.

CASE STUDY 19-2

In the intensive care unit, the cardiac monitor alarm goes off and the monitor displays this rhythm:

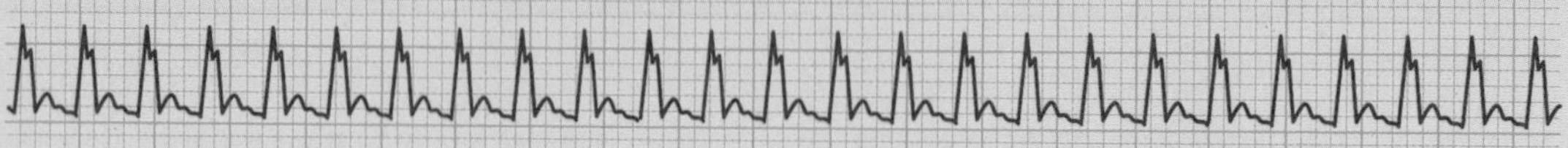

Questions

1. Analyze the rhythm strip and discuss its clinical implications.
2. What types of clinical information is needed?

TABLE 19-13 **Factors that affect heart rate**

Increase Heart Rate	Decrease Heart Rate
Circulating catecholamines	Vagal stimulation
Sympathomimetic medications	Long-term, high-intensity exercise
Parasympatholytic medications	Sedatives
Stress	Myocardial infarction
Pain	Intracranial tumors
Fear	Digitalis
Low blood volume	

TABLE 19-14 **Factors that affect preload**

Factor	Influences on Factor
Venous return	Venomotor tone, pumping action of skeletal muscle, circulating blood volume
Ventricular compliance	Ventricular hypertrophy, myocardial scarring, ventricular enlargement
Duration of diastole	Heart rate, premature ectopic beats
Atrial contraction	Atrial fibrillation, atrial flutter

Stroke volume is the net result of three factors: preload, afterload, and contractility (see Chapter 6).

In general, the higher the **preload** is (i.e., the stretching of the ventricle before the next contraction), the stronger the subsequent contraction will be. However, once the myocardial fibers are stretched beyond a certain point, even though preload continues to increase, the force of contraction deteriorates.

The amount of stretching is determined by the volume of blood in the ventricles at the end of diastole and is reflected in ventricular end-diastolic pressure. Changes in end-diastolic volume alter preload, such that an increase in preload raises stroke volume. End-diastolic volume is influenced by several factors, including venous return, ventricular compliance, duration of diastole, and atrial contraction (Table 19-14).

Increases in venous return to the heart increase preload. Factors that increase venous return are increased venomotor tone, pumping action of the skeletal muscles, and greater circulating blood volume. When the ventricles are less compliant (e.g., ventricular hypertrophy or myocardial scarring due to an infarction), preload is reduced because of lower end-diastolic volumes. At slower heart rates, the longer diastolic filling time allows for greater end-diastolic volume and thus improves preload. Atrial contraction at the end of diastole contributes 25–30% of total ventricular filling. Therefore, the loss of atrial contraction decreases the end-diastolic volume and preload. In patients with decreased ventricular compliance (e.g., postmyocardial infarction or ventricular hypertrophy), atrial contraction is extremely important to maintain adequate ventricular filling.

TABLE 19-15 **Factors that affect afterload**

Factor	Increase	Decrease
Blood volume and viscosity	Polycythemia	Anemia
Vascular resistance	Arterial hypertension, pulmonary hypertension, vasoconstrictors	Arterial hypotension, pulmonary hypotension, vasodilators
Cross-sectional area of vascular bed	Valvular stenosis	

Afterload is the force against which the ventricles must work to pump blood; in other words, afterload is the resistance to flow from the ventricle. As the resistance increases (e.g., in hypertension or valvular stenosis), stroke volume may decrease. On the other hand, as the resistance decreases (e.g., in sepsis or exercise), stroke volume may increase. Afterload is reflected in the arterial systolic pressure because blood pressure equals cardiac output times vascular resistance (Table 19-15).

Factors that tend to increase afterload are:

- Hypertension.
- Semilunar valve stenosis.
- Polycythemia.
- Vasoconstrictor medications.

Factors that typically decrease afterload are:

- Hypotension.
- Anemia.
- Vasodilator medications.

Contractility is the intrinsic vigor of contraction of the myocardial fibers; that is, it is the force generated by the shortening of the myocardial muscle fibers. Whenever contractility increases (*positive inotropism*) or decreases (*negative inotropism*), stroke volume and therefore cardiac output also increase or decrease.

TABLE 19-16 **Factors that affect contractility**

Increase	Decrease
Sympathetic stimulation	Hypoxemia
Circulating catecholamines	Hypercapnia
Positive inotropic agents:	Acidosis
Epinephrine	Myocardial ischemia
Digitalis	Myocardial infarction
Isoproterenol	Negative inotropic agents:
Dopamine	Procainamide
Dobutamine	Beta-blockers
Amrinone	Calcium channel blockers
Milrinone	Anesthetic agents

Many factors influence contractility (Table 19-16), including:

- Sympathetic stimulation.
- Metabolic abnormalities.
- Heart rate.
- Pharmacological agents.

EVALUATION

Evaluating the hemodynamic status of a patient can take the form of a brief noninvasive physical assessment or of a more complex procedure involving invasive catheters. If the patient's condition is critical, a rapid assessment should be completed, focusing on the parameters that provide evidence of tissue perfusion:

- Heart rate and rhythm.
- Presence and quality of pulses.
- Capillary refill.
- Color of skin and mucus membranes.
- Skin temperature.
- Level of consciousness.
- Urine output.
- Neck veins.

Typically, in the presence of decreased tissue perfusion, the *heart rate* increases. However, when assessing a patient's heart rate and rhythm, the respiratory therapist needs to evaluate more than just the rate and rhythm from the cardiac monitor. In addition to determining the number of beats per minute, listen to heart sounds to ensure that the valves open and close with the electrical events. If arrhythmias are present, ascertain the hemodynamic tolerance for this rhythm disturbance. (For example, can the patient maintain an adequate blood pressure with this rhythm?) Auscultating for the quality of heart sounds, presence of murmurs, and gallop rhythms aids in detecting the early onset of congestive heart failure.

Rate and rhythm are further evaluated by checking the upper and lower extremity *pulses* for rate, regularity, and pulse volume. Pulse volume is evaluated by assessing the strength of each beat. Typically, shorter cardiac cycles produce a weak pulse, whereas longer cardiac cycles produce a stronger pulse. Premature beats are usually not felt because of reduced ventricular filling secondary to the shortened ventricular filling time, the lack of atrial contraction, and the distorted ventricular contractility. These extrasystolic beats are often referred to as *nonperfusing beats* because the pressure generated by the contracting ventricles is not enough to eject blood.

Pulse volume changes with alterations in cardiovascular function. Patients with a hyperdynamic circulation (e.g., fever, anemia, excited state, pregnancy) have increased pulse volume, whereas those with significant tachyarrhythmias or hypodynamic circulation (e.g., left ventricular failure, hypovolemia) will have decreased pulse volume.

Capillary refill is assessed by pressing the patient's nailbed to squeeze blood from the underlying capillary bed. If tissue perfusion is normal, color returns to the nailbed within 2 seconds. In states of reduced tissue perfusion (e.g., shock, heart failure), the return of color takes longer than 2 seconds.

In circulatory failure, blood is shunted to the major organs; therefore, the *skin* becomes cool and pale. This change in color and temperature begins distally and moves toward the trunk as the hemodynamic status deteriorates. Cyanosis is possible, but it is not a reliable indicator of tissue perfusion.

Level of consciousness is a sensitive indicator of cerebral perfusion and therefore of hemodynamic status. Early signs of underperfusion are the inability to think or perform complex mental tasks, restlessness, apprehension, uncooperativeness or irritability, and loss of short-term memory.

Urine output is another sensitive indicator of tissue perfusion. Decreased urine output in adequately hydrated patients indicates hypoperfusion and may occur long before other signs of impaired perfusion.

Examining the *neck veins*, specifically the jugular veins, provides information regarding the hemodynamic status of the right heart. The neck veins are examined with the patient lying supine, with the head elevated approximately 30°, and with the head and neck relaxed. The external jugular vein is relatively easy to identify because it lies superficially and can be seen just above the superior border of the midclavicle. Pressing gently on the superior border of the midclavicle allows the external jugular vein to fill and makes it easy to identify. In the patient with

TABLE 19-17 Causes of elevated venous pressure

Cardiac Causes	Noncardiac Causes
Right ventricular failure secondary to left ventricular failure, right ventricular infarction, cor pulmonale	Superior vena cava obstruction, thoracic tumor, hematoma
Tricuspid or pulmonic stenosis	Increased blood volume
Pericardial effusion or tamponade	Increase intrathoracic pressure, positive pressure mechanical ventilation, Valsalva maneuver, COPD, tension pneumothorax
Restrictive cardiomyopathy	Increased intra-abdominal pressure, pregnancy, obesity, ascites
Constrictive pericarditis	
Space-occupying lesions of the right heart, right atrial thrombus or tumor	

good right heart function, the vein quickly collapses after compression is released. The internal jugular vein is more difficult to identify because it lies deep within the neck lateral to the carotid arteries. However, internal jugular vein pulsation can be seen at the base of the neck just lateral to the head of the sternocleidomastoid. Distention of the jugular veins indicates elevated venous pressure. High venous pressure can be due to cardiac or noncardiac abnormalities (Table 19-17).

If upon completion of the physical assessment, it has been determined that the tissues are not being adequately perfused, further hemodynamic monitoring may be necessary. Important hemodynamic parameters that can be measured directly are:

- Oxygenation.
- Cardiac output/cardiac index.
- Central venous pressure.
- Pulmonary artery pressure.
- Pulmonary capillary wedge pressure.
- Arterial pressure.

Important derived hemodynamic parameters are:

- Mean arterial pressure.
- Systemic vascular resistance.
- Pulmonary vascular resistance.
- Ventricular stroke work index.

MONITORING OXYGENATION

Oxygen delivery (DO_2) is calculated by multiplying the cardiac output (CO) by the oxygen content of arterial blood (C_AO_2). The amount of oxygen delivered to tissues is regulated by the metabolic needs of each organ system. The normal response to increased oxygen demand by the tissues is to increase oxygen supply by increasing cardiac output.

Arterial oxygen content (C_AO_2) is the total amount of oxygen carried in arterial blood, which is equal to the oxygen bound to hemoglobin (Hb) plus the oxygen dissolved in plasma. Normal values for C_AO_2 are 18–20 mL O_2/dL blood. Normal values for venous oxygen content (C_VO_2) are 14–16 mL/dL blood.

A gross indicator of tissue perfusion is the arterial-venous oxygen content difference [$D(a - v)O_2$], which is normally 3–5.5 mL/dL blood. Typically, as cardiac output falls owing to poor ventricular function, the $D(a - v)O_2$ increases. This increase is secondary to a large drop in C_VO_2 as the tissues extract more oxygen from the hemoglobin molecule.

One method of monitoring oxygenation is to measure arterial oxygen saturation (S_aO_2). Normal values for S_aO_2 are 9–100%. Arterial oxygen saturation can be:

- Estimated on the basis of arterial oxygen tension (P_aO_2).
- Measured noninvasively via a pulse oximeter (S_PO_2).
- Measured invasively via a light source in the arterial catheter.

The S_aO_2 is the percentage of *total* hemoglobin that combines with oxygen; that is, it is a measure of oxyhemoglobin plus carboxyl and methemoglobin. Therefore, pulse oximetry is not accurate in the presence of dysfunctional hemoglobin or poor distal perfusion (e.g., shock, vasoconstrictor agents).

Arterial oxygen saturation provides information regarding the patient's pulmonary function and oxygenation, but the venous oxygen saturation (S_VO_2) indicates whether oxygen supply is meeting oxygen demand. Venous oxygen saturation reflects the amount of oxygen consumed by the tissues. Normal S_VO_2 is 60–80%; however, S_VO_2 varies depending on the organ system it serves (e.g., the kidney and skin have a higher S_VO_2, owing to high flow, than the heart).

Decreased cardiac output is the most common cause of decreased S_VO_2; however, S_VO_2 can also decrease because of a lowered C_aO_2, decreased Hb, or increased oxygen consumption. Patient movement, agitation, pain, shivering, seizure activity, or increased body temperature all raise oxygen demand. Changes in S_VO_2 usually precede hemodynamic changes and therefore signal the need to reassess the patient's status. Cardiac output should be measured to confirm the presence of underperfusion.

MONITORING CARDIAC OUTPUT/CARDIAC INDEX

Cardiac Output. Cardiac output is the amount of blood ejected by the heart per unit of time; it is reported in liters per minute (Lpm). Reasons for cardiac output monitoring are:

- Assessment of left ventricular function.
- Assessment of perfusion status.
- Evaluation of hemodynamic status.
- Evaluation of response to medical therapy.
- Calculation of cardiac index, vascular resistance, and ventricular stroke work index.

Cardiac output monitoring is routinely measured at the bedside by means of a pulmonary artery catheter and the *thermodilution technique,* which measures the temperature change of blood after an injection of a solution colder than body temperature. A specified quantity of cold saline (iced or at room temperature) is injected rapidly into the proximal (right atrium) port of a thermodilution pulmonary artery catheter. The temperature drop, measured at the distal tip of the catheter, is plotted against time to produce a *thermodilution curve*. The cardiac output is then calculated by computer.

- The *normal* curve should have a smooth rapid upstroke with an even downslope.
- In cases of *high* cardiac output, the area under the curve is small.
- *Low* cardiac output produces a longer downslope with a greater area under the curve.
- An *uneven* upslope indicates poor injection technique (i.e., perhaps the solution was not injected quickly and evenly).

The following protocol should be used to ensure the accuracy of cardiac output measurements:

1. Repeat the procedure three times.
2. Wait 1.5–2 minutes between injections.
3. Calculate the average of all three measurements (if all are within 10% of each other).
4. Repeat the procedure a fourth time if one measurement is greater than 10% of the others.

Normal cardiac output is 4.0–8.0 Lpm, but this value varies. Variables that affect cardiac output are:

- Metabolic rate and oxygen demand.
- Gender. (Females have lower CO than males.)
- Age. (CO is highest in childhood and diminishes with age.)
- Posture. (CO measured in the supine position decreases by approximately 20% when the person stands up.).
- Body size. (Larger people have a greater CO.)

Cardiac Index. The effect of body size can be corrected by calculating the *cardiac index* (*CI*). This index is determined by dividing the cardiac output by the patient's body surface area (BSA), and it is expressed in units of liters per minute per square meter (Lpm/m^2). The cardiac index provides a greater clinical value than cardiac output because it is a more precise indicator of hemodynamic status and tissue perfusion.

A normal cardiac index of 2.5–4.2 Lpm/m^2 indicates good cardiac function.

- An increase in CI is normally seen during exercise or in patients with mild tachyarrhythmias.
- Reduced CI is seen in patients with an abnormal heart rate, preload, or afterload; decreased contractility; and arrhythmias.
- A cardiac index of 1.8–2.1 Lpm/m^2 indicates moderate cardiac depression and impending deterioration.
- A cardiac index of 1.7 Lpm/m^2 or less indicates severe cardiac depression with a poor prognosis.

MONITORING CENTRAL VENOUS PRESSURE

Central venous pressure (*CVP*) monitoring provides measurement of right atrial (RA) pressures, which are reflective of changes in right ventricular (RV) function and cardiovascular status. The purposes of CVP monitoring are to:

- Assess blood volume status.
- Administer fluids.
- Sample blood.
- Measure S_VO_2.
- Assess right ventricular preload.

The central venous catheter is typically inserted via the subclavian, internal jugular, or external jugular vein, with the distal tip of the catheter positioned in the superior vena cava just above the right atrium.

The graphic waveform recorded by the CVP catheter is the same as a right atrial pressure curve, with the classic a-wave, c-wave, and v-wave configuration.

- The *a-wave* is an increase in pressure due to RA contraction.
- The *c-wave,* which is not always seen, is a brief "bump-up" in pressure due to the tricuspid valve's closing.
- The *v-wave* is a gradual rise in pressure caused by the right atrium's filling during ventricular systole.
- The *x-descent* is the downward slope of the a-wave, representing right atrial relaxation.

- The *y-descent* is the downward slope of the v-wave, representing right ventricular relaxation and right atrial emptying.

The normal CVP is 0–7 mm Hg, with the a-wave slightly higher than the v-wave. This is a mean value because systolic and diastolic pressures are not recorded. Since the CVP values vary with intrathoracic pressures, CVP measurements should be made at end-expiration to minimize the effect of respiratory variations on pressures.

High CVP readings occur normally during spontaneous expiration or during positive pressure inspiration. However, increased CVP may indicate:

- Increased right ventricular preload, which may be due to fluid overload, a left-to-right shunt, or tricuspid valve regurgitation.
- Increased right ventricular afterload, which may be due to chronic left ventricular failure, cor pulmonale, pulmonary embolism, COPD, hypoxemia, or positive pressure ventilation (especially with PEEP).
- Decreased right ventricular contractility, which may be due to **cardiac tamponade** (compression of the heart caused by a large volume of fluid in the pericardium), cardiomyopathy, constrictive **pericarditis** (inflammation of the pericardium), right ventricular infarct, or right ventricular failure.
- Other problems, such as tricuspid valve stenosis, catheter tip migrated into the RV, patient position change, transducer position change, or a clot in the monitoring line.

Low CVP readings occur normally during spontaneous inspiration or positive pressure expiration. However, low CVP readings may indicate:

- Hypovolemia.
- Positional changes in patient or transducer.

Clinically, trends in CVP measurements are more important than absolute values. The CVP measurements are most useful in monitoring blood volume, venous return, and right ventricular function. When a change in CVP is noted, however, the respiratory therapist should assess additional hemodynamic parameters to determine the cause of that change. A pulmonary artery pressure measurement may be necessary to further evaluate the patient's hemodynamic status because the CVP is not useful for monitoring left ventricular function.

MONITORING PULMONARY ARTERY PRESSURE

Pulmonary artery pressure (*PAP*) monitoring utilizes a flow-directed, balloon-tipped catheter to provide hemodynamic information regarding right and left ventricular function. The pulmonary artery (PA) catheter is inserted via a peripheral vein (internal or external jugular, subclavian, basilic, or femoral) and advanced through the heart into the pulmonary artery. A balloon at the distal tip of the catheter is inflated to allow the catheter to advance itself with the flow of blood. The PAP catheter allows the following hemodynamic parameters to be measured and assessed:

- Pulmonary artery pressures (systolic, diastolic, mean)
- Right ventricular preload (via RA pressure)
- Right ventricular afterload (via PA systolic pressure)

As the catheter is advanced from the right atrium to the pulmonary artery, a pressure waveform is generated. As the catheter tip enters the right atrium, the pressure waveform looks like a CVP waveform (i.e., low pressure with a-wave, c-wave, and v-wave configuration). The normal right atrial mean pressure is 0–7 mm Hg.

The catheter then advances through the tricuspid valve into the right ventricle. The RV waveform displays a steep upstroke to *peak right ventricle systolic pressure* (*RVSP*), followed by a sharp downstroke to the *right ventricular end-diastolic pressure* (RVEDP). The normal RVSP is 15–25 mm Hg, and the normal RVDP is 0–7 mm Hg. The RVEDP is roughly the same as the right atrial mean pressure (in the absence of tricuspid valve disease) and reflects right ventricular preload. In the case of tricuspid stenosis, RVEDP is less than the right atrial mean pressure because the valve obstructs the blood flow and causes pressure to increase in the right atrium.

From the right ventricle, the catheter is advanced through the pulmonic valve into the pulmonary artery. The PA waveform displays a steep upstroke to peak *pulmonary artery systolic pressure* (*PASP*) and is followed by a sharp downstroke to *pulmonary artery diastolic pressure* (*PADP*). This downstroke is interrupted by the *dicrotic notch*, which is caused by the pulmonic valve's closing. The normal PASP is 15–25 mm Hg; the normal PADP is 8–15 mm Hg; pulmonary artery mean pressure is 10–20 mm Hg.

The catheter is advanced to the pulmonary capillary wedge position by slowly inflating the balloon while observing the PAP waveform. The balloon catheter floats out toward the pulmonary capillaries until the balloon becomes "wedged" in the smaller vessel. At this point, the pressure waveform changes, measuring the pressure distal to the tip of the catheter, that is, the *pulmonary capillary wedge pressure* (*PCWP*). Since there are no valves between the pulmonary capillaries, pulmonary veins, and left atrium (LA), the

PCWP measures pressure changes in the left atrium and therefore the left ventricular preload.

The PCWP waveform displays low-amplitude oscillations similar to the right atrial waveform, with the a-wave (atrial contraction)–v-wave (atrial filling) configuration. The normal mean PCWP is 4–15 mm Hg. The PCWP is equal to *left ventricular end-diastolic pressure* (*LVEDP*) in the absence of mitral valve disease and reflects left ventricular preload.

The pulmonary artery diastolic pressure is typically used as a reflection of left ventricular end-diastolic pressure, instead of pulmonary capillary wedge pressure, because the PADP and PCWP are nearly equal. The pulmonary artery systolic pressure is roughly the same as right ventricular systolic pressure in the absence of pulmonary valve disease. Both pulmonary artery systolic and diastolic pressures decline during spontaneous inspiration; therefore, pulmonary artery and pulmonary capillary wedge pressures should be measured at end-expiration. For continuous monitoring purposes, the balloon should always be left deflated, with the catheter tip in the pulmonary artery as evidenced by the waveform. The balloon should be deflated passively by opening the valve; never aspirate the balloon.

Arrhythmias cause the pulmonary artery pressure to vary. For example, in the presence of atrial fibrillation, the pulmonary artery pressure varies with the heart rate. In other words, with slower ventricular response, the ventricular filling time is longer (increased preload), causing an increase in both PASP and PADP. Conversely, premature ventricular contractions cause the pulmonary artery pressure to drop owing to reduced stroke volume (secondary to reduced ventricular filling). Therefore, pressure measurements should exclude ventricular ectopic beats.

Elevated pulmonary artery pressures are due to one of four factors:

- Increased pulmonary vascular resistance (e.g., pulmonary disease, pulmonary hypertension, pulmonary embolus, hypoxemia, or acidosis).
- Increased pulmonary venous pressure (e.g., mitral valve stenosis or left ventricular failure).
- Increased pulmonary blood flow (e.g., hypervolemia, left-to-right shunt).
- Cardiac tamponade.

Decreased pulmonary artery pressures are typically associated with hypovolemia owing to either vasodilator therapy or dehydration. However, when the pulmonary artery pressure is reduced, the therapist must ensure that it is not a damped pressure curve. The **damped pressure curve** both changes the shape of the waveform and decreases the pressure measurements. The waveform loses its sharp definition and becomes rounded out, the upstroke of systole slows, and the dicrotic notch disappears. Damping of the pulmonary artery pressure curve can be due to several factors, which can be easily checked and corrected (Table 19-18).

TABLE 19-18 **Causes of a damped pressure curve**

Cause	Remedy
Fibrin at the catheter tip	Gently aspirate, and then flush catheter.
Tip of catheter against vessel wall	Reposition catheter.
Air bubbles in the tubing system	Gently aspirate, and then flush catheter.
Kinks in catheter or tubing	Reposition catheter or tubing.

MONITORING PULMONARY CAPILLARY WEDGE PRESSURE

Because the pulmonary artery diastolic pressure closely reflects changes in the left ventricular end-diastolic pressure and the left ventricular preload, it can be continuously monitored instead of the pulmonary capillary wedge pressure. In certain conditions, however, the PCWP must be measured directly. An increase in pulmonary vascular resistance increases PADP measurements, while the PCWP measurements are normal or low. Pulmonary vascular resistance can be increased by:

- Pulmonary embolism.
- Hypoxia.
- COPD.
- Acute respiratory distress syndrome (ARDS).

In addition, in the presence of tachycardia, PADP may be falsely elevated owing to the shortened diastolic filling period.

An *elevated* pulmonary capillary wedge pressure indicates an increase in left ventricular preload and can be due to several factors: left ventricular failure, mitral valve stenosis or regurgitation, cardiac tamponade, constrictive pericarditis, or volume overload. A PCWP of 18–20 mm Hg usually produces mild pulmonary congestion and shortness of breath as fluid moves from the capillaries into the alveoli. As the PCWP approaches and exceeds 30 mm Hg, acute pulmonary edema is present.

In a patient with normal cardiac function, a *low* PCWP (less than 5 mm Hg) indicates hypovolemia. In a patient with compromised cardiac function, however, hypovolemia may be present despite normal or high

PCWP measurements; therefore, cardiac output must be measured. If measuring cardiac output directly is not possible, calculate the $D(a - v)O_2$. If the $D(a - v)O_2$ is increased, the patient has poor cardiac function.

Pulmonary capillary wedge pressure should be monitored every 2–4 hours or whenever a change in pulmonary artery pressure or S_VO_2 is noted, but the catheter should never be left in the wedge position because it can cause a pulmonary infarction. The balloon should be deflated within 15 seconds or a maximum of five breaths. Once the balloon is deflated, the PA waveform should reappear immediately.

To ensure accurate PCWP measurements, verify that the catheter is positioned properly by observing the pressure waveform. The pulmonary artery waveform flattens to a left atrial waveform with a pressure drop once the balloon is inflated. The pulmonary capillary wedge pressure mean should be less than the pulmonary artery mean. A PCWP that is greater than the PADP, an artifact known as **overwedging**, indicates a problem with catheter position and must be corrected. Overwedging is caused by overinflation or eccentric inflation of the balloon. Either may produce artificially elevated, damped, and inaccurate pressure readings. To correct this problem, deflate the balloon, reposition the catheter, and reinflate the balloon.

Other common artifacts seen with PCWP monitoring that can lead to abnormal pressure measurements are a damped pressure curve and mixed PA-PCWP waveforms.

- *Damping* of the pressure curve produces a rounded-out appearance of the curve, with a lack of clearly defined a-waves and v-waves. To correct this problem, deflate the balloon, aspirate, and gently flush the distal port of the catheter. Never flush the distal port with the catheter in the wedge position.
- A *mixed PA-PCWP waveform* occurs because of incomplete wedging of the catheter tip. The waveform varies with respiration such that, during inspiration, a PA curve is present, but, during expiration, a PCWP curve is present. Slight advancement of the catheter usually corrects the problem.

The respiratory therapist must be aware of several clinical pitfalls to obtain accurate PA/PCWP measurements.

- The first is body position relative to the pressure transducer. For accurate pressure measurements, the transducer-air interface must be level with the patient's heart—that is, at the patient's midaxillary line. Pressure measurements must be made with the transducer and patient in the same position each time. If the transducer is higher than the level of the patient's heart, the pressure reading will be falsely low. Conversely, if the transducer is lower than the patient's heart, the pressure reading will be falsely high because of the effects of gravity on the transducer-air interface. Also, the patient should be in the supine position, with the head elevated no more than 20 degrees. With the head elevated greater than 20 degrees, measurements will be inaccurate, but that position is acceptable for monitoring trends in pressure changes rather than absolute numbers.
- Second, a phenomenon known as **catheter whip** ("fling") artifact is the excessive movement of the catheter tip, as seen as a spike superimposed on the PA pressure waveform. Pressure measurements are inaccurate because the artifact causes an overestimation of systolic pressure and an underestimation of diastolic pressure. Catheter whip artifact can be due to the catheter tip's being too close to the pulmonic valve. This problem can be corrected by slightly advancing the catheter farther into the pulmonary artery. This artifact can also be due to external noise (such as shivering or patient movement). Keeping the patient still and comfortable usually eliminates the problem. A hyperdynamic heart (e.g., early sepsis or excessive catecholamines) can also cause catheter whip artifact. This cause is not easily corrected, so only trends in the pressure measurements can be observed, not absolute numbers.
- Third, in certain types of cardiac dysfunction, pulmonary capillary wedge pressure does not equal left atrial pressure or left ventricular end-diastolic pressure. In cases of decreased left ventricular compliance (e.g., acute myocardial infarction, aortic regurgitation, cardiac tamponade, or constrictive pericarditis), the PCWP is lower than the LVEDP. Typically, when the LVEDP is greater than 25 mm Hg, the pressure is not adequately reflected back to the pulmonary capillary bed.
- Finally, the PCWP is greater than the LVEDP for a number of reasons:
  - Whenever there is an obstruction between the pulmonary artery and the left ventricle, there is increased resistance. This type of finding typically occurs with patients with pulmonary disease (e.g., acute respiratory distress syndrome, COPD, and pulmonary emboli).
  - PCWP can be greater than LVEDP secondary to increased pulmonary artery pressure in patients receiving positive pressure ventilation or CPAP.

- Other causes are tachycardia (heart rate over 125 bpm), hypovolemia, hypoxemia, mitral valve stenosis, pulmonary venous obstruction, and left atrial myxoma.

The position of the catheter tip in the pulmonary artery relative to the lungs can have an impact on the accuracy of the PA-PCWP pressures. (The position of the catheter tip may be identified by a lateral chest X-ray.)

- Pulmonary artery pressures increase progressively toward the base of the lungs, such that at the apexes (*zone 1*) the alveolar pressure (P_{alv}) is greater than the pulmonary artery systolic and diastolic pressures (P_A) and the pulmonary venous pressure (P_V) (i.e., $P_{alv} > P_A > P_V$). Therefore, in zone 1, the vessel is closed, and no vessel is open to the left atrium. As a result, the catheter tip is sensing P_{alv}, the PCWP waveform is damped, and the pressure measurement is equal P_{alv}, not LA pressure.
- As the catheter tip moves toward the middle of the lungs (*zone 2*), P_A is greater than P_{alv}, and P_{alv} is greater than P_V (i.e., $P_A > P_{alv} > P_V$). As a result, the vascular channel is open intermittently. The vessel is open during systole because P_A systolic pressure is greater than P_{alv}; therefore PCWP is accurately measuring LA pressure. During diastole, the vessel is closed off because PA diastolic pressure is less than P_{alv}, and PCWP is recording alveolar pressure, not LA pressure. Therefore, hemodynamic measurements are not accurate when the catheter tip is in zone 2 of the lungs.
- With the catheter tip placed at the base of the lung (*zone 3*), PA systolic and diastolic pressures are greater than P_V, and P_V is greater than P_{alv} (i.e., $P_A > P_V > P_{alv}$). The vessel remains open throughout the cardiac cycle, and the PCWP is accurately measuring LA pressure. Therefore, for accurate PCWP measurements, the catheter tip must be placed in zone 3. When the patient is supine, the majority of the lung is zone 3. However, zones 1 and 2 enlarge with positive pressure ventilation, especially with PEEP or air trapping (as in asthma or COPD), secondary to the increases in alveolar pressure. A drop in arterial and venous pressure, as seen with hypovolemia, hemorrhage, or diuresis, also enlarges zones 1 and 2.

To perform a zone placement check, observe the PA and PCWP waveform (Table 19-19). The catheter is in zone 3 if:

- The PA diastolic pressure is greater than the mean PCWP.

TABLE 19-19 **Determining zone placement**

Zone 1 or 2	Zone 3
PADP < PCWP	PADP > PCWP
PCWP curve damped with smooth contour	PCWP curve displays clear a-, c-, and v-waves
An increase in PEEP causes PCWP to increase to more than half the PEEP change	An increase in PEEP causes PCWP to increase to less than half the PEEP change

- The PCWP-waveform exhibits clear a-, c-, and v-waves.
- With a change in positive end-expiratory pressure (PEEP), the PCWP mean is less than half the change in PEEP.

In addition, placement of the catheter in zone 3 can be confirmed by the presence of the catheter tip below the left atrium on the chest X-ray.

The catheter is in zone 1 or 2 if:

- The PA diastolic pressure is less than the PCWP.
- The PCWP-waveform is damped with a smooth contour.
- With a change in PEEP, the PCWP mean is greater than half the change in PEEP.

On a chest X-ray, the tip of the catheter is shown at or above the left atrium.

The PCWP tracing and therefore measurements are affected by ventilation. During normal spontaneous breathing, the PCWP is minimally affected by changes in intrathoracic pressures. In general, during inspiration PCWP drops slightly, whereas during exhalation it increases slightly. As spontaneous breathing becomes more labored, the PCWP and PAP become greatly affected. Inspiration causes a large decrease in PCWP, and expiration causes a large increase in PCWP.

Mechanical positive pressure ventilation (PPV) has several physiological effects, and therefore it affects PCWP and PA pressure measurements.

- During PPV, inspiration causes an increase in PCWP secondary to increased alveolar, intrathoracic, and intravascular pressures.
- In addition, the increased alveolar and intrathoracic pressures decrease venous return, thereby reducing cardiac output.
- The sizes of zones 1 and 2 increase with PPV secondary to alveolar pressures increased to greater than PA pressures.
- The cardiovascular effects of PPV are directly proportional to the increase in intrathoracic

pressures (i.e., level and mode of ventilation as well as lung compliance). Patients with preexisting depressed cardiac function or hypovolemia are highly susceptible to the pressure changes. Therefore, hemodynamic measurements should be made at end-expiration, when pressure changes are minimal.

The use of PEEP exaggerates the effects of PPV on PCWP measurements. In general:

- With a PEEP of 0–10 cm H_2O, the PCWP is approximately equal to LA pressure and LVEDP. However, with PEEP greater than 10 cm H_2O, there is an increased disparity between PCWP and left heart pressures.
- The exaggeration of PCWP measurements with PEEP is most pronounced in lungs with increased compliance. However, the effects of PEEP are not as significant in patients with decreased lung compliance because the increased pressures are not well transmitted to the pulmonary vasculature.

The use of PPV and PEEP almost always results in an overestimation of the actual PCWP. However, these measurements are still useful clinically to determine the patient's hemodynamic status. Keeping the patient on PPV and PEEP while taking pressure measurements is preferable because doing so provides the clinician with valuable information regarding the patient's hemodynamic status during mechanical ventilation.

MONITORING ARTERIAL PRESSURE

Arterial pressure monitoring allows the constant monitoring of arterial blood pressure via an intra-arterial catheter, which is indicated when the patient's blood pressure is unstable. In addition, continuous arterial monitoring is used to assess the patient's response to therapeutic interventions and for arterial blood sampling.

Note: Arterial lines are not indicated for medication administration or fluid maintenance.

The most common site for arterial catheter insertion is the radial artery because this site provides good accessibility, good collateral circulation, low injury risk at insertion, good patient comfort and mobility, and easy access to control or observe bleeding. Other sites for arterial catheter insertion are the axillary, brachial, femoral, and dorsalis pedis arteries.

The *arterial pressure waveform* reflects the function and pressure changes in the left ventricle and systemic vascular resistance. The pressure waveform generated by the intra-arterial catheter closely resembles the pulmonary artery pressure waveform: a steep upstroke to peak systolic pressure (BP_{sys}), followed by a sharp downstroke to diastolic pressure (BP_{dia}). This downstroke is interrupted by the dicrotic notch, which is caused by the aortic valve's closing.

The normal BP_{sys} is 100–140 mm Hg and reflects left ventricular systolic pressure (in the absence of aortic stenosis). Arterial systolic pressure increases in the distal vessels, such that the BP_{sys} in the femoral artery is 20–50 mm Hg greater than the BPsys in the brachial artery.

The normal BP_{dia} is 60–80 mm Hg and indicates the distal runoff of arterial blood and the elastic recoil of the arteries. Arterial diastolic pressure decreases slightly or remains the same in the distal vessels. Arterial diastolic pressure is greatly affected by heart rate: a longer diastole (as occurs with bradycardia) allows the BP_{dia} to decline further, whereas faster heart rates increase BP_{dia} secondary to a shorter diastole. In addition, BP_{dia} greatly affects coronary perfusion pressure (CPP), because most of coronary blood flow occurs during diastole. Therefore, heart rate also affects CPP. A CPP of less than 50 mm Hg indicates poor myocardial perfusion and threatens cardiac performance. Myocardial perfusion can be improved by increasing BP_{dia} or decreasing PCWP, or both.

Normal *mean arterial pressure* (*MAP*) is 70–95 mm Hg and reflects cardiac output (CO) and systemic vascular resistance (SVR). The MAP is the same in the distal vessels and represents the average arterial pressure throughout the cardiac cycle. Since the diastolic period (approximately two-thirds of the cardiac cycle) is longer than the systolic period, the MAP is calculated by the following equation:

$$MAP = \frac{BP_{sys} + (2\ BP_{dia})}{3}$$

Pulse pressure, calculated by subtracting BP_{dia} from BP_{sys}, reflects changes in stroke volume and arterial compliance. Wide pulse pressures are associated with a large stroke volume (e.g., aortic valve regurgitation or hypervolemia) or with an increase in ejection velocity due to medications (e.g., dobutamine, dopamine, isoproterenol). Narrow pulse pressures, on the other hand, are associated with low stroke volume (e.g., heart failure or shock) or an increase in ejection time (e.g., aortic valve stenosis).

Increased arterial pressures are typically seen with specific diseases or disorders such as aortic valve regurgitation, arteriosclerosis, and systemic hypertension. Aortic valve regurgitation allows blood to leak back into the left ventricle during diastole, thereby increasing preload and consequently increasing stroke volume. As a result, the BP_{sys} rises while BP_{dia} drops, and the pulse pressure increases. Medications that increase systemic vascular resistance (SVR), such as positive inotropic agents and vasopressors, also increase arterial pressures.

Low arterial pressures are typically associated with arrhythmias (e.g., atrial fibrillation, premature ventricular contractions) and decreased stroke volume. The effect of atrial fibrillation on arterial pressure is highly variable, but, because of the loss of atrial kick, stroke volume is usually diminished in the presence of atrial fibrillation. Premature ventricular contractions also decrease stroke volume secondary to the lack of diastolic filling, and therefore reduce arterial pressure. Other disorders that decrease stroke volume are left ventricular failure, shock, cardiac tamponade, and left ventricular outflow tract obstruction (e.g., aortic valve stenosis).

There are several variations to the arterial pressure curve, each of which indicates a change in the patient's hemodynamic status: pulsus alternans, pulsus bisferiens, pulsus paradoxus, and pulsus parvus.

- **Pulsus alternans** is a regular waveform pattern in which, on every other beat, the amplitude and therefore the pressure are larger. This irregularity occurs because of alternating ventricular contractility associated with arrhythmias or left ventricular failure.
- **Pulsus bisferiens** is an arterial pressure curve that displays two systolic peaks. One peak may be higher than the other, or the two peaks may be equal. The first peak is due to early systolic rapid ejection, followed by a brief drop in pressure. The second peak is due to forward blood flow later in systole. This type of pressure waveform is indicative of aortic valve regurgitation, hypertrophic cardiomyopathy, or hyperthyroidism.
- With **pulsus paradoxus**, BP_{sys} falls by more than 10 mm Hg during spontaneous inspiration despite a regular heart rate. This finding is most commonly seen in patients with cardiac tamponade. Other causes of pulsus paradoxus include COPD, pulmonary embolus, hypovolemic shock, severe asthma, and constrictive pericarditis. A reverse pulsus paradoxus, in which the BP_{sys} rises by more than 10 mm Hg, can occur during positive pressure ventilation. Reverse pulsus paradoxus is usually caused by hypovolemia.
- **Pulsus parvus** is a weak pulse seen on the arterial pressure curve as a low BP with decreased pulse pressure. Pulsus parvus is indicative of decreased cardiac output caused by aortic valve stenosis, left ventricular failure, or shock.

Other variations of the arterial pressure curve may be due to mechanical abnormalities rather than physiological changes: damping, catheter whip (fling) artifact, and inaccurate zeroing or calibration.

A small rounded arterial pressure curve with a slow upstroke, no clear dicrotic notch, decreased BP_{sys}, and decreased BP_{dia} indicates pressure *damping*, which may be caused by:

- Air bubbles in the pressure tubing or catheter.
- A partial clot in the catheter.
- Inadequate pressure on the IV flush bag.
- Loss of infusion solution.
- The catheter's being lodged against the vessel wall.
- Loose connections in the tubing.

To correct for pressure damping, follow this procedure:

1. Aspirate the catheter and flush the system.
2. Make sure all connections are tight and the tubing is not kinked.
3. Check for proper pressure on the IV flush bag and to ensure there is enough IV solution in the bag.
4. Recheck zeroing or calibration.

Catheter whip (fling) artifact is an erratic, or "noisy," pressure curve with sharp negative or positive waves. This type of abnormality is usually associated with excessive movement of the catheter tip, excessive connecting tubing, rapid heart rates, or some combination of those. To correct for this problem, limit patient movement, reposition the catheter tip, or use a frequency filter. Some monitoring equipment comes with a filter to eliminate this type of high-frequency artifact.

Spotlight On

The Pulse Oximeter

There is a new use for a common monitoring tool: the pulse oximeter. In the February 1999 issue of *Chest*, T. V. Hartert and colleagues identified a use of pulse oximetry in critically ill patients with severe airway obstruction. They suggested that the respiratory variation of the baseline pulse-oximetry waveform, termed RWV (respiratory waveform variation), is an indicator of severe airway obstruction. Monitoring the baseline pulse oximetry variation during breathing identifies the presence of pulsus paradoxus. It is already known that pulsus paradoxus is positively correlated with severe air trapping in critically ill asthmatic and COPD patients. Improvement in the number of millimeter change from the baseline waveform can be used as a noninvasive measure of clinical improvement.

Source: Hartert TV, Wheeler AP, Sheller JR. Use of pulse oximetry to recognize severity of airflow obstruction in obstructive airway disease: correlation with pulsus paradoxus. Chest. *1999;115:475–481.*

SYSTEMIC VASCULAR RESISTANCE

Systemic vascular resistance (SVR) is the force that the left ventricle must overcome to maintain systemic blood flow. Hence, SVR is a measure of left ventricular afterload. This important hemodynamic parameter cannot be measured directly, but it can be derived from pressure measurements and cardiac output by the following equation:

$$SVR = \frac{MAP - CVP_{mean}\ (mm\ Hg) \times 80}{CO\ Lpm}$$

Resistance to flow is the ratio of the mean pressure drop across the system to the flow through the system. In the cardiovascular system, the pressure drop across the system is measured from the proximal end (i.e., the aorta) to the distal end [i.e., the right atrial or central venous pressure (CVP)] of the system, and flow is cardiac output. The correction factor of 80 is used to convert millimeters of mercury to dynes per square centimeter and liters per minute to cubic centimeters per second to yield units of dyne·s·cm^{-5}. The normal SVR is 900–1400 dyne·s·cm^{-5}.

Under normal hemodynamic conditions, the cardiovascular system rapidly adjusts SVR in response to changes in body position, activity, or stress to maintain stroke volume and a narrow blood pressure range. Therefore, in a normal heart, stroke volume remains constant with fluctuations in SVR, and myocardial oxygen consumption (VO_2) is directly related to SVR, such that an increase in SVR increases myocardial VO_2 and vice versa. However, in the presence of cardiac disease, as the left ventricule fails and cardiac output drops, stimulation of baroreceptors causes vasoconstriction, and SVR rises in an attempt to maintain blood pressure. The increased SVR increases afterload and further burdens the already failing heart, thereby decreasing stroke volume even more. In cases of myocardial dysfunction, stroke volume is inversely related to SVR, whereas myocardial oxygen consumption is directly related to SVR. That is, an increase in SVR decrease stroke volume while increasing myocardial VO_2, and vice versa. With afterload-reducing medications, SVR is decreased, thereby improving stroke volume and decreasing myocardial VO_2 without a significant drop in blood pressure.

Regulation of SVR, according to Poiseuille's law, is a function of the length of the vessel, the viscosity of the blood, and the radius (R) of the vessel:

$$SVR = \frac{(8 \times \text{length}) \times \text{viscosity}}{\pi - R^4}$$

Because the length of the vessel does not change significantly once growth is complete and the viscosity of the blood remains relatively constant (except in cases of dehydration, polycythemia, or significant temperature changes), vessel radius is the primary determinant of SVR. Causes of changes in systemic vascular resistance are summarized in Table 19-20.

TABLE 19-20 **Causes of changes in systemic vascular resistance**

Increase	Decrease
Vasoconstriction	Vasodilation
Decreased cardiac output	Vasodilator therapy
Excessive catecholamine secretion	Shock (anaphylactic, hyperdynamic sepsis, neurogenic)
Hypertension	Other
Hypothermia	Anemia
Hypovolemia	Aortic regurgitation
Stress response	Cirrhosis
Vasopressors	
Decreased distensibility of vessels	
Aortic stenosis	
Atherosclerosis/arteriosclerosis	

PULMONARY VASCULAR RESISTANCE

Pulmonary vascular resistance (PVR) is the force that the right ventricle must overcome to maintain pulmonary blood flow; that is, PVR is a measure of right ventricular afterload. To calculate PVR, measure the mean pressure difference across the pulmonary capillary bed and divide by the flow:

$$PVR = \frac{PA_{mean} - PCWP_{mean}\ (mm\ Hg) \times 80}{CO\ Lpm}$$

The normal PVR is 20–120 dyne·s·cm^{-5}. Under normal conditions PVR is low; approximately one-sixth of SVR. When the right ventricle is faced with an increase in afterload (PVR), it dilates as a compensatory mechanism to maintain stroke volume (i.e., Frank-Starling mechanism). However, the thin-walled right ventricle is not able to withstand high afterload for very long before it begins to fail. As the right ventricle begins to fail, its stroke volume falls while myocardial oxygen consumption increases.

A change in PVR can be assessed by monitoring the pulmonary artery pressure. Increased pulmonary artery systolic, diastolic, and mean pressures indicate increased PVR. When PVR increases, pulmonary artery

TABLE 19-21 Causes of increased pulmonary vascular resistance

Pulmonary arteriolar constriction
Sympathetic nervous system stimulation
Acidosis
Hypercarbia
Hypoxemia
Drugs (epinephrine, norepinephrine)
Obstruction of pulmonary vascular bed
Pulmonary emboli
Pulmonary stenosis
Positive pressure ventilation/PEEP
Adult respiratory distress syndrome (ARDS)
Alveolar septal destruction
Surgical lung resection
Pulmonary edema

pressures rises while the pulmonary capillary wedge pressure remains normal. Therefore, in these types of patients, PCWP must be measured to determine the left ventricular end-diastolic pressure because the PCWP does not reflect changes in PVR. A drop in pulmonary artery systolic, diastolic, and mean pressures indicates a decrease in PVR.

The regulation of PVR is primarily accomplished via vasoconstriction and vasodilation. An increase in PVR can result from either pulmonary arteriolar constriction or obstruction of the pulmonary vascular bed. Factors that lead to an increase in PVR are listed in Table 19-21.

Decreases in PVR typically indicate hypovolemia or pulmonary vasodilation due to medications (e.g., captopril, diltiazem, hydralizine, isoproterenol, nifedipine, nitroprusside, and nitrous oxide).

VENTRICULAR STROKE WORK INDEX

Calculating the *ventricular stroke work index* provides an indirect evaluation of contractility and therefore of ventricular function. The right ventricular stroke work index (RVSWI) and the left ventricular stroke work index (LVSWI) are calculated separately using the calculated stroke index (SI) and pressure measurements:

$$\text{LVSWI} = \text{SI} \times (\text{MAP} - \text{PCWP}_{\text{mean}} \text{ mm Hg}) \times 0.0136$$

$$\text{RVSWI} = \text{SI} \times (\text{PA}_{\text{mean}} - \text{CVP}_{\text{mean}} \text{ mm Hg}) \times 0.0136$$

The factor of 0.0136 is used to convert units of pressure to units of work, that is, millimeters of mercury to grams per square meter per beat. The normal LVSWI is 40–70 g/m^2/beat, and the normal RVSWI is 7–12 g/m^2/beat.

Stroke volume (SV) is the volume of blood ejected by the ventricles with each contraction. The stroke volume is simply the difference between the ventricular volume at the end of diastolic filling and the ventricular volume at the end of systolic ejection. At the bedside, the stroke volume, in milliliters per beat, is calculated by dividing cardiac output (Lpm) by heart rate (bpm):

$$\text{SV} = \frac{\text{CO Lpm}}{\text{HR bpm}}$$

The stroke index (SI), in units of milliliters per beat per square meter, is calculated to account for the effects of body size on stroke volume. It is calculated by dividing stroke volume (SV) by the patient's body surface area (BSA):

$$\text{SI} = \frac{\text{SV}}{\text{BSA}}$$

The normal stroke volume is 60–120 mL/beat, and the normal stroke index is 30–60 mL/beat/m^2. Factors affecting stroke volume and stroke index are preload, afterload, contractility, and muscular synchrony (as previously discussed).

In the presence of a low or dropping cardiac output, calculating RVSWI and LVSWI can help in identifying the cause. A fall in cardiac output can be due to low preload, excessive afterload, or diminished ventricular contractility. Preload and afterload can be evaluated by monitoring pressures (CVP, PA, PCWP, and MAP) and vascular resistance. In the presence of stable preload and afterload with a decrease in cardiac output, altered contractility should be considered, and LVSWI and RVSWI should be calculated.

Decreased LVSWI and RVSWI can occur secondary to hypovolemia or myocardial ischemia or infarction or with the use of certain pharmacological agents (e.g., verapamil and beta-blockers). Ventricular contractility, and therefore LVSWI and RVSWI, can be increased with the use of positive inotropic agents (e.g., digoxin, dopamine, dobutamine, isoproterenol). Recall that an increase in contractility is associated with an increase in myocardial oxygen consumption. In the presence of compromised myocardial blood flow (e.g., ischemia or infarction), this increase in oxygen demand can be detrimental. Therefore, for these patients, administering medications that reduce contractility (e.g., beta-blockers) is often more beneficial. In shock patients, inotropic agents should be titrated to maintain an LVSWI greater than 55 g/m^2/beat.

Summary

Managing the critically ill patient in the clinical setting requires a complete assessment of the patient's cardiac status. Noninvasive assessment includes determining the patient's heart rate and rhythm and correlating them with the presence and quality of peripheral pulses. In addition, a quick check of the patient's capillary refill, skin color and temperature, level of consciousness, urine output, and neck veins determines whether further invasive monitoring is necessary. With the use of invasive catheters, important hemodynamic parameters can be measured directly: oxygenation, cardiac output, central venous pressure, pulmonary artery pressure, pulmonary capillary wedge pressure, and arterial pressure. With the information obtained from the invasive catheters, additional parameters can be calculated (mean pressures, vascular resistance, and ventricular stroke work index), allowing for the optimal use of medications to maintain hemodynamic stability.

Study Questions

REVIEW QUESTIONS

1. What is the normal time range for the P-R interval?
2. What is the landmark on the patient's chest for the placement of lead V_4?
3. Name the seven steps in dysrhythmia recognition.
4. Identify the following dysrhythmia:

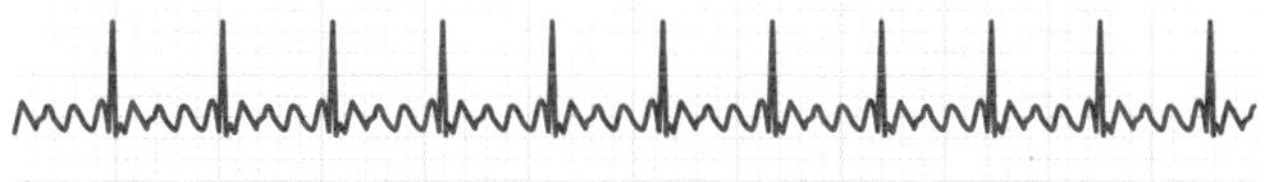

5. If the R-R interval is regular and each R-wave hits on the every second large square line, what is the calculated rate?
6. What is the most common symptom of atrial tachycardia?
7. What factors increase venous return and can result in an increase in preload to the heart?
8. Using a cardiac output of 5 Lpm, a hemoglobin of 14.8 gm/dL, a P_aO_2 of 100, and an S_aO_2 of 98%, calculate oxygen delivery.
9. What is the most common cause of a decrease in S_VO_2?
10. What substance is used to measure cardiac output using the thermodilution technique?

MULTIPLE-CHOICE QUESTIONS

1. The action potential of a single cell is described as
   a. depolarization.
   b. repolarization.
   c. one electrical cycle of depolarization and repolarization.
   d. a wave of electrical current.
2. Which electrode of the ones used in the Einthoven triangle is considered the ground or neutral electrode?
   a. right leg
   b. left leg
   c. right arm
   d. left arm
3. Which wave or time interval represents ventricular depolarization on an ECG?
   a. P-wave
   b. QRS complex
   c. T-wave
   d. ST segment
4. Which of the following dysrhythmias is considered the most life threatening?
   a. sinus tachycardia
   b. sinus brachycardia
   c. atrial flutter
   d. ventricular fibrillation
5. If an AV block results from digitalis toxicity, which AV block would you *not* see?
   a. first-degree block
   b. type I second-degree block
   c. type II second-degree block
   d. third-degree block
6. Which type of AV block is also called the Wenckebach phenomenon?
   a. first-degree block
   b. type I second-degree block
   c. type II second-degree block
   d. third-degree block
7. Which type of ventricular dysrhythmia does *not* have any effective cardiac output associated with it?
   a. ventricular escape
   b. accelerated idioventricular rhythm
   c. premature ventricular contraction
   d. ventricular fibrillation
8. Which of the following categories of PVC is not considered a serious condition?
   a. multifocal PVCs
   b. couplets of PVCs
   c. three or more PVCs in a row
   d. R on T PVCs
9. What is one unable to do with a central venous pressure invasive line?
   a. administer fluids
   b. assess blood volume status
   c. sample blood
   d. measure S_aO_2

10. If a patient had a blood pressure of 160/100 mm Hg, what is the estimated mean arterial pressure?
    a. 80 mm Hg
    b. 100 mm Hg
    c. 120 mm Hg
    d. 140 mm Hg
11. What are the ECG characteristics of Mobitz type I second-degree AV block?
    a. constant PR intervals, and constant QRS intervals
    b. variable PR intervals, and variable QRS intervals
    c. variable PR intervals and constant QRS intervals
    d. constant PR intervals and variable QRS intervals
12. What is the physiologic mechanism of paroxysmal supraventricular tachycardia?
    a. increased automaticity
    b. decreased conduction through the AV node
    c. the initiation of a reentry pattern
    d. decreased automaticity
13. In which of the following cardiac emergencies will the patient's ECG show a life-sustaining ECG pattern but the patient may have no pulse?
    a. ventricular fibrillation
    b. ventricular tachycardia
    c. PEA
    d. asystole
14. Which of the following dysrhythmias may have a rate of 42?
    a. sinus bradycardia
    b. junctional escape rhythm
    c. third-degree heart block
    d. a and b
    e. a, b, and c

References

1. Huszar RJ. *Basic Dysrhythmias*. Rev, 3rd ed. St. Louis: Mosby Jems; 2007.
2. Beachy W. Cardiac Electrophysiology. In: *Respiratory Care Anatomy and Physiology*. St. Louis: Mosby-Yearbook; 1998:267–281.
3. Beachy W. The electrocardiogram and cardiac arrhythmias. In: *Respiratory Care Anatomy and Physiology*. St. Louis: Mosby-Yearbook; 1998: 282–303.
4. Ellis KM. *EKG Plain and Simple*. Upper Saddle River, NJ: Prentice Hall; 2002:59–71.
5. Van Hare GF, Dubin AM. The normal electrocardiogram. In: Moss AJ, et al., eds. *Moss and Adams' Heart Disease in Infants, Children and Adolescents.* 7th ed. Philadelphia: Lippincott Williams & Wilkins; 2007:253–268.
6. Ibid.
7. Prystowsky E, Pritchett E, Gallagher J. Origin of the atrial electrogram recorded from the esophagus. *Circulation*, 1980;61,5:1017–1023.
8. Fletcher G, Froelicher V, Hartley L, Haskell W, Pollock M. Exercise standards. A statement for health professionals from the American Heart Association. *Circulation*. 1990;82,6:2286–2322.
9. Akinpelu D, Gonazalez JM. Treadmill and pharmacologic stress testing. eMedicine Specialties, Cardiology and Cardiovascular Syndromes in Systemic Diseases; 2008.
10. Wiederhold R. The 12-lead electrocardiogram. In: Wiederhold, R. *Electrocardiography, the Monitoring and Diagnostic Leads*. 2nd ed. Philadelphia: W.B. Saunders Co; 1999:103–116.
11. Catalano JT. *Guide to ECG Analysis*. 2nd ed. Philadelphia: Lippincott Williams & Wilkins; 2002.
12. Goldenberg I, Moss AJ, Wojciech Z. QT Interval: how to measure it and what is "normal." *J Cardiovasc Electrophysiol*. 2006;17:333–336.
13. Bollinger B, Heidenreich J. Cardiac arrhythmias. In: Stone C, Humphries R, eds. *CURRENT Diagnosis and Treatment, Emergency Medicine.* 6th ed. New York: McGraw-Hill; 2008:Chapter 33.
14. Kastor JA. Supraventricular tachyarrhythmias. In: Kastor JA, ed. *Arrhythmias*. Philadelphia: WB Saunders; 2000:39–276.
15. Kastor JA. Atrioventricular block. In: Kastor JA, ed. *Arrhythmias*. Philadelphia: WB Saunders; 2000:509–565.
16. Marriott HJ. *ECG/PDQ*. Baltimore: Williams & Wilkin; 1987.
17. Kastor JA. Ventricular arrhythmias. In: *Arrhythmias*. Philadelphia: WB Saunders; 2000:277–308.

Suggested Readings

Ahrens T. Hemodynamic monitoring. *Crit Care Nurs North Am*. 1999;11:19–31.

Guilbeau JR, Applegate AR. Thermodilution: an advanced technique for measuring continuous cardiac output. *DCCN-Dimens Crit Care Nurs*. 1996;15:25–30.

Headly J. Invasive hemodynamic monitoring: applying advanced technologies. *Crit Care Nurs Q*. 1998;21:78–83.

Heger JW, Niemann JT, Roth RF, Criley JM. Arrhythmias. In: Heger JW, Niemann JT, Roth RF, Criley JM, eds. *Cardiology*. 4th ed. Baltimore, MD: Williams & Wilkins; 1998:33–80.

Ignatavicius D, Workman M. *Medical-Surgical Nursing*. 5th ed. St. Louis, MO: Elsevier Saunders; 2006:698–705, 708, 226–244.

Lippincott Manual of Nursing Practice. 7th ed. Philadelphia: Lippincott Williams & Wilkins; 2001:105–103, 319–395.

Lodato R. Use of the pulmonary artery catheter. *Semin Respir Crit Care Med.* 1999:20:29–42.

Porth C. *Essentials of Pathophysiology Concepts of Altered Health States.* 2nd ed. Philadelphia: Lippincott Williams & Wilkins; 2007:311–349.

Ramsey J, Tisdale L. Use of ventricular stroke work index and ventricular function curves in assessing myocardial contractility. *Crit Care Nurs.* 1995;15:61–67.

Rieter MJ, Rieffel JA. Importance of beta blockade in the therapy of serious ventricular arrhythmias. *Am J Cardiol.* 1998;82:91–191.

Sarubbi B, Jucceschi VD, Andrea A, Liccardo B, Santangelo L, Iacono A. Atrial fibrillation: what are the effects of drug therapy on the effectiveness and complications of electrical cardioversion? *Can J Cardiol.* 1998;14:1267–1273.

Thaler MS. *The Only EKG Book You'll Ever Need.* 3rd ed. Philadelphia: Lippincott Williams & Wilkins; 1999.

SECTION IV

Essential Therapeutics

CHAPTER 20

Oxygen and Medical Gas Therapy

Jodi Green and Victoria Frain

OBJECTIVES

Upon completion of this chapter, the reader should be able to:

- Describe the physical characteristics of medical gases.
- Summarize the production and storage methods for medical gases.
- Categorize the responsibilities of the various agencies involved in the regulation of medical gases.
- Describe the characteristics of oxygen regulation devices.
- Describe the causes, assessment, and treatment of hypoxemia.
- Identify the goals, indications, and hazards of oxygen therapy.
- Differentiate between high- and low-flow oxygen delivery systems.
- Choose the proper method of oxygen delivery and treatment, given specific patient data.
- Describe the invasive and noninvasive methods of monitoring oxygen therapy.
- Identify the methods of operation for the various types of oxygen analyzers.
- Describe the therapeutic uses of gas mixtures.

CHAPTER OUTLINE

(continues)

(continued)

KEY TERMS

carbogen
fraction of inspired oxygen (F_IO_2)
fractional saturation
functional saturation
heliox
high-flow oxygen system
hyperbaric oxygen therapy (HBO)
hypercapnea
hypoxemia
hypoxia
hypoxic drive
low-flow oxygen system
plethysmography
polycythemia
shunt effect
specific gravity
spectrophotometry
transcutaneous monitoring
true shunt

Oxygen and medical gas therapy is the very foundation of respiratory care. Equipment for oxygen administration ranges from the simplest nasal catheter to the most sophisticated mechanical ventilator. The respiratory therapist (RT) must have a clear understanding of all aspects of medical gases, from their production and regulation to their proper administration and monitoring. The RT's skills must range from simple motor skills to complex assessment of the effects of medical gases on the cardiopulmonary system and other body systems.

Many institutions have adopted the use of protocols, care plans, and practice guidelines for the administration of medical gases. This development represents a great advance for the respiratory care profession; however, caution must be taken. Protocols and guidelines must *never* be used as cookbook recipes for treatment. They actually *increase* the responsibility of the respiratory therapist. The importance of critical thinking and assessment skills cannot be overemphasized.

Physical Characteristics of Medical Gases

Gases are categorized according to their fire risk. Although most institutions provide training in fire safety to their employees, this training rarely includes the fire risks imposed by specific medical gases. Table 20-1 groups the common medical gases according to whether they are *nonflammable* (will not burn), *nonflammable but will support combustion*, or *flammable* (will readily burn, may be explosive).

TABLE 20-1 **Fire risk for medical gases**

Nonflammable	Support Combustion	Flammable
Carbon dioxide	Oxygen	Most anesthetic gases
Nitrogen	Air	
Helium	Nitrous oxide	
	Oxygen–nitrogen	
	Oxygen–carbon dioxide	
	Helium–oxygen	
	Nitric oxide	

OXYGEN

Oxygen (O_2) is a colorless, odorless, tasteless, transparent gas. It constitutes 20.95% of the atmosphere, exerting a partial pressure of 159 mm Hg at the normal sea level barometric pressure of 760 mm Hg. It is slightly heavier than air, having a density of 1.429 g/L and a specific gravity of 1.108, compared with the 1.29 g/L density and 1.0 specific gravity of air. These physical characteristics of oxygen are at *standard temperature and pressure, dry (STPD)*, which is 0°C (32°F) and 760 mm Hg without the presence of water vapor. **Specific gravity** is a ratio of the density of one substance to the density of a standard substance, which, for gases, is air (see Chapter 3). The physical characteristics of oxygen are summarized in Table 20-2.

TABLE 20-2 **Characteristics of oxygen (O_2)**

General	Colorless, odorless, tasteless, transparent
Fire risk	Supports combustion
Percentage of atmosphere	20.95%
Partial pressure	159 mm Hg
Density	1.429 g/L
Specific gravity	1.108
Critical temperature	−118.8°C
Critical pressure (at critical temperature)	50 atm
Solubility coefficient	0.0244 (mL/mL H_2O)

TABLE 20-3 **Composition of air**

Gas	Fractional Concentration in Atmosphere (%)	Partial Pressure at Sea Level (mm Hg)
Nitrogen (N_2)	78.08	593.0
Oxygen (O_2)	20.95	159.0
Carbon dioxide (CO_2)	0.03	0.2
Argon (Ar) and trace gases	0.93	7.0

AIR

Air is the naturally occurring atmospheric gas mixture composed of nitrogen, oxygen, carbon dioxide, argon, and trace gases. The composition of atmospheric air is summarized in Table 20-3. Air has a density of 1.29 g/L (STPD) and a specific gravity of 1.0.

Compressed air has various medical applications. It is used to power pneumatically driven medical equipment and is commonly used as a source carrier gas when oxygen is not indicated or is contraindicated.

CARBON DIOXIDE

Carbon dioxide (CO_2) is a colorless and odorless gas. It is nonflammable and does not support combustion. Carbon dioxide constitutes a miniscule percentage of our atmospheric air (0.03%), exerting a partial pressure of only 0.2 mm Hg. The specific gravity of CO_2 (STPD) is 1.53, making it 1.5 times as heavy as air. The solubility coefficient of CO_2 is 0.592, showing much more solubility in water than oxygen (0.0244). On the basis of both Henry's and Graham's laws (see Chapter 3), CO_2 is approximately 20 times more diffusible in water than O_2.

Most medical uses for carbon dioxide are for laboratory purposes, such as diagnostics and equipment calibration. A mixture of carbon dioxide and oxygen (carbogen) is occasionally used for specific pulmonary disorders. The therapeutic use of carbogen is limited (discussed later in the chapter).

> **Best Practice**
>
> For safety reasons mixtures of oxygen and other gases meant for inhalation should never contain less than 20% oxygen. Common He/O_2 mixtures are 70% He/30% O_2 and 80% He/20% O_2.

HELIUM

Helium (He) is an odorless, tasteless, nonflammable gas. At STPD, helium's density is only 0.1785 g/L. It is one of the lightest of all gases, second only to hydrogen. Helium is present only in minute quantities in the atmospheric air.

Because of its low density, a combination of helium and oxygen *(Heliox)* is used therapeutically as a transport agent to carry oxygen distal to airway obstructions. Therapeutic uses of heliox are discussed later in the chapter.

NITROUS OXIDE

Nitrous oxide (N_2O) is nonflammable but, like oxygen, supports combustion. It is a colorless gas and slightly sweet in odor and taste.

Inhaled nitrous oxide must always be mixed with at least 20% oxygen. It is used clinically as an anesthetic agent because of its depressant effect on the central nervous system. True anesthesia is achieved only with dangerously high levels of N_2O; therefore, it is almost always used in combination with other anesthetic gases.

NITRIC OXIDE

Nitric oxide (NO) is nonflammable, but it supports combustion. It is a colorless, toxic gas. When combined with air, this gas is a strong irritant. If inhaled, it can cause a strong chemical inflammation, pulmonary edema, or death.

Nitric oxide has been FDA approved for some disorders. In very low concentrations, it is found to dilate pulmonary blood vessels. Therapeutically, nitric oxide has potential in the treatment of pulmonary hypertension owing to its vasodilating properties. This use of NO is discussed later in the chapter.

Production and Regulation of Medical Gases

Gases that are used for medical purposes—for obvious reasons—must meet much higher standards of production and stricter regulations than those produced for general industry. The U.S. Food and Drug Administration (FDA) requires an oxygen purity of at least 99.0%.

PRODUCTION OF MEDICALLY SAFE GASES

Oxygen is commercially produced for medical purposes by two main methods: fractional distillation and physical separation.

Fractional distillation is the most common and cost-effective method of oxygen production. Atmospheric air is first filtered, removing water, carbon dioxide, and pollutants. The resulting air is then compressed to high pressure, liquefying the mixture, and cooled by rapid expansion. The mixture (oxygen, nitrogen, and trace gases) is then heated slowly in a distillation tower, causing gases to escape in the order of their boiling points. Nitrogen escapes first, followed by the various trace gases. Liquid oxygen remains. The liquid oxygen is stored in cryogenic storage containers, to be converted to gas for later use or for storage in high-pressure cylinders. Fractional distillation produces oxygen that is 99.5% pure, exceeding FDA standards.

The *physical separation* of oxygen is accomplished by two methods, resulting in very different concentrations of oxygen.

- The *molecular sieve* method of separation incorporates the use of inorganic mineral pellets that absorb nitrogen and water vapor, allowing oxygen to pass through. The resulting oxygen concentration is approximately 90% at flows of 1–2 Lpm. The oxygen concentration decreases with an increase in flow rate.
- The second method uses a *permeable plastic membrane*, through which gases diffuse at different rates. Oxygen and water vapor pass through the membrane at a faster rate than nitrogen. The result is humidified oxygen at an approximate concentration of 40%. This concentration remains constant, regardless of flow rate.

The physical separation of oxygen production is used almost exclusively for oxygen concentrators in the home care setting. The effect of flow rate on oxygen concentration must be fully understood by the respiratory therapist. Figure 20-1 shows a typical oxygen concentrator used in the home.

Medical-grade air is produced by filtering and compressing atmospheric air. The air must be dry and free of oil and particulates. Drying is accomplished by cooling to produce condensation. Freedom from oil and particulates is accomplished through the use of inlet filters and Teflon piston rings. Air compressors can be large enough to provide the compressed air source for an entire institution or compact enough to provide medication nebulization at the bedside, whether in the hospital or at home.

There are three main types of air compressors.

- *Piston compressors* (Figure 20-2) use a reducing valve to reduce the high pressure down to a working pressure of 50 psig (pounds per square inch gauge).
- *Diaphragm compressors* (Figure 20-3) cannot generate large amounts of compressed air, so they should not be used as a power source for large medical equipment.
- *Centrifugal compressors* (Figure 20-4) can be small enough to be incorporated into a mechanical ventilator or large enough to provide the compressed air source to an entire hospital.

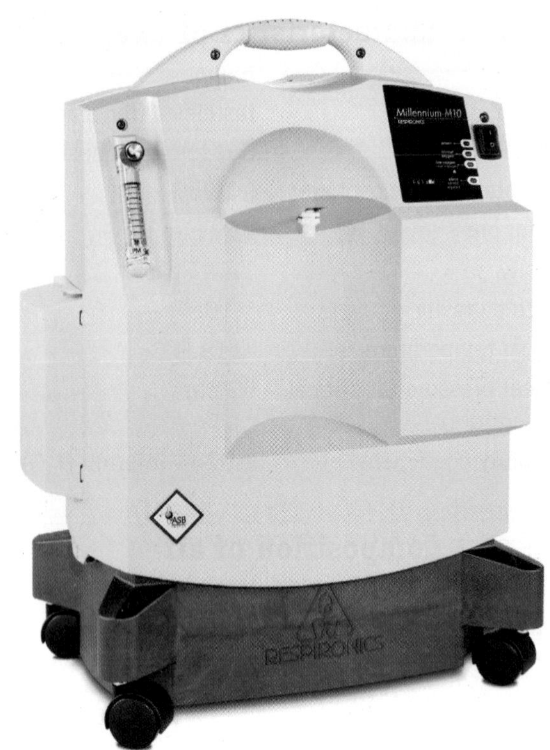

FIGURE 20-1 Oxygen concentrator.
Courtesy of Philips Respironics

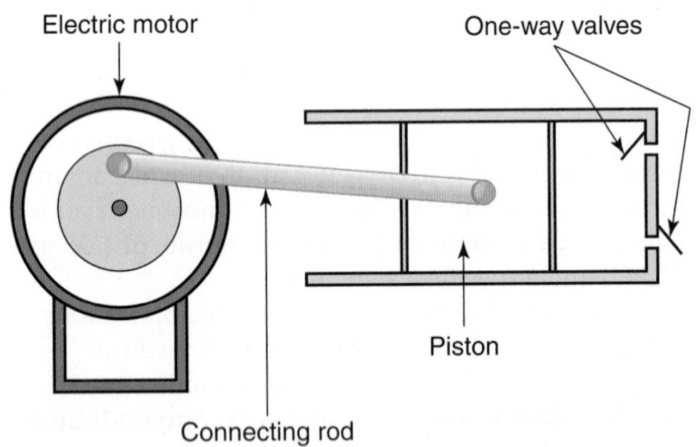

FIGURE 20-2 A functional diagram of a piston compressor.

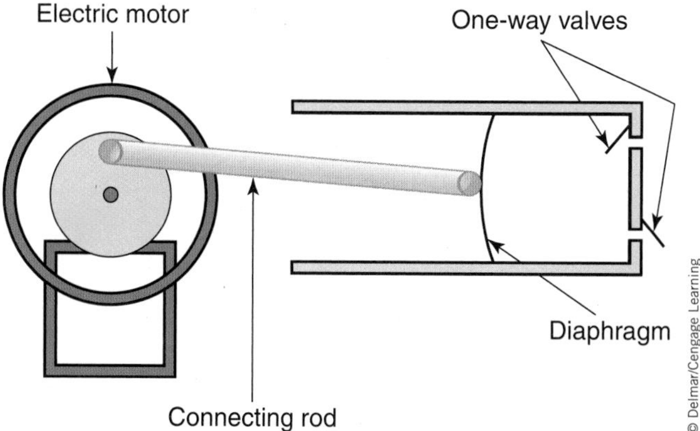

FIGURE 20-3 A functional diagram of a diaphragm compressor.

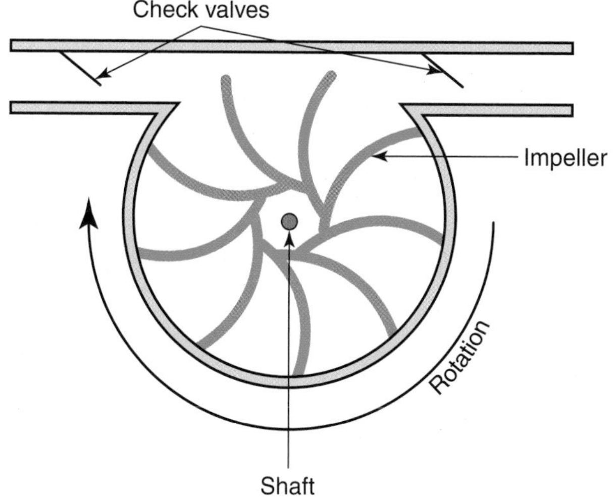

FIGURE 20-4 A functional diagram of a centrifugal compressor.

Other medical gases are produced in alternate ways:

- *Carbon dioxide* is usually produced by heating water-contacted limestone. The gas is liquefied by cooling and compression. The resulting carbon dioxide meets the FDA purity standards of 99.0%.
- *Helium* is produced by the liquefaction of natural gas. Purity standards are at least 95.0%.
- *Nitrous oxide* is produced by thermal decomposition of ammonium nitrate.
- *Nitric oxide* is produced by the oxidation of ammonia at high temperatures with the aid of a catalyst. When combined with air, the resulting nitrogen dioxide (NO_2) is toxic.

TABLE 20-4 **Responsibilities of governmental and nongovernmental agencies in gas regulation**

Agency	Responsibilities
U.S. Department of Transportation (DOT)	Compressed gas cylinders: shipping, marking, filling, labeling, purity levels
U.S. Food and Drug Administration (FDA)	Identification tags, precaution statements
Occupational Safety and U.S. Health Administration (OSHA)	Occupational safety related to medical gases
Compressed Gas Association (CGA)	Compressed gas cylinders: handling, storage, piping, fittings, markings
National Fire Protection Association (NFPA)	Codes and safety recommendations for storage of flammable and oxidizing gases
International Standards Organization (ISO)	Technical standards for manufacture terminology and testing procedures
American National Standards Institute (ANSI) Z-79 Committee	Coordination of standards for health devices

REGULATION OF MEDICAL GAS SAFETY

Various governmental and nongovernmental agencies regulate medical gas safety. The responsibilities of these agencies include overseeing:

- The production of compressed gas cylinders and bulk systems.
- The inter- and intrastate transportation of gases.
- The handling, storage, and labeling of medical gases.
- Gas safety, purity, precautions, education, and occupational safety.

Table 20-4 summarizes the responsibilities of the main agencies involved in the regulation of medical gases.

Storage and Distribution of Medical Gases

Medical gases are stored in one of three types of storage containers: compressed gas cylinders, liquid oxygen cylinders, and bulk storage systems.

COMPRESSED GAS CYLINDERS

Compressed cylinders are a convenient method for the storage and delivery of oxygen. Manufactured in various sizes, the smaller cylinders are portable and easy to transport. Compressed oxygen cylinders are a high-pressure storage system that requires a reduction in pressure down to a *working pressure* of 50 psig before delivery to a patient.

Cylinder Construction. Oxygen cylinder construction is strictly regulated by the U.S. Department of Transportation (DOT). Medical gas cylinders are seamless, spun into shape while the steel is still hot. DOT type 3A cylinders are manufactured from carbon steel, and DOT type 3AA cylinders are manufactured from heat-treated, high-strength steel. Type 3AL indicates aluminum construction. Aluminum cylinders are popular because they are lighter.

Hydrostatic Testing. The DOT requires hydrostatic testing of cylinders every 5 or 10 years. The test is a measure of the cylinder's elasticity. Cylinders are pressurized to five-thirds of their service pressure. Cylinder expansion, leakage, and wall stress are measured. "EE" followed by a number indicates the cylinder's *elastic expansion*. A cylinder that has been approved by the DOT for 10-year testing has a star next to the test date. A plus sign (+) indicates that the cylinder can be filled to 10% above its service pressure.

Cylinder Markings and Identification. Identification and markings of medical gas cylinders appear as metal stamps on their shoulder. Typically, the front of the cylinder has the letters "DOT" or, for older cylinders, "ICC" (Interstate Commerce Commission). On the same line are the cylinder classification (3A, 3AA, or 3AL) and the service pressure. Below this line are the cylinder letter size (not present on all cylinders), the serial number, the ownership mark, and the manufacturer's mark.

The rear of the cylinder contains hydrostatic test information and may also include the cylinder's elastic expansion rating. The type of steel used and the spinning process may be listed. Hydrostatic retest dates are listed vertically, along with the inspector's mark. The exact location of identification marks may vary. All cylinders are also color coded and labeled to identify their contents. Figure 20-5 shows the front and back cylinder markings.

Cylinder Color Coding and Sizes. The Compressed Gas Association (CGA) has developed a system of color coding for medical gas cylinders. The color code used in the United States differs slightly from the international code. The FDA requires that cylinders also be labeled to identify their contents. The label and the color code must match, or the cylinder should not be used. Table 20-5 compares the U.S. color-coding system with the international system.

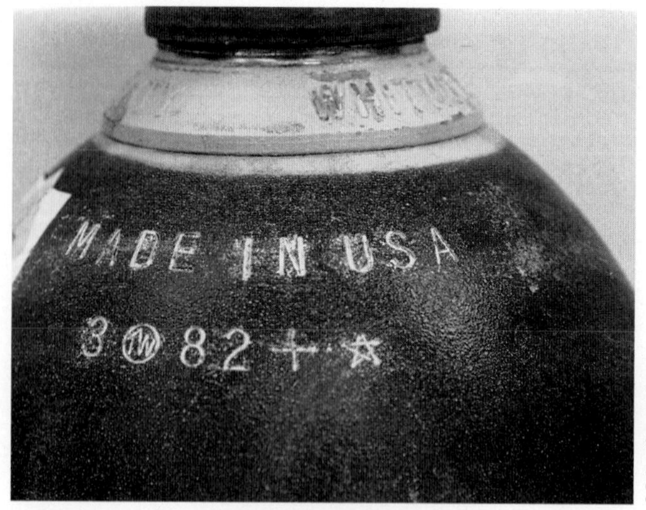

(A)

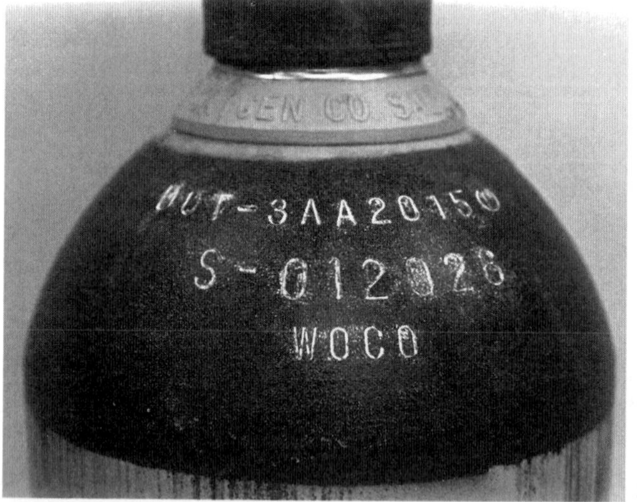

(B)

FIGURE 20-5 Markings on the front (A) and on the back (B) of an oxygen cylinder.

TABLE 20-5 **Color coding for medical gas cylinders**

Medical Gas	United States	International
Oxygen	Green	White
Air	Yellow	Black/white
Carbon dioxide	Gray	Gray
Carbon dioxide–oxygen	Gray/green	Gray/white
Helium	Brown	Brown
Helium–oxygen	Brown/green	Brown/white
Nitrogen	Black	Black
Nitrous oxide	Blue	Blue
Nitrogen–oxygen	Black/green	Pink
Cyclopropane	Orange	Orange
Ethylene	Red	Red

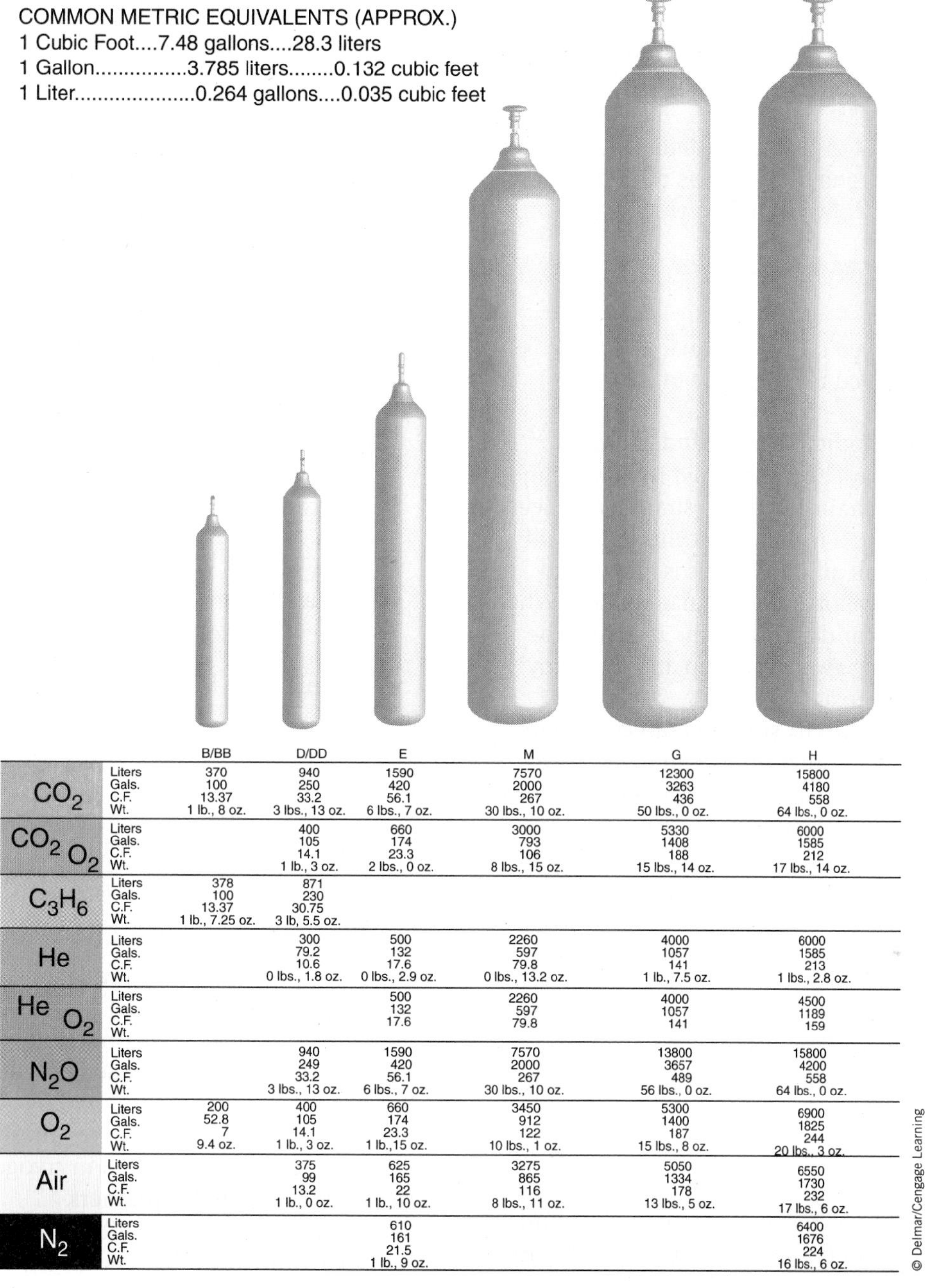

Gas		B/BB	D/DD	E	M	G	H
CO_2	Liters	370	940	1590	7570	12300	15800
	Gals.	100	250	420	2000	3263	4180
	C.F.	13.37	33.2	56.1	267	436	558
	Wt.	1 lb., 8 oz.	3 lbs., 13 oz.	6 lbs., 7 oz.	30 lbs., 10 oz.	50 lbs., 0 oz.	64 lbs., 0 oz.
CO_2 O_2	Liters		400	660	3000	5330	6000
	Gals.		105	174	793	1408	1585
	C.F.		14.1	23.3	106	188	212
	Wt.		1 lb., 3 oz.	2 lbs., 0 oz.	8 lbs., 15 oz.	15 lbs., 14 oz.	17 lbs., 14 oz.
C_3H_6	Liters	378	871				
	Gals.	100	230				
	C.F.	13.37	30.75				
	Wt.	1 lb., 7.25 oz.	3 lb, 5.5 oz.				
He	Liters		300	500	2260	4000	6000
	Gals.		79.2	132	597	1057	1585
	C.F.		10.6	17.6	79.8	141	213
	Wt.		0 lbs., 1.8 oz.	0 lbs., 2.9 oz.	0 lbs., 13.2 oz.	1 lb., 7.5 oz.	1 lbs., 2.8 oz.
He O_2	Liters			500	2260	4000	4500
	Gals.			132	597	1057	1189
	C.F.			17.6	79.8	141	159
	Wt.						
N_2O	Liters		940	1590	7570	13800	15800
	Gals.		249	420	2000	3657	4200
	C.F.		33.2	56.1	267	489	558
	Wt.		3 lbs., 13 oz.	6 lbs., 7 oz.	30 lbs., 10 oz.	56 lbs., 0 oz.	64 lbs., 0 oz.
O_2	Liters	200	400	660	3450	5300	6900
	Gals.	52.8	105	174	912	1400	1825
	C.F.	7	14.1	23.3	122	187	244
	Wt.	9.4 oz.	1 lb., 3 oz.	1 lb.,15 oz.	10 lbs., 1 oz.	15 lbs., 8 oz.	20 lbs., 3 oz.
Air	Liters		375	625	3275	5050	6550
	Gals.		99	165	865	1334	1730
	C.F.		13.2	22	116	178	232
	Wt.		1 lb., 0 oz.	1 lb., 10 oz.	8 lbs., 11 oz.	13 lbs., 5 oz.	17 lbs., 6 oz.
N_2	Liters			610			6400
	Gals.			161			1676
	C.F.			21.5			224
	Wt.			1 lb., 9 oz.			16 lbs., 6 oz.

FIGURE 20-6 Gas cylinder sizes, factors, and conversions.

Medical gas cylinders are manufactured in various sizes, designated by letters.

- Sizes AA–E are small cylinders, typically used for patient transport. Small cylinders have a unique valve and yoke connection.
- The larger cylinders, F–K, use a threaded valve connection.
- The sizes most commonly used in the hospital setting are E and H cylinders. E cylinders are used for patient transport and ambulation. Although most large institutions use a central piping system, H cylinders are still used in older institutions and in older areas of the hospital.

Figure 20-6 provides condensed information on gas cylinder sizes and includes cylinder factors and conversions.

Filling Methods for Medical Gas Cylinders. A cylinder is filled according to its service pressure, which is usually 2000–2015 psi. A cylinder that has passed hydrostatic testing, as signified by the plus sign (+), can be filled to 10% above its service pressure. For

Best Practice

Storage Temperature

Because of thermal expansion, cylinders stored in a very cold environment, such as outdoors, should be allowed to warm before cracking and use.

Best Practice

Duration of Flow

For safety considerations, use 500 psig as a buffer when calculating how long a cylinder will last. To do so, simply subtract 500 psig from the starting cylinder pressure.

example, if an approved cylinder's service pressure is 2000 psi, it can be filled to a pressure of 2200 psi.

Safety Factors for Medical Gas Cylinders. Gas cylinders should always be transported in a stand and kept in place with a chain or other restraining device. Before it is attached to a regulator, a cylinder should be *cracked*, that is, a small amount of gas is allowed to escape to free the valve of any particulate matter. When cracking the cylinder and attaching the regulator, be sure the valve is facing away from you and from any other persons in the area.

Cylinders should not be stored in direct sunlight. An increase in temperature results in an increase in pressure inside the cylinder. In very high temperatures, such as during a fire, the cylinder may explode. Therefore, cylinders are equipped with high-pressure relief valves. Of the several types of relief valves, all are designed to vent gas from the cylinder in order to prevent an excessive build-up of pressure.

Duration of Cylinder Gas Flow. The practitioner must be able to estimate how long a cylinder will last for circumstances such as patient transport. The duration of gas flow from a cylinder can be estimated if the following factors are known: cylinder size, starting pressure, and gas flow.

- First, the volume, in cubic feet, of a full cylinder must be converted to liters. There are 28.3 L in one cubic foot. For a full cylinder, the *cylinder factor* is derived by dividing the volume, in liters, by the pressure (psig). Cylinder factors are constant; they are calculated from full cylinder volume and pressure.

$$\text{cylinder factor (L/psig)} = \frac{\text{cubic feet (full cylinder)} \times 28.3}{\text{pressure (full cylinder)}}$$

$$\text{H cylinder} = \frac{244\ \text{ft}^3 \times 28.3\ \text{L/ft}^3}{2200\ \text{psig}}$$

$$\text{H cylinder factor} = 3.14\ \text{L/psig}$$

$$\text{E cylinder} = \frac{22\ \text{ft}^3 \times 28.3\ \text{L/ft}^3}{2200\ \text{psig}}$$

$$\text{E cylinder factor} = 0.28\ \text{L/psig}$$

- The next step is to find the contents of the cylinder in liters by multiplying the cylinder factor by the existing gauge pressure.
- The duration of flow, in minutes, is then determined by dividing the contents by the existing gas flow (liters per minute).

$$\text{duration of flow (minutes)} = \frac{\text{gauge pressure} \times \text{cylinder factor}}{\text{flow (LPM)}}$$

For example, how long will an E cylinder last, if it has 1000 psig pressure and a flow rate of 4 Lpm?

$$\text{duration of flow} = \frac{1000\ \text{psig} \times 0.28\ \text{L/psig}}{4\ \text{LPM}}$$

$$\text{duration of flow} = 70\ \text{minutes, or } 1.16\ \text{hours}$$

LIQUID OXYGEN CYLINDERS

Oxygen gas occupies a volume that is 861 times that of liquid oxygen per cubic foot. Therefore, liquid oxygen containers are much more practical when large amounts of oxygen are needed or when oxygen is running at a constant high-liter flow. Because maintaining oxygen in its liquid state requires very low temperatures, liquid oxygen is stored in cryogenic, insulated, vacuumized thermal containers.

Liquid containers are filled to a *filling density* rather than to a filling pressure. The filling density is the ratio of the weight of liquid gas to the weight of water that the container could contain. The gauge pressure indicates only the pressure of the vapor above the liquid. This pressure remains constant as long as liquid is remaining in the container. When all the liquid is gone from the container, the gauge pressure begins to drop according to the volume of gas remaining. At this point, rapid falls in gauge pressure can occur. Although a liquid container is a relatively low-pressure system compared with a gas container, a small amount of vapor above the liquid is constantly venting. Therefore, the only accurate way to measure liquid contents is to weigh the container.

Liquid oxygen systems are very popular in the home care setting, especially when a continuous flow

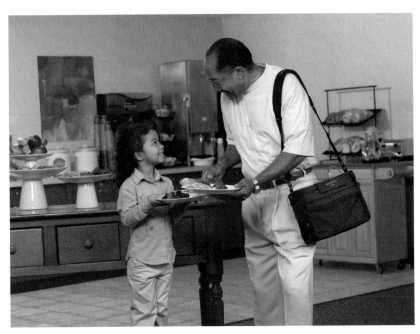

FIGURE 20-7 Portable oxygen concentrator.
Courtesy of Philips Respironics

of oxygen is needed. The systems include floor and portable models. Portable units often include a shoulder bag, which is an advantage for patients who are not confined to the home (Figure 20-7).

BULK STORAGE SYSTEMS

A *bulk oxygen storage system* holds a minimum of 13,000 ft^3 of oxygen gas. Bulk oxygen is stored in either liquid or gaseous form. Liquid storage is more common and convenient as an oxygen source for facilities that use large volumes of oxygen because they vastly reduce the space requirements for bulk storage (1 ft^3 liquid oxygen = 861 ft^3 gaseous oxygen).

Keeping liquid oxygen from reverting to its gaseous state requires storage below its critical temperature of −118.8°C. The construction of the storage container is similar to that of a thermos insulated bottle, with inner and outer steel shells separated by a vacuum space. This construction enables liquid oxygen to be stored without the need for refrigeration. Figure 20-8 illustrates a typical liquid bulk storage system.

Bulk liquid oxygen systems have several advantages over gas cylinders.

- Liquid systems operate at much lower pressures, approximately 250 psig, rather than the 2200 psig pressures of compressed gas cylinders.
- The delivery pressures of bulk liquid systems are regulated centrally, eliminating the need for pressure-reducing valves at individual outlets. In any event, all medical gas systems are reduced to a working pressure of 50 psig at the final outlet.

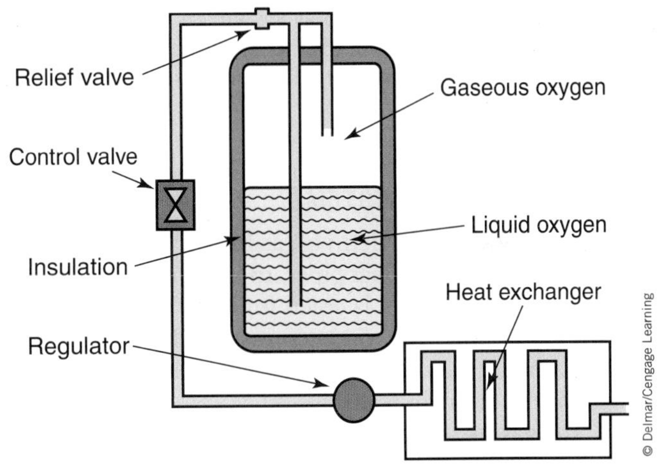

FIGURE 20-8 A bulk liquid oxygen storage and supply system.

Gas bulk oxygen systems are usually large cylinders linked together in a manifold system. Manifold systems have two banks of cylinders, a primary bank and a reserve bank.

The National Fire Protection Association (NFPA) sets the safety standards for bulk oxygen systems. A key NFPA requirement is the presence of a reserve back-up gas supply. This supply must be equal to the hospital's average daily gas use. Figure 20-9 illustrates the reserve systems for three bulk storage systems.

The distribution of medical gases takes place via central piping systems, connector systems, and oxygen regulation devices.

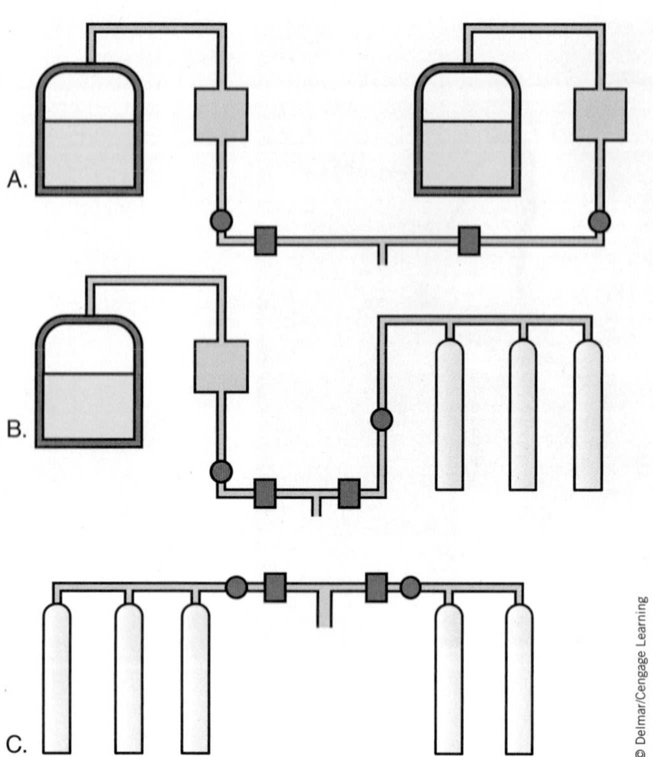

FIGURE 20-9 Bulk oxygen supply systems. (A) Liquid primary and liquid reserve. (B) Liquid primary and cylinder reserve. (C) Cylinder primary and cylinder reserve.

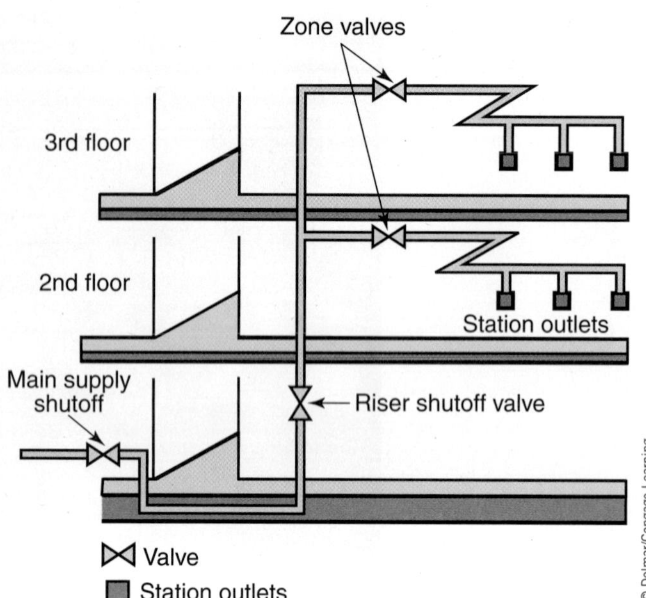

FIGURE 20-10 Zone valve placement in a central piping system.

CENTRAL PIPING SYSTEMS

A *central piping system* delivers gas from the bulk storage area, via seamless copper pipes, to its various points of use. The piping system is tested for leaks by pressurizing it to 1.5 times its working pressure. This pressure is maintained for 24 hours. To pass final inspection, the system must remain leak free.

The gas pressure is reduced to the normal working pressure of 50 psig at the bulk storage location. Sensors are placed at various locations in the piping system to continuously monitor pressure. Alarms are included to alert personnel of pressure drops in the system caused by leaks or gas depletion.

Zone valves are located at strategic points. These permit the gas to be shut off to certain areas in the event of a fire. Respiratory therapists must be able to identify the locations of the zone valves. Of course, in the event of a shutoff, all oxygen patients must be provided with supplemental oxygen from cylinders. Figure 20-10 illustrates the zone valve placement in a central piping system.

CONNECTOR SYSTEMS

The Compressed Gas Association (CGA) developed not only a system of color coding for medical gas cylinders, but also a connector system. Indexed safety systems make it virtually impossible to connect one gas source to a system designed to deliver another. For example, connecting an oxygen delivery system to a cylinder of carbon dioxide is impossible.

The *American Standard Safety System* (*ASSS*) provides standards for threaded systems. These are the high-pressure connections (>200 psig) between large compressed gas cylinders (F–K) and their attachments. Figure 20-11 depicts typical ASSS connections.

The *Pin-Index Safety System* (*PISS*) was designed for the valve outlet of small cylinders (A–E). Small cylinders use a yoke connection. The two pins on the connector must fit precisely into the pin index holes of the cylinder valve. There are six pinhole positions and a

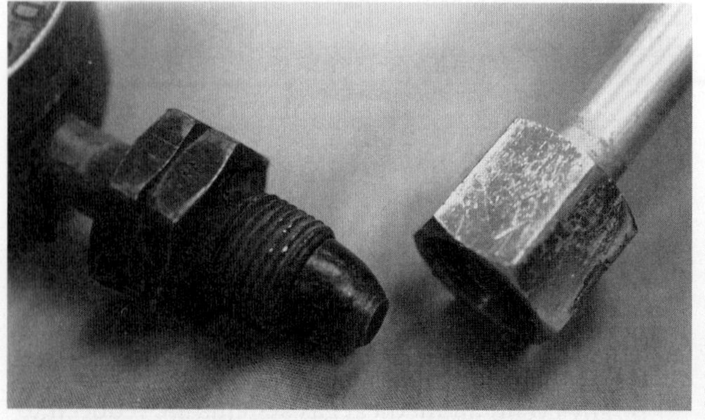

FIGURE 20-11 Two-thread ASSS connections.

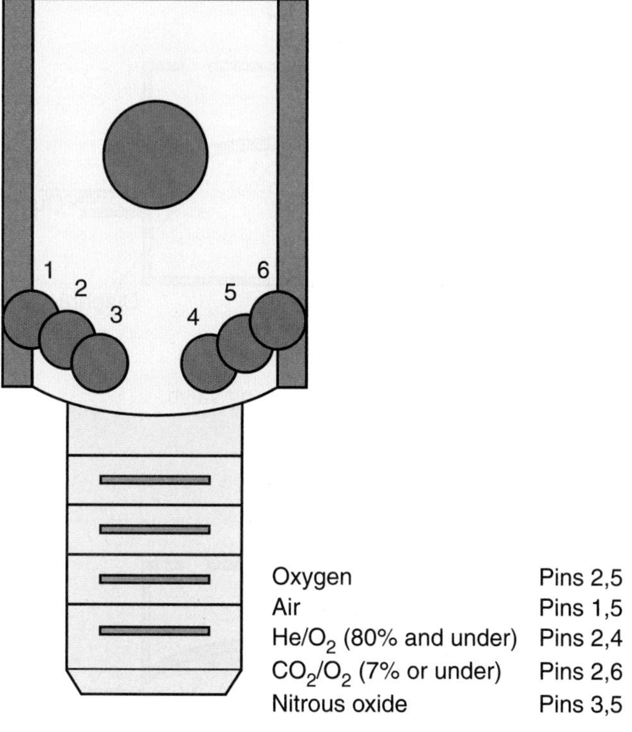

FIGURE 20-12 Six different pin index positions for medical gases.

number of possible combinations. For example, the pin index position for oxygen is 2–5. Only the yoke connection pins for an oxygen delivery system precisely correspond to the pin index holes of a small oxygen cylinder valve. Figure 20-12 illustrates six pin index positions.

The *Diameter-Index Safety System (DISS)* also prevents the interchange of medical gas connectors. The DISS system, however, is designed specifically for low-pressure connections, that is, when the pressure has already been reduced to under 200 psi, usually to a working pressure of 50 psi. DISS connections are usually found at the station outlets of the central piping system and at the inlets of pneumatic equipment such as flowmeters, humidifiers, nebulizers, and mechanical ventilators. DISS systems incorporate check valves to prevent gas loss when the system is not in use.

Quick-connect systems, a variation of the DISS connection, are also designed for low-pressure connectors. Each medical gas has a differently shaped connection and fitting. Quick-connect systems are convenient, and they provide easy and rapid connection and disconnection of equipment. Unlike DISS connections, the design of quick-connect systems varies among manufacturers. The variation should not pose a problem as long as the facility is standardized on a specific system.

OXYGEN REGULATION DEVICES

Gas contained in cylinders is under high pressure, usually 2200 psi when the cylinder is full. Cylinder valves and reducing valves are necessary to regulate gas pressure and for the safe attachment of pneumatic equipment. Specialized regulation devices are also needed to control gas flow and oxygen concentration.

Cylinder Valves. There are two types of cylinder valves: direct-acting cylinder valves and diaphragm cylinder valves.

- The *direct-acting cylinder valve* (Figure 20-13) is a needle valve that opens and closes the valve seat directly. When the valve seat opens, gas flows through the valve from the high-pressure interior of the cylinder to the lower outside pressure.
- A *diaphragm cylinder valve* (Figure 20-14), as its name suggests, uses a diaphragm to open or close the valve seat. Gas pressure displaces the diaphragm, allowing the gas to flow from the cylinder.

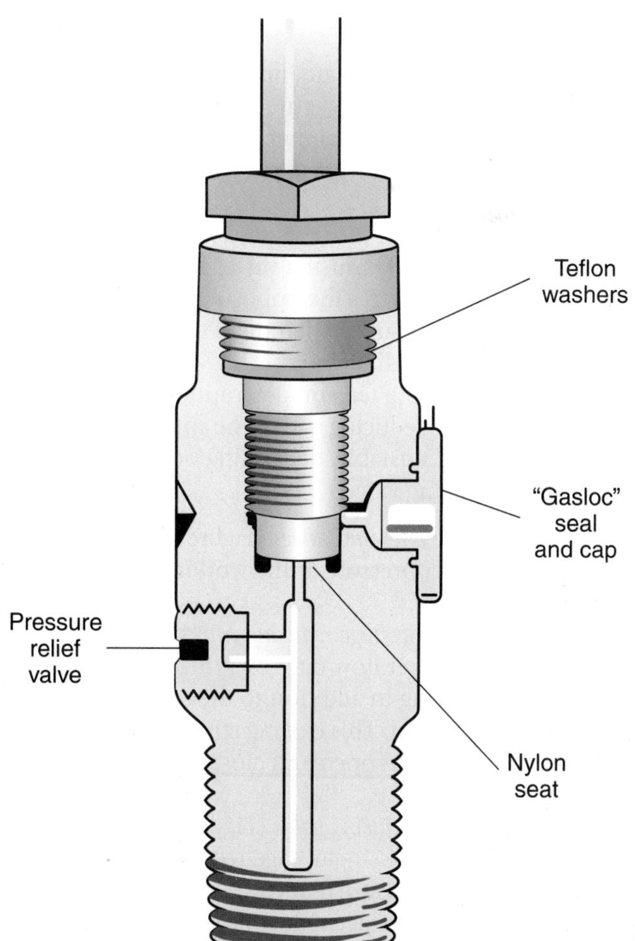

FIGURE 20-13 A direct-acting cylinder valve.

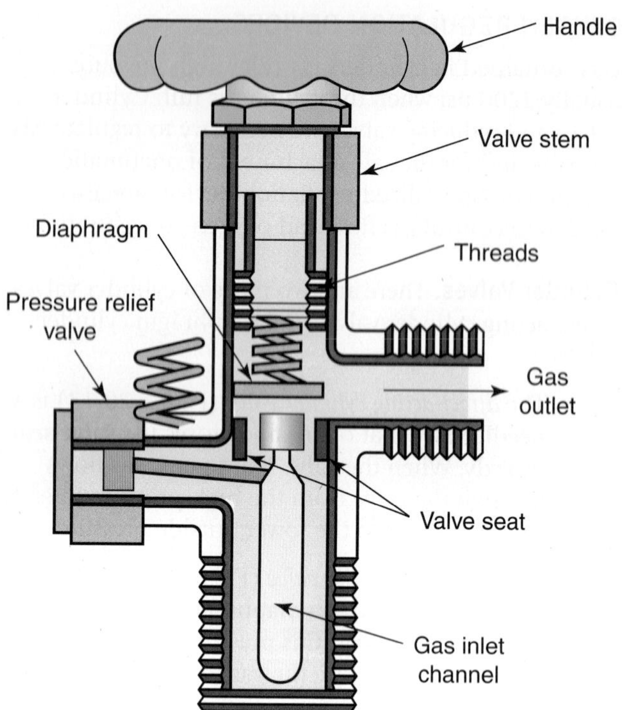

FIGURE 20-14 A diaphragm cylinder valve.

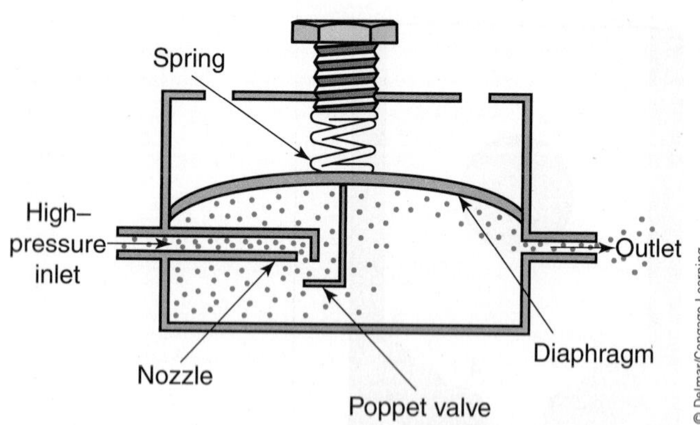

FIGURE 20-15 A single-stage reducing valve.

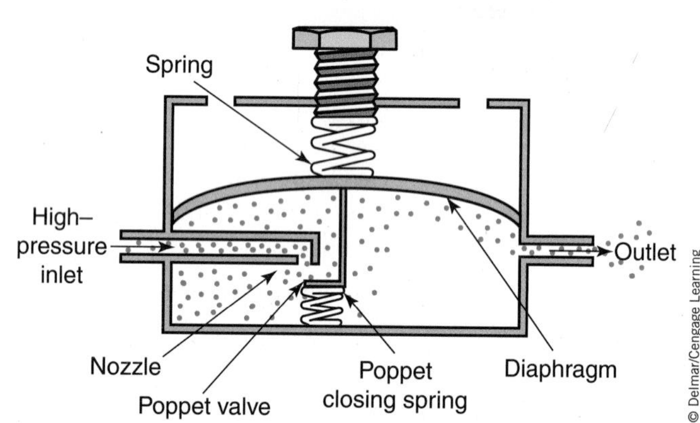

FIGURE 20-16 A modified single-stage reducing valve.

Pressure relief devices are incorporated into cylinder valves. These devices are designed to open if either the pressure or the temperature rises beyond safe limits; their opening prevents the cylinder from rupturing.

Reducing Valves. All reducing valves have a flexible diaphragm that separates the opposing forces of spring tension and gas pressure. When these two opposing forces are equal, the diaphragm is flat and the poppet valve is closed. Spring tension determines the outlet pressure from the reducing valve. The spring tension may be fixed or adjustable, depending on the construction of the reducing valve.

- *Single-stage reducing valves* (Figure 20-15) reduce the cylinder pressure to the working pressure in one step.
- *Modified single-stage reducing valves* (Figure 20-16) provide greater flow rates by utilizing a poppet closing spring in addition to the spring above the diaphragm. This closing spring allows the poppet valve to open and close much more rapidly.
- A *multistage reducing valve* (Figure 20-17) consists of two or more single-stage reducing valves in a series. The pressure reduction is accomplished in steps. The first stage reduces the pressure to approximately 200 psi. The second stage reduces this pressure to a normal working pressure, usually 50 psi. Each stage of a multistage reducing valve operates independently of the others. Multistages allow for more precise pressure regulation and greater flow rates, such as those required for operating mechanical ventilators.

Each stage of a reducing valve incorporates a *pressure relief valve*, or *pop-off valve*, for safety in the event of excessive pressure build-up. The relief valve is designed to vent the excess pressure, preventing the reducing valve from rupturing. The reducing valve inlet is indexed with either the ASSS or the PISS. The valve outlet is indexed with the DISS.

Regulators. A *regulator* is a combination of a reducing valve and a flowmeter in a single unit. This unit not only reduces gas pressure but also regulates gas flow to the patient. Regulators are much more convenient than separate reducing valves and flowmeters. Only one high-pressure connection is required.

Proportioners (Air-Oxygen Blenders). *Air-oxygen blenders* (Figure 20-18) are devices that mix air and oxygen in precise proportions, resulting in very accurate and stable oxygen concentrations. Blenders

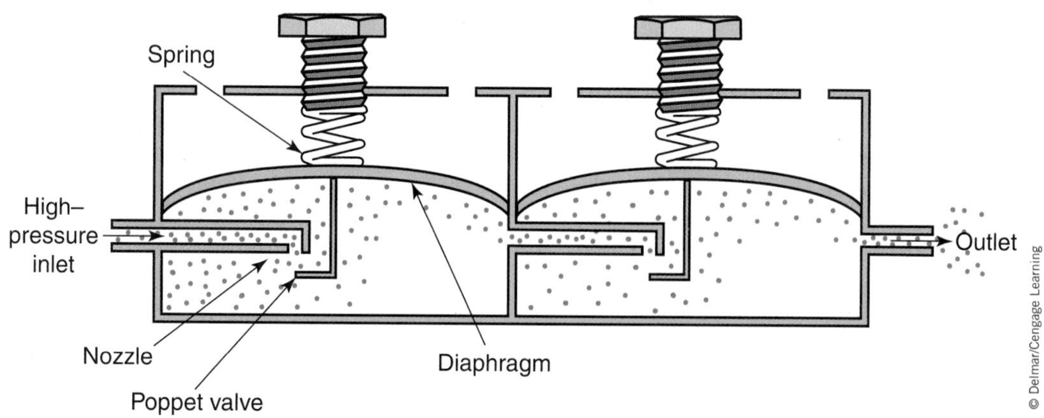

FIGURE 20-17 A multistage reducing valve (two stages).

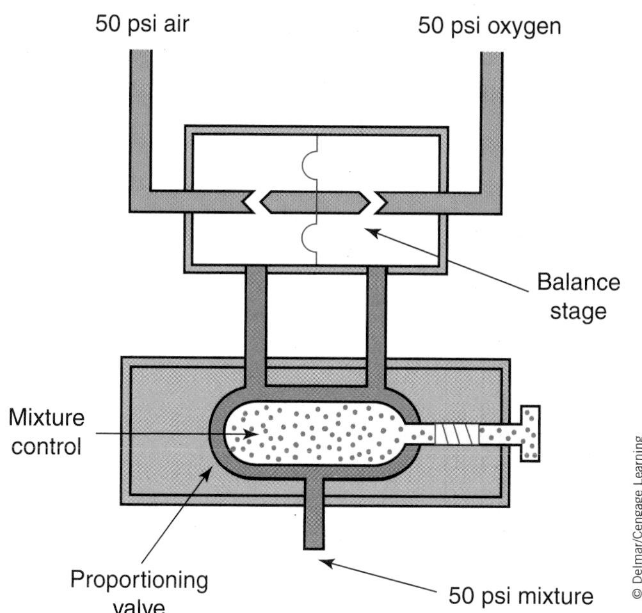

FIGURE 20-18 A functional diagram of an air-oxygen blender.

require a 50-psi source of air and oxygen and provide a 50-psi source of blended gas. Be aware that changes in gas densities can affect mixing ratios.

Air and oxygen, occupying two separate chambers, enter the blender separately. A regulator is incorporated to ensure that the pressures of the two gases are equal. Each gas passes through a proportioning valve. As the control is adjusted to allow more of one gas, the valve closes proportionally to the other gas. For example, if a higher concentration of oxygen is desired, dialing for this higher concentration not only opens the valve for more oxygen but also closes the valve to air, proportionally, allowing less air to exit.

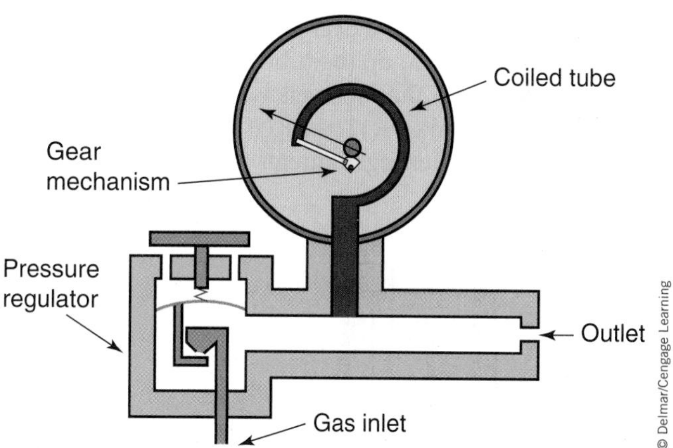

FIGURE 20-19 A Bourdon gauge flowmeter.

Most blenders are equipped with an alarm to signal a pressure drop in either the air or the oxygen supply line in the regulator.

Note: The oxygen concentration from a blender should always be verified by analysis.

Flowmeters. There are two major types of oxygen flowmeters: the Bourdon gauge flowmeter, and the Thorpe tube flowmeter.

The *Bourdon gauge flowmeter* (Figure 20-19) is a fixed-orifice type of flowmeter that uses a Bourdon gauge and an adjustable reducing valve. As pressure increases between the reducing valve outlet and the fixed orifice, the coiled copper tube in the Bourdon gauge uncurls and begins to straighten out. Although the Bourdon gauge actually measures pressure, it is calibrated to illustrate flow rather than pressure.

An advantage to the Bourdon gauge is that it is not gravity dependent; therefore, an accurate reading can be obtained in any position. This flowmeter is very convenient for patient transport situations when the tank cannot remain upright.

Caution must be taken when using the Bourdon gauge flowmeter. Any increase in pressure distal to the fixed orifice, such as that caused by kinks in the oxygen tubing, causes the flowmeter to read inaccurately. The presence of back-pressure may cause this flowmeter to indicate a *higher* flow than is actually being delivered. In fact, this gauge may indicate flow even if the outlet is completely occluded!

The *Thorpe tube flowmeter* can either be uncompensated or compensated.

In the *uncompensated* Thorpe tube flowmeter (Figure 20-20A), the needle valve is *proximal* to the Thorpe tube. The pressure in the tube is equal to ambient pressure. The Thorpe tube gradually increases in diameter from the bottom to the top of the tube. The ball float indicates flow rate. As the needle valve is opened, the gas pressure overcomes the force of gravity, pushing the ball float up the tube. The higher the ball float is in the tube, the more gas is needed to flow around the float in order to keep it in a stable position because of the widening diameter of the tube. The needle valve adjusts the flow rate. As it is opened, more gas flows into the tube.

The uncompensated Thorpe tube flowmeter reads inaccurately in the presence of back-pressure. If pressure exists distal to the Thorpe tube, as it would if the oxygen tubing had a kink, the Thorpe tube becomes pressurized. This effect decreases the pressure gradient between the top and the bottom of the ball float, causing the float to drop in the tube. The indicated flow rate may be *lower* than the flow rate actually being delivered.

In a *back-pressure-compensated* Thorpe tube flowmeter (Figure 20-20B), the needle valve is positioned *distal* to the Thorpe tube. The pressure in the tube is equal to working pressure (50 psi) when the flowmeter is connected to a gas source, rather than to ambient pressure as in the uncompensated tube. Back-pressure applied distal to the tube does not affect the performance of the Thorpe tube. Further back-pressure restricts the flow rate, but this restriction is indicated by the position of the ball float. Even in the presence of back-pressure, the compensated Thorpe tube flowmeter reads *accurately*.

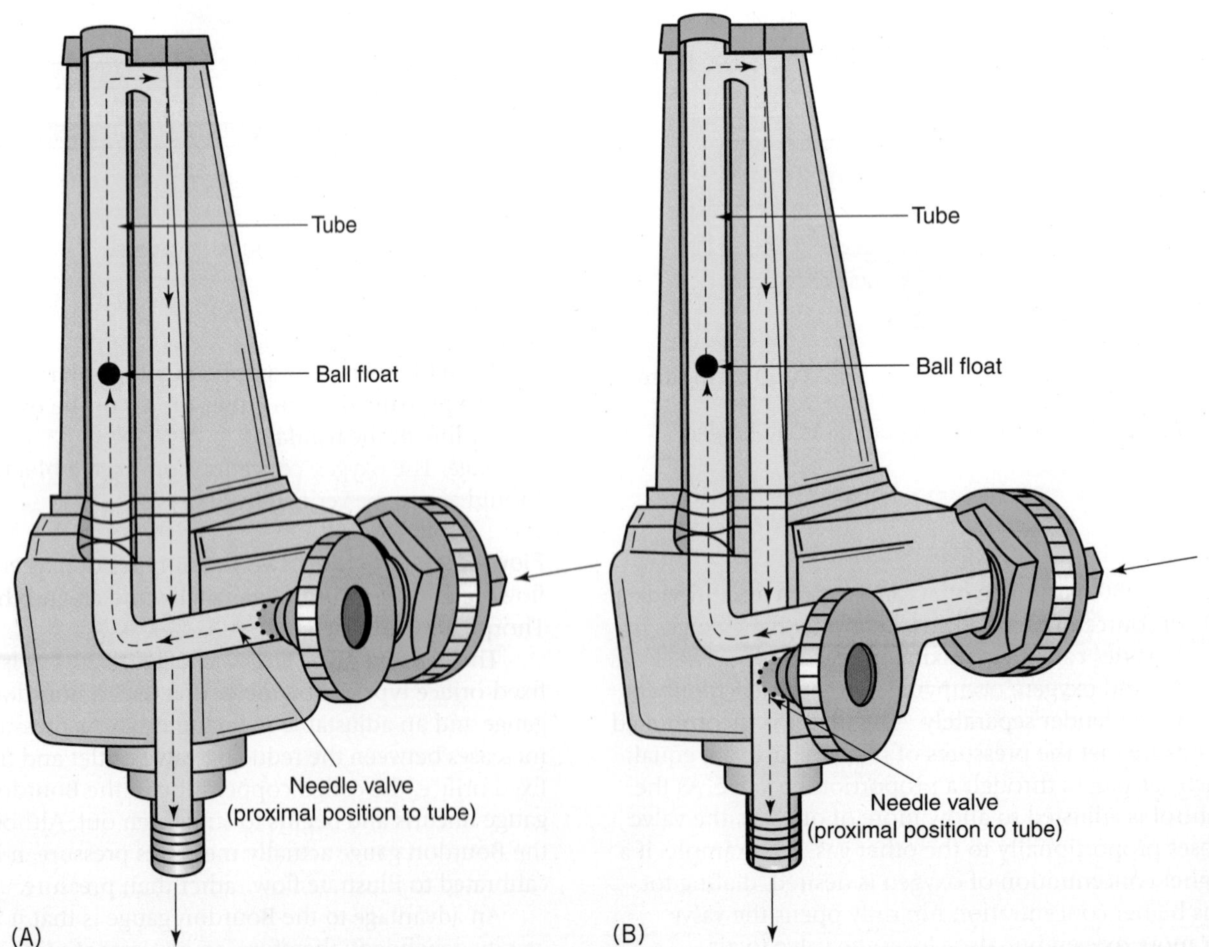

FIGURE 20-20 Thorpe tube flowmeters: (A) Uncompensated. (B) Back-pressure-compensated. (*continues*)

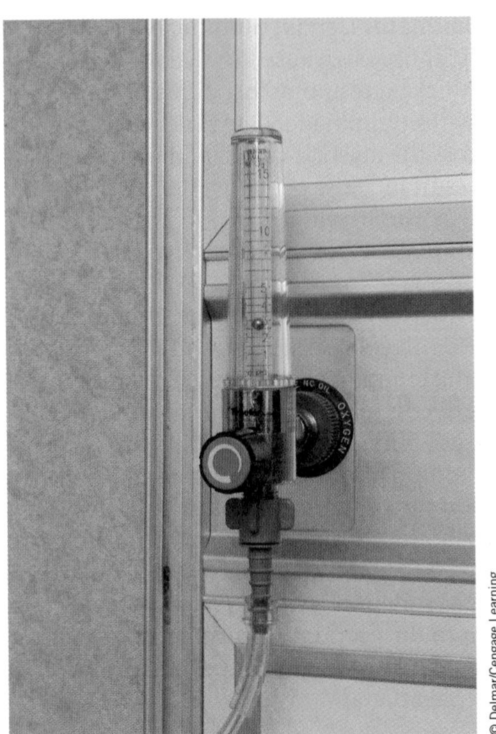

(C)

FIGURE 20-20 *(continued)* (C) The Thorpe flowmeter.

© Delmar/Cengage Learning

Best Practice

Identifying a Back-Pressure-Compensated Flowmeter

The following three methods should be used to identify a back-pressure-compensated Thorpe tube flowmeter (Figure 20-20 C):

- Check the label for one of two statements: "Calibrated at 760 mm Hg, 70°F, 50 psig inlet and outlet pressure" or "pressure compensated."
- Connect the flowmeter to the gas source with the needle valve closed. The ball float rapidly jumps up the tube if it is back-pressure compensated.
- Completely occlude the tubing or outlet after turning on the flowmeter. The flowmeter should read 0.

Technically, if the needle valve is distal to the Thorpe tube, the flowmeter is back-pressure compensated. However, determining the position of the needle requires dismantling the flowmeter.

Therapeutic and Diagnostic Uses of Oxygen

The respiratory therapist needs to be well versed in both the therapeutic and diagnostic uses of oxygen. The practitioner must be able to assess the need for oxygen therapy and to recognize the indications and hazards of therapy. Monitoring the patient during oxygen therapy and assessing its outcome are equally important.

GOALS AND OBJECTIVES OF OXYGEN THERAPY

The broad goal of oxygen therapy is to maintain adequate tissue oxygenation. Specific objectives of oxygen therapy are to:

- Correct acute hypoxemia.
- Alleviate the symptoms associated with chronic hypoxemia.
- Decrease the workload of the cardiopulmonary system.

Correction of Acute Hypoxemia. **Hypoxemia** is the term used to describe a low level of oxygen in the arterial blood. Table 20-6 lists the three levels of hypoxemia according to P_aO_2.

Increasing the concentration of inspired oxygen usually increases the level of oxygen in the blood. Exceptions are discussed later in the chapter.

Alleviation of Symptoms of Chronic Hypoxemia. The dyspnea that occurs with both obstructive and restrictive lung disease can be somewhat alleviated with oxygen therapy. The alleviation of dyspnea may result in a decreased work of breathing and, over time, an improved tolerance to exercise.

Decrease in the Work of the Cardiopulmonary System. The cardiac system compensates for hypoxemia by increasing cardiac output. Because of the low blood oxygen level, the heart must pump more blood to maintain tissue oxygenation. The results are heightened blood pressure and heart rate. Increasing the blood oxygen level with oxygen therapy decreases the work of the left ventricle.

Chronic hypoxemia, over time, causes certain physiological changes. One physiological effect of

TABLE 20-6 **Levels of hypoxemia (adult values)**

Level	P_aO_2
Mild	60–80 mm Hg
Moderate	40–60 mm Hg
Severe	< 40 mm Hg

hypoxemia is constriction of the pulmonary arterioles, which leads to pulmonary hypertension and eventually cor pulmonale (right ventricular failure). Continuous low-flow oxygen therapy may alleviate the vasoconstriction, decreasing the work of the right ventricle.

Another physiological change of chronic hypoxemia is **polycythemia**, an excess or increased number of red blood cells. Although polycythemia has various causes, when it results from chronic hypoxemia, it is a compensatory response. Oxygen that is carried in the blood is either dissolved, as indicated by the P_aO_2, or bound to hemoglobin (a constituent of red blood cells), as indicated by the S_aO_2. Red blood cells carry almost all transported oxygen in its bound form. Chronic hypoxemia stimulates the bone marrow to increase production of red blood cells by the release of erythropoietin (EPO) by the kidneys. This is a compensatory mechanism designed to increase the oxygen-carrying capacity of the blood. This increase in red blood cells increases the viscosity of the blood, presenting as an increase in hematocrit (Hct, see Chapter 6). More driving pressure is needed to pump high-viscosity blood, resulting in an increase in work of both the right and left ventricles, and increasing afterload. Polycythemia can be alleviated by increasing the blood oxygen level with oxygen therapy, thereby decreasing the work of the heart.

CAUSES OF HYPOXEMIA

Hypoxemia, a low oxygen concentration in the arterial blood, must be differentiated from **hypoxia,** an inadequate amount of oxygen available for cellular metabolism at the tissue level. Tissue hypoxia can be categorized as hypoxic, anemic, circulatory, or histotoxic. The broad category of tissue hypoxia is discussed in Chapter 6. The focus here is on hypoxic hypoxia, or hypoxemia.

There are four major causes of hypoxemia: low alveolar PO_2 (P_AO_2), diffusion impairment, ventilation/perfusion mismatch ($\dot{V}/\dot{Q}$), and true shunt.

Low Alveolar PO_2. The arterial blood level of oxygen depends on the alveolar level of oxygen. If the alveolar level of oxygen (P_AO_2) is low, the result is a low arterial level of oxygen (P_aO_2). A low P_AO_2 can be caused by hypoventilation (such as from a drug overdose), COPD, neuromuscular disease, or the effects of anesthesia. Other causes include ascent to high altitudes where the partial pressure of oxygen is lower than 159 mm Hg, and breathing gas mixtures less than 21% oxygen, as occurs during a fire.

Hypoxemia caused by a low P_AO_2 readily responds to oxygen therapy. In most cases, an increase in the P_AO_2 results in an increase in the P_aO_2.

Diffusion Impairment. Certain pulmonary diseases, such as interstitial fibrosis, cause the alveolar-capillary membrane to thicken, resulting in a diffusion impairment. This may result in inadequate time for oxygen to equilibrate across the alveolar-capillary membrane. Diseases that result in a loss of surface area for diffusion, such as emphysema, also result in a diminished transfer of oxygen from the alveoli to the blood.

Ventilation/Perfusion Mismatch. When pulmonary perfusion exceeds alveolar ventilation ($\dot{Q} > \dot{V}_A$), low ventilation/perfusion ratio exists, producing a shunt effect. **Shunt effect** is a condition in which the PaO_2 is decreased because pulmonary perfusion is greater than alveolar ventilation. This effect can be caused by an accumulation of mucus, bronchospasm, or any cause of uneven distribution of ventilation. In shunt effect, the pulmonary perfusion is in contact with ventilated alveoli, but the ventilation is inadequate to provide enough oxygen to the blood. $\dot{V}/\dot{Q}$ mismatch is the most common cause of hypoxemia. Shunt effect readily responds to oxygen therapy.

True Shunt. True shunt (absolute shunt) is a condition in which ventilation is *absent* to certain alveoli or to a section of the lung (see Chapter 6). True shunt is caused by conditions such as alveolar collapse, atelectasis, or consolidation. In this condition, pulmonary perfusion is in contact with alveoli that are not ventilated at all. The perfusion that is in contact with normal alveoli cannot pick up more oxygen because the blood is already fully saturated. For these reasons, true shunt conditions are *refractory* (not responsive) to oxygen therapy.

ASSESSMENT OF HYPOXEMIA

The assessment of hypoxemia and of the need for oxygen therapy is accomplished by a thorough patient assessment, combined with laboratory data indicating hypoxemia. Table 20-7 lists the common physical signs and laboratory findings of hypoxemia.

TABLE 20-7 **Clinical signs of hypoxemia**

Respiratory	Cardiac	Neurological	Laboratory
Dyspnea	Tachycardia	Headaches	Decreased PaO_2
Tachypnea	Hypertension	Restlessness	Decreased SaO_2
Cyanosis*		Confusion	Decreased CaO_2
			Polycythemia

Cyanosis presents as a pale or bluish tint of the lips and extremities, caused by 5 or more grams of unbound hemoglobin.

INDICATIONS FOR OXYGEN THERAPY

Obviously, the primary indication for oxygen therapy is documented hypoxemia. According to the American Association for Respiratory Care clinical practice guideline for oxygen therapy in the acute care hospital, the level of hypoxemia that indicates the need for oxygen therapy is a P_aO_2 below 60 mm Hg or an S_aO_2 below 90%.[1] Other indications for oxygen therapy include acute myocardial infarction, trauma, postoperative recovery, and any condition in which hypoxemia is suspected.

> **Best Practice**
>
> ### Chronic Hypercapnea and Hypoxemia
>
> COPD patients, or any patients with suspected chronic hypercapnea and hypoxemia, should have an arterial blood gas performed to verify P_aO_2 and P_aCO_2. These patients should be placed on an oxygen delivery system that ensures practitioner control of the F_IO_2 and should be maintained at an F_IO_2 just high enough to ensure adequate oxygenation. Oxygen levels should be titrated to achieve acceptable baseline values for these patients.

HAZARDS OF OXYGEN THERAPY

There are four major hazards of oxygen therapy: absorption atelectasis, ventilatory depression, oxygen toxicity, and retinopathy of prematurity. All are related to a high **fraction of inspired oxygen (F_IO_2)**, prolonged exposure to a high F_IO_2, or a high P_aO_2.

Absorption Atelectasis. *Absorption atelectasis* occurs as a result of nitrogen washout. Two factors increase the risk for absorption atelectasis: a high F_IO_2 (greater than 0.50) and the presence of partially obstructed alveoli. Nitrogen exists in equilibrium in the alveoli and in the blood, acting as a filler gas. When a person is breathing high concentrations of oxygen, the nitrogen is rapidly washed out of the alveoli and replaced by oxygen. A pressure gradient for oxygen exists between the alveoli and the blood; therefore, oxygen diffuses into the blood. However, owing to a partial or full obstruction, the oxygen is diffusing into the blood *faster* than it is being replaced in the alveoli. The alveolar pressure falls, deflating the alveoli in the areas of obstruction.

Ventilatory Depression (Oxygen-Induced Hypoventilation). Ventilation is controlled primarily by central chemoreceptors that respond indirectly to a rise in P_aCO_2 and by peripheral chemoreceptors that respond directly to a low P_aO_2. The *central chemoreceptors* are located in the medulla oblongata; the *peripheral chemoreceptors* are in the aortic arch and the carotid artery.

The normal physiological stimulus to breathe is a rising P_aCO_2; the secondary stimulus is a low P_aO_2. As the P_aCO_2 rises, the concentration of H^+ in the cerebrospinal fluid (CSF) increases. The increase in H^+ stimulates the central chemoreceptors, resulting in an increase in ventilation. The P_aCO_2 of some patients with COPD or neurological disorders is chronically high. Bicarbonate (HCO_3) eventually buffers the increase in H^+ in the blood and cerebrospinal fluid in order to normalize the pH (see Chapter 4). This buffering blunts the central chemoreceptors. So, in the patient with chronic **hypercapnea** (increased P_aCO_2), the peripheral chemoreceptors, responding to hypoxemia, are the primary stimulus to breathe. These patients are breathing on what is termed **hypoxic drive**. Peripheral chemoreceptors are significantly activated when the P_aO_2 is below 60 mm Hg, resulting in an increase in ventilation. Patients with a chronic P_aCO_2 above 50 mm Hg and a P_aO_2 below 60 mm Hg are at risk of oxygen-induced hypoventilation if administered an F_IO_2 that results in a P_aO_2 above 60 mm Hg. Although oxygenation should never be compromised, these patients need to be treated with caution.

Oxygen Toxicity. During the normal metabolism of oxygen, O_2 splits and forms oxygen free radicals. In response, the body produces enzymes and antioxidants in defense against the free radicals. However, prolonged exposure to a high F_IO_2 can overwhelm the body's natural defenses. Alveolar cell damage occurs, especially to type I pneumocytes (see Chapter 6), which are primarily responsible for alveolar wall integrity. Thickening of the alveolar-capillary membrane and interstitial edema follow. Eventually, pulmonary fibrosis develops. In response to the cellular damage, the immune system is activated, releasing neutrophils and macrophages (see Chapter 6). The chemical mediators of these immune cells actually worsen the damage and release free radicals of their own. Lung compliance, diffusing capacity, and vital capacity all decrease. Worsening of the $\dot{V}/\dot{Q}$ mismatch occurs as pulmonary shunting increases. These effects, in turn, worsen the hypoxemia, creating the need for an even higher F_IO_2.

Retinopathy of Prematurity. *Retinopathy of prematurity (ROP)*, previously known as retrolental fibroplasia (RLF), is a condition that sometimes occurs in

Best Practice

Limiting High F_IO_2 Exposure

Try to limit exposure to 100% oxygen to fewer than 24 hours. Strive to keep the F_IO_2 below 0.50 while maintaining adequate oxygenation. Consider balancing F_IO_2 with the application of positive pressure in the form of continuous positive airway pressure (CPAP) for spontaneously breathing patients or positive end-expiratory pressure (PEEP) for mechanically ventilated patients. These methods aid in keeping the F_IO_2 as low as possible.

Age-Specific Competency

Values for Infants

In infants, maintain a P_aO_2 between 50 and 80 mm Hg or an S_aO_2 of 88–92%. Attempt to avoid wide fluctuations in P_aO_2. F_IO_2 should be kept below 0.50.

premature infants receiving supplemental oxygen (see Chapter 29). In this case, a high P_aO_2 or a wide fluctuation in P_aO_2, more than the F_IO_2, causes the hyperplasia of the retina.[2] High blood levels of oxygen cause constriction of the blood vessels in the retina. These blood vessels eventually turn necrotic, and new vessels form (a process called *neovascularization*). The new vessels tend to hemorrhage and cause scarring behind the retina, which can result in blindness. The infant is at risk for this condition until about 1 month of age. At that time, the arteries of the retina are mature.

OXYGEN DELIVERY SYSTEMS

Oxygen delivery systems are commonly categorized as high-flow, low-flow, reservoir, or enclosure systems. Categorization as high- or low-flow does not refer to the liter flow of the device but rather to whether the outflow of the device satisfies the entire inspiratory demands of the patient.

High-Flow Systems. High-flow oxygen systems use various methods to entrain room air. The air then mixes with the source gas, and the system delivers enough gas to completely satisfy the patient's inspiratory flow needs. *The total flow of a high-flow oxygen delivery system meets or exceeds the patient's total inspiratory flow requirements.* The actual flow rate that the patient receives is much higher than that indicated on the flowmeter. The amount of air entrained by a high-flow system is controlled by the delivery device, which is set by the practitioner, making the delivered F_IO_2 *fixed*. Air is entrained into a high-flow system by the viscous shearing that occurs at the jet orifice of the system. Viscous shearing and Bernoulli's and Venturi's principles are discussed in Chapter 3.

The F_IO_2 is changed by varying the size of the entrainment ports or the jet size. In most systems, the jet size is fixed by the manufacturer, but the practitioner can vary the size of the entrainment ports. Simply stated:

- The *larger* the air entrainment port is, the *more* air is entrained—the *lower* the F_IO_2, the *higher* the total flow.
- Conversely, the *smaller* the air entrainment port is, the *less* air is entrained—the *higher* the F_IO_2, the *lower* the total flow.

The patient's inspiratory flow needs must be approximated to determine whether a system is delivering gas flow in excess of the patient's inspiratory needs. A patient breathing at a tidal volume of 500 mL, a breathing rate of 20 bpm, and an I/E ratio of 1:2 (see Chapter 6), has the following inspiratory flow requirements:

$$\text{cycle time} = \frac{60 \text{ seconds}/20 \text{ bpm}}{3 \text{ seconds}}$$

$$\text{I:E} = 1:2$$

$$\text{I time} = 1 \text{ second}$$

$$0.5 \text{ L } (V_T) \times 60 \text{ seconds}$$

$$30 \text{ Lpm}$$

- Although the patient's minute ventilation ($\dot{V}_E$) is 10 Lpm, expiration constitutes two-thirds of the ventilatory cycle. Ten liters is only one-third of the total flow required. A minimum flow of 30 Lpm is required to satisfy the patient's *peak inspiratory flow requirements*.
- Next, the total flow of the system must be known. The first step in this process is to compute the air-to-oxygen ratio. The following equation is applied:

$$\text{air:oxygen ratio} = \frac{\text{liters of air entrained}}{\text{liters of oxygen}} = \frac{1.0\ (100\%) - F_IO_2}{F_IO_2 - 0.21\ (21\%)}$$

Using an F_IO_2 of 0.50, substitutions are made:

$$\text{air:oxygen ratio} = \frac{1.0 - 0.50}{0.50 - 0.21}$$

$$\text{air:oxygen ratio} = \frac{0.50}{0.29} = \frac{1.7}{1.0}$$

TABLE 20-8 **Air-to-oxygen ratios for common F_IO_2s**

F_IO_2	Air/Oxygen
0.24	25:1
0.28	10:1
0.30	8:1
0.35	5:1
0.40	3:1
0.50	1.7:1
0.60	1:1
1.00	0:1

- The air-to-oxygen ratio of a device set at 50% is 1.7:1. In other words, for every liter of oxygen from the input source, 1.7 L of air is entrained. Table 20-8 lists the air-to-oxygen ratios for common F_IO_2s from 0.24 to 1.0.
- To calculate the total flow from the system, simply add the air and oxygen parts and multiply by the source oxygen input flow. Again, using an F_IO_2 of 0.50 and an oxygen input flow rate of 10 Lpm:

  1.7 parts air + 1 part oxygen = 2.7 total parts

  2.7×10 Lpm = 27 Lpm

This system is providing a total flow of only 27 Lpm. This is not enough to satisfy the patient's inspiratory flow needs, which are a minimum of 30 Lpm. The source input flow rate must be increased, or a double system or specialized nebulizer must be employed.

A less commonly used calculation, but one included for completeness, is calculating the resulting F_IO_2 from a fixed air/oxygen ratio. A device having a fixed air/oxygen ratio of 5:1 delivers the following F_IO_2:

$$F_IO_2 = \frac{(\text{air parts} \times 0.21) + (\text{oxygen parts} \times 1.0)}{\text{total parts}}$$

$$F_IO_2 = \frac{(5.0 \times 0.21) + (1.0 \times 1.0)}{6.0}$$

$$F_IO_2 = \frac{2.05}{6.0}$$

$$F_IO_2 = 0.34$$

A device with a fixed air-to-oxygen ratio of 5:1 will deliver gas at an approximate F_IO_2 of 0.34.

Examples of high-flow systems are aerosol masks, trach collars, trach tubes, and mist tents.

Air Entrainment Masks *High airflow with oxygen entrainment (HAFOE) masks,* by the principle of viscous shearing, utilize specific combinations of entrainment ports and jet sizes to deliver specific F_IO_2s. Although commonly called *Venturi masks,* or *venti-masks,* the name "Venturi" is really a misnomer. These devices do not use a Venturi tube to entrain gas; rather they utilize the principle of viscous shearing (described in Chapter 3). Figure 20-21 depicts a Venturi mask. Although the mask contains side exhalation ports, room air is not entrained by the patient as long as the total flow exceeds the patient's peak inspiratory needs. There is little concern at F_IO_2s of 0.35 or less, but at higher F_IO_2s, total flow drops significantly.

Best Practice

Peak Inspiratory Flow Requirements

A quick and easy method used to approximate a patient's peak inspiratory flow requirements is to multiply the patient's $\dot{V}_E$ by 3: 10 Lpm $\times$ 3 = 30 Lpm, the minimum flow required.

Best Practice

Minimum Total Flow

It is common practice to ensure a minimum total flow of 60 Lpm for a high-flow system.

Air Entrainment Nebulizers Air entrainment nebulizers have a fixed jet orifice. Air entrainment and F_IO_2 are adjusted by varying the size of the entrainment port. These nebulizers have the added options of delivering additional humidification in the form of an aerosol and of delivering heat. For these reasons, air entrainment nebulizers are commonly used for patients with intact upper airways and those with artificial airways. For patients with intact upper airways, the desired F_IO_2 is delivered via an aerosol mask or face tent. For patients with artificial airways, such as a tracheostomy or an endotracheal tube, oxygen is delivered via a tracheostomy collar or a T-tube (see Chapter 20).

Most nondisposable air entrainment nebulizers (Figures 20-22 and 20-23) have preset, fixed F_IO_2 settings, such as 0.40, 0.70, and 1.0. Most disposable nebulizers have a much wider or a continuous range.

- Because of the function of aerosol production, the jet size of most air entrainment nebulizers is very small. Consequently, they are designed to function properly at a limited range of source flows, usually between 10 and 15 Lpm, depending on the manufacturer. Although increasing the source input flow rate is not an option to

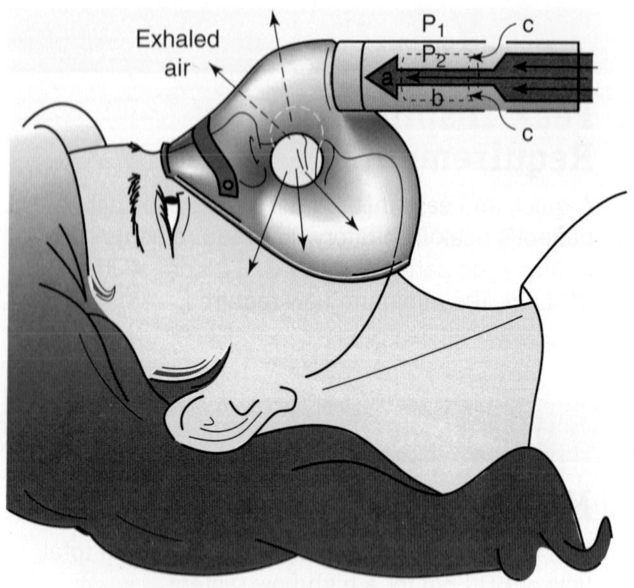

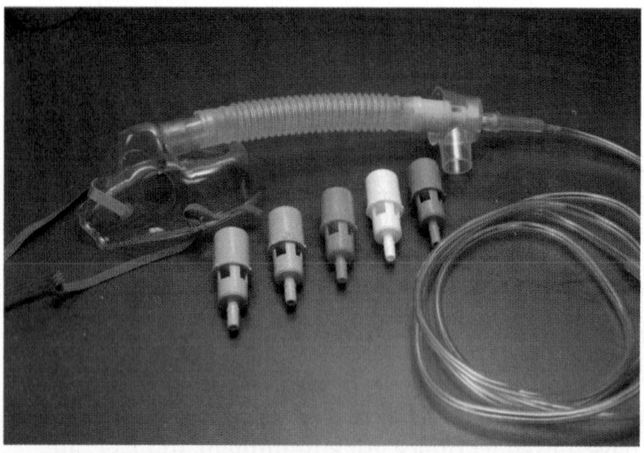

FIGURE 20-21 A venturi mask: (a) High-velocity jet. (b) Area of viscous shearing (c) Air entrainment.

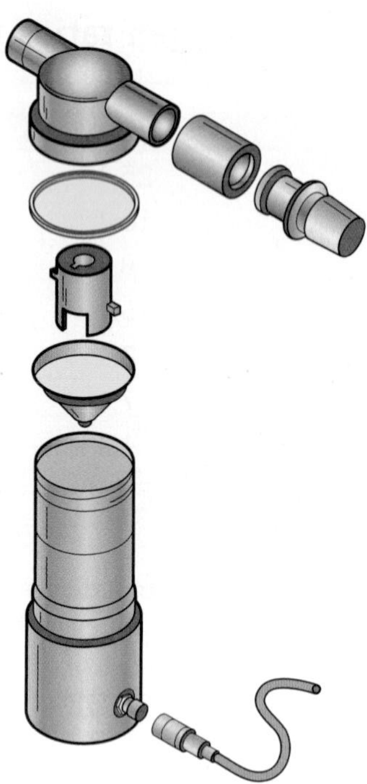

FIGURE 20-22 A drawing of the EasyNEb.

Image used by permission from Nellcor Puritan Bennett LLC, Boulder, Colorado, part of Covidien.

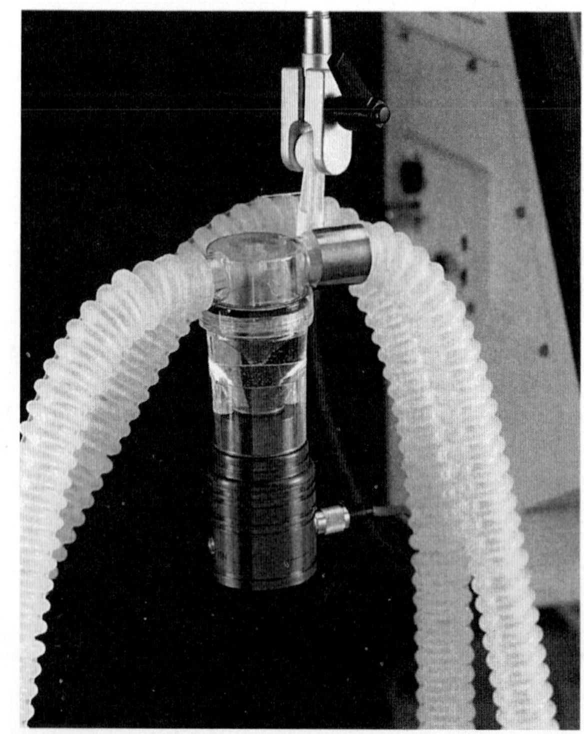

FIGURE 20-23 EasyNeb.

Image used by permission from Nellcor Puritan Bennett LLC, Boulder, Colorado, part of Covidien.

increase total flow, there is rarely a problem at F_IO_2s of 0.35 and below because of the relatively large air entrainment port opening. However, increasing the F_IO_2 decreases the size of the entrainment port, decreasing the total flow. At F_IO_2s above 0.35, the system must be assessed to ensure that it is meeting the patient's peak inspiratory flow needs. To make this assessment, calculate the patient's inspiratory flow needs and the total flow from the system, making sure that the system flow exceeds the patient's requirements. A quick and simple method of assessing adequate flow is by visual inspection.

The total flow can be increased in several ways.

- One method is to connect 50–150 mL of aerosol tubing, which acts as a reservoir, to the expiratory side of the system. This method is routinely used, but it can be used only with a T-tube.
- Another method is to install a 6-in. (50–75-mL) length of large-bore corrugated tubing in the exhalation holes of an aerosol mask. These "tusks" provide a 100–150-mL reservoir.
- A third common method is to connect two nebulizers, both set at the prescribed F_IO_2. This

Best Practice

Assessing the Flow of an Air Entrainment Nebulizer

Observe the aerosol mist at the exhalation area of the system. If the mist is continuous *throughout the patient's inspiration*, the flow is adequate and the delivered F_IO_2 is stable. If the aerosol mist is broken during the inspiratory cycle, the system flow is inadequate. The patient is entraining an *uncontrolled* amount of room air, and the delivered F_IO_2 is *lower* than the F_IO_2 setting.

Age-Specific Competency

Pediatric Air Entrainment Masks

Air entrainment masks are also available in pediatric sizes; however, they are not recommended for children younger than 3 years of age.

setup doubles the total flow delivered to the patient (see Chapter 21).

- A fourth method is to set the nebulizer to a lower F_IO_2 than prescribed and bleed in supplemental oxygen. The lower F_IO_2 setting on the nebulizer increases the size of the air entrainment port, increasing the total flow. The bled-in oxygen compensates for the lower F_IO_2 setting. Although the F_IO_2 of the system is being monitored via oxygen analysis, the system can be adjusted to deliver the prescribed F_IO_2 with enough flow to exceed the patient's inspiratory flow requirements. Care should be taken to document the settings that ensure adequate flow and an accurate F_IO_2, assuming the patient's ventilatory pattern remains constant. All staff should be notified that both flowmeters are supposed to be running.
- A fifth method is to use a specialized nebulizer such as the Misty Ox Hi-Fi nebulizer or the Misty Ox Gas Injection nebulizer (GIN).[4] Both nebulizers are designed to provide a high total flow output that exceeds the patient's peak inspiratory requirements at any F_IO_2. The Misty Ox Hi-Fi nebulizer uses air entrainment as the mechanism for increasing total flow. The Misty Ox Gas Injection nebulizer is not an entrainment device but a closed system that uses two gas sources and gas injection. Both nebulizers can provide high total flows at high F_IO_2s. These nebulizers are discussed in more detail in Chapter 21.

Low-Flow Oxygen Systems. Low-flow oxygen systems *provide only part of the patient's inspiratory flow requirements.* The remainder of the flow is room air that is entrained *by the patient.* The amount of air entrained by the patient cannot be controlled; thus, the delivered F_IO_2 varies with changes in the patient's ventilatory pattern. Delivered F_IO_2 is dependent on the patient's tidal volume, respiratory rate, and peak inspiratory flow rate. In a typical low-flow system, supplemental oxygen is delivered directly to the patient's airway, commonly at liter flows of 6 Lpm or less. Because low-flow systems do not satisfy the patient's entire inspiratory demands and require room air entrainment by the patient, the F_IO_2 is *variable* (but it can be estimated). Some low-flow systems incorporate a reservoir system that collects oxygen.

- For a patient with a low tidal volume, a higher percentage of each breath is delivered by the system, resulting in a higher F_IO_2.
- Conversely, a patient with a large tidal volume has a smaller percentage of each breath delivered by the system and a larger amount of room air being entrained, resulting in a lower F_IO_2.

High respiratory rates and high inspiratory flow rates also result in a lower F_IO_2 owing to more room air entrainment by the patient. Examples of low-flow systems are nasal cannulas, simple O_2 masks, and partial-rebreathing and nonrebreathing masks.[1]

Nasal Cannula The *nasal cannula* (Figure 20-24) is a disposable plastic device with two curved prongs that

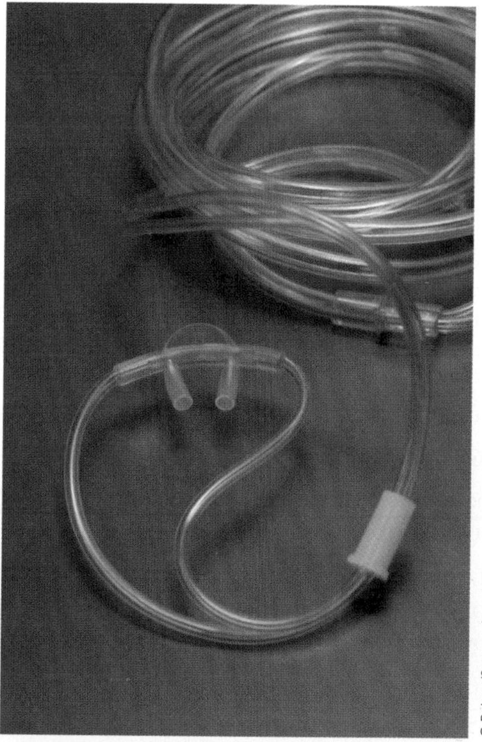

FIGURE 20-24 Nasal cannula.

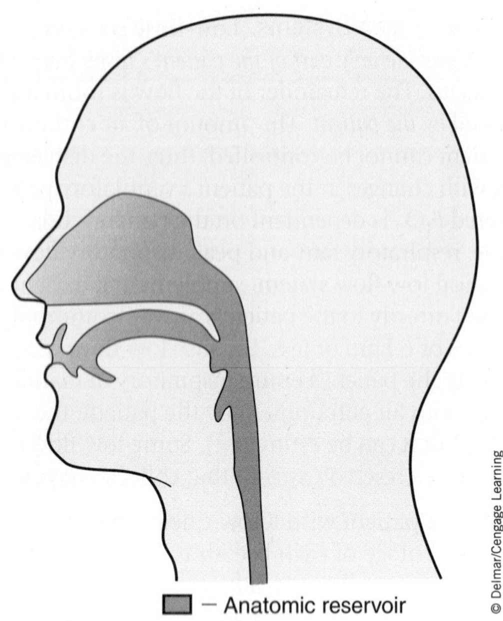

FIGURE 20-25 The anatomic reservoir.

are positioned in the nasal passage. The cannula rests on the upper lip, and the tubing is connected directly to the flowmeter or to a bubble humidifier. Humidification is typically used at liter flows above 4 Lpm. Humidification is discussed in Chapter 21.

The nasopharynx and the oropharynx constitute the anatomic reservoir, as illustrated in Figure 20-25. This reservoir has a volume of approximately 50 mL in a normal adult. During the normal pause between expiration and inspiration, this reservoir fills with 100% oxygen. Therefore, at the beginning of the next inspiration, the patient receives 50 mL of 100% oxygen. The remainder of the inspiration consists of oxygen mixed with room air. For example, a patient on a nasal cannula at 5 Lpm has an inspired tidal volume of 500 mL. Of the 500 mL, 50 mL is 100% oxygen from the anatomic reservoir. The liter flow of 5 Lpm is converted to seconds as follows:

$$\frac{5000 \text{ mL}}{60\text{s}} = 83 \text{ mL/s}$$

Assuming a 1-second inspiratory time, 83 mL of 100% oxygen is added to the breath. The remaining 367 mL of the inspiration is room air at 21%, adding an additional 77 mL of oxygen to the breath.

$$367 \text{ mL} \times 0.21 = 77 \text{ mL}$$

This patient is receiving approximately 42% oxygen, computed as follows:

50 mL (oxygen from anatomic reservoir) + 83 mL (oxygen from source flow) + 77 mL (oxygen from room air) = 210 mL of 100% oxygen

$$\frac{210 \text{ mL of 100\% oxygen}}{500 \text{ mL tidal volume}} = 0.42\ F_IO_2$$

TABLE 20-9 Approximate F_IO_2s from a nasal cannula

Liters of 100% Oxygen per Minute	Approximate F_IO_2
1	0.24
2	0.28
3	0.32
4	0.36
5	0.40
6	0.44

Table 20-9 lists approximate F_IO_2s according to liter flow from a nasal cannula. Note that each additional liter per minute adds 0.40 to the F_IO_2. The F_IO_2s are *approximations* only and are contingent on the patient's tidal volume, respiratory rate, and inspiratory flow rate being consistent and within normal range.

Nasal Catheter A *nasal catheter* is a disposable plastic tube with small holes at its tip. It is inserted through the nostril until the tip is visualized behind and slightly above the uvula. The catheter is then taped to the bridge of the nose for stabilization. If the catheter is inserted too deeply, it stimulates the gag reflex and thus can increase the risk of aspiration. Figure 20-26 illustrates the proper placement of a nasal catheter. Oxygen is delivered directly into the oropharynx. F_IO_2s

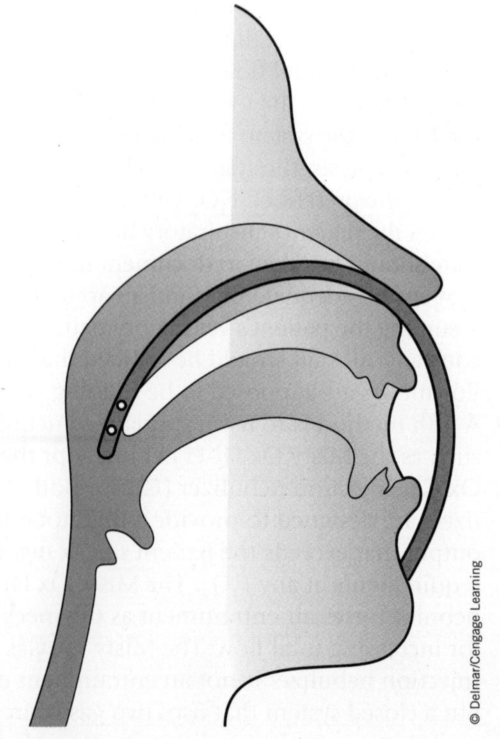

FIGURE 20-26 The placement of a nasal catheter.

and liter flows are similar to those of the nasal cannula. Nasal catheters are rarely used for simple oxygen administration and have mostly been replaced by nasal cannulas.

Transtracheal Catheter A *transtracheal catheter* is a Teflon catheter that is surgically inserted directly into the trachea at the second cartilaginous ring (also referred to as *transtracheal oxygenation*). In addition to the upper airway, the anatomic reservoir now includes part of the trachea, necessitating much less oxygen flow. Compared with the nasal cannula, approximately 50% less oxygen is needed; in fact, some patients need as little flow as 0.25 Lpm to maintain adequate oxygenation. Cosmetically, the catheter is much less obtrusive than the nasal cannula. Another advantage, especially for the mobile patient, is that the time that a portable system lasts between changes is greatly extended, in some cases, quadrupled.

However, great care needs to be taken in patient selection. Rigorous patient education is needed because this system requires much care, maintenance, and preventive measures. Hazards are infection, subcutaneous emphysema, catheter obstruction, decannulation, and hemoptysis (expectoration of blood). Figure 20-27 illustrates the transtracheal catheter and its anatomic placement.

New Devices Nasal cannulas have been an available option since 1956 for the delivery of oxygen. However, the cannulas do not come without their own

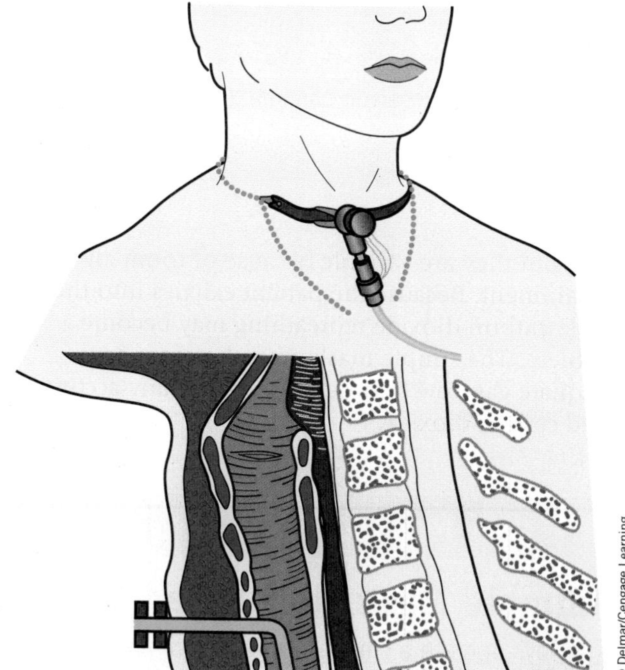

FIGURE 20-27 A transtracheal catheter and its placement.

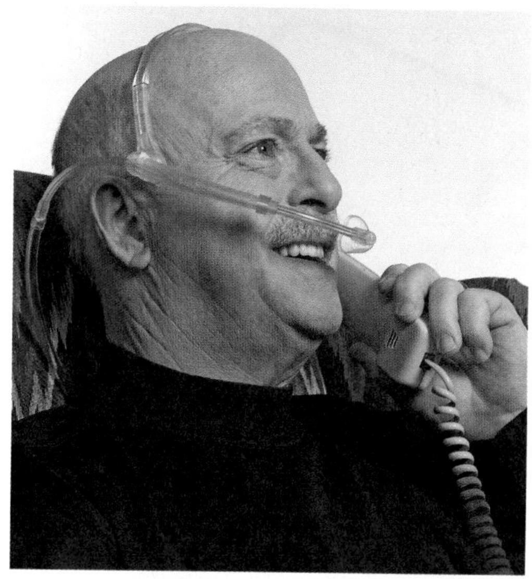
FIGURE 20-28 OxyArm.
Courtesy of Southmedic, Inc

comfort-related complications, such as nasal dryness and irritation. Several options have become available in the last few years, including the Oxy-Arm and the Oxy-View.

- The *Oxy-Arm* is an oxygen delivery device that looks like a telephone operator's headset (Figure 20-28). It delivers oxygen flow to the tip of the device, called the *diffuser*, and creates a so-called oxygen cloud in front of the patient. The range of liter flow is 1–15 Lpm. There is no physical contact between the patient and the device.[4]
- The *Oxy-View* is a pair of eyeglasses with tubes that curl downward and loop into each nostril in a J-shape (Figure 20-29). This range is also 1–15 Lpm. Both options can be connected to a patient's current oxygen source.

Reservoir Systems. *Reservoir systems* incorporate a small reservoir that collects and holds oxygen. The patient draws on this reservoir during inspiration whenever the inspiratory flow demand is greater than that supplied by the source flow. This system reduces air entrainment, resulting in an overall higher F_IO_2. Reservoir systems also conserve oxygen use because comparable F_IO_2s can be achieved with lower flows. Examples of such systems are reservoir cannulas and pendants, simple masks, and partial and nonrebreathing masks.

Reservoir and Pendant Oxygen Cannulas Reservoir and pendant cannulas store approximately 20 mL of oxygen during the expiratory cycle. This gas is available for use during inspiration, resulting in lower flows needed for a given F_IO_2. Figure 20-30 depicts a reservoir and a pendant cannula. The cannula is very noticeable, and

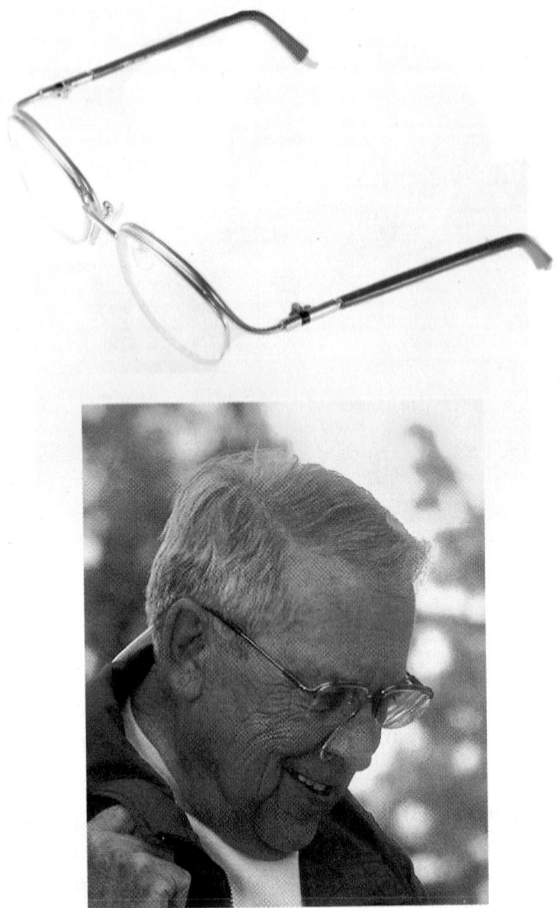

FIGURE 20-29 Oxy-View.
Courtesy of Oxy-View, Inc.

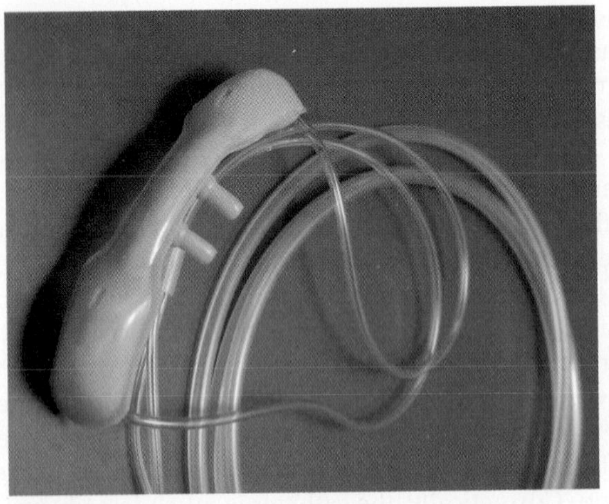

(A)

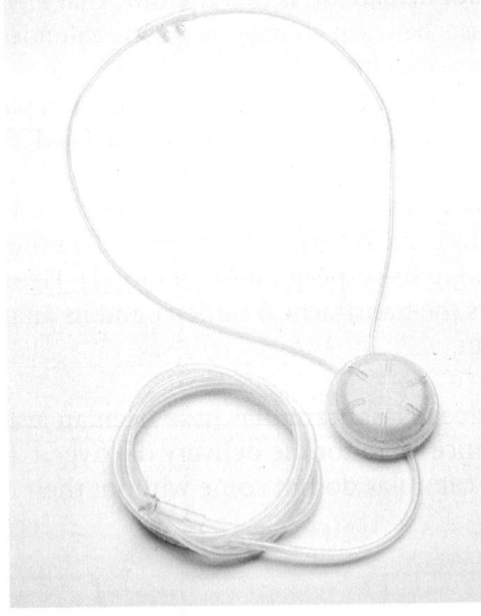

(B)

FIGURE 20-30 (A) Reservoir cannula. (B) Pendant cannula.
Courtesy of Chad Therapeutics

some patients object to using one because of its appearance. The reservoir pendant can be concealed beneath the clothing, but the weight of the pendant may put pressure on the ears.

Simple Mask A simple mask (Figure 20-31) is a plastic unit designed to fit over both the nose and mouth, with open ports on both sides of the mask. These openings serve as air entrainment ports for the amount of inspiratory flow gas not provided by the source. They also serve as exhalation ports and function as an access for inspiration should flow to the mask cease.

The body of the mask serves as a reservoir, filling with oxygen between breaths. The oxygen is then available to the patient during the next inspiration. During the beginning of inspiration, most of the gas inspired is high-F_IO_2 gas that has filled the reservoir. During the later part of inspiration, room air is entrained through the side ports of the mask.

Simple masks are designed to operate at liter flows of 6–12 Lpm. Typical F_IO_2s range from 0.35 to 0.55, but they are variable because of room air entrainment. Because the patient exhales into the mask, carbon dioxide rebreathing may become a problem. The simple mask must therefore have adequate gas flow in order to flush out any accumulated carbon dioxide.

Best Practice

Simple Mask Flow Rate

Always operate a simple mask at a *minimum* flow rate of 6 Lpm in order to flush out the reservoir.

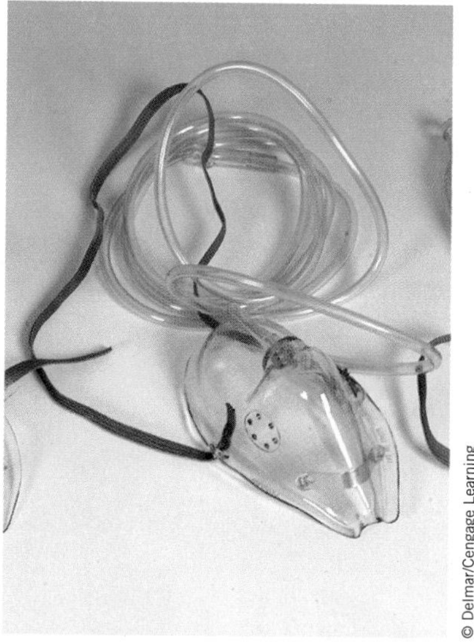

FIGURE 20-31 Simple oxygen mask.

Partial Rebreathing Mask The partial rebreathing mask (Figure 20-32) is a mask with a 1-L reservoir bag. During inspiration, oxygen from the gas source enters the mask via the small-bore tubing. During expiration, source oxygen fills the reservoir bag. Because there is no valve to separate the mask and the reservoir bag, the first third of the patient's exhaled gas also enters the bag. Although the patient rebreathes this gas (hence the name, partial rebreather), the level of carbon dioxide is negligible. The first third of the patient's expiration consists of the high-F_IO_2 gas that filled the anatomic reservoir at the end of the previous inspiration. As the reservoir bag is filled with this gas, plus oxygen from the source, the last two-thirds of the patient's expiration, which is high in carbon dioxide, exits through the side ports of the mask. As long as the flow rate of the source gas is high enough to prevent the reservoir bag from collapsing, safe operation is ensured, and carbon dioxide rebreathing is negligible. Because of air dilution from the exhalation ports and from the loose fit of the mask itself, the F_IO_2 is variable, with an upper limit of approximately 0.60 being delivered.

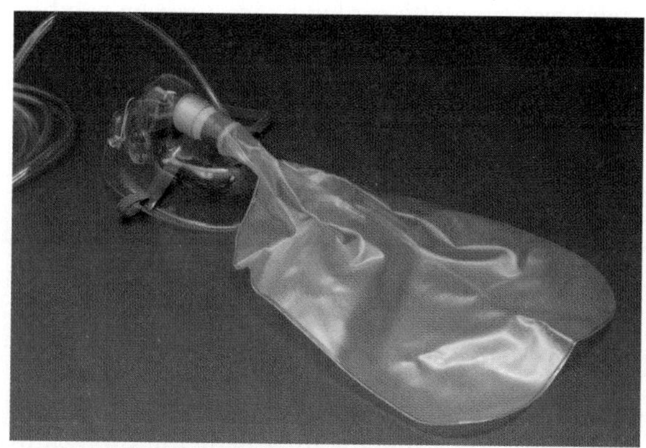

FIGURE 20-32 Partial rebreather mask.

Nonrebreathing Mask The nonrebreathing mask is similar in design to the partial rebreather. The nonrebreather also has a 1-L reservoir bag that collects and stores oxygen, but it also has strategically placed, one-way leaf valves to prevent rebreathing.

- A one-way valve between the reservoir bag and the mask allows gas to flow in one direction only, *from* the bag *to* the mask.
- Another valve, covering one of the exhalation ports on the outside of the mask, allows gas to flow only *from* the mask *to* the outside.

During inspiration, the valve between the reservoir bag and the mask opens, allowing gas delivery to the patient. The patient's inspiratory effort closes the valve on the expiration port, preventing air entrainment from that port. During expiration, the valve on the expiration port opens, allowing the patient's exhaled gas to exit. At the same time, the valve between the reservoir bag and the mask closes because of the slight back-pressure created by the patient's expiratory effort. The closing of this valve prevents any exhaled gas from entering the reservoir bag. One of the side expiration ports is commonly left open as a safety feature, to ensure an access for inspiration should the source gas fail.

The addition of the two one-way leaf valves increases the delivered F_IO_2. However, owing to the air dilution resulting from the open exhalation port and the loose fit of the mask itself, realistically, the delivered F_IO_2s are in the range of 0.70.

Oxygen Enclosures. *Oxygen enclosures* are environmentally controlled head- or body-surrounding reservoir systems. Surrounding the head or the entire body with oxygen-enriched air was one of the first approaches to oxygen therapy. Currently, these systems are used primarily with infants and children.

Best Practice

Nonrebreathing Masks

On both the partial and the nonrebreathing systems, always maintain a high enough source gas flow rate to ensure that the reservoir bag does not collapse. Proper functioning of the system is verified by the visualization of slight fluctuations in the reservoir bag during inspiration.

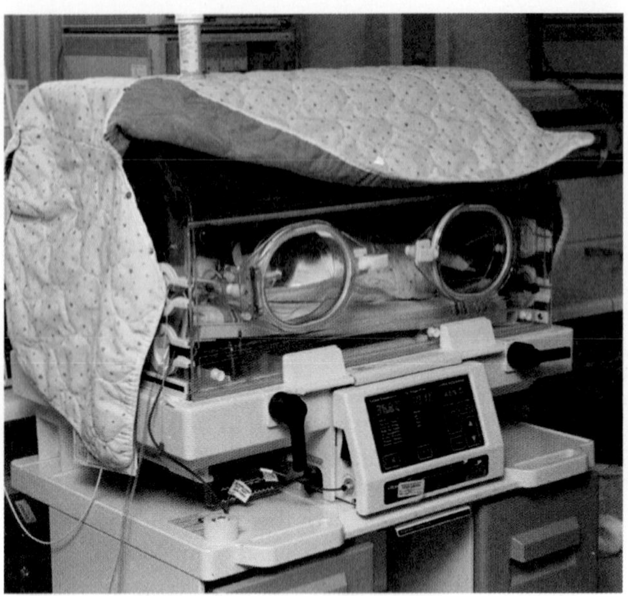

FIGURE 20-33 An incubator.

Incubators An *incubator* (Figure 20-33), or Isolette, is a total body enclosure that provides convection heat with supplemental oxygen (see Chapter 29). Supplemental humidity is also provided by an external heated humidifier or nebulizer. A neutral thermal environment is important because cool gas over the infant's face significantly increases oxygen consumption, and incubators are the best choice to ensure a neutral thermal environment. The incubator is directly connected to an oxygen flowmeter by way of the humidifier or nebulizer.

Because the incubator is opened often to administer care to the infant, delivered F_IO_2s are variable and generally less than 0.40. If a controlled or high-F_IO_2 is required, an Oxyhood can be used inside the incubator.

Oxyhoods An *Oxyhood* (Figure 20-34) is a transparent box designed to enclose the infant's head (see Chapter 29). It can be used alone or inside an incubator. The Oxyhood leaves the infant's body free for nursing care without disturbing the delivered F_IO_2. The gas that enters the Oxyhood is premixed, humidified, and heated. A minimum total flow of 7 Lpm should be set to prevent the accumulation of carbon dioxide inside the hood.

When an Oxyhood is in use:

- Analyze the oxygen concentration at the infant's face, near the bottom of the hood. At higher F_IO_2s, the hood has a layering effect on oxygen, with the highest concentration at the bottom of the hood. The difference in F_IO_2s at the top and the bottom of the hood can be as much as 20%.

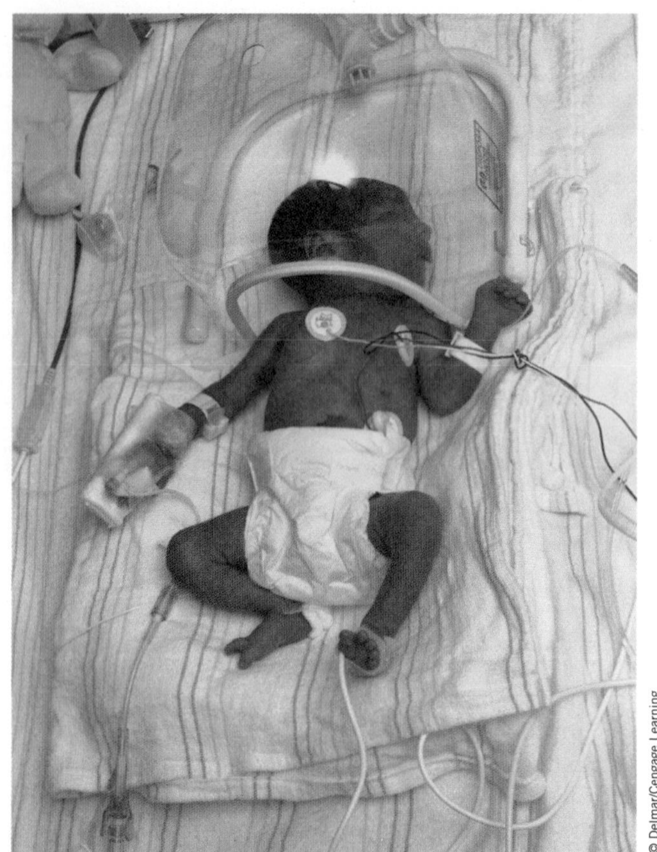

FIGURE 20-34 An oxygen hood.

- Also monitor the infant's oxygenation status. Oxygenation can be monitored continuously with either pulse oximetry or transcutaneous monitoring.

Mist Tents As its name suggests, a mist tent is generally used to administer aerosol therapy (see Chapter 21). *Mist tents*, or croupettes, are plastic tents that are large enough to enclose a child, usually powered with a high-output aerosol device, and air-conditioned. Older models were generally cooled by ice. Oxygen can be bled in from a flowmeter or another nebulizer. F_IO_2s are variable and generally low owing to constant leaks and opening of the tent.

Mist tents are primarily used to provide aerosol therapy to children with croup or cystic fibrosis. Fire safety measures must be strictly adhered to because mist tents pose a significant fire hazard.

OXYGEN-CONSERVING DEVICES

The primary goal of *long-term oxygen therapy* (*LTOT*) is to treat hypoxemia, thereby increasing the survival in hypoxic patients with COPD and, in turn, leading to a decreased number of hospitalizations and/or lengths of stay. Very often this goal is obtainable, but only through the continuous use of this oxygen therapy after the patients return to their homes.

Many options are available to make sure the needs of each and every patient are individually met. In addition to the longstanding oxygen concentrator or liquid vessels, today's options include a number of *oxygen-conserving devices* (OCDs):

- *Pulse dose oxygen delivery devices* (PDOD)
- *Demand oxygen delivery systems* (DODS)
- *Portable oxygen concentrators* (POC)
- Liquid filling oxygen concentrators.

The PDOD and DODS are electronic or pneumatic (mechanical) devices that are used with the compressed cylinders or liquid vessels to extend their usable time. Portable oxygen concentrators, such as the Sequal Eclipse, Inogen One, Air Sep Lifestyle, and Respironics' EverGo, are more limiting; however, when appropriate, they allow users the freedom to travel and ambulate as they did prior to the initiation of therapy.[3]

The portable concentrators offer patients the ability to manage their power options rather than their oxygen contents. All are available with AC power supply, mobile power charger (to be used in cigarette lighter outlet), and an internal battery for unlimited options due to the fact that they are also FAA (Federal Aviation Administration) approved. Users must be aware of each manufacturer's limitations. For instance, some portable oxygen concentrators offer only pulse dose flows, and others offer continuous along with pulse dose but only up to a limited liter flow. The options certainly benefit patients' quality of life, but they need to be used in connection with a knowledgeable home care company that will accommodate each's specific needs.

HYPERBARIC OXYGEN THERAPY

Hyperbaric oxygen therapy (HBO) is the exposure of a patient to a pressure greater than one atmosphere (1 atm) while breathing 100% oxygen either continuously or intermittently. Clinically, this exposure is accomplished by means of a *compression*, or *hyperbaric, chamber*. Pressures used in hyperbaric medicine are expressed in multiples of *atmospheric pressure absolute* (*ATA*): 1 ATA is equal to 760 mm Hg, normal sea level barometric pressure.

Physiological Effects. The physiological effects of hyperbaric oxygen therapy are caused by either increased pressure or increased oxygen tensions in the body fluids and tissues. Although very little oxygen can be added to the bound portion of the blood once saturation is 97%, the quantity of *dissolved* oxygen rises linearly with increases in P_aO_2.

- *Bubble reduction.* Any trapped gas bubbles decrease in size when exposed to an increase in pressure, an effect supported by Boyle's law. This effect accounts for the success of hyperbaric therapy in treating disorders such as decompression sickness, commonly known as the bends. Nitrogen bubbles form in the blood and tissues when a diver ascends too quickly from an area of high pressure (the depths) to an area of low pressure (the surface). The rapid decrease in pressure causes the bubbles to form as gas expands. The increase in pressure that results from hyperbaric oxygen therapy decreases the size of the bubbles, and the increase in oxygen tension helps flush nitrogen from the body. Gas embolism that occurs from central line placement or other procedures can be treated in the same manner.
- *Supersaturation of blood and tissues.* Vast increases in P_aO_2 can occur during hyperbaric oxygen therapy. Under hyperbaric conditions, the P_aO_2 can get as high as 1500 mm Hg. This increase greatly improves oxygen transport even to areas of poor perfusion.
- *Generalized vasoconstriction.* Although vasoconstriction may decrease perfusion, the decrease is offset by the greatly increased P_aO_2. Vasoconstriction may help reduce tissue edema in conditions such as burns.
- *Elimination of other gases.* Nitrogen and carbon monoxide can be eliminated from the body more quickly with high oxygen pressures. Carbon monoxide has a strong affinity for hemoglobin and, once bound, unbinds very slowly. The half-life of carbon monoxide when a person is breathing room air is over 5 hours. Under hyperbaric conditions of 3 ATA, this half-life is reduced to 23 minutes.
- *Enhanced immune function.* The increase in available oxygen may help the white blood cells

Age-Specific Competency

Oxygen Delivery to Infants

Blended, humidified gas is the preferred method of oxygen delivery for infants rather than air entrainment nebulizers. Nebulizers should be avoided because they produce an aerosol particle that increases the risk of bacterial contamination and infection, especially if the aerosol is heated. In addition, nebulizers can generate excessive noise levels, which can further stress an infant.

TABLE 20-10 **Indications for hyperbaric oxygen therapy**

Gas Diseases	Vascular Insufficiency States	Infections	Defects in Oxygen Transport
Decompression sickness Gas embolism	Radiation necrosis of bone or soft tissue Severe acute anemia or hemorrhage Diabetic microangiopathy Crush wounds Ischemic skin grafts or tissue transplants Acute traumatic ischemias Thermal burns	Clostridial myonecrosis (gas gangrene) Necrotizing soft tissue infections Chronic refractory osteomyelitis Refractory anaerobic infections	Carbon monoxide poisoning Cyanide poisoning

perform their immune functions. The high P_aO_2 aids in wound healing.

- *Neovascularization*. Hyperbaric oxygen therapy promotes neovascularization (the formation of new capillary beds) to poorly perfused tissues. The increased oxygenation promotes the formation of osteoblasts, fibroblasts, granulocytes, and collagen, which, in turn, promote capillary budding. This physiological effect is beneficial in treating conditions such as gas gangrene and difficult-to-heal wounds.

Indications. The indication for hyperbaric oxygen therapy is any condition that would benefit from an increase in ambient pressure or in oxygen tension. Table 20-10 summarizes the conditions that benefit from hyperbaric oxygen therapy.

Mode of Administration. A specialized chamber is required to administer hyperbaric oxygen therapy. The chamber is either a multiplace chamber or a monoplace chamber.

Multiplace Hyperbaric Chamber The *multiplace hyperbaric chamber* is large enough to accommodate more than one patient. The chamber is pressurized with air, and oxygen is delivered to the patients individually by way of a nonrebreather mask or other oxygen administration device. Oxygen is delivered via a closed system because O_2 leakage into a pressurized chamber poses a significant fire hazard. The multiplace chamber has the advantage of being large enough to accommodate the patients and the health care team (who must take care to avoid decompression sickness). Multiplace chambers are very expensive to purchase and maintain.

Monoplace Hyperbaric Chamber The monoplace hyperbaric chamber (Figure 20-35) accommodates only one patient. Because the chamber is pressurized with 100% oxygen, the patient does not have to wear a mask. However, 100% oxygen throughout the entire pressurized chamber greatly increases the fire hazard and the need for strict precautions. Another disadvantage of the monoplace chamber is the necessity to depressurize the chamber in order to manage an emergency situation.

Complications and Hazards. The complications and hazards of hyperbaric oxygen therapy are related to:

- High pressures, causing barotrauma.
- The effects of oxygen toxicity.
- Decompression.
- Fire.

Table 20-11 summarizes the hazards of hyperbaric oxygen therapy.

Safety Considerations. The risk of fire is great with the use of hyperbaric chambers because of the vast increase in the partial pressure of oxygen, which supports combustion. Safety considerations during hyperbaric oxygen therapy are directed toward fire prevention:

- Use only cotton materials.
- Prevent static electricity.
- Use no alcohol- or oil-based products.
- Patients and health care workers are not to wear make-up, deodorant, hair sprays, or jewelry.
- Use adequate fire suppression systems.

MONITORING OXYGEN THERAPY

Objective outcomes must be measured and documented to ascertain whether oxygen therapy is effective. Monitoring oxygen therapy can be accomplished by both invasive and noninvasive methods.

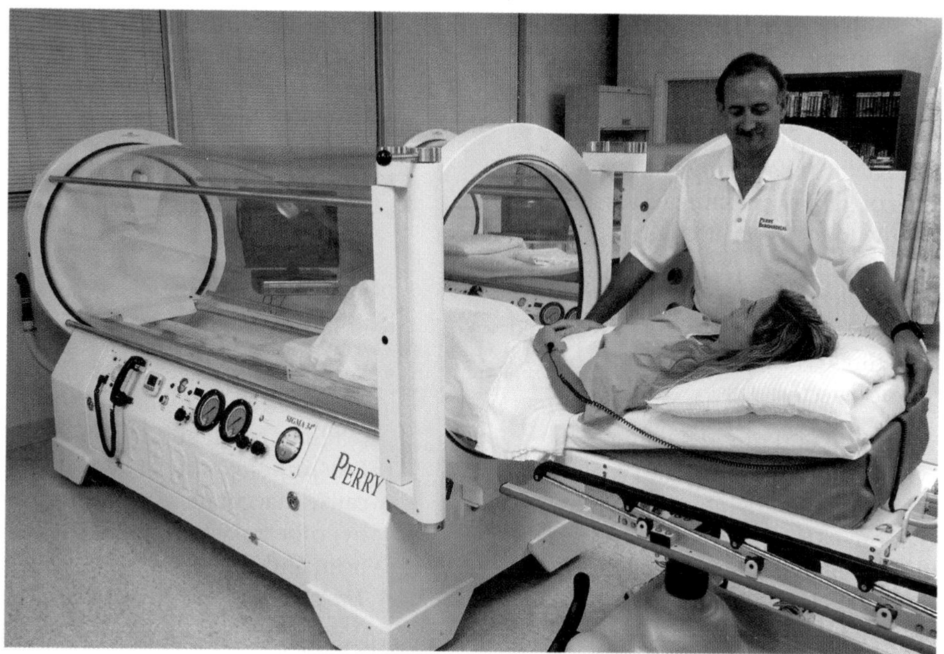

FIGURE 20-35 Hyperbaric chamber.
Courtesy of Perry Baromedical

TABLE 20-11 Hazards of hyperbaric oxygen therapy

Oxygen Toxicity	Barotrauma	Other
Pulmonary toxic reaction	Sinus trauma Tympanic membrane rupture	Fire
Central nervous system toxic reaction	Pneumothorax Air embolism	Sudden decompression

Invasive Methods. The most accurate assessment of oxygenation status is the arterial blood gas analysis, which not only gives a direct measurement of P_aO_2, but also data needed to derive values for S_aO_2 and C_aO_2. S_aO_2 and C_aO_2 can be measured directly by co-oximetry, which is also used to measure total hemoglobin and to recognize and quantify dyshemoglobins (discussed in the following section, where it is contrasted to pulse oximetry). Although arterial blood gas analysis is more accurate than noninvasive means, it is an isolated and static measurement. It cannot reflect continuous changes in oxygenation status.

An *indwelling arterial line* (*A-line*) has certain advantages over the arterial puncture. An arterial line spares the patient from having to undergo repeated punctures, and, when connected to a monitor, it provides a continuous display of arterial blood pressure and heart rate. (Arterial blood gas sampling and analysis are discussed in greater detail in Chapter 16.)

In general, invasive methods of monitoring carry a much greater risk of complications than noninvasive monitoring.

Noninvasive Methods. Although noninvasive methods of monitoring oxygenation status may not be as accurate as arterial blood gas analysis, they have certain advantages.

- The most obvious advantage is patient comfort.
- The risk of complications is minimal.
- Noninvasive monitoring can provide the practitioner with a *continuous* display of the patient's oxygenation status, rather than isolated static measurements.

Pulse Oximetry Pulse oximetry is the most common noninvasive method to monitor a patient's oxygenation status, either intermittently or continuously. *Oximetry* is a technique used to measure the oxygen saturation of hemoglobin in the blood by absorption of different wavelengths of light.

Principles of Operation The principles of operation of pulse oximetry are spectrophotometry and plethysmography.

- **Spectrophotometry** is the generation of light at a known intensity going into a solution and the measurement of the intensity of light that leaves the solution. The solution in this instance is the arterial blood.

- **Plethysmography** is the study of changes in the shape or size of an organ. It is used to separate static from dynamic components; in other words, plethysmography measures *pulsatile* waves.

These two principles enable pulse oximeters to measure different wavelengths of light in pulsatile waves, giving them the specific ability to focus on arterial, or pulsatile, blood.

Modern pulse oximeters use two wavelengths of light: red and infrared. The wavelengths are transmitted from a light-emitting diode (LED) through the body part (artery) to a photodetector.

- At the wavelength of 660 nm, red light passes through oxyhemoglobin (HbO_2) and is absorbed by reduced hemoglobin (RHb), or deoxyhemoglobin ($RHbO_2$).
- At the wavelength of 940 nm, infrared light passes through reduced hemoglobin and is absorbed by oxyhemoglobin.

Pulse oximeters compare oxyhemoglobin and reduced hemoglobin, using the two wavelengths of light:

$$\frac{HbO_2}{RHbO_2 + HbO_2} \times 100$$

This is a measure of **functional saturation**.

Pulse oximetry *does not* take into account the presence of dyshemoglobin. *Dyshemoglobin* is an abnormal type of hemoglobin, such as carboxyhemoglobin (COHb), methemoglobin (MetHb), or sulfhemoglobin (SulfHb). Dyshemoglobins interfere with the binding of oxygen, greatly decreasing the oxygen-carrying capacity of hemoglobin and significantly lowering the arterial oxygen concentration (C_aO_2). Because the hemoglobin is bound in the presence of dyshemoglobin, the pulse oximeter reading is falsely high.

Co-oximetry must therefore be used to obtain a truly accurate measurement of oxygen saturation. Co-oximetry uses four wavelengths of light and *does* measure dyshemoglobins. The co-oximetry result is a measure of **fractional saturation**. Oxyhemoglobin is compared with *total* hemoglobin.

$$\frac{HbO_2}{HbO_2 + RHbO_2 + COHb + Met\ Hb} \times 100$$

Unfortunately, an arterial blood sample must be obtained; therefore, this is an invasive procedure. Co-oximetry is usually performed in conjunction with arterial blood gas analysis.

Limitations The limitations of pulse oximetry are both technological and physiological. *Technological factors* that can cause inaccurate readings are:

- Motion artifact.
- Sources of ambient light, such as xenon lamps and fluorescent and infrared lights.
- Optical shunting (light passes from the LED to the photodetector by passing around the body part rather than through it).
- Vascular dyes, such as methylene blue or cardiogreen.
- Deeply pigmented skin.
- Nail polish, especially dark colors such as black, blue, or green.

Physiological factors that can cause inaccurate readings are:

- *Very low saturations*. False high readings can be produced at S_aO_2s below 80%, and inaccurate readings result at S_aO_2s below 65%.
- *Low-perfusion states*. Low-perfusion states that can cause inaccurate readings include cardiac arrest, hypothermia, peripheral shunting, vasoconstriction, and shock.
- *The presence of dyshemoglobin*.

Also, the oxyhemoglobin dissociation curve flattens out at P_aO_2s above 60 mm Hg ($S_aO_2 > 90\%$). There is a wide range of P_aO_2s between 60 and 100 mm Hg with relatively little change in S_aO_2. For this reason, arterial blood gas analysis is more accurate than pulse oximetry.

Clinical Applications The clinical applications of pulse oximetry are:

- Continuous monitoring of oxygenation during anesthesia.
- Adjusting F_IO_2 or titrating oxygen liter flow during oxygen therapy
- Documenting S_aO_2 during long-term oxygen therapy for purposes of Medicare requirements, reimbursement, or disability benefits.
- Continuous monitoring of oxygenation during weaning from mechanical ventilation.
- Prevention of retinopathy of prematurity (ROP) in neonates, although transcutaneous monitoring is more sensitive.
- Monitoring oxygenation during diagnostic procedures such as bronchoscopy, sleep studies, and exercise testing.

Transcutaneous Monitoring **Transcutaneous monitoring** measures the partial pressures of the gases that are diffusing through the skin. The transcutaneous partial pressures of both oxygen (T_cO_2) and carbon dioxide (T_cCO_2) can be measured simultaneously by incorporating the *Clark electrode* for measuring PO_2 and the *Severinghaus pH electrode* for measuring PCO_2 into the same probe. The probe is secured to the skin and connected to a monitor for continuous readings. A heater and a thermistor inside the probe are connected to an external heat source to control skin temperature.

Principles of Operation The skin is heated to 44°–45°C to promote vasodilation of the capillary bed and to increase perfusion to the area. The increased perfusion increases the diffusion of oxygen and carbon dioxide. The resulting T_cO_2 and T_cCO_2 measurements should be positively correlated with P_aO_2 and P_aCO_2, assuming conditions are optimal.

T_cO_2 Correlation with P_aO_2 Correlation of transcutaneous values with arterial blood gas values are currently limited to PO_2 measurements. Various factors determine how well T_cO_2 is correlated with P_aO_2:

- *Skin thickness.* The thicker the skin, the larger the diffusion pathway for oxygen. The correlation is not accurate; the T_cO_2 is *lower* than the actual P_aO_2.
- *Oxygen consumption.* Regional oxygen consumption in the area of the sensor site affects correlation. The T_cO_2 is *lower* than the P_aO_2.
- *Perfusion status.* Adequate perfusion, or even hyperperfusion, must exist for an accurate correlation. This is the rationale behind heating the skin. In low-perfusion states—such as a decreased cardiac output, vasoconstriction, or hypothermia—the T_cO_2 is substantially *lower* than the P_aO_2. If adequate perfusion exists (a cardiac index of 2 Lpm/m^2), the T_cO_2:P_aO_2 ratio is 70% ± 12%.
- *Temperature.* If the skin temperature is too low, adequate peripheral perfusion is not present, and the T_cO_2 is *lower* than the P_aO_2. If the skin temperature is too high, the T_cO_2 is higher than the P_aO_2 (as temperature increases, pressure increases).
- *Age.* Transcutaneous monitoring is used almost exclusively in neonates and newborns. Their skin is much thinner than an adult's, so the diffusion pathway is smaller. Under proper conditions, the correlation of T_cO_2 and P_aO_2 is excellent. T_cO_2 can actually equal P_aO_2 if the proper temperature is maintained, adequate perfusion exists, and the infant is younger than 2 weeks old. This positive correlation decreases with age.

Clinical Applications Transcutaneous monitoring of PO_2 is typically used to monitor oxygenation status and oxygen therapy in neonates and newborns. It is much more sensitive than pulse oximetry.

Transcutaneous monitoring of PO_2 can also serve to reflect cardiopulmonary compromise. Whenever the T_cO_2 is decreased, an arterial blood gas should be drawn. If the P_aO_2 is normal but the T_cO_2 is decreased, a perfusion or circulatory impairment should be suspected. A decrease in both the T_cO_2 and the P_aO_2 reflects a pulmonary impairment.

Hazards The most important hazard of transcutaneous monitoring is burns caused by the sensor. The risk of burns increases greatly during conditions of low perfusion because the diminished blood flow prevents adequate dissipation of the heat.

OXYGEN THERAPY PROTOCOLS

Advances in noninvasive monitoring and bedside patient assessment make oxygen therapy well suited for a therapist-driven protocol. Protocols ensure that immediate changes can be made in oxygen delivery without the lapse time involved in contacting the physician for an order change. Protocol-based therapy ensures that the patient receives bedside assessments, individual treatment based on need, and the timely discontinuance of therapy when it is no longer

Best Practice

Transcutaneous Probe

These precautions help prevent burns:

- The sensor site for the transcutaneous probe *must* be rotated every 2–4 hours.
- The probe should *never* be placed over a bony area.

Age-Specific Competency

Monitoring Oxygenation in Neonates

Transcutaneous monitoring is the preferred method of monitoring oxygenation status in infants younger than 2 weeks of age. The skin composition is such that the correlation of T_cO_2 and P_aO_2 is excellent. Transcutaneous monitoring is more sensitive than pulse oximetry. There is a much wider range in P_aO_2 relative to S_aO_2. Pulse oximetry is unable to reflect hyperoxia, because a large increase in P_aO_2 presents only as a small increase in S_aO_2 above a P_aO_2 of 80 mm Hg. Transcutaneous monitoring is a great benefit in preventing conditions such as ROP, for which oxygenation should be monitored continuously.

Source: From American Association of Respiratory Care. AARC clinical practice guideline: transcutaneous blood gas monitoring for neonatal and pediatric patients. Respir Care. *1994;39:1176–1179.*

required. The oxygen protocol in Figure 20-36, for example, was adopted by Saint Clare's Hospital (Denville, New Jersey).[5]

ANALYZING OXYGEN CONCENTRATIONS

An integral part of oxygen therapy is the analysis of oxygen concentration. Oxygen analysis is the only way to verify that the desired F_IO_2 is being delivered to the patient.

All oxygen analyzers should be calibrated before use. Calibration is accomplished by exposing the sensor to a source of 100% oxygen and then to a source of 21% oxygen (room air), making slight adjustments as necessary. After calibration, if the analyzer does not function to within ± 2% at both the 21% and 100% points, the equipment should not be used.

Oxygen systems should be analyzed as close to the patient's airway as possible. Although analyzing the system near its source verifies the *system* F_IO_2 delivery, it does not indicate leaks in the system or air entrainment *by the patient.*

Physical Oxygen Analyzers. Physical oxygen analyzers utilize the principle of *paramagnetism* to measure oxygen concentrations. If a gas is paramagnetic, its molecules align themselves with the north-south lines in a magnetic field. Diamagnetic gases do not. Oxygen is a paramagnetic gas, so it responds to a magnetic field.

The physical oxygen analyzer (Figure 20-37) consists of two magnets separated by a dumbbell filled with nitrogen. The dumbbell is suspended by a thin quartz wire. As oxygen is drawn into the sensor, its molecules align themselves with the magnetic field. The dumbbell rotates, and its degree of rotation is proportional to the oxygen partial pressure. The analyzer measures partial pressure but displays both partial pressure and F_IO_2.

Electrical Oxygen Analyzers. Electrical oxygen analyzers (Figure 20-38) utilize the principle of *thermoconductivity* to measure oxygen percentages. A molecule with a large mass conducts more heat than a molecule with a smaller mass. Oxygen has a greater mass than nitrogen, which is the main gas in ambient air. Therefore, the more oxygen there is in a mixture, the greater the heat transfer will be. The electrical oxygen analyzer utilizes a special electrical circuit known as a *Wheatstone bridge,* which can detect small changes in resistance. The small change in resistance causes a measurable change in current. One limb of the Wheatstone bridge is exposed to ambient air, and the other limb is exposed to the sample gas. The side with the greater oxygen concentration cools, causing a current change that is proportional to the oxygen concentration. The electrical oxygen analyzer can measure only air–oxygen combinations. It does not work with other gases because the reference wire is limited to comparisons with room air.

Electrochemical Oxygen Analyzers. Electrochemical oxygen analyzers produce a current from a chemical reaction. There are two types of electrochemical oxygen analyzers: galvanic and polarographic.

Galvanic Oxygen Analyzers The *galvanic oxygen analyzer* (Figure 20-39) utilizes the reduction reaction that occurs when oxygen combines with water and electrons from the cathode (negative electrode), forming hydroxyl ions (OH^-). These ions migrate to the anode

SAINT CLARE'S HOSPITAL

RESPIRATORY CARE SERVICES

POLICY AND PROCEDURE MANUAL

OXYGEN PROTOCOL

POLICY

It is the policy of Saint Clare's Hospital to administer oxygen, utilizing the Oxygen Protocol, based on the following guidelines.

Goals of Oxygen Therapy

Correct documented or suspected hypoxemia
Relieve or prevent dyspnea
Decrease symptoms associated with chronic hypoxemia
Decrease workload imposed on the cardiopulmonary system by hypoxemia

PROCEDURE

I. DECISION MAKING (Refer to the Oxygen Protocol Flowchart)

1. After receiving an order for oxygen therapy or oxygen protocol, the patient is evaluated for oxygen needs and type of device, based on:
   a. Relevant medical history
   b. Baseline assessment
   c. Degree of consciousness, alertness
   d. Stability of minute ventilation and airway
   e. SpO_2 obtained via pulse oximetry
   f. PaO_2 / $PaCO_2$ obtained via arterial blood gas
   g. Severity/cause of hypoxemia
   h. Chronic CO_2 retention
2. High-flow vs. low-flow oxygen therapy devices:

⇒ High-flow systems provide a flow of oxygen sufficient to meet and/or exceed the patient's inspired flow rate needs; therefore the F_IO_2 is predictable and stable.

⇒ Low-flow systems provide a flow which supplements the pateint's inspired flow rate needs; therefore the F_IO_2 is variable, depending on the patient's size, minute volume, and respiratory pattern.

FIGURE 20-36 Oxygen protocol. (*continues*)
Reprinted with permission from Saint Clare's Hospital, Denville, New Jersey

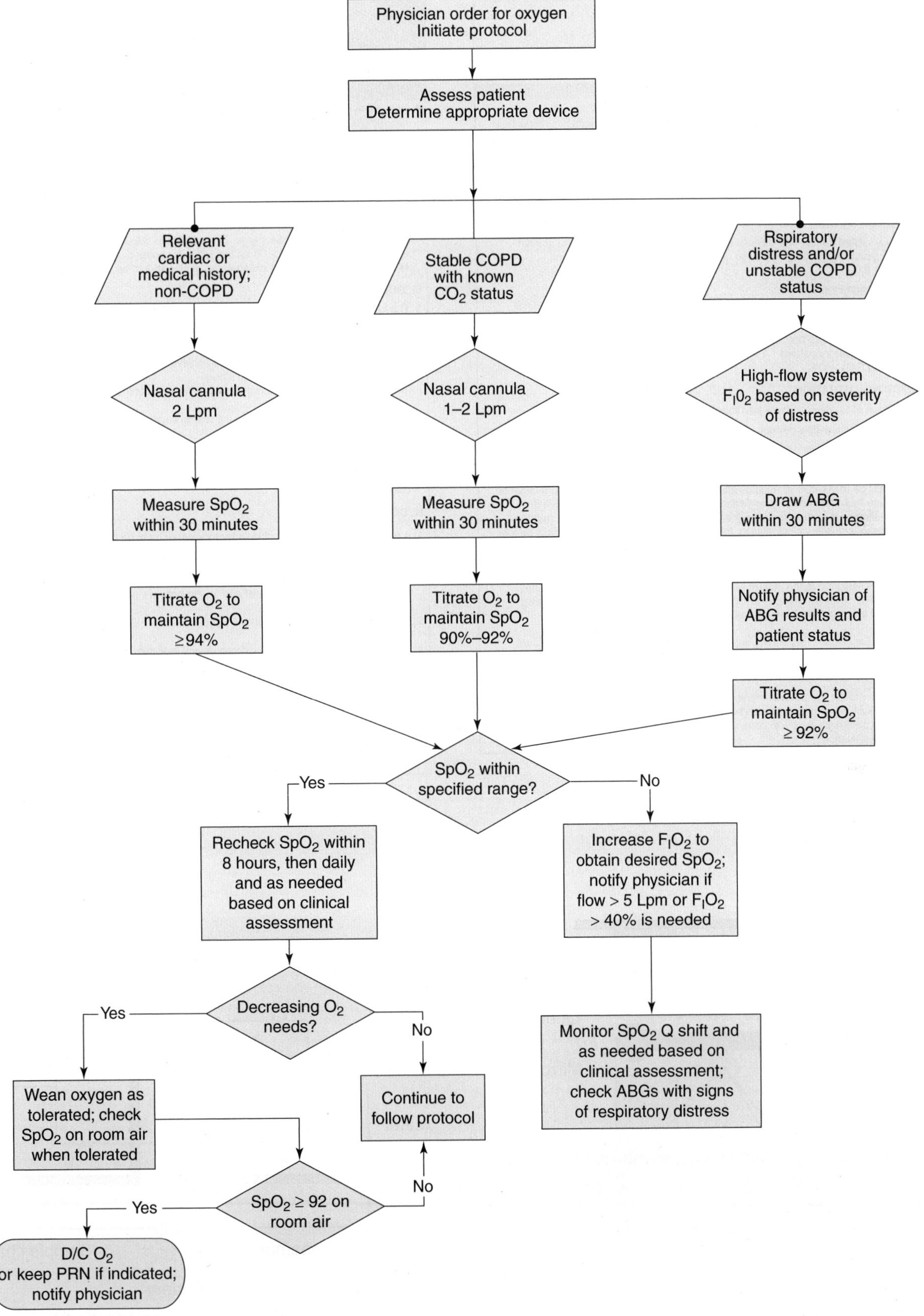

FIGURE 20-36 Oxygen protocol. (*continues*)

Saint Clare's Hospital

RESPIRATORY CARE SERVICES
POLICY AND PROCEDURE MANUAL

OXYGEN PROTOCOL

3. Classification of Oxygen Devices:

Device	Flow Range (Lpm)	F_IO_2 Range(%)	Flow Type
Nasal cannula	$\frac{1}{4}$–6	22–45	Low
Simple mask	5–12	35–50	Low
Partial rebreather	6–10	35–60	Low
Nonrebreather	10–15	55–95	Low/High
Air entrainment mask	Variable	24–50	High
Large-volume nebulizer	10–15	28–100	High

Note: The F_IO_2s listed for low-flow devices are approximate and are based on normal breathing patterns. Settings on these devices should be reported in Lpms, not as an F_IO_2.

4. Low-Flow vs High-Flow Criteria:

Low-Flow Criteria	High-Flow Criteria
a. Tidal volume: 300–700 mL	a. Tidal volume: <300 mL
b. Respiratory rate: <25 bpm	b. Respiratory rate: >25 bpm
c. Regular ventilatory pattern	c. Alveolar hypoventilation/CO_2 retention
d. Required F_IO_2 <40%	d. Required F_IO_2 >40%

II MONITORING / TITRATION

1. Upon initiation of O_2 device, titrate liter flow/F_IO_2 to meet targeted SpO_2 range:
   a. Patients utilizing low-flow devices <6 Lpm will be titrated in increments of 1 Lpm.
   b. Patients utilizing low-flow devices >6 Lpm or high-flow devices will be titrated in 5%–10% increments.

2. The SpO_2 will be measured 30 minutes after the initiation of an O_2 device for evaluation of appropriate F_IO_2, liter flow and/or device. Arterial blood gases will be drawn if respiratory distress is noted. *Clinical signs of respiratory distress include tachypnea, use of accessory muscles of ventilation, tachycardia, erratic or excessively high minute ventilation, cyanosis, alterations in level of consciousness.*

3. Once an appropriate device has been selected and SpO_2 is within an acceptable range, the RN assigned to the patient will be notified of the patient's oxygen status. This should also occur as changes are made in the device or liter flow/F_IO_2 setting. Arterial blood gas results will be reported to the physician.

4. In a stable patient who is responding appropriately to the device selected, SpO_2 will be reevaluated within 8 hours, and then on a daily basis. SpO_2 can be reevaluated as needed, based on clinical evaluation.

5. In an unstable patient, or one with increasing oxygen needs, SpO_2 will be monitored a minimum of once per shift and as-needed based on clinical evaluation. Arterial blood gases should be reevaluated with continuing signs of respiratory distress to confirm adequacy of ventilation.

Saint Clare's Hospital

RESPIRATORY CARE SERVICES
POLICY AND PROCEDURE MANUAL

OXYGEN PROTOCOL

6. In a stable patient with decreasing oxygen needs, oxygen may be weaned as tolerated, unless specified otherwise by the physician. Oxygen may be discontinued on a patient who maintains a satisfactory SpO_2 on room air and shows no signs of increased work of breathing or respiratory distress. *Oxygen may need to be kept PRN in the following situations: a history of COPD, congestive heart failure, chest pain, nocturnal dyspnea, dyspnea on exertion.*

7. In a patient who will be discharged with oxygen for use in the home, the goal may not necessarily be to discontinue the oxygen device, but to optimize the level of oxygen needed prior to discharge. *The inability to maintain an SpO_2 > 88% on room air, at the time of discharge, is an indication for home oxygen therapy.* If the physician is not already aware of this situation, he or she should be notified.

III. GUIDELINES

1. The physician must be notified in the following circumstances:

⇒ a. Abnormal ABGs: pH <7.30 or >7.50 ; $PaCO_2$ <30 mm Hg or >50 mm Hg; PaO_2 <55 mm Hg
⇒ b. F_IO_2 >40% or >5 Lpm is required to achieve targeted SpO_2
⇒ c. Unexpected changes in clinical status
⇒ d. Patient remains in respiratory distress after appropriate level of oxygen has been initiated
⇒ e. Patient is being discharged and still needs supplemental O_2 to maintain an adequate SpO_2

2. If oxygen has been discontinued and patient presents with a change in status indicating a need for oxygen, the Oxygen Protocol may be reinstituted based on the original order.

IV. DOCUMENTATION

1. A written order and/or standing order for oxygen must be on the patient's chart on a physician's order sheet.

2. The device, flow rate, and/or F_IO_2 will be documented on the patient's chart on the Respiratory Care Graphic Sheet and on the patient's pathway sheet if applicable.

3. SpO_2 results will be charted on the Respiratory Care Graphic Sheet.

4. A sticker will be placed on the oxygen device indicating the current liter flow and/or F_IO_2 setting.

5. A sticker will be placed in the Progress Notes section of the chart notifying the physician when the oxygen is discontinued.

Reviewed: **Value-based Content ☐ Date Reviewed:**
Revised:
Prepared by: Sharon Shenton, RRT 4/99

FIGURE 20-36 Oxygen protocol. (*continued*)

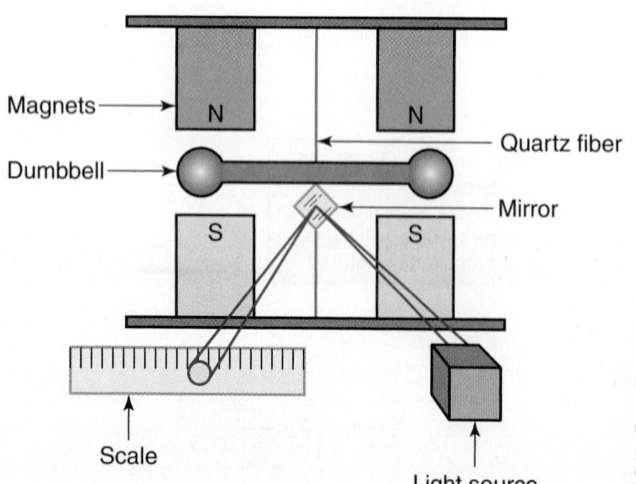

FIGURE 20-37 A physical oxygen analyzer.

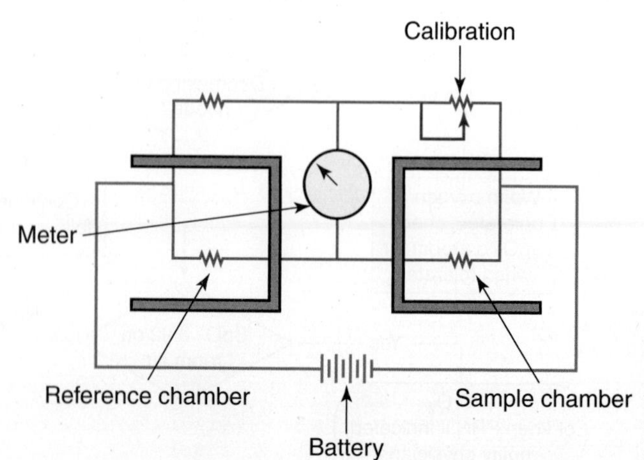

FIGURE 20-38 A schematic of an electrical oxygen analyzer.

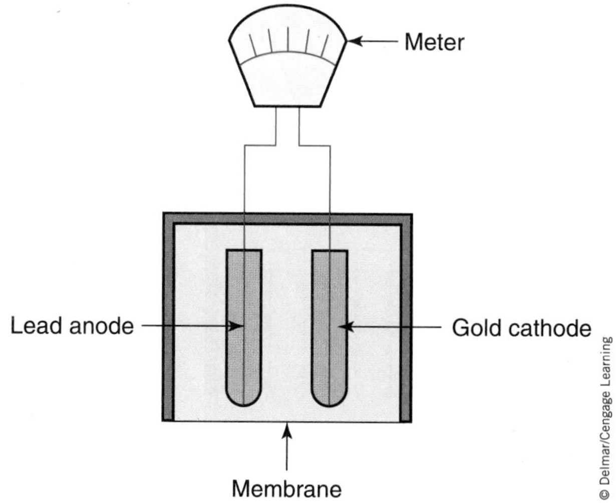

FIGURE 20-39 A schematic of a galvanic electrochemical oxygen analyzer.

Best Practice

Calibrating an Oxygen Analyzer

When analyzing a system with a high F_IO_2, such as 0.80, use 100% as the final calibration point. When analyzing a system with a low F_IO_2, such as 0.35, use 21% as the final calibration point. An F_IO_2 of 0.60 can be used as the point of change.

CASE STUDY 20-1

R. T. was admitted to the hospital through the emergency room. Mr. T. is a 56-year-old male who was in apparent good health until 3 days ago, when he developed a fever, chills, chest pain, and a cough productive of thick yellow sputum.

Upon arrival in the emergency room, Mr. T. was dyspneic and tachypneic and had a temperature of 103°F. An arterial blood gas analysis, a complete blood count, and a sputum specimen were obtained. Mr. T. was started on IV therapy with broad-spectrum antibiotics and placed on a nonrebreathing mask.

The complete blood count revealed most values within normal range, with the exception of the white blood cell count, which was greatly elevated. Arterial blood gas values were as follows:

pH: 7.47
P_aO_2: 44 mm Hg
PCO_2: 30 mm Hg
HCO_3: 24 mEq/L

Mr. T was admitted to the hospital. The sputum culture revealed pneumococcal pneumonia. Mr. Tyler's antibiotics were changed to a narrow-spectrum antibiotic according to the sensitivity results. He was kept on a nonrebreather mask. The next set of ABGs revealed the following results:

pH: 7.40
P_aO_2: 100 mm Hg
PCO_2: 35 mm Hg
HCO_3: 24 mEq/L

Mr. T.'s oxygen therapy orders were changed to an aerosol mask at an F_IO_2 of 0.60. The respiratory therapist set up the aerosol mask as ordered and analyzed the system at the nebulizer outlet. Oxygen analysis confirmed an F_IO_2 of 0.60.

Two hours later Mr. T. was again dyspneic and tachypneic. Another ABG was obtained with the following results:

pH: 7.45
P_aO_2: 60 mm Hg
PCO_2: 30 mm Hg
HCO_3: 24 mEq/L

Mr. T.'s F_IO_2 was increased to 0.70, with orders for another ABG to be obtained in 1 hour. Mr. T. continued to be dyspneic and tachypneic. One hour later, ABG results were as follows:

pH: 7.45
P_aO_2: 50 mm Hg
PCO_2: 30 mm Hg
HCO_3: 24 mEq/L

Questions

1. Were the respiratory therapist's actions in setting up the aerosol system and analyzing the system correct? Explain your answer.
2. How can you explain the drop in the patient's P_aO_2 after an increase in the F_IO_2?
3. What would you have done differently with regard to Mr. Tyler's oxygen therapy?

(positive electrode) through a semipermeable membrane that allows only oxygen to pass through. The change in current is proportional to the partial pressure of oxygen. Although the analyzer measures partial pressure, it displays the percentage of oxygen.

Polarographic Oxygen Analyzers The *polarographic oxygen analyzer* (Figure 20-40) utilizes the same principle of operation and the same chemical reaction as the galvanic oxygen analyzer. The polarographic oxygen analyzer, however, uses a battery to polarize the system; polarizing speeds up the reduction reaction, resulting in a faster response time. Like the galvanic analyzer, the polarographic oxygen analyzer measures the partial pressure of oxygen and displays it as the percentage of oxygen. Polarographic oxygen analyzers can be used for continuous oxygen analysis, such as in-line with a mechanical ventilator.

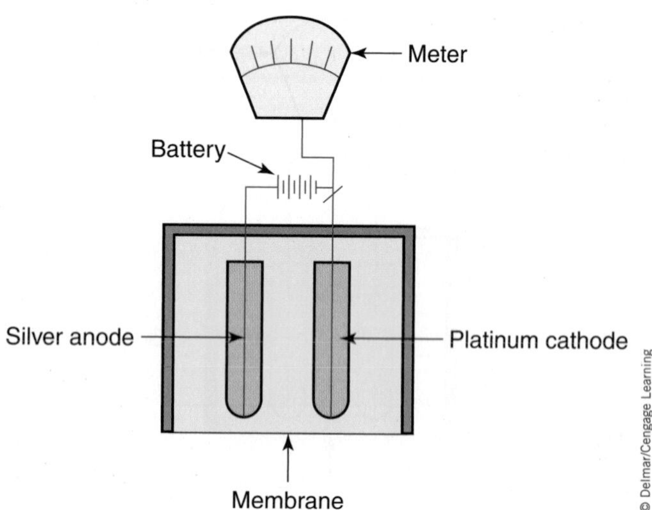

FIGURE 20-40 A schematic of a polarographic electrochemical oxygen analyzer.

CASE STUDY 20-2

E. G., a 65-year-old woman, arrived in the emergency room with acute shortness of breath. She had a history of COPD. Mrs. G. had a respiratory rate of 30 bpm; she was using accessory muscles and pursed-lip breathing. A complete blood cell count and arterial blood gas analysis were performed. The results of the CBC were within normal range, and the ABG results were as follows:

pH: 7.40
P_aO_2: 50 mm Hg
PCO_2: 68 mm Hg
HCO_3: 38 mEq/L

A diagnosis of exacerbation of COPD was made. Mrs. G. was placed on 100% oxygen via a nonrebreathing mask. Her oxygen saturation improved, as confirmed by continuous pulse oximetry, and her respiratory rate dropped to 16 bpm. Arterial blood gases on 100% oxygen were as follows:

pH: 7.32
P_aO_2: 80 mm Hg
PCO_2: 78 mm Hg
HCO_3: 38 mEq/L

Mrs. G. became lethargic and hard to rouse. Her respiratory rate decreased even further, to 10 bpm.

Questions

1. Was the oxygen therapy order appropriate? Explain your answer.
2. Explain the resulting P_aCO_2, respiratory rate, and neurological reaction.
3. Suggest an alternative method of oxygen delivery.

Therapeutic Use of Gas Mixtures

Certain gases can be combined with oxygen in specific concentrations and administered to treat a variety of conditions: carbon dioxide–oxygen, helium–oxygen, and nitric oxide therapy.

CARBON DIOXIDE AND OXYGEN (CARBOGEN)

At a concentration of less than 10%, carbon dioxide acts as a respiratory stimulant; indeed, the rise in carbon dioxide acts as the normal stimulus to breathe. This is the rationale for using carbon dioxide–oxygen **(carbogen)** mixtures to treat hypoventilation and to augment lung inflation. However, this approach has been found to be ineffective for hyperinflation because most patients treated with it preferentially increase their respiratory rate rather than their tidal volume.

Carbon dioxide–oxygen mixtures have also been used to treat *singulation* (hiccups), although the efficacy is questionable. Singulation is the spastic contraction of the diaphragm. Increased PCO_2 levels increase phrenic nerve discharge (the phrenic nerve innervates the diaphragm). Increasing the discharge of the phrenic nerve may improve the coordination of diaphragmatic contractions.

More modern uses of carbogen include:

- Early treatment of central retinal artery occlusion.
- In biology, to research in vivo oxygen and carbon dioxide flows.[6]
- To increase cerebral blood flow by dilating the cerebral blood vessels. However, most patients respond by hyperventilation in an attempt to normalize the PCO_2 because the brain indicates an increase in CO_2 as a decrease in O_2.[7]

Normally, the concentration of the administered carbon dioxide–oxygen mixture is 5% CO_2/95% O_2 for 10–15 minutes. Although low concentrations of carbon dioxide are a respiratory stimulant, concentrations above 10% result in respiratory *depression*.

Side effects of carbon dioxide–oxygen therapy include headache, palpitations, hypertension, dizziness, muscle tremors, and mental depression. Do not leave the patient unattended during this treatment.

HELIUM AND OXYGEN (HELIOX)

The benefit of helium as a therapeutic adjunct is based on its low density. In areas of turbulent flow, higher driving pressures are needed to maintain a given flow (see Chapter 3). Turbulent flow exists in the larger airways. In the presence of large airway obstructions, a patient, especially one compromised by pulmonary disease, has a greatly increased work of breathing (WOB). Administering a gas of lower density, such as helium, lowers the driving pressure needed to maintain gas flow. A helium–oxygen mixture **(heliox)** can substantially reduce a patient's work of breathing.[8] The density of an 80:20 helium–oxygen mixture is only 0.429 g/L as compared with the 1.29 g/L density of air. Keep in mind that helium–oxygen mixtures are effective only in large airways, where turbulent flow exists. There is no benefit in small airways because the flow in these areas is laminar; density is not a factor.

Helium is inert; it must always be mixed with at least 20% oxygen. The most commonly used mixture is 80% helium and 20% oxygen. A mixture of 70% helium and 30% oxygen can be used for patients with hypoxemia.

When administering helium–oxygen mixtures, remember that the oxygen flowmeter is inaccurate. Oxygen flowmeters are calibrated for the density of oxygen. Helium's density is lower; therefore, more gas exits the source than the flowmeter indicates. The correction factor for an 80:20 helium–oxygen mixture is 1.8. This means that for every liter of flow indicated on the flowmeter, 1.8 L is actually being delivered. For example, if 10 Lpm of the mixture is needed, the flowmeter should be set at 5.6 Lpm (10 ÷ 1.8). The correction factor for a 70:30 helium/oxygen mixture is 1.6. Also, due to its low density, helium–oxygen must be administered via a closed system to prevent gas escape.

Side effects of helium–oxygen therapy are directly related to its low density: distorted voice pitch and impaired cough. The helium should be washed out before the patient performs the cough maneuver. The lower density of the gas also reduces its aerosol-carrying capacity.

NITRIC OXIDE THERAPY

Although nitric oxide therapy is no longer in the investigation stage as a therapeutic modality, extensive clinical trials have been performed with successful results. FDA approval was obtained in December 1999.

Physiological Effects of Nitric Oxide. The benefits of nitric oxide are due to its physiological effect of capillary smooth muscle relaxation. By improving blood flow to ventilated alveoli, it:

- Improves $\dot{V}/\dot{Q}$ relationships.
- Decreases pulmonary vascular resistance and pulmonary pressures.
- Improves arterial oxygenation.

Indications and Potential Uses for Nitric Oxide Therapy. Indications for nitric oxide therapy are conditions that would benefit from its physiological effects. Table 20-12 summarizes the indications and

TABLE 20-12 **Indications and potential uses for nitric oxide therapy**

Pulmonary	Newborn/Pediatric	Other
Primary pulmonary hypertension	Congenital heart disease	Heart transplant
Chronic pulmonary hypertension	Pulmonary hypertension of the newborn	Lung transplant
Pulmonary fibrosis	Hypoxemic respiratory distress of the newborn	Sepsis
Pulmonary embolism	Pediatric chronic lung disease	Sickle-cell disease
Adult respiratory distress syndrome		

TABLE 20-13 **Adverse and toxic effects of nitric oxide therapy**

Direct Effects	Effects Due to By-Products
Paradoxical response	Cell damage
Worsening hypoxemia	Hemorrhage
Platelet inhibition	Pulmonary edema
Increased left ventricular filling pressures	Formation of methemoglobin
Pulmonary hypertension	Formation of peroxynitrite

potential uses that are currently being investigated for inhaled nitric oxide therapy.[2,9,10]

Dose and Mode of Delivery. Effective doses of nitric oxide have been reported in the range of 2–20 ppm (parts per million), with an optimal dose of 10 ppm. Doses less than 20 ppm show minimum adverse effects.[2,10]

Nitric oxide can be inhaled spontaneously by nonintubated patients, but therapy is more commonly delivered by mechanical ventilation. A nitric oxide injector and flow sensor are incorporated into the inspiratory limb of the ventilator circuit.[2]

Adverse and Toxic Effects of Nitric Oxide Therapy. Adverse and toxic effects of nitric oxide therapy can be due to its direct action or to its chemical by-products. Nitrogen dioxide (NO_2), which is produced whenever nitric oxide is exposed to oxygen, has very toxic effects at concentrations greater than 10 ppm.[2] Table 20-13 lists the adverse and toxic effects of nitric oxide therapy.

Discontinuation of Nitric Oxide Therapy. Withdrawing nitric oxide therapy must be done carefully to prevent rebound effect. Take the following steps when withdrawing a patient from nitric oxide therapy.[5]

- Decrease the nitric oxide level to the lowest effective dose, optimally at 5 ppm or less.
- Confirm that the patient is able to maintain adequate oxygenation on an I_IO_2 of 0.40 or lower.
- The patient should be hyperoxygenated before discontinuing nitric oxide.

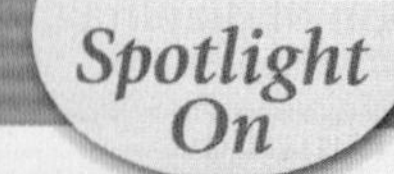

I-NOvent

The I-NOvent delivery system (INO Therapeutics) is the only commercially available nitric oxide (NO) delivery system that has FDA approval. However, the hospital must have an Investigational New Drug Number for INO administration. It is designed for mechanically ventilated patients.

The injection module is between the ventilator output and the humidifier in the inspiratory circuit. Nitric oxide is injected in proportion to the sensed inspiratory flow, providing the desired dose of NO. The concentration of NO remains accurate over a wide range of ventilator flows and desired NO concentrations.

Source: From Hess DR, Hurford WE. Journal conference on inhaled nitric oxide. Respir Care. *1999;44.(3);241–384.*

Summary

Medical gas therapy is an integral part of respiratory care practice. The competent, skilled practitioner is well versed in all aspects of therapy. Patient assessment and critical thinking skills are vital, as are skills in equipment selection and troubleshooting. The goals, indications, physiological effects, hazards, and side effects of therapy must always be considered and recognized. These factors, along with documented outcomes assessment, reflect not only a competent practitioner but also a professional one who is able to interact successfully with other members of the health care team and to contribute actively to the diagnosis, treatment, and recovery of the patient.

Study Questions

REVIEW QUESTIONS

1. List the indications for oxygen therapy.
2. List and briefly explain the hazards of oxygen therapy.
3. List and briefly explain the causes of hypoxemia.
4. Describe the indications for a liquid oxygen delivery system versus gaseous oxygen.
5. Differentiate between a noncompensated and a back-pressure compensated Thorpe tube.
6. Differentiate between a high- and a low-flow oxygen delivery system.
7. Describe the physiological effects of hyperbaric oxygen therapy.
8. Differentiate between functional and fractional oxygen saturation.
9. Describe the physiological effects of the following medical gas mixtures: carbon dioxide–oxygen, helium–oxygen, nitric oxide.

MULTIPLE-CHOICE QUESTIONS

1. The regulatory agency that is responsible for the purity levels of medical gases is the:
   a. DOT.
   b. OSHA.
   c. FDA.
   d. CGA.
2. Which of the following is not a low-flow delivery device?
   I. Venturi mask
   II. nasal cannula
   III. high-volume nebulizer
   IV. simple mask
   a. I and II
   b. II and III
   c. II and IV
   d. I and III
3. When checking on a patient wearing a nonrebreathing mask, the respiratory therapist notices that the reservoir bag is deflating almost completely during inspiration. The appropriate action is to:
   a. leave the system as is.
   b. increase the flow of source oxygen.
   c. decrease the flow of source oxygen.
   d. change the patient to a simple mask.
4. The best oxygen delivery device to administer the highest F_IO_2 as quickly as possible is a:
   a. Venturi mask.
   b. simple mask.
   c. partial rebreather.
   d. nonrebreather.
5. A COPD patient requires an oxygen delivery system that provides a moderate concentration of oxygen. The patient has a history of chronic hypoxemia and carbon dioxide retention. The most appropriate system for oxygen delivery is a:
   a. simple mask.
   b. nasal cannula.
   c. Venturi mask.
   d. partial rebreather.
6. A patient is wearing a HAFOE device set at an F_IO_2 of 0.50. When the therapist analyzes the system at the patient's airway, the analyzer reads 35%. What is the most likely reason for the large difference in concentrations?
   a. The analyzer is malfunctioning.
   b. The patient is breathing very shallowly.
   c. The source gas outlet is faulty.
   d. The patient is entraining room air.
7. In an adult with proper skin temperature and adequate perfusion, the T_CO_2 should be:
   a. 20–30% of the P_aO_2.
   b. equal to the P_aO_2.
   c. 70–80% of the P_aO_2.
   d. higher than the P_aO_2.
8. The measurement that is taken by the use of two wavelengths of light to compare oxyhemoglobin with deoxyhemoglobin is known as the:
   a. fractional saturation.
   b. wavelength saturation.
   c. functional saturation.
   d. hemoglobin saturation.
9. Which of the following factors may cause an erroneous pulse oximetry reading?
   a. hyperperfusion
   b. hyperthermia
   c. an S_aO_2 of 78%
   d. the presence of carboxyhemoglobin
10. The type of oxygen analyzer that utilizes oxygen's property of paramagnetism is:
    a. physical.
    b. electrical.
    c. galvanic.
    d. polarographic.

CRITICAL-THINKING QUESTIONS

1. A patient suffering from smoke inhalation is admitted to the emergency room. His P_aO_2 on arrival is 42 mm Hg. He is placed on a nonrebreathing mask at 100%; his P_aO_2 rises to 80 mm Hg and his S_aO_2 via pulse oximetry is 95%. There is no apparent cyanosis; in fact, the patient's coloring seems quite good. The patient remains tachypneic and lethargic despite the fact that his P_aO_2 and S_aO_2 are within normal range. Discuss the reason for the discrepancy between the patient's normal blood values and his poor respiratory and neurological status. Describe how you would treat and monitor this patient.
2. A patient with COPD is suffering from an acute exacerbation of her condition. Arterial blood gas analysis reveals a P_aO_2 of 48 mm Hg and a P_aCO_2 of 62 mm Hg. Describe how to treat and monitor this patient.
3. A patient is on a high-volume nebulizer and aerosol mask at an F_IO_2 of 0.60. Oxygen analysis at the patient's airway reads 30%. Why is there a discrepancy? Discuss appropriate alternative methods of delivering an F_IO_2 of 0.60.

References

1. American Association for Respiratory Care. AARC clinical practice guideline: oxygen therapy in the acute care facility-2002 Revision & Update. *Respiratory Care*. June 2002; 47(6);717–720.

2. Scanlon CL, et al. *Egan's Fundamentals of Respiratory Care.* 9th ed. Philadelphia: Mosby; 2008.
3. American Association for Respiratory Care. AARC clinical practice guideline: oxygen therapy in the home or alternate site health care facility-2007 Revision & Update. *Respiratory Care.* August 2007; 52(1)1063–1068.
4. White GC. *Equipment Theory for Respiratory Care.* 3rd ed. Clifton Park, NY: Delmar Cengage Learning; 1999.
5. Shenton S. Oxygen protocol. *Policy and Procedure Manual.* Denville, NJ: Saint Clare's Hospital; 1999.
6. Arnold JF, Kotas M, Fidler F, Pracht ED, Flentje M, Jakob PM. Quantitative regional oxygen transfer imaging of the human lung. *Journal of Magnetic Resonance Imaging.* 2007; 26,3:637–645.
7. Walsh, RN. *Higher Wisdom: Eminent Elders Explore the Continuing Impact of Psychedelics.* Albany, NY: State University of New York Press; 2005.
8. Chevrolet J-C. Helium oxygen mixtures in the intensive care unit. *Crit Care.* 2001;5,4:179–181.
9. Hsu C-W, et al. The initial response to inhaled nitric oxide treatment for intensive care unit patients with acute respiratory distress syndrome. *Respiration.* 2008; 75:288–295.
10. Hess DR, Hurford WE. Journal conference on inhaled nitric oxide, *Respir Care.* 1999;44.

Suggested Readings

American Association for Respiratory Care. AARC clinical practice guideline: in vitro pH and blood gas analysis and hemoximetry. Respir Care. 1993;38:505–510.

American Association for Respiratory Care. AARC clinical practice guideline: selection of an oxygen delivery device for neonatal and pediatric patients, *Respir Care.* 1996;41:637–646.

Burton GG, Tietsort JA. *Therapist-Driven Protocols, A Practitioner's Guide.* Los Angeles: Academy Medical Systems Inc; 1993.

Eubanks DH, Bone RC. *Principles and Applications of Cardiorespiratory Care Equipment.* Philadelphia: Mosby; 1994.

McPherson SP. *Respiratory Care Equipment.* 5th ed. Philadelphia: Mosby; 1995.

White GC. *Basic Clinical Lab Competencies for Respiratory Care, An Integrated Approach.* 4th ed. Clifton Park, NY: Delmar Cengage Learning; 2003.

CHAPTER 21

Humidity and Aerosol Therapy

Dianne A. Adams

OBJECTIVES

Upon completion of this chapter, the reader should be able to:

- Differentiate between the physical properties of humidity and aerosol.
- Explain the understanding of physiologic mechanisms for airway hydration.
- Recognize the effect of underhydration and overhydration on the respiratory system.
- Evaluate the function and effectiveness of devices that provide supplemental humidification to the respiratory system.
- Evaluate the function and effectiveness of devices that deliver aerosol particles to the respiratory system.
- Identify the appropriate clinical application of devices used to provide humidity and aerosol to patients who require supplemental hydration or aerosol therapy.

CHAPTER OUTLINE

KEY TERMS

absolute humidity (AH)
aerosol
body humidity (BH)
body temperature pressure saturated (BTPS)
deposition
homeostasis
humidifier
humidity
humidity deficit
hygrometer
hygroscopic
hypertonic
hypotonic
isotonic
nebulizer
relative humidity (RH)
stability
tonicity
water vapor content
water vapor pressure

The body's systems require a certain amount of hydration to maintain **homeostasis**, a state of relatively constant conditions. The respiratory system is no exception. Hydrating the body is necessary to maintain adequate cellular function and is usually associated with water or fluid consumption. External signs of dehydration are evident to us: chapped lips, flaky skin, dry cracked elbows and heels. Hydration of the respiratory system is rarely a concern until signs of dehydration appear: crusty nasal drainage, nosebleeds, dry mouth, scratchy throat, a dry hacking cough. Overhydration can also cause problems and lead to conditions associated with excess fluid retention. Maintaining hydration of the mucociliary lining of the airway and subsequent humidification of inspired air are primary functions of the upper airway. However, when an optimal balance cannot be met because of pathology or environmental conditions, compromise of respiratory function is likely. Therefore, maintaining these conditions during altered states is the primary goal of humidity and aerosol therapy. This requires an understanding of humidification concepts and their effect on airway function.

Concepts of Humidity

"Humidity" is a familiar term. The humidity of the atmosphere affects people's comfort whether they are out- or indoors. In this section, humidity is defined and ways of quantifying it are discussed, both in the atmosphere and in the respiratory system.

DEFINING HUMIDITY

Humidity is the amount of water vapor present in an environment or substance. Water vapor (water in its molecular, or gaseous form) enters the atmosphere through evaporation and leaves it through condensation. *Evaporation* occurs when water changes from its liquid form to its gaseous form; *condensation* occurs when water changes from its gaseous to its liquid form. Both processes are temperature dependent, as is a carrier gas's water-carrying capacity.

The **water vapor content** (the amount of water vapor present) of a given volume of a gas depends on both the temperature of the carrier gas and the gas's water-carrying capacity. Water vapor content is expressed as the mass of water in a volume of gas, in either milligrams of water suspended in a liter of gas (mg/L) or in grams per cubic meter (g/m^3). As the temperature of a gas increases, the amount of water vapor the gas can carry also increases. When the water vapor content is at the maximum possible at a given temperature, the gas is considered *fully saturated*. As a gas cools, its capacity to hold water vapor decreases. This decrease causes condensation, in which the vapor turns back into liquid form and "rains out" of the gas. Humidity, then, can be explained as the cumulative effect of the evaporation of moisture into the air and the condensation of moisture out of the air. A comparison of water vapor content in the atmosphere at given temperatures is shown in Table 21-1.

Absolute humidity (AH) is the actual amount of water present in a given volume of gas, and it is usually expressed in the same terms as water vapor content (mg/L or g/m^3). Because water vapor is in a gaseous state and behaves like any gas, absolute humidity can also be expressed by the amount of pressure exerted by the water molecules, or **water vapor pressure**, in millimeters of mercury (mm Hg). The water vapor content of fully saturated air at 21°C is 18.4 mg/L and exerts a pressure of 18.6 mm Hg (Table 21-1). Therefore, one could refer to the AH of that air sample as 18.4 mg/L or as 18.6 mm Hg.

Relative humidity (RH) compares the actual amount of water present in a given volume of gas (content, or AH) with the amount the gas is capable of holding at that temperature (capacity). It is always expressed as a percentage. The following formula illustrates the relationship:

$$\%RH = \frac{\text{absolute humidity}}{\text{capacity}} \times 100$$

When the AH of a gas equals the capacity, the gas is fully saturated, and RH is 100%. If the AH of a gas at

TABLE 21-1 Water vapor content and pressure of a fully saturated air sample at various temperatures

Temperature (°C)	Water Vapor Content (mg/L)	Water Vapor Pressure (mm Hg)
20	17.3	17.5
21	18.4	18.6
22	19.4	19.8
23	20.6	21.0
24	21.8	22.3
25	23.0	23.7
26	24.4	25.1
27	25.8	26.7
28	27.2	28.3
29	28.8	29.9
30	30.4	31.7
31	32.0	33.6
32	33.8	35.5
33	35.6	37.6
34	37.6	39.8
35	39.6	42.0
36	41.7	44.4
37 (body temperature)	*43.9*	*47.0*
38	46.2	49.5
39	48.6	52.3
40	51.1	55.1

21°C is 9.2 mg/L and its capacity at that temperature is known to be 18.4 mg/L, the RH is 50%.

$$\%RH = \frac{9.2 \text{ mg/L}}{18.4 \text{ mg/L}} \times 100 = 50\%$$

Understanding the different ways of expressing humidity and the underlying concepts helps the respiratory therapist (RT) appreciate the differences in capabilities of humidifying devices. These same expressions also explain concepts of humidity as related to the respiratory system.

MEASURING HUMIDITY

In terms of our environment, relative humidity is a familiar method of measuring and reporting the amount of moisture present in the air and is used to monitor outdoor as well as indoor humidity levels. The RH expresses how close the air is to becoming fully saturated. As RH reaches 100%, the rate of evaporation is equal to the rate of condensation. Depending on the season or geographic region, a dehumidifier might be used to remove excess water vapor from the air, such as in a damp, cool basement during the spring. Or a room humidifier might be run to increase the water vapor in air that is dry due to home heating systems during the winter months. Relative humidity can be measured in such conditions with a **hygrometer**.

EFFECT OF TEMPERATURE ON HUMIDITY

The temperature of a carrier gas plays an important role in determining the amount of water vapor a gas is capable of carrying. At a given temperature, a gas has its individual capacity to carry a certain amount of moisture (Table 21-1). As the temperature increases, the gas has a greater capacity for holding water vapor; at lower temperatures, its water-holding capacity and thus its water vapor content decrease. If the water vapor content is kept at a constant volume, an increase in temperature decreases RH because the higher temperature increases the gas's water-holding capacity. Comparing its content with its new capacity at the increased temperature would then decrease RH, as shown in the following situations.

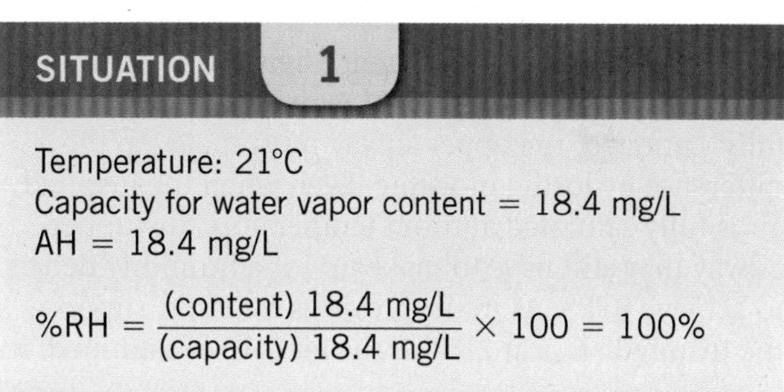

SITUATION 1
Temperature: 21°C
Capacity for water vapor content = 18.4 mg/L
AH = 18.4 mg/L
%RH = (content) 18.4 mg/L / (capacity) 18.4 mg/L × 100 = 100%

SITUATION 2

Temperature = 26°C
Capacity for water vapor content = 24.4 mg/L
AH = 18.4 mg/L

$$\%RH = \frac{\text{(content) } 18.4 \text{ mg/L}}{\text{(capacity) } 24.4 \text{ mg/L}} \times 100 = 75\%$$

The role of temperature on humidity must be understood to appreciate the effect of body temperature on inspired air. Using this knowledge of AH and the capacity of a gas to hold moisture helps in the explanation of how temperature affects humidity and airway function.

BODY HUMIDITY

The concepts of absolute and relative humidity can also be applied to conditions of inspired gases and humidity in alveolar air. **Body humidity (BH)** is the water vapor content required to fully saturate alveolar air at normal body temperature, expressed as a percentage. At 37°C (normal body temperature), the capacity for water vapor content is 43.9 mg/L, or 47 mm Hg, which represents normal BH. If the BH of inspired air is 100%, the air is fully saturated. The condition of fully saturated alveolar air at normal body temperature and at barometric (atmospheric) pressure (760 mm Hg) is called **body temperature pressure saturated (BTPS)**. However, BH may not be 100% if the AH of an inspired air sample is low. Suppose the room temperature is 22°C and the water vapor content of the room is 14 mg/L. The following formula shows that BH is 32%:

$$\%BH = \frac{\text{content at } 22°C}{\text{capacity at } 37°C} \times 100$$

$$\%BH = \frac{14 \text{ mg/L}}{43.9 \text{ mg/L}} \times 100 = 32\%$$

At the room temperature in this example, the air is not fully saturated because the capacity for water vapor content at 21°C is 18.4 mg/L. Furthermore, as the air is inspired, the temperature changes to 37°C, increasing the capacity to 43.9 mg/L. These circumstances create a **humidity deficit**, or a difference between the BH and the AH of inspired gas. If the inspired air is to become fully saturated, the upper airway must make up the difference by losing moisture. Even when the inspired air is fully saturated at room temperature, the upper airway may still have to make up for a humidity deficit to achieve BTPS. As in the previous example, suppose the inspired air is at 21°C. If the air is fully saturated, its AH is 18.4 mg/L. The formula for BH shows a BH of 42%:

$$\%BH = \frac{18.4 \text{ mg/L}}{43.9 \text{ mg/L}} \times 100 = 42\%$$

Determining the humidity deficit with the following formula shows how much moisture the body has to give up to reach BTPS.

$$\text{Humidity deficit} = \text{BH (mg/L)} - \text{AH (mg/L)}$$
$$\text{Humidity deficit} = 43.9 \text{ mg/L} - 18.4 \text{ mg/L}$$
$$= 25.5 \text{ mg/L}$$

This difference becomes clinically significant as the deficit increases over an extended period of time. Maintaining normal physiological function through proper hydration or by artificial administration of supplemental humidity helps in avoiding a humidity deficit and in restoring normal airway function. Table 21-2 summarizes terms describing humidity concepts and their mathematical expression.

Physiological Mechanisms of Airway Humidification

Humidification of the airways occurs naturally under ideal conditions. The physiological mechanisms set in place by the cellular layer and mucus blanket that make up the mucosal lining are designed to maintain a balance of moisture and heat exchange. Any alteration in this state causes airway dysfunction and eventually pulmonary compromise. The specific indications and devices for humidity therapy are discussed later in this chapter. Here are some of the basic principles of humidification.

TABLE 21-2 **Humidity terms and their mathematical expressions**

Term	Definition	Mathematical Expression
Absolute humidity	The actual amount of water vapor in a gas	Content = mg/L Pressure = mm Hg
Relative humidity	The actual amount of water vapor in a gas compared with the amount necessary to cause 100% saturation, multiplied by 100	$\%RH = \frac{AH}{\text{capacity}} \times 100$
Body humidity	The absolute humidity of inspired gas saturated at body temperature	$\%BH = \frac{AH}{\text{capacity at } 37°C} \times 100$
Humidity deficit	The difference (usually in mg/L) between the water vapor content of gas at BTPS (fully saturated air at normal body temperature and pressure) and the water vapor content of inspired gas	Humidity deficit = BH – AH

MAINTAINING ADEQUATE HUMIDIFICATION

The upper airway is designed to prepare inspired air for gas exchange and to maintain efficient pulmonary function by filtering and heating the inspired air to 37°C and providing 100% RH, or BTPS. This optimal gas conditioning continues from the initial inhalation by nose or mouth through the pharynx and usually has been completed before the air reaches the trachea, the beginning of the lower airways. The primary layers of the airway mucosa responsible for gas conditioning are the *cellular layer* (epithelial lining) and the *aqueous sol layer* and *mucus gel layer*, which make up the mucus blanket (Chapter 6). A change in either the temperature or the moisture of the inspired air affects the function of each layer.

The aqueous sol layer is a low-viscosity fluid that bathes the cilia. When the cilia are fully extended, microhooks at their tips reach through the aqueous sol layer to engage the mucus gel layer above. With each stroke, the mucus gel layer is moved toward the pharynx. The depth of this aqueous layer is the result of the amount of water evaporation that occurs during inspiration and water condensation that occurs with exhalation.

- When air that is less than BTPS is *inspired*, water evaporates from the mucus gel layer in an attempt to reach full saturation at 37°C. This phenomenon is part of what is known as *insensible water loss* and under normal conditions amounts to a net loss of 250 mL of water and 35 kcal of heat from the lungs each day.[1] Water that is lost in this layer is replaced by the secretory cells found in the cellular layer.
- Conversely, during *exhalation*, some heat and moisture are given back to the mucosal lining, preparing the lining for the next inspiration. Condensation during exhalation occurs when gas exiting the airways comes into contact with the mucosal lining, which is now cooler as a result of heat loss during inspiration.

Likewise, heat is transferred from the exhaled gas, warming the mucosal lining for the next inspiration. Under certain conditions, water gained by condensation can increase the depth of this fluid layer, thus decreasing the function of the mucociliary transport. The activity of the cilia is also dependent on the gas temperature and the RH. When the temperature of the inspired gas is not at 37°C and the RH is less than 100%, the beat frequency is affected. These conditions may occur because of changes in the viscosity of the gel layer above the mucosal lining or as a result of the change in depth of the aqueous sol layer. The depth of the aqueous sol layer represents an equilibrium between water loss and water gain and greatly determines the ability of the mucociliary transport system to function adequately.[2]

The mucus gel layer is composed of mucus secreted by goblet cells and submucosal glands. Mucus is 95% water and 5% glycoproteins and lipids. The complex bonding of these substances is critical in determining the viscosity of mucus and thereby its ability to be propelled by the cilia and function in mucociliary transport. Any alteration, such as water loss or gain, disturbs this delicate balance and impairs the mobility of mucus.

The upper airway is responsible for conditioning the inspired air and for maintaining clearance of contaminants. Under normal circumstances, such as breathing room air that is 22°C and has an RH of 50%, gas conditioning occurs by reaching 31–33°C and 59–73% RH at the larynx, 34°C and 77% RH in the trachea, and 37°C and 100% RH in the mainstem bronchi. These conditions can be achieved only when the body and the respiratory system are adequately hydrated. Depleting the body of the needed water—whether a result of improper oral intake, exposure to dry gases, or artificial bypass of the upper airway—can lead to detrimental consequences, as can excessive water accumulation in the respiratory tract.

CONSEQUENCES OF UNDERHUMIDIFICATION

When the respiratory tract is exposed to anhydrous gases, physiological changes occur in the primary layers of the airway mucosa. The degree of decreased humidity and the length of exposure time to dry gases determine the severity of these changes.

As cool, dry gas is inspired, heat and moisture are given up by the mucus gel layer and then by the aqueous sol layer, leading to changes in the system.

- The most noticeable change begins with the thickening of the mucus gel and the retention of secretions. The mucociliary transport is greatly compromised owing to the change in viscosity of the gel layer and depletion of the fluid layer.
- The beat frequency of the cilia is also affected by the decreased temperature of the gas, adding to the inability of the cilia to participate in secretion movement.[2]
- As the dehydrated state continues, the mucus blanket becomes encrusted, increasing the likelihood that mucus will plug smaller airways. Plugging of the airways may lead to atelectasis and impaired pulmonary function.
- Exposure to cold, dry air may be responsible for the impairment of pulmonary function and bronchoconstriction among asthmatic patients.[3]
- Histological changes that occur with prolonged impairment of the mucociliary transport include

the destruction of cilia, damage to mucus glands, and the destruction of the epithelial lining and basement membrane.

Of all the changes that occur in the airway as a result of underhumidification, thickening and retention of secretions are the hallmark signs of dehydration of the respiratory tract.

CONSEQUENCES OF OVERHUMIDIFICATION

The airways can also be overhumidified. Too much humidity occurs when the insensible water loss decreases, such as when either the temperature of the inspired gas is higher than body temperature or inspired gas contains aerosols (droplets). Both of these conditions can lead to excess body fluid retention and intoxication.

When the inspired gas *temperature* is higher than 37°C and the gas is 100% saturated:

- Condensation rather than evaporation occurs, adding water to the mucosal lining.
- As exhaled gas passes over the mucosal lining, condensation continues to reduce the amount of normal insensible water loss and results in an increase in the depth of the aqueous sol layer.

Inspired air that contains *aerosols* can lead to overhumidification:

- The presence of aerosols increases the risk of adding water to the mucosal lining. The change in depth affects the efficiency of the cilia because their microhooks can no longer reach the mucus gel layer above and propel it forward.
- The mucus gel layer is also affected because the balance between its substances has now changed, resulting in a less viscous layer that cannot be cleared with the rhythmic motion of the cilia.[2]
- Added moisture may also dilute surfactants at the alveolar level, leading to decreased surface tension and thereby affecting pulmonary function.
- Histologically, degeneration and adhesion of cilia result.

Eventually these changes lead to increases in secretions, decreases in ventilation, and compromise of oxygenation. The hallmark signs of overhumidification are weight gain in neonates, crackles on auscultation, and radiographic changes that suggests pulmonary congestion.

Concepts of Aerosols

Humidification therapy often involves aerosols. This section explains how aerosols can be used in the respiratory system and what effect they have on airway function. The therapeutic use and design of aerosol-generating devices are discussed later in the chapter.

DEFINING AEROSOL

An **aerosol** is any liquid or solid particle that is suspended in a gas. Whereas humidity involves water in its molecular (gaseous) form, aerosols contain actual droplets of liquid water. Thus, aerosols are visible to the naked eye. Aerosols can occur naturally in the external environment (e.g., fog), can be a result of a chemical reaction (e.g., a by-product of combustion), or can be artificially created. Smoke and smog are composed of solid particles suspended in a gas; they result from combustion. Liquid aerosols are in aerosolized cleaning solutions, spray deodorants, and hair sprays. Likewise, in medical use, aerosols are created as a delivery system for medication or for hydration to a desired location. Producing aerosols for this purpose requires an in-depth understanding of them and the delivery systems used to deposit the aerosol particles at the intended site.

CHARACTERISTICS OF AEROSOLS

How an aerosol behaves is determined by factors such as the physical nature and activity of the particle.

The size of an aerosol particle and its ability to remain in suspension dictate whether the aerosol reaches the intended site in the airways and thus affects how therapeutic the aerosol administration will be. Size depends on several factors. Ambient conditions, such as temperature and RH, determine whether an aerosol particle gets larger, gets smaller, or remains the same size in its suspended state.

- If aerosol particles are introduced to a cooler and less humid gas stream, the aerosol particle evaporates and decreases in size as the gas warms.
- If introduced to a warmer gas stream that is more humid, small aerosol particles coalesce, forming fewer, but larger, particles.
- Ideally, to maintain a steady size, aerosol particles should be introduced into a main gas stream that has the same temperature and humidity as the carrier gas.

Aerosols that absorb moisture from the surrounding environment are called **hygroscopic**. Aerosols can absorb moisture when they are exposed to a humidified environment such as that within ventilator circuits. The **tonicity** of an aerosol is its tendency to absorb water.

- **Hypertonic** aerosols, such as hypertonic saline solutions, have a greater tonicity than body fluids, so they absorb water from the surrounding tissues and increase in size.

- **Hypotonic** aerosols have less tonicity than body fluids and tend to evaporate and decrease in size.
- An **isotonic** aerosol is one that neither gains nor loses water but maintains a steady size.

Because of the way they are created, therapeutic aerosols contain a range of particle sizes. The design of equipment that produces aerosols determines the initial size. How the equipment is powered (gas or ultrasonic) and the use of structural objects (baffles) can produce a variety of particle sizes.

In the clinical setting, the concern is to create an aerosol that delivers an average-sized particle that guarantees distribution to the intended site. The term *mass median aerodynamic diameter* (*MMAD*) describes the average size of aerosol particles generated, expressed in micrometers (μm). MMAD divides the range of aerosol particles generated in half. If the MMAD of an aerosol device is 5 μm, 50% of the aerosol particles produced are smaller than 5 μm and have less mass, and 50% of the aerosol particles are larger than 5 μm and have greater mass.

Knowing that aerosol particle size is affected by the temperature and RH of the gas, the tonicity of the particle, and the equipment design helps the respiratory therapist to choose appropriate devices, set correct temperatures, and select the proper solutions to achieve the desired results.

The ability of an aerosol particle to remain suspended in a gas is its **stability**. Aerosol stability is influenced by several factors such as size, activity, and concentration.

- The *size* of the aerosol particle determines how much influence gravity imposes because a large particle is more affected by gravity than a small one is; it has a greater tendency to fall out of its carrier gas and be deposited on the surface. The effect of particle size on deposition is summarized in Table 21-3.

TABLE 21-3 **Particle deposition in the respiratory tract**

Particle Size (μm)	Deposition Site
>50	Is filtered out before it enters the respiratory tract
5–50	Mouth, nose, pharynx
2–5	Respiratory tract proximal to alveolar ducts
0.5–3	Lung parenchyma: alveoli
<0.5	Remains in suspension and is exhaled

- The *kinetic activity* of the aerosol affects when **deposition** (the landing of the particle on a surface) occurs. All molecules are in continuous motion and often collide with one another. These collisions cause even more rapid, random motion, referred to as *Brownian movement*, which mainly involves particles of less than 0.1 μm. As an aerosol particle decreases in size, it becomes more subject to Brownian movement and to collisions with other molecules. The collisions cause particles to coalesce (join together) and eventually fall out of suspension.
- As the *concentration* of aerosol particles increases, the chances are greater that the particles collide, coalesce to form larger particles, and fall out of suspension.

EFFECT OF AEROSOLS ON AIRWAY FUNCTION

Aerosol delivery is designed to target three specific areas: the upper airway, the lower airways, and the lung parenchyma. The aerosols may be categorized as either bland aerosols or pharmacologically active (medicated) aerosols. The site of deposition and the type of aerosol administered determine the effect of the aerosol on airway function.

The initial size of the aerosol being generated usually determines the approximate area for deposition (the site of aerosol action). The first step in ensuring appropriate deposition in the airway is knowing the location of aerosol deposition according to particle size and the MMAD production of the available aerosol-generating device, or **nebulizer**.

Although the choice of aerosolized agent is usually the responsibility of the physician, the respiratory therapist must still know the various agents available and understand their use as therapeutic or diagnostic adjuncts to respiratory care. Aerosolized agents can be *bland* (not containing medication) or *pharmacologically active* (containing medication designed to elicit a biological effect when topically applied in aerosol form to the airways). Bland aerosols can be sterile water and hypotonic, isotonic, or hypertonic saline; they can also be either cooled or heated. Successful results require that the respiratory therapist be familiar with the solution agents, delivery devices, and desired site of deposition. Table 21-4 summarizes the uses of bland and pharmacologically active (medicated) aerosols. Pharmacologic agents are discussed further in Chapter 7.

Therapeutic Use of Humidifying Devices

The decision to use clinical humidifying devices (**humidifiers**) is typically left to the discretion of the respiratory therapist. More often than not, a

TABLE 21-4 **Uses of bland and medicated aerosols**

Type of Nebulizer	Type of Solution	Desired Effect
Cool bland aerosols		
Small-volume nebulizer (SVN), ultrasonic nebulizer (USN)	Hypotonic saline	Induce sputum without added sodium
SVN, USN	Isotonic saline	Induce sputum
SVN, USN	Hypertonic saline	Induce sputum
Large-volume nebulizer (LVN), Babbington	Sterile water	Reduce upper airway swelling
Heated bland aerosols		
LVN	Sterile water	Reduce humidity deficit
Medicated aerosols		
Dry powder inhaler (DPI), metered-dose inhaler (MDI), SVN	Bronchoactive agents	Reduce smooth muscle spasm
SVN	Mucokinetic agents	Promote clearance of secretions
MDI, SVN	Glucocorticoids	Reduce airway inflammation
MDI, SVN	Anti-asthmatics	Prevent allergic airway reactions
SVN, small-particle aerosol generator (SPAG)	Antimicrobial agents	Reduce and inhibit microbial growth

Best Practice

Choosing a Nebulizer

A particle's deposition in the respiratory tract depends on its size. To optimize delivery of aerosol particles to the targeted site, choose a nebulizer for the particle size range it produces.

- If the targeted site is the nasal cavity, choose a nebulizer that generates particles in the size range of 5–50 µm, according to Table 21-3.
- If the desired site is the lower airway, the particle size range should be 2–5 µm, and the device of choice would have an MMAD of 2–5 µm.
- In some cases, deposition must occur at the alveolar level to promote systemic absorption. The particle size required for this location is 0.5–3 µm.

The response to aerosol administration depends on the deposition site of the particle and on the activity—bland or medicated—of the agent.

- If deposition occurs in the upper airway, as is the intended site when using nasal sprays, the activity of the aerosol is then directed to the mucosal lining or to the vasculature of the nasal cavity.
- When aerosol deposition occurs in the lower airways, the activity is directed to the mucus layer, submucosal cells, or nerve endings.
- Aerosols whose site of action is the lung parenchyma stimulate a response through systemic absorption of a pharmacologic agent.

physician's order for humidity is not forthcoming. Hospital policy on the application of these devices varies from institution to institution; therefore, the decision to provide supplemental humidity requires that the respiratory therapist be proficient in this treatment modality. The respiratory therapist must be able to recognize the need for humidity therapy and to choose the most appropriate device for the patient.

INDICATIONS FOR HUMIDITY THERAPY

Clinical indications for providing humidity therapy include the administration of dry medicated gases and altered BTPS. When a patient is breathing dry gas supplied from a cylinder or central supply system, a humidity deficit may result, causing further respiratory complications for the already compromised patient. Humidity therapy is not limited to patients whose upper airway is bypassed; it must also be considered

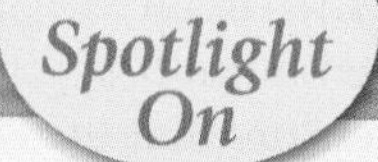

Aerosol Delivery of Macromolecules

Until recently, injection or ingestion was thought to be necessary for delivering drugs to the systemic circulation because most bioengineered drugs consist of macromolecules too large for entry in any other way. Currently, aerosolizing devices are being designed to provide inhalation delivery of these drugs for systemic therapy.

- Inhaling macromolecules provides a direct route of entry for systemic absorption without the problems associated with traditional drug therapy, such as inconvenience, pain, and gastrointestinal upset, all of which result in poor patient compliance.
- Aerosol therapy provides a more rapid onset of the desired results. Macromolecules that are currently being tested for administration by inhalation are insulin, morphine, hormones, calcitonin, and vaccines.

Device design appears to be the key to the effective delivery of these drugs to the lung periphery. Currently, several companies are conducting clinical and preclinical trials of aerosol devices to deliver macromolecules. The development of systemic drug delivery by inhalation will dramatically change the way medication is delivered for many patients.

Source: Corkery K. Inhalable drugs for systems therapy. Respir Care. *2000;45:831–835.*

for the spontaneously breathing patient receiving medicated gas therapy. The type of gas flow device also indicates whether supplemental humidity is necessary:

- A *low-flow device,* such as a nasal cannula, can be humidified in an attempt to supplement a spontaneously breathing patient's humidity level. But, because the room air and humidity are being entrained with each breath on these devices, supplemental humidity may not be required.
- A *high-flow device,* such as a mechanical ventilator, requires supplemental humidity delivery to meet BTPS because the gas delivered is fully supplied by the medical gas system, which is anhydrous.

Hospital policies on humidity therapy attempt to set guidelines for the respiratory therapist to follow. For example, a hospital's policy may state that supplemental humidity is not necessary with oxygen devices at flows of less than 3 Lpm. However, the respiratory therapist must recognize signs and symptoms of inadequate humidification and the need for humidity therapy. If a spontaneously breathing patient on oxygen therapy presents with a dry nonproductive cough, nasal bleeding, and complaints of throat dryness or discomfort, a lack of humidity may be the cause. the respiratory therapist has the responsibility of providing an appropriate humidification device.

The RT must also recognize whether a patient with a mechanically ventilated artificial airway is receiving poorly humidified gas. Evidence of the need for increased hydration for such patients is thick tenacious secretions, mucus plugging, increased airway resistance, and increased work of breathing.[4] A patient who presents with any of those signs requires delivery of humidified gas at a temperature of at least 30 °C, according to the relevant American Association for Respiratory Care (AARC) clinical practice guideline (CPG) for providing humidity to a patient during mechanical ventilation.[5] Standards for the humidity output of any humidifying device for medical use have been established by the American National Standards Institute (ANSI). Their report states that:

- The minimum output of 10 mg/L is the lowest acceptable humidity level for devices that deliver gas to the upper airway.
- A minimum output of 30 mg/L is necessary when gas delivery bypasses the upper airway.[6]

HAZARDS

In addition to the physiological hazards associated with under- and overhumidification, the technical hazards associated with humidity therapy are related to the functioning of the humidity devices.

- Unheated humidification devices, such as bubble humidifiers and heat and moisture exchangers, are simple in their design and require minimal assembly. The respiratory therapist should inspect these devices for cracks or manufacturing defects before setting them up.

- Once a device has been connected to the oxygen delivery device, it must be checked for proper functioning, and the patient must be assessed for any discomfort or adverse effects.
- Heated units that provide humidification to patients receiving medicated gas therapy can impose a risk if they are incorrectly set up or improperly monitored.

Before connecting a patient to any electrical humidity device, the respiratory therapist should inspect the humidifier for damaged or worn parts to reduce the risk of electrical shock.

- Equipment that is powered by electricity must meet the Underwriters Laboratory (UL) compliance for power specifications, conduction, and leakage current before being approved for medical use.
- The power plug should be grounded, intact, and unmodified.
- The device should have an up-to-date inspection label from the hospital's biomedical engineering department, which certifies that the equipment has passed the minimum standards for electrical safety as set by the National Fire Protection Association (NFPA). The NFPA 1999 norms require that electrical leakage be less than 300 microamps and that the electrical ground be less than 0.5 ohms.[7]
- The device should be cleaned and properly packaged to discourage cross-contamination.
- Once a heated humidifier is in place, the RT's responsibility is to monitor its functioning.

The respiratory therapist has other responsibilities when using humidifying equipment.

- Most of the humidity devices used today are fully disposable or have disposable components, such as the humidity chamber used with heated humidifiers. The respiratory therapist must inspect all disposable as well as nondisposable equipment to avoid risks associated with defective or damaged parts.
- Continuous water feed systems and the level of water in the humidifier chamber must be checked, and the amount of condensation occurring in the circuit must be monitored. Any build-up of water in the circuit can cause an increase in the patient's work of breathing and add to the risk of inadvertent lavage of the patient's airway when the circuit or the patient is repositioned.
- The temperature of the chamber and of the circuit proximal to the airway must be monitored to prevent overheating or underheating the patient's airway. If heated wire circuits are used in conjunction with a heated humidifier, the respiratory therapist must ensure that the temperature settings are correct and that the circuit is properly eliminating excess condensation.

General Principles of Humidifying Devices

Many humidifying devices are available, and they have a variety of designs and offer a range of humidity capabilities. The respiratory therapist needs to be familiar with the basic designs and to know how each affects performance in order to make appropriate selections in various clinical situations.

FACTORS AFFECTING EFFECTIVENESS

Several factors determine the effectiveness of a humidity device. The goal may be to achieve the same RH as that of the ambient air when delivering dry medicated gases to a spontaneously breathing patient or to provide heated humidity that is near BTPS when bypassing the upper airway. Whatever the goal, the humidification system has to meet certain requirements:

- It should comply with ANSI standards.
- The humidity output is determined, in part, by the temperatures of the water and of the carrier. Heating the water increases the gas's water-carrying capacity. Thus, a heated humidifier is much more effective at achieving BTPS than is a cool humidifier.
- The length of time that the water and gas are in contact with each other also affects humidity output. Exposing the gas to water for a longer period of time gives the water molecules a better chance of being picked up by the carrier gas. So, if the time a gas is in contact with water is increased, the water vapor content is increased.
- Contact time is regulated by the liter flow of gas through a humidifying device. So, as liter flow is increased through a humidifying device, the exposure time is decreased and the less saturated the gas is when it reaches the patient.
- Humidifier design, such as depth of the water reservoir, also affects exposure time.
- The surface area between the gas and the water has its effect. The greater the surface area is of the gas-liquid interface, the greater is the chance of increasing humidity levels. Devices that encourage increased surface area can deliver fully saturated gases.

TYPES OF HUMIDIFIERS

Humidifiers can be categorized according to the type of gas flow system with which they are used.

- *Low-flow humidifiers* are used with low-flow oxygen-delivery devices and are limited in the amount of humidity they provide. Because a patient on a low-flow oxygen device still entrains room air with each breath, the low-flow humidifier is only partially providing humidification. In these systems, the volume of dry medical gas that is being humidified represents only a portion of the patient's total inspired volume of air; the remainder is entrained from the surrounding room air.
- *High-flow humidifiers* are used with high-flow oxygen-delivery devices and are responsible for providing the total volume of inspired gas going to the patient. Therefore, they should meet the patient's total needs for RH.

Table 21-5 lists the devices available for use with low-flow and high-flow systems.

Bubble Humidifier. The *bubble humidifier* is designed to create bubbles below the surface of water; the bubbles increase the contact time and surface area of the liquid-gas interface. It is the most commonly used disposable humidifier with low-flow devices. Several designs are available; all achieve an RH range of about 33–40%.

All bubble humidifiers incorporate a capillary tube submerged in a reservoir of water.

- The reservoir bottle cap is fitted with a connector that attaches to a gas source, such as a flowmeter.
- Gas flows through the capillary tube and is directed to the bottom of the bottle, where bubbles are created.
- As the bubbles travel upward, they pick up water vapor, which is released at the surface of the water and carried on to the patient via a low-flow oxygen-delivery device, usually a nasal cannula.

TABLE 21-5 **Types of humidifiers by flow delivery**

Low-flow humidifiers
Bubble humidifier
Diffuser humidifier
Jet humidifier
High-flow humidifiers
Passover humidifier
Heated, high-flow, high-humidity device
Wick humidifier
Heat and moisture exchanger

The design of the capillary tube may vary and affect the amount of RH delivered. The simplest of bubble humidifier designs and the lowest in humidity output is the capillary tube with an open end. RH is also affected by the liter flow of the gas and the temperature of the room. As flow rates are increased or room temperature is increased, the RH of the gas delivered to the patient is decreased.

Diffuser Humidifier. The *diffuser humidifier* is based on the principles of the bubble humidifier but has a different capillary tube design. The diffuser humidifier's capillary tube has a plastic or porous metal diffuser at the end. The diffuser increases the number of bubbles created below the water surface, thereby increasing the surface area of the liquid-gas interface. Because of the larger surface area of the liquid-gas interface, this humidifier is more efficient in providing humidity with a low-flow oxygen device than is the bubble humidifier (Figure 21-1A and B).

Jet Humidifier. The *jet humidifier*, available as a nondisposable or disposable bubble humidifier, applies Bernoulli's principle (Chapter 3) with an underwater jet. The capillary tube is designed to direct gas to the bottom of the reservoir bottle, passing through the jet and creating an aerosol. The bubbles containing the aerosol droplets now pass through a diffuser before floating to the surface and being carried to the patient. This design enhances the efficiency of this type of humidifier by increasing both the time and amount of the gas and water interface. The jet humidifier is designed for use with a low-flow device.

Passover Humidifier. The *passover humidifier*, a high-flow humidifier, is the simplest in design. As its name implies, gas simply passes over the surface of a container of water. The gas is not diverted beneath the water to increase the amount of contact time, nor is the gas-liquid interface surface area increased. Humidification occurs through simple evaporation; molecules of water simply move from the surface of the water into the gas flowing above it. This type of humidifier has a very low efficiency and cannot provide gas at BTPS. The humidity output from a passover humidifier is not suitable for humidification when the upper airway has been bypassed. Furthermore, humidity can be increased only by reducing the flow, or heating the water, or both.

Wick Humidifier. Modifications to the earlier design of the simple passover humidifier have led to several

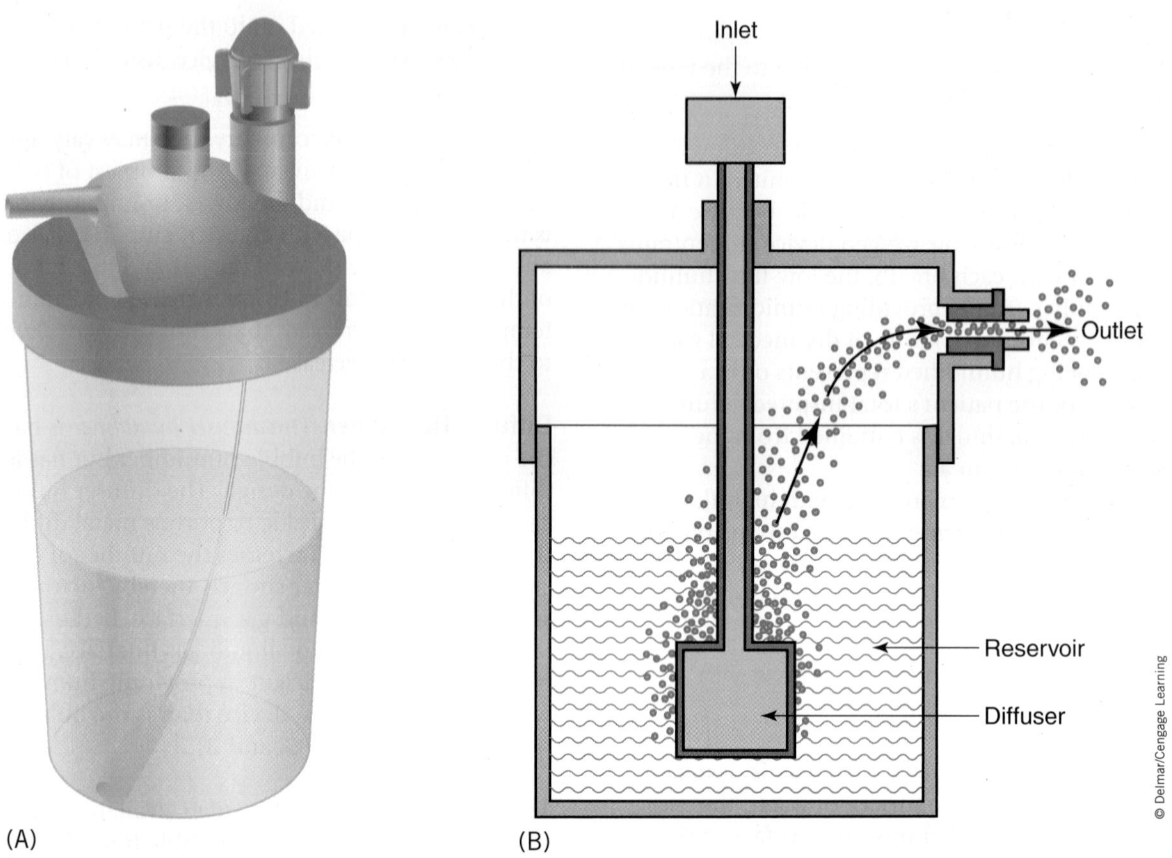

FIGURE 21-1 (A) Bubble humidifier with diffuser. (B) Schematic of a diffuser humidifier.

CASE STUDY 21-1

The night shift therapist in a 200-bed community hospital has just been called to the third floor to assess a patient who is complaining of breathing discomfort.

T. S. is a 65-year-old female who was admitted two nights ago through the emergency department with a diagnosis of acute exacerbation of COPD. A review of her chart for current respiratory orders reveals an order for oxygen therapy at 2.5 Lpm via a nasal cannula. She is also receiving bronchodilator therapy every 3 hours. The last treatment was given 1 hour ago.

Her most recent arterial blood gas analysis shows pH 7.37, P_aCO_2 60 and P_aO_2 58, HCO_3^- 34, S_aO_2 89% when on a nasal cannula at 2 Lpm.

Upon entering the room, the therapist notes that Ms. Simpson appears mildly short of breath. The nasal cannula is directly connected to the nipple adaptor on the flowmeter, which is set at 2.5 Lpm. Her respiratory rate is 25 breaths per minute, and her breathing is mildly labored. The therapist introduces himself while taking note of the pulse oximetry readings, which show a pulse of 110 and an S_pO_2 of 91% (S_pO_2 is oxygen saturation as measured by a pulse oximeter). The RT observes dried bloody secretions around her nares and on the nasal cannula. Her breath sounds are diminished but free of wheezing or rhonchi. When asked to cough, she explains that her throat is very dry and irritated and that it hurts to cough.

Questions

1. On the basis of the RT's assessment, what is causing Ms. Simpson's breathing discomfort?
2. According to the hospital policy, oxygen orders for flow rates of less than 3 Lpm do not require additional humidification. On the basis of this policy, what do you recommend?

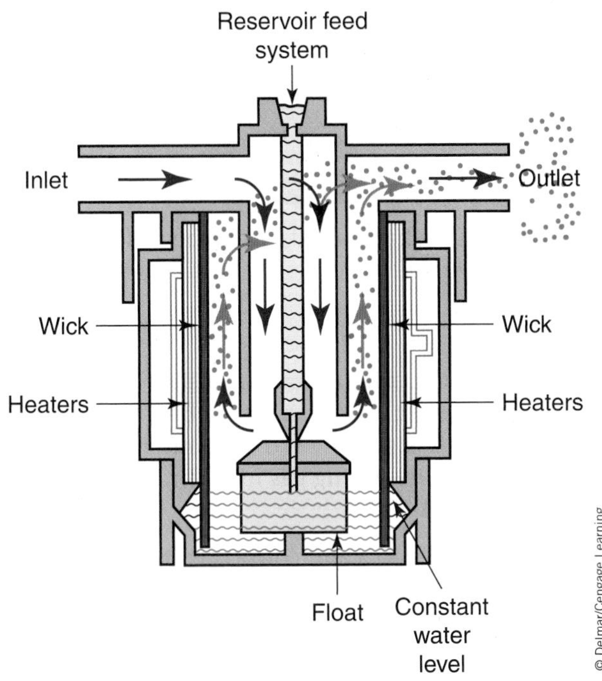

FIGURE 21-2 A Bird wick humidifier.

models of humidifiers that provide greater humidity outputs and higher RH, making them ideal for use with mechanical ventilation when the upper airway is bypassed.

The so-called *wick humidifiers* are designed for high-flow devices. The addition of heat from an electrical plate or heating element increases the water-carrying capacity of the dry gas, which enters the wick chamber. Porous absorbent paper or water-saturated cloth in the chamber provides greater surface area and good conditions for humidifying dry gas (Figure 21-2). The Inspiron Vapor-Phase humidifier, for example, uses a hydrophobic wick that allows only water vapor to pass through it and efficiently provides 100% RH. The liquid chamber remains separate from the gas chamber, preventing any water from passing through the wick. This design offers some protection against microbial growth.

Other wick humidifiers are designed for use with wick paper that is fully saturated with water. A continuous water feed system keeps the paper wick moist, thereby providing continuous humidity to the airways. The Fisher & Paykel Model MR 850 heated humidifier is a wick humidifier with these features; it can provide 100% RH (Figure 21-3).

Some wick humidifiers also include spiral vanes to increase surface area and to enhance humidification capabilities (Figure 21-4). The Bear VH-820 humidifier uses this spiral design to increase the surface area and contact time of water to gas in the chamber, enabling this humidifier to provide 100% RH.

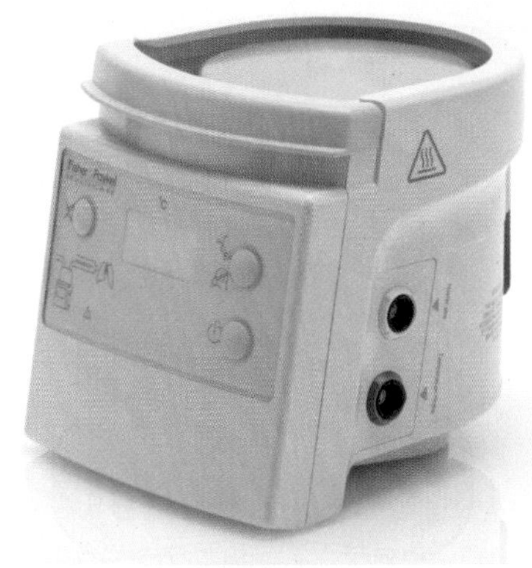

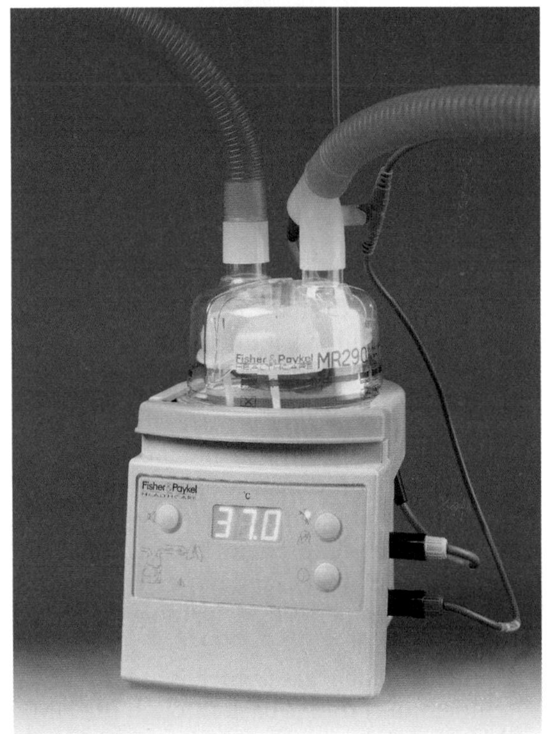

FIGURE 21-3 Heated wick humidifier.

Courtesy of Fisher & Paykel Healthcare, Inc.

All these units incorporate nondisposable heating elements with servocontrols to regulate temperature and disposable humidification chambers.

Heat and Moisture Exchanger. *Heat and moisture exchangers* (*HMEs*) use the effects of airway physiology to provide humidification with high-flow systems to patients with an artificial airway. Sometimes referred to as *passive humidifiers* or artificial noses, HMEs mimic the airway's exchange of heat and moisture during inspiration and expiration. An HME is placed close to

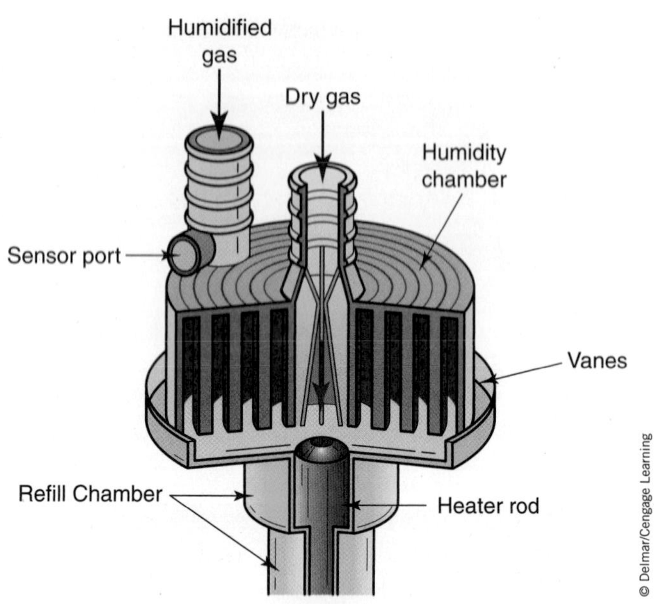

FIGURE 21-4 A wick humidifier with spiral vanes.

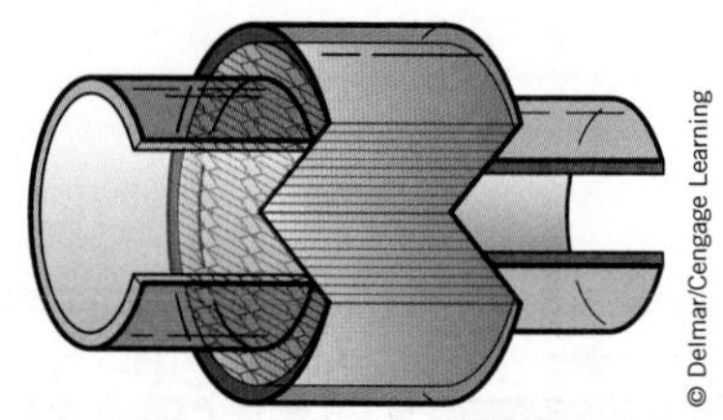

FIGURE 21-5 A heat and moisture exchanger (HME).

the patient's artificial airway in line with a high-flow device. As gas travels from the high-flow device and through large-bore tubing, it must pass through the HME before being delivered to the patient.

- During *inspiration*, as gas passes through the HME, it picks up the heat and moisture produced by the previously exhaled breath, thereby warming and humidifying the dry gas coming from the high-flow system. The gas delivered to the patient is at 30°C and has as high as 100% RH at this temperature, depending on the design of the HME.
- Upon *exhalation*, gas (which is at body temperature) travels back through the HME, this time giving up heat to the cooler HME. At the same time, water condenses, or rains out, of the exhaled gas because of the cooler temperature and is absorbed by the HME. Thus the HME is prepared to heat and humidify the cool, dry incoming gas for the next inspiration (Figure 21-5).

A study by Vitacca and coworkers showed that HME use improves the viscosity of secretions and reduces bacterial colonization in chronically tracheostomized patients who breathe spontaneously.[8] Use of these devices during mechanical ventilation, however, is contraindicated in certain situations, according to the AARC CPG for humidification during mechanical ventilation.[5]

Heat and moisture exchangers are available in four basic designs:

- The one that uses the physical principles of heat and moisture exchange as just described is simply called an *HME*.
- Another, called a *hygroscopic condenser humidifier* (*HCH*), includes hygroscopic material.
- The design that functions as a filter is known as a *heat and moisture exchanging filter* (*HMEF*).
- The fourth design incorporates both hygroscopic properties and filtration: the *hygroscopic condenser humidifier filter* (*HCHF*).[9]

Table 21-6 compares terms that identify the different types of HMEs by material and by function.

TABLE 21-6 **Terminology for heat and moisture exchanger devices**

Type of Device	Classified by Material Used	Classified by Function
A device that uses physical methods to exchange heat and moisture	Heat and moisture exchanger (HME)	Heat and moisture exchanger (HME)
A device that uses material treated hygroscopically	Hygroscopic condenser humidifier (HCH)	Hygroscopic heat and moisture exchanger (HHME)
An HME device with a filter	Heat and moisture exchanging filter (HMEF)	Heat and moisture exchanging filter HMEF)
An HCH device with a filter	Hygroscopic condenser humidifier filter (HCHF)	Hygroscopic heat and moisture exchanging filter (HHMEF)

Best Practice

Contraindications to HME Use

The use of a heat and moisture exchanger during mechanical ventilation is or may be contraindicated for patients with:

- Thick, copious, or bloody secretions.
- An expired tidal volume of less than 70% of the delivered tidal volume.
- A body temperature of less than 32°C.
- A high spontaneous minute volume (>10 Lpm).

Best Practice

HMEs with Inline Nebulizers

Heat and moisture exchanger devices must be removed from the ventilator circuit during aerosol drug therapy when the nebulizer or metered-dose inhaler (MDI) is placed inline. Otherwise, the HME filters and traps the aerosol, resulting in little if any deposition of aerosolized medication to the airway and interference with the therapeutic effect.

HEATING SYSTEMS

Adjuncts to heated humidifiers are heating elements, temperature control units, and heated wire circuits. Their combined use improves the humidity output of any humidifying device and reduces condensation in the tubing.

Heating Elements. Several types of electrical heating sources are available for heating the water contained in the humidifier's reservoir. Three basic designs are described in terms of their location.

- *Immersion heaters* extend a heating element into the water reservoir.
- Other heating elements, such as the Hudson RCI Concha, wrap around the humidity chamber. In this design, an aluminum cylinder (the Concha-Column) that contains a column of water is surrounded by a heating element.
- In other designs, heating plates located at the base of a heating chamber provide the heat, which is transferred by conduction between the heating plate and the base of the aluminum humidifying chamber. Whether the heat source is immersed, wrapped around, or beneath the humidifying chamber, an RH of 100% can be achieved.

Still other types of heating systems provide heat and hydration with high-flow air or oxygen by nasal cannula. Traditionally, the use of a nasal cannula implied low-flow delivery of supplemental oxygen in connection with a bubble humidifier. (These devices are not heated and not capable of producing high humidification.) However, advances in humidification technology and cannula design have led to the development of humidification systems that combine the advantage of 100% RH at body temperature with the comfort of a nasal cannula.

In 2002, Vapotherm introduced the first high-flow humidification system that accomplished this. Their newest device—Precision Flow, shown in Figure 21-6—is capable of delivering a set temperature of 33–43° C at gas flows of 1–40 Lpm with the use of a triple-lumen

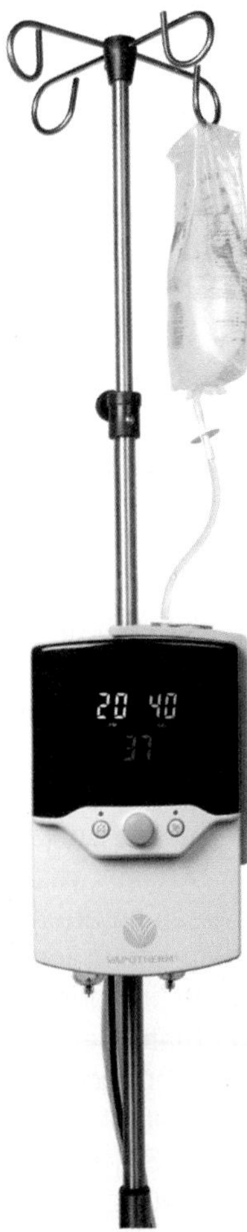

FIGURE 21-6 Vapotherm Precision Flow.
Courtesy of VapoTherm Precision Flow™

patient delivery tube and integrated nasal cannula. Humidification is supplied using a continuous feed reservoir of sterile water to a membrane cartridge that incorporates a permeable membrane. Molecular water vapor is permitted to pass into the gas stream, producing an output of 95–100% RH. The triple-lumen patient delivery tube maintains gas temperature and minimizes condensation in the nasal cannula. Similarly, Smith's Medical AquinOx high-flow system provides heated humidified oxygen therapy at flows of 15–35 Lpm. This system utilizes a heating unit that mounts directly to bottled sterile water. The particulate recovery system reclaims large particles and returns them to the humidification system, so only molecular humidity reaches the patient through a nasal cannula. Both systems vary in alarm features and digital monitoring, but only the Vapotherm device allows the use of flows between 1 and 8 Lpm with the use of their low-flow cartridge, which is suitable for neonatal and pediatric use.[10]

Temperature Control Units. The temperature of these heating elements is regulated by either servocontrolled or nonservocontrolled units.

- A *servocontrolled unit* is a microprocessor closed-loop system that allows a set parameter, such as temperature, to be compared with a measured parameter and that makes an automatic adjustment to maintain the preset value. Power to the heating element is adjusted when a difference exists between the set and measured temperatures. Temperature probes are placed as close to the airway connection as possible on the inspiratory limb of the ventilator circuit so that the monitored temperature reflects the conditions closest to the patient.
- *Nonservocontrolled units* are capable of monitoring the temperature of the heater but are not influenced by the temperature at the patient's airway. In these units, power to the heating element will shut off if the temperature reaches 40°C. The temperature at the patient's airway can be monitored with an external probe, but the respiratory therapist is responsible for adjusting the temperature of the heating element.

Both servocontrolled and nonservocontrolled units incorporate heater alarms to alert the RT of temperature changes in the heating chamber, in addition to an alarm-activated heater shutdown.

Heated Wire Circuits. The advancement of humidifier design has led to improvements in humidity output through heating systems but has increased condensation in the ventilator circuits tubing. As gas leaves the humidifying chamber, it begins to cool because of the ambient temperature on the outside of the tubing. The distance between the heating chamber and the patient connection can be more than 5 feet, which allows for significant cooling before the gas reaches the patient. The heating chamber temperature may be set as high as 39°C, a temperature that allows for some cooling while still providing gas near body temperature when it

CASE STUDY 21-2

The day-shift therapist is assigned to the surgical intensive care unit (SICU). The patient in room 4 has been mechanically ventilated for the past 3 days.

B. C. is a 55-year-old male who was admitted to the SICU after a right upper lobectomy that required postoperative mechanical ventilation. He has a history of emphysema and congestive heart failure. His chart reveals a 50-pack-year smoking history. He has failed two weaning attempts and remains on the ventilator with an endotracheal tube in place.

Respiratory orders include daily weaning parameters and ventilator settings to be adjusted according to weaning protocol.

The morning arterial blood gases reveal pH 7.38, P_aCO_2 45, P_aO_2 88, HCO_3^- 28, and S_aO_2 95%, and an F_IO_2 of 50%. (S_aO_2 is the oxygen saturation of arterial blood. F_IO_2 is the fractional concentration of oxygen; see Chapter 3.)

During the morning assessment, the therapist notes that the patient's heart rate is 100, total respiratory rate is 16 (10 mechanical breaths and 6 spontaneous breaths), breath sounds reveal rhonchi bilaterally, and the S_pO_2 is reading 96%. When the RT attempts to suction, the secretions are thick, yellow, and difficult to clear from the airway. Inspection of the ventilator reveals that the humidifier has been bypassed, and an HME is in line with the ventilator circuit. The daily ventilator flow sheet shows that an HME has been used since the patient was received in the SICU 3 days ago.

Questions

1. What immediate action should you take to rehydrate this patient's airway?
2. When is it appropriate to use an HME device?

reaches the patient's airway. However, the drop in temperature decreases the capacity of the gas to carry water vapor thus causing water molecules to rain out within the tubing.

Heated wire circuits attempt to maintain the set temperature throughout the circuit, preventing any cooling and rainout in the tubing. Heating wires wrapped inside the ventilator circuit are electrically connected to the heating unit close to where the tubing leaves the heating chamber, and they continue to the patient connection so that the tubing is unaffected by the ambient temperature. Servocontrol guarantees regulation of the set temperature throughout the circuit. Reducing the condensation in the tubing eliminates the need for frequent draining and lessens the risk of infection for the patient and the respiratory therapist.

Therapeutic Use of Aerosol-Generating Devices

Aerosol-generating devices, called *nebulizers*, are selected for the delivery of bland or medicated aerosols. The choice of nebulizer is usually made by the ordering physician because of the varying therapeutic effects of such devices. A bland aerosol with sterile water can be administered for 15 minutes every 4 hours with an ultrasonic nebulizer, or it can be delivered by continuous administration with a large-volume nebulizer. Both would provide hydration to the airway; however, the deposition and thus the therapeutic effect of the two devices differ significantly.

A physician who writes a request for aerosolized medication should state the method of delivery preferred for the patient. In some cases, hospital policy on the type of nebulizing devices used may allow the respiratory therapist to convert a patient from the initial device ordered to one that is equal in therapeutic outcome or more clinically appropriate. As shown on Table 21-4, bland or medicated aerosols can be created with a variety of nebulizing devices. Although the respiratory therapist may not make the initial selection of the aerosol-generating device, the RT is responsible for knowing the indications for use of each device in a given situation and whether another device is more appropriate and must be capable of evaluating a patient's response to the therapy selected.[11,12]

INDICATIONS FOR AEROSOL THERAPY

The clinical indications for aerosol therapy are best explained on the basis of the type of agents used for aerosolization.

Bland aerosols can be delivered as either cool or heated aerosols on a continuous or intermittent basis. Both are primarily used to deliver water that is in aerosol form to the patient who presents with upper airway swelling or who has a humidity deficit. Sterile water is the solution of choice for continuous bland aerosols, whether cool or heated.

A cool, bland aerosol with sterile water is usually indicated when upper airway swelling is present. It has been shown that breathing cool air causes a decrease in airway mucosal blood flow, resulting in vasoconstriction and reduction in swelling that may occur postextubation, or with upper airway disorders such as croup.[13] In this situation, the cool aerosol is the most efficient if delivered continuously.

Heated, bland aerosol is primarily used when a humidity deficit exists or during hypothermic situations.

Current practice has promoted the use of continuous bland aerosols with sterile water to promote secretion thinning and spontaneous removal of secretions through coughing or suctioning. However, studies to determine the efficacy of continuous bland aerosol delivery have concluded that there is no scientific evidence that bland aerosol therapy aids in the removal of airway secretions.[14] The AARC CPGs for bland aerosol administration and humidification during mechanical ventilation support these findings and recommend use of cool bland aerosol for upper airway swelling and heated bland aerosol for situations in which a humidity deficit may occur.[5,13]

Aerosolized saline administered intermittently is primarily indicated for sputum induction or as a diluent for aerosolizing pharmacologic agents. The AARC CPG for bland aerosol administration recommends hypotonic or hypertonic salines for inducing sputum specimens.[12] Isotonic or normal saline is used as a diluent, with medication being delivered in aerosol form. In this situation, the saline, which is added to the medication in the appropriate aerosol-generating device, acts as a carrier for the medication. Because dosages of respiratory drugs are so small, the saline extends the aerosol delivery time and promotes deposition to the lower airway.

Medicated aerosols deliver drugs that:

- Reduce inflammation of the mucosal lining.
- Decrease bronchospasm of the airway smooth muscle.
- Prevent allergic response by inhibiting mediator release.
- Restore airway patency by promoting expectoration and clearance of secretions.
- Treat infectious processes through absorption of anti-infectious drugs.

Most medicated aerosols are delivered intermittently and require fewer than 10 minutes to nebulize. Other therapeutic modalities require continuous nebulization of certain drugs by means of special devices. Furthermore, medicated aerosol delivery to the upper and lower airway is far more desirable than systemic delivery because it allows for rapid onset of the desired results without much of the systemic side effects that occur with oral or intravenous routes. The selection of a device that delivers aerosolized medication to the lung parenchyma should be based on the ability of the device to produce aerosol particles with an MMAD of 0.5–3 μm.[15]

HAZARDS

Infection from contamination should always be a concern for the respiratory therapist but especially when aerosol therapy is administered.

Aerosols can carry microorganisms to the patient and deposit them in the airway. Therefore:

- The RT must follow aseptic technique when handling aerosol equipment during the initial set-up and when refilling the nebulizer reservoir.
- Tubing should be drained away from the nebulizer to prevent any microorganisms from contaminating the sterile water inside the reservoir.
- Water traps placed at the dependent portion of the tubing encourages drainage of excess water away from the patient and away from the nebulizer, and they can aid in removal without contamination.

Hazards associated with aerosol therapy may also occur as a result of the agent being aerosolized or the nebulizer being employed. Aerosolization of bland agents delivers additional water to the airway's mucosal lining. The amount of water delivered is based on the output of the nebulizer and the duration of exposure, which is related to the incidence of hazards. When deposition occurs in airways with dried retained secretions, the dried secretions tend to absorb water, causing the mucus to swell. This swelling usually does not pose a problem if measures are taken to promote mobilization and expectoration of the secretions after aerosol therapy:

- Proper coughing techniques
- Postural drainage and percussion
- Possibly aspiration of secretions from the airway

The continuous inhalation of aerosols with sterile water and normal saline presents possible hazards.

- It can lead to overhydration, fluid weight gain, and electrolyte imbalance. Patients especially at risk are infants, patients with existing fluid imbalances such as those in renal or congestive heart failure, and patients in pulmonary edema.
- The administration of bland aerosols can also lead to increased airway resistance due to bronchoconstriction in patients with preexisting respiratory disease, such as asthma. Because the airways of asthmatic patients are hyper-reactive, the mere administration of aerosol particles can induce bronchospasm.
- Cool aerosols tend to cause more airway reactivity than heated aerosols, presumably by the same mechanism that causes exercise-induced bronchospasm.
- Furthermore, aerosolized hypertonic saline is known to be irritating to the airway and responsible for inducing bronchospasm in asthmatic patients.[16] A pretreatment administration of a bronchodilator medication to reduce the likelihood of bronchospasm is recommended.

Hazards associated with medicated aerosols are related to the side-effects of the specific drugs. Respiratory therapists must be aware of the pharmacologic effect of any drug they administer on airway function, cardiovascular response, onset, duration, clearance, and compatibility with other drugs. See Chapter 7 for specific drug information.

Electrical hazards exist with electrically powered nebulizers. The respiratory therapist is responsible for inspecting the device and monitoring its operation, as with any electrical device.

General Principles of Aerosol-Generating Devices

Aerosol generators are available in a variety of designs that determine the physical features, including the particle size, of the aerosol. Nebulizer performance, airway integrity, and the patient's breathing pattern affect how and where the aerosol is deposited in the airway and thus determine the efficacy of the therapeutic intervention.[17]

FACTORS AFFECTING AEROSOL DISTRIBUTION

Several factors are involved in determining the distribution of aerosol particles in the respiratory system.

- Patient-related factors are the patient's ventilatory pattern and airway integrity.
- Device-related factors are nebulizer design and type of delivery device.
- The nature of the aerosol particles and the effect of the RH of the carrier gas determine aerosol stability and the effect on distribution in the lungs.

A very important factor in the distribution of aerosols in the lungs is the *ventilatory pattern* of the spontaneously breathing patient. In the ideal breathing pattern, inspiration is slow and deep, lasts 3–4 seconds, and is twice the normal tidal volume; at the end of the inspiration, there is a 3–5-second breathhold followed by a passive exhalation. The breathhold slows the forward movement of the aerosol, making deposition into the distal airways possible. This pattern, although ideal, is difficult to achieve with a patient who is short of breath, but the RT can achieve it with mechanical manipulation of an artificially ventilated patient.

The type of *flow* created during inspiration is an aspect of the ventilatory pattern that affects distribution.

- A *laminar flow*, which is achieved with slower flow rates, promotes deeper deposition and better distribution of aerosols.
- A *turbulent flow*, which is achieved with faster flow rates, causes inertial impaction of larger aerosols into the upper airways.

Airway integrity also determines the distribution of aerosols in the lungs. A decrease in the lumen of the airway restricts inspiratory flow, causing aerosol deposition to occur in the upper airways, and hinders lower airway distribution. Airway size may be decreased in bronchospasm, in inflammation of the mucosal lining, or in the presence of excess secretions. The respiratory therapist can encourage lower airway deposition by first assessing the airways for signs of increased production of mucus. By employing methods for secretion clearance and following an ideal breathing pattern, the RT can enhance aerosol distribution even when bronchospasm is present.

Nebulizer design determines the initial size range of the aerosols. Certain nebulizers are designed to create particles between 2 and 5 MMAD, thereby delivering aerosols primarily to the lower airway. The internal design of some nebulizers includes structures such as baffles, which shatter the aerosol particles into smaller and smaller sizes, thereby preventing larger particles from entering the main stream of gas flow to the patient. The effect is to promote distribution in the lower airway.

The *delivery device* used also affects aerosol distribution. These devices deliver aerosols through the mouth, the nose and mouth, or an artificial airway.

- Mouth breathing is encouraged because it lacks the filtering effects of the nasal cavity and thereby prevents the filtering out of the aerosols that would occur if the patient were breathing through the nose. Mouth breathing is usually accomplished with a mouthpiece. If necessary, noseclips are used to guarantee breathing entirely through the mouthpiece.
- Patients who are unable to use a mouthpiece, such as small children or unresponsive patients, may require a face mask, which delivers the aerosols to the airway but cannot eliminate nose breathing.
- A face tent or blow-by delivery device delivers aerosols to the immediate space surrounding the patient's mouth, but the patient inhales a much smaller amount of aerosol than with a mouthpiece because the device is open to the room, allowing aerosol to escape.
- When the aerosol is delivered to an artificial airway, the gas flows directly into the patient's lungs. In this situation, the filtering effects of the nose are bypassed as is any potential rainout in the oropharynx.

The performance of the nebulizer and the delivery device in which the aerosol particle is introduced to the airway is enhanced by the respiratory therapist's *interaction with the patient*. Although the initial choice of nebulizer may be the responsibility of the physician, appropriate breathing instructions and the correct choice of a delivery device are the sole responsibility of the respiratory therapist.

TYPES OF AEROSOL GENERATORS

Aerosols can be generated from nebulizers that are pneumatically, electrically, or manually powered. A range of particle sizes can be produced from the various types of nebulizers. The nebulizer reservoir size varies from a small, 5-mL container to one large enough to hold 1000 mL. Knowing how each nebulizer operates and understanding the clinical use for each help the respiratory therapist to properly administer aerosol therapy to the patient who requires respiratory care.

Bulb Nebulizer. The *bulb nebulizer* has earned its place in history as the first hand-held nebulizer that is

Best Practice

Ideal Breathing Pattern

When administering aerosol therapy, the respiratory therapist should encourage the patient to follow an ideal breathing pattern by instructing the patient to:

- Inhale slowly and deeply through the mouth for 3–4 seconds.
- Hold the breath for 3–5 seconds.
- Exhale.

manually powered. To use this nebulizer, the patient must be able to squeeze a rubber bulb that forces airflow through a jet in the reservoir, which contains the medicated solution. This action produces an aerosol that is directed out of the reservoir through the mouthpiece and to the patient. This nondisposable device is designed for single-patient use and is ideal for home use. Patient instruction and coordination are important. The bulb nebulizer has lost popularity since the introduction of smaller devices, such as metered-dose inhalers, which eliminate the need for mixing solutions and are capable of producing smaller particles. Its use today is limited mostly to the nasal or oropharyngeal application of medications.

Dry Powder Inhaler. *Dry powder inhalers* (*DPIs*) are small, portable, manual nebulizing devices that are activated by the patient's inspiratory effort. Medication supplied in a powder capsule is inserted into the DPI container. The DPI is designed to break the capsule open so that, when the patient places the mouthpiece into the mouth and begins to inhale, the powdered medication is available for delivery (Figure 21-7). This device produces particles of 2–6 μm. The patient must generate enough inspiratory flow (greater than 1 L per second) to guarantee delivery of medication to the lower airways. These devices are especially popular for home use and are ideal for patients who cannot coordinate activation and inspiration, as is necessary in other devices.

Age-Specific Competency

Dry Powder Inhalers

The dry powder inhaler is appropriate for patients who can achieve an inspiratory flow greater than or equal to 50 Lpm. Because children under the age of 6 cannot achieve this inspiratory flow, the use of a DPI for this age group is not recommended.

Source: American Association for Respiratory Care. AARC clinical practice guideline: selection of an aerosol delivery device for neonatal and pediatric patients. Respir Care. *1996;40:1325–1335.*

Metered-Dose Inhaler. *Metered-dose inhalers* (*MDIs*) are small pressurized canisters that are manually activated to release medication suspended in a gas propellant. The canister contains 80–300 doses of medication. When the patient depresses the canister, a valve opens, releasing the medication particles with an MMAD of 2–4 μm (Figure 21-8). The gas propellant used until recently was chlorofluorocarbon (CFC), but, because of environmental concerns, CFC has been replaced with other propellants such as hydrofluoroalkanes (HFAs). Once released from the canister, the propellant that carries the medication evaporates into the air, leaving the medication suspended as an aerosol.

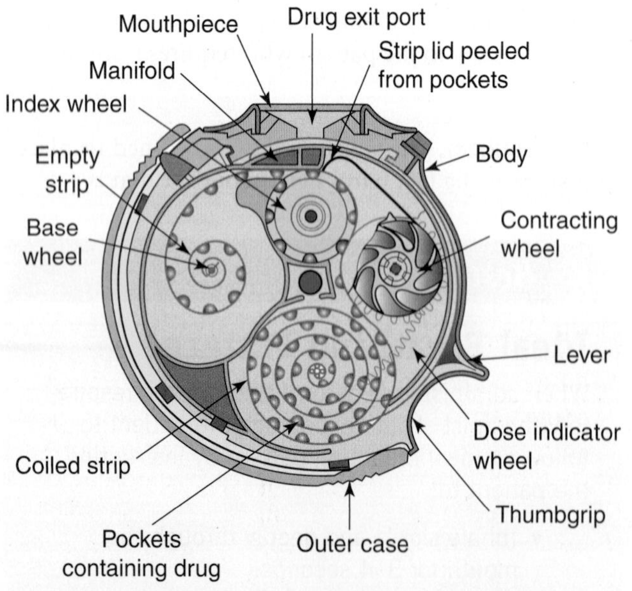

FIGURE 21-7 A cross-section of the discus inhaler, a commonly used dry powder inhaler.

Reprinted with permission of Glaxo Wellcome

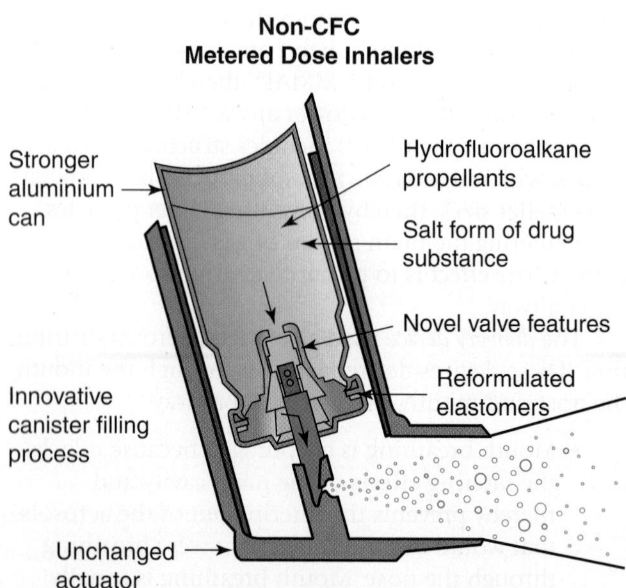

FIGURE 21-8 The functional design of a non-CFC metered-dose inhaler.

Reprinted with permission of Glaxo Wellcome

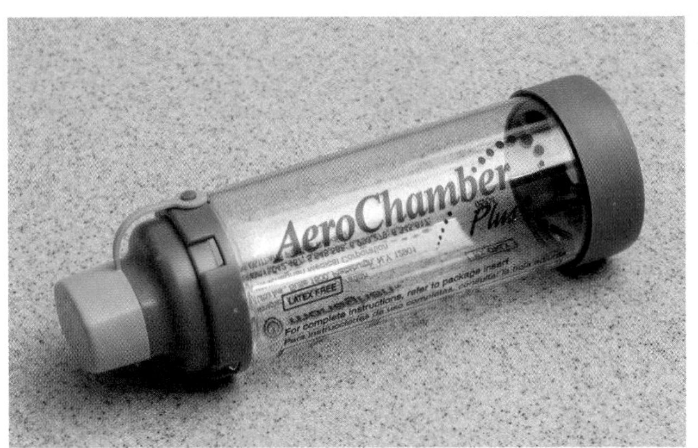

FIGURE 21-9 Spacer used with a metered dose inhaler.

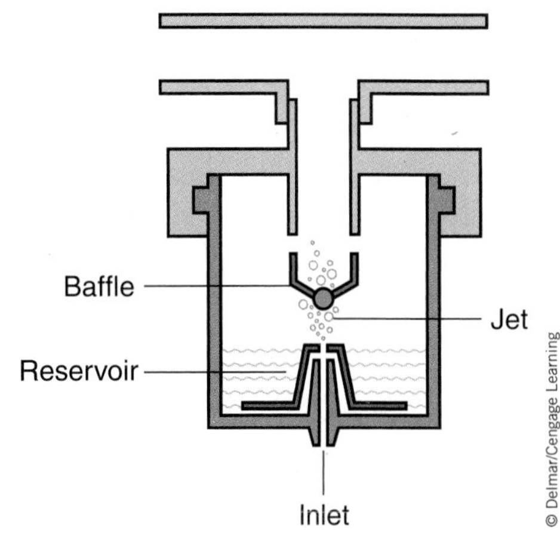

FIGURE 21-10 A small-volume nebulizer.

The use of MDIs for spontaneously breathing patients requires proper patient instruction and coordination of inspiration and activation to achieve optimal deposition. Additional devices, referred to as *spacers* or *chambers*, create a reservoir in which the aerosol particle is held until being inspired by the patient (Figure 21-9). Spacers eliminate the need for synchronizing inspiration and activation. Most spacers incorporate a one-way valve to ensure the flow of medication from the canister through the reservoir to the patient. Some have a signaling device that alerts the patient to reduce inspiratory flow to prevent deposition in the upper airway. Because MDIs are often needed for mechanically ventilated patients, some spacers are made for use with ventilator circuits.

Small-Volume Nebulizers. *Small-volume nebulizers (SVNs)* come in a variety of designs that produce an aerosol with a particle size range of 1–5 μm. They are primarily used in short-term intermittent delivery of aerosolized medication, but they can also be used for delivery of bland aerosols such as hypotonic saline for sputum induction. SVNs require a pneumatic source either from a central piping system or a cylinder to a flowmeter or from an electrical air compressor. Flow rates of 6–8 Lpm are recommended to achieve optimal particle size and aerosol output. Directing the gas flow through a jet within the 5–6-mL reservoir container causes a shearing effect of the liquid solution, producing an aerosol that enters the mainstream of gas flow to the patient (Figure 21-10). They are used in both clinical and home settings.

An SVN can be used as a handheld nebulizer for a spontaneously breathing patient or incorporated into a ventilator circuit for delivery to a patient requiring mechanical breaths. Additionally, SVNs are available as *breath-actuated devices (BANs)*, such as the AeroEclipse II Nebulizer by Monahan Medical. These devices are

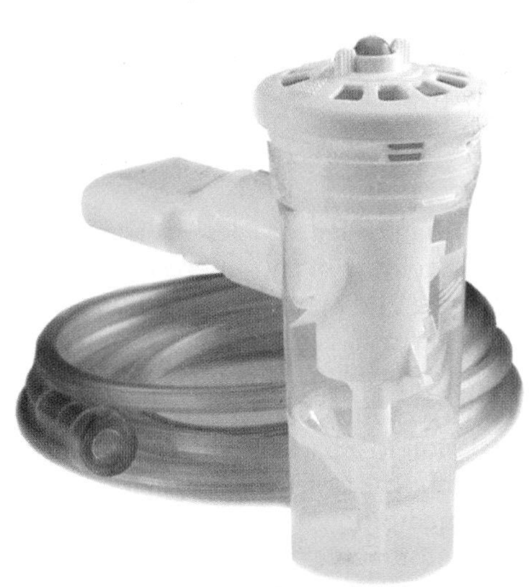

FIGURE 21-11 Aero Eclipse II Breath Actuated Nebulizer.
Courtesy of Monaghan Medical Corporation

designed to decrease aerosol waste during exhalation with the use of a one-way valve that directs gas flow away from the nebulizer chamber. This design prevents medication from being nebulized rather than the traditional practice of using an extension reservoir tubing to trap medication during exhalation. BANs nebulize only when the patient inhales, making them ideal for reduction in therapy time and wasted medication (Figure 21-11).[18] SVNs can be used for the patients of any age—from neonatal to geriatric patients. Common delivery devices are a mouthpiece attached to a Briggs T-adaptor, aerosol face mask, aerosol face tent, trach collar, and inline adaptation for IPPB and ventilator circuits.

The Marquest Respigard II is an SVN that is designed to create a particle size with an MMAD of 0.93 μm, which deposits more deeply in the lung

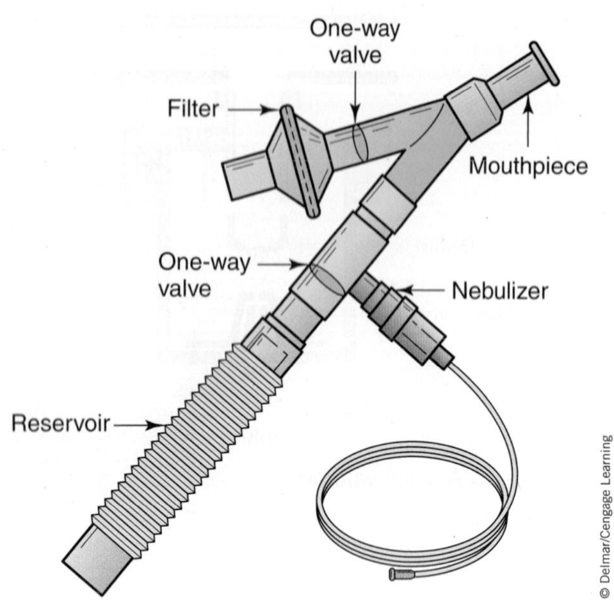

FIGURE 21-12 The small-volume nebulizer assembly of the Marquest Respirgard II.

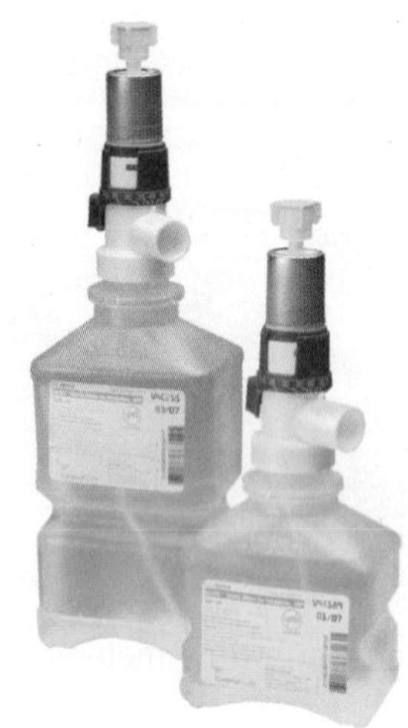

FIGURE 21-13 Large-volume nebulizer.
Courtesy of CareFusion

parenchyma than larger particles do. The SVN's design is ideal when delivery of anti-infectious agents is required (Figure 21-12). Within its nebulizer reservoir, this SVN produces an aerosol that is directed to the patient through a circuit containing one-way valves. The valves act as baffles to trap large particles and to direct exhalation to a bacteria-filtering system on the expiratory limb. The system is designed to prevent any aerosolized medication from escaping into the surrounding environment.

Large-Volume Nebulizers. *Large-volume nebulizers (LVNs)* are designed to provide long-term and continuous nebulization of cool or heated bland aerosols as well as medicated aerosols. A variety of designs are available, all with a large reservoir capable of holding 240–1000 mL of solution. Most LVNs are designed for use with large-bore tubing connected to an aerosol delivery device such as an aerosol mask, face tent, tracheostomy collar, or Briggs T-adaptor. Disposable nebulizers are available for use with or without sterile water, such as the Air*Life* Prefilled Nebulizer or the Portex Unfilled Nebulizer (Figure 21-13).

The oxygen percentage varies among devices. Some provide a range of 40–100%; others provide a range of 21–100%. A flow rate that exceeds the patient's inspiratory flow rate is required for adequate aerosol delivery and to meet the desired F_IO_2, usually above 25 Lpm. The total flow through an LVN that incorporates a jet venturi uses flow from the source gas (oxygen flowmeter) plus room air that is being entrained. The two gases are mixed to provide a precise fractional oxygen concentration (F_IO_2; see Chapters 3 and 20) to the patient. Air-to-oxygen ratios are fixed for each oxygen percentage. For example, the air-to-oxygen ratio for delivering an F_IO_2 of 40% is 3:1. This F_IO_2 setting allows 3 parts of air to be entrained for every 1 part of oxygen. If the oxygen flowmeter is set at 10 Lpm, the amount of room air being entrained is 30 Lpm, making a total flow of 40 Lpm. Table 21-7 lists air-to-oxygen ratios of commonly used F_IO_2s.

Bland aerosol delivery is the most common use for LVNs. Most LVNs incorporate a jet venturi to entrain gas from the oxygen source and room air, allowing precise mixing to achieve the desired F_IO_2. Medical Molding Corporation's Misty Ox Hi-Flo nebulizer is an example of a disposable LVN capable of meeting flow rates of 42–77 Lpm at F_IO_2 ranges of 60–90% (Figure 21-14). The nebulizer is designed to fit a standard reservoir bottle. Depending on the flow rate

TABLE 21-7 **Air-to-oxygen ratios at commonly used fractional oxygen concentrations**

Room Air/Oxygen Ratio	Fractional Oxygen Concentration (%)
25:1	24
10:1	28
8:1	30
5:1	35
3:1	40
1.7:1	50
1:1	60
0:1	100

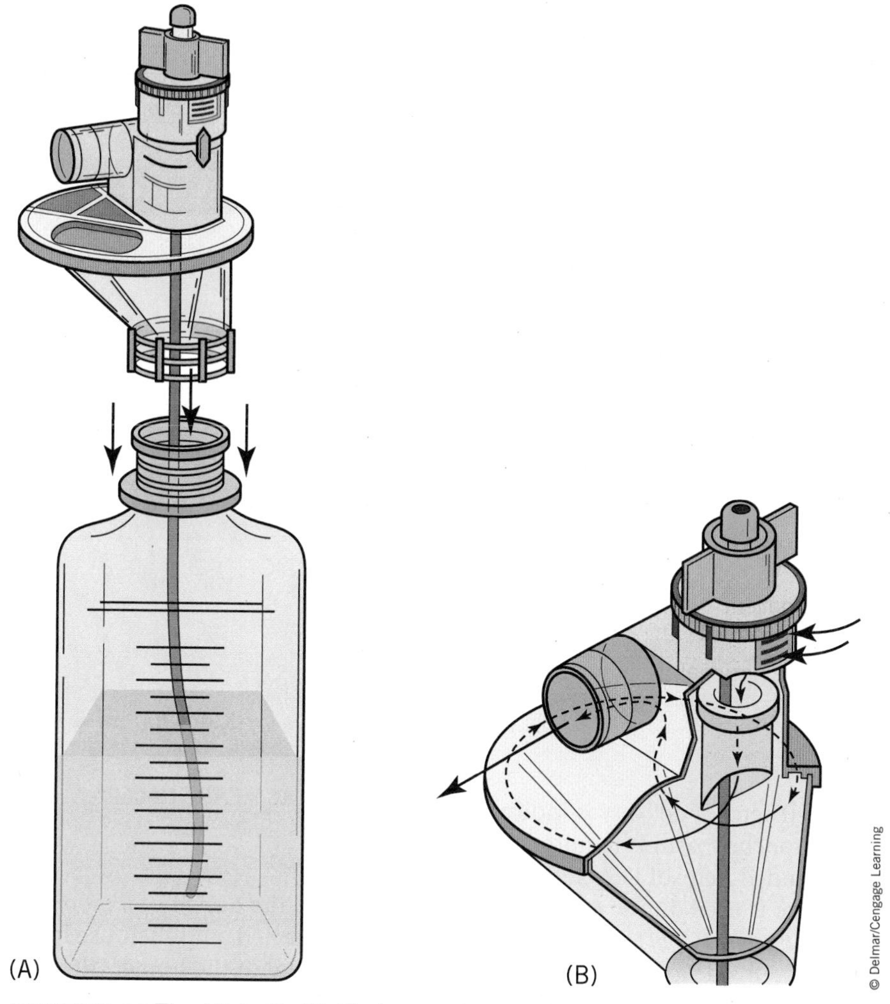

FIGURE 21-14 The Misty Ox Hi-Flo large-volume nebulizer: (A) Assembly. (B) Functional diagram.

and the set F_IO_2, this LVN can provide an aerosol output of 30–50 mg/L with an MMAD of 3 µm.

In certain situations, one nebulizer may not be enough to meet a patient's inspiratory demand. If the patient's inspiratory demand is being met, the aerosol continually flows from the delivery device even when the patient increases inspiratory volume. If the aerosol disappears when the patient inhales, there is not enough gas flow through the device, and the patient draws from the surrounding room air to meet inspiratory needs. The patient's needs for humidification and for oxygen are affected.

A solution to this situation, while maintaining the same F_IO_2 setting, is to pair two oxygen flowmeters and two LVNs with large-bore tubing that is connected to a wye adaptor. Large-bore tubing is then attached to the third port of the wye, and the delivery device of choice can be used at the proximal end of the tubing. This arrangement is referred to as a *tandem set-up* (Figure 21-15). The two flowmeters should be set at the same flow rate, and the two LVNs must be set at the same F_IO_2.

Age-Specific Competency

Nebulizer Interfaces

Depending on a patient's age, which determines ability and coordination, various devices can be used in conjunction with the SVN and MDI to optimize drug delivery. These devices, referred to as *interfaces*, are spacers, accessory devices with mouthpieces, and face masks. Patients younger than 3 years of age may not be able to use a mouthpiece; therefore, a face mask with a spacer device for MDI use or a face mask for SVN use may be necessary. Cooperative children over the age of 3 can receive aerosol therapy via an SVN with a mouthpiece and extension reservoir or via an MDI with a mouthpiece and spacer.

Source: American Association for Respiratory Care. AARC clinical practice guideline: selection of an aerosol delivery device for neonatal and pediatric patients. Respir Care. *1995;40:1325–1335.*

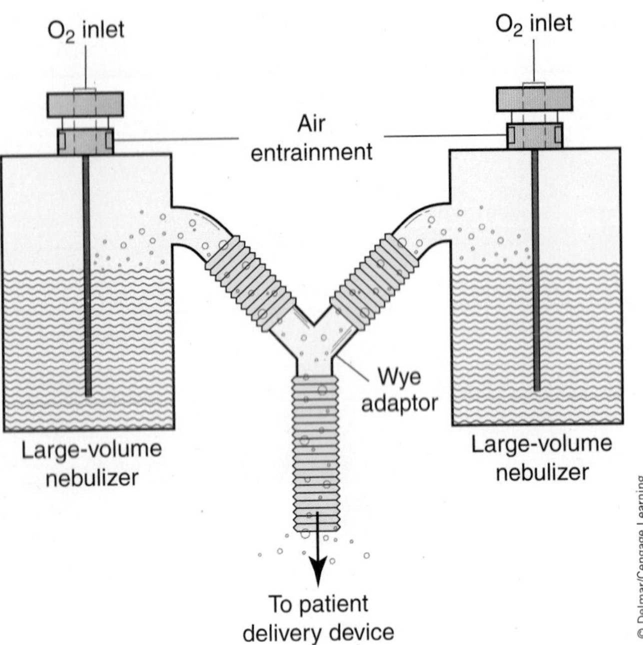

FIGURE 21-15 Assembly and functional design of a tandem large-volume nebulizer set-up.

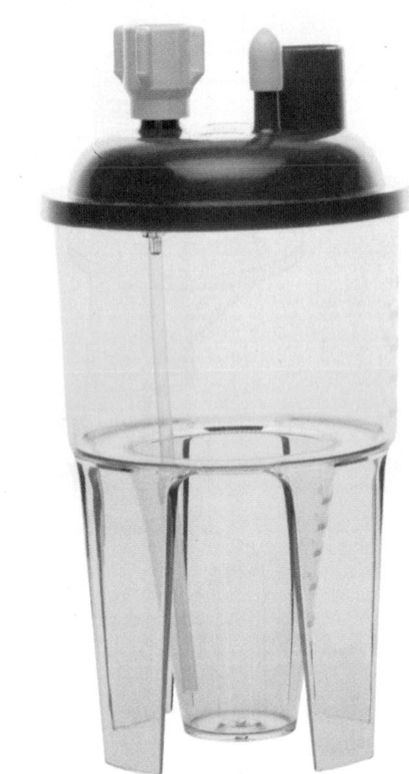

FIGURE 21-16 HEART Nebulizer.
Reprinted with permission of Westmed, Inc.

Continuous medicated aerosol delivery is indicated when aggressive care of bronchospasm is required. The Vortran High Output Extended Aerosol Respiratory Therapy (HEART) nebulizer is used during *continuous bronchodilator nebulization therapy* (*CBNT*). The medication and solution are placed inside a standard reservoir container capable of holding 240 mL. A mini unit with a 30-mL reservoir is also available. The HEART nebulizer produces an aerosol particle size of 3.5–2.2 MMAD, which is optimal for the continuous delivery of aerosols to the lower respiratory tract for up to 8 hours (Figure 21-16), if the flow rate is set at 10 Lpm.

Albuterol with normal saline solution is the recommended bronchodilator for CBNT. Medical centers with the highest emergency room discharge rate and the lowest length of stay for patients treated for moderate to severe asthma are using the following dosages of albuterol:

- 3 mL or more per hour for status asthmaticus cases
- 2 mL per hour for severe asthma cases
- 1 mL per hour for moderate asthma[19]

The patient should be reevaluated 1 hour after initiation of CBNT for improvement in bronchospasm and pulmonary mechanics. The physician's order must include dosage, medication, flow rate, and duration of treatment.

Ultrasonic Nebulizer. The use of ultrasonic sound waves to produce aerosols began in the 1960s. Since that time, the design of *ultrasonic nebulizers* (*USNs*) has been perfected, and their use has been expanded from the hospital to the home. Ultrasonic nebulizers are used in the hospital setting to deliver bland aerosols on an intermittent basis. Smaller, more portable units are available for medication delivery in the home.

The USN is an electrically powered device that sends electrical current to a radio frequency generator. The generator produces electromagnetic energy, which is conducted to a transducer through a shielded cable. In the transducer, a piezoelectric crystal converts electrical energy from the radio frequency to mechanical energy in the form of sound waves. These high-frequency sound waves travel through a water-filled chamber that acts as a medium for the sound waves, transmitting them to the surface of water in the nebulizer chamber, where they break the water into a fine aerosol (Figure 21-17).

Particles generated by a USN can range from 1 to 10 μm with an MMAD of 3 μm. The aerosol output from a USN can range from 60 to 100 mg/L. A fan in the USN creates the gas flow necessary to move the aerosol from the nebulizing chamber to the patient through large-bore tubing attached to a delivery device, usually an aerosol mask or a mouthpiece. To increase the aerosol output, adjust the amplitude of the sound waves by selecting an appropriate setting on the dial. The frequency of the sound waves, which determines

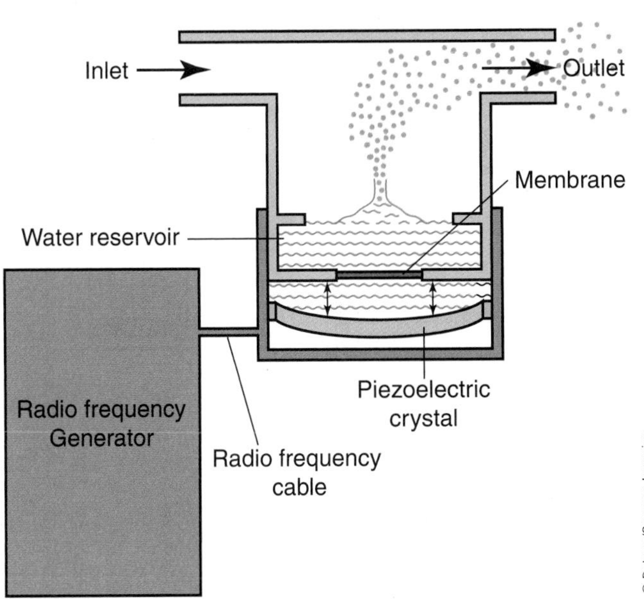

FIGURE 21-17 An ultrasonic nebulizer.

the particle size produced, is preset by the manufacturer and cannot be adjusted. The DeVilbiss Ultra-Neb 99 is a USN used in the hospital setting for intermittent use. Its fine aerosol and high-density output make it ideal for lower respiratory tract hydration of dried retained secretions and for sputum induction (Figure 21-18).

Babbington Nebulizer. The *Babbington nebulizer*, designed for long-term continuous use with aerosol tents, is a pneumatically powered nebulizer that incorporates a pressurized glass sphere. As the sphere is

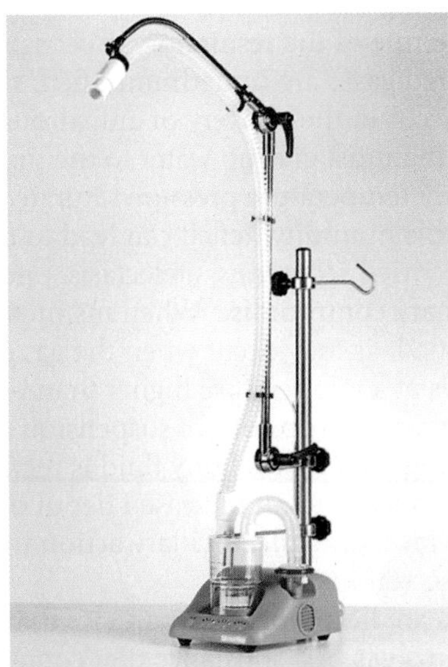

FIGURE 21-18 UltraNeb.

Courtesy of DeVilbiss Healthcare, Inc., Somerset, Pa.

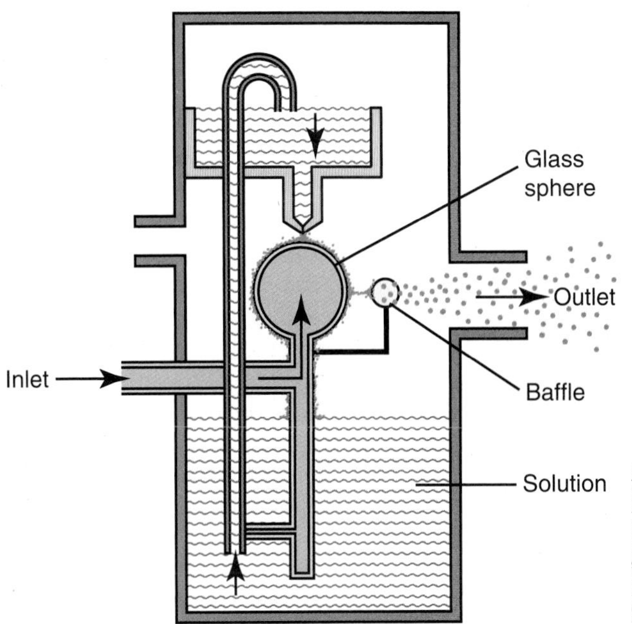

FIGURE 21-19 A Babbington nebulizer.

continually bathed with a bland solution from the reservoir above, an aerosol is produced (Figure 21-19). Gas enters the hollow sphere from an inlet connected to a 50-psig (pounds per square inch gauge) source. The pressure in the inlet channel activates a siphoning system in an adjacent channel that draws liquid in the form of small bubbles up a capillary tube to the reservoir above the glass sphere. The bubble escalator continually fills the reservoir and bathes the surface of the sphere with the solution to be aerosolized. Gas pressure exits the sphere through a very small hole, rupturing the thin sheet of water that coats the sphere, creating a fine aerosol. A baffle positioned in the flow of the aerosol further reduces the particle size.

The Maxi Cool nebulizer uses two glass spheres to produce a high-density output of 60–70 mg/L with an MMAD of 4 μm. Flow rates generated by the Maxi Cool can be as high as 250 Lpm, making the unit ideal for providing a moisture-rich enclosed environment, such as a croup tent, while flushing out heat and exhaled carbon dioxide.

Small-Particle Aerosol Generator. The *small-particle aerosol generator* (*SPAG*) is a nebulizer specifically designed for the administration of ribavirin, an antiviral medication used in the treatment of *respiratory syncytial virus* (*RSV*). This pneumatically powered nebulizer is used in conjunction with an aerosol tent, hood, or mask or in conjunction with a mechanical ventilator. The source gas flows into a regulator set at 26 psig, and the regulator is connected to two flowmeters. One flowmeter directs gas into the nebulizer flask,

CASE STUDY 21-3

The respiratory therapist is covering a medical step-down unit in a university hospital. One of the patients has been successfully weaned from mechanical ventilation and is currently on a 60% LVN to a tracheostomy collar.

The patient, M. W., is a 60-year-old male who was admitted 3 months ago in respiratory failure due to Guillain-Barré syndrome. He was intubated and placed on mechanical ventilation at that time. He required a tracheostomy after 2 weeks of mechanical ventilation. After a slow weaning process, he was placed on a 60% continuous bland aerosol with an LVN to a tracheostomy collar 24 hours ago.

The respiratory orders state that the patient is to remain on a 60% LVN as tolerated. The physician wants to be notified if the respiratory therapist feels that an increase in F_IO_2 is necessary.

The patient's morning arterial blood gas analysis revealed pH 7.39, P_aCO_2 50, P_aO_2 55, HCO_3^-29, S_aO_2 88%.

During the morning assessment, the RT notices that Mr. W. appears to be short of breath and has a respiratory rate of 30 breaths per minute. His pulse oximetry readings show a pulse rate of 102 and an S_pO_2 of 88%. Although the LVN is set up correctly, all of the aerosol disappears from the exhalation port of the tracheostomy collar when the patient inhales. The therapist calculates the total flow from the LVN based on the air-to-oxygen ratio of 1:1 at a flow rate of 15 Lpm.

Questions

1. What is the total flow being delivered to the patient? Is the flow meeting the patient's inspiratory demand?
2. How can the RT maintain the same F_IO_2 setting and guarantee a flow rate that meets the patient's inspiratory demand?

which holds approximately 300 mL of the medication solution. Here, the aerosol particles are produced and travel to a drying chamber. The other flowmeter directs gas into the drying chamber, which functions to dehumidify and reduce the size of the aerosol particle to approximately 1.3 μm within the drying chamber. The aerosol is then directed through large-bore tubing to the delivery device (Figure 21-20).

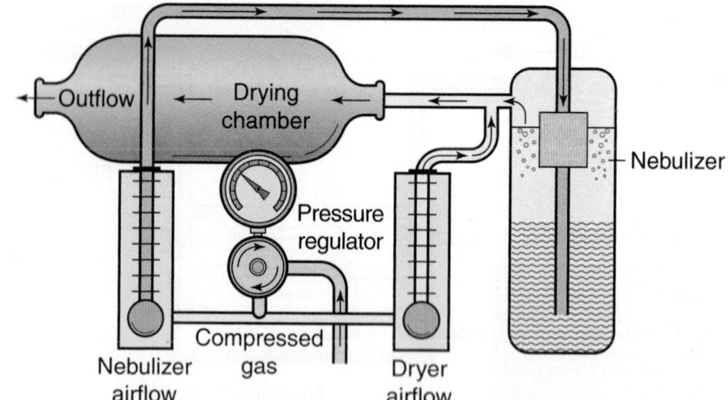

FIGURE 21-20 The functional design of a small-particle aerosol generator.

Summary

Humidity is described in terms of its presence in our environment as absolute humidity (AH) and relative humidity (RH), according to the amount of water vapor present and expressed as water vapor content or water vapor pressure. Temperature affects a gas's ability to carry moisture: As temperature increases, a gas can carry more water vapor; as a gas cools, its capacity to carry water vapor decreases and condensation, or rainout, occurs.

This relation also pertains to inspired gas as it travels through the respiratory system. Humidity in our respiratory system, body humidity, is the water vapor content required to fully saturate alveolar air at normal body temperature. The difference between the body humidity and the absolute humidity of inspired air is called the *humidity deficit*.

Maintaining adequate humidity in the respiratory system is the role of the respiratory mucosal lining. When inspired gases are underhumidified, such as those that occur in the delivery of anhydrous gases, the mucosal lining must give up water to the inspired gas to reach body temperature pressure saturated (BTPS). Over time, this humidity deficit can lead to the retention of thick dried secretions, atelectasis, pneumonia, and pulmonary compromise. When inspired gas is overhumidified, as may occur when the gas contains aerosols or is at a temperature higher than body temperature, water drops out of suspension onto the mucosal lining, and excess body fluid is retained. This fluid retention leads to an increased depth of the aqueous sol layer and affects ciliary action in the removal of secretions.

Aerosols are liquid or solid particles that are suspended in a gas or a substance that contains such particles. Aerosols can occur naturally in the environment or in a chemical reaction, or they can be created

CASE STUDY 21-4

The respiratory therapist is called to the emergency room of a large university hospital for a patient diagnosed as status asthmaticus. When the RT arrives, the nurse assigned to the patient advises that the patient received three bronchodilator treatments by SVN while in transit to the hospital.

Ms. K. M. is a 40-year-old woman with a long history of asthma who has required two intubations in the past 2 years. Ms. M. is unable to speak because of her extreme shortness of breath, but the nurse states that the patient uses her MDI bronchodilator four times a day. She stopped using her corticosteroid inhaler 2 weeks ago because she felt she didn't need it.

The emergency room physician has asked the RT to measure peak flows pre- and postbronchodilator and to administer an aerosol treatment with a bronchodilator via an SVN every 30 minutes.

No lab orders are available.

The patient is obviously unable to perform a peak flow maneuver. As the therapist begins administration of the aerosolized medication, the patient is taking rapid shallow breaths at a rate of 40 per minute. Her breath sounds are very diminished, with posterior lower lobe wheezing bilaterally. The patient's cough is weak, dry, and nonproductive. Before it is time for the next treatment, the nurse calls the RT again, explaining that the patient is extremely short of breath. The patient's dsypnea is slightly relieved during the second treatment, but the bronchospasm persists, and the physician calls for another treatment.

Questions

1. What alternative treatment should the therapist suggest at this time?
2. What equipment is needed to administer a CBNT, and what information should the physician's order include?

artificially. How long an aerosol particle can remain in suspension depends on its size. Size, in turn, is affected by the temperature and RH of the carrier gas and by the tonicity of the solution being aerosolized. Equipment design determines the mass median aerodynamic diameter (MMAD) of the artificially created aerosol, thus determining its initial size. Aerosol stability is also influenced by the kinetic activity of the aerosol particle and the concentration of the particles. The instability of an aerosol particle in the respiratory tract leads to deposition in the upper or lower airway or in the lung parenchyma. Where deposition occurs and the type of agents being used determine the therapeutic effectiveness of the aerosolized solution.

The use of humidity devices in the clinical setting is the responsibility of the respiratory therapist and must be considered when administering dry medical gases. Supplemental humidity in low-flow systems that deliver gas to the upper airway should provide a minimum output of 10 mg/L, whereas a high-flow system delivering gas that bypasses the upper airway should provide a minimum of 30 mg/L. Hazards of humidity therapy include excessive delivery of heat and moisture, electrical malfunctions, and risk of infection. The effectiveness of humidity devices depends on the temperature of the water and gas, the length of contact time, and the surface area of the liquid-to-gas interface.

The types of low-flow humidity devices are various types of bubble humidifiers such as the diffuser and jet humidifier. High-flow devices are the passover and wick humidifiers and the heat and moisture exchangers. These systems can deliver humidity that is cool or heated using heating elements that are servocontrolled or nonservocontrolled. Systems such as the Vapotherm and Aquinox are high-flow, high-humidity, heated systems designed for use with a nasal cannula. Heated wire circuits are an adjunct to humidification systems that attempt to eliminate the excess condensation due to changes in temperature within the ventilator circuit.

The use of aerosol-generating devices in the clinical setting requires a physician's order in most hospitals or a respiratory care department protocol to allow the respiratory therapist to choose the type of nebulizer that will meet the patient's needs. Aerosols are delivered as bland solutions or as medicated solutions, for intermittent therapy or continuous therapy, to achieve a variety of desired effects. Hazards of aerosol therapy are contamination, overhydration, swelling of dried secretions, medication side effects, and shock from electrically powered devices. Aerosol deposition in the airway is determined by the patient's ventilatory pattern, the integrity of the airway, nebulizer design, and delivery device. The types of aerosol generators are bulb nebulizers, dry powder inhalers, metered-dose inhalers, small-volume nebulizers, large-volume nebulizers, ultrasonic nebulizers, Babbington nebulizers, and small-particle aerosol generator (SPAG) units.

The respiratory therapist must understand the principles of hydration of the respiratory tract to maintain a humidity balance in a patient's airways and must determine the need for medication delivery to the airways of the compromised patient. In aerosol and humidity therapy, selecting the most appropriate device, monitoring the functioning of the device, assessing the patient, and making any necessary changes are the responsibilities of the respiratory therapist.

Study Questions

REVIEW QUESTIONS

1. What are the differences between providing humidification and delivering an aerosol to a patient's airway?
2. When dehydration of the mucosal lining occurs, what conditions may result?
3. Which low-flow humidification device provides the greatest amount of relative humidity?
4. Which aerosol device provides the greatest amount of absolute humidity?
5. What are the benefits of providing supplemental humidity to a patient receiving oxygen therapy?
6. What are the benefits of administering aerosolized medication via the inhaled route?

MULTIPLE-CHOICE QUESTIONS

1. Which of the following heating devices could be used to increase the temperature of water in a nondisposable large-volume nebulizer?
   a. hot plate
   b. immersion rod
   c. heating chamber
   d. heated wire circuit
2. Which aerosol delivery device cannot be used to administer medication?
   a. small-volume nebulizer
   b. metered-dose inhaler with spacer
   c. ultrasonic nebulizer
   d. Babbington nebulizer
3. Which of the following devices is capable of delivering 100% RH with the use of a nasal cannula?
   a. bubble humidifier
   b. ultrasonic nebulizer
   c. Vapotherm hydration system
   d. Fisher & Paykel wick humidifier
4. Heated wire circuits are used with mechanical ventilation for all of the following reasons except to:
   a. reduce the amount of condensation in the tubing.
   b. maintain an even temperature from the exit port of the humidifier to the patient connection.
   c. prevent overhydration.
   d. eliminate the need for frequent drainage of excess water in the circuit.
5. If inspired gas in the lower airway contains 43.9 mg/L water vapor and the absolute humidity of the room at 21°C is 9 mg H_2O/L, what is the humidity deficit between the alveolar and ambient air?
   a. 43.0 mg H_2O/L
   b. 34.9 mg H_2O/L
   c. 52.9 mg H_2O/L
   d. 61.2 mg H_2O/L
6. What is the RH if the water vapor content of room air at 24°C is 21.8 mg/L and the AH is 12.8 mg H_2O/L?
   a. 50%
   b. 55%
   c. 59%
   d. 60%

CRITICAL-THINKING QUESTIONS

1. J. A. is a frequently admitted patient with a long history of cystic fibrosis. His current chief complaint is an increased production of thick secretions that he is unable to clear. The physician would like to supplement his oxygen on the basis of an oxygen saturation of 88%. What device would you recommend?
2. J. A.'s condition deteriorates, and he requires a higher F_IO_2. The physician orders an oxygen concentration of 60% but does not order a specific device. What devices could deliver a 60% F_IO_2? Which device would the RT recommend, and why?
3. J. A. now requires intubation and mechanical ventilation. What devices can be used in conjunction with a mechanical ventilator, and which device would be most suited for this patient?
4. After selecting a humidification device to be used with mechanical ventilation, what should the RT inspect? What precautions should the RT take before connecting this device to the patient?

References

1. Jackson C. Humidification in the upper respiratory tract: a physiological overview. *Intensive Crit Care Nurs.* 1996;12:27–32.
2. Williams R, Rankin N, Smith T, Galler D, Seakins P. Relationship between the humidity and temperature of inspired gas and the function of the airway mucosa. *Crit Care Med.* 1996;24:1920–1929.
3. Omari C, Schofield BH, Mitzner W, Freed AN. Hyperpnea with dry air causes time-dependent alterations in mucosal morphology and bronchovascular permeability. *J Appl Physiol.* 1995;78:1043–1051.

4. Ronnestad I, Thorsen E, Segadal K, Hope A. Bronchial response to breathing dry gas at 3.7 Mpa ambient pressure. *Eur J Appl Physiol*. 1994;69:32–35.
5. American Association for Respiratory Care. AARC clinical practice guideline: humidification during mechanical ventilation. *Respir Care*. 1992;37: 887–890.
6. Chatburn R, Primiano FP. A rational basis for humidity therapy. *Respir Care*. 1987;32:249–254.
7. National Fire Protection Association. *NFPA 1999: Standard for Health Care Facilities*. Quincy, MA: American National Standards Institute/National Fire Protection Association; 1999.
8. Vitacca M, Clini E, Foglio K, Scalvini S, Marangoni S, Quadri A, Ambrosino N. Hygroscopic condenser humidifiers in chronically tracheostomized patients who breathe spontaneously. *Eur Respir J*. 1994;7:2026–2032.
9. Branson R. Humidification for patients with artificial airways. *Respir Care*. 1999;44:630–641.
10. Walsh, B. Comparison of High Flow Nasal Cannula Devices. *Respir Care*. 2006 AARC Open Forum Abstract.
11. American Association for Respiratory Care. AARC clinical practice guideline: selection of device, administration of bronchodilator, and evaluation of response to therapy in mechanically ventilated patients. *Respir Care*. 1999;44:105–113.
12. American Association for Respiratory Care. AARC clinical practice guideline: selection of an aerosol delivery device. *Respir Care*. 1992;37:891–897.
13. LeMere C, Kim H, Chediak AD, Wanner A. Airway blood flow responses to temperature and humidity of inhaled air. *Respir Physiol*. 1996;105:235–239.
14. American Association for Respiratory Care. AARC clinical practice guideline: bland aerosol administration. *Respir Care*. 1993;38:1196–1200.
15. American Association for Respiratory Care. AARC clinical practice guideline: selection of a device for delivery of aerosol to the lung parenchyma. *Respir Care*. 1996;41:647–653.
16. Makker HK, Walls AF, Goulding D, Montefort S, Varley JJ, Karrol M, Howarth PH, Holgate ST. Airway effects of local challenge with hypertonic saline in exercise-induced asthma. *Am J Respir Crit Care Med*. 1994;149:1012–1019.
17. Dolovich M. Influence of inspiratory flow rate, particle size and airway caliber on aerosolized drug delivery to the lung. *Respir Care*. 2000;45:597–608.
18. Hess, D. Aerosol delivery devices in the treatment of asthma. *Respir Care*. 2008:53:699–715
19. Ferrante S, Painter E. Continuous nebulization: a treatment modality for pediatric asthma patients. *Pediatr Nurs*. 1995;21:327–331.

Suggested Readings

American Association for Respiratory Care. AARC clinical practice guideline: selection of an aerosol delivery device for neonatal and pediatric patients. *Respir Care*. 1995;40:1325–1335.

Branson RD, Davis Jr K. Evaluation of 21 passive humidifiers according to the ISO 9360 standard: moisture output, dead space, and flow resistance. *Respir Care*. 1996;41:736–743.

Branson RD, Davis Jr K, Brown R, Rashkin M. Comparison of three humidification techniques during mechanical ventilation: patient selection, cost, and infection considerations. *Respir Care*. 1996;41: 809–816.

Branson RD, Campbell RS, Johannigman JA, Ottaway M, Davis Jr K, Luchette FA, Frame S. Comparison of conventional heated humidification with a new active hygroscopic heat and moisture exchanger in mechanically ventilated patients. *Respir Care*. 1999;44:912–917.

Chatbaurn, R. A new system for understanding nebulizer performance. *Respir Care*. 2007:52:1037–1050

Corkery K. Inhalable drugs for systemic therapy. *Respir Care*. 2000;45:831–835.

Dhaud R, Fink J. Dry powder inhalers. *Respir Care*. 1999;44:940–951.

Dolovich M, MacIntyre NR, Anderson PJ, Camargo CA, Chew N, Cole CH, Dhand R, Fink JB, Gross NJ, Hess DR, Hickey AJ, Kim CS, Martonen TB, Pierson DJ, Rubin BK, Smaldone GC. Consensus statement: aerosols and delivery devices. *Respir Care*. 2000;45:589–596.

Fink J, Dhand R. Technology at the bedside: aerosol therapy in respiratory care. *Respir Care*. 1995;44: 24–25.

Mitchell JP, Nagel MW, Rau J. Performance of large-volume versus small-volume holding chambers with chlorofluorocarbon-albuterol and hydrofluoroalkane-albuterol sulfate. *Respir Care*. 1999;44:38–44.

Whitaker KB. *Comprehensive Perinatal & Pediatric Respiratory Care*. 3rd ed. Clifton Park, NY: Delmar Cengage Learning; 2001.

White G. *Equipment Theory for Respiratory Care*. 4th ed. Clifton Park, NY: Delmar Cengage Learning; 2004.

CHAPTER 22

Hyperinflation Therapy

John A. Rutkowski

OBJECTIVES

Upon completion of this chapter, the reader should be able to:

- State the physiological basis for hyperinflation therapy.
- List the indications for and discuss the appropriateness of the three hyperinflation therapy modalities: sustained maximal inflation, continuous positive airway pressure, and intermittent positive pressure breathing.
- Identify the hazards and contraindications of the various modalities used for hyperinflation therapy.

OUTLINE

KEY TERMS

atelectasis
biofeedback
collateral ventilation
continuous positive airway pressure (CPAP)
elastic recoil
functional residual capacity (FRC)
glossopharyngeal breathing (GPB)
hyperinflation
incentive spirometry (IS)
inspiratory capacity (IC)
intermittent positive pressure breathing (IPPB)
pleural pressure
positive airway pressure (PAP)
surface tension
sustained maximal inflation (SMI)
total lung capacity (TLC)

Periodic deep breaths are essential for maintaining adequate bronchial hygiene. A normal breathing pattern incorporates periodic deep breaths called *sighs*. Patterns of shallow, monotonous tidal ventilation without deep breaths lead to a gradual collapse of alveoli, beginning within an hour. If the pattern is maintained for several hours, gross atelectasis develops, and reinflation may be difficult.[1] The collapse of alveoli leads to impaired gas exchange and retention of secretions. If allowed to progress, pneumonia may result.

This chapter reviews therapeutic modalities collectively referred to as **hyperinflation** therapy. Most patients can achieve adequate hyperinflation without assistance. Some patients may achieve better results with the use of a biofeedback device; others may require the assistance of a device capable of generating positive pressure. The selection of appropriate interventions based on patient assessment in conjunction with multidisciplinary care plans is a vital role of the respiratory therapist.

Unfortunately, these interventions are all too often considered routine. Effective hyperinflation therapy demands that patients are assessed and appropriate interventions initiated, coached to achieve the best results, and monitored to determine clinical impairment and adjustments in care plans. Positive outcomes may shorten length of stay, reduce admission or readmission to critical care units, improve patient satisfaction, and contribute to reduced expenses.

Although hyperinflation therapy has application in bronchial hygiene, this chapter generally addresses the prophylaxis and treatment of alveolar collapse. Because airway obstructions can result in the development and progression of atelectasis, bronchial hygiene therapies often play a significant role in the prophylaxis and treatment of alveolar collapse.

Key Definitions, Concepts, and Professional Standards

A *hyperinflation maneuver* is a breathing pattern that emphasizes an inflation to **total lung capacity (TLC)** and maintenance of a normal **functional residual capacity (FRC)**. Ideally, high alveolar inflating pressure is exerted for a long period of time, resulting in the largest possible inhaled tidal volume.[1] The alveolar inflating pressure can be achieved with positive or negative pressure. The inhaled volume should be measured with either method.

The relationship among three forces determines the functional residual capacity.[2]

- Pulmonary **atelectasis** is the collapse of lung tissue.
- The **elastic recoil** of the lungs and chest wall, combined with **surface tension,** tends to cause collapse of the lung.
- **Pleural pressure** (normally negative) provides a countering force that tends to expand the lung.

These concepts are illustrated in Figure 22-1.

Atelectasis may occur owing to decreases in distending pressure (compressive atelectasis) or as the result of airway obstruction (obstructive atelectasis).

- *Compressive atelectasis* is seen in patients who have suffered pleural effusion, pneumothorax, hemothorax, or similar conditions.
- *Obstructive atelectasis* is the result of a complete obstruction of an airway.

Atelectasis is associated with increased physiologic shunting and reduced FRC. Although atelectasis has a number of causes, it is frequently associated with the postsurgical period. If atelectasis is caused by mucus obstruction of the airway, the techniques utilized to enhance the removal of secretions (see Chapter 23) may be helpful in correcting conditions that lead to lung collapse.

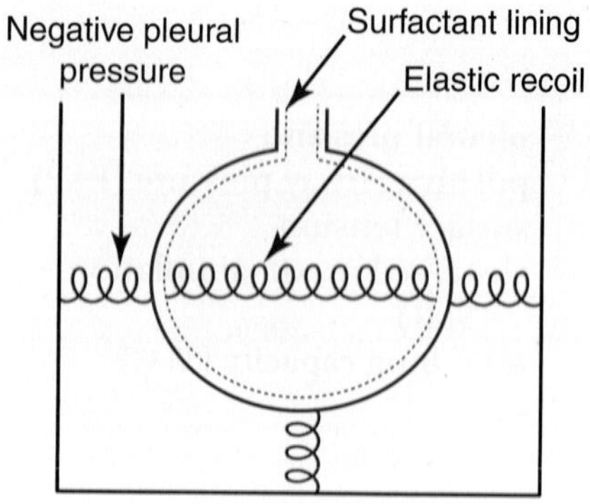

A. Forces in the normal lung

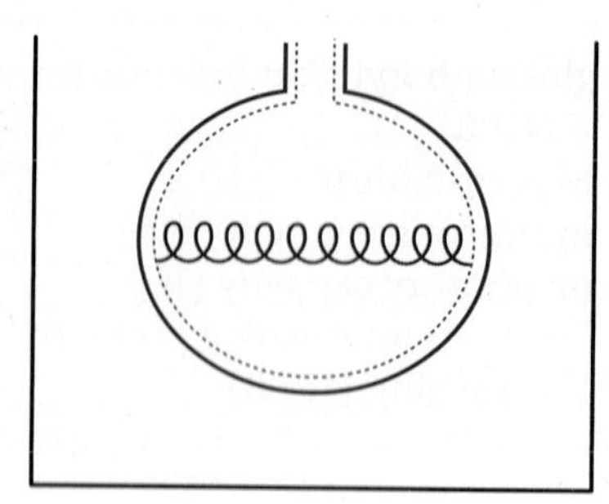

B. Lack of distending forces on the lung

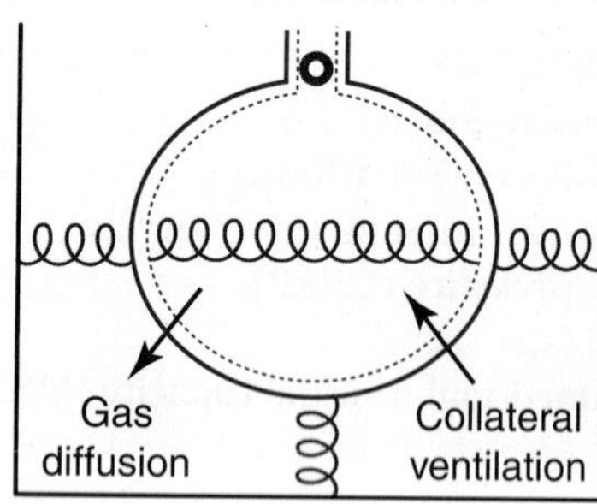

C. Localized airway obstruction

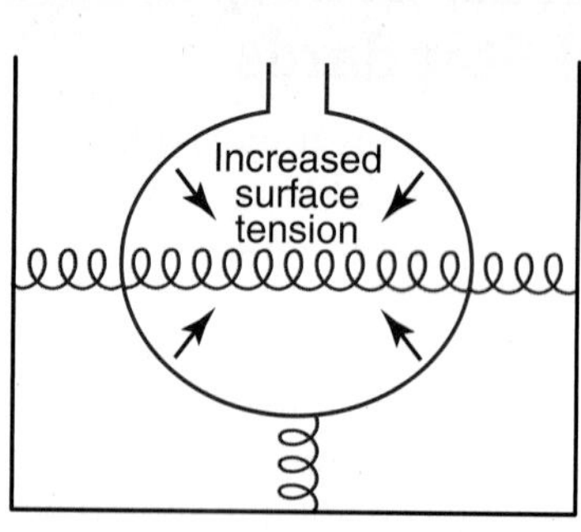

D. Insufficient surfactant

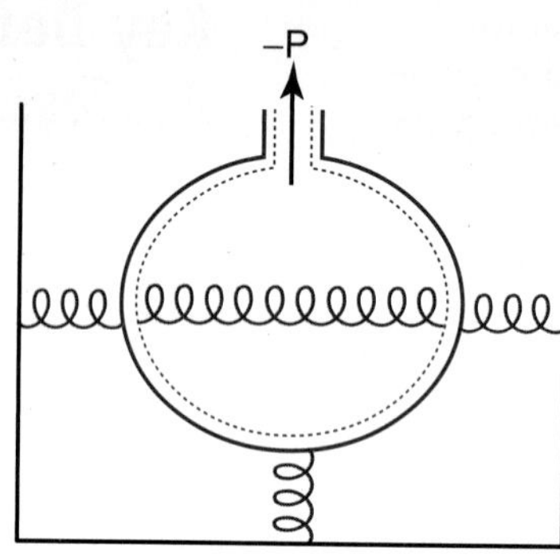

E. Negative airway pressure

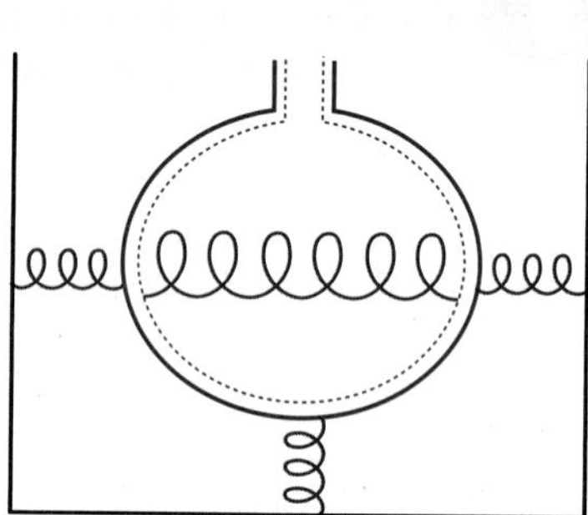

F. Increased lung elastic recoil

FIGURE 22-1 Models illustrating mechanisms involved in pulmonary atelectasis.
Courtesy of Respiratory Care, Dallas, Texas

AMERICAN ASSOCIATION FOR RESPIRATORY CARE CLINICAL PRACTICE GUIDELINES

A *clinical practice guideline* (*CPG*) is a systematically developed statement to help practitioners deliver appropriate care in specific clinical circumstances. The guidelines serve to improve consistency and appropriateness of care and as guides for education and research.[3] CPGs dealing with hyperinflation therapy include the following:

- Directed Cough[4]
- Incentive Spirometry[5]
- Use of Positive Airway Pressure Adjuncts to Bronchial Hygiene Therapy[6]
- Intermittent Positive Pressure Breathing[7]
- Perspectives in Disease Prevention and Health Promotion Update: Universal Precautions for Prevention of Transmission of Human Immunodeficiency Virus, Hepatitis B Virus, and Other Bloodborne Pathogens in Health Care Settings[8]

The guidelines review indications, contraindications, hazards/complications, and assessment of outcomes.

Historical Perspectives

Over the years, a number of approaches have been taken to prevent or reverse lung collapse. These techniques include:

- Rebreathing of carbon dioxide or breathing of gas mixtures with concentrations of carbon dioxide great enough to stimulate increased minute ventilation. The inhalation of gases with increased carbon dioxide levels induces hyperventilation but primarily with increased respiratory rate.
- Resistive breathing devices (blow bottles), as shown in Figure 22-2.[9] The patient must exhale with sufficient force to move the water from the first container to the second. Resistive breathing devices are more likely to be successful if a deep breath and a prolonged exhalation are incorporated into the maneuver.[9]

DEVELOPMENT OF POSITIVE PRESSURE BREATHING

Intermittent positive pressure breathing (IPPB) was introduced into clinical practice in 1947.[10] In the

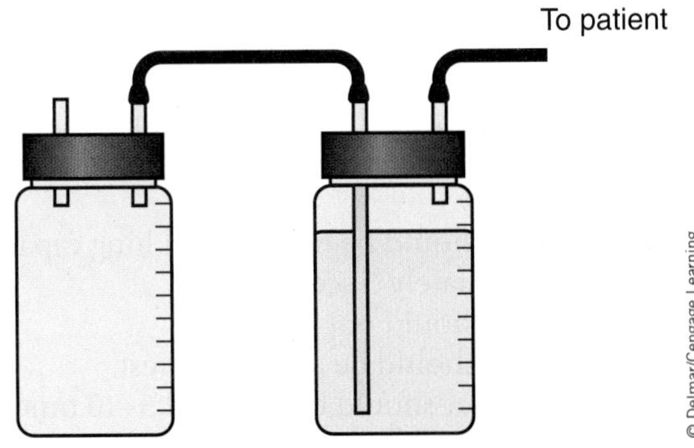

FIGURE 22-2 System to create resistance breathing.

years after its introduction, it attained broad acceptance, and its application increased with little regard for its appropriateness. In 1974 at the Conference on the Scientific Basis for Respiratory Therapy (the so-called Sugarloaf Conference),[11] it was generally concluded that the clinical evidence could not support the widespread use of IPPB, and the participants recommended continued investigation into its effectiveness and appropriateness. A few years later, at a conference on the use of in-hospital respiratory therapy,[12] IPPB was again identified as overused.

Subsequently, the Respiratory Care Committee of the American Thoracic Society[13] released guidelines for the use of IPPB, and the American Association for Respiratory Care provided an assessment of its effectiveness[14] and clinical practice guidelines[7] for its use.

Hyperinflation Therapy

Hyperinflation therapies are utilized primarily for the prevention and treatment of pulmonary atelectasis.

PHYSIOLOGIC BASIS

The physiologic basis for lung reexpansion or for the prevention of atelectasis depends on the relationship between distending pressure and the resulting change in lung volume. The key factor in preventing atelectasis or in the reexpansion of small areas of collapsed lung appears to be a deep, prolonged inspiratory effort.[15] This factor should be included when preparing treatment plans for the prevention or reversal of lung collapse.

COLLATERAL CHANNELS

Alternate pathways for the movement of air in the lung may be provided by:

- Interalveolar communications such as the pores of Kohn (Figure 22-3).

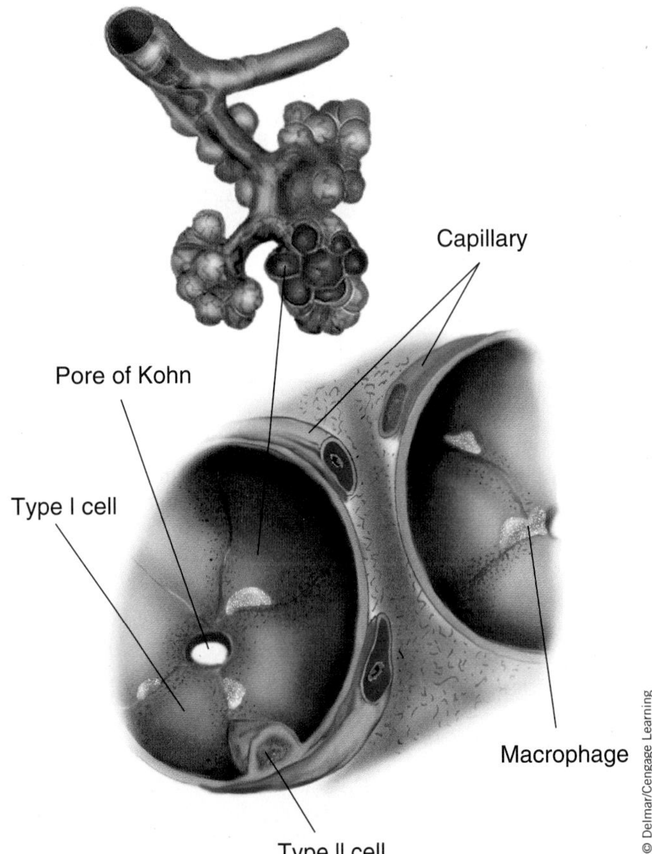

FIGURE 22-3 Collateral ventilation channels: pores of Kohn.

- Bronchiole-alveolar channels called the canals of Lambert (Figure 22-4).
- Interbronchiolar communications.

A number of investigators have related that complete obstruction of an airway is not always followed by alveolar collapse and that ventilation and gas exchange distal to an obstruction could be well preserved by **collateral ventilation.**[16]

Deep Breathing Techniques

Essential elements of most care plans aimed at the prevention or resolution of pulmonary atelectasis are deep breathing techniques. In most instances when patients have a reduced lung compliance or shallow breathing patterns, they are at risk for atelectasis and the retention of secretions. These problems can often be reversed by voluntary or assisted lung expansion, provided the large airways remain patent. Spontaneous deep breathing using the diaphragm and chest wall tends to better expand the dependent areas of the lung where atelectasis is likely to occur.[17]

How the deep breathing is carried out may also be important. Multiple short, deep breaths have little

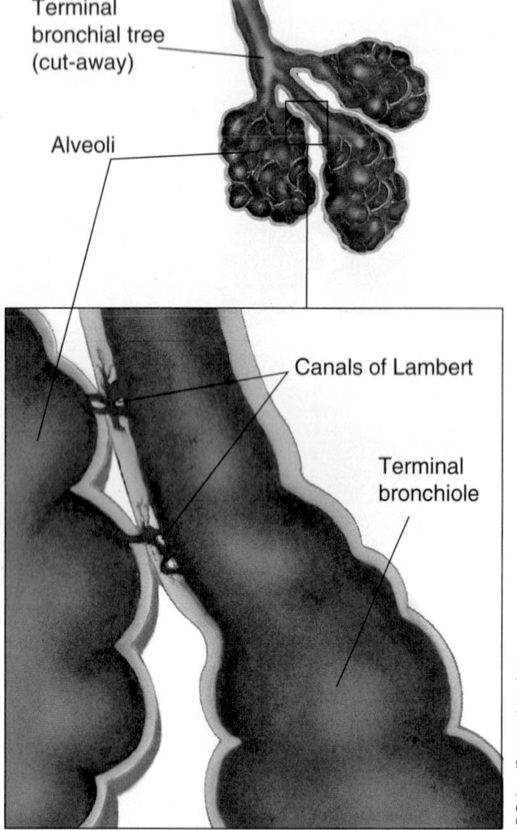

FIGURE 22-4 Collateral ventilation channels: canals of Lambert.

effect on altering lung volume and function; sustained inspiratory efforts are more effective.

- The patient should be coached to inspire slowly from the normal end-expiratory level to total lung capacity.
- The breath should be held at total lung capacity for approximately 5 seconds.
- Exhalation should not be forced.
- The patient should be allowed to rest.
- The maneuver should be repeated 5–10 times each hour.

Age-Specific Competency

Deep-Breathing Exercises

Young children can be taught to perform deep-breathing exercises. Many activities can be utilized to encourage lung expansion and can also be enjoyable for the patient.[18] Providing the child with a surgical glove, which can be easily inflated, makes the sessions more enjoyable. As the child inflates the toy or glove, the caregiver should coach the child to take deep inspirations with an inspiratory hold prior to inflating the glove. If the child is to have elective surgery, deep breathing instruction and practice should occur prior to surgery. Also, provide adequate supervision and avoid potential hazards for aspiration (small balloons or broken pieces).

Best Practice

Deep-Breathing Exercises

When indicated, sequential deep breaths (5–10) are necessary to increase compliance. Each breath should be held at or near total lung capacity for 5 seconds to allow inflation of poorly ventilated areas through collateral ventilation channels. Exhalation should not be forced and should end at the normal end-expiratory level (not continued into the FRC). This sequence should be repeated once every hour while the patient is awake. After thoracic or upper abdominal surgery, the management of pain during the postoperative period is important in maximizing success with voluntary deep breathing exercises. Preoperatively, the respiratory therapist should instruct the patient in the splinting of incisions, as well as in the sustained maximal inflation maneuver and use of incentive spirometer when indicated.

CASE STUDY 22-1

E. D., a 65-year-old woman, was admitted to the hospital for treatment of cholecystitis. On the second day of her hospital stay, a cholecystectomy was performed. The surgery and recovery were uneventful, and she was returned to her room for postoperative care. On the second day after surgery, the nurse observed that her heart rate and respiratory rate were increased and that she had an increased temperature. Auscultation revealed a decrease in breath sounds in the bases and inspiratory crackles.

Questions

1. What clinical process(es) might have brought about the sudden change in this patient's vital signs?
2. How should the RT assess this patient?
3. What elements would the RT include in the plan of care?

Glossopharyngeal Breathing

Glossopharyngeal breathing (GPB) (sometimes referred to as *frog breathing* or *glossopharyngeal insufflation*) is a method of increasing the lung volume at end-inspiration (Figure 22-5). This method utilizes the muscles of the mouth and pharynx to add additional air to the volume already inspired by gulping boluses of air into the lungs. GPB was first described in the 1950s when it was used by patients with weak inspiratory muscles to augment tidal volumes and to prolong the time they were able to remain off mechanical ventilator support.[19]

The technique may be useful in patients with a reduced vital capacity due to inspiratory muscle paralysis or weakness. It is a form of positive pressure ventilation produced by the patient's voluntary muscles, in which boluses of air are forced into the lungs. To breathe in, a series of pumping strokes are produced by the action of the lips, tongue, soft palate, pharynx, and larynx. Air is held in the chest by the larynx, which acts as a valve, as the mouth is opened for the next gulp.[20]

An alternative to glossopharyngeal breathing for patients who have glottis dysfunction is passive lung insufflation with breath stacking. This is accomplished using a manual resuscitator with a closed expiratory port. The closed expiratory port mimics a closed glottis (Figure 22-6). Expanding the lungs beyond inspiratory capacity:

- Increases lung distention.
- Improves the ability to cough.
- Can decrease atelectasis.
- Can improve lung compliance.[21]

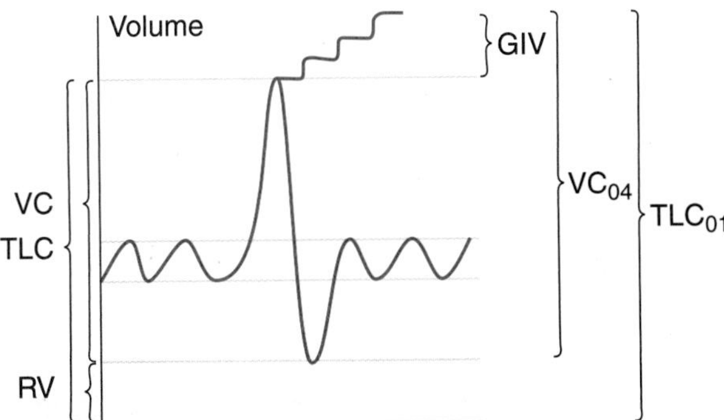

FIGURE 22-5 Schematics of lung volumes (*V*) achieved with normal breathing (TLC, RV, and vital capacity, VC), and with glossopharyngeal insufflation and GI (glossopharyngeal insufflation volume, GIV). GI adds air to lungs. The individual steps in the GIV represent separate boluses of air injected with each cycle. Volume (*V*), total lung capacity (TLC).

Modified from Lindholm P, et al. A fluoroscopic and laryngoscopic study of glossopharyngeal insufflations and exsufflation. Respiratory Physiology and Neurobiology. *2009:167:189–194.*

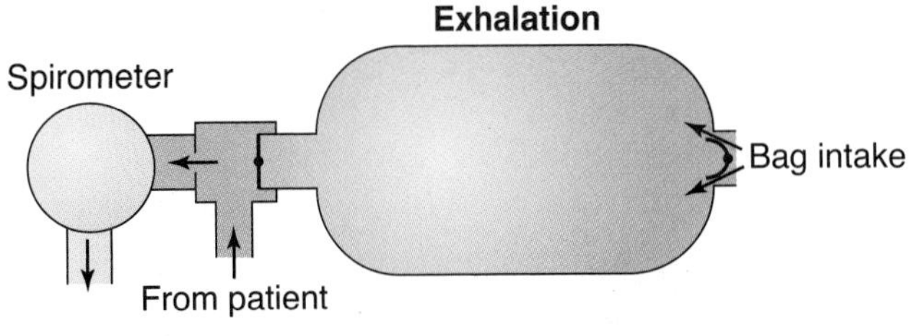

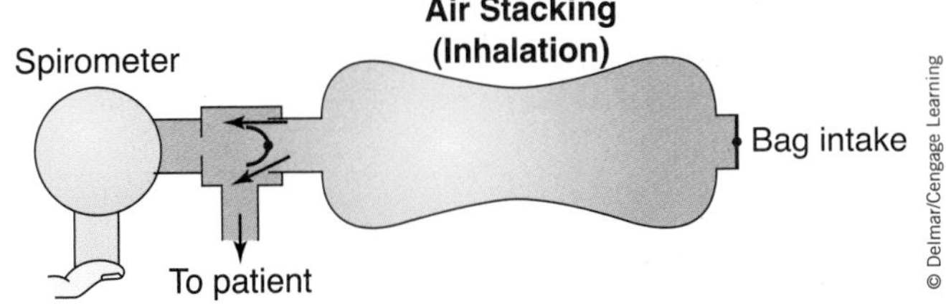

FIGURE 22-6 Air is delivered via the manual resuscitator (bottom) to full lung expansion, with the exhalation port of the spirometer manually covered so that the insufflated air does not exit the patient (or enter the spirometer) until its exhalation port is uncovered at maximally tolerated lung inflation (top).

Sustained Maximal Inflation (Incentive Spirometry)

The rationale for using **sustained maximal inflation (SMI)**, or **incentive spirometry (IS)**, is precisely the same as for spontaneous deep breathing. The incentive spirometer is an adjunct device to improve patient success in accomplishing the maneuver.

PROCEDURE

Sustained maximal inflation (SMI) with incentive spirometry is a modality that depends on the patient's ability to generate an adequate hyperinflation maneuver. Recall that the ideal maneuver generates a high inflating pressure (40–60 cm H_2O) over a long period of time (5–15 seconds), resulting in the largest possible inhaled volume (6–10 times tidal volume).[1]

The incentive spirometer gives an indication of the inspired volume and provides **biofeedback** to the patient. Commonly available devices utilize the flow of inhaled air and volume displacement (Figure 22-7 A and B). The use of an incentive spirometer provides the patient and caregiver with immediate feedback regarding the ability to accomplish the maneuver. The incentive spirometer also provides an objective assessment of the patient's progress or regression and may provide guidance as to the need for more aggressive therapy. The use of a prediction nomogram (Table 22-1) for inspiratory capacity is useful in setting goals for patients and as an indicator that more aggressive therapy is needed (that is, intermittent positive pressure breathing).

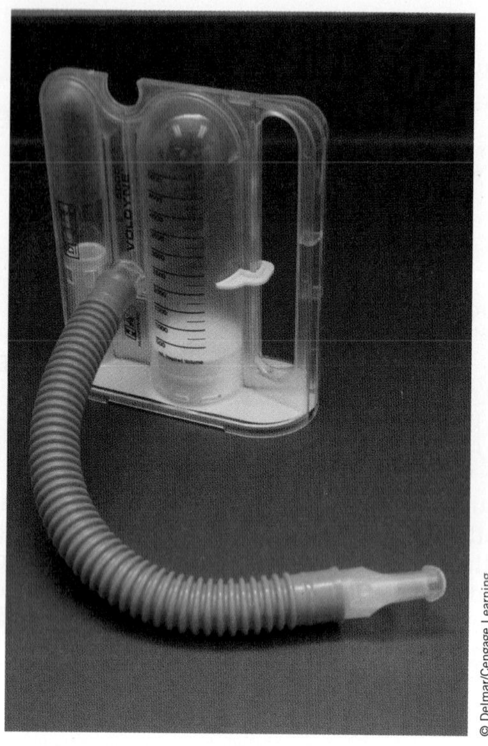

(A)

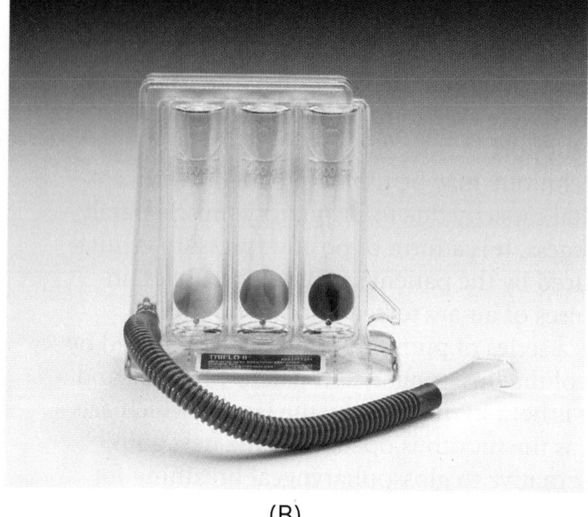

(B)

FIGURE 22-7 (A) Incentive spirometer with "volume" indication markings (B) In-Flow Incentive Spirometer
Courtesy of Teleflex Incorporated

Flow-dependent incentive spirometers provide a visual indication of activity only until flow ceases. The incentive to hold the breath, an essential element of the maneuver, is negated and must be emphasized in other ways; a spirometer is required to assess vital capacity or inspiratory capacity.

Typical incentive spirometers with volume displacements of approximately 4 L may not get the best results when working with children. Generally, children respond better when smaller volume displacements result in greater movement of the indicators. Pediatric incentive spirometers require about half the volume displacement and therefore provide the patient with increased satisfaction and motivation.

SPECIFIC INDICATIONS

Indications for the use of incentive spirometry are:

- The presence of any condition that predisposes a patient to atelectasis.
- The presence of atelectasis.

CONTRAINDICATIONS

Patient cooperation is essential for the effective utilization of this modality. Consider other modalities if:

- The patient cannot be instructed or is unwilling or unable to cooperate.
- The patient's vital capacity is less than 10 mL/kg or the inspiratory capacity is less than one third of predicted capacity.

HAZARDS AND COMPLICATIONS

If performed correctly, the maneuver is relatively safe. The patient should be observed and coached not to maintain the hyperinflation by closing the glottis and contracting the expiratory muscles. This is a Valsalva-like maneuver.

Positive Airway Pressure

A widely recognized and significant mechanism leading to postoperative pulmonary complications is the reduction in *functional residual capacity* (*FRC*) that occurs during the postoperative period. The FRC reduction leads to the collapse of peripheral airways in dependent areas of the lung and atelectasis.[22] **Positive airway pressure (PAP)** may be added to treatment plans for the prevention or resolution of atelectasis. The various methods of application differ owing to the method by which positive pressure is generated:

- *Positive expiratory pressure* (*PEP*) therapy. The patient exhales against a fixed orifice resistor

TABLE 22-1 **Inspiratory capacity prediction nomogram**

	Male Height										
Age	58 in. 147 cm	60 in. 152 cm	62 in. 158 cm	64 in. 163 cm	66 in. 168 cm	68 in. 173 cm	70 in. 178 cm	72 in. 183 cm	74 in. 188 cm	76 in. 193 cm	78 in. 198 cm
20	2.35	2.55	2.70	2.90	3.05	3.25	3.40	3.55	3.75	3.90	4.10
25	2.30	2.50	2.65	2.85	3.00	3.20	3.35	3.55	3.70	3.90	4.05
30	2.30	2.45	2.60	2.80	2.95	3.15	3.30	3.50	3.65	3.85	4.00
35	2.25	2.40	2.60	2.75	2.95	3.10	3.30	3.45	3.65	3.80	4.00
40	2.20	2.35	2.55	2.70	2.90	3.05	3.25	3.40	3.60	3.75	3.95
45	2.15	2.35	2.50	2.70	2.85	3.05	3.20	3.35	3.55	3.70	3.90
50	2.10	2.30	2.45	2.65	2.80	3.00	3.15	3.35	3.50	3.70	3.85
55	2.10	2.25	2.40	2.60	2.75	2.95	3.10	3.30	3.45	3.65	3.80
60	2.05	2.20	2.40	2.55	2.75	2.90	3.10	3.25	3.45	3.60	3.80
65	2.00	2.15	2.35	2.50	2.70	2.85	3.05	3.20	3.40	3.55	3.75
70	1.95	2.15	2.30	2.50	2.65	2.85	3.00	3.15	3.35	3.50	3.70
75	1.90	2.10	2.25	2.45	2.60	2.80	2.95	3.15	3.30	3.50	3.65
80	1.90	2.05	2.20	2.40	2.55	2.75	2.90	3.10	3.25	3.45	3.60
	Female Height										
Age	58 in. 147 cm	60 in. 152 cm	62 in. 158 cm	64 in. 163 cm	66 in. 168 cm	68 in. 173 cm	70 in. 178 cm	72 in. 183 cm	74 in. 188 cm		
20	2.25	2.40	2.55	2.75	2.90	3.05	3.20	3.35	3.50		
25	2.20	2.35	2.50	2.65	2.80	2.95	3.10	3.25	3.40		
30	2.10	2.25	2.40	2.60	2.75	2.90	3.05	3.20	3.35		
35	2.05	2.20	2.35	2.50	2.65	2.80	2.95	3.10	3.25		
40	1.95	2.10	2.25	2.45	2.60	2.75	2.90	3.05	3.20		
45	1.90	2.05	2.20	2.35	2.50	2.65	2.80	3.00	3.10		
50	1.80	1.95	2.10	2.30	2.45	2.60	2.75	2.90	3.05		
55	1.75	1.90	2.05	2.20	2.35	2.50	2.65	2.80	2.95		
60	1.65	1.82	1.95	2.15	2.30	2.45	2.60	2.75	2.90		
65	1.60	1.75	1.90	2.05	2.20	2.35	2.50	2.65	2.80		
70	1.50	1.65	1.80	2.00	2.15	2.30	2.45	2.60	2.75		
75	1.45	1.60	1.75	1.95	2.05	2.20	2.35	2.50	2.65		
80	1.35	1.50	1.65	1.85	2.00	2.15	2.30	2.45	2.60		

Source: Courtesy of DHD Healthcare, Wampsville, New York.

(Figure 22-8A and B). The pressure returns to ambient on inspiration.

- *Expiratory positive airway pressure (EPAP)* therapy. The patient exhales against a threshold resistor (Figure 22-9). The pressure returns to ambient on inspiration.
- **Continuous positive airway pressure (CPAP)** therapy. Positive pressure is maintained during inspiration and expiration (Figure 22-10).

All three appear to be effective in increasing FRC in spontaneously breathing patients. CPAP appears to be more effective in increasing FRC.[22]

When PEP or EPAP therapy is used appropriately, the positive pressure on exhalation encourages collateral ventilation. The positive pressure is developed when the patient exhales against a resistance. The pressure generated on exhalation ranges from 10 to 20 cm H_2O. PEP or EPAP therapy can be self-administered if the

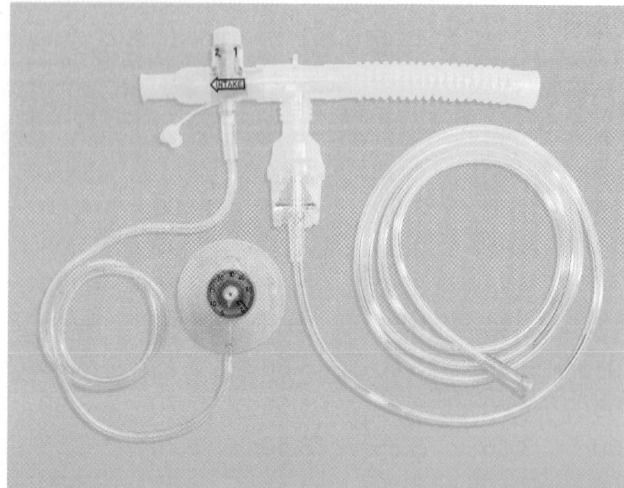

(A)

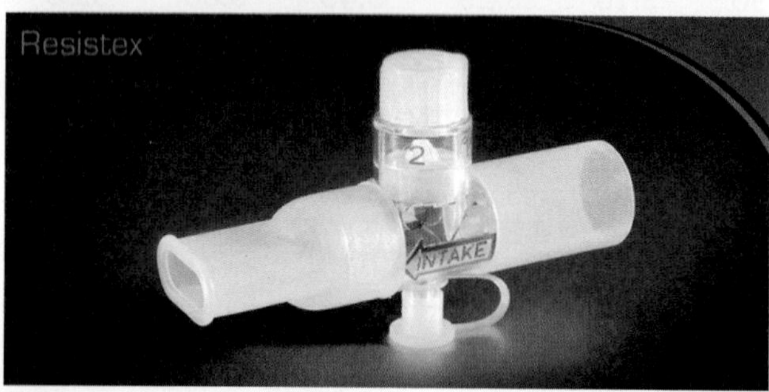

(B)

FIGURE 22-8 (A) PEP device with small volume aerosol nebulizer. (B) PEP device close-up showing flow direction and selected PEP level.

Courtesy of Mercury Medical

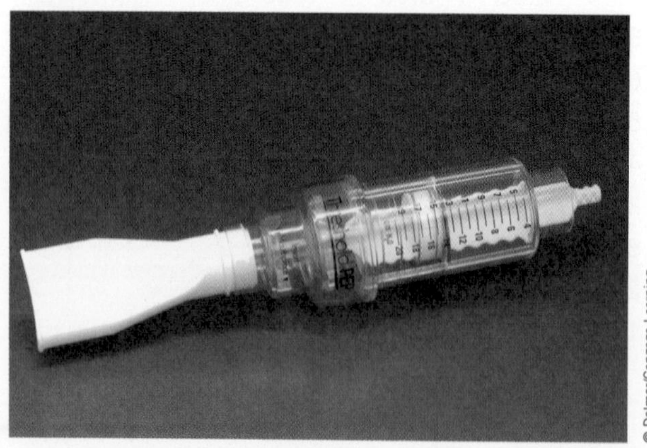

FIGURE 22-9 Threshold devices incorporate flow-independent one-way valves to ensure consistent resistance and feature adjustable specific pressure settings.

patient is given proper instruction. When used with directed cough techniques, secretion removal may also be enhanced. Small-volume nebulizers may also be used to simultaneously deliver and perhaps improve the distribution of medications throughout the lungs (Figure 22-10).

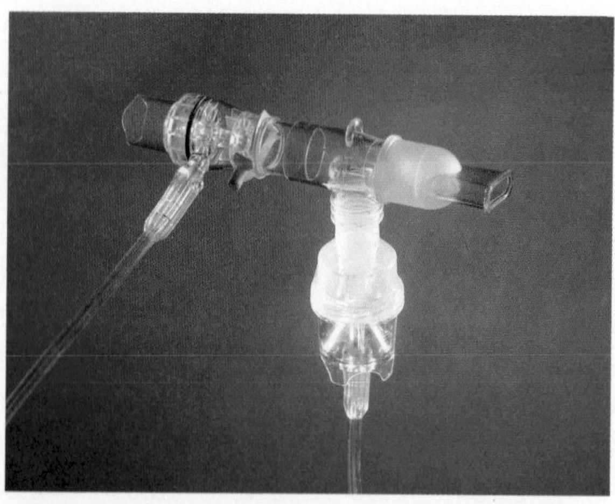

FIGURE 22-10 Ez PAP Positive Airway Pressure with nebulizer.

Courtesy of Smiths Medical

The effectiveness of CPAP in increasing FRC seems well documented, and CPAP may increase collateral ventilation.[23] Both phenomena should be beneficial in the resolution of atelectasis. Positive airway pressure techniques should incorporate diaphragmatic breathing with significantly increased inspiratory volumes and long exhalation times. The increased tidal volumes assist in the recruitment of collapsed alveoli. The expiratory pressure assists in keeping the recruited alveoli inflated.

PROCEDURE

Intermittent CPAP can be applied to the airway by using a face mask. The patient breathes through a pressurized circuit against a threshold resistor capable of developing 5–20 cm H_2O. Effective administration requires a gas flow sufficient to maintain the desired inspiratory pressure. F_IO_2 should be regulated according to the patient's needs.

The frequency of therapy ranges from once per hour to twice per day for 10 minutes or more. It may be beneficial for the patient to take two or three maximal inhalations periodically during the CPAP sessions.

CONTRAINDICATIONS

As noted in the AARC clinical practice guidelines, there are no absolute contraindications to the administration of positive pressure therapy; however, this modality should be used with careful evaluation in the following situations:

- Patients unable to tolerate the therapy due to increased work of breathing.
- Elevated intracranial pressure.
- Hemodynamic instability.

- Facial trauma.
- Acute sinusitis.
- Hemoptysis.
- Nausea.
- Middle ear pathology.
- Untreated pneumothorax.
- Esophageal surgery.

HAZARDS AND COMPLICATIONS

Although therapy is generally benign and well tolerated, several complications may arise, which should be monitored, and therapy should be modified if possible. The documented complications are:

- Hypoventilation and hypercarbia secondary to increased work of breathing.
- Increased intracranial pressure.
- Decreased venous return and myocardial ischemia secondary to cardiovascular compromise.
- Gastric insufflation.
- Claustrophobia.
- Skin irritation and breakdown from the mask.
- Pulmonary barotrauma.

LIMITATIONS

CPAP requires additional equipment and skilled personnel. Other methodologies, if appropriate, would have a lower cost. Additionally, patients must be able to breathe effectively without mechanical assistance.

Intermittent Positive Pressure Breathing

Intermittent positive pressure breathing (*IPPB*) is utilized to provide short-term ventilatory support in an effort to:

- Augment lung expansion.
- Improve delivery of aerosolized medication when other methodologies have been ineffective.
- On occasion, assist ventilation.

Few modes of therapy have been more controversial than IPPB. Most of the criticism has been due to its overuse, especially with regard to the belief that aerosol medication administration improved with the addition of IPPB. An indication that appears to respond to effective IPPB administration is pulmonary atelectasis when bronchial obstruction has been excluded.[24] The effectiveness of IPPB may be the direct result of its potential to inflate the lungs to volumes greater than what the patient could achieve without mechanical assistance.

The use of IPPB to provide large inspiratory volumes when patients will not or cannot take a deep breath has been found to be beneficial in the management of atelectasis where other approaches have failed to correct the problem.[24] The use of an end-inspiratory hold or expiratory retard may have a positive impact on the results achieved with IPPB.[15]

IPPB treatments can be administered either passively or actively. Most of the literature characterizes the routine therapy session as passive.

- During *passive* IPPB, the patient initiates inspiration and is coached to relax and allow the "machine" to fill the lungs. The patient should be instructed to hold the inspired volume in for several seconds before exhaling without force.
- During an *active* therapy session, the patient is required to inhale to maximum inflation. Peak pressure is increased gradually as tolerated. Active therapy sessions appear to result in the greatest post-treatment **inspiratory capacity (IC)**.[25]

The effectiveness of IPPB requires a tidal volume greater than is possible for the spontaneously breathing patient. Tidal volumes and pressure should be monitored during therapy and incorporated into assessments. The increased tidal volumes achieved with IPPB necessitate that the respiratory rate be reduced to maintain a normal minute ventilation for the patient and to avoid side effects that hyperventilation may cause.

IPPB should not be the therapy of first, or only, choice for lung expansion or aerosol delivery. Generally, patients who can demonstrate a vital capacity greater than 10 mL/kg might not benefit from IPPB.

IPPB therapy is generally more costly to administer than other therapies. It requires additional equipment, supplies, monitoring, and time for instruction of patients; however, when appropriate, it must be included in care plans. At this time, one device is being manufactured and sold for single-patient use (Figure 22-11).

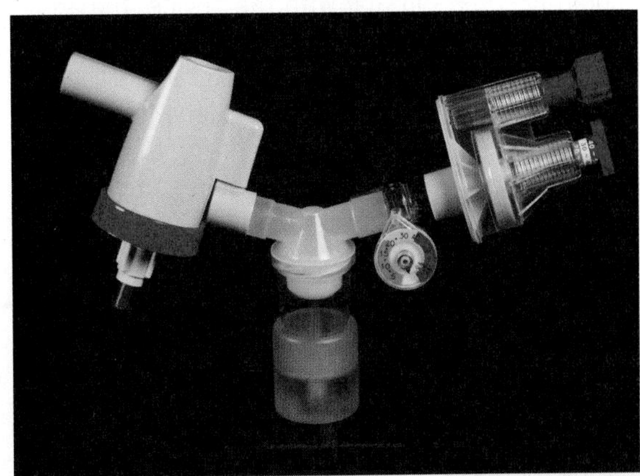

FIGURE 22-11 Single patient-use IPPB device.

VORTRAN® Medical Technology1, Inc., Sacramento, California

PROCEDURE

- The patient should be seated comfortably in a chair or in bed. Avoid a slouched position, which limits diaphragmatic excursions.
- Vital signs and breath sounds should be recorded.
- The patient should be encouraged to relax and breathe slowly through the mouth. If a mouthpiece is used, it should be positioned between the teeth with the lips sealed tightly around the mouthpiece. Nose clips may be used, if required, to minimize air leak.
- Inspiratory pressure should be initiated at low pressure. The pressure should be increased gradually until the desired volume is achieved (10–15 mL/kg of body weight). Auscultation should reveal improved expansion of the dependent areas of the lungs.
- The patient should be coached to perform 2 to 3 inspiratory holds periodically.
- Pulse rate should be measured periodically. If the heart rate changes to greater than 20% of , discontinue the therapy and reassess.
- If signs of hyperventilation are present (dizziness, nausea, tingling), suspend therapy and reevaluate.
- At midway and at the end of the session, the patient should be instructed to rest, and then deep breathe and cough.
- At the completion of the session, vital signs and breath sound data should be collected and the outcome assessed.

Age-Specific Competency

IPPB Treatment

IPPB may be effectively taught to young children. If necessary, and when possible, the patient should become familiar with the device, the procedure, and the caregivers prior to surgery. The child should be encouraged to handle the equipment to reduce fear and anxiety. If possible, observation of another child receiving a treatment can be very effective in gaining cooperation. Uncooperative patients and patients who are unable to cooperate must never be forced to undergo the procedure. For small children, the equipment used should have the smallest mechanical deadspace (rebreathed gas) possible. The treatments should always be initiated at minimal pressure. The pressure can be increased gradually until adequate tidal volumes are achieved.

SPECIFIC INDICATIONS

IPPB is the most useful when:

- The patient's ability to take deep breaths or to generate an effective cough is impaired due to pathology or the inability to cooperate fully.
- Other methods of lung expansion have not been effective in preventing or correcting atelectasis.

IPPB may be valuable for:

- The administration of aerosolized medications in patients with muscle weakness or conditions that limit the effectiveness of breathing patterns important to the effective deposition of aerosolized medication.
- Short-term support of ventilation as an alternative to tracheal intubation and continuous mechanical ventilatory support.[25–26]

CONTRAINDICATIONS

In addition to the relative contraindications noted for CPAP, the AARC clinical practice guidelines recommend a careful evaluation prior to initiating IPPB therapy for patients who have any of the following:

- Active untreated tuberculosis.
- Evidence of bleb on X-ray.
- Singultation (hiccups).

HAZARDS AND COMPLICATIONS

In addition to the complications that may be associated with CPAP, the AARC clinical practice guidelines note that careful monitoring of the patient should include observation for the following:

- Hospital-acquired infection.
- Hemoptysis.
- Impaction of dessicated secretions.
- Cardiovascular embarrassment.
- Air trapping and overdistention of alveoli.
- Increased mismatch of ventilation and perfusion.
- Psychological dependence.

LIMITATIONS

The effectiveness of the IPPB therapy is short-lived. If the patient returns to an ineffective pattern of ventilation, lung collapse begins within an hour after the therapy session.

Outcomes Assessment

Post-treatment assessment should be made in two steps.

- First, evaluate the therapy session, comparing breath sounds, vital signs, and mental status to the baseline assessment. Note any unexpected or undesirable.

- Second, collect post-treatment data to evaluate progress toward meeting the goal(s) of therapy.

Post-treatment and daily progress should include references to the following:

- Sputum production and characteristics.
- Breath sounds.
- Patient's subjective response.
- Vital signs.
- Chest radiograph.
- Oxygen saturation.

Best Practice

Atelectasis

Atelectasis can be the result of multiple factors. Evaluation of patients for all factors that place them at risk for the development and progression of atelectasis must be thorough. Hyperinflation therapy alone may not be effective in the prevention or reinflation of atelectasis. The factors that predispose the patient to atelectasis must be addressed in the treatment plan. Control and removal of excessive secretions, adequate pain control, and other appropriate interventions must be considered.

CASE STUDY 22-2

A day after initiating SMI therapy with an incentive spirometer and cough instruction, the respiratory therapist is called to evaluate E. D., a postop cholecystectomy patient. On arrival you note that Ms. D. is awake and oriented. The patient complains of dyspnea, and inspiratory capacity is decreased to 800 mL. The respiratory rate is 28/min and heart rate is 120/min, both increased from an earlier visit. She is febrile. Auscultation reveals diminished breath sounds in the bases and inspiratory crackles. S_pO_2 is 92% on 6 Lpm of oxygen via nasal cannula.

Questions

1. What is the RT's assessment after the first day of treatment?
2. What changes in the treatment plan should the RT suggest?

Summary

Pulmonary atelectasis is a condition characterized by areas of the lung that have collapsed. Although atelectasis is generally associated with upper abdominal and thoracic surgery, it can occur anytime when lung expansion is limited. Factors that predispose a patient to atelectasis are obesity, general anesthesia, and preexisting pulmonary disease. Atelectasis can result from three mechanisms that may act independently or in combination: inadequate lung distending forces, airway obstruction, and loss of pulmonary surfactant.

Patients must be assessed for the presence of any of the risk factors prior to surgery, before procedures that require sedation, or before procedures that result in extended periods of immobilization. The RT must also assess when possible therapy should begin preoperatively when risk factors are present. Appropriate therapy should continue postoperatively until the patient is ambulating. The patient's condition and effectiveness of the treatment plan must be assessed often and therapy adjusted accordingly.

Study Questions

REVIEW QUESTIONS

1. What are the general indications for hyperinflation therapy?
2. What is atelectasis? Differentiate between compressive and obstructive atelectasis.
3. What are the key factors for the prevention or reversal of atelectasis?
4. Under what circumstances would IPPB be recommended as an alternative to incentive spirometry?

MULTIPLE-CHOICE QUESTIONS

1. What inspiratory capacity goal should be set for a male patient 45 years old and 5 feet 8 inches tall?
   a. at least 500 mL
   b. at least 1000 mL
   c. approximately 3000 mL
   d. approximately 5000 mL
2. Incentive spirometry is most effective if the maneuver is performed at least:
   a. twice/day for 10 repetitions each session.
   b. four times/day for 10 repetitions each session.
   c. at least every hour for 10 repetitions each session.
   d. Frequency and repetitions have no relationship to effectiveness.

3. Key factors in the prevention or correction of atelectasis include:
   a. depth of inspiration and duration of inspiration.
   b. depth of inspiration and respiratory rate.
   c. maximum inspiratory flow rate and tidal volume.
   d. F_IO_2 and vital capacity.
4. CPAP is valuable in the correction of atelectasis because of its ability to:
   a. increase tidal volume.
   b. increase functional residual capacity.
   c. increase inspiratory capacity.
   d. decrease residual volume.
5. Which of the following may be an indication of a patient's inability to tolerate intermittent CPAP therapy?
   a. a 10% reduction in respiratory rate
   b. a 10% reduction in heart rate
   c. a 10% increase in tidal volume
   d. a 25% increase in heart rate
6. An IPPB treatment should be stopped and reevaluated if:
   a. during the first 5 minutes of the session the patient has no improvement of aeration to the posterior basal lung fields.
   b. during the treatment session, the patient's heart rate increases significantly, the patient complains of dyspnea, and distant breath sounds can be heard in the left upper lobe.
   c. the patient's exhaled tidal volume increases by 10% without a change in peak inspiratory pressure.
   d. the patient expectorates 5 mL. of tenacious purulent secretions.
7. All of the following are important to improved collateral ventilation except:
   a. canals of Lambert.
   b. pores of Kohn.
   c. sustained maximum inflation maneuvers.
   d. eustachian tube.
8. During properly coached active IPPB therapy sessions:
   a. functional residual capacity should remain unaffected.
   b. inspiratory capacity is likely to be increased after the therapy session.
   c. heart rate should always be increased by 15%.
   d. coughing and expectoration of secretions should never be encouraged.

CRITICAL-THINKING QUESTIONS

1. Discuss the relationship between distending pressure, surface tension, and elastic recoil of the lungs as they relate and interact to determine functional residual capacity.
2. Develop a rational approach to decision making with regard to recommendations of modality for the prevention or correction of atelectasis.
3. When coaching a patient to perform sustained maximal inflation maneuvers, the therapist notes that the inspiratory capacity being achieved has decreased by 500 mL since the previous day. Is this significant? Discuss the RT's assessment of the therapy.
4. When coaching a patient to perform sustained maximum inflation maneuvers, the respiratory therapist notes that the patient coughs with each attempt, has a rapid shallow breathing pattern, poor quality of breath sounds on auscultation of the basal lung fields, and increased oxygen requirements. What should the RT recommend to the physician?

References

1. Bartlett RH, Gazzaniga AB, Geraghty TR. Respiratory maneuvers to prevent postoperative pulmonary complications. *JAMA*. 1973;224:1017–1021.
2. Johnson NT, Pierson DJ. The spectrum of pulmonary atelectasis: pathophysiology, diagnosis, and therapy. *Respir Care*. 1986;31:1107–1120.
3. Hess D. The AARC clinical practice guidelines. *Respir Care*. 1991;36:1398–1401.
4. American Association for Respiratory Care. Directed cough. *Respir Care*. 1993;38:495–499.
5. American Association for Respiratory Care. Incentive spirometry. *Respir Care*. 1991;36:1402–1405.
6. American Association for Respiratory Care. Use of positive airway pressure adjuncts to bronchial hygiene therapy. *Respir Care*. 1993;38:516–521.
7. American Association for Respiratory Care. Intermittent positive pressure breathing. *Respir Care*. 2003;48(5):540–546.
8. Centers for Disease Control. Perspectives in disease prevention and health promotion update: Universal precautions for prevention of human immunodeficiency virus, hepatitis B virus, and other bloodborne pathogens in health care settings. *MMWR*. 1988;37:377–388.
9. Colgan FJ, Mahoney MC, Fanning GL. Resistance breathing (blow bottles) and sustained hyperinflations in the treatment of atelectasis. *Anesthesiology*. 1970;32:543–550.
10. Motley HL, Werko L, Cournand A, and Richardo DW. Observations on the clinical use of intermittent positive pressure. *J Aviation Med*. 1947;18:417.
11. Pierce AK, Saltzman HA. Conference on the scientific basis for respiratory therapy. *Am Rev Respir Dis*. 1974;110.
12. Pierce AK. Scientific basis of in-hospital respiratory therapy. *Am Rev Respir Dis*. 1980;122.

13. The Respiratory Care Committee of the American Thoracic Society. Guidelines for the use of intermittent positive pressure breathing. *Respir Care.* 1980;25:365.
14. American Association for Respiratory Care. The pros and cons of IPPB. *AARC Times.* 1986;10:48.
15. Martin RJ, Rogers RM, Gray BA. The physiologic basis for the use of mechanical aids to lung expansion. *Am Rev Respir Dis.* 1980;122:105–107.
16. Menkes HA, Traystman RJ. Collateral ventilation. *Am Rev Respir Dis.* 1977;116:287–309.
17. Donohue WJ. Postoperative pulmonary complications. *Postgraduate Medicine.* 1992;91:157–165.
18. Lester MK, Flume PA, Airway clearance guidelines and implementation. *Respiratory Care,* 2009:54(6)733–753.
19. Lindholm P, et al. A fluoroscopic and laryngoscopic study of glossopharyngeal insufflations and exsufflation. *Respiratory Physiology and Neurobiology.* 2009:167:189–194.
20. Pryor JA, et al. Physiotherapy for airway clearance in adults. *European Respiratory Journal.* 1999:14,6:1420.
21. Bach JR, et al. Lung insufflations capacity in neuromuscular disease. *American Journal of Physical Medicine and Rehabilitation.* 2008;87(9):720–725.
22. Ingwersen UM, et al. Three different mask physiotherapy regimens for prevention of post-operative pulmonary complications after heart and pulmonary surgery. *Intensive Care Med* (1993) 19:294–298.
23. Pontoppidan H. Mechanical aids to lung expansion in non-intubated surgical patients. *Am Rev Respir Dis.* 1977;109–119.
24. O'Donahue WJ. Maximum volume IPPB for the management of pulmonary atelectasis. *Chest.* 1979;76:683–687.
25. Welch MA, Shapiro BJ, Mercurio P, Wagner W. Methods of intermittent positive pressure breathing. *Chest.* 1980;78:463–467.
26. De Troyer A, Deisser P. The effects of intermittent positive pressure breathing on patients with muscle weakness. *Am Rev Respir Dis.* 1981;124:132–137.

Suggested Readings

Farzan F. *A Concise Handbook of Respiratory Disease.* 2nd ed. Reston, VA; Reston; 1985.

Shapiro BA, Kacmarek RM, Cane RD, et al. *Clinical Application of Respiratory Care.* 4th ed. St. Louis: Mosby-Yearbook; 1991.

White GC. *Equipment Theory for Respiratory Care.* 3rd ed. Clifton Park, NY: Delmar Cengage Learning; 1999.

Wilkins RL, Dexter JR. *Respiratory Disease: Principles of Patient Care.* Philadelphia: FA Davis; 1993.

CHAPTER 23

Pulmonary Hygiene and Chest Physical Therapy

John A. Rutkowski

OBJECTIVES

Upon completion of this chapter, the reader should be able to:

- Understand the rationale for pulmonary hygiene and chest physical therapy.
- Identify diseases and conditions for which pulmonary hygiene and chest physical therapy might be appropriate.
- Assess the need for pulmonary hygiene and chest physical therapy.
- Assess the results of pulmonary hygiene and chest physical therapy.
- List and describe the characteristics and limitations of various pulmonary hygiene modalities.

CHAPTER OUTLINE

KEY TERMS

active cycle breathing (ACB)
autogenic drainage
collateral ventilation
continuous lateral rotation therapy (CLRT)
elasticity
high-frequency chest wall oscillation (HFCWO)
high-frequency oscillation (HFO)
intrapulmonary percussive ventilation (IPV)
mucociliary escalator
mucokinesis
mucostasis
percussion
proprioceptive
rheology
spinnability
transudate
vibration
viscosity

The word "hygiene" is derived from the Greek word for "healthful." It is a general reference to the science of health and the prevention of disease or conditions and procedures promoting or preserving health. *Pulmonary*, or *bronchial, hygiene* is the promotion or preservation of healthy lungs. Exercise, nutrition, avoidance of airborne pollutants, and immunization are all vital components of bronchial hygiene and the maintenance of pulmonary health.

An understanding of how pulmonary hygiene might be achieved requires an awareness of the natural mechanisms for maintaining lung health. Normal airway clearance requires that two processes operate optimally and in coordination: (1) mucus manufacture and transport and (2) an effective cough.

Submucosal glands and the goblet cells produce pulmonary secretions with contributions from the Clara cells and tissue fluid **transudate**. The diaphragm, intercostals, and abdominal muscles generate the forces required for the effective movement of air and the generation of forceful coughs. The brain is responsible for coordination of all of the events required for clearance of the airways.

Key Definitions, Concepts, and Professional Standards

Bronchial hygiene therapies have been collectively referred to as *chest physical therapy* (*CPT*), which is usually a reference to *postural drainage, percussion, and vibration* (*PDPV*). Recently, new techniques have expanded the capabilities and requirements placed on caregivers and further complicated decision making regarding the application of therapy.

In 1990 the American Association for Respiratory Care began the development of clinical practice guidelines. The guidelines provide a broad, but limited, context within which specific departmental procedures, policies, and protocols can be developed.[1] The first five guidelines were published in the December 1991 issue of *Respiratory Care*. Periodic additions and revisions continue to occur on an annual basis. The guidelines with application to bronchial hygiene are:

- Directed cough.
- Postural drainage, percussion, and vibration therapy.
- Humidification during mechanical ventilation.
- Incentive spirometry.
- Use of positive airway pressure adjuncts to bronchial hygiene therapy.

Goals and Objectives of Pulmonary Hygiene and Chest Physical Therapy

The goals of treatment with all airway clearance methods are to improve the removal of secretions, thereby decreasing obstruction of the airways with the hope of improving the distribution of ventilation and gas exchange.[2]

Normal Mucociliary Clearance

The clearance of mucus from the airways is normally achieved by a combination of factors, most important of which are the **mucociliary escalator** and cough.[3] In healthy individuals, estimates for the volume of mucus secreted are 10–100 mL per day. When the rate of mucus production or the characteristics of the mucus produced change, clearance mechanisms become less effective, mucus accumulates in airways, and respiratory function is impaired. **Mucostasis** is a frequent complication of such diseases as bronchitis, pneumonia, cystic fibrosis, and bronchiectasis.

FUNCTIONS OF AIRWAY MUCUS

Under normal circumstances, the secretion of mucus into the airway serves as a defense against inhaled irritants that are breathed in to the lungs. Inhaled

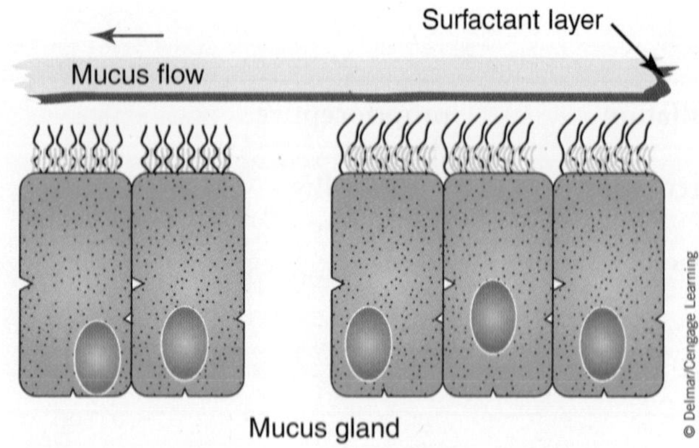

FIGURE 23-1 Physiology of airway mucus clearance.

irritants, including dust, microbes, and gases, may damage the airway epithelium. After entrapment in the airway mucus, the irritants are removed through a process termed *mucociliary clearance*. These alterations can result in the retention of secretions in the lungs and subsequent increased work of breathing and other complications.[4]

CHARACTERISTICS OF MUCUS

Respiratory airway mucus is a complex mixture of glycoproteins, proteoglycans, lipids, other proteins, and sometimes DNA. The glycoproteins and proteoglycans associate closely to form the main structural component of the viscoelastic hydrophylic mucus gel. The lipids interacting with the glycoproteins also contribute to the formation of a viscoelastic gel. Other proteins that are present have a role in protection against microorganisms. [5] The mucus blanket consists of two layers, separated by a layer of surfactant.[3] The layer adjacent to the epithelium, the sol layer, is less viscous than the gel layer (Figure 23-1).

MUCOCILIARY ESCALATOR

The transport of mucus depends on the mechanical forces of cilia beating and airflow.[6] Normally the cilia move through the sol layer in a wavelike fashion with the tips striking the lower surface of the gel layer at rates of 8–15 Hz.[6] As the cilia penetrate the viscous gel layer, they propel it toward the larger bronchi.

Tidal breathing and forced exhalation also propel mucus cephalad.[6] During normal breathing, the diameter of flexible airways increases during inspiration and narrows during exhalation. The narrowing of the airways during exhalation increases the velocity of exhaled air, assisting with the movement of mucus.[7]

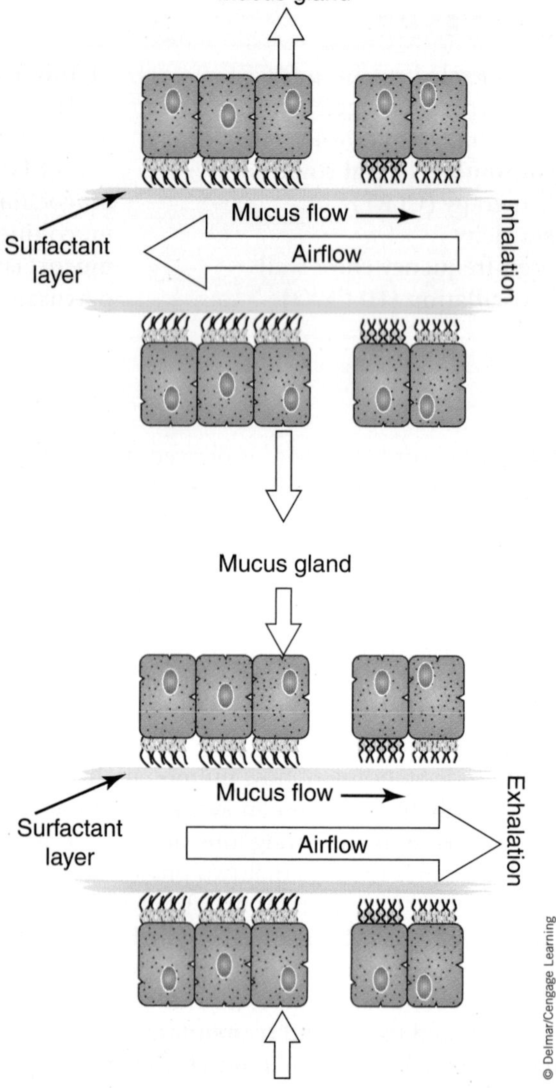

FIGURE 23-2 Cephalad airflow bias: With normal mucociliary function, greater energy is applied to the mucus layer during expiration than during inspiration, because of airway narrowing during expiration.

Factors having a significant role in bronchial hygiene and its effectiveness are:

- The **rheologic** (ability to flow or be deformed) properties of the mucus layers.
- The various factors that can alter those properties.
- The functional status of the cilia and airflow (Figure 23-2).

COUGH

Cough is an important defense mechanism that helps to clear excessive secretions and foreign material from the airways. The effectiveness of a cough depends on its

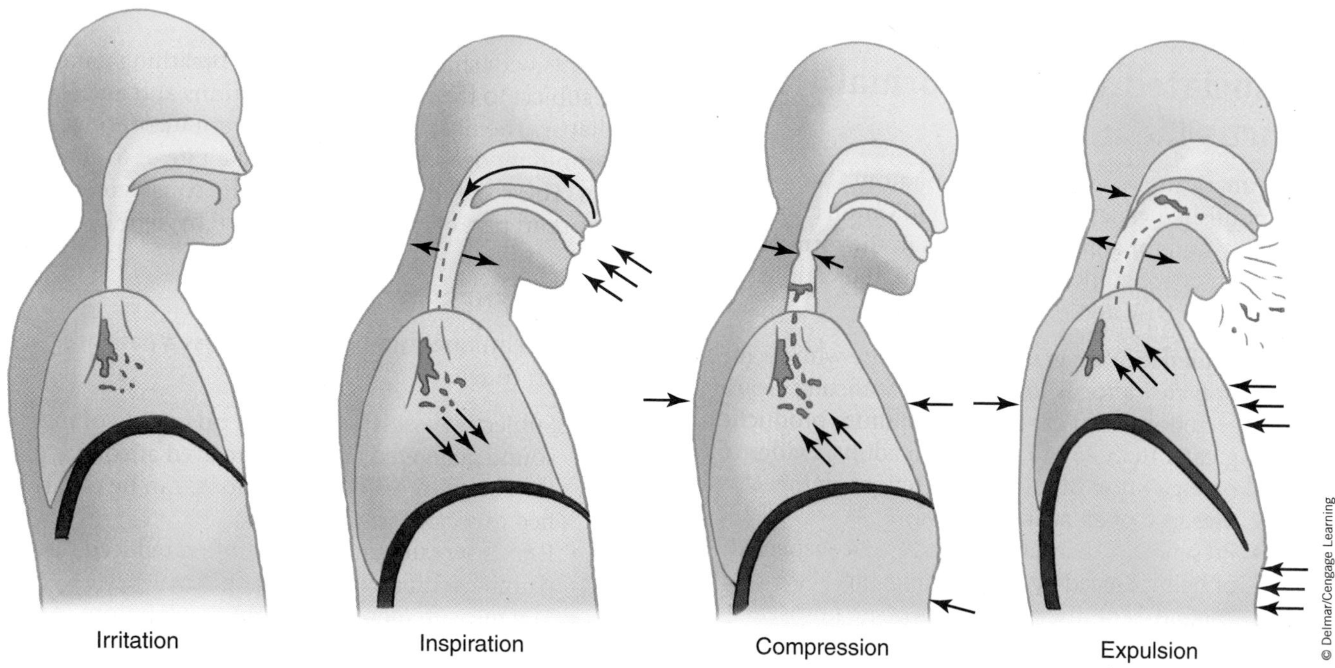

FIGURE 23-3 The four phases of a normal cough.

ability to achieve high gas flows and velocities through the airways. The sequence of events during a typical cough have been well described.[4–8]

There are four phases of the cough mechanism (Figure 23-3):

- A deep inspiration.
- A pause at peak-inspiration to improve the distribution of inspired air.
- A compressive phase, which is the closure of the glottis, accompanied by active contraction of the expiratory muscles.
- The expiratory phase, which is the opening of the glottis with an explosive release of air from the lungs.

An ineffective cough can result from any condition that interferes with the inspiratory or expiratory phases of cough:

- Pain.
- Weakness.
- Neuromuscular disorders.
- Artificial airways.
- Pulmonary diseases that reduce expiratory flow.

Cough can be a symptom of an underlying problem that requires treatment. Cough can have a beneficial effect on bronchial hygiene, and directed coughing may have a significant role in therapy. If the cause of a cough is unknown or if the coughing has no beneficial function, the complications that might result from the coughing may represent a potential hazard, and symptomatic treatment should be considered.[4–8]

Potential hazards and complications of cough that have been identified in the literature and listed in the AARC clinical practice guidelines for directed cough are:

- Reduced coronary artery perfusion.
- Reduced cerebral perfusion.
- Incontinence.
- Fatigue.
- Headache.
- Paresthesia or numbness.
- Bronchospasm.
- Muscular damage or discomfort.
- Spontaneous pneumothorax, pneumomediastinum, subcutaneous emphysema.
- Cough paroxysms.
- Chest pain.
- Rib or costochondral junction fracture.
- Incisional pain, evisceration.
- Anorexia, vomiting, and retching.
- Visual disturbances, including retinal hemorrhage.
- Central line displacement.
- Gastroesophageal reflux.

Coughing is a source of droplet nuclei and is associated with the transmission of airborne pathogens, including tuberculosis. Risk of exposure to these airborne pathogens must be minimized. The most effective method for reducing the transmission of droplet nuclei is to have patients cover their mouths with a tissue or handkerchief when coughing. Personal protective equipment and effective air exchange systems should also be used.

Diseases and Conditions Associated with Abnormal Mucus Clearance

The American Association for Respiratory Care (AARC) has published generally accepted indications for CPT or PDPV and for adjunctive devices in the form of clinical practice guidelines. In general, indications for CPT or PDPV are:

- Evidence or suggestion of difficulty with secretion clearance as indicated by: Difficulty clearing secretions with expectorated sputum production greater than 25–30 mL/day in adults. Evidence or suggestion of retained secretions in the presence of an artificial airway.
- Presence of atelectasis caused by, or suspected of being caused by, mucus plugging.
- Diagnosis of diseases such as cystic fibrosis, bronchiectasis, or cavitating lung disease.

Assessment of Pulmonary Hygiene

Assessment of the need for and the effectiveness of pulmonary hygiene generally focuses on the ability of the patient to cough effectively and expectorate secretions. Factors that alter the effectiveness of coughing include the characteristics of the mucus, the breathing pattern, and the mechanics of the cough.

MUCUS

Mucokinesis (mucus movement) depends on two factors: ciliary activity and the production of mucus.

Ciliary dyskinesis, or *abnormal ciliary function*, may be the result of many pulmonary and nonpulmonary stresses. Examples are smoking, high oxygen concentrations, dehydration, and general anesthesia. Mucus **rheology** (or movement) can be adversely impacted by many other factors:

- Inflammatory processes involving the pulmonary epithelium.
- Abnormalities of the serous or mucus secreting glands.
- Dehydration.

Inadequate humidification of inspired air when artificial airways are used can lead to desiccation of secretions.[10]

Bronchial hygiene is dependent on adequate mucokinesis. Any abnormality in the production or transport of mucus can result in the retention of secretions with the potential for further complications.

BREATHING PATTERN

Patients with shallow, monotonous breathing patterns are subject to the retention of secretions and alveolar collapse. The normal breathing pattern incorporates intermittent deep breaths (sighs) at a rate of 6–10 per hour. These sigh breaths are generally considered an important part of adequate bronchial hygiene.

EFFECTIVENESS OF COUGH

Several techniques can be used to assess a patient's ability to cough.

- Subjective assessment, based on quality of the sound generated and the perceived adequacy of the cough to dislodge secretions, can be classified as weak or strong.
- Peak flow rates and FVC are often reduced in patients with an ineffective cough.
- The measurement of maximum expiratory pressure (MEP) at the mouth appears to be an excellent indicator for the capacity to generate peak flow transients.[11] The MEP should be measured at total lung capacity and repeated until reproducible results are achieved.

Although subjective assessment and FVC measurements are routinely used to evaluate patients, the findings presented by Szeinberg and colleagues suggest that MEP is a more accurate measurement of cough strength. Patients with an MEP value of 60 cm H_2O or more are able to generate transients of peak flow during coughing and should be able to cough effectively. Evidence suggests that a *peak cough flow* (*PCF*) of at least 160 L/min is the minimum required to clear airway debris. Peak cough flows of greater than 270 L/min may be necessary to prevent upper respiratory tract infections.[12]

Improving Pulmonary Hygiene

Efforts to improve pulmonary hygiene are generally focused on two primary objectives: altering the physical properties of mucus and improving the distribution of air in the lungs.

- *Alterations in the physical properties of mucus.* Mucus transport can be altered by changes in the physical properties of mucus. **Viscosity** (resistance to flow in a fluid), **elasticity** (tendency to return to original shape), and **spinnability** (the capacity to form threads under traction) are considered to be the most important of the properties. Decreases in viscoelasticity and spinnability have been shown to correlate with increases in secretion mobilization. Maintaining adequate hydration, the administration of mucolytic agents, and the utilization of techniques and devices discussed later in this chapter can all have positive impacts on the characteristics of mucus.

- *Alterations in airflow and air distribution.* Abnormal patterns of ventilation and distribution of air in the periphery of the lungs can lead to retention of secretions. Effective air distribution is essential for the clearing of mucus from the respiratory tract. Techniques that improve volume and distribution of inspired air are an important factor in prophylaxis and therapy of secretion retention.

COUGHING

An effective cough is essential for clearing mucus from the airway. Coughing may be ineffective when the mucus blanket is abnormal or when the essential mechanical components necessary to generate an effective cough are not intact. If necessary, cough may be encouraged, simulated, or assisted mechanically. In postoperative patients, the incision site must be supported to minimize the stress that an adequate cough exerts on the wound. Proper support of an incision minimizes pain and reduces the complications that might occur owing to stress at the incision site.

Chest Physical Therapy

Chest physical therapy consists of a group of generally accepted procedures to improve airflow and distribution of air in the lungs that utilizes gravity and a variety of physical maneuvers to assist in the movement and expectoration of mucus.

BREATHING RETRAINING

When performed effectively, breathing exercises can greatly assist patients in obtaining the best possible lung function. The patients are instructed and coached with the purpose of:

- Promotion of a normal, relaxed pattern of breathing.
- Minimizing the effort required to breathe.
- Assisting the removal of secretions.
- Aiding the reexpansion of lung tissue.
- Mobilizing the thoracic cage.

The effectiveness of these techniques requires the frequent and regular performance of the exercises. The patient should be advised to carry out each of the exercises 18–24 times in groups of 6, resting between groups to avoid hyperventilation. The exercises should be repeated 2 to 5 times a day, depending on the patient's condition.[13]

Diaphragmatic breathing is taught and coached with the patient in a relaxed position. The patient is seated, with the head and neck well supported; if in bed, the patient is semirecumbent with the knees slightly flexed and supported. The therapist's hands rest lightly on the anterior-costal margins to stimulate and palpate the costal movement.

- The upper chest and shoulders are relaxed. Instructions should be short and precise. Do not confuse the patient with a complicated series of commands. Demonstrating the technique is beneficial.
- Instruct the patient to breathe out quietly, relaxing the shoulders and chest.
- Then tell the patient to breathe in gently and "feel the air coming in around the waist" or to "push away the therapist's hands." A method that may encourage the early movement of the diaphragm is to have the patient initiate inspiration by sniffing.

The therapist should observe a normal sequence of inspiratory muscle movements:

- The diaphragm contracts, resulting in the upper abdomen rising.
- Lateral-costal expansion occurs.
- The upper chest expands.

The inspiration occurs in a 1-2-3 sequence with the upper chest wall moving slightly, if at all. If the upper chest wall moves, it should move after the diaphragm contracts and lateral-costal expansion occurs. Observe the patient to note and correct some common errors:

- Forced expiration should be avoided.
- Prolonged expiration should be discouraged.
- The patient should not be "bloating" the abdomen or arching the back to give the appearance of abdominal expansion.
- Overuse of the upper chest and accessory muscles should be discouraged.

The exercises can be gradually advanced to include the necessary use of other skeletal muscles. A good progression is moving from the bed to sitting to standing to walking to climbing stairs.

The techniques used in the training of the diaphragm can also be applied to improve the movement of the rib cage and can assist further in the removal of secretions. These exercises, often referred to as *localized expansion exercises, segmental breathing exercises,* or *lateral-costal breathing,* may be valuable when addressing specific problem areas in the lungs. Examples are atelectasis, pneumonia, muscle splinting from pain often observed after cardiothoracic surgery, tight chest walls, or kyphoscoliosis.[14]

The therapist's hand is placed over the area of the chest wall to be emphasized. The hand is used to provide **proprioceptive** input for the selected muscle movement. At the end of exhalation, hand pressure is increased slightly and the patient is instructed to push up against the therapist's hand. Some resistance to inspiration may encourage the patient to inhale more completely.

The areas that are most often selected to encourage segmental expansion are:

- Lateral-costal, unilateral or bilateral, anterior at the lower ribs.
- Posterior at the lower chest and midchest for the lower lobes.
- Midaxillary for the right middle lobe and lingula.

Repeated contractions should be encouraged, along with deep breathing and an end-inspiratory breath-hold. During the breath-hold phase, the patient is encouraged to breathe deeper, deeper, deeper to provide a stretch. A technique suggested by Frownfelter that may be helpful in teaching the stretch is to ask the patient to mimic a sneeze. The patient can usually relate to the deep breath, holding it, and then ah-ah-ah-ah-choo!

These exercises can be helpful if done several times prior to coughing to increase the distribution of ventilation and to promote the movement of secretions.

POSTURAL DRAINAGE, CHEST WALL PERCUSSION, AND CHEST WALL VIBRATION

This group of techniques is often collectively referred to as *chest physical therapy* (*CPT*), or *postural drainage, percussion, and vibration* (PDPV). In general, these techniques are employed to improve mucociliary clearance, increase expectorated sputum volume, and improve airway function.

An analogy for the fundamental concepts of PDPV is getting ketchup out of a bottle. The first step in the procedure is to position the bottle with the open end down; next the bottle gets a few thumps on its , followed by some vigorous shaking. If there is any ketchup in the bottle, some may be deposited on the dinner plate.[15]

PDPV utilizes a combination of gravity and mechanical energy in the form of percussion and vibration to assist the natural movement of secretions from the periphery of the lung to the larger segmental bronchi. When the secretions are transported to the segmental bronchi, they can then be expectorated by coughing.

Postural Drainage. The postural drainage component of CPT is an attempt to make the best use of gravity. This is analogous to turning the open end of the ketchup bottle down. There is a recommended position for each of the segmental bronchi and its corresponding area of the lung (Figure 23-4). Nine different positions are employed to assist in the drainage of secretions from the segmental bronchi (Figure 23-5).

Questions that should be answered prior to initiating therapy are:

- Which area(s) of the lung are to be emphasized during therapy sessions?
- What is the patient's general condition?

Also before beginning therapy, the respiratory therapist:

- Gathers sufficient information to determine which areas of the lung should be emphasized by thoroughly examining the patient's chest, conferring with the physician, and reviewing the medical record for chest X-ray reports and other notes.
- Considers any cardiopulmonary instability, the ability of the patient to cooperate and tolerate the therapy, and coexisting conditions that might limit the positioning of the patient.
- Determines the best time for the administration of therapy. (The RT avoids therapy sessions immediately after meals, including tube feedings. If the patient is experiencing pain, therapy sessions should be coordinated after the administration of pain medications.)

Each of the positions employed should be maintained for 5–10 minutes or longer if the patient can tolerate the time and has a large volume of secretions or thick secretions.

Age-Specific Competency

CPT or PDPV Sessions

Children and infants may be positioned effectively by supporting them on the upper legs or cradling them in the arms of the caregiver. Older children may benefit by performing CPT or PDPV independently; however, some assistance is advisable to treat some of the segments.

CPT or PDPV sessions have an additional benefit for children. The regular sessions can often provide a "special time" for the child. This time may be enhanced if the sessions are scheduled to coincide with a favorite television program. A favorite tape or CD can be played, or a game can be played or created to make the sessions more enjoyable.

These techniques may also be beneficial with adolescents and adults. The sessions can be quality time for the patient and caregiver.

Right lung		Left lung	
Upper lobe		Upper lobe	
Apical	1	Upper division	
Posterior	2	Apical/Posterior	1 & 2
Anterior	3	Anterior	3
Middle lobe		Lower division (lingular)	
Lateral	4	Superior lingula	4
Medial	5	Inferior lingula	5
Lower lobe		Lower lobe	
Superior	6	Superior	6
Medial basal	7	Anterior medial basal	7 & 8
Anterior basal	8	Lateral basal	9
Lateral basal	9	Posterior basal	10
Posterior basal	10		

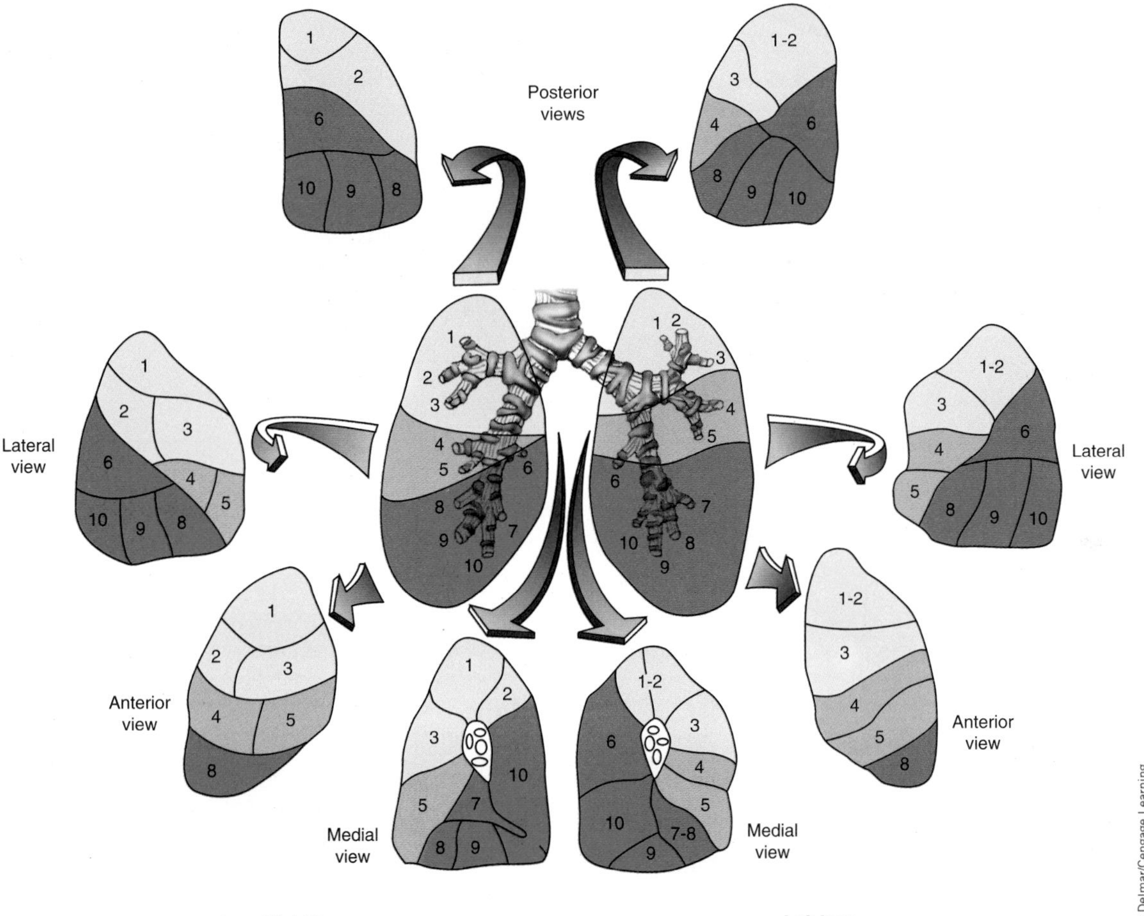

FIGURE 23-4 Lung segments.

Percussion. **Percussion**, or clapping, is performed with a *cupped hand* (Figure 23-6) over the area of the chest corresponding to the segment being drained. The purpose of the percussion is to loosen and mobilize secretions that are adhering to the bronchial walls. Percussion is analogous to the thumping of the ketchup bottle.

- The cupped hand must be formed in a manner that traps a cushion of air, which can be compressed and then used to transmit a wave of mechanical energy through the chest wall and into the lung parenchyma.
- The percussion should be applied rhythmically and vigorously throughout inspiration and expiration.
- The percussion should not be painful or result in erythema and should not be applied over bare skin or bony prominences.

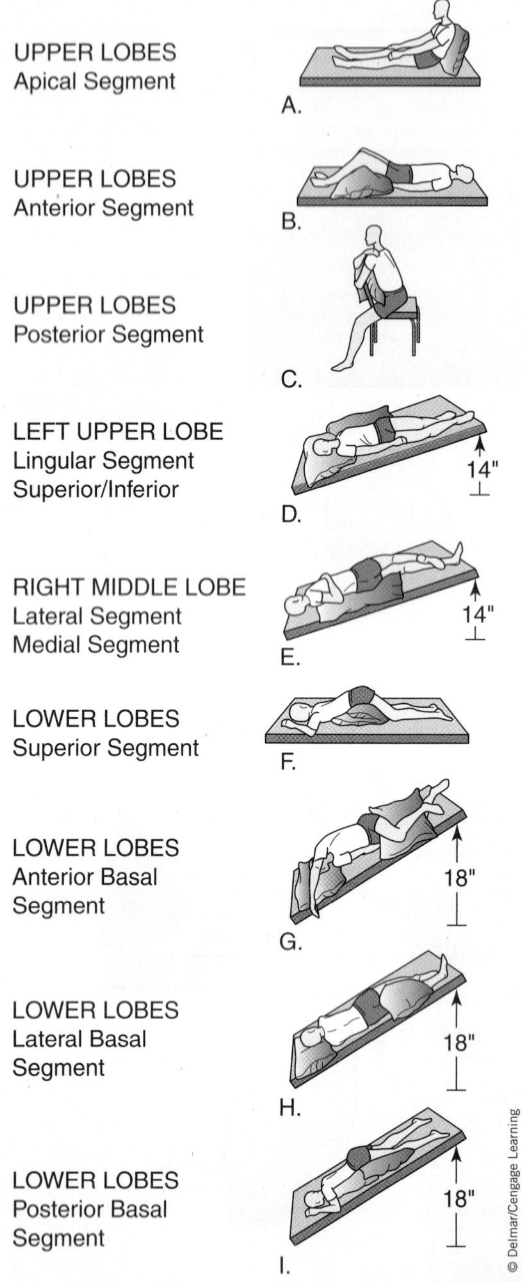

FIGURE 23-5 Segmental bronchial drainage positions.

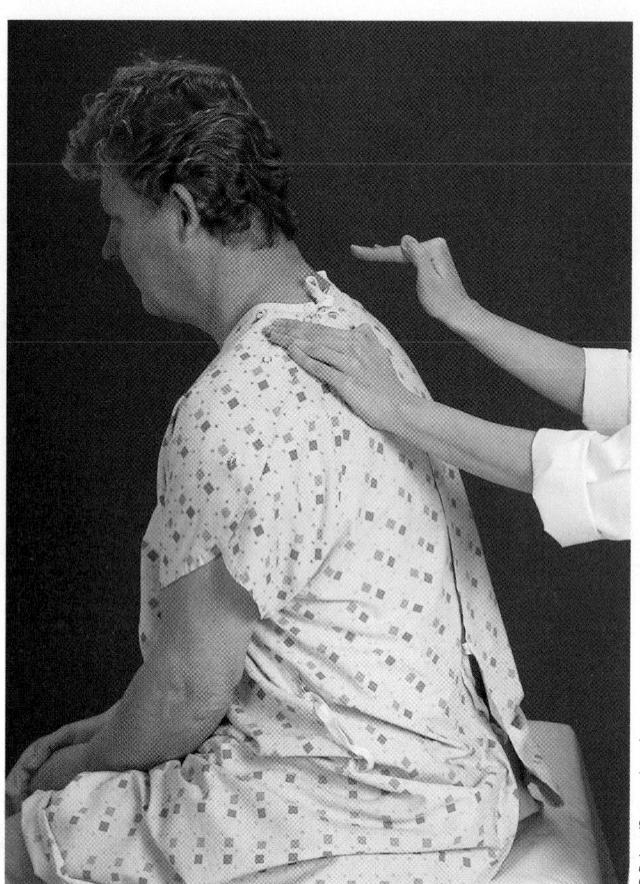

FIGURE 23-6 Cupped hand for manual percussion.

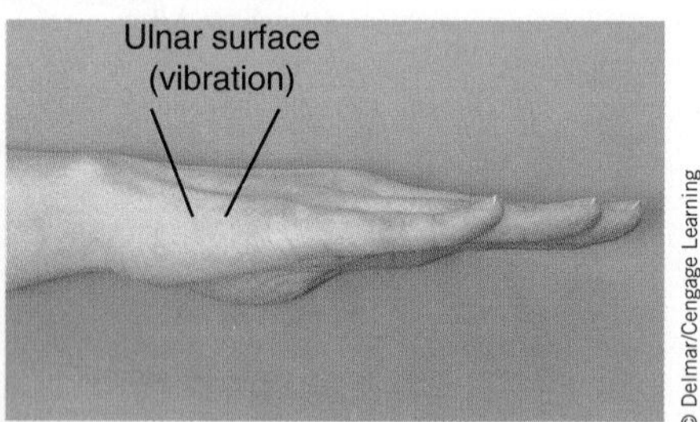

FIGURE 23-7 Flat hand for vibration.

- The percussion should be applied for 3–5 minutes continuously in each of the positions utilized.

Vibration. Vibration is also a technique that may stimulate the movement of secretions.

- The therapist places a hand firmly on the chest wall over the lung segment being treated and tenses the muscles from the shoulders to the hands, producing vibrations. Some therapists may be more comfortable placing one hand over the other, pressing the upper hand and lower hand into each other for vibration.
- The therapist presses the hands firmly against the chest wall, sending the vibrations to the chest wall and through to the lung parenchyma by pressing.
- The hands are flattened and contoured to the chest wall (Figure 23-7), not cupped as in percussion.
- The vibrations are applied at the end of inspiration and continuously throughout a prolonged and complete exhalation.

- The therapist should be mindful of the normal movement of the rib cage and follow the rib cage movement when applying the vibrations.

PDPV can be followed with deep breathing and coughing to assist the movement and expectoration of secretions.

FORCED EXHALATION TECHNIQUE

The *forced exhalation technique* (*FET*) consists of:

- One or two huffs (forced expirations), from midlung volume to low lung volume, followed by a period of relaxed, controlled diaphragmatic breathing.
- Bronchial secretions mobilized to the upper airways are then expectorated.
- The process is repeated until maximal bronchial clearance is obtained.
- The patient can reinforce the forced expiration by self-compression of the chest wall, using a brisk adduction movement of the upper arm.[16]

ACTIVE CYCLE BREATHING

Active cycle breathing (**ACB**) incorporates the FET and two additional components: thoracic expansion exercises and diaphragmatic breathing. The three components are combined in a set cycle:

1. Relaxation and breath control
2. Three to four thoracic expansion exercises (possibly with percussion, vibration, chest compressions)
3. Relaxation and breathing control
4. Three to four thoracic expansion exercises (possibly with percussion, vibration, chest compressions)
5. Relaxation and breathing control
6. One or two forced expirations (huffs)
7. Relaxation and breathing control

Theoretically, the ACB technique includes the benefit of the FET and the improvement of alveolar aeration. Benefits of ACB are:

- Independence for patients who are capable of performing the maneuver.
- The absence of desaturation, or physical compromise during its performance.
- No need for costly equipment.

The technique is not useful for infants, young children, and others who cannot follow instructions or who are otherwise unable to perform the maneuver.

AUTOGENIC DRAINAGE

Autogenic drainage is a breathing training technique that theoretically improves airflow in the small airways, facilitating the movement of mucus. The method allows for improved airflow at lower lung volumes than would be utilized for coughing and active breathing. The patient is trained to breathe at three lung volumes in phases (Figure 23-8):

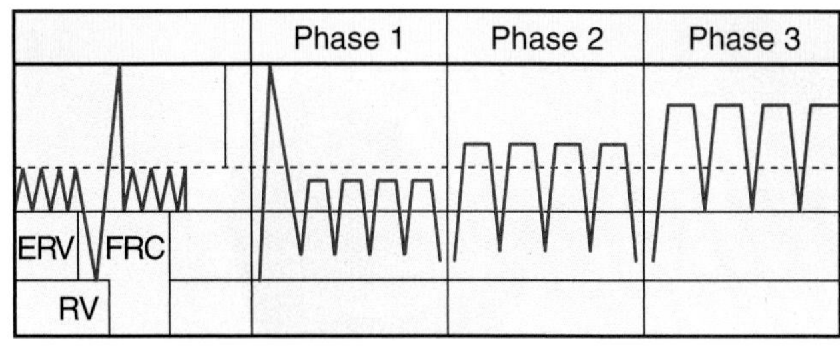

FIGURE 23-8 Spirogram of lung volumes during phases of autogenic drainage: Phase 1, unstuck: phase 2, collect; phase 3, evacuate.

From Hardy KA. A review of airway clearance: new technologies, indications, and recommendations. Respir Care. *1994:39:446.*

- Breathing at low lung volume to loosen secretions.
- A series of breaths at midlung volumes to move secretions to larger airways.
- Then a series of high-volume breaths to expel secretions.

The patient must be instructed to balance maximal expiratory flows against collapse of unstable airways. The goal is to achieve a mucus rattle, not a wheeze. Auditory, visual, and tactile feedback are essential to the effective teaching of this technique.

Biofeedback and Breathing Retraining. One of the concerns regarding the use of these techniques is the difficulty in teaching the breathing patterns to patients. *Biofeedback* devices may be useful in achieving adequate performance of the maneuvers and in coaching patients who may not be able to pay attention during therapy sessions. Biofeedback technology adds additional cost to therapy sessions; however, the long-term outcomes may improve enough to offset this added cost.

MECHANICAL ADJUNCTS TO CHEST PHYSICAL THERAPY

A wide variety of devices are useful adjuncts to CPT. Mechanical percussors, vibrators, and positioning appliances allow for improved consistency and may increase compliance with the plan of care.

Mechanical Percussion and Vibration. Traditionally, PDPV has been performed using manual techniques for percussion and vibration. Some of the negatives of manual percussion and vibration are fatigue and

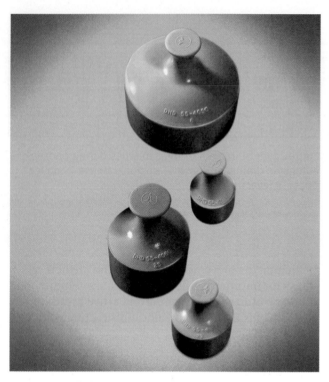

FIGURE 23-9 Palm cup percussors.
Courtesy of Smiths Medical

inconsistencies in application when different therapists provide the therapy. Partial solutions include the use of mechanical adjuncts to supplement the PDPV.

A number of devices are available and used as mechanical adjuncts to PDPV. These devices are generally referred to as *percussors* and *vibrators*. *Percussors* are motor-driven (electrical or pneumatic) pistons to which a cushioned rubber cup is attached. There are also manual models (Figure 23-9). The percussor can be applied in the usual PDPV positions.

Tilt Table. A drainage table or board may provide an advantage in positioning patients. These commercially available devices are constructed to adjust angles and heights for optimal therapy sessions. They are also helpful in achieving comfortable positioning of the patient and the caregiver. When these are not convenient, pillows, foam wedges, or cushions can be used to optimize positioning.

POSITIVE AIRWAY PRESSURE ADJUNCTS TO BRONCHIAL HYGIENE THERAPY

Positive airway pressure adjuncts are used to mobilize secretions and to treat atelectasis. They include continuous positive airway pressure (CPAP) and positive expiratory pressure (PEP), with or without vibration. These techniques are used with cough techniques and other bronchial hygiene therapies.

Continuous Positive Airway Pressure. During *continuous positive airway pressure* (*CPAP*) therapy, the patient breathes through a system that is capable of maintaining positive pressure throughout the breathing cycle. There should be very little fluctuation in airway pressure during inhalation and exhalation. The primary goal of CPAP therapy is to achieve a normal functional residual capacity (FRC). The improved FRC is usually accompanied by an increase in P_aO_2, decreased intrapulmonary shunt, work of breathing, and oxygen consumption. CPAP increases collateral ventilation to collapsed lung regions and assists in the inflation of collapsed regions and removal of secretions.[17]

Positive Expiratory Pressure Therapy. After its introduction in Scandinavia in the late 1970s, *positive expiratory pressure* (*PEP*) therapy has gained wide acceptance in Europe, Canada, and the United States. The original application was for patients who had difficulty clearing secretions, and it is now used as an alternative or adjunct to traditional bronchial hygiene modalities.

When used appropriately, PEP therapy can improve airway patency and airflow into and out of partially obstructed airways. The improved airflow enhances mucus clearance. The positive pressure during exhalation encourages **collateral ventilation**, which allows air to enter collateral ventilation channels and open airways behind mucus obstructions (Figure 23-10).

An additional effect of the positive pressure during exhalation is the splinting (Figure 23-11) of airways, which acts to oppose the premature collapse of airways. With the airway splinted open, the expiratory airflow can move secretions into larger airways, from which they can be coughed.

The positive expiratory pressure is developed when the patient exhales against a resistance, provided by either a fixed-orifice resistor or a threshold resistor. The pressures generated during expiration range from 10 to

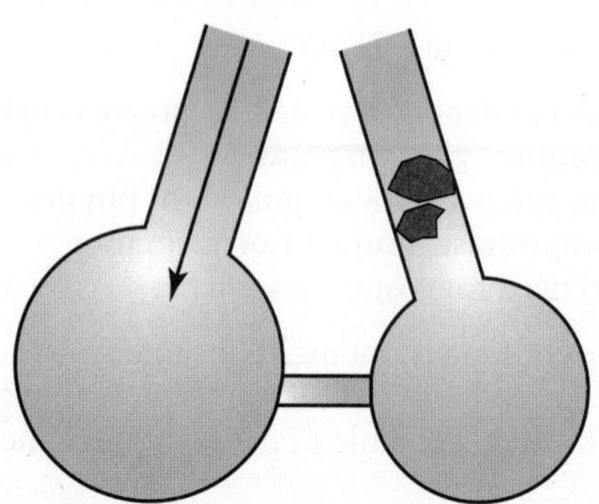

FIGURE 23-10 Collateral ventilation.
Courtesy of DHD Healthcare. Canastota, New York

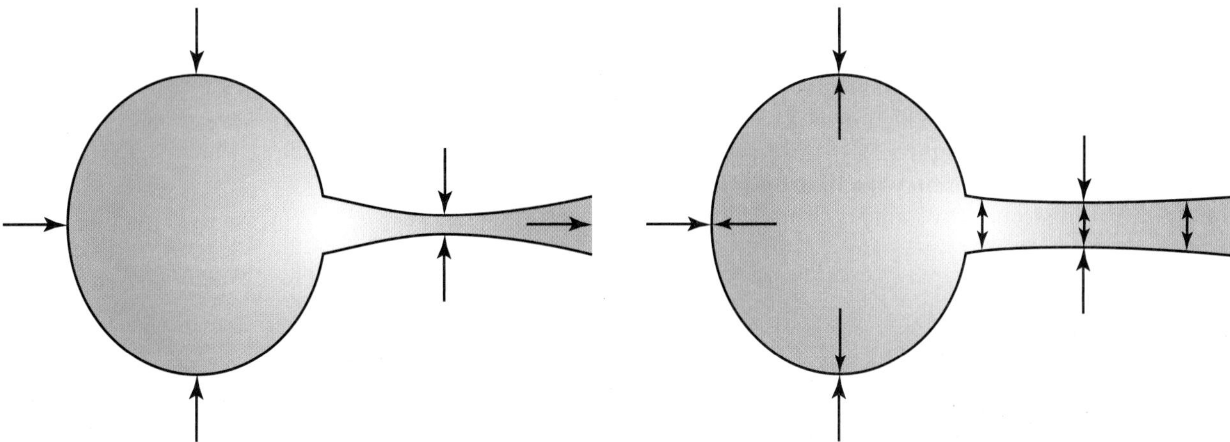

Elevated intrathoracic pressure can compress unstable airways during exhalation.
Pursed-lips breathing (or use of a fixed orifice resistor such as a PEP device) creates back pressure that splints the airway open during exhalation.

FIGURE 23-11 Splinting of airways during exhalation with PEP.
Courtesy of DHD Healthcare, TheraPEP® PEP Therapy System

20 cm H_2O; additionally, no pressurized gas source is required.

A distinct advantage to PEP therapy as an adjunct or alternative to traditional therapy is that it can be self-administered. It is not as time-consuming as traditional therapies and does not require precise positions that are often uncomfortable or painful for the patient. When used in conjunction with FET, or huff coughing, it appears to be an effective therapy for enhancing secretion removal (Figure 23-12).

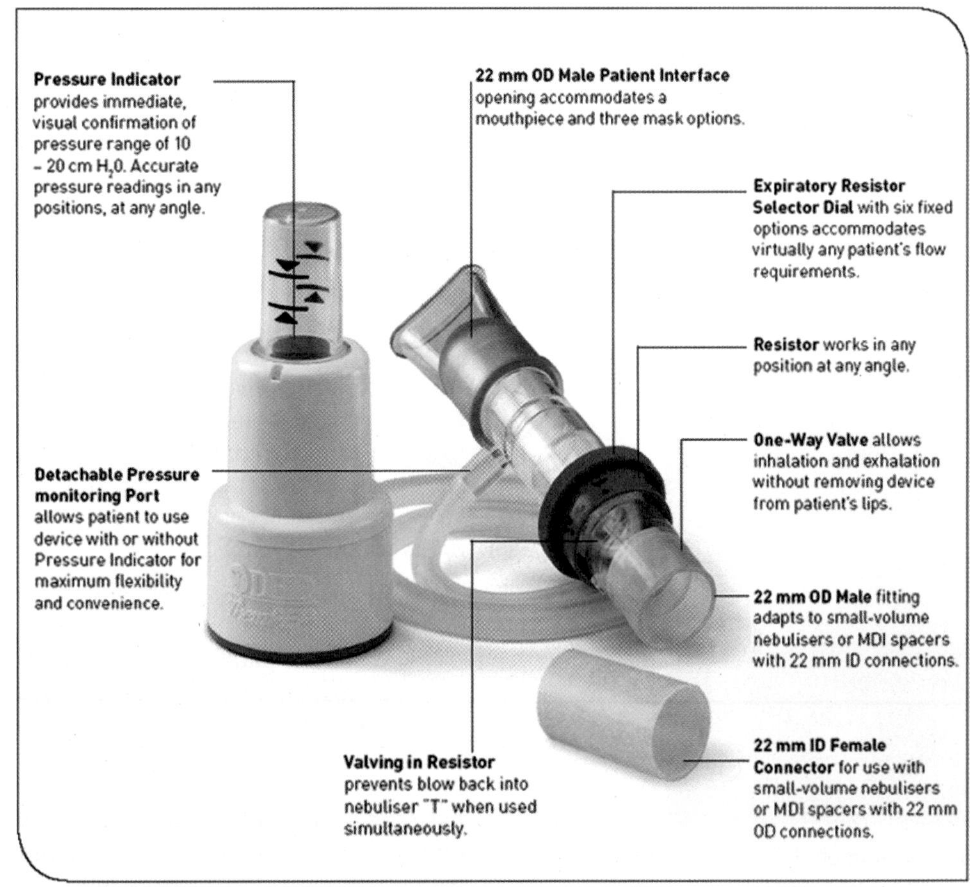

Pressure Indicator provides immediate, visual confirmation of pressure range of 10 - 20 cm H_2O. Accurate pressure readings in any positions, at any angle.
22 mm OD Male Patient Interface opening accommodates a mouthpiece and three mask options.
Expiratory Resistor Selector Dial with six fixed options accommodates virtually any patient's flow requirements.
Resistor works in any position at any angle.

Detachable Pressure monitoring Port allows patient to use device with or without Pressure Indicator for maximum flexibility and convenience.
22 mm OD Male fitting adapts to small-volume nebulisers or MDI spacers with 22 mm ID connections.
Valving in Resistor prevents blow back into nebuliser "T" when used simultaneously.
22 mm ID Female Connector for use with small-volume nebulisers or MDI spacers with 22 mm OD connections.

FIGURE 23-12 TheraPEP® Therapy System.
Courtesy of Smiths Medical

Positive Expiratory Pressure with High-Frequency Oscillation (Vibratory Positive Expiratory Pressure Therapy). Two commercially available devices, the Flutter® (Axcan Scandipharm) (Figure 23-13) and the Acapella® Smiths Medical (Figure 23-14) incorporate PEP therapy and **high-frequency oscillation (HFO)** and deep breathing to improve mucus clearance. The addition of oscillation at frequencies 6–20 Hz theoretically vibrates the airways to loosen secretions.

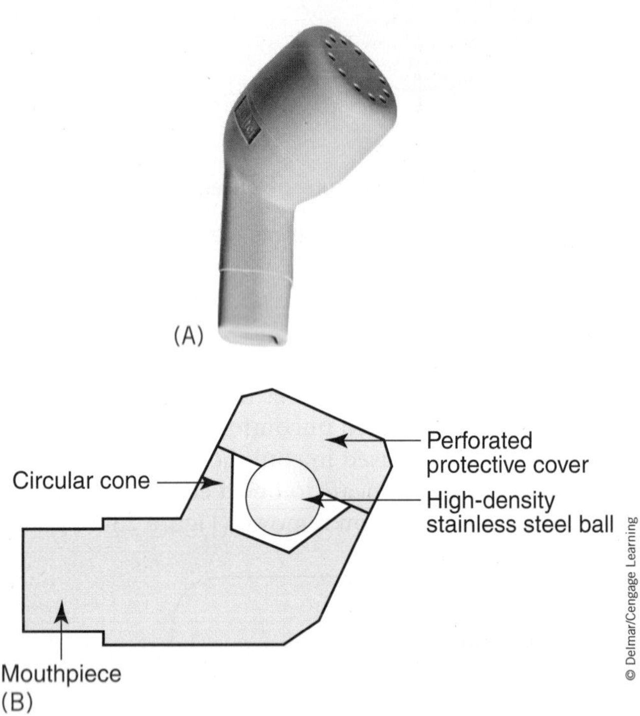

FIGURE 23-13 (A) Flutter valve. (B) Schematic of flutter valve.

(A) Courtesy of CareFusion

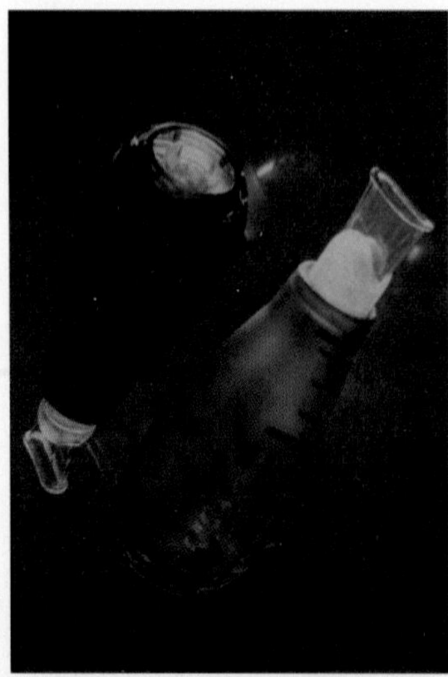

FIGURE 23-14 Acapella Vibratory PEP Therapy System (green for high flow and blue for low flow).

Courtesy of Smiths Medical

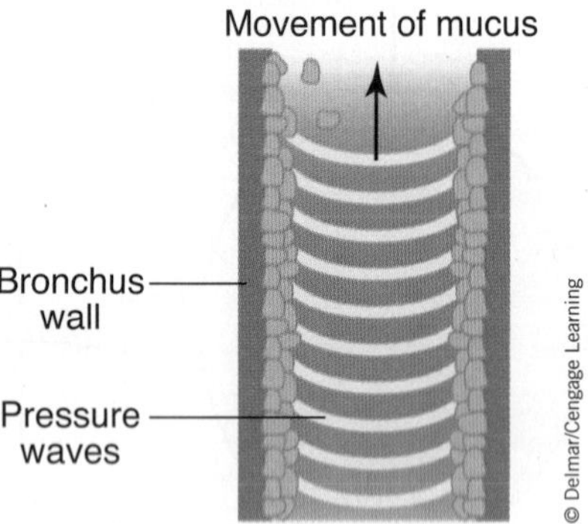

FIGURE 23-15 Vibration of airway with loosening of mucus.

- The *Flutter* device consists of a hardened plastic pipe with a mouthpiece at one end and a steel ball resting in a cone at the other end. As the patient exhales through the Flutter, the steel ball rolls and bounces up and down. The motion of the ball and the resultant intermittent opening and closing of the tube cause oscillations that resonate and are amplified in the airways (Figure 23-15).
- The *Acapella* device directs exhaled air through an opening that is periodically closed by a pivoting cone. As air passes through the opening, the cone alternately closes and opens the airflow path. The result is a vibrating pressure waveform. Acapella is available in two flow rate ranges for patients who can achieve greater than 15 Lpm. The other device is available for patients who are capable of achieving less than 15 Lpm. The frequency of vibration can be adjusted by turning a dial on the exhalation port.

Intermittent Positive Pressure Breathing. After gaining wide acceptance without benefit of controlled studies,[18] the *intermittent positive pressure breathing (IPPB)* mode of therapy is now infrequently used. However, in some conditions it is considered a useful intervention:

- In disease states in which the patient's inspiration is limited.
- When the patient's vital capacity is less than 15 mL/kg, owing to an acute illness or chronic condition that has caused a temporary deterioration in the patient's overall respiratory state.[19]

Assisted Cough Techniques. Pulmonary complications are major causes of morbidity and mortality for patients with severe expiratory muscle weakness. The vital capacity, forced vital capacity, and peak cough

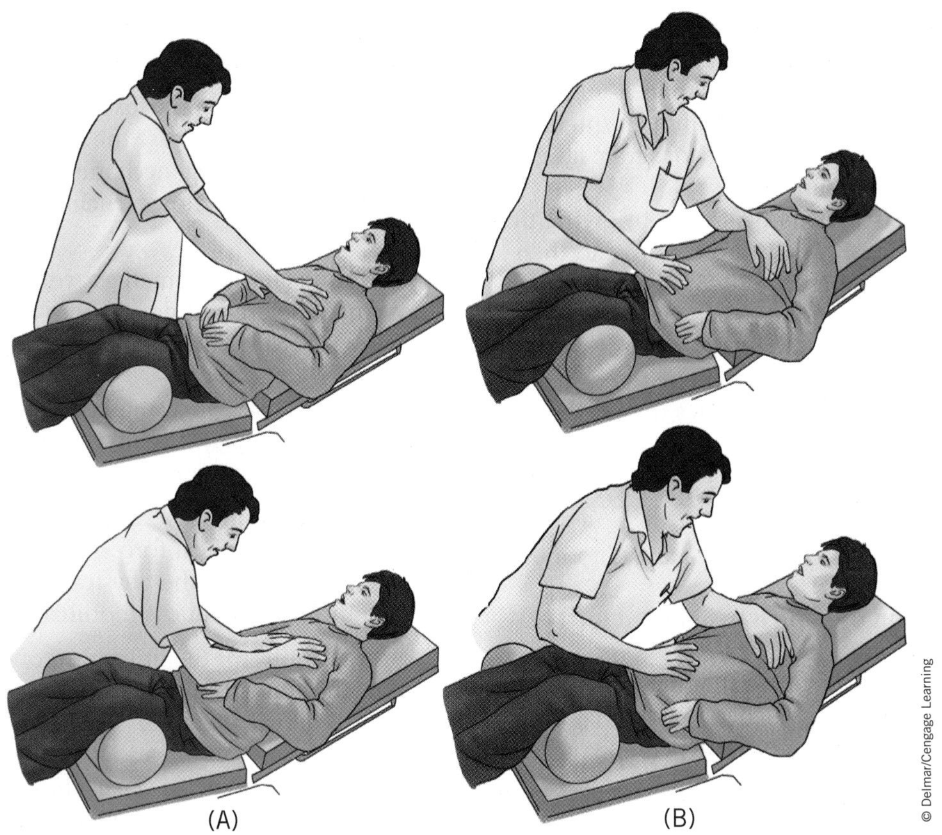

FIGURE 23-16 (A) Manually assisted cough via thoracic compression. (B) Manually assisted cough via abdominal thoracic compression.

expiratory flows are diminished during respiratory tract infections because of fatigue, weakening of inspiratory and expiratory musculature, and mucus plugging. PDPV techniques are often problematic or ineffective in patients with severe musculotedinous contractures, skeletal injury, or limited mobility[20] (Figure 23-16).

Cough efforts can be improved with devices and techniques that simulate natural coughing. Manual thrusts applied to the anterior chest wall or abdominal thrusts may be adequate to prevent pulmonary complications. However, these techniques must be used with caution in patients with fragile chest walls and indwelling abdominal or pelvic catheters. They should not be used on patients with Greenfield filters.[20]

Manual ventilators have also been utilized to simulate the cough mechanism. The manual ventilator is used to deliver a deep breath and inspiratory hold. A sudden release of pressure allows expiration at higher velocities than what the patient may develop without assistance. The positive pressure on inspiration may also be applied with intermittent positive pressure breathing devices.

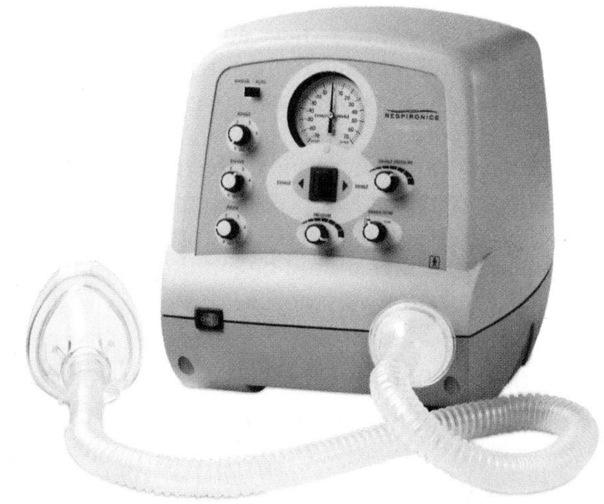

FIGURE 23-17 Philips Respironics Cough Assist device.
Courtesy of Philips Respironics

Mechanical Insufflation and Exsufflation with Negative Pressure. The Philips Respironics Cough Assist (Figure 23-17) is used to assist patients in clearing retained bronchopulmonary secretions by gradually applying a positive pressure to the airway, and then rapidly shifting to a negative pressure [*mechanical insufflation* and *exsufflation with negative pressure* (*EWNP*)]. This rapid shift in pressure produces a high expiratory flow rate from the lungs, simulating a cough.

The indication for the use of this device is the inability to cough or clear secretions effectively owing to reduced peak expiratory flow (less than 5–6 Lps). This indication is often associated with high spinal cord injuries, neuromuscular deficits, or severe fatigue associated with intrinsic lung disease.

The Cough Assist is usually applied by giving the patient 4–5 coughing cycles in succession, and then allowing the patient to rest for 20–30 seconds. The resting period helps avoid the hyperventilation that may result from the cough cycles. During the resting period, any visible secretions should be removed. The cycles can be repeated 6–10 times for a full treatment.

- Pressures are allowed to build up slowly over 2–3 seconds.
- Then the device is switched to "exhale" to induce cough.
- The exhalation pressure is maintained for 1–2 seconds.
- The machine can be left in the "neutral" position for a few seconds or switched to positive pressure for another cough cycle, depending on the patient's preference.

Individual patients require special settings for maximum positive and maximum negative pressures. For patients using the device for the first time, begin with lower pressures to let them get the feel of EWNP. Subsequent treatment pressures can then be increased as necessary to achieve adequate secretion clearance. Maximum positive pressure with the device is 60 cm H_2O, and maximum negative pressure is 60 cm H_2O.

Potential contraindications to the use of EWNP are bullous emphysema, susceptibility to pneumothorax or pneumomediastinum, and recent barotrauma. Patients with cardiac instability should be monitored for pulse and oxygen saturation very closely.

High-Frequency Chest Wall Oscillation. **High-frequency chest wall oscillation (HFCWO)** is also referred to as:

- External chest wall oscillation (ECWO).
- External oscillation of the chest.
- High-frequency chest compression (HFCC).
- High-frequency chest wall compression (HFCWC).
- High-frequency transthoracic ventilation (HFTV).

In 1966, Beck demonstrated the effectiveness of so-called thoracic vibrocompression in chronic bronchial asthma and emphysema.[21] Further investigations have documented the effectiveness of HFCWO and its ability to enhance mucus clearance. Possible mechanisms for the improvement in mucus clearance have been proposed. Most are associated with:

- An increase in mucus-airflow interaction that appears to decrease the sputum viscosity.
- And a shearing mechanism resulting from the oscillatory airflow, which loosens and mobilizes secretions.

During HFCWO, small gas volumes alternately flow into and are withdrawn from an inflatable vest (Figure 23-18) by an air-pulse generator at user-controlled frequencies of 5–25 Hz. These pressure pulses are superimposed on a small positive pressure background (0.0125 psi). The mean pressure exerted on the chest wall is also user controlled. HFCWO produces:

- Transient increases in airflow.
- Coughlike shear forces.
- Alterations in the physical properties of mucus.
- Increases in mucus mobilization.

Indications for the utilization of HFCWO generally follow the guidelines established by the AARC for airway clearance therapies. The decision to utilize HFCWO therapy requires a patient-specific assessment of the potential benefits versus the potential risks.

Absolute contraindication to the use of HFCWO are:

- Head and/or neck injury not yet stabilized.
- Active hemorrhage with hemodynamic instability.

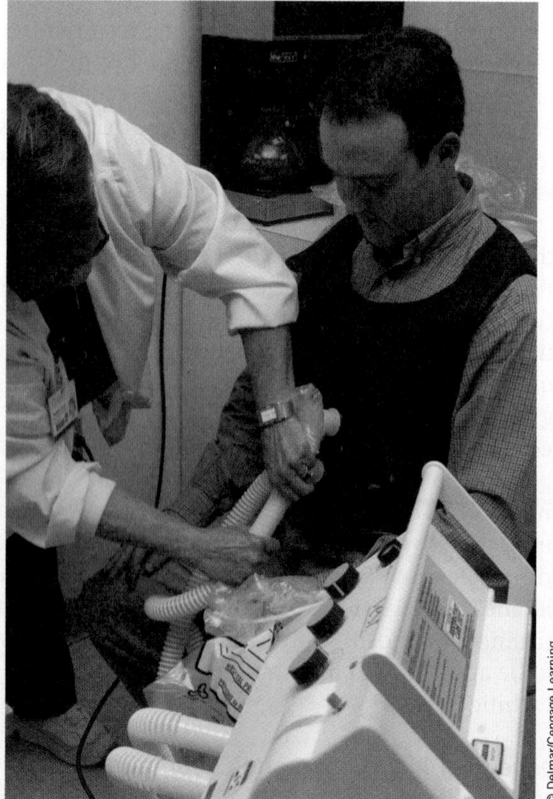

FIGURE 23-18 Vest airway clearance system.

Relative contraindications are:

- Subcutaneous emphysema.
- Recent skin grafts on the thorax.
- Burns, open wounds, and skin infections of the thorax.
- Recently placed transvenous or subcutaneous pacemaker.
- Suspected pulmonary tuberculosis.
- Lung contusion.
- Complaint of chest wall pain.

Therapy should be reevaluated and/or modified if the following circumstances are present:

- Pulmonary hemorrhage.
- Hypoxemia.
- Increased intracranial pressure.
- Vomiting and aspiration.
- Acute hypotension during the procedure.
- Bronchospasm.
- Pain or injury to muscles, ribs, or spine.
- Dysrhythmias.

INTRAPULMONARY PERCUSSIVE VENTILATION THERAPY

Intrapulmonary percussive ventilation (IPV) is a form of physical therapy administered to the airways by a pneumatic device called a *percussionator* or *intrapulmonary percussive device.*

- The patient breathes through a mouthpiece and the percussionator delivers high-flow-rate bursts of gas into the lungs 100–300 times per minute.
- During the percussive bursts of gas into the lungs, continuous positive pressure is maintained while the pulses progressively dilate the airways.
- At the end of the percussive interval (5–10 seconds), a deep exhalation is performed with resultant mucus transport; then the cycle is repeated. Coughing is performed as necessary to clear secretions.

The therapy period lasts approximately 20 minutes.

The device is also capable of delivering a medicated or nonmedicated aerosol.

A recently introduced device, the MetaNeb System, (Hill-Rom Services, Inc.) is capable of providing lung expansion with medicated aerosol and continuous positive pressure, or secretion clearance with medicated aerosol while oscillating the airways with continuous pulses of pressure. The device can also automatically alternate between these modes.

A single-patient device capable of delivering high-frequency intrapulmonary percussive ventilation with simultaneous administration of medicated aerosols is also available. The PercussiveTech HF is designed to oscillate primarily on exhalation. Please note that in general the devices discussed above also oscillate as the patient exhales. The PercussiveTech HF provides intrapulmonary percussion at 360–840 cycles per minute at a maximum pressure of 20 cm H_2O when operated according to the manufacturer's instructions (Figure 23-19).

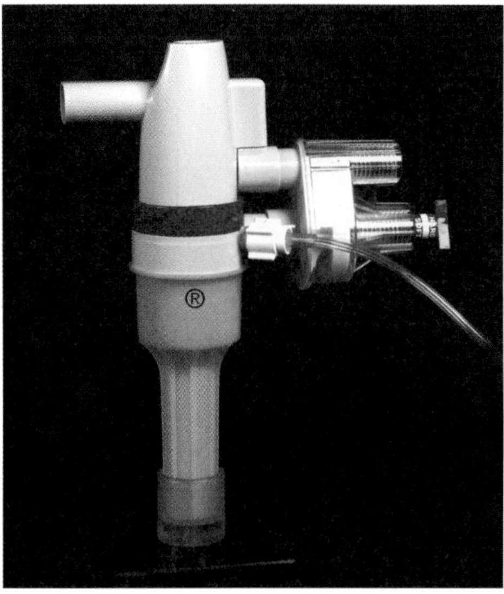

FIGURE 23-19 Percussive Tech HF device.
VORTRAN® Medical Technology1, Inc., Sacramento, California.

COMBINED MECHANICAL AND ACOUSTICAL VIBRATION

The Frequencer is described as a digitally controlled electroacoustical transducer device. It has a control unit (digital frequency generator and amplifier) and a transducer that applies mechanical and acoustical stimulation to the chest wall. Typical frequency of vibration is 30–70 Hz depending on the patient needs (see Figure 23-20).

The manufacturer has set a default frequency at 30 Hz. However, the recommendation is to find the "best" setting by adjusting the volume and frequency to a level that the patient finds comfortable. Indications

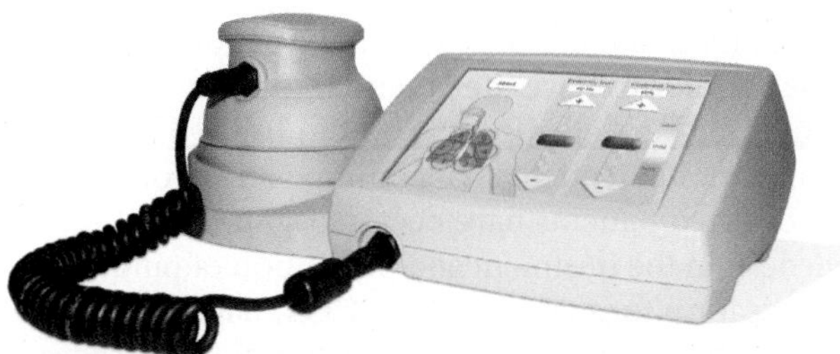

FIGURE 23-20 Frequencer.
Courtesy of Dymedso, Inc.

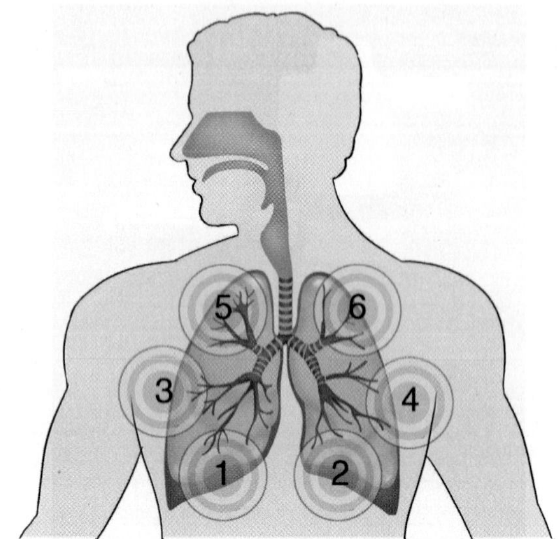

FIGURE 23-21 Placement of device for frequencer.
Courtesy of Dymedso, Inc.

CASE STUDY 23-1

B. T. is an 8-year-old girl who was hospitalized for the sixth time in the past 8 months. All of the previous admissions were for the treatment of various pneumonias. The X-ray on admission is consistent with bronchiectasis and atelectasis of the lower lobes. Traditional methods of CPT or PDPV have resulted in minimal improvement of the patient's pulmonary status.

Questions

1. Evaluate the effectiveness of the therapy provided.
2. What, if any, alternatives to traditional CPT or PDPV might be considered?
3. How else might bronchial hygiene be improved in this case?

that optimal frequency is being reached are a desire to cough and a change in voice. Since sound moves better through relaxed muscle, the patient is instructed to relax the shoulder and chest muscles. The patient should also take deeper breaths than usual, exhale through pursed-lips and use abdominal muscles to increase diaphragm excursion slightly. The transducer is applied to the six regions, as shown in Figure 23-21. The default treatment time is set at 20 minutes, after which the device automatically stops. The default treatment time can be adjusted to accommodate physician prescription or patient comfort. The Frequencer can be applied in either a seated or reclining position.

Airway clearance devices generating vibrations that can penetrate into the airways have the ability to alter mucus rheology. The Frequencer is capable of generating higher frequencies than other devices (30–70 Hz). Theoretically, the more mucus that is agitated, the more liquid it becomes.

CONTINUOUS LATERAL ROTATION (KINETIC) THERAPY

Immobilization is associated with hypoxemia, pooling of secretions, and atelectasis in the dependent lung. These conditions have the potential to promote pneumonia, and all appear to be diminished by mobilization. Frequent changes in position for immobilized patients have been recognized as beneficial in the treatment and prevention of pulmonary complication for many years. In 1954, Baker noted its value in the treatment of poliomyelitis.[22] For decades, half-hour rotations to alternating lateral positions have been a standard of care in postoperative care and care of immobilized patients. This movement ensures that one lung is raised above the other. The constant changes in position may enhance secretion clearance, resulting in effective therapy for the treatment and prevention of pulmonary complications. There may also be some benefit with respect to the prevention of thrombophlebitis, pulmonary embolus, and decubitus ulcer.

In recent years, specialty beds have become available that can rotate patients several times an hour at angles up to 67 degrees from the horizontal.[23] This mechanical turning of the body to 40 degrees or greater on each side is known as **continuous lateral rotation therapy (CLRT)**, or kinetic therapy (KT). CLRT is a method of providing constant turning of patients who have decreased mobility and who are unable to reposition themselves (Figure 23-22).

SELECTION OF MUCOCILIARY CLEARANCE TECHNIQUE

Selection of the mode, or combination of modes, of therapy is largely based on a thorough evaluation of the patient's respiratory status. The primary indication for pulmonary hygiene therapy must be defined.

- Is the indication for prophylaxis?
- Is the location of the pulmonary problem central or peripheral?
- Can the patient cough and deep breathe?
- Can the patient cooperate to improve the effectiveness of therapy?

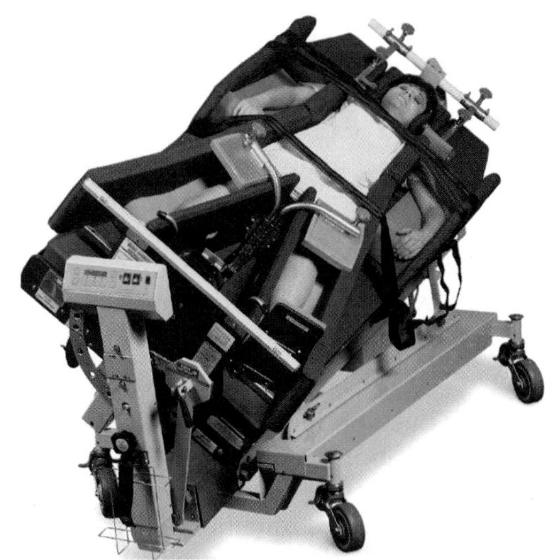

FIGURE 23-22 Roto Rest.
RotoRest™ Delta Advanced Kinetic Therapy System. Courtesy of KCI Licensing, Inc.

- Does the patient have complicating or limiting factors that question the appropriateness of some modes of therapy?

All such questions should be answered prior to initiating therapy (Tables 23-1 and 23-2).

Respiratory therapists should also consider that individual patient responses to therapy are extremely variable and that there is no evidence yet that any single treatment is superior to another. It may be necessary to try several airway clearance techniques to find the one that works well for the

TABLE 23-1 **Factors to be considered when selecting an airway clearance technique**

- Motivation
- Patient's goals
- Physician's/caregiver's goals
- Effectiveness (of considered technique)
- Patient's age
- Patient's ability to concentrate
- Ease (of learning and of teaching)
- Skill of therapists/teachers
- Fatigue or work required
- Need for assistants or equipment
- Limitations of technique based on disease type and severity
- Costs (direct and indirect)
- Desirability of combining methods

Source: From Hardy KA. A review of airway clearance: new techniques, indications, and recommendations. Respir Care. *1994; 39:449.*

TABLE 23-2 **Recommendations for airway clearance techniques in specific conditions***

Condition	Recommendation
Cystic fibrosis, cilial syndromes, bronchiectasis (require ACT)	Infants—PDPV 3–12 years—exercise, PEP, PDPV, ACB, HFCC (HFao or flutter valve) > 12 years—exercise, ACB, AD, PEP, PDPV, HFCC
Atelectasis, abdominal surgery	PEP, PDPV
Prevention of postoperative atelectasis	PEP, ACB
Asthma (with mucus plugging but without airleak)	PEP, PDPV
Neurologic abnormalities (spasticity, bulbar palsy, aspiration-prone)	PDPV, suction
Musculoskeletal weakness (muscular dystrophy, myasthonia, poliomyelitis)	PEP, negative and positive-assist devices

**ACT = airway clearance technique; PDPV = postural drainage, percussion, and vibration; PEP = positive expiratory pressure; ACB = active cycle of breathing; HFCC = high-frequency chest wall compression; HFao = high-frequency compression at the airway opening; and AD = austogenic drainage*

Source: From Hardy KA. A review of airway clearance: new techniques, indications, and recommendations. Respir Care. *1994; 39:450.*

Best Practice

Bronchial Hygiene

In addition to determining the most effective technique for clearing secretions, the patient's underlying problems must also be considered. Techniques or therapies that benefit the underlying problems often enhance the effectiveness of bronchial hygiene. The coordination of other appropriate therapies can also benefit the patient. For example:

- Dehydration has a negative effect on the mobilization of secretions, and a bronchodilator, if indicated, can help in this respect.
- Physical therapy and rehabilitation might be more effective if the patient has cleared secretions prior to the session.
- Sleep patterns should be considered when preparing a schedule for therapy sessions.

A rational approach to all relevant aspects of patient care must be a part of the treatment plan.

CASE STUDY 23-2

M. S., a 20-year-old patient, was admitted to the emergency department after a high-speed motor vehicle accident. On his arrival, the injuries noted were a fractured right femur and right forearm. There were no complaints of difficulty breathing, and his level of consciousness did not appear to be altered. Mark later complained of increasing breathing difficulty. The attending physician suspected a fat embolism.

During the ensuing two weeks. Mark's condition deteriorated and required mechanical ventilation. A tracheostomy was performed to improve pulmonary hygiene and airway care. Mark was noted to have atelectasis.

Questions

1. Evaluate the effectiveness of the therapy provided.
2. What recommendations might optimize pulmonary hygiene?
3. How else might bronchial hygiene be improved in this case?

individual patient. The RT must also recognize that individual patients may prefer to utilize airway clearance techniques that are self-administered.[24]

COMPLICATIONS AND ADVERSE EFFECTS OF CHEST PHYSICAL THERAPY

Complications that may be the result of cough efforts have already been noted. Adverse effects that may be related to PDPV are:

- Bronchospasm.
- Transient hypoxemia.
- Increased intracranial pressure.
- Hypotension.
- Pain.
- Vomiting.
- Dysrhythmias.

In the event of a significant change in clinical status during therapy:

- Stop the session.
- Return the patient to the prior or a comfortable position.
- Contact the physician.
- If necessary, consider increasing the inspired oxygen concentration, and call for assistance if needed.

Most of the hazardous situations noted are the result of the position required for optimal CPT or PDPV. Patients who have responses to CPT or PDPV that are unexpected or that may limit its effectiveness may benefit from techniques that are not position dependent (PEP therapy with/without vibration, high-frequency chest wall oscillation, and the like).

When utilizing modalities that require pressure to augment lung expansion, the respiratory therapist has to consider additional complications and hazardous situations.

- Tension pneumothorax is the only absolute contraindication cited with regularity.
- Cardiovascular side effects that are often associated with increased intrathoracic pressure are reduced venous return, reduced cardiac output, and tachycardia.
- Increased intracranial pressure is also a concern.
- Pulmonary barotrauma is a potential complication of positive pressure generation.

Summary

Under normal conditions pulmonary hygiene is ongoing, and individuals are generally unaware of the processes involved. When chronic or debilitating illnesses develop, patients often need assistance to maintain pulmonary hygiene, ranging from education and encouragement to complex devices and regimens.

The chapter reviewed a number of techniques and devices that are used to promote the removal of retained secretions and to reduce the likelihood of progressive worsening of pulmonary function. Proper nutrition and fluid balance, as well as the incorporation of physical conditioning into the care plan, should not be neglected. The use of pharmacologic agents to improve air distribution and alter the physical characteristics of mucus must also be considered when appropriate. Additionally, the caregiver must be prepared to remove secretions by performing tracheal aspiration when necessary.

The selection of therapy modalities and development of a care plan must be based on the nature of the problems being addressed; the patient's ability or desire to comply with proposed regimens, and the complexity of equipment and associated expenses.

Study Questions

REVIEW QUESTIONS

1. List the three general indications for CPT or PDPV.
2. An analogy often used to illustrate the concept of CPT or PDPV is the ketchup bottle. Discuss the

similarities between getting ketchup out of the bottle and mucus clearance.

3. List the four phases of an effective cough. Give one illustration of a disorder that would compromise each of the four phases.
4. Discuss the rationale for continuous lateral rotation therapy (CLRT) or kinetic therapy (KT).

MULTIPLE-CHOICE QUESTIONS

1. An ineffective cough is often associated with:
   a. maximum expiratory pressures greater than 80 cm H_2O.
   b. weakened abdominal muscles.
   c. vital capacity greater than 80% of predicted vital capacity.
   d. inspiratory capacity greater than 80% of predicted inspiratory capacity.
2. Percussion of the chest wall should *always*:
   a. be performed with a cupped hand, or mechanical adjunct.
   b. be performed over bare skin.
   c. be performed for a maximum of 30 seconds to 1 minute in each position.
   d. be performed during inspiration only.
3. Drainage of the posterior basal segments is best accomplished with the patient in which of the following positions?
   a. the foot of the bed elevated 30 degrees, lying on the abdomen, head down
   b. the foot of the bed elevated 15 degrees, lying on the back, head down
   c. the head of the bed raised to a 30-degree angle, lying on back
   d. the bed flat, lying on the abdomen
4. Indications for CPT or PDPV include all of the following except:
   a. difficulty expectorating secretions with expected sputum production greater than 25 mL/day in adults.
   b. presence of an artificial airway and evidence of retained secretions.
   c. bilateral pleural effusions.
   d. cystic fibrosis.
5. When instructing a patient to cough effectively during the immediate postoperative period, you should instruct the patient to:
   a. support the incision with a pillow.
   b. inspire at low tidal volumes to control pain.
   c. minimize abdominal muscle contraction during exhalation.
   d. minimize movement of the rib cage during inspiration.
6. Active cycle breathing is sometimes described as a combination of the FET maneuver and:
   a. diaphragmatic breathing and intrapulmonary percussive ventilation (IPV).
   b. thoracic expansion exercises and PEP therapy
   c. intrapulmonary percussive ventilation (IPV) and postural drainage (PD).
   d. thoracic expansion exercises and diaphragmatic breathing.
7. PEP therapy may be helpful in promoting the expectoration of mucus by:
   a. allowing peripheral airways to collapse during exhalation.
   b. improving air distribution with positive pressure during inhalation.
   c. minimizing collateral ventilation.
   d. generating a slight increase in pressure during inspiration.
8. Continuous lateral rotation therapy (CLRT):
   a. is a method of providing constant turning of patients to minimize complications that might result from immobilization.
   b. has no application in preventing pulmonary complications in immobilized patients.
   c. has its greatest effect on secretion clearance if the rotation is limited to less than 20 degrees from horizontal.
   d. should *never* be used with patients who have decreased mobility.

CRITICAL-THINKING QUESTIONS

1. A patient presents with a consolidation of the left lower lobe. The respiratory therapist auscultates the chest and hears bronchial breath sounds over the left posterior basal region. A recent chest X-ray indicates the presence of an air bronchogram. How would the RT develop a bronchial hygiene plan for this scenario?
2. The therapist receives an order to perform CPT or PDPV on a child. The right middle lobe appears to be one of the regions that needs to be addressed. How would the RT develop a bronchial hygiene plan? What postural drainage position(s) would be utilized?
3. A patient presents with a consolidation of the right lower lobe. The therapist auscultates the chest and hears coarse crackles over the right posterior basal region. A recent chest X-ray indicates that no air bronchogram is present. How would the RT develop a bronchial hygiene plan for this scenario?

4. A physician asks the respiratory therapist for input on developing a bronchial hygiene plan for a patient. The patient is expected to be immobilized for a prolonged period of time owing to injuries suffered in a motor vehicle accident. How would the RT proceed in developing a bronchial hygiene plan for this scenario?

References

1. Hess D. The AARC clinical practice guidelines. *Respir Care*. 1991;36:1398–1401.
2. Hardy AH. A review of airway clearance: new techniques, indications, and recommendations. *Respir Care*. 1994;39:440–452.
3. Sleigh MA, Blake JR, Liron N. The propulsion of mucus by cilia. *Am Rev Respir Dis*. 1988;137: 726–741.
4. Rodgers DF. Physiology of airway mucus secretion and pathophysiology of hypersecretion. *Respir Care*. 2007;52:1134–1146.
5. Rubin BK. The physiology of mucus clearance. *Respir Care*. 2002: 761–768.
6. van der Schans CP. Bronchial mucus transport. *Respir Care*. 2007;52:1150–1158.
7. Fink JB. Forced expiratory technique, directed cough and autogenic drainage. *Respir Care*. 2007;52:1210–1223.
8. Irwin RS, Rosen MJ, Braman SS. Cough: A comprehensive review. *Arch Intern Med*. 1977;137: 1186–1191.
9. Shapiro BA, Kacmarek RM, Cane RD, et al. *Clinical Application of Respiratory Care*. 4th ed. St. Louis: Mosby-Yearbook; 1991.
10. Judson MA, Sahn SA. Mobilization of secretions in ICU patients. *Respir Care*. 1994;39:213–227.
11. Szeinberg A, Tabachnik E, Rashed N, et al. Cough capacity in patients with muscular dystrophy. *Chest*. 1988;94:1232–1235.
12. Bach JR, Ishikawa Y, Heakyung K. Prevention of pulmonary morbidity for patients with Duchenne Muscular Dystrophy. *Chest* 1997;112:1024.
13. Gaskell DV, Webber BA. *The Brompton Hospital Guide to Chest Physiotherapy*. 2nd ed. London: Blackwell Scientific Publications; 1973.
14. Frownfelter DL. *Chest Physical Therapy and Rehabilitation: An Interdisciplinary Approach*. Chicago: Year Book Medical Publishers; 1978.
15. Murray JF. The ketchup bottle method. *N Eng J Med*. 1979;300:1155–1157.
16. Pryor JA, Webber BA, Hodson ME, Batten JC. Evaluation of the forced expiration technique as an adjunct to postural drainage in treatment of cystic fibrosis. *Br Med J*. 1979;2:417–418.
17. Branson RD, Hurst JH, DeHaven CB. Mask CPAP: State of the art. *Respir Care*. 1985;309:846–857.
18. Pierce AK, Saltzman HA. Conference on a scientific basis for respiratory therapy. *Am Rev Resp Dis*. Supp. 1974:110.
19. Peruzzi WT, Smith B. Bronchial hygiene therapy. *Critical Care Clinics*. 1995;11:79–96.
20. Bach JR. Mechanical insufflation-exsufflation: comparison of peak expiratory flows with manually assisted and unassisted coughing techniques. *Chest*. 1993;104:1553–1562.
21. Beck GJ. Chronic bronchial asthma and emphysema: Rehabilitation and use of thoracic vibrocompression. *Geriatrics*. 1966;21:137–158.
22. Baker AB. Poliomyelitis: treatment. *Neurology*. 1954;4:379–392.
23. MacIntyre NR, Helms M, Wunderink R, Schmidt G, Sahn SA. Automated rotational therapy for the prevention of respiratory complications during mechanical ventilation. *Respir Care*. 1999;44: 1447–1457.
24. Main E, Prasad A, van der Schans CP. Conventional chest physiotherapy compared to other airway clearance techniques for cystic fibrosis (Review). *Cochrane Database of Systematic Reviews* 2009;2.

Suggested Readings

Bills GW, Soderberg RC. *Principles of Pharmacology for Respiratory Care*. 2nd ed. Clifton Park, NY: Delmar Cengage Learning; 1998.

Sorenson HM, Thorson JA. *Geriatric Respiratory Care*. Clifton Park, NY: Delmar Cengage Learning; 1998.

Whitaker K. *Comprehensive Perinatal and Pediatric Respiratory Care*. 3rd ed. Clifton Park, NY: Delmar Cengage Learning; 2001.

White GC. *Equipment Theory for Respiratory Care*. 3rd ed. Clifton Park, NY: Delmar Cengage Learning; 1999.

CHAPTER 24

Airway Management

Doug McIntyre

OBJECTIVES

Upon completion of this chapter, the reader should be able to:

- List and describe the two basic classifications of airway obstructions.
- List the indications for artificial airways.
- Describe a Carlens tube.
- List the advantages and disadvantages of the oroendotracheal tube versus the nasoendotracheal tube.
- Describe the difficult airway and identify the equipment and techniques used to manage the difficult airway.
- Differentiate between a tracheostomy and a laryngectomy.
- Describe the Passy-Muir valve, and define the function of the valve.
- Differentiate between low-volume, high-pressure cuffs and high-volume, low-pressure cuffs.
- List the complications associated with airway suctioning.
- Explain the suction technique for the Trach Care suction device.
- Describe how to safely handle patients with artificial airways.

CHAPTER OUTLINE

KEY TERMS

airway obstruction
airway suctioning
artificial airways
blind nasotracheal intubation
cricothyrotomy
cuff
difficult airway
emergency airway adjuncts
endotracheal intubation
fiberoptic intubation
tracheostomy tube

The upper airway does most of the conditioning of the ambient air; cleaning, warming and humidifying, before it reaches the *carina*. They condition the inspired air by correcting the temperature and humidity and by cleansing it. Think of the temperature of ambient air on a dusty road in a desert being 112°F with a 10% relative humidity. Without conditioning, ambient air with those characteristics would destroy the respiratory system. The upper airway filters out the dust, cools the air-to-body temperature, and humidifies the air-to-body humidity.

The vocal cords are responsible for generating the sounds of vocalization, and the upper airways are responsible for phonation. The structure and movement of the upper airways actually form the quality of the sounds that we use to communicate by speaking, singing, screaming, whispering, and making other sounds.

The most important function of the upper airway is conducting air to and from the lower airways. *Ventilation* is defined as the mass movement of air to and from the lower airways.

This chapter focuses on the upper airway when function is impaired. Impaired function necessitates the use of artificial airways and adjunct therapy to mimic normal function. Discussed in this chapter are the numerous types of special-purpose artificial airways and their applications.

Airway Management

The goal of airway management is to maintain an open airway to ensure adequate ventilation.

There are two basic classifications for **airway obstructions**, or blockage: partial and complete.

- With *partial* airway obstruction, some air is allowed to move, and the patient can cough and produce breath sounds.
- *Complete* airway obstruction differs in that there is no movement of air, even with marked inspiratory efforts.

The causes of airway obstruction are:

- The tongue occluding the airway (the most common cause).
- Aspiration of foreign objects.
- Thick mucus in the airway.
- Laryngeal edema.
- Laryngospasm.
- Glottic edema.
- Subglottic edema.

Airway obstruction of the unconscious patient is usually the result of loss of muscle tone in the tongue, allowing the tongue to fall back and occlude the airway.

When acute airway obstruction occurs, the airway has to be opened.

ARTIFICIAL AIRWAYS

Artificial airways are indicated for:

- The prevention or relief of airway obstruction.
- Providing an access to the airway for the purpose of suctioning.
- Prevention of aspirating foreign substances into the airway.
- Creating a closed system for mechanical ventilation.

Several different types of artificial airways are in use today. Each type has a specific application in airway management.

Nasopharyngeal Airways. *Nasopharyngeal airways* (Figure 24-1) are designed with a flared proximal tip, much like a trumpet. They are sometimes referred to as a *nasal trumpet*. Nasopharyngeal airways are commonly manufactured from a soft flexible polyvinyl chloride material that contours to the nasopharyngeal structure.

Nasopharyngeal airways are indicated for the conscious patient who has difficulty maintaining a patent upper airway or who needs frequent suctioning. The airway must be properly sized with the outside diameter smaller than the nasal passage and well lubricated for insertion to prevent trauma to the nasal mucosa. The advantages of the nasopharyngeal airway are as follows:

- It provides relief for upper airway obstruction.
- It is better tolerated than the oropharyngeal airway.
- It provides an easily accessible route for suctioning with less trauma to the nasal mucosa.

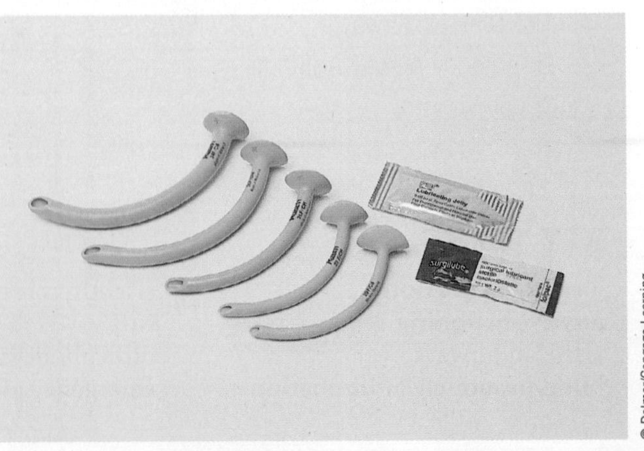

FIGURE 24-1 Nasopharyngeal airways.

Best Practice

Opening the Airway

The preferred technique for opening the airway is the head lift with the anterior movement of the jaw by chin lift and jaw thrust, if indicated (Figures 24-2 and 24-3). The jaw thrust is performed by placing the fingers behind the mandible while the hands are on each side of the patient's face and then thrusting the jaw forward. If neck injury is suspected, begin with the chin lift without the head tilt. If the airway is still obstructed, the head tilt is gradually and very slowly incorporated until the airway opens. Safety Note: Don't use techniques that rotate or extend the head until the "head and neck are cleared"; that is it is determined that there are no head or spinal injures.

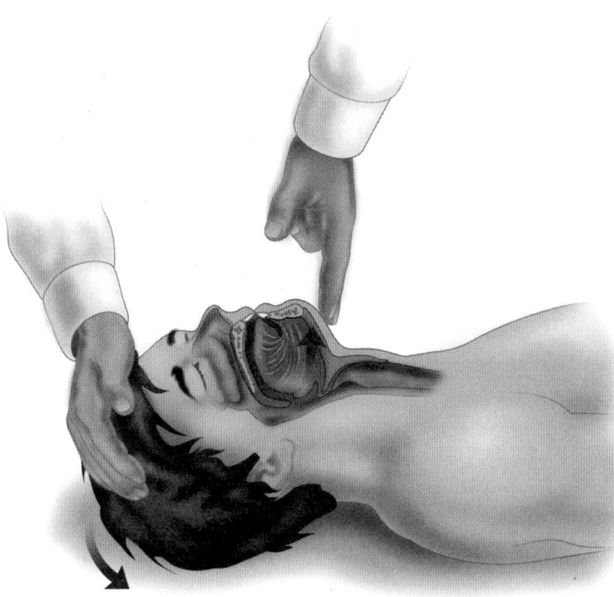

FIGURE 24-2 Head tilt, chin lift maneuver.

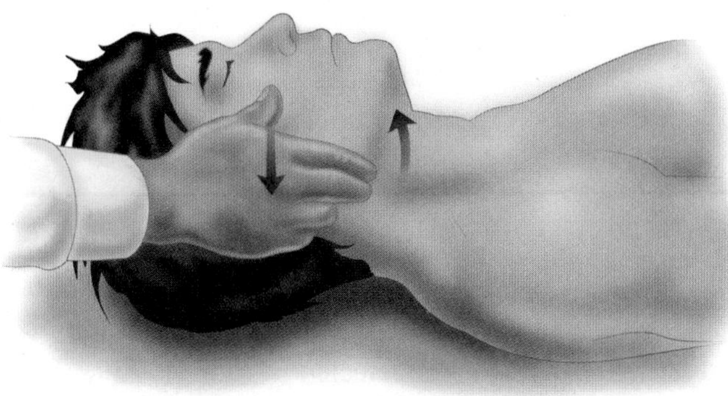

FIGURE 24-3 Jaw thrust maneuver.

The disadvantages of the nasopharyngeal airway are as follows:

- It is difficult to insert.
- It should be alternated between the nares every 24 hours.
- Drainage for sinuses and eustachian tubes can be obstructed, potentially causing congestion or infection.

Oropharyngeal Airways. *Oropharyngeal airways* (Figure 24-4) are available in two basic designs: the Berman airway and the Guedel airway.

- The *Berman airway* has two horizontal plates connected by one ridge in the center of the airway. Each side of the ridge serves as a channel to pass a suction catheter through to the laryngopharynx. The two horizontal plates provide a flat surface for the teeth to contact. The smooth rounded tip prevents trauma to the soft tissue of the upper airway.
- The *Guedel airway* is designed with one smooth channel through the center. Suction catheters are passed through the center channel into the laryngopharynx.

Oropharyngeal airways are indicated for the unconscious or nonresponsive patient who has difficulty maintaining a patent upper airway. The size of the airway to be inserted is determined by measuring from the angle of the jaw to the tip of the chin.

The advantages of the oropharyngeal airway are that:

- It may be used with endotracheal tubes to prevent problems associated with biting the tube.
- It can be used with seizure patients to prevent the tongue from being bitten.

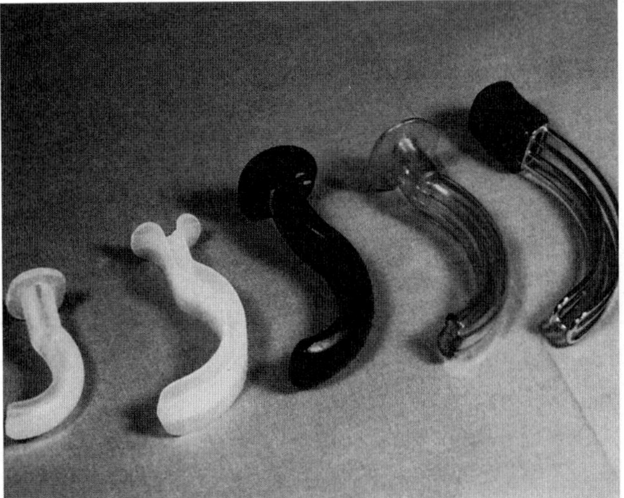

FIGURE 24-4 Oropharyngeal airways.

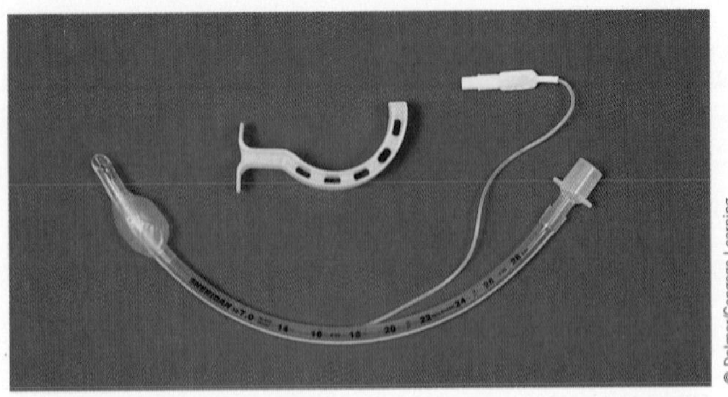

FIGURE 24-5 Endotracheal tube.

The disadvantage of the oropharyngeal airway is that conscious patients have difficulties tolerating it because of the gag reflex.

Endotracheal Airways. *Endotracheal tubes* (Figure 24-5) are probably the most commonly used artificial airways. Historically, endotracheal tubes were manufactured using red rubber. The cuff was supplied separately and required installation by the user. These cuffs were all low-volume, high-pressure cuffs inflated with high pressures at low volumes by design. The invention of a clear *polyvinyl chloride* (*PVC*) endotracheal tube brought with it the advantage of being able to visualize secretions in the tube. Originally, the cuff on the PVC tube was also low volume, high pressure. The high-volume, low-pressure cuff (i.e., high inflation volume at low pressures) was introduced shortly after the advent of the PVC endotracheal tube.

Endotracheal Intubation **Endotracheal intubation** is the introduction of an endotracheal tube into the trachea, by either the oral or the nasal route. The oral route is used most commonly in the acute situation. A laryngoscope (Figure 24-6), an instrument that consists of a handle and a curved or straight blade, is used to aid in the insertion by the oral route and sometimes by the nasal route. The blade is gently inserted through the mouth into the oropharynx until the vocal cords are visualized. A light at the distal tip of the blade facilitates vocal cord visualization. Then the endotracheal tube is guided through the vocal cords and into the trachea.

Verification of Placement Immediate verification of endotracheal placement in the trachea is still a problem. Verification is often necessary before an X-ray machine is on the scene.

- The most common method is by auscultation of the thorax for bilateral and equal breath sounds. When breath sounds are unequal and present on one side only, main stem intubation must be suspected. The tube must be withdrawn until breath sounds are present on both sides.
- Auscultation of the thorax should be concurrent with auscultation of the stomach. If sounds of air are being introduced into the epigastrium and not into the lungs, esophageal intubation must be suspected.

The introduction of *disposable colorimetric CO_2 detectors* provides another method of placement verification (Figure 24-7). The presence of CO_2 turns the media in the detector yellow. The color change must be consistent with each exhalation because the detectors are not 100% accurate. CO_2 may not be present in sufficient quantities to change the color if cardiac output is insufficient to provide adequate pulmonary circulation.

The introduction of *radiopaque lines* placed in endotracheal tubes changed the standard for verification of tube placement (see Chapter 14). The radiopaque line should be in place from the proximal end to the distal

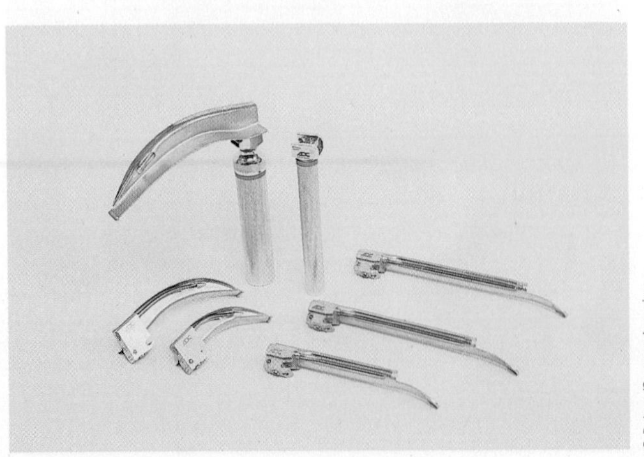

FIGURE 24-6 Laryngoscope and blades.

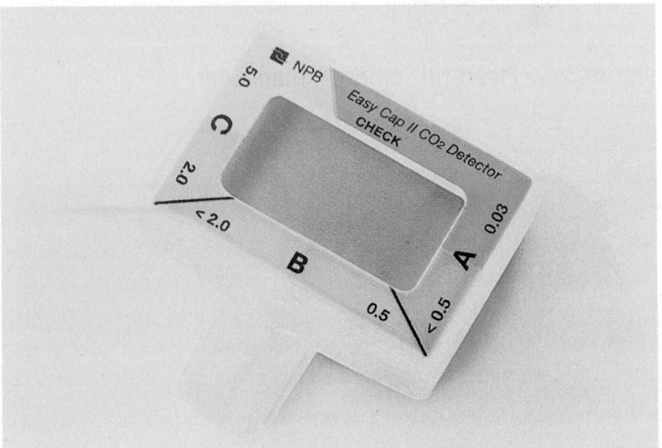

FIGURE 24-7 End-tidal CO_2 detector.

Image used by permission from Nellcor Puritan Bennett LLC, Boulder, Colorado, doing business as Covidien.

tip and centered in the posterior curve of the endotracheal tube. The use of a simple radiographic examination of the chest became, and continues to be, the standard. With radiographic examination of the chest, the radiopaque line can be visualized to determine the placement of the distal tip of the endotracheal tube. The radiopaque line has been incorporated into the design of other devices used for insertion into the body. It improves the clinician's ability to ascertain the appropriate placement of tubes and other medical devices.

Tube Securing Methods Accidental extubation is a common problem when the tube is not secured properly. The therapist must therefore secure endotracheal, tracheostomy, and laryngectomy tubes after the proper placement is verified.

Securing tubes has been accomplished in a number of ways. The widespread and first method ever used is taping endotracheal tubes in place.

- One-inch-wide tape, sufficient in length to reach around the patient's head with each end extending 6 inches past the tube, is used to secure the tube.
- Another length of tape, sufficient to reach from ear to ear behind the patient's head, is placed in the center of the first length of tape. This makes a non-stick surface for the tape behind the patient's head that does not adhere to the patient's hair.
- The tape is placed around the patient's head, and both ends are split in the middle. One half of the split tape, on each side, is secured across the patient's upper lip under the nose or across the chin, and the other split is wrapped around the tube, with the sticky side to the tube.

Patients who are conscious and alert should not be taped across the chin to avoid inadvertent extubation by movement associated with the chin.

Best Practice

Endotracheal Intubation

Sometimes endotracheal intubation may take several attempts before the tube is properly placed. The attempts must not exceed 30 seconds without reoxygenating the patient. If the person attempting the intubation is unsuccessful after two attempts, the patient should be returned to 100% oxygen bag-and-mask ventilation, and another rescuer should attempt the intubation.

Other considerations are as follows:

- Cloth tape performs better than silk or some of the newer types of tape.
- The endotracheal tube should be retaped each shift.
- If the skin is extremely moist, tincture of benzoin is sometimes useful to ensure a secure bonding between the skin and the tape.
- Care must be taken to monitor the skin for signs of sensitivity and reactions to the tape. The tube should be moved from one side of the mouth to the other during retaping to avoid tissue breakdown in the corner of the mouth.

Manufactured securing devices are available for securing an endotracheal tube during a code. The Advanced Cardiac Life Support Standards recommends several of such devices, which come in some creative styles and configurations. Most are effective; some are better than others.

Twill ties have been the mainstay of securing methods for tracheostomies and laryngectomies.

Tube Holders

Several tube holders that have become available in recent years vary in design and methodology.

- One of these uses a piece of Velcro, which is secured on the tube at the level of the lip. The neckband attaches directly to the tube via the Velcro fastening method.
- Another holder secures the tube by placing the holder component of the device to the chin with adhesive. The tube is placed in the holder and secured with a tying band that resembles a plastic electrician tie.
- Still another has a bite block incorporated into the holder and is secured with rubber straps.

Holders for tracheostomies and laryngectomies are also available. Most of them are designed with a neckband made of soft material. On each end is a tab, manufactured from Velcro-like material, that threads through the tracheostomy tube plate and folds back to attach to the neckband. Even though the neckband stretches for comfort and safety, the tabs can be removed and reattached repeatedly due to the Velcro-like material.

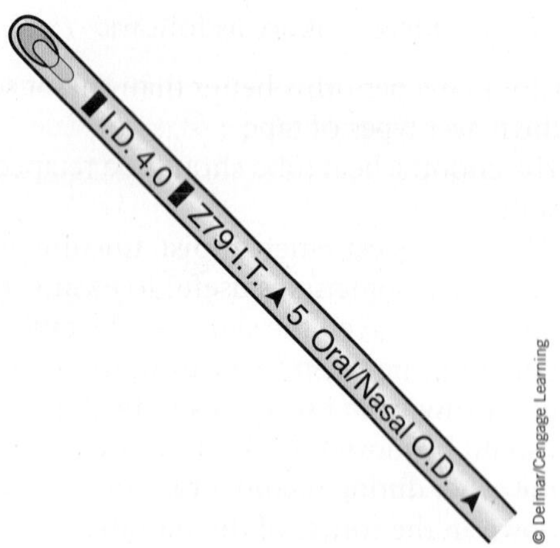

FIGURE 24-8 Tube markings.

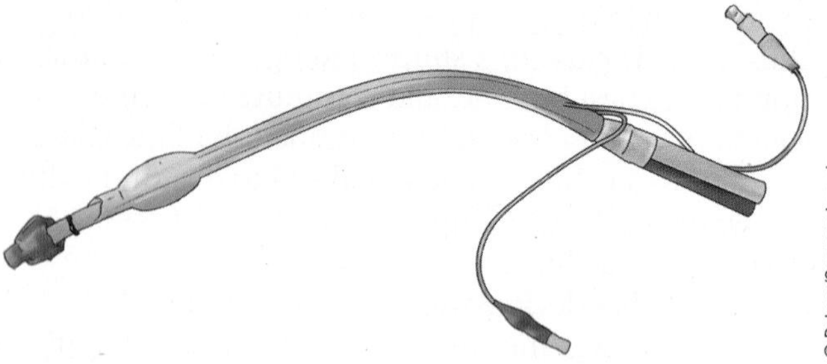

FIGURE 24-9 Double-lumen endobronchial tube.

Endotracheal Tubes Markings on an endotracheal tube may include the following (Figure 24-8):

- *IT* indicates that the material used to manufacture the tube has been implant-tested in living tissue for toxic reactions.
- *Z79* indicates that the tube meets the standards established by the American Materials Standard Institute's Z79 committee.
- *Centimeter markings* are used as a guide to determine how far the distal tip is inserted into the airway.
- *The size of the endotracheal tube in millimeters* is expressed in terms of internal diameter (ID) and outside diameter (OD).
- *The name of the manufacturer.*

Endotracheal tubes are manufactured to maintain a curvature that resembles the curvature of the upper airway, which aids in the intubation procedure. However, sometimes a small stylet, a thin rodlike device, must be placed in the lumen of the tube to change the curvature to facilitate a difficult intubation.

Specialty endotracheal tubes, designed for specific uses, are also available. The *double lumen endobronchial sometimes refer to as a Carlen's tube.* (Figure 24-9) tube has a double lumen design complete with two cuffs and two pilot balloons. It is used to intubate the right mainstem bronchus with the distal cuff resting inflated in the right mainstem bronchus above the right upper lobe bronchial opening. The second cuff rests inflated in the distal end of the trachea. The purpose is to perform independent lung ventilation. These tubes are also available in a left mainstem bronchial orientation. Both versions of these tubes have a carinal hook that straddles the carina and prevents overly deep insertion of the tube and the blockage of segmental or lobar bronchi openings.

Age-Specific Competency

Endotracheal Tube Sizes

Endotracheal tubes are available in sizes ranging from 2.5 to 9.5 mm in diameter. The tube size and cuff application are determined by the patient's age and size (Table 24-1).

Stylet The *stylet* is a smooth, malleable metal or plastic rod that is placed inside an endotracheal tube to adjust the curvature, typically into a the shape of a J or hockey stick to allow the tip of the endotracheal tube to be directed through a poorly visualized or unseen glottis (Figure 24-10).[1] To avoid potential airway injury, the stylet must not project beyond the end of the endotracheal tube.

Gum Elastic Bougie The *gum elastic bougie* is a blunt-ended, malleable rod that may be passed through the poorly visualized or nonvisualized larynx by putting a J-shaped bend at the tip and passing it blindly in the midline upward beyond the base of the epiglottis. The endotracheal tube can then be advanced over the bougie, which is then withdrawn.

Lighted Stylet The *lighted stylet* is a malleable fiberoptic light source on which an endotracheal tube can be

TABLE 24-1 **Endotracheal tube sizes**

Age Recommended	Internal Diameter (mm)
Premature infant	2.5–3.0 uncuffed
Full-term infant	3.0–3.5 uncuffed
6 months–1 year old	3.5–4.5 uncuffed
1–6 years old	4.5–5.5 uncuffed
6–10 years old	5.5–6.5 uncuffed or cuffed
10 years old–adolescent	6.5–8.0 cuffed
Adolescent–adult	7.0–9.0 cuffed

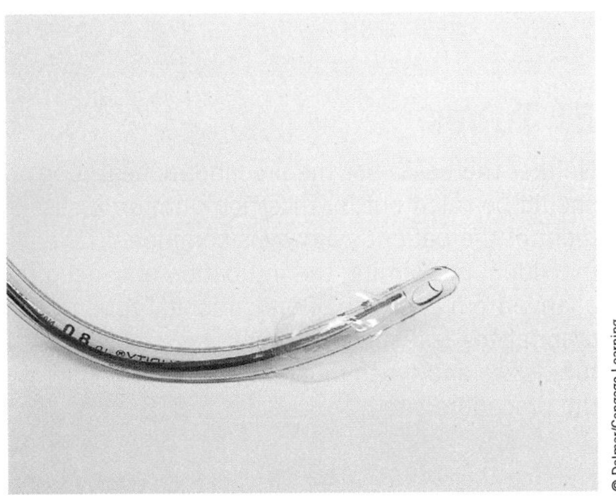

FIGURE 24-10 Malleable stylet.

mounted and subsequently advanced into the trachea when the light source has passed beyond the glottis. The result is a greater intensity of light visible through anterior soft tissues of the neck as the light source passes beyond the vocal cords. The lighted stylet facilitates blind tracheal intubation by distinguishing the tracheal lumen from the (more posterior) esophagus.[2]

A potential disadvantage is the need for low ambient light, which may not be desirable (or easily achieved) in a critical care setting. Light wand devices may be contraindicated in patients with known abnormal upper airway anatomy and those in whom detectable transillumination is unlikely to be adequately achieved.[3]

Endotracheal Tube Insertion Routes With appropriate training, endotracheal intubation can be performed, and it is not restricted to use in the hospital environment. There are two routes of insertion: nasoendotracheal (nasal) and oroendotracheal tubes (oral). When the two are compared, each has its advantages and disadvantages.

The *advantages of the nasoendotracheal tube* are that:

- It can be inserted without the aid of a laryngoscope in some instances.
- Once inserted, it can be stabilized easily.
- It is tolerated better by the patient because it does not pass through the mouth.
- The patient can close the mouth and swallow.
- It is easier to provide oral hygiene.
- Communication is better because the patient can form words with the mouth.
- Connection to a ventilator or other equipment is easier.
- Turning and nodding pressures on the trachea are less likely.
- Inadvertent extubation is less likely.

The *disadvantages of the nasoendotracheal tube* are that:

- The individual inserting the tube must exhibit a high degree of skill to attempt the procedure.
- Size limitations of the nasal passage require the use of a tube at least 0.5 mm smaller than for oral intubation.
- The curvature of the tube is greater owing to the insertion path.
- The size limitation and the increased curvature of the tube makes it more difficult to suction the patient, increases the work of breathing, and raises airway resistance.
- Tissue necrosis may occur in the nasal passage owing to the pressure exerted by the tube.
- Though less likely than with oral intubation, vagal stimulation still occurs.
- Drainage for sinuses and eustachian tubes can be obstructed, potentially causing congestion or infection.
- Laryngeal trauma is possible, just as is true for oral intubation.

The *advantages of the oroendotracheal tube* are that:

- It is the airway of choice in an emergency situation because of ease of insertion.
- Size limitations are not as limiting as with the nasal route, thus allowing a tube at least 0.5 mm larger.
- The curvature of the tube is not as great as with nasal insertion because of the increased size of the insertion path (the complications associated with suctioning, work of breathing, and airway resistance are of less significance than with nasal intubation).
- There is no interference with drainage from the sinuses and eustachian tubes.

The *disadvantages of the oroendotracheal tube* are that:

- A laryngoscope is required for insertion, increasing the possibility of lacerating the lip or breaking teeth if the procedure is improperly performed.
- Tube stabilization is more difficult than with the nasal route, with occasional resultant skin irritation or trauma.
- Patients conscious enough to realize the presence of the tube have a very low tolerance for the tube because of gag reflex, dry mouth, and general discomfort associated with having a secured foreign object in the oral cavity.
- The patient's mouth cannot be closed completely, and swallowing becomes difficult.
- Oral hygiene is extremely difficult to provide.
- Communication is difficult because of difficulty in forming words with the mouth.

- Vagal stimulation is more common than with nasal intubation.
- The tube may become dislodged more easily than with nasal intubation.
- Inadvertent extubation is more common with oral intubation.
- Ventilator and equipment connection and stabilization is often more difficult.
- The tube forms a channel for secretions from the mouth to travel into the area above the cuff and hence to the lungs, causing aspiration pneumonia.[4]

Endotracheal Tube Removal When the endotracheal tube is no longer needed for ventilation, airway stability, or secretion management, it can be removed. Before extubation occurs, the patient's airway above and below the cuff must be suctioned well to remove any secretions that may migrate into the lung when the tube is removed. If secretions are already present in the lungs, care must be taken to remove as many of the secretions as possible before removing the tube.

Then perform the following steps rapidly:

- Remove the endotracheal securing device.
- Oxygenate the patient well.
- Insert a suction catheter.
- Apply suction.
- Deflate the cuff while instructing the patient to cough.
- Remove the endotracheal tube.

Once the patient is extubated, remember that cuff pressures low enough to prohibit the necrosis of the trachea might be high enough to reduce the normal flow of the lymphatic system. The glottic and subglottic edema associated with these pressures may create problems when the tube is removed.

- If the patient experiences difficulties, the first action is to start humidified oxygen to prevent resultant hypoxemia.
- If there is no sign of improvement or if worsening is noted, it may become necessary to administer racemic epinephrine 2.25% and normal saline in a small volume nebulizer. Racemic epinephrine has a vasoconstriction action and produces shrinkage of the tissue in the larynx and vocal cords to reduce airway resistance.
- Should symptoms of the edema persist, be prepared to reintubate the patient.

After extubation, the patient may exhibit hoarseness, sore throat, and vocal cord trauma or paralysis.

Best Practice

ET Tubes

Neither the naso- nor the oroendotracheal tube should be ruled out for insertion until an assessment of the patient's airway is completed. The individual performing the intubation may need to change from one type of endotracheal tube to the other at the last second. Therefore, a variety of tube sizes and types must be readily available at the procedure site.

Specialized Endotracheal Tubes Several types of specialized endotracheal (sometimes called *endobroncheal tubes*) are used for specific purposes, one of which is used for differential lung ventilation. In differential lung ventilation, each lung is ventilated differently than the other. These differences may result in different volumes, in different pressures, or perhaps in no ventilation at all in one lung while the other lung is being ventilated mechanically or manually. The *Carlen's tube* (a type of endobroncheal tube) is a double-lumen, double-cuffed endobrocheal tube with two pilot balloons, two inflation lines, and two cuffs. In addition to the double lumens and double cuffs, Carlen's tubes differ from other endotracheal tubes in that they come with either a right or a left orientation, each of which has color-coded inflation lines, pilot balloons, and lumen shafts as a safety measure to prevent accidental misconnections.

Due to its unique structure, the Carlen's tube provides the opportunity to perform procedures that would be otherwise impossible, extremely dangerous, or even life-threatening to the patient. Table 24-2 lists some of the indications for and contraindications of use of a Carlen's tube.

The Laryngeal Mask Airway The *laryngeal mask airway (LMA)* (Figure 24-11) is a small mask with an inflatable rim on the end of a tube. Developed in 1982 by Archie Brain, MD and approved for use in the US by the FDA in 1991, it comes in four sizes.[5] It is inserted blindly with the mask facing the tongue until resistance is met. The mask is then inflated to cover the opening of the trachea, providing a route for ventilation.

The LMA works well in approximately 90% of cases. However, it is not without limitations, which include the following:

- Ventilation may not be adequate because the cuff fails to seal the larynx, the tongue pushes over the larynx, or the epiglottis flips over the larynx.

TABLE 24-2 **Indications and contraindications for Carlen's tubes**

Lung isolation (separate access to each lung)
Indications:
Infection (prevent contamination of the nonaffected lung)
Pulmonary hemorrhage
Control of the distribution of ventilation
Prevent air volume loss through the fistula due to bronchopleural fistula
Prevent air volume loss through the fistula due to bronchopleural cutaneous fistula
Surgical opening of major conducting airway
Giant unilateral cyst or bulla
Life-threatening hypoxemia from unilateral pulmonary process
Unilateral bronchopulmonary lavage
Relative indications:
Surgical exposure (strong indication)
Thoracic aortic aneurysm
Pneumonectomy
Upper lobectomy
Mediastinal exposure
Thoracoscopy
Surgical exposure (moderate indication)
Middle and lower lobectomy
Subsegmental resection
Esophageal resection
Procedures on the thoracic spine
Post-C-P bypass status after removal of totally occluding chronic unilateral pulmonary emboli
Severe hypoxemia from unilateral pulmonary process
Requirement for differential ventilation for critical care
Contraindications
Absolute contraindications:
Patient refusal
Airway (especially laryngeal or tracheal) mass that may be occluding, dislodged, traumatized, or hemorrhaging
Relative contraindications:
Patients requiring rapid intubation to prevent aspiration of gastric contents
Patients who are likely to be difficult to intubate

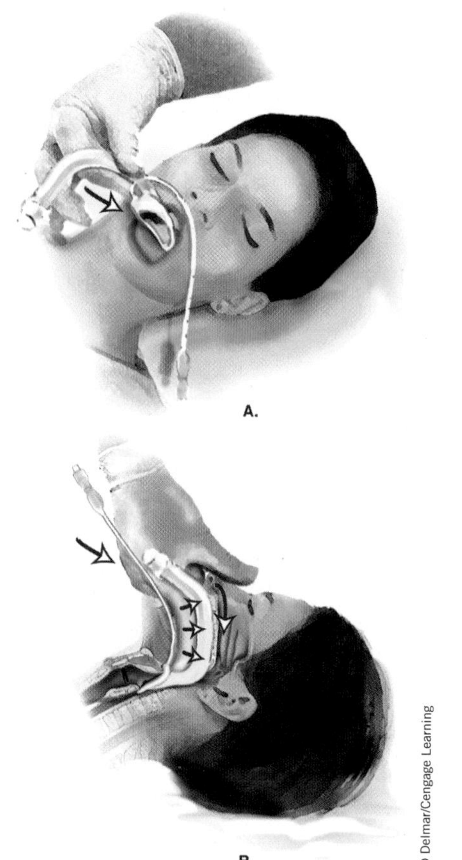

FIGURE 24-11 Insertion and placement of the laryngeal mask airway.

- Laryngospasm can occur when the mask is inserted or removed without adequate anesthesia.
- It cannot protect against aspiration of gastric content. (The operator must remember this.)

Esophageal-Tracheal Combitube The *esophageal-tracheal combitube* (*ETC*) (Figure 24-12) is a double-lumen tube that is blindly inserted into the pharynx. One lumen is open to the end, similar to an endotracheal tube. The other lumen ends blindly with holes that wind up in the vicinity of the opening of the larynx when the tube is inserted into the esophagus. Once the tube is inserted, the operator inflates the small balloon on the end of the tube and the large, 100 mL balloon, which occludes the pharynx. Verification of placement in the trachea is determined by the operator. If it is determined to be properly placed, the tube can then be used for ventilation much like the endotracheal tube.

If the tube is determined to be in the esophagus, ventilation can be accomplished by using the other opening.

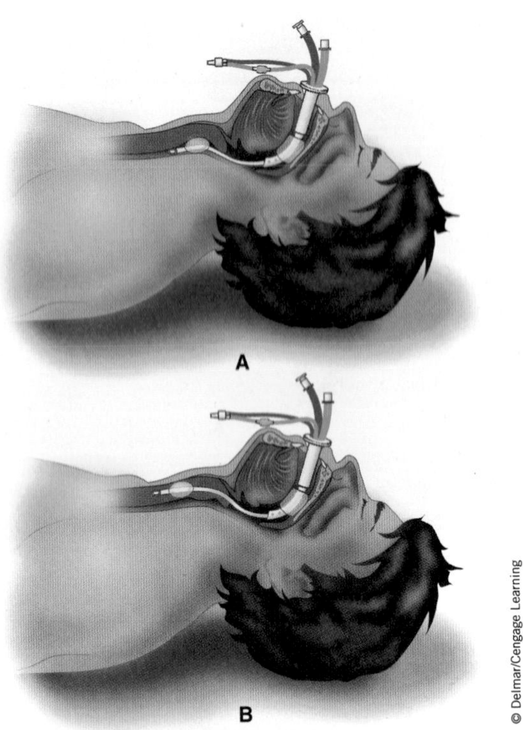

FIGURE 24-12 (A) Combitube in the esophageal position. (B) Combitube in the tracheal position.

Sealing the esophagus with the small balloon allows the evacuation of gastric contents through that lumen. The ETC thus provides ventilation similar to that accomplished with the endotracheal tube while preventing gastric content aspiration.

The ETC has two major limitations:

- It comes in one size, which limits the application to adults.
- The trachea is not accessible for suctioning if the tube is in the esophagus.

Fiberoptic Intubation. The fiberoptic scope can be used in the unanticipated difficult airway but only if it is readily available and the operator is skilled.[6] **Fiberoptic intubation** is usually more straightforward through the nasal route instead of the oral route. The scope is advanced to the midtracheal level, and the carina is visualized. The endotracheal tube may then be placed carefully through the nasal cavity and into the trachea. Occasionally, passing the endotracheal tube through the vocal cords is difficult. Withdrawing the endotracheal tube, rotating it 90 degrees counterclockwise, and readvancing it usually allows passage with less difficulty. The endotracheal tube should be positioned approximately 3 cm above the carina.[7]

Blind Nasotracheal Intubation. Blind nasotracheal intubation is especially valuable for intubating spontaneously breathing patients but is contraindicated for patients with bleeding disorders. The nasal mucosa should be prepared with phenylephrine or oxymetazolone (Afrin) prior to the procedure. Local anesthesia should be considered, especially in the awake, sedated patient. The procedure is as follows:

- Place the patient's head and neck in the "sniffing position," if it is not contraindicated.
- The appropriate tube size for the nasal intubation route is the same as used for the oral route. Position the naso endotracheal tube connector in a position that corresponds to the curvature of the endotracheal tube to provide a reference for guiding the endotracheal tube.
- Slowly advance the endotracheal tube along the floor of the nose. Using the endotracheal tube connector as a reference, guide the endotracheal tube toward the larynx. This is slightly to the opposite side of the nares that a tube is entering (i.e., left for the right nares and right for the left nares).
- Listen for breath sounds as the tube is advanced.
- When the tube is correctly positioned in the trachea, breath sounds will continue and the patient will cough through the tube.
- Auscultate the breath sounds bilaterally, confirm tube placement and secure the tube. The absence of breath sounds and cough through the tube, while the tube is still being advanced, indicates that the tube is inappropriately placed in the esophagus.[8]

THE DIFFICULT AIRWAY

The **difficult airway** can result from:

- An inability to open the mouth.
- Abnormal facial anatomy.
- Cervical immobility,
- Pharyngeal abnormality.
- Laryngeal abnormality.

All can contribute to difficult tracheal intubation.

Difficult tracheal intubation is tracheal intubation that requires multiple intubation attempts. It may result from difficulty in visualization of the larynx, a situation termed *difficult direct laryngoscopy*.[9] Visualization of the larynx is described using the Cormack and Lehane grades (Table 24-3).[10] Grades 3 and 4 indicate difficult direct laryngoscopy, and a nondirect laryngoscope may be required to obtain an airway.

Nondirect techniques are available. However, the clinician must have the necessary equipment and supplies to perform them. The recommended items for a difficult airway cart are listed in Table 24-4.

TABLE 24-3 Grades of Difficult Laryngoscopy

		Mallampati airway scale
Grade I	Most of glottis is seen.	
Grade II	Only posterior portion of glottis can be seen.	
Grade III	Only epiglottis may be seen (none of glottis seen).	
Grade IV	Neither epiglottis nor glottis can be seen.	

Source: Cormack and Lehane

TABLE 24-4 Recommended items for difficult airway cart

- Bag mask ventilator with oxygen supply source
- Oropharyngeal airways, various sizes
- Nasopharyngeal airways, various sizes
- Endotracheal tubes, various sizes
- Endotracheal tube stylet
- Lighted stylet, if available
- Gum elastic bougie
- Laryngoscope with various type and size blades
- Laryngeal mask airway, various sizes
- Esophageal-tracheal Combitube, various sizes
- Endotracheal tube carbon dioxide detectors
- Cricothyroidotomy kit
- Tracheostomy mini kit
- Oxygen supply source with required connectors and supply tubing
- Suction catheters and Yankauer suction device
- Spare bulbs and batteries as required

Endotracheal Tube Removal in Patients with a Difficult Airway. Patients with a difficult airway can be problematic when it is time to remove the endotracheal tube. If there is a need for reintubation, the difficulty level is higher than the initial intubation. Reintubating these patients can be exceptionally difficult. The procedure for removing the endotracheal tube from the difficult airway patient is similar to removal from a patient intubated without difficulty. The difference is that a plan must be in place in the event that the patient requires reintubation. And the plan should include a difficult airway cart and skilled staff capable of reestablishing the airway.

EMERGENCY AIRWAY ADJUNCTS

Approximately 30 years ago a category of devices was created to fill the void presented when circumstances made it impractical or impossible to insert an endotracheal tube. The category is known as **emergency airway adjuncts**, and it includes the esophageal obturator airway and the esophageal gastric tube airway.

Esophageal Obturator Airway. The *esophageal obturator airway* (*EOA*) (Figure 24-13) is a tube that looks a lot like an endotracheal tube with a mask attached. It has a cuff with small holes above the cuff and is designed to be inserted into the esophagus, not the trachea. Once inserted, the cuff is inflated to block the esophagus, the mask seals the patient's airway, and air blown into the tube passes through the holes in the tube into the patient's lungs, not the stomach.

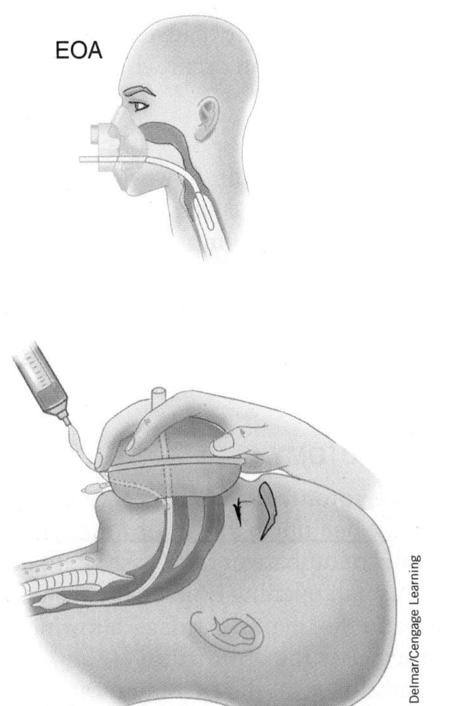

FIGURE 24-13 Esophageal obturator airway.

Best Practice

Esophageal Obturator Airway

The end of the airway tube is sealed. If inadvertent intubation of the trachea occurs, the patient cannot breathe. Also, tracheal intubation must be done before the esophageal obturator airway is removed to prevent aspiration when the patient regurgitates.

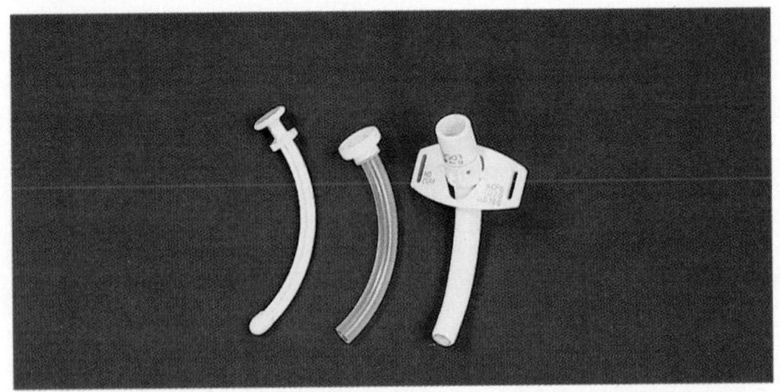

FIGURE 24-14 Tracheostomy tubes.

The esophageal obturator airway is used primarily by health care providers outside the hospital setting when intubation efforts have failed or when personnel cannot intubate because of licensure or training limitations. The advantages of the esophageal obturator airway are:

- Ease of insertion.
- Security of the airway from the aspiration of gastric juices.
- Prevention of gastric distention from air introduced into the stomach.

The disadvantages of the esophageal obturator airway are as follows:

- It is indicated for short-term use only.
- Esophageal trauma is possible.
- The trachea can be inadvertently intubated.
- Regurgitation can occur when the tube is removed.

Esophageal Gastric Tube Airway. The *esophageal gastric tube airway* (EGTA) has a gastric tube lumen in the center to permit decompression of the stomach after bag and mask ventilation. Its use is compared with the that of the EOA. The level of ventilation provided by these devices is generally less than that provided by intubation of the patient.

CRICOTHYROTOMY

The **cricothyrotomy** is an emergency airway procedure performed when upper airway obstruction renders it impossible to intubate or otherwise ventilate the patient. A small opening is made between the cricoid cartilage and the thyroid cartilage, allowing the patient to breathe below the obstruction.

The advantage of the cricothyrotomy is that an airway can usually be established quickly when other efforts fail.

The disadvantages are the potential for:

- Hemorrhage.
- Thyroid, vocal cord, and esophageal tissue trauma.
- Pneumothorax and subcutaneous emphysema related to the incorrectly performed procedure.
- The increase of airway resistance due to the small diameter of the airway.[11]

TRACHEOSTOMY TUBES

Tracheostomy tubes (Figure 24-14) were common before a nucleus of professionals became adequately trained to insert endotracheal tubes. A tracheostomy is primarily performed for use in long-term ventilation or in the case of permanent upper airway obstruction.

Nontoxic soft materials such as Teflon, silicone rubber, nylon, and PVC are used in the construction of tracheostomy tubes and other artificial airways. PVC is the most common material in tracheostomy and endotracheal tubes. The Z79 committee of the American Materials Standards Institute establishes the standards for the composition of the materials that manufacturers use in the construction of medical products.

The advantages of tracheostomies are that:

- Suctioning is much easier than it is with endotracheal tubes.
- Trauma to the larynx is not a concern.
- The tube is secured easily, using ties around the neck.
- Communication is facilitated.
- The oropharynx is free of foreign objects, which allows the patient to eat or drink. thus making it more tolerable.

The disadvantages of tracheostomies are twofold:

- Problems associated with the surgical tracheotomy procedure, such as:
  - Bleeding.
  - Damage to the thyroid.
  - The possibility of pneumothorax, subcutaneous emphysema, and air embolism associated with air leaks.
- Problems that occur after the stoma is completely healed, such as:
  - Infection.
  - Tracheal esophageal fistula.
  - Erosion of the innominate artery.
  - Hemorrhage.
  - Obstruction from mucus plugs.
  - Inadvertent insertion into the subcutaneous tissue.
  - Often constipation associated with the inability to increase abdominal pressures influenced by the vocal cords, which are bypassed.

Under normal circumstances, tracheostomy tubes should need to be changed only once a week. The tube may need to be changed if the cuffed tube is too small, the cuff develops a leak, or the tube becomes obstructed. Cleaning should be daily, and the ties are to be cleaned or changed when they become soiled. Ties are not too tight or loose if you can place two fingers between the ties and the neck.

Tracheostomy tubes are designed for specific functions. Most have:

- An outer cannula with a neck plate to affix ties for stability in the stoma.
- An obturator used to guide the tube into the stoma.
- An inner cannula, usually with a standard 15 mm connector. The inner cannula can be removed for cleaning or eliminating obstruction without removing the outer cannula.

The most common tracheostomy tube is the *cuffed tracheostomy tube* designed with the standard 15-mm connector for ease of connecting equipment or ventilators. A low-profile tracheostomy tube is available for the active patient concerned about cosmetic appearance.

Fenestrated Tracheostomy Tube. Another type is the fenestrated tracheostomy tube (Figure 24-15), designed with a fenestration (hole) in the outer cannula of the tube that aligns with the tube's distal opening. Removing the inner cannula and plugging the outer cannula allow the patient to breathe around the tube and through the fenestration. This allows breathing through the oropharynx and aids in the weaning process from the tracheostomy tube.

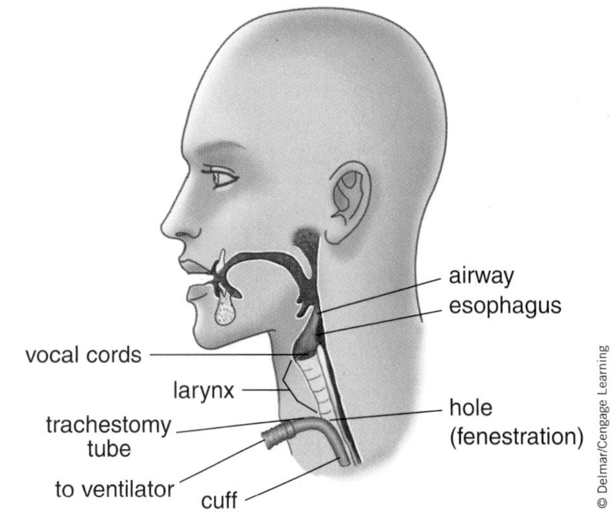

FIGURE 24-15 Fenestrated trach tube.

Best Practice

Fenestrated Tracheostomy Tubes

Fenestrated tracheostomy tubes equipped with cuffs must have the cuff deflated before the plug is inserted into the outer cannula.

Silver Tracheostomy Tube. A number of *silver tracheostomy tubes* are still in use. It is constructed of sterling silver and has an inner cannula matched to the individual tube. A cuff must be installed externally when a cuff is indicated. A fenestrated version of the silver tracheostomy tube is also manufactured.

The disadvantages of the silver tracheostomy are that:

- Its rigid construction contributes to patient discomfort and pressure necrosis.
- The metal can be irritating to the skin and contribute to the production of secretions.

Laryngectomy Tubes. The laryngectomy tube (Figure 24-16), designed much like the tracheostomy tube, is shorter and usually has a larger internal diameter. It is intended for use after a laryngectomy to maintain a patent airway. The most important thing to remember about the laryngectomy tube is that it cannot be plugged. The larynx is absent, and the patient cannot breathe through the oropharynx.

A respiratory therapist is a good resource for providing instructions for appropriate care. Some health care organizations provide support groups that

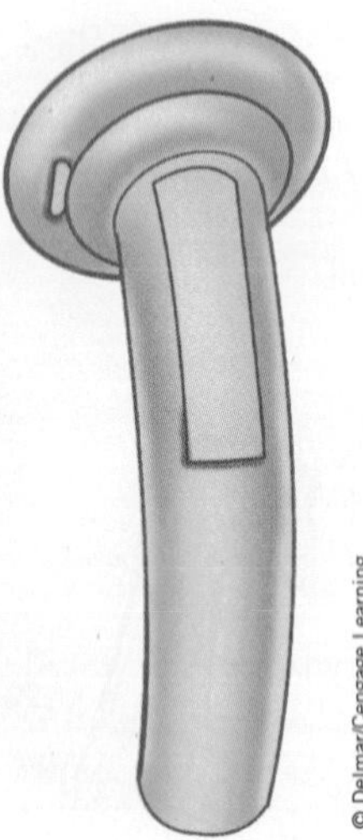

FIGURE 24-16 Laryngectomy tube.

are beneficial to patients. Additional information is available from the American Lung Association and the American Cancer Society.

Airway Adjuncts for Tracheostomy Patients. Airway adjuncts for tracheostomy patients are available for different functions.

Best Practice

Laryngectomies

Patients with newly acquired laryngectomies or permanent tracheostomies must receive appropriate instructions related to communicating, eating, and caring for the new airway.

Trach-Button The Trach-Button (Figure 24-17) is a self-retaining prosthesis for the maintenance of the tracheal stoma. The Trach-Button is indicated for long- or short-term patients who:

- May need to reinstate the use of a tracheostomy in an emergency.
- Require repeated tracheostomies for conditions such as myasthenia gravis, quadriplegia, poliomyelitis, COPD, and sleep disordered breathing.
- Must be evaluated during decannulation for ability to cough and to manage secretions of the respiratory tract.

An expansion lock on the proximal end makes the Trach-Button self-retaining. Ties are not required to secure the unit. The "petals" on the end of the cannula

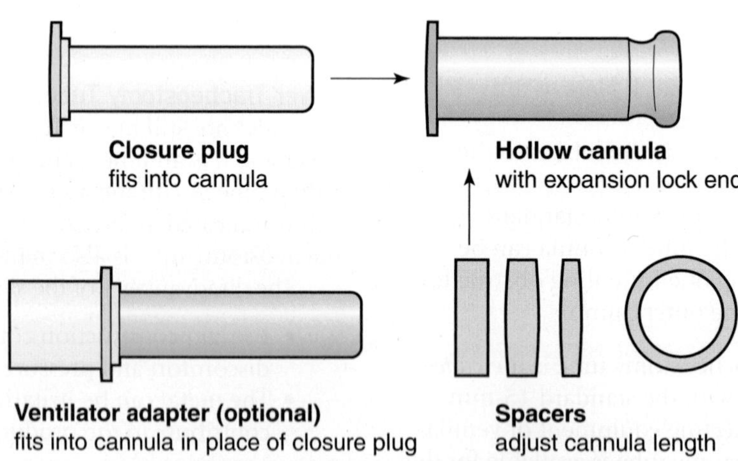

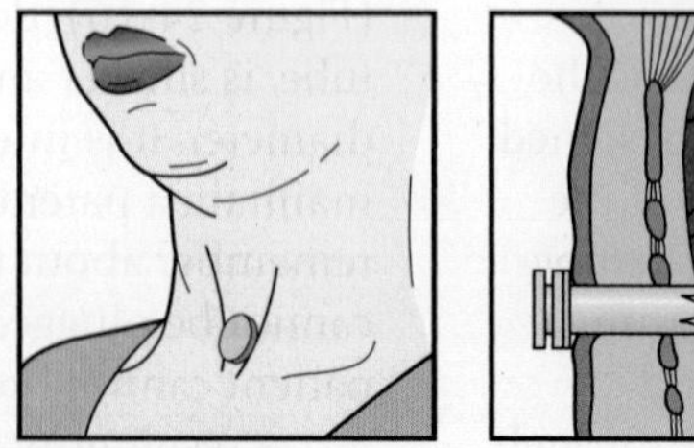

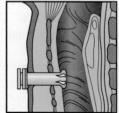

FIGURE 24-17 Trach-Button®.

Courtesy of Olympic Medical, Seattle, Washington

expand against the anterior wall of the trachea when the closure plug is inserted into the hollow cannula. This unique lock eliminates the danger of the unit being ejected during violent coughing spells or hyperextension of the sternocleidomastoid muscles. The cannula locks flush against the tracheal wall and does not protrude into the tracheal lumen, allowing the patient to breathe through the mouth and nose, speak normally, and expectorate more readily.

The patient can be easily and conveniently suctioned with the closure plug removed. A standard 15-mm fitting is available to replace the closure plug if mechanical ventilation becomes necessary.

The Trach-Button is available in sizes of 9–14 mm in diameter and 15–40 mm in length. The length is adjustable by using the spacers provided by the manufacturer, thus allowing adjustments as the length of the stoma changes. The device is constructed of Teflon and is comfortable, nonirritating, and well tolerated in long-term use. The external end of the device is small and cosmetically unobtrusive.[12]

Speech Aids Special speech aids are available to enable the tracheostomy patient to speak without having to cover the tube with a finger. Indications for the use of special speech aids include but are not limited to:

- Neuromuscular disease.
- Quadriplegia.
- Head trauma.
- COPD.
- Tracheomalacia.
- Mild tracheal stenosis.
- Mild laryngeal stenosis.
- Vocal cord paralysis without airway obstruction.
- Nonobstructive laryngeal tumors.
- Tracheostomized sleep apnea patient, used instead of plugging while awake.
- Patients who cannot tolerate tracheal plugging, either psychologically or physically.

Trach-Talk Valves The Trach-Talk (Figure 24-18) allows the patient to speak normally and cough more effectively. The device attaches directly to any standard tracheostomy tube. The principal mechanism of the device is a one-way valve that is held in the open position by a stainless steel spring.

The valve remains open except during exhalation. The force of expiration closes the valve, allowing the

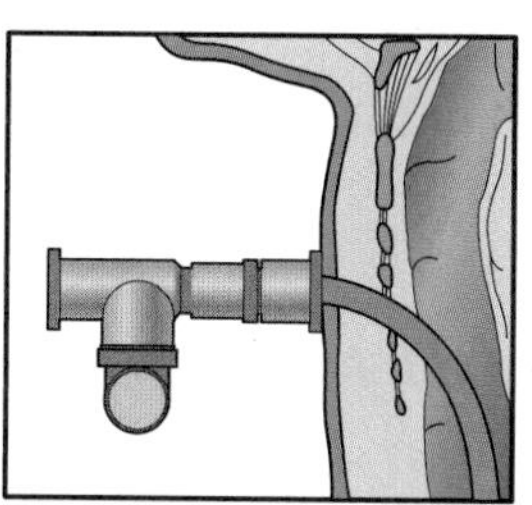

• Attaches to any trach tube.
• Patient does not have to cover tube in order to speak.
• Triggered by patient's breathing.

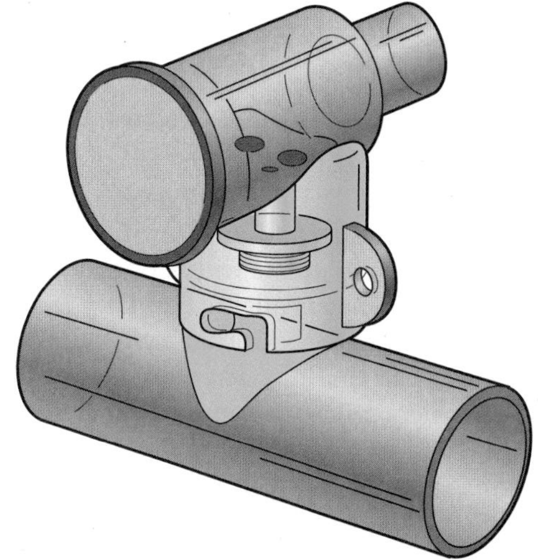

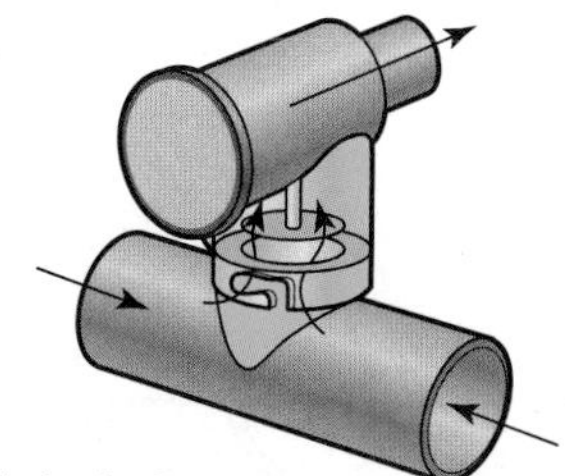

Inhalation
Spring-loaded, one-way valve remains open during inhalation.

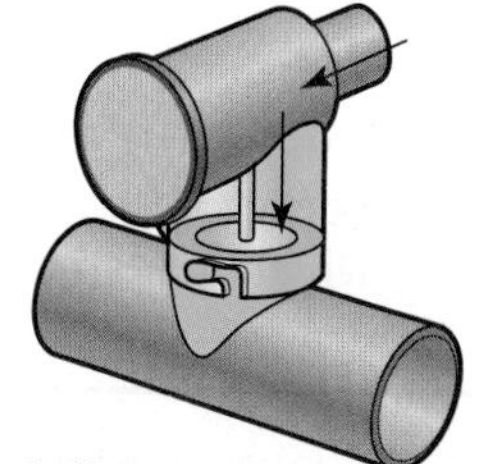

Exhalation
One-way valve closes, forcing air and mucus up trachea and past vocal cords.

FIGURE 24-18 Trach-Talk®.

Courtesy of Olympic Medical, Seattle, Washington

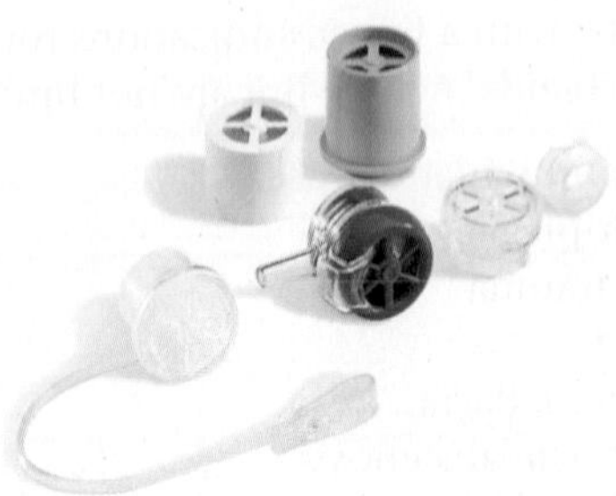

FIGURE 24-19 Passy-Muir® tracheostomy and ventilator speaking valve.
Courtesy of Passy-Muir Inc., Irvine, California

expired air to flow through the larynx and enabling the patient to speak. When exhalation stops, the spring forces the valve into the open position again.

The use of Trach-Talk is indicated when mechanical ventilation is no longer required and the patient is beyond the acute phase. It is not necessary to remove the unit for suctioning, administering oxygen, or humidifying the inspired gases. Removing the cap from the distal end allows a suction catheter to be passed into the tracheostomy for suctioning. Oxygen or humidity may be administered by connecting a large-bore tubing to the inlets provided for this purpose.[13]

Passy-Muir Valve The Passy-Muir tracheostomy and ventilator speaking valve (Figure 24-19) is likewise designed to eliminate the necessity of having to cover the tube with a finger to speak.[14] The Passy-Muir valve is designed for use by both short- and long-term adult, pediatric, and neonatal patients with a tracheostomy or ventilator dependence. Patients must be awake and alert and have adequate airflow around the tracheostomy tube during exhalation. The valve can be connected to the standard 15 mm connector of tracheostomy tubes in adults, pediatrics, and neonates, including fenestrated, nonfenestrated, cuffless, metal, and air-filled cuffed with the cuff completely deflated.

The application of the Passy-Muir valve is contraindicated in the following situations:

- Unconscious or comatose patients.
- Inflated tracheostomy tube cuff.
- Foam-filled cuffed tracheostomy tube.
- Severe airway obstruction, which may prevent sufficient exhalation.
- Thick and copious secretions.
- Severely reduced lung compliance that may cause air trapping.
- Endotracheal tubes.

The Passy-Muir valve is a lightweight, one-way valve, available in four configurations. It is designed with positive closure that maintains a bias closed position except during inspiration. When the patient breathes in, the valve opens, allowing air to enter the airway. At the end of inspiration, the valve closes and remains closed during the complete expiratory phase. When the patient breathes out, the air is directed through the larynx and pharynx, allowing the patient to speak as air passes through the vocal cords and the oral and nasal cavities. The positive closure design creates a column of air in the tracheostomy tube, inhibiting secretions from entering the valve. The normally closed position of the valve allows for a nearly normal closed respiratory system. The resultant restoration of subglottic pressure facilitates a more normal swallow, permits a stronger and more effective cough that allows expectoration of secretions orally, and may reduce aspiration.

The advantages of the valve are that it:

- Restores a closed respiratory system.
- Improves speech production.
- Improves swallowing.
- Improves olfaction.
- Facilitates secretion management.
- Facilitates weaning.
- Reduces aspiration in some patients.
- Promotes hygiene.
- Is ventilator applicable.

Ventilator dependency is an indication only for the Passy-Muir valve. Trach-Talk valves are not suitable for use with mechanically ventilated patients.

ARTIFICIAL AIRWAY CUFFS

Cuffs (Figure 24-20) are commonly used with some artificial airways in certain applications. A **cuff** is a balloonlike device consisting of three parts:

- The pilot balloon.
- The pilot balloon tubing.
- The cuff.

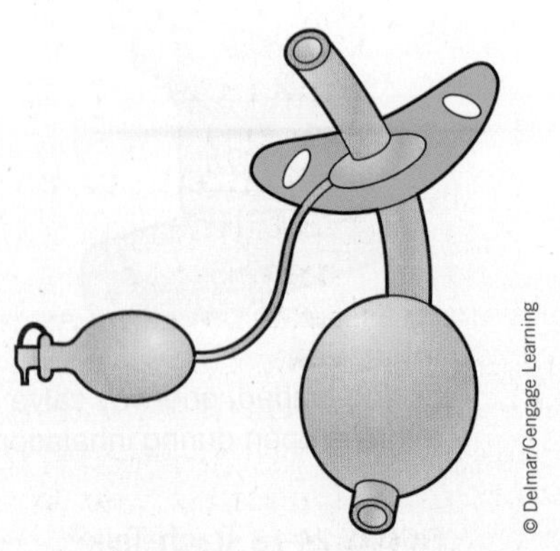

FIGURE 24-20 Artificial airway cuff.

Best Practice

Patient Assessment Before Using a Speaking Valve

The respiratory therapist must perform a thorough assessment of the patient before using any special speech aids. The assessment should consider the following:

- The patient must be awake, alert, and making an effort to communicate.
- Lung mechanics must be sufficient to exhale around the tracheostomy tube.
- The patient must be able to tolerate having the cuff deflated.
- There must be adequate space in the airway around the tracheostomy tube.
- There must not be thick and copious secretions.
- Vital signs, work of breathing, breath sounds, and any change in the patient's color or responsiveness to questions or commands.

Assessment for the ventilator-dependent patient includes the preceding list, plus assessments, before and after, placement of the valve:

- All ventilator settings.
- Alarm settings.
- Airway pressure levels.

The cuff surrounds the distal end of the artificial airway to provide an airway seal. Air is injected with a syringe into it through the pilot tubing that runs the length of the endotracheal tube or tracheostomy tube to the cuff.

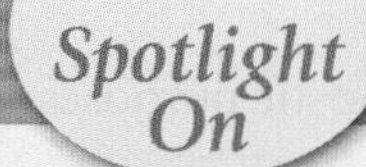

Speaking Valve

A new Passy-Muir tracheostomy tube speaking valve was recently introduced in 1985. The new low-profile valve is intended for use by both short-term and long-term adult, pediatric, and neonatal non-ventilator-dependent tracheostomized patients. It can be used with the Bivona non-foam-filled and Pilling-Weck metal Jackson tracheostomy tubes.

Most cuffs are classified as either high-volume, low-pressure cuffs or as low-volume, high-pressure cuffs.

- The *high-volume, low-pressure cuff,* the cuff of choice, requires a larger volume of air to inflate and has a larger surface area that comes into contact with the trachea, thus requiring less pressure to seal the airway. It is often referred to as the *floppy cuff* because of the soft pliable and loose-fitting material that surrounds the artificial airway.
- Conversely, the *low-volume, high-pressure cuff* requires a smaller volume of air to inflate and has a smaller surface area, which requires higher pressures to seal the airway.

Cuffs originally were supplied separately from the tubes and installation was the user's responsibility. This was not an easy task, and many ingenious methods of installation were attempted. Hemostats, Magill forceps, and all types of lubricants were used to make the task easier. Many times, a seemingly successful attempt would result in producing a small hole in the cuff. Of course, the leak went undetected until it was the last available cuffed tube.

Cuff Types. Low-volume, high-pressure cuffs were the only types available until manufacturers began to listen and respond to users. In the interim, a multitude of different low-volume, high-pressure designs were introduced in hopes of solving the problems. The list included double-cuffed tubes with the ability to inflate either or both cuffs to alternate pressure sites on the trachea.

The advent of the high-volume, low-pressure cuffs eliminated most of the problems. This classification of cuff includes two basic designs.

- The *air-filled cuff* still sets the standards by being the most commonly used.
- The *foam-filled cuff* reverses the methodology of inflation. Before inserting the tube, a syringe is employed to withdraw all air from the cuff. Once the tube is inserted, the pressure in the cuff is allowed to return to ambient pressure, causing the foam to expand to its original size. This allows the cuff to expand to the wall of the trachea, sealing the airway.

The first generation of foam-filled cuffs had difficulties.

- Some cuffs developed leaks while in the airway.
- Air could not be withdrawn from the cuff, and consequently removal of the tube became a problem.

Subsequent design improvements reduced the recurrence of these problems.

The three primary reasons to use cuffed artificial airways are to:

- Provide a sealed airway for the application of mechanical ventilators.
- Prevent aspiration of foreign materials into the lungs.
- Maintain the artificial airway in the center of the trachea.

Cuff Pressure Management. The cuff of a permanent artificial airway is usually deflated and inflated as needed for eating or for connecting to a mechanical ventilator. Conversely, cuffs used in the acute care setting are usually inflated most of the time. There are two commonly used methods of cuff inflation.

- The *minimal leak method* is used when it is not essential to maintain high levels of PEEP or peak inspiratory pressures. This is accomplished by adding air to the cuff until no leak can be heard during the inspiratory phase and withdrawing air until a minimal leak can be heard.
- The *minimal occlusion method* is used during the use of high PEEP and peak inspiratory pressures. This is accomplished by adding air to the cuff during the inspiratory phase until no leak can be heard, withdrawing air until a leak is present, and gradually adding air until no leak can be heard.

Cuff Complications. The RT must be aware of possible complications:

- Cuff pressures greater than 5 mm Hg reduce lymphatic flow.
- Pressures greater than 18 mm Hg reduce venous flow.
- Pressures greater than 30 mm Hg reduce arterial flow of the trachea.
- Sustained high cuff pressures cause ischemia of the mucosa, hemorrhage, and ultimately stenosis of the trachea.
- Other complications are related to the esophagus and its position against the soft tissue of the trachea, specifically, aerophagia (air swallowing) and dysphasia (difficulty swallowing).

Cuff Monitoring. Cuff pressures can be measured by means of a simple pressure manometer with an adapter to fit the fill port of the cuff or any one of the devices specifically designed for measuring cuff pressures to the clinician can feel the pilot balloon while observing the pressure on a cuff pressure monitor and estimate the pressure in the cuff. This manual technique is useful to approximate cuff pressures when a pressure monitor is not available. Monitoring of cuff pressures is always indicated but especially with the minimal occlusion inflation method. Cuff pressures and cuff filling volumes should be included in the routine documentation of airway management when a cuff is employed.

Common problems identified with cuff pressure monitoring are leaking cuffs and tubes that are too small for the patient.

- If the cuff pressure is unaffected by adding more and more air, the cuff is leaking.
- Conversely, if the pressure is higher with additional air and the leak around the cuff continues, the tube is undersized for the patient.

In both cases, the tube must be changed.

Best Practice

Airway Cuffs and Hyperbaric Procedures

An important exception to the filling of cuffs with air is in hyperbaric procedures. Normal saline is used to fill the cuffs of the tracheostomy and endotracheal tubes. If air is used, the increased pressure compresses the air, decreasing the cuff volume. Normal saline is essentially incompressible and maintains the required volume.

AIRWAY SUCTIONING

Airway suctioning is indicated for patients who are unable to eliminate accumulated secretions without assistance. Airway suctioning is performed to:

- Maintain a patent airway by removing secretions and other foreign objects.
- Stimulate a cough in patients who are unable or unwilling to cough.
- Collect specimens for diagnostic purposes.

Complications associated with airway suctioning are:

- Hypoxemia associated with the removal of oxygen from the lungs.
- Lung collapse associated with the removal of air from the lungs.
- Airway occlusion with suction catheters greater than one half the diameter of the artificial airway.
- Arrhythmia associated with resultant hypoxemia.
- Mucosal stripping associated with poor catheter design or greater-than-required vacuum levels.
- Cardiac arrest associated with vagal stimulation.

Best Practice

Suction Catheters

Always remember that each millimeter is equal to approximately three French units. To determine the appropriately sized suction catheter for use with an 8-mm artificial airway, divide the size of the artificial airway by 2 and then multiply the answer by 3 (i.e., 8 mm ÷ 2 = 4, 4 × 3 = 12). In this example, a 12 French suction catheter is appropriate for use with the 8-mm artificial airway. Equally important, use the largest suction catheter allowable to facilitate the removal of secretions in the least amount of suctioning time.

Airway suctioning to maintain a patent airway can be accomplished by using several devices.

- Straight suction catheters
- The Yankauer Suction Device
- Trach Care

Straight Suction Catheters. Suction catheters (Figure 24-21) are most commonly used for the removal of secretions from the airway. Three of the numerous suction catheter designs available are:

- Whistle tip
- Argyle airflow
- Coudé Suction

Whistle Tip Catheter The *whistle tip suction catheter* (Figure 24-21A) is the most commonly used design in the clinical setting. It has a rounded distal tip with a hole in the center of the tip and a series of holes along the sides of the tip. Manufacturers have made several modifications to the whistle tip with little functional change from the original design.

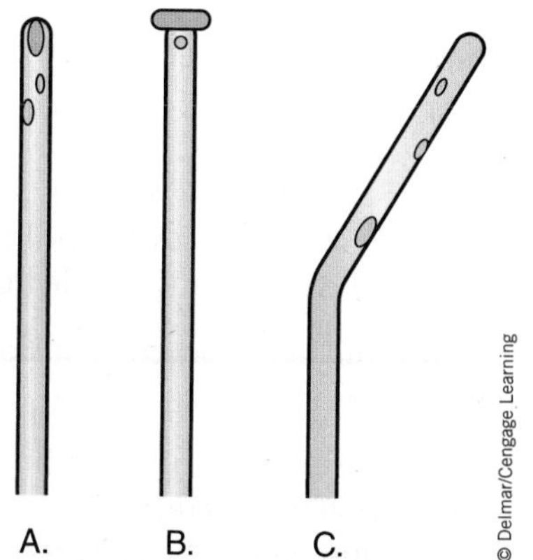

FIGURE 24-21 Types of suction catheters: (A) Whistle tip. (B) Argyle airflow. (C) Coudé directional.

Argyle Airflow Catheter The Argyle *airflow suction catheter* (Figure 24-21B) is designed with a doughnut-shaped tip on the distal end. It differs from other suction catheters because one of the suction ports in the distal end is in the center, and several are on the proximal side of the doughnut. The port placement is part of the design to prevent contact with the mucosa of the airways.

Coudé Suction Catheter The distal tip of most suction catheters inserted for the purpose of secretion removal, however, enters the right mainstem bronchus. The *Coudé directional suction catheter* (Figure 24-21C) is designed with a fixed-angle distal tip, which allows the operator to rotate the proximal end of the suction catheter using reference marks to guide the distal tip in order to direct it into the left mainstem bronchus. The Coudé directional suction catheter can be a useful device to facilitate the removal of accumulated secretions from the left mainstem bronchus.

Characteristics of Suction Catheters Characteristics of good suction catheters are that:

- They must be manufactured from materials that are nonirritating to the airway mucosa.
- They must be of sufficient length to extend past the distal tip of the artificial airway, usually 20–22 inches.
- They must be manufactured from a material that does not produce frictional resistance on the airway when inserted.
- The finger port on the proximal end (Figure 24-22) should be of sufficient size to minimize aspiration of air from the unoccluded lung.
- The tip of the catheter and all openings should be molded and free of sharp edges to prevent mucosal trauma.

Catheter Size Suction catheters must be less than one half the diameter of the artificial airway being suctioned to prevent excessive removal of oxygen and potentially lung collapse. Determining the appropriately sized suction catheter is sometimes difficult when artificial airways are measured in millimeters and catheters are measured in French units.

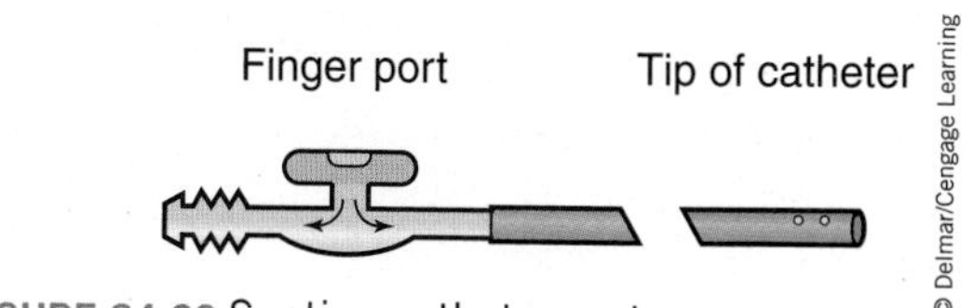

FIGURE 24-22 Suction catheter port.

Suctioning should be performed for need only. It should not be performed on a schedule except to obtain a specimen for analysis.

Suction Technique An appropriate suction technique should include the following:

- Use a sterile technique using sterile equipment, gloves, and sterile rinse solutions.
- Set vacuum pressure within a range of 80–120 mm Hg for adults.
- Oxygenate the patient well before, during, and after the airway suction procedure.
- Insert the catheter into the artificial airway without applying suction.
- Advance the catheter until resistance is felt.
- Withdraw it slightly.
- Remove the catheter, slowly applying suction.
- Release the suction if resistance is felt, withdraw slightly, and reapply suction.
- Oxygenate the patient well, allowing a brief resting period, if possible, before repeating the procedure.

The application of suction to the airway should never exceed 15 seconds in adults.

Yankauer Suction Device. The *Yankauer suction device* (Figure 24-23) is especially effective for the removal of secretions accumulated in the oropharyngeal cavity. Sometimes referred to as the *tonsil suction device,* the Yankauer is rigid and designed to conform to the angle of the oropharyngeal anatomy. The distal end has a ball-shaped tip with a hole in the center large enough to facilitate thick copious secretion removal. Insertion is enhanced by the rigid design, and the smooth rounded distal tip reduces trauma to the oropharyngeal cavity.

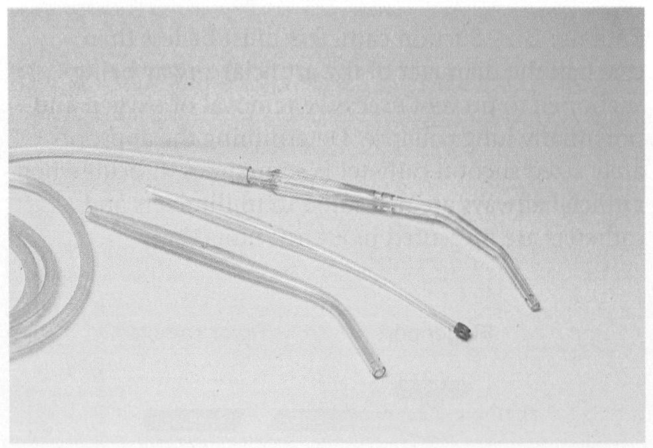

FIGURE 24-23 Yankauer and tonsil tip suction catheters.

Specimen Collection. Airway suctioning is indicated for the purpose of specimen collection for sputum analysis. The most common is specimen collection for microbiological culture and sensitivity to determine the pathogen causing the disease process and the antibiotic sensitivity of the organism cultured. The technique for suctioning for sputum specimen collection differs only by the incorporation of a sterile inline suction trap, between the suction catheter and the vacuum supply line, to collect the specimen.

Trach Care Suctioning System. The Trach Care Closed Tracheal Suction System is a self-contained device that can be incorporated into the mechanical ventilator circuit or continuous flow circuit.[15] Trach Care is used for suctioning of the airway when a patient has a tracheostomy or an endotracheal tube.

The Trach Care incorporates a self-contained suction catheter, enclosed in a clear plastic sleeve, which passes through a modified T-piece into the airway. The lockable external suction control on the suction catheter allows the application of suction only when the thumb control valve is depressed. The thumb piece requires a 180-degree rotation from the locked position to operate; the lock prevents the inadvertent application of suction. There is an irrigation port to instill fluid through to lavage the airway.

Here is the suctioning procedure for the Trach Care:

- Grip the T-piece with one hand.
- Advance the catheter with the other hand to the desired depth.
- Depress the control valve to apply suction.
- Withdraw the catheter slowly until the black marking on the catheter is visible on the back-side of the T.

This is the procedure to lavage the airway:

- Insert the catheter approximately 4–5 inches into the endotracheal tube or 1–2 inches into a tracheostomy tube.
- Instill fluid through the irrigation port.
- Continue to advance the catheter to the desired depth.
- Depress the control valve to apply suction.
- Withdraw the catheter slowly until the black marking on the catheter is visible behind the T.

The therapist must keep several considerations in mind during these procedures:

- Do not apply suction while instilling the fluid during the lavage procedure.
- After suctioning, flush the catheter by depressing the control valve and then slowly instill fluid through the irrigation port.

Best Practice

Safe Suctioning

Patient safety considerations should be paramount from the first signs and symptoms of respiratory insufficiency until normal breathing is restored.

Best Practice

Artificial Airways and Ventilator-Associated Pneumonia

The use of artificial airways, especially endotracheal tubes, in mechanically ventilated patients is strongly related to ventilator-associated pneumonia (VAP).

- The thumb piece should be turned 180 degrees to the locked position on the control valve until safely in the off position.
- The Trach Care has a cap on one side of the T-piece to provide a sealed system for mechanical ventilation. The cap must be removed from the Trach Care before continuous flow therapy is applied.

The advantages of the Trach Care are that the use of gloves is not indicated and sterile technique is ensured; a new catheter is not necessary for every set-up. The manufacturer recommends not to resterilize the Trach Care and not to use the unit for more than 24 hours. However, some studies indicated no reduction of infection secondary to increased change intervals.

ARTIFICIAL AIRWAYS AND PATIENT SAFETY

Patient safety considerations should be paramount from the first signs and symptoms of respiratory insufficiency until normal breathing is restored. Every precaution must be adhered to including:

- Maintaining ventilation before the introduction of an artificial airway.
- Safely establishing a patent artificial airway.
- Securing the artificial airway.
- Using caution to prevent the inadvertent obstructing or removal of the artificial airway.
- Determining the appropriate time for safely removing the artificial airway.

TABLE 24-5 **Actual published cases and monetary awards for injury and death as a result of lack of caution**

"Premature Extubation Following Gastric Bypass Surgery—Respiratory Distress and Tracheotomy—Tracheotomy is permanent–$1 Million Verdict."[16]
"Failure to Maintain Airway for Appendectomy—Brain Damage with Significant Disability–$35 Million Settlement."[17]
"Failure to Properly Monitor Woman in ICU—Self-Extubation With Cardiac Arrest and Death–$1 Million Verdict"[18]

Most of these precautions are sufficiently addressed elsewhere in this chapter or textbook.

Especially important, however, is taking steps to prevent the inadvertent obstruction or removal of the artificial airway. The volume of references to the subject is relatively small in medical literature. One study reported 96 intubated ICU patients who underwent 101 episodes of unplanned extubation. Of these, 85% were self-extubation and 15% were accidental. Overall, 57% required reintubation, and most were reintubated within the first hour. Difficulty with reintubation was common, and one patient who could not be reintubated died.[19] The medical literature usually chronicles the aftermath resultant from the lack of caution. Unfortunately, almost as much is found in legal journals publishing the monetary awards for injury or death as a result of the lack of caution (Table 24-5).

Safety concerns for patients with artificial airways should include:

- Adequate staffing.
- Alarms.
- Secretions and diaphoresis.
- Airway securing devices.
- Restraining devices.

Adequate Staffing. Enough staff should be available to accomplish any procedure safely anytime a patient with an artificial airway, especially a mechanically ventilated patient, is:

- Pulled up in the bed or turned for a position change.
- Rolled for bathing or linen change.
- Lifted to be weighed.
- Transferred to another bed or stretcher.
- Transported on a bed or stretcher.
- Subjected to any movement that may compromise the airway.

In most cases, the respiratory therapist should be assisted by at least two nursing service staff members.

The respiratory therapist should monitor and maintain the airway during the procedures.

Alarms. Alarms on mechanical ventilators are there to alert the staff that something is not right with the patient's ventilatory status. The most common alarm indicates that the patient is not receiving adequate ventilation, and usually the patient needs suctioning. However, the alarm can also be warning of a problem with the artificial airway, such as a kinked endotracheal tube. *Regardless of the reason, when the alarms sound, they are not to be ignored. The alarm may be a false one, but it may also mean the patient is at risk of injury or death.*

CASE STUDY 24-1

J. C. is a 68-year-old white male with a history of COPD, CHF, and noncompliance. Additionally, in the past 10 months, he has been intubated and ventilated a total of 36 times for respiratory failure resultant from his COPD and CHF and noncompliance.

On this admission (at 0115, 03-23-2011) he presented with, as before, labored breathing, profuse sweating, slight cyanosis, four-plus pitted edema, wet breath sounds bilaterally, and nonresponsiveness to verbal stimulus. ABG results on the aerosol treatment with oxygen as the driving gas; P_aO_2 94 mm Hg, P_aCO_2 118 mm Hg, and pH 7.01.

He was intubated orally with an 8.0 endotracheal tube and taped at the 25-mm mark on the tube at the lip. Radiographic examination of the chest verified proper tube placement.

A PB 7200 mechanical ventilator was set up with settings as follows: CMV, Rate 12, VT 800, F_IO_2 1.0, PEEP 10, PIP 45 (cm H_2O). Lasix 40 mg was administered IV × 2, 40 mg on arrival and 40 mg 15 minutes after the first dose. (This drug and dose had been determined effective for this patient during the previous ER admits.)

0200: The patient was transferred to the intensive care unit. Ventilator: CMV, Rate 12 vent/5 pt, V_T 800, F_IO_2 1.0, PEEP 10, PIP 34. ABG results: P_aO_2 359, P_aCO_2 44, pH 7.37. Ventilator changes: SIMV 12, pressure support 10, V_T 800, F_IO_2 0.40, PEEP 10.

0400: The Lasix has produced 1 L of urine. Pulmonary status markedly changed. Breath sounds: scattered crackles especially in bases. Moderate amount of oral secretions. Ventilator: SIMV, Rate 12 vent/6 pt, V_T 800 vent/ 560 pt., F_IO_2 .40, PEEP 10. ABG results: P_aO_2 150, P_aCO_2 42, pH 7.39. Ventilator changes: SIMV 6, PS 10, V_T 800, F_IO_2 0.30, PEEP 5.

0600: The Lasix has produced another 500 mL of urine. The patient was somewhat more restless and anxious. Ventilator: SIMV, Rate 6 vent/25 pt, V_T 800 vent/ 300 pt, F_IO_2 .40, PEEP 5, PIP 49. ABG results: P_aO_2 78, P_aCO_2 56, pH 7.30. Pulmonary status has worsened. Breath sounds: crackles and slight rales on the right and markedly diminished on the left.

This patient historically was weaned and extubated within 8–10 hours after being intubated. It is unusual for his ABGs to have worsened after improving. All parameters were reassessed.

The following was observed after reassessing the endotracheal tube. The tape securing the tube in place was wet because of the oral secretions. The endotracheal tube's 29-mm mark was now at the patient's lip.

The problem: The patient's endotracheal tube was taped at the 25-mm mark on the tube at the patient's lip. The moderate amount of oral secretions moistened the tape and reduced its ability to hold the tube in place. The endotracheal tube advanced farther into the lung until the tip was in the right mainstem bronchus. In this position, the left lung was deprived of ventilation.

The solution: The patient was placed on a F_IO_2 of 1.0, the airway was suctioned with the Trach Care suction unit, and the oropharynx was suctioned thoroughly with a Yankauer. With his airway thoroughly cleared, the endotracheal cuff was deflated, the endotracheal tube was withdrawn to the 25-mm mark at the lip, the cuff was reinflated, and the tube was resecured. Breath sounds returned to bilateral and equal. Weaning was continued.

1030: The patient was extubated successfully.

Questions

1. What could the respiratory therapist do to prevent the endotracheal tube from slipping into the right mainstream bronchus?
2. If a patient has had to be intubated 36 times over the last 10 months, what should the respiratory therapist recommend?
3. When the patient was initially intubated, what kind of intubation would have been the easiest to maintain during the patient's short period of intubation?

Secretions and Diaphoresis. Patients who have copious amounts of secretions, either oral or nasal, and/or diaphoresis should be monitored very closely. Both conditions contribute to the problems associated with securing artificial airways, arterial lines, IVs, as well as with attaching devices for monitoring equipment. The moisture can interfere with the bonding between the patient and the adhesive utilized to secure them.

Airway Securing Devices. Airway securing devices designed to prevent unplanned or inadvertent extubation sometimes are contributing factors in the act they were designed to prevent. Usually the cause is that the device is firmly attached to the endotracheal tube and inappropriately attached to the patient. Copious amounts of secretions or extreme diaphoresis can prevent the device from attaching securely. Under these conditions, the patient is vulnerable to unplanned or self-extubation. The therapist must closely monitor the patient and ensure that the securing device is equally well attached to the patient and to the endotracheal tube.

Restraining Devices. Just the mention of restraining devices for patients should raise a red flag. Legal, ethical, medical and moral issues arise with the application of both chemical (drugs) or physical restraints to the patient's freedom of motion and movement. In most jurisdictions in the United States and Canada, restraint orders must be renewed daily and restraints themselves must be frequently checked for comfort, appropriateness, and safety by the appropriate personnel. The respiratory therapist must exercise extreme caution with the use of any type of patient-restraining device. Soft restraints on the patient's upper extremities become necessary for most patients requiring mechanical ventilation. Even though some conscious and alert patients do not intentionally self-extubate, they may fall asleep and unknowingly do so. If soft restraints are employed, the physician's orders have to be in compliance with standards set forth by regulatory agencies and clearly written on the patient's chart.

Summary

Airway management is one of the areas of care that respiratory therapists perform so routinely that they sometimes overlook its importance. With the artificial airways, emergency airway adjuncts, airway adjuncts, and speech aids for tracheostomy patients, as well as suctioning capabilities, all constantly improving, RTs have the tools to be ever more effective with airway management. Their duty is to be the most informed member of the health care team and match the appropriate patient with the most effective modalities. Numerous devices and techniques have not been changed significantly since they were introduced to clinical practice. The reason is that they are useful as introduced and they blend in with the new technologies to provide the tools necessary for airway management.

Study Questions

REVIEW QUESTIONS

1. List and describe two basic classifications of airway obstruction.
2. List the indications for artificial airways.
3. Describe the double lumen endobronchial tube.
4. Differentiate between a tracheostomy tube and a laryngectomy.
5. Describe the Passy-Muir valve, and define the function of the valve.
6. List the complications associated with airway suctioning.
7. Explain the suction technique for the Trach Care suction device.
8. Define difficult tracheal intubation.
9. Describe the gum elastic bougie.

MULTIPLE-CHOICE QUESTIONS

1. The most common cause of airway obstruction is:
   a. the tongue occluding the airway.
   b. aspiration of foreign objects.
   c. laryngeal edema.
   d. thick mucus in the airway.
2. The radiopaque line is used to:
   a. measure the distance for endotracheal intubation.
   b. measure the diameter of the trachea using X-ray.
   c. determine proper placement of endotracheal tube cuffs.
   d. determine proper placement of the distal tip of the endotracheal tube.
3. Endotracheal tube markings include all of the following except:
   a. Z79 committee.
   b. centimeter markings.
   c. inhalation therapy (IT).
   d. serial number.

4. Before removing an EOA, the respiratory therapist must:
   I. suction the oral cavity well.
   II. suction above the cuff before deflating.
   III. ensure that the endotracheal tube is properly in place.
   IV. ensure the proper deflation of cuff.
   a. all of the above
   b. II and III
   c. III only
   d. I and IV
   e. I only
5. In an emergency situation in a hospital, the airway of choice is:
   a. Guedel.
   b. Berman.
   c. oroendotracheal tube.
   d. nasoendotracheal tube.
6. The length of a oropharyngeal airway can best be determined by measuring:
   a. from the tip of the nose to the angle of the jaw.
   b. from the tip of the nose to the ear lobe.
   c. from the center of the nare to the tip of the ear lobe.
   d. from the jaw to the Adam's apple.
7. The most appropriate artificial airway for the conscious patient is the:
   a. Guedel.
   b. Berman.
   c. nasopharyngeal.
   d. esophageal obdurator airway.
8. The surgical procedure making an incision into the trachea is a:
   a. cricothyrotomy.
   b. tracheostomy.
   c. laryngectomy.
   d. appendectomy.
9. The most commonly used material in the manufacture of artificial airways is:
   a. silicone.
   b. Teflon.
   c. nylon.
   d. polyvinyl chloride.
10. The tracheostomy tube that is still manufactured but that can be irritating to the skin is:
    a. fenestrated.
    b. silver.
    c. foam filled.
    d. plastic.
11. The Trach-Button does not allow the tracheostomized patient to:
    a. breathe through the nose and mouth.
    b. speak normally.
    c. expectorate more normally.
    d. breathe through the stoma.
12. The Trach-Talk valve is indicated in all of the following patients except:
    a. head trauma.
    b. neuromuscular disease.
    c. ventilator dependency.
    d. tracheomalacia.
13. Passy-Muir valve is indicated in all of the following patients except:
    a. quadriplegia.
    b. tracheomalacia.
    c. mild tracheal stenosis.
    d. a comatose patient.
14. Contraindications for use of the Passy-Muir valve include:
    I. conscious patients.
    II. endotracheal tubes.
    III. foam-filled tracheostomy cuff.
    IV. deflated tracheostomy tube cuff.
    V. fenestrated tracheostomy tube.
    a. I and II
    b. II and III
    c. I and IV
    d. III and V
    e. all of the above
15. The cuff of choice is:
    I. hydrofilled.
    II. foam filled.
    III. high volume, low pressure.
    IV. low volume, high pressure.
    V. floppy.
    a. I and II
    b. II and III
    c. I and IV
    d. III and V
    e. all of the above
16. Cuff pressures should be monitored and should not exceed:
    a. 5–10 cm H_2O pressure
    b. 11–15 cm H_2O pressure
    c. 16–20 cm H_2O pressure
    d. 22 cm H_2O pressure
17. The following are characteristics of a good suction catheter except:
    I. construction from nonirritating material
    II. constructed from materials with low frictional qualities
    III. maximum length of 12–15 inches
    IV. proximal finger port small enough to apply suction at all times
    V. molded catheter tip and openings
    a. I and II
    b. III and IV
    c. II and V
    d. III and V
    e. none of the above

18. The suction device design most suitable for oropharyngeal suctioning is:
    I. whistle tip catheter.
    II. tonsil suction device.
    III. Argyle airflow catheter.
    IV. Yankauer suction device.
    V. modified oropharyngeal airway.
    a. I and II
    b. III and IV
    c. II and IV
    d. IV
    e. V
19. The most appropriate set vacuum pressure for airway suctioning in adults is:
    a. 60–100 mm Hg.
    b. 80–120 mm Hg.
    c. 90–140 mm Hg.
    d. 100–180 mm Hg.
20. The Trach Care closed suction device is designed for suctioning:
    a. the nasopharyngeal airway.
    b. a tracheostomy.
    c. the endotracheal tube.
    d. b and c.

CRITICAL-THINKING QUESTIONS

1. How would you determine whether to use an oropharyngeal airway or a nasopharyngeal airway?
2. In what situation should adjunct airways be considered for ventilation?
3. What should be monitored closely about cuffs when they are in use, and how can they be monitored best?
4. When should patient safety with artificial airways be considered?
5. Under which circumstances should safety precautions be exercised for patients with artificial airways?

References

1. Finucane BT, Santora AH. Difficult intubation. In: *Principles of Airway Management*, 3rd ed. St. Louis, MO: Mosby-Yearbook, 2009.
2. Mehta S. Transtracheal illumination for optimal tracheal tube placement. A clinical study. *Anaesthesia* 1989;44:970–972.
3. Hung OR, Stewart RD. Lightwand intubation: a new lightwand device. *Can J Anaesth.* 1995; 42:820–825.
4. Kacmarek, R. *The Essentials of Respiratory Care.* 4th ed. St. Louis, MO: Mosby; 2005.
5. Brain A I J. The Laryngeal Mask—A New Concept in Airway Management. *Br J Anaesth* 1983;55,8:801–5.
6. Morris IR. Continuing medical education: fibreoptic intubation. *Can J Anesth.* 1994;41: 996–1008.
7. Jolliet P, Chevrolet JC. Bronchoscopy in the intensive care unit. *Intensive Care Med.* 1992;18:160–169.
8. Burkle CM, Walsh MT, Harrison BA, et al. Airway management after failure to intubate by direct laryngoscopy: outcomes in a large teaching hospital. *Can J Anaesth.* 2005;52: 634–640.
9. Benumof, J. Management of the difficult airway. *Anesthesiology*. 75:1087–1210.
10. Cormac RS, Lehane J. Difficult tracheal intubation in obstetrics. *Anaesthesia.* 1984; 39:1105–1111.
11. Cricothyrotomy. In: Finucane BT, Santora AH, eds. *Advanced Cardiac Life Support Manual.* Dallas, TX: American Heart Association; 1997:2–13.
12. Trach-Button [product literature]. Seattle, WA: Olympic Medical; 1999.
13. Trach-Talk [product literature]. Seattle, WA: Olympic Medical; 1999.
14. Passy-Muir tracheostomy and ventilator speaking valves. *Instruction Manual.* Irvine, CA: Passy-Muir Inc.;1–14.
15. Trach Care closed suction system [product literature]. Des Moines, IA: Ballard Inc;1998.
16. *Medical Malpractice—Verdicts, Settlements & Experts.* 2006;22,7:3–4.
17. *Medical Malpractice—Verdicts, Settlements & Experts.* 2006;22,7:4–5.
18. *Medical Malpractice—Verdicts, Settlements & Experts.* 2006;22,7:21.
19. Christie JM, Dethlefsen M, Cane RD. Unplanned ETT extubation in the ICU unit. *J Clinical Anesthesia.* 1996;8,4:289–293.

Suggested Readings

American Association for Respiratory Care. AARC clinical practice guidelines: management of airway emergencies. *Respir Care.* 1995;40(7): 749–760.

American Heart Association adjuncts for airway control and ventilation. *Circulation* 2005;112:IV-51–IV-57. Originally published online November 28, 2005. http://circ.ahajournals.org/cgi/content/full/112/24_suppl/IV-51

American Heart Association. Advanced cardiac life support. www.americanheart.org/presenter.jhtml?identifier=3011775

ASA practice guidelines for management of the difficult airway. *Anesthesiology* 2003; 98:1269–1277.

Endotracheal suctioning of mechanically ventilated patients with artificial airways. *Respir Care.* 2010;55(6):758–764.

Gavin GL, McCloskey BV. The difficult airway in adult critical care. *Crit Care Med.* 2008;36,7:2163–2173. Posted August 12, 2008. http://www.medscape.com/viewarticle/578622

In-hospital transport of the mechanically ventilated patient, 2002 revision & update. *Respir Care.* 2002;47(6):721–723.

Nasotracheal suctioning, revision & update. *Respir Care.* 2004;49(9):1080–1084.

Patient-ventilator system checks. *Respir Care.* 1992;37(8):882–886.

Removal of the endotracheal tube, 2007 revision & update. *Respir Care.* 2007;52(1):81–93.

Suctioning of the patient in the home. *Respir Care.* 1999;44(1):99–104.

CHAPTER 25

Physiological Effects of Mechanical Ventilation

Chad J. Pezzano

OBJECTIVES

Upon completion of this chapter, the reader should be able to:

- Describe the difference between transairway, transpulmonary, and transthoracic pressures and how they affect the process of gas movement through the pulmonary system.
- Explain the difference between intra-alveolar and intrapleural pressures.
- Discuss the difference between negative pressure ventilation, positive pressure ventilation, and high-frequency ventilation.
- Describe the difference between static and dynamic lung compliance.
- Describe airway resistance and how it relates to the mechanically ventilated patient.
- Summarize the concept of time constants for mechanically ventilated patients.
- Discuss the complications that are associated with mechanical ventilation and how to minimize them.

CHAPTER OUTLINE

KEY TERMS

barotrauma
dynamic compliance
high-frequency ventilation
intra-alveolar pressure
intrapleural pressure
lung compliance
negative pressure ventilation
positive pressure ventilation
static compliance
time constant
transairway pressure
transpulmonary pressure
transthoracic pressure
volutrauma

Mechanical ventilation assists individuals who are suffering from conditions that impair their ability to maintain adequate ventilation and/or oxygenation. Even with mechanical ventilation, complications may arise in the form of physiological side effects that occur with the application of positive pressure ventilation. The hemodynamic, renal, neurological, and pulmonary systems may all be at an increased risk. The respiratory therapist who is providing mechanical ventilation must be aware of the potential side effects and limit any ill consequences that may result from the application of positive pressure ventilation.

Pulmonary and Thoracic Pressure Gradients

Invasive mechanical ventilation is based on different physiological principles from those of spontaneous breathing. Spontaneous respirations are initiated by means of a complicated series of nerve stimuli and muscle contractions. Stimuli are sent from the medulla oblongata in response to a physiological change, such as an increase in carbon dioxide levels, a rise in hydrogen ions (acidosis), a decrease in pH, or a lowered oxygen level. When the medulla oblongata senses a physiological change, a stimulus is sent through the phrenic nerve to the diaphragm to begin the process of inspiration. This nerve signal causes the diaphragm to contract, creating changes in the pressure gradients associated with respiration.[1]

Spontaneous breathing depends on many physiological and physical changes occurring both in the pulmonary system and the thorax. During inspiration and expiration, pressure gradient changes result, such as transairway pressure, transpulmonary pressure, and transthoracic pressures. These are responsible for some of the physiological changes that deliver fresh gas to the lower respiratory system and that remove expired gases.

TRANSAIRWAY PRESSURE

Transairway pressure (P_{ta}), also known as airway pressure, is the change in pressure gradient between the barometric pressures at the mouth (P_m) and at the alveoli (P_{alv}). Transairway pressure is the driver of the physiological movement of air from the upper respiratory system to the conductive airways (Figure 25-1).[2]

$$P_{ta} = P_m - P_{alv}$$

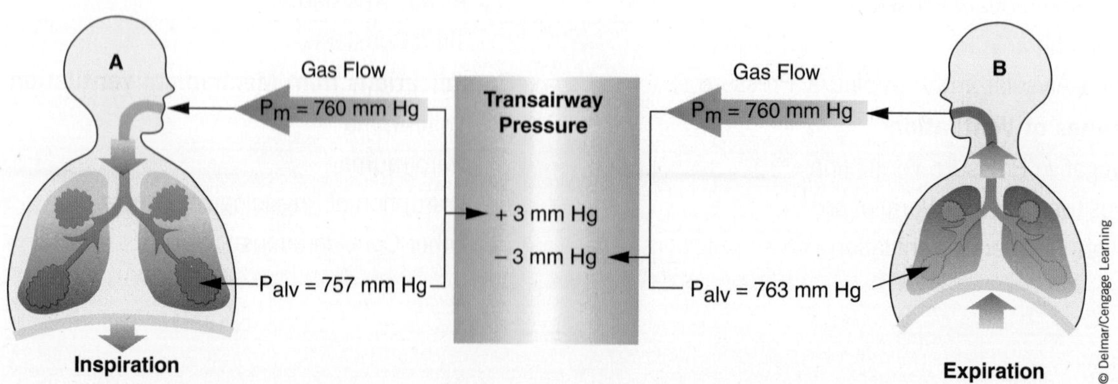

FIGURE 25-1 Transairway pressure: The difference between the pressure at the mouth (P_m) and the alveolar pressure (P_{alv}). Even though the gas is moving in opposite directions in A and B, the transairway pressure is 3 mm Hg in both examples. In this illustration, the pressure at the mouth (P_m) is equal to the barometric pressure (P_B).

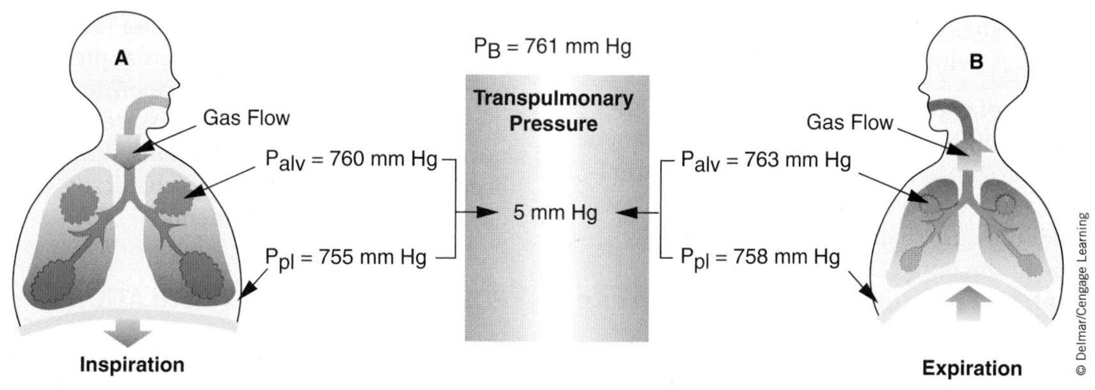

FIGURE 25-2 Transpulmonary pressure: The difference between the alveolar pressure (P_{alv}) and the pleural pressure (P_{pl}). This illustration assumes a barometric pressure (P_B) of 761 mm Hg.

TRANSPULMONARY PRESSURE

Transpulmonary pressure (P_{tp}) is the change in alveolar pressure (P_{alv}) and pleural pressure (P_{pl}) of the lungs, basically the change inside the lung versus outside it (Figure 25-2).

$$P_{tp} = P_{alv} - P_{pl}$$

Transpulmonary pressure is often referred to as alveolar distending pressure. All of the processes of assisted mechanical ventilation attempt to increase the transpulmonary pressure. During negative pressure ventilation, such as ventilation through a chest cuirass, the ventilator attempts to decrease transpulmonary pressure to enable a larger gas volume to reach the lungs. During positive pressure ventilation, the mechanical ventilator likewise attempts to increase the transpulmonary pressure by delivering a volume of gas to the alvoli.[2,3]

TRANSTHORACIC PRESSURE

The last pressure gradient involved in respiration is **transthoracic pressure** (P_{tt}), which represents the difference between alveolar pressure (P_{alv}) and body surface pressure (P_{bs}) (Figure 25-3).

$$P_{tt} = P_{alv} - P_{bs}$$

Transthoracic pressure is the pressure required to dilate and contract both the chest wall and the lungs simultaneously during the respiratory cycle. Transthoracic pressure changes based on the patient's weight, restrictive disease processes, and during situations that create a decrease in chest wall compliance.[2,3]

INTRA-ALVEOLAR AND INTRAPLEURAL PRESSURE

The action of ventilation requires several changes in the characteristics of the thoracic system. Intra-alveolar and

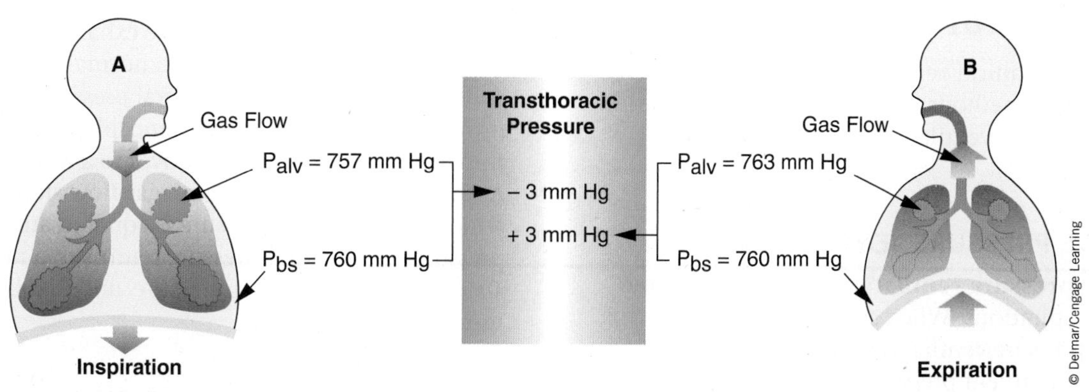

FIGURE 25-3 Transthoracic pressure: The difference between the alveolar pressure (P_{alv}) and the body surface pressure (P_{bs}). In this illustration, the body surface pressure (P_{bs}) is equal to the barometric pressure (P_B).

intrapleural pressures change as a result of positive and negative pressures being applied to the thoracic cavity.

- **Intra-alveolar pressure** is the pressure in the alveoli during ventilation. This pressure changes from approximately +1 cm H_2O during expiration to −1 cm H_2O during inspiration.[3] Intra-alveolar pressure changes in response to a change in the intrapleural pressure.
- **Intrapleural pressure** is the pressure difference between the visceral and parietal pleura. The intrapleural pressure at end-expiration is approximately −2 cm H_2O; during inspiration, it can reach anywhere from −6 to −8 cm H_2O.[3]

All of theses changes in pulmonary and thoracic dynamics play a crucial role in the process of spontaneous respirations.

During *inspiration* in a spontaneously breathing patient, the diaphragm and rib cage begin to increase the volume of the thoracic cavity. The result is a decrease in intrapleural pressure and a resulting decrease in intra-alveolar pressure. The negative intrapleural pressure results in a pressure difference (gradient) across the lung. Since atmospheric pressure is higher than intra-alveolar pressure, air flows into the lung. Once the necessary inspiratory volume is reached and the thorax stops expanding, the difference between atmospheric and intra-alveolar pressure becomes zero and gas flow into the lungs stops.

Expiration is a passive process. The elastic property of the lung and thorax become prominent once the muscular effort of the diaphragm and thoracic muscles ceases. This results in a positive intrapleural pressure and consequently an increase in intra-alveolar pressure. A pressure difference between the alveoli and atmosphere now exists. Intra-alveolar pressure is greater than atmospheric pressure and air begins to move out of the lung until the pressure gradient once again becomes zero. [2,3]

Modalities of Ventilation

Artificial mechanical ventilation can be administered through three methods: negative pressure ventilation, positive pressure ventilation, and high-frequency ventilation.

NEGATIVE PRESSURE VENTILATION

Negative pressure ventilation attempts to mimic normal respirations. When an individual is receiving negative pressure ventilation, the upper airway is exposed to ambient pressure while the thoracic cavity is placed in an airtight environment. When negative pressure is applied to this airtight environment, the thoracic cavity pressure drops and becomes a negative pressure environment. In response to the change in thoracic pressure, the intra-alveolar pressure becomes negative as a result of a negative pressure generated at the upper airway.[2] Negative pressure ventilation mimics normal physiological respirations, though it has not been commonly used as a mechanically ventilated device since the polio epidemic.

POSITIVE PRESSURE VENTILATION

Positive pressure ventilation is currently one of the most common methods of artificial ventilation. During positive pressure ventilation, the ventilator delivers a volume of gas through either an endotracheal tube or a noninvasive nasal or face mask to the patient's lungs to assist in ventilation. The volume of gas that the ventilator delivers to the lungs causes changes in the alveolar pressure, making the alveolar pressure gradient a positive pressure environment. This positive pressure is transmitted throughout the lungs, and gas exchange results.

During expiration, the ventilator stops delivering flow, and gas passively exits the lungs. The pressure at the endotracheal tube or mask during expiration returns to baseline. However, alveolar pressure remains in a positive pressure state in response to positive end-expiratory pressure and ventilator pressure change.

When a person requires the assistance of mechanical ventilation, the physiological process of respiration undergoes significant changes. As a breath is mechanically delivered to the patient, intra-alveolar and intrapleural pressures both increase above the atmospheric pressure.[1,2,3] The diaphragm is pushed downward in response to the breath being delivered by the mechanical ventilator. Once the ventilator has delivered the mechanical breath, a no-gas state occurs in which both the intra-alveolar and intrapleural pressures are both greater than atmospheric pressure in response to the volume, or pressure, of gas delivered to the individual.[1,2,3] Diaphragmatic movement ceases at the end of inspiration during mechanical ventilation.

Expiration for the mechanically ventilated patient is a passive process in which the exhaled air causes intra-alveolar pressure drops to normalize with atmospheric pressure. [1,2,3] Intrapleural pressure likewise drops to a static level below atmospheric pressure, and the diaphragm relaxes and moves to a resting position. At the end of expiration, a no–gas-flow state exists in which intra-alveolar pressure is equal to atmospheric pressure. Intrapleural pressure returns to a negative state below atmospheric pressure, and diaphragmatic movement ceases.

HIGH-FREQUENCY VENTILATION

High-frequency ventilation provides ventilation that delivers a tidal volume less than deadspace and respiratory rates anywhere between 60 and 900 breaths per minute.[4] The three types of high-frequency ventilation are high-frequency oscillation ventilation, high-frequency jet ventilation, and high-frequency flow interruption ventilation.

High-Frequency Oscillation Ventilation. During *high-frequency oscillation ventilation* (*HFOV*), the oscillating ventilator delivers a bulk flow of gas to the airways, which provides fresh gas to the airways for ventilation. Coupled with a high respiratory rate, the HFOV delivers tidal volumes that are less then deadspace; thus the pressure delivered to the lungs is attenuated by the time it reaches the alveolar space.[5] The mean airway pressure is constant throughout ventilation to keep the alveoli distended and the lungs inflated in order to allow ventilation to occur.

HFOV relies on a number of physiological principles for effective ventilation and oxygenation such as the principles of Taylor dispersion (an effect in fluid mechanics in which a shear flow can increase diffusivity), molecular diffusion, bulk flow gas convection, Pendelluft effect (the movement of air back and forth between the lungs), gas flow streaming, and cardiogenic mixing.[4,5] HFOV is the only form of ventilation in which active exhalation occurs; the bellows, located in the oscillator, actively pulls the gas out of the lungs. Because expiration is active, the mean airway pressure needs to be maintained to keep the alveoli open; if the mean airway pressure is decreased too much, atalectasis occurs, causing a disturbance in ventilation and oxygenation.

HFOV is commonly used for:

- Infant respiratory distress syndrome.
- Acute respiratory distress syndrome.
- Pulmonary interstitial emphysema.
- Air leak syndromes.

High-Frequency Jet Ventilation. *High-frequency jet ventilation* (*HFJV*), like HFOV, delivers tidal volumes of 1–5 mL/kg with very high respiratory rates.[4] Similar gas law principles apply to HFJV: Taylor dispersion, molecular diffusion, bulk flow gas convection, Pendelluft effect, gas flow streaming, and cardiogenic mixing.[4,5] There are a few differences between HFJV and HFOV.

- HFJV can utilize additional support from a conventional ventilator to prevent atelectasis.
- HFJV uses passive exhalation instead of active exhalation, as HFOV does.
- Passive exhalation makes HFJV a good choice for ventilation when hemodynamic status is of concern for the patient.

High-Frequency Flow Interruption Ventilation. *High-frequency flow interruption ventilation* (*HFFIV*) is similar to HFJV in that they both stream gas flow into the patient's lungs. In the HFFI ventilator is a ball that interrupts the flow of gas, which causes this streaming of gas into the airway.[6] Respiratory rates can reach as high as 600 breaths per minute. This form of mechanical ventilation is not as commonly used today with the advent of HFOV and HFJV.

Pulmonary Dynamics

The lungs, in and of themselves, have characteristics that vary from patient to patient and that play important roles in how effectively mechanical ventilation can be delivered. Lung compliance and airway resistance are two of the most important concepts that a respiratory therapist must be aware of during mechanical ventilation.

LUNG COMPLIANCE

When a volume of gas is being delivered to the lungs, that air is working to open a lung unit against the force of the thoracic cavity.[7] **Lung compliance** relates to how elastic the lungs are when a volume of gas is applied to them. Lung compliance (C_L) relates to the change in volume (ΔV) in liters (L) over the change in pressure (ΔP) in centimeters of water pressure (cm H_2O).[8] This can be represented in the following expression $C_L = \Delta V \div \Delta P$.

Two types of compliance can be measured: dynamic compliance and static compliance.

Dynamic compliance (C_{dyn}) measures the changes in volume and pressure in the nonelastic airways. The normal dynamic compliance for a nonintubated patient is 30–40 mL/cm H_2O.[8] When a patient is intubated and mechanically ventilated, the practitioner managing the patient should consider using serial measurements to trend any changes occurring in the nonelastic airways. Dynamic compliance is measured by taking the corrected tidal volume from the patient in milliliters and dividing that factor by the difference in *peak inspiratory pressure* (*PIP*) subtracted by the *positive end-expiratory pressure* (*PEEP*).

$$C_{dyn} = \frac{V_t}{(\text{PIP} - \text{PEEP})}$$ [7]

A second type of compliance that measures the elastic properties of the lungs, is known as **static compliance** (C_{st}). The normal static compliance of a person who is spontaneously breathing and not receiving mechanical ventilation is 0.05–0.17 L/cm

H_2O (50–170 mL/cm H_2O).[2] These normal values can be affected by a variety of factors:

- Mental status
- Patient position
- Abdominal girth
- Change in thoracic compliance such as burns
- Any factors that impede the work of the thoracic system

When an artificial airway is used to provide respiratory assistance, compliance changes in relation to the positive pressure ventilation and to the increase in airway resistance created by the artificial airway (dynamic compliance (Cdyn)).[7] In males who are intubated and receiving mechanical ventilation, compliance can range from 40 to 50 mL/cm H_2O and at times, based on lung pathology such as ARDS, can reach as high as 100 mL/cm H_2O.[2] Females who are intubated and receive mechanical ventilation have lung compliances ranging from 35 to 45 mL/cm H_2O and, as in males, can have lung compliance as high as 100 mL/cm H_2O.[2]

To calculate the static compliance of a patient receiving mechanical ventilation, the respiratory therapist has to obtain a static lung hold, that is, cause a plateau hold a state of no flow at the end of inspiration before exhalation begins. The static lung hold (measured as plateaus pressure) can then be inserted into the equation of lung compliance

$$C_{st} = \frac{V_t}{(P_{plateau} - \text{PEEP})}$$ [8]

AIRWAY RESISTANCE

Airway resistance, also known as transairway pressure, is the difference between the pressures at the mouth and at the alveoli.[7] Airway resistance informs the respiratory therapist of the resistance created by the airway when a volume of gas is delivered through the patient's conducting airway systems. Normal airway resistance of a nonintubated patient varies from 0.6 to 2.4 cm H_2O/L/sec if the patient has a spontaneous flow rate of 0.5 L/sec.[2] An artificial airway increases airway resistance; thus an intubated patient may have airway resistance from 6 cm H_2O/L/sec and higher based on artificial airway diameter.[2] Mechanically ventilated patients should have airway resistance trended to ascertain any changes when the patient receives bronchodilator therapy, has an artificial airway suctioned, or undergoes any other procedure that may improve airflow.[8] Airway resistance (R_{aw}) equals the peak airway pressure in centimeters of water pressure (cm H_2O, (PIP)) subtracted from the plateau pressure in centimeters of water pressure (cm H_2O, $P_{plateau}$) divided by flow rate in liters per second (L/sec).[8]

$$R_{aw} = \frac{(\text{PIP} - P_{plateau})}{\text{flow}}$$ [8]

> **Best Practice**
>
> **Lung Mechanics**
>
> Monitoring static compliance, dynamic compliance, and airway resistance in the mechanically ventilated patient assists the health care provider in determining improvement or deterioration in pulmonary status. Static compliance, dynamic compliance, and airway resistance should be monitored postintervention, such as suctioning and bronchodilator therapy, to examine whether improvements occurred.

Airway resistance in the intubated patient can vary for a variety of reasons, such as the diameter of the artificial airway, airway secretions, bronchospasm, pulmonary edema, chronic obstructive pulmonary disease, surfactant deficiency, and any other pathology that creates a high pressure environment in the lungs.[2,7] To decrease airway resistance, the clinician needs to correct the problem causing the restriction in the lungs.

> **CASE STUDY 25-1**
>
> A 35-year-old male is intubated in the intensive care unit for septic shock and respiratory failure. He is intubated with an 8.0-mm endotracheal tube, and mechanical ventilation is initiated. The current ventilator settings are: assist control with a corrected tidal volume of 600 mL, a PEEP of +5 cm H_2O, set respiratory rate of 12 breaths per minute, a flow rate of 60 L/min (1 L/sec), and an F_IO_2 of 40%. On these ventilator settings, he is reaching a peak inspiratory pressure of 40 cm H_2O and a plateau pressure of 35 cm H_2O.
>
> ***Questions***
>
> 1. What is the static compliance for this ventilated patient?
> 2. What is the dynamic compliance for this ventilated patient?
> 3. What is the calculated airway resistance on these current ventilator settings?

CASE STUDY 25-2

A 60-year-old female has been intubated for chronic obstructive pulmonary disease exacerbation (COPD exacerbation) and placed on mechanical ventilation in the intensive care unit. She is placed on assist control ventilation with a tidal volume of 450 mL, a PEEP of +8 cm H_2O, a set respiratory rate of 20 breaths per minute, a flow rate of 40 L/min (0.67 L/sec), and a F_IO_2 of 80%. On these ventilator settings she has a peak inspiratory pressure of 35 cm H_2O and a plateau pressure of 28 cm H_2O.

Questions

1. What is the static lung compliance for this ventilated patient?
2. What is the dynamic lung compliance for this patient?
3. What is the calculated airway resistance for this ventilated patient?

TIME CONSTANTS

Lung compliance and airway resistance change constantly during respiration, and, as a result, lung units open and close at different intervals. Lung units with high areas of airway resistance or areas of decreased compliance require a longer time to inflate. The constant related to the amount of time it takes to inflate a lung unit is the **time constant** (t), which indicates the amount of time required to fill a lung unit to approximately 60% of its total filling capacity. One time constant is equal to compliance of the lung unit multiplied by the airway resistance of the lung unit:

$t = C \times R_{aw}$[7]

In a healthy individual:

- One time constant should fill approximately 60% of a lung unit.[2,9]
- Two time constants should fill approximately 87% of a lung unit.
- Three time constants should fill approximately 95% of a lung unit.[2,9]
- Four time constants should fill approximately 98% of a lung unit.
- Five time constants should fill approximately 99% of a lung unit.[2,9]

As airway resistance increases, it takes longer for the lung unit to inflate during ventilation. The amount of increased airway resistance increases the time constant by a proportional ratio of 1:1; therefore if airway resistance increases by 3, the lungs will take three times longer to inflate.

Changes in lung compliance, on the other hand, affect time constants in a contrasting manner. As compliance decreases, the time constant likewise decreases. With a decrease in compliance and time constant, the lung unit loses the potential for reaching its total filling capacity. This concept is important in the newborn with surfactant deficiency, because lung compliance is decreased in relation to surfactant deficiency. The lung cannot fully inflate and ventilate effectively. To assist the newborn child with surfactant deficiency, it is necessary to provide surfactant therapy to increase the lung compliance to assist in fully ventilating the child.[9]

Time constants are an important factor in mechanical ventilation; they assist the respiratory therapist in selecting the initial inspiratory time and expiratory time to suit the patient's clinical condition. The normal time constant varies from 0.42 to 0.7 seconds in adults and from 0.25 to 0.75 seconds in infants. Delivering the fully set tidal volume to the patient should take approximately three time constants. If inspiratory time is too short, the lung units do not have enough time to open; conversely, if the inspiratory time is too long, inadequate exchange of gas may occur, which can result in increased carbon dioxide levels.

Likewise, expiratory time needs to be set to meet the patient's pulmonary condition. If expiratory time is too short, air trapping and autogenic PEEP can occur. Expiration can take more than five time units to provide the adequate removal of gas. The respiratory therapist should routinely examine time constants in relation to the patient's condition. As compliance and airway resistance change, time constants are affected and ventilator adjustments need to be made.

Complications from Mechanical Ventilation

Mechanical ventilation is utilized for individuals who have impairments of the pulmonary, thoracic, neurological, and/or cardiac systems. The goal of mechanical ventilation is to correct the underlying pathological condition while preventing further injury from being on mechanical ventilation. Invasive or noninvasive mechanical ventilation is physiologically abnormal. Individuals who receive positive pressure ventilation are at risk from ventilator-induced injuries that relate to the volume, the pressure, and the physiological reactions that occur as a response to a change in homeostasis.

Best Practice

Complications of Mechanical Ventilation

The main objective for mechanical ventilation is to correct the associated problems that lead to the need for mechanical ventilation and to minimize the potential physiological effects to the cardiac, renal, neurological, and associated body systems. The respiratory therapist needs to be aware of the associated complications with mechanical ventilation in order to reduce the risk of complications.

VOLUTRAUMA

Volutrauma is a condition that occurs when too much tidal volume is delivered to the lungs. This large amount of tidal volume has the potential to cause an overdistension of the lungs that results in lung injury. Overdistension can result in the stretching of the alveolar spaces, which can lead to an inflammatory mediator release that further injures the lungs.[2,10] In May 2000, the National Institute of Health and the National Heart Lung Blood Institute published a large study that examined adult patients with acute respiratory distress syndrome and the optimal strategies for preventing injury that may occur as a result of ventilation. The results of the study demonstrated that patients with acute lung injury or ARDS had an improved chance of survival with the use of tidal volumes ranging from 4 to 8 mL/kg ideal body weight when compared to the traditional 10–15 mL/kg of body weight.[11]

The low–tidal-volume-ventilation strategy also utilizes a titration of inspired oxygen and positive end-expiratory pressure to ensure that the patient receives adequate alveolar distending pressure when the lungs are in a low lung compliance state (Table 25-1).[11] The goal of oxygenation is to have a P_aO_2 of 55–80 mmHg or S_pO_2 of 88–95%.[11] The minimal positive end expiratory pressure is 5 cm H_2O with a maximum level of 24 cmH_2O.[11] There are two strategy limbs in the oxygen and PEEP titrations:

- One limb utilizes a lower PEEP level and higher F_IO_2.[11]
- The second limb utilizes a higher PEEP level with a lower F_IO_2.[11]

Either limb has been found acceptable in the treatment of alveolar stabilization and oxygenation for a patient who has acute lung injury or acute respiratory distress syndrome.[11]

TABLE 25-1 **Oxygen and PEEP titration strategies**

Lower PEEP/ Higher F_IO_2	
F_IO_2	PEEP
0.3	5
0.4	5
0.4	8
0.5	8
0.5	10
0.6	10
0.7	10
0.7	12
0.7	14
0.8	14
0.9	14
0.9	16
0.9	18
1.0	18–24

Higher PEEP/ Lower F_IO_2	
F_IO_2	PEEP
0.3	5
0.3	8
0.3	10
0.3	12
0.3	14
0.4	14
0.4	16
0.5	16
0.5	18
0.5–0.8	20
0.8	22
0.9	22
1.0	22
1.0	24

Source: Adapted from Ventilation with lower tidal volume as compared to traditional tidal volume for acute lung injury and the acute respiratory distress syndrome. N Engl J Med. *2000;18:342:1301–1308.*

The low–tidal-volume strategy concluded early because of the significantly higher survival rate among patients who received a lower tidal volume than the traditional tidal volumes.[11] The strategy has been effective in decreasing the mortality of patients with acute lung injury and acute respiratory distress syndrome, but currently no clinical data support the use of the low–tidal-volume-ventilation strategy for all patients who receive mechanical ventilation.

Best Practice

Mechanical Ventilation Strategies

Mechanical ventilation is a lifesaving procedure and should be utilized to assist patients in the recovery from pulmonary-related illnesses. While providing medical therapy that is in the best interest of the patient, the respiratory therapist must refer to the most current medical literature on treatment guidelines. Current medical literature suggests the use of a low–tidal-volume-ventilation strategy to treat adult patients with the diagnosis of acute respiratory distress syndrome and acute lung injury. Target tidal volumes for an adult patient with ARDS or acute lung injury, based on the low tidal volume study should range from 4 to 8 mL/kg ideal body weight.[11]

BAROTRAUMA

Barotrauma results from a high level of positive pressure, causing air to escape from the alveolar areas.[2,10] Barotrauma results in airleak syndromes such as pneumothorax or pulmonary interstitial emphysema, as well as free air in the thoracic cavity. When plateau pressures rise above the level of 30 cm H_2O, lung injury occurs as a result of high airway pressures. To prevent barotraumas, the clinician should attempt to decrease plateau pressures to a level of <30 cm H_2O. Ventilator parameters should be adjusted according to the specific patient condition in order to decrease the plateau pressures. Plateau pressures can be lowered by:

- Decreasing the tidal volume.
- Decreasing the positive end-expiratory pressure.
- Suctioning the patient if the high pressure is a result of secretions.
- Providing bronchodilators if bronchospasm is present.
- Manipulating the inspiratory time. (Any manipulation should be specific to the patient's condition.)

DISRUPTION OF PHYSIOLOGICAL FUNCTIONS

Mechanical ventilation can disrupt the normal physiological functions of the body. Positive pressure ventilation can cause discord among the cardiac, pulmonary, neurological, and renal systems, to name a few. For example:

- When a positive pressure environment is introduced to the thoracic system, changes in cardiac and hemodynamic statuses can result. These changes can lead to hypotension and tissue hypoxia as a direct result of limited blood flow perfusion in tissues.
- Positive pressure ventilation can be attributed to a decrease in cardiac output. Cardiac output decreases because heightened intrathoracic pressure limits the amount of blood returning to the heart, decreasing venous return to the right heart.[2,10] During the expiratory phase of ventilation, venous return increases in a response to the decreasing of intrathoracic pressure.[2,10]
- Positive pressure ventilation can also be attributed to an increase in pulmonary vascular resistance, which rises in response to an increase in alveolar pressure that occurs when positive end-expiratory pressure is present during mechanical ventilation. As a result of the increase in pulmonary vascular resistance, cardiac output and left ventricular filling pressure both drop. In response to an increase in right ventricular afterload, the effect can be right ventricular hypertrophy, which can cause discord with left ventricular function.[2,10]
- Patients who receive positive pressure ventilation through high-frequency ventilation can be at greater risk for hemodynamic compromise due to the high levels of mean airway pressure that is present in the lungs.[12,13,14] High-frequency ventilation can cause overdistension of the lungs, which can lead to further decreases in venous return and, in turn, to increases in pulmonary vascular resistance. Thus cardiac output is further reduced.[12]

To minimize the cardiovascular effects of mechanical ventilation, the respiratory therapist must ventilate the patient with the lowest possible mean airway pressure, positive end-expiratory pressure, and tidal volumes in order to prevent compression of the vascular structures in the thoracic cavity.[12] Some patients may require the assistance of fluid resuscitation and cardiac medication support to improve hemodynamic status. Medical management should be made on a case-by-case basis and meet the medical needs of the patient.

Renal dysfunction can also result from positive pressure ventilation in a variety of ways.

- When intrathoracic pressure increases and cardiac output is decreased, less perfusion is available to the kidneys.[2,10]
- There is a release of antidiuretic hormones from the pituitary glands in response to the change in intrathoracic pressure.[2,10]
- An imbalance of pH, P_aCO_2, and P_aO_2 can lead to renal dysfunction.[2,10]

To prevent edema and third spacing, the therapist has to closely monitor the fluid status of the patient receiving mechanical ventilation.

Patients with closed head injuries are at risk for complications:

- One risk is of decreased cerebral perfusion in response to the hemodynamic changes during mechanical ventilation.[2,10] Positive end-expiratory pressure and high mean airway pressures, in conjunction with decreased venous return can impede the blood flow to the brain.[2,10] High levels of positive end-expiratory pressure and high mean airway pressures should be avoided, when possible, to allow adequate perfusion to the brain.
- With the patient who has a closed head injury, controversy surrounds the use of hyperventilation, which may cause compromise to the uninjured areas of the brain. The patient with a closed head injury should be ventilated to prevent any further injury to the brain as well as to meet the ventilatory needs of the patient.

Hyperoxia-related injuries occur when patients are exposed to high levels of oxygen ($> 60\%$ F_IO_2) for prolonged periods of time.[2,10] Side effects of high oxygen levels are:

- Retrolental fibroplasia.
- Mucociliary dyskinesis.
- Oxidative stress lung injury.
- Pulmonary tissue injury.[2,10]

If patient conditions permit, the oxygen concentration should be lowered to a level that prevents lung injury. One way to do this is to increase the positive end-expiratory pressure to allow more time for the gas exchange to take place. Oxygen should be set at an appropriate level to meet the needs of the patient. It is currently not known what exposure time to oxygen causes lung injury. In neonatal patients during post-birth resuscitation, using low levels of oxygen to prevent oxidation injury is acceptable, but the optimal level has not yet been determined.[15]

OTHER CONSIDERATIONS

Other considerations related to mechanically ventilated patients are:

- Prevention of ventilator associated pneumonias.
- Maintaining adequate nutritional status.
- Preventing injuries associated with the artificial airway.
- Assisting the patient in communication needs.
- Taking care of the psychological well-being of the long-term mechanically ventilated patient.

Best Practice

Managing Oxygenation

Other important considerations for managing oxygenation relate to the titration of positive end-expiratory pressure and inspired oxygen. To assist in alleviating any ill effects of high oxygen concentrations, the practitioner should consider using positive end-expiratory pressure at the lowest possible oxygen concentration to increase the surface area for gas exchange.

Summary

Mechanically ventilated patients are at risk for a number of complications associated with the physiological effects of positive pressure ventilation. To effectively provide positive pressure ventilation while alleviating the potential hazards of mechanical ventilation, the respiratory therapist needs to understand the physiological changes that result from mechanical ventilation. Early recognition of the potential effects enables the therapist to prevent further complications.

Study Questions

REVIEW QUESTIONS

1. How do transairway, transpulmonary, and transthoracic pressure interact during the process of respiration?
2. Name the two types of lung compliances.
3. Describe airway resistance and ways of improving high airway resistance.
4. Discuss time constants and the importance they play with mechanical ventilation.
5. What is the difference between volutrauma and barotrauma?
6. List some of the complications associated with mechanical ventilation.

MULTIPLE-CHOICE QUESTIONS

1. What is the normal static lung compliance of a nonmechanically ventilated patient?
   a. 40–60 mL/cm H_2O
   b. 30–40 mL/cm H_2O
   c. 20–30 mL/cm H_2O
   d. 10–20 mL/cm H_2O

2. How many time constants are required to fill 60% of a lung region?
   a. three
   b. five
   c. two
   d. one
3. Which pressure gradient describes the difference between the alveolar pressure and body surface pressure?
   a. transairway pressure
   b. transthoracic pressure
   c. transpulmonary pressure
4. What complications may occur if too large a tidal volume and high ventilator pressures are consistently delivered to a patient on mechanical ventilation?
   a. volutrauma
   b. barotrauma
   c. pneumothorax
   d. all of the above
5. Cardiac output decreases as a result of which of the following factors during mechanical ventilation?
   a. increased intrathoracic pressure
   b. decreased venous return to right heart
   c. high mean airway pressures
   d. all of the above
6. What is the static compliance for a patient with a tidal volume of 500 mL, a respiratory rate of 10, positive end-expiratory pressure of + 5 cm H_2O, a flow of 50 Lpm, and an F_IO_2 set at 30%? The patient's peak airway pressure is 30 cm H_2O with a plateau pressure of 20 cm H_2O.
   a. 50 mL/cm H_2O
   b. 33.3 mL/ cm H_2O
   c. 15.8 mL/cm H_2O
   d. 25.5 mL/cm H_2O

CRITICAL-THINKING QUESTIONS

1. How can time constants be useful in the initial phases of ventilation?
2. What pulmonary changes occur to a newborn child who has respiratory distress and who receives surfactant therapy?
3. How can early extubation or noninvasive ventilation curtail the ill effects associated with mechanical ventilation?

References

1. Jardins T. *Cardiopulmonary Anatomy & Physiology.* 5th ed. Clifton Park: Delmar Cengage Learning; 2007.
2. Pilbeam S. *Mechanical Ventilation—Physiological and Clinical Applications.* 4th ed. St. Louis: Mosby; 2006.
3. Ward JPT, Ward J, Leach RM, Wiener CM. *The Respiratory System at a Glance.* 2nd ed. Chichester: Blackwell Publishing; 2006.
4. dos Santos CC, Slutsky AS. Overview of high-frequency ventilation modes, clinical rationale, and gas transport mechanisms. *Respir Care Clin N Am.* 2001;7:4.
5. Mildner R, Cox P. The preclinical history of high-frequency ventilation. *Respir Care Clin N Am.* 2001;7:4.
6. Hess D, Mason S, Branson R. High frequency ventilation, *Respir Care Clin N Am.* 2001;7:4.
7. West JB. *Respiratory Physiology: The Essentials.* 8th ed. New York: Lippincott Williams & Wilkins; 2008,
8. Chang DW. *Respiratory Care Calculations*, 2nd ed.: Clifton Park Delmar Cengage Learning.; 1998.
9. Goldsmith JP, Karotkin EH. *Assisted Ventilation of the Neonate.* 4th ed. Philadelphia: Saunders; 2003.
10. Hess DR, Kacmarek RM. *Essentials of Mechanical Ventilation.* 2nd ed. New York: McGraw-Hill; 2002.
11. Ventilation with lower tidal volumes as compared with traditional tidal volumes for acute lung injury and the acute respiratory distress syndrome. *N Engl J Med.* 2000;342,18:1301–1308.
12. Cotton M, Clark RH. The science of neonatal high-frequency ventilation. *Respir Care Clin N Am.* 2001;7:4.
13. Priebe GP, Arnold JH. High-frequency oscillatory ventilation in pediatric patients. *Respir Care Clin N Am.* 2001;7:4.
14. Mehta S, MacDonald R. Implementing and troubleshooting high-frequency oscillatory ventilation in adults in the intensive care unit, *Respir Care Clin N Am.* 2001;7:4.
15. Kattwinkel J. *Textbook of Neonatal Resuscitation.* 5th ed. Elk Grove Village, IL: American Academy of Pediatrics; 2006.

CHAPTER 26

Initiation, Monitoring, and Discontinuing Mechanical Ventilation

Bethene L. Gregg

OBJECTIVES

Upon completion of this chapter, the reader should be able to:

- Describe the essential events of initiating mechanical ventilation.
- Interpret changes in peak, plateau, and mean airway pressures
- Identify changes in scalar and/or loop waveforms indicating a leak, air trapping, or patient-ventilator dyssynchrony.
- Describe PEEP and its application in contrast to auto-PEEP.
- Discuss the hazards and complications of mechanical ventilation including ventilator-associated pneumonia.
- Describe the purpose of ventilator checks in preventing potential complications.
- State the appropriate actions to take in correcting respiratory acidosis, alkalosis, or ventilator dyssynchrony.
- State how changes in the ventilator controls affect volume delivery and mean airway pressure.
- Explain the appropriate course of action when multiple alarms are activated and the patient's condition has suddenly deteriorated.
- Discuss methods of weaning, and list two important considerations for extubation.

CHAPTER OUTLINE

KEY TERMS

alveolar recruitment	baseline pressure	peak pressure
barotrauma	mean airway pressure	plateau pressure

Continuous mechanical ventilation typically refers to positive pressure ventilation, in which the patient-ventilator interface is an artificial airway, usually an endotracheal or tracheostomy tube. This chapter focuses on the initiation, monitoring/management, and discontinuation of mechanical ventilation in adults.

Indications for Mechanical Ventilation

Initiate mechanical ventilation in cases of:

- Apnea.
- Acute ventilatory failure.
- Oxygenation failure.
- Impending ventilatory failure.

Any condition that impairs the physiologic pathway of breathing may lead to apnea or *acute ventilatory failure,* which is the failure of the thorax to pump air. Depression of the respiratory centers in the brain, spinal cord injury, neuromuscular dysfunction, and diaphragmatic fatigue can all impair the movement of the thorax. The inability of the thorax to move air reduces alveolar ventilation and results in alveolar hypoventilation and respiratory acidosis. Hypoxemia is secondary to hypercarbia. Mechanical ventilation delivers 14–16 tidal volumes per minute that restores adequate alveolar ventilation and corrects the arterial blood gases by lowering the P_aCO_2 to normal values. A normalized P_aCO_2 raises the P_aO_2 and the pH.

On the other hand, *oxygenation failure* is the failure of the lungs to provide gas exchange. A ventilator provides the bulk movement of gas into the lungs: It does not bring about gas exchange. An *extracorporeal membrane oxygenator* (*ECMO*) allows the exchange of O_2 and CO_2 in the blood but does not provide ventilation. Oxygenation failure produces severe hypoxemia that is refractory to oxygen therapy; that is, the P_aO_2 does not increase by at least 10 mm Hg with each increase of 0.20 in F_IO_2.[1] Hypoxemia stimulates the peripheral chemoreceptors, in turn *increasing* alveolar ventilation.[2] The result is alveolar hyperventilation and respiratory alkalosis. Since ventilation is not impaired per se, mechanical ventilation is less effective in oxygenation failure, which may progress to *acute respiratory distress syndrome* (*ARDS*).

The respiratory therapist (RT) understands why mechanical ventilation alone does not improve arterial oxygen tensions in oxygenation failure. Oxygenation failure is due to pulmonary shunting, in which pulmonary capillary blood passes by collapsed, flooded, or underinflated alveoli.[3] Alveoli may also collapse at the end of a tidal breath and contribute to shunt. The distribution of ventilation dictates that inspiratory gas goes to the areas of the lung that are the most easily expanded (compliant) and that have the least airway resistance. A tidal breath may not inflate the affected areas at all and therefore does little to reduce shunt and improve oxygenation.

The volume of the lung as a whole must increase; specifically, the *functional residual capacity* (*FRC*) must increase. The increase in FRC is typically accomplished by applying *positive end-expiratory pressure* (*PEEP*). PEEP holds pressure in the lung and increases the end-tidal lung volume. Because the principles governing the distribution of ventilation for this added lung volume still apply, PEEP may not reexpand a localized area of atelectasis. However, if collapsed, flooded, or underinflated alveoli are more diffuse throughout the lung, PEEP may open collapsed alveoli and prevent the end-tidal collapse of others when it is applied early in the course of acute lung injury or respiratory insufficiency. The reopening of collapsed alveoli is called **alveolar recruitment**.

A critical care ventilator is not needed to apply PEEP; less complicated devices can provide it. However, all critical care ventilators are capable of providing PEEP.

When applied to patients who are breathing in a *spontaneous* mode of ventilation or who are independent of a mechanical ventilator, PEEP is referred to as *continuous positive airway pressure* (*CPAP*). Treating cases of oxygenation failure with CPAP only can present a problem. If CPAP is applied too late, the expiratory work of breathing at the elevated pressure may become excessive and cause respiratory muscle fatigue. Once fatigue occurs, mechanical ventilation becomes necessary. For this reason, a patient in oxygenation failure is often intubated to protect the airway and to provide mechanical ventilation. In some cases, however, early intervention with mask CPAP may increase FRC, improve oxygenation, and avoid intubation.

To identify impending ventilatory failure, physiologic function is often measured to determine the adequacy of a patient's capacity to maintain spontaneous breathing. Variables such as vital capacity, negative inspiratory pressure, and maximum voluntary ventilation are typically measured in addition to arterial blood gases (ABG). There are critical thresholds or limits beyond which physiologic function becomes incompatible with sustained spontaneous breathing. These values are as follows:

- Partial pressure of oxygen in arterial blood (P_aO_2) < 50 mm Hg
- Frequency (f) > 35 bpm
- Tidal Volume (VT) < 5 mL/kg
- Negative inspiratory force or pressure (NIF, NIP) < −20 cm H_2O
- Vital Capacity (VC) < 10 mL/kg

In general, indicators such as inadequate arterial blood gases, coupled with the signs and symptoms of acute respiratory distress, identify the patient who requires intubation and mechanical ventilation. The notable exception is the patient with *chronic airflow obstruction* (*CAO*). A trial of medical treatment, including oxygen therapy and bronchodilators, is indicated in this case before intubation and mechanical ventilation. Also, the use of noninvasive ventilation has gained support in emergent situations such as exacerbation of CAO. Noninvasive ventilation is discussed in more detail in Chapter 28.

Initiation of Mechanical Ventilation

Use the following guidelines to initiate mechanical ventilation:

- Verify ventilator function, select the humidifier type, and connect the humidifier, calibrate the sensors, set the high airway pressure alarm limit on 40 cm H_2O for *volume control* (*VC*) or on 35 cm H_2O for *volume-targeted pressure control* (*VTPC*). Also for VTPC, set the high tidal volume alarm limit equal to 10 mL/kg.
- Set a tidal volume (V_T) of 8 mL/kg of *predicted body weight* (*PBW*) at a rate of 15 breaths per minute (bpm). If the **plateau pressure** is greater than 30 cm H_2O when the ventilator is connected to the patient (low compliance), use 6 mL/kg of PBW V_T and a rate of 20 bpm. If the plateau pressure is still greater than 30 cm H_2O, drop the tidal volume to 4 mL/kg of PBW (minimum tidal volume) and increase the rate to 30 bpm (maximum 35 bpm).
- Set a peak flow of 50 Lpm or a flow in milliliters per minute equal to V_T mL × bpm × $(I + E)$
- Set the primary disconnect alarm, the high tidal volume alarm limit, and the apnea ventilation parameters, if available.
- Set a flow trigger of 2 Lpm.
- Set 5 cm H_2O PEEP.
- Connect the ventilator in volume control mode to the patient and:
  - Check that the patient's chest expands (that the ventilator delivered a breath).
  - Reduce tidal volume if the high pressure alarm is activated; check that the plateau pressure is less than or equal to 30 cm H_2O in VC.
  - Check the flow/time waveform that the expiratory flow returns to baseline; that is, there's no air trapping.
  - Check for signs of patient-ventilator asynchrony; that is, adjust the peak flow to meet the patient's inspiratory demand.
- Perform a ventilator check.

A ventilator should be on standby, ready for use, and it should have had proper preventative maintenance by qualified staff. Attach a ventilator circuit and connect an appropriate humidification system. Connect the ventilator to a power and gas source. Before the ventilator is connected to the patient, its operation must be verified and the patient values entered on the control panel. Most ventilators require the selection of the type of humidification system, either a heated wet humidifier or a heat and moisture exchanger (HME), during the initial ventilator start-up when the patient's weight is entered. The initial start-up is also when flow and oxygen sensors are calibrated and when the neonatal, pediatric, or adult patient range is selected. During this time, the patient is being ventilated with a manual resuscitator or transport ventilator.

Ventilators vary in their operation verification procedures. These programmed self-tests may take several minutes and result in ventilator failure if performed too quickly. Some of the current ventilators have a short leak test, and it should be used. This test creates a pressure hold that checks for leaks, exhalation valve function, and tubing compliance factor. Failure to perform the manufacturer's recommended performance check may cause the ventilator to malfunction during patient use.

Best Practice

Checking Ventilator Function

Always verify the proper functioning of the ventilator according to the manufacturer's recommendations before connecting the unit to the patient.

For older ventilators or for those without a short self-test, check for leaks by observing that the ventilator holds pressure during an inspiratory pause with the patient wye occluded.

- Set a long pause time and a small tidal in volume control.
- Adjust the high airway pressure alarm to maximum.
- The patient wye is aseptically occluded, and a breath is manually initiated.
- Observe the airway pressure monitor to check that the ventilator holds pressure during the pause.

A falling pressure during the pause indicates a leak. All connections should be rechecked and an inspiratory pause repeated until the system holds pressure. The high-pressure alarm, pause time, and tidal volume must be readjusted when setting the control panel for the patient.

For older ventilators, the pause pressure generated during the leak test may be used to calculate the circuit compliance or tubing compliance factor.

- Divide the tidal volume by the pause pressure to calculate the tubing compliance factor.
- Use this factor to calculate the volume that is compressed in the circuit during a volume-controlled inspiration and that is therefore not delivered to the patient.
- After the ventilator is connected to the patient, multiply the pressure during a pause (minus any PEEP) by the tubing compliance factor to find the compressible volume loss to the circuit.
- Subtract the compressible volume from the exhaled tidal volume to calculate the tidal volume that the patient actually receives.

Most current critical care ventilators automatically calculate tubing compliance during the performance verification test.

A common but not as safe verification practice is to:

- Check that the ventilator is in the proper mode to deliver a breath.
- Block the patient wye,
- Manually trigger a breath to observe that pressure builds up during inspiration and activates the high airway pressure alarm.

Although this practice serves several functions, it does not always detect a leak or a malfunctioning exhalation valve. It does:

- Verify that gas is actually exiting the ventilator and that the high pressure alarm functions.
- Check the patient disconnect alarm if the patient wye is then opened.

This procedure is not recommended, however.

Respiratory therapists must know which ventilators automatically perform self-tests when first powered on and which tests the operator may initiate. Some tests are not to be performed at the bedside. For example, most ventilators, with the exception of the Puritan Bennett (PB) 840, may be powered on, and then the patient wye can be aseptically blocked. The PB 840 must *not* have the patient wye blocked when it is powered on. If the patient wye is inadvertently blocked when the PB 840 is powered on, the ventilator switches to a second microprocessor in the breath delivery unit and provides safety ventilation. The ventilator needs to be shut off and restarted.

INITIAL VENTILATOR SETTINGS

After verifying ventilator operation, adjust the control settings based on the patient's ideal or predicted body weight. *Predicted body weight* (*PBW*) may be estimated as:

Men (in kilograms)	= 50 + 2.3 per inch over 5 feet
Women (in kilograms)	= 45.5 + 2.3 per inch over 5 feet
Men (in pounds)	= 110 + 5 per inch over 5 feet
Women (in pounds)	= 100 + 5 per inch over 5 feet

The current recommended initial settings are V_T = 8 mL/kg of the patient's ideal body weight and 15 breaths per minute (bpm). Before the first delivered breath, the high airway pressure alarm should be set on 40 cm H_2O. This setting allows a quick check on the patient's compliance with the first volume-controlled breath.

Best Practice

High Airway Pressure Alarm

Check that the high airway pressure alarm is set on 40 cm H_2O before connecting the unit to the patient.

Age-Specific Competency

Pediatric Settings

Ventilator settings vary for infants and children. For example, airway pressure alarms should be less than 30 cm H_2O for infants.

For example, if the patient weighs 70 kg and the set tidal volume is 560 mL, the high-pressure alarm is activated if the patient's compliance is severely reduced to around 20 mL/cm H_2O, assuming approximately 10 cm H_2O from airway resistance.

- Should the high-pressure alarm activate with the first delivered breath or if the target tidal volume is not delivered, adjust the tidal volume to 6 mL/kg and increase the bpm to 20. Check that the plateau pressure is less than 25, and add 5 cm H_2O PEEP.
- If the plateau pressure is over 25 cm H_2O, drop the tidal volume to 4 mL/kg before adding 5 cm H_2O of PEEP.
- If the plateau pressure is over 30 cm H_2O with the addition of PEEP at a tidal volume of 4 mL/kg, change the mode to *airway pressure release ventilation* (*APRV*). Set high pressure on 30 cm H_2O and low pressure on 0 cm H_2O. Set a high time of 4 seconds and a low time of 0.5 seconds. (The management of APRV and the application of PEEP for patients with ARDS are discussed in more detail later in this chapter.)

The patient must be adequately sedated when small tidal volumes (4–6 mL/kg) are delivered in volume control or the result of either volume-targeted pressure control or *pressure-controlled* (*PC*) ventilator breaths. If the patient increases inspiratory effort in an attempt to take larger breaths, the increased effort may generate more negative swings of intrathoracic pressure that could exacerbate pulmonary edema. Lung protective strategies favor the use of VTPC or PC breaths to reduce the work of breathing from increased patient demand for flow, provided the pressure does not exceed 30 cm H_2O. [4] Since most ventilators in VTPC mode do not allow the pressure to come within 5 cm H_2O of the high airway pressure alarm, the high pressure alarm should be set on 35 cm H_2O. Because both VTPC and PC breaths are time cycled, the inspiratory time must be set appropriately, usually 1.0 second for adults. Inspiratory time may be readjusted after connecting the ventilator to the patient and observing flow/time waveforms.

When the tidal volume and beats per minute have been determined in volume control, the flow rate and flow pattern need to be set. Both peak flow rate and flow pattern determine the length of inspiration, or *inspiratory time*. The inspiratory flow must be high enough to meet the patient's inspiratory demand and to limit the length of inspiration in order to allow adequate time for exhalation. Expiratory time is a function of the beats-per-minute control. At any given inspiratory time, increasing the number of breaths per minute lower the time allowed for exhalation. *Inspiratory/expiratory ratios* (*I/Es*) of 1:3 or 1:4 are usually an adequate starting point. Calculate the peak flow setting in milliliters per minute as:

$$V_T(\text{mL}) \times \text{bpm} \times (\text{I} + \text{E})$$

For example, 560 mL × 15 × 4 = 33,600 mL per minute or 33.6 Lpm; therefore, set 34 Lpm for the peak flow for an I/E ratio of 1:3 if the tidal volume is 560 mL and the frequency setting is 15 bpm.

The peak flow calculated with this formula is lower than what is generally used and appropriate as long as the patient is not triggering every breath. Typically, a starting peak flow of 50 Lpm is used initially and adjusted after the ventilator has been connected to the patient. If the pressure fails to increase immediately during a patient inspiration, the peak flow is not high enough and must be increased.

Use a descending ramp flow waveform in volume control, if available, because a ramp waveform provides the highest **mean airway pressure** at the lowest **peak pressure**. Increasing mean airway pressure improves oxygenation as long as cardiac output does not decrease. The change in flow waveform from a rectangular to a descending ramp increases the inspiratory time and produces a larger I/E ratio (closer to 1:1); so verify that there is adequate expiratory time after changing to a ramp flow waveform in VC mode.

There is no documented advantage to initiating ventilation in PC mode over volume control mode if the patient is apneic, provided the precautions just discussed are followed. No studies document an advantage to VTPC over PC or VC. [5] Initiating volume control is more efficient, provided the high airway pressure alarm is appropriately set, and provides better control of lung-protective tidal volumes. [6] To initiate ventilation in pressure control, ideally the respiratory therapist needs to be able to adjust the level of pressure control rapidly with the turn of a knob.

A tidal volume of 8 mL/kg and a set rate of 15 bpm is still desirable. However, in PC and in VTPC, the tidal volume is a function of the pressure level, the patient's pulmonary compliance, and the patient's airway resistance. If the patient's compliance is not known, a level of 15 cm H_2O of PC is an appropriate starting point, provided a high tidal volume limit alarm is available and set to a volume equal to 10 mL/kg.[7]

- In *VTPC* modes, the ventilator initially delivers a volume-controlled breath for the purpose of calculating the patient's compliance and resistance. Then the ventilator automatically adjusts the PC level until the target tidal volume is achieved.

TABLE 26-1 **Adaptive pressure control modes**

Dräger Evita 4 and XL	AutoFlow®
Engström Carestation	Pressure controlled, volume guaranteed
Hamilton Galileo	Adaptive pressure ventilation
Maquet 300, 300A, Servo*i*	Pressure-regulated volume control
Puritan Bennett 840	Volume control plus
Newport E500	Volume-targeted pressure control
Viasys/Pulmonetics PalmTop	Pressure-regulated volume control
Viasys Avea	Pressure-regulated volume control

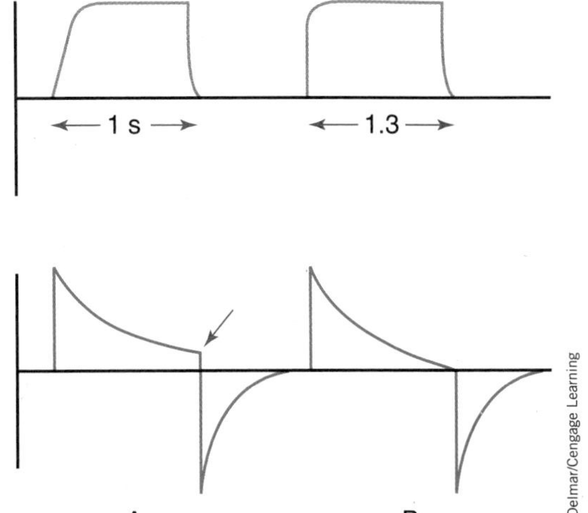

FIGURE 26-1 (A) The arrow indicates flow above baseline at the end of inspiratory time. (B) The longer inspiratory time shows flow returning to the baseline.

- In *PC*, the respiratory therapist needs to adjust the PC level until the target tidal volume is achieved. The inspiratory pressure level should not exceed 30 cm H_2O.

The names of volume-targeted pressure control modes, also called adaptive pressure control[5] modes, for various ventilators are listed in Table 26-1.

The inspiratory time should be fixed in pressure control, rather than by fixing the I/E ratio. Fixing the inspiratory time may help prevent excessively large swings in tidal volume in the event of a change in beats per minute. For example, if the I/E ratio is fixed and then the set frequency is decreased from 20 to 15 bpm, the increase in inspiratory time could deliver excessively large tidal volumes. Fixing the I/E ratio is more appropriate when providing inverse ratio ventilation (discussed later in the chapter).

An inspiratory time of 1.0 second may be used initially in PC or VTPC and then adjusted according to the flow waveform. Flow waveforms are monitored to maximize volume delivery for any level of pressure control. In Figure 26-1A, the inspiratory time ends before flow has returned to baseline. Increasing the inspiratory time to 1.3 seconds increases the volume delivered, as shown in Figure 26-1B, where the flow returns to baseline before inspiration ends. Any further increase in tidal volume requires an increase in the level of pressure control. The inspiratory time may need to be adjusted in VTPC as well. The ventilator automatically adjusts the level of pressure in VTPC, but not the inspiratory time.

Because flow has returned to baseline in Figure 26-1B, there is a period of no flow at end-inspiration. To estimate the patient's compliance under this condition, divide the tidal volume by the level of pressure control (minus PEEP). The compliance is then used to determine the level of pressure control (x) for any desired tidal volume.

$$\frac{500\text{ mL}}{x\text{ H}_2\text{O } 30} = 30\text{ mL } 500 = x = 17\text{ cm H}_2\text{O of PC}$$

If the compliance is 30ml/cm H_2O and the desired tidal volume is 500ml, the pressure required is 500ml/30 ml/cm$_2$O = 17 cm H_2O.

In VTPC, the ventilator automatically adjusts or adapts the level of pressure control *between* breaths to maintain the target tidal volume because pressure is the variable controlled by the ventilator during inspiration. The control variable may also be switched *within* a breath. *Within-breath changes* are typically changes from pressure control to volume control during the same breath. Pressure augmentation on the Bear and volume-assured pressure support (VAPS) on the Bird 8400STi and Tbird essentially provide volume-supported breaths (that may be time triggered) as long as the target tidal volume is delivered before the inspiratory flow falls to the peak flow setting. In this case, there is no change in control variable (Figure 26-2A).

However, if inspiratory flow falls to the set peak flow level *before* the tidal volume has been delivered, the control switches to flow (volume control), and gas delivery continues at the peak flow rate setting to complete volume delivery (Figure 26-2B). When the control switches to flow, airway pressure increases over the set inspiratory pressure limit. Ventilation then resumes in volume support (that may be time triggered) with the next breath. The patient can also receive a larger tidal volume than the target setting (Figure 26-2C).

Pressure-limited ventilation on the Dräger Evita4 and EvitaXL is one of the few modes that has a

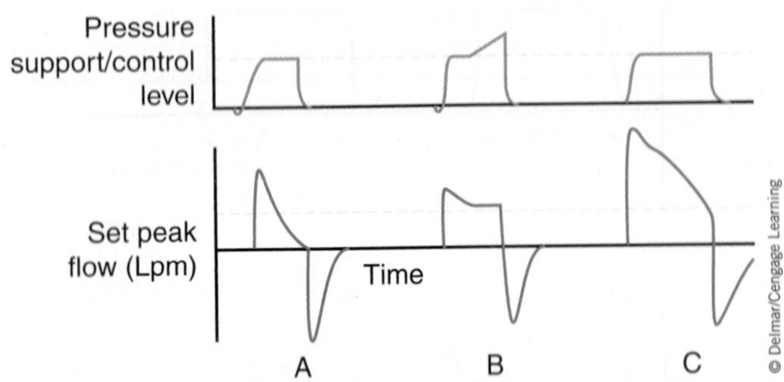

FIGURE 26-2 Pressure augmentation (Bear 1000, Bear Medical, Riverside, California) and volume-assured pressure support (Bird 8400ST, Bird Corp., Palm Springs, California) work the same way: (A) A target tidal volume is delivered; no switch in control variable. (B) The flow falls to the peak flow setting before the target volume is delivered; control variable switches to volume control. (C) A greater patient inspiratory effort allows a larger tidal volume than the target volume.

within-breath change from volume to pressure control. A pressure-limited breath starts in volume control but switches to pressure control if the airway pressure reaches the set maximum pressure (P_{max}). Inspiration at P_{max} continues until the set tidal volume is delivered.[8] If the tidal volume is delivered before inspiratory time ends, inspiratory flow falls to zero, and an inspiratory pause ensues for the remaining inspiratory time.

For patients with relatively normal compliance, either *assist-control* (*A/C*) or *synchronized intermittent mandatory ventilation* (*SIMV*) mode may be used initially as long as full ventilatory support is provided. SIMV has several advantages over A/C mode. SIMV prevents excessive triggering of machine breaths that could lead to hyperventilation and respiratory alkalosis, air-trapping, or patient-ventilator dyssynchrony. When SIMV is used, set to the pressure support for any spontaneous breaths taken in between mandatory (machine) breaths to minimize the patient's work of breathing. An initial pressure support level of 5 cm H_2O is usually sufficient to overcome most of the resistance from the circuit and an endotracheal tube with an inner diameter of 8.0–8.5 mm. The level of pressure support should be reevaluated after the patient is connected.

A variation of pressure support, volume-targeted pressure support or volume support, is also available on some ventilators. Both pressure support and volume support are considered spontaneous breathing modes because the patient must initiate the breath and determine when the flow-cycled breath ends. On some ventilators. the flow cycle variable for terminating pressure or volume supported breaths is adjustable.[2]

In addition to pressure support, several ventilators have another option to reduce the resistive inspiratory work of breathing through an endotracheal tube for the spontaneously breathing patient. *Automatic tube compensation* (*ATC*) (Dräger XL) or *tube compensation* (*TC*) (PB 840) automatically applies a level of pressure support that is proportional to the resistance across the endotracheal or tracheostomy tube during inspiration. The pressure level depends on the calculated value for tracheal pressure. Tracheal pressure is calculated as the proximal airway pressure minus the product of the known resistance of the tube, multiplied by the squared flow. The flow is measured instantaneously throughout inspiration. ATC can also decrease the patient's expiratory work of breathing by reducing the PEEP as needed to partially compensate for resistance of the endotracheal tube during exhalation.[10] The expiratory compensation feature may be turned off.

A variation on A/C or SIMV mode is *Adaptive Support Ventilation* (*ASV*), available on the Galileo Gold (Hamilton Medical, Reno, Nevada) that provides VTPC time-triggered mandatory breaths or volume support for patient-triggered spontaneous breaths. ASV automatically selects the ventilator values for respiratory rate, inspiratory time, I/E ratio, and pressure limit on the basis of the patient's required minute volume. The clinician inputs the patient's body weight, and the minute volume is determined as 100 mL/min/kg. The percentage of the minute volume to be supplied can be adjusted from 10% to 350%.[11] The ventilator delivers test breaths to calculate compliance, resistance, and intrinsic or auto-PEEP ($PEEP^i$). It then automatically adjusts the frequency and tidal volume to minimize the elastic and resistive loads according to the minimal work of breathing equation described by Otis and associates in 1950. The ventilator algorithm for ASV is designed to prevent apnea, volutrauma (injury to the lung parenchyma from alveolar overexpansion and shear stress), $PEEP^i$, or rapid shallow breathing. The flow cycle variable for VS breaths can be adjusted from 10% to 40% of the initial peak flow.[11]

For patients with severely reduced compliance, bilevel ventilation may be initiated. Essentially, bilevel ventilation allows a high and low CPAP setting. The patient can breathe spontaneously with or without pressure support at two different pressure levels (Figure 26-3). The difference between bilevel ventilation and PC with PEEP is that, on bilevel, the patient is able to exhale during the high-pressure period. Exhalation is possible at the higher pressure level because the exhalation valve is active or floating and allows exhalation without terminating the inspiratory phase.[12] During a PC inspiration, the exhalation valve is closed, preventing exhalation because PC is time cycled. Table 26-2 summarizes bilevel modes.

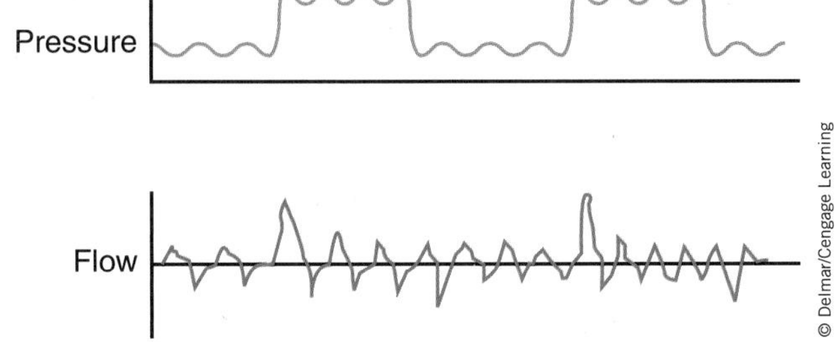

FIGURE 26-3 Bilevel ventilation allows spontaneous breathing at two levels of pressure. Pressure-supported breaths are also an option in bilevel (not shown).

Theoretically, less sedation is required with bilevel ventilation because the patient is free to initiate breaths at any time during the high or lower levels of pressure. In bilevel ventilation, the patient's actual inspiratory time is not limited by the ventilator. The ventilator's control of time simply determines how much time is allowed at the high CPAP level (T_H) versus the time allowed at the lower pressure level (T_L). APRV typically refers to a minimal T_H of 4–6 seconds for adults (2–3 seconds for neonates) and a low CPAP time of 0.2–0.8 seconds for adults (0.2–0.4 seconds for neonates) for an T_H/T_L ratio of 8:1 or more.[13] Ideally, the low pressure time is set according to the peak expiratory flow. The low pressure time is set to end-expiratory time at 50–75% of the peak expiratory flow observed from a flow-time waveform or flow-volume loop. Carbon dioxide elimination is facilitated by a greater difference between the high and low CPAP levels and by more frequent cycles, or releases, from the high to the low pressure levels. Typical APRV pressure settings are 30 cm H_2O for the high pressure and 0 cm H_2O for the low pressure. Sixty divided by the sum of T_H plus T_L equals the number of releases per minute. For example, a T_H of 4.5 seconds and a T_L of 0.5 seconds produces 12 releases per minute.

Whichever mode is used in an intensive care unit depends on:

- The needs of the patient.
- The type of ventilator available.
- The qualifications and experience of the respiratory care staff.
- The restraints placed on the RCP by the medical staff's ventilator knowledge or lack thereof.

All modes have advantages and disadvantages that must be considered in light of the clinical situation.[14]

All modes include a patient trigger setting. The patient may initiate a breath by creating a drop in pressure or a drop in flow. A flow trigger setting of 2–3 Lpm for adults (1–2 Lpm for infants) is preferable to a pressure trigger for critical care ventilators, except in the case of an unavoidable leak in the system. A leak equal to or greater than the flow trigger mimics a patient's inspiratory effort and initiates breaths. A baseline or bias flow is available automatically on most current ventilators with a flow trigger. The flow trigger is usually not more than half of the baseline flow. The ventilator begins baseline flow delivery through the circuit when at least half the patient's exhalation has occurred. The Babylog 8000*plus* (Dräger, Telford, Pennsylvania) is an infant ventilator with a flow trigger that allows different expiratory and inspiratory flow rate settings. Activating *VIVE* (*variable inspiratory variable expiratory*) allows the user to independently set the expiratory baseline flow rate. A lower baseline expiratory flow reduces the infant's expiratory work of breathing.

In addition to a flow or pressure trigger, a patient can now initiate a breath from the change in electrical activity of the diaphragm. *Neurally adjusted ventilatory assist* (*NAVA*) applies pressure in proportion to the strength of a diaphragmatic contraction. Inspiration is also terminated or cycled by a decrease in the electrical activity of the diaphragm.[15] NAVA on the Maquet Servo^i was approved by the FDA in 2007 and requires a specially designed nasogastric (NG) tube. The NG tube is embedded with microelectrodes and has a cable that transmits the signal to the Servo^i. NAVA improves patient-ventilator synchronicity by reducing the number of *missed breaths*, that is, breaths that the patient attempts to initiate but that the ventilator fails to allow. NAVA also has the potential to reduce the patient's work of

TABLE 26-2 **Bilevel modes**

Bilevel	840 (Puritan Bennett, Pleasanton, California)
Bivent	Servo^i (Maquet, Bridgewater, New Jersey)
Bilevel airway pressure ventilation	Engström Carestation (GE Healthcare, Chalfont St. Giles, UK)
Airway pressure release ventilation (APRV)	Evita XL (Dräger, Telford, Pennsylvania) Galileo Gold (Hamilton Medical, Reno, Nevada) Viasys Avea (Cardinal Health, Dublin, Ohio)

breathing by ending a breath when the neural signal diminishes.[16]

Before connecting the patient to the ventilator, set the primary disconnect alarm if one is available. The disconnect alarm is usually the low inspiratory pressure alarm or low tidal or minute volume alarm. After connecting to patient, the low inspiratory pressure alarm should be set on 10 cm H_2O and readjusted to 5–10 cm H_2O below the peak pressure. Many ventilators set the low inspiratory pressure alarm automatically. The low minute volume alarm should be set appropriately less than the set minute volume, usually 20% less. If using VTPC, set the high tidal volume limit alarm to 10 mL/kg of the patient's PBW. Any ventilator with a volume-targeted pressure control or support mode should have a high tidal volume limit alarm. If oxygenation status is unknown, an F_IO_2 of 1.0 (100%) oxygen should be used initially and the low F_IO_2 alarm set on 95%. A quick check and adjustment of all other alarms completes the process. If the ventilator has apnea ventilation, set the apnea ventilation controls. Several ventilators allow only parameter adjustment of apnea ventilation when the selected mode permits spontaneous breathing. A spontaneous breath by definition must be triggered and cycled by the patient.[8–9]

Finally, connect the ventilator circuit to the patient.

- Immediately upon connection, observe that the patient receives a ventilator breath and that chest expansion occurs.
- Breath sounds should be clear, equal, and bilateral.
- Set a level of 5 cm H_2O PEEP for an adult.
- Adjust alarm settings.
- Complete a ventilator check.
- Record the endotracheal tube insertion depth in centimeters at the teeth. The endotracheal tube should be inserted to a depth of approximately 23 cm at the incisors in men, 21 cm in women.[1,17]
- Note the peak inspiratory pressure and the plateau pressure during a pause.
- Calculate the tidal volume, corrected for compressible volume loss as appropriate.
- Calculate the patient's effective compliance as exhaled tidal volume over (plateau – PEEP).
- In volume control with rectangular flow waveforms, calculate airway resistance as (peak pressure minus plateau pressure) over peak flow in liters per second (Lps).
- Ensure that the patient appears comfortable on the ventilator and is not triggering breaths at a rate over 25/min.
- Observe the flow-time waveform and check that the expiratory flow returns to baseline *before* the start of the next inspiration to verify the absence of air trapping.
- Observe the pressure-time waveform for an immediate increase in pressure during inspiration.
- Check the volume-time waveform to verify that the expiratory limb returns to baseline, indicating that there are no leaks in the system.
- Note the pulse oximetry saturations and the F_IO_2.
- After 15 minutes, obtain an arterial blood gas (ABG). After drawing the ABG, suction the patient and measure cuff inflation pressure. An appropriate suction catheter size in French equals half the endotracheal tube inner diameter times 3. Cuff inflation pressure should be 20–30 cm H_2O to seal the airway and to prevent secretions immediately above the inflated cuff from inadvertently passing down around the cuff into the lower airway.[18]
- Airway stability is also important. An endotracheal tube that is not properly secured is a problem waiting to happen.
- A manual resuscitator connected to oxygen with an appropriately sized mask should be kept available at the bedside under aseptic conditions.[19]

An initial PEEP/CPAP setting of 5 cm H_2O for adults, 2–3 cm H_2O for infants, helps in maintaining FRC and counteracts the loss of end-expiratory lung volume that results from placement of the endotracheal tube through the glottis. In cases of ARDS, the level of PEEP should coincide with the pressure that maintains alveolar recruitment. Some practitioners believe this pressure is represented by the lower inflection point of the patient's pressure-volume

Best Practice

Disconnect Alarm

Know the primary patient disconnect alarm and what conditions activate preprogrammed alarms.

Best Practice

Verify Chest Expansion

Always verify chest expansion from a ventilator breath when the patient is first connected to the ventilator and listen for bilateral breath sounds.

CASE STUDY 26-1

The respiratory therapist is ready to connect the patient to the ventilator and sets the controls for volume control: A/C. The high pressure alarm limit is on 40 cm H_2O. Immediately after the patient is connected, the high pressure limit alarm activates.

Question

1. The patient is not triggering breaths or biting on the tube. What should you do first?

CASE STUDY 26-2

The ventilator is connected to a conscious and alert patient. The respiratory therapist notices that the airway pressure hesitates around zero before rapidly increasing at the end of inspiration. The patient looks agitated and uncomfortable. The RT is in volume control with a rectangular flow waveform.

Question

1. What is most likely the problem?

relaxation curve. Other practitioners advocate an optimal PEEP level that maximizes alveolar recruitment. The end-expiratory pressure is set above the point where significant alveolar destabilization occurs, usually determined during decremental deflation from an alveolar recruitment maneuver.[20,21] When pressure-volume curves are not measured, increase PEEP as high as possible without exceeding a plateau pressure of 28–30 cm H_2O to improve oxygenation without overdistension and to keep tidal volume equal to 6 mL/kg of predicted body weight.[22] Overdistension is measured as a decrease in effective compliance.

SUMMARY OF INITIATING MECHANICAL VENTILATION

- Verify ventilator function, connect humidification system, calibrate sensors.
- Set patient parameters:
  - VT 8 ml/kg at a rate of 15 bpm
  - Peak flow of 50 Lpm or a flow in mL equal to VT × bpm × (I + E)
  - Flow trigger of 2 Lpm
  - PEEP of 5 cm H_2O
- Set alarms:
  - Primary disconnect
  - High airway pressure alarm: 40 cm H_2O for VC; 35 cm H_2O for VTPC
  - High tidal volume limit
  - Apnea ventilation, if available
- Connect the ventilator to the patient and:
  - Check that the patient's chest expands (that the ventilator delivers a breath).
- Reduce tidal volume if the high pressure alarm is activated for VC or the volume is not constant alert given for VTPC. Check that the plateau pressure is less than or equal to 30 cm H_2O in VC. Possibly increase frequency to maintain $\dot{V}E$.
- Check the flow/time waveform that expiratory flow returns to baseline; that is, there's no air trapping.
- Check for signs of patient-ventilator asynchrony if the patient is triggering breaths.
  - Are the patient's inspiratory efforts failing to initiate inspiration? Check the trigger setting and the presence of intrinsic PEEP.
  - Does the inspiratory pressure fail to rise immediately? Is the peak flow adequate to meet patient's inspiratory demand (in VC)?
  - Is the patient working to exhale? Shorten the inspiratory time, reduce or eliminate the pause time.
  - Is there air trapping? Shorten the inspiratory time, increase the peak flow, reduce the number of machine breaths by changing to SIMV mode.
- Perform a ventilator check

Patient Monitoring

After mechanical ventilation has been established, the patient's ventilation, oxygenation, circulation, and perfusion are assessed to determine the appropriateness of the ventilator settings and to prevent complications. Arterial blood gases are drawn soon after initiating ventilation and then after changes in the patient's condition or ventilator settings. In general, change one ventilator parameter at a time in order to assess its effect and wait at least 15 minutes after interrupting ventilation or after endotracheal suctioning to obtain a blood gas. Although pulse oximetry can monitor oxyhemoglobin saturation, it cannot measure arterial PCO_2 or pH. The P_aCO_2 is the best assessment of alveolar ventilation. Pulse oximetry is useful for trending and detecting hypoxemia, but it does not warn of hyperoxic conditions. The arterial PO_2 blood gas is a better assessment of oxygenation when the F_IO_2 is considered. The P_aO_2/F_IO_2 (*P/F*) ratio, which should be greater than 300, can also be used to predict a lower F_IO_2 when the P_aO_2 is greater than 100 mm Hg.

Mean airway pressure provides a measure of the overall effect of the ventilator settings on oxygenation. Oxygenation improves when the mean airway pressure increases, unless cardiac output is compromised. If a higher mean airway pressure decreases venous return to the right atrium, the cardiac output decreases, especially in a seriously ill patient whose compensatory mechanisms for maintaining blood pressure are already compromised. A decrease in cardiac output and therefore of lung increases alveolar deadspace and decreases the expired PCO_2 and the volume of expired CO_2 in mL/min.[23] *Capnography*—the graphic display of expired CO_2 over time or per volume during a respiratory cycle—may be used to monitor lung perfusion to optimize oxygenation when setting PEEP. Increasing PEEP is usually the best method of increasing mean airway pressure. Monitoring the fraction of expired CO_2 and CO_2 volume allows the calculation of deadspace and alveolar ventilation and, with the temporary addition of a rebreathing circuit, cardiac output.[24] Ventilator settings may then be adjusted to minimize deadspace and maximize alveolar ventilation.

The shape of the capnogram also provides information. A continually rising CO_2 pattern in place of a relatively flat plateau shape indicates that a significant proportion of lung units are emptying slowly due to their long time constants. Observing the capnogram for a dip in the exhaled CO_2 tracing, sometimes referred to as the *curare cleft*, indicates a patient's inspiratory attempt and alerts the clinician to the patient's waning level of sedation. Capnography does not eliminate the need for arterial blood gases because the (a-ET)PCO_2 gradient must be measured to accurately interpret expired PCO_2.

CASE STUDY 26-3

The respiratory therapist has just received a blood gas back on a ventilator patient. The patient is on 100% oxygen with the arterial PO_2 of 210 mm Hg.

Question

1. What oxygen concentration can be safely used avoid complications of oxygen toxicity?

VENTILATOR CHECK

Every hour for the first day and then every two hours thereafter, a *ventilator check sheet* is filled out with the ventilator settings and patient values. It can be done by hand or electronically by a data capture system. The respiratory therapist has to remember how the patient values are determined, especially if a data capture system is used. Valuable patient information can be missed if the captured data are not scrutinized for error. For example:

- I/E ratios are displayed for mandatory or ventilator-defined breaths only, not for spontaneous breathing.
- Exhaled tidal volumes may be from either mandatory or spontaneous breaths, depending on the mode of ventilation.
- The displayed respiratory rate usually includes both mandatory and spontaneous breaths.
- A peak inspiratory pressure is displayed in most modes, but a plateau pressure may require the volume control mode and a set pause time. Check the displayed or captured lung compliance value by dividing the mandatory exhaled tidal volume by the plateau minus PEEP pressure.
- Recording the difference between peak and plateau pressure as a measure of airway resistance is appropriate only when the inspiratory flow is constant (i.e., a volume control mode with a rectangular flow waveform).
- If the ventilator does not display auto-PEEP, the clinician can initiate an end-expiratory pause to measure its presence. Prior observance that the expiratory limb of the flow-time waveform fails to return to baseline indicates the presence of air trapping and therefore the need to initiate an expiratory hold to measure auto-PEEP.

Check that the *alarms* are set appropriately. Critical care ventilators have extensive alarm systems that monitor flow, pressure, exhaled volume, and time. Life-threatening situations are usually detected by more than one audiovisual alarm. Alarm conditions are usually based on the monitored patient parameters, such as exhaled volume or airway pressure.

Apnea and ventilator disconnection are two of the most life-threatening situations that alarms are designed to detect. In most modes currently available, the ventilator is able to detect whether a breath has been taken. Flow and pressure sensors measure changes in inspiratory flow and pressure as well as the length of time when flow or pressure changes are absent. If no inspiration has been detected within a certain period of time, usually called the *apnea interval*, the ventilator activates an apnea alarm. When the apnea alarm is activated, some ventilators automatically switch to an apnea ventilation mode that delivers a preset tidal volume at a preset rate.

Apnea ventilation is usually available for spontaneous modes, but not all ventilators have apnea ventilation. For example:

- Pressure support mode on the Servo 300 (Maquet, Bridgewater, New Jersey) has an apnea alarm but does not switch to apnea ventilation.
- Automode on the Servo 300A and Servo^i automatically switches from pressure support to pressure control mode at the set rate if apnea occurs.
- The Automode feature automatically switches back to the spontaneous mode when a patient-triggered breath is detected on the Servo^i.
- The Servo 300A requires two consecutive patient-triggered breaths before switching.
- If the patient is in volume support mode and experiences apnea, the Servo 300A and Servo^i automatically switch to either PRVC or VC, depending on which mode is set.

Ventilator disconnect alarms usually sense *low inspiratory pressure*. Low inspiratory pressure alarms may be adjusted by the clinician, or they are automatically determined by the ventilator manufacturer. A low inspiratory pressure alarm activates if the pressure during inspiration does not go above the alarm setting. Low exhaled tidal volume or minute volume alarms also detect a ventilator disconnection but usually require a drop in the running breath average exhaled volume; so they require a longer period of time before activation. Adjustable low inspiratory pressure alarms are typically set at 10 cm H_2O below the peak inspiratory pressure.

High airway pressure alarms activate when the peak airway pressure equals the high pressure alarm setting. Inspiration is usually terminated when the high pressure alarm is activated. Low inspiratory pressure or low exhaled tidal volumes are monitored to detect a leak in the system or a disconnection of the patient from the ventilator. Ventilator error or inoperative alarms are also common on critical care

Best Practice

Understanding Alarms

Respiratory care practitioners must know what conditions activate the various alarms for their ventilators.

Best Practice

The Patient First

In the event of a ventilator alarm, the first action should be to *look at the patient* to verify that the patient is still connected to the ventilator.

ventilators. It is crucial that alarm volumes are set loud enough to be detected by care givers.

Regardless of which alarm is activated:

- The number 1 rule when an alarm occurs is to *look at the patient!* Make sure the patient is still connected to the ventilator.
- The second rule is to ensure adequate ventilation and oxygenation for the patient in the event of a ventilator problem, by disconnecting the patient from the ventilator and initiating manual ventilation. Do not spend minutes searching the ventilator for the problem while the patient is inadequately ventilated. Guarantee adequate ventilation while troubleshooting the ventilator system.

WAVEFORMS

The assessment of breathing involves not only auscultating breath sounds but also evaluating the quality of the breath.

- Is the ventilator responding to the patient's inspiratory effort fast enough?
- Is the patient getting enough flow during inspiration?
- Does breathing appear to be labored?
- Is the patient fighting the pattern of breathing set by the machine?

One of the ways to evaluate the quality of breathing is to observe the patient's waveforms. The graphic representation of pressure, flow, and volume over time can provide information about the quality of ventilator breaths that is not as easily recognized otherwise. Ventilator settings can be tailored to the patient's demand. Volume–over-pressure curves may be used to determine optimal PEEP levels and to estimate the imposed work of breathing.

Figure 26-4A is an example of a volume-controlled breath in which the peak flow setting is too low to meet the patient's inspiratory demand. This situation may lead to dyssynchrony between the timing of the inspiratory flow delivered by the ventilator and the initiation of inspiration by the patient. Eventually, this results in the patient trying to exhale while the

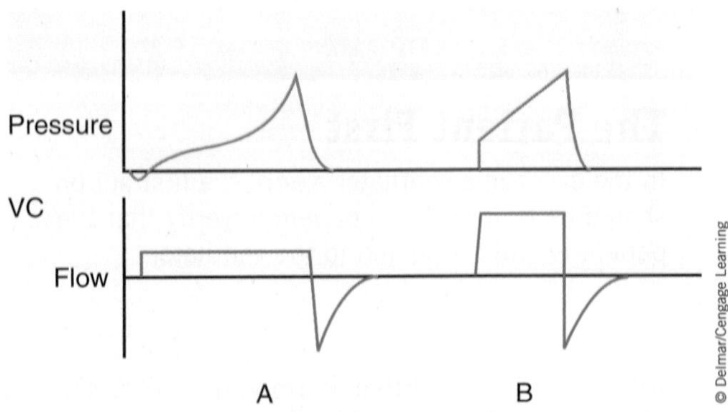

FIGURE 26-4 (A) Flow is not adequate to meet the patient's inspiratory demand. (B) A higher peak flow rate allows a steady rise in pressure. In VC, a higher peak flow shortens the time of inspiration.

ventilator is still delivering flow. The increase in airway pressure may activate the high-pressure alarm, ending inspiration. The set tidal volume is not delivered, contributing to the patient's sensation of air hunger and the desire to trigger breaths more frequently. Inadequate inspiratory flow is the most common reason for a patient to fight the ventilator in volume control. Figure 26-4B shows the effect of an increase in the peak flow. As the patient's inspiratory flow demand is met, the entire tidal volume is delivered, the patient's anxiety subsides, and the respiratory rate decreases.

Pressure-volume (P/V) curves performed under static conditions may identify two points where the patient's compliance changes on the inflation curve, especially in the early phase of ARDS. As shown in Figure 26-5A, the first point (point A) represents an improvement in compliance represented by an increase in the slope of the curve. Some clinicians believe that this point, called the *lower inflection point,* occurs when adequate alveolar recruitment has occurred. Numerous studies have reported that the lower inflection point generally falls between 10 and 15 cm H_2O in patients

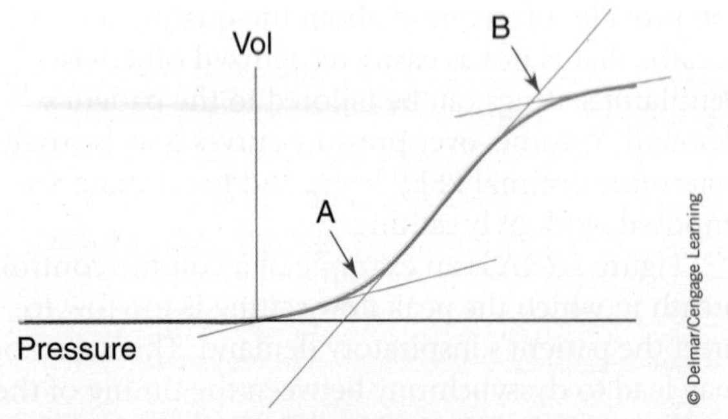

FIGURE 26-5 Static pressure-volume curve measured with the patient sedated and paralyzed. (A) The lower inflexion point. (B) The upper inflexion point.

who meet the criteria for ARDS. With this approach, the level of PEEP should be 2 cm H_2O more than the pressure at the inflection point. However, not all patients with ARDS have a lower inflection point, particularly during the later phase of ARDS.

Figure 26-5 also shows the second point of change in compliance (point B) that occurs when the lungs become overinflated. The point or pressure at which the compliance decreases is called the *upper inflection* or *deflection point* on an inflation static pressure-volume curve. It represents the plateau pressure that should not be exceeded. Overinflation creates a pressure spike on a dynamic P/V curve.

Few studies have compared the inflection point measured with a dynamic pressure-volume waveform with that obtained by the static method. Lu and coworkers found that resistive properties are reduced when a flow rate of 9 Lpm is used to measure a dynamic P/V curve.[25] The P/V 2 tool on the Galileo Gold (Hamilton Medical, Reno, Nevada) uses a low peak flow to generate dynamic inflation and deflation pressure-volume curves. A time cursor can then be scrolled along the curves to display respiratory system compliance at any given point, which is particularly useful in identifying the greatest change in compliance on the deflation curve (Figure 26-6). The upper inflection pressure on the *deflation curve* after a recruitment maneuver has been suggested as the optimal PEEP setting to maintain recruited alveoli.[20,21]

Waveforms can help detect a problem as well. A leak in the system is easily observed on a volume-time waveform. The ascending portion represents the inspiratory volume, and the descending leg is the expiratory volume. If the exhaled volume is less than the inspiratory volume, the descending leg does not return to

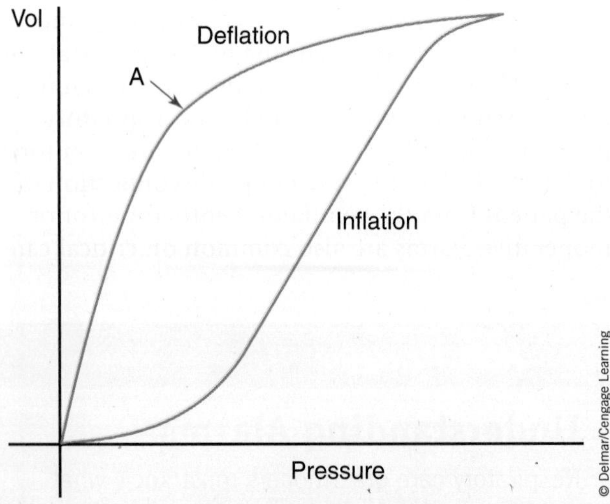

FIGURE 26-6 A dynamic pressure volume curve measured during a recruitment maneuver: Point A is the maximal curvature on the deflation limb.

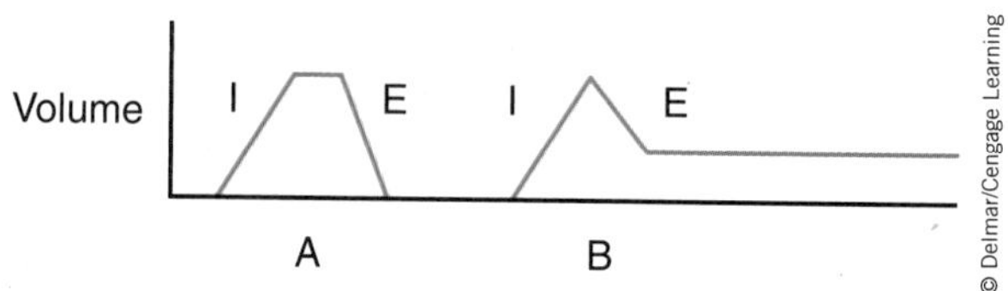

FIGURE 26-7. (A) A leak has reduced the exhaled volume returning to the ventilator. (B) A volume-time waveform showing an inspiratory pause.

baseline (Figure 26-7A). A leak also causes a difference in the ventilator's patient data displays between the inspiratory or set volume and the patient's exhaled tidal volume. If a pause is used, it creates a flattop on the volume-time waveform, as shown in Figure 26-7B.

The presence of an air leak may cause the ventilator to self-trigger if a flow trigger is used. The leak causes a drop in flow similar to a patient's inspiratory effort. A flow trigger should not be used in this case. A leak in the system may also prevent inspiration from ending in a flow-cycled mode. In pressure support, inspiration ends when the flow rate falls to 25% of the highest flow that occurred during the inspiration or to some preset level such as 5 Lpm, depending on the ventilator. A few ventilators have the option of adjusting the flow-cycle threshold for pressure-supported breaths. The liter flow of the leak may be observed in a flow-time waveform. The flow- cycle threshold could then be adjusted to a higher flow rate than the leak to end-inspiration (Figure 26-8).

A flow-time waveform detects the presence of airtrapping by showing that the expiratory flow does not return to baseline by the time the next breath starts (Figure 26-9). When this is observed, produce an end-expiratory pause to measure the end-expiratory pressure. Any end-expiratory pressure during a pause

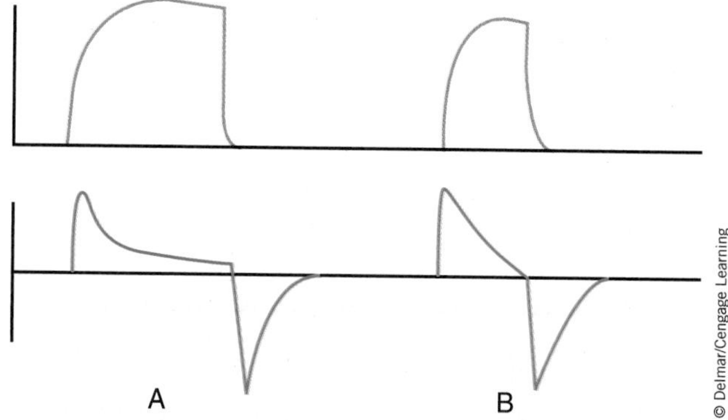

FIGURE 26-8 (A) Inspiration is prolonged owing to a leak in the system. (B) The flow-cycle level has been increased to a flow rate greater than the leak. Inspiration ends appropriately.

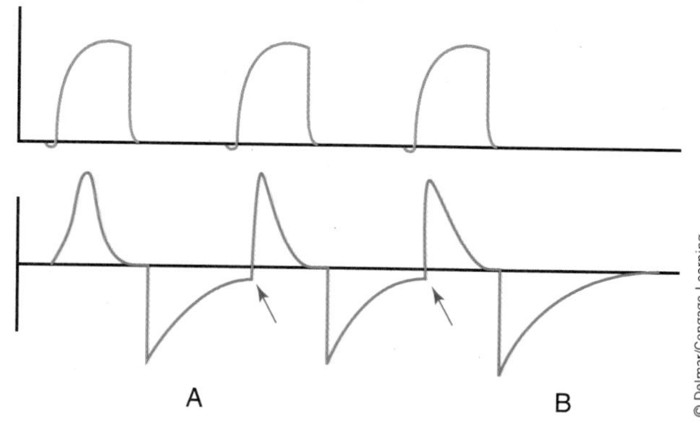

FIGURE 26-9 (A) Arrows indicate air trapping. An end-expiratory pause is needed to measure the actual auto-PEEP; however, patient-triggered breaths make this inaccurate. (B) The patient has been sedated, and expiratory flow shows no evidence of air trapping.

that is greater than **baseline pressure** is auto-PEEP. Applied PEEP or CPAP should equal the level of auto-PEEP to maintain a given pressure trigger. For example, a pressure trigger set on −2 when 5 cm H_2O of auto-PEEP is present requires the patient to actually exert an inspiratory effort of −7 cm H_2O. The problem in compensating for auto-PEEP, however, is that it varies with the time allowed for exhalation. Higher patient-triggered respiratory rates increase the level of auto-PEEP by decreasing the time left for exhalation. Any compensation by increasing the applied PEEP may be overkill if the patient's respiratory rate slows down.

If waveforms are not available on the ventilator, a comparison of ventilator settings with the patient's exhaled values can provide clues. For example, an air leak in the ventilator circuit, either around the patient's endotracheal tube or out through chest tubes, results in a loss of exhaled volume, lowers peak airway pressures, and possibly leads to the loss of end-expiratory pressure. If the patient is in a flow-trigger setting, the air leak may trigger ventilator breaths in rapid succession, as discussed previously. The loss of volume and

CASE STUDY 26-4

A patient's flow-time waveforms appear to indicate air trapping. The patient is somewhat agitated and not in synchrony with the ventilator. The respiratory therapist knows that auto-PEEP often leads to patient-ventilator dyssynchrony.

Question

1. What should the RT do?

Best Practice

Inadequate Ventilation

Whenever adequate ventilation of the patient is in question, remove the patient from the ventilator and ventilate with a manual resuscitator.

pressure may activate alarms. Whenever adequate ventilation of the patient is in question, remove the patient from the ventilator and ventilate with a manual resuscitator.

WORK OF BREATHING

Work of breathing (*WOB*) is the respiratory muscle energy or force used to move a tidal volume of air. Work is defined in physics as the force times distance. In fluid systems, however, breathing work is measured in terms of pressure times volume (e.g., inspiratory pressure × tidal volume displaced). The units of WOB are kilogram-meters (kg · m) or joules, with 0.1 kg · m equal to 1 joule. WOB is usually expressed as either joules per liter of ventilation or joules per minute. *Work per liter of ventilation* (j/L) is a better indication of the patient's breathing capacity when the patient has pulmonary disease.[26] Normal WOB in healthy individuals is 0.3–0.8 j/L. In patients with CAO, breathing workloads over 1.3 j/L are associated with ventilator dependence. Patients with marginal ventilatory reserves do not tolerate spontaneous breathing even if the workload is only moderately increased. The WOB is excessive any time the demand placed on the respiratory muscles exceeds their capacity or ability to function.

Lung disease that leads to expiratory flow limitation causes air trapping and lung hyperinflation. Hyperinflation shortens the inspiratory muscles, thereby reducing their capacity to contract farther and generate force. The reduction in contractile force decreases inspiratory muscle strength and the maximal inspiratory pressure. Patients with respiratory muscle weakness may find even small increases in the pressure or effort needed to breathe (increased demand) to be intolerable. The presence of auto-PEEP creates such a situation. The patient must generate enough inspiratory muscle effort to overcome the elevated alveolar pressure before the pressure at the mouth can drop below the ambient pressure level to create a pressure gradient for gas flow.

Diseases or disorders that increase airway resistance (increased inelastic or resistive force) or that decrease compliance (increased elastic force) of the lungs or chest wall increase the intrinsic work of breathing. Equipment added to the patient that increases WOB is *extrinsic* or *imposed work*. The endotracheal tube, the demand flow valve, the ventilator circuit, and the humidifier may all be sources of resistance to gas flow that the patient must overcome to take in a breath from the ventilator. In addition, the expiratory WOB may increase if exhalation valves or PEEP valves create resistance that makes the patient work harder to exhale.

Best Practice

Breathing Workloads

Breathing workloads over 1.3 j/L may be excessive for patients with CAO and compromise their ability to breathe spontaneously, particularly through an ETT. Recognize and limit the factors that may increase the work of breathing.

HUMIDIFICATION OF MECHANICAL VENTILATION

Gas delivered by a ventilator must be monitored for adequate humidity. Ensuring adequate humidity levels requires an appropriate humidifier with adequate water levels and monitoring of the inspiratory gas temperature at the patient wye. Temperatures should be maintained between 31° and 35°C.[27] As long as the humidifier is functioning properly, the appropriate inspiratory gas temperature reflects the delivery of an adequate absolute humidity level when using a ventilator circuit without heated wires. There are two exceptions to letting the inspiratory gas temperature guide proper humidity delivery: use of heat and moisture exchangers/hygroscopic condenser humidifiers (HME/HCH) and heated wire ventilator circuits.

When using *heat and moisture exchangers* or *hygroscopic condenser humidifiers* (*HMEs* or *HCHs*):

- Measuring inspiratory airway temperatures is not useful.
- It is, however, important to monitor secretions, minute ventilation, and differences between inhaled and exhaled tidal volumes. Thick, copious secretions are a contraindication for HME/HCH methods of humidification, as are minute volumes over 10 Lpm and a 30% loss in volume during exhalation.
- High minute volumes exceed the capacity of most HME/HCHs to provide a minimum of 70% relative humidity at body temperature. When the exhaled tidal volume is less than 70% of the inspiratory tidal volume, an inadequate amount

of exhaled moisture is available for the next inspiration.

- HME/HCHs should not be used in the presence of large air leaks through chest tubes or air leaks around the artificial airway. HME/HCHs should be removed or bypassed when delivering aerosol therapy.[28]

With the use of *heated-wire ventilator circuits* comes the added responsibility of monitoring the relative humidity (RH). The purpose of heated-wire circuits is to prevent cooling of the gas in the tubing as it travels from the heated wet humidifier to the patient connection. Expiratory limb heated wires serve the same purpose for exhaled gas from the patient to the exhalation valve. Maintaining temperature prevents the gas from cooling, which would produce condensation in the tubing, or *rainout*. With some brands of heated-wire circuits, the circuit temperature can be higher than the humidifier temperature to the point of lowering the delivered relative humidity. In infant ventilation, the respiratory therapist has to ensure an adequate RH by noting the presence of beads of moisture at the patient wye or at the ventilator circuit connection to the patient's endotracheal or tracheostomy tube.[29] Failure to monitor the RH leads to inspissated secretions, mucus plugging, and arterial hypoxemia.

COMPLICATIONS OF MECHANICAL VENTILATION

The underlying purpose of monitoring is to ensure patient safety and comfort by anticipating the potential problems of any ventilator patient's situation. Recognizing the onset of anticipated problems provides time to intervene and possibly prevent the complications from becoming life-threatening. Potential problems of mechanical ventilation may be classified as patient, patient-ventilator interface, and ventilator complications.

Patient Complications. *Patient complications* are associated with the delivery of positive pressure. The most common patient complication with the delivery of positive pressure ventilation is an alteration in blood circulation from a decrease in cardiac output or from a redistribution of blood flow through major organs. If the mean positive airway pressure transmitted across the lung to structures in the thorax is high enough, it decreases venous return and therefore cardiac output. A drop in cardiac output causes a decrease in blood pressure because the normal compensatory mechanisms responsible for maintaining blood pressure are often compromised in the critically ill patient. The decrease in blood pressure reduces or redistributes perfusion of the brain, heart, lungs, kidneys, liver, and gut, leading to multiple organ dysfunction. Therefore, all attempts to improve oxygenation by increasing mean airway pressure must be closely monitored for possible hemodynamic repercussions. A reduction in cardiac output offsets any gain from an increase in arterial oxygen tension, thereby reducing oxygenation.

For example, an increase in PEEP is generally the best method for increasing mean airway pressure, but there is a limit to the amount of PEEP that can improve oxygenation. Excessive PEEP increases the volume of the more compliant alveoli. As an alveolus overexpands, its pulmonary capillary is stretched; the stretching increases alveolar-capillary permeability and reduces the lumen of the capillary. An increase in alveolar-capillary permeability leads to interstitial pulmonary edema, which reduces the compliance of the alveoli. Stretched and narrowed pulmonary capillaries from overinflated alveoli, in combination with vasoconstricted capillaries of hypoxemic collapsed alveoli, increase pulmonary vascular resistance (PVR). An increase in PVR decreases the blood pressure gradient for venous return to the heart. A reduction in blood returning to the heart reduces cardiac output. Increased alveolar pressure that adversely affects cardiac output and reduces oxygen delivery does not improve oxygenation, despite an increase in P_aO_2. Oxygen delivery is the cardiac output multiplied times the oxygen content of the arterial blood. The small increase in oxygen content from an increase in P_aO_2 does not increase oxygen delivery enough to counterbalance even a small reduction in cardiac output. The challenge in providing mechanical ventilation with PEEP is therefore to increase alveolar pressure and volume effectively without causing alveolar overinflation or compromising the circulatory system.

A reduction in systemic circulation alters perfusion and impairs the function of the brain, lungs, kidneys, liver, and gut.

- The brain and kidneys are especially sensitive to alterations in perfusion. Inadequate cerebral perfusion causes disorientation, confusion, and loss of consciousness.
- A drop in cardiac output redistributes perfusion of the kidney and causes a decrease in urine output.

Best Practice

Humidification

When heated wire circuits are used:

- Ensure that the patient receives adequate humidity to prevent inspissated secretions, mucus plugging, and arterial hypoxemia.
- Check for beads of moisture at the patient wye.

- Reduced perfusion of the lung increases alveolar deadspace and decreases expired CO_2.
- Mucosal ischemia of the gut reduces absorption of nutrients and increases the gut's susceptibility to infection and bleeding.
- An elevation of venous blood pressure, resulting from positive pressure, impairs venous drainage of the brain and may lead to an increase in intracranial pressure.
- Elevated venous pressure impairs liver function.

Patient-Ventilator Interface Complications. Complications associated with the *patient-ventilator interface* relate to the use of endotracheal or tracheostomy tubes. Ventilator disconnection from the artificial airway and pulmonary infection are two such important complications.

- The incidence of *accidental ventilator disconnection* is reduced when the patient is immediately observed at the time of any ventilator alarm or monitor problem. Ventilator disconnection may also allow the collapse of alveoli and small airways in patients with ARDS.
- The endotracheal or tracheostomy tube provides a direct route of transmission of *infectious agents* to the lower airway. Despite controversies concerning the frequency of ventilator circuit changes, essential measures of infection control are aseptic technique during endotracheal tube suctioning or when the patient-ventilator system is interrupted, the proper disinfection of ventilator circuit components, and making appropriate ventilator circuit changes.[30]

Part of the controversy in establishing definitive guidelines for ventilator circuit changes involves the difficulty in diagnosing *ventilator-associated pneumonia* (*VAP*), generally defined as pneumonia that develops 48–72 hours after intubation.[31–33] Diagnosis is difficult in patients with respiratory failure, especially those with ARDS who have bilateral diffuse infiltrates on chest radiographs.[34] In a recent multicenter study, VAP was diagnosed in 36.5% of the patients with ARDS compared to 23% in ventilator patients without ARDS.[35] Sixty-five percent of the episodes of VAP occurred after the fifth day of mechanical ventilation. There was no difference in mortality rate (58%) in ARDS patients with or without VAP. The survivors with VAP were on mechanical ventilation twice as long as the survivors without VAP.

Several risk factors for VAP were analyzed, but frequency of ventilator circuit change was not reported. Currently, routine ventilator circuit changes are not recommended more often than once a week or when the circuit is visibly soiled or malfunctioning.[36] The Centers for Disease Control and the American Thoracic Society guidelines recommend a so-called VAP Bundle to prevent VAPs:

- Keep the head of the patient's bed elevated between 30° and 45°.
- Use closed suction systems.
- Create frequent "sedation vacations" to evaluate the continued need for mechanical ventilation.
- Use aseptic technique with an emphasis on alcohol-based hand rubs.
- Give routine oral care, including nonabsorbable antibiotics.

Continuous aspiration of subglottic secretions (CASS) from above the cuff requires a specially designed endotracheal tube (Hi-Lo Evac tube, TYCO Healthcare/Mallinckrodt, St Louis, Missouri, distributed by Nellcor Puritan Bennett, Pleasanton, California). ATS recommends CASS, *if available*.[33] The ATS also recommends that "endotracheal tube cuff pressure should be maintained at greater than 20 cm H_2O."

Ventilator Complications. Complications related to the ventilator are inadequate humidification leading to mucus plugging and airway obstruction, ventilator malfunction, operator error, and ventilator-induced lung injury (VILI).

Inadequate humidification may be avoided by following the AARC clinical practice guidelines for humidification during mechanical ventilation. An appropriate airway temperature of inspired gas, humidifier, and percentage relative humidity when using heated wire circuits prevents desiccation of airway secretions. An adequate percentage relative humidity greater than 70% when using heated wire circuits may be monitored by the presence of beads of moisture at the patient-ventilator connection.[29] Heat and moisture exchangers (HMEs) can also be monitored by observing beads of moisture at the patient connection.[37]

Adherence to the preventive maintenance schedule published by the ventilator manufacturer aids in preventing *ventilator malfunction*. In many cases, ventilator malfunction is actually operator error.

Ventilator changes made by health care personnel inadequately trained in ventilator application—*operator error*—are more often the cause of problems in

Best Practice

Humidification

To prevent complications associated with inadequate humidity, monitor the patient-circuit connection for beads of moisture.

Best Practice

Proper Training

Only individuals with extensive training in the function and operation of critical care ventilators should make changes in ventilator settings. Respiratory care practitioners are the only hospital personnel so qualified.

Best Practice

Protective Lung Strategies

Protective lung strategies of ventilation use tidal volumes of 4–6 mL/kg and PEEP levels that produce plateau pressures <30 cm H_2O.

ventilation than mechanical failure of the ventilator itself. Improper use of ventilator modes may force the patient to assume more of the work of breathing than the patient can provide. Patient-ventilator dyssynchrony from inadequate peak flow in VC, excessively long inspiratory times, and inappropriate rise time % or slope settings for pressure breaths all increase the patient's work of breathing.[38]

Ventilator-induced lung injury (*VILI*) in ARDS occurs when regions of the lung are overinflated or strained (*volutrauma*) and from the shear stress associated with repeated opening and closing of terminal airways (*atelectrauma*).[39,40] Approximately one-third of the lung is open in ARDS with collapsed, noncompliant alveoli adjacent to open compliant alveoli.[41] Applying tidal volumes over 9 mL/kg of predicted body weight to patients with ARDS overexpands the compliant alveoli and creates tissue strain as they attempt to pull away from their less compliant neighbors.[42]

Shear stress is also generated by the repetitive opening and end-tidal collapse of small airways. These mechanisms combine to cause diffuse alveolar damage marked by increased epithelial and endothelial permeability, interstitial pulmonary edema, and alveolar flooding.[43–44] Alveolar damage triggers the inflammatory response, which aggravates the alveolar-capillary injury (*biotrauma*).[39] There is evidence to suggest that microorganisms present in the alveoli may enter the systemic circulation via the damaged pulmonary capillaries and cause *multiple organ dysfunction syndrome* (*MODS*).[41]

The landmark ARDSnet clinical trial[45] found approximately 25% fewer deaths among patients receiving 6 mL/kg tidal volumes as compared to those receiving 12 mL/kg volumes. The study protocol required that tidal volumes be adjusted to keep plateau pressures between 25 and 30 cm H_2O in the intervention group. This study was the first to provide conclusive evidence that small tidal volumes of 6 mL/kg improve mortality for patients with ARDS. The importance of plateau pressures <30 cm H_2O is less clear since the control group had mean plateau pressures <33 cm H_2O. The two groups also had similar levels of PEEP (10 cm H_2O). Since volutrauma occurs when tidal volume and the level of PEEP excessively increase end-inspiratory lung volume, mechanical ventilation should be applied in a manner that protects the lung. Low tidal volumes should be used in conjunction with PEEP since low tidal volumes alone are associated with atelectasis.[46]

Barotrauma is another type of ventilator-associated lung injury that is more closely related to regional lung distention than to absolute airway pressure. Excessive transpulmonary pressure (alveolar minus pleural pressure) can allow air to enter the interstitial tissue and dissect along the bronchovesicular sheath to the mediastinum to cause:

- Pneumomediastinum.
- Pneumothorax.
- Pneumopericardium.
- Subcutaneous emphysema.
- Pulmonary interstitial emphysema.[46]

Ventilator Management

Ideally, (therapist-driven) ventilator management protocols are initiated from the moment the patient is placed on mechanical ventilation. Management priorities are determined by the reason for ventilatory support. In general, the pulmonary functions of patients requiring mechanical ventilation fall into one of three categories: restrictive, obstructive, or relatively normal. Potential problems associated with the application of positive pressure in each condition should be anticipated and monitored accordingly.

MECHANICAL VENTILATION IN OXYGENATION FAILURE

The therapeutic objectives for patients with ARDS are to promote alveolar recruitment and to prevent alveolar overinflation. The standard method of opening alveoli is to increase alveolar pressure and then provide PEEP to maintain alveolar expansion. Atelectatic lung requires approximately 30–40 cm H_2O over 7–8 seconds to reopen.[47] There is evidence to support the use of small tidal volumes, but less support for setting PEEP levels 2 cm H_2O above the lower inflection point.[48] The level of PEEP may need to be even higher to prevent alveolar derecruitment, particularly when chest wall compliance is reduced from an increased intra-abdominal pressure, often associated with the extrapulmonary type of ARDS.[49] It is also recognized that limiting inspiratory plateau pressure to less than 30 cm H_2O may not prevent alveolar overinflation.[50] Therefore, the problem becomes one of how to reexpand the lung without overdistension.

Recruitment Maneuvers. At this time, there is no optimal method for performing alveolar recruitment maneuvers (RMs).[51] Ventilators that provide so-called sighs in the form of higher PEEP levels for two consecutive ventilator breaths may not apply the pressure for a long enough period of time. Giving two consecutive sighs per minute by increasing the PEEP from 9 to 16 cm H_2O in volume-controlled ventilation did not improve oxygenation over volume-controlled ventilation at a constant level of 16 cm H_2O PEEP.[52] Lim and coworkers found that high pressure control and PEEP levels (45/16 cm H_2O for 2 minutes at an I/E ratio of 1:2) were equivalent to a 40-second sustained maneuver of 45 cm H_2O CPAP in three different porcine models of acute lung injury.[53] Patients with pulmonary ARDS or late-stage extrapulmonary ARDS typically do not respond favorably to any type of alveolar recruitment maneuver.

In patients with ARDS Amato et al. (1998) used a recruitment maneuver (RM) of 35-40 cm H_2O CPAP for 30–40 seconds before initiating protective ventilation.[54,55] The same pressure range has been applied successfully for 20 seconds.[56] Kacmarek and colleagues recommend a more conservative approach of 30 cm H_2O CPAP for 30–40 seconds. The maneuver needs to produce a passive inflation, which usually requires sedation of the patient. The patient should also be preoxygenated with an F_IO_2 of 1.0 for 5–10 minutes. If oxygenation does not improve after the first recruitment period but the patient tolerated the procedure, repeat the RM in 15–20 minutes at a CPAP of 35–40 cm H_2O. A third maneuver at 40 cm H_2O may be required to produce a positive response in some patients. A P_aO_2/F_IO_2 ratio > 300 indicates effective recruitment. To maintain recruited lung after the maneuver, set a PEEP of 20 cm H_2O and reduce the F_IO_2 until the S_pO_2 is around 92%.[57] The benefit from the recruitment maneuver is lost if a low level of PEEP is then set and adjusted up. The PEEP of 20 cm H_2O can then be reduced by 2 cm H_20 every 30 minutes until desaturation occurs.[57] The PEEP level before desaturation is the level that prevents derecruitment. Set PEEP at that level after repeating RMs to reopen the lung. The practice of using low tidal volumes of 6 mL/kg and setting the PEEP as just described after a recruitment maneuver has been referred to as the *open lung ventilation strategy*.[58] The F_IO_2 should be ≤ 0.45 before attempting to decrease the PEEP. Interruptions in ventilation require repeated RMs.[59]

> *Best Practice*
>
> **PEEP Settings**
>
> Set PEEP at a high enough pressure (20 cm H_2O) after recruitment maneuvers to keep the lung open. Titrate PEEP down to determine the derecruitment point. After repeating recruitment maneuver, set PEEP at the level immediately before derecruitment occurred.

Measurement of functional residual capacity (FRC), such as end-expiratory lung volume (EELV), could track improvements in lung volume following recruitment maneuvers and/or the application of PEEP. The gas module on the Engström Carestation ventilator (Datex-Ohmeda, Inc. of GE Healthcare) allows a simplified measurement of the patient's FRC at the bedside. The FRC measurement uses a modified multiple-breath nitrogen washout/washin technique that requires inspiratory and expiratory analyses of oxygen and carbon dioxide and a change in F_IO_2 of just 10%. Chiumello and colleagues found that the EELV measured by the modified nitrogen washout/washin technique of the Engström Carestation correlated well with the EELV measured via computed tomography scanning.[60] Two 20-breath measurements are required for a single FRC procedure. The FRC measurement may take up to 10 minutes to achieve the required steady-state condition. The FRC INview™ function also allows the scheduling of a series of FRC procedures at specified intervals. The PEEP INview™ function automatically measures FRC at incremental levels of PEEP. The clinician sets the number of steps to be made between the start and stop PEEP levels. Each PEEP level is held for 5 minutes, and the FRC-at-PEEP values are plotted on a graph and displayed numerically.[61] FRC measurements may aid in quantifying recruited lung volume and lung overinflation.

Prone Ventilation. The mechanical ventilation of ARDS patients in the prone position improves oxygenation in roughly 50–75% of cases. The improvement in oxygenation persists after returning to the supine position. The prone position theoretically creates a more uniform distribution of ventilation that enhances the expansion of dorsal lung units that were previously compressed by the weight of edematous ventral lung units.[62] Pelosi and coworkers found that changes in oxygenation from prone positioning were associated with a reduction in chest wall compliance but not related to elevations in end-expiratory lung volume or improvement in lung compliance.[63] Regional changes in ventilation/perfusion ratios were given as the only explanation for improved oxygenation. Prone positioning can be expected to improve oxygenation only in patients who have severe inflammatory pulmonary edema, and to date no study has been properly designed to determine the impact of prone positioning on survival in this specific population.[64]

Inverse Ratio Ventilation. When inspiratory time exceeds expiratory time, the I/E ratio is inverse. Lengthening the time of inspiration increases mean airway pressure and improves oxygenation up to the point of hemodynamic compromise. Inverse ratio ventilation (IRV) may be instituted in either pressure-control or volume-control ventilation. If VC is used, a ramp flow waveform is preferred. In either case, limiting the inspiratory or plateau pressure results in lower tidal volumes. Because low tidal volumes and prolonged inspiratory times are uncomfortable, the patient needs to be sedated and paralyzed. Tidal volumes of less than 5 mL/kg require RMs and appropriate PEEP levels to prevent atelectasis. The respiratory rate can be increased to maintain minute ventilation, but this reduces the time available for exhalation. Incomplete emptying of the lung causes air trapping. Air trapping creates auto-PEEP that raises mean airway pressure, but that pressure favors overdistension of the more compliant lung units. Yanos and coworkers found that auto-PEEP from IRV increased mean airway pressure but was less beneficial for improving gas exchange.[65] Certainly APRV is preferable to IRV in most cases and has the added benefit of greater patient comfort with less sedation by allowing spontaneous breathing. Spontaneous breathing in APRV eliminates the inverse ratio component of IRV while achieving a comparable increase in mean airway pressure.

Permissive Hypercapnia. If the increase in respiratory rate is not enough to maintain minute ventilation in IRV, P_aCO_2 rises. As long as this change occurs gradually and the pH is 7.25 or higher, the effects of hypercapnia are not serious.[66] However, increased P_aCO_2 and the associated decrease in pH cause cerebral vasodilation. The increase in cerebral blood flow and in intracranial pressure is detrimental if cerebral edema is a concern.

Inhaled Nitric Oxide. Endogenous nitric oxide (NO), first identified in 1987, is synthesized by vascular endothelial cells, able to diffuse rapidly across cell membranes, and relaxes vascular smooth muscle. Nitric oxide administered as an *inhaled agent* (*iNO*) is a potent and selective pulmonary vasodilator. It improves oxygenation in ARDS by vasodilating the capillaries adjacent to well ventilated alveoli. Increased blood flow to ventilated alveoli reduces perfusion to poorly ventilated alveoli. The vasodilator response to iNO occurs in 5–15 minutes. Once inhaled, it is rapidly inactivated by binding to hemoglobin to form methemoglobin. At doses of iNO below 20 ppm, methemoglobin levels are generally less than 3%.

The administration of iNO requires special equipment. Since gaseous NO reacts with oxygen to form nitrogen dioxide (NO_2), a toxic gas, iNO is stored in nitrogen and bled into the ventilator circuit. Scavenger systems and NO_2 analyzers must ensure that the level of NO_2 is kept to less than 2 ppm. In the form administered to patients, iNO is also potentially toxic as a free radical when it reacts with other free radicals such as superoxide. In combination, NO^- and superoxide form peroxynitrate ($ONNO^-$), an oxidizing compound thought to cause acute lung injury.[67]

Despite numerous studies of the effects of iNO, there have been no large randomized clinical trials demonstrating its efficacy in reducing morbidity or mortality in patients with ARDS.[68] Only one study has demonstrated that it improves oxygenation after the first day. Inhaled nitric oxide administration should be considered experimental.

High-Frequency Oscillation Ventillation. In 2001, the Food and Drug Administration approved the SensorMedics 3100B high-frequency oscillatory ventilator (Yorba Linda, California) for use in patients whose actual body weight is more than 35 kg. *High-frequency oscillatory ventilation* (*HFOV*) has been used for decades to treat respiratory distress syndrome in neonatal and pediatric patients, successfully preventing ventilator-induced lung injury.

Theoretically, the very small tidal volumes produced with HFOV protect the lungs, and the relatively high mean airway pressures facilitate alveolar recruitment and maintenance of restored end-expiratory lung volume to improve oxygenation. However, the actual guidelines for HFOV application to adults favor amplitude and frequency settings that produce larger tidal volumes to maximize CO_2 clearance.[69] The recommended starting amplitudes (ΔP) of 20 + P_aCO_2 (~ 60 cm H_2O) and low frequencies (5–6 Hertz) produce larger tidal volumes with greater potential for lung injury. Proponents of HFOV recommend higher amplitudes of 90 cm H_20 at the highest possible frequency (well over 6 Hz) to reduce tidal volumes and protect the lungs.[69] The problem then becomes the relatively high mean airway pressures that may be required to improve oxygenation.[70] A mean airway pressure of 45 cm H_2O is not expected to offer much protection against volutrauma and is more likely to compromise circulation. There is no evidence to date that HFOV improves patient outcomes when compared to low tidal volume strategies.[71]

MECHANICAL VENTILATION IN CHRONIC AIRFLOW OBSTRUCTION (CAO)

Ventilation of a patient with CAO requires a very different approach than for patients with ARDS. The concerns are less about oxygenation and more about ventilation, the work of breathing, and reducing auto-PEEP from hyperinflation.[72] In many cases of CAO exacerbation, noninvasive positive pressure ventilation provides effective treatment and reduces the need for intubation. Obstructive airway disease requires attention to the appropriateness of the minute ventilation, maintaining airway patency, and allowing adequate expiratory time to reduce hyperinflation. The least amount of ventilation should be provided while ensuring that flow rates meet the patient's inspiratory demand. Higher inspiratory flow rates allow a longer time for expiration and reduce auto- or intrinsic PEEP.[73] Also, low levels of applied PEEP/CPAP may be required to unload the respiratory muscles in the presence of auto-PEEP.[74] Sedation may be required to prevent patient-ventilator dyssynchrony and auto-PEEP because patient-triggered respiratory rates over 15 bpm may be sufficient to increase air trapping. Minute ventilation should be titrated to the pH, not to P_aCO_2.[75]

These patients may experience dyspnea even when the P_aO_2 is adequate. A possible explanation is that the hyperinflated condition of the thorax places the respiratory muscles at a mechanical disadvantage. The force generated by the inspiratory muscles is disproportionately large for the minimal change in muscle length (i.e., inspiratory volume that is achieved). This imbalance is sensed by proprioreceptors in the lung and contributes to the sensation of dyspnea. High respiratory rates, causing inadequate expiratory time, increase auto-PEEP and hyperinflation. The challenge is to provide adequate ventilation at inspiratory flow rates high enough to meet the patient's inspiratory demand and allow adequate time for exhalation.

The mode of ventilation for patients with CAO must also be considered in terms of their work of breathing. Patients with a limited ventilatory reserve have little tolerance for excessive workloads. After a period of respiratory muscle rest for ventilatory failure due to respiratory muscle fatigue, the mode must allow the use of the patient's respiratory muscles without imposing an excessive load. In the past, SIMV with pressure support and CPAP were thought to provide a way to balance the work of breathing between the patient and the ventilator. Limiting the number of machine breaths in SIMV theoretically reduces the risk of air trapping. Now we know the patient's work of breathing may vary little between machine and supported breaths. There is evidence to suggest that patients do not reduce their work of breathing with pressure support immediately but rather that they allow pressure support to increase the efficiency of breathing.[76]

Pressure support increases breathing efficiency if patient-ventilator dyssynchrony from delays in triggering (initiating) and cycling (terminating) breaths is avoided. Trigger delays are reduced by correcting the auto-PEEP from dynamic hyperinflation. Cycle delays may contribute to dynamic hyperinflation and should be minimized by increasing the Inspiratory Cycle-off % or Esen % setting to achieve a higher cycle flow rate. The cycle flow rate should be high enough to terminate a pressure-supported breath immediately before the patient attempts to exhale. An active expiratory effort toward the end of a pressure-supported, or pressure-controlled, inspiration creates a spike in pressure. as indicated by the arrow in Figure 26-10.[73] To end the breath before the spike occurs, either

> **Best Practice**
>
> **The CAO Patient**
>
> Because of the high expiratory airway resistance in patients with CAO, the time allowed for exhalation generally needs to be three to four times longer than the length of time for inspiration.

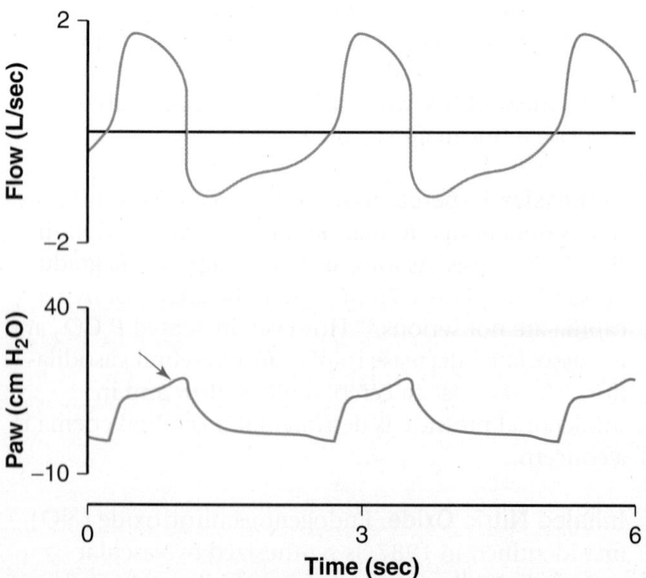

FIGURE 26-10 Arrow points to airway pressure spike toward the end of a pressure-supported inspiration, indicating the patient's attempt to exhale.

increase the cycle flow rate for pressure support, or decrease the inspiratory time for pressure control. Terminating the breath before the pressure spike relieves cycle delays, decreases the inspiratory period, increases the time available for exhalation, and thereby reduces dynamic hyperinflation.

Mechanical ventilation with a helium-oxygen mixtures (heliox) may be indicated for some patients with refractory asthma to reduce airway resistance and P_aCO_2s.[77] The Viasys Avea™ (Cardinal Health, Dublin, Ohio) simplifies Heliox delivery by allowing an 80/20 heliox gas input connection in place of the medical air. The special connector that flows heliox signals the ventilator to automatically correct all delivered and displayed volumes. Increasing the oxygen percentage on the ventilator to 30% delivers a 70/30 heliox mix. The benefits from breathing the lower density Heliox are lost with mixtures less than 60/40. Heliox has been documented to:

- Increase ventilation.
- Reduce peak pressures.
- Increase peak expiratory flows.[78]

MECHANICAL VENTILATION IN NEUROMUSCULAR DISEASE

Patients with neuromuscular disease requiring mechanical ventilation have relatively normal lung compliance. Neuromuscular disease results in respiratory muscle weakness that reduces the patient's capacity to take deep breaths and cough effectively. Ventilator management for these patients should include larger tidal volumes, higher inspiratory flow rates, and aggressive management of secretions. Oxygenation is usually not a problem for this group, so low PEEP levels are adequate.[75] Noninvasive ventilation plays a more important role in neuromuscular disease.

INDEPENDENT LUNG VENTILATION

Independent lung ventilation is indicated when the pulmonary problem is primarily unilateral. Large bronchopleural fistulas or air leaks are typically an indication that oxygenation and ventilation should be maintained by the uninvolved lung. A double-lumen endotracheal tube isolates each lung and allows independent ventilation. Each lung has its own ventilator, and the ventilatory pattern may be different between the two. The injured lung may be on CPAP or high-frequency ventilation while the functional lung is ventilated more conventionally. When two ventilators are used in this situation, one ventilator is designated as the primary and the other as the secondary. The primary ventilator establishes the timing of the respiratory cycle that the secondary ventilator follows. The aim is to avoid the inflation of one lung while the other is in exhalation. A see-saw ventilatory pattern would be counterproductive.

Ventilator Discontinuance

The transition from ventilator-supported breathing through an artificial airway to breathing without the need of either the ventilator or the artificial airway is generally referred to as *ventilator discontinuance*. The process can be rapid or require weeks, months, or even years. After the indication for mechanical ventilation has greatly improved or resolved, patients who do not tolerate a period of spontaneous breathing need to be weaned from the ventilator. In the past, weaning was the process of gradually reducing support provided by the ventilator until the patient could maintain spontaneous breathing on minimal support. Clinical studies have failed to demonstrate that a gradual withdrawal of ventilator support through a periodic reduction in the SIMV rate is superior to other weaning methods.

SHORT-TERM VENTILATION DISCONTINUANCE

Most patients do not require weaning postoperatively. They are extubated when the effects of the anesthesia have dissipated, the patient's condition has stabilized, and the gag reflex is functional. Because the protective reflexes of the upper airway return in an ascending order, the presence of the gag reflex means that the laryngeal and tracheal protective reflexes are also functional. Readiness for extubation requires assessment of the patient's ability to provide and protect a patent upper airway as well as to maintain adequate gas exchange during spontaneous breathing. These needs should be assessed separately.

Factors affecting airway patency and protection are related to the patient's medical condition, airway anatomy, and neurologic function. Abnormalities may compromise the patient's ability to clear secretions, increase the risk of pulmonary aspiration, or may heighten the potential of airway obstruction. A *negative inspiratory pressure* or *force* (*NIF*) of -20 cm H_2O is correlated with a vital capacity of 15 mL/kg, a minimally acceptable volume for an effective cough in subjects with relatively normal pulmonary function. However, in a study of healthy volunteers who were given muscle relaxants, an NIF of -25 cm H_2O was associated with adequate minute ventilation, even though the muscles that protect the airway were still nonfunctional. The AARC clinical practice guideline for the removal of an endotracheal tube recommends a negative inspiratory force of greater than -30 cm H_2O.[79]

The NIF is the peak negative pressure measured during a patient's maximal inspiratory effort and reflects the strength of the ventilatory muscles. The negative pressure measured after the first 100 milliseconds of a patient's inspiratory effort is the airway occlusion pressure ($P_{0.1}$) and reflects ventilatory muscle strength *and* central ventilatory drive.[80] A high ventilatory drive is associated with a greater ventilatory demand and a greater WOB. A normal $P_{0.1}$ at rest is -2 to -4 cm H_2O. Values more negative than -4.5 cm H_2O have been associated with poorer extubation rates.[81] However, the accurate interpretation of $P_{0.1}$ values may be difficult in the presence of neuromuscular impairment, respiratory muscle weakness or altered resting end-expiratory lung volume.[82]

Patients at risk of developing edema leading to airway obstruction during the postextubation period are those who have had either head or neck surgery or smoke inhalation injury. The *cuff leak test* assesses the presence of edema while the tube is still in place. When the patient is able to breathe spontaneously without ventilatory support, the cuff on the endotracheal tube (ETT) is deflated. The ETT is then manually occluded, and the patient's ability to breathe around the tube is evaluated. If the patient is able to breathe around the ETT, there is a good chance that extubation will be successful.

Obviously, failure of the cuff leak test does not prohibit extubation. The test may be sensitive only for patients with obvious neck or airway involvement. Partial airway obstruction due to glottic edema may produce stridor that presents within minutes after extubation. Rapidly developing stridor indicates a serious compromise of the airway and the need for reintubation. Stridor that occurs after an hour is usually not a serious problem and should respond to aerosolized racemic epinephrine, which is used for its vasoconstrictive properties to reduce mucosal edema.

Engoren used a different version of the cuff leak test in 531 cardiac surgery patients before extubation.[83] The patient was left on the ventilator in assist/control mode, and the cuff was deflated. The difference between inspiratory and exhaled tidal volumes defined the leak. A leak of 110 mL or less was considered a positive test. None of the 20 patients with a positive test developed stridor. The three patients who did develop stridor all had leaks of more than 350 mL around the tube. There was no mention of head or neck reasons to suspect stridor in this population, but 4% had problems not detected by this method.[83] In a retrospective study by Shin and colleagues, four trauma patients (10%) who had a good leak test of more than 10% of the tidal volume required reintubation.[84] None of the patients with a poor cuff leak test required reintubation.

All extubations should be performed by clinicians capable of providing mask and bag ventilation should the need arise. Although rare, laryngeal spasm following extubation should be treated immediately by the application of a constant low pressure via mask and bag until muscle relaxants are given and reintubation is performed. Under extreme conditions, the loss of airway patency may require cricothyrotomy or transtracheal catheter ventilation. The extubation of patients at risk of developing airway obstruction should be attempted only if personnel skilled in intubation and ventilatory support are immediately available.

Extubation should be considered when the indication for mechanical ventilation is no longer present. Protocols typically call for frequent screening of the patient to assess oxygenation status, alveolar ventilation, acid-base balance, sputum production, and mechanics of ventilation. The patient should have a minimal need for vasopressors or sedatives and an acceptable nutritional status. The screening criteria that may be included in an extubation protocol are as follows:

- P/F > 150
- PEEP < 5
- NIF > -20
- $S_pO_2 > 90$
- ABGs
- VE < 15 L/m
- RR < 30
- VT/RR < 105 (better predictive value if patient is not on PS/CPAP[85])
- VR $> 50\%$

Patients with acceptable screening values are given a trial of spontaneous breathing for 30 minutes on 5 cm H_2O CPAP, CPAP and pressure support (PS), or T-tube. If the patient tolerates the trial of spontaneous breathing, extubation is in order. Signs that the patient is not tolerating the trial are:

- Agitation.
- Diaphoresis.
- Decreased mental status.
- Frequency of more than 35 bpm or an increase in frequency of 50%.
- Increase in heart rate or systolic blood pressure of 20%.
- Or a drop in oxyhemoglobin saturation to $< 90\%$.

If the screening values are unacceptable or if the patient cannot tolerate spontaneous breathing after repeated trials, the patient is placed on a weaning protocol.

LONG-TERM VENTILATION DISCONTINUANCE

Of the variety of modes and strategies used to wean patients from mechanical ventilation, no single method has been proven to be superior. In a recent systematic review of the literature, Butler and colleagues suggest that the method in which the mode is applied has a greater impact on the duration of mechanical ventilation and weaning outcome than the mode itself.[86] The mode of ventilation during the weaning process must not place excessive demands on the respiratory system of the patient with a marginal respiratory reserve due to preexisting impairment of cardiopulmonary or neurological function. Excessive demands on the respiratory system may be caused by:

- High pressure loads due to abnormal mechanics of ventilation.
- Increased ventilatory load from elevated minute ventilation.
- Or workloads imposed by the ventilator system.

Any method that promotes respiratory muscle fatigue prolongs the duration of mechanical ventilation and extends the weaning process.

There is valid evidence to support that weaning protocols implemented by respiratory therapists and nurses reduce the duration of mechanical ventilation and that the protocols should include a daily screening of the patient's respiratory function.[87,88] The screening values are similar to those for the extubation protocol criteria:

- P/F > 150
- PEEP < 7.5
- NIF > -20
- Small or moderate amount of sputum
- VE < 20 Lpm
- RR < 30 bpm
- Minimal vasopressors and sedative agents
- Acceptable nutritional status

If the patient meets the criteria, a trial of spontaneous breathing is indicated. Most clinicians favor pressure-supported breathing trials over T-piece breathing to eliminate the work of breathing imposed by the endotracheal tube. However, in a recent study by Mehta and associates, there was no significant difference in the work of breathing (j/L) during 5 cm H_2O of PS, 5 cm H_2O of CPAP, or T-piece breathing trials.[89] Tidal volumes on both pressure support and CPAP overestimated postextubation tidal volumes, but tidal volumes on T-piece did not. The work of breathing for any of the three trial methods was significantly less than the work of breathing measured at 15 and 60 minutes postextubation.[89] Ishaaya and colleagues also reported an increased work of breathing after extubation in their patients that was not due to tracheal or laryngeal factors. They speculated that upper airway narrowing may have been due to pharyngeal soft tissue edema.[90] Straus and coworkers found the work of breathing through an endotracheal tube to mimic postextubation work of breathing.[91]

Proportional assist ventilation (*PAV*) was designed to unload the respiratory system in a predictable fashion and improve patient comfort. Theoretically, PAV can unload elastic and inelastic (resistive) components of the work of breathing by adjusting volume-assist or flow-assist. Ventilatory support is provided in proportion to the patient's inspiratory effort. Greater inspiratory effort on the part of the patient results in higher inspiratory pressure. The work provided by the ventilator is set as a percentage of support. A few small studies have favored PAV over PS, but PS remains the primary method of improving ventilation during spontaneous breathing trials.[92]

The sample weaning protocol presented in this section calls for a 2-hour trial. However, Esteban and coworkers found no difference in the reintubation rate when the spontaneous breathing trial was reduced from 120 to 30 minutes.[93] Longer trials may offer more reassurance for the weaning team than benefits for the patient. In a recent study by Mokhlesi and coworkers, 13% of 122 patients who were extubated following a successful 2-hour spontaneous breathing trial had to be reintubated within 48 hours.[94] The patients who required reintubation had, during their spontaneous breathing trials:

- Significantly more secretions.
- A Glasgow Coma Scale score of 10 or less.
- P_aCO_2s of 44 mm Hg or more.

There is some evidence that automated weaning approaches may shorten weaning time to a spontaneous breathing trial or to extubation.

- Automode, available on the Servo 300A and Servo^i, automatically switches the patient to a spontaneous breathing mode with the patient's first triggered breath in an assist/control mode (300A requires two consecutively triggered breaths).
- Should the patient become apneic for the interval set by the Trigger Timeout limit, Automode returns the patient to the assist/control mode. An indicator illuminates when the patient is breathing in the spontaneous mode.
- The clinician can track the respiratory rates, tidal volumes, and time periods of the patient's spontaneous breathing in the trends display to decide whether the patient should be screened for extubation.

Hendrix and coworkers found that Automode on the 300A reduced the time to extubation by 2 hours, when compared to their standard extubation protocol of assist/control to SIMV to CPAP, in a small group of

20 postoperative coronary artery bypass graft (CABG) patients. The study was underpowered, however, and the difference of 2 hours was not significant ($p = 0.069$).[95]

Petter and coworkers compared Adaptive Support Ventilation to SIMV in a slightly larger patient group ($n = 34$) and found no difference between the two methods in time to extubation or in time in the intensive care unit (ICU). However, there were fewer manipulations of the ventilator controls and fewer alarms in the ASV group. Gruber and colleagues found that ASV resulted in shorter mechanical ventilation time and less time to extubation, when compared to PRVC and Automode, for 48 postoperative CABG patients.[96]

In a 2006 study, Lellouche and coworkers compared frequent screenings for spontaneous breathing trials (SBTs) to a closed-loop knowledge-based system for driving pressure support (SmartCare, EvitaXL, Dräger, Telford, Pennsylvania) in 144 ICU patients on mechanical ventilation for at least 24 hours.[97] They found that SmartCare significantly reduced the time to extubation, the time of mechanical ventilation, and the length of ICU stay.

SmartCare automatically adjusts the level of pressure support to keep the patient's frequency, tidal volume, and end-tidal CO_2 values within a specific range, or so-called comfort zone. Three comfort zones are defined according to the patient's actual body weight: 15–35 kg, 36–55 kg, and >55 kg. Each body weight range has predetermined criteria for acceptable tidal volume, frequency, and $etCO_2$

SmartCare compares the patient's initial frequency, tidal volume, and $etCO_2$ to the acceptable criteria and assigns the patient's ventilation to one of eight categories:

- Normal
- Insufficient
- Hypoventilation
- Central hypoventilation
- Tachypnea
- Severe tachypnea
- Hyperventilation
- Unexplained hyperventilation

Each category is defined by frequency, tidal volume, and $etCO_2$ criteria. For patients weighing over 55 kg, normal ventilation is defined as a spontaneous frequency between 15 and 30 breaths per minute, a tidal volume over 300 mL, and an $etCO_2$ below 55 mm Hg. Insufficient ventilation is classified as an acceptable frequency, but the $etCO_2$ is too high *or* the tidal volume is too low. Hypoventilation, on the other hand, is considered to be an acceptable tidal volume but the $etCO_2$ is too high *and* the frequency is too low. The remaining categories are similarly delineated.[98]

The initial setup screen for SmartCare allows the user to select Neurological Disorder, COPD, or both under Medical History. Selecting Yes for neurological disorder increases the higher-frequency limit to 34 bpm for body weights of 36 kg and over. Selecting the COPD setting sets the high $etCO_2$ limit to 65 mm Hg. Ventilator alarms for $etCO_2$, high frequency, and tidal volume need to be set according to the selected Medical History limits, because activation of a ventilator alarm interrupts SmartCare. Once interrupted, the unit needs to be manually restarted.

Ventilation classified as not in the normal range for that patient prompts an increase or decrease in pressure support by 2 or 4 mbar (1 mbar $\times$ 1.02 = 1 cm H_2O), depending on which parameter limit is violated. If SmartCare changes the level of pressure support, reclassification of ventilation takes 5 minutes. If there is no change in the level of pressure support, SmartCare analyzes ventilation every 2 minutes. The goal is to obtain a target level of pressure support that indicates the patient may be discontinued from the ventilator. The target PS is 5–12 cm H_2O, depending on the type of airway and type of humidifier. For example, the target pressure support for ventilator discontinuance is 12 cm H_2O for the patient with an endotracheal tube and an HME humidifier. The SC program conducts a spontaneous breathing test when the target PS has been obtained, providing the PEEP is 5 cm H_2O or less. If the test is successful, a message is displayed indicating that the patient may be discontinued from the ventilator.

Summary

The initiation and management of a patient on mechanical ventilation require a thorough understanding of the function of various ventilator modes and how changes in the patient's compliance and resistance affect gas delivery. Respiratory therapists need to be able to determine the primary control variable during the inspiratory phase to make sense of the ventilator manufacturer's mode terminology. For example, it's important to clarify what is actually meant by the term "spontaneous breathing" when it is used to describe any given mode. Knowledge of how a specific ventilator breath is triggered, limited, and cycled, coupled with basic cardiopulmonary physiology, provides the foundation for appropriate patient application, management, and subsequent discontinuation of mechanical ventilation.

REVIEW QUESTIONS

1. Describe the classification system for mechanical ventilators using the following terms: trigger, control, cycle, and limit.
2. State the advantages and disadvantages of the following modes: VC or PC CMV, VC or PC SIMV,

MMV, PS, VS, PRVC (AutoFlow, VC+), Automode, Proportional Assist Ventilation, Adaptive Support Ventilation, and CPAP.

3. Discuss the advantages and disadvantages of the different waveforms, and interpret the peak, plateau, and mean airway pressures in each type.
4. Describe PEEP and its application in contrast to auto-PEEP.
5. Discuss the hazards and complications of mechanical ventilation.
6. Describe the purpose of ventilator checks in preventing potential complications.
7. State the appropriate actions to take in correcting respiratory acidosis, alkalosis, or ventilator dyssynchrony.
8. State how changes in the ventilator controls affect volume delivery and mean airway pressure.
9. Explain the special considerations in the initiation and management of mechanical ventilation in given patient cases.
10. Discuss methods of weaning and list two important considerations for extubation.

MULTIPLE-CHOICE QUESTIONS

1. Which of the following creates a greater difference between the peak and plateau pressures with a constant flow mandatory breath?
   a. pneumothorax
   b. atelectasis
   c. pleural effusion
   d. bronchospasm
2. Which of the following increases the plateau pressure with a constant flow mandatory breath?
   a. atelectasis
   b. bronchospasm
   c. increased peak flow rate
   d. both b and c
3. In a pressure support or pressure control mode of ventilation, the inspiratory flow to the patient is the highest at:
   a. the beginning of inspiration.
   b. midinspiration.
   c. end-inspiration.
   d. none of the above.
4. Which one of the following statements describes the pressure-regulated volume control (PRVC) mode on the Servo^i ventilator?
   a. Inspiratory flow is constant (rectangular waveform).
   b. Pressure is constant (rectangular waveform).
   c. Inspiration is volume cycled.
   d. Inspiration is flow cycled.
5. Which one of the following statements describes the AutoFlow mode on the Evita XL ventilator?
   a. Inspiratory flow is constant (rectangular waveform).
   b. Pressure is constant (rectangular waveform).
   c. Inspiration is volume cycled.
   d. Inspiration is flow cycled.
6. (Peak – Plateau)/peak flow estimates airway resistance only for which flow pattern in VC?
   a. rectangular
   b. descending ramp
   c. decelerating
   d. sine
7. Which term does not create essentially two levels of CPAP?
   a. APRV
   b. bilevel
   c. bivent
   d. AutoFlow
8. What is a patient-triggered breath in Adaptive Support Ventilation?
   a. pressure support
   b. volume support
   c. PRVC
   d. PC-CMV
9. All of the following modes provide volume targeted pressure controlled breaths except:
   a. AutoFlow.
   b. PRVC.
   c. VC+.
   d. ATC.
10. Which one of the following ventilator conditions may increase the work of breathing for the patient?
    a. Inspiratory flow is too low in volume control mode.
    b. The pressure trigger level is set on −8 cm H_2O.
    c. Inspiration is prolonged in pressure support.
    d. All of the above are correct.

CRITICAL-THINKING QUESTIONS

1. How would respiratory therapists determine the ventilator's response to a change in the patient's compliance and resistance for a new mode that they have never worked with before?
2. Under what circumstances can one estimate the patient's lung compliance in a pressure-controlled mode?
3. In volume control mode with a rectangular flow waveform, the difference between peak and plateau

pressure reflects the patient's airway resistance. Why is this difference in pressure not reflective of the patient's airway resistance in volume control with a descending ramp flow waveform?

4. In the management of a ventilator on a patient with chronic airflow obstruction, what are important considerations?
5. In the management of a ventilator on a patient with acute respiratory distress syndrome, what are important considerations?
6. What should always be considered in pressure support mode when adding nebulizer treatments or when there is a leak in the system?

References

1. Shapiro BA, et al. *Clinical Application of Respiratory Care*. 4th ed. St. Louis, MO: Mosby; 1991.
2. Mines AH. *Regulation of Breathing*. 3rd ed. Respiratory physiology. New York: Raven Press, Ltd; 1993:107–139.
3. Musch G, et al. Relation between shunt, aeration, and perfusion in experimental acute lung injury. *Am. J. Respir. Crit. Care Med.* 2008;177,3: 292–300.
4. Kallet R., et al. Exacerbation of acute pulmonary edema during assisted mechanical ventilation using a low-tidal volume, lung-protective ventilator strategy. *Chest.* 1999;116:1826–1832.
5. Branson RD, Chatburn RL. Should adaptive pressure control modes be utilized for virtually all patients receiving mechanical ventilation? *Respir Care.* 2007;52,4:478–485.
6. Kallet RH, et al. Work of breathing during lung-protective ventilation in patients with acute lung injury and acute respiratory distress syndrome: a comparison between volume and pressure-regulated breathing modes. *Respir Care*. 2005; 50,12:1623–1631.
7. Gajic O, et al. Ventilator-associated lung injury in patients without acute lung injury at the onset of mechanical ventilation. *Crit Care Med.* 2004;32,9: 1817–1824.
8. Chatburn RL. Classification of ventilator modes: Update and proposal for implementation. *Respir Care.* 2007;52,3:301–323.
9. Branson R, Campbell R, Davis K. Update on respiratory critical care. In: Bigatello L, Hess D, eds. *New Modes of Ventilatory Support*. Vol. 37. Philadelphia: Lippincott Williams & Wilkins; 1999:103–125.
10. Fabry B, et al. Breathing pattern and additional work of breathing in spontaneously breathing patients with different ventilatory demands during inspiratory pressure support and automatic tube compensation. *Inten Care Med.* 1997;23: 545–552.
11. Hamilton-Medical-AG. Adaptive Support Ventilation: user's guide. Switzerland; 2006.
12. Jiao G.-Y, Newhart JW. Bench study on active exhalation valve performance. *Respir Care.* 2008;53,12:1697–1702.
13. Habashi NM. Other approaches to open-lung ventilation: airway pressure release ventilation. *Critical Care Medicine.* Supp. 2005;33,3:S228–S240.
14. Branson RD, Johannigman JA. What is the evidence base for the newer ventilation modes? *Respir Care.* 2004;49,7:742–760.
15. Sinderby C, et al. Inspiratory muscle unloading by neurally adjusted ventilatory assist during maximal inspiratory efforts in healthy subjects. *Chest.* 2007;131,3:711–717.
16. Beck J, et al. Improved synchrony and respiratory unloading by neurally adjusted ventilatory assist (NAVA) in lung-injured rabbits. *Pediatric Research.* 2007;61,3:289–294.
17. Ashton RW, Burkle CM. Endotracheal intubation by direct laryngoscopy. 2004 [cited 2009 February 8]. http://www.thoracic.org/sections/clinical-information/critical-care/atlas-of-critical-care-procedures/procedures/endotracheal-intubation-by-direct-laryngoscopy.cfm
18. Diaz E, Rodrıguez AH, Rello J. Ventilator-associated pneumonia: issues related to the artificial airway. *Respir Care.* 2005;50,7:900–906.
19. Hess DR, et al. Care of the ventilator circuit and its relation to ventilator-associated pneumonia. *Respir Care.* 2003;48,9:869–879.
20. Hickling KG. Best compliance during a decremental, but not incremental, positive end-expiratory pressure trial is related to open-lung positive end-expiratory pressure . A mathematical model of acute respiratory distress syndrome lungs. *Am. J. Respir. Crit. Care Med.* 2001;163,1:69–78.
21. DiRocco JD,. Carney DE, Nieman GF. Correlation between alveolar recruitment/derecruitment and inflection points on the pressure-volume curve. *Intensive Care Med.* 2007;33,7:1204–1211.
22. Gattinoni L, Caironi P. Refining ventilatory treatment for acute lung injury and acute respiratory distress syndrome. *JAMA.* 2008;299,6:691–693.
23. Cheifetz IM, Myers TR. Should every mechanically ventilated patient be monitored with capnography from intubation to extubation? *Respir Care.* 2007;52,4: 423–438.
24. Hofer CK, Ganter MT, Zollinger A. What technique should I use to measure cardiac output? *Current Opinion in Critical Care.* 2007;13:308–317.
25. Lu, Q., et al. A simple automated method for measuring pressure-volume curves during

mechanical ventilation. *Am. J. Respir. Crit. Care Med.* 1999;159,1:275–282.

26. Fleury B, et al. Work of breathing in patients with chronic obstructive pulmonary disease in acute respiratory failure. *Am Rev Respir Dis.* 1985;131: 822–827.
27. American Association for Respiratory Care. AARC Clinical practice guideline: humidification during mechanical ventilation. *Respir Care.* 1992;37,8: 887–890.
28. American Association for Respiratory Care. AARC Clinical practice guideline: selection of device, administration of bronchodilator, and evaluation of response to therapy in mechanically ventilated patients. *Respir Care.* 1999;44,1:105–113.
29. Miyao H, Hirokawa T, Miyasaka K. Relative humidity, not absolute humidity, is of great importance when using a humidifier with a heated wire. *Crit Care Med.* 1992;20:674–679.
30. Tablan OC, et al. CDC Guidelines for preventing health-care-associated pneumonia. Health and Human Services, Centers for Disease Control and Prevention; 2003:15–24.
31. Cook D, Mandell L. Endotracheal aspiration in the diagnosis of ventilator-associated pneumonia. *Chest.* 2000;117,4:195S–197S.
32. Wunderink R. Clinical criteria in the diagnosis of ventilator-associated pneumonia. *Chest.* 2000;117,4: 191S–194S.
33. ATS guidelines for the management of adults with hospital-acquired, ventilator-associated, and healthcare-associated pneumonia. *Am. J. Respir. Crit. Care Med.* 2005;171,4:388–416.
34. Meduri G. Ventilator-associated pneumonia in patients with respiratory failure. *Chest.* 1990;97,5: 1208–1218.
35. Markowicz P, et al. Multicenter prospective study of ventilator-associated pneumonia during acute respiratory distress syndrome. *Am J Respir Crit Care Med.* 2000;161:1942–1948.
36. Branson RD. The ventilator circuit and ventilator-associated pneumonia. *Respir Care.* 2005;50,6: 774–785.
37. Ricard J, et al. Bedside evaluation of efficient airway humidification during mechanical ventilation of the critically ill. *Chest.* 1999;115:1646–1652.
38. Hess DR. Ventilator waveforms and the physiology of pressure support ventilation. *Respir Care.* 2005. 50,2:166–183.
39. Marini JJ and Gattinoni, L. Ventilatory management of acute respiratory distress syndrome: a consensus of two. *Crit Care Med.* 2004;32,1:250–255.
40. Gattinoni, L, et al. Physical and biological triggers of ventilator-induced lung injury and its prevention. Eur Respir J, 2003;22,47_suppl:15s–25.
41. Artigas A, et al. The American-European Consensus Conference on ARDS, Part 2: ventilatory, pharmacologic, supportive therapy, study design strategies and issues related to recovery and remodeling. *Intensive Care Med.* 1998;24:378–398.
42. International consensus conferences in intensive care medicine: ventilator-associated lung injury in ARDS. This official conference report was cosponsored by the American Thoracic Society, The European Society of Intensive Care Medicine, and The Societe de Reanimation de Langue Francaise, and was approved by the ATS Board of Directors, July 1999. *Am J Respir Crit Care Med.* 1999;160,6: 2118–2124.
43. Matthay MA. Conference summary: acute lung injury. *Chest.* 1999;116,90001:119–126.
44. Dreyfuss D, Saumon G. Ventilator-induced lung injury: lessons from experimental studies. *Am J Respir Crit Care Med.* 1998;157:294–323.
45. The acute respiratory distress syndrome network, ventilation with lower tidal volumes as compared with traditional tidal volumes for acute lung injury and the acute respiratory distress syndrome. *N Engl J Med.* 2000;42,18:1301–1308.
46. Slutsky A. Lung injury caused by mechanical ventilation. *Chest.* 1999;116:9S–15S.
47. Rothen H, et al. Dynamics of re-expansion of atelectasis during general anesthesia. *Brit J Anes.* 1999;82:551–556.
48. Mergoni M, et al. Impact of positive end-expiratory pressure on chest wall and lung pressure-volume curve in acute respiratory failure. *Am. J. Respir. Crit. Care Med.* 1997;156,3:846–854.
49. Pelosi P, Caironi P, Gattinoni L. Pulmonary and extrapulmonary forms of acute respiratory distress syndrome. *Seminars in Respiratory and Critical Care Medicine.* 2001;22,3:259–268.
50. Bersten AD. Measurement of overinflation by multiple linear regression analysis in patinets with acute lung injury. *Eur Respir J.* 1998;12:526–532.
51. Sessler CN. Mechanical ventilation of patients with acute lung injury. *Crit Care Clinics.* 1998;14,4: 707–729.
52. Foti G, et al. Effects of periodic lung recruitment maneuvers on gas exchange and respiratory mechanics in mechanically ventilated acute respiratory distress syndrome (ARDS) patients. *Intensive Care Med.* 2000;26:501–507.
53. Lim SC, et al. Intercomparison of recruitment maneuver efficacy in three models of acute lung injury. *Crit Care Med.* 2004;32,12:2371–2377.
54. Gattinoni L, et al. Physiologic rationale for ventilator setting in acute lung injury/acute respiratory distress syndrome patients. *Crit Care Med.* Supp. 2003;31,4:S300–S304.

55. Amato M, et al. Effect of protective-ventilation strategy on mortality in the acute respiratory distress syndrome. *N Engl J Med.* 1998;338,6: 347–354.
56. Lapinsky S, et al. Safety and efficacy of a sustained inflation for alveolar recruitment in adults with respiratory failure. *Inten Care Med.* 1999; 25: 1297–1301.
57. Girgis K, et al. A decremental PEEP trial identifies the PEEP level that maintains oxygenation after lung recruitment. *Respir Care.* 2006;51,10: 1132–1139.
58. Kallet RH, Branson RD. Do the NIH ARDS clinical trials network PEEP/FIO2 tables provide the best evidence-based guide to balancing PEEP and FIO2 settings in adults? *Respir Care.* 2007;52,4:461–475.
59. Kacmarek R. Lung recruitment-setting PEEP in ARDS. In: *Issues in Critical Care*. Kansas City, KS; 2000.
60. Chiumello D, et al. Nitrogen washout/washin, helium dilution and computed tomography in the assessment of end expiratory lung volume. *Critical Care.* 2008;12,6:R150.
61. Mathews P, Gregg B. University of Kansas equipment review: The Engstrom Carestation critical care ventilator. In: *Focus Journal*. Rhinebeck, NY: Bob Miglino, 2007:52–53.
62. Blanch L, et al. Short-term effects of prone position in critically ill patients with acute respiratory distress syndrome. *Intensive Care Med.* 1997;23: 1033–1039.
63. Pelosi P, et al. Sigh in acute respiratory distress syndrome. *Am J Respir Crit Care Med.* 1999;159,3: 872–880.
64. Gattinoni L, Protti A. Ventilation in the prone position: for some but not for all? *CMAJ.* 2008;178,9:1174–1176.
65. Yanos J, Watling S, Verhey J. The physiologic effects of inverse ratio ventilation. *Chest.* 1998;114:834–838.
66. Girard TD, Bernard GR. Mechanical ventilation in ARDS: a state-of-the-art review. *Chest.* 2007;131,3: 921–929.
67. Greene J, Klinger J. The efficacy of inhaled nitric oxide in the treatment of acute respiratory distress syndrome. *Crit Care Clin.* 1998;14,3:387–409.
68. Sokol J, Jacobs SE, Bohn B. Inhaled nitric oxide for acute hypoxic respiratory failure in children and adults: a meta-analysis. *Anesth Analg.* 2003;97,4: 989–998.
69. Fessler HE, Hager DN, Brower RG. Feasibility of very high-frequency ventilation in adults with acute respiratory distress syndrome. *Crit Care Med.* 2008;36,4:1043–1048.
70. Fessler HE, et al. A protocol for high-frequency oscillatory ventilation in adults: results from a roundtable discussion. *Crit Care Med.* 2007;35,7: 1649–1654.
71. Fessler HE, Hess DR. Does high-frequency ventilation offer benefits over conventional ventilation in adult patients with acute respiratory distress syndrome? *Respir Care.* 2007;52,5:595–605.
72. Koh Y. Ventilatory management in patients with chronic airflow obstruction. *Critical Care Clinics.* 2007;23,2:169–181.
73. Dhand R. Ventilator graphics and respiratory mechanics in the patient with obstructive lung disease. *Respir Care.* 2005;50,2:246–261; discussion 259–261.
74. Munoz J, et al. Interaction between intrinsic positive end-expiratory pressure and externally applied positive end-expiratory pressure during controlled ventilation. *Crit Care Med.* 1993;21,3: 348–356.
75. Slutsky A. Consensus conference on mechanical ventilation—January 28–30, 1993. *Intensive Care Med.* 1994;20,5:378.
76. Viale J, et al. Time course evolution of ventilatory responses to inspiratory unloading in patients. *Am J Respir Crit Care Med.* 1998;157:428–434.
77. Marik PE, Varon J, Fromm JR. The management of acute severe asthma. *J Emerg Med.* 2002;23,3: 257–268.
78. Hurford WE, Cheifetz IM. Should heliox be used for mechanically ventilated patients? *Respir Care.* 2007;52,5:582–591.
79. Durbin C, Campbell R, Branson R. Removal of the endotracheal tube: AARC clinical practice guideline. *Respir Care.* 1999;44,1:85–90.
80. MacIntyre NR. Respiratory mechanics in the patient who is weaning from the ventilator. *Respir Care.* 2005;50,2:275–286; discussion 284–286.
81. Grinnan DC, Truwit JD. Clinical review: respiratory mechanics in spontaneous and assisted ventilation. *Critical Care.* 2005;9,5:472–484.
82. Sassoon CS. Blunted response to hypercapnia: Synonymous with depressed respiratory drive? *Respir Care.* 2008;53,8:1006–1007.
83. Engoren M. Evaluation of the cuff-leak test in a cardiac surgery population. *Chest.* 1999;116: 1029–1031.
84. Shin SH, et al. The cuff leak test is not predictive of successful extubation. *Am Surg.* 2008;74,12: 1182–1185.
85. Eskandar N, Apostolakos MJ. Weaning from mechanical ventilation. *Critical Care Clinics.* 2007;23,2:263–274.
86. Butler R, et al. Is there a preferred technique for weaning the difficult-to-wean patient? A systematic review of the literature. *Crit Care Med.* 1999;27,11: 2331–2336.

87. AHRQ summary. *Criteria for weaning from mechanical ventilation.* In: *Summary, Evidence Report/Technology Assessment: Number 23.* Rockville, MD: Agency for Healthcare Research and Quality; 2000.
88. Alia I, Esteban A. Protocol-guided weaning: a key issue in reducing the duration of mechanical ventilation. *Intensivmed.* 1999;36:429–435.
89. Mehta S, et al. Predictions of post-extubation work of breathing. *Crit Care Med.* 2000;28,5:1341–1346.
90. Ishaaya A, Nathan S, Belman M. Work of breathing after extubation. *Chest.* 1995;107:204–209.
91. Straus C, et al. Contribution of the endotracheal tube and the upper airway to breathing workload. *Am. J. Respir. Crit. Care Med.* 1998;157,1:23–30.
92. Grasso S, et al. Compensation for increase in respiratory workload during mechanical ventilation: pressure-support versus proportional assist ventilation. *Am J Respir Crit Care Med.* 2000;161,3 Pt 1:819–826.
93. Esteban A, et al. Effect of spontaneous breathing trial duration on outcome of attempts to discontinue mechanical ventilation. *Am. J. Respir. Crit. Care Med.* 1999;159,2:512–518.
94. Mokhlesi B, et al. Predicting extubation failure after successful completion of a spontaneous breathing trial. *Respir Care.* 2007;52,12:1710–1717.
95. Hendrix H, et al. A randomized trial of automated versus conventional protocol-driven weaning from mechanical ventilation following coronary artery bypass surgery. *Eur J Cardiothorac Surg.* 2006;29,6: 957–963.
96. Gruber PC, et al. Randomized controlled trial comparing adaptive-support ventilation with pressure-regulated volume-controlled ventilation with automode in weaning patients after cardiac surgery. *Anesthesiology.* 2008;109,1:81–87.
97. Lellouche F, et al. A multicenter randomized trial of computer-driven protocolized weaning from mechanical ventilation. *Am J Respir Crit Care Med.* 2006;174,8:894–900.
98. Dragger Medical, SmartCare™/PS Operating Instructions: EvitaXL Software 6.0 or higher. Telford, PA; 2005.

Suggested Readings

Artigas A, Bernard G, et al. The American-European Consensus Conference on ARDS, Part 2: ventilatory, pharmacologic, supportive therapy, study design strategies and issues related to recovery and remodeling. *Intensive Care Med.* 1998;24: 378–398.

Greene J, Klinger J. The efficacy of inhaled nitric oxide in the treatment of acute respiratory distress syndrome. *Crit Care Clin.* 1998;14,3:387–409.

International Consensus Conferences in Intensive Care Medicine. Ventilator-associated Lung Injury in ARDS. *Am J Respir Crit Care Med.* 1999;160,6: 2118–2124.

Slutsky, A. Lung injury caused by mechanical ventilation. *Chest.* 1999;116: 9S–15S.

CHAPTER 27

Mechanics and Modes of Mechanical Ventilation

Tina Wellman

OBJECTIVES

Upon completion of this chapter, the reader should be able to:

- Identify the benefits of using real-time ventilator graphics to manage patient-ventilator interactions.
- Utilize ventilator graphics to differentiate pressure and volume control ventilation.
- Utilize ventilator graphics to differentiate modes of ventilation.
- Explain the effect of clinically significant changes in airway resistance and lung compliance on ventilator graphics.
- Identify common clinical problems using ventilator graphics.

CHAPTER OUTLINE

KEY TERMS

airway resistance (R_{aw})
autocycling
auto-PEEP
flow-volume loop
I/E ratio
inspiratory cycle off
inspiratory pause
inspiratory rise time
intrinsic PEEP
mean airway pressure (MAP)
peak inspiratory pressure
plateau pressure ($P_{plateau}$)
positive end expiratory pressure (PEEP)
pressure ventilation
pressure-volume loop
scalar
static compliance
volume ventilation

Respiratory therapists working in intensive care units (ICUs) today are fortunate to be using ventilators with graphic displays that are capable of presenting a variety of waveforms. In fact, purchasing a modern ICU ventilator without graphic displays would be difficult because all manufacturers and end users recognize the need for this monitoring tool. Many currently available ventilators are designed with graphic displays that also serve as the user interface. This design allows for the graphics to be monitored continuously while at the patient bedside. Some of these ventilators are included in this chapter as examples, including the Draeger Evita XL, VIASYS Avea, Puritan Bennett 840, and the Maquet Servo^{i}. The reason continuous monitoring of graphics has become so important is that the graphics provide an immediate display of the patient-ventilator interaction on which clinicians have come to rely.[1] Much like pulmonary function testing, a clinician can learn and use pattern recognition to detect and evaluate a patient's normal and abnormal breathing patterns while on the ventilator.[2]

Ventilator graphics (waveforms) provide important data in real time at the bedside. They can help in:

- Forming a clinical diagnosis.
- Providing information about the patients' pulmonary mechanics and patient-ventilator interaction.
- Determining the appropriateness of the ventilator settings, including triggering, synchrony, and flow.
- Troubleshooting.
- Trending patient progress.
- Quickly recognizing patient changes.[2,3]

Mastering ventilator waveform interpretation is a skill that takes time and commitment. This skill, however, is a-proficiency that can help a clinician recognize many problematic clinical situations and ultimately improve the care provided to the patient.[4]

Waveforms

Three primary variables are assessed with waveforms: pressure, volume, and flow. These specific waveforms are commonly referred to as **scalar**. The term scalar means that the waveform is related to either pressure, volume, or flow and is plotted against time. They are always represented as pressure versus time, volume versus time, or flow versus time. Time is always plotted on the horizontal, or *x*, axis and the variable being measured on the *y* axis. A few typical shapes or waveforms are seen in scalars during mechanical ventilation (Figure 27-1).[4,5]

- *Square*—The square scalar waveform is generated by a constant flow rate throughout inspiration. The waveform can also be referred to as a *rectangular* or *constant flow rate wave.*
- *Decelerating*—The decelerating waveform is generated by flow that begins at peak and decreases in a linear manner until the end of inspiration. This waveform is also known as a *descending waveform*.
- *Accelerating*—The accelerating waveform is generated by flow that begins with a low level and then increases throughout inspiration. This waveform has also been called an *ascending waveform*.
- *Sinusoidal*—The sinusoidal waveform is generated by flow that increases to a peak and then decreases. At times only half of this curve may be present.
- *Decay*—The exponential decay waveform is generated by flow that begins at peak and decreases.
- *Rise*—The exponential rise waveform is generated by flow that begins at a low level and then increases gradually throughout inspiration.

Interaction of Pressure, Volume, and Flow over Time

The interaction of the three measured variables of pressure, volume, and flow over time is what the ventilator uses to calculate and draw the waveforms. The interaction includes a number of components of mechanical ventilation in order to create the waveform displays:

- *Tidal volume* (V_t) delivered depends on the flow rate used and the inspiratory time allowed: flow rate (Lpm) × inspiratory time (s) = tidal volume (mL).[3]
- The lungs inflate as the result of a *pressure gradient*. If the pressure on the outside of the lungs (the ventilator circuit) is higher than the pressure inside the lungs, the lungs inflate. The larger the gradient is, the higher the generated flow rates are and the faster the lungs inflate. The flow is measured as the volume change per unit

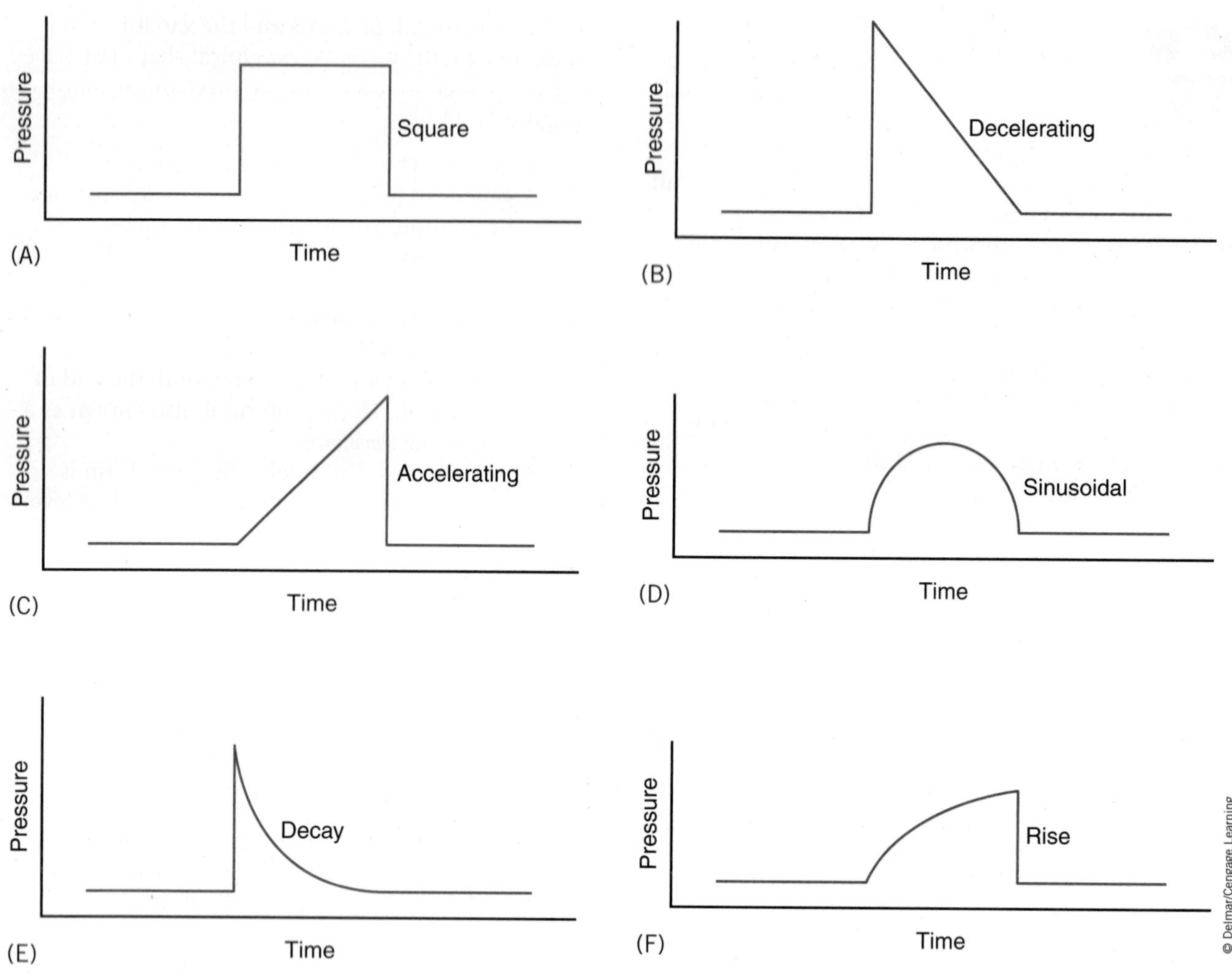

FIGURE 27-1 (A) A square scalar waveform. (B) A decelerating waveform. (C) An accelerating waveform. (D) A sinusoidal waveform. (E) An exponential decay waveform. (F) An exponential rise waveform.

of time: tidal volume ÷ inspiratory time = flow rate (in volume control modes only).[4]

- The amount of pressure required to inflate the lungs depends on the lung compliance. *Compliance* is the distensibility of an elastic structure, such as the lung, and is defined as the change in volume of the structure produced by a change in pressure across that structure. If the lungs are healthy and inflate easily (compliant), not much pressure is needed. If the lungs are very stiff (low compliance), however, a large amount of pressure may be needed to inflate the lungs.
- *Airway resistance*, another factor related to pressure in mechanical ventilation, is the opposition to flow caused by the forces of friction. It is defined as the ratio of driving pressure to the rate of air flow. Resistance to flow in the airways depends on whether the flow is laminar or turbulent, on the dimensions of the airway, and on the viscosity of the gas. If the airway diameter is large with low resistance, the greater the flow is that can move through the airways. If the airway diameter is narrow (constricted), the greater the resistance is, and therefore the lower the flow rate is that can move through the airways.[3] The resistance through the airways can greatly affect the pressures, whether set or created on the ventilator, and cause specific variations in the waveforms.
- Another important factor in looking at waveforms is total cycle time (Figure 27-2). The *total cycle time* (*TCT*) is the total respiratory cycle, that is, the time required for both inspiration (T_i) and expiration (T_e) and the events that occur during that time.[6]

$$TCT = T_i + T_e$$

Minute	Respiratory Rate	TCT
60 sec	60	1
60 sec	30	2
60 sec	20	3
60 sec	15	4
60 sec	12	5
60 sec	10	6
60 sec	6	10

If the T_i is set the T_e must change.

FIGURE 27-2 Total cycle time.

THE I/E RATIO

The **I/E ratio** is simply a proportion of the inspiratory and expiratory time in a respiratory cycle.[6] To figure out the I/E ratio, refer to the TCT in Figure 27-2 ($TCT = T_i + T_e$). The TCT cycle time must be divided between the two portions. A normal I/E ratio is 1:2 or 1:3 (T_i to T_e), giving the patient more time for exhalation than inhalation. If the ratio is changed to be 2:1 or 3:1, it is called an *inverse ratio*. This is done at times to improve oxygenation in a sick patient but is not considered normal.[3]

In Figure 27-3A, the ventilator is set for a respiratory rate (RR) of 8 breaths per minute with an inspiratory time of 1 second. The TCT in this case is 7.5 seconds (60 seconds ÷ 8 RR = 7.5 TCT). The I/E ratio is 1:6.5. The yellow line on the graph is showing the period of time between breaths. If the inspiratory time remains constant while the ventilator respiratory rate is changed, the expiratory time and I/E ratio must change.

In Figure 27-3B, the ventilator is set with a respiratory rate of 15 breaths per minute and a 1-second inspiratory time. The yellow line in this example is tracing the period of time between breaths. There is much less time between breaths than seen in Figure 27-3A with a respiratory rate of 8 breaths per minute. With the set rate of 15 breaths per minute and a 1-second inspiratory time, the I/E ratio is 1:3 and the TCT is only 4 seconds.

In Figure 27-3C, the ventilator is set with a respiratory rate of 20 breaths per minute and a 1-second inspiratory time. The yellow line is tracing the period of time between breaths, which is even shorter. The TCT in this example is only 3 seconds with an I/E ratio of 1:2. The higher the respiratory rate gets with the same inspiratory time, the less time the patient has to exhale.

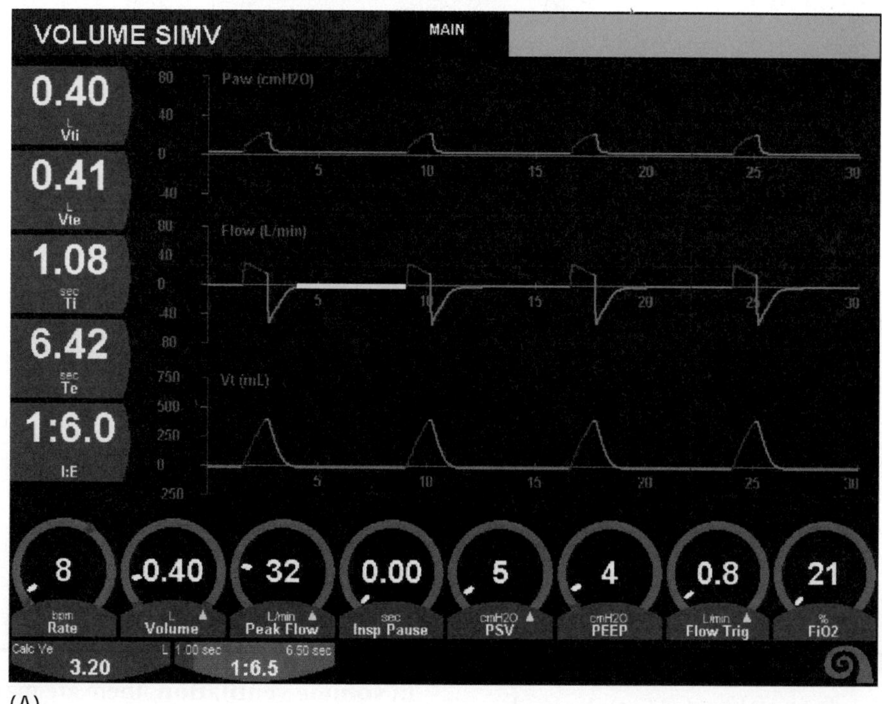

(A)

FIGURE 27-3 If the inspiratory time remains constant while the ventilator respiratory rate is changed, the expiratory time and I/E ratio must change. (A) I/E of 1:6.5, (B) I/E of 1:3, (C) I/E of 1:2. (*continues*)

Courtesy of CareFusion

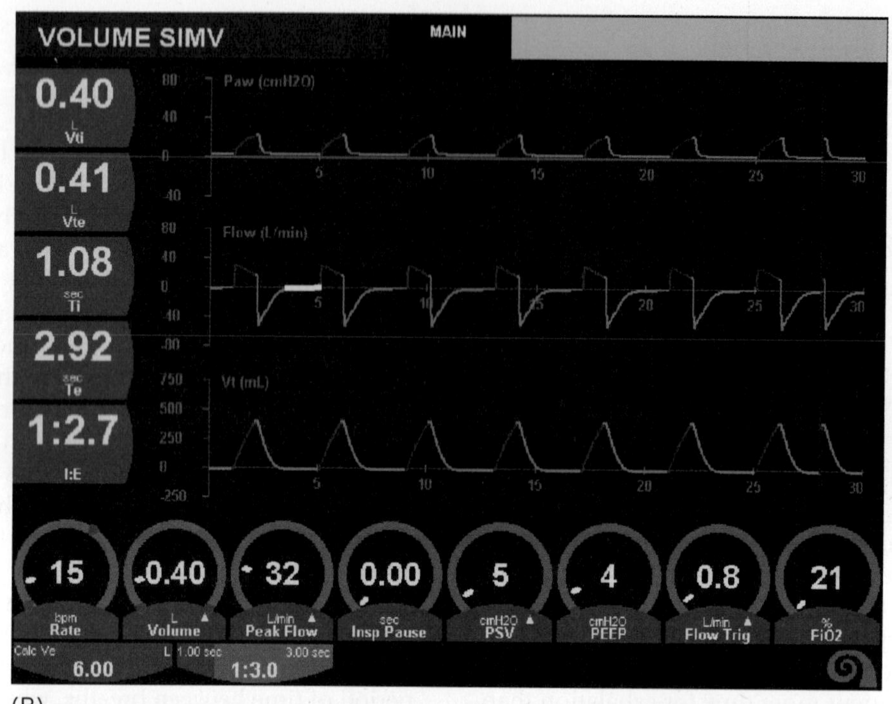

(B)

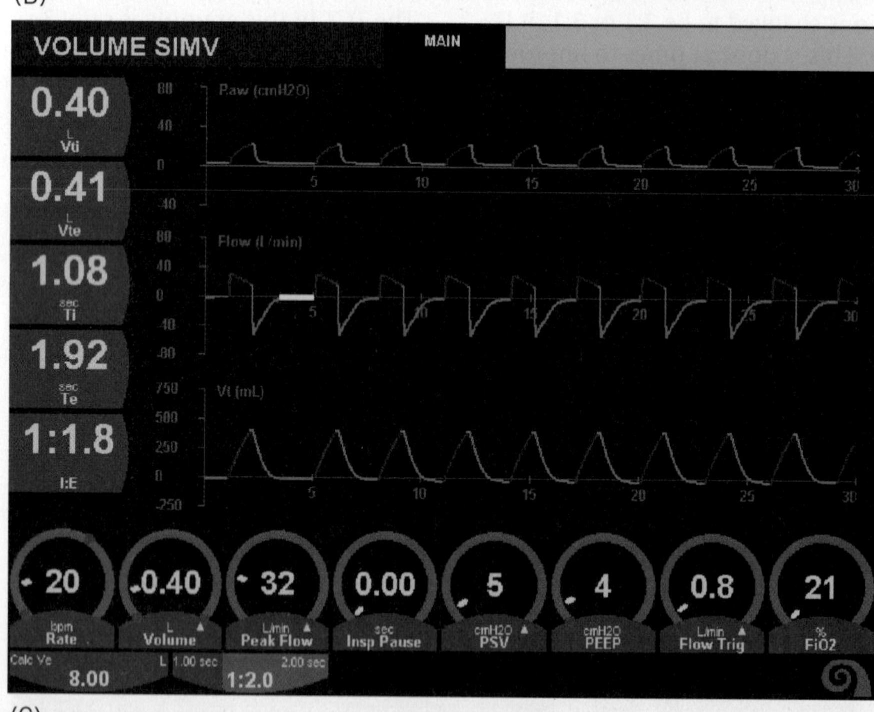

(C)

FIGURE 27-3 *(continued)*

Types of Ventilation

There are only two fundamental types of mechanical ventilation. The patient is ventilated either with pressure or with volume ventilation. Understanding these principles makes understanding ventilator waveforms very easy. All the modes of ventilation on any ventilator fall under one of these two categories.

VOLUME VENTILATION

In **volume ventilation**, there are many active parameters on the ventilator. However, a few operator-set parameters affect the ventilator waveforms in predictable ways:

- Tidal volume (V_t)
- Inspiratory time (T_i)

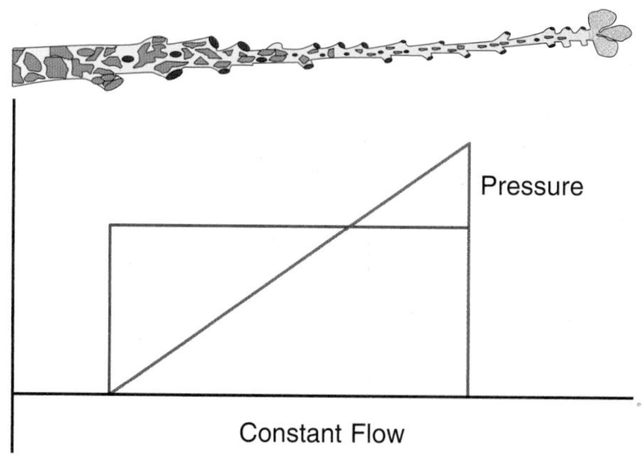

FIGURE 27-4 Typical volume ventilator breath.
Courtesy of Maquet Inc.

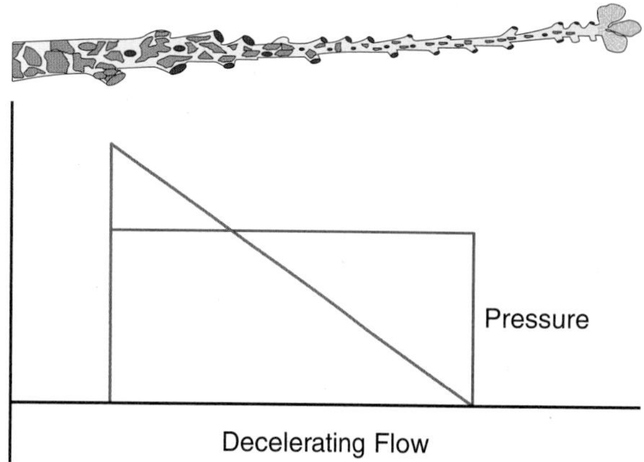

FIGURE 27-5 Typical pressure-ventilated breath.
Courtesy of Maquet Inc.

- Respiratory rate
- Rise time
- Flow rate
- **Positive end-expiratory pressure (PEEP)**, the positive pressure at the end of exhalation during spontaneous breathing or mechanical ventilation[4]

These settings generate an accelerating inspiratory pressure.

Figure 27-4 shows a typical volume ventilator breath. The breath begins at a low flow and quickly increases to the set amount, where it is maintained at that constant rate until the end of the inspiratory phase (green line). Then exhalation occurs. This figure shows that, with a constant flow rate in volume ventilation, the pressure tracing generated is accelerating.

This outcome is due to the anatomy of the lung. When a constant flow rate is applied to the lung, the pressure generated increases as it travels to the smaller airways. The resistance is higher in the small airways than in the larger airways. The increase in resistance generates higher pressures, which in turn cause the pressure tracing associated with volume-ventilated breaths to accelerate. Volume ventilation breaths guarantee the set tidal volume delivery regardless of changes in the lung characteristic such as compliance and resistance. This can be an asset if control of P_aCO_2 is needed by guaranteeing a set minute ventilation (V_e). Minute ventilation is the product of respiratory rate and tidal volume: $V_e = RR \times V_t$.

PRESSURE VENTILATION

In **pressure ventilation**, a few set parameters affect the waveform. There is a set/constant **peak inspiratory pressure** or ventilating pressure (P_{eak}). Peak inspiratory pressure is the highest pressure achieved during inspiration on positive pressure ventilation.[4] Set times—inspiratory time (T_i), rise time, respiratory rate, and PEEP—give the patient a variable tidal volume and a decelerating inspiratory flow rate.

Figure 27-5 shows a typical pressure ventilated breath. The breath begins at peak flow and decreases in a linear fashion until the end of inspiration. Exhalation occurs passively at the end of the inspiratory time. The constant pressure in the ventilator circuit is depicted in the Figure 27-5 as a square wave. During inspiration, pressure continuously increases in the periphery of the lung. This results in a continuous diminishing of the pressure gradient across the lung until there is none. Without a pressure gradient, there can be no flow into the lung. Inspiration ends when the preset inspiratory time (T_I) is reached, as shown in the figure as a decelerating flow rate.[5]

The square inspiratory pressure waveform that is produced during a pressure-ventilated breath not only limits airway pressure, but also gives constant pressure throughout the inspiratory phase. Because of the initial high peak flow at the beginning of the breath, the preset pressure is achieved quickly and remains at this level until the set inspiratory time is achieved. In pressure ventilation, the inspiratory flow and the T_I are independent of one another. The RCP sets the inspiratory time according to the patient's particular needs, and the decelerating inspiratory flow pattern provides a more even distribution of air to the alveoli regardless of compliance.[7]

Ventilator Modes

Ventilator modes correlate to either pressure or volume. Within the two categories (pressure and volume) are four modes: controlled modes, assist-controlled modes, support modes, and combination modes. Understanding the type of mode being used is important in optimizing synchrony. Knowing the type of mode helps in identifying normal versus abnormal breathing patterns displayed on the graphics.

- *Controlled modes.* In controlled modes, the ventilator starts the breath, controls the inspiratory gas delivery, and ends inspiration with no input from the patient.[6] With each breath is a guaranteed delivery of either a preset pressure or tidal volume that is controlled by the ventilator.
- *Assist-controlled mode.* Assist-controlled modes are identical to controlled modes except that the patient is able to trigger the ventilator by exerting respiratory muscles.
- *Support modes.* In support modes, where the patient is breathing spontaneously, the patient initiates the breath and controls the depth of the breath and the flow rate at which the breath is delivered.[3]
- *Combination mode.* The combination modes include both types of breaths (control and support). It is primarily used to provide partial mechanical support. The patient can take some spontaneous breaths but may also receive some mandatory or control breaths as well.

Table 27-1 provides examples of common modalities that may be seen on modern ventilators.

TABLE 27-1 **Categories pressure and volume with designated ventilator modes**

Category	Mode
Volume Category	
Volume control (VC)	Controlled mode
Synchronized intermittent mandatory ventilation (VC-SIMV)	Combination mode
Pressure Category	
Pressure control (PC)	Controlled mode
Pressure support (PSV)	Assist-control or support mode
PC-SIMV	Combination mode
Volume support	Assist-control or support mode
Pressure-regulated volume control (PRVC)	Controlled mode
SIMV-PRVC	Combination mode
Airway pressure release ventilation (APRV)	Combination mode

Interpretation of Ventilator Graphics

Figure 27-6 is a representative graphics display of volume ventilation for the VIASYS Avea ventilator.

- The top waveform represents the *pressure scalar* waveform. The measured pressure is shown in cm H_2O.
- The middle waveform represents the *flow scalar*. The measured flow is shown in liters per min (Lpm).
- The bottom waveform represents *volume scalar* and the measured volume is shown in milliliters (mL).

These are the three main waveforms that are monitored on all ventilators in the ICU. When interpreting ventilator graphics, follow a set of steps.

STEP 1: DETERMINE THE TYPE OF VENTILATION

First, identify what type of ventilation the patient is on: pressure or volume. To decipher a volume mode from a pressure mode, look at the flow scalar first, then the pressure scalar.

Volume Ventilation. Recall that the flow scalar for a volume breath should be square or constant flow. The flow rate may vary in a predictable fashion if a flow pattern is "set" on the ventilator controls. This is shown in Figure 27-6. The pressure increases at a constant rate due to the constant, or square, flow pattern. The pressure increases as the volume being delivered inflates the lung. This is what a typical pressure scalar waveform looks like in volume ventilation.

Pressure Ventilation. In Figure 27-7, the top scalar on this ventilator is the pressure scalar, and it is displaying a square, or constant, pressure pattern. The bottom scalar is the flow scalar, which has a decelerating flow pattern. This pattern is consistent with pressure ventilation.

STEP 2: DETERMINE THE MODE OF VENTILATION

After determining the type of ventilation, ascertain whether the mode is a controlled, assist-controlled, support, or a combination. To do this, first look at the breaths to see whether they all look exactly alike.

- Are they the same size?
- Are they the same shape?
- Do they come at a regular and marchable frequency?

If these questions can be answered positively, the mode is most likely controlled or assist-controlled.

- In both *controlled and assist-controlled modes*, the inspiratory time, or flow rate, is set by

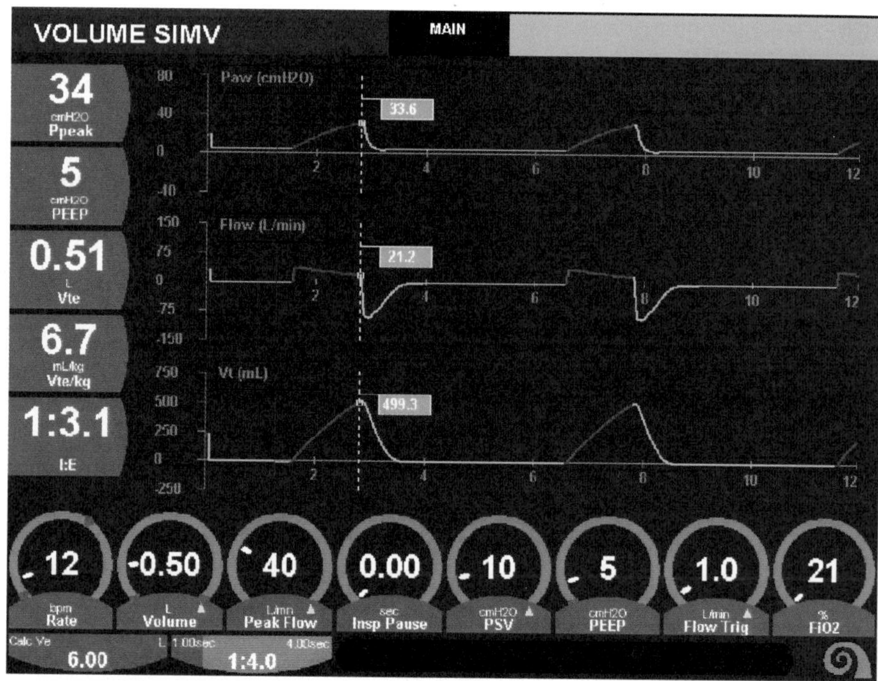

FIGURE 27-6 Typical waveforms in a volume ventilation.
Courtesy of CareFusion

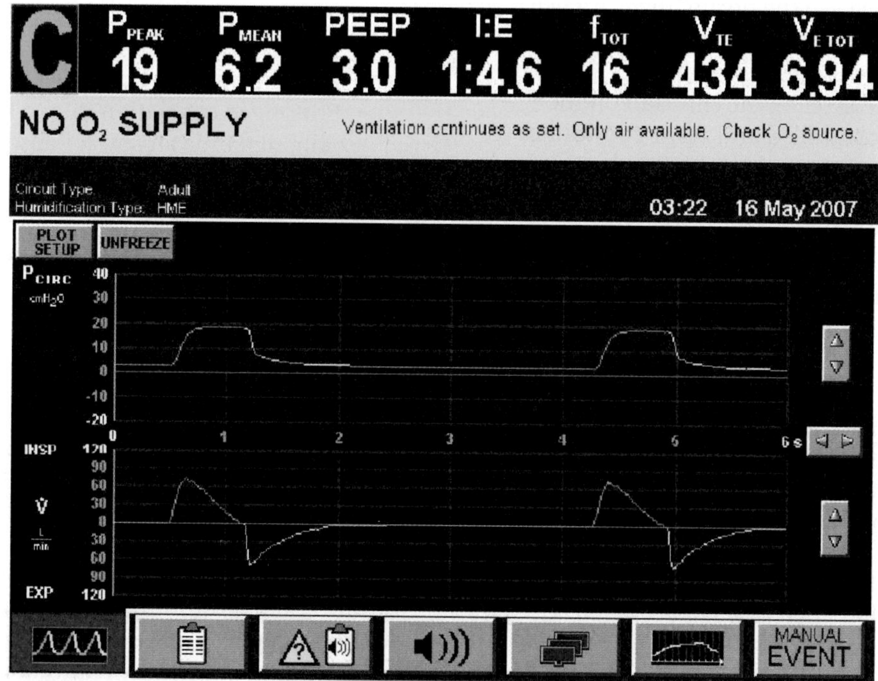

FIGURE 27-7 Typical waveforms in a pressure ventilation.
Reprinted by permission from Nellcor Puritan Bennett LLC, Boulder, Colorado, part of Coviden

the operator of the ventilator. In that case, each breath has exactly the same inspiratory time.

- In *spontaneous modes*, the inspiratory time is controlled by the patient and therefore has some variability.
- In *combination modes*, some breaths are exactly the same while others are varied.

If the inspiratory times and the "shape" of inspiration are consistent from breath to breath, then the breaths are identical. To understand the concept of

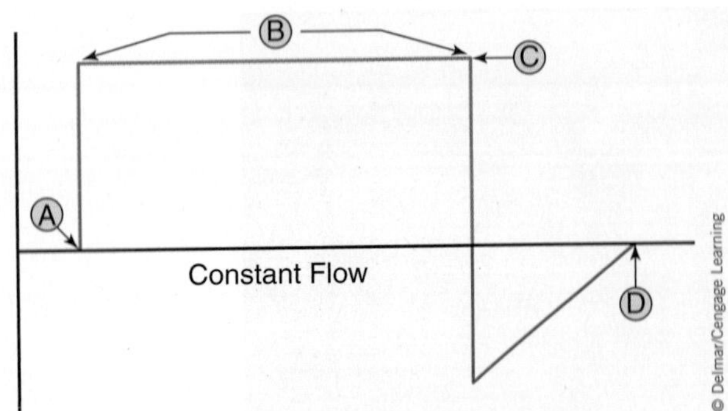

FIGURE 27-8 Parts of the breath on a waveform: (A) The beginning of inspiration. (B) Inspiration, or inspiratory time. (C) The end of inspiration and the beginning of exhalation. (D) The end of exhalation.

shaping inspiration, the respiratory therapist must be able to distinguish the parts of the breath on the waveform. In Figure 27-8:

- (A) is the *beginning of inspiration*. Inspiration can be initiated by the ventilator or by the patient, depending on the mode of ventilation. If the patient has triggered the breath, there is a negative deflection just prior to the mechanical breath.
- (B) represents *inspiration or inspiratory time*. This period of time is set by the clinician on the ventilator in controlled and assist-controlled modes. During inspiration of a volume breath, the flow is constant [that is, the flow pattern is predictable (a set parameter)], and the pressure develops at a rate that depends on the characteristics of the lung and the ventilator settings.
- (C) represents the *end of inspiration and the beginning of exhalation*. Exhalation is passive and commences upon the ventilator's opening of the expiratory valve.
- (D) is the *end of exhalation*. In a normal breath, exhalation should return to baseline before the next breath begins. The characteristics of the lung, as well as parts of the ventilator circuit (such as smaller endotracheal tubes and clogged expiratory filters) can slow patient exhalation.

Volume Ventilation. Figure 27-9A shows a volume-control mode that is not being assisted by the patient. On the flow scalar (middle) waveform, the first arrow represents the beginning of inspiration. The second arrow represents the inspiratory time for this breath. Based on the inspiratory time for all three breaths on the graph, the breaths appear to be identical. This is a volume control mode, and no assisted breaths are being delivered to the patient. If the patient had triggered a breath, a negative deflection would appear just prior to the mechanical breath in either the pressure or flow scalar depending on the ventilator setup with regard to trigger sensitivity. The negative deflection indicates a patient-initiated breath. Once the breath has been started, it is generally shaped by the set parameters. If the flow rate, and/or volume, are not set appropriately patient/ventilator dysynchrony is likely to result.

In Figure 27-9B, the first arrow on the flow scalar represents the beginning of exhalation, where inspiration ends and exhalation begins. The second arrow represents the end of exhalation. When the patient is finished exhaling, the breath comes all the way back to baseline between breaths. This is what a normal breath looks like upon complete exhalation. If the waveform does not return to baseline between the breaths, it is abnormal and results in auto-PEEP, or **intrinsic PEEP**. **Auto-PEEP** is abnormal and is usually undetected above the atmospheric pressure remaining in the alveoli at the end of exhalation due to dynamic air trapping.[3] Auto-PEEP, or air trapping, may result from:

- Inadequate expiratory time.
- Too high a respiratory rate.
- Long inspiratory times.
- Prolonged exhalation due to bronchoconstriction, dynamic airway collapse, small endotracheal tubes, and clogged expiratory filters, or similar disorders.[4,8]

In Figure 27-9C, the first two arrows on the pressure scalar represent the patient's set PEEP. The waveform remains above zero cm H_2O (blue arrow). For this patient, the operator has set a therapeutic PEEP level. The third arrow represents the peak pressure being generated. Notice it occurs at the end of inspiration when the patient's lungs are the most inflated.

Figure 27-9D provides a closer look at the volume scalar. The waveform is divided into two unequal pieces: The first half is inspiration, and the second half is exhalation. This is an example of a normal volume scalar. Volume scalar waveforms generally look the same regardless of the mode or type of ventilation. In a normal breathing pattern, the tracing in a volume scalar should come to baseline between breaths.

The volume scalar may appear differently in two instances.

- One is in the face of a *leak* in the system, either in the ventilator circuit, around the cuff of the artificial airway, or in the ventilator itself.

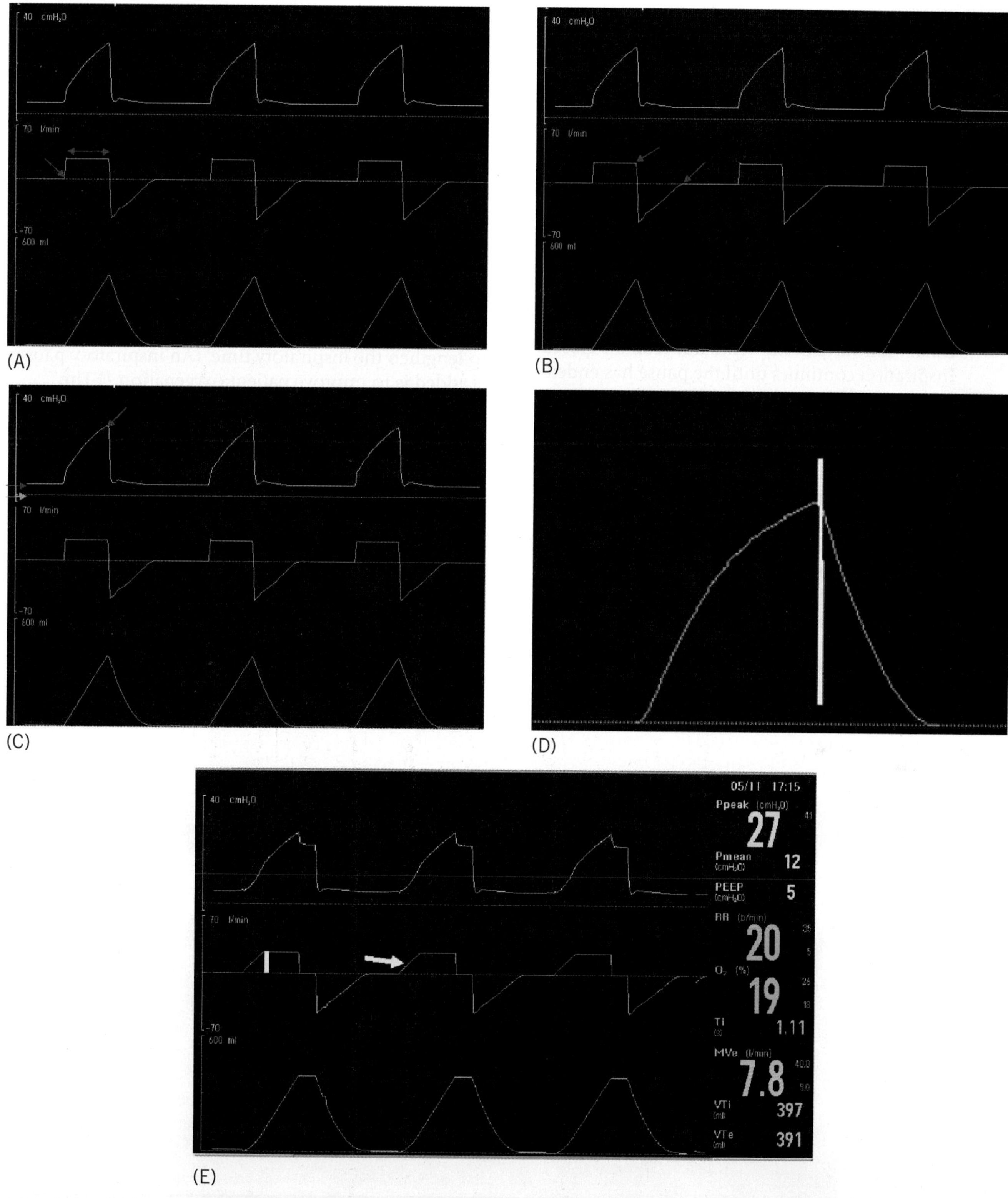

FIGURE 27-9 (A) A volume-control mode that is not being assisted by the patient. (B) A normal breath with complete exhalation. (C) PEEP setting. (D) A normal volume scalar. (E) A change in setting showing inspiratory pause and inspiratory rise time.

Courtesy of Maquet Inc.

- The other is if the patient is forcibly exhaling instead of allowing the normal passive exhalation. If a patient is forcibly exhaling, the waveform appears steeper due to the speed of the volume changing, and the area between breaths might dip below the baseline.

Inspiratory Pause and Inspiratory Rise Time In Figure 27-9E, this is still volume ventilation, but a couple of settings have been changed.

- All the breaths look identical, but an inspiratory pause has been set. An **inspiratory pause** is just an extension of the inspiratory time where the exhalation valve of the ventilator remains closed. Inspiration continues until the pause has ended and then exhalation begins.[4] Inspiratory pause results in plateaus on all the scalars.
- A second new setting affects **inspiratory rise time**. *Rise time* is a setting on a ventilator that allows a clinician to control the rate at which the ventilator disperses the initial gas burst from the ventilator. In volume ventilation, the gas normally comes out of the ventilator very quickly and rises to the set constant flow rate, where it remains until exhalation. The clinician can slow down the initial gas burst using rise time. An appropriately set rise time should result in greater patient comfort and a more laminar flow, decreasing resistance.

When setting rise time, the therapist must remember that patient effort and work of breathing are known to be affected by the ventilator's ability to meet the patient's peak inspiratory demand. If the inspiratory flow does not meet the demand, then patient-ventilator dyssynchrony results. In Figure 27-9E, it is apparent that a substantial rise time is set. In the first breath of the flow scalar (green), the white line represents how the breath would look without rise time—a very sharp and square breath. In the second breath, the arrow marks the very sloped and gradual climb to the set constant flow rate. This is what a volume breath with a significant amount of rise time looks like.

In Figure 27-10, an inspiratory pause has been set to lengthen the inspiratory time. (An inspiratory pause is added is to improve patient oxygenation.[4]) The arrows on all three scalar waveforms point out the same characteristic. During an inspiratory pause, there is no additional flow from the ventilator into the patient's lungs. This is a static maneuver.

- So the *flow scalar* shows a drop in flow that is held at zero until exhalation begins.
- The *pressure scalar* also shows a decrease in pressure from the peak pressure to the plateau pressure. The **plateau pressure ($P_{plateau}$)** is the pressure measured in the patient's circuit of a ventilator during an inspiratory hold maneuver, in addition to the added pressure to overcome the elastic component of the lungs (static

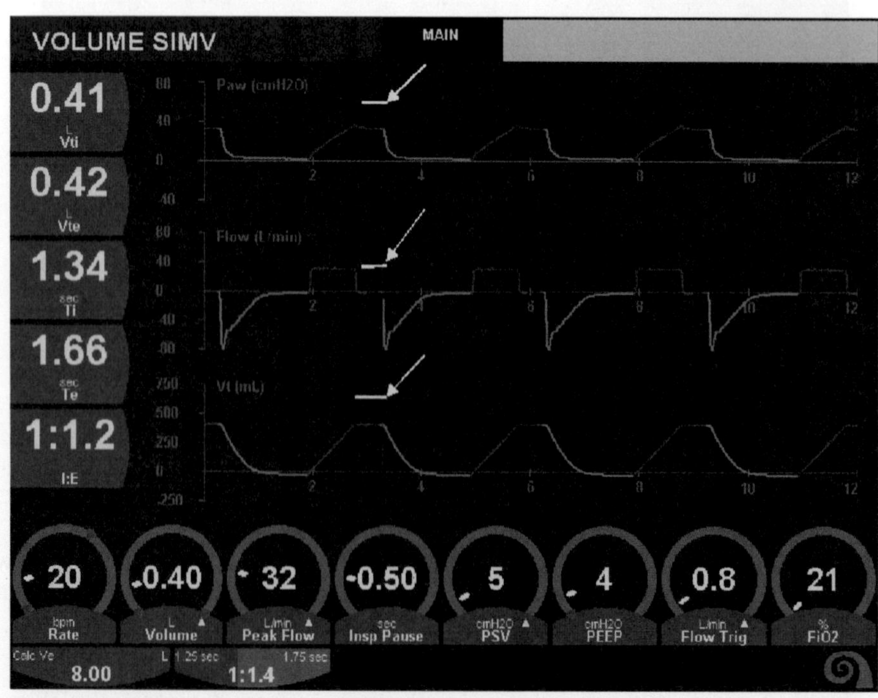

FIGURE 27-10 An inspiratory pause set to lengthen the inspiratory time.
Courtesy of CareFusion

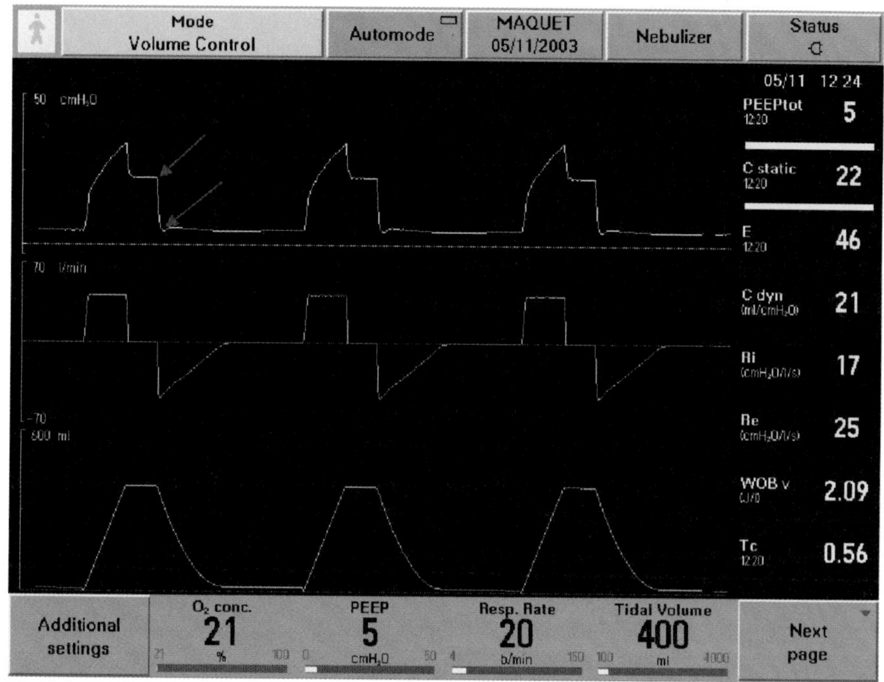

FIGURE 27-11 A calculation for compliance uses data from exhaled tidal volume divided by the plateau pressure minus the PEEP.

Courtesy of Maquet Inc.

compliance) during breath delivery.[6] Differences between peak pressure and plateau pressure are the result of resistance to inspiratory flow.

- Finally, the tip of the *volume scalar* has flattened out from its traditional triangular top. During the inspiratory pause, when no additional flow is entering the patient, no additional volume is added.

Static Compliance *Compliance* is equal to a volume change divided by a pressure change.[4] **Static compliance** is a compliance measurement done under conditions of no gas flow, and it can be trended over time using waveforms. Most modern ICU ventilators allow for an inspiratory pause to be set briefly in order to gain data, or it can be added to every mandatory breath to improve oxygenation. In Figure 27-11 the two arrows are pointing out the plateau pressure and the PEEP. The ventilator uses a formula to calculate the compliance using exhaled tidal volume divided by the plateau pressure minus the PEEP. Over time this data can be used as a trend to see whether the patient's lungs are becoming more or less compliant. The greater the difference is between plateau pressure and PEEP, the lower the compliance of the patient will be.

Airway Resistance Using the same trending technique, **airway resistance (R_{aw})** can also be monitored. *Resistance* is:

- The frictional force associated with ventilation due to the anatomical structure of conduit airways.
- The resistance to gas flow through the airways.
- The viscous resistance of the lungs and the adjacent tissues and organs as the lungs expand and contract.[4]

In Figure 27-12, the two arrows are pointing to the peak and plateau pressures. In trending airway resistance on a ventilator, these are the two parameters to monitor. If the plateau pressure remains constant, there is a directly related increase in the airway resistance with every increase in the peak pressure. This is a dynamic measurement. Table 27-2 demonstrates the relationship between compliance and resistance.

As another example of determining compliance change versus resistance change, see Figure 27-13. The pressure scalar makes it apparent that this is volume ventilation with an inspiratory pause set on each breath. A line drawn across the captured plateau pressures makes clear that these plateau pressures have remained the same. The peak pressures, however, show a significant reduction in pressure from the first breath to the second. This pattern is consistent with a decrease in R_{aw}. This type of reduction in R_{aw} could come from suctioning the patient or administering a bronchodilator.

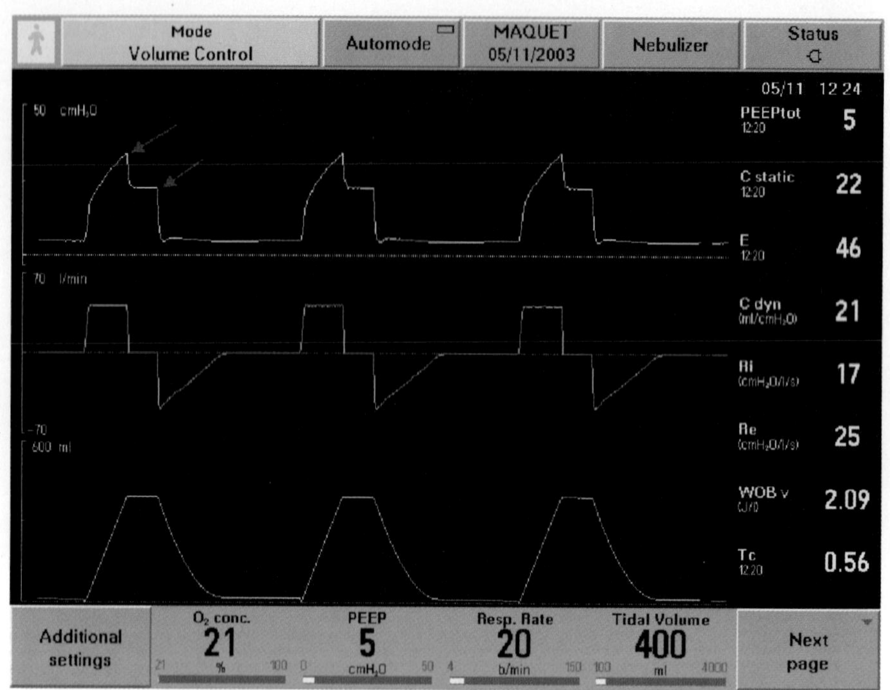

FIGURE 27-12 With every increase in the peak pressure, there is a directly related increase in the airway resistance if the plateau pressure remains constant.
Courtesy of Maquet Inc.

TABLE 27-2 **Compliance and resistance**

Peak pressure	Plateau pressure	Indicates
Increases	Remains the same	Increased RAW
Decreases	Remains the same	Decreased RAW
Remains the same	Increases	Decreased compliance
Remains the same	Decreases	Increased compliance
Increases	Increases	Decreased compliance and increased RAW
Decreases	Decreases	Increased compliance and decreased RAW

Figure 27-14 presents a change in airway resistance. The horizontal green line drawn over the pause of each breath shows that the plateau pressure has remained the same while the peak pressure has decreased. This pattern indicates a decrease in R_{aw}.

Synchronized Intermittent Mandatory Ventilation. *Synchronized intermittent mandatory ventilation* (*VC-SIMV*) is another type of volume ventilation; however, it is typically used with the addition of *pressure support ventilation* (*PSV*), which is a pressure type of ventilation. PSV is a patient-triggered, pressure-limited, flow-cycled mode of ventilator support that allows the patient control of the respiratory frequency, inspiratory time, and inspiratory flow rate.[9]

Figure 27-15 shows an example of a VC-SIMV with PSV. The third and seventh breaths, shown with arrows on the flow scalar, are clearly volume-type breaths with a set pause. However, the rest of the breaths look considerably different. The patient initiated these breaths. Because they are pressure support breaths, they have a decelerating flow pattern, and they are controlled by the patient throughout the entire cycle. This is a combination mode designed to be used for weaning.

Pressure Control Ventilation. As noted, pressure breaths look different from volume breaths. Figure 27-16 shows a breath under pressure type ventilation.

- (A) is the *beginning of inspiration*. Inspiration can be initiated by the ventilator or the patient depending on the mode of ventilation. If the patient has triggered the breath, a negative deflection appears just prior to the mechanical breath.

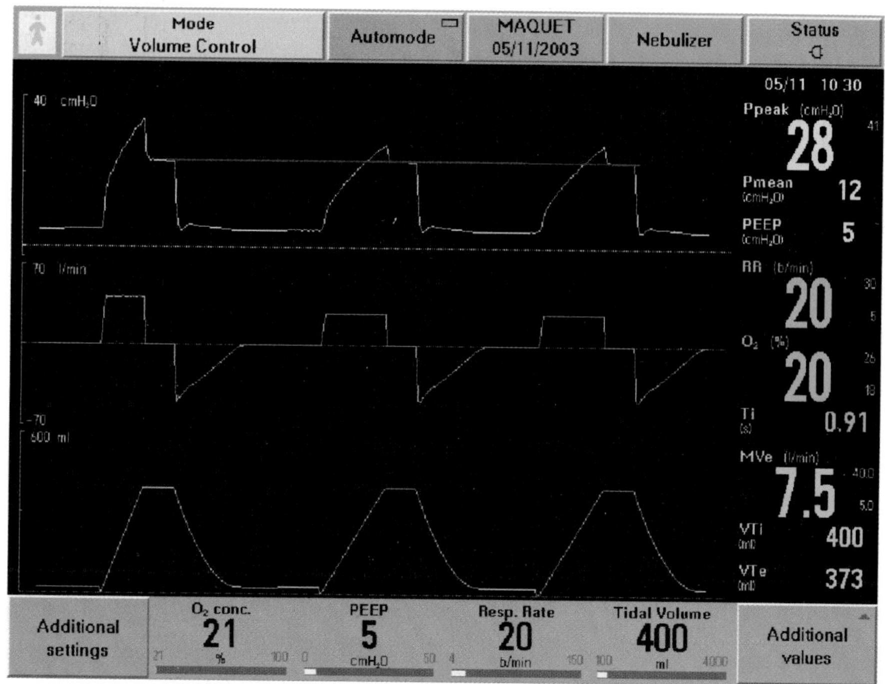

FIGURE 27-13 A significant reduction in pressure from the first breath to the second is consistent with a decrease in R_{aw}.
Courtesy of Maquet Inc.

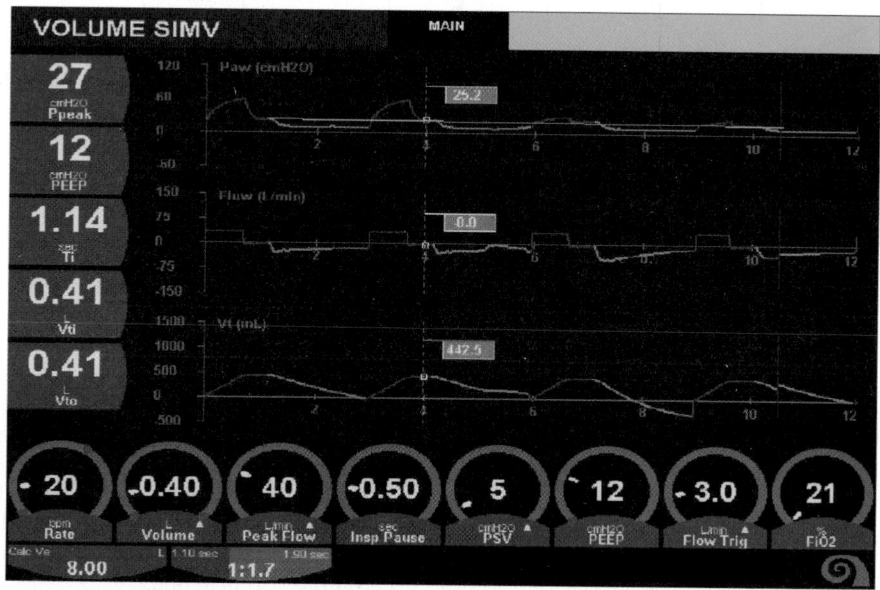

FIGURE 27-14 The plateau pressure has remained the same while the peak pressures mean has decreased, indicating a decrease in R_{aw}.
Courtesy of CareFusion

- (B) represents *inspiration or inspiratory time*. This period of time is set by the clinician on the ventilator. During the inspiratory portion of a pressure-controlled breath, the pressure is constant and the flow rate decelerates.
- (C) is the *end of inspiration* and the *beginning of exhalation*. Exhalation is passive and commences upon ventilator's opening the expiratory valve.
- (D) is the *end of exhalation*. In a normal breath, exhalation should return to baseline before the next breath begins. Characteristics of the lung can slow patient exhalation, as well as parts of the ventilator circuit, such as smaller endotracheal tubes and clogged expiratory filters.

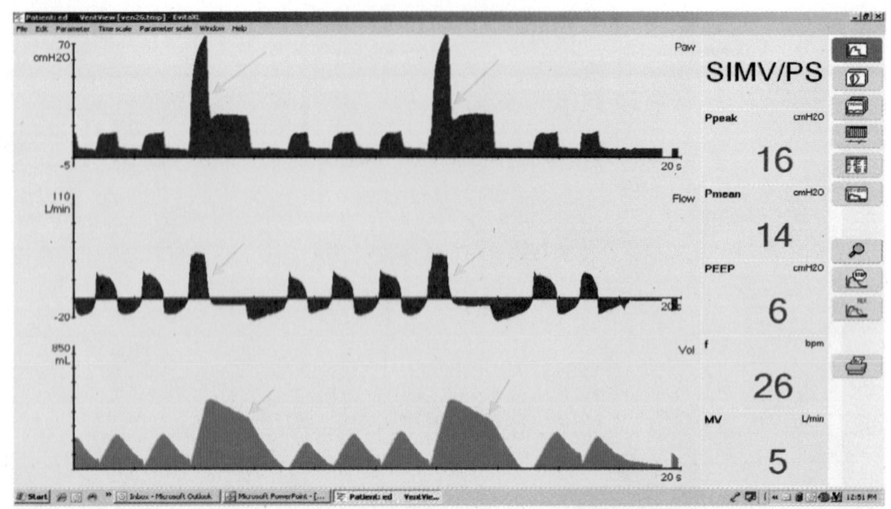

FIGURE 27-15 The third and seventh breaths, shown with arrows on the flow scalar, are volume-type breaths with a set pause; the remaining are pressure support breaths with a decelerating flow pattern, controlled by the patient throughout the entire inspiratory cycle.

Courtesy of Draeger Medical

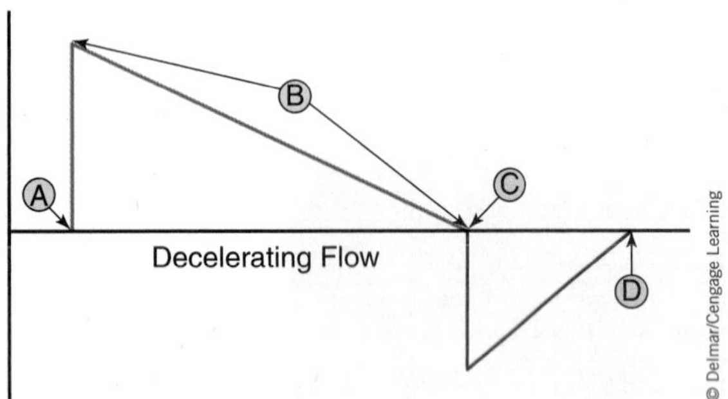

FIGURE 27-16 Pressure ventilation: (A) The beginning of inspiration. (B) Inspiration or inspiratory time. (C) The end of inspiration and the beginning of exhalation. (D) The end of exhalation.

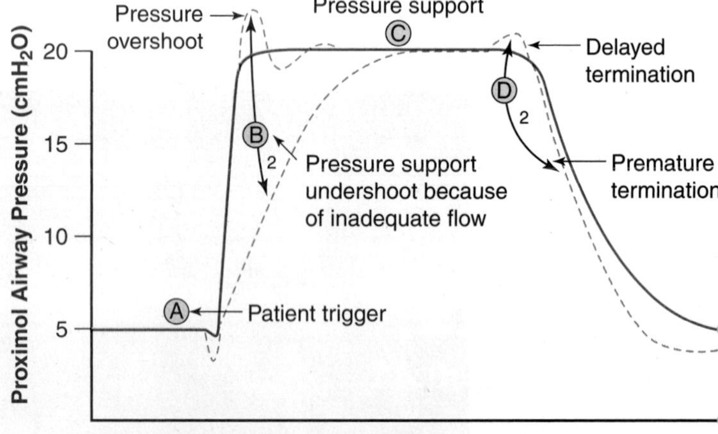

FIGURE 27-17 Pressure support breath: (A) The normal triggering of a spontaneous pressure support breath. (B) The rapid increase in pressure to the set pressure level. (C) The set inspiratory pressure level. (D) Inspiration terminates when the inspiratory flow decreases to the specific threshold of the system, allowing the pressure to drop back to baseline.

The most important facet of pressure support ventilation is the delivery of flow and responding pressures. Figure 27-17 presents the components that make up a pressure support:

- (A) represents the *normal triggering* of a spontaneous pressure support breath.
- (B) represents the rapid *increase in pressure* to the set pressure level (C). The tapered dotted line represents a scenario where the flow may be inadequate to meet the inspiratory demand of the patient. The patient may outstrip the available flow. The pressure overshoot can occur as a result of the quickly increasing pressure colliding with a small ETT or an obstructed airway. This pressure overshoot can also occur if the flow exceeds the patient's demand usually for a brief period before the pressure settles again to the set level.
- (C) represents the set inspiratory pressure level.
- In (D), inspiration terminates when the inspiratory flow decreases to the specific threshold of the system, allowing the pressure to drop back to baseline. Delayed termination can happen when a dysynchronous patient attempts to end the breath early.

Figure 27-18 presents the parts of the waveforms in pressure ventilation. In Figure 27-18A, the arrows on both breaths of the flow scalar (bottom waveform)

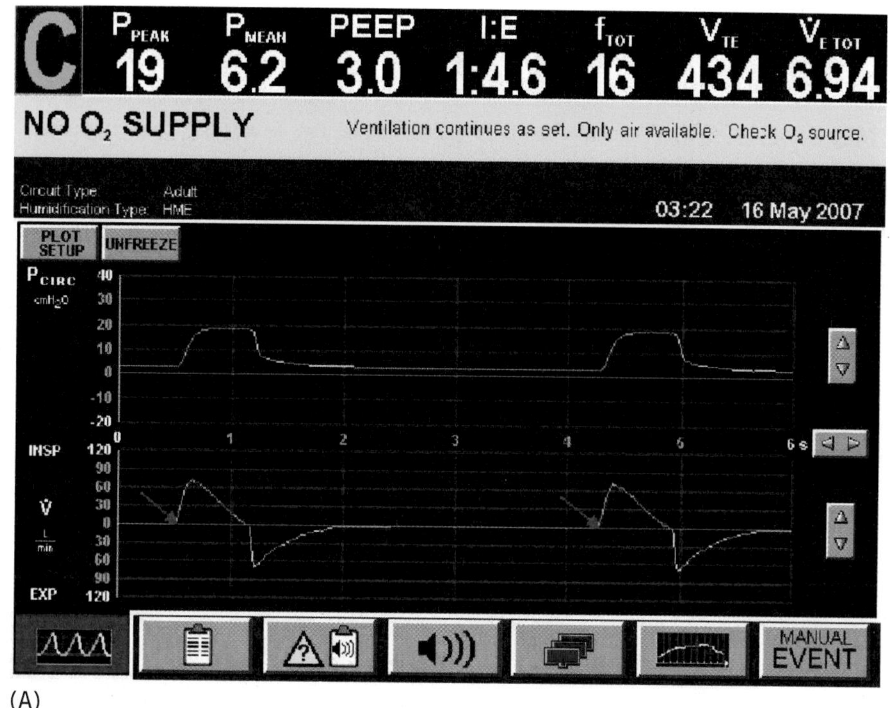

(A)

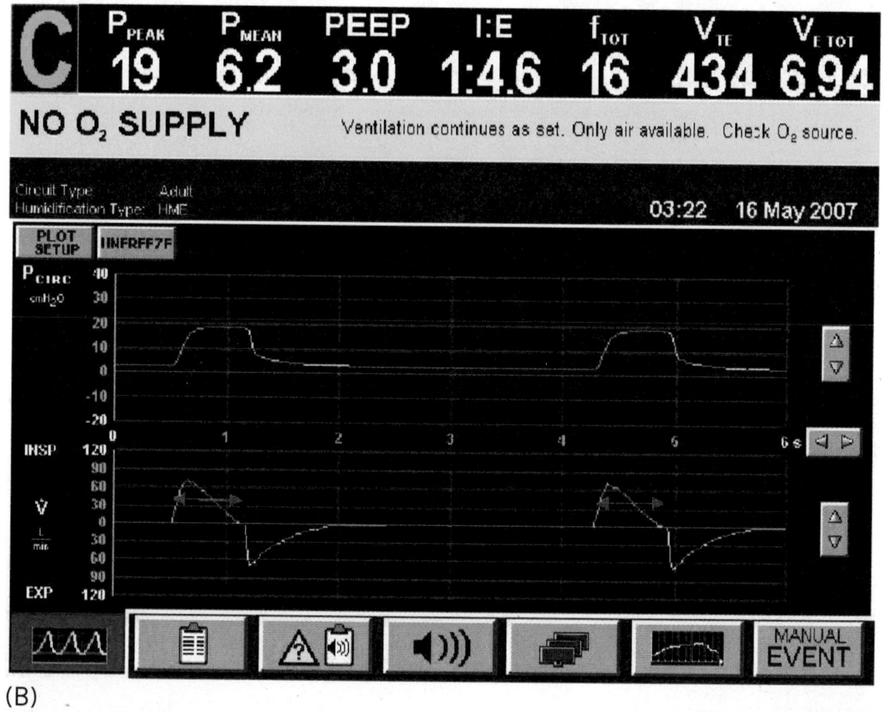

(B)

FIGURE 27-18 (A) The arrows on the flow scalar of both breaths indicate the beginning of inspiration of pressure type breaths. (B) A control mode of ventilation. (C) The first arrow on the first breath represents the beginning of exhalation; the second arrow represents the end of exhalation. This is an example of a normal breath with complete exhalation. (D) The red arrow represents the space between breaths. (*continues*)

Reprinted by permission from Nellcor Puritan Bennett LLC, Boulder, Colorado, part of Coviden

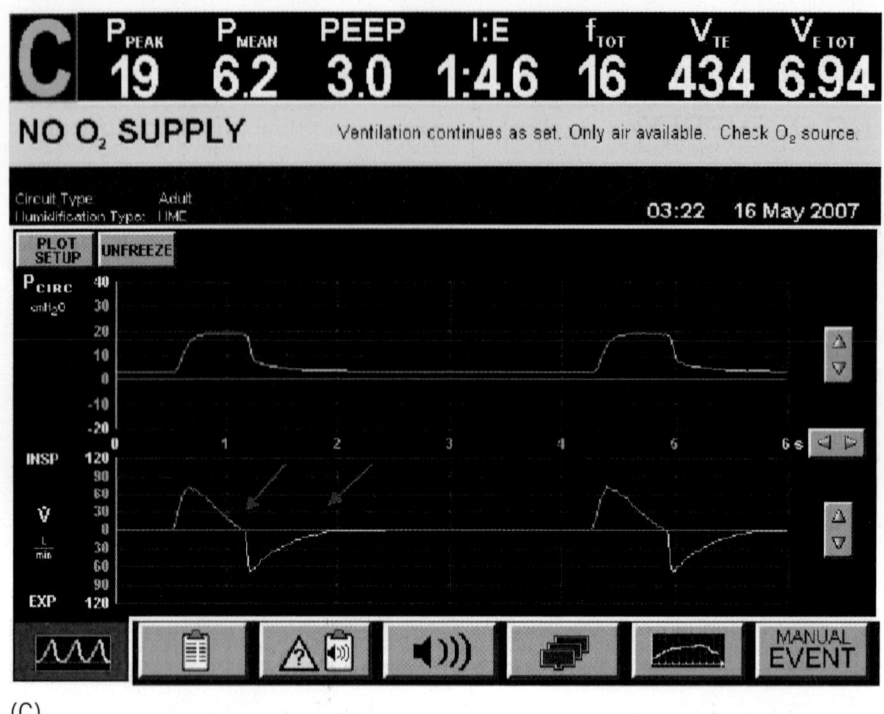

(C)

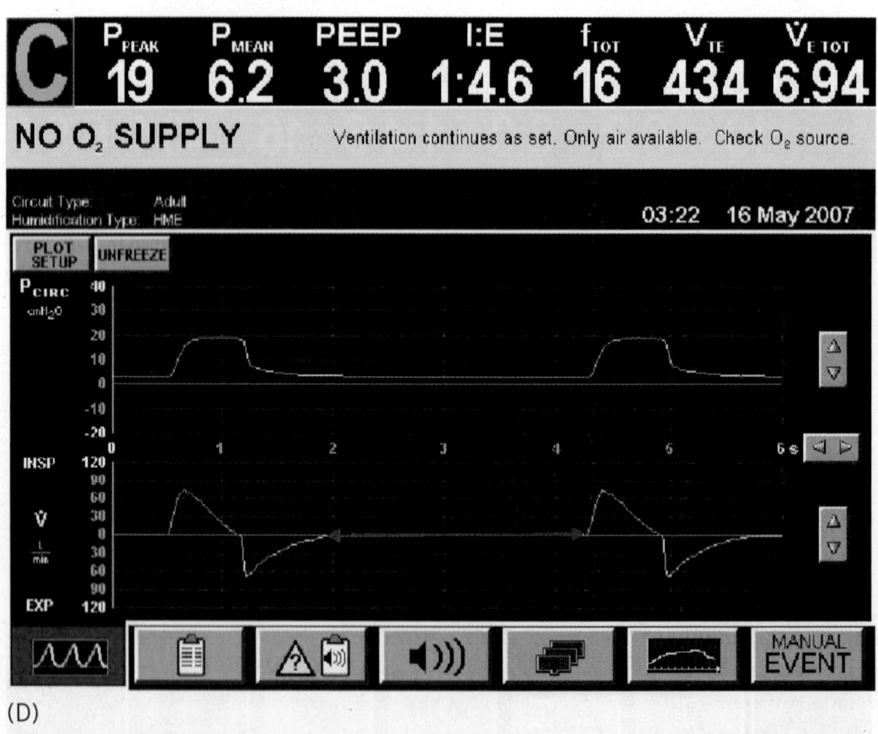

(D)

FIGURE 27-18 (*continued*)

indicate the beginnings of inspiration of these pressure type breaths. The inspiratory time is set by the clinician on the ventilator in controlled modes of ventilation.

Determining whether the mode is controlled, assist-controlled, support, or combination is the second step in interpreting waveforms. To determine the mode, examine the inspiratory time of all the breaths.

- Are they the same length?
- Do the breaths appear to be the same size and shape?

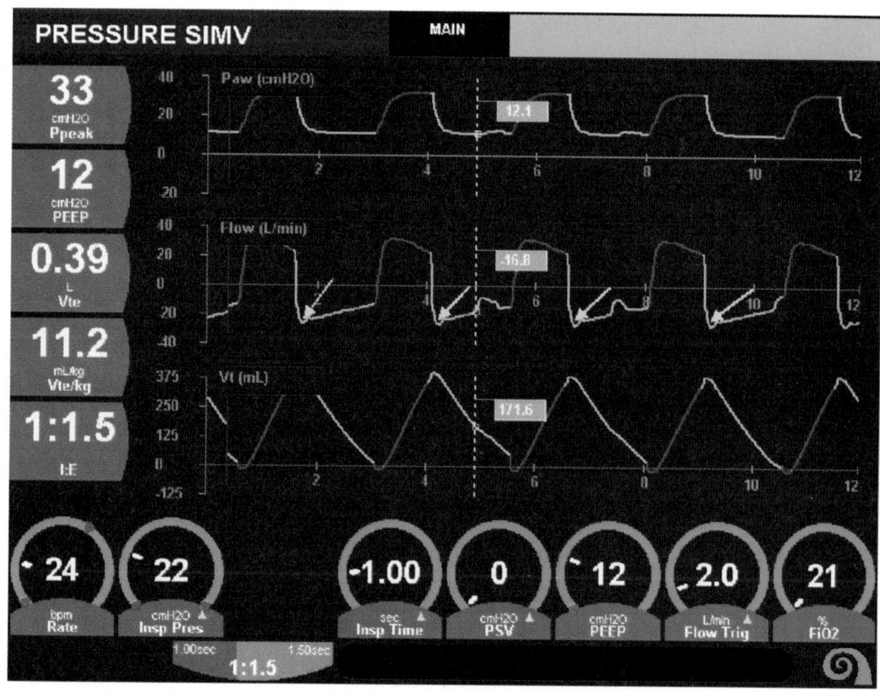

FIGURE 27-19 On each breath in the flow scalar, the arrow points to the beginning of inspiration for the following breath. The exhalation of each of these breaths is cut short by the patient's next breath, causing the patient to generate significant auto-PEEP over time.

Courtesy of CareFusion

If the answer is yes to these questions, as in the case of Figure 27-18B, the mode is controlled. In both support modes and combination modes, there would be some variability in the inspiratory times, sizes, and shapes of the breaths.

The first arrow on the first breath of the flow scalar of Figure 27-18C represents the beginning of exhalation. The second arrow represents the end of exhalation. Notice that when this patient is finished exhaling, the breath returns to baseline between breaths. This is an example of a normal breath with complete exhalation. If the tracing does not return to baseline, the patient did not completely exhale, indicating auto-PEEP.

In Figure 27-18D, the red arrow represents the space between breaths. This space is very important. For the patient to be able to completely exhale, the breath must return to the baseline for a period of time before the next breath begins. If this does not occur the patient generates auto-PEEP. The management of this space between breaths and ensuring that the breath returns to baseline is done by the precise control of the I/E ratio.

The Figure 27-19 graphic is from the VIASYS Avea ventilator. The screen is set up with the pressure scalar on top, the flow scalar in the middle, and the volume scalar on the bottom. This graphic is an example of pressure type ventilation where the exhaled breath does not return to baseline. On each breath in the flow scalar, the arrow points to the beginning of inspiration for the following breath. The exhalation of each of these breaths is cut short by the patient's next breath, causing the patient to generate significant auto-PEEP over time.

Looking at the end of exhalation observe that in the best scenario the patient's breath should return to baseline between breaths. Now examine the beginning of inspiration again and see how rise time can affect a pressure type breath.

Earlier in this chapter, Figure 27-9D illustrated the effects of rise time on the waveform of volume type ventilation. Rise time has a similar effect graphically in pressure type ventilation, but it can be slightly more difficult to see. Figure 27-20A presents an example of pressure type ventilation. In looking at the flow scalar it is observed that by comparing the ventilator waveform to the drawn in line that there is a slight difference. Typically, with decelerating waveforms in pressure type ventilation, the flow starts at peak and then decreases in a linear manner. There is a slight delay in this graphic in reaching peak flow. This is rise time, and it allows the clinician to slow the initial gas flow to meet the needs of the patient. The clinician has a range of choices depending on the ventilator being used. Faster

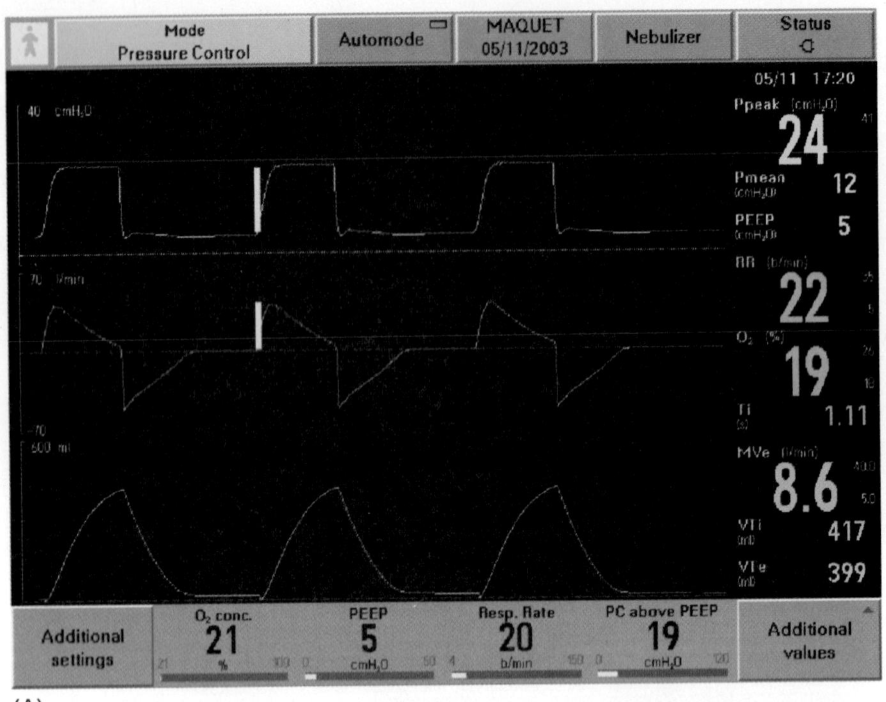

(A)

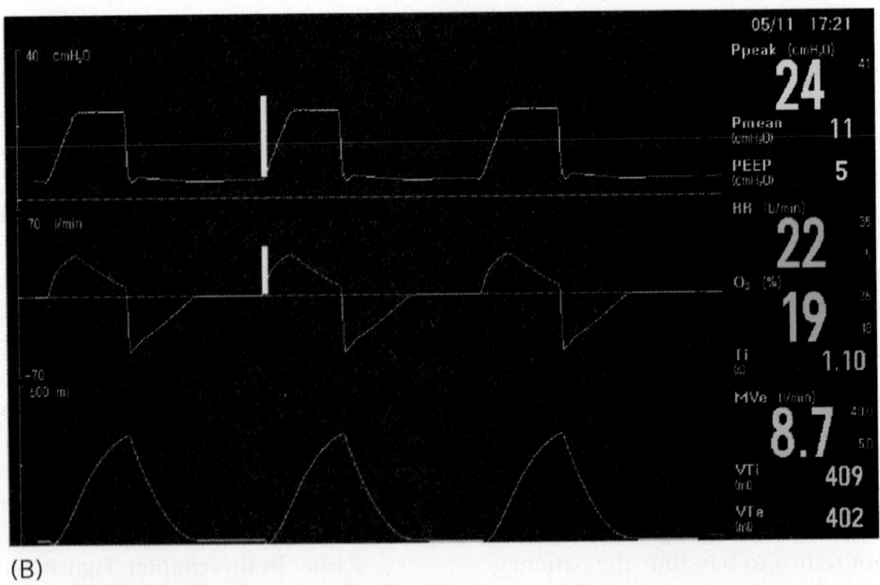

(B)

FIGURE 27-20 (A) Comparing the ventilator waveform to the drawn line shows a slight difference; the delay in reaching peak flow is rise time. (B) This patient has a set rise time, as illustrated by comparing the drawn line and the actual waveforms. (C) On the second breath, an arrow points to the end of inspiration. This same point is also the beginning of exhalation. In this example, the end of inspiration is exactly correct for this patient. (*continues*)

Courtesy of Maquet Inc.

rise times allow for more available flow and can decrease the work of breathing for the patient. If the rise time slows the flow too much, it can be inadequate for the patient, making the patient flow starved and dyssynchronous. The flow waveform should smoothly reach peak flow and then gradually decrease.[10]

In Figure 27-20B, a comparison of the drawn line and the actual waveforms shows that this patient has a set rise time. The delay is much more significant than in the last example in Figure 27-20A. In this scenario, the flow takes longer to reach peak. This setting is used mostly for patient comfort and to improve synchrony

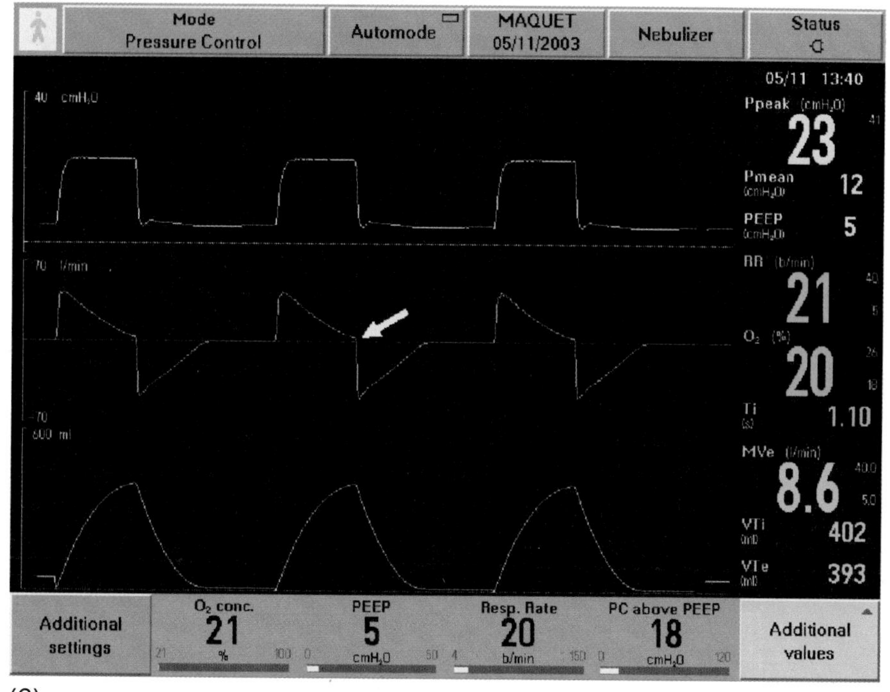

(C)

FIGURE 27-20 (*continued*)

with the ventilator. However, it affects both the ability of the ventilator to meet the patient's flow demands and the **mean airway pressure (MAP)**,[11] which is the average pressure occurring in the airway during the complete respiratory cycle.[6] Although rise time does not change, the set inspiratory time does change the amount of time the peak flow/pressure is applied to the airways. This can affect the MAP by decreasing it overall.[12]

We have looked at the end of exhalation and the beginning of inspiration so far. It is time to look at the end of inspiration. Due to their respective flow waveforms, it is much more important to look at the end of inspiration in pressure type ventilation than it is in volume ventilation. In volume ventilation, the square flow waveform gives no graphic indication of an optimized inspiratory time. In pressure ventilation, however, there is a decelerating flow waveform. This waveform is the most similar to a normal, unventilated breathing pattern (negative pressure), and it can be seen graphically if there are optimal settings for the inspiratory time.

Figure 27-20C shows a pressure type ventilation. In the flow scalar for the second breath, an arrow points to the end of inspiration. This same point is also the beginning of exhalation. In this example, the end of inspiration is exactly correct for this patient. It should decelerate linearly until it reaches the baseline, after which exhalation immediately follows. Inspiratory time, or flow rate, can be set only in controlled and assist-controlled modes of ventilation. In spontaneous modes, the patient controls the entire inspiratory cycle. In combination modes, the T_i, or flow rate, can be set only on the mandatory breaths, and often the inspiratory time is set incorrectly. It is a setting or parameter on the ventilator that should be checked frequently because the requirements may change for a patient several times throughout a day.

Figure 27-21 is an example of pressure ventilation where the inspiratory time is significantly shorter than optimal. On the flow scalar for the first breath, a red arrow indicates where inspiration has been prematurely ended. On the flow scalar for the second breath, a red dotted line represents the plane the tracing should have followed if the T_i had been optimally set.

Figure 27-22 also shows the end of inspiration. In the flow scalar (middle waveform), the arrows show that inspiration ends long before the breath reaches baseline. The inspiratory time is too short and therefore not optimized for this patient. Optimizing this T_i means that it is increased until the breath tracing reaches the baseline, thereby increasing the inspiratory time and the MAP. Increasing the MAP is a technique often used to increase the patient's oxygenation.[12]

Figure 27-23 demonstrates pressure type ventilation. On the flow scalar (middle waveform), the inspiratory times are not all the same for the three breaths shown. In the first breath on the flow scalar, the inspiratory time is set too long; note the arrow. The breath returns to the baseline and continues to follow the baseline for a period of time before allowing the patient to exhale. This is not an optimized inspiratory

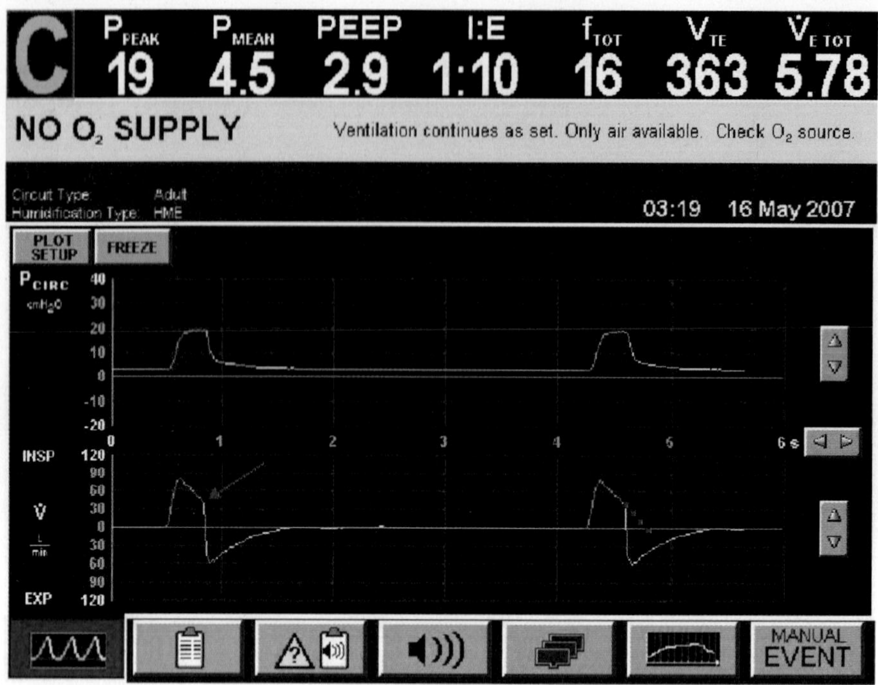

FIGURE 27-21 On the flow scalar for the first breath, a red arrow indicates where inspiration has been prematurely ended. On the flow scalar for the second breath, a red dotted line represents the plane the tracing should have followed if the T_i had been optimally set.

Reprinted by permission from Nellcor Puritan Bennett LLC, Boulder, Colorado, part of Coviden

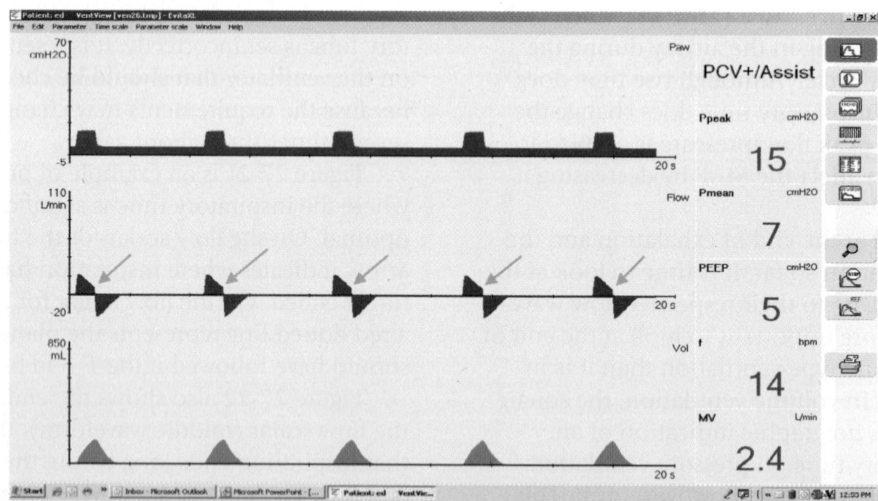

FIGURE 27-22 In the flow scalar (middle waveform), the arrows show that inspiration ends long before the breath reaches baseline. The inspiratory time is too short and therefore not optimized for this patient.

Courtesy of Draeger Medical

time. Although it is longer and increases the MAP, it can also increase asynchrony between the patient and the ventilator. At times, increasing the inspiratory time to beyond optimal is a technique used to increase oxygenation and may be an inverse ratio type of ventilation. This is not considered a normal inspiratory time.

Figure 27-24 is an example of pressure type ventilation with an inappropriately set inspiratory time. Notice the second breath on the flow scalar. The inspiratory portion of the breath returns to the baseline and then follows the baseline for an extended period of time. The inspiratory portion of this breath should have ended sooner. In response to this extended

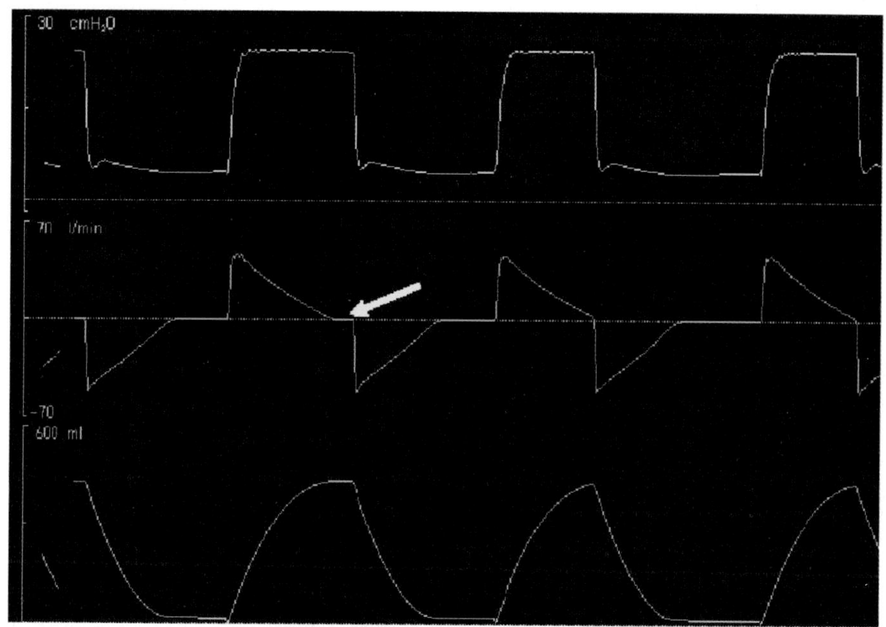

FIGURE 27-23 On the flow scalar (middle waveform), the inspiratory times are not all the same for the three breaths shown; the arrow indicates a inspiratory time that is set too long.

Courtesy of Maquet Inc.

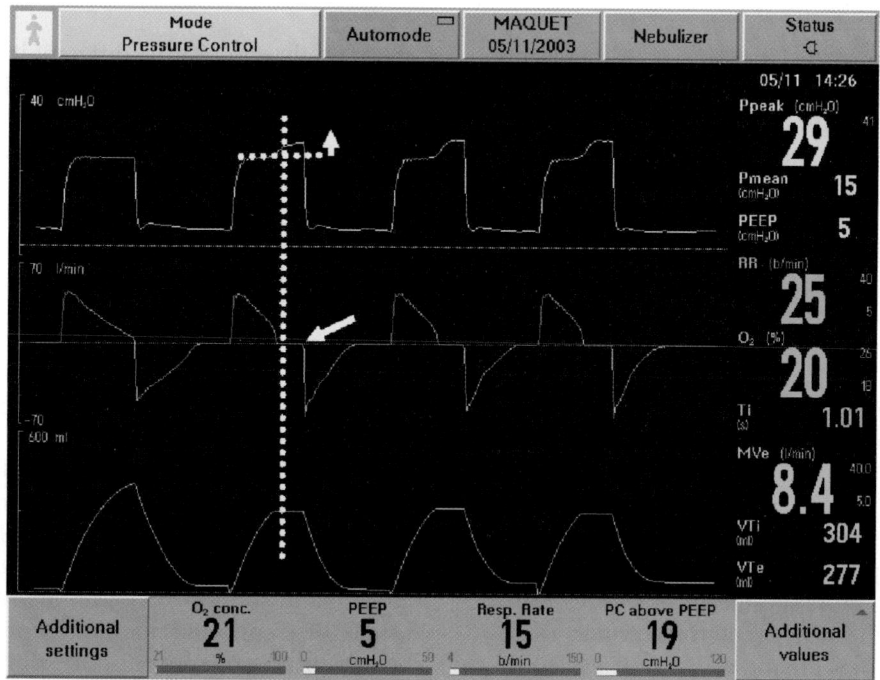

FIGURE 27-24 This is an example of asynchrony due to inappropriately set inspiratory time.

Courtesy of Maquet Inc.

inspiratory time, the patient begins to experience some asynchrony. Line up the pressure scalar (top waveform) with the point on the flow scalar where the inspiratory time should have ended (dotted vertical line), and note the corresponding increase in pressure directly following. This pressure increase is due to the patient attempting to exhale against the closed expiratory valve, which is closed due to the set inspiratory time. This is an example of asynchrony due to an inappropriately set inspiratory time. Learning to set an appropriate inspiratory time is one of the most beneficial aspects of mastering waveform analysis.

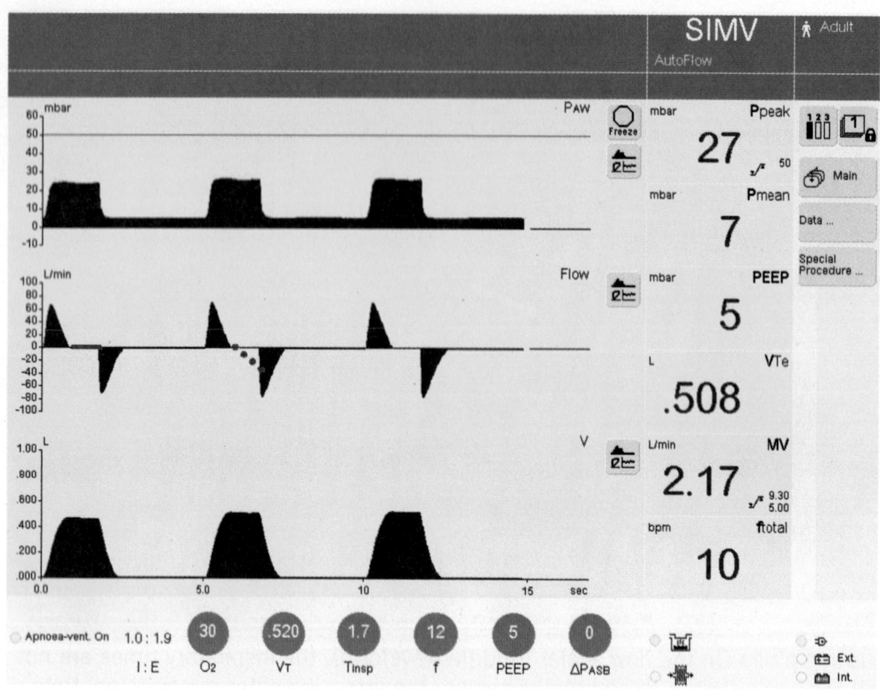

FIGURE 27-25 An example of an extended inspiratory time.
Courtesy of Draeger Medical

Figure 27-25 (from the Draeger Evita XL) presents another example of an extended inspiratory time. The top scalar of this ventilator is pressure versus time. The middle scalar is flow versus time, and the bottom scalar is volume versus time. The first breath on the flow scalar (the red line) is the portion of the inspiratory time where no additional flow is being added. The patient however, is unable to exhale due to the set T_i. The second breath in the flow scalar (the red dotted line) is the path that a more optimally set inspiratory time would follow. On the volume scalar, the typical triangular shape is not present. The top of the triangle is flattened out, signaling that a long inspiratory time or a pause is set.

Combination Mode Pressure Ventilation. Figure 27-26 presents another type of pressure ventilation. It is a combination mode, more specifically PC-SIMV with PSV. Again, follow the steps of interpretation to determine the type of ventilation.

Is it pressure or volume ventilation? The flow scalar is a decelerating flow waveform, which is generally indicative of pressure ventilation. In this case, every breath is a pressure type breath.

Is this is a controlled, support, or combination mode? Examine the inspiratory time, size, and shape of the breath. Are they all the same? In this example, not all the breath waveforms are identical. This must be either a support or combination mode, in which case some variability in inspiratory times is expected. There are not only significantly different inspiratory times, but also large volume and pressure differences between breaths. However, some of the breaths seem to follow a pattern and have similarity. The waveform begins with a mandatory pressure control breath, and then the next breath is a pressure support, patient-initiated breath. This pattern continues throughout the example. This is a combination mode pressure control synchronized intermittent mandatory ventilation (PC-SIMV).

The next step is to determine whether the mandatory breaths are optimized. Look closely at the inspiratory time of the mandatory breaths. The tops of the waveforms (note the arrows) appear to be somewhat flattened. Unless an inspiratory hold is clinically desired, the inspiratory time may be too long. This conclusion is confirmed by the slightly flattened tops of the volume tracings. When the control and support pressures are set close to each other, differentiating mandatory pressure control breaths from pressure support spontaneous breaths in the combination mode can be difficult—especially when the patient is initiating some or all of the mandatory breaths.

Pressure Support Ventilation. Figure 27-27 depicts pressure support ventilation (PSV). In this pressure type of ventilation, the waveform is characterized by a decelerating flow pattern. This is not a controlled mode. All breaths are initiated by the patient and may vary considerably in terms of their inspiratory times,

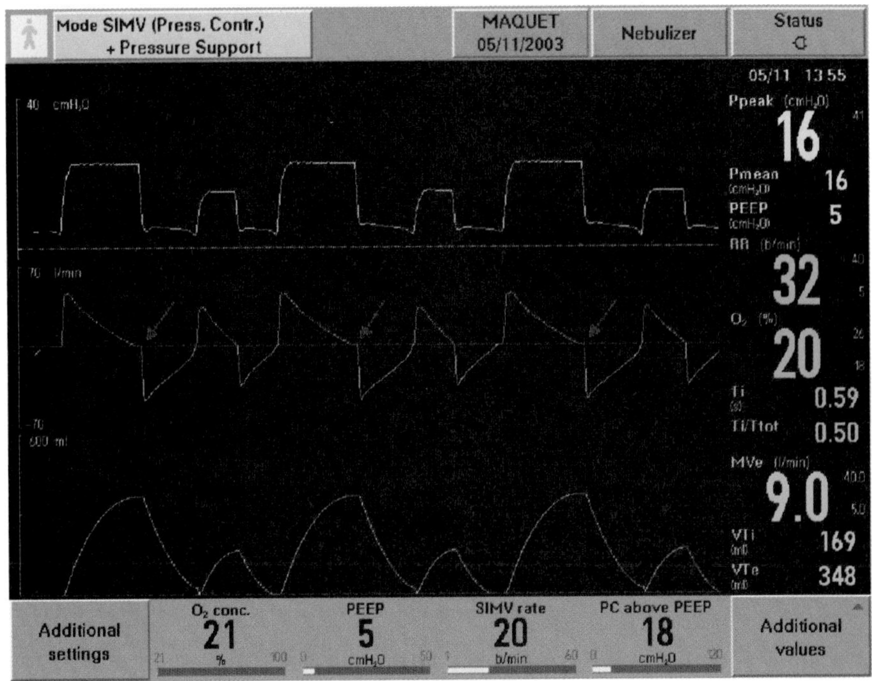

FIGURE 27-26 An example of a combination mode, more specifically PC-SIMV with PSV.

Courtesy of Maquet Inc.

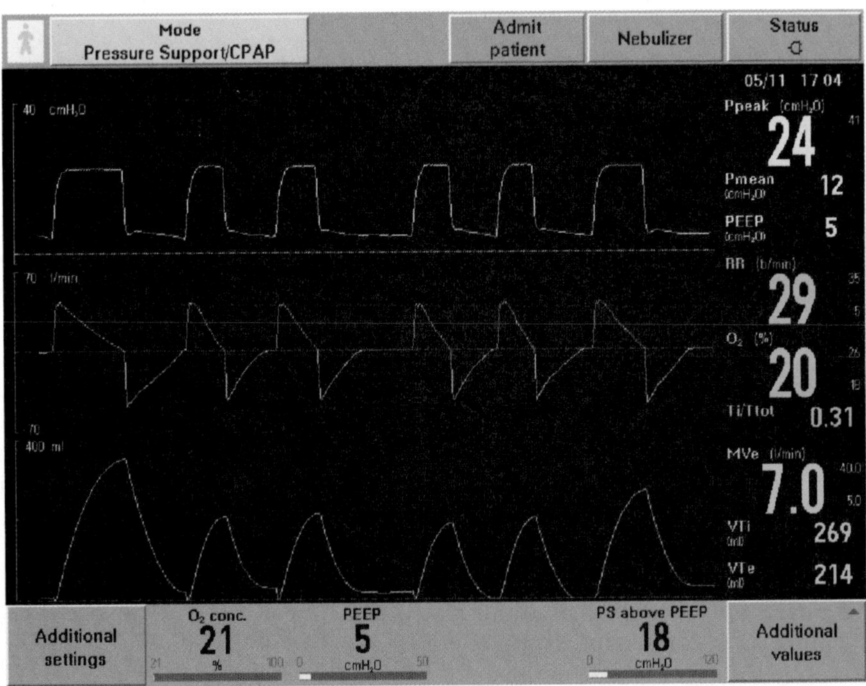

FIGURE 27-27 A pressure support ventilation.

Courtesy of Maquet Inc.

volumes, and shapes. To differentiate between a combination mode and a support mode, look at the volume and pressure delivered. The amount of pressure displayed on the pressure scalar remains consistent while there is a wide range of delivered volume. In this mode, the clinician sets an inspiratory pressure, but the tidal volume can vary greatly depending on patient effort and lung physiology.

Note that the patient has triggered each breath. The ventilator used to generate the waveform in Figure 27-27 notifies the clinician of patient triggering by turning the flow scalar from green to pink upon initiation of the

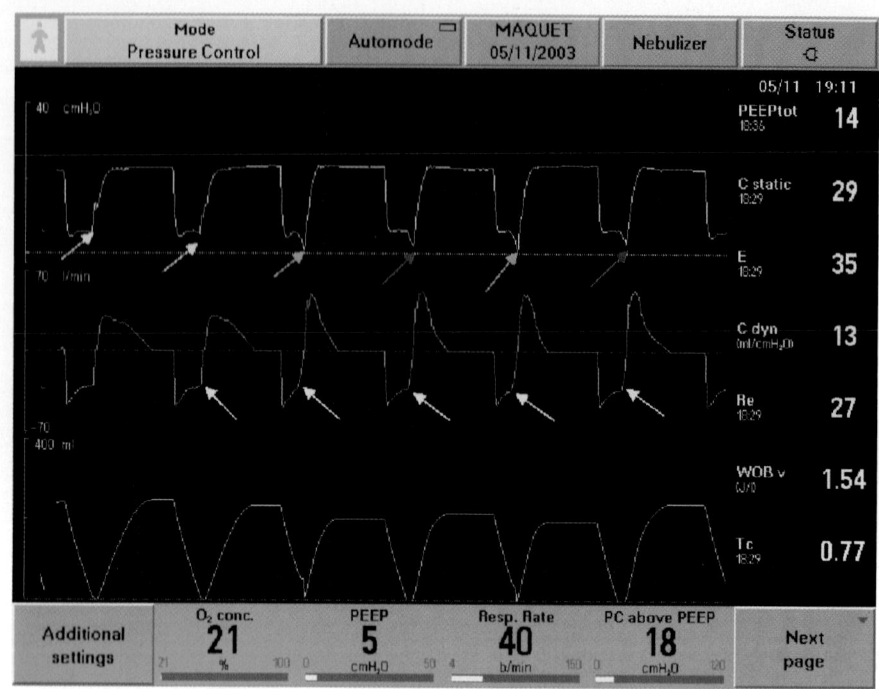

FIGURE 27-28 A pressure control ventilation in which the patient is attempting to trigger some of the pressure controlled breaths.

Courtesy of Maquet Inc.

breath. PSV is patient triggered and pressure limited. The ventilator can be initiated by either a pressure or a flow trigger.

- For the patient effort to be detected in pressure triggering, the patient must be able to decrease the airway pressure from the end-expiratory level to the predetermined negative pressure set on the ventilator (pressure sensitivity).
- Flow triggering is similar. The patient effort is detected by a flow change in the ventilator circuit beyond a predetermined parameter level set on the ventilator (flow sensitivity).

Triggering plays a large role in patient-ventilator synchrony. In addition to using a flow or pressure trigger, a patient can initiate a breath from the change in electrical activity of the diaphragm. *Neurally adjusted ventilatory assist* (*NAVA*) applies pressure in proportion to the strength of a diaphragmatic contraction. Inspiration is also terminated or cycled by a decrease in the electrical activity of the diaphragm.[13]

Auto-PEEP can have a negative impact on triggering. Patients must exert enough effort to first overcome the auto-PEEP before they can change flow or pressure enough to trigger the ventilator. The amount of effort it takes to overcome the auto-PEEP can be much greater than the effort needed to trigger the ventilator.[14,15]

In patients who are experiencing auto-PEEP, look for failed trigger attempts graphically. If this condition is found, clinicians can try to improve synchrony by making ventilator changes.

Figure 27-28 depicts pressure control ventilation. The patient is attempting to trigger some of the pressure controlled breaths. This patient has a significant amount of auto-PEEP (note the white arrows in the flow scalar). As a result, the patient is having difficulty triggering the ventilator (Servo^{i}), which has a flow trigger set as a parameter. The clinician is made aware of that because the flow scalar on some of the breaths has turned from green to pink, indicating patient triggering. If the ventilator were set for pressure triggering, this color change would be taking place in the pressure scalar when the patient initiated the breath. On the pressure scalar, the patient's trigger attempts are both successful and failed at times.

- In the first two breaths of the pressure graph, the patient did not attempt to take a breath; the breaths were mandatory breaths from the ventilator. There is no observable negative deflection just prior to the mechanical breath, which would indicate patient triggering. The corresponding flow scalar for these two breaths did not turn pink, indicating no patient effort.
- In the third breath on the pressure scalar, a blue arrow points to a decrease in pressure that reached baseline. This is a successful trigger by the patient. The effort was sufficient to decrease

the pressure enough to trigger the ventilator, even though the patient had to overcome the auto-PEEP. For the corresponding breath on the flow scalar, the tracing changed from green to pink, indicating a successful patient trigger.

- In the fourth breath on the pressure scalar, a red arrow points to a decrease in pressure that does not reach baseline. This is a failed trigger attempt. The patient was unable to generate enough effort to overcome the auto-PEEP and trigger the ventilator. In the corresponding breath in the flow scalar, there is no color change, indicating no registered effort by the patient.

Dyssynchrony caused from failed trigger attempts can be very fatiguing for the patient. Clinicians can adjust the sensitivity parameters to promote patient synchrony, but this can be a difficult task. A setting not sensitive enough can make the patient use considerable muscle effort, whereas a setting that is too sensitive can cause **autocycling**[3,10,14] (autotriggering), which occurs when the ventilator triggers a breath without a patient effort.[4] Autocycling can result from patient movement, a leak in the system, water in the ventilator circuit, or cardiogenic occilations.[10,13] Another common form of trigger asynchrony is double triggering or breath stacking. *Double triggering* happens when a patient has a continued inspiratory effort that causes a change in pressure or flow below the predetermined level that triggers a second breath prior to the set time frame.[10]

Figure 27-29 is an example of autocycling due to a leak in the system. The ventilator is cycling one breath after another without any delay or effort from the patient. Leaks are common in mechanical ventilation. Depending on its cause and size, the leak can be rather problematic in mechanical ventilation. In dealing with a leak, the first step is to identify the source and try to correct it. In some cases, the clinician is unable to completely correct the leak.

Figure 27-30 demonstrates a pressure support waveform with a leak. In the first breath on the flow scalar, the yellow arrow indicates a normal PSV breath. The inspiratory portion of the breath is a normal decelerating waveform that comes all the way to the baseline before the patient exhales. The second and the third breaths in the flow scalar, red arrows, show an abnormal waveform. On both breaths, the inspiratory portions begin to come toward the baseline, but, instead of going into exhalation, the tracing starts to travel upward again. The point at which the flow tracing turns upward and continues on is due to the leak.

This pattern is echoed in the volume tracing. In the first breath, the blue arrow shows a normal breath. The second and third breaths, however, do not have the characteristic shape expected with a pressure support breath (a triangle tipped to the right.) The white arrows point to the portion of the tracing that shows the leak. The tracing is showing that the volume delivered is not returning to the baseline. Instead of the lungs filling and the patient ending inspiration, thereby signaling the ventilator to end inspiration, the volume continues to be delivered and is lost to the leak.

The ventilator, of course, cannot tell the difference between an excessively long inspiration and a leak. If the leak is large, it can cause dyssynchrony at times because the patient is unable to end inspiration. In

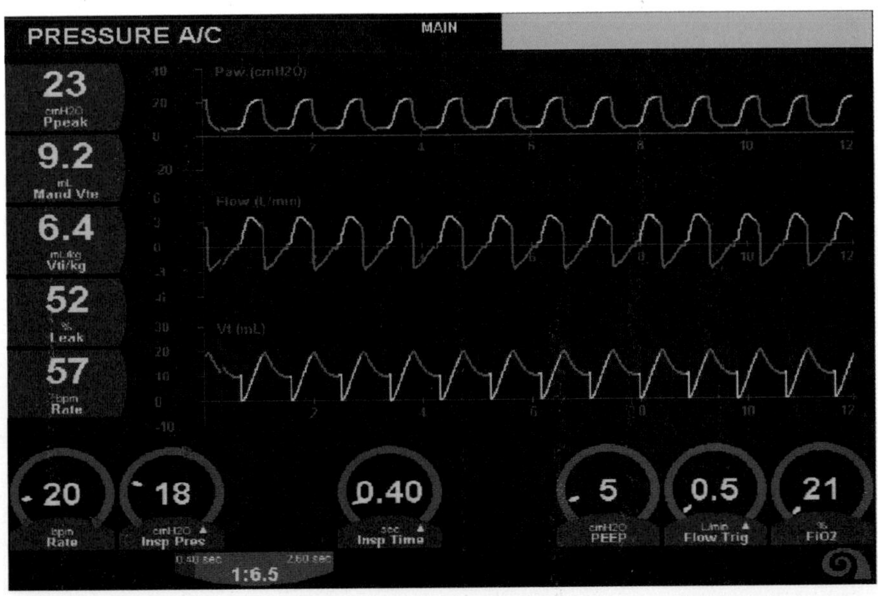

FIGURE 27-29 Autocycling due to a leak in the system.

Courtesy of Maquet, Inc.

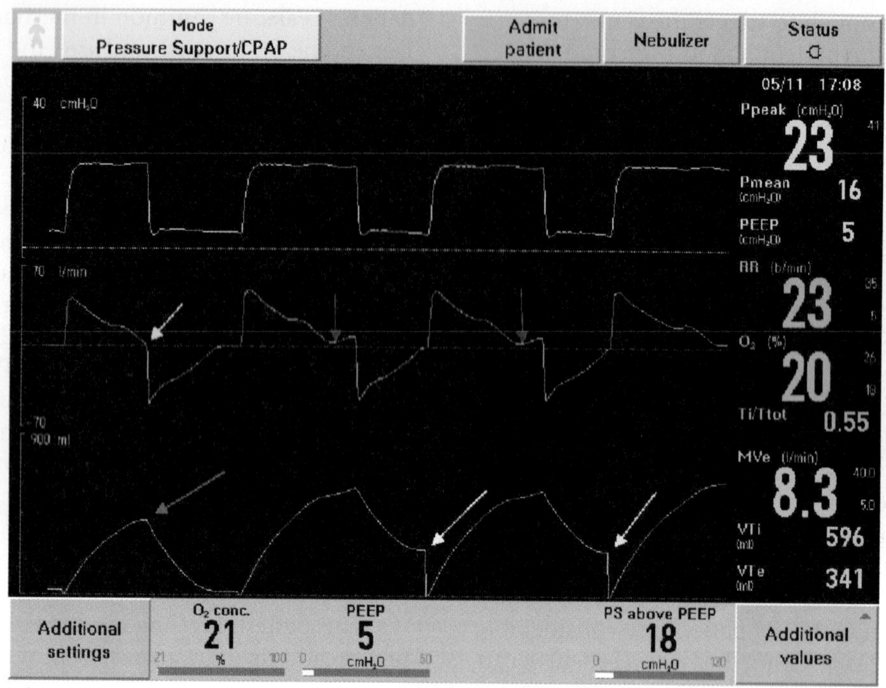

FIGURE 27-30 A pressure support waveform with a leak.
Courtesy of Maquet Inc.

support modes, ventilators have a built-in time threshold for inspiration that tells them to stop inspiration for safety purposes. (In support modes, the patient is in control of the entire breath cycle.) If a leak occurs in a support mode, the patient may not be able to control inspiration due to inadequate respiratory muscle strength. Some ventilators also have a parameter, called **inspiratory cycle off**, that allows the clinician to decide when inspiration should end based on graphics in pressure support. In controlled modes, the inspiratory time is already the limit; there is no need for a further parameter control. Inspiratory cycle off allows the clinician to end inspiration before the leak.

Figure 27-31 is another example of a leak. The dotted yellow line shows where the leak is occurring.

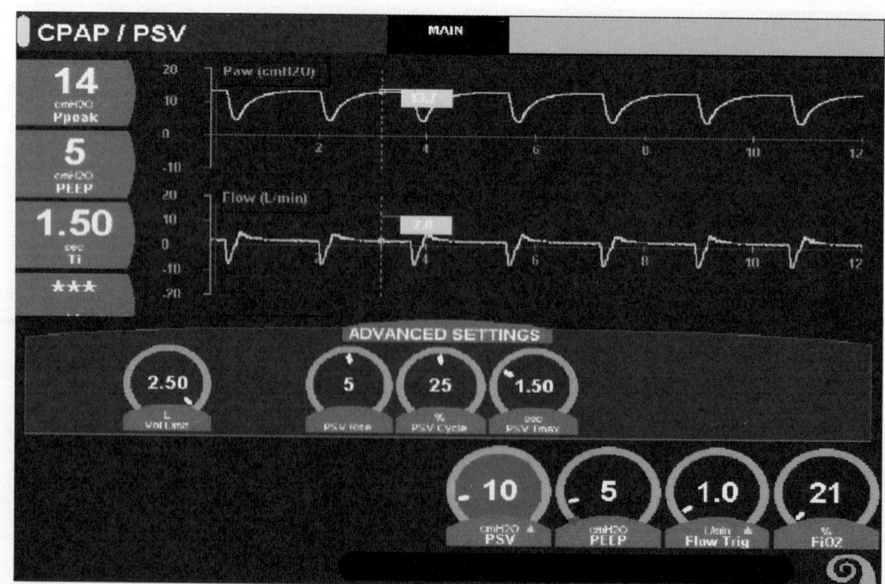

FIGURE 27-31 A leak: The dotted yellow line shows where the leak is occurring.
Courtesy of CareFusion

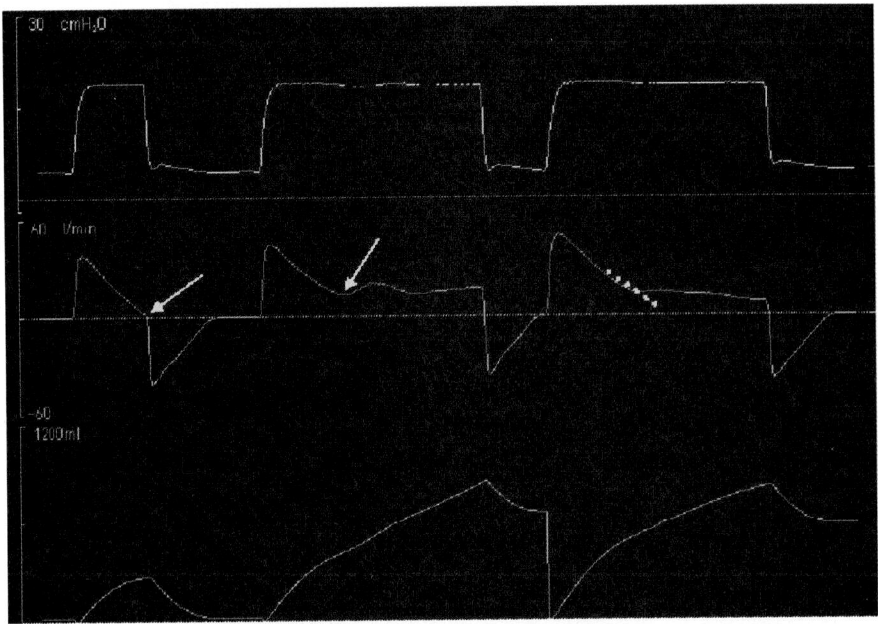

FIGURE 27-32 A pressure support ventilation with a leak.
Courtesy of Maquet Inc.

Figure 27-32 demonstrates a pressure support ventilation with a leak. The first breath in the flow scalar is a normal breath. The second breath is showing a leak. The yellow arrow points to where the leak is beginning and where the breath should be cycled off by the clinician, using the parameter inspiratory cycle off. The third breath in the flow scalar also shows the same leak. The drawn line through the breath shows the path the breath should have followed without the leak. This is also the path the breath will take once the breath has been cycled off.

Figure 27-33 is a pressure support with the additional setting page of the Servo^i ventilator open. This patient had a leak that was treated by setting inspiratory

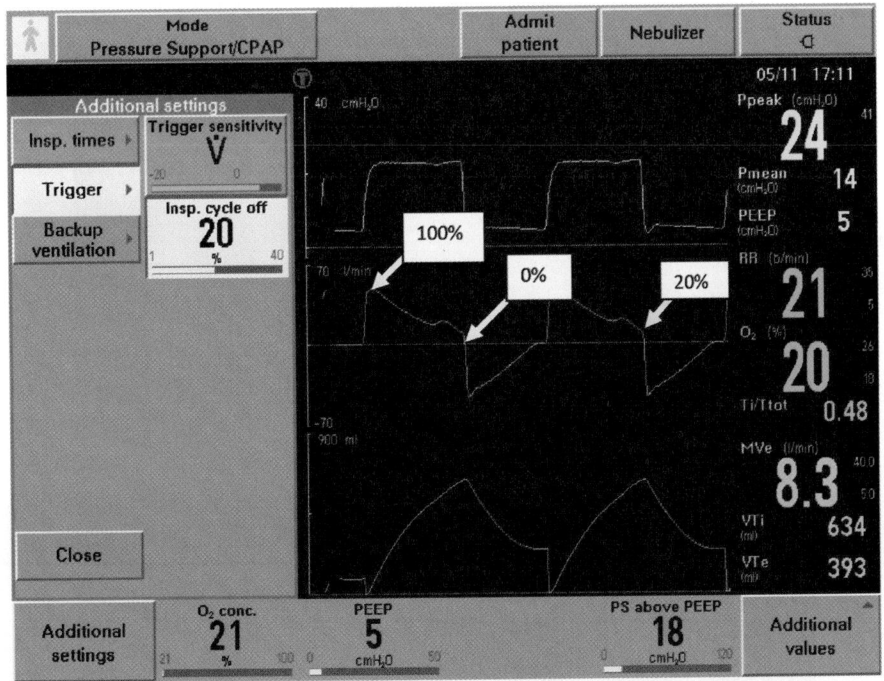

FIGURE 27-33 A pressure support with the additional setting page of the Servo^i ventilator open.
Courtesy of Maquet Inc.

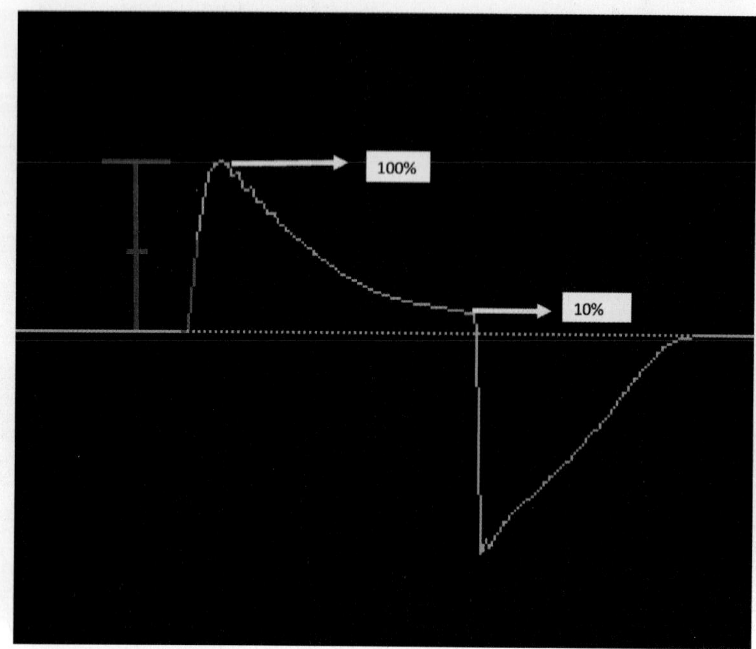

FIGURE 27-34 A pressure support breath being cycled off at 10% of peak flow.

Courtesy of Maquet Inc.

cycle off. In the first breath on the flow scalar, two white arrows point out 100% of peak flow and baseline, or 0%, of peak flow. The goal of setting the inspiratory cycle off is to set the terminal flow level higher than the leak in order to stop the extended inspiratory time. The second breath of the flow scalar has a yellow arrow pointing to the 20% point, where the inspiratory cycle off is set. The inspiratory flow off allows the patient to begin exhalation, thereby improving synchrony. Figure 27-34 demonstrates a pressure support breath cycled off at 10% of peak flow.

Figure 27-35 shows a pressure support breath with a leak. The breath is being cycled off at 60% using the inspiratory cycle off parameter. This is a large leak.

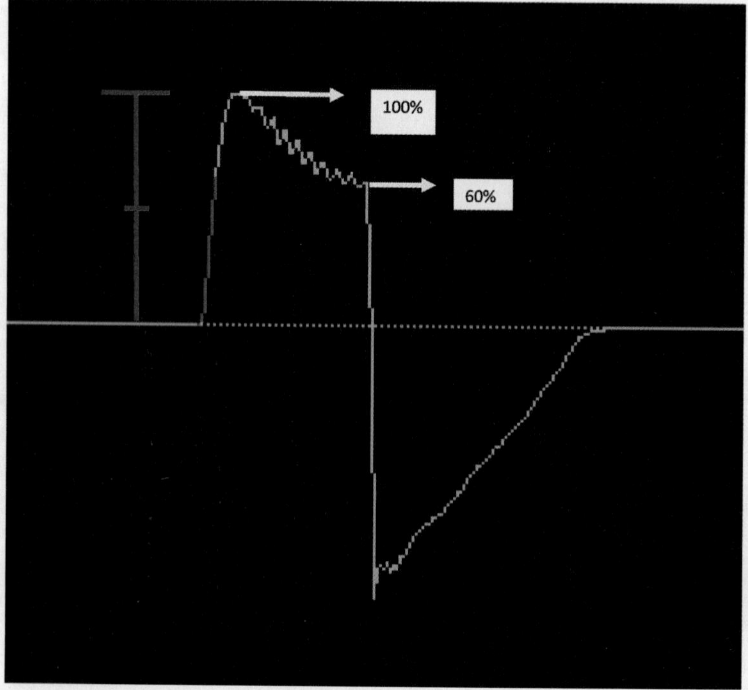

FIGURE 27-35 A pressure support breath with a leak.

Courtesy of Maquet Inc.

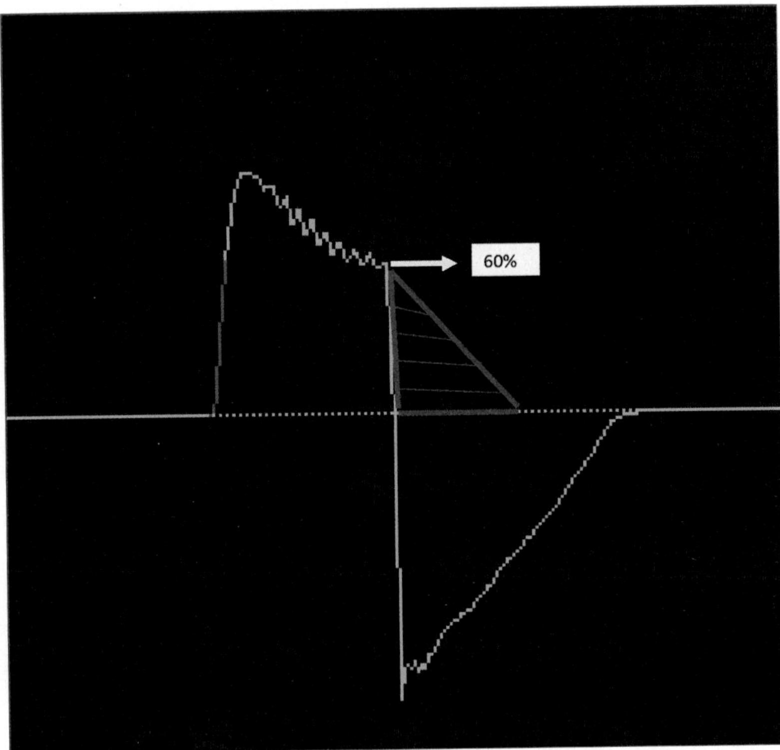

FIGURE 27-36 A pressure support breath that has been cycled off at 60% due to a large leak.
Courtesy of Maquet Inc.

When patients have large leaks like this one, the clinician must be aware that the patient is losing a lot of tidal volume. Every effort should be made to determine where the leak is and, to the extent possible, eliminate it.

Figure 27-36 shows a pressure support breath that has been cycled off at 60% due to a large leak. The red shaded area approximates the volume being lost by cycling this breath off so early in the inspiratory phase. This volume would also be lost to some degree should the leak remain uncorrected. In addition, the patient would have considerable dyssynchrony, and perhaps discomfort, if such a large leak were left untreated. The amount of loss to the leak can be calculated as follows:

$$\text{leak percentage} = \frac{\text{inspiratory volume} - \text{expiratory volume}}{\text{inspiratory volume}} \times 100$$

Loops

Clinicians can use loops much as they use scalar waveforms. The patterns are recognizable and can aid in diagnosing and trending changes in the patient's lung characteristics. Two types of loops are discussed here: a pressure-volume loop and a flow-volume loop (Figure 27-37). Both types of loops are made up of inspiratory and expiratory phases that are connected but not related to time. The easiest way to interpret loops is to become familiar with what the normal loops look like for both types.

PRESSURE-VOLUME LOOPS

Figure 27-38 demonstrates a normal **pressure-volume loop** in mechanical ventilation that traces changes in pressures and corresponding changes in volume. Normal pressure-volume loops should sit at a 45° angle within the two axes, the vertical axis being volume and the horizontal being pressure. This loop is often referred to as football shaped, but in reality it rarely has equal or symmetrical halves for inspiration and expiration. In this example, the upper half is expiration, and the lower half is inspiration.

Inspiration begins from the FRC level and terminates when the preset parameter (volume or pressure) is achieved. The tracing continues during expiration and returns to FRC at end of exhalation. Peak inspiratory pressure and delivered tidal volume are readily obtained from the pressure-volume loop.[16] The pattern is drawn counterclockwise with each breath. The points marked with 1 and 2 indicate the inflections during inspiration (point 1) and exhalation (point 2) of this breath.

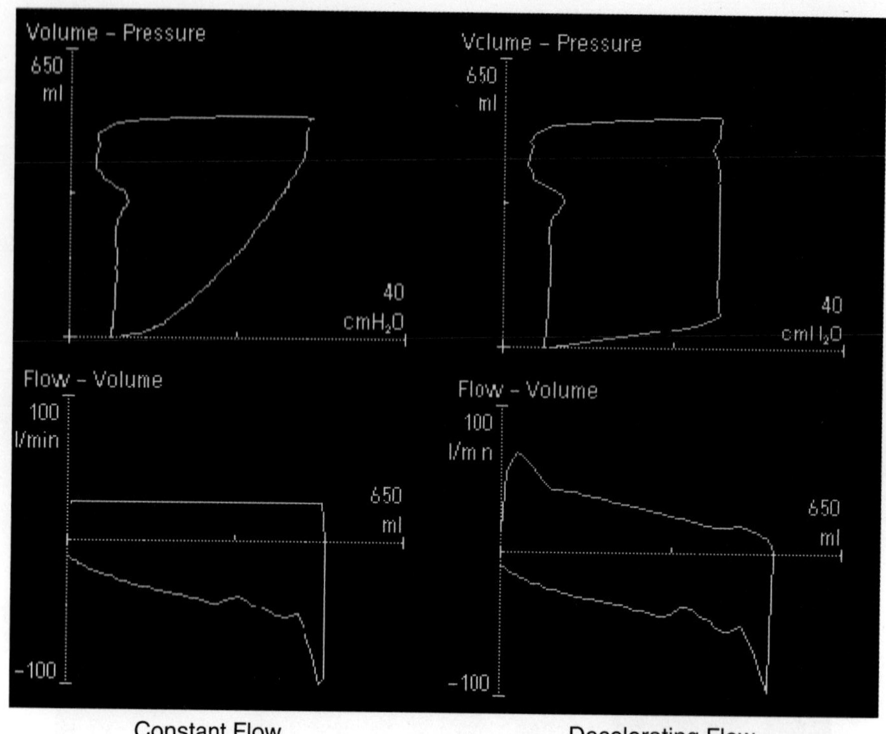

FIGURE 27-37 Examples of loops.

Courtesy of Maquet Inc.

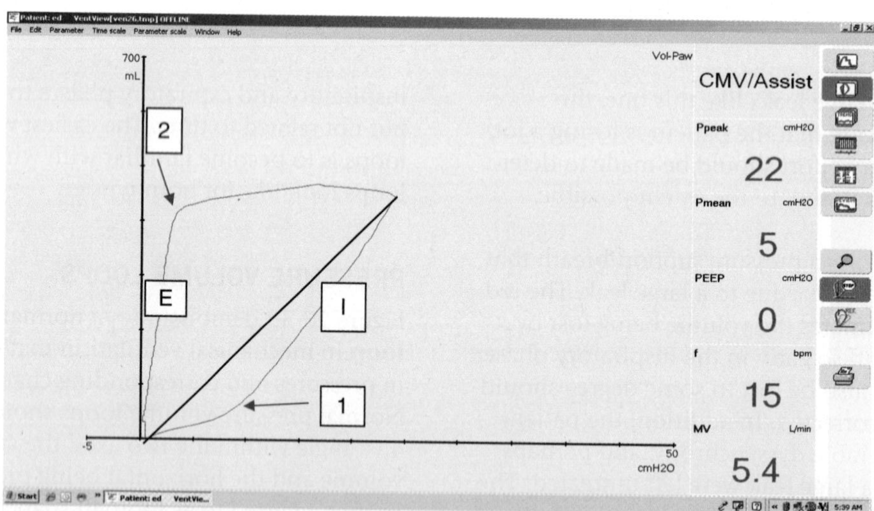

FIGURE 27-38 A normal pressure-volume loop in mechanical ventilation that traces changes in pressures and corresponding changes in volume.

Courtesy of Draeger Medical

Historically, these inflection points have been thought to represent the onset of recruitment of the alveoli during inspiration and the derecruitment of alveoli during exhalation. More recently it has been found that recruitment can occur throughout inflation at a wide range of pressures.[17] It is also thought that an upper inflection point during inspiration can be used as a reference for overdistension (Figure 27-42). The idea is that the best compliance for a patient is between the two inflection points and that ventilating the patient using pressures within the zone limited by the upper and lower inspiratory inflection points may prevent damage to the lung tissue.[17,18]

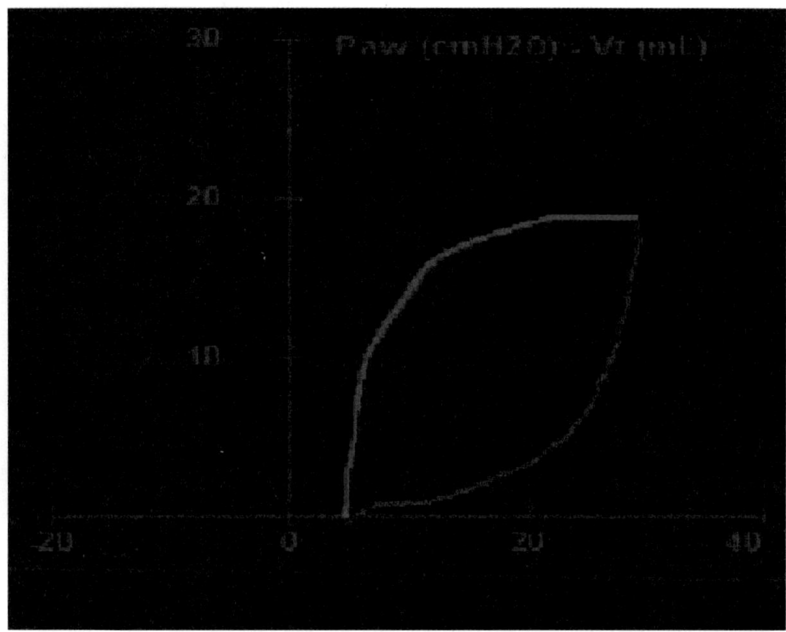

FIGURE 27-39 A volume-pressure loop with normal compliance.
Courtesy of CareFusion

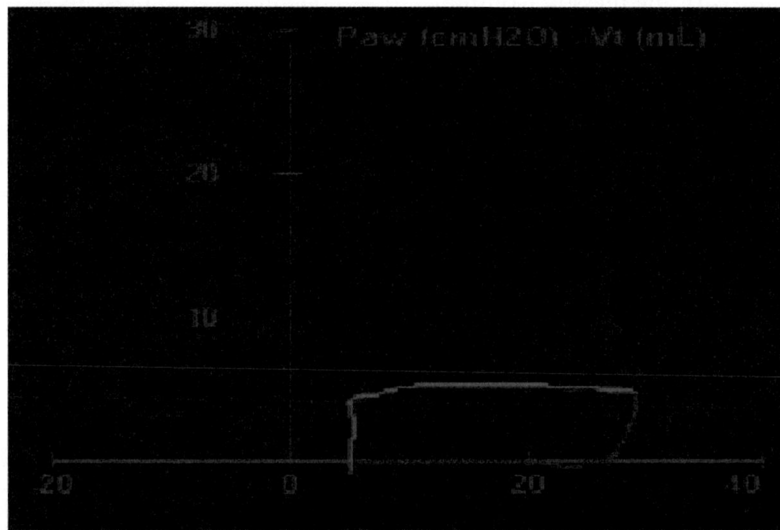

FIGURE 27-40 A volume-pressure loop with very poor compliance, or stiff lungs.
Courtesy of CareFusion

Using the pressure-volume loop to assess lung compliance changes can be done relatively quickly and easily. Normally, the slope of the loop is 45° and is an indication of the patient's lung compliance. The slope of the loop can change greatly as compliance increases or decreases.

Figure 27-39 demonstrtates a volume-pressure loop with normal compliance. The loop is sitting at a 45° angle and is football-shaped.

Figure 27-40 demonstrates a volume-pressure loop with very poor compliance, or stiff lungs. The typical result of stiff lungs is for the loop to shift to the right. If the patient had overly compliant lungs, the loop can tip from normal in the opposite direction (left) as well.[16]

Airway resistance can also be detected using pressure-volume loops. During pressure-regulated modes of ventilation, the increased airway resistance

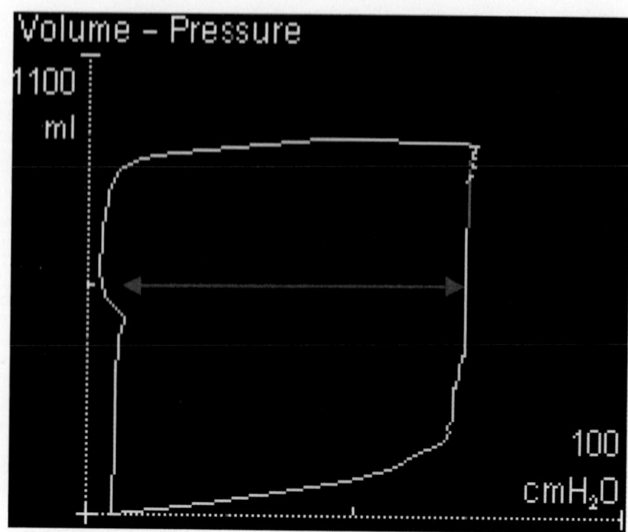

FIGURE 27-41 The pressure-volume loop is widened, showing increased airway resistance.

Courtesy of Maquet Inc.

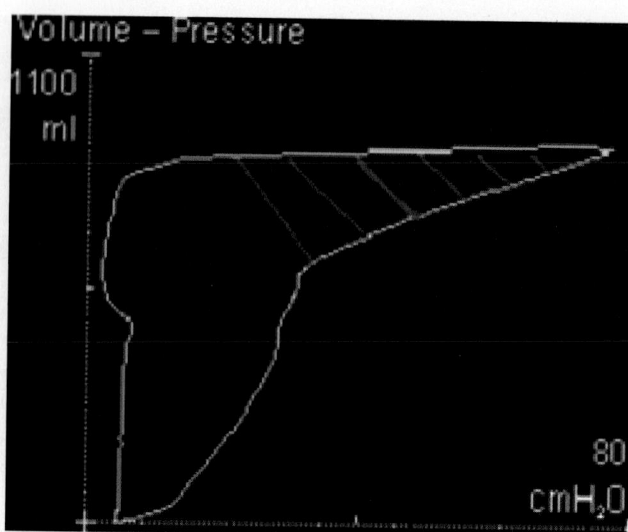

FIGURE 27-42 A volume pressure loop that is showing overdistension.

Courtesy of Maquet Inc.

causes flow rates to slow down and pressure to increase. The slower flow rate causes the change in volume to be less in relation to the change in pressure, a phenomena called *hysteresis*.[16] In Figure 27-41, the pressure-volume loop is widened due to increased airway resistance. Higher pressures are reached with a comparatively small change in volume, and the controlled pressure remains constant until the end of inspiration. Inspiratory time may have to be increased in order to deliver the desired volume.

Figure 27-42 is a volume pressure loop that is showing overdistension. The ventilator is continuing to add pressure to the patient's lungs without gaining significant added volume. The lungs are overdistended and cannot accept any more gas volume. The cross-hatched area graphically depicts the overdistension. Increasing the pressure has no further volume benefit beyond the plateau. This phenomenon is often referred to as *beaking* because the graph shape resembles a bird's beak.[4,16]

Figure 27-43 represents the work of breathing in a positive pressure breath. The red area represents the work associated with overcoming the elastic resistance of the lungs during inspiration. The crossed-hatched area represents the work associated with overcoming airway resistance during exhalation.[4,16] The sum of adding both pieces of a breath together is the total amount of work associated with that breath. The work of breathing can be performed by the ventilator, by the patient, or by both.

Figure 27-44 provides an example of a leak. The area denoted by the red marker (volume leaked) indicates that the inspiratory and expiratory tidal volumes are not equal.

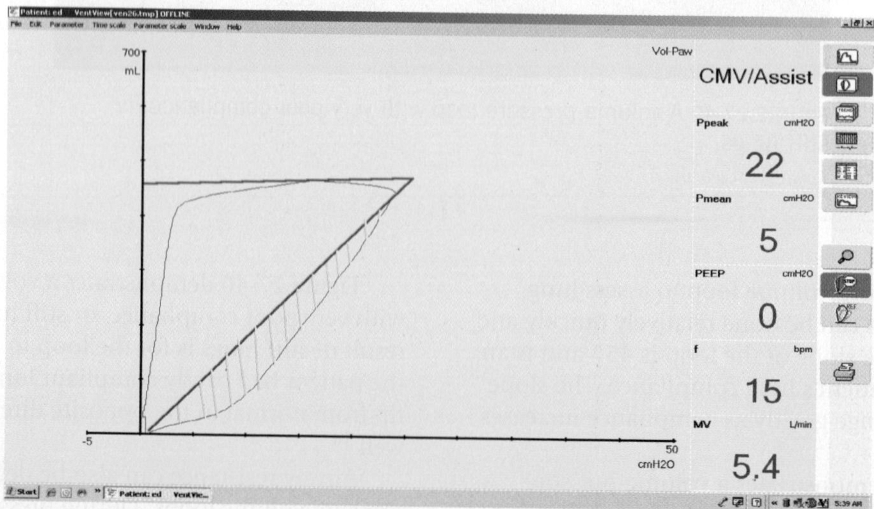

FIGURE 27-43 The work of breathing in a positive pressure breath.

Courtesy of Draeger Medical

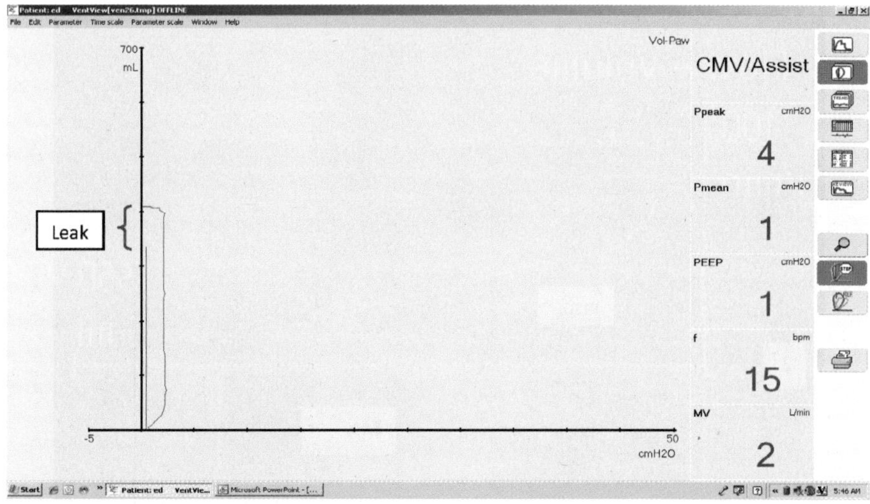

FIGURE 27-44 An example of a leak.
Courtesy of Draeger Medical

FLOW-VOLUME LOOPS

Figure 27-45 shows a normal **flow-volume loop** (FVL) of a mechanically ventilated breath. The shape of the loop can look differently depending on the mode set on the ventilator and pressure-volume ventilation. Although this loop may look familiar—similar to pulmonary function testing—the orientations of inspiration and expiration may be different depending on the equipment being used.

There are other differences. In pulmonary function testing, the patient is breathing spontaneously and is asked to give a maximal inspiratory and expiratory effort (FVC) when creating an FVL. A ventilated patient is unable to do this maneuver and generally exhales passively. In mechanical ventilation, the loop is based on the patient's tidal breathing. In addition, a mechanically ventilated patient is also breathing through an ETT or tracheostomy, which creates far more airway resistance than a nonventilated patient has. This is why the traditional ranges used for the classification of mild, moderate, and severe obstruction in pulmonary function testing do not correlate with mechanically ventilated patients' loops.

Figure 27-46 demonstrates an abnormal FVL. In this example, the top half is representing inspiration while the bottom half is exhalation. The loop exhibits flow limitation throughout both inspiration and exhalation, but the limitation is more prominent on exhalation. The normal pattern for the expiratory flow is linear, showing that the lung is reacting the same

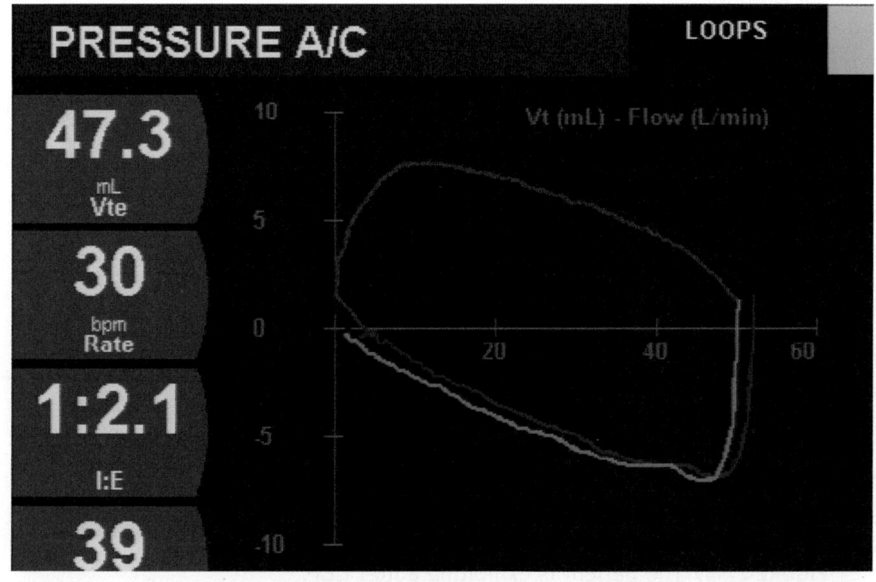

FIGURE 27-45 A normal flow-volume loop (FVL) of a mechanically ventilated breath.
Courtesy of CareFusion

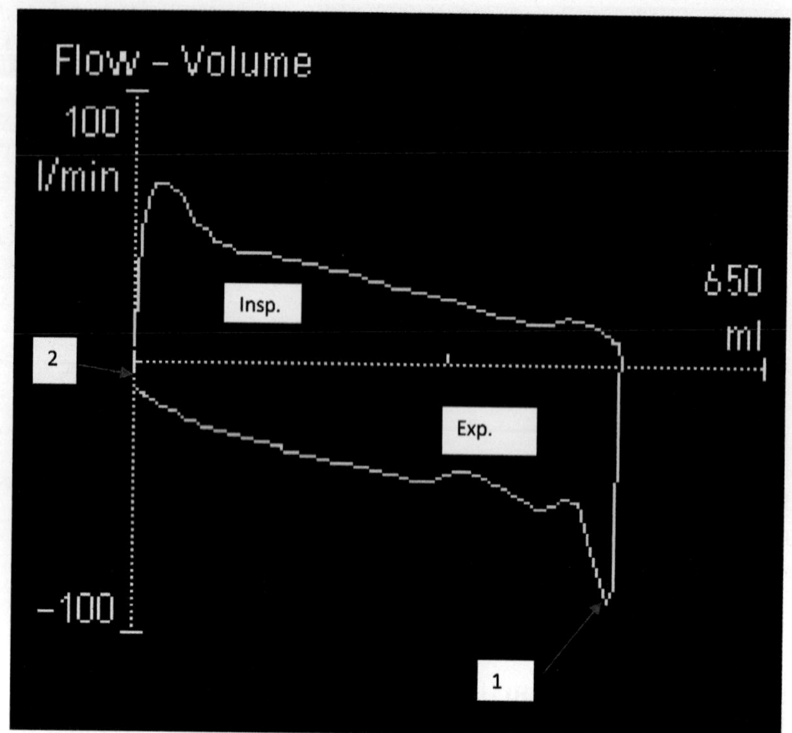

FIGURE 27-46 An abnormal FVL.
Courtesy of Maquet Inc.

throughout (homogenous lung), during exhalation. When lung disease is present, as in this example, there is a less linear tracing throughout exhalation, showing that some areas of the lung behave differently than others during exhalation. This example is consistent with a diagnosis of COPD. Arrow 1 in the figure shows a very high flow at the onset of exhalation due to the exhaled gases being compressed in the patient's ventilator circuit. Arrow 2 points to air trapping, or auto-PEEP, which is also common in COPD. Notice that the expiratory flow does not return to baseline.[4,18]

In Figure 27-47, the patient is exhibiting auto-PEEP. Inspiration is beginning before exhalation is complete, as depicted by the arrow.

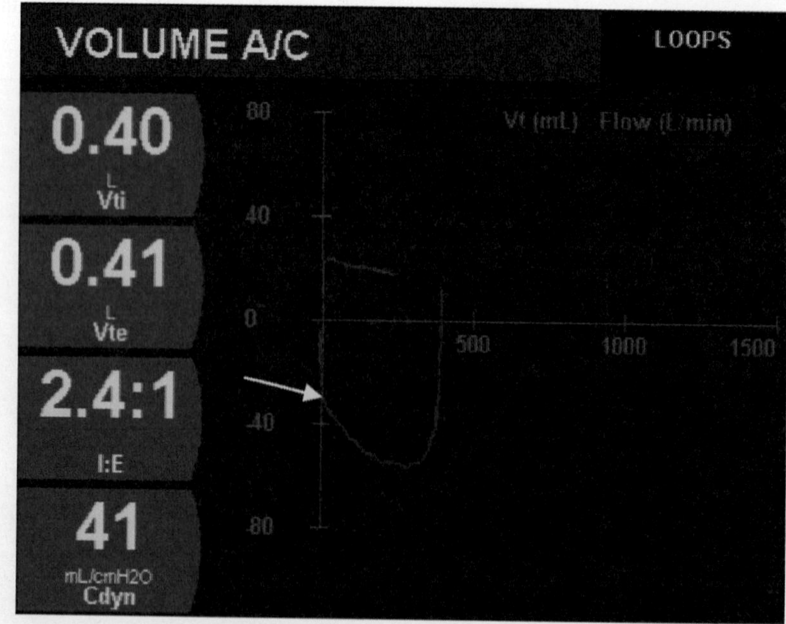

FIGURE 27-47 The patient is exhibiting auto-PEEP.
Courtesy of CareFusion

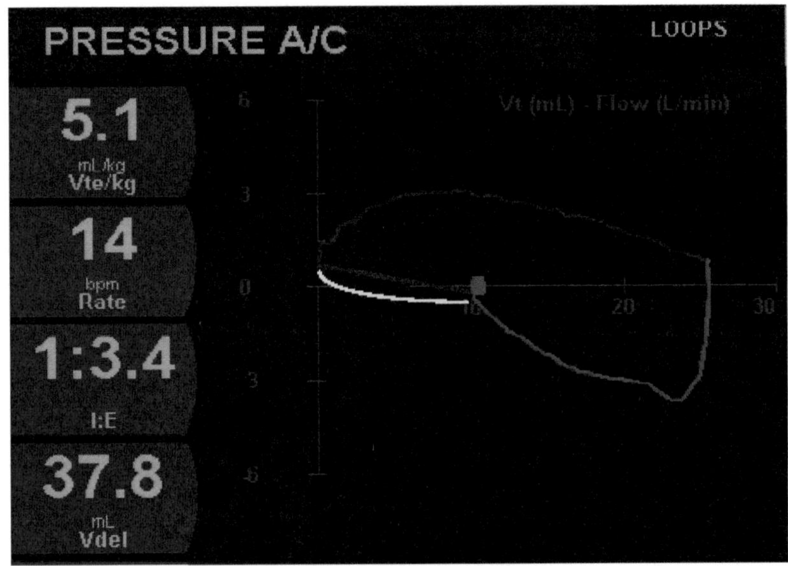

FIGURE 27-48 An example of a leak in the system.

Courtesy of CareFusion

Figure 27-48 is an example of a leak in the system. On this ventilator, the inspiratory portion of the breath is red, and the expiratory portion is blue. Notice how the expiratory portion does not return to baseline at the end the breath. The area traced in yellow is the lost volume from the leak.

In Figure 27-49, the flow volume loops show a pre- and postrepresentation of the effect of suctioning. In the first FVL, there is a lot of irritability in the tracing of the loop. This is the result of the gas flowing through airway secretions and creating a lot of turbulence in the breath. In the second FVL, after the patient has been suctioned, there is much more laminar flow, which results in a smoother tracing. The pre- and post-FVL technique is also used in mechanical ventilation to measure response to bronchodilators. The expectation is to see a bigger loop, representing more volume and improved peak flow following bronchodilator administration.

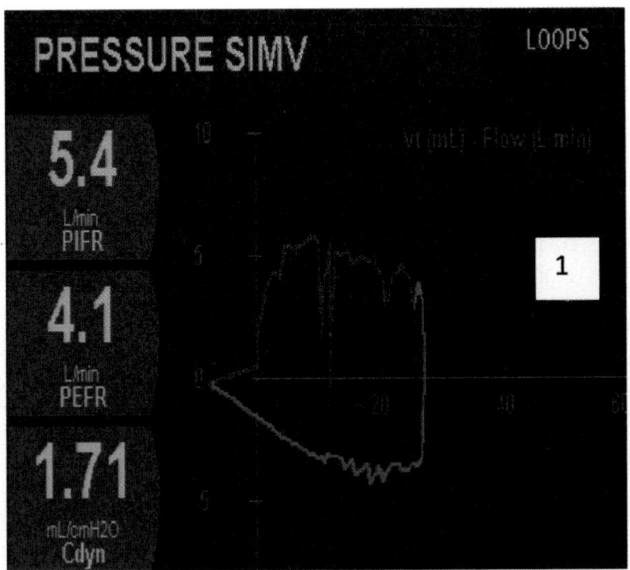

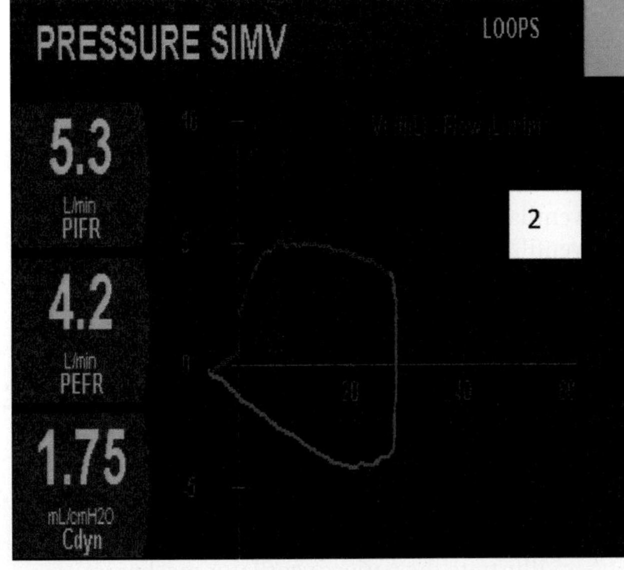

FIGURE 27-49 A pre- and postrepresentation of the effect of suctioning.

Courtesy of CareFusion

Summary

Currently available mechanical ventilators that are designed for use in critical care have ventilator graphic displays (or at a minimum options to include ventilator graphics). Ventilator graphics have provided the respiratory therapist with a clinically significant tool for managing patient-ventilator interactions, monitoring pulmonary mechanics, and detecting clinically significant issues with the ventilator system.

Mastering the interpretation of ventilator graphics can be challenging for the respiratory therapist, but understanding ventilator graphics is an important element in the improvement of patient care in critical care and other patient care areas.

This chapter provides a fundamental approach to understanding the information that ventilator graphics provide and the analysis of that information. Some of the commonly observed abnormal patterns have been discussed in this chapter. However, not every clinical situation and/or every available ventilator could be included. Respiratory therapists are challenged to continue to improve their understanding and utilize ventilator graphics as a tool to enhance patient care and management of patient-ventilator interactions. Follow-up suggested readings are included at the end of the chapter, and manufacturers' representatives and Web sites can provide equipment-specific information. Experienced colleagues can also be a valuable resource by sharing their accumulated knowledge.

Study Questions

REVIEW QUESTIONS

1. List the three primary variables that are plotted against time during mechanical ventilation.
2. Discuss the use of ventilator graphics in monitoring changes in compliance.
3. Discuss the use of ventilator graphics in monitoring changes in airway resistance.
4. How is patient inspiratory effort observed on a ventilator graphic display during mechanical ventilation?
5. Describe patient-ventilator dyssynchrony.
6. What is an inflection point?

MULTIPLE-CHOICE QUESTIONS

1. Ventilator graphics can do all of the following except:
   a. provide information on ventilator-patient interaction.
   b. determine the patient's clinical diagnosis.
   c. illustrate the patient-ventilator mechanics.
   d. present graphic interpretation triggering pressure, synchrony, and flow-volume relationships.
2. The scalar functions of the ventilator graphics relate pressure, flow, and volume to what?
   a. compliance
   b. each other
   c. time
   d. mechanical and patient resistance
3. Resistance to flow in the lung is dependent on:
   I. type of flow (turbulent or laminar).
   II. airway diameter.
   III. types and distribution of tissue.
   IV. gas viscosity.
   a. I and II
   b. II and III
   c. I, II, and IV
   d. I and III
4. TCT = $T_i + T_e$:
   a. only when R_{aw} is low.
   b. True.
   c. False.
   d. Only during low-volume ventilation.
5. If TCT = 5 seconds and T_i = 1.5 seconds, what does T_e = ?
   a. 1.5 seconds
   b. 2.0 seconds
   c. 4.5 seconds
   d. 3.5 seconds
6. In the previous question, what is the respiratory rate (RR)?
   a. 12/minute
   b. 10/minute
   c. 15/minute
   d. Not enough data was given.
7. In constant flow volume ventilation, the ventilator graphic indicates which scalar form?
   a. decelerating
   b. sinusoidal
   c. square
   d. accelerating
8. During pressure ventilation, the initial flow _____ in a linear fashion to maintain the set pressure.
   a. decelerates
   b. remains constant
   c. increases
   d. varies in a sinusoidal manner
9. Failure of the graphic to reach baseline at the end of expiration may result from:
   I. a small diameter ET tube.
   II. kinked ventilator tubing.
   III. clogged expiratory filter(s).
   IV. patient chewing on ET tube.
   a. I, II, III, and IV
   b. II and III
   c. I and III
   d. II and IV

10. Failure to meet the patient's inspiratory demand is reflected in:
    a. increased rise time.
    b. ventilator dyssynchrony.
    c. increased expiratory time (T_e).
    d. increased respiratory rate (RR).
11. Airway resistance (R_{aw}) can be approximated by which formula?
    a. plateau pressure (P_{plat}) - peak pressure (P_{peak})
    b. $V_t - P_{peak}$
    c. peak flow (F_{peak}) $\div P_{peak}$
    d. $P_{peak} - P_{plat}$
12. In a pressure-volume curve, the inspiratory portion of the curve moves:
    a. upward to the left.
    b. downward to the right.
    c. upward to the right.
    d. downward to the left.

CRITICAL-THINKING QUESTIONS

1. Using ventilator graphic displays, differentiate between constant flow and constant pressure ventilation.
2. How might inflection points be used to identify a "safe" inspiratory pressure?
3. How might inflection points be used to set PEEP?
4. How might a respiratory therapist use a ventilator graphic display to observe a partially obstructed endotracheal tube?
5. How can ventilator graphics be used to detect auto-PEEP?
6. How can ventilator graphics be used to detect a leak in the ventilation system?

References

1. Lucangelo U, Bernabe F, Blanch L. Respiratory mechanics derived from signals in the ventilator circuit. *Respir Care.* 2005;50:50.
2. Dhand R. Ventilator graphics and respiratory mechanics in the patient with obstructive lung disease. *Respir Care.* 2005;50:246.
3. Nilsestuen JO, Hargett BS. Managing the patient-ventilator system using graphic analysis: an overview and introduction to graphics corner. *Respir Care.* 1996;41:1105.
4. Pilbeam SP, Cairo JM. *Mechanical Ventilation: Physiologic and Clinical Applications.* 4th ed. St. Louis, MO: Mosby; 2006.
5. Rau JL. Inspiratory flow patterns: the shape of ventilation. *Respir Care.* 1993;38:132.
6. Pilbeam SP. Introductions to ventilators. In: Cairo JM, Pilbeam SP, eds. Mosby's respiratory care equipment. St Louis, MO: Mosby; 1999.
7. Shortall S, Oakes D. Practical uses of pressure control ventilation. *Focus Journal for Respiratory Care and Sleep Medicine.* 2005;(2):64.
8. Blanch L, Bernabe F, Lucangelo U. Measurement of air trapping, intrinsic positive expiratory pressure, and dynamic hyperinflation in mechanically ventilated patients. *Respir Care.* 2005;50:110.
9. Branson RD. Enhanced capabilities of current ICU ventilators: do they really benefit patients. *Respir Care.* 1991;36:362.
10. Nilsestuen JO, Hargett KD. Using ventilator graphics to identify patient-ventilator asynchrony. *Respir Care.* 2005;50:202.
11. Chatmongkolchart S, Williams P, Hess D, Kaczmarek R. Evaluations of inspiratory rise time and inspiration termination criteria in new generation mechanical ventilators: a lung model study. *Respir Care.* 2001;46:666.
12. Holt T. Physics and physiology of ventilator support. In: Scanlan CJ, Wilkins RL, Stoller JK, eds. Egan's Fundamentals of Respiratory Care. St. Louis, MO: Mosby; 1999.
13. Sinderby C, et al. Inspiratory muscle unloading by neurally adjusted ventilatory assist during maximal inspiratory efforts in healthy subjects. *Chest.* 2007;131,3:711–717.
14. Hess D. Ventilator waveforms and physiology of pressure support ventilation. *Respir Care.* 2005;50:166.
15. Sasson CSH, Mahutte CK. What you need to know about the ventilator in weaning. *Respir Care.* 1995;40:249.
16. Waugh JB, Deshpande VM, Harwood RJ. *Rapid Interpretation of Ventilator Waveforms.* Upper Saddle River, NJ: Prentice Hall; 1999.
17. Hess D, Kaczmarek R. Advanced pulmonary mechanics. In: Hess D, Kaczmarek R, eds. *Essentials of Mechanical Ventilation.* New York: McGraw Hill Professional; 2002.
18. Chatburn RL. Fundamentals of mechanical ventilation: a short course in the theory and application of mechanical ventilators. Cleveland Heights, OH: Mandu Press Ltd; 2003.

Suggested Readings

Ouellet P. *Waveform and Loop Analysis in Mechanical Ventilation.* Solna, Sweden: Siemens-Elema; 1997.

Rittner F, Doring M. *Curves and Loops in Mechanical Ventilation.* Telford, PA: Draeger Medical; 1996.

Waugh J, Deshpande V, Harwood R. *Rapid Interpretation of Ventilator Waveforms.* Upper Saddle River, NJ: Prentice Hall; 1999.

CHAPTER 28

Noninvasive Mechanical Ventilation

Bethene L. Gregg

OBJECTIVES

Upon completion of this chapter, the reader should be able to:

- Describe the advantages of noninvasive positive pressure ventilation (NPPV).
- State which patients in acute respiratory failure may benefit the most from noninvasive positive pressure ventilation according to the recommendations of the 2001 International Consensus Conferences in Intensive Care Medicine: noninvasive positive pressure ventilation in acute respiratory failure and the 2009 42nd Respiratory Care Journal Conference Noninvasive ventilation in acute care: controversies and emerging concepts, Parts I and II.
- Identify the advantages and disadvantages of using critical care versus home care positive pressure ventilators for NPPV.
- Describe the patient interface for NPPV.
- Explain the function of the major settings on the ventilators discussed.
- Describe how pressure support may be cycled for some critical care ventilators.
- Describe a common complication of NPPV delivered via face mask.
- Explain when NPPV should be discontinued.
- List one advantage and one disadvantage of negative pressure ventilators.

CHAPTER OUTLINE

Noninvasive Positive Pressure Ventilation
- Indications for Use Acute Care
- Contraindications
- Application
- Initial Ventilator Settings
- Monitoring
- Complications
- Limitations
- Ventilators Used
- Continuous Positive Airway Pressure Units

Long-Term Use

Negative Pressure Ventilation
- Types
- Physiologic Effects
- Ventilators
- Indications for Use

KEY TERMS

castle port
continuous positive airway pressure (CPAP)
expiratory positive airway pressure (EPAP)
extrathoracic
inspiratory positive airway pressure (IPAP)
nasal mask
negative pressure ventilation (NPV)
noninvasive positive pressure ventilation (NPPV)
oronasal mask
pressure support (PS)
rise time percentage
shape signal
spontaneous mode
spontaneous or timed (S/T) mode

Noninvasive mechanical ventilation includes both positive and negative pressure ventilator applications that do not require the placement of an endotracheal or tracheostomy tube. Short-term noninvasive ventilatory support to treat acute respiratory failure in adults is discussed in this chapter. Long-term noninvasive ventilatory support in home care is also discussed briefly.

Noninvasive positive pressure ventilation (NPPV) is a treatment for hypercapnic respiratory failure in which the ventilator-patient interface is typically a **nasal mask** or an **oronasal mask** (a mask that covers the nose and mouth). In **negative pressure ventilation (NPV)**, the ventilator is applied to the thorax and abdomen or to the entire body from the neck down, and no ventilator apparatus is in contact with the face. In both types of noninvasive ventilation, gas flows through the upper airway and into the lungs.

The purpose of noninvasive ventilation is to provide adequate gas exchange while avoiding the complications associated with endotracheal intubation and invasive ventilation. For example:

- The incidence of ventilator-associated pneumonia is reduced with NPPV.[1,2]
- Nourdine and colleagues found that NPPV reduced the risk of ventilator-associated pneumonia and hospital-acquired infection when compared with intubated ventilation, regardless of the severity of illness.[2,3]
- Noninvasive ventilation also eliminates the problems associated with an increased work of breathing through an endotracheal tube that may prolong the weaning process.[4–6]

Noninvasive Positive Pressure Ventilation

Noninvasive positive pressure ventilation (NPPV) dates to the first reports of mouth-to-mouth resuscitation. Successful use of it in the mid-1700s led to the first bag-mask device, introduced by Chaussier in 1780. In 1887, Dr. George Fell applied a bellows ventilator using a face mask.[7] Barach and associates pioneered the application of **continuous positive airway pressure (CPAP)** breathing, which was used as a method of delivering oxygen to pilots flying at high altitudes during World War II. In the mid-1940s, V. Ray Bennett expanded the clinical application of positive pressure breathing when he engineered a device to deliver oxygen under pressure during inspiration via intermittent positive pressure breathing (IPPB).[8] IPPB via face mask was used extensively in the 1950s and 1960s to treat patients with acute respiratory failure (ARF).

The successful use of NPPV was limited by technology. The rubber face mask did not seal properly unless applied with a great deal of pressure. Skin injury from the mask was a common complication. Full-face masks, which were opaque, concealed the presence of oral secretions or emesis. Aspiration was frequently cited as a complication. Leaky IPPB devices used in the 1960s and 1970s did not function well. Interest in NPPV declined in the late 1960s, when volume-cycled ventilators became available and endotracheal tubes were improved.

After 20 years of use of volume-limited ventilators and endotracheal tubes, NPPV was reconsidered as a way of treating ARF to avoid endotracheal intubation and its associated complications and costs. **Pressure support (PS)** and pressure control ventilation available on the Siemens Servo 900C (Siemens Medical Systems, Inc., Danvers, Massachusetts) renewed interest in the application of pressure ventilation. (In pressure support, exhalation starts when the patient's airway pressure approaches the inspiratory target pressure, causing a decrease in inspiratory flow to the patient. When the flow drops to the cycle threshold, inspiration ends.) The use of mask CPAP to treat obstructive sleep apnea prompted the design of better masks and CPAP devices. Noninvasive positive pressure ventilation found increased use in home care to support ventilator-dependent individuals. In the 1980s, there were numerous clinical studies in the use of pressure support applied by face mask or nasal mask to treat ARF.

During the 1990s, the efficacy of NPPV in treating ARF was well established, particularly for patients with acute exacerbation of COPD. In 1996 the American Association for Respiratory Care (AARC), the American Respiratory Care Foundation, and the Respiratory Care Journal convened the Consensus Conference on Noninvasive Positive Pressure Ventilation (AARC Consensus Conference) to clarify terminology and describe the appropriate application of NPPV in various clinical settings.[9] Then, in 1997, the federal government effectively curtailed the use of long-term NPPV in the United States through the Balanced Budget Act (BBA), which redefined which health care costs are covered by Medicare (discussed later in this chapter).

INDICATIONS FOR USE IN ACUTE CARE

In cases of acute respiratory failure, NPPV provides adequate gas exchange and decreased respiratory muscle work without the need for an endotracheal tube or when intubation is undesirable. When applied properly, NPPV of patients with acute exacerbation of COPD reduces mortality and length of intensive care stay.[10] NPPV also reduces the intubation rate in patients with more severe COPD exacerbations.[11] The successful application of NPPV requires the patient to be able to clear secretions effectively.

A trial of NPPV is indicated for patients with COPD when they fail to respond to standard medical care. According to the AARC Consensus Conference, NPPV is indicated when at least two of the following criteria are present:

- Respiratory distress with moderate to severe dyspnea, use of accessory muscles, and abdominal paradox
- pH < 7.35 with $P_aCO_2 > 45$ mm Hg
- A respiratory rate ≥ 25 bpm

In one study, patients treated successfully with NPPV had a higher level of consciousness (LOC) initially and improved LOC, P_aCO_2, and pH values after 1 hour.[12] Results from numerous clinical studies indicate that intubation can be avoided in 50–75% of patients in acute ventilatory failure supported with NPPV. Postextubation application of NPPV also has been successful in avoiding reintubation, especially in COPD patients with hypercapnic respiratory insufficiency.[13,14] For patients with neuromuscular disease, NPPV has been effective when swallowing was not severely impaired and assisted cough flows were greater than 160 Lpm.[15] There is also substantial evidence that CPAP and NPPV improve physiologic variables and reduce the intubation rate for patients with acute cardiogenic pulmonary edema.[16,17] However, there is little evidence that NPPV is superior to CPAP in terms of intubation rate or mortality for these patients.[18] There is enough evidence to recommend a trial of NPPV in immunocompromised patients with ARF and bilateral pulmonary infiltrates.[11]

Evidence does not support the use of NPPV when refractory hypoxemia is the primary cause of respiratory failure, as in acute respiratory distress syndrome (ARDS).[11] There is also inadequate evidence to support the *routine* use of NPPV for patients with community-acquired pneumonia, asthma, or blunt chest trauma.[19,20]

CONTRAINDICATIONS

Absolute contraindications for NPPV are listed in Table 28-1. Noninvasive ventilation is contraindicated for respiratory arrest and circulatory collapse. Signs of imminent respiratory arrest include altered level of consciousness, the presence of respiratory muscle fatigue, obvious exhaustion, quiet chest. diaphoresis, and hemodynamic instability (systolic BP < 90 mm Hg). Such patients require endotracheal intubation.[21]

Relative contraindications that may lead to unsuccessful NPPV are also listed in Table 28-1. Additional factors that reduce the chance of successful NPPV are excessive secretions and a high acute physiologic and

TABLE 28-1 **Absolute and relative contraindications for noninvasive positive pressure ventilation**

Absolute Contraindications	Relative Contraindications
Facial burns, facial or skull trauma	Altered level of consciousness
Hemodynamic instability	ARDS
Need for airway protection—vomiting, etc.	Excessive secretions
Respiratory arrest (need for immediate intubation)	Extreme anxiety
Uncooperative patient	Massive obesity

Source: From Bach JR. Consensus statement: noninvasive positive pressure ventilation. Paper presented at the Consensus Conference IV: Noninvasive Positive Pressure Ventilation. Vail, Colorado; 1997

chronic health evaluation (APACHE) score.[9] The APACHE score, comprised of physiologic variables, is used to estimate the probability of hospital mortality for adult ICU admissions.

APPLICATION

The application of NPPV requires a ventilator, an appropriate circuit, and a patient interface.

- The patient interface for short-term NPPV is a nasal mask (Figure 28-1) or an oronasal mask (Figure 28-2), held in place by head straps. Oronasal masks specifically designed for NPPV are more effective than face masks used with manual resuscitators.
- Full-face masks (Figure 28-3) are also an option.
- The helmet (Figure 28-4) is an option.[22,23]

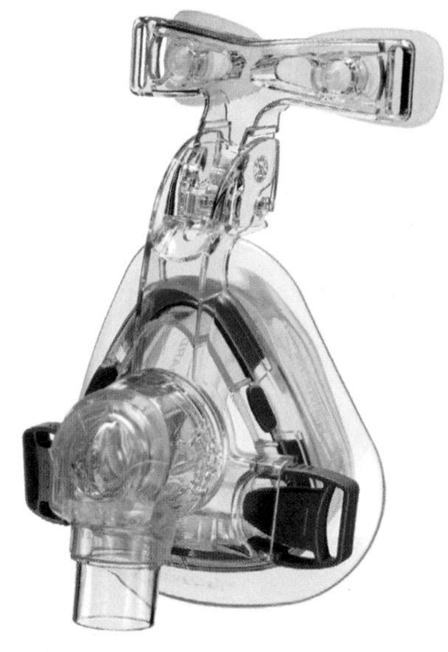

(A)

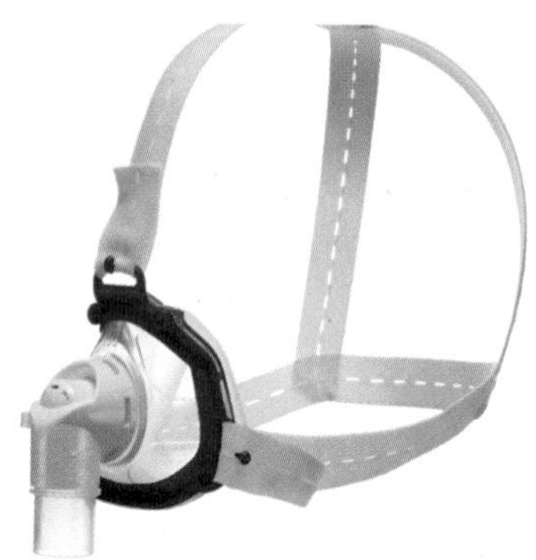

(B)

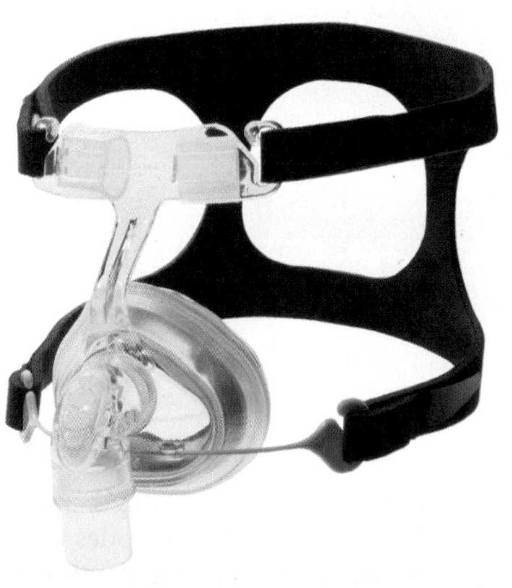

(C)

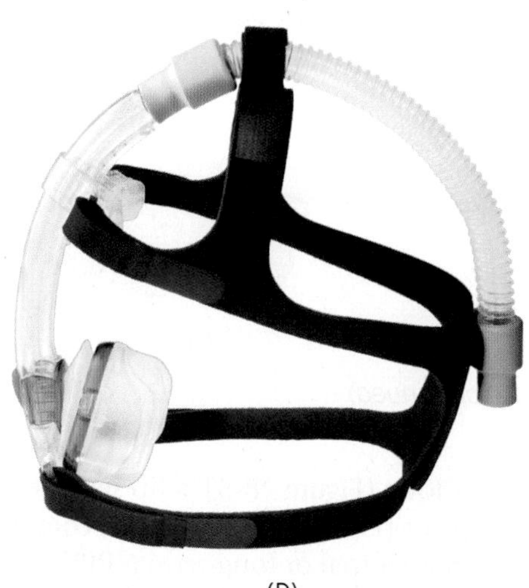

(D)

FIGURE 28-1 Nasal masks: (A) Activa (© ResMed 2010 Used with permission). (B) Mirage Micro (© ResMed 2010 Used with permission). (C) FlexiFit™ 405 Nasal Mask (Used with permission Fisher and Paykel). (D) DreamFit (Image used by permission from Nellcor Puritan Bennett LLC, Boulder, Colorado, part of Covidien). (E) Comfort Gel (Courtesy of Philips Respironics). (F) Comfort Curve (Courtesy of Philips Respironics). (G) Comfort Fusion (Courtesy of Philips Respironics). (H) Comfort Lite 2 (Courtesy of Philips Respironics). (I) Simplicity (Courtesy of Philips Respironics). *(continues)*

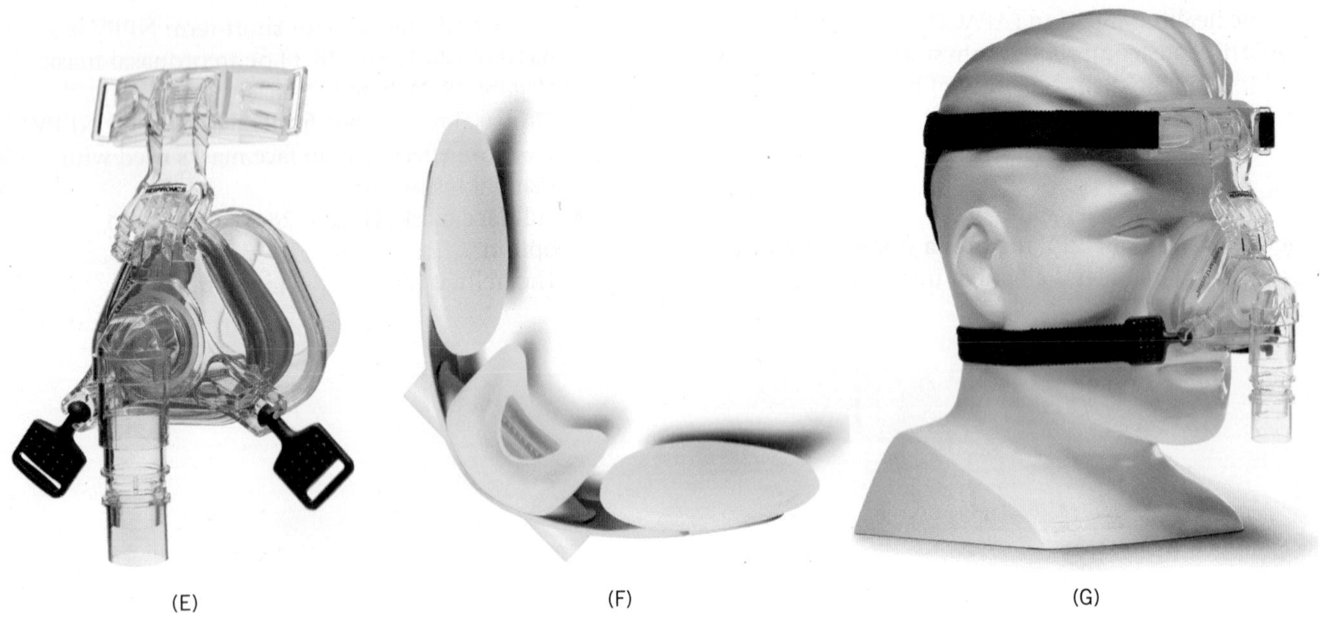

(E) (F) (G)

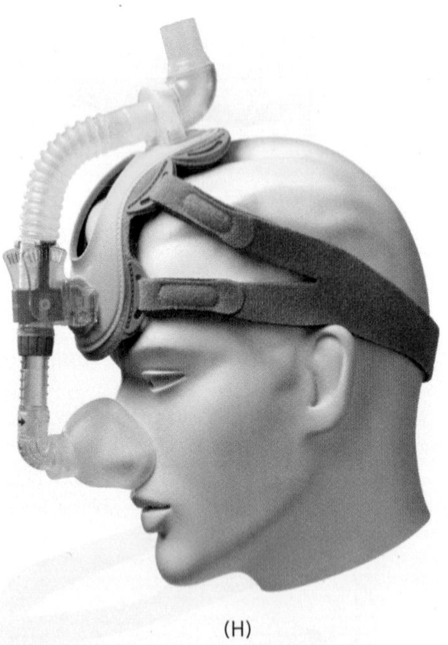

(H)

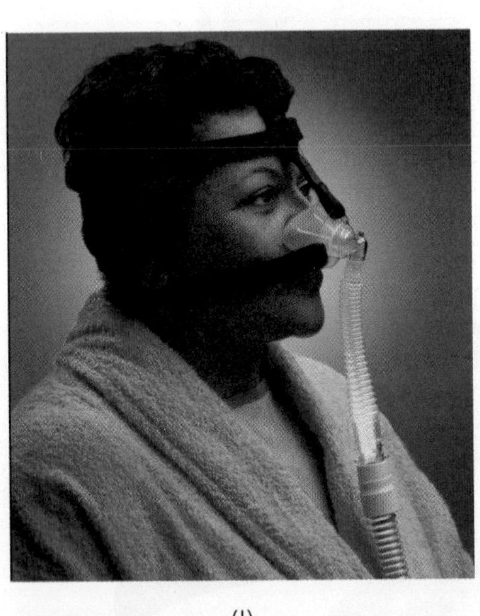

(I)

FIGURE 28-1 *(continued)*

- Nasal pillows (Figure 28-5), a lip seal, or a mouthpiece (Figure 28-6) are more commonly used for nocturnal or long-term NPPV.

The wide variety of patient interfaces currently available increase the likelihood of achieving effective NPPV.[24]

Ventilators specifically designed for NPPV provide **inspiratory positive airway pressure (IPAP)** and **expiratory positive airway pressure (EPAP)**. IPAP is flow or time triggered, pressure limited, and flow or timed cycled. IPAP and EPAP are modes on the BiPAP and Vision ventilatory support devices (Philips Respironics Inc., Murrysville, Pennsylvania). Home care ventilators may be indicated if the patient requires higher pressures or volume control ventilation.[25] Critical care ventilators are also commonly used to deliver short-term NPPV in the emergency department or intensive care unit, and they usually work best with oronasal masks.

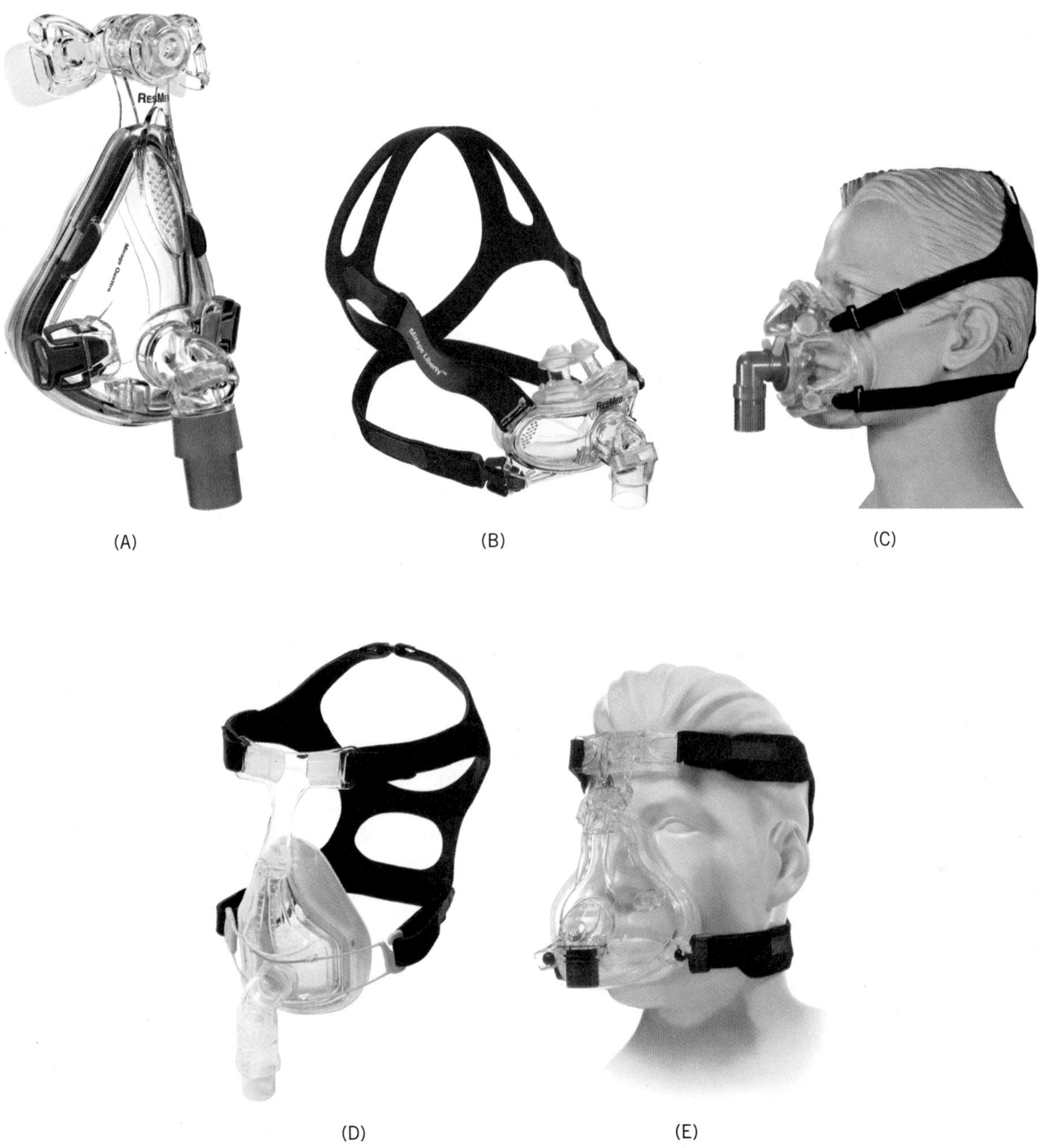

FIGURE 28-2 Oronasal masks: (A) Mirage Quattro (© ResMed 2010 Used with permission). (B) Mirage Liberty (© ResMed 2010 Used with permission). (C) Disposable 6500 Tri-Glide (Courtesy of Hans Rudolph, Inc). (D) Forma™ Full Face Mask (Fisher and Paykel). (E) ComfortFull (Courtesy of Philips Respironics).

Fitting the Mask. Successful NPPV depends on the selection of the proper interface as much as it does on the appropriate ventilator settings.[26] If the mask is too uncomfortable, the patient does not tolerate NPPV. Masks that are sized and positioned well do not need to be strapped on too tightly for patient comfort.[10] The clinician should be able to slide two fingers under the straps of the head harness for an appropriate fit. Overly tight masks are likely to cause skin abrasions. Nasal masks may be better tolerated than full-face masks, provided there is no excessive leak at the mouth or partial obstruction of the nasopharynx. A chinstrap may keep the mouth closed sufficiently. Nasal polyps or a deviated septum may increase upper airway resistance and patient discomfort with nasal masks.

The goal is to get patients accustomed to wearing a mask that is blowing air into their nose or face while they are deciding on the proper mask size. For example, using ventilator settings of 8 cm H_2O of IPAP and 0 cm H_2O of EPAP, hold the mask in place to assess

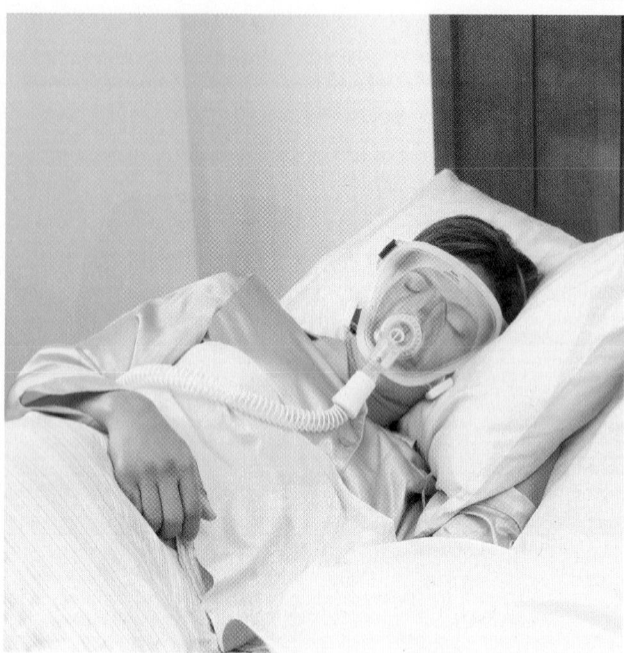

FIGURE 28-3 Full-face masks: FitLife Total Face Mask.
Courtesy of Philips Respironics

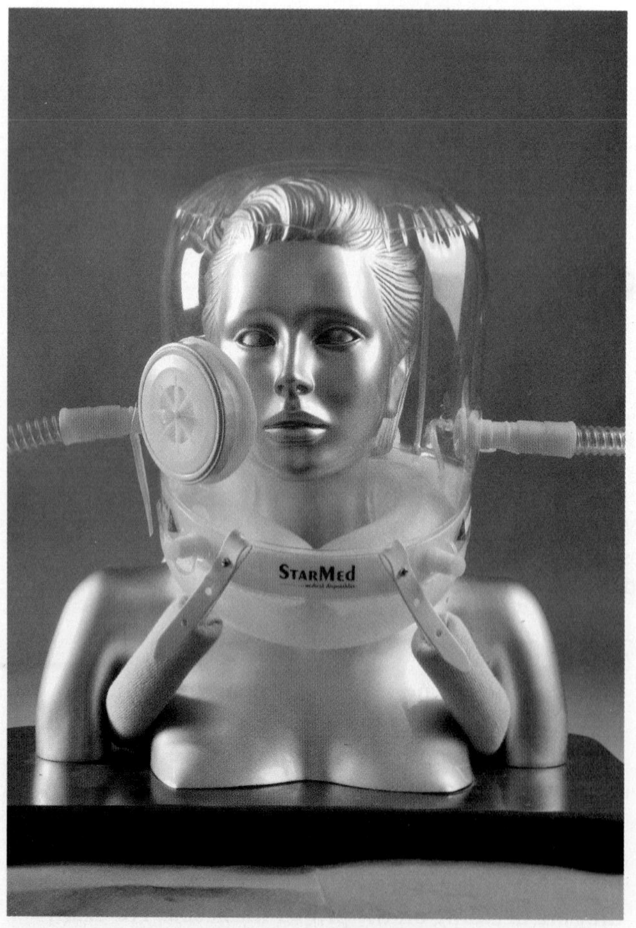

FIGURE 28-4 StarMed Castar R helmet.
Courtesy of STARMED SpA

Best Practice

Mask Fit

To prevent leaks, having the nasal mask a little too small is better than having one that is too large.

Age-Specific Competency

Reducing Patient Anxiety

The indications for NPPV use are based on clinical studies of elderly patients with chronic lung disease. Chronic dyspnea and past experiences with face masks may predispose some patients to feel extremely anxious when masks are applied. Reassurance and encouragement are key factors that influence patient tolerance of mask ventilation.

the fit.[27] The top of a mask should fit halfway down the bridge of the nose to prevent excessive leaks or damage to the eyes. Nasal masks should be large enough to barely clear the sides of the nose. Figure 28-7 shows the use of a nasal mask gauge to size Philips Respironics nasal masks. Mask-size cutouts are also included as part of the mask packaging. In Figure 28-7 the medium-wide size barely clears the sides of the nose at (A) but may extend too high up the bridge of the nose (B). In this example, if a medium-wide mask is used, the leak at the top of the mask might be excessive. A nasal mask that is too small is better than one that is too large. A variety of mask styles should be available to increase the likelihood of finding a mask that seals properly. A synthetic covering, such as Duoderm (Bristol-Myers Squibb, New York, New York), may be applied over the bridge of the nose to prevent skin damage.

INITIAL VENTILATOR SETTINGS

Initial ventilator settings depend on whether volume or pressure ventilation is used and on the type of ventilator. With ventilators specifically designed for NPPV that provide pressure support with positive end-expiratory pressure (PEEP), inspiratory pressures are increased as needed to achieve a respiratory frequency of less than 25 bpm and a tidal volume of 6–7 mL/kg body weight. Inspiratory pressures over 20 cm H_2O may be required but result in a greater leak.[6,28]

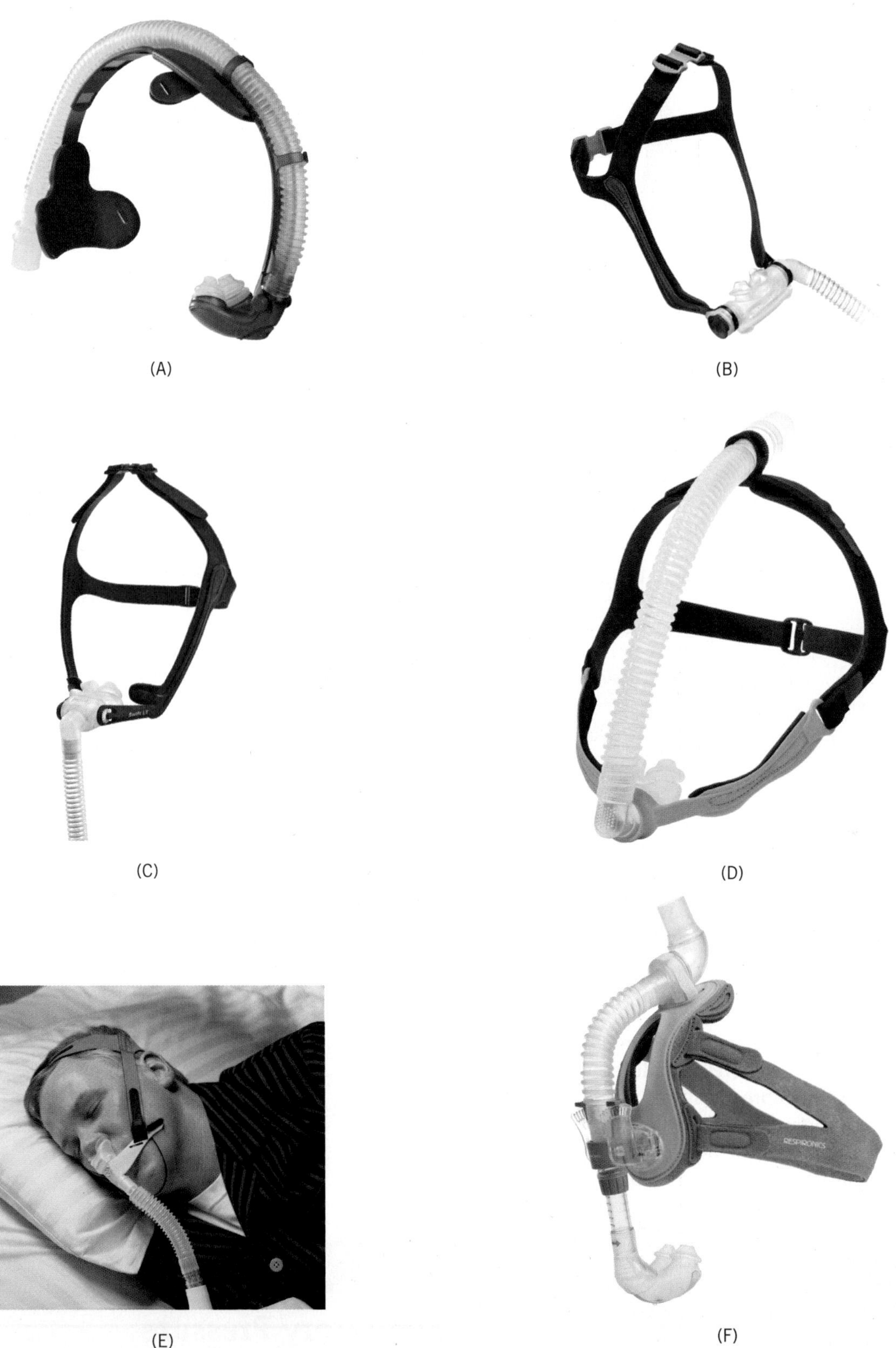

FIGURE 28-5 Nasal pillows: (A) Breeze (Image used by permission from Nellcor Puritan Bennett LLC, Boulder, Colorado, part of Covidien). (B) Mirage Swift II (© ResMed 2010 Used with permission). (C) Swift LT. (© ResMed 2010 Used with permission). (D) Opus™ 360 Nasal Pillows Mask (Courtesy of Fisher and Paykel). (E) OptiLife (Courtesy of Philips Respironics). (F) ComfortLite 2 (Courtesy of Philips Respironics).

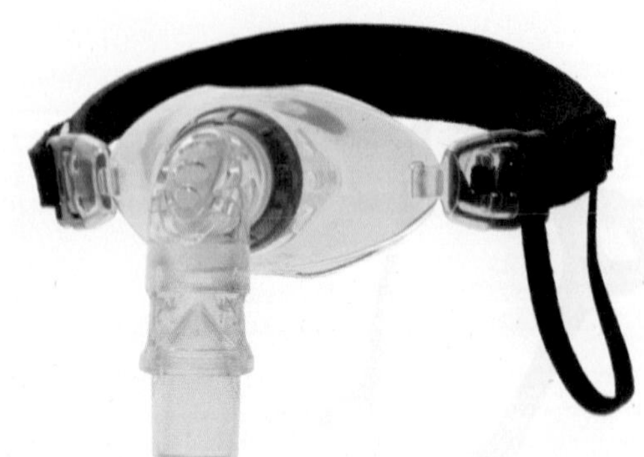

FIGURE 28-6 Oral interfaces: Oracle Oral Mask.
Fisher and Paykel

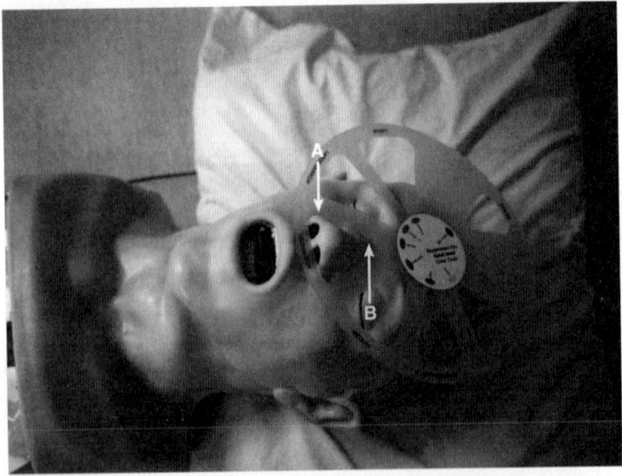

FIGURE 28-7 A nasal mask gauge may be used to determine the proper size of a nasal mask. In this example, the medium-wide size barely clears the sides of the nose at (A) but may extend up too high on the bridge of the nose (B).

Expiratory pressures are generally 4–8 cm H_2O. The risk of rebreathing at EPAP levels is reduced at least 4 cm H_2O. Although some rebreathing occurs, it may not be as clinically important, given the flow delivery systems of current ventilators designed for NPPV. Rebreathing may be more of a problem with oronasal masks. Check that the exhalation port in the circuit is not blocked. In most cases, the circuit must be specified by the ventilator manufacturer.

When pressure support and CPAP are being compared with bilevel ventilation, pressure support corresponds to the difference in pressure between IPAP and EPAP, or the *pressure gradient*. To increase the tidal ventilation, increase the pressure gradient by increasing the IPAP pressure. An increase in the EPAP level without the same adjustment in IPAP reduces the pressure gradient and, as a consequence, reduces the tidal volume. Expiratory pressures of 4–8 cm H_2O help in reducing air trapping, which may be considerable in COPD patients. However, higher EPAP pressures may create more of a leak around the mask.

Most devices designed specifically for NPPV are blower driven; so if supplemental oxygen is required, it must be added. Oxygen is added to a mask port or placed in-line between the exhalation port and the mask. The delivered oxygen concentration vary with the oxygen liter flow, the pressure gradient, and the EPAP level.[29] In addition, when oxygen is added to the ventilator outlet, oxygen concentrations may be higher at the outlet than at the mask port.[30] However, oxygen added to the ventilator outlet is close to the blower intake and constitutes a fire hazard. Oxygen should be added as described in the ventilator's operation manual. The BiPAP Vision (Philips Respironics) can deliver set oxygen concentrations when connected to a 50-psig oxygen source.

NPPV should not be given continuously. Most patients respond within 1–2 hours, but some may take up to 20 hours. After the patient has been stabilized, NPPV should be interrupted and the mask should be removed for rest periods of 10–15 minutes.[9] If NPPV is initiated in the emergency department and the patient stabilizes, consider transporting the patient to the ICU on oxygen alone. Reestablish NPPV and reduce the time of ventilation as tolerated with the same amount of rest time. One of the advantages of NPPV is that the patient knows it can be interrupted periodically.

Aerosol therapy may be given in-line with various pressure support units. The BiPAP manual recommends

Best Practice

Inspiratory Airway Pressure

Airway pressures greater than 20 cm H_2O may be required but may create a greater leak. If higher pressures are needed, check that the mask is the appropriate size.

Best Practice

Expiratory Pressure

An EPAP pressure of at least 4 cm H_2O reduces the amount of rebreathing. Higher tidal volumes may require a higher level of EPAP to reduce rebreathing. Do not block the exhalation port, and direct it away from the patient's face.

adding the nebulizer between the mask and exhalation port.[31] There should be a main-flow bacteria filter at the ventilator outlet. A mouthpiece is recommended in place of the mask for the duration of the treatment. An adapter for a metered-dose inhaler can also be added to the circuit. If the patient is stable, NPPV may be interrupted for the treatment.

MONITORING

Noninvasive ventilatory support requires attentive monitoring of the patient's initial response and comfort.

- Assess clinical signs of the patient's work of breathing for improvement: reduced use of accessory muscles, respiratory rate < 25 bpm, and reduced distress.
- Patient-ventilator asynchrony may be difficult to detect with a ventilator that does not display pressure, flow, and volume waveforms.
- Titrate inspiratory pressures or volumes according to arterial blood gases.
- The estimated tidal volumes displayed on pressure support devices may be more than 200 mL less than actual volumes but are useful for trending purposes.[32]
- After establishing adequate ventilation, titrate oxygen flow rate to achieve pulse oximeter saturations over 90%.

Patients require continued coaching and reassurance during NPPV. If respiratory care staffing dictates only periodic checks after initial stabilization, the task of patient comfort falls to the nursing staff. All personnel involved in providing NPPV must be trained in the goals, techniques, complications, and patient comfort aspects of NPPV.

COMPLICATIONS

Many of the problems encountered with NPPV are related to improper mask fit. A mask strapped on too tightly for prolonged periods damages the skin. Conjunctivitis may occur if the mask rides too high on the bridge of the nose or is loose and slips out of position.[33] Excessive leaking leads to patient-ventilator dyssynchrony and inadequate tidal volumes.[34] Progressive hypercapnia is a reason to terminate NPPV and intubate. Masks that reduce most complications if they are fitted properly are available. For example, the Profile mask by Philips Respironics has a gel cushion that conforms to the contours of the face.

The second most common problem associated with NPPV is patient intolerance. Several types of patient interfaces should be available to increase the likelihood of finding one that the patient can tolerate. The sensation of relatively high flow rates applied

Best Practice

Pressure Gradient

The pressure gradient between IPAP and EPAP determines the tidal volume. If EPAP is increased, increase the IPAP by the same amount.

Best Practice

Oxygen Hazard

Oxygen added to the ventilator outlet is close to the blower intake and is a fire hazard. Add oxygen as described in the ventilator's operation manual to either a mask port or placed in-line between the exhalation port and the mask.

Best Practice

Personnel

All personnel involved in providing NPPV must be trained in the goals, techniques, complications, and patient comfort aspects of NPPV. Key personnel should be included in the training program and in establishing a protocol for the initiation and management of NPPV.

Spotlight On

The Profile Lite

The Profile Lite nasal mask (Philips Respironics Inc.) has a gel cushion that can be formed to fit the contour of the patient's face. The mask is submerged in boiling water for 4 minutes and then cooled in cold water for 10 seconds. The mask is then attached to the spacer and headgear, and it is worn for 5 minutes to allow time for the gel cushion to conform to the face. The mask retains its shape when removed and can be reshaped by repeating the process.

nasally may be too uncomfortable. Ventilators that allow the adjustment of the initial flow rate with a rise time percentage control may increase comfort. Nasal or oral dryness may also contribute to discomfort and can be alleviated by adding a heated passover-type humidifier.

LIMITATIONS

Rebreathing of carbon dioxide (CO_2) has been reported to increase frequency, minute volume, and the work of breathing by 50%.[35] Use of a nonrebreathing exhalation valve increases the time required for flow to reach peak value and increases resistance during exhalation.[36] Increased resistance also decreases tidal volume. Ferguson and Gilmartin (1995) found that the Sanders NRV-2 nonrebreather valve or the Plateau Exhalation Valve, both from Philips Respironics, with the BiPAP prevented exhaled CO_2 from entering the ventilator circuit when compared to the fixed-resistance exhalation port of the Whisper-Swivel. They found that, with the Whisper-Swivel, an EPAP level of 8 cm H_2O was needed to prevent rebreathing when an IPAP of 20 cm H_2O provided tidal volumes of approximately 1200 mL. Eight cm H_2O of EPAP provided enough flow to flush the exhaled volume out the exhalation port (Figure 28-8).[37] High EPAP may increase the leak around the mask to an unacceptable level. Some ventilatory support devices are not compatible with a nonrebreathing exhalation valve. The additional flow required to maintain expiratory pressures favors the use of at least 4 cm H_2O EPAP to reduce rebreathing.

CASE STUDY 28-1

I. O., a 64-year-old man with COPD, is treated in the emergency department for respiratory distress. His initial blood gas values are pH 7.30, P_aCO_2 63 mm Hg, P_aO_2 52 mm Hg, S_pO_2 86%, and HCO_3^- 29 mEq/L. He receives standard medical care, including inhaled bronchodilators, oxygen, antibiotics, systemic corticosteroids, intravenous aminophylline, and diuretics. After 20 minutes on 2-Lpm oxygen via nasal cannula, his blood gas values are pH 7.29, P_aCO_2 67 mm Hg, P_aO_2 56 mm Hg, and S_pO_2 88%. His respiratory rate has dropped from 34 to 31 bpm.

Questions

1. Why is this patient a candidate for a trial of NPPV?
2. What initial settings would be used on the BiPAP S/T?
3. How is the tidal volume adjusted after the patient accepts the mask and it is strapped in place?
4. Where should oxygen be added and how much?

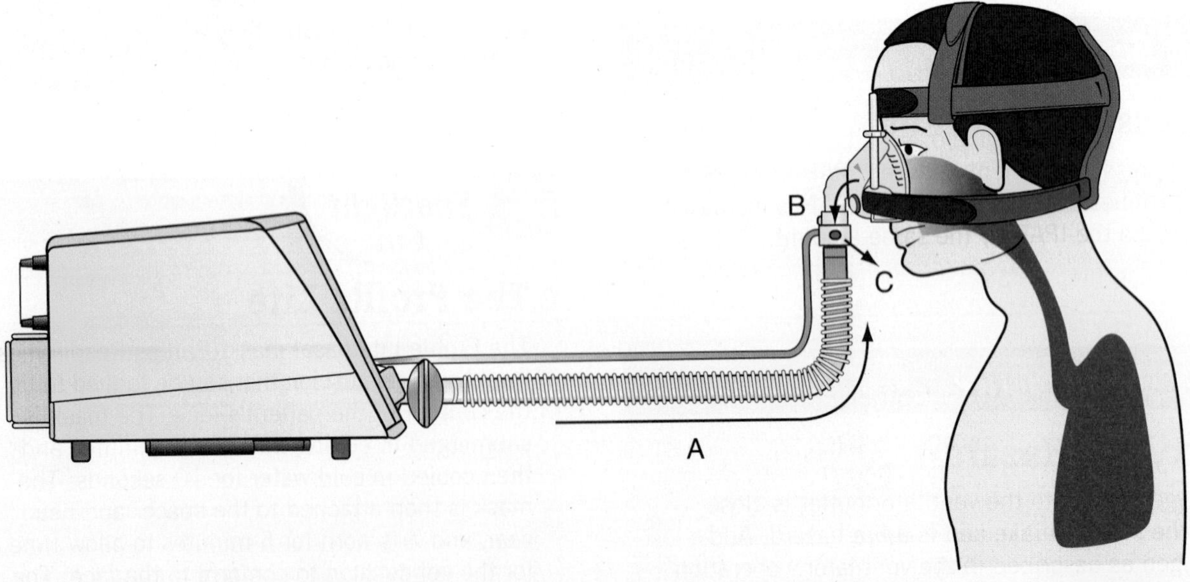

FIGURE 28-8 The flow rate required to maintain EPAP (A) is equal to or greater than the patient's exhaled flow rate (B), CO_2 is flushed from the circuit through the exhalation port (C).

Modified from the Vision Clinic Manual. Courtesy of Philips Respironics Inc., Pittsburgh, Pa.

CASE STUDY 28-2

M. C., a patient treated in the emergency department for acute exacerbation of COPD, is now in stable condition on nasal mask NPPV. She is going to be transferred to the respiratory intensive care unit (RICU).

Questions

1. How should the patient be transferred to the RICU?
2. What are now important factors for this patient on NPPV?

Best Practice

Setting the bpm Rate for Pressure-Supported Breaths

For Servo 300A ventilators that limit the time of a pressure-supported breath to 80% of the total cycle time (TCT), use the following formula to determine the breaths per minute rate to set:

Desired T_I/0.8 = TCT

60/tct = bpm setting

For example, start with a desired inspiratory time of 1.2 seconds. The formula becomes 1.2 ÷ 0.8 = 1.5 and 60 ÷ 1.5 = 40 bpm. The rate should be set on 40 bpm to time cycle pressure-supported breaths after 1.2 seconds. Time cycle a pressure-supported breath if the leak is too much and the inspiratory cycle off threshold cannot be adjusted high enough.

VENTILATORS USED

Critical care and home care ventilators have been used to provide NPPV, in either pressure control or volume control mode. Some ventilators are designed specifically for NPPV that provide pressure support or pressure control and PEEP.

Advantages of critical care ventilators are:

- The delivery of a precise oxygen concentration.
- Greater flexibility in modifying the breathing pattern.
- Graphic display of waveforms.
- More accurate monitors.
- Extensive alarm systems.
- An exhalation valve to prevent rebreathing of expired CO_2.

The primary disadvantage of critical care ventilators in the past was that few were designed to function in the presence of a leak. Several critical care ventilators now have a mask or noninvasive option. For most critical care ventilators, a pressure-supported inspiration ends when the flow falls to a specific threshold, usually 5 Lpm or 25% of the peak flow achieved during inspiration.

In NPPV a leak at the mask may exceed the flow cycle threshold of pressure-supported breaths and prolong inspiration. Prolonged inspirations unresponsive to the patient's breathing pattern promote asynchrony and reduce patient tolerance of NPPV. Several critical care ventilators have an adjustable flow cycle threshold for pressure-supported breaths. The expiratory sensitivity percentage (E_{sens} %) on the Puritan Bennett 840 (Nellcor Puritan Bennett LLC) and the inspiratory cycle off on the Servo^i (Maquet, Bridgewater, New Jersey) allows the clinician to adjust the terminal flow rate to a value greater than the leak flow rate.

For ventilators lacking an expiratory sensitivity adjustment, the pressure control mode may be used with a set inspiratory time of less than 1 second. The inspiratory time should be adjusted to match the patient's breathing pattern. In addition, some critical care ventilators, such as the Servo 300A, limit the duration of a pressure-supported breath to 80% of the total cycle time. The total cycle time is the period of time equal to 60 over the set breaths per minute. The breaths per minute control can be adjusted to time-cycle a pressure-supported breath in synchrony with the patient's breathing pattern.

Home care ventilators are traditionally volume controlled. Larger tidal volumes can generally compensate for the leak with NPPV. Slow responding pressure triggers on these ventilators make them better suited for patients with neuromuscular disease who tolerate time-triggered inspirations. The fixed inspiratory flow pattern delivered by most home care ventilators may not meet the inspiratory flow required by patients in acute respiratory failure who have a high respiratory rate.

Patient-triggered breaths should be monitored closely because the presence of a leak affects the

Best Practice

Mask Leaks

Mask ventilation in volume control may require larger tidal volumes to compensate for the leak. The leak may also compromise the patient's ability to trigger breaths.

ventilator's sensitivity to the patient's inspiratory efforts. Pressure-triggered breaths are more difficult to initiate. The use of a flow trigger may result in autotriggering. In either case, ventilator-patient asynchrony may increase the patient's work of breathing and reduce patient tolerance of mask ventilation.

Pressure ventilation, sometimes referred to as bilevel ventilation in NPPV, usually means providing pressure support or pressure control and PEEP. BiLevel (a trademark mode for the Puritan Bennett 840) is basically two levels of CPAP called High PEEP and Low PEEP. An active exhalation valve in BiLevel allows spontaneous breathing at either level of pressure. Spontaneous breaths are also pressure supported. The breathing time allowed at each pressure level is adjustable, and the changeover from one level of pressure to the other is synchronized with the patient's inspiratory effort.

In general, most pressure ventilators designed specifically for NPPV are similar in design.

- They are electrically powered, blower driven, microprocessor controlled, flow triggered, pressure limited, and flow cycled.
- Internal components consist of a blower, flow sensor, pressure-regulating valve, and pressure transducer.
- Controls allow the selection of the mode, the inspiratory and expiratory pressures, breaths per minute, and inspiratory time percentage.
- Some ventilators include a **rise time percentage** control that allows a gradual increase to the set pressure limit, thereby reducing the initial blast of flow. Pressure and flow waveforms in Figure 28-9 illustrate the effect of increasing rise time percentages. Reducing the initial blast of flow increases patient comfort but may also reduce the tidal volume for any given level of pressure support or control. Rise time percentage is available for both pressure support and pressure control breaths on most ventilators.

Most units use continuous flow from the blower to control inspiratory and expiratory pressures. The ventilator's microprocessor measures the known or

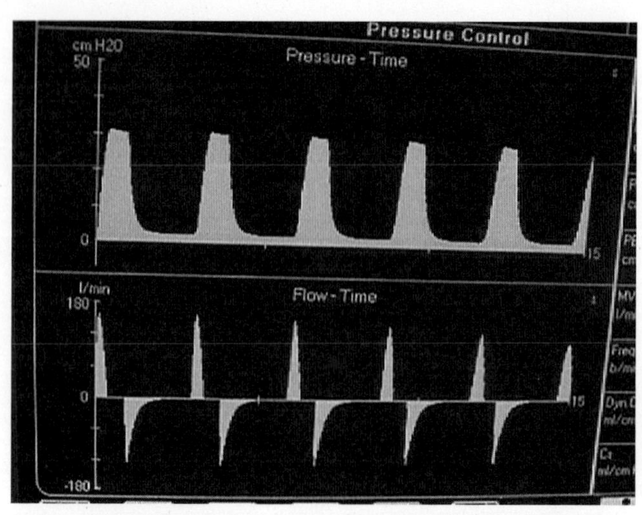

FIGURE 28-9 Pressure-time and flow-time waveforms as the rise time percentage is increased: The peak flow decreases as the rise time percentage increases. The front edge of the pressure-time waveform rounds off as more inspiratory time is taken to reach the pressure limit.

intentional leak out of the exhalation port during the initial setup and performance check. When the baseline leak is established, additional leak at the mask can be recognized and compensated for by adjusting flow to maintain the preset pressure limits. Many ventilator circuits do not include a standard exhalation valve. Exhalation is a function of the size of the leak in the circuit's exhalation port at the patient interface. As noted, rebreathing is possible and could prevent adequate alveolar ventilation if EPAP levels of <4 cm H_2O are used. Long inspiratory times, low inspiratory pressures, or large tidal volumes tend to increase the level of CO_2 rebreathing. In these cases, Philips Respironics recommends the use of the Plateau Exhalation Valve instead of the Whisper Swivel to reduce the level of CO_2 rebreathing for their ventilators. Both the Whisper Swivel II and the Plateau Exhalation Valve are reusable; the **castle port** comes with the disposable circuit. All BiPAP circuits must have one of these three types of exhalation devices.

Best Practice

Increasing Rise Time

Increasing the rise time percentage may make inspiration more comfortable but could reduce tidal volume. A long rise time may lead to patient-ventilator dyssynchrony.

BiPAP. The BiPAP S/T-D (Philips Respironics) has IPAP, EPAP, **spontaneous mode, spontaneous or timed (S/T) mode**, and timed modes. When either the IPAP or EPAP mode is selected, the patient is receiving CPAP. In spontaneous mode, the IPAP setting should be set higher than the EPAP pressure level or PEEP. The initiation of inspiration depends on the patient's respiratory effort. The patient triggers inspiration when the flow sensor measures an increase in flow of 40 mL per second over the leak flow for 30 ms. The minimum IPAP time is 180 ms. After 180 ms have elapsed, the unit flow cycles when the inspiratory flow equals the leak flow.[31]

In S/T mode, a breaths-per-minute rate may be set to ensure time-triggered breaths in addition to setting the IPAP and EPAP pressure levels. The patient is still able to trigger inspiration. In timed mode, the addition of the inspiratory time percentage control is added to determine the length of time that the IPAP pressure is applied. The patient's respiratory efforts cannot influence a changeover in the inspiratory or expiratory phase in the timed mode.

The monitor on the detachable control panel allows selection of IPAP, EPAP, estimated tidal volume (V_T in milliliters), or estimated leak (Lpm) for the LED display. A similar control panel is located under the back cover of the unit. In the estimated V_T position, the display flashes when the tidal volume is inaccurate because the estimated leak has changed by 15 Lpm.

- A display of "000" indicates that there has not been a change in flow for 20 seconds.
- When less than 1.0 cm H_2O is sensed by the pressure transducer, "OFL" is displayed in any of the selected positions.

The battery-powered *airway pressure monitor* (*APM*) should be turned on whenever the unit is on. The Inadvertent Off alarm activates if the APM is not turned on and the airway pressure is over 5 cm H_2O. There are also adjustable high- and low-airway-pressure alarms.

- The low-airway-pressure alarm activates if the airway pressure does not exceed the alarm setting within the adjustable delay time.
- The audible low-pressure-alarm can be silenced for either 20 or 60 seconds. The silence time is set by a switch located inside the device.
- A Replace Battery alarm warns when the batteries to the APM need replacing.

To check the operation of the BiPAP before use:

- Connect the circuit without the mask attached.
- Completely block the tubing outlet without blocking the exhalation port.

Best Practice

Reducing CO_2 Rebreathing

Long inspiratory times, low inspiratory pressures, or large tidal volumes tend to increase the level of CO_2 rebreathing. In these cases, Philips Respironics recommends the use of the Plateau Exhalation Valve instead of the Whisper Swivel to reduce the level of CO_2 rebreathing for its ventilators.

Best Practice

Inspiratory Flow

Inspirations are flow triggered and flow cycled when using the BiPAP ventilator in the spontaneous mode. To flow-trigger a breath, the patient's inspiratory effort must increase the flow by 40 mL per second over the leak flow for 30 ms. The unit flow cycles when the inspiratory flow equals the leak flow after 180 ms have elapsed.

- Set the IPAP at 8 cm H_2O and the EPAP at 5 cm H_2O and wait for 5 seconds.
- The Vest (estimated leak) display should be 20 Lpm or less.

Also check the APM by creating each of the alarm conditions and checking for alarm activation.

BiPAP Vision. Philips Respironics also makes the BiPAP Vision with CPAP and S/T modes.

In the *S/T mode*, a rate of 4–40 bpm may be set for time-triggered inspirations. In clinical practice, a set rate of 10 bpm is appropriate for most adults because the patient should trigger inspiration. The inspiratory time control determines the duration of inspiration or cycle time for timed-triggered, pressure control breaths. The patient triggers and cycles inspiration as long as the respiratory rate is greater than the breaths per minute control setting.

The user interface is as follows:

- A liquid crystal control panel displays waveforms, patient settings, F_IO_2, and alarm values.
- Four hard keys change the main screen to display monitoring, parameters, mode, or alarms values.
- The monitoring screen displays the current operating mode, parameters, and waveforms for pressure, flow, and volume.
- The main screen automatically returns to the monitoring view if no key is pressed for 3 minutes.

Best Practice

Verifying BiPAP Performance

The performance verification of the BiPAP is a check of the estimated leak. Block the circuit outlet, and set the IPAP on 8 cm H_2O and the EPAP on 5 cm H_2O. The estimated leak displayed should be 20 Lpm or less.

- Ventilator settings are adjusted by pressing the parameter hard key.
- The parameter screen displays the selected settings by pressing the soft key next to the displayed variable. The selected value can then be adjusted by turning a knob. Each click of the knob changes the value by 1, regardless of the variable.
- The same process applies for changing the mode and alarm values.

The BiPAP Vision can respond to changes in unintentional leaks at the patient interface by automatically adjusting its trigger and cycle criteria. Unintentional leaks are recognized as a change in the expiratory flow rate at 5 seconds or as the difference between inspiratory and expiratory tidal volumes. In either case, the baseline flow rate previously allowed for the intentional leak through the exhalation port is reset to include the flow from the unintentional leak. Intentional leak may also be manually reset by pressing Learn Base Flow. Learn Base (baseline) Flow should be pressed whenever gas flow from an external source is added to the circuit, for example, to power an inline medication nebulizer.

The trigger on the BiPAP Vision is either a 6-mL volume trigger or a shape signal. The **shape signal** is described as a graphic representation of the patient's actual flow pattern that is delayed by 300 ms and reduced by 15 Lpm (Figure 28-10). When the patient's actual flow signal crosses the shape signal:

- Inspiration begins. (The shape signal is sensitive to changing ventilatory patterns and circuit leaks.)
- The shape signal can also cycle spontaneous breaths.

Inspiration ends when the patient's:

- Inspiratory flow falls to 75% of the peak flow achieved during inspiration (spontaneous expiratory threshold).
- Inspiratory time exceeds 3 seconds.
- Or the flow toward the end of inspiration suddenly increases (flow reversal).

A rise time control can be set at either 0.05, 0.1, 0.2, or 0.4 second. Increasing the rise time lengthens the time required to reach the pressure limit and reduces the blast of gas flow that the patient experiences at the start of inspiration.

The oxygen module on the Vision adds oxygen to the air from the blower, allowing set oxygen concentrations up to 100%. The delivered oxygen concentration is within ±3% of the set percentage in concentrations of 30% or less, and it should be within ±10% of the set oxygen concentration in concentrations of over 30%.

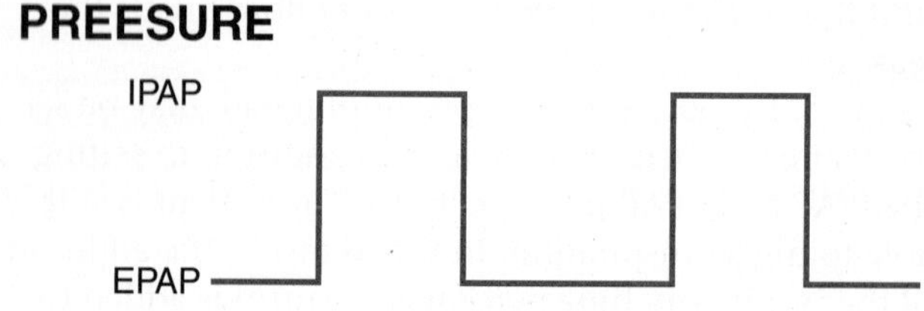

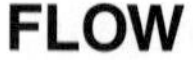

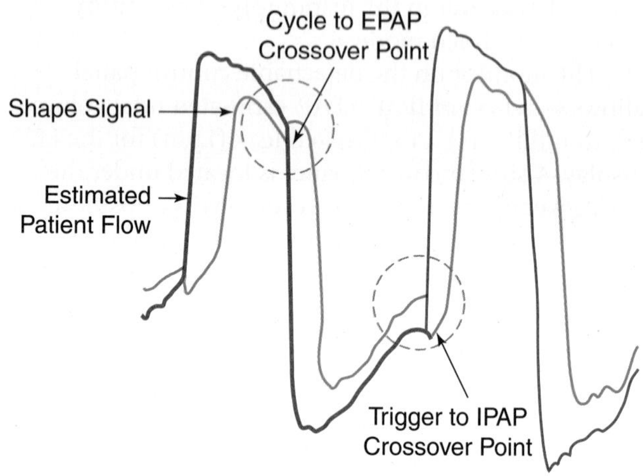

FIGURE 28-10 Inspiration is triggered and cycled when the actual flow pattern crosses the delayed flow pattern.
Courtesy of Philips Respironics

The performance verification of the Vision includes a check of the battery-powered Ventilator Inoperative alarm, exhalation port test, mode function, and alarms. When the Vision is powered on, a 60-second self-test is initiated. The setup screen then displays the soft key to run the exhalation port test. With the circuit connected and the circuit outlet occluded, start the test. The exhalation port test allows the unit to measure the leak at the exhalation port over the complete pressure range. This intentional leak information is stored in memory and used in leak calculations and in estimating the displayed tidal volume. If the exhalation port test is performed, the Patient's Leak % is displayed next to the minute ventilation. If the circuit is connected to the patient without running the exhalation port test, the Total Leak % is displayed. After the leak test is complete, press the monitoring hard key to begin operation with the last settings used before the unit was turned off. Verify mode, control, and alarm function before applying the flow to the patient.[38]

BiPAP-AVAPS[39]. Philips Respironics recently introduced the BiPAP-AVAPS (Figure 28-11). Activation of the average volume-assured pressure-support (AVAPS) feature provides volume-targeted pressure-support/control breaths in all modes except CPAP. The modes are CPAP, spontaneous (PS/CPAP),

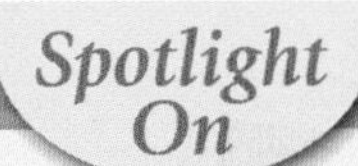

Shape Signal

The BiPAP Vision maintains trigger sensitivity despite changes in the patient's ventilatory pattern and circuit leaks by using a shape signal. A shape signal is a duplication of the patient's actual flow pattern, delayed by 300 ms and reduced by 15 Lpm. Inspiration begins or ends whenever the actual flow pattern crosses the shape signal.

Best Practice

BiPAP Vision Performance Test

Run the *exhalation port test* (*EPT*) as the performance check for the BiPAP Vision. The EPT establishes the leak at the exhalation port over the entire pressure range. This intentional leak information is stored in memory and used to track leaks and to estimate displayed tidal volumes during ventilation.

CASE STUDY 28-3

J. R., a patient treated in the emergency department with NPPV, has received nasal mask ventilation with the BiPAP S/T-D for 2 hours. Ventilator settings for the last 30 minutes in S/T mode are IPAP 20 cm H_2O, EPAP 5 cm H_2O, respiratory rate 10 bpm, and total respiratory rate 17 bpm. The patient's P_aCO_2 has remained elevated but consistently between 65 and 69 cm H_2O since admission. The S_pO_2 has been between 90% and 92% with oxygen added at 8 Lpm.

The respiratory therapist notices that J. has lost consciousness and his blood pressure has started to fall. He is no longer triggering inspiration. S_pO_2 has dropped to 85%.

Questions

1. What action is now indicated?
2. What ventilator settings would be appropriate?
3. Why would not the appropriate action have been to maintain NPPV and change the mode on the BiPAP to timed mode with an inspiration time of 25%?

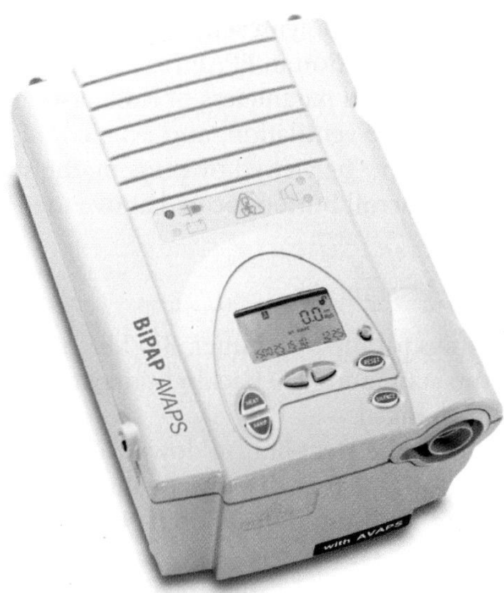

FIGURE 28-11 BiPAP® *AVAPS*™

Courtesy of Philips Respironics, Murrysville, Pennsylvania

spontaneous/timed, timed and pressure control. All breaths in the CPAP and spontaneous modes are patient triggered and cycled by the Digital Auto-Trak system previously described for the Vision. Breaths are time triggered in S/T mode if the patient fails to initiate a breath within the set total cycle time window that equals 60/bpm. Machine-triggered breaths are time cycled. The patient's inspiratory efforts do not trigger a breath in the Timed mode, in which all breaths are time triggered and cycled. In pressure control mode, breaths may be patient or machine triggered, but all breaths are time cycled.

When the unit is first connected to power with the side pressure button off:

- The screen lights up and begins to scroll through self-test, software version, blower hours, and standby screens. The standby screen displays the enable features: patient, apnea, light, and whether Encore SmartCard is inserted. The Encore SmartCard records compliance data, short-term and long-term ventilation trends, and ventilation statistics.
- Setup is displayed in the upper right corner if the unit is in Provider mode, which allows access to settings that are not available to the patient.
- The numbers on the standby screen indicate the hours of use at pressure.
- Pressing the pressure button displays the monitoring screen.
- The monitoring screen displays the mode and actual pressure Activation of FLEX or AVAPS will allow a Bi-FLEX reduction of the IPAP at end-inspiration and drops the EPAP during active exhalation to improve patient comfort. Bi-FLEX

settings are 0–3, with setting 3 creating the greatest reduction in EPAP (to zero pressure).

- The measured parameters of leak, respiratory rate, minute ventilation, and exhaled tidal volume may be viewed by pressing the small circular Scroll button located above the Reset button.

In the User mode:

- Settings for the humidifier, Bi-FLEX, rise time, ramp start, and LED backlight may be viewed and changed.
- Holding the Heat button down in the standby or monitoring screen displays the humidifier setting screen. The humidifier is on if "HEAT" appears on the screen.
- The Bi-FLEX setting appears only in the spontaneous mode and only if the IPAP is set on 20 cm H_2O or less.
- Rise time can be changed if the mode is not CPAP and if the Bi-FLEX setting is zero.
- The ramp start may be adjusted from 4 cm H_2O to the EPAP pressure setting.
- Backlighting of the control buttons may be turned on or off.

When the AVAPS feature is activated:

- The provider sets the target tidal volume, the IPAPmax at 25–30 cm H_2O, the IPAPmin at EPAP + 4 cm H_2O, and EPAP. The unit automatically adjusts IPAP to provide the target tidal volume.
- The unit must be in the Provider mode to activate AVAPS or change AVAPS settings. To access the Provider mode when the unit is in the User mode, press and hold down the Right and Silence buttons simultaneously for 2 seconds. A short audible alarm indicates access to the Provider mode.
- Use the Heat or Ramp button to select a mode.
- When the desired mode is displayed, press the Right user button to activate AVAPS.
- Use the Heat or Ramp button to display a 1 to activate AVAPS or a 0 to deactivate it.
- With AVAPS activated, press the Right user button to set the parameters: target volume, IPAPmax, IPAPmin, EPAP, bpm, inspiratory time, ramp length in seconds, ramp start pressure, rise time, apnea interval, patient disconnect alarm in seconds, low minute ventilation alarm, and low tidal volume alarm.
- Use the Heat button to increase or the Ramp button to decrease the value for each setting.

Inspiratory time and bpm settings are not available in spontaneous mode.

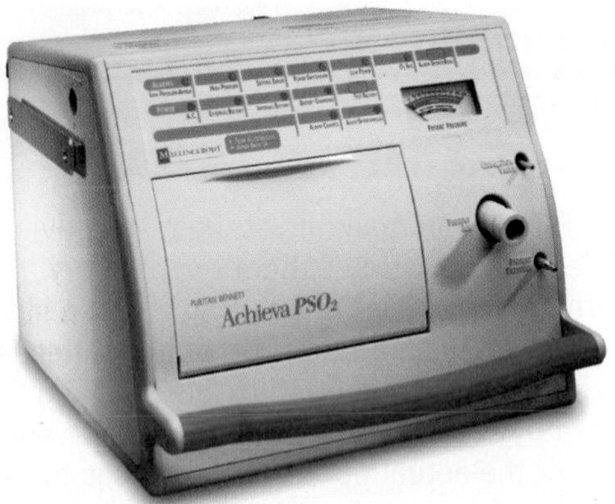

FIGURE 28-12 AchievaPS.

Image used by permission from Nellcor Puritan Bennett LLC, Boulder, Colorado, part of Covidien

PB AchievaPS. The AchievaPS (Covidien Puritan Bennett, Boulder, Colorado) is a portable ventilator intended for use with adult and pediatric patients in the subacute and home care settings (Figure 28-12). The ventilator is piston driven and microprocessor controlled, with download capabilities to a computer or modem. The AchievaPS provides both volume-limited and pressure-limited A/C, volume-limited SIMV with pressure support, and a spontaneous mode of pressure support with CPAP. There is no backup ventilation in the spontaneous mode. Pressure-limited ventilation is activated in A/C mode by setting an inspiratory pressure level. In volume-limited A/C, tidal volumes can be adjusted from 50 to 2200 mL at frequencies of 1–80 bpm. The AchievaPS has an internal PEEP valve and an internal oxygen blender. A fully charged internal battery lasts approximately 1 hour during high load operation and 4 hours under minimal load.

The three buttons along the top of the inside front panel are Standby, Ventilate, and Menu/Esc.

- Pressing the Start/Enter switch powers the ventilator on in Standby mode.
- While in Standby mode, an operation verification test can be initiated through the Menu/Esc key.
- After setting the controls, initiate ventilation by pressing Ventilate. Indicators light, and a nonadjustable audible alarm sounds.
- Allow three ventilator breaths to check the low inspiratory alarm function. The circuit must be disconnected from the patient to set the low pressure alarm. The pressure trigger setting flashes in the display for verification.
- Flow trigger settings are continuously displayed under the sensitivity. Breaths are flow or pressure triggered, depending on which trigger condition occurs first. Pressure triggering is recommended when using PEEP.[40]

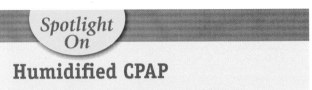

Humidified CPAP

The HC200 Series Humidified CPAP System supplies a built-in heated humidifier with the CPAP system. A warm-up mode gradually increases the pressure to allow the patient to fall asleep.

CONTINUOUS POSITIVE AIRWAY PRESSURE UNITS

The devices just described for NPPV can also deliver CPAP. However, if the patient requires only nocturnal CPAP, a less expensive CPAP unit is indicated. CPAP and its use in the home care setting for obstructive sleep apnea are discussed elsewhere in this text. Both NPPV and CPAP devices share common patient interfaces, as well as the problem of providing adequate humidification. An unheated passover humidifier can be added to most CPAP systems. Certain heated humidifiers may also be used in the home care setting.

HC200 Series Humidified CPAP System. The HC200 Series Humidified CPAP System (Fisher & Paykel, Auckland, New Zealand) is a CPAP device with a built-in heated humidification system. The humidity system of the HC200 ensures adequate humidification overnight. Set pressure varies at 3–18 cm H_2O. The warm-up mode allows a gradual increase in airflow and pressure as the heater plate reaches the set temperature,

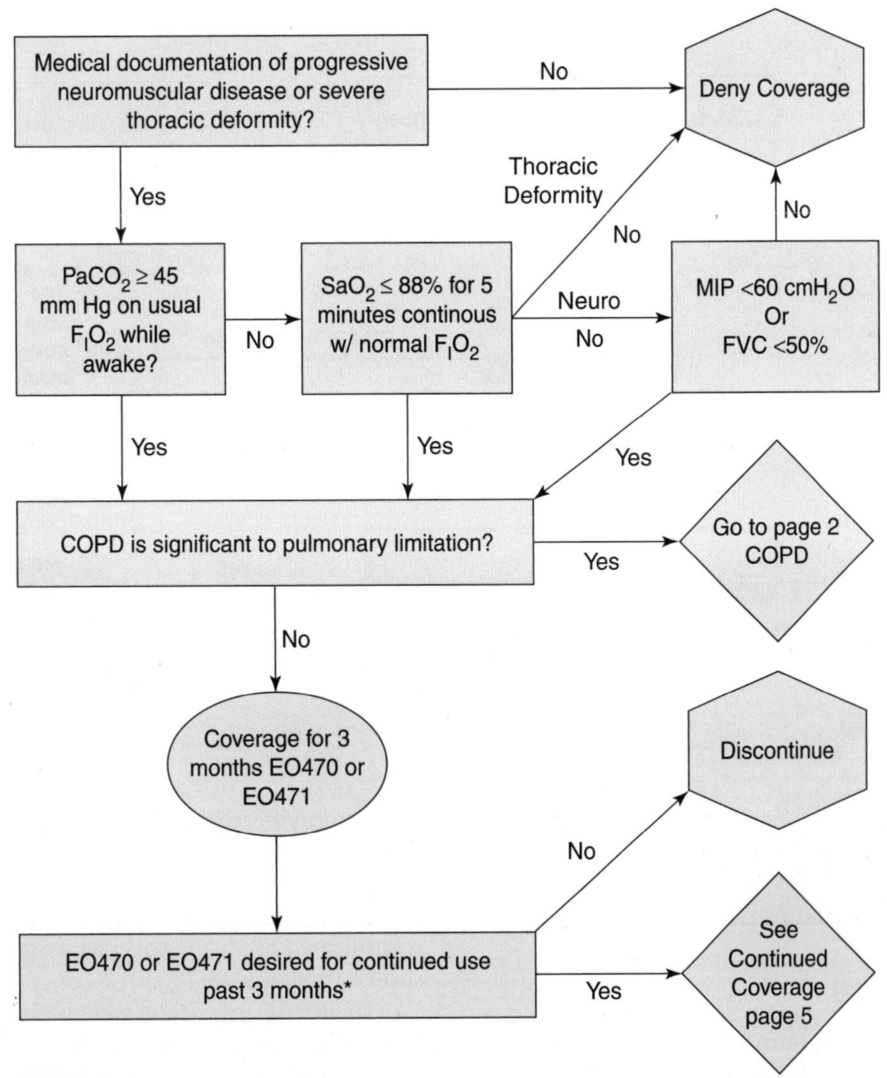

FIGURE 28-13 Medicare flowchart of coverage criteria for NPPV. (*continues*)

Reprinted with permission from Hill KF. NPPRA revisited. American Association of Respiratory Care Home Care Bulletin. *2000:1–3*

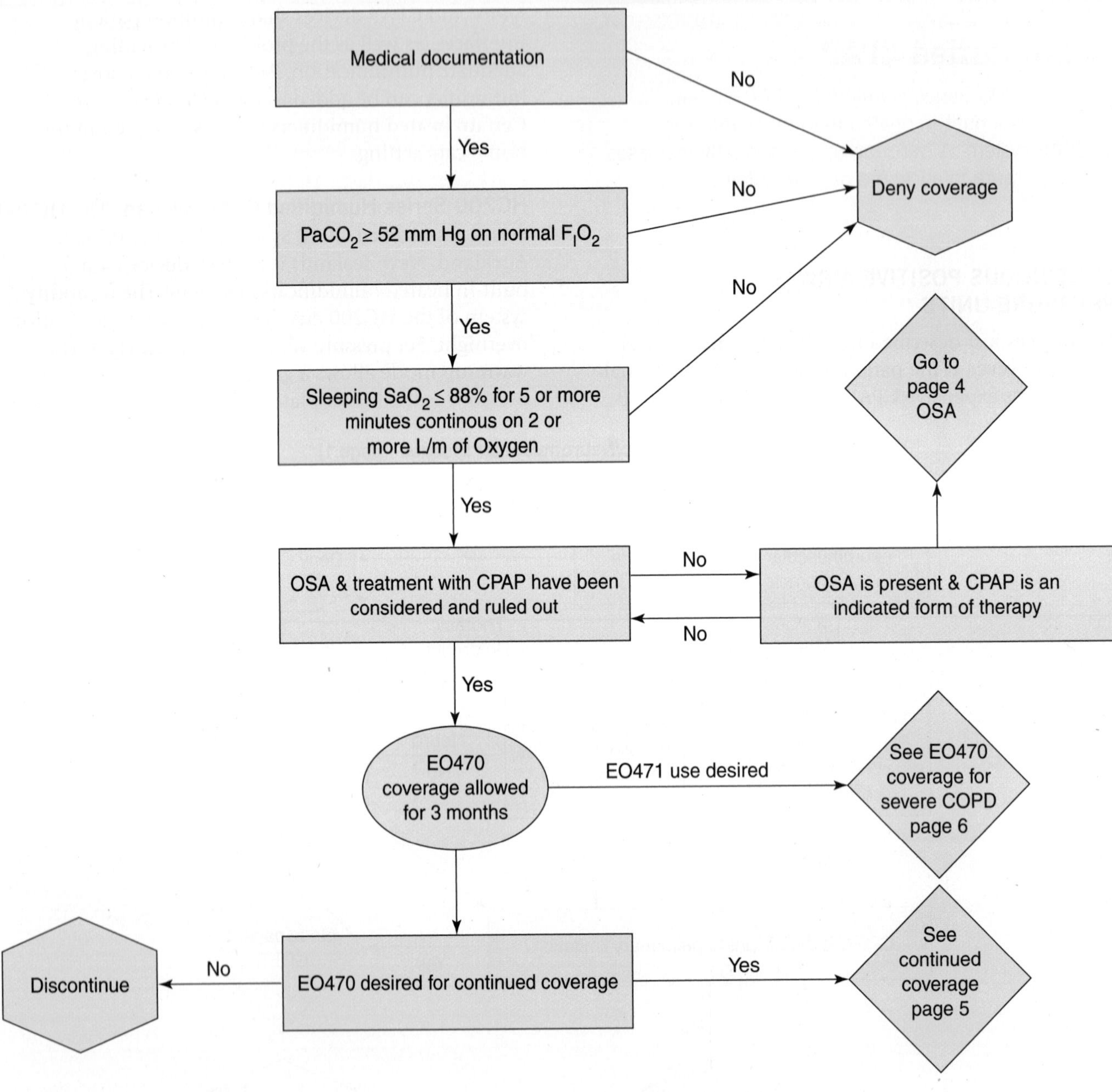

FIGURE 28-13 *(continues)*

which is adjustable by the user. The unit can also be switched from warm-up mode to the full set pressure in the Test mode. The power supply can use either 110 or 240 V for international travel.

Long-Term Use

Medicare coverage of long-term NPPV for patients with COPD is essentially limited to patients without obstructive sleep apnea, as documented by a multichannel sleep study, or to cases where nocturnal CPAP has been ineffective. Medicare policy refers to the bilevel units specifically designed for NPPV as respiratory assist devices (RAD) to provide noninvasive positive pressure respiratory assist (NPPRA). The complicated Medicare coverage criteria for RAD are shown in Figure 28-13.[41]

The Medicare criteria were based in part on the recommendations from the 1998 Consensus Conference on indications for nasal NPPV, convened by the National Association for Medical Direction of Respiratory Care (NAMDRC). The conference was held at the

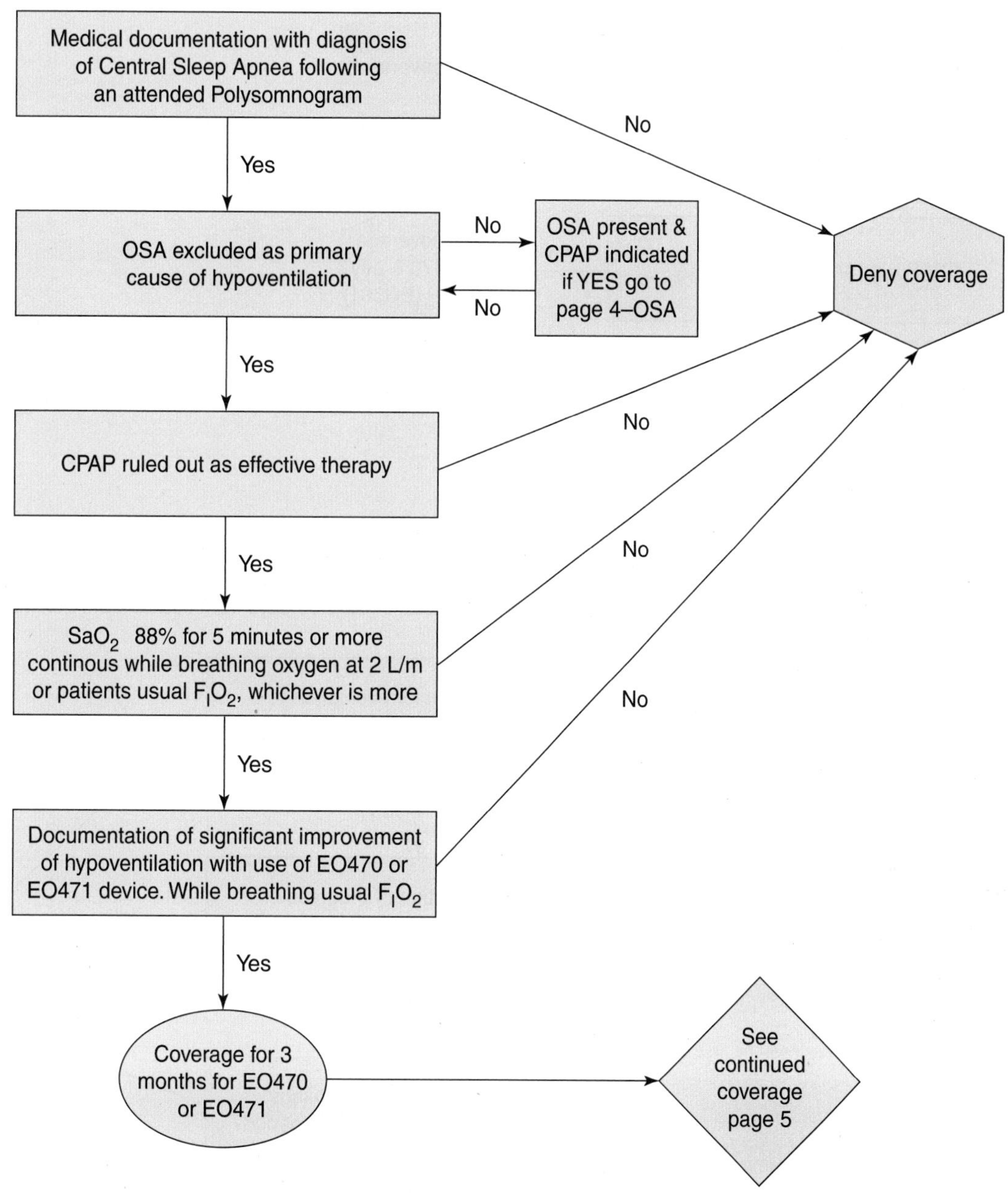

FIGURE 28-13 (*continues*)

request of the Centers for Medicaid & Medicare Services (CMMS), which pays for the services and equipment provided to Medicare beneficiaries. Reimbursement for NPPV devices that did not have a backup rate control was approximately $240 per month for up to 15 months in 1998. These devices were not categorized as mechanical ventilators. The NPPV device was classified as a mechanical ventilator with reimbursement of approximately $550 per month for as long as the device was being used if it incorporated a backup rate control.[42] To provide their patients with quality respiratory care services in the home that were otherwise not covered under Medicare, some physicians prescribed NPPV devices with backup rates. CMMS saw the rapid increase in the use of nasal NPPV with mechanical ventilators as an abuse of the system. Rather than recognizing that respiratory care services are an important element in quality home care and worthy of reimbursement, CMMS simply changed the rules of reimbursement for NPPV. The guidelines

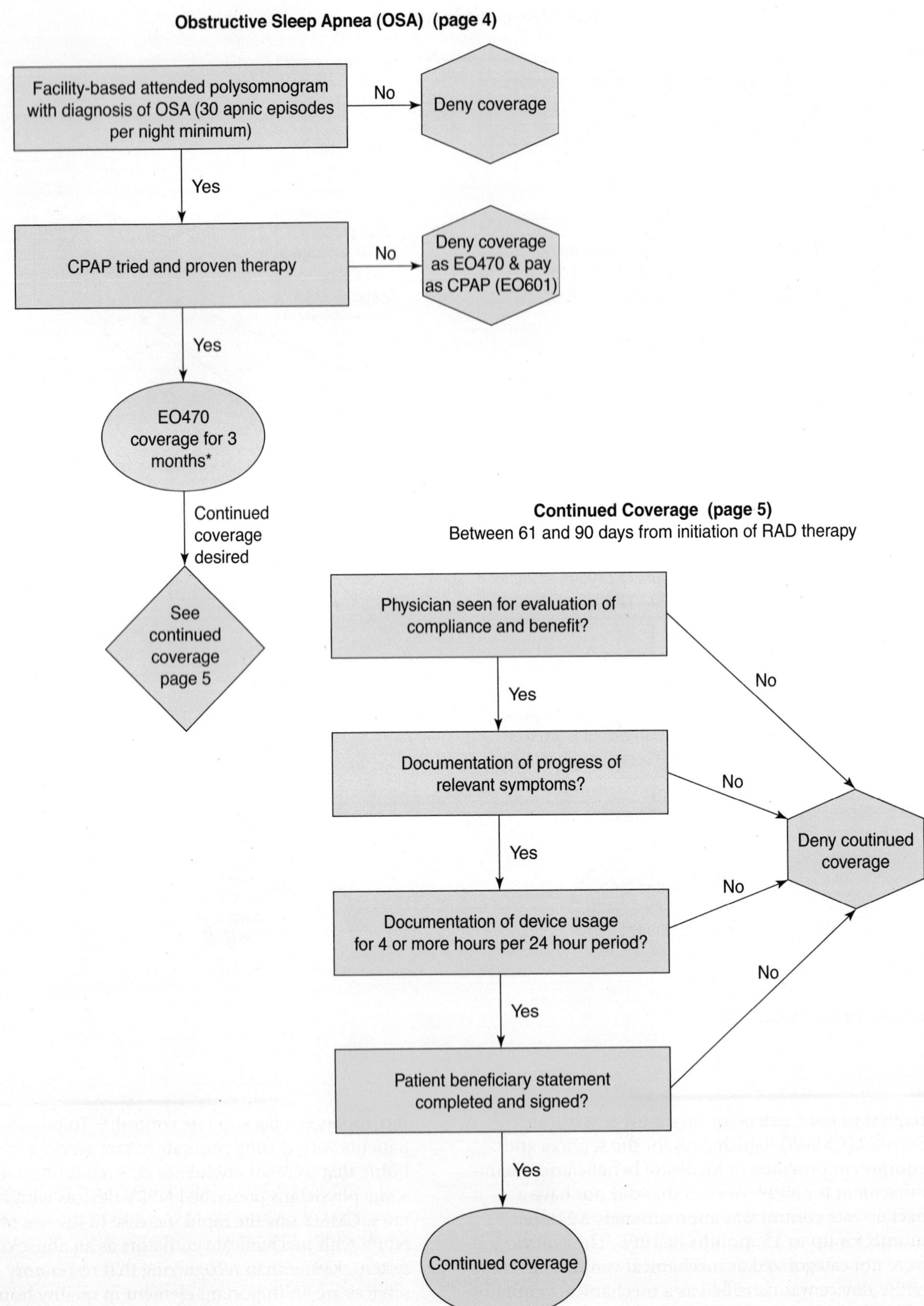

FIGURE 28-13 (*continues*)

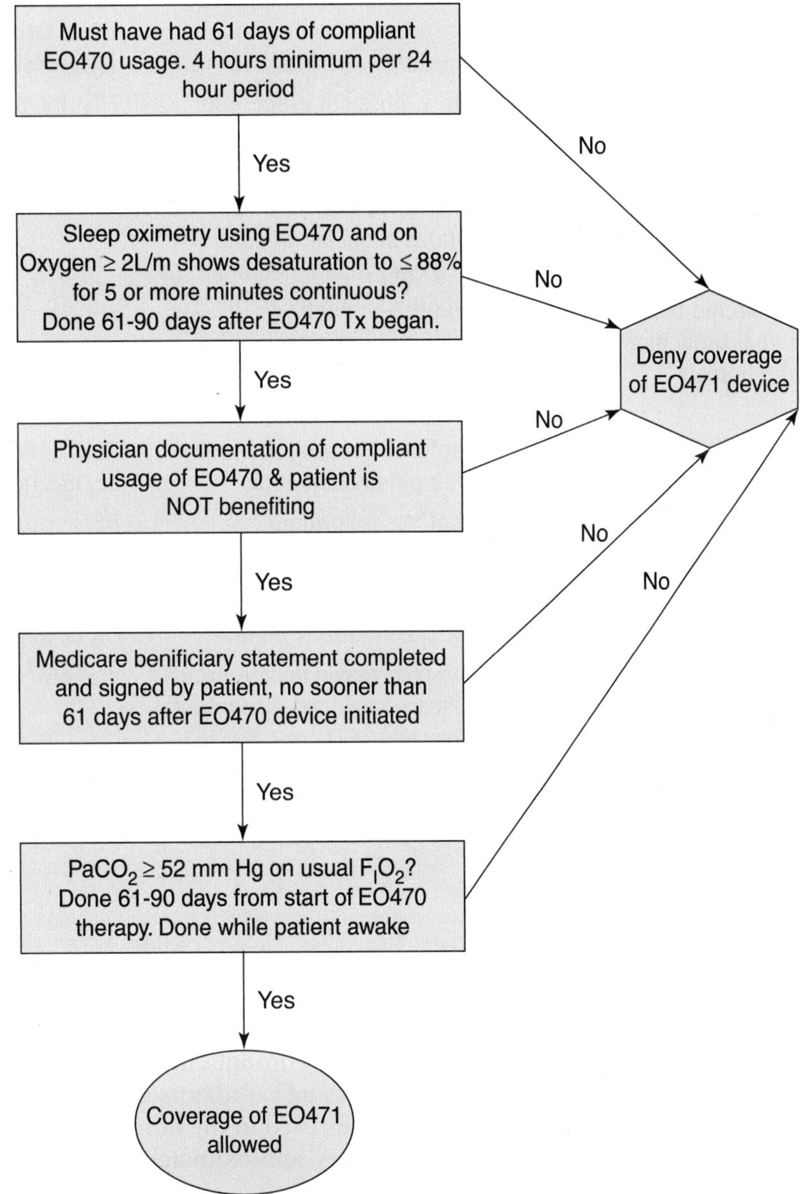

FIGURE 28-13 (*continued*)

from the conference proceedings are listed in Table 28-2. There are some discrepancies between the conference guidelines and the Medicare flowcharts. Medicare coverage changed again in 2006 when certain RADs that had been classified as durable medical equipment (DME) requiring frequent servicing were reclassified as capped rental DME items. The covered rental payment drops after 3 months, and the patient takes over ownership of the device after 13 months.

Negative Pressure Ventilation

Negative pressure ventilators date back to the 1800s, when inventors in the United States and Europe were independently developing similar devices. J. Dalziel described the first tank ventilator in 1832.[43] In 1928, P. Drinker and L. Shaw produced the first practical model of the tank ventilator, dubbed the iron lung. J. H. Emerson Co. (Cambridge, Massachusetts) modified the design and made the iron lung commercially available.

TABLE 28-2 **NAMDRC guidelines for nasal NPPV for restrictive thoracic disorders, COPD, and nocturnal hypoventilation**

	COPD	Restrictive Thoracic Disorders	Nocturnal Hypoventilation from Other Than COPD or Neuromuscular Disease
Disease	History, physical exam, and diagnostic tests Optimal management and management of underlying disorders; sleep study if indicated Includes chronic bronchitis, emphysema, bronchiectasis, and cystic fibrosis	History, physical exam, and diagnostic tests; optimal management of underlying disease; sleep study if indicated Includes sequelae of polio spinal cord injury, neuropathics, myopathics, and dystrophics, amyotrophic lateral sclerosis, chest wall deformities, and kyphoscoliosis	History, physical exam, and polysomnogram for diagnosis of OSA; CPAP trial unless previous trial unsuccessful
Indications for use	Symptoms: fatigue, dyspnea, morning headache, etc. One of the following: • $P_aCO_2 \geq 55$ mm Hg • P_aCO_2 50–54 mm Hg and nocturnal desaturation (S_pO_2) ≤ 88% for 5 continuous minutes on ≥2 Lpm O_2 • P_aCO_2 50–54 mm Hg and hospitalization related to recurrent (≥2 in 12 months) episodes of hypercapnic respiratory failure	Symptoms: fatigue, dyspnea, morning headache, etc. One of the following: • $P_aCO_2 \geq 45$ mm Hg • Nocturnal desaturation ≤88% for 5 continuous minutes • For progressive neuromuscular disease, maximal inspiratory pressure <60 cm • H_2O or FVC <50% predicted	Polysomnography (PSG) criteria of OSA not responsive to CPAP PSG criteria for mixed sleep apnea not responsive to CPAP Central sleep apnea Other forms of nocturnal hypoventilation

Source: Goldberg A, Legar P, Hill N, et al. Clinical indications for noninvasive positive pressure ventilation in chronic respiratory failure due to restrictive lung disease, COPD, and nocturnal hypoventilation—a consensus conference report. Chest. *1999;116: 521–534. Reprinted with permission*

For the next 20 years. the iron lung was used extensively to provide both acute and long-term ventilatory support. The polio epidemics of the 1930s and 1940s put hundreds of patients with respiratory muscle paralysis in iron lungs.[44]

During a particularly severe polio outbreak in Denmark in 1952, the iron lung supply was quickly depleted, and over 2000 cases of respiratory failure were managed with manual positive pressure ventilation. The success of positive pressure ventilation in Denmark sparked a fervor of research and development of positive pressure ventilators. The advance of the Salk polio vaccine in 1955, however, marked a dramatic decline in new cases of respiratory muscle paralysis from polio.

Intubation and positive pressure ventilation were widely accepted as best practice by the mid-1960s. In the 1980s, the nocturnal use of negative pressure ventilation gained attention as a way to improve daytime oxygen and carbon dioxide levels for patients with neuromuscular disease and COPD. Positive pressure ventilators still outnumber negative pressure units used in the home. Currently in the United States, approximately 50 individuals are using the

Best Practice

Negative Pressure Ventilation Support

Negative pressure can support ventilation in four ways: during inspiration, continuously, continuously with additional pressure during inspiration, and as negative pressure during inspiration with positive pressure applied during exhalation. Continuous negative pressure can provide the same increase in lung volume as CPAP.

Emerson iron lung. However, several pulmonary rehabilitation centers in Europe predominantly use negative pressure ventilators. Recent studies report the use of tank ventilators for patients with acute respiratory failure.[9,43,45–47]

TYPES

Negative pressure ventilation can be applied during inspiration to provide adequate tidal volumes:

- Intermittent negative pressure ventilation (INPV) to continuously increase lung volume during spontaneous breathing
- Continuous negative extrathoracic pressure (CNEP) for the same increase in lung volume as CPAP
- Intermittent negative pressure, superimposed on continuous negative pressure breathing
- A negative pressure during inspiration and positive pressure during exhalation

PHYSIOLOGIC EFFECTS

A tank ventilator can provide adequate alveolar ventilation for a patient with little or no spontaneous inspiratory effort. Negative pressure ventilation has been used to treat hypercapnic respiratory failure in patients with COPD. In a study that compared positive pressure ventilation with negative pressure ventilation in 26 pairs of patients with COPD, there was no significant difference in mortality, complications, or the median number of days in the hospital.[48] The duration of mechanical ventilation in the group ventilated with negative pressure was significantly shorter.

There is some evidence that NPV can effectively rest the respiratory muscles in patients with COPD. In two studies, respiratory muscle strength increased, and P_aCO_2 decreased after a week in which either a tank or Pulmo-Wrap device was used for 6 hours continuously or for 8 hours intermittently each day.[49,50] In another report, the electromyographic activity of the respiratory muscles of patients with COPD decreased dramatically during NPV when compared with spontaneous breathing.[51]

A major concern with NPV is its effect on the upper airway. NPV may decrease the caliber of the upper airway at the glottic or subglottic level. When NPV is applied during sleep, normally coordinated respiratory activity between the pharyngeal, laryngeal, and inspiratory muscles may be abolished and result in upper airway obstruction. Negative pressure ventilation may also cause lower esophageal dysfunction and increase the risk of regurgitation and aspiration.

Tank ventilators also have the same adverse effects on hemodynamics as do positive pressure ventilators. The Pulmo-Wrap and cuirass may have less of an effect on cardiac output because the applied negative pressure is less effective in expanding the lungs compared with tank ventilators.

VENTILATORS

These devices apply subambient pressure to the body surface. As the chest wall moves outward, alveolar pressure drops below ambient pressure, creating a pressure gradient for gas flow into the lungs. When the negative **extrathoracic** pressure is released, the elastic recoil of the lungs increases alveolar pressure, reversing the pressure gradient for exhalation. Tank ventilators apply subambient pressure to the entire body from the neck down. Chest shells like the cuirass or Pulmo-Wrap fit over the thorax and abdomen or only over the thorax.[52] There is no need for an artificial airway in either case, but the natural upper airway must be patent.

Negative pressure devices use a vacuum pump to generate negative pressure. The peak negative inspiratory pressure control determines the tidal volume. A square or rectangular negative pressure waveform produces a greater tidal volume than does a sine waveform. Most devices have inspiratory and expiratory time controls or an inspiratory time and rate setting. Most can provide CNEP. Some units can be flow triggered via a nasal sensor. Tank ventilators are the most efficient, followed by the Pulmo-Wrap and then the chest cuirass. Less efficient ventilators require higher negative pressures to achieve tidal volumes similar to those from a tank ventilator.[53] Peak negative pressure is adjusted on the basis of tidal volumes measured at the mouth by a handheld respirometer.

INDICATIONS FOR USE

Negative pressure ventilation may be an option for patients who are able to maintain a patent upper airway but who are unable to tolerate NPPV or for patients who find tracheostomies undesirable. There is inadequate evidence to support the use of negative pressure ventilation for patients with acute exacerbation of COPD.[9]

Best Practice

Adjusting Peak Negative Pressure

During NPV, the peak negative pressure is adjusted on the basis of tidal volumes measured at the mouth by a handheld respirometer.

CASE STUDY 28-4

A therapist working in the Unita di Terapia Intensiva Respiratoria in a hospital in Firenze, Italy, was called to the emergency room. G. S., who has a chest wall deformity, was admitted for acute ventilatory failure. The physician ordered negative pressure ventilation for Mr. S., and he was is placed in a Porta-Lung tank ventilator.

Questions

1. What control determines the tidal volume?
2. What negative pressure setting should be used initially?
3. How is the tidal volume monitored?
4. How should the breaths per minute and I/E ratio be adjusted?

Although NPV has been used successfully over the years to support patients in respiratory failure from a variety of etiologies, no randomized controlled trials have demonstrated its superiority over positive pressure ventilation. There are enough concerns about airway integrity during NPV to restrict its use to selected patients.

Summary

Although noninvasive ventilation is not new, the technology associated with noninvasive positive pressure ventilation (NPPV) ventilation has improved since the 1990s. In the acute care setting, NPPV may be an alternative to intubation and invasive ventilation in 75% of the patients with acute exacerbation of COPD. Long-term NPPV is an option for select patients with COPD who meet Medicare's coverage criteria. The use of negative pressure ventilation in the same patient population is not currently supported by the results of clinical trials but may be useful in patients unable to tolerate mask ventilation. Finally, CPAP or NPPV application represents the current standard of care in cases of acute cardiogenic pulmonary edema.

Study Questions

REVIEW QUESTIONS

1. What are the advantages of noninvasive positive pressure ventilation?
2. According to the recommendations of the AARC Conference on Noninvasive Positive Pressure Ventilation, which patients in acute respiratory failure may benefit the most from noninvasive positive pressure ventilation?
3. What are the advantages and disadvantages of using critical care versus home care positive pressure ventilators for NPPV?
4. What are the various types of patient interfaces used in noninvasive positive pressure ventilation?
5. What are the primary settings on the BiPAP S/T-D ventilator?
6. What is an alternative method of cycling pressure support for some critical care ventilators?
7. What is a common complication of NPPV delivered via face mask?
8. Under what circumstances should NPPV be discontinued?
9. What is one advantage and one disadvantage of negative pressure ventilators?

MULTIPLE-CHOICE QUESTIONS

1. Which of the following is not associated with NPPV?
   a. head straps
   b. endotracheal tube
   c. nasal mask
   d. nasal pillows
2. Which of the following are complications of NPPV?
   I. aspiration
   II. vocal cord paralysis
   III. eye irritation or conjunctivitis
   IV. skin abrasions on the nose
   a. I, II, III, and IV
   b. I and IV only
   c. II only
   d. I, III, and IV only
3. Which of the following have occurred for patients with acute respiratory failure due to exacerbation of COPD who have been treated with NPPV?
   I. decreased mortality
   II. decreased duration of mechanical ventilation
   III. reduced incidence of ventilator-associated pneumonia
   IV. decreased need for endotracheal intubation
   a. I, II, III, and IV
   b. I and IV only
   c. III and IV only
   d. IV only
4. Which of the following are contraindications (absolute or relative) for the use of NPPV in patients with acute respiratory failure due to exacerbation of COPD?
   I. respiratory arrest
   II. excessive secretions
   III. increased P_aCO_2 level
   IV. severe claustrophobia
   a. I, II, III, and IV
   b. IV only
   c. I, II, and IV
   d. I only

5. Which *pressure support* ventilator allows the user to set an oxygen concentration?
   a. BiPAP S/T-D
   b. BiPAP AVAPS
   c. BiPAP Vision
   d. none of the above
6. Which of the following alters the oxygen concentration delivered when supplemental oxygen is added to the circuit?
   I. a change in the pressure gradient (IPAP – EPAP)
   II. an increase in IPAP alone
   III. an increase in EPAP alone
   IV. a change in the percentage inspiratory time
   a. I, II, III, and IV
   b. I and III only
   c. II and IV only
   d. I only
7. Which one of the following types of negative pressure ventilation has the same effect as CPAP?
   a. negative pressure during inspiration only
   b. negative pressure during inspiration and positive pressure during exhalation
   c. continuous negative extrathoracic pressure with a greater negative pressure superimposed during inspiration
   d. continuous negative extrathoracic pressure

CRITICAL-THINKING QUESTIONS

1. What is one way to determine the IPAP level for a patient in acute or chronic respiratory failure?
2. Why is it important to check the pressure support ventilators by occluding the circuit?
3. Why would 4 cm H_2O EPAP probably be appropriate for most patients?
4. Under what circumstance would negative pressure ventilation be inappropriate?

References

1. Confalonieri M, et al. Acute respiratory failure in patients with severe community-acquired pneumonia. *Am J Respir Crit Care Med.* 1999;160: 1585–1591.
2. Hess DR. Noninvasive positive-pressure ventilation and ventilator-associated pneumonia. *Respir Care.* 2005;50,7:924–929.
3. Nourdine K, et al. Does noninvasive ventilation reduce the ICU nosocomial infection risk? A prospective clinical survey. *Intensive Care Med.* 1999. 25,6:567–573.
4. Girault, C., et al. Noninvasive ventilation as a systematic extubation and weaning technique in acute-on-chronic respiratory failure: a prospective, randomized controlled study. *Am J Respir Crit Care Med.* 1999;160,1:86–92.
5. Nava S, et al. Noninvasive mechanical ventilation in the weaning of patients with respiratory failure due to chronic obstructive pulmonary disease. A randomized, controlled trial. *Ann Intern Med.* 1998;128,9:721–728.
6. Kallet RH, Diaz JV. The physiologic effects of noninvasive ventilation. *Respir Care.* 2009;54,1:102–115.
7. Pierson DJ. Noninvasive positive pressure ventilation: history and terminology. In: *Consensus Conference IV: Noninvasive Positive Pressure Ventilation*. Vail, Colorado: Daedalus Enterprises, Inc.; 1997.
8. Mushin W, et al. *Historical Background to Automatic Ventilation*. 3rd ed. A.V.o.t. Lungs. St. Louis, MO: Blackwell Mosby; 1980.
9. Bach JR. Consensus statement: noninvasive positive pressure ventilation. In: *Consensus Conference IV: Noninvasive Positive Pressure Ventilation*. Vail, Colorado: Daedalus Enterprises, Inc.; 1997.
10. Brochard L. Noninvasive ventilation in acute respiratory failure. *Respir Care.* 1996;41,5: 456–446.
11. Keenan SP, Mehta S. Noninvasive ventilation for patients presenting with acute respiratory failure: the randomized controlled trials. *Respir Care.* 2009; 54,1:116–126.
12. Anton A, et al. Predicting the result of noninvasive ventilation in severe acute exacerbations of patients with chronic airflow limitation. *Chest.* 2000;117,3: 828–833.
13. Hilbert G, et al. Noninvasive pressure support ventilation in COPD patients with postextubation hypercapnic respiratory insufficiency. *Eur Respir J.* 1998;11,6:1349–1353.
14. Ferrer M, et al. Early noninvasive ventilation averts extubation failure in patients at risk: a randomized trial. *Am J Respir Crit Care Med.* 2006;173,2: 164–170.
15. Boles JM, et al. Weaning from mechanical ventilation. *Eur Respir J.* 2007;29,5:1033–1056.
16. Mehta S, Al-Hashim AH, Keenan SP. Noninvasive ventilation in patients with acute cardiogenic pulmonary edema. *Respir Care.* 2009;54,2: 186–195; discussion 195–197.
17. Winck J, et al. Efficacy and safety of noninvasive ventilation in the treatment of acute cardiogenic pulmonary edema-a systematic review and meta-analysis. *Critical Care.* 2006;10,2:R69.

18. Hess DR, Fessler HE. Should noninvasive positive-pressure ventilation be used in all forms of acute respiratory failure? *Respir Care.* 2007;52,5: 568–578.
19. Medoff BD. Invasive and noninvasive ventilation in patients with asthma. *Respir Care.* 2008;53,6: 740–748; discussion 749–750.
20. Soroksky A, Stav D, Shpirer I. A pilot prospective, randomized, placebo-controlled trial of bilevel positive airway pressure in acute asthmatic attack. *Chest.* 2003;123,4:1018–1025.
21. Jain S, Hanania NA, Guntupalli KK. Ventilation of patients with asthma and obstructive lung disease., In: Tharratt, RS, ed. *Critical Care Clinics*. Philadelphia: W. B. Saunders Co: 1998: 685–705.
22. Costa R, et al. Comparative evaluation of different helmets on patient-ventilator interaction during noninvasive ventilation. *Intensive Care Med.* 2008;34,6:1102–1108.
23. Navalesi P, et al. Noninvasive ventilation in chronic obstructive pulmonary disease patients: helmet versus facial mask. *Intensive Care Medicine.* 2007;33,1:74–81.
24. Hess DR. How to initiate a noninvasive ventilation program: bringing the evidence to the bedside. *Respir Care.* 2009;54,2:232–243; discussion 243–245.
25. Chatburn RL. Which ventilators and modes can be used to deliver noninvasive ventilation? *Respir Care.* 2009;54,1:85–101.
26. Nava S, Navalesi P, Gregoretti C. Interfaces and humidification for noninvasive mechanical ventilation. *Respir Care.* 2009;54,1:71–84.
27. Hotchkiss JR, Marini JJ. Noninvasive ventilation: an emerging supportive technique for the emergency department. *Ann Emerg Med.* 1998; 32,4:470–479.
28. Schettino, G.P., et al. *Mask mechanics and leak dynamics during noninvasive pressure support ventilation: a bench study. Intensive Care Med.* 2001;27,12:1887–1891.
29. Waugh JB, Kler RMD. Inspiratory time, pressure settings, and site of supplemental oxygen insertion affect delivered oxygen fraction with the Quantum PSV NPPV. *Respir Care.* 1999;5,44: 520–523.
30. Waugh JB, Kler RMD. Titration of delivered FiO_2 using incremental changes in supplemental oxygen in the Quantum PSV noninvasive positive pressure ventilator. *Respir Care.* 1996:955. http://www.rcjournal.com/abstracts/1996/?id=A00001273
31. BiPAP Clinical Manual: S/T and S/T-D. Murrysville, PA: Respironics, Inc.; 1990.
32. Lattin C, et al. *Noninvasive Bias Flow Pressure Support Ventilation Device Estimates of Tidal Volume.* Detroit, MI: Wayne State University; 1998.
33. Rabatin JT, Gay PC. Noninvasive ventilation. *Mayo Clin Proc.* 1999;74,8:817–820.
34. Gay PC. Complications of noninvasive ventilation in acute care. *Respir Care.* 2009;54,2:246–257; discussion 257–258.
35. Lofaso F, et al. Evaluation of carbon dioxide rebreathing during pressure support ventilation with airway mangement system (BiPAP) devices. *Chest.* 1995;108:772–778.
36. Lofaso F, et al. Home versus intensive care pressure support devices: experimental and clinical comparison. *Am J Respir Crit Care Med.* 1996;153: 1591–1599.
37. Ferguson GT, Gilmartion M. CO_2 rebreathing during BiPAP ventilatory assistance. *Am J Respir Crit Care Med.* 1995;151:1126–1135.
38. Vision clinical manual. Murrysville, PA: Respironic, Inc.; 1998.
39. BiPAP AVAPS ventilatory support system. Murrysville, PA: Respironics, Inc; 2007.
40. Achieva ventilator user's manual. Mallinckrodt, St. Louis MO: Nellcor Puritan Bennett; 1999.
41. Hill KF. *NPPRA revisited.* [online] 2000 [cited 2000 Jan/Feb]; Available from: www.aarc.org/sections/sections_index.html.
42. Goldberg A, et al. Clinical indications for noninvasive positive pressure ventilation in chronic respiratory failure due to restrictive lung disease, COPD, and nocturnal hypoventilation—a consensus conference report. *Chest.* 1999;116,2: 521–534.
43. Corrado A, et al. Negative pressure ventilation in the treatment of acute respiratory failure: an old noninvasive technique reconsidered. *Eur Respir J.* 1996;9:1531–1544.
44. Morch ET. History of mechanical ventilation. In: *Mechanical Ventilation.* New York: Churchill Livingstone; 1985.
45. Bonekat HW. Noninvasive ventilation in neuromuscular disease. In: *Critical Care Clinics*. Tharratt RS, ed. Philadelphia: W.B. Saunders Co; 1998: 775–797.
46. Jackson M, et al. The effects of five years of nocturnal cuirass-assisted ventilation in chest wall disease. *Eur Respir J.* 1993;6:630–635.
47. Bach JR. Update and perspective on noninvasive respiratory muscle aids. *Chest.* 1994;105,4: 1230–1240.
48. Corrado A, et al. Negative pressure ventilation versus conventional mechanical ventilation in the treatment of acute respiratory failure in COPD patients. *Eur Respir J.* 1998;12:519–525.

49. Corrado A, et al. Respiratory muscle insufficiency in acute respiratory failure of subjects with severe COPD: treatment with intermittent negative pressure ventilation. *Eur Respir J.* 1990;3:644–648.
50. Montserrat J, et al. Effect of negative pressure ventilation on arterial blood gas pressure and inspiratory muscle strength during an exacerbation of chronic obstructive lung disease. *Thorax.* 1991; 46:6–8.
51. Gigliotti F, et al. Suppression of ventilatory muscle activity in healthy subjects and COPD patients with negative pressure ventilation. *Chest.* 1991;99: 1186–1192.
52. Hill NS. Clinical applications of body ventilators. *Chest.* 1986;90,6:897–905.
53. Make BJ, Hill NS, Goldberg AI. Mechanical ventilation beyond the intensive care unit. In: *Report of a Consensus Conference of the American College of Chest Physicians.* 1997: *Chest.* 1998;114(6):1794–1795.

Suggested Readings

Bonekat HW. Noninvasive ventilation in neuromuscular disease. *Critical Care Clinics.* 1998;14:775–797.

Hill, NS. Noninvasive mechanical ventilation. In: MacIntyre NR, Branson RD, eds. *Mechanical Ventilation.* 2nd ed. St. Louis, MO: Saunders, an imprint of Elsevier Inc.; 2009:366–391.

Keenan SP, Brake D. An evidence-based approach to noninvasive ventilation in acute respiratory failure. *Critical Care Clinics.* 1998;14:359–372.

Padman R, Lawless ST, Kettrick RG. Noninvasive ventilation via bilevel positive airway pressure support in pediatric practice. *Crit Care Med.* 1998; 26:169–173.

Sittig SE. Transport, home care, and alternative ventilatory devices. In: Cairo JM, Pilbeam S, eds. *Mosby's Respiratory Care Equipment.* 8th ed. St. Louis, MO: Mosby; 2009:744–778.

SECTION V

Levels of Care Delivery

CHAPTER 29

Neonatal and Pediatric Respiratory Care

John Salyer and Robert DiBlasi

OBJECTIVES

Upon completion of this chapter, the reader should be able to:

- List the common neonatal respiratory disorders.
- List common pediatric respiratory disorders.
- List the effects of prematurity on the neonatal lung.
- Describe fetal blood flow and the transition to adult circulatory pathways.
- Describe the components of a respiratory assessment of neonatal and pediatric patients.
- List the key steps and techniques related to the resuscitation of a newborn.
- Describe the factors that influence the performance of pulse oximeters in infants and children.
- Describe the appropriate device selection for oxygen delivery and aerosolized medication delivery to a pediatric patient.
- Describe the basics of CPAP administration in infants and children

CHAPTER OUTLINE

(continues)

(continued)

Technology of Pediatric and Neonatal Respiratory Therapy
- Manual Resuscitators
- Monitoring
- Pulse Oximetry
- Conventional Ventilators
- High-Frequency Ventilators
- Continuous Positive Airway Pressure
- Nasal CPAP Systems
- Oxygen Delivery
- Aerosol Delivery

KEY TERMS

conduction
convection
diaphragmatic hernia
evaporation
meconium
neonatal
pediatric

Some of the most widely used technological advances in the treatment of respiratory failure were first developed in neonatal and pediatric practice and then introduced into adult populations. These include continuous positive airway pressure, intermittent mandatory ventilation, high-frequency ventilation, inhaled nitric oxide therapy, and extra corporeal membrane oxygenation.[1,2] The clinician who is considering practicing in units and hospitals specializing in the treatment of neonatal and pediatric patients will enter an environment with a history of innovation and research and one in which new technologies are continuously being developed.

Through the steady accumulation of a solid base of scientific evidence, improvements in the quantity and quality of training, as well as the introduction of new technologies, remarkable improvements in outcomes have been accomplished over the last four decades.[3] Respiratory therapists have played a vital role in this steady progress.[4]

The Practice of Neonatal and Pediatric Respiratory Care

The terms "neonatal" and "pediatric" are used throughout this chapter because, functionally, these are fairly distinct populations of patients (although there is some overlap).

- **Neonatal** is from the Greek *neos* for "new" and the Latin *natus* for "born." Thus, the term "newborn" is often substituted for neonatal.
- **Pediatric** is from the Greek *pais* for "child" and *iatreia* for "treatment."

More specifically, "neonatal" typically refers to the period from birth through the first four weeks of life, and "pediatric" refers to the period from 1 month to 18 years of age. However, most pediatric hospitals admit a small number of patients over 18 years of age, some as old as 23 years. These are typically patients with a chronic disease who have been managed all their lives by pediatric subspecialists.

Many misconceptions surround the care of neonates and pediatric patients. It is important to dispel these myths about the care of these populations in order to learn how to properly care for them.

- Misconception: *Neonatal and pediatric practice is harder or more demanding than respiratory care for adult populations.*
  Truth: These respective practice environments are simply different. So, to practice effectively in most neonatal and pediatric populations, the respiratory therapist needs different preparation, training, and experience than respiratory therapists who treat adult populations.
- Misconception: *Pediatric patients are small adults, and neonates are smaller pediatric patients.*
  Truth: Nothing could be further from the truth. For example, a premature neonate is indeed very small but *also* has tissues and organ systems in various stages of development. Depending on the patient's gestational age at birth, some organ systems can be very underdeveloped, particularly the lungs in babies born under 35 weeks of gestation. In general, the airways form early in gestational life (by about 17 weeks) and grow by enlargement. At the same time, the alveoli

TABLE 29-1 **Distinctions between the adult and the neonatal and pediatric respiratory tract**

1. Prior to 28 weeks of gestation the premature lung has no real alveoli. Instead the airways end in saccules, which are larger, and thicker walled than true alveoli. Some gas exchange can probably occur in these units.
2. Elastin and collagen (important connective tissues that lend stability to lung structures) are nearly absent during late gestation and at birth. This may be why it is relatively easy to rupture the air spaces of the premature lung (air leak).
3. The development of airways, the vasculature and alveoli are adversely affected by chronic hypoxia.
4. The young lung lacks elastic recoil; as a result, airways are less well supported, leading to greater airway closure and the development of patchy atelectasis frequently observed in the child under school age.
5. Airway walls of young lungs may be thicker. This, combined with reduced elastic recoil, favors greater airway narrowing for any degree of smooth muscle contraction.
6. The chest wall is relatively more compliant in the young child and stiffens with increasing age. As a result, the infant can develop paradoxical respiration. Diaphragmatic movement during inspiration, and the resulting negative intra-thoracic pressure can produce inward displacement of the rib cage, contributing to increased work of breathing for a given level of ventilation. Chest wall-abdominal paradox may be normal in the premature infant during REM sleep but not in the older child or adult.
7. Infants and children from large families or those who attend day care have frequent respiratory tract infections. It may be that the profuse secretions are aspirated and with a shorter path length to peripheral airways, the epithelium lining these structures becomes infected. Because of complex structural differences with adults, the effects of any degree of airway smooth muscle contraction will be exaggerated and contribute to the uneven ventilation and perfusion and modest hypoxemia observed in so many children with respiratory tract infections.
8. The rate of mucociliary clearance is less in infants than adults.
9. The infants' airway has a higher ratio of mucus glands than adults.

Source: Wohl, M. E. B. Developmental physiology of the respiratory system. In: Chernick, V.C., Boat, T.F., Wilmott, R.W., Bush, A., eds. Kendig's Disorders of the Respiratory Tract in Children. *7th ed. Philadelphia. Saunders Elsevier, 2006: 23–28.*

develop late in gestational life and early childhood and grow by forming new structures. At term, the healthy newborn has approximately 150 million alveoli, although this number is highly variable. Apparently, new alveolar structures are added throughout the first few years of life (for a total of about 274–790 million[5]), and further lung growth takes place by enlargement of the existing structure.[6] Other important distinctions between the neonatal/pediatric and adult respiratory system are listed in Table 29-1. See Wohl's excellent summary of developmental physiology of the respiratory system.[7]

Preparation to become a neonatal and pediatric respiratory therapist (RT) includes all of the customary classroom and clinical education for any RT. But RTs can undertake some additional training and credentialing that better prepares them for neonatal and pediatric practice (Table 29-2). *Having* the credential is not nearly as valuable as *obtaining* the credential. The value is in the journey. The work done to pass these examinations and simulations helps the clinician be a better neonatal and pediatric RT. These credentials are becoming increasingly recognized and indeed required to get and keep employment in some pediatric hospitals.

Epidemiology

In 1862, a paper was submitted to the British National Social Science Association entitled, "Excessive Infant-Mortality: How Can It Be Stayed?" The author, M. A. Baines, reported the following:

> Of the deaths in England in 1859, no less than 184,264—two in every five of the deaths of the year—were of children under five years of age; and above half of these—105,629—had scarcely seen the light, and never saw one return of their birthday. . . . from 43 to 45 infant deaths take place in every 100 births—45 percent! Almost half of the children who are born, die—perish miserably! And this is far from representing the whole mass of pain and suffering, which it is the calamity of children to endure.

TABLE 29-2 **Preparations for becoming a neonatal and pediatric respiratory therapist**

Credential	Issued by	Comments
Neonatal Pediatric Specialist (NPS)	National Board for Respiratory Care	This advanced practice credential is well respected in the neonatal and pediatric community. It is obtained by passing a written test.
Neonatal Resuscitation Program (NRP)	American Academy of Pediatrics	This training program is a combination of didactic training and laboratory simulation that focuses on the resuscitation of newborns. This is essential training for anyone who will be attending deliveries or transporting neonates.
S.T.A.B.L.E.*	The S.T.A.B.L.E.® Program	Specialized training in postresuscitation/pre-transport stabilization care of sick infants.
Pediatric Advanced Life Support (PALS)	American Academy of Pediatrics	The pediatric equivalent of Advanced Cardiac Life Support for adult patients (ACLS). Anyone who will be attending code blues or working in a pediatric intensive care unit should have PALS.

**McCraine-Taylor, R., Price-Douglas, W. The S.T.A.B.L.E.® Program: Post-Resuscitation/Pre-transport Stabilization, Care of Sick Infants.* J Perinat Neonat Nurs, *2008:22(2):159–165.*

Worldwide infant mortality at one year of life is *now* about 8 per 1000 live births. Baines reports 45 infant deaths per 100 live births, or 450 per 1000 live births. When we malign the problems and dislocations of modern life, we might do well to remember that we live in an unprecedented time in human history.

More than 500,000 babies (one in eight) are born prematurely each year in the United States.[8] Most of these infants are cared for in neonatal intensive care units, of which there are about 700 nationally, comprising 16,000 beds.[9] Approximately 337 hospitals in the United States have dedicated pediatric critical care beds, and about one-half of all U.S. hospitals admit pediatric patients, but they do not have specialized pediatric beds or units.[10] U.S. hospitals receive about 30 million emergency visits from the population under 18 years of age, which is about one-fourth of all patients cared for in emergency departments.[11]

Common Neonatal Respiratory Diseases and Conditions

TRANSITION FROM INTRA-UTERINE TO POST NATAL CIRCULATION

Normally, blood flow through the fetal heart and lungs is different when in the uterus than in the neonatal after delivery. During the delivery and in the immediate postnatal period, the newborn must transition from having gas exchange supported mostly by the mother's cardiac output to completely independent breathing and adult patterns of blood flow. Failure to make a rapid transition can result in life-threatening conditions, such as persistent pulmonary hypertension of the newborn.

In utero, the fetal requirements for oxygen and nutrients are supplied by the oxygenated blood flowing from the placenta to the fetus through the umbilical vein. Figure 29-1 illustrates the fetal circulatory pathways. Carbon dioxide is removed from the fetal blood when it flows back out to the placenta via the umbilical arteries. Fetal cardiac and pulmonary blood flows are different because the fetus needs little blood flow through the lungs. In utero, the resistance to blood flow in the lungs is higher than resistance to blood flow in the rest of the fetus. This causes the majority output of the right ventricle to shunt past the lung directly to the left or somatic side of the cardiac circulation.

There are three major sites of shunting: the foramen ovale, the patent ductus arteriosus, and the ductus venosus.

- The *foramen ovale* is a flaplike opening between the right and left atria, allowing blood flow only from the right to the left side of the heart under normal conditions.
- The *ductus arteriosus* is a connection between the ascending aorta and the pulmonary artery.
- The *ductus venosus* connects the umbilical vein directly to the inferior vena cava, allowing most blood to bypass the liver.

Normal fetal P_aO_2 is 25–35 mm Hg. This is possible because the fetus is in a nearly motionless state and in a neutral thermal environment; it needs less oxygen to maintain body temperature and muscle activity. Also, a fetus has predominantly *fetal* hemoglobin. This variant of adult hemoglobin has a higher affinity for oxygen at lower P_aO_2s. This *fetal* hemoglobin is normally replaced by adult hemoglobin shortly after birth.

After the clamping of the umbilical vessels, the low-resistance circulatory system of the placenta is removed from the fetal circulation.

- As the lungs inflate and gas exchange occurs, an increase in P_aO_2 causes dilation of the pulmonary arterial bed, resulting in a reduction in pulmonary vascular resistance (PVR).
- Blood pressure in the right (or pulmonary) side of the heart decreases relative to the blood pressure in the left or somatic side of the heart.
- The pressure in the aorta increases and becomes greater than the pressure in the pulmonary artery. This decreases the amount of right-to-left shunting through the ductus arteriosus and foramen ovale.

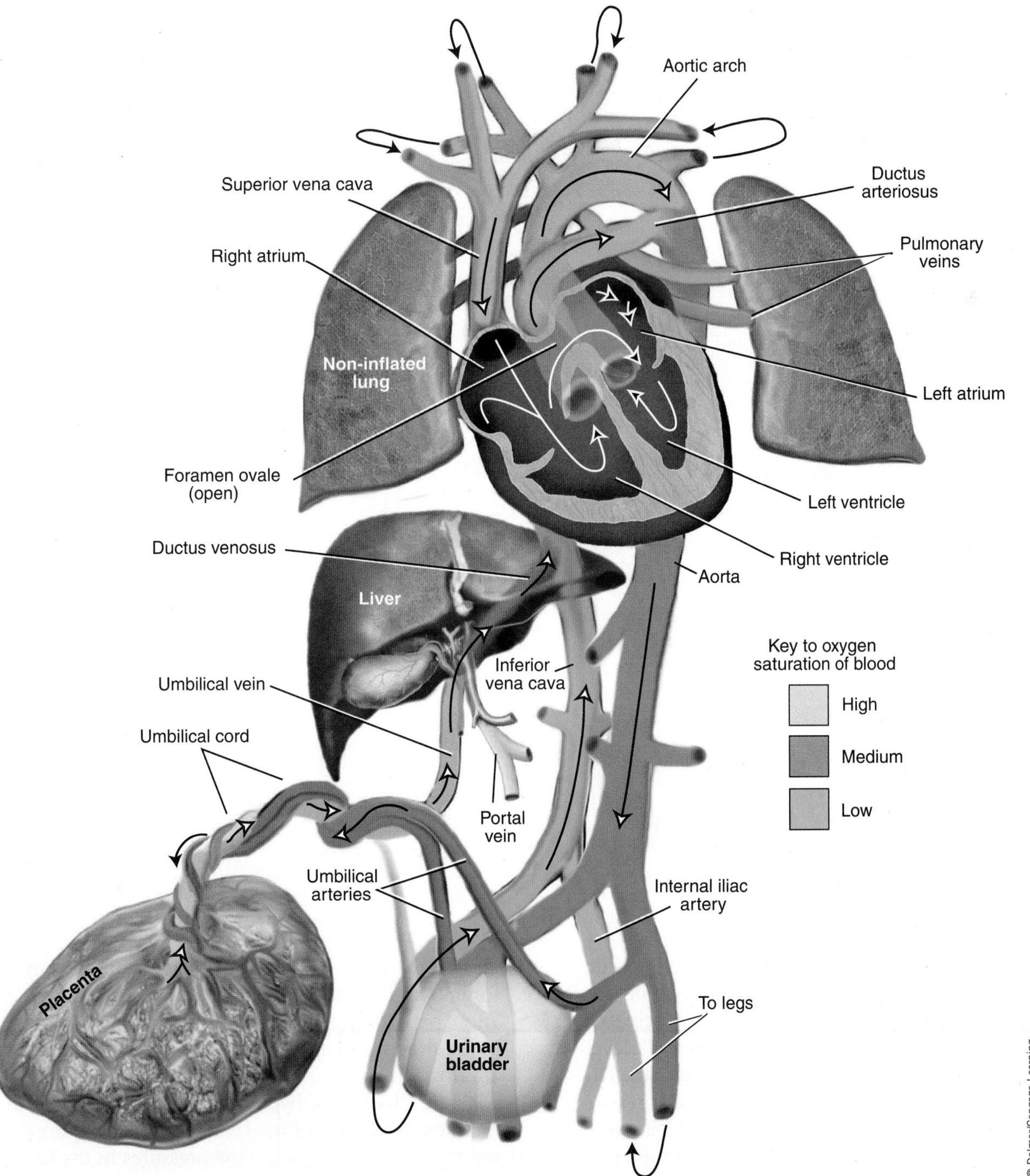

FIGURE 29-1 Fetal circulatory pathways and transition to extra-uterine circulatory pathways. *(continues)*

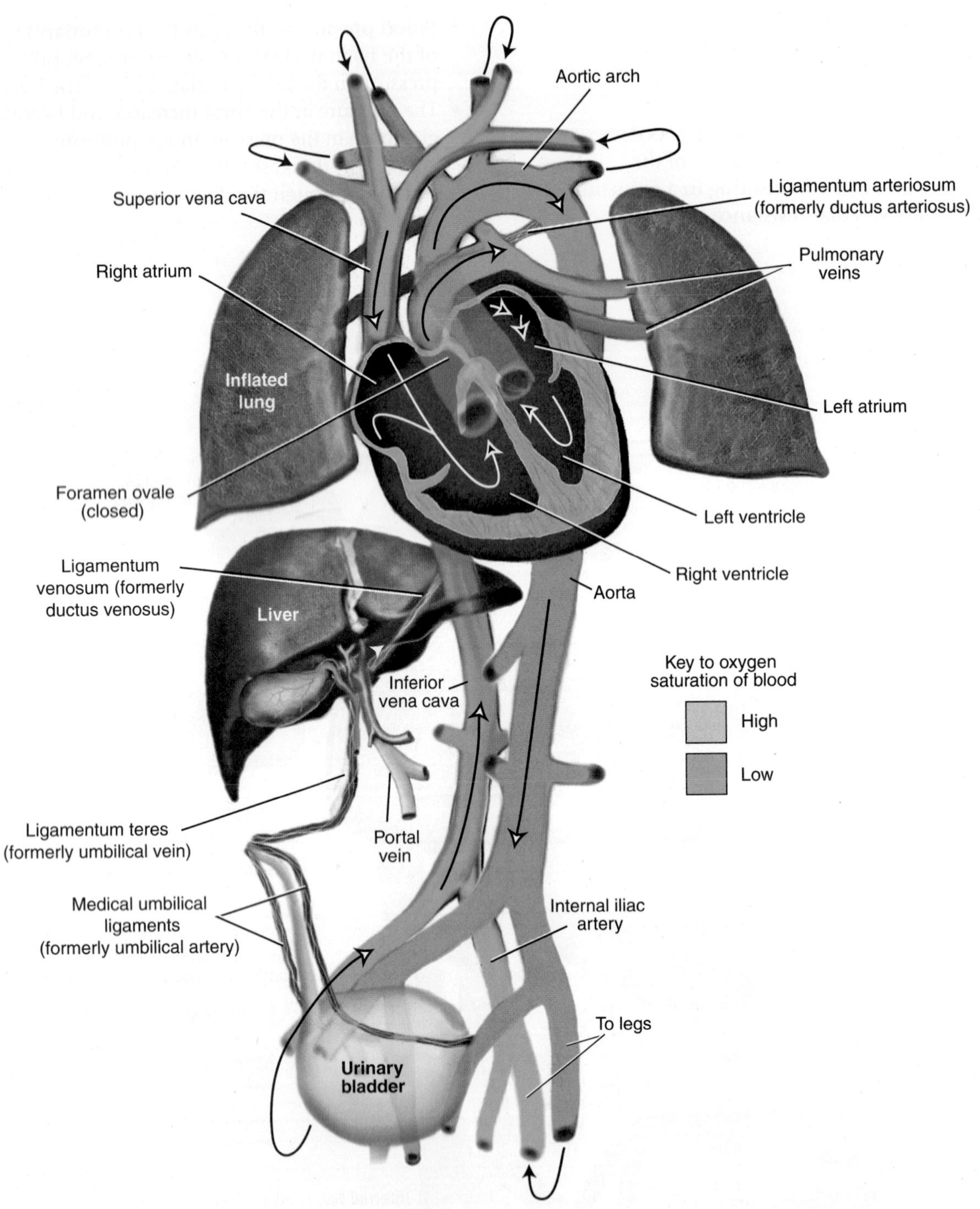

FIGURE 29-1 (*continued*)

- Closure of the ductus arteriosus usually occurs within the first 24 hours to 2 weeks of life, except in the premature infant, in whom musculature of the ductus arteriosus may not be well developed and its ability to constrict is limited. The PVR is lower than the systemic vascular resistance (SVR), and blood flows into the lungs from the systemic circulation (left to right).

The ductus arteriosus may not close completely in some term infants (e.g., in meconium aspiration). These patients may experience very high PVR, and blood then flows from right to left through the ductus arteriosus from the pulmonary circulation to the systemic circulation, bypassing the lungs. Because the foramen ovale flap allows blood to flow only from right to left, it closes when the pressures in the LA become greater than those in the RA. If the foramen ovale lacks a flap-like structure or has a defective one, the opening begins to function as an *atrial septal defect* (*ASD*).

NEWBORN RESUSCITATION

Proper care and resuscitation of the newborn begin in the delivery suite and are essential to the transition to extra-uterine life. RTs who attend deliveries can greatly enhance their preparation by getting the NRP credential, which focuses on the resuscitation of newborns. Table 29-3 describes the basic equipment and steps of newborn resuscitation; Table 29-4 is a guide to selecting the appropriate endotracheal tube size based on birth weight.

Two circumstances are important during the resuscitation of newborns: diaphragmatic hernia and the presence of meconium in the amniotic fluid.

- In newborns presenting with a **diaphragmatic hernia**, consider the following:
  Avoid positive pressure ventilation with a mask; this can force air into the stomach. The stomach and or small intestines may be extruding into the chest through the defect in the diaphragm. If air is forced into the bowel, the portion of the bowel in the chest cavity can expand and compress other structures in the chest, including the heart, lungs, and great vessels. If positive pressure ventilation is needed (which is likely in diaphragmatic hernia), the patient should be intubated as soon after delivery as possible to avoid distension of the bowel.
- A newborn might have **meconium** in the amniotic fluid at delivery: Meconium is a thick, dark, viscous fluid that is a waste product of the fetal bowel and that normally occurs in trace amounts in the amniotic fluid. It is nearly sterile but can be chemically irritating to the lung. When the infant is stressed during labor and delivery, the bowel can evacuate in utero and the amniotic fluid can contain varying amounts of meconium, which can then be aspirated into the infant's upper airway. If it is, it can cause obstruction of the airways and chemical irritation of the airways and lung tissue (*meconium aspiration syndrome*). This syndrome, in its severe forms, can be life-threatening. During labor, the amniotic fluid is examined and tested for meconium staining. If thick meconium is present, the clinician who delivers the infant should suction the upper airway when the head is delivered, prior to delivery of the rest of the infant's body. After delivery of the rest of the body, the infant is intubated and immediately suctioned—if possible, before initiating the first breath by the infant. If the meconium staining is mild, it is usually necessary only to thoroughly suction the upper airway.

There is considerable debate about how to use oxygen (O_2) in the resuscitation of newborns. For most of the modern history of resuscitation of newborns, 100% O_2 was used during the immediate postdelivery resuscitation. But evidence has steadily grown that O_2 use has toxic effects in newborns, particularly low-birth-weight infants (discussed late in this chapter in "Retinopathy of Prematurity"). Recent findings suggest that even a brief O_2 exposure during resuscitation is potentially more toxic than had been previously thought. There are even suggestions that resuscitation of the newborn with room air is better than using O_2. Stola and colleagues report:

> Clinical studies have shown that delivery room resuscitation with 100% oxygen when compared with room air is associated with a lower 5-min Apgar score, a prolonged time to first cry and breath, increased neonatal mortality, increased oxidative stress that persisted for at least 4 weeks after birth in one study, increased myocardial and kidney injury and also with a higher risk for childhood leukemia and cancer. These studies were largely undertaken in underdeveloped countries and primarily involved term babies.[12]

These findings and others have led to the widespread practice of using air-oxygen blenders with resuscitators during delivery. Finer[13] summarizes the current state of knowledge and recommends:

> Until the results of further studies are available, a reasonable approach to resuscitation would include initial resuscitation with 30–40% oxygen for very preterm infants using targeted S_PO_2 values and blended oxygen during the first 10 minutes. For ongoing management of preterm infants, S_PO_2 targets of 85–93% seem to be most appropriate . . .

TABLE 29-3 Guide to newborn resuscitation

1) Deliveries that should be considered high risk:
   a) Thick meconium after maternal membranes ruptured
   b) Fetal distress
   c) "Crash" C-section
   d) Premature birth
   e) Prenatally diagnosed congenital anomalies, such as but not limited to:
      i) Congenital diaphragmatic hernia
      ii) Congenital heart disease
      iii) Abdominal wall defects
      iv) Neural tube defects
2) Equipment to be gathered:
   a) Self-inflating bag with reservoir attached to 100% oxygen source
   b) Appropriate size mask
   c) Bulb syringe
   d) Wall suction
   e) Warmer bed and blankets
   f) Intubation equipment
   g) Meconium aspirator
3) Initial step: warm and dry infant
   a) Place infant under radiant heat warmer bed and dry infant vigorously. This helps prevent cold stress and provides stimulation to assist the infant with transition.
4) Initiate ABC's
   a) Airway: position head in neutral position and suction the nares first, then the mouth.
   b) Breathing: assisted ventilation with a manual resuscitator if necessary. See below.
   c) Circulation: assess heart rate by:
      i) Auscultating an apical pulse,
      ii) Palpate an umbilical or brachial pulse.
5) Evaluate infant for:
   a) Color:
      i) Peripheral cyanosis (acrocyanosis) is normal and typically does not require supplemental oxygen.
      ii) If centrally cyanotic give infant supplemental oxygen.
   b) Signs of Respiratory distress:
      i) Increased work of breathing
      ii) Nasal flaring
      iii) Grunting
      iv) Tachypnea
6) Manual Ventilation (if necessary)
   a) Indications for manual ventilation
      i) Apnea
      ii) Heart rate less than 100 breaths per min
   b) Manual ventilation with a mask
      i) Self-inflating bags are preferred because of ease of use and more consistent tidal volume and PEEP delivery.
      ii) Careful attention required to ensure good mask fit and patent airway.
      iii) Rate = 40–60 breaths per min
      iv) Ventilating pressures
         (1) A pressure manometer should be used
         (2) Initial breath after delivery
            (a) Normal delivery = 15–20 cmH_2O
            (b) Diseased Lungs = 20–40 cmH_2O
7) Chest Compressions:
   a) Indications: If after approximately 30 s of positive pressure ventilation with 100% F_IO_2 the heart rate is below 60 breaths per min or between 60–80 breaths per min and not increasing
   b) Technique:
      i) Use two fingers placed one finger's breadth below nipple line
      ii) 1/2 to 3/4 inch compression depth accompanied by ventilations,
         (1) Frequency of compressions = 90/min
         (2) Ratio of compressions to breaths is 3:1
8) Intubation:
   a) Indications:
      i) If heart rate does not increase to > 100 beats per min within 5 min
      ii) Apnea
      iii) Inability to adequately oxygenate
   b) See Table 29-4 for guide to selecting endotracheal tubes.

TABLE 29-4 **Guidelines for selection of endotracheal tube and associated size suction catheter for intubation of newborns**

Birth Weight	ETT Size	Suction Catheter Size
<1000 g	2.5 mm	5–6 French suction catheter
1000–2000 g	3.0 mm	6 French suction catheter
2000–3000 g	3.5 mm	8 French suction catheter
>3000 g	4.0 mm	8 French suction catheter

Spotlight On

Dr. Virginia Apgar

Dr. Virginia Apgar has been described as the founder of neonatology. She was an anesthesiologist who specialized in pediatrics. She carried resuscitation equipment with her everywhere she went. She explained, "Nobody, but nobody, is going to stop breathing on me!"

Best Practice

Avoid Unnecessary Complexity

Sometimes clinicians are fooled into thinking they are giving newborns supplemental oxygen when they are not. This is because the attachment of the resuscitator to a blender is set on room air. Sometimes this happens because the blender is not mounted clearly within the line of site of the bedside clinicians.

Note: The addition of blenders to the delivery room enhances the potential for mishaps associated with clinicians' ventilating the patient with an "unintended" F_IO_2.[1]

[1] We know of multiple episodes of care where clinicians were manually resuscitating infants with what they thought was 100% oxygen, only to discover that the blender was not set on 100%. Sometimes the visual environment is very complex, and blenders can be mounted in places at the bedside that cannot readily seen by the clinicians.

APGAR SCORING

Clinical scoring systems now abound in the hospital. There are asthma scores, bronchiolitis scores, coma scores, and trauma scores. All these scores help in bringing a degree of sorely needed standardization to the way clinicians evaluate patients. A pioneer in this field in the early 1950s, Dr. Virginia Apgar created a simple yet reliable and effective method of assessing the cardio respiratory status of infants at delivery and to assess the effectiveness of resuscitation efforts.[14]

Apgar scores are typically assessed at 1 and 5 minutes after delivery by the respiratory therapist, nurse, or doctor participating in the resuscitation. The scoring is done by evaluating the patient for five signs; heart rate, color, respiratory effort, muscle tone, and reflex irritability, which is related to how the infant reacts to stimuli. An ordinal score of 0, 1, or 2 is assigned to each of these categories and then totaled. Table 29-5 lists the details of the Apgar score.

PREMATURITY

Infants are considered premature if they are born under 37 weeks, or the *estimated gestational age* (*EGA*). The

TABLE 29-5 **Apgar Infant Scoring System**

	Score		
Sign	0	1	2
Heart rate	Absent	Under 100 beats per min	Over 100 beats per min
Respiratory effort	Absent	Slow (irregular)	Good crying
Muscle tone	Limp	Some flexion of extremities	Active motion
Reflex irritability	No response	Grimace	Cough or sneeze
Color	Blue, pale	Pink body, blue extremities	All pink

1. A score of 8–10 is excellent, 4–7 is guarded, 0–3 is critical. This lets you know how the baby is doing and if he/she is going to need extra assistance.
2. Reflex irritability is the newborn response to stimulation. This is often assessed as the response of the child to bulb suctioning of the nose.

gestational age is estimated because the exact date of conception is often not known. Infants of the same EGA can have different levels of maturity depending on their exposure to factors and conditions that can accelerate or slow their maturation process. For most of human history, premature babies had little chance of survival. The earliest infants to have survived are in the 23–24-week gestational age range, although survival at this level of prematurity is rare. Figure 29-1 shows the survival in different birth weight groupings. With increasing prematurity, there is also an increased risk of temporary or permanent morbidities and complications that can cause physical and/or neurodevelopment disabilities. Respiratory therapists play an important role in helping to prevent or minimize these risks. Table 29-6 lists some common complications.

TABLE 29-6 **Morbidities and complications of premature birth**

Intraventricular hemorrhage (IVH)[1]	IVH of the newborn is bleeding into the fluid-filled areas (ventricles) surrounded by the brain. The condition is most often seen in premature babies. Infants born before 30 weeks of pregnancy are at highest risk for such bleeding. The smaller and more premature the infant, the higher the risk for IVH. This is because blood vessels in the brain of premature infants are not yet fully developed and are extremely fragile. IVH is more common in premature babies who have had physical stress, such as respiratory distress syndrome, pneumothorax, or high blood pressure. IVH falls into four groups, called grades. The higher the grade, the more severe the bleeding. Grades 1 and 2 involve a small amount of bleeding and do not usually cause long-term problems. Grades 3 and 4 involve more severe bleeding, which presses on or leaks into brain tissue. Blood clots can form and block the flow of cerebrospinal fluid, leading to increased fluid in the brain (hydrocephalus).
Periventricular leukomalacia (PVL)[2]	PVL is caused by a lack of oxygen or blood flow to the periventricular area of the brain, which results in the death or loss of brain tissue. The periventricular area—the area around the spaces in the brain called ventricles—contains nerve fibers that carry messages from the brain to the body's muscles. Although babies with PVL generally have no outward signs or symptoms of the disorder, they are at risk for motor disorders, delayed mental development, coordination problems, and vision and hearing impairments. PVL can lead to cerebral palsy. The disorder is diagnosed by ultrasound of the head. Extremes in circulating P_aCO_2 levels have been implicated as contributing to the development of cerebrovascular injury in neonates.[3] Besides the obvious effects of hyper- or hypocarbia on pH, extremes also affect cerebral blood flow. Thus, sudden large swings are to be avoided. These can occur when a new mode of ventilation is introduced, such as high frequency oscillatory ventilation. The clinician is cautioned to take care not to over ventilate the patient as well as under ventilate.
Bronchopulmonary dysplasia (BPD)[4]	BPD is a structural malformation. It is an arrest of lung maturation, with or without ventilator induced lung injury (VILI). Other features are a halt in alveolarization, abnormal capillary bed development, presence of antioxidants, and lack of surfactant.[5] BPD is characterized by the need for supplemental oxygen at 36 weeks of postmenstrual age. It affects nearly one third of surviving infants born at less than 1000 grams, but also occurs in infants born weighing over 1250 grams or more than 30 weeks gestational age. The etiology of BPD is multifactorial. Lung immaturity, oxygen therapy, and mechanical ventilation have major roles. Meconium aspiration, pneumonia, and in-utero cytokine release also are implicated.
Retinopathy of prematurity (ROP)[5,6]	Retinopathy of prematurity (ROP) is a potentially blinding eye disorder that primarily affects premature infants born weighing <1250 grams or < 31 weeks of gestation. The disorder is caused by giving infants too much oxygen. The smaller a baby is at birth, the more likely that baby is to develop ROP. We now know that restricting P_aO_2 or S_aO_2 levels helps reduce the risk of ROP, although the optimal range of oxygenation levels to achieve this remains controversial. Until better information is developed, typical target ranges are P_aO_2 50–90 mm Hg or S_aO_2 88–93%

(continues)

TABLE 29-6 **Morbidities and complications of premature birth (*continued*)**

Hydrocephalus[7]	The term hydrocephalus is derived from the Greek words "hydro" meaning water and "cephalus" meaning head. As the name implies, it is a condition in which the primary characteristic is excessive accumulation of cerebrospinal fluid in the brain that is caused by IVH. The excessive accumulation results in an abnormal widening of spaces in the brain called ventricles. This widening creates potentially harmful pressure on the tissues of the brain. Hydrocephalus can permanently damage the brain, causing problems with physical and mental development. If untreated, it is usually fatal. With treatment, many people lead normal lives with few limitations. Treatment usually involves surgery to insert a shunt that drains the excess cerebrospinal fluid from the brain to the peritoneum.
Necrotizing enter colitis (NEC)[8]	NEC occurs when the lining of the intestinal wall dies and the tissue falls off. NEC is the most common gastrointestinal emergency in the neonatal intensive care unit and can be life threatening. It affects approximately 6% to 10% of very low birth weight (VLBW) infants and a case fatality rate as high as 20% to 40%.[5] The etiology of NEC is not clearly established but appears to be multifactorial, involving enteral feeding, vascular or perfusion-related gastrointestinal compromise, and bacterial invasion. Those with a higher risk for this condition include: • Premature infants • Infants who are fed concentrated formulas • Infants in a nursery where an outbreak has occurred • Infants who have received blood exchange transfusions Treatment includes surgical excision of necrotic bowel segments.

1 *National Institute of Health. http://www.nlm.nih.gov/medlineplus/ency/article/007301.htm. Accessed May 23, 2009.*

2 *National Institute of Health. http://www.nlm.nih.gov/medlineplus/ency/article/007232.htm. Accessed May 23, 2009.*

3 *McCrea HJ, Ment LR. The diagnosis, management, and postnatal prevention of intraventricular hemorrhage in the preterm neonate. Clin Perinatol. 2008;35(4):777–92.*

4 *Ikagami AM. Mechanism initiating lung injury in the preterm infant. In: Goldsmith JP, Karotkin EH. Editors. Assisted Ventilation of the Neonate. Philadelphia, PA: Saunders: 2003:347.*

5 *National Eye Institute. http://www.nei.nih.gov/health/rop/. Accessed May 25, 2009.*

6 *Askie LM, Henderson-Smart DJ, Ko H. Restricted versus liberal oxygen exposure for preventing morbidity and mortality in preterm or low birth weight infants. Cochrane Database Syst Rev. 2009 Jan 21;(1):CD001077.*

7 *National Institute of Neurological Disorders and Stroke. http://www.ninds.nih.gov/disorders/hydrocephalus/detail_hydrocephalus.htm. Accessed May 25, 2009.*

8 *Meinzen-Derr J, Morrow AL, Hornung RW, Donovan EF, Dietrich KN, Succop PA. Epidemiology of necrotizing enterocolitis temporal clustering in two neonatology practices. J Pediatr. 2009 May;154(5):656–61.*

Preventing premature delivery has been under investigation for decades, but premature birthrates have actually been increasing. Since 1981 there has been a 31% increase in the premature birthrate in the United States, with the rate now at approximately 12%.[15] This has been attributed to the increase in the number of multiple births related to the use of fertility drugs. There are persistent ethnic differences in premature birth rates, with African American infants having twice the premature birth rate of Caucasian or Hispanic infants.[16]

Maternal factors that can lead to premature birth include:

- High blood pressure of pregnancy, also known as *pre-eclampsia* or *toxemia* of pregnancy.
- Infections of the fetal/placental tissues, vagina, or urinary tract.
- Drug use.
- Abnormal uterine morphology.
- The inability of the cervix to stay closed during pregnancy (also known as *cervical incompetence*).

Factors involving the pregnancy include:

- Abnormal or decreased function of the placenta.
- Low lying position of the placenta, called *placenta previa*.
- Early detachment from the uterus, called *placental abruption*.
- Premature rupture of the amniotic sac (membranes).
- Abnormally low or high amounts of amniotic fluid (oligohydramnios and polyhydramnios, respectively).

NEUTRAL THERMAL ENVIRONMENT, INSENSIBLE WATER LOSS, AND MINIMAL STIMULATION

Low-birth-weight infants are fragile and delicate. They do not tolerate excessive handling well. They are very sensitive to changes in ambient temperature. They have very little physiologic reserve; when stressed, they can have a profound response, which usually manifests itself in hypoxemia and/or bradycardia. Newborns and particularly premature infants are at risk of severe physiologic insult if careful attention is not paid to maintaining their body temperature.

Neutral Thermal Environment. Unlike adults, premature infants have poor mechanisms for self-regulation of body temperature. The ratio of body surface area to body mass increases with decreasing birth weight. This makes the newborn more prone to heat loss, which occurs by means of three mechanisms in newborns: convection, conduction, and evaporation.

- **Convection** is the principle by which heat is transferred from food in a refrigerator or freezer. As cool air is circulated around the food, heat is transferred from the warmer food to the cooler air. So a newborn can lose heat if air circulating around it is lower than body temperature.
- **Conduction** occurs when the newborn's skin comes in direct contact with objects that are lower than body temperature.
- Finally, **evaporation** is a natural cooling mechanism by which sweat and other liquids on the surface of the skin transition from liquid to the vapor phase, absorbing heat as they do.

Complications and consequences of neonatal hypothermia are:

- Increased rate of basal metabolism. which leads to higher glucose consumption and hypoglycemia.
- Peripheral vasoconstriction and the resulting decreased peripheral perfusion, tissue ischemia, and possibly metabolic acidosis.
- Vascular changes in the lungs resulting in decreased ventilation, increased demand for oxygen, and worsening of respiratory distress.
- Acidosis and hypoxia, predisposing to pulmonary hemorrhage, and disseminated intravascular coagulation.
- Effects on liver function, resulting in hyperbilirubinemia.

Thus newborns must be quickly dried at birth and swaddled in blankets. Premature newborns are soon placed under radiant warmers or in incubators, which limit heat loss by providing a neutral thermal environment around the patient.

Insensible Water Loss. Evaporation on the newborn's skin also causes insensible water loss. In very low-birth-weight infants, this effect can be so pronounced that it can become very difficult to maintain fluid balance in the patient, particularly because water loss cannot be directly measured. Thus some low-birth-weight infants are placed in environments to limit water loss, such as hoods that go over the whole infant into which heated humidified ambient gas is circulated and incubators into which heated humidified gas is circulated. Very low-birth-weight infants are also sometimes ensconced in a small framework that is covered with plastic wrap (the same found in kitchens) to provide a moisture barrier.

Minimal Stimulation. It is now well-known that the intensive care environment can be injurious to the neurodevelopment and physical growth of low-birth-weight infants.[17,18] The principal culprit is the often nonstop visual and auditory stimulation in the ICU environment. These stimulations, when added to the unavoidable noxious stimulation of manipulating the patient, taking blood samples, inserting catheters, bathing, weighing, suctioning, and many other interventions, can create an environment where there is little chance for quiet or sleep. However, when environmental factors are modified, care is coordinated, and interventions are developed to minimize the number and duration of these kinds of stimulations, improvements have been considerable, including:[19]

- Requiring less ventilator support.
- Less supplemental oxygen.
- Earlier discharge.
- Lower intraventricular hemorrhage rates.
- Improved weight gain.

A list of methods for ensuring minimal stimulation can include:

- Providing for long periods of reduced lighting.
- Minimizing loud talking at the bedside and throughout the unit.
- Frequent drainage of ventilator tubing if excessive water accumulates, causing bubbling.
- Minimizing alarm volumes, including various monitors and ventilator alarms. Alarms that are hooked to a remote system allow the volume in patient rooms to be kept low, while having the alarms higher in the rest of the unit.

- Using care to quietly open/close isolette portholes and doors.
- Utilizing isolette covers on all isolettes.
- Avoiding use of the isolette roof as a shelf or writing table.
- Removing the bedside phone or turning the ring to its lowest level.
- Transitioning the infant from the warming table to the isolette as soon as possible.
- Utilizing continuous monitoring to assess vital signs rather than the laying on of hands.
- Posting a "minimal handling" sign on the patient's bed to notify team members of the protocol.
- Careful coordination of care between respiratory therapy, nursing, and medicine. This requires the RT and RN to collaborate and plan their respective interventions so as to minimize the number of times the infant is disturbed.

RETINOPATHY OF PREMATURITY

One of the most common causes of vision loss in childhood is *retinopathy of prematurity* (*ROP*).[20] This disorder occurs mostly in newborns weighing $\leq$1250 g and/or $\leq$31 weeks of gestation. The risk of developing ROP is inversely related to birth weight and gestational age. ROP results from the abnormal growth and spread of blood vessels throughout the retina. The fragility of these abnormal blood vessels can lead to leakage, which can scar the retina. The scarring can pull the retina out of position, and in its most severe form can cause retinal detachment and severe loss of vision or even blindness.

First described in 1942, ROP emerged as hospital nurseries began using high levels of oxygen in incubators to save the lives of premature infants. During this period, measurement of serum oxygen level was not available, and there was little if any ability to control F_IO_2. Clinicians were giving oxygen to relieve cyanosis. Consequently, an epidemic of ROP ensued in the 1940s and 1950s. In 1954, scientists determined that the relatively high levels of oxygen routinely given to premature infants at that time were an important risk factor and that reducing the level of oxygen given to premature babies reduced the incidence of ROP. With newer technology and methods to monitor the oxygen levels of infants, oxygen use as a risk factor has diminished in importance.

Annually about 14,000–16,000 of these infants are affected by some degree of ROP, with 1100 to 1500 infants developing ROP that is severe enough to require medical treatment. Approximately 400–600 infants each year in the United States become legally blind from ROP. In milder cases, the disease improves and leaves no permanent damage. About 90 percent of all infants with ROP are in the milder category and do not need treatment.

The causes of ROP are multifactorial, and oxygenation derangement alone does not explain the pathology. But oxygen therapy plays a major role, and the RT treating the low-birth-weight/premature infant has an important role in keeping blood oxygen levels within a "safe" range to reduce the risk of ROP. Generally accepted treatment guidelines include keeping P_AO_2 in the range of 50–90 mm Hg or S_PO_2 in the 88–94%.

RESPIRATORY DISTRESS SYNDROME

One of the most common conditions in the NICU is neonatal *respiratory distress syndrome* (*RDS*), which is also known as idiopathic respiratory distress syndrome or hyaline membrane disease. This condition is primarily caused by an insufficient amount of pulmonary surfactant and immature cell and vascular development in the newborn lung. *Pulmonary surfactant* is a soapy, slippery, protective phospholipid substance that lines the alveolar and terminal airways and helps to reduce surface tension at the air/fluid interface. Type II pneumocytes produce surfactant, but they develop late in gestation. Thus, the more premature the lung is, the higher the risk is of RDS. Risk is highest in infants >28–30 weeks, and RDS is very uncommon in term infants.

With insufficient surfactant, the alveoli and small airways become unstable and tend to collapse at the end of exhalation, leading to widespread atelectasis. This results in loss of functional residual capacity, decreased pulmonary compliance, increased airway resistance, hypoxemia, and hypercarbia. The resultant respiratory acidosis and hypoxemia can lead to increased pulmonary vascular resistance and increased right-to-left shunting of blood at the site of the patent ductus arteriosis and foramen ovale, thus increasing hypoxemia and acidosis, which can lead to lung injury and thus even less surfactant production.

Mortality associated with RDS is approximately 10% of cases, but at one time was as high as 100%.[21] The disease affects more than 20,000 infants per year, with significant differences in incidence and mortality among ethnic groups.

The infant presenting with RDS may have the following signs:

- *Grunting*: Infants make this sound while exhaling against a partially closed epiglottis. It has been described as the infant's attempt to maintain back-pressure in the lungs and thus create a sort of self-administered PEEP.

- *Nasal flaring*: The dilation of the nares on inspiration has been described as a sign of air-hunger. This is an attempt by the infant to reduce airway resistance by dilating the nasal opening
- *Retracting*: The chest walls of newborn infants and children are more compliant than those of adults. When the diaphragm contracts, creating negative intrathoracic pressure, the more compliant chest collapses slightly because it lacks rigidity. Retractions can be seen between the ribs (intercostal) and at the suprasternal notch (sometimes called tracheal tugging). Typically, the more severe the retractions, the more severe the respiratory disease.
- *Head bobbing*: This occurs when the sternocleidomastoid muscles (accessory respiratory muscles) constrict to overcome poor compliance and high airway resistance. These muscles also serve to lift and rotate the head. Thus when they constrict to aide in respiration, they also pull the head up and forward.
- *Tachypnea*: Normal respiratory rates in newborns are in the range of 30–60 per minute. Normal respiratory rates adjusted for increasing age can be found in Table 29-7.
- *Atelectasis*: RDS usually produces a diffuse bilateral atelectasis on X-ray, often referred to as a ground glass.
- *Hypoxemia*: $P_aO_2 < 50$ mm Hg (arterial), or < 35 mm Hg (capillary), or $S_aO_2 < 88\%$.
- *Hypercarbia*: $P_aCO_2 > 50$ mm Hg (arterial or capillary).

TABLE 29-7 **Normal respiratory rates in sleeping and awake pediatric patients**

	Range	
	Sleeping	Awake
6–12 months	22–31	58–75
1–2 yr	17–23	30–40
2–4 yr	16–25	23–42
4–6 yr	14–23	19–36
6–8 yr	13–23	15–30
8–10 yr	14–23	15–31
10–12 yr	13–19	15–28
12–14 yr	15–18	18–26

Source: Schellhaese, D. E. Examination and assessment of the pediatric patient. In: Walsh, B.K., Czervinske, M.P., Diblasi, R.M., eds. Perinatal and Pediatric Respiratory Care. *3rd ed. St. Louis, MO: Saunders Elsevier, 2010: 261–272.*

- *Rales or crackles on auscultation*: Rales, also called crackles or crepitations, are the fine, crackling noises heard on auscultation. They have been described as being similar to the sound of rolling human hairs between the fingers held close to the ear. The word "rales" comes from the French word *râle* meaning "rattle." These sounds are caused by the "popping open" of small airways and alveoli collapsed by fluid, exudate, or lack of aeration during expiration, all of which are typical in the premature surfactant-deprived lung.

This list of signs describes most infants in respiratory distress, whether the cause is surfactant deficiency (as in neonatal respiratory distress syndrome) or other diseases. The key difference in presentation between diseases is often the breath sounds, such as wheezing in asthma or rales and wheezing in bronchiolitis.

The treatment of neonatal RDS was revolutionized with the introduction of artificial surfactant in the 1990s. This treatment can cause rapid and remarkable improvements in compliance and oxygenation by reducing alveolar surface tension and decreasing atelectasis. Table 29-8 lists the basic procedural steps and considerations for surfactant administration.[22]

Supplemental oxygen therapy, *nasal continuous positive airway pressure* (*NCPAP*), and mechanical ventilation are also frequently used to treat RDS. NCPAP is used to reduce the atelectasis associated with RDS and can frequently help in avoiding intubation in neonates. More severe cases can require intubation and mechanical ventilation. In severe cases, high tidal volumes and ventilating pressures can be required to maintain acceptable blood gases. With increasing levels of ventilatory support comes increasing risk of iatrogenic lung injury. In neonates

Neonatal Blood Gases

Views about what constitutes acceptable ranges for neonatal blood gases are divergent. P_aO_2 is normally lower in the newborn infant, and this fact is widely understood and accepted. But for a long time, clinicians attempted to normalize P_aCO_2 and pH. Clinicians eventually learned that this was not necessary and that the increased tidal volumes and ventilating pressures required to do so contribute to lung injury in the neonate. This point is discussed more later in this chapter.

TABLE 29-8 **Surfactant administration: steps and considerations**

Preterm infants first dose	• Infants with RDS should receive surfactant as a bolus and handling during administration should be minimized • Infants < 27 weeks gestation should be automatically intubated, immediately after birth and given prophylactic surfactant in the delivery room or as soon as possible after intubation • Infants > 27 weeks and < 30 weeks gestation should receive prophylactic surfactant as soon as possible if low exposure to antenatal steroids • Infants > 30 weeks gestation should receive surfactant therapy if they have a diagnosis of RDS
Preterm Infants Additional Doses:	• Infants < 30 weeks gestation with the diagnosis of RDS should receive a second dose of surfactant as a bolus 6–12 hr after the first dose if they continue intubated on mechanical ventilation, regardless of the inspired oxygen concentration • Infants > 30 weeks gestation with the diagnosis of RDS should receive a second dose of surfactant as a bolus 6–12 hr after the first dose if they continue intubated on mechanical ventilation and require an $F_IO_2 > 0.3$. If the infant remains intubated with an F_IO_2 0.21–0.29, one should consider a second dose of surfactant. • One may consider continued treatment with additional doses of surfactant (total of 4 doses maximum) for preterm infants with RDS and worsening oxygenation 6–12 hr after the s dose
Dosage	• 4mL/kg Survanta every 6 hr times 4, if indicated
Equipment	• 10-mL syringe • Adapter for ETT • Surfactant vial(s) • Multi Access Catheter (MAC) of appropriate size • 19-gauge needle
Preparation	• Surfactant should be inspected visually for discoloration. Color should be off-white to light brown • Swirl vial gently (Do Not shake) if settling occurs • Should be warmed by standing at room temperature for at least 20 min or warmed in hand at least 8 min • Unused, unopened warmed vials may be returned to refrigerator within 8 hr of warming only once • Using sterile technique, aspirate appropriate dose into syringe
Procedure	1. Patient will be intubated and hand-bagged during administration. 2. Suction prior to administration. 3. Obtain a Trach Care Multi Access Catheter (MAC). 4. Obtain matching Y adapter for endotracheal tube. 5. Attach adapter to endotracheal tube. 6. Determine the measurement where endotracheal tube is cut and add 4.5 cm and note marking on catheter. This will place catheter at end of endotracheal tube. 7. Attach syringe of medication to end of MAC catheter. 8. Advance catheter until measured mark has been reached. 9. Instill ½ dose slowly; pull out catheter after small amount has been given. Then keep instilling small amounts until the full ½ dose has been given. Administer drug over a period of 5–20 min. 10. Turn infant 45 degrees to the right after administration of the first ½ dose. Hold in this position for 30 s. 11. Return infant to midline. Repeat procedure with the second ½ dose. 12. Turn to left 45 degrees and hold for 30 seconds. 13. After completion, return infant to midline. Remove syringe and replace with inline suction. 14. Store remaining surfactant in refrigerator for up to 12 hr after labeling with patient name, date/time.

(continues)

TABLE 29-8 **Surfactant administration: steps and considerations (*continued*)**

Monitoring	1. The following should be monitored during and 30 min after dose administration: a. Heart rate b. Color c. Tidal volume d. Pulse oximetry 2. If HR slows, the infant becomes dusky or agitated, oxygen saturations fall more than 15%, or surfactant backs up in ETT, dosing should be slowed or halted, and, if necessary, ventilatory support gently increased until the patient returns to baseline. 3. Special care must be taken to keep tidal volumes in "safe" range during or immediately after surfactant administration. This is typically in the range of 5–7 mL/Kg (some centers use 6–8 mL/Kg). As compliance improves, tidal volume will increase in pressure limited modes. The PIP must be quickly weaned to limit the risk of lung injury cause by over-distention. 4. Avoid suctioning for at least one hr (preferably two to four hr) after surfactant administration, unless clinical deterioration is evident and patient is nonresponsive to other measures.

this often manifests itself in various forms of so-called air-leak syndrome.

AIR LEAK SYNDROME

Pulmonary *air leak syndrome* is the leakage and dissection of air out of the normal pulmonary airspaces. In this context, dissection means that the air leaks into non-air spaces and moves along the perivascular sheaths to other pulmonary structures. The site of leakage is visually represented in Figure 29-2. The distance the air travels and the amount of air leakage contribute to which type of air leak is present: pulmonary interstitial emphysema, pneumomediastinum, pneumopericardium, pneumoperitoneum, and pneumothorax.

- *Pulmonary interstitial emphysema* is the leakage of gas into the pulmonary interstitium, lymphatics, or subpleural space. One or both lungs may be involved. If dissection of air is severe and widespread enough, it can cause the lung to stiffen, that is, reduce lung compliance, making ventilation more difficult. This condition can often be a precursor to the development of bronchopulmonary dysplasia. If one lung is significantly more involved than the other, the infant can benefit from being placed in the lateral recumbent position with the more affected lung down. This causes more compression of the bad lung thereby decreasing air leakage and perhaps improving ventilation of the better (elevated) lung.
- *Pneumomediastinum* is the leakage of air into connective tissue of the mediastinum. This can be asymptomatic or, in its severe forms, may compress lung tissue.

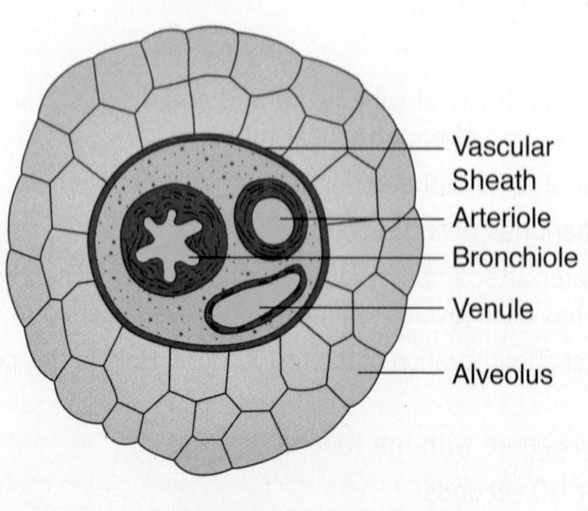

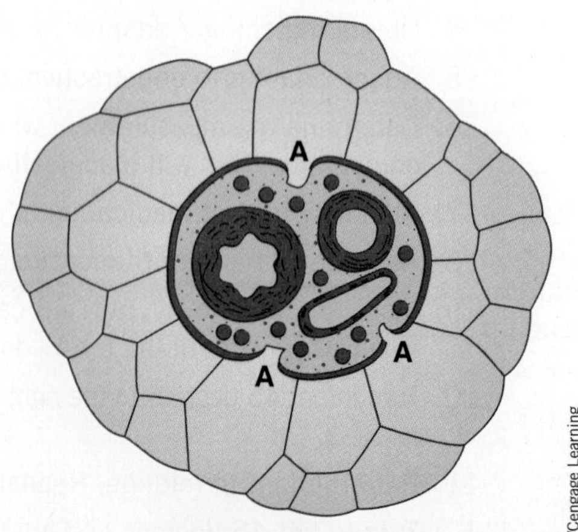

FIGURE 29-2 Schematic representation of possible sites of air leak in the newborn lung. This cross sectional view is of the terminal respiratory unit.

- *Pneumopericardium* is the dissection of air into the pericardial sac. If sufficient air leaks into the sac, it can restrict the movement and refilling of the heart, a condition called *cardiac tamponade*.
- *Pneumoperitoneum* is the dissection of air into the peritoneum and is seen almost exclusively in extremely severe cases of air leak.
- *Pneumothorax* is leakage and dissection of air into the pleural space. If air continues to accumulate, causing significant compression of adjacent lung tissues and vascular structure, it is called a tension pneumothorax. Small pneumothoraces may resolve spontaneously, but larger pneumothoraces require evacuation of the air in the pleural cavity via chest tube. A tension pneumothorax happens almost exclusively during positive pressure ventilation. During inspiration, the positive pressure forces air out through the site(s) of the leak. It is assumed that during exhalation, these leak sites close so that this pressurized air accumulates in the pleural space with each successive breath. Untreated, the tension pneumothorax may be immediately life-threatening because it can grow to such a large size that it compresses lung tissue and vascular structures in the thorax.

CONGENITAL DIAPHRAGMATIC HERNIA

During intra-uterine lung development, a defect or hole can occur in the diaphragm. This is called *congenital diaphragmatic hernia (CDH)*. If large enough, the defect allows the abdominal contents (loops of bowel or the stomach) to enter the chest cavity. These abdominal structures can then press on the developing lung and hinder lung growth. The limitation of lung growth is called *pulmonary hypoplasia*. In more severe cases, an entire side of the lung cavity can be occupied by bowel and result in the development of only one functional lung, which may also be hypoplastic. Lung hypoplasia can involve significant reductions in lung volumes and severe diffusion defects that can make it very difficult to make the transition to extra-uterine life. CDH occurs in 1 of every 3000 to 5000 live births.[23,24] Mortality from CDH is typically described in the 40% range[25] but has been reported as high as 68%.[26]

About 90% of the hernias affect the left side of the diaphragm, although they can occur on either side or both sides. The majority of hernias are diagnosed prenatally, and so the clinician knows about it at the time of delivery. Prenatal diagnosis significantly improves the chances for survival.

Ventilation during neonatal resuscitation using positive pressure ventilation via facemask should be avoided with CDH. During positive pressure ventilation with a mask, gas often enters the stomach under pressure and can cause distension of the stomach or bowel. If parts of the bowel or the stomach are in the thoracic cavity and are distended by gas, the distended organs can press more on lung tissue, making ventilation even more difficult. It ventilatory support is required at the time of delivery, intubation should be accomplished immediately.

The treatment of diaphragmatic hernia involves mechanical ventilation and cardiovascular support until and after the hernia can be surgically corrected. Because the lung can be very hypoplastic, lung volumes are often significantly decreased in these infants. Pneumothorax is a typical complication of mechanical ventilation in CDH patients, occurring in as many as 25% of cases. The presence of a pneumothorax is a risk factor for death, and thus great efforts are taken to avoid lung overdistension. Practice from center to center varies considerably. Some groups use early high-frequency oscillatory ventilation to keep tidal volumes very small. Others use conventional ventilators run at very high rates with shortened inspiratory times and low peak inspiratory pressures and little or no set PEEP (sometimes called *gentle-a-tion*). The theory is that this approach minimizes volumetric lung distension. The very high rates probably create inadvertent PEEP because expiratory times are too short to allow complete exhalation. Thus the set PEEP is kept at zero, on the assumption that the patient is getting inadvertent PEEP.

Spotlight On

PEEP

Inadvertent PEEP has also been creatively and variously called occult PEEP, hidden PEEP, or intralung PEEP. A conviction among some is that PEEP that cannot be measured with a proximal airway pressure measurement needs to be hunted down and stamped out. Of course, during some forms of high-frequency ventilation, intralung PEEP is an important therapeutic goal. Intralung PEEP can be measured by occluding the airway at the end of inspiration and noting whether airway pressure returns to zero or rises slightly (a sign of PEEP).

Common Pediatric Respiratory Diseases and Conditions

ASTHMA

Pediatric asthma is one of the most prevalent diseases affecting children.[27] Childhood asthma has been increasing, and 14 million children in the United States under the age of 18 have been diagnosed at one time or another to have had asthma (about 14%).[28] There are disparities in asthma prevalence and impact among ethnic groups and economic strata. There are approximately 335,000 hospitalizations per year in the United States for asthma among children 2–17 years of age.[29]

A recent large survey conducted to study the scope and impact of asthma in the lives of children and their families revealed that:

- 54% of children four to 18 years of age with asthma missed school (or daycare) in the past year as a result of their disease.
- An estimated 21 million school days are lost per year due to asthma.
- Nearly 9% of children with asthma missed more than two weeks of school in the past year as a result of their condition.
- More than a third of parents missed work in the past year as a result of their child's asthma, and 11% missed more than a week of work in the past year.
- An estimated 5 million workdays are lost per year for parents of children with asthma.

(These data are from a survey of over 41,000 homes conducted by GlaxoSmithKline and published on the world wide web at http://www.asthmainamerica.com/children_survey.html. Survey findings were then extrapolated to the entire population of U.S. children.)

Asthma is an inflammatory disease of the lungs. It has been the subject of a great deal of work at the national level to develop standardized and widely accepted definitions, descriptions, and treatment guidelines. Under the auspice of the National Institute of Health, the National Heart Blood and Lung Institute created the National Asthma Education and Prevention Program. The "Expert Panel Report 3: Guidelines for the Diagnosis and Management of Asthma" is one of the products of this work and offers an excellent tool for the clinician interested in a thorough understanding of the nature and treatment of this disease.[30] In the report, asthma is defined as follows:

> Asthma is a chronic inflammatory disorder of the airways in which many cells and cellular elements play a role: in particular, mast cells, eosinophils, neutrophils. . . . T-lymphocytes, macrophages, and epithelial cells. In susceptible individuals, this inflammation causes recurrent episodes of coughing (particularly at night or early in the morning), wheezing, breathlessness, and chest tightness. These episodes are usually associated with widespread but variable airflow obstruction that is often reversible either spontaneously or with treatment.

The principal mechanisms of this airflow obstruction are illustrated in Figure 29-3 and can include any or all of the following:

- *Mucosal edema*. The inner lumen of the airways is narrowed as the mucosal lining of the airways becomes swollen.
- *Excessive mucus secretion*. The inner lumen of the airways can become completely or partially obstructed by accumulated mucus, which is secreted in abnormally large amounts when the airways are inflamed.
- *Bronchoconstriction*. The smooth bronchial muscles that surround the airways respond to inflammation by constricting and narrowing the lumen of the airway.

A prominent clinical feature of asthma is wheezing. However, the lack of wheezing on auscultation does not indicate an absence of airflow obstruction or of asthma. In a severe attack, asthmatic children can appear to have almost no wheezing on auscultation. This can be an ominous sign because it can indicate not enough air is moving into the lung to create a wheeze. Also, the lungs can be significantly inflamed even though no wheezing is heard. Conversely, the presence of wheezing does not always indicate asthma. Other causes of wheezing in children are:

- Infections like bronchitis or bronchiolitis.
- Foreign bodies or lesions in or outside the airway.
- Congenital or acquired malformations of the airways.

Asthma is typically difficult to diagnose in children under 3–5 years old, owing to the inability of these patients to cooperate with airflow measurement maneuvers. Thus, some infants and toddlers diagnosed with other respiratory disorders like bronchiolitis are actually pre-emergent asthmatics. This can lead to the mistaken observation that bronchodilators seem to work in bronchiolitis (which has been disproven). The pre-emergent asthmatics are responding to bronchodilators (which do work in asthma for short-term relief).

The primary treatment for asthma is pharmacological. The rapid relief of acute symptoms and long-term asthma control are the two mainstays of asthma treatment.

- Short-acting inhaled or oral ß2-agonists, short-course oral or intravenous corticosteroids, and

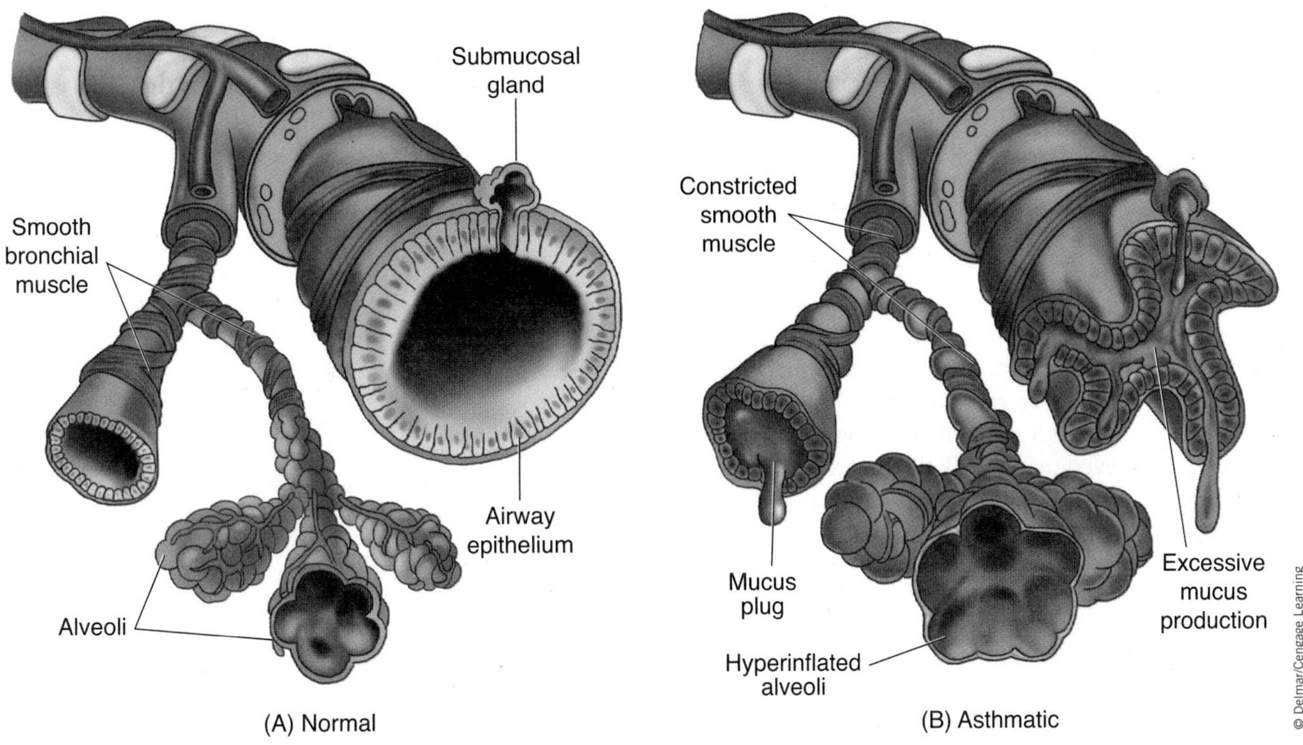

FIGURE 29-3 Illustration of normal versus asthmatic airways and terminal respiratory units.

ipratropium bromide are recommended for quick relief.

- Long-term control involves the use of cromolyn sodium, inhaled and oral corticosteroids, leukotriene modifiers, long-acting ß2-agonists, nedocromil sodium, and sustained-release theophylline.
- A typical clinical quality measure for the treatment of pediatric asthmatics in emergency rooms is the elapsed time from arrival to first dose of steroids, highlighting the importance of anti-inflammatory drugs in the treatment of asthma.
- Typically, inpatient treatment involves short-term relief with inhaled albuterol and supportive measures like hydration and oxygen, until the steroids can kick in and reduce lung inflammation.

For severe asthma attacks, other treatments are sometimes used, including intubation and mechanical ventilation, although this approach is becoming rarer as the understanding of how to manage asthma improves. Intubation should be avoided in asthmatics if possible because the introduction of the endotracheal tube can act as an irritant to an airway that is already hyper-responsive. To this end, some clinicians have used noninvasive positive pressure ventilation to avoid intubation.[31,32]

Mixtures of oxygen and helium (heliox) have been used as a treatment for asthma in children. This therapy replaces nitrogen with helium as the inert carrier gas that is mixed with oxygen. Helium has one-third the density of nitrogen, and theoretically this less dense gas mixture is easier to breath because the patient does not have to work as hard to move the same volume of gas through narrowed airways.[33] Heliox is administered via simple mask or cannula, or it is used to drive nebulizers or administered through a mechanical ventilator. Heliox typically comes from the supplier in concentrations of approximately 80% helium and 20% oxygen. F_IO_2 can be increased by adding more oxygen via bleed-in or with specially modified blender setups. A rule of thumb is that heliox therapy is of little value if the $F_IO_2 > 0.40$ because the smaller overall amount of helium does not reduce work of breathing enough to make a difference.

There are a limited number of studies on the utility of this therapy in children,[34,35] and the results are conflicting. It is not clear that heliox really alters outcomes for asthma patients, although for some patients it clearly offers immediate, visible relief. The utilization of heliox varies widely with some hospitals hardly ever using it, while others employ it frequently.[36] Heliox can be given to intubated asthmatics via a mechanical ventilator. Most ventilators are not designed for this, and so the therapist must make special adaptations of the blender-ventilator system to safely control the amount of heliox the patient receives.

Whenever heliox is used, the respiratory therapist must remember that the lower density gas makes most flow meters and flow measurement devices inaccurate. To estimate actual flow rate when using heliox, take the visual reading from a typical flow meter and multiply times 1.8. Some pediatric neonatal ventilators are specifically designed to allow the use of heliox. Their intrinsic measurement and flow control systems are programmed in such way to allow for accurate operation in the presence of heliox. (At the time of writing, three widely used ventilators have the built-in capacity to operate accurately with heliox: Viasys Avea, Hamilton G5, and Maquet Servo*i*.)

The diagnosis of asthma involves physical examination, history, and assessment of airflow obstruction. In children older than 5 years of age, diagnosis can typically be achieved using peak flow meters at the bedside or spirometry before and after bronchodilator treatment. In younger children, the measurement of airflow obstruction is more difficult and is typically not routinely used in the assessment of asthma severity or response to therapy.

The respiratory treatment of inpatient asthmatics is often now guided by the use of asthma clinical scores. These are typically composite scores constructed by assessing or scoring patients on several variables. Their basic design is similar to APGAR scores. Table 29-9 shows a typical asthma clinical score that was studied and shown to have a high agreement between different providers scoring the same patient.[37] The patient's clinical score is used to guide the need for bronchodilators, dosage and frequency, and periodicity of reassessment. In many facilities, the respiratory care of asthmatics is guided by a standardized protocol. The respiratory therapist and nurses administer the asthma clinical score and use it to guide the intensity of bronchodilator therapy.

BRONCHIOLITIS

Pediatric bronchiolitis is a disease caused by viral lower respiratory tract infection. It is characterized by acute airway inflammation, edema, and necrosis of epithelial cells lining the small airways. Generalized interstitial swelling, combined with inhibition of pulmonary surfactant function, leads to the narrowing of airways. The net result is increased secretion production and decreased secretion clearance due to the compromise of the mucociliary elevator. Brochoconstriction may be present, but generally it is not the principal cause of airway obstruction, which is usually the airway edema and accumulated secretions. This explains the failure of bronchodilators to work in most of these patients. Signs and symptoms are typically rhinitis, tachypnea, wheezing, cough, crackles, use of accessory muscles, and/or nasal flaring.

Each year there is a near pandemic in the United States (and other countries) of viral lower respiratory tract infections in infants and children. About two-thirds of this bronchiolitis is caused by *respiratory syncitial virus* (*RSV*), a ubiquitous virus that infects over 90% of children by age 2. In previously healthy infants, the disease typically has a short course (3–5 days) and very mild to moderate symptoms. However, in more severe cases, hospitalization is required. Bronchiolitis causes more than180,000 hospitalizations per year in children $<$ 1 year of age at a cost of almost $2.5 billion annually.[38] The reasons for hospitalization include the need for:

- Close observation.
- Supplemental oxygen therapy.
- Bronchodilator treatments.
- Frequent nasal suctioning.
- Rehydration.
- Treatment for apnea.

Uncomplicated bronchiolitis in previously healthy infants is typically a self-limited illness with few interventions that actually substantially alter the course of the disease. However, multiple interventions are frequently used, including corticosteroids, antibiotics, ribavirin, the repeated use of bronchodilators, and chest physical therapy in the form of postural drainage and percussion. However, when these interventions have been tested in controlled scientific studies designed to measure their impact on outcomes, they have almost universally failed to demonstrate any efficacy.[39,40] This evidence[41,42] (or lack thereof) notwithstanding, there continues to be considerable variation in how bronchiolitics are treated when inpatients. There continues to be widespread use of bronchodilators in this population in spite of repeated studies showing a lack of efficacy. Chest physiotherapy, antibiotics, and steroids are also prone to overutilization in this group.

Spotlight On

Bronchiolitics

Patients admitted to the hospital typically expect that their conditions can be cured or their suffering can be minimized. So they expect caregivers to intervene, that is, do *something* for them or to them to help them. This is particularly true for parents of pediatric cases. In bronchiolitis care, this expectation creates pressure among clinicians to do something to help these sick children. The authors believe that this pressure contributes to the overuse of these ineffective interventions in bronchiolitics.

TABLE 29-9 **A clinical asthma scoring tool.***

Variable	0 point	1 point	2 points	3 points
Respiratory rate (breaths/min)				
<2 mo		≤60	61–69	≥70
2–12 mos		≤50	51–59	≥60
1–2 yr		≤40	41–44	≥45
2–3 yr		≤34	35–39	≥40
4–5 yr		≤30	31–35	≥36
6–12 yr		≤26	27–30	≥31
> 12 yr		≤23	24–27	≥28
Retractions	None	Subcostal or intercostal	2 of the following: subcostal, intercostal, substernal, *or* nasal flaring (infants)	3 of the following: subcostal, intercostal, substernal, suprasternal, supraclavicular, *or* nasal flaring or head bobbing (infants)
Dyspnea				
0–2 yr	Normal feeding, vocalizations, and activity	1 of the following: difficulty feeding, decreased vocalization, *or* agitated	2 of the following: difficulty feeding, decreased vocalization, *or* agitated	Stops feeding, no vocalizations, *or* drowsy or confused
2–4 yr	Normal feeding, vocalizations, and play	1 of the following: decreased appetite, increased coughing after play, hyperactivity	2 of the following: decreased appetite, increased coughing after play, hyperactivity	Stops eating or drinking, stops playing, *or* drowsy or confused
≥ 5 yr	Counts to ≥ 10 in one breath	Counts to 7–9 in one breath	Counts to 4–6 in one breath	Counts to ≤ 3 in one breath
Auscultation (as it relates to wheezing)	Normal breathing; no wheezing present	End-expiratory wheeze only	Expiratory wheeze only (greater than end-expiratory wheeze)	Inspiratory and expiratory wheeze *or* diminished breath sounds *or* both

**Scores range from 0–12. Scores <5 are considered mild, while scores >9 are severe. Respiratory rate should be counted for a full min while patient is awake*

In our experience, a small number of infants—typically about 20% of presenting bronchiolitics—with uncomplicated bronchiolitis appear to respond to bronchodilators. The conventional wisdom holds that these are pre-emergent asthmatics, who appear to be more susceptible to bronchiolitis. Thus, most bronchiolitis treatment protocols include a trial of bronchodilators.[43,44] Only if the patient clearly responds to the drug are the treatments continued.

Response is assessed using clinical bronchiolitis scores, some of which are similar to asthma clinical scores. Table 29-10 shows one such bronchiolitis score.[45] Typically infants are scored (assessed), their upper airways are cleared, and then they are reassessed. If the scores significantly improve, then further treatment with bronchodilators is deemed unnecessary. If upper airway clearance does not improve the score, then a bronchodilator treatment is given, then the patient is rescored. If the scores improved, bronchodilators therapy is continued with frequent reassessment. If the score does not improve, bronchodilator therapy is discontinued because it did not seem to help the patient. Figure 29-4 is an algorithm for the management of bronchodilators. This algorithm and bronchiolitis score were developed at Primary Children's Medical Center in Salt Lake City and were very successful in reducing the unnecessary utilization of interventions.[46]

An essential part of bronchiolitis care is the use of *nasal pharyngeal suctioning*. This technique is sometimes mistakenly referred to as deep suctioning. Usually, deep suctioning is reserved for when an attempt is made to insert the suction catheter all the way to the epiglottis and even into the trachea. The technique

TABLE 29-10 **Bronchiolitis Score**

Score Assigned	Respiratory Rate	Wheezing	Retractions
0	<30	no wheezing with good air exchange	none
1	31–45	late expiratory with stethoscope only	mild
2	46–60	entire expiratory or inspiratory phase with stethoscope only	moderate
3	>60	loud wheezes without stethoscope or no wheezing in the presence of severely diminished gas exchange	severe

0–1 = normal; 2–3 = mild; 4–6 = moderate; 7–9 = severe

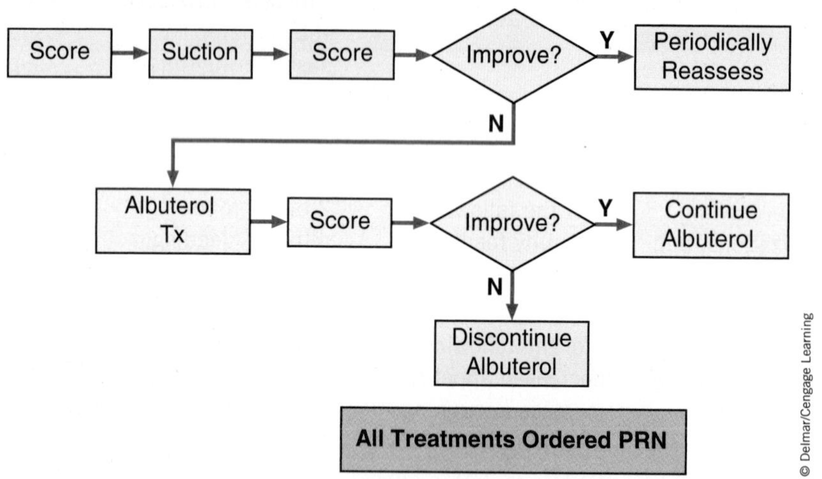

FIGURE 29-4 Algorithm for managing bronchodilator use in bronchiolitics. In this particular protocol, nasal pharyngeal suctioning through both nares into the hypopharynx was used on all infants with bronchiolitis prior to giving bronchodilators.

includes the passing of an appropriately sized catheter through each nare into the hypopharynx. This clearing of the upper airway reduces work of breathing and often reduces symptom severity and resource consumption.[47,48] Some clinicians have argued that it is too traumatic to routinely use nasal pharyngeal suctioning on infants, but in our experience, when the staff are properly trained and experienced, nasal pharyngeal suctioning was safe and effective. Also, some clinicians have suggested that olive tip style of suctioning is sufficient, but we find this technique less effective in clearing the upper airway.

ACUTE RESPIRATORY DISTRESS SYNDROME (ARDS)

Acute respiratory distress syndrome (*ARDS*) is a condition that results from overwhelming inflammation, increased alveolar capillary permeability, and consequent pulmonary edema. Pediatric ARDS can be caused by aspiration, near-drowning, smoke inhalation, lower respiratory tract infections, trauma, and multisystem organ failure.[49,50]

It has been estimated that there are 190,600 cases of ARDS in all age groups, involving 74,500 deaths and

> *Best Practice*
>
> **Suctioning**
>
> In children, passing a catheter through the nose and blindly entering the trachea is all but impossible. However, simply passing the catheter down into the hypopharynx is usually sufficient to cause a strong cough reflex in the patient, which in the end is usually a good thing to do in patients with secretion problems.

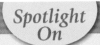

Statistical Data

Statistics can be misleading. The adult data include *all* hospital days, whereas the pediatric data report only PICU days. This is often the case in broad studies of disease epidemiology and impact. Data from different studies are sliced up in different ways.

3.6 million hospital days per year.[51] For pediatric ARDS,[52] there is an estimated 7700 cases, 1400 deaths, and 6200 pediatric intensive care days per year.

ARDS is characterized by reduced lung compliance, increased airway resistance, refractory hypoxemia, and respiratory acidosis. These factors can cause severe respiratory failure, which often results in intubation and mechanical ventilation.

In adults, mortality from ARDS has been reported to be approximately 39%.[51] The incidence of mortality in pediatric ARDS has been reported as 18%.[52]

ARDS often follows a severe physiologic insult like trauma or sepsis and presents with:

- An acute onset.
- Severe arterial hypoxemia refractory to oxygen therapy alone (P_aO_2/F_IO_2 ratio $\leq$ 200 mm Hg).
- Diffuse bilateral pulmonary infiltrates on chest radiograph.[53]

Some pediatric clinicians prefer the use of the S_pO_2/F_IO_2 ratio in infants and children as a surrogate marker to diagnose ARDS since arterial blood gas sampling can be challenging in infants and children. In fact, an $S_pO_2/F_IO_2 < 275$ corresponds well with the predefined P_aO_2/F_IO_2 criteria of < 200 for ARDS.[54]

In the last decade, the pediatric community has adopted the successful application of adult lung-protective ventilation strategies. These strategies have developed out of the growing understanding that the application of mechanical ventilation itself can be injurious to the acutely ill lung. This is true for neonatal, pediatric, and adult scenarios. It was long held that high airway pressures were the chief cause of ventilator-induced lung injury. *Excessive lung volumes, not excessive airway pressures, are the chief cause of ventilator-induced lung injury* (discussed later in this chapter). The basic premise is that limiting tidal volume is more important than limiting pressures in the prevention of injury.[55]

Conventional mechanical ventilation is generally designed to allow permissive hypercapnea (pH>7.20 and P_aCO_2 55–65), lower tidal volumes and alveolar distending pressures (plateau pressures).[56] Typically, tidal volumes are kept in the 4–6 mL/kg or lowest tidal volume possible while keeping plateau pressures <30 cm H_2O. PEEP is set according the level of required F_IO_2. Once the oxygenation improves, aggressive attempts are often made to reduce the F_IO_2 to minimize the risk of toxic effects from exposure to high oxygen levels in the lung. Table 29-11 lists some guidelines for setting up and managing the mechanical ventilatory for a child with ARDS.

Respiratory Assessment in the Neonatal and Pediatric Patient

A common duty of the neonatal pediatric RT is to evaluate the respiratory status of a child. The two principal parts of this respiratory assessment are a visual inspection and auscultation. In addition to the previously described signs associated with assessing respiratory failure in infants, a special consideration for the respiratory assessment of infants and children is the use (or lack of use) of blood gases. For the presenting infant or child, blood gas sampling can be very difficult because of the technical challenges of doing an arterial stick on an infant or small child. In addition, the lack of patient cooperation can make arterial blood gases difficult to get. Finally, parents are understandably reluctant to see their children subjected to a lot of pain.

Consequently, blood gases are usually obtained only when significant respiratory distress is evident from other signs. When blood gases are needed, venous and capillary samples are sometimes used to avoid the need for percutaneous arterial sampling. Capillary sticks are less painful for children. Venous samples are usually easier because the patients are getting venipuncture for other laboratory work being done, and additional blood is drawn for blood gases. In general, venous and capillary blood gases are suitable for determining the level of ventilation and acid-base balance, but they have limited value in determining oxygenation status. Pulse oximetry is the tool most often used for assessing oxygenation. Table 29-12 describes normal blood gas and pulse oximetry ranges in neonates and children.

Another important issue in neonatal and pediatric assessment is the *lack of reserve* that some sick infants and children exhibit. An infant or child in respiratory distress can very quickly worsen, and the pulmonary assessment of these patients is in part dependent on learning how to determine whether these patients are on the edge of a sudden deterioration. By way of example, a P_aCO_2 of 46 mm Hg might not bother you at all in most infants, children, or adults. But if this blood gas comes from a 4-year-old asthmatic who is

TABLE 29-11 Guidelines for pediatric ARDS ventilator management

1) *Initial ventilator tidal volume and rate adjustments*
   a) *Calculate predicted body weight (PBW)*
      i) Male = 50 + 2.3 [height (inches) – 60] or 50 + 0.91 [height (cm) –152.4]
      ii) Female = 45.5 + 2.3 [height (inches) – 60] or 45.5 + 0.91 [height (cm) –152.4]
   b) *Mode: Volume Assist-Control or PRVC Assist-Control*
      i) Set initial tidal volume to 8 ml/kg PBW
      ii) Reduce tidal volume to 7 mL/kg after 1–2 hr and then to 6 mL/kg PBW after 1–2 hr
      iii) Set initial ventilator rate to maintain baseline min ventilation (not > 35 bpm)
2) Subsequent tidal volume adjustments
   a) Plateau pressure goal: ≤ 30 cm H_2O
   b) If plateau pressure > 30 cm H_2O, decrease tidal volume by 1 mL/kg PBW steps to 5 or if necessary to 4 mL/kg PBW.
   c) If plateau pressure < 25 cm H_2O and tidal volume < 6 mL/kg, increase tidal volume by 1 mL/kg PBW until plateau pressure at > 25 cm H_2O or tidal volume = 6 mL/kg.
   d) If breath stacking or severe dyspnea occurs, tidal volume may be increased (not required) to 7 or 8 mL/kg PBW if plateau pressure remains ≤ 30 cm H_2O.
3) *Arterial oxygenation*
   a) Goal: P_aO_2 55–80 mm Hg or S_pO_2 88–95%
   b) Use the F_IO_2/PEEP combinations in the table to the right to achieve oxygenation goal.
4) Respiratory Rate (RR) and pH (arterial)
   a) *pH Goal: 7.30–7.45 (arterial)*
   b) Acidosis Management:
      i) *If pH 7.15—7.30:* Increase set RR until pH > 7.30 or P_aCO_2 < 25 mm Hg
      ii) Maximum Set RR = 35 bpm
      iii) If set RR = 35 bpm and pH < 7.30, $NaHCO_3$ may be given (not required)
      iv) *If pH < 7.15:*
         (1) Increase set RR to 35 bpm.
         (2) If set RR = 35 and pH < 7.15 and $NaHCO_3$ has been considered, tidal volume may be increased in 1 mL/kg PBW steps until pH > 7.15 (plateau pressure target may be exceeded).
   c) Alkalosis Management: (pH > 7.45):
      i) Decrease set RR until patient RR > set RR
      ii) Minimum set RR = 6 bpm
   d) I/E ratio
      i) Goal: 1:1.0 to 1:3.0
      ii) Adjust flow rate and inspiratory flow waveform to achieve goal.

Best Practice

PEEP Guidelines: These include recommendations for a lower or higher PEEP strategy, which remains controversial

F_IO_2	Low PEEP	High PEEP
0.3	5	5–14
0.4	5–8	14–16
0.5	8–10	16–18
0.6	10	20
0.7	10–14	20
0.8	14	20–22
0.9	14–18	22
1.0	18–24	22–24

TABLE 29-12 Normal (reference) ranges for blood gases and pulse oximetry

Age	Range	Neonatal		Pediatric	
Source	Arterial	Venous	Capillary	Arterial	Venous
pH	7.35–7.45	7.31–7.41	7.31–7.47	7.35–7.45	7.31–7.41
pCO_2	35–45 mm Hg	41–51 mm Hg	29–49 mm Hg	35–45 mm Hg	41–51 mm Hg
pO_2	50–90 mm Hg	30–40 mm Hg	33–61 mm Hg	80–100 mm Hg	30–40 mm Hg
S_pO_2	92–94%	NA		>95%	NA

Source: Capillary values are from Cousineaua, J., Anctilb, S., Carcellerb, A., Gonthierb, M., Delvin, E. E. Neonate capillary blood gas reference values. Clin Biochem *2005;38(10):905–907.*

very tachypnic, has labored breathing, and is wheezing loudly on inspiration and expiration, this is an ominous blood gas. Pediatric asthmatics can decompensate very rapidly, and it is concerning that this patient is working so hard to maintain such a marginal P_aCO_2. This sign could be a portent of a sudden deterioration, and close monitoring and escalation of care is in order.

The other key factors in respiratory assessment are:

- Respiratory rate.
- Grunting.
- Flaring.
- Retracting.
- Level of consciousness.
- Level of irritation.

The typical child in respiratory distress presents tachypnic, agitated, or highly irritable with exaggerated work of breathing.

Technology of Pediatric and Neonatal Respiratory Therapy

A wide array of technical tools are available to the RT in the pediatric setting. Mastering the application of these devices is essential to practicing successfully. Some RTs have been practicing long enough to have seen this amazing transition to a much more complex technological environment. In this long passage, they have also noticed that this amazing technical wizardry can make them lose sight of the patient amid all the monitors, catheters, tubes, masks, and machines. *The respiratory technician must avoid the black box preoccupation* that occurs when the RT at the bedside becomes overly focused on the readings of the various machines and monitors. The first and most important indication of how well the patient is doing is a physical examination; this fact can be forgotten in the swirl of bedside technology. The technology scenario can be visually very poignant with infants and small children, who can be dwarfed by the size and number of devices and monitors at the bedside.

Consider the patient on a mechanical ventilator, extracorporeal life support, various infusions of fluids, antibiotics, vasopressors, inotropes, a cardiorespiratory monitor, pulse oximetry, and capnography. Some 15 to 20 different screens may be in the room presenting digital data in numeric and or graphical form. Along with the obvious opportunity to commit errors of commission or omission in this visually complex environment, the patient tends to be lost amid the clutter.

There is also a tendency to not really understand the limitations of the devices being used. *Respiratory therapists must understand that all measurements are erroneous*. Even the best clinical instruments have intrinsic measurement errors under the best of conditions of $\pm 5\%$ of the absolute reading. Many are worse. Some measurement devices have severe limitations under certain conditions, and some of these limitations are more pronounced in neonatal/pediatric populations. Clinicians must have a deep understanding of these limitations to make informed decisions about the quality of the data they produce. Also, some of the respiratory therapy technology that is suitable for adults has serious limitations in neonates and children.

MANUAL RESUSCITATORS

Today, newborns require resuscitation more frequently than any other patient population, and one of the common features of this resuscitation is the application of positive pressure ventilation (PPV) using manual resuscitators.[57] Nearly 10 million newborns per year require some type of resuscitation worldwide.[58] Along with the resuscitation of newborns in the delivery suite, manual resuscitators are widely used in the intensive care unit for PPV during disconnection from the mechanical ventilator and during intra- and interhospital transport. The most commonly used manual resuscitators fall into two categories: flow-inflating bags and self-inflating bags.

Flow-inflating bags (*FIBs*) require a constant (though adjustable) flow of source gas to operate (SIBs can operate without a flow of source gas). Positive end-expiratory pressure (PEEP) is maintained by partially occluding excess flow out of the bag through a small hole or an adjustable flow-resisting valve at the tail of the bag. The thumb is used to partially occlude the hole in the bag. Adjusting the flow and maintaining PEEP with this type of resuscitator requires a relatively advanced degree of both experience and skill.[59] However, many less skilled and trained clinicians end up using these bags owing to turnover of staff and the constant flow of newly graduated clinicians into our hospitals.

With *self-inflating bags* (*SIBs*), the elastic recoil of the bag draws in the gas, which may be ambient or supplemental oxygen, depending on the bag's configuration. The design allows the bag to operate even with a loss of source gas. Certain brands of SIBs have valve mechanisms that allow gas to be directed to the patient during inhalation. If PEEP is desired, typically an add-on spring-loaded variable orifice PEEP valve is attached to the exhalation port of the bag.

There is a great deal of so-called conventional wisdom about the (*alleged*) relative merits of both types of resuscitators:

- FIBs are made of softer material, allowing the clinician to feel changes in lung compliance better than with an SIB.[60,61]

- FIBs deliver blow-by O_2 more effectively than an SIB. In this context, *blow-by* refers to the practice of holding the resuscitator bag (with or without a mask) close to the face.
- When using an SIB for blow-by O_2 delivery, the bag must be squeezed to deliver O_2 to a spontaneously breathing patient.[8]
- SIBs cannot give as high an F_IO_2 as FIBs.
- SIBs are easier to use, more suitable for inexperienced personnel, do not require a compressed gas source, have a lower incidence of gastric inflation, and provide more consistent ventilation and PEEP.[10–14]

Research by the authors and others has disproved most of these assumptions:[62–63]

- SIBs produce more consistent tidal volumes than FIBs.
- SIBs produce more consistent PEEP than FIBs.
- Clinicians do not feel changes in compliance more with either style of bag.
- SIBs can effectively be used for blow-by oxygen if configured properly.

During manual ventilation, the importance of limiting tidal volume to minimize volutrauma and the maintenance of appropriate levels of PEEP atelectrauma in limiting iatrogenic lung injury[64] should not be forgotten. Low-birth-weight infants with surfactant-depleted, fluid-filled, underdeveloped lungs are at particularly higher risk for developing lung injury and consequent chronic lung disease. Cellular mediators that signal lung inflammation have been measured in the lungs of premature infants after brief manual resuscitation, suggesting that even short-term ventilation can be injurious to the lungs.[65] Thus, when all factors are considered, SIBs are better for use during the manual ventilation of infants and small children.

New technology may offer advantages over either FIB or SIB with regard to limiting ventilation variability. The Neopuff (Fisher and Paykel, Auckland, New Zealand) is a neonatal resuscitator that allows a fixed inspiratory flow rate and pressure-limiting neonatal resuscitator. The operator controls inspiratory time with a thumb, and the peak inspiratory pressure is controlled via a pressure relief mechanism in the device. The obvious advantage is that the flow and inspiratory pressures are more carefully controlled than during bagging. The apparent result is more consistent ventilating pressures and limited excessive overpressures or high PEEP levels.[66] Of course, tidal volume can still vary considerably, probably as a result of variations in the inspiratory time created by the operator's thumb and a poor face seal with a mask.[67]

However, investigators have reported dangers of higher-than-desired PIP with the Neopuff if the flow is not set at the recommended levels.[68] In another report, McHale and colleagues report large variations in tidal volume when members of various clinical disciplines with varying levels of experience ventilated a neonatal mannequin with the Neopuff. Also reported were large variations in mean airway pressures and tidal volumes that were independent of experience. More research needs to be done to determine whether the Neopuff really offers neonates an advantage.

MONITORING

Continuous and intermittent monitoring of respiratory status and/or the performance of respiratory support devices has become a very large part of the duties of respiratory therapists. *RTs should be experts on the principles of operation and limitations of every monitoring and treatment device they operate.* It is to the benefit of the sick children they care for to become expert on how these devices really work and on the strengths and limitations of each. As clinicians, RTs spend a significant portion of their time at the bedside interpreting monitoring data and trying to determine whether to change therapeutic interventions. The way to become expert is to thoroughly digest the operating manuals and a textbook on the topic.

PULSE OXIMETRY

The pulse oximeter can (under ideal conditions) estimate the level of oxygenation saturation of hemoglobin and heart rate. Newer pulse oximeter technology also allows for the noninvasive determination of various other types of hemoglobin, including carboxyhemoglobin, methemoglobin, and total hemoglobin.[69] A more detailed description of the operation of oximeters is beyond the scope of this chapter but can be found elsewhere.[70]

In pediatric and neonatal applications, conditions are often not ideal. The oximeter has difficulty continuously producing reliable and accurate data due to three circumstances: motion artifact, low peripheral perfusion and elevated levels of dyshemoglobins, explained in detail in Table 29-13. All three of these circumstances can be prevalent in certain neonatal and pediatric populations. There has been a great debate about the comparative performance of various brands of oximeters. Conventional wisdom holds that most oximeter brands work sufficiently well on about 80% of patients they are used on. But on certain patient types and under certain conditions, performance differences are more notable, particularly in pediatric

TABLE 29-13 Circumstances affecting the reliability of pulse oximeter readings in neonatal and pediatric applications

Circumstance	Affect on Measurement Principle	Clinical Impact
Motion artifact	When the tissue bed being measured is distorted by movement, this can create very small changes in the absorption of the light emitted by the pulse oximeter.	Many brands and models of oximeters (especially older versions) simply "drop-out," or fail to show a reading. Other brands freeze the reading. Sometimes a reading is displayed, but the reading can be profoundly inaccurate.[1] Infants and toddlers are prone to motion and thus this can be problematic in this population. However, some models of oximeters have demonstrated improved performance during motion artifact.[2]
Low peripheral perfusion	The signal processing in most oximeters requires the detection of pulsatile changes in absorption that occurs as a result of systole. During low perfusion states it is very hard for the oximeter to detect these pulsatile changes. Also, poor peripheral perfusion can lead to oxygenation readings of the peripheral blood that is really not representative of systemic oxygenation.	This also can result in "drop-outs," freezes, and false alarms. Often you simply cannot get a reading at all. Children with congenital cardiac disease can be prone to poor peripheral perfusion. Also, cardiac patients who have had their body cooled down for surgery can be difficult to monitor in the immediate post-operative period. Again, there are important performance differences between oximeter brands under these conditions.[3]
Elevated levels of dyshemoglobins	Hemoglobin exists in a number of variants under normal conditions. Some of these are called "dyshemoglobins" because they are unable to carry oxygen and thus are dysfunctional. They include carboxyhemoglobin and methemoglobin. The standard two wavelength pulse oximeters (currently all brands except one) can distinguish these dyshemoglobins from oxygenated hemoglobin.	Elevated levels of dyshemoglobins causes most pulse oximeters to display a falsely high S_PO_2. Thus the clinician can believe that patient's blood is carrying much more oxygen than it really is. There can be significant hypoxia while the pulse oximeter continues to display normal levels of S_PO_2. Currently only one brand of pulse oximeter measures more than two wavelengths of light and thus can distinguish these dyshemoglobins.[4] Carboxyhemoglobin can be present when the patient inhales elevated levels of carbon monoxide, e.g., smoke inhalation or inhaling the exhaust from internal combustion engines. There is now a commercially available pulse oximeter that can measure total hemoglobin (g/dL) noninvasively.[5,6]

[1] *Van de Louw A, Cracco C, Cerf C, Harl A, Duvaldestin P, Lemair F, et al. Accuracy of pulse oximetry in the intensive care unit. Intensive Care Med. 2001:27:1606–1613.*

[2] *R Sahni, A Gupta, K Ohira-Kist, T S Rosen Motion resistant pulse oximetry in neonates. Arch Dis Child Fetal Neonatal Ed 2003;88:F505–F508.*

[3] *Kawagishi T, Kanaya N, Nakayama M, Kurosawa S, MD, Namiki A. A comparison of the failure times of pulse oximeters during blood pressure cuff-induced hypoperfusion in volunteers. Anesth Analg. 2004;99:793–6.*

[4] *Barker SJ, Curry J, Redford D, Morgan S. Measurement of carboxyhemoglobin and methemoglobin by pulse oximetry: a human volunteer study. Anesthesiology. 2006;105:892–897.*

[5] *Macknet MR, Norton S, Kimball-Jones P, Applegate R, Martin R, Allard M. Continuous non-invasive measurement of hemoglobin via pulse oximetry. Anesth Analg. 2007;104:S–117.*

[6] *Macknet MR, Norton S, Kimball-Jones P, Applegate R, Martin R, Allard M. A prospective study to validate continuous non-invasive measurement of hemoglobin via pulse CO-oximetry.*

and neonatal populations who are prone to movement and poor peripheral perfusion.

A dizzying array of claims and counterclaims are made about oximeter brands. But a careful review of the scientific literature indicates important performance differences among the brands. As of this writing, one technology in particular appears to perform better under the challenging conditions of pediatric care. (Of course, this could change as more peer-reviewed scientific literature is published on the latest generation of oximeter signal processing.) Signal extraction technology (Masimo Inc., Irvine, California) uses a proprietary combination of filtering and statistical treatment of the pulse oximeter signal. This device produces saturation readings that are less prone to dropout and false desaturations.[71,72] *False alarms and false desaturations are a major problem with pulse oximetry, particularly in pediatrics.* It is reported in two studies that:

- 44–63% of all critical care alarms were caused by pulse oximeters.
- 94% of oximeter alarms were considered clinically unimportant.
- 71% were false alarms.[73,74]

At the bedside, RTs spend a lot of time trying to analyze monitoring data and to use it to make care decisions about patients.

Typically, the pulse oximeter is used to ensure that patients have a minimal level of oxygen saturation. There are two exceptions: neonatal patients and patients with certain types of congenital cardiac defects. In neonatal patients, RTs need to ensure both minimal and maximal allowable levels of oxygenation to reduce the risk of retinopathy of prematurity (as explained earlier in this chapter). Thus, both upper and lower alarm limits are set. Opinions are divergent about the best limits to set to reduce the risk. Currently, a typical recommendation is 88–93% in neonates.[75] This is a sea-level recommendation, and care must be taken to adjust for hospitals at higher altitudes.

CONVENTIONAL VENTILATORS

As far as I am concerned the whole area of ventilation of infants with respiratory distress syndrome is one of chaos. Claims and counterclaims about the best and least harmful method of ventilating the premature infant make me light-headed. I can't wait for the solution or solutions to premature birth, and I look forward to the day when all this gadgetry will come to an end and the neonatologist will be retired. (Gellis SS. *1977 Yearbook of Pediatrics*. In Gellis SS, ed. London: YB Medical Publishers; 1978.)

Since the time of this famous quote, the gadgetry has not come to an end and indeed has increased and become more complex. The claims and counterclaims have also continued. There are several camps in the neonatal community regarding mechanical ventilation, and exploring them all in depth is beyond the scope of this chapter. The interested student is cautioned that, in the area of mechanical ventilation, very few claims and counterclaims have ever been thoroughly tested and or proven to be efficacious.[76] Further details about the state of the evidence base for mechanical ventilation of neonates can be found in the writing of Donn.[77,78]

The general ventilation goal of sustaining gas exchange that is compatible with life is balanced with the goal of minimizing the patient's chance of being injured by the ventilator. These injuries fall into three basic categories: mechanical injury (lung overdistension), biochemical injury (oxygen toxicity), and infection injury (ventilator associated pneumonias). At the risk of oversimplification, these can be loosely categorized as four "schools" of ventilation: pressure-limited, volume-targeted, noninvasive, and high-frequency. These categories are not mutually exclusive; they represent a general focus.

- The *pressure-limited* focus holds that the best way to minimize the risk of overdistension is by carefully limiting airway pressure.
- The *volume-targeted* adherents suggest that the careful control of tidal volumes is the best way.
- The *noninvasive* school advocates the avoidance of intubation whenever possible through the use of various noninvasive ventilation techniques, such as nasal continuous positive airway pressure, to minimize the risk of lung injury and infection.
- Advocates of early intervention with *high-frequency* ventilation maintain this is a less risky (in terms of lung injury) technique than conventional positive pressure ventilation.

There is tremendous variation in the use of these techniques among neonatal and pediatric practice groups. At this point in time, a consensus has not yet developed about the best ways to use these interventions.

The many claims and counterclaims about the best modes of ventilation include the time-triggered, flow-triggered, pressure-triggered, time-cycled, flow-cycled, volume-cycled, and single- and dual-control modes. Yet there has historically been surprisingly little evidence that any one mode is any better than others in terms of the effect of the ventilation on morbidities and mortality conference.[79]

In the early 1970s, technology was developed that allowed *time-triggered, time-cycled, pressure-limited infant (TCPL) ventilation*. This revolutionized neonatal respiratory care and, along with surfactant replacement therapy, contributed to a 50% reduction in the infant mortality rate in the 20 years that followed.[80]

Improvements in ventilator capabilities now provide better ways for neonatal and pediatric patients to synchronize their breathing efforts with those generated by the ventilator using a mode called *synchronized IMV (SIMV)*.

Another important advance in neonatal and pediatric ventilators has been the development of the accurate measurement of airflow and tidal volumes in very small patients. This is generally accomplished by using proximal airway sensors that measure airflow at the connection of the ventilator's circuit and the patient's artificial airway. It has been shown that ventilators that do not measure tidal volume with a sensor at the proximal airway produce tidal volume measurements that are insufficiently accurate for use in managing the ventilator in neonates and infants.[81,82] Thus, the best neonatal and pediatric ventilators have proximal airway flow sensors for the accurate determination of inhaled and exhaled tidal volumes.

The overall goals for managing pediatrics using mechanical ventilation are to:

- Maintain adequate lung volume and alveolar ventilation.
- Support gas exchange.
- Improve lung mechanics.
- Reduce the work of breathing.
- Minimize lung injury.

Pediatric patients receiving mechanical ventilation are different from adults on many levels.

- Pediatric patients decompensate more quickly than adults and respond to hypoxia by becoming bradycardic, whereas adults typically become tachycardic.
- Airway resistance is greater and compliance is lower in infants than in adults.
- Small endotracheal tubes can kink and become occluded with secretions easier than do larger ones.

However, like all mechanically ventilated patients, pediatrics and adults alike, the clinician must be well aware of changes in the lung pathophysiology by carefully monitoring and assessing the patient's airway and respiratory status.

Table 29-14 shows some general initial guidelines for implementing ventilation in neonatal and pediatric patients.

The management of the endotracheal tube is also a particular challenge among infants and children. The small tubes and the lack of patient cooperation in this population make accidental extubations an ongoing problem. Loss of the airway can be a life-threatening event, and much work goes into securing endotracheal tubes. Of the wide range of taping techniques, few have actually been tested. One technique that has shown particular promise involves the use of modified umbilical clamps to help hold the ETT in place. This technique has been shown to reduce accidental extubations.[83]

HIGH-FREQUENCY VENTILATORS

The U.S. Food and Drug Administration (FDA) defines a *high-frequency ventilator* (HFV) as a device that provides respiratory frequencies under 150 breaths/min. High-frequency ventilators can apply high frequencies (150–900 breaths/min) while using smaller-than-normal tidal volumes. High-frequency ventilation has been applied to patients using a number of devices, including high-frequency jet ventilation, high-frequency low interrupter ventilation, and high-frequency oscillatory ventilation.[84]

High-frequency oscillatory ventilation is the most commonly used modality in neonatal and pediatrics today. This approach differs from the other modes in that it uses a rapidly oscillating piston diaphragm. So gas is forced into the lung under positive pressure and pulled from the lung during exhalation with an equal amount of negative pressure. Thus, this mode is said to have *active exhalation.*

For reasons that are not entirely understood, gas exchange and lung recruitment are often enhanced when very diseased lungs are switched from conventional to high-frequency ventilation. In some ways, the physical principles and mechanisms of gas exchange are similar to those of conventional ventilation (convection and molecular diffusion), but some principles are believed to be inherently different when using an HFV: asymmetric velocity profiles, pendeluft ventilation, augmented diffusion, bulk alveolar ventilation, and cardiogenic gas mixing.[85] It has also been speculated that the improvements in gas exchange and lung

TABLE 29-14 **Initial mechanical ventilator settings**

	Premature Infant	Infant	Toddler	Small Child	Child	Adolescent
Frequency (bpm)	40–60	25–40	20–35	20–30	18–25	12–20
V_T (mL/Kg)	4–6	5–8	5–8	6–9	7–10	7–10
T_I (s)	0.25–0.4	0.3–0.4	0.6–0.7	0.7–0.8	0.8–1.0	1.0–1.2
PEEP (cm H_2O)	3–5	5	5	5	5	5
F_IO_2	Start 0.10 higher than preintubation oxygen requirement					

Frequency = respiratory rate set on ventilator, V_T = tidal volume, T_I = inspiratory time, PEEP = positive end expiratory pressure, F_IO_2 = fraction of inspired oxygen. Adapted from Walsh, B. K., DiBlasi, R. M. Mechanical ventilation of the neonate and pediatric patient. In Walsh, B. K., Czervinske, M., DiBlasi, R.M., edi. Perinatal and Pediatric Respiratory Care, *3rd ed. St. Louis, MO: Elsevier; 2009: 325.*

recruitment are related to higher mean airway pressure that are obtainable during HFV without the cardiovascular and lung injury consequences of achieving these higher pressures with a conventional ventilator.

High-frequency oscillatory ventilation (*HFOV*) has been described simply as CPAP with wiggles and in many ways may be simpler to operate than conventional mechanical ventilation. The reason is that this mode allows the clinician separate controls for managing oxygenation and ventilation. During HFOV, the primary adjustments for oxygenation are F_IO_2 and mean airway pressure, and for ventilation (CO_2 removal) it is the amplitude and frequency settings.

The *mean airway pressure* (*MAP*) can be compared to a super CPAP setting that is applied continuously to the airway. MAP is adjusted upward in increments of 1–2 cm H_2O to augment lung volume and improve oxygenation. Amplitude (power) is typically set to achieve adequate shaking (or wiggling) from the shoulder to the umbilicus in infants and from the shoulder to the midthigh in larger pediatrics. Typically, the clinician increases the amplitude in response to hypercarbia and reduces the amplitude in response to hypocapnea. Amplitude can be thought of as analogous to tidal volume, although actual tidal volumes during HFOV are not known.

Relatively high *amplitudes* can be set in pediatrics without causing lung injury. One reason for this is that high frequencies, combined with the small internal diameter of neonatal and pediatric endotracheal tubes, cause the pressure signal to be significantly attenuated. Thus, only a fraction of the pressure swing measured at the airway is actually transmitted into the lung.

The hertz setting controls the *frequency* (set respiratory rate) by which these pressure oscillations occur. The frequency is usually set and not adjusted much unless the patient is exhibiting poor ventilation responses as a result of adjusting the amplitude. Frequency during HFOV is inversely proportionate to the CO_2 level. Unlike conventional ventilation, a lower frequency results in a lower P_aCO_2, and vice versa. Decreasing the frequency permits more time for the airway pressures to equilibrate with the lung; thus, airway pressure oscillations have more time to penetrate deeper into the lung.

In pediatrics, high-frequency ventilation has traditionally been used for children failing conventional ventilation. Concerns about ventilator-induced lung injury have led many clinicians to favor HFOV over conventional ventilation in pediatric applications and to move sooner to HFOV. However, practices continue to vary widely. This variation is contributed to by the divergent literature on HFOV use in infants and children. Some studies seem to support early intervention in neonatal and pediatric patients.[86,87] However, other studies of both neonates and pediatric patients have failed to find compelling evidence to suggest that HFOV produces better outcomes than conventional ventilation.[88,89] We look forward to the day when widely accepted standardized, evidence-based approaches to mechanical ventilation are in place.

A probable reason for the divergent findings in the literature is a lack of established standards for managing HFOV. Table 29-15 lists some basic guidelines for the management of HFOV.

CONTINUOUS POSITIVE AIRWAY PRESSURE

Continuous positive airway pressure (*CPAP*) is a form of respiratory support that is used primarily in spontaneously breathing patients with lung disease and apnea. NCPAP applies a continuous distending pressure to the nasal airway during inhalation and exhalation. CPAP was first described and used in neonates by Gregory and colleagues in 1971.[90] In theory, the technique simulates the physiologic effects of grunting in intubated newborns. It was speculated that neonates with respiratory distress grunted to create a slight back-pressure at the end of exhalation. The back-pressure is believed to be a form of self-administered CPAP that prevents widespread alveolar collapse with each breath. This collapse is a consequence of insufficient surfactant production and performance in the premature lung. Since CPAP seemed to be self-administered, the assumption was that artificially administered CPAP might be beneficial.

Infants have been described as being obligatory nasal breathers, and therefore nasal CPAP is effective in providing a continuous pressure to the lungs. However, there is considerable debate about the ability of newborns to breathe through their mouths when their noses are occluded.[91] Whether infants are true obligate nose breathers or preferential nose breathers is not clear. While this debate may seem arcane, it is actually very important when physiologists attempt to explain whey NCPAP and heated high-flow nasal cannula appear to work in some neonates.

The most common indication for NCPAP is for premature infants with RDS and apnea; however, NCPAP has been used successfully in supporting newborn infants with nearly all types of restrictive and obstructive lung disorders. In larger patients, NCPAP is used in intubated patients as an adjunct for weaning or to relieve upper airway obstruction using a nasal mask.

NCPAP has many potentially beneficial effects:[92]

- Increasing the functional residual capacity
- Improving gas exchange
- Reduced work of breathing.
- Reducing airway resistance by holding (or stenting) the airways open during exhalation (under certain conditions, as some theorize)

TABLE 29-15 **Guidelines for HFOV management**

1) Initial HFOV Settings
   a) Oxygenation
      i) The main determinant of oxygenation during HFOV is the MAP this is generally initiated at 5–8 cm H_2O above the MAP on conventional ventilation in large patients and 2 cm H_2O in premature patients.
      ii) Brief hypotension after initiation of HFOV is usually managed with a trial of fluid boluses to improve preload.
      iii) F_IO_2 is usually set at 100% on initiation of HFOV, and then tapered using pulse oximetry guidance to maintain SpO_2 of ≥ 88% in pediatric patients, and 88–94% in neonates.
      iv) If S_pO_2 or P_aO_2 has not improved enough to allow weaning of F_IO_2 %, the MAP is increased by 3–5 cm H_2O increments at 30–60 min intervals in hopes of improving lung recruitment. Incremental increases are less in neonatal patients.
      v) Some patients may slowly improve oxygenation only after a period of several hr. Vigilance and patience are required during the early phase of treatment.
   b) Ventilation
      i) The main determinants of P_aCO_2 removal are the pressure amplitude of oscillation (which is controlled by the power setting) and the frequency setting (Hz).
      ii) Increasing the amplitude and decreasing the frequency (Hz) increases the delivered tidal volume and conversely decreasing the amplitude and increasing the frequency (Hz) decreased the delivered tidal volume and allows P_aCO_2 to rise.
      iii) The amplitude is usually initiated at a value where the patient has good visual chest wall vibration (wiggle). For neonates this "wiggle" should be visible to the mid-abdominal level. For the larger pediatric patient this wiggle should be visible to the mid thigh level.
      iv) The initial frequency is set at 6–8 Hz for pediatric patients. This frequency is titrated upward for smaller neonatal patients to the point where neonates < 1000 g should have a frequency of approximately 15 Hz.
      v) Aggressive action is required for a rapidly rising P_aCO_2 during initiation of HFOV because improvements in P_aCO_2 do not occur quickly as is noted when changes are made to conventional ventilators.
      vi) An ABG should be obtained 15 to 20 min after starting HFOV to determine the trend of the P_aCO_2; subsequent ABGs are generally obtained at 30–60 min intervals until stabilization occurs. In neonates, where vascular access to arterial blood is limited, transcutaneous carbon-dioxide should be monitored throughout the period when the patient is on HFOV.

- Reduced incidence and severity of apneic episodes in infants by providing improvements in oxygenation and nasal airflow stimulation
- Reduced need for surfactant administration, endotracheal intubation, and mechanical ventilation
- Avoidance or minimization of the risk factors associated with intubation and mechanical ventilation, including infection, accidental extubation, and ventilator-induced lung injury
- Decreased lung injury and promotion of better lung growth and development
- Association with improved survival and reduced incidence and severity of BPD when compared with infants managed using mechanical ventilation as the primary form of respiratory support

Infants are supported initially using 4–6 cm H_2O of CPAP. The CPAP level can be increased if oxygenation is marginal. However, NCPAP levels greater than 10 cm H_2O are usually reserved for infants with obstructive airway lesions that are prone to collapse (i.e., tracheal malacia). Infants showing signs of excessive end-expiratory lung volume (hyperinflation) warrant lower CPAP levels.

The monitoring of the patient's respiratory status using blood gases, pulse oximetry, and chest X-rays are essential to the successful management of infants supported by NCPAP. The frequent monitoring of the nasal prong patency, the proper fit of prongs, and the proper adjustment of the fixation being used to secure the prongs in place are essential. If done properly, the amount of bedside care required by infants receiving CPAP is similar to or greater than that of a mechanically ventilated patient.

Unfortunately, not all infants can be supported using NCPAP alone. Infants failing CPAP typically present with increased grunting, nasal flaring, retractions, worsening oxygenation (P_aO_2 <50 mm Hg on

F_IO_2 >0.60), worsening ventilation (P_aCO_2 > 65 mm Hg and PH <7.20), and increased episodes of apnea and bradycardia. Approximately 40–50% of premature infants supported initially with NCPAP fail and require intubation and mechanical ventilation for surfactant administration. Nearly 30% of infants supported with CPAP following extubation require reintubation related to poor gas exchange and severe apneic episodes (stefanescu). Therefore, other types of noninvasive support, including noninvasive positive pressure ventilation, are focused in an area of intense clinical research.

NASAL CPAP SYSTEMS

The nasal CPAP system consists of a nasal prong or nasal mask interface, heated humidified gas source, patient circuit, and a pressure-generating device. CPAP systems also incorporate pressure-monitoring (manometer) and pressure relief mechanisms (Pop-off). CPAP is generated using a number of devices, including mechanical ventilators, fluidic devices (Infant Flow and Airlife), and a water-seal column (bubble CPAP). Each of these devices has its advantages and disadvantages, but there is insufficient evidence to support the concept that one device is better than another for reducing mortality or incidence of BPD.

The complications of NCPAP are similar to those reported using all forms of positive pressure ventilation (air leak, decreased cardiac output, and so on). The most prevalent and frequently reported complication with NCPAP is gastric insufflation, which can be relieved using an orogastric catheter. Because infants are being supported longer with NCPAP, nasal breakdown, erosion, and nasal distortion are frequently reported. These problems put the infant at a greater risk for infections. These problems can be lessened by ensuring proper prong size and fixation and by frequently assessing areas prone to nasal damage.

OXYGEN DELIVERY

In newborn infants, hypoxemia is indicated when P_aO_2 is <60 mm Hg. The exception to this is the infant with a congenital cardiac defect. In certain varieties of these defects, more profound hypoxia is acceptable and in some cases even desirable. In older pediatrics, hypoxemia is indicated when P_aO_2<80 mm Hg. Patients presenting with hypoxia typically manifest with tachypnea, nasal flaring, retractions, tachycardia, bradycardia, and cyanosis. Prolonged hypoxia can lead to severe metabolic acidosis from anaerobic metabolism. If not treated, persistent hypoxia can also lead to severe neurologic sequela and death.

Oxygen therapy can be administered using a number of oxygen delivery devices that are chosen based on the patient's size and oxygen requirement. Table 29-16 shows the range of oxygen delivery devices, flow ranges, and the approximate F_IO_2 levels. Oxygen is typically applied using either a low-flow meter (0.125–3.0 Lpm) or a standard flow meter to provide 100% oxygen through the device. Air-oxygen blenders are commonly found in NICU settings and provide precise adjustments in F_IO_2. The delivered F_IO_2 to the patient may be very different from what is set on the blender or what is coming from the flow meter. Pulse oximetry is an extremely useful clinical tool for monitoring the effectiveness of oxygen delivery and weaning.

TABLE 29-16 **Traditional estimated oxygen delivery capabilities during *pediatric* applications**

Device	Flow rate (L/min)	F_IO_2*
Nasal cannula	0.01–6	0.24–0.44
Blow-by oxygen	10	0.3–0.4
Oxygen hood	7–15 L/min	0.21–1.0
Simple mask	5–8	0.35–0.55
Air-entrainment mask	2–10	0.24–0.50
Nonrebreather mask	6–10 L/min	0.6–0.8

Source: Adapted in part. Pilbeam and Cairo text. Walsh and Grenier 2009 Respiratory Care. Walsh and Diblasi. 2002 CPG guidelines for administering oxygen to children.

The F_IO_2 can be highly variable using a nasal cannula. Changes in inspiratory flow, tidal volume and respiratory rate affect the rate of air entrainment, which can cause fluctuations in F_IO_2. However, the conventional wisdom that only a low F_IO_2 is possible with nasal cannula has been shown to be most probably untrue (see Table 29-16). In larger patients, the flow used to adjust the F_IO_2 is 0–6 Lpm; however, conventional wisdom holds that the maximum flow rate should be limited to 2 Lpm in infants and newborns.

A common practice is the intermittent administration of oxygen via free-flow or blow-by. This practice has oxygen blown by the face in an uncontrolled and highly variable fashion using a variety of techniques:

- A simple oxygen mask held near the face
- A flow-inflating manual resuscitator with the patient connection held close to the face
- A self-inflating bag equipped with a corrugate reservoir tube that is held near the patient's face

This method of oxygen delivery to children is discouraged because it is highly variable and the clinician has no idea how much oxygen the patient is actually receiving. The oxygen requirement of these patients is an important indication of the severity of respiratory symptoms.

AEROSOL DELIVERY

The selection of devices for delivering inhaled medications in children has historically not been well described in the literature. Inertia and tradition have contributed to a widespread belief that small-volume and large-volume pneumatic nebulizers are the preferred method of delivering inhaled medications to infants and children. However, a growing body of literature has led to an evolving practice. Conventional wisdom dictated that *metered dose inhalers* (*MDIs*) could not be effectively used in infants and children because of children's inability to cooperate or even to have sufficient hand-eye coordination to allow the effective operation of an MDI.

The authors' work has shown that, when used with the appropriately valved holding chamber and mask, MDIs are very efficient and effective methods of delivering inhaled medications to children.[93] The authors now use an MDI with a valved holding chamber (VHC) to administer nearly 90% of all inhaled albuterol to inpatients and have reduced our albuterol delivery costs by 21%. The source of these savings has been a reduction in the time required to give an MDI versus a small-volume nebulizer. It has been repeatedly shown that using an MDI with a VHC for inhaled medication administration in infants and children produces outcomes that are equivalent to and sometimes better than those produced by using small-volume nebulizers.[94,95]

The authors place no age limitations on the use of MDI-VHC, using it to give medications to infants, toddlers, and larger children. An internal panel of experts arrived at a dosing equivalency:

- A nebulizer dose of 2.5 mg of albuterol is equivalent to 4 puffs via MDI-VHC.
- A 5-mg nebulizer dose is equivalent to 8 puffs via MDI.

The authors have largely eliminated the use of the blow-by technique for aerosol medication delivery in children. In this widespread practice, the therapist holds the output of a nebulizer near the face, blowing toward the nose and mouth. The procedure has been largely discredited,[96] although it is still probably widely used.[97]

Summary

Respiratory care of the pediatric patient presents clinicians with unique challenges. An understanding of the diseases and pathologies related to infants and children are essential to craft effective respiratory care for this population. The size and complexity of some pediatric patients present special challenges when using technology in their treatment. Some techniques that work well in adult scenarios perform differently in these populations, such as oxygen delivery, aerosol delivery, mechanical ventilation, and airway management. Recently, certain practices have been exposed as ineffective or inefficient, including blow-by oxygen or aerosol delivery and the use of pneumatic (jet) nebulizers for the delivery of aerosolized medications.

Study Questions

REVIEW QUESTIONS

1. What are the three distinctions between the respiratory tract of neonatal/pediatric patients and that of adults?
2. What are the three sites of cardiac shunting during fetal circulatory pathways?
3. What special considerations should be taken when resuscitating a newborn with diaphragmatic hernia?
4. Describe several techniques to ensure minimal stimulation of premature infants.
5. Identify four signs of respiratory distress in infants.
6. Describe the role of nasopharyngeal suctioning in the treatment of bronchiolitis.

MULTIPLE-CHOICE QUESTIONS

1. The chief cause of ventilator-induced lung injury in pediatric ARDS is:
   a. excessive airway pressures.
   b. excessive lung volumes.
   c. malpositioned endotracheal tube.
   d. inappropriate modes of ventilation.
2. Which of the following statements is true about flow-inflating and self-inflating manual resuscitators?
   a. Clinicians cannot feel changes in compliance better with flow-inflating bag.
   b. Self-inflating resuscitators produce more consistent tidal volumes than flow-inflating resuscitators.
   c. Flow-inflating resuscitators produce more variable PEEP than self-inflating resuscitators.
   d. Self-inflating bags can be used for blow-by\ oxygen if configured properly.
   e. All of the above
3. What is a typical recommended range for maintaining S_pO_2 in neonates?
   a. 88–93%
   b. >95%
   c. 90–98%
   d. 92–98%

4. Which of the following is not a potential benefit of nasal continuous positive airway pressure for neonatal patients?
   a. increasing the functional residual capacity
   b. improving gas exchange
   c. reduced work of breathing
   d. improved cerebral blood flow
5. Which interventions have been proven to be efficacious in uncomplicated bronchiolitis in infants?
   a. aerosolized bronchodilators
   b. chest physical therapy
   c. inhaled corticosteroids
   d. antibiotics
6. Which of the following statements is true?
   a. Small-volume nebulizers are typically a better way to give bronchodilators to nonintubated infants and children.
   b. Metered dose inhalers should usually not be used in infants and children because of the patients' inability to coordinate actuation of the inhaler with inspiration.
   c. Metered dose inhalers with valved holding chambers are a more expensive way to give inhaled bronchodilators compared to small-volume nebulizers.
   d. Metered dose inhalers with spacers/holding chambers have been shown to be as effective or better than small-volume nebulizers at delivering inhaled medication to children.
7. What size endotracheal tube should an RT recommend for a 1500-g infant?
   a. 2.0 mm
   b. 2.5 mm
   c. 3.0 mm
   d. 3.5 mm
   e. 4.0 mm
8. Which of the following situations does *not* cause increased risk for intraventricular hemorrhage in low-birth-weight infants?
   a. physical stress
   b respiratory distress syndrome
   c. pneumothorax
   d. high inspired oxygen concentration
   e. high blood pressure.
9. Which of the following is a limitation of the pulse oximeters in children?
   a. inaccuracy in the presence of elevated levels of dyshemoglobins
   b. inaccuracy due to elevated body temperature
   c. motion artifact
   d. false alarms and data dropout
10. During mechanical ventilation of pediatric patients with acute respiratory distress syndrome, what level of positive end-expiratory pressure is recommended if the F_IO_2 is 0.50 using a high-PEEP strategy?
   a. 18–24 cm H_2O
   b. 16–18 cm H_2O
   c. 10–12 cm H_2O
   d. 8–10 cm H_2O

CRITICAL-THINKING QUESTIONS

1. How are the lungs and airways of adults different from infants and children?
2. Describe the important design and performance differences between child manual and infant resuscitators and how the differences might affect the ventilation of infants and children.
3. Describe the mechanisms of airway obstruction in asthma, including the role of inflammation, in this disease process.
4. What is minimal stimulation of neonates, and why is it important.
5. Discuss the role of tidal volume measurement and targeting in preventing ventilator-induced lung injury in neonates.

References

1. Phillips AGS. Evolution of Neonatology. *Pediatr Res.* 2005;58,4:799–815.
2. Neonatology on the Web. History of neonatology. http://www.neonatology.org/tour/history.html
3. Meadow W, Lee G, Lin K, Lantos J. Changes in mortality for extremely low birth weight infants in the 1990s: implications for treatment decisions and resource use. *Pediatrics.* 2004; 113,5:1223–9.
4. Birenbaum HJ, Dentry A, Cirelli J, et al. Reduction in the incidence of chronic lung disease in very low birth weight infants: results of a quality improvement process in a tertiary level neonatal intensive care unit. *Pediatr.* 2009;123,1:44–50.
5. Ochs M, Nyengaard JR, Jung A, Knudsen L, Voigt M, Wahlers T, et al. The number of alveoli in the human lung. *Am J Respir Crit Care Med.* 2004;169:120–124.
6. Balinotti JE, Tiller CJ, Llapur CJ, Jones MH, Kimmel RN, Coates CE, et al. Growth of the Lung Parenchyma Early in Life. *Am J Respir Crit Care Med.* 2009;179:134–137.
7. Wohl MEB. Developmental physiology of the respiratory system. In: Chernick VC, Boat TF,

Wilmott RW, Bush A, eds. *Kendig's Disorders of the Respiratory Tract in Children.* 7th ed. Philadelphia: Saunders Elsevier; 2006:23–28.

8. Centers for Disease Control and Prevention. Premature birth. http://www.cdc.gov/Features/PrematureBirth/
9. Howell EM, Richardson D, Ginsburg P, Foot B. MS de-regionalization of neonatal intensive care in urban areas. *Am J Public Health.* 2002;92:119–124.
10. Odetola FO, Clark SJ, Freed GL, Bratton SL, Davis MM. A National Survey of Pediatric Critical Care Resources in the United States. *Pediatr.* 2005;115:e382–e386. www.pediatrics.org/cgi/doi/10.1542/peds. 2004–1920.
11. McCaig LF, Burt CW. National Hospital Ambulatory Medical Care Survey: 2003 emergency department summary. Advance data from vital and health statistics; no 358. Hyattsville, MD: National Center for Health Statistics; 2005.
12. Stola A, Schulman J, Perlman J. Initiating delivery room stabilization/resuscitation in very low birth weight (VLBW) infants with an F_IO_2 less than 100% is feasible. *Journal of Perinatology.* 2009; 29:548–552.
13. Finer N, Leone T. Oxygen saturation monitoring for the preterm infant: the evidence basis for current practice. *Pediatr Res.* 2009:65:375–380.
14. Apgar V. A proposal for a new method of evaluation of the newborn infant. *Anesth Analg.* 1953;32:260.
15. Saigal S, Doyle LW. An overview of mortality and sequelae of preterm birth from infancy to adulthood. *Lancet.* 2008;371,9608:261–269.
16. Alexander GR, Kogan M, Bader D, Carlo W, Allen M, Mor J. US birthweight/gestational age-specific neonatal mortality: 1995–1997 rates for whites, Hispanics, and blacks. *Pediatr.* 2003; 111: e61–e66.
17. Als H, Lawhon G, Duffy FH, et al. Individualized developmental care for the very low-birth-weight preterm infant. Medical and neurofunctional effects. *JAMA.* 1994;272:853–858.
18. Fleischer BE, Vandenberg K, Constantinou J, et al. Individualized developmental care for very-low-birth-weight premature infants. *Clin Pediatr.* 1995;34:523–529.
19. Als H. Developmental care in the newborn intensive care unit. *Current Opinion Pediatr.* 1998;10:138–142.
20. National Eye Institute: National Institute of Health. Retinopathy of prematurity. http://www.nei.nih.gov/health/rop/
21. American Lung Association. Lung disease at a glance: respiratory distress syndrome. http://www.lungusa.org/site/c.dvLUK9O0E/b.327819/k.D93E/Lung_Disease_Data at_a_Glance_Respiratory_Distress_Syndrome_RDS.htm
22. Engle W. The Committee on Fetus and Newborn. Surfactant-replacement therapy for respiratory distress in the preterm and term neonate. *Pediatr.* 2008;121,2:419–432.
23. Philip N, Gambarelli D, Guys JM, Camboulives J, Ayme S. Epidemiological study of congenital diaphragmatic defects with special reference to aetiology. *Eur J Pediatr.* 1991;150:726–9.
24. Langham Jr MR, Kays DW, Ledbetter DJ, Frentzen B, Sanford LL, Richards DS. Congenital diaphragmatic hernia. Epidemiology and outcome. *Clin Perinatol.* 1996; 23: 671–688.
25. Gallot D, Boda C, Ughetto S, Perthus I, Robert-Gnansia E, Francannet C, et al. Prenatal detection and outcome of congenital diaphragmatic hernia: a French registry-based study. *Ultrasound Obstet Gynecol.* 2007;29,3:276–283.
26. Colvin J, Bower C, Dickinson JE, Sokol J. Outcomes of congenital diaphragmatic hernia: a population-based study in Western Australia. *Pediatr.* 2005;116,3:e356–e363.
27. Centers for Disease Control and Prevention. FastStats; Asthma. http://www.cdc.gov/nchs/fastats/asthma.htm
28. National Center for Health Statistics Summary Health Statistics. Centers for Disease Control and Prevention. Summary health statistics for U.S. children, provisional report: National Health Interview Survey, 2008. Vital and Health Statistics Series 10, Number 244.
29. Stranges E, Merrill CT, Steiner CA. Hospital stays related to asthma for children, 2006. Health Care Cost and Utilization Project Statistical Brief #58. August 2008. Agency for Health Care Quality Research. http://www.hcup-us.ahrq.gov/reports/statbriefs/sb58.pdf
30. National Heart, Lung, and Blood Institute National Asthma Education and Prevention Program Expert Panel report 3: guidelines for the diagnosis and management of asthma. Full Report 2007. NIH Publication Number 08-5846. October 2007. http://www.nhlbi.nih.gov/guidelines/asthma/asthsumm.pdf
31. Akingbola OA, Simakajornboon N, Hadley Jr EF, Hopkins RL. Noninvasive positive-pressure ventilation in pediatric status asthmaticus. *Pediatr Crit Care Med.* 2002;3:181–184.
32. Ram FS, Wellington S, Rowe B, Wedzicha JA. Noninvasive positive pressure ventilation for treatment of respiratory failure due to severe acute exacerbations of asthma. *Cochrane Database Syst Rev.* 2005;3:CD004360.
33. Levine DA. Novel therapies for children with severe asthma. *Curr Opin Pediatr.* 2008;20:261–265.
34. Kim IK, Phrampus E, Venkataraman S, Pitetti R, Saville A, Corcoran T, et al. Helium/oxygen-driven

albuterol nebulization in the treatment of children with moderate to severe asthma exacerbations: a randomized, controlled trial. *Pediatr.* 2005; 116:1127–1133.

35. Piva JP, Menna Barreto SS, Zelmanovitz F, et al. Heliox versus oxygen for nebulized aerosol therapy in children with lower airway obstruction. *Pediatr Crit Care Med.* 2002;3:6–10.
36. Joshi G, Tobias JD. A five-year experience with the use of BiPAP in a pediatric intensive care unit population. *J Intensive Care Med.* 2007;22:38–43.
37. Liu LL, Gallaher MM, Davis RL, et al. Use of a respiratory clinical score among different providers. *Pediatr Pulmonology.* 2004;37:243–248.
38. Leader S, Kohlhase K. Recent trends in severe respiratory syncytial virus (rsv) among US infants, 1997 to 2000. *J Pediatr.* 2003;143:S127–S132.
39. Turner TWS, Evered LM. Are bronchodilators effective in bronchiolitis? *Ann Emerg Med.* 2003;42:709–711.
40. Subcommittee on Diagnosis and Management of Bronchiolitis. Diagnosis and management of bronchiolitis. *Pediatr.* 2006;118,4:1174–1793.
41. Ralston S, Hartenberger C, Anaya T, Qualls C, Kelly HW. PharmD randomized, placebo-controlled trial of albuterol and epinephrine at equipotent beta-2 agonist doses in acute bronchiolitis *Pediatr Pulmonol.* 2005;40: 292–299.
42. King VJ, Viswanathan M, Bordley WC, Jackman AM, Sutton SF, Lohr KN, Carey TS. Pharmacologic treatment of bronchiolitis in infants and children: a systematic review. *Arch Pediatr Adolesc Med.* 2004;158:127–137.
43. Adcock PM, Sanders CL, Marshall GS. Standardizing the care of bronchiolitis. *Arch Pediatr Adolesc Med.* 1998;152,8:739–744.
44. Conway E, Schoettker PJ, Moore A, Britto MT, Kotagal UR, Rich K. Empowering respiratory therapists to take a more active role in delivering quality care for infants with bronchiolitis. *Respir Care.* 2004;49,6:589–599.
45. McKinley G, Ballard J, Salyer J. The effect of NP suctioning on symptom scores in bronchiolitis patients. *Respir Care.* 2001;46:1071.
46. Ballard J, Salyer J. The use of a bronchiolitis symptom scoring system in infants. *Respir Care.* 2001;47:1118.
47. Bennion K, Ballard J, Salyer J. The interaction of nasopharyngeal suction and albuterol in the treatment of bronchiolitis: a two year comparison. *Respir Care.* 2001;46:1072.
48. Bennion K, Ballard J, Salyer J. The use of chest x-ray in the treatment of bronchiolitis patients. *Respir Care.* 2001;46:1108.
49. Lyrene RK, Truog WE. Adult respiratory distress syndrome in a pediatric intensive care unit: predisposing conditions, clinical course, and outcome. *Pediatr.* 1981;67,6:790–795.
50. Randolph AG. Management of acute lung injury and acute respiratory distress syndrome in children. *Crit Care Med.* 2009;37,8: 2448–2454.
51. Rubenfeld GD, Caldwell E, Peabody E, Weaver J, Martin DP, Neff M, Stern EJ, Hudson LD. Incidence and outcomes of acute lung injury. *N Engl J Med.* 2005;353:1685–1693.
52. Zimmerman JJ, Akhtar SR, Caldwell E, Rubenfeld GD. Incidence and outcomes of pediatric acute lung injury. *Pediatr.* 2009;124,1:87–95.
53. Bernard GR, Artigas A, Brigham KL, Carlet J, Falke K, Hudson L, Lamy M, Legall JR, Morris A, Spragg R. The American-European consensus conference on ARDS. Definitions, mechanisms, relevant outcomes, and clinical trial coordination. *Am J Respir Crit Care Med.* 1994;149,3,Pt 1: 818–824.
54. Khemani RG, Patel NR, Bart 3rd RD, Newth CJ. Comparison of the pulse oximetric saturation/ fraction of inspired oxygen ratio and the PaO_2/ fraction of inspired oxygen ratio in children. *Chest.* 2009;135,3:662–668.
55. Dreyfuss D, Soler P, Basset G, Saumon G. High inflation pressure pulmonary edema. Respective effects of high airway pressure, high tidal volume, and positive end-expiratory pressure. *Am Rev Respir Dis.* 1988;137,5:1159–1164.
56. Acute Respiratory Distress Syndrome Network. Ventilation with lower tidal volumes as compared with traditional tidal volumes for acute lung injury and the acute respiratory distress syndrome. *N Engl J Med.* 2000;342,18:1301–1308.
57. Goldsmith JP, Karotkin EH. Introduction to assisted ventilation. In: Goldsmith JP, Karotkin EH, eds. *Assisted Ventilation of the Neonate.* 4th ed. Philadelphia, PA: Saunders; 2003:1–14.
58. Wistwell TE. Neonatal resuscitation. *Respir Care.* 2003;48:288–294.
59. Hussey SG, Ryan CA, Murphy BP. Comparison of three manual ventilation devices using an intubated mannequin. Archives of disease in childhood: *Fetal and Neonatal Edition.* 2004;89: 490–493.
60. Spears RS, Yeh A, Fisher DM, Zwass MS. The educated hand: can anesthesiologists assess changes in neonatal pulmonary compliance manually? *Anesthesiology.* 1991;75:693–696.
61. Egbert LD, Bisno D. The educated hand of the anesthesiologist: A study of professional skill. *Anesth Analg.* 1967;46:195–200.

62. Keenan J, Salyer JW, Ashby T, Withers J, Bee N. Manual ventilation technique variability in a pediatric lung model. *Respir Care.* 1999;44: 1252.
63. Salyer JW. Manual resuscitators: some inconvenient truths. *Respir Care.* 2009;54,12:1638-1643.
64. The Acute Respiratory Distress Syndrome Network. Ventilation with lower tidal volumes as compared with traditional tidal volumes for acute lung injury and the acute respiratory distress syndrome. *N Eng J Med.* 2000;342,18:1301–1308.
65. Nilson C, Grossman G, Robertson B. Lung surfactant and the pathogenesis of neonatal bronchiolar lesions induced by artificial ventilation. *Pediatr Res.*1978;12:249–255.
66. Finer NN, Rich W Craft A, Henderson C. Comparison of methods of bag and mask ventilation for neonatal resuscitation. *Resuscitation.* 2001;49: 299–305.
67. O'Donnell CPF, Davis PG, Lau R, Dargaville PA, Doyle LW, Morley CJ. Neonatal resuscitation 2: an evaluation of manual ventilation devices and face masks. *Arch Dis Child Fetal Neonatal Ed.* 2005;90:F392–F396.
68. Hawkes CP, Oni OA, Dempsey EM, Ryan CA. Potential hazard of the Neopuff T-piece resuscitator in the absence of flow limitation *Arch Dis Child Fetal Neonatal Ed.* 2009 Apr 8. [Epub ahead of print] http://fn.bmj.com/cgi/rapidpdf/adc .2008.155945v1
69. Masimo receives FDA clearance for Masimo Rainbow SET[R] acoustic respiration rate monitoring. *Biotech Week.* Farmington Hills, MI: Gale Group, 2009.
70. Salyer JW. Neonatal and pediatric pulse oximetry. *Respir Care.* 2003;48,4:386–396.
71. Poets CF, Urschitz MS, Bohnhorst B. Pulse oximetry in the neonatal intensive care unit (NICU): detection of hyperoxemia and false alarm rates. *Anesth Analg.* Supp, 2002;94,1:S41–S43.
72. Goldman JM, Petterson MT, Kopotic RJ, Barker SJ. Masimo signal extraction pulse oximetry. *J Clin Monit Comput* .2000;16,7:475–483.
73. Lawless ST. Crying wolf: false alarms in a pediatric intensive care unit. *Crit Care Med.* 1994;22,6: 981–985.
74. Sabar R, Zmora E. Nurse's response to alarms from monitoring systems in NICU (abstract). *Pediatr. Res.* 1997;41:174A.
75. Finer NN, Mannino FL High-flow nasal cannula: a kinder, gentler CPAP? *J Pediatr.* 2009;154,2: 160–162.
76. Branson RD, Johannigman JA. What is the evidence base for the newer ventilation modes? *Respir Care.* 2004;49,7:742–760.
77. Donn SM, Sinhab SK. Can mechanical ventilation strategies reduce chronic lung disease? *Seminars in Neonatology.* 2003;8:441–448.
78. Donn SM, Boon W. Mechanical ventilation of the neonate: should we target volume or pressure? *Respir Care.* 2009;54,9:1236–1243.
79. Branson RD, Johannigman JA. What is the evidence base for the newer ventilation modes? *Respir Care.* 2004;49,7:742–760.
80. Singh GK, Yu SM. Infant mortality in the United States: trends, differentials, and projections, 1950 through 2010. *Am J Public Health.* 1995;85,7: 957–964.
81. Cannon ML, et al. Tidal volumes for ventilated infants should be determined with a pneumotachometer placed at the endotracheal tube. *Am J Respir Crit Care Med.* 2000;162:2109–2112.
82. Salyer JW, Jackson C. Accuracy of tidal volume (VT) displayed during volume targeted ventilation in neonatal ventilators. *Respir Care.* 2005; 50:149.
83. Loughead JL, Brennan RA, DeJuilio P, Camposeo V, Wengert J, Cooke D. Reducing accidental extubation in neonates. The Joint Comm Jl Qual Pat Safety. 2008;34,3:164–170.
84. Mildner R, Cox P, The pre-clinical history of high-frequency ventilation. *Respir Care Clin North America.* 2001;7:523–534.
85. Chang HK. Mechanisms of gas transport during ventilation by high-frequency oscillation. *J Appl Physiol.* 1984;56:553–563.
86. Ben Jaballah N, Mnif K, Khaldi A, Bouziri A, Belhadj S, Hamdi A. High-frequency oscillatory ventilation in term and near-term infants with acute respiratory failure: early rescue use. *Am J Perinatol.* 2006;23,7:403–411.
87. Courtney SE, Durand DJ, Asselin JM, et al. High-frequency oscillatory ventilation versus conventional mechanical ventilation for very-low-birth-weight infants. *N Engl J Med.* 2002;347:643–652.
88. Bollen CW, Uiterwaal CSPM, Vught AJV. Cumulative meta-analysis of high-frequency versus conventional ventilation in premature neonates. *Am J Respir Crit Care Med.* 2003;168:1150–1155.
89. Johnson AH, Peacock JL, Greenough A: United Kingdom Oscillation Study Group. High-frequency oscillatory ventilation for the prevention of chronic lung disease of prematurity. *N Engl J Med.* 2002;347:633–642.
90. Gregory GA, Kitterman JA, Phibbs RH, Tooley WH, Hamilton WK, Treatment of the idiopathic respiratory-distress syndrome with continuous positive airway pressure. *N Engl. J Med.* 1971;284,24:1333–1340.

91. Bergeson PS, Shaw JC. Are infants really obligatory nasal breathers? *Clin Pediatr.* 2001;40,10:567–569.
92. Diblasi RM. Nasal continuous positive airway pressure (CPAP) for the respiratory care of the newborn infant. *Respir Care.* 2009 Sep;54,9:1209–1235.
93. Salyer JW, DiBlasi RM, Crotwell DN, Cowan CA, Carter ER. The conversion to metered-dose inhaler with valved holding chamber to administer inhaled albuterol: a pediatric hospital experience. *Respir Care.* 2008;53,3:338–345.
94. Delgado A, Chou KJ, Silver EJ, Crain EF. Nebulizers vs. metered dose inhalers with spacers for bronchodilator therapy to treat wheezing in children aged 2 to 24 months in a pediatric emergency department. *Arch Pediatr Adolesc Med.* 2003;157,1:76–80.
95. Castro-Rodriguez JA, Rodrigo GJ. Beta-agonists through metered dose inhaler with valved holding chamber versus nebulizer for acute exacerbation of wheezing or asthma in children under 5 years of age: a systematic review with meta-analysis. *J Pediatr.* 2004;145,2:172–177.
96. Rubin BK. Bye-bye blow-by. *Respir Care.* 2007; 52 ,8:981.
97. Everard ML, Clark AR, Milner AD. Drug delivery from jet nebulisers. Arch Dis Child. 1992;67,5: 586–591.

CHAPTER 30

Geriatric Applications

Melaine Head Giordano and Helen M. Sorenson

OBJECTIVES

Upon completion of this chapter, the reader should be able to:

- Describe the changing demographics of the U.S. population.
- Address issues related to the current cost of health care for elders.
- Identify and explain the major components of a comprehensive geriatric assessment.
- Discuss the fundamental elements involved in the functional assessment of older adults.
- Discuss pharmacodynamics and pharmacokinetics in the older adult.
- Identify clinical interventions to promote medication compliance.
- Explain ways to improve communication with older adult patients.

CHAPTER OUTLINE

Demographic Changes in the United States
Health Care Venues
The Cost of Health Care
Assessment of the Older Patient
- Physical Assessment
- Functional Assessment
- Environmental Assessment
- Socioeconomic Assessment
- Cognitive Assessment
- Assessment of Medication Use

Communicating with Older Patients

KEY TERMS

activities of daily living (ADLs)
adherence
aphasia
centenarian
chronic
cohort
comorbid
geriatrics
iatrogenic
instrumental activities of daily living (IADLs)
life expectancy
life span
Medicaid
Medicare
ototoxicity
pharmacodynamics
pharmacokinetics
polypharmacy

At the beginning of the twenty-first century, the United States faces many complex challenges associated with the unprecedented increase in the growth of the older population (defined as age 65 and older). Among those challenges is the provision of social services, adequate housing, and financial assistance. Because of the increased incidence of health problems, however, one of the most crucial areas in preparing for the growth of this **cohort** (a group of individuals having a statistical factor in common in a demographic study) is the challenge of providing for their health care needs.

The dramatic increase in life expectancy, coupled with technological advances in medicine, will increase the need for long-term care. The appropriate delivery of care for older adults with chronic disease will be the greatest challenge. (**Chronic** refers to an illness that lasts for more than 3 months.) This will require an enormous amount of health care, social, financial, familial, and community support. Historically, U.S. health care systems were designed around acute care models. As the population ages, this system will soon be outdated due to the increased numbers of chronically ill. Health care will increasingly need to be provided in alternative care sites such as the home, assisted-living facilities, nursing homes, congregate housing, outpatient settings, and rehabilitation hospitals.

One other challenge presented by the so-called gray explosion is the provision of health care professionals who are educated in **geriatrics** (a specialized branch of medicine that deals with the diseases of later life and the provision of health care for older people). Unfortunately, the aging citizens in the United States, according to a new report from the Institute of Medicine (IOM) are relying on a health care workforce that is too small and unprepared to meet their needs.[1]

Demographic Changes in the United States

Demographic changes, owing to the lowered birth rates during the Great Depression (1929–1939), have been gradual. As the baby boomers (individuals born between 1946 and 1964) reach 65, between 2010 and 2030 (Figure 30-1), there will be a dramatic increase (10,000 individuals per day) in the older adult population.

One of the fastest growing segments of the older population are minorities. Identified as members of the non-European population: Native Americans, African Americans, Asian Americans, Pacific Islanders, and Latinos. Minorities represent about 10% of the older population; by 2020, they will account for more than 15%. By 2050, it is estimated that more than 38% of the older population will be minorities.[2] The health care implications of the growing number of older minorities are immense because these groups experience a significantly higher incidence of morbidity and mortality than older whites.[3] The higher incidence of health problems among minority populations is attributed to risk factors such as smoking, poor nutrition, limited access to health care services, and inadequate housing.

Not only is the older population growing in size, but they are also living longer. In addition to the minorities, another rapidly growing segment of the older population in the United States are people over 85. According to the Census 2000 Summary File, in 2000 over 4.2 million adults were 85 and older, and an astonishing 337,000 were 95 and older.[4] Unfortunately, many of the oldest-old (persons over 85) do not enjoy good health and may require assistance with basic self-care activities.

Life expectancy (the number of years that an individual is expected to live, determined by statistics) in the United States increased from 49 years in 1900 to over 78 years in 2005.[5] The increase in life expectancy can probably be attributed to advances in the prevention and treatment of infectious diseases, as well as to improvements in nutrition, basic health care, education, and technology. Women have a longer life expectancy than men (Table 30-1). The gender disparity is attributed to differences in lifestyle and health behaviors of the two sexes. It probably will diminish in the future, as women increasingly adopt lifestyle and health behaviors that have traditionally been associated with men.

Despite the statistics indicating that health declines with age, individuals enjoy healthy, productive lives well into their eighties and nineties, and a few are still active and healthy beyond their 100th birthday. In 2006, there were 67,000 **centenarians** (adults 100 years and older) in the United States, and this number has been projected to be 580,000 by 2040.[6]

There is a limit, however, to just how old a person can get. The human **life span** (the length of time an organism or species can be expected to survive) is approximately 120 years old. One thing is certain; the aging process is very individual. It is not uncommon to observe a 75-year-old who appears to be in her early sixties or a fifty-year-old who appears to be in his sixties.

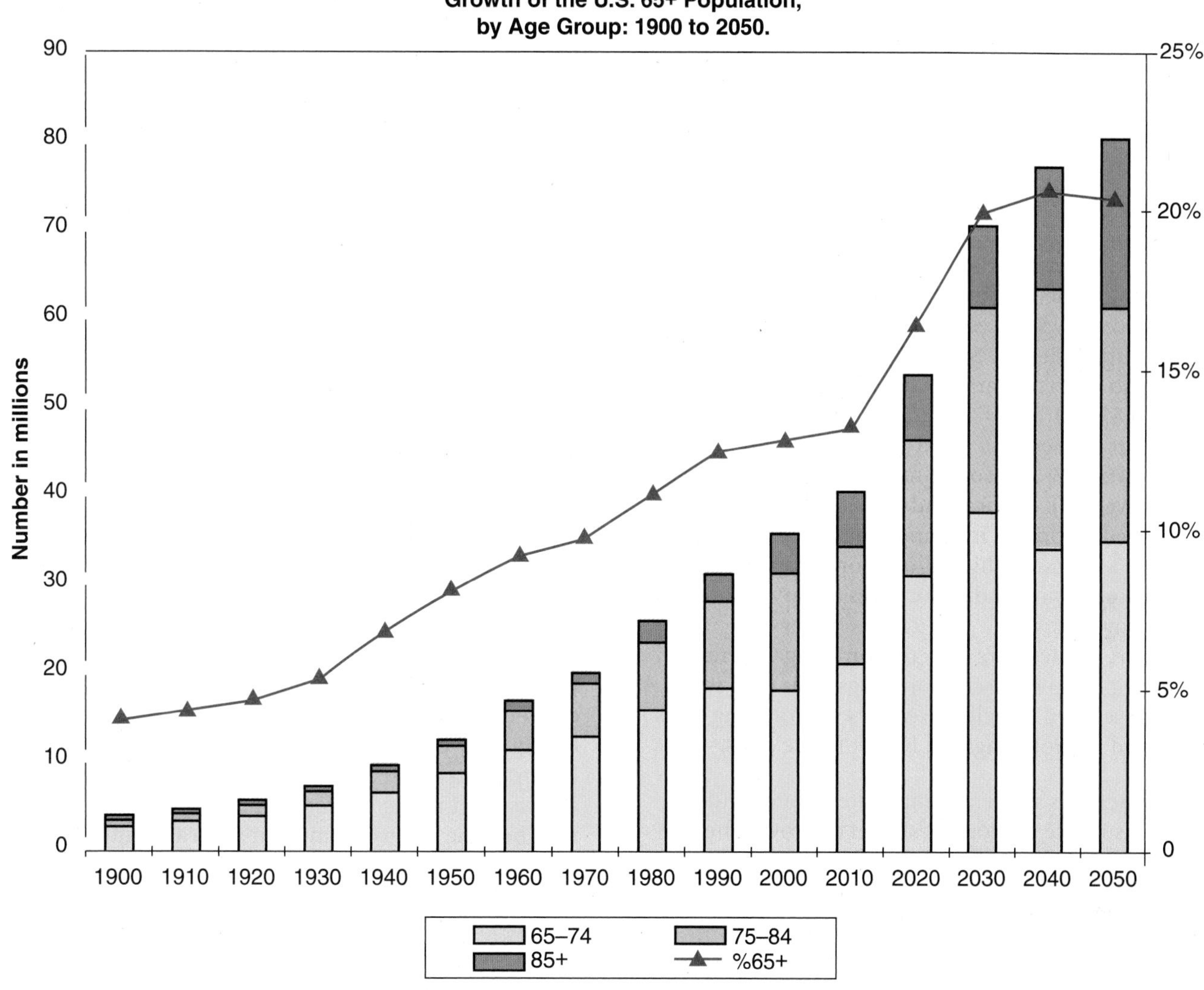

FIGURE 30-1 Growth of the U.S. 65+ population by age group: 1900–2050.

Courtesy of National Center for Health Statistics, Hyattsville, Maryland

TABLE 30-1 **Life expectancy in selected regions, by gender, 2006**

Countries	Male	Female
Australia	79.2	83.9
Belize	65.3	73.6
Brazil	68.4	75.1
Canada	78.3	82.9
Central African Republic	48.3	47.8
Denmark	76.2	81.3
Haiti	59	63.4
Japan	79.2	85.9
United Kingdom	77	81.3
United States	75.5	80.4

Source: World Health Organization Life Tables for WHO Member States, 2006. WHO Statistical Information System. www.who.int/reseach/en/-cached

Health Care Venues

Because of the chronic nature of respiratory disease, the respiratory therapist encounters older patients in all health care venues. Today, 60% of acute care patients, 80% of home care patients, and 90% of nursing home patients are 65 years or older. Advances in medical technology, expedient hospital discharges, a demand for cost-efficient health care services, and the growing number of older adults have contributed to a phenomenal growth in the home health care industry (see Chapter 35), along with the utilization of subacute and long-term care facilities (Chapter 34) and rehabilitation facilities (Chapters 34 and 36).

The Cost of Health Care

Reimbursement for health care services for the aging population comes from three sources: Medicare, Medicaid (see Chapter 1), and private out-of-pocket payments.

Medicare provides health insurance for people age 65 or older, adults under 65 with certain disabilities, and individuals of any age with end-stage-renal disease (permanent kidney failure requiring dialysis or a kidney transplant). Medicare has four different parts:

- *Part A.* Hospital insurance, also covers skilled nursing facilities, hospice, and home health care under certain conditions.
- *Part B.* Medical insurance, helps cover medically necessary services like physician's services and outpatient care. Some preventative services are also covered. Part B requires a monthly premium of $115.40 as of 2011.
- *Part C.* Medicare Advantage Plus, combines Parts A, B, and sometimes D (prescription drug coverage). Medicare Advantage Plans are managed by private insurance companies approved by Medicare, which allows for copayments, coinsurance, and deductibles to vary among providers.
- *Part D.* Medicare Prescription Drug Coverage, helps cover prescription drugs. This plan was developed to help lower prescription drug costs and to protect against higher future costs.[7]

Medicaid is a federally mandated, state-funded health insurance program designed to provide health care services to the poor and disabled. As of 2002, about 41 million people in the United States were on Medicaid. Low-income parents and children make up 73% of all Medicare recipients, but they account for only 27.5% of all Medicaid expenses. The elderly, disabled, and mentally challenged collectively comprise only 27% of Medicaid recipients, but account for 72.5% of all expenditures.[8]

Medicaid is the single largest payer of nursing home charges in the United States and for many, is the last resort when there are no other means of paying for long-term care. Medicaid, however, will pay for nursing home care only if provided in a facility certified by the government to provide services to Medicaid recipients.[9]

Older adults may qualify for both the Medicare and Medicaid programs. Dual-eligible beneficiaries are determined on the basis of financial need. Those who typically qualify for dual eligibility are the older-old (85 or older), ethnic minorities, females, and persons living in rural areas.

The health care financing system is complex and confusing for people of any age. For an older person with physical and financial limitations, it can be impenetrable. Many organizations and agencies can help. For a list of some resources for patients and professionals, see Resources at the end of this chapter.

Assessment of the Older Patient

One of the most daunting aspects of caring for older individuals is addressing the multitude of age-related issues they face. These may include Alzheimer's disease or other memory disorders, chronic illnesses, mobility difficulties, caregiver dilemmas, complex medication issues, sensory deficits, and nutritional inadequacies.

To provide efficient and effective geriatric care, the clinician must assess the older person in a systematic manner. A *comprehensive geriatric assessment* (CGA), while time-consuming, offers the clinician the best tool to systematically evaluate the overall health status of an older adult. As caregivers for so many elderly patients, respiratory therapists (RTs) must think outside of the pulmonary system and assess older patients in a more holistic manner. Because CGAs are multidisciplinary evaluations in which the multiple health issues of the older adult are uncovered, described, and explained, RTs may reasonably take their place at the table.

The American Geriatrics Society, in its Comprehensive Geriatric Assessment Position Statement (updated in August 2005), promulgated the CGA as a cost-effective intervention that improves quality of life, quality of health, and quality of social care.[10] Unfortunately, the application of the CGA is not always used in the United States. The assessment itself may be time intensive and impractical in most primary care settings. Adding to the problem is that, of the 650,000 licensed physicians practicing in this country, fewer than 9,000 of them are geriatricians.[11] When viewed as a multidisciplinary task, however, and approached as a comprehensive health screening, coordinated care plans can be developed that address individual patient needs.

A comprehensive assessment does not have to conform to a single format. CGAs have been effective in a number of settings: inpatient geriatric evaluation units, inpatient geriatric consultation, ambulatory geriatric assessment clinics, and in-home geriatric assessment programs.[12] One series of interventions that has shown great promise is a combination of:

- An initial CGA.
- Followed by providing recommendations to the older patient/family members.
- And a follow-up home visit to see if the recommendations are being implemented.

The ultimate goal is to identify older adults at high risk for functional decline and follow-up with programs combining rehabilitation and coordinated care. When decline is inevitable, the CGA can result in an improved quality of life by mobilizing available medical, psychological, and social resources. Although this may sound simplistic, there is enough interest in healthy aging, as well as an adequate supply of very old adults, to make some iteration of the CGA possible in every community.

How does this relate to respiratory therapists? RTs make up one of the multidisciplinary components of coordinated care planning for older adults. We care for older patients with cardiopulmonary disease, both in the hospital and after discharge; so we need to be educated about our role in the CGA.

The following are core elements of a multidisciplinary comprehensive geriatric assessment:

- Physical assessment
- Functional assessment
- Environmental assessment
- Socioeconomic assessment
- Cognitive (mental) assessment
- Medication assessment (Meducation)

CASE STUDY 30-1

Mrs A. is an 86-year-old Latino woman who has been a widow for 20 years. She lives alone (in publicly funded housing), and her sources of income are a small pension and a monthly Social Security check for a total of $540 a month. Her rent, utilities, and Medicare premiums average $425 a month. She finances her medical expenditures through Medicare Parts A and B and has obtained nutritional assistance by means of food stamps and Meals on Wheels. Six months ago, Mrs. A. rated her health as good, and if it were not for arthritis and diminished vision, she would have rated her health as excellent.

Last week, Mrs. A. was diagnosed with congestive heart failure (CHF) and asthma, and she was prescribed three new medications at a monthly cost of $80. This new expense is a challenge for Mrs. A.; the cost of the additional medications is more than half of her disposable income.

Questions

1. Would a Managed Medicare program help Mrs. A.?
2. How could Mrs. A. get help with the expense of her medication?
3. Identify professionals who could assist Mrs. A. in meeting her financial and health care needs.

PHYSICAL ASSESSMENT

Physical well-being, or the lack of it (frailty), is a major issue. Unfortunately, many health care professionals assume that aging is parallel to a disease process and that signs and symptoms of disease are simply a part of getting old.

Any clinician assessing an older person's physical health must be familiar with normal age-related physiological changes in order to distinguish them from signs and symptoms of disease processes (Table 30-2).

The physical evaluation of an older person takes more time. Standard procedures may have to be modified to accommodate the special circumstances of the older adult. Breath sounds are softer, pulses and respiration more irregular, body temperature may be lower, and the cough reflex may be weaker. Older patients may find it more difficult to move around in bed, and getting them in an optimal position for patient assessment is often time-consuming.

Review the patient's past medical records before performing the physical assessment. This reduces the time

Best Practice

Health Care Characteristics of Older Patients

Chronological age is not a good indicator of physiological age or organ system functioning. The rate of age changes is distinctively individualized, and the assessment must reflect the uniqueness of each person. However, when assessing older persons (especially those over 75) the practitioner should keep in mind their health care characteristics and vulnerability. Older patients tend to:

- Exhibit greater medical complexity and vulnerability than younger patients.
- Have illnesses with atypical or obscure presentations.
- Suffer major cognitive, affective, and functional problems.
- Be especially vulnerable to **iatrogenic** diseases or symptoms (induced by examinations or treatments).
- Be socially isolated and economically deprived.
- Be at high risk for premature or inappropriate institutionalization.

TABLE 30-2 **Normal age-related physiological changes**

System	Increase	Decrease
Pulmonary	Residual volume increases almost 50% by age 70	Vital capacity, both slow and forced (32 mm/yr for men; 25 mm/yr for women)
	Functional residual capacity	Peak expiratory flow rate
		Inspiratory capacity
		Forced expiratory flow rate (25–75%)
		Forced expiratory volume (32 mm/yr for men; 25 mm/yr for women)
		Diffusing capacity (20% over the course of adult life)
		Arterial partial pressure of oxygen, although not as much as previously thought (Resting P_aO_2 can be estimated: $P_aO_2 = 104 - [\text{age} \times 0.42]$ supine position and $P_aO_2 = 104 - [\text{age} \times 0.27]$ sitting position.)
		Mucocilliary clearance
		Elasticity
Cardiovascular	Left ventricular wall size	Elasticity in the large arteries and aorta
	Peripheral vascular resistance	Serum albumin
		Maximal O_2 consumption during exercise (men about 10% and women about 7.5% with each decade of life)
Renal		Renal blood flow (10% with each decade)
		Renal mass
		Glomerular filtration rate (50% from age 30 to 90)
		Total number of glomeruli (30–40% by age 80)
		Tubular secretion
Hepatic		Liver mass
		Blood flow (40–50%)
		Enzyme activity
Gastrointestinal	pH	Acid
		Blood flow to stomach (30–40%)
		Motility
		Absorption
Body	Fatty tissue (15–18%)	Muscle mass
	Skin dryness	Body water
		Height (2–3 in.)
		Elasticity of skin
Vital signs		Core temperature (96°–98.6°F; 35.6°–37°C)

spent in asking questions and allows the therapist to focus on key events in the history that need clarification. The medical record is a useful tool for identifying high-risk health care patterns such as repeated hospitalizations or emergency room visits, noncompliance with prescribed medication regimes, and inadequate support systems.

Having a family member present (if the patient agrees) during the history portion of the physical examination may be helpful because family members can supply supplemental information. However, ask assistance of the family member only after giving the patient sufficient time to respond.

TABLE 30-3 **Chronic conditions most frequently reported by older adults**

Condition	Percentage (%) of Elderly (>65 years old)
1. Arthritis	50
2. Hypertension	36
3. Heart disease	32
4. Cataracts	17
5. Hearing impairment	16
6. Orthopedic impairments	16
7. Sinusitis	15
8. Diabetes	10

Illness in older people is generally characterized as being chronic. On average, most older adults report having one to three chronic diseases (Table 30-3). Arthritis, reported by 50% of older adults, is very common. The multiplicity of complaints, related to **comorbid** (coexisting) disease processes, make it difficult to discern the true nature of the current complaint. It is extremely important for therapists, to assess each patient individually without any preconceived expectations based solely upon the age of the patient.

Another complication of geriatric care is that diseases in older adults may have atypical presentations. For example, the classic signs of pneumonia (fever, chills, cough, dyspnea, and sputum production) are commonly absent in the older person. Older patients with pneumonia may present with vague and atypical symptoms such as abdominal pain and confusion. They are often afebrile, have no elevation of white blood cells, and do not have a cough; their chest X-rays are inconclusive. Unfortunately, other disease processes such as myocardial infarction, pulmonary embolism, and atelectasis can also present in the same atypical manner.[3]

CASE STUDY 30-2

G. A., a 76-year-old male, was admitted to the local community hospital emergency room on December 16. He was complaining of loss of appetite and malaise. He was extremely confused, and he had fallen twice in the last 2 days. Mr. A. was accompanied by his wife. Because of his altered mental state, it was difficult to obtain the necessary medical information from Mr. A. Mrs. A. reported that he had been in relatively good health until this current episode. She stated that Mr. A.'s symptoms had come on gradually over the past 3 or 4 days. She stated further that her growing concern over her husband's increasing confusion had caused her to seek hospital assistance.

Vital signs for Mr. A. are heart rate 110, respiratory rate 30, temperature 98°F, and blood pressure 130/92. His laboratory results and chest X-ray were unremarkable.

Questions

1. On the basis of his confusion, vital signs, laboratory results, and chest X-ray, what might the RT assume is Mr. A.'s problem?
2. What is another possible diagnosis, and which of Mr. A.'s presentations indicate which of the possible diagnoses is correct?

Best Practice

Pneumococcal Immunization

Respiratory therapists should educate older patients concerning the importance of pneumococcal immunization. Each year, pneumococcal disease accounts for an estimated 500,000 cases of pneumonia and approximately 40,000 deaths in adults aged 65 and older. Healthy People 2010 had a goal of vaccinating 90% of adults over the age of 65 with Pneumovax. In 2002, 54% were vaccinated. Current recommendations are that every adult over age 65 should receive a pneumococcal vaccine. Revaccination is indicated if the first vaccination was before the age of 65 and more than 5 years has elapsed since the initial immunization.

Source: From MMWR (Morbidity Mortality Weekly Report) April 1, 2005;54,RR05: 1–11.

FUNCTIONAL ASSESSMENT

Chronic diseases, are not always curable; so the focus of care is to restore or maintain the functional status of the older patient. The loss of physical, mental, and social function can result in the inability to perform self-care and seriously impair an older adults' ability to live independently. The *functional assessment* is a methodical evaluation of an individual's ability to perform tasks that are necessary for independent living, and it serves as a benchmark to monitor the patient's functioning over time. A functional assessment should routinely be performed in all health care environments and should be well documented in the patient's records.

Some functional decline may not be reversible; progressive functional loss often accompanies patients with degenerative joint disease, Parkinson's disease, dementia, heart failure, and cancer. Other chronic illnesses including exacerbation of COPD or cardiovascular disease, although acute infections and joint replacements may respond well to rehabilitation and a recovery of function.

Many instruments and methods are available for conducting a functional assessment. Commonly used instruments evaluate **activities of daily living (ADLs)** and **instrumental activities of daily living (IADLs)**. ADLs are basic self-care activities and can be evaluated following the guidelines described in Table 30-4. The likelihood of institutionalization is extremely high for persons who have difficulty performing ADLs. According to a recent meta-analysis predicting nursing home admission, a person with three or more ADL dependencies, cognitive impairment, and prior nursing home use are the strongest predictors of nursing home admission.[13]

IADLs are activities that require both physical and cognitive functioning. To evaluate a person's IADLs, follow the guidelines presented in Table 30-5. If individuals lose the ability to perform IADLs, they should be assessed to determine the cause. A recent loss of functional ability (both ADLs and IADLs) should alert the therapist to an underlying disease process, an exacerbation of a chronic condition, alterations in cognitive function, or some combination of those. When identified early, loss of the ability to perform IADLs should trigger the implementation of appropriate clinical or community interventions that put off or prevent the onset of deficits and premature institutionalization.

The level of function in older adults depends on their sensory perception (auditory, visual, olfactory, and tactile) and dexterity. Any impairment in sensory perception can be disabling and can affect the older person's health status.

TABLE 30-4 Activities of daily living

Dressing. Inquire if any assistance is needed in dressing, including fastening buttons or zippers and tying shoes.
Grooming. Determine ability to trim nails (feet and hands), shave, brush teeth, and brush hair.
Bathing. Inquire if any assistance is needed in bathing in tub or shower, such as preparing bathwater, getting into or out of tub or shower, and washing all body parts.
Toileting. Determine if help is needed in using the toilet.
Mobility. Inquire if the client has difficulty ambulating in the home, such as getting into and out of bed, lowering to or rising from a chair, walking, climbing stairs, reaching for items in cupboards, and opening doors.
Eating. Ask if any help is needed in eating, such as using the utensils, cutting food, and putting food in mouth.

TABLE 30-5 Instrumental activities of daily living

Laundry. Inquire as to the ability to do one's own laundry with machine or by hand.
Telephone. Determine ability to read numbers, dial the phone, hear the phone ring, and hear conversation over the phone.
Housekeeping. Inquire if any assistance is needed in performing housekeeping chores, such as making bed, cleaning house, washing dishes, and taking out trash.
Access to community. Determine access to transportation, such as taking the bus or driving a car to shop, go to the doctor, and perform other necessary functions outside the home.
Food preparation. Determine ability to plan, prepare, and serve adequate meals independently.
Medication. Determine ability to take medications in the right dose at the right time.
Managing money. Determine ability to plan, budget, write checks or money orders, and exchange currency or coins. Includes ability to count and to open and post mail.

Vision Assessment. Age-associated changes in the eyes can result in impaired vision. Studies vary in the magnitude of this problem, but most agree that the degree of impaired or lost vision is significant in the older adult population. The most common causes of visual impairment are presbyopia, cataract, glaucoma, diabetic retinopathy, and macular degeneration. Visual disorders can result in decreased mobility, poor orientation, feelings of vulnerability, isolation, poor hygiene, the inability to manage medication delivery, and loss of independence. The *Snellen Eye Chart* is a useful screening tool. Referral to a specialist is recommended when visual acuity is worse then 20/40 and the impairment is interfering with daily activities.[14]

Respiratory therapists who care for elderly patients can appropriately implement clinical interventions to compensate for visual deficits that certainly are an asset to the patient and the health care team.

- If the patient wears glasses, make sure they are clean and accessible.
- If the loss of vision impairs their ability to distinguish MDIs, help patients come up with creative solutions to distinguish between their long-acting and rescue inhalers. Some practical suggestions: a short length of flex tubing, rubber bands, puff paint, and/or Velcro dots can all be used to enhance tactile ability. Ideally this intervention takes place before the patient leaves the hospital, allowing therapists to modify misconceptions.
- If the patient's vision loss makes it difficult for them to distinguish pills, suggest that they use a piece of black felt (which provides contrast and keeps pills from rolling around) to sort the pills before placing them into a dated pill container. Having a family member double-check the accuracy of their pills is an excellent idea.
- In the hospital, patients with vision loss are adept at moving around their room as long as the furniture is not moved without their knowledge. Even moving a wastebasket to a location more suitable for the therapist may create a stumbling block for the patient.
- If written instructions need to be sent home with the patient, assure that the font is large enough (14 font), the font color is black, the paper is white (for contrast), and the writing is double-spaced.

Cataracts Cataracts are the most common cause of poor vision in older adults. A *cataract* is a clouding of the eye's lens that causes loss of vision. A cataract starts out small, at which point it has little effect on vision (like looking through a cloudy piece of glass). As the cataract gets bigger and begins to cloud more of the lens, vision becomes increasingly yellowed. The yellowish tint distorts the eye's color vision; blues and greens are particularly hard to see. Cataracts can cause images to appear hazy and out of focus, and double vision is possible. The eyes become overly sensitive to light and glare, making night driving difficult.

Age-Related Macular Degeneration *Age-related macular degeneration* (*AMD*) affects central vision. It is a common cause of vision loss among people over 60. Because only the central vision is affected, people rarely go blind from the disease. A person with AMD gradually loses the ability to see things clearly. Objects may appear to be the wrong shape or size, or straight lines may appear to be wavy or crooked. Color vision is gradually lost, and ultimately a dark area occupies the center of the field of vision, as if the person were looking through a camera with a spot on the center of the lens. Peripheral vision generally remains intact.

Glaucoma *Glaucoma* is a group of diseases that can lead to damage to the optic nerve and result in blindness. It is a result of increased pressure in the eye. At first, glaucoma has no symptoms. Unless the pressure at the front of the eye is controlled, however, it can eventually damage the optic nerve and cause blurred vision, loss of peripheral vision, and the appearance of colored rings around lights. If glaucoma goes untreated, the remaining forward vision may decrease until none is left.

Diabetic Retinopathy *Diabetic retinopathy* is a potentially blinding complication of diabetes that damages the retina of the eye. It occurs when diabetes damages the tiny blood vessels in the retina. At first, most people do not notice any change in vision. As the disease progresses, fragile blood vessels grow along the retina. These blood vessels can bleed, clouding vision and destroying the retina. In extreme cases, a person is able to tell only light from dark. Large hemorrhages tend to happen more than once, often during sleep.

Additional Clinical Interventions for Patients with Visual Disorders

- Encourage regular eye examinations.
- Clean the patient's glasses.
- Avoid the use of pastel colors; reds, yellows, and oranges are easier to see than are blues and greens.
- Apply red nail polish or colored tape to identify different medication bottles.
- Use elastic bands to indicate the daily number of doses; each time a pill is taken, a band is removed. At the end of the day the bands are replaced.
- Make sure that lighting is bright and at a constant level, with glare and reflection eliminated as much as possible.

Best Practice

Diabetic Retinopathy

Diabetic retinopathy is particularly prevalent among Hispanics, African Americans, and Native Americans. Diabetic patients in those groups should be checked frequently.

- Ensure adequate lighting on stairwells, hallways, and steps and in the bedroom. Use a night-light if necessary.
- Use large-button phones and remote controls.
- Place textured warning strips or brightly colored tape at changes in floor level.
- Paint door frames in colors that contrast with that of the walls.
- Supplement teaching with audiotapes.
- Organize a list of emergency numbers (in large bold type), and preprogram the telephone for emergency numbers.

Auditory Assessment. Many elders have hearing problems. They mistake words in a conversation, miss musical notes at a concert, or leave ringing doorbells or telephones unanswered. Hearing problems can be small (missing certain sounds) or large (total deafness).

Some adults may not admit they have trouble hearing. Older people who cannot hear well may become depressed or withdraw from others to avoid the frustration or embarrassment of not understanding what is being said. They may become suspicious of or angry at relatives, friends, or health care providers who "mumble" or "don't speak up." It is easy to mistakenly identify behaviors caused by hearing deficits as confusion, unresponsiveness, or lack of cooperation. Some obvious indications, however, that a person is experiencing hearing loss are as follows:

- Difficulty hearing telephone conversations
- Turning up the volume on the television or radio
- Difficulty understanding women and children talking
- Appearing to be straining to understand conversations

Hearing Loss

- *Presbycusis*, the most common hearing impairment in older adults, is a progressive high-frequency hearing loss. This auditory impairment decreases the ability to hear what others are saying, thereby hindering communication.
- *Conductive hearing loss* occurs when sound waves are not properly conducted to the inner ear. Sounds seem to be muffled. Ear wax in the ear canal, fluid in the middle ear, abnormal bone growth, or a middle ear infection can cause this loss.
- *Sensorineural hearing loss* occurs when there is damage to the inner ear or auditory nerve. Sound waves reach the inner ear but are not properly converted into a message that the brain can understand. Sounds are distorted. In general, low-pitched tones are easier to hear than high-pitched tones.

Clinical Interventions for Patients with Hearing Loss

To help patients with hearing deficits:

- Check to see that the hearing aid is functioning properly.
- Face the patient when speaking.
- Have the patient put on a stethoscope to amplify your voice and speak into the bell.
- Carry a writing pad to use when clarification is needed.
- Lower the tone of your voice, and do not shout at the patient.
- Use facial expressions and hand gestures.
- Decrease extraneous noise.
- Encourage the use of visuals (e.g., a flashing light), as well auditory alerts for smoke alarms, security systems, doorbells, and telephones.

Nutritional Assessment. Because malnutrition and undernutrition are common in the geriatric population, assessment of this problem and intervention are important considerations. Additionally, the prevalence of malnutrition in ill elderly is cited at up to 60%.[15] A compromised nutritional status delays healing and prolongs hospital stays. Therapists may notice some of the signs of malnutrition in their patients (Table 30-6). For community-dwelling elders, the Nutritional Health Screen is simple to administer and may help prevent problems in at-risk older adults. Malnutrition has serious consequences in older patients, thus nutritional assessment, followed by appropriate interventions, may save a life.

Dexterity Assessment Older adults commonly have arthritis, as well as difficulty bending, kneeling, and stooping. Normal aging changes, such as decreased muscle mass, strength, and joint flexibility, greatly affect the older person's agility, mobility, and dexterity. Other factors that adversely affect dexterity are medications,

TABLE 30-6 **Signs of malnutrition in elderly patients**

An emaciated appearance, 15–20% below ideal body weight (IBW)
Muscle wasting, loss of subcutaneous fat
Poor coordination
Muscle weakness, fatigue
Dry, brittle thinning hair, or hair loss
Dry skin, poor coloring
Dry cracked lips
Swollen red tongue

alcohol, medical procedures, disease processes, and lack of exercise. Lack of mobility and dexterity can lead to falls. Comprehensive risk assessments for falls can include two simple evaluations:

- The *one-leg balance* (ability to stand unaided on one leg for 5 seconds)
- The *get-up-and-go test* (rise from a sitting position, walk 10 feet, return to the chair and sit)

Both are easy to administer. If completion of the get-up-and-go test takes longer than 16 seconds, the patient may be at increased risk for falling.

ENVIRONMENTAL ASSESSMENT

Accessible housing enables older adults to live their lives independently. Many homes and commercial environments, however, are full of potential booby traps for the older adult. As in exercise, imagine your home, a health care facility, or a patient's home. Picture an older person who is suffering from functional impairments walking through this environment. How many physical barriers must the person overcome? How many hazards must the person avoid?

A thorough environmental assessment and appropriate environmental adaptations promote safety, reduce accidents, reduce visits to the emergency room and subsequent hospital stays, and improve the quality of life for the older adult. The most efficient way to perform an environmental assessment is to evaluate the exterior access to the house or facility and then evaluate each room in it. Home care therapists may be the first to note the need for such an evaluation. Although environmental assessments are outside the scope of the RT's practice, therapists can contact social workers who can make arrangements for such an evaluation.

Exterior Access Evaluation. Outside things to look for:

- Adequate nonglare lighting
- Handrails on *both* sides of the steps and extending the full length of the stairs
- Filling in potholes and irregular surfaces on driveways and sidewalks
- Appropriate flooring and surfaces: ramps, reflector tape to indicate level changes, nonskid texturing on stairs and surfaces that get wet, color (no blues, greens, or pastels) to highlight entrances and signage
- Lightweight doors with lever handles
- Deadbolt locks and wide-angle peepholes (installed at the appropriate height for the person)

Interior Evaluation. Assess the kitchen for the following:

- Control knobs for the stove toward the front, and large control knobs for stove and oven
- The refrigerator temperature set to 40°F or lower to prevent food spoilage
- Nonglare lighting in all work and living areas to help reduce the incidence of cuts, burns, and falls
- Lightweight pots and pans to reduce the occurrence of spills and burns
- Removal of all throw rugs

Assess the bedroom for the following items:

- Fire alarms
- A telephone with large buttons within arm's reach of the bed
- Night-lights with red bulbs (the aging eye can more readily accommodate to red light than to white light)
- The elimination of heating devices—electric blankets, portable heaters, and heating pads
- "No Smoking" signs clearly posted in bedrooms to discourage smoking in bed or near a supplemental oxygen supply

Assess the bathrooms for presence of safety precautions:

- Ground circuit interrupters to protect against accidental shock
- Hot water heaters set to 120°F or below
- Nonskid bath mats
- Grab bars installed around toilets, in dressing areas, and in the bathing area

SOCIOECONOMIC ASSESSMENT

Historically in America in the early 1900s, the problem of old age was primarily a problem of poverty. Few organizations had any provisions or safety nets for older adults at retirement age. In 1910, only 9 of the nation's 56 largest cities (<2%) had pension plans for their teachers, police officers, or firemen.[16] Even in 1935, when Social Security was first enacted, little help was provided to the indigent or poor. Not until 1965, when Medicare and Medicaid were passed, was major help provided for adults over age 65. Over the years, many revisions of the Social Security Act have made it more equitable and a source of steady income for our elderly citizens. In 2000, Social Security was the major source of income for older adults, but it was not their only resource. On average, according to the 2000 Social Security Fact Sheet, fewer than 22% of older adults cited Social Security as their only income.[17]

Does poverty still exist among the elderly in America? Will we see patients who cannot afford

Best Practice

Need for Financial Assistance

If someone does not have enough money to buy food and to pay rent, what are the odds of the patient purchasing three newly prescribed MDIs? Simply asking the patient if the cost of medications, housing, or food causes financial strain gives the patient the opportunity to communicate the need for financial assistance.

health care? Unfortunately, the answer to both questions is yes. A growing concern today is about the rising cost of living and the rising cost of health care expenditures. To those on fixed incomes, to those living below the poverty level, and to the indigent, medical care may be substandard. Financial insecurity affects an older person's ability to seek medical assistance, to purchase prescribed drugs, to satisfy minimal nutritional requirements, and to maintain adequate housing. Because many aspects of the social situation can affect functional ability, therapists should inquire about any recent changes that have occurred in their patients' living arrangements, activities, or financial support. Home care therapists may be in the best position to do this, but any therapist assisting a patient with hospital discharge has an opportunity to intervene. Patients may be eligible for assistance provided by caregivers, and many patients are still unaware of the resources available to them. As uncomfortable as doing so may be, the respiratory therapist must assess the financial means of the older patient.

COGNITIVE ASSESSMENT

Cognitive impairments can greatly restrict an older person's ability to live independently, manage financial affairs, adhere to medical regimens, and interact socially. Typically, older adults experience alterations in mental functioning such as a decreased ability to think abstractly, decreased short-term memory, reduced attention span, and alterations in the ability to concentrate. Due to the increased incidence of Alzheimer's disease, impaired cognition, and other dementias in this population, the yield of screening for cognitive impairment increases with age. The Mini-Mental State exam, which consists of 30 questions, can be used to assess several dimensions of cognitive function.[18] The Clock Drawing Test (CDT), as well as the recall of items on this test using either a 10-point or 18-point clock drawing scoring system, are also validated screening instruments and easier to incorporate into clinical practice.

Communicating with cognitively impaired elders may be challenging also. Instead of walking away in frustration, try some of the following interventions for more successful communication:

- Identify yourself by approaching the patient from the front, calling the patient by name and limiting distractions.
- Speak slowly and distinctly; choose words carefully, using short simple sentences. Avoid vague words and confusing expressions.
- Avoid sudden movements. Use friendly facial expressions and maintain eye contact.
- Ask one question at a time. Give the patient time to reply. Repeat information. Turn questions into answers. Offer a guess if the patient used the wrong word and cannot find the right one.
- Give simple directions and simple explanations, offer pictures if available.
- Try a written note when spoken messages seem too confusing. Encourage unspoken communication such as pointing or gesturing.
- Be patient and supportive. Avoid criticizing or correcting. Offer comfort and reassurance.

ASSESSMENT OF MEDICATION USE

Studies have estimated that 40–70% of older adults do not take their medication as prescribed (at the right time or in the right amount).[19] Adherence to a drug regimen may be challenging for older adults for a variety of reasons. A study conducted on patients two weeks after

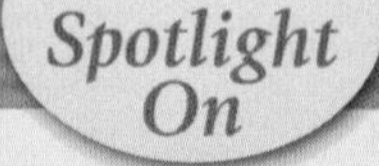

Geriatric Assessment

The geriatric assessment should be applied at each encounter with an older patient. The systematic approach of the geriatric assessment guides the clinician through the complex multidisciplinary nature of illness in older adults and promotes a thorough assessment of the older individual. Thinking through the six components of the geriatric assessment enables the clinician to detect and evaluate signs or symptoms that affect the health and well-being of the older patient.

hospital discharge to home revealed that 49% of the elderly patients were noncompliant with their drugs, either over- or undermedicating themselves.[20] An alarming number of nursing home admissions are due, at least in part, to the persons' inability to take medications correctly. A recent systematic review revealed that, compared to the prevalence of hospital admissions associated with an adverse drug reaction (ADR) in children of 4.1%, for the elderly the admission rate was 10.7%.[21]

Because older adults frequently suffer from comorbid disease processes, they are likely to have three or four physicians *independently* treating the disease processes. Each of these physicians prescribes medications to treat a particular disease process, and often physicians are unaware of the prescribing practices of the other physician.

- **Polypharmacy** (the use of multiple medications), age-related physiological changes, and comorbid disease processes have a direct effect on the pharmacokinetics and pharmacodynamics of medication in the older adult. Polypharmacy may harm the patient or nullify medication benefits because of drug interactions, and determining which medication is causing undesired affects becomes difficult.
- **Pharmacokinetics** is the body's absorption, distribution, hepatic metabolism, and renal clearance of a drug. Because of age-related changes in the renal, hepatic, and gastrointestinal systems and in muscle mass and fatty tissue (see Table 30-7), drugs may not have their intended effects. Disease states may also affect pharmacokinetics.
- **Pharmacodynamics** (a drug's mechanism of action) can be affected by age-related changes in the systems just listed as well as in the cardiovascular, nervous, and endocrine systems. In addition, many prescription and over-the-counter preparations are contraindicated in patients with respiratory disorders (Table 30-8).
- **Adherence** to a medication regimen is a multidimensional phenomenon. The World Health Organization defines it as the extent to which a person's behavior in taking their medication corresponds with agreed recommendations from a health care provider.[22] Failure to take drugs as recommended is defined as *nonadherence*.

TABLE 30-7 **Disease states that affect pharmacokinetics**

Malabsorption
Pancreatitis
Gastric surgery
Congestive heart failure
Hepatic or renal insufficiency
Congestive heart failure
Thyroid disease
Cancer
Volume depletion
Chronic renal insufficiency

Factors that contribute to adverse drug reactions and nonadherence with medication regimes are:

- Use of nonprescription medications.
- Use of alcohol and caffeine.
- Nutritional deficits.
- Dexterity limitations.
- Use of vitamin and herbal preparations.
- Sensory impairment.
- Alterations in cognitive function.
- Financial difficulties (including lack of insurance).
- Impairment of swallowing ability.
- Health care professionals' inadequate knowledge of geriatric pharmacology.
- Lack of appropriate patient education.

Unfortunately, no medication regimen is without risk. All medications, including herbal compounds, have the potential to cause side effects, some minor and some fatal.

Educating the patient about medications and medication regimens is, without exception, the greatest factor in improving adherence to medication regimes. To promote safe and effective pharmacological treatment of the older patient, the practitioner must ensure that the patient understands the answers to the following questions for each medication prescribed:

- What is the medicine's name, and what is it supposed to do?
- How, when, and for how long must it be taken?
- While the patient is taking this medicine, what should be avoided:
  - Certain foods and dietary supplements?
  - Caffeine, alcohol, and other beverages?
  - Other medicines (prescription or over-the-counter)?
  - Certain activities (such as driving or smoking)?
- What are the side effects, and what should the patient do if they occur?
- Will this medicine affect sleep or activity level?
- What should be done if the patient misses a dose?

TABLE 30-8 **Nonasthma medications with increased potential for adverse effects in the older patient with asthma**

Medication	Comorbid Conditions for Which Drug is Prescribed	Adverse Effect	Comment
Beta-adrenergic blocking agent	Hypertension Heart disease Tremor Glaucoma	Worsening asthma Bronchospasm Decreased response to bronchodilator Decreased response to epinephrine in anaphylaxis	Avoid when possible; when must be used, use a highly beta-selective drug
Nonsteroidal anti-inflammatory drugs	Arthritis Musculoskeletal diseases	Worsening asthma Bronchospasm	Not all older patients with asthma have nontolerance of NSAIDs, but they are best avoided if possible.
Non-potassium sparing diuretics	Hypertension Congestive heart failure	Worsening cardiac function or dysrhythmias due to hypokalemia	Additive effect with antiasthma medications that also produce potassium loss (steroids, beta-agonist); older patients also likely to be receiving drugs (e.g., digitalis) that increase the likelihood of hypokalemia
Certain nonsedating antihistamines (terfenadine and astemizole)	Allergic rhinitis	Worsening cardiac function or ventricular arrhythmias	
Cholinergic agents	Urinary retention Glaucoma	Bronchospasm Bronchorrhea	Some over-the-counter asthma medications contain ephedrine, which can aggravate urinary retention, glaucoma.
ACE inhibitors	Heart failure	Increased incidence of cough	Hypertension

Source: From National Asthma Education and Prevention Program. Considerations for diagnosing and managing asthma in the elderly. Washington, DC: National Heart, Lung, and Blood Institute, National Institutes of Health; February 1996. NIH Publication No 96-3662.

Best Practice

Medication History

The respiratory therapist must record a thorough and accurate medication history in the patient record and update the record as needed. The medication history should include *all* prescription and over-the-counter medications.

When discussing medication adherence with older adults:

- Present the information in a clear and concise manner.
- Keep it simple; eliminate medical jargon.
- Provide information in small segments, and reinforce teaching with each patient encounter. It often is helpful to coordinate medication administration times with activities of the day (e.g., mealtime, bedtime, and awakening).

Best Practice

Medication Education

To promote the understanding and retention of medication education, you must employ clinical interventions that minimize the effects of sensory, cognitive, and functional impairments. Plan to take extra time when educating the older adult because often repetition and reinforcement of information are needed.

CASE STUDY 30-3

T. W. is a 76-year-old widow who lives alone in the home she and her husband purchased 50 years ago. Her medical problems include COPD, congestive heart failure, arthritis, hyperlipidemia, cataracts, and insomnia. She has been hospitalized for the past 6 days because of an exacerbation of her COPD. She is in stable condition, and, except for the fact that she fractured her right clavicle 2 nights ago after slipping on her IV tubing, her stay has been unremarkable. Her physician plans to discharge her in 2 days. Mrs. W.'s discharge orders include:

Continuous home oxygen therapy: 2 Lpm
Albuterol metered-dose inhaler: 2 puffs Q4
Corticosteroid metered-dose inhaler:
 2 puffs qd
Prednisone: 10 mg qd
Diazepam: 10 mg HS PRN
Digoxin: 0.25 mg qd
Cipro: 500 mg BID
Hydrochlorothiazide: 25 mg qd
Theophylline: 400 mg TID
Home physical therapy twice a week

Questions

1. What, if any, complications or potential problems do you see with Mrs. W.'s current prescription medications?
2. Describe how you would educate Mrs. W., and prioritize your teaching.
3. What environmental concerns do you have for Mrs. W.? Which interventions would be beneficial for her?

- Make sure patients understand the teaching by asking them questions to assess their understanding of the drug's actions and side effects.
- Give them a sheet of instructions containing the phone numbers of their physician and pharmacist.

Communicating with Older Patients

Communication implies two things: a message delivered and a message understood. When caring for older adults, therapists must be cognizant of some potential barriers to communication.

- Simply telling patients who you are and what therapy the physician wants you to deliver does not guarantee that they have processed the information. Hearing deficits are not uncommon in older adults, especially older male patients. If there is noise in the room—television, radio, equipment humming, noise from the hallway, or noise from construction outside the hospital—patients may not hear the message.
- Some drugs can cause **ototoxicity**, a damaging effect on the eighth cranial nerve, resulting in transient or permanent hearing impairment.
- Patients who are depressed may hear the therapist speak but may disconnect from the message.
- Poststroke patients who suffer from **aphasia** may have lost the power of speech and/or comprehension of the spoken word. This does not mean that they did not receive the message, but rather, because they do not respond, therapists may assume that the message was not delivered.
- Dementia, as in Alzheimer's disease, is always a challenge. The patient may not remember who you are, or your instructions 5 minutes after you leave the room.
- In addition to potential pathology-related lack of communication, the RT has to remember that hearing loss may simply be part of the normal aging process. As stated by Robinson and coworkers, "at a time when older patients have the greatest need to communicate with their doctors [and caregivers] life and physiologic changes make it the most difficult."

The following communication tips are similar to those suggested for use with hearing impaired individuals:

- Make a connection physically and emotionally with the patient; smiling may remove the fear factor or lessen the "white coat" increase in blood pressure.

- Allow a little extra time to deliver therapy to older patients. If therapists appear rushed, irritated, or disinterested, communication may not happen at all.
- Avoid distraction if possible, and let the patient know that your time in the room is their time, even if it is only 7–10 minutes.
- Maintain eye contact and listen to their responses, comments, or questions. Research indicates that physicians listen to patients for an average of 18 seconds before they interrupt, causing them to miss the message the patient is trying to deliver.
- Deliver one message at a time, speaking clearly and loudly enough for them to hear (not shouting) and making sure they can see your lips clearly. Multiple instructions given as you are multitasking is a recipe for miscommunication.
- When teaching a new technique and using good communication skills, ask the patient for a return demonstration. If they cannot do what you taught them and or if they leave out steps, the whole message was not understood.

Communication is a learned activity, often referred to as the art of communication. There is no exact science to delivering an understandable message. Sometimes the strategies work; sometimes they are unsuccessful. Patients respond if the effort is sincere, and, over time, they will understand enough of the basics to participate in therapeutic endeavors.

Summary

In 2002, a document titled "Ten Reasons Why America is Not Ready for the Coming Age Boom" was published by the Alliance for Aging Research. Their statistics are compelling, their message even more so. Despite increased numbers of older adult patients, physicians trained in geriatrics will be woefully lacking. The same goes for allied health professionals; there will be more older patients, but fewer therapists (occupational therapy, physical therapy, respiratory therapy) will be trained in bedside geriatric care. The approaching and very real geriatric gap has the potential to overwhelm the health care system.

It does not have to be that way. The graying of America will offer superior job security to those who are competent in the skills and knowledge required to care for the aging population. The aged patient will challenge the therapist to look beyond the obvious answers. Therapists will need to use all their clinical skills, senses, intuition, reasoning, and common sense to provide safe and competent care. Change can take place only if there is a determined effort to turn the corner and embrace geriatric educational initiatives. The older adult patient population will be available, the time to train is now.

Study Questions

REVIEW QUESTIONS

1. What challenges will the gray explosion present to the health care system?
2. What population of older adults derives the greatest benefit from a comprehensive geriatric assessment? Why?
3. What is the value of the functional assessment? List the components of a functional assessment. Who can do the assessments?
4. Medications can be hazardous to the health of an older adult. Why? How can older adults be made more aware of the benefits and hazards of drug therapy?
5. How can the clinician promote medication compliance among older adults?
6. Describe ways that therapists can communicate more effectively with older patients when delivering therapy.

MULTIPLE-CHOICE QUESTIONS

1. Which of the following factors is not associated with hospital readmission for the older population?
   a. limitations in ADLs
   b. polypharmacy
   c. low economic status
   d. male gender
2. Which statement is true concerning illness in the older person?
   a. The assessment of activities of daily living and instrumental activities of daily living is not a reliable indicator of failing health.
   b. Most older persons who are ill require acute health care.
   c. Most older adults have at least one chronic condition, and many have multiple conditions.
   d. Most older persons have an average of 10 chronic conditions.
3. One of the fastest growing segments of the U.S. aging population consists of:
   a. baby boomers.
   b. the 65–75 age group.
   c. the 75–85 age group.
   d. the 85-plus age group.

4. Activities of daily living are:
   a. useful in identifying individuals who are at risk for institutionalization.
   b. fundamental self-care tasks essential to maintaining independence.
   c. beneficial in identifying exacerbation of disease processes.
   d. physical exercises older patients perform on a daily basis.
5. All of the following interventions help the cognitively impaired retain learning material except:
   a. presenting material slowly.
   b. introducing small amounts of new information.
   c. keeping reading level of written information at the tenth grade level.
   d. repetition.
6. What is pharmcokinetics?
   a. the concurrent use of different medications
   b. an adverse effect of medication
   c. what the body does with a drug
   d. the inert chemical compounds found in medications
7. What is an appropriate font size for literature designed for an older adult with a visual disorder?
   a. 14 point
   b. 10 point
   c. 16 point
   d. 8 point
8. What percentage of older adults cite Social Security as their only income?
   a. 22%
   b. 32%
   c. 42%
   d. 52%
9. The geriatric assessment is designed:
   a. to provide a systematic diagnostic tool for the treatment of acutely ill older adults.
   b. to be multidisciplinary in nature and used by all health care professionals in any health care setting.
   c. for older patients who do not have comorbid disease processes.
   d. to allow the health care practitioner to independently assess each component separately.
10. Which of the following is not a characteristic of disease in old age or of an older patient?
   a. tendency to get angry at people who mumble
   b. belief that the medical condition is just a part of the aging process
   c. atypical presentation of disease states
   d. having more muscle mass than when younger

CRITICAL-THINKING QUESTIONS

1. What changes in the present health care system are most beneficial to the older patient as well as to the economy?
2. How has Medicare Part D impacted older adults on a variety of medications?

ACTIVITIES

1. Visit a health care facility and describe the design features of the facility. Comment on its best and worst design features. How does the physical environment accommodate and present obstacles to the older patient?
2. Interview a person over 70 years old. Write a summary of the interview, including the subject's age, gender, and level of independence. Have them answers the following questions: How has the world changed since you were young? What are some positive aspects of aging? What are some negative aspects of aging? What do you enjoy now that you did not enjoy in your younger years?

References

1. Institute of Medicine. Retooling for an aging America: building the health care workforce. Washington, DC: National Academies Press; Available: April 14, 2008. www.iom.edu/CMS
2. Yancy CW. The prevention of heart failure in minority communities and discrepancies in health care delivery systems. *Medical Clinics of North America.* 2004;88,5:1347–1368.
3. U.S. Department of Health and Human Services: What are health disparities: www.omhrc.gov Content last modified 11/18/2005.
4. Census 2000 Summary File 1 (SF1). http://factfinder.census.gov/servlet/DatasetMainPageServlet?_lang=en
5. National Center for Health Statistics. U.S. life expectancy hits new high of nearly 78 years. September 2007. www.cdc.gov/nchs
6. U.S. Census Bureau. Facts for features. March 2006. www.census.gov/Press-Release/www/releases/archives/facts_for_features_special_editions/ 006537.html
7. Centers for Medicare& Medicaid Services. *Medicare and you, 2008*. Department of Health and Human Services CMS Publication #10050; January 2008.
8. Feldstein PJ. *Health Care Economics*. 6th ed. Clifton Park, NY: Delmar Cengage Learning; 2005.
9. Centers for Medicare & Medicaid Services, U.S. Department of Health and Human Services. Nursing homes: paying for care. March 27, 2008. www.medicare.gov/Nursing/Payment.asp

10. Comprehensive Geriatric Assessment Position Statement. (Special thanks to Dr. Paul Mulhausen.) New York: AGS Public Policy Committee, May 2005.
11. Alliance for Aging Research: Executive Summary. Medical never-never land: ten reasons why America is not ready for the coming age boom. February 2002. www.agingresearch.org
12. Osterweil D. Comprehensive geriatric assessment: lessons in progress. *Israel Medical Association Journal (IMAJ)*. 2003;5:371–374.
13. Gaugler JE, Duval S, Anderson KA, Kane RL. Predicting nursing home admission in the US: A meta-analysis. *BMC Geriatrics.* 2007;7:13.
14. Miller KE, Zylstra RG, Standridge JB. The geriatric patient: a systematic approach to maintaining health. American Family Physician. February 15, 2000. http://www.aafp.org/afp/20000215/1089.html
15. Seiler WO. Clinical pictures of malnutrition in ill elderly subjects. *Nutrition*. 2001;17:496–498.
16. Fischer DH. *Growing Old in America*. New York: Oxford University Press; 1975.
17. Social Security Administration. Income of the population 55 or older, 2000. Washington, DC: Government Printing Office, 2002.
18. Wagenaar DB. Communicating with the elderly. *Dialogue and Diagnosis*. April 2007. www.do-online.org/pdf/pub_dd0407wagenaar.pdf
19. Salzman C, Kupfer DJ Medication compliance in the elderly. *The Journal of Clinical Psychiatry*. Supp. 1.1995;56:18–23.
20. Gray SL, Mahoney JE, Blough DK. Medication adherence in elderly patients receiving home health services following hospital discharge. *The Annals of Pharmacotherapy.* 2001;35:539–545.
21. Kongkaew C, Noyce PR, Ashcroft DM. Hospital admissions associated with adverse drug reactions: a systematic review of prospective observational studies. *The Annals of Pharmacotherapy*. 2008;32,7:1017–1025.
22. Sabate E, ed. *Adherence to Long-Term Therapies: Evidence for Action*. Geneva: World Health Organization; 2003.

Resources

COMMUNITY AND HEALTH RESOURCES

Centers for Medicare & Medicaid Services, formerly the Health Care Finance Administration (Medicare and Medicaid information): http://www.hcfa.gov/

Eldercare Locator (a nationwide directory designed to help older persons and caregivers locate support services): Call1-800-677-1116 or contact the local area agency on aging.

Medicare Fraud and Abuse: 1-800-HHS-TIPS (1-800-447-8477)

Medicare Information: 1-800-318-2596

Nursing Home Database (information about nursing homes, including results of recent surveys): http://www.medicare.gov/coverage/home.asp

VISION INFORMATION AND RESOURCES

American Foundation for the Blind: 1-212-502-7661 or afbinfo@afb.org

American Optometric Association: 1-314-991-4100

Lighthouse National Center for Vision and Aging: 1-800-334-5497

National Eye Care Project of the Americas of the American Academy of Ophthalmology (a help line to refer callers to local ophthalmologists who will volunteer to provide needed medical care): 1-800-222-EYES

National Eye Institute: http://www.nih/gov/publications

National Institute on Aging: 1-800-222-2225 or 1-800-222-4225 (text telephone)

The National Library Service for the Blind and Visually Handicapped (provides free medical services to people with vision problems and offers braille and large-print materials and recorded books): 1-800-424-8567

Vision Foundation (publishes the Vision Resource List, which includes information on special products and services for people with visual impairments): 1-617-926-4232

AUDITORY INFORMATION AND RESOURCES

American Academy of Otolaryngology—Head Neck Surgery, Inc.: 1-703-836-4444 or 1-703-519-1585 (text telephone)

American Speech-Language-Hearing Association: 1-800-638-8255 (voice/text telephone)

National Information Center on Deafness: 1-202-651-5051 or 1-206-651-5052

National Institute on Aging: 1-800-222-2225 or 1-800-222-4225

National Institute on Deafness and Other Communication Disorders: 1-800-241-1044 or 1-800-241-1055

Self-Help for Hard of Hearing People, Inc.: 1-301-657-2248 or 1-301-657-2249 (text telephone)

ENVIRONMENTAL RESOURCES

Abledata: The National Database for Assistive Technology Information 8455 Colesville Road, Suite 935, Silver Spring, MD 20910-3319; 1-800-227-0216 or 1-301-427-0277(voice/text telephone) http://www.abledata.com

American Association for Retired Persons (AARP): *The Do-Able Renewable Home*. AARP publication, online access: http://www.usc.edu/go/hmap/library/drhome/

CHAPTER 31

Emergency Respiratory Care

Robert R. Fluck Jr.

OBJECTIVES

Upon completion of this chapter, the reader should be able to:

- Highlight the importance of ABCs in any patient situation.
- Describe manual methods of maintaining airway patency.
- Describe the equipment and techniques for maintaining airway patency.
- Describe the management of the first 10 minutes of an adult cardiac arrest.
- Describe the priorities in the management of cardiac arrest in a child.
- Differentiate priorities between infant and adult resuscitation.
- Describe situations under which airway adjuncts other than an endotracheal tube are used.

CHAPTER OUTLINE

Basic Life Support
- Components of Basic Life Support
- Adult Airway Obstruction
- Child Airway Obstruction
- Infant Airway Obstruction

Advanced Cardiovascular Life Support
- Ventricular Fibrillation (VF), and Pulseless Ventricular Tachycardia (v-tach)
- Asystole
- Pulseless Electrical Activity
- Bradycardias
- Tachycardias
- Acute Coronary Syndromes (ACS)
- Defibrillation

Pediatric Advanced Life Support
- Broselow Tape
- Initial Patient Assessment and Prevention
- Fluid Therapy and Drugs
- Resuscitating the Newborn Outside the Delivery Room
- Cardiac Rhythm Disturbances
- Pediatric Trauma

Neonatal Resuscitation Program
- Primary Versus Secondary Apnea
- Changes in Lungs and Circulation at Birth
- Ventilation
- Circulation
- Intubation
- Drug and Volume Therapy During Resuscitation

Emergency Airway Adjuncts
- Esophageal Obturator Airway/Esophageal Gastric Tube Airway
- Esophageal Tracheal Combitube
- Laryngeal Mask Airway

KEY TERMS

advanced cardiovascular life support (ACLS)
automatic external defibrillator (AED)
basic life support (BLS)
esophageal obturator airway (EOA)/esophageal gastric tube airway (EGTA)
esophageal tracheal combitube (ETC)
laryngeal mask airway (LMA)
neonatal resuscitation program (NRP)
pediatric advanced life support (PALS)
ventricular fibrillation (VF)
ventricular tachycardia (v-tach)

In nearly every emergency situation, the respiratory therapist (RT) is a valuable player. The therapist's expertise lies in the area of maintaining the airway, breathing, and circulation—the ABCs of resuscitation. Regardless of the etiology or circumstances of the emergency, the victim's airway must be secured, breathing assured, and circulation supported. Whether one looks in burn, neurosurgery, or orthopedic literature, the first measures are the same: Take care of ABCs and worry about the injuries later. The proper actions must be taken in the proper order *and* in a timely fashion. If the actions are not proper and timely, the result is almost invariably what is euphemistically termed in medicine an unfavorable outcome: The patient dies or worse, survives in a persistent vegetative state. The ability of a respiratory therapist to assess the patient rapidly and just as rapidly institute the appropriate life-saving or -sustaining treatment puts the RT at the head of the bed when the patient is in trouble. The reader should note that the guidelines for resuscitations are updated every five years and should therefore stay abreast of these changes. The techniques specified in this chapter are recommended as of the time of this writing (2011).

Basic Life Support

Basic life support (BLS) encompasses all the actions that can be accomplished without adjunctive equipment. In spite of the fact that it is *basic*, it is indeed vital; advanced treatments become meaningless (and ineffective) without well performed BLS. According to the American Heart Association, in the adult patient in cardiac arrest, the time to cardiopulmonary resuscitation (CPR) is one of the two determinants of survival after an arrest (ACLS Instructor's Manual, 2010).

COMPONENTS OF BASIC LIFE SUPPORT

In performing BLS, the rescuer must first ascertain that the patient is indeed in need of resuscitation. The *shake and shout maneuver* (shaking the victim's shoulders vigorously and shouting, "Are you OK?") provides both tactile and audible stimuli to the patient to attempt to elicit a response. If the patient is able to speak, the ABCs are confirmed in one step. However, if there is no response, it is next appropriate to call for help. Rarely, if ever, does the single rescuer complete a resuscitation singlehandedly.

If the patient is in a bed with the head elevated, the rescuer has two choices:

- The bed can be quickly lowered to the flat position. If the rescuer chooses to leave the patient on the bed, the head of the bed can be removed (the head of *every* hospital bed comes off) and then used for a firm surface under the patient's back to facilitate compressions.
- The other option is to move the patient to the floor (if the rescuer has been trained to do so without sustaining an injury or injuring the patient).

The rescuer should then check for no more than 10 seconds for the presence of a pulse. If there is no

Best Practice

Defibrillation

The vast majority of adults who suffer cardiac arrest have **ventricular fibrillation (VF)** or, less commonly, **ventricular tachycardia (v-tach)** as their initial rhythm. The only treatment for fibrillation is *defibrillation.* Therefore, in contrast to what we have all learned, the priority in an adult arrest is acquiring a monitor to determine the patient's rhythm and then defibrillating that rhythm if doing so is appropriate. Therefore the action taken first depends on location and on the available equipment. In a hospital, head for the **automatic external defibrillator (AED)**, which is at every nursing station and which all respiratory therapists have been trained to use. On a medical-surgical floor in a hospital without an AED, begin BLS until the arrival of someone who can use the manual monitor-defibrillator (unless the RT is authorized by the hospital to use the manual unit). So it comes down to priorities versus resources: If it is possible to defibrillate, do so at the earliest time. If not, wait until the trained people get there.

pulse, begin chest compressions with a depth of at least 2 inches (on an adult) at a rate of >100 per minute. If alone, the rescuer delivers cycles of 30 compressions followed by 2 ventilations. If two (or more) people are performing the resuscitation, the person performing compressions should deliver 30 (counting out loud while doing so to cue the person performing ventilations) and then pause for the delivery of two breaths. After 5 cycles of 30 compressions and two breaths, the rescuers should change positions due to the strenuous nature of the performance of compressions. That change should ideally take less than 5 seconds. The airway should be opened using the head tilt-chin lift method unless the rescuer suspects potential C-spine trauma (Figure 31-1A). In that case, he should use the jaw thrust; however, should the jaw thrust not provide a patent airway, the rescuer should use the head tilt-chin lift, as ventilation is a priority at this time (Figure 31-1B). If there is an airway obstruction, the rescuer should continue to perform cycles of 30 compressions and 2 breaths, checking the mouth for the presence of a foreign body before every two breaths. In a hospital scenario, the presence of a meal tray should alert the rescuer to a possible airway obstruction. The rescuer(s) should continue the sequence of 30 compressions to 2 ventilations until:

- Someone confirms the presence of a DNR and the resuscitation can be stopped.
- A physician determines that further resuscitation attempts are futile and should be stopped.
- Someone relieves the rescuer.
- Or spontaneous circulation alone or both spontaneous circulation and breathing return. If only spontaneous circulation returns, the rescuer should deliver one breath every 6–8 seconds or approximately 8–10 per minute. It should be noted that the American Heart Association now recommends that lay persons (non-professionals) performing CPR should administer only compressions (a procedure known as "hands-only CPR," which can be performed by any rescuer for the *first 5 minutes* of a *witnessed adult* cardiac arrest) and not attempt any ventilations.

As compressions are now determined to be the more important action in CPR, there should be minimal interruption of compressions, even for the delivery of breaths. "Push hard and push fast" is the new mantra for resuscitation. In addition, the American Heart Association recommends avoiding excessive ventilation. This is a significant departure from past practice when therapists were encouraged to hyperventilate the patient. There are two physiologic reasons for limiting ventilation. For one, positive pressure

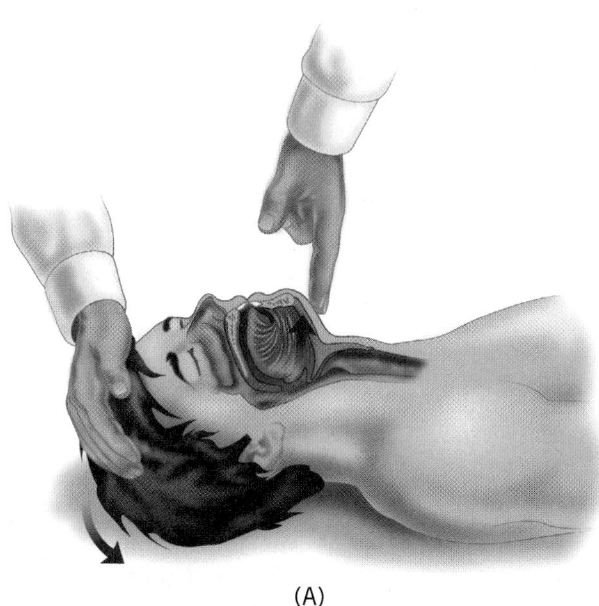

(A)

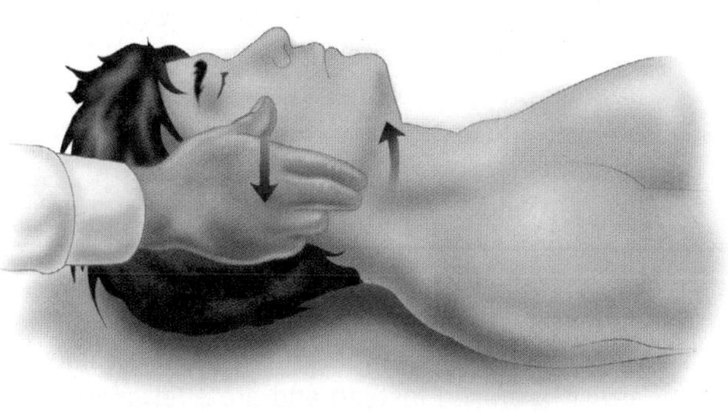

(B)

FIGURE 31-1 (A) Head tilt, chin lift maneuver. (B) Jaw thrust maneuver.

Best Practice

Terminating Resuscitation Efforts

Modern ethicists have agreed that stopping a medical treatment (in this case cardiopulmonary resuscitation) is no different from not beginning it at all. Formerly, almost all hospital personnel believed that once you started some treatment, stopping it was more difficult than not having begun. For example, if someone were intubated and placed on mechanical ventilation in an emergency situation, extubating that person required him to be weaned from mechanical ventilation. The reality now is that once a valid DNR is found for someone, resuscitation can cease immediately.

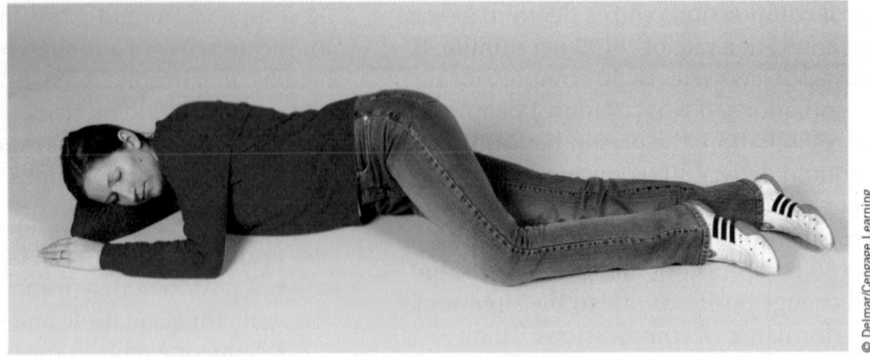

FIGURE 31-2 The recovery position, used when the victim has spontaneous breathing and circulation: The position allows maintenance of the airway and lets secretions drain from the mouth by gravity.

ventilation increases mean intrathoracic pressure. This impedes venous return and thus cardiac output since the venous-intrathoracic pressure gradient is the main determinant of venous return in the arrest situation. In addition, excessive ventilation decreases PCO_2, resulting in a left shift of the oxyhemoglobin dissociation curve. This decreases the availability of oxygen to the tissues.

If the victim is breathing spontaneously at least 10 or more times per minute, then the victim should be placed in the *recovery position*, technically known as the *lateral decubitus position* (Figure 31-2). The victim is placed on a level surface on his or her side with the inferior arm extended straight up. The position of the arm provides several benefits:

- It helps to cushion the head.
- It helps position the head to maintain a patent airway.
- It keeps the mouth tilted down to let secretions or vomitus drain out, thus minimizing the likelihood of aspiration.

Age-Specific Competency

Performing Basic Life Support

Several techniques for basic life support are different for children and infants. The American Heart Association defines an infant as someone younger than 1 year old. A child is between 1 and 8 years old.

- Ventilation rates for both infants and children are the same as for adults: 8–10 per minute or one every 6–8 seconds.
- Ventilation for the infant, however, is effected by mouth–to-mouth-and-nose ventilation due to the small size of the infant's mouth.
- Compression depth generally one-half of the anteroposterior diameter of the thorax. This depth is estimated at 1.5 inches for infants and 2 inches for children.
- Compressions are performed with the index and middle fingers or by the two hands encircling technique using both thumbs in an infant and the heel of one hand in a child. As with adults, the ratio of compressions to ventilations for infants and children for one rescuer is also 30:2. However, if there are two rescuers for children and infants, the ratio is 15 compressions:2 ventilations.
- The pulse is palpated at the brachial artery on an infant because the infant's neck is short, a fact that makes palpating the carotid artery more difficult in infants.

The airway obstruction sequence in infants and children differs somewhat from that of adults also.

- In both cases, the finger sweep is never automatic. The rescuer inspects the child or infant's pharynx for the presence of a foreign body. If one is actually seen, then the rescuer attempts removal with a finger.
- In an infant, because of the anatomy and the likelihood of damaging the liver, abdominal thrusts (the Heimlich maneuver) are not done; chest compressions, done exactly as though one were performing them in cardiac arrest, are used instead and are alternated with back blows (Table 31-1).

TABLE 31-1 **Specifications for CPR performance**

Ventilation Rate	Compression Rate	Compression Depth
Adults	8–10 per minute (every 6–8 seconds) > 100 per minute	At least 2 inches
Child	8–10 per minute (every 6–8 seconds) > 100 per minute	2 inches
Infant	8–10 per minute (every 6–8 seconds) > 100 per minute	1.5 inches

The victim's knees should be bent to maintain stability on the side. The rescuer should continue to monitor the adequacy of breathing and be prepared to assist ventilation if the respiratory rate drops to fewer than 10 per minute.

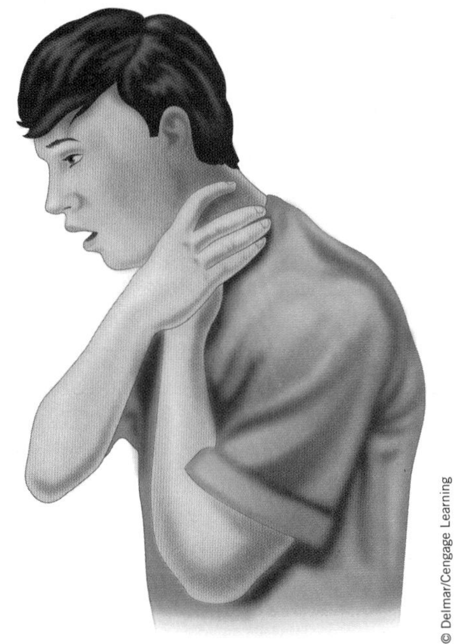

FIGURE 31-3 The "official" sign for choking.

ADULT AIRWAY OBSTRUCTION

The one circumstance in which the rescuer's efforts (if successful) are rewarded almost immediately is in the case of the conscious person with a complete upper airway obstruction. For adults, the risk factors for this situation include:

- Alcohol ingestion.
- Talking while eating.
- Ill fitting dentures (a condition which causes the person to cut progressively larger pieces of meat and attempt to swallow with minimal chewing).

The adult with a complete upper airway obstruction may look surprised and be unable to make a sound. The victim may (or may not) be giving the "official" choking sign of placing the thumb and forefingers of both hands around the neck (Figure 31-3). First confirm complete obstruction by asking the victim whether he or she is choking. If the victim is able to cough forcefully and is not cyanotic, he or she should be allowed to continue to try to expel the obstruction without assistance.

If, however, there is poor air exchange or cyanosis, the victim needs assistance. Take a position directly behind the victim, turned 90° to the victim. In this position, should the victim lose consciousness and fall, the rescuer can control the victim's descent to the floor without anyone's being injured. The rescuer can support the weight of the victim on the closer thigh simply by guiding the victim with the arms, at the same time moving backward and lowering the victim gently to the floor. In the conscious victim, the rescuer should then deliver the Heimlich maneuver (abdominal thrusts) until either the foreign body is expelled or the victim loses consciousness.

Note: For someone who is pregnant or obese, the rescuer should perform chest thrusts instead of abdominal thrusts.

If the victim loses consciousness, the rescuer should call for help and then begin the sequence of CPR, with one change: The rescuer should inspect the victim's mouth for the presence of a foreign body each time before attempting to deliver ventilation.

By the time a patient needs either ventilation or both compressions and ventilation, the therapist has missed a golden opportunity (or a number of them). The motto in health care today is health promotion/disease prevention. In other words, keeping people healthy is less expensive than treating them once they become ill. The concept parallels preventive maintenance in an automobile. The problem is that we deal with individuals who may or may not do the things that prolong their lifespan, especially if the actions are inconvenient—even though who would not want to live longer given the chance?

CHILD AIRWAY OBSTRUCTION

The sequence for treating a complete upper airway obstruction in a child is exactly the same as that for an adult. The only difference is that chest thrusts are not performed on a child.

Best Practice

Health Promotion/Disease Prevention in Adults

The respiratory therapist must try to teach people healthful behaviors, for both themselves and also their children, for whom they have responsibility. For adults, the behaviors are best described as heart healthy behaviors and address the cardiac risk factors that can be modified. In 2004, the Report of the Surgeon General identified smoking as the main cause of coronary artery disease (CAD) and that cessation of smoking by adults would probably have the most significant effect of any behavior on the rate of CAD in the United States. Helping people stop smoking should be high on the priority list for respiratory therapists. To assist in this endeavor, the Tobacco-Free Lifestyle Roundtable of the American Association for Respiratory Care has created a pamphlet that the respiratory therapist can give to patients to reinforce the stop-smoking message.

Hypertension is another cause of CAD. The first step in controlling blood pressure knows what it is. An easy way to have blood pressure taken several times a year is to donate blood! A person can donate blood every 56 days (American Red Cross, 2010) and can therefore have blood pressure taken in a relatively no-stress environment as many as seven times each year, while performing a significant public service. Continuing to take prescribed medication is the most important step in controlling hypertension. Of course, if people do not feel ill, they frequently stop taking prescribed medication for any condition.

INFANT AIRWAY OBSTRUCTION

In dealing with an infant with complete upper airway obstruction, the completeness of the obstruction needs to be inferred by the lack of sound coming from a small person whose face and body language show extreme anxiety. A risk factor for upper airway obstruction for infants, as well as for small children, is the presence of small objects that the infant or child can reach and then place in the mouth. Once a complete obstruction has been confirmed, the rescuer should:

- Place the infant face down over his or her arm with the head lower than the hips.
- Administer up to 5 back blows (Figure 31-4A).
- Turn the infant supine while carefully supporting the head with the head lower than the

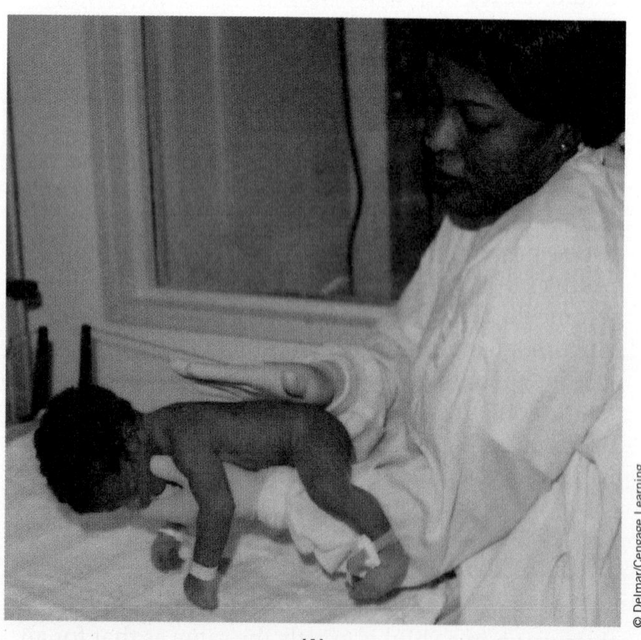

(A)

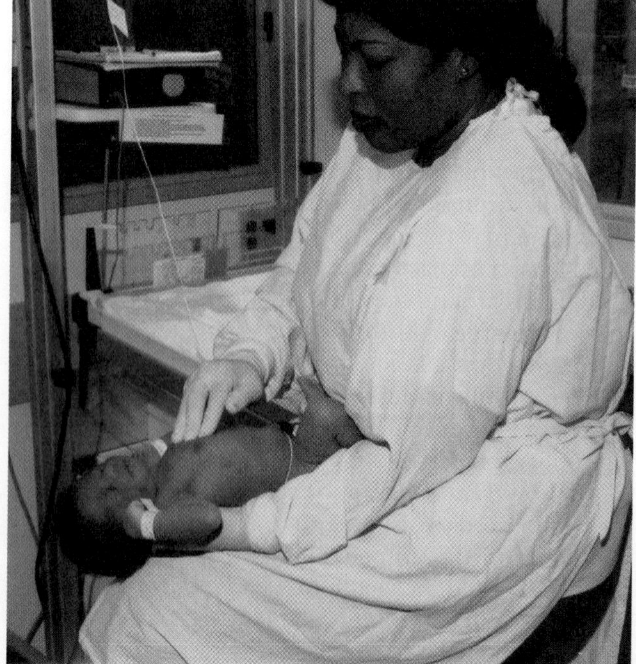

(B)

FIGURE 31-4 (A) Back blows for removal of a foreign body airway obstruction. (B) Chest thrusts.

Best Practice

Critical Incident Stress Debriefing

We frequently forget the stress which resuscitation places on the professionals providing the resuscitation. Whereas on television about 80% of victims are resuscitated successfully, in real life 80% of resuscitations are *unsuccessful*. Prehospital care includes a process called *critical incident stress debriefing* (*CISD*). The CISD gathers all those involved in a rescue or resuscitation a few days after the incident and allows them to talk about their performance and especially their feelings following an incident that goes beyond everyday events. An example of an especially stressful incident might be the fire department whose emergency responder finds that one of the victims of a fatal automobile collision is one of their own members. A professional is brought in to conduct the CISD. Health care givers in the hospital tend to neglect taking care of their own mental health. People can develop post-traumatic stress disorder if they are not allowed to work through their feelings after a particularly stressful resuscitation in the hospital such as the attempted resuscitation of a child, which is always a stressful situation.

hips and administer up to 5 chest thrusts (Figure 31-4B).

- Repeat this sequence until either the obstruction is removed or the infant loses consciousness.

If the infant becomes unconscious, the rescuer should have someone activate the emergency response system. The infant should be placed on a hard surface, and the rescuer should begin CPR with compressions with the same caveat as that for adults–inspect the mouth for a foreign body each time prior to delivering breaths.

Advanced Cardiovascular Life Support

Advanced Cardiovascular Life Support (ACLS) encompasses the tasks and techniques used in cardiac resuscitation that go beyond what a rescuer can do with the hands and mouth (or pocket mask). ACLS includes (but is not limited to):

- Endotracheal intubation or other means of securing the airway.
- Administration of drugs and fluids by IV, IO, and (with some limitations), intra-tracheal.
- Monitoring of cardiac rhythm.
- Electrical therapy, which includes defibrillation, cardioversion, and pacing.

Upon completing an ACLS course, the participant should be able to direct the resuscitation for the first 10 minutes of a cardiac arrest. Although other situations are included in the course, competency in management of the full cardiopulmonary arrest is the key. Most adults are found in VF when they suffer cardiac arrest as a result of a medical problem (as opposed to a traumatic arrest); in children and infants, the cardiac arrest is more likely secondary to a respiratory problem. The two important areas that therapists might not be managing but should know how to treat are acute stroke and acute coronary syndromes (ACS). The time-dependent nature of the treatments for both of these situations requires that someone suffering from either of these illnesses have access to medical care as soon as possible. (The window for treatment of stroke is only 3 hours *from the onset of signs and symptoms*.) The therapist, knowing the signs and symptoms of stroke and ACS, is in a position to expedite that medical care for friends and relatives.

A reasonable question is why RTs should take ACLS training when most hospitals do not allow them to intubate, defibrillate, or administer drugs via IV, IO, or endotracheal routes. The reality is that the respiratory therapist may be the best trained and educated person at the scene of a cardiac arrest. For example, the nurses on most medical-surgical floors might see one cardiac arrest in a calendar year. They might not quickly remember where the electrodes are supposed to be placed on the patient. Yet respiratory therapists go to every cardiac arrest in the hospital. For example, the author was at work when a cardiac arrest was paged. Upon responding, he found a female in full arrest with the monitor already connected showing v-tach. No one was doing anything, even though the correct action at that point was defibrillation as soon as possible. Even if forbidden to perform a particular action, the RT can indicate the correct action to take and encourage a credentialed person to take it.

Three other points about ACLS are important.

- First, ACLS is worth little without *excellent* BLS. The ABCs of resuscitation encompass ensuring an adequate airway, providing adequate breathing, and augmenting circulation as appropriate. People become enamored of the gadgets for use in ACLS and forget the importance of BLS in the overall picture. Do not fall short on the basic skills.

- Second, ACLS is driven by rhythm algorithms. Each rhythm has an algorithm giving the procedure for resuscitating that rhythm. If the rhythm changes, then the therapist changes to the appropriate algorithm.
- Third, the title of the publication containing all the procedures for resuscitation is *Guidelines for Cardiopulmonary Resuscitation and Emergency Cardiac Care* (American Heart Association, 2010). When first published, the title of the publication contained the word "standards." However, realizing the legal and medical implications, the American Heart Association changed that word to "guidelines." The change indicates that, practically, a clinician may deviate from the stated protocols when doing so is appropriate and warranted based on the situation and the patient's condition. Do not be overly concerned when a resuscitation effort does not follow the American Heart Association script exactly.

VENTRICULAR FIBRILLATION (VF), AND PULSELESS VENTRICULAR TACHYCARDIA (V-TACH)

In the latest guidelines, VF, v-tach, asystole, and PEA are grouped together in the *Cardiac Arrest* algorithm. The big picture of the difference is that VF and v-tach should receive electrical therapy (defibrillation) while there is no electrical therapy for PEA and asystole. The most common initial rhythm for the adult in cardiac arrest is ventricular fibrillation. Thus, the respiratory therapist should be facile in diagnosing and treating this rhythm. The following case study highlights the important aspects of treating this dysrhythmia.

CASE STUDY 31-1

John S. is a registered respiratory therapist with a current ACLS card who is working the night shift in Progressive Community Hospital. He arrives to administer aerosol bronchodilator therapy to Mr. C. J., a patient who was just admitted to a medical-surgical floor with an acute exacerbation of COPD. He enters the room and cheerily greets Mr. C. J., who is in semi-Fowler's position in his hospital bed with his eyes closed. Receiving no response, John puts on gloves and gives Mr. J. a shake and calls to him quite loudly. Still getting no response, John goes to the hallway and calls out, "I've got a code here—Room 1313!" He returns to the room and grabs the pocket mask off the cork board at the foot of the bed. He then lowers the bed to the flat position as low as possible. He checks for a pulse for no more than 10 seconds.

Feeling no pulse, he removes the head of the bed and places it behind Mr. J.'s back. He delivers 30 compressions. John S. then applies the pocket mask and delivers two slow breaths over one second each. Just then the patient's nurse and the charge nurse enter the room with the crash cart. John asks one of them to take over ventilation and the other to attach the electrodes to Mr. J.'s chest. The other night shift therapist arrives and assumes compression duties from John. John notes that the rhythm displayed on the monitor is VF (Figure 31-5). He opens the gel pads and places one to the right of Mr. J.'s sternum and the other on the left side of his chest at the apex of the heart, about 22 cm (9 in) below the axilla. He sets the defibrillator to 200 joules and charges the paddles. He places the paddles on Mr. J.'s chest over the gel pads with good pressure (25 pounds is the listed value), chants in a loud voice (while scanning the bed to assure that there is no one in contact with either the bed or the patient), "I'm clear. You're clear. We're all clear. Defibrillating!" He discharges the paddles. He advises the team performing compressions to resume CPR. The nursing supervisor arrives and begins to record the events.

Note: Older defibrillators deliver energy in what is known as a monophasic waveform (current travels

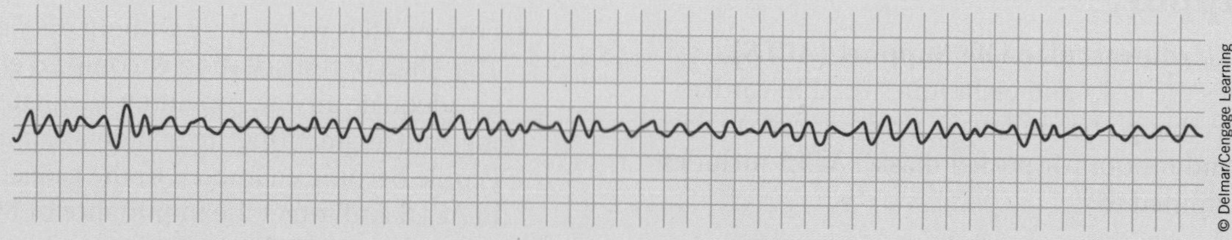

FIGURE 31-5 EKG showing ventricular fibrillation.

(*continues*)

(continued)

in only one direction). Newer defibrillators (including AEDs) deliver energy in a biphasic waveform (current travels in both directions). These biphasic defibrillators have been found to be more effective at terminating VF or v-tach at lower energy doses than monophasic defibrillators. This is advantageous since the less energy delivered to the myocardium, the less likely it is to be damaged in the process.

John requests the charge nurse to start an IV and administer 1 mg of epinephrine every three to five minutes once she has established the line, while he prepares and checks his equipment for endotracheal intubation. Once he has intubated the patient, he confirms the position of the endotracheal tube by a number of means.

Once the intubation is accomplished, the therapist documents (charts):

- The date and time.
- The size, and type (Miller or Macintosh) of blade used.
- The size tube.
- The ease of visualization of the cords.
- All indicators that were checked to confirm proper placement of the tube.
- The distance mark in cm at the corner of the mouth.

By this time, things should have settled down. The RT is working with the minimum number of people needed to perform such a resuscitation properly. There should be one person each to:

- Ventilate.
- Perform compressions.
- Administer drugs and defibrillate.
- Record the chronology of events (the scribe).
- Lead the group.

Having a clearly designated leader is important. (Some hospitals place a white hard hat on the code cart; whoever is wearing it is in charge.) Clear leadership is especially critical in hospitals with medical students and house officers; failure to designate who is in charge can lead to confusion and a less than optimal resuscitation.

Questions

1. If the RT were unable to lower the bed to the flat position, what alternatives would he have to position Mr. J. properly for CPR?
2. What are the hazards of placing insufficient pressure on the defibrillator paddles?
3. Who has a greater role in carbon dioxide elimination when a patient is in cardiac arrest: the person ventilating or the one performing compressions?

Best Practice

Confirmation of Endotracheal Tube Placement

Confirmation of proper endotracheal tube placement should be done by a number of means:

- Auscultation of equal breath sounds
- Lack of gurgling auscultated over the epigastrium (referred breath sounds might be heard just below the diaphragm!).
- Inspection of equal thoracic expansion.
- Visualization of condensation on the inside of the tube
- Seeing the tube pass between the vocal cords.
- The use of an esophageal detector device (EDD, described later in this chapter).

The respiratory therapist asks the nursing supervisor to request a STAT portable chest X-ray. Although a chest X-ray is the gold standard for ensuring the proper location of an endotracheal tube, a clinical determination of proper position has to be done long before the chest film is read. Otherwise, other efforts might be futile. In a patient with at least spontaneous circulation (though not necessarily spontaneous breathing), the use of a CO_2 detector is the best technique. The detector can be electronic, as is common in the operating room, or colorimetric, which is more convenient for the resuscitation cart (Easy Cap™). The colorimetric detector is placed between the manual resuscitator and the patient's endotracheal tube. It is purple when there is no carbon dioxide and turns tan and then yellow with increasing concentrations of carbon dioxide (Figure 31-6).

Normally in the body, carbon dioxide is present as a gas only in the lungs. But what if the person has eaten pretzels and drunk beer before being intubated in the esophagus? According to the manufacturer, if the endotracheal tube is accidentally placed

(continues)

(continued)

into the esophagus, four or five breaths will wash out any such carbon dioxide. Then the Easy Cap™ will read zero carbon dioxide (purple). The problem in this case is that 5 L or more of air has been insufflated into the stomach, and such air is looking for a route out of the stomach, bringing other gastric contents with it, a situation which complicates airway management. At the very least, that much distension of the stomach will impede subsequent efforts to ventilate the patient. So the rescuer must ensure proper placement of the endotracheal tube at the outset.

If the patient has no spontaneous circulation (full cardiopulmonary arrest), the excretion of carbon dioxide is determined more by the adequacy of compressions (and thus circulation) than by the adequacy of ventilations. In these situations, the rescuer should use another device, called the *esophageal detector device* (*EDD*). This consists of either a 60-mL syringe with a catheter tip (commonly referred to as a Toomey syringe) or a rubber bulb; either one has an endotracheal tube connector (Figure 31-7). If a *bulb* is used, the bulb is squeezed and then attached to the endotracheal tube.

- If the tube is in the trachea, the bulb rapidly reinflates as the trachea is held open by its cartilaginous rings.
- If the tube is in the esophagus, the bulb reinflates slowly if at all, because the esophagus collapses around the end of the tube.

If the EDD has the *syringe*, the rescuer pulls rapidly back on the syringe.

- If the tube is in the trachea, the syringe pulls back easily to full capacity.
- If it is in the esophagus, the syringe stops quickly—as little as 10 mL.

If the tube is determined to be in the esophagus:

- Remove it immediately.
- Reventilate the patient for 2 minutes.
- Reintubate.

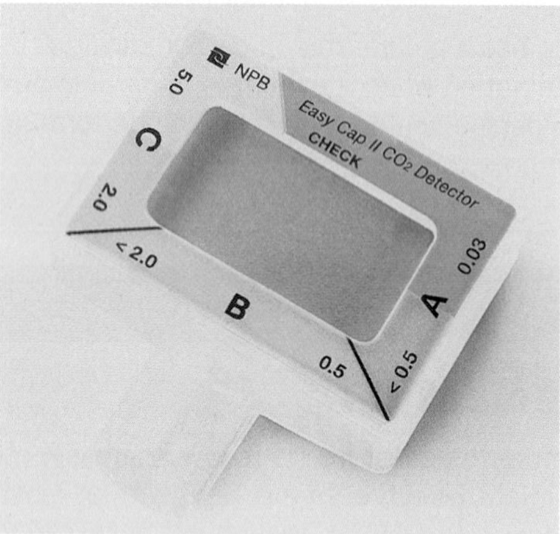

FIGURE 31-6 The Easy Cap™ colorimetric CO_2 detector is purple at <0.5% CO_2, tan from 0.5 to <2% CO_2, and yellow at >2% CO_2.

Image used by permission from Nellcor Puritan Bennett LLC, Boulder, Colorado, doing business as Covidien.

Drug Sequence for VF/Pulseless v-tach. Suppose, in the preceding case, the monitor still shows VF after 5 cycles of 30 compressions and 2 ventilations. Here is what might happen:

- John defibrillates at 200 joules; CPR is resumed immediately after.
- He asks the med nurse to administer 300 mg of amiodarone. (Refer to Table 31-2 for a synopsis of drugs used in adult resuscitation.)

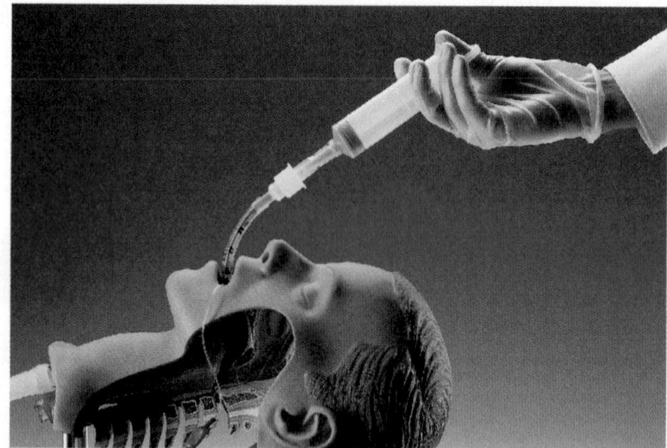

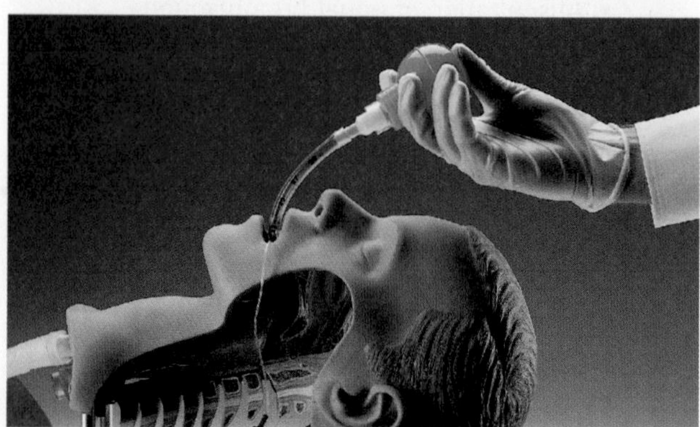

FIGURE 31-7 Termed an **E**sophageal **D**etector **D**evice **(EDD)**, a 60-mL syringe with a catheter tip or a rubber bulb can be used to determine endotracheal tube placement.

Courtesy of Ambu, Inc., Linthicum, Maryland

TABLE 31-2 **Drugs most commonly used in adult resuscitation delivered by either IV or IO route**

Drug	Classification	Action	Dosage
Epinephrine	Sympathomimetic	α, β_1, β_2 stimulator	1 mg q 3–5 minutes
Lidocaine	Antiarrhythmic	Decreases ventricular irritability	1–1.5 mg/kg; max 3.0 mg/kg/24 hours
Amiodarone	Antiarrhythmic	Decreases ventricular irritability	300 mg second dose of 150 mg
Magnesium Sulfate	Antiarrhythmic for torsades de pointes	Decreases ventricular irritability	1–2 g over 10 min
Procainamide	Antiarrhythmic	Decreases ventricular irritability (also used in supraventricular dysrhythmias)	20–30 mg/min to a max of 17 mg/kg
Atropine	Parasympatholytic	Parasympathetic blocker	1 mg/dose to max 3 mg
Bicarbonate	Alkalinizing agent	Buffers acids	Calculated from base excess and vascular volume)—½ this dose is given initially
Narcan (naloxone)	Narcotic antagonist	Blocks narcotic receptor sites	2 mg repeated as necessary
Vasopressin	Sympathomimetic	α, β_1, β_2 stimulator	40 mg—may replace first or second dose of epinephrine

Note: Lidocaine may be used instead of amiodarone as an antiarrythmic. Initial dose of lidocaine is 1–1.5 mg/kg with subsequent doses of 0.5–0.75 mg/kg up to a maximum of 3 mg/kg.

- After about another 2 minutes of CPR, seeing that the rhythm is unchanged, John again defibrillates a 200 joules.
- Another 1 mg of epinephrine is followed by one more defibrillation after five cycles of CPR, assuming the rhythm is unchanged.
- A dose of 150 mg of amiodarone is delivered, followed by 5 cycles of CPR and then defibrillation if the rhythm is unchanged.
- Five cycles of CPR are delivered following another 1 mg dose of epinephrine; defibrillation is again performed at 200 joules if the rhythm remains unchanged.
- The sequence continues with five cycles of CPR followed by a rhythm check and defibrillation if warranted. (Note: The therapist has 23 seconds to deliver 30 compressions and 10 seconds of off-the chest time to deliver two breaths. Thus, five cycles should take approximately 165 seconds or two minutes and 45 seconds. The American Heart Association persists in saying "5 cycles or two minutes of CPR".)
- Should the resuscitation reach this point, the next drug delivered is magnesium sulfate: 1–2 g in 50 mL of normal saline—and *only* if the rhythm is torsades de pointes or there is measured or suspected hypomagnesemia.

Best Practice

Scribe

The scribe is critical to have on the resuscitation team. The epinephrine is given every 3 to 5 minutes throughout *any* cardiac arrest. In this case, it is given between one of two antiarrhythmic drugs. Without someone watching the clock and logging each therapeutic intervention, the resuscitation could get out of control. It is also very difficult, if not impossible, to accurately reconstruct the chronology of events during a resuscitation after the fact. This post hoc reconstruction is, however, common in patients in cardiac arrest who have been resuscitated in the field and brought in by ambulance, since there is not enough room in the back of an ambulance for the full resuscitation team.

The reality is that things rarely reach this stage. The VF or pulseless v-tach usually resolves, either into some sort of perfusing rhythm or into asystole, with no further cardiac response to the resuscitation efforts.

- The magnesium sulfate is followed by five cycles of CPR and then defibrillation at 200 joules, if indicated.
- Finally, procainamide may be given (the only drug given as an infusion during complete cardiac arrest) at 20 mg/min up to 17mg/kg. For an 80 kg person, then, infusing this amount at this rate would take over 45 minutes! (The procainamide may be infused at 50 mg/min, which in this example would reduce the time needed to 18 minutes.)

Thirty-five years ago, sodium bicarbonate (bicarb) was administered every 5 minutes, just like epinephrine. However, bicarb has fallen out of favor for routine use in a full cardiopulmonary arrest. To understand its banishment, the RT needs to understand the rating system for drugs and treatments that the American Heart Association has adopted.

- Class I is definitely helpful.
- Class IIa is acceptable, *probably* helpful.
- Class IIb is acceptable, *possibly* helpful.
- Class III is not indicated, may be harmful.

The American Heart Association also mentions drug overdoses, especially with tricyclic antidepressants as additional appropriate times for bicarbonate administration; in a full arrest, this does not seem pertinent.

Within this system:

- For a hypoxic lactic acidosis, bicarb is considered Class III.
- For a known preexisting bicarbonate sensitive acidosis (such as someone in renal failure), it is Class IIa.
- If the patient is intubated and the resuscitation has been proceeding for some time, or if the patient has had ROSC after a prolonged interval, bicarb is deemed Class IIb.

Bicarb can have seven adverse effects on the body, all of which should be given consideration when it is administered during a full arrest (American Heart Association, 1992).

- Bicarbonate shifts the oxyhemoglobin dissociation curve to the left, inhibiting the release of oxygen to the tissues.
- It has not been shown to enhance the ability to defibrillate or to improve survival rates in animal models.
- It can induce hyperosmolarity and hypernatremia.
- It causes other adverse effects due to the extracellular alkalosis that it causes.
- It exacerbates central venous acidosis.
- It may deactivate catecholamines (specifically epinephrine), which are administered at the same time.
- Finally, bicarb produces carbon dioxide when it buffers acids. This respiratory acidemia may result in a paradoxical tissue acidosis due to the reverse diffusion of carbon dioxide, especially in the cardiac and cerebral circulations. Therefore, adequate ventilation must be assured before bicarbonate administration.

Termination of Resuscitative Efforts. When should resuscitation be stopped? Of course, if a valid DNR appears, then resuscitation should be stopped immediately.

Otherwise, the general answer is when there is no further response from the cardiovascular system. As long as the patient can be successfully defibrillated, the resuscitation continues even though the patient periodically reverts to VF. However, it is clearly medically futile to continue resuscitating the patient, and the effort should be terminated if:

- The patient has been in asystole with no response to therapy for a period of time.
- All potential causes have been ruled out (see the asystole algorithm).
- And the entire algorithm has been run.

ASYSTOLE

Probably the next most common rhythm that rescuers see is asystole. Of course, "asystole usually is a confirmation of death rather than a rhythm to be treated" (American Heart Association ACLS Instructor's manual). So respiratory therapists must be able to recognize indications for ending the resuscitation. Asystole (known in lay terms as *flatline*) is easy to recognize (Figure 31-8). To be sure of the diagnosis of asystole, it should be confirmed that all electrodes are firmly attached to the patient. (People often inappropriately and imprecisely refer to them as *leads*, but a *lead* is the potential difference between two electrodes.)

The lead most commonly monitored in emergencies is lead II (the right arm and left leg). This lead is popular because it is the limb lead that provides the best P-waves. In fact, when most monitor/defibrillators are turned, on they are in lead II, but the operator can switch to lead III (left arm and left leg), lead I (left arm and right arm), or paddles.

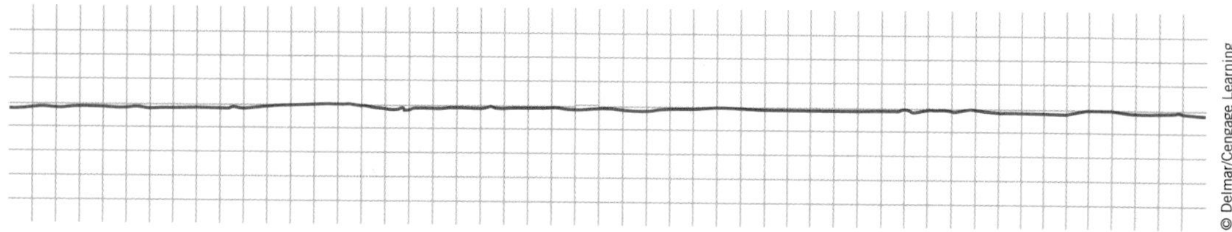

FIGURE 31-8 EKG showing asystole.

Definitive Therapy. Once pulselessness has been determined, it is time to begin compressions, intubation, and obtaining an IV access. One mg of epinephrine is given via IV/IO or 2 mg via the endotracheal tube once access is available.

Causes of Cardiac Arrest. The rescuer has to run down the list of possible causes of cardiac arrest to determine whether there is any immediately correctable one. This list can be remembered as the 6 Hs and 5 Ts.

- Certainly *hypoxia* (1) can be immediately addressed. Check the basics: Is the resuscitation bag connected to an oxygen source? Is that source actually turned on? Is there adequate ventilation, as judged by breath sounds and chest rise? Obtaining an arterial blood gas is probably not a useful exercise during a full cardiac arrest for three reasons: (1) the time involved in obtaining the results, (2) the controversy over exactly what constitutes good arterial blood gas values in the context of full cardiopulmonary arrest, and (3) because of the venous pulsations in the femoral vein secondary to cardiac compressions, blood may be mistakenly sampled from the vein instead of the artery. Besides, hypoxia denotes insufficient oxygen delivery to the tissues; arterial blood gas values give us only the ability to determine content and not the transport or delivery in the absence of a value for cardiac output (see Chapters 16 and 19). Some people, in fact, feel that venous blood gases (not necessarily mixed venous from the pulmonary artery) provide a better picture of the metabolic conditions at the tissue and cellular level.

> **Best Practice**
>
> ## Drug Administration
>
> What if IV is not an option? What if, for instance, an elderly diabetic has no visible peripheral veins? Intubating the trachea takes priority over starting an IV if only one person has to do both. The endotracheal tube provides both airway control and a means for administering some drugs. Five liquid and one gaseous drug can be given by means of an endotracheal tube. The gaseous one is, of course, oxygen. The others go by the acronym of LEAN-V (or LANE-V): lidocaine, epinephrine, atropine, narcan, and vasopressin. The dose of any drug administered through the endotracheal tube should be 2–2.5 times that given intravenously. The one caveat is that a volume of no more than 10 mL should be instilled down the endotracheal tube at one time. To avoid having the drug expelled into your face, the best plan is to give 5 mL, bag a few times, and administer another 5 mL. Note that the optimal doses of these drugs given via the endotracheal tube have not been determined; IV/IO delivery is preferred because there is more reliable drug delivery and pharmacologic effect.

- Two other conditions—*hypo-* and *hyperkalemia* (2)—would be known ahead of time by means of routine lab tests:
  - If the patient is determined to be hyperkalemic, the resuscitation effort could pretty much be ended at that time. Lowering the serum potassium of someone in cardiac arrest is not really feasible.
  - If the patient is hypokalemic, potassium could be administered to raise the serum level.

If the patient has a preexisting *acidosis* (excess *hydrogen ions*) (3), buffering with bicarbonate is indicated. To estimate the base deficit, use the following formula:

$$\text{total base deficit} = 0.25\ \text{L/kg} \times \text{base deficit mEq/L (from an ABG)} \times \text{body weight (kg)}$$

The factor of 0.25 estimates the volume of extracellular fluid. Bicarbonate typically is in preloaded syringes with about 45 mEq in 50 mL. Because this calculation is an approximation, administer one-half of the calculated amount and reevaluate the patient's acid-base status.

Hypothermia (4) is probably the one condition whose presence would lead to the prolongation of the resuscitation efforts. This becomes more common as outside temperatures fall. As the saying goes, "You are not dead until you are warm and dead!" The patient's core temperature should be 30–32°C before it is determined that the person is dead. In fact, at lower temperatures, surface (skin) electrodes may reveal no electrical activity in the heart; needle electrodes may be necessary to determine the cardiac rhythm. The rewarming process may take some time, as external rewarming is inappropriate in any setting, whether prehospital or in the hospital. Internal rewarming can be accomplished by:

- Warm gastric, peritoneal, colonic, and bladder lavage.
- The provision of humidified gas warmed above body temperature for ventilation.
- The use of warmed IV fluids.

Cardiopulmonary bypass can also be used if the following conditions are all met:

- All else fails.
- There is optimism for the patient's recovery if rewarmed.
- And the procedure is available.

In the case of hypothermia, the team should stop electrical therapy and hold any further drug therapy until the body temperature is at least 30°C.

- *Hypovolemia* (5) can be empirically determined by delivering a bolus of 250–500mL of normal saline or lactated Ringers. Any response to this should cause the delivery of another fluid challenge bolus. The bolus should be infused fairly rapidly. Remember that IV pumps have a maximum infusion rate of 999 mL/hour; the infusion of 500 mL would take a half hour via a pump. It is faster, therefore, simply to run the IV wide open and watch the bag closely.

- *Hypoglycemia* (6) (serum glucose < 70 mg/dL in adults or < 40 mg/dL in infants) is more a potential problem in infants and neonates.

- If the patient had taken a *drug overdose* (*toxins*) (1), such as tricyclic antidepressants, digoxin, β blockers, or calcium channel blockers. Suspect a drug overdose in the patient with a history of psychiatric problems who is taking one of these drugs. There may be little to do in these cases as removal of that drug from the blood would be as difficult as treating hyperkalemia. There needs to be some circulation for the drug to be metabolized or excreted. There are a few types of drugs for which there are direct antidotes, such as narcotics (naloxone/Narcan) and benzodiazepenes (romazicon/Flumazenil). Certainly, if there is an antidote, it should be administered at that time.

- To determine of the presence of *cardiac tamponade*, (2) insert a needle into the pericardium and aspirate. Of course, this procedure is the province of a physician. If cardiac tamponade is the cause, the improvement in the patient's condition should be immediate.

- The respiratory therapist should be able to rapidly to assess the presence of a *tension pneumothorax* (3), but there would have to be some suspicion that this is a problem. A typical patient at increased risk for tension pneumothorax:

- Is postoperative lobectomy.
- Has severe bullous disease.
- Has been generating high peak pressures on mechanical ventilation.
- Or has had a subclavian line recently inserted.

There is no time for an X-ray. Diagnosis and treatment must be immediate or the patient will die. The signs of a tension pneumothorax include:

- Breath sounds are decreased or absent over the affected side.
- There is decreased movement of the affected side.
- If the RT can judge the percussion note, there would be hyper-resonance over the affected side as well.
- A late sign is tracheal displacement away from the effected side due to movement of the entire mediastinum

Treatment is simple and within the purview of the respiratory therapist (assuming the RT has been credentialed by the hospital to perform the procedure): needle decompression.

- Find the second or third intercostal space in the midclavicular line (straight laterally from the angle of Louis or sternal notch).
- Insert a 14- or 16-gauge IV catheter over the superior edge of the inferior rib (to avoid the neurovascular bundle that runs in a groove in the inferior edge of the superior rib) (Figure 31-9).
- The clinician may hear a rush of air.
- The needle is left in place as you have now changed a tension pneumothorax into an open pneumothorax, not an ideal situation but a better one.

This results in rapid improvement if tension pneumothorax is the problem.

- *Massive pulmonary embolism* (*thrombosis*) (4) needs to be suspected by recent clinical history. The common denominator in pulmonary embolism is

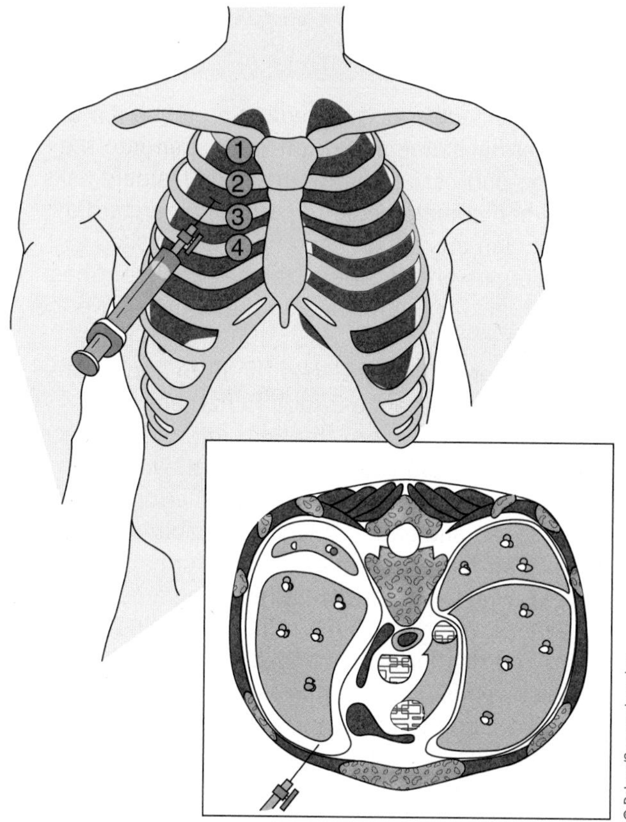

FIGURE 31-9 Proper location for needle decompression for tension pneumothorax at the second or third intercostal space, hugging the superior edge of the inferior rib.

inactivity. (Even otherwise healthy individuals have developed pulmonary emboli after prolonged airplane trips without physical activity.) Added risk factors are smoking, recent surgery, phlebitis, the use of birth control pills, cardiovascular disease, obesity, pregnancy, trauma, and polycythemia (with smoking and birth control pills being a particularly bad combination). If the embolism is so massive as to result in cardiac arrest, it is likely fatal in that the only treatment is surgical embolectomy.

• Acute *myocardial infarction* (*MI*) (*thrombosis*) (5). This would be suspected from the patient's medical history, including:

- A history of coronary artery disease (CAD).
- Previous MI.
- Family history of MI (especially at or before the age of 55).
- The reason for admission to hospital.
- Previous coronary revascularization surgery or percutaneous coronary intervention (PCI).
- Cardiac catheterization reports.
- EKG changes.
- Medications.

PULSELESS ELECTRICAL ACTIVITY

Pulseless electrical activity (*PEA*), which can be associated with a variety of rhythms, used to be called electromechanical dissociation (EMD). However, a variety of situations can produce electrical activity in the absence of a pulse; hence the name change.

The key in treating PEA is to eliminate the potential causes in a methodical fashion. (See the list following the section on asystole on p.866.)

BRADYCARDIAS

For an adult, the official definition of bradycardia is a heart rate less than 60 beats per minute. However, highly conditioned athletes may have a resting heart rate in the forties; a person in congestive heart failure may have a resting heart rate of 110 per minute just to maintain minimal perfusion. The important determination is whether the patient has serious signs and symptoms associated with this heart rate such as:

- Chest pain
- Shortness of breath
- Altered level of consciousness
- Low blood pressure
- Signs of shock
- Pulmonary congestion (crackles auscultated in lung bases)
- Congestive heart failure
- Acute MI

If the bradycardia is symptomatic, regardless of the rate, then the therapist should intervene. The RT should, of course, examine the electrocardiogram (EKG) (see Chapter 19). If there is third-degree AV heart block, the patient needs a transcutaneous pacer as temporizing therapy on the floor. A physician can insert a transvenous pacer to stabilize the heart rate until the patient can be taken to the OR and a permanent pacer installed. In the case of type II second-degree AV block (Mobitz II) with the absence of serious signs and symptoms, a pacer is still a good idea because the condition may progress to third-degree AV heart block. Once the therapist has determined that intervention is appropriate, the intervention should proceed through the following sequence.

Definitive Treatment. Initially, atropine should be administered. If the person had a heart transplant, atropine has no effect on the denervated heart. Atropine should be administered in increments of 0.5 mg up to a maximum of 3 mg. It should be administered as rapid IV push; slow administration or administration of a bolus of less than 0.5 mg can cause a paradoxical *decrease* in heart rate. The limitation of administering medication as a bolus is that the effect

CASE STUDY 31-2

A 50-year-old woman is hospitalized on a medical-surgical floor for chemotherapy for breast cancer following a course of radiation therapy. She has just had a triple lumen subclavian line placed for central venous access. Jan, the respiratory therapist, is called to her room because she has been found unconscious, apneic, and pulseless. Jan quickly begins compressions after lowering the head of the bed and placing the head of the bed under the patient for a firm surface. Once the code cart arrives with a monitor, a nurse places three electrodes (one under each clavicle at the midclavicular line and one at the left costal margin at the midaxillary line) and turns on the monitor, displaying sinus rhythm. Jan requests an 8-mm endotracheal tube and the intubation equipment. Jan also requests 1 mg of epinephrine to be administered into the patient's central line.

Another therapist arrives and intubates the trachea. (Note: Given the new emphasis on delivering excellent compressions without interruption, intubation is not a high priority if adequate ventilation can be easily delivered via a face mask.) Once intubation is completed and the proper tube placement is confirmed, the medical admitting resident enters the room and confers with Jan. The three possibilities are:

- Iatrogenic tension pneumothorax (from insertion of the central subclavian line).
- Pericardial tamponade from radiation therapy or metastases.
- Hypovolemia.

In this setting, all three potential causes can be addressed simultaneously.

The resident asks the medication nurse to hang 1 L of normal saline and run it wide open into the 16-gauge port of the central line. The resident asks for a 5-inch spinal needle to perform a pericardiocentesis. Jan auscultates and finds diminished breath sounds on the side of the central line. Chest excursion also is diminished on that side. Above the chaos that is typical in a resuscitation in a patient's room, the percussion note is difficult to appreciate. Jan asks for a 14-gauge 2-inch IV catheter. She quickly preps the area of the third intercostal space with an alcohol prep pad and inserts the catheter perpendicular to the chest, hugging the top of the fourth rib. As she enters the plural space, she hears a hiss as air leaves the thorax. Jan informs the resident, who pauses before attempting a pericardiocentesis. Nearly 500 mL of normal saline have run in. The rhythm is unchanged, but Jan asks the therapist who is doing compressions to stop. She feels for a carotid pulse and finds a weak one. The resident requests another 500-mL fluid bolus and a blood pressure. The initial pressure Jan obtains is 90/40 mmHg.

Questions

1. In someone with end-stage renal disease, what cause for cardiac arrest is uppermost in Jan's mind?
2. In someone with no blood flow (except as performed by external cardiac compression), can drug overdose or hyperkalemia, as causes of cardiac arrest, realistically be treated such that the patient can recover? Why?

can be difficult to predict and cannot be modified once the drug is given. Additionally, if no further therapies are instituted, the heart rate will decrease in about 15 minutes to what it was initially.

After atropine, transcutaneous pacing is the intervention of choice. Place the pacer pads in the same location as for defibrillation. Note: Insure that the pads are specified as able to be used for pacing.

- Once the RT turns the pacer on and starts it, the unit marks each QRS, usually with a bright dot or line on or above the QRS.
- The rate should be set at 80/min.
- The current is increased in 10 mA increments until capture occurs (usually over 70-80 mA)—that is, each pacer spike is followed by a wide QRS.
- Next, the current is decreased in 5-mA increments until capture is just lost and then returned to the last level to minimize the current being delivered. Remember that the patient may not be entirely grateful; transcutaneous pacing is a painful procedure. Analgesia and sedation may be appropriate. Confirmation of the presence of a pulse along with the electrical activity should not be done at the carotid artery as the muscle movement which accompanies transcutaneous pacing can be misconstrued to be a pulse. Note: A patient who has undergone transcutaneous pacing will be very sore the following day due to contraction of large numbers of skeletal muscles because of the cutaneous delivery of current.

Best Practice

Oxygen Therapy

For anyone who suffers the sudden onset of signs or symptoms suggesting a cardiovascular problem, the first interventions are O2-IV-monitor. In the emergency situation, there is no such thing as too much oxygen. Thus, a nonrebreather or a high-flow, high-concentration aerosol system should be applied to the patient. For those concerned about potential depression of the hypoxic stimulus to breathe in patients with chronic obstructive pulmonary disease (COPD), remember two important facts:

- Only a small minority of patients with COPD are actually carbon dioxide retainers whose breathing is stimulated due to lack of oxygen (Scanlan, et al., 1999).
- If someone's breathing is depressed, the RT can intubate and mechanically ventilate. To quote one of the pioneers in oxygen therapy, John Haldane: "Hypoxia not only stops the machine, it wrecks the machinery" (Haldane, 1919). In other words, the worst thing that can happen to the patient is to become hypoxic. Respiratory therapists should do their utmost to ensure that this does not happen.

Intravenous access should be obtained while the patient is as stable as possible. Starting an IV becomes very difficult if there is a decrease in blood flow to the extremities. An alternative is IO access. Finally, ACLS treatments are based on algorithms determined by the cardiac rhythm. All three interventions can be effected in just a few minutes and provide the basis for everything that follows.

If pacing does not have the desired effect, continue the drug sequence. In order, the drugs and dosages are:

- Dopamine in an infusion of 5–20 μg/kg/min (a Class IIb intervention).
- Epinephrine in an infusion of 2–10 μg/min (a Class IIb intervention).

TACHYCARDIAS

Probably the most complex of all the ACLS algorithms is for tachycardias. Although it is initially a fairly daunting piece, just take it step by step.

Under any circumstances, assess ABCs first, and deal with any defects found. As with any potential cardiac problem, the rescuer should:

- First apply O2-IV-monitor.
- Then obtain vital signs (including what some are now calling the fifth vital sign: pulse oximetry).
- Set up a 12-lead EKG.
- Perform a physical examination.
- Obtain a chest radiograph.
- Review the patient's history.

Stable or Unstable? The first determination is whether the patient is stable or unstable. As soon as the therapist finds indications of instability, the assessment should be interrupted to treat the problem. As with the bradycardias, serious signs and symptoms are:

- Chest pain.
- Shortness of breath.
- Decreased level of consciousness.
- Low blood pressure.
- Indications of shock, pulmonary edema, or acute MI.

If the patient is unstable, then the therapist should prepare for immediate cardioversion. A heart rate of >150 implies instability; the therapist should proceed directly to cardioversion.

Cardioversion. *Cardioversion* is the synchronized delivery of electrical energy to the heart to change a rhythm. If the cardioversion is elective, then the patient could be premedicated with (usually) a benzodiazepine (such as midazolam or Versed) or a barbiturate (such as methohexital or Brevital) plus a narcotic for analgesia. However, if the patient is unstable, then this becomes an urgent procedure—taking the time to administer drugs delays the application of the electrical therapy to restore effective circulation; in addition, most sedatives and analgesics have adverse effects on the cardiovascular system. At any rate, the therapist should make provisions for securing the patient's airway should this procedure become necessary. In other words, a manual resuscitator with mask should be connected to oxygen and intubation supplies should be at the bedside and checked beforehand.

The patient is connected to the monitor/defibrillator with EKG electrodes in the standard monitoring positions (just below each clavicle at the midclavicular line and at the left costal margin at the midaxillary line).

- The therapist turns on the defibrillator and activates the synchronizer. The device begins to indicate in some way that it is finding R-waves. This can simply be a flashing light (as on PhysioControl LifePack 5) or a bright dot on the R-wave and a flashing "SYNC" on the monitor screen (as on PhysioControl LifePack 10). The rescuer should be aware of the function of his hospital's particular model because some defibrillators disable the synchronizer after each delivery of energy; others remain in the synchronized mode until it is turned off.
- The initial energy level should be selected: 50 to 200 joules (watt-seconds) depending upon the presenting rhythm.

There are two techniques used to cardiovert. In the past, the therapist took paddles and applied them with about 25 pounds of pressure to the patient's thorax with gel pads or conductive gel (which looks like toothpaste) just as for defibrillation. The safer and thus preferred method is the *hands-off technique*.

- For hands-off cardioversion, connect the electrodes to the cable (if necessary—some come preconnected) *before* attaching the electrodes to the patient because it is often difficult to connect the cable once the electrodes are on the patient's skin.
- Large electrodes are attached to the patient by their adhesive border in one of two locations: either to the right of the sternum and at the apex (as previously described for defibrillation) or at the front midsternum and back. The location is specified by the manufacturer and marked both on the outside of the foil packet containing the electrodes and on the electrodes themselves. (There are two alternative locations for the pads underneath the scapula on either side.)
- Once the patient is connected to the defibrillator and the initial energy level is selected, the therapist charges the unit.
- Then the RT places the paddles on the patient (if using paddles) and chants: "I'm clear, you're clear, we're all clear. Shocking!" During this announcement, the operator is scanning the stretcher for someone who is not paying attention. The therapist has to be sure that he or she is also clear because the operator is the one most often shocked during defibrillation or cardioversion.
- The therapist holds down both buttons on the paddles (it is somewhat awkward to do) or pushes the "discharge" button on the machine itself if using hands off until the machine discharges (listen for the relay click inside). It may take a second or so before the machine confirms an R-wave and discharges. The delay can be disconcerting if one is expecting an immediate discharge as happens when defibrillating.
- If the initial cardioversion is unsuccessful, the therapist should increase the energy level (from 50 to 100 or from 100 to 200 joules) and attempt cardioversion again. Remember that the synchronizer may need to be turned on again; otherwise you are delivering an unsynchronized shock which may cause the rhythm to deteriorate into v-fib.

Drug and Nondrug Treatments. If the patient is determined to be stable, the therapist can move a little more slowly. With all the preliminary investigations completed, it is time to treat the rhythm.

- Patients in chronic atrial fibrillation should also be anticoagulated because it has been found that they have more than five times greater risk of stroke than someone not in that rhythm (Harvard Health Letter, 1998).
- If the rhythm displays a wide QRS (>0.12 seconds) and *only* if it is regular and monomorphic, then adenosine can be considered. If the rhythm has a wide QRS but is not regular, the therapist should consider an antiarrythmic infusion.

Antiarrhythmic infusions for stable wide-QRS tachycardia:

Procainamide infused at 20–50 mg/min until one of four situations occurs: the arrhythmia is suppressed, hypotension occurs, the QRS width increases > 50%, or the maximum dose of 17 mg/kg has been delivered.

Amiodarone 150 mg delivered over 10 minutes; repeat as needed if VF or v-tach recurs; follow up with an infusion of 1 mg/min for 6 hours.

Sotalol 1 to 1.5 mg/kg: Although package insert recommends slow infusion, the literature supports infusion of the maximum dose over 5 minutes or less.

If the QRS is narrow, *vagal maneuvers* lead the therapeutic parade. The therapist can ask the patient to bear down (Valsalva maneuver). An alternative is carotid sinus massage. The therapist should auscultate first before performing this maneuver because this is contraindicated in those with a bruit, which indicates the presence of partial obstruction due to peripheral vascular disease. It is also best to do only one side at a time because bilateral carotid sinus massage has been known to lead to cardiac arrest due to greatly increased vagal tone.

If the vagal maneuvers do not "break" the rhythm, the next rung on the therapeutic ladder is adenosine. Each dose of adenosine is given by *rapid* IV push; the first is 6 mg. The therapist should immediately flush it with 20 mL of normal saline. The therapist should also understand that the first rhythm after administration of adenosine is asystole. The good news is that the half-life of adenosine is only about 5 seconds, so it goes away very quickly. A second dose at double the initial dose is given after 2–3 minutes if the initial one has no effect.

- If the complex is still narrow and the patient remains stable, a beta blocker or calcium channel blocker is the next drug of choice.

All pathways ultimately lead to cardioversion if traveled all the way. Under these circumstances, assuming the patient remains stable, premedicate the patient. A short-acting benzodiazepine such as Versed (midazolam) is the drug of choice. It provides mild sedation and is also an amnesiac; its short duration allows the patient to recover more quickly.

ACUTE CORONARY SYNDROMES (ACS)

The key to dealing with what are now grouped as acute coronary syndromes is the urgency of treatment. For coronary reperfusion (percutaneous coronary intervention or PCI) or thrombolytic therapy) to minimize the size of the myocardial infarct, the patient has to have the intervention in less than 12 hours after the onset of symptoms. Since denial causes people to delay seeking medical attention in the first place, they use up valuable time. The emergency department must have a system already in place to deal with the patient who is complaining of chest pain.

The key drugs used in treating acute coronary syndromes are:

- Oxygen.
- Morphine.
- Nitroglycerine.
- Aspirin.
- Heparin.
- β-blockers.
- Thrombolytic agents.
- Angiotensin-converting enzyme (ACE) inhibitors.

The mechanical intervention is *percutaneous coronary intervention* (PCI). The American Heart Association emphasizes the initial treatment by saying: "MONA (morphine, oxygen, nitroglycerine, aspirin) greets all patients with chest pain" (ACLS Instructor's Manual, 2010). The reader may wonder what role the respiratory therapist might play in the emergency treatment of acute coronary syndromes. As in many situations, and in the previous example, knowing what to do may be as important as being able to do it. If the person with the suspected ACS is a friend or relative, having the person chew one adult (325 mg) or two (formerly children's) 81 mg non enteric-coated aspirin may be life saving.

Initial Assessment and Connection of Patient to AED. Prior to attaching the AED, the rescuer needs to confirm that the victim is unresponsive, apneic, and pulseless. The AED should not be attached to the victim who does not meet all three criteria.

- The rescuer should place the AED next to the left side of the victim's head.
- The pads should be connected to the cable (if they are not already connected in the package). Where the pads should be placed is indicated on the outside of the package and on the pads themselves (just as pads used for transcutaneous pacing have their location noted). The pads are placed in the same locations as for manual

Best Practice

Decisions Involving Resuscitative Care

The bottom line is delivering the best patient care possible. Who actually delivers the care or who determines the appropriate care to give is not important. If a therapist knows the right thing to do, then the therapist can help the patient achieve a better outcome (live rather than die). Never be hesitant to make suggestions or to voice an opinion.

For example, the respiratory therapist arrives at a code that has just been called. Moving to the head of the bed to ventilate, he discovers that the floor nurses have already attached the patient to a monitor, which is showing v-tach. The patient's nurse confirms that the patient has no pulse. There is no coronary certified nurse on the scene yet; the hospital does not credential respiratory therapists to perform defibrillation. The medical resident has just walked into the room. What is the appropriate treatment right now? Of course, it is defibrillation. The therapist quickly summarizes the situation to the resident ("We have an unresponsive, apneic, pulseless woman in v-tach who needs to be defibrillated") and asks the nurses to find the gel pads for the defibrillator. The therapist has expedited the delivery of the appropriate treatment to this patient, possibly saving her life. If the therapist knew nothing about ACLS, he would have simply continued to ventilate or perform compressions.

Spotlight On

Automatic External Defibrillation

An automatic external defibrillator (AED) is a device that requires minimal training to operate. The operator does not have to know how to interpret an EKG (although some have EKG display screens). The device actually talks the operator through the proper sequence of actions (Figure 31-10).

defibrillation, that is, to the right of the sternum and at the apex of the heart; they can also be placed anteriorly and posteriorly.

- A towel, a razor, a pair of gloves, and a pocket mask should be included in the AED kit. The towel is used to dry off the wet or diaphoretic victim; the razor is used to shave the chest if necessary. An alternative to shaving (assuming there is more than one set of electrodes) is to place one set of electrodes firmly on the chest and then forcefully remove them, thus removing the hair. (Good skin contact is important to avoid arcing and possible skin burns. Most people have seen a patient after a resuscitation with paddle-shaped burns on the chest.) The adhesive pads achieve energy delivery comparable to handheld paddles without the pressure because these pads are flexible and the entire surface is sticky. The pads therefore can contact a larger surface area than the metal paddles can.

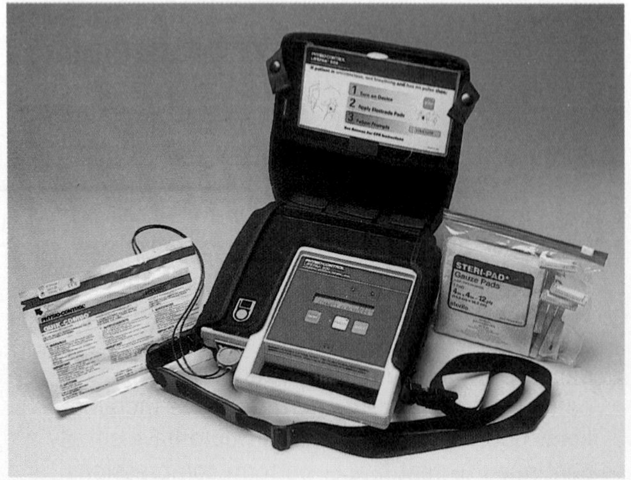

FIGURE 31-10 An automated external defibrillator (AED).

Sequence of Operation.

- The AED should now be turned on. (Some AEDs automatically turn on when the cover is raised.) At this point, the victim needs to be completely still; the AED cannot analyze the rhythm if the patient is moving. (CPR must be stopped or, if the patient is in the back of an ambulance, the vehicle must be pulled off the road and stopped.)
- Depending on the model, the AED may automatically go into analyze mode, or the rescuer may have to push the "Analyze" button.
- The AED responds to only one of two rhythms, VF or v-tach, usually with a rate of >150. If either of these rhythms are present, the AED usually makes a decision quickly. A long pause after the AED begins analyzing the rhythm usually indicates that the rhythm is not treatable with defibrillation. If the AED decides it is a defibrillatable rhythm, it begins to charge. Once charged, it indicates "Shock Advised—Push Button to Shock." Some completely automatic models analyze, charge, and defibrillate without any action by the operator, but these are in the minority.
- Just as with a manual defibrillator, the operator should chant "I'm clear! You're clear! We're all clear! Shocking," while scanning the victim to ensure no one is in direct contact before defibrillating. If the victim is on metal seats (such as at a stadium), the rest of the people in that row should be asked to stand during defibrillation.
- Once the shock is delivered, the rescuers should immediately begin CPR for another 5 cycles. The AED will time this and inform the rescuers when 2 minutes have elapsed.
- This sequence of CPR-rhythm evaluation-defibrillation continues as long as the victim remains in v-tach or VF; a nondefibrillatable rhythm may be NSR, v-tach with a slow rate, asystole, or indeed any rhythm but VF or v-tach. Return of spontaneous circulation (ROSC) is the best indication to stop AED use. However, the pads should remain in place as the therapist continues to monitor the pulse in case defibrillation becomes necessary again.

American Heart Association AED Initiative. The American Heart Association has a major initiative to increase awareness and use of AEDs by people who are not medically trained. The first-priority group consists of people such as police officers, firefighters, personnel in sports stadiums, and managers of large apartment buildings who are likely to come across job situations in which there is need to defibrillate. Next in line are people with relatives who have conditions that might result in the need for defibrillation. (Unfortunately, the literature does not demonstrate increased survival among those with home defibrillators.) Ultimately, the AHA vision is that an AED will be located anywhere there is a fire extinguisher or telephone. The reason is that the two most important determinants of survival in adult cardiac arrest are time to CPR and time to defibrillation. The success rate for defibrillation is 90% after 1 minute, but it falls to zero after about 10 minutes. Thus, speed is of the essence in determining the need for defibrillation and actually defibrillating.

AEDs also clearly have a place in the hospital. One may question the wisdom of buying *more* defibrillators when every crash cart has one and people are around who can use them. Think about the sequence of events during a cardiac arrest in the hospital outside the critical care units. A nurse who finds a patient in cardiac arrest must alert someone to page a code. That person calls the code phone number, and the operator then pages the code team. When their beepers sound, the members of the code team (including the CCU or ICU nurse) must stop whatever they are doing and get to the location of the arrest. Thus, several minutes have elapsed before someone who is credentialed to operate the manual defibrillator arrives, significantly lowering the chances for a successful defibrillation.

The timing is very different with an AED at the nursing station and all nurses trained to use it (about a 2-hour class for people with medical backgrounds). Upon discovering a patient in full cardiac arrest, the nurse shouts for someone to bring the AED. After delivering 5 cycles of 30 compressions and 2 breaths, the nursing staff can deliver the first (and possibly only) shock. With the cost of AEDs falling, it is only a matter of time before they will appear at general nursing stations. Presently, many manual monitor/defibrillators are able to function in AED mode. Thus, there does not have to be a separate AED purchased.

One place where AEDs have special significance is aboard an airplane. If a passenger suffers a full cardiac arrest while on an airplane, landing is not even an option as far as treatment goes. It could take as long as a half hour under the best of circumstances before the plane arrives at the gate of an airport. More airlines are placing AEDs on their planes as time passes. (Qantas was the first; American, Hawaiian, and Air Zimbabwe, among others, also have them.)

DEFIBRILLATION

Defibrillation was briefly described in the scenario of the patient in persistent VF. The therapist can determine the patient's initial rhythm in one of two ways: Attach the electrodes as was done in the scenario or use the paddles for a so-called quick look. It is better to attach the standard monitoring electrodes first rather than acquiring the EKG through the paddles for three reasons.

- First, it is easy to forget to switch from paddles back to lead II and think the patient is in asystole, thus not defibrillating the patient at the earliest possible time.
- Second, the electrodes are needed anyway, and attaching them takes only a few seconds.
- Last, with the high epinephrine level in the therapist's blood due to the excitement of the situation, some muscle tremor may result, which mimics v-fib on the monitor.

If the therapist decides to use the paddles:

- The lead selector switch on the monitor/defibrillator is set on "Paddles."
- The paddles are applied to the patient's chest with good pressure over gel pads and the rhythm is analyzed. If it is VF or v-tach, defibrillation can be carried out immediately.

Enhancing Conduction. To achieve good contact with the patient's chest and to avoid burns to the skin, the therapist should use something to enhance conduction between the paddles and the skin. Probably the messiest is *electrode cream* applied to the paddles. The downside of using electrode cream is that the patient's chest is very slippery following application of the paddles, and performing compressions is difficult unless the chest is wiped off, further delaying the resumption of compressions.

Next in terms of convenience is *saline-soaked 4 × 4s*. Their advantages are:

- They are not slippery.
- They cling to the chest wall.
- The ingredients are readily available everywhere in the hospital and are inexpensive.

They do tend to leak saline, however.

Last on the list of conduction enhancers are *gel pads*. They are probably the most expensive conduction enhancement but the most convenient. They cling to the thorax, are not slippery, and do not drip.

Hands-Off Versus Paddles. The other decision in defibrillation is whether to use hands-off versus using paddles. Everyone is familiar with the paddles the rescuer holds on the victim's chest (with 25 pounds of pressure). The rescuer presses the buttons on the paddles to discharge them for either cardioversion or defibrillation. The major danger with this technique is electric shock, and the operator is the one most likely to be shocked. There is special danger if the therapy is performed in a moving ambulance because the ambulance could lurch in an unpredictable way, throwing the rescuer into contact with the metal stretcher frame.

To obviate some of the danger of using the paddles for electrical therapy, use the hands-off technique. For this technique, the rescuer needs to connect the pads to the monitor/defibrillator in the receptacle where the paddles are connected.

- The electrodes are placed on the patient's thorax, either to the right of the sternum (about at the middle) and at the apex (in the midaxillary line on the lower third of the thorax) or anterior and posterior. The pads and the foil package in which the pads come both have line drawings showing the proper placement of the pads.
- Defibrillation or cardioversion is then accomplished by pressing the button on the monitor/defibrillator at a safe distance from the patient. The rescuer still chants "I'm clear! You're clear! We're all clear! Shocking!" and scans the patient for anyone who is not paying attention.

Conscious Sedation. As in the case of tachycardia, some procedures (which include cardioversion and transcutaneous pacing as well as bronchoscopy) require conscious sedation. This involves administering drugs to provide:

- Pain relief—generally narcotics such as morphine sulfate or fentanyl.
- And sedation—generally benzodiazepines such as Versed (midazolam) or Ativan (alprazolam) or as an alternative Diprivan (propofol) are used while maintaining the patient in an arousable state. Benzodiazepines are also amnesiacs so the conscious patient will not remember the cardioversion.

This state is specifically differentiated from general anesthesia, in which the patient is unconscious and pain free. During the administration of conscious sedation, the respiratory therapist must monitor the patient; the key phrase is patient *assessment*. The person monitoring the patient should have no other responsibilities, including delivering electrical therapy or assisting during bronchoscopy. Especially during electrical therapy, adverse changes in the patient's cardiovascular system may occur, and the RT needs to be prepared to intubate. The intubation equipment should be readily at hand; no one should have to look for it.

- The most important functions to monitor are airway, breathing, and circulation (as always).
- Pulse oximetry gives the therapist a pulse indication as well as oxygenation monitoring.
- Heart rate and blood pressure should be monitored every 5 minutes.
- Finally, at least one EKG lead should be displayed, preferably lead II, which provides the best P-waves (lead II is the difference between the right arm and the left leg). An alternative is V_1, modified V_1, or MCL_1 (modified chest lead 1)—all different names for the same chest or precordial lead. These chest leads use the V_1 position as the positive electrode (located in the fourth intercostal space just to the right of the sternum) with one of the other electrodes as the negative. This chest lead similarly gives the best P-waves as does lead II of the precordial leads.
- Monitoring level of consciousness or responsiveness also enhances the clinical picture.

Of course, this whole scenario assumes that the hospital permits the therapist to administer these kinds of drugs and intubate. Such authorization requires a number of factors. First is state licensure (everywhere but Alaska) that allows the therapist to administer these drugs under the respiratory therapy scope of practice. Next is a medical director who is supportive of the enhanced responsibilities. Very importantly, the department leader must embrace these activities. Then the staff have to be willing to learn new duties and be eager to expand their responsibilities. Lastly, the medical board must be forward thinking enough to entrust such advanced duties to respiratory therapists.

Pediatric Advanced Life Support

An important age-specific competency for respiratory therapists is **pediatric advanced life support (PALS)**. The basic concept of PALS is stated in the old saying that "children are not just little adults." For instance, a fluid challenge for an adult is typically 250–500 mL, which turns out to be about 3–6 mL/kg; that for a child is 20 mL/kg.

BROSELOW TAPE

One piece of essential equipment for use in pediatric resuscitation is the *Broselow tape*. The therapist measures the supine victim from crown to heel with the tape. Based on where the victim's height falls on the tape, the RT can read precalculated drug doses and the size of endotracheal tube and suction catheter. These values are calculated based on the 50th percentile for weight based on height in a population of 20,000 children. Use of this tape can bring order to the determination of drug dosages and tube sizes in pediatrics.

There is no good ALS without good BLS. So the first requirement of PALS, just as in ACLS, is that the participants can perform excellent BLS, especially ventilation with bag and mask. Refer to the beginning of this chapter with age-specific competencies for specifics on child (age 1–8 years) and infant (age less than 1 year) BLS, including relief of foreign body airway obstruction.

INITIAL PATIENT ASSESSMENT AND PREVENTION

As in many situations, the prevention of respiratory or cardiac arrest is preferable to the need for resuscitation once the child has arrested. The basic preventive measure is assessing the patient for the signs and symptoms of impending respiratory failure and circulatory shock and initiating the appropriate treatments. The therapist should look at:

- *General appearance.* Does the child appear comfortable or ill, active or flaccid?
- *Respiratory rate.* A rate over 60 is always abnormal; irregular respirations are also a poor sign. Tachypnea relative to the age group may be the first sign of respiratory distress. A rate below 10 in an ill or injured child is a poor prognostic sign.
- *Skin color and temperature.* The skin should be pink, warm, and dry. Pallor, mottling, or cyanosis (also of mucus membranes) or a fall in oxyhemoglobin saturation indicates inadequate oxygen delivery, blood flow, or both. Diaphoresis is indicative of sympathetic discharge in cardiovascular emergencies.
- *Evidence of increased respiratory effort.* Nasal flaring, grunting, use of accessory muscles, tracheal tug, and intercostal and suprasternal retractions all indicate increased respiratory effort.
- *Connection with environment.* The child should regard the speaker when addressed and, if old enough, respond to questions. Infants may be looking around and babbling and cooing. Unusual irritability or lethargy or the failure to respond to painful procedures are poor signs in the infant.
- *Adequacy of tidal volume.* Inspection and auscultation should reveal subjectively sufficient movement of the thorax with each breath.
- *Rate and quality of peripheral pulses.* The rate for the awake infant or child should be age specific within normal limits: up to 3 months, 85–205/minute; 3 months to 2 years, 100–190/minute; 2–10 years, 60–140/minute. Pulses should be readily palpable.
- *Capillary refill.* This should be less than 2 seconds in a warm environment and extremities should be warm.
- *Urine output (if available).* This should be 1–2 mL/kg/hr.
- *Blood pressure.* Systolic should be age specific within normal limits: 0–1 month, 60 mm Hg; 1 month–1 year, 70 mm Hg; 1–10 years, 90 + (2 × age in years).
- *Level of consciousness (LOC).* The LOC can rapidly be determined by the AVPU scale (**A**lert, responds to **V**oice, responds to **P**ain, **U**nresponsive).

This whole evaluation should take only a minute or so.

Should the rapid assessment reveal problems, treatment needs to be quickly initiated.

- If the therapist determines that the child is in *possible respiratory failure,* the child should be allowed to assume a position of comfort with a caregiver. Repositioning minimizes oxygen demand and helps in maintaining the airway. Oxygen should also be provided as tolerated, monitored with pulse oximetry.
- If the therapist determines that *respiratory failure is probable,* the child should be removed from the caregiver, the airway secured, and ventilation assisted with 100% oxygen. In addition, cardiac monitoring should be initiated and vascular access obtained.
- If the child is in *shock,* either compensated or decompensated, the therapist should ensure an adequate airway, ventilate with 100% oxygen, obtain vascular access, and provide volume expansion. Vasoactive drugs may be necessary.

FLUID THERAPY AND DRUGS

Vascular access is necessary as part of most resuscitations for the delivery of fluids for volume resuscitation, drugs or both. The routes for administering drugs can be a central vein, peripheral vein, intraosseous, or endotracheal. In a child younger than 6 years old, the therapist should not waste time establishing a peripheral vascular line if access is difficult. An intraosseous line can be used for administration of anything deliverable via intravenous line, including volume replacement, because blood from the bone marrow of the tibia passes into the central circulation via the popliteal vein.

Fluids for resuscitation are normal saline or lactated Ringer's solution. Unless hypoglycemia has been determined, solutions containing glucose are not appropriate due to an association between hyperglycemia and poor neurologic outcome. When vascular access cannot be immediately obtained, drugs that can be delivered via the endotracheal tube indicated by the mnemonic LEAN (or LANE).

Drugs other than epinephrine are given much less frequently during pediatric resuscitation.

- Atropine is useful in symptomatic bradycardia.
- Narcan (naloxone) is given for the infant with respiratory depression caused by narcotics. The clinician should be aware that naloxone has a shorter half-life than narcotics, so one may need to repeat its administration.
- Sodium bicarbonate should be given only later in the resuscitation, once adequate ventilation is established with documented severe metabolic acidosis, hyperkalemia, or tricyclic antidepressant overdose. (Contrast this to the situation 25 years ago when sodium bicarbonate was routinely given every 5 minutes during an arrest.)
- Calcium used to be administered after every other drug had been given during a resuscitation without effect. Now, calcium is given *only* for documented hypocalcemia, hypermagnesemia, hyperkalemia, or calcium channel blocker overdose.

Shock: A Flow Definition. Adequate perfusion to the body relies on three things:

- A *pump* that can supply adequate flow, because cardiac output is never great enough to supply everywhere simultaneously.
- A *vascular bed* that is able to change size to allocate blood flow.
- Sufficient fluid (*blood*) to fill the system.

Every type of shock causes a problem with one (or more) of these conditions. For example:

- Cardiogenic shock involves a malfunctioning pump.
- Septic shock results from the inability of the body to constrict the arterioles to allocate blood flow.
- Hypovolemic shock results from insufficient blood volume to fill the vascular space due to excessive blood or fluid loss.

The human body has no flow sensors in the vascular system; the sensors are baroreceptors or pressure sensors. The priority of the system is to maintain arterial pressure to perfuse the circulations that matter the most: the brain and the heart. Because both organs extract a large amount of oxygen from the blood passing by, maintaining pressure is of paramount importance in the continued performance of both organs. However, in shock, perfusion is inadequate. In the infancy of critical care, practitioners thought that, since the body worked to maintain pressure, so should they. However, when the body has already effected significant vasoconstriction, adding vasoconstrictors is detrimental in two ways:

- Although arterial pressure may actually increase, the net effect on the patient's condition is negligible.
- The increase in systemic vascular resistance (SVR) may actually decrease cardiac output because an overloaded heart is unable to eject blood against the increased afterload.

Thus, clinicians sometimes tread a fine line between maintaining sufficient pressure to perfuse the cerebral and coronary circulations adequately while maintaining flow to the remainder of the organs, which are sensitive to ischemia in varying degrees.

In treating any type of shock, the first priority is to be sure that "the tank is filled"—that there is enough fluid (blood) to circulate. This is especially true in septic shock, in which volume expansion is the first-line therapy. In children and infants, the tank can be relatively large. As noted, the fluid challenge for a child is 3–6 times that of an adult (on a weight basis, 20 mL/kg as opposed to 3–6 mL/kg). Children who are very hypovolemic or in severe septic shock may need more than 60 mL/kg. The clinician must be sure that sufficient volume is on board (the patient is *euvolemic*).

At that point, the clinician may start thinking about positive inotropes, of which three are commonly used. Once their use has been optimized, it is time for vasopressors as a last resort.

Epinephrine may be the inotrope or vasopressor of choice in several clinical circumstances. It is useful in symptomatic bradycardia, anaphylactic shock, hypotension, and cardiac arrest. Its use may be limited by the development of tachycardia or tachydysrhythmias. At doses less than 0.3 μg/min, it is primarily a positive inotrope; at higher doses, the vasoconstrictor effect predominates.

Dobutamine is useful in the child in cardiogenic shock with normal blood pressure. Its vasodilatory effects may cause a fall in blood pressure or failure to increase an already low pressure. Its dosage range is from 2–10 μg/kg/min. *Dopamine* at low doses (2 μg/kg/min) increases renal and splanchnic flow; at high doses ($>$ 10 μg/kg/min), it is a vasoconstrictor. In the middle range (2–10 μg/kg/min) it adds positive inotropy to the increased renal blood flow. Because it causes the release of endogenous catecholamines, it may not work in the patient who is in chronic congestive heart failure (CHF) or shock. The clinician would see this if a dose of $>$ 20 μg/kg/min has no effect. In this case, epinephrine is the better choice.

RESUSCITATING THE NEWBORN OUTSIDE THE DELIVERY ROOM

Everything else being equal, it is best to resuscitate newborns in the delivery suite, where all the equipment and people with special skills in this area reside. However, from time to time, a newborn needs to be resuscitated in other venues. As an example, the pregnant mother in her third trimester who is in the intensive care unit gives birth unexpectedly. The objectives for infant resuscitation, regardless of where it takes place, are to:

- Eliminate preventable morbidity.
- Restore effective ventilation, perfusion, and oxygenation.
- Maintain body heat by reducing heat loss to the environment (a major consideration in the newborn).

Maintaining a neutral thermal environment is of paramount importance in resuscitating the newborn for two reasons:

- Neonates are wet when born, and the wetness enhances evaporative cooling.
- Neonates have a large surface area-to-volume ratio, which enhances radiation cooling.

If a radiant warmer is not available, the therapist can use warmed towels, aluminum foil, or warmed IV bags (there is always a microwave around) wrapped in towels. It should go without saying that all involved in a neonatal resuscitation should observe standard precautions during the entire procedure. As in many situations, it pays to be prepared. Before it is needed, equipment for neonatal resuscitation should be gathered and conveniently organized. Part of preparation is anticipating the situations in which resuscitation might be expected. For a list of such situations, see Table 31-3.

Directed History. The respiratory therapist should obtain a directed resuscitation-oriented history. Four items may affect the initial resuscitation:

- Is the infant premature? Immature lungs increase the likelihood that resuscitation will be needed.
- Are there multiple fetuses? These will require multiple resuscitation teams.
- Has the mother received narcotics in the last 4 hours? The administration of narcotics raises the likelihood of respiratory depression in the newborn.
- Is the amniotic fluid meconium-stained? The newborn will require rapid suctioning to remove meconium from the airway.

Initial Interventions. An inverted pyramid, proceeding from basic to advanced, illustrates the relative

TABLE 31-3 **Risk factors indicating potential need for neonatal resuscitation**

Antepartum Factors
Mother's age > 35 years
Post-term gestation
Maternal diabetes
Multiple gestation
Pregnancy-induced hypertension
Pre-eclampsia
Size-dates discrepancy
Chronic hypertension
Anemia or isoimmunization
Previous fetal or neonatal death
Drug therapy such as:
Lithium carbonate
Magnesium
Adrenergic blocking drugs
Bleeding in second or third trimester
Maternal infection
Maternal substance abuse
Hydramnios
Fetal malformation
Oligohydramnios
Diminished fetal activity
Premature rupture of membranes
No prenatal care
Intrapartum Factors
Emergency cesarean section
Nonreassuring fetal heart patterns
Breech or other abnormal presentation
Use of general anesthesia
Prolonged rupture of membranes (more than 24 hours before delivery)
Narcotics administered to mother within 4 hours of delivery
Precipitous labor
Meconium-stained amniotic fluid
Prolonged labor (more than 24 hours)
Prolapsed umbilical cord
Prolonged second stage of labor (more than 2 hours)
Abruptio placenta
Placenta previa

frequency with which interventions are needed in resuscitating neonates.

- Starting at the top of the pyramid, every newborn needs to be dried and warmed.
- Next, the infant should be positioned supine with the head in a neutral position. (Hyperextension of the neck can result in occlusion of the airway.) This position can be achieved by placing a towel or blanket to elevate the torso 0.5 inch.
- Finally, the therapist should stimulate the infant, beginning with gentle flicking of the soles or gently rubbing the back. In most cases, there should be a vigorous response from the neonate (crying).
- If the infant is breathing adequately but cyanotic, the respiratory therapist should administer blow-by oxygen.
- If, on the other hand, the infant is not breathing adequately or at all, has a heart rate <100, or remains cyanotic despite oxygen administration, the therapist should immediately begin bag-mask ventilation. A rate of 40–60 per minute should be used, with assessment of efforts by the adequacy of chest expansion, the presence of good bilateral breath sounds, and improvement in heart rate and color.
- If there is no improvement in the infant's condition after a brief trial, then it is time to intubate.

Next down the pyramid is chest compressions.

- Once adequate bag-mask ventilation is established and done for about 30 seconds, the therapist determines the need for circulatory assistance. Frequently, the infant heart rate increases with good ventilation.
- However, if the heart rate is less than 60 or is 60–80 with no increase (see neonatal normals for heart rate), then the respiratory therapist begins compressions. The complete absence of a pulse is not necessary. The neonatal heart is relatively unable to increase its stroke volume; cardiac output is therefore very much dependent on rate.
- The compressions should be performed with two thumbs with the hands encircling the chest at a rate of 120 per minute, with ventilations interspersed at a ratio of 3:1.
- Once the heart rate rises above 80 per minute, compressions can be stopped.

In contrast to adult resuscitation, neonatal resuscitation depends mostly on adequate ventilation. The only drug routinely used is epinephrine. Epinephrine can be given via the IV, endotracheal tube (ETT), or intraosseous route (IO). (See Table 31-4 for doses of these drugs.) Bicarbonate is used to adjust acid-base status once the infant has stabilized. Another "medication" is volume expanders, either normal saline or blood.

Once the neonate has been stabilized, the therapist continues to monitor the newborn's condition. Four problems, indicated by the mnemonic DOPE, can cause subsequent deterioration in the resuscitated infant:

- Displaced endotracheal tube (This is easy to do with such a short trachea; simply moving from full flexion to full extension may displace the tube.)
- Obstructed endotracheal tube
- Pneumothorax (from overzealous ventilation)
- Equipment failure

In addition, the therapist should be on the lookout for gastric distension (almost guaranteed after positive pressure ventilation with a mask) and inadequate ventilatory support (it is easy to become complacent, but vigilant monitoring must be continuous).

This is now the time for a more complete evaluation of the neonate.

- A chest X-ray after the intubation
- Routine lab studies, especially glucose
- Maintenance of the neutral thermal environment
- Determination and adjustment of acid-base status

CARDIAC RHYTHM DISTURBANCES

Rhythm changes are not the usual primary cause of cardiac arrest in neonates. Most cardiac arrests are the result of hypoxia, acidosis, or both, and they are secondary to ventilatory problems. The first decision is whether the neonate is stable or unstable. A neonate is

TABLE 31-4 **Drugs most commonly used in neonatal resuscitation**

Drug	Classification	Action	Dose
Epinephrine	Sympathomimetic	$\alpha\ \beta_1,\ \beta_2$ stimulator	*Initial dose:* IV/IO: 0.01 mg/kg ET: 0.1 mg/kg, *Subsequent doses:* IV/IO/ET: 0.1 mg/kg
Bicarbonate	Alkalinizing agent	Buffers acids	1–2 mEq/kg only for prolonged resuscitation

unstable if he or she has a rhythm either that may deteriorate to cause shock or that is actually causing shock (either compensated or decompensated) or circulatory arrest. To keep things simple, these unstable rhythms fall into one of three categories:

- Bradyarrhythmias if they are too slow
- Tachyarrhythmias if they are too fast
- Collapse rhythms if there is cardiac arrest (anything with no pulse)

Because cardiac output in neonates is very rate dependent, the bradycardia simply does not provide a sufficient number of stroke volumes per minute for adequate cardiac output. The tachycardia interferes with ventricular filling by shortening diastole too much, resulting in a decreased stroke volume.

Treatment options for pediatric patients are relatively simple.

For the tachycardia with a narrow QRS:

Vagal maneuvers should initially be considered but should not delay other treatment.

- Adenosine is the drug of first choice at 0.1 mg/kg with the maximum dose of 6 mg. Adenosine should be delivered by rapid push immediately followed by a rapid flush of 5–10 mL NS. A second dose is given at 0.2 mg/kg, with the maximum dose 12 mg.
- If there is a regular monomorphic wide-complex tachycardia (possibly ventricular tachycardia), the therapist should first administer adenosine at the doses given above for a narrow-complex tachycardia. Should that fail, expert consultation is advised; drugs potentially administered are *either* amiodarone at a dose of 5 mg/kg over 20–60 minutes **or** procainamide15 mg/kg over 30–60 minutes.

Age-Specific Competency

ECGs in Neonatal/Pediatric Arrhythmias

A tachyarrhythmia with a narrow complex is likely to be either sinus tachycardia or supraventricular tachycardia. Using the rate as an initial guide, the rate for a sinus tachycardia is likely to be less than 220 for an infant and 180 for a child. Also, variability in R-R interval is more likely in sinus tachycardia, although at these high rates the variability may be difficult to discern without the use of calipers. A wide complex tachycardia is almost always ventricular in origin in children (as opposed to a supraventricular tachycardia with aberrant conduction in adults).

(*Note:* These two drugs should not routinely be administered together.)

- Should these treatments fail to convert the rhythm, synchronized cardioversion is the next step.

For symptomatic bradycardia:

- Epinephrine is the drug of first choice. The RT must remember to treat the patient, not the monitor. The rate, whether fast or slow, is not as important as its effect.
- The next drug for children is atropine. Atropine must be pushed rapidly, or its administration may result in a paradoxical slowing of heart rate.

(Refer to Table 31-4 for drug dosages.)

The group of collapse rhythms consists of asystole, VF, pulseless v-tach, and pulseless electrical activity (PEA), formerly called electromechanical dissociation).

In the case of collapse rhythms, the priorities are:

- Initiating chest compressions.
- Securing the airway and insuring adequate ventilation.
- Obtaining vascular access, either IV or IO.
- Giving epinephrine every 3–5 minutes.

Treatment for ventricular fibrillation is parallel to that for adults.

First, 5 cycles of 30 compressions to 2 ventilations for one rescuer or a ratio of 15:2 for two rescuers

- An initial shock, with 2 joules/kg, 4 joules/kg for the second one, and subsequent shocks at >4 joules/kg up to 10 joules/kg or adult dose. As with adults, each defibrillation is immediately followed by 5 cycles of compressions and ventilations.
- Epinephrine, given to everyone in cardiac arrest, at a dose of 0.01 mg/kg IV/IO or 0.1 mg/kg down the endotracheal tube if there is no IV/IO access.
- If v-tach or v-fib persists, amiodarone is the next drug, given as a bolus of 5 mg/kg; it may be repeated twice more if v-tach or VF persists. Lidocaine is an alternative antiarrhythmic drug.
- Defibrillate between each drug administration. Be sure to perform 2 minutes of CPR after each defibrillation before assessing rhythm.
- If ventricular fibrillation or ventricular tachycardia recurs after resuscitation, a lidocaine drip may be started. If a dose has not been given in 15 minutes, the therapist should administer a loading dose of 1 mg/kg and then start a drip of 20–50 μg/kg/min.

For PEA, the treatment runs exactly parallel to that for an adult. The therapist:

- Starts compressions, intubates the trachea, and secures vascular access.
- Gives epinephrine every 3–5 minutes (although most clinicians lean toward 3-minute intervals).
- Investigates and treats possible causes. (See the list under asystole for adults.)

PEDIATRIC TRAUMA

"Injury is the leading cause of death and disability in children" (AHA PALS Instructor Manual, 2010). Having a system already in place for handling trauma cases improves outcomes.

Boys are injured more often than girls. The average pediatric trauma patient is 7 years old and weighs about 50 pounds. Head injuries account for nearly 6 out of 10 cases, with injuries to extremities following at

CASE STUDY 31-3

A 2-year-old boy, weighing about 12 kg, has just been removed from a pond in front of his grandparents' house after an unknown immersion time. He is unresponsive, apneic, and pulseless. An advanced life support ambulance is requested via the 911 system. The grandfather initiates CPR in a somewhat clumsy fashion. A neighbor who is a nurse hears the grandmother's cries and responds, beginning effective CPR.

The ambulance arrives after 5 minutes and applies monitor electrodes; the initial rhythm is asystole. One paramedic intubates the child with a 4.5-mm endotracheal tube. The second searches for a vein and readily acquires intravenous access via an antecubital vein. They give an initial dose of epinephrine. Within a minute, there is an organized rhythm with narrow complexes accompanied by a faint pulse. The paramedics administer a saline bolus of 240 mL (20 mL/kg), which results in a stronger pulse. The rhythm is now clearly sinus tachycardia with a rate of 130. The child, unfortunately, responds only to painful stimuli presently. He is cut out of his wet clothes, dried, and wrapped in blankets. He is placed in a heated ambulance and transported to the regional pediatric specialty hospital. He receives an additional 240 mL fluid bolus in response to another dip in systolic blood pressure. By arrival at the hospital, he is beginning to take a few spontaneous breaths but still responds only to painful stimuli.

The paramedics report to the hospital staff, who congratulate them on a successful textbook resuscitation.

Caregivers at the hospital should:

- Start with ABCs, just as the paramedics did.
- Confirm the proper tube position by clinical criteria (breath sounds, bilateral chest expansion, good color, tube taped at the appropriate level).
- Order a chest X-ray.
- Monitor with pulse oximetry and vital signs.
- Because *any* ventilation using a mask or mouth-to-mouth insufflates gas into the stomach, place a nasogastric or orogastric tube to decompress the stomach and facilitate ventilation.
- Continue monitoring cardiac rhythm—an important part of this child's care.
- Order an arterial blood gas to determine acid-base status and adequacy of ventilation.
- Place the child on mechanical ventilation, beginning with A/C (or whatever mode is most familiar) with 90% oxygen, a rate of 20, 4 cm H_2O PEEP, and a tidal volume of 100 mL (8 mL/kg) and adjusted as appropriate.
- Determine whether they will need to sedate this child to ventilate him appropriately.
- Send blood off for a complete blood count (CBC) and basic electrolyte panel (including sodium, potassium, chloride, total CO_2, BUN, creatinine, and, especially important in children, glucose).

Because this child will likely require critical care for a period of time, additional vascular access is appropriate via a large line, either peripheral or central.

Questions

1. What is the usual cause for cardiac arrest in children? How does this differ from the cause in adults?
2. What effect does water immersion have on outcome?
3. What additional considerations must be addressed for this victim of near drowning?

1 out of 4 (AHA PALS Instructor Manual, 2007). The two main reasons children die after traumatic events are airway compromise and unrecognized bleeding.

Three injuries can affect priorities in resuscitating the injured child: potential cervical spine injuries, hemorrhage, and chest trauma. Initially, a rapid survey of the ABCs should be done. D should be added for disability (rapid neurologic evaluation, such as Glasgow Coma Scale), and E should be added for exposure (maintenance of body heat). A secondary survey covers head to toe once the therapist has dealt with the things discovered in the primary survey that can rapidly lead to death if not treated.

Neurologic Evaluation. The respiratory therapist should be familiar two methods of neurological evaluation: the AVPU scale (discussed earlier in this chapter) and the Glasgow Coma Scale. The Glasgow Coma Scale (Figure 31-11) enables the therapist to hone in more closely on the exact level of neurological function. The total possible score ranges from 3, representing the unconscious unresponsive person to 15, which is normal. Some clinicians suggest that the totals for each section should be specified if the value is less than 15 to provide even more detail.

Fluid Resuscitation. The therapist should also be familiar with fluid resuscitation for the child in hemorrhagic shock. The estimated circulating volume for a child is 80 mL/kg, slightly more than the 70 mL/kg used for estimating circulating volume in an adult.

- Fluid boluses are given at 20 mL/kg of crystalloid, or roughly 25% of the circulating volume.
- After reassessment, this may be done two more times.
- Plan on replacing lost blood with crystalloids at a 3:1 ratio because only about one-third of crystalloids remains in the vascular space.
- After three 20-mL/kg boluses, if further fluid resuscitation is necessary, consider packed red blood cells, initially 10 mL/kg and then 20 mL/kg if further volume is needed. (Remember that normal saline has very little oxygen-carrying capacity compared to any fluid containing red blood cells.)

Eye Opening	Spontaneous	4
	To voice	3
	To pain	2
	None	1
Verbal Response	Oriented	5
	Confused	4
	Inappropriate words	3
	Incomprehensible words	2
	None	1
Motor Response	Obeys commands	6
	Localizes pain	5
	Withdraws to pain	4
	Flexion to pain	3
	Extension to pain	2
	None	1

FIGURE 31-11 Glasgow Coma Scale.

Neonatal Resuscitation Program

The **neonatal resuscitation program (NRP)** is a joint effort of the American Academy of Pediatrics and the American Heart Association. The NRP textbook is actually a self-learning text, with clear objectives at the beginning of each of the six lessons and quizzes as the learner progresses through each chapter. Therapists who feel they are conversant with the material covered in any given chapter can simply proceed to the quizzes for self-evaluation. However, the text clearly states that the successful completion of the course does not imply that the therapist is competent in neonatal resuscitation. Supervised clinical experience (a preceptorship) is needed before actually taking sole responsibility for any component of a neonatal resuscitation.

PRIMARY VERSUS SECONDARY APNEA

Neonatal apnea is a primary cause for neonatal resuscitation. Two types of apnea are seen in newborns: primary and secondary.

- The infant in *primary apnea* may initiate adequate spontaneous ventilation with just stimulation and exposure to supplemental oxygen.
- The neonate in *secondary apnea* has already progressed through primary apnea and is showing a fall in heart rate, blood pressure, and oxygen saturation. Unless ventilation is promptly initiated, the infant in secondary apnea will continue to rapidly spiral down to death.

There are two complications, however: First, the infant may progress through primary apnea in utero and be in secondary apnea at birth. Second, clinically differentiating between primary and secondary apnea can be difficult. Therefore, the therapist should assume the worst and immediately begin aggressive resuscitation measures. Should the infant respond and begin spontaneous ventilation, then efforts can be reduced.

CHANGES IN LUNGS AND CIRCULATION AT BIRTH

Major physiologic and anatomic changes occur in the lungs and in the circulation at birth. In utero, the primary gas exchange organ for the fetus is the placenta. The lungs are filled with amniotic fluid and only about 10% of the total cardiac output goes to the lungs to provide for growth and metabolism (as contrasted with 100% after birth). At birth, two changes must occur within the first few breaths.

First, the fluid must be removed from the lungs and be replaced with air. There are three mechanisms for removing the fluid. During the passage through the birth canal, the thorax is squeezed, expelling some of the fluid out the airway. The infant who is born by Cesarean section is therefore denied this mechanism for fluid removal. The rest of the fluid is absorbed and carried away by both the pulmonary lymphatics and the pulmonary circulation, mechanisms two and three.

Second, there must be a significant increase in blood flow through the pulmonary blood vessels. This is accomplished by a significant decrease in the pulmonary vascular resistance (PVR). Again, three factors reduce PVR. First, when the fluid is removed from the lungs, the external pressure on the pulmonary blood vessels is reduced, allowing them to increase in size. Second, the inflation of the previously airless lungs straightens out the pulmonary blood vessels, decreasing their resistance. Finally, the introduction of air into the lungs raises the alveolar PO_2, reversing the hypoxic vasoconstriction. To further ensure two series circuits (the blood passes first through the pulmonary circulation, then the systemic circulation in order), the bypass valves for the pulmonary circulation, must close. The closure of the *ductus arteriosus* is facilitated by the release of bradykinin from the lung with the first breath and also with the increase in P_aO_2. The closure of the *formen ovale,* a one-way flap valve opening from right to left, occurs because left atrial pressure will now exceed right atrial pressure because of the increased blood return to the left atrium from the lungs.

If any of these events does not occur in due course, the infant is unable to transfer enough oxygen from the atmosphere into the blood and becomes progressively asphyxiated. This failure of change mechanisms maintains the fetal circulatory pattern with its resultant insufficient pulmonary circulation. Intervention must be prompt if the infant is to survive.

As in any resuscitation, it pays to be prepared. The equipment and personnel must be in the delivery room at every birth. Once the neonate is born and needs resuscitation, it is too late to assemble the team and the necessary equipment.

The first step in preparation is anticipating the need for resuscitation. Many antepartum and intrapartum factors suggest that the about-to-be-born fetus will need more than the normal care immediately after birth (refer again to Table 31-3). All the necessary equipment must be present *and* operational in the delivery room, with one set of equipment for each neonate anticipated. Someone who is able to perform a complete resuscitation must be present at *every* birth; that person must have no other responsibilities and cannot therefore also care for the mother. As with equipment, there must be at least one resuscitator for each expected birth. When ante- or intrapartum factors suggest the delivery of an asphyxiated infant, at least one team of two persons should be present at the delivery for every infant expected: a deliverer and a resuscitator.

Once the infant is born, the first important need is to *prevent heat loss*. Newborns, especially preterm infants, rapidly lose heat to their surroundings. One reason is that they have relatively little subcutaneous tissue and a thin epidermis. In addition, they have a high ratio of body surface area to mass ratio compared to adults. Finally, as previously mentioned, newborns are wet when born, a condition that accelerates evaporative heat loss. The therapist should place the neonate on a preheated radiant warmer and dry him or her with a warmed towel. This drying provides the added benefit of gentle stimulation, which may begin or help continue respirations.

With the infant dry and under the warmer, positioning is the next important step for facilitating the maintenance of a *patent airway and breathing*. The proper position is on the back (supine) with the neck *slightly* extended. In an adult, maximum hyperextension of the neck is the position for establishing a patent airway. In the infant, however, hyperextension obstructs the airway because of its flexibility. The position of slight extension can be established by placing a small roll under the shoulders to lift the neonate off the mattress about 0.75–1 inch. If there is a large volume of secretions, turn the infant's head to the side.

The next step depends on whether the amniotic fluid is stained with meconium, especially with pieces of meconium, or if the amniotic fluid has the appearance of pea soup. In either case, the deliverer should intubate the infant to remove meconium from the lower airway. If the infant is active, suctioning of the mouth and nose is not recommended.

At this point, there is a major change from normal *suctioning* procedures. Suctioning is usually

Best Practice

Converting from Millimeters to French

A common problem is conversion from millimeters (the normal units for an endotracheal tube inner diameter) to French (the normal units for the outer diameter of suction catheters). The simple rule of thumb is to divide French by 3 to arrive at the actual diameter in millimeters. Thus, our 5 French suction catheter is 5/3 or about 1.67 millimeters in diameter.

accomplished with a catheter passed through the endotracheal tube. For endotracheal tubes less than 4 mm in diameter, the suction catheter should then be 5 French (less than one-half the internal diameter of the endotracheal tube). This is the smallest suction catheter made.

Trying to suction meconium through a small suction catheter is an exercise in futility. A special adapter is placed on the endotracheal tube to connect it to the wall by suction once the infant's trachea has been intubated. The therapist:

- Applies suction as the endotracheal tube is withdrawn.
- Repeats the process of intubating and suctioning until no more meconium is aspirated.
- Inserts the tube and uses a suction catheter to remove any small amount of meconium remaining.

For most infants, suctioning is as far as the interventions go. Nonetheless, the therapist should now proceed with a rapid cardiopulmonary assessment of the infant. The scheme is simple.

- If respirations are inadequate, then ventilation with a manual resuscitator is indicated.
- If respirations appear to be adequate, then the therapist checks the heart rate.
- If the heart rate is less than 100, the RT begins ventilation; if it is greater than 100, the RT assesses color.
- If the neonate is pink, no treatment is indicated. If the neonate has central cyanosis, then oxygen should be administered. It can be given with a simple mask applied to the infant's face or as blow-by with green oxygen tubing held between the thumb and forefinger in a cupped hand. In either case, the flow should be at least 5 Lpm; for this short time, the therapist should not worry about delivering too much oxygen because hypoxia is the worst thing that can happen to the neonate. As the infant's condition improves, the oxygen can be gradually withdrawn.

Should the drying and suctioning (if needed) not provide sufficient tactile stimulation to initiate breathing in the newborn, two other methods of stimulation are recommended. The first is either slapping the sole of the foot with one's hand or flicking the heel with a finger. The second is rubbing the back. These techniques should be done only once or twice; if there is no response, the therapist should start ventilating. Continuing to provide tactile stimulation without any response now simply wastes time and decreases the likelihood of a successful resuscitation.

VENTILATION

Ventilation of the neonate can be accomplished with two different types of devices. One is an anesthesia bag, which requires gas flow to inflate it. The other is a self-inflating resuscitator.

- The *anesthesia bag* should have an initial flow of 5–8 Lpm of oxygen. A pressure manometer helps in judging lung compliance. Many anesthesia bags have a pressure popoff that can be set to limit the pressure delivered to the infant's lungs. Of course, if compliance or resistance changes, then the delivered tidal volume changes too; the RT is delivering manual pressure-cycled ventilation in this case. Thus, the therapist must maintain a good airway by keeping the neonate's head tilted properly, while monitoring ventilation of the infant by chest expansion, color, and adequacy of breath sounds.
- The *self-inflating resuscitator* should have a reservoir to allow delivery of a concentration of oxygen as close to 100% as possible. The therapist is delivering manual volume-cycled ventilation in this case. Changes in compliance or resistance can be monitored by the pressure needed to deliver the tidal volume via the attached manometer. The self-inflating resuscitator also has a popoff valve that is preset, usually to 40 cm H_2O. The therapist needs to pay attention to this to ensure that the infant is being ventilated, not the room. The reality is that it is difficult to hear the popoff amid the noise of the delivery suite. Consequently, the therapist has to keep careful watch on the pressure manometer. If it is indicating the same pressure each time, part of the tidal volume is probably being vented to the room.

For either ventilating device, the interface between the device and the newborn is the mask. A proper size mask covers both the mouth and nose easily. The too-large mask interferes with the neonate's eyes; the too-small mask may not cover the face properly and may even push down on the nose, partially occluding it. Both ventilating units should be checked for proper function before they are needed as follows:

- The *self-inflating resuscitator* should be squeezed once and released, then checked for rapid reinflation. Then, the mask should be blocked with the hand and the bag squeezed again to check both the bag's ability to deliver pressure and also the function of the popoff.
- To check the *anesthesia bag*, turn the flowmeter on to 5–8 L/min, occluding the mask with a hand and ensuring inflation of the bag. Then squeeze the bag to check that the popoff is set to somewhere between 30 and 40 cm H_2O.

Ventilation can now begin. Once the quick check of the ventilation device is performed, ventilate the infant for 15–30 seconds at a rate of 40–60 per minute, watching for the rise and fall of the chest. After this initial period, evaluate the infant's heart rate.

- If it is greater than 100 and the infant has spontaneous respirations, stop ventilation.
- If the heart rate is between 60 and 100 and increasing, continue ventilation.
- If the heart rate is 60–100 and *not* increasing, evaluate what is being done.
  Is the chest rising and are breath sounds good?
  Is the resuscitation device used actually attached to a flowmeter delivering oxygen? (Always check the simple things!)
- If using an anesthesia bag connected to a blender, is the blender set at 100%?
- If the heart rate is less than 80, the therapist should begin chest compressions.
- If the heart rate is less than 60, the therapist should evaluate the preceding items in addition to immediately beginning chest compressions. (Remember that the infant's cardiac output is very rate dependent.)

Most of the time, initial ventilation can be effected with bag and mask. However, if the neonate has a known or suspected congenital diaphragmatic hernia (CDH), the better plan is to intubate the trachea. The reason is that bag-and-mask ventilation invariably results in some amount of insufflation of air into the stomach. If any part of the GI tract is in the thorax, this air further compromises ventilation. In fact, the insufflated gas can impede ventilation of even the normal neonate by:

- Directly forcing the diaphragm up, decreasing lung compliance.
- Moving into the intestines, continuing to apply pressure to the diaphragm.
- Causing gastric contents to be forced into the pharynx, from where they can be aspirated or forced into the lungs.

Thus, *any* infant who is ventilated in this fashion should have an orogastric or nasogastric tube inserted.

CIRCULATION

Once the airway has been opened and ventilation has been ensured, the therapist should, of course, evaluate circulation if this has not already been done. Whereas chest compressions should be performed on adults only in the absence of a pulse, chest compressions should be performed on infants if their heart rate drops below 80 per minute (or is 60–80 per minute and not increasing). (Again, infants depend on heart rate to maintain adequate cardiac output.)

Chest compressions on neonates are preferentially performed by encircling the thorax with both hands with the thumbs on the sternum. Pressure should be delivered to the sternum, not to the ribs. As with any performance of CPR, the person doing compressions should count out loud to allow the one doing ventilation to easily coordinate the ventilation with the compressions.

INTUBATION

The next major step in neonatal resuscitation is intubation of the trachea. For the neonate, there are five indications for endotracheal intubation:

- Ineffective bag-and-mask ventilation
- The need for prolonged positive pressure ventilation
- A known or suspected diaphragmatic hernia
- The need for suctioning of a meconium-stained neonate
- Infants weighing less than 1000 g at birth (due to the very high likelihood they will require positive pressure ventilation)

Prior to intubating, estimate the size tube needed by referring to the chart in Table 31-5. If the therapist opts to use a stylette, a practice that is strongly recommended, it should be secured in the tube so that it does not project beyond the tip and cannot advance any farther during insertion. A straight laryngoscope blade (Miller) is preferred for infants and children for two reasons:

- The epiglottis in an infant and child is longer and floppier than that of the adult. Thus, the use

TABLE 31-5 **Endotracheal tube sizes for neonates**

Tube ID (mm)	Weight (g)	Gestational Age (weeks)	Insertion Depth from Upper Lip (cm)
2.5	<1000	<28	6.5–7
3.0	1000–2000	28–34	7–8
3.5	2000–3000	34–38	8–9
3.5–4.0	>3000	>38	>9

of the curved (Macintosh) blade may not allow the therapist to visualize the larynx adequately.
- Lifting in the vallecula (as is done with the curved blade) can move the larynx anteriorly out of view of the operator.

The operator should check the laryngoscope to be sure that the light is bright and that the bulb is screwed in tightly. The therapist should also be sure to have *working* suction available because it is too late if the RT discovers it is needed. Finally, a manual resuscitator, attached to a *running* source of oxygen, should be quickly checked as previously described.

During the intubation procedure, the therapist may find it useful to enlist the aid of an assistant, who might have many duties before, during, and after intubation:

- Preparation and checking of the equipment used in intubation
- Stabilizing the infant's head
- Handing equipment and suction to the operator
- Providing pressure over the larynx
- Monitoring the infant and notifying the operator of deterioration in the infant's condition
- Timing the intubation attempt and notifying the operator if it exceeds 20 seconds
- Assisting with bagging between intubation attempts
- Checking for proper tube placement
- Securing the tube

Here is the procedure:

- The proper position for intubating an infant, in contrast to that for an adult, is exactly the same as that for ventilating with a mask: slight extension of the neck.
- The therapist inserts the blade to the base of the tongue and then *lifts* along the long axis of the handle. Prying not only does not provide proper visualization of the larynx but also may harm tooth formation.
- When introducing the tube, the operator inserts it in the *right* side of the infant's mouth. The tendency is to follow the straight blade down to the larynx. The problem with this technique is that it obstructs the view of the larynx and then the therapist cannot see whether the tube passes through the vocal cords.
- If the larynx cannot be visualized adequately with just the blade, the therapist may apply gentle pressure (or ask the assistant to apply pressure) to the larynx to move it posteriorly into view.
- The tube should be inserted until the cord marker (the black band near the bottom of the tube) passes through the vocal cords. That the position is appropriate can be determined by adding 6 to the infant's weight in kilograms and confirming that the tube marker at the upper lip corresponds to that number (see Table 31-5).
- Once the tube has been placed, the therapist should *immediately* confirm proper position by:
  Auscultating over the apices for equal, bilateral breath sounds.
  Visualizing adequate chest excursion.
  Visualizing lack of stomach distension.
  Hearing no air entry into the stomach.
- Once proper position has been confirmed, the therapist notes the depth of the tube at the upper lip and tube diameter, then secures the tube to the infant.
- Finally, the therapist should chart the intubation procedure.

DRUG AND VOLUME THERAPY DURING RESUSCITATION

Medications can be administered via four different routes: umbilical vein (preferred), peripheral vein, intraosseous, or endotracheal tube instillation. Endotracheal administration of medications has not been fully studied in infants, and intravenous administration is the preferred route. There are two general indications for medication administration in infants:

- The heart rate remains less than 80 despite adequate ventilation and 30 seconds of chest compressions.
- The heart rate is 0.

A limited number of medications is useful in neonatal resuscitation: epinephrine, sodium bicarbonate, 10% dextrose (D_{10}), and volume expanders.

- The normal dose of *epinephrine,* if administered endotracheally, should be increased to 0.05–0.1 mg/kg in 0.1–1.2 mL total volume. Although some infants may respond to intravenous doses as high as 0.2 mg/kg, the use of this high a dose of epinephrine is not recommended.
- If the resuscitation is prolonged once vital signs are restored, *sodium bicarbonate* may be tried. The bicarbonate should be administered over 1–2 minutes in a concentration of 0.5 mEq/mL (one-half normal strength) to minimize the chance of intraventricular hemorrhage.
- Additionally, when vital sign are restored following a prolonged resuscitation, 10% dextrose (D_{10}) can be administered for a blood glucose < 40 mg/dL. The bolus is followed by an infusion of 5 mL/kg/hr either IV or IO.

(Refer to Table 31-5 for other dosages for these drugs.)

Two possible volume expanders can be used in neonates: whole blood or normal saline. Either of these is given when there is an indication of hypovolemia, as evidenced by:

- Pallor that persists after oxygenation.
- Low blood pressure (if it is available).
- Weak pulse with an adequate heart rate.
- Poor response to resuscitative efforts.

The dose is 10 mL/kg IV/IO given over 5–10 minutes. After giving the volume expander, the therapist should see the pallor improve, the pulse strength increase, and some response to the resuscitative efforts.

CASE STUDY 31-4

Mrs. L., who is pregnant with a fetus of 30 weeks gestational age, has had problems with gradually increasing blood pressure and proteinuria. At her latest prenatal visit, due to her increasing peripheral edema, 4+ proteinuria, and a blood pressure of 160/110 torr (all signs of severe pre-eclampsia), her obstetrician decided to perform an urgent Cesarean section. Mrs. L. is at risk for delivering an asphyxiated infant because of her pregnancy-induced hypertension and the somewhat emergent nature of her Cesarean section. Of course, there is also concern about the maturity of the infant's lungs.

Because of the possible problems, Jim, a neonatal specialist from respiratory care and Dr. Carson, a neonatologist, are present at the delivery. Mrs. L. is brought to the delivery suite where an anesthesiologist establishes epidural anesthesia along with oxygen by cannula and continuous pulse oximetry monitoring. The obstetrician delivers a somewhat limp, pale female in about 10 minutes and hands her to the neonatologist. Dr. Carson places her in a prewarmed radiant warmer, dries her off, and positions her on her back with slight extension of her head. Because she still shows little movement, Jim begins bagging her with a Mapleson (flow-inflating) bag and 100% oxygen.

The neonatologist announces the 1 minute Apgar score as 4 and prepares the intubation equipment. Jim asks one of the nurses to set the suction regulator to 60 mm Hg. As Dr. Carson is intubating, he asks Jim for some laryngeal pressure and then easily intubates. Jim confirms equal bilateral breath sounds with no sound over the epigastrium and adequate bilateral chest movement. One of the nurses bags while he tapes the tube. Dr. Carson is now cannulating the umbilical vein. Jim continues ventilation at a rate of 60 per minute. The infant's pulse is 60 and weak; the EKG monitor shows sinus bradycardia. The nurse begins chest compressions on Baby L., who weighs about 1500 g.

After 1 minute, the neonatologist asks the nurse to stop compressions to assess the progress of the resuscitation. Because the heart rate is still 60, a nurse administers 0.015 mg of epinephrine. After another minute of chest compressions, Baby L.'s heart rate is now 100, but her pulse is still very hard to palpate. Dr. Carson draws up 15 mL of normal saline (10 mL/kg fluid challenge) and infuses it slowly into the umbilical vein line. Her color begins to improve, and her pulse becomes stronger. A pulse oximeter shows Baby L.'s saturation to be 90% during ventilation with 100% oxygen. Jim suggests a chest X-ray to assess the infant prior to moving her to the neonatal intensive care unit. Once the chest film has been taken, the team moves Baby L. to the neonatal ICU.

Questions

1. How could the maturity of the infant's lungs be predicted prior to delivery?
2. How does the necessity of drug administration during an infant resuscitation affect the possible outcome?

If the infant does not improve following a couple of fluid challenges, it is time to consider *dopamine* starting at 5 μg/kg/min and titrating to effect up to a maximum of 20 μg/kg/min.

Emergency Airway Adjuncts

In the emergency situation, the airway of choice is the oral endotracheal tube. It is readily inserted by properly trained medical professionals and provides an open airway, airway protection (although it is not a guarantee against aspiration), a route for secretion removal, and a connection for positive pressure ventilation. If the endotracheal tube is not needed for one of these reasons during a resuscitation and ventilation is easily performed using a bag and mask, endotracheal intubation is not a priority and can be delayed to the postresuscitation time. However, in some circumstances it is either not practical or possible to insert an oral endotracheal tube. In these cases, other devices can provide some of the functions of the endotracheal tube: esophageal obturator airway (EOA)/esophageal gastric tube airway (EGTA), esophageal-tracheal combitube (ETC), and the laryngeal mask airway (LMA).

ESOPHAGEAL OBTURATOR AIRWAY/ESOPHAGEAL GASTRIC TUBE AIRWAY

The **esophageal obturator airway (EOA)** and **esophageal gastric tube airway (EGTA)** were designed about 30 years ago for when there was no one skilled in endotracheal intubation. The EOA, a tube about 25 cm long and 1 cm in diameter, is inserted blindly into the esophagus; it comes in only one size for adults (Figure 31-12). Once it is in place, a large cuff is inflated, which occludes (obturates) the esophagus. Proper placement is verified by auscultation of breath sounds and auscultating over the epigastrium.

A major disadvantage of the EOA is that the rescuer still must maintain a seal of the mask on the victim's face. It is not intended for use when someone is available who can intubate the trachea. Nor it is it intended for use for people who:

- Are shorter than 5 feet tall.
- Are breathing spontaneously.
- Are not completely unconscious (as it would stimulate vomiting).
- Have esophageal disease or have swallowed caustic materials.
- Require resuscitation for prolonged periods of time.

Before the EOA is removed, the trachea must be intubated. The removal of the EOA is frequently accompanied by gastric contents, which can then be aspirated or forced into the lungs by positive pressure breathing.

The EGTA has a gastric tube lumen in the middle to permit decompression of the stomach after bag-and-mask ventilation by means of the insertion of a gastric tube (Figure 31-13). Its use is otherwise similar to that of an EOA. The level of ventilation and oxygenation provided by either an EOA or EGTA is generally less than that provided when the patient's trachea is intubated.

ESOPHAGEAL TRACHEAL COMBITUBE

The **esophageal tracheal combitube (ETC)** is a double-lumen tube that is blindly inserted into the pharynx. One lumen is like an endotracheal tube (open to the end), and the other lumen ends blindly with holes that wind up in the vicinity of the opening for the larynx if the tube is placed in the esophagus (like an EOA). Once the tube is inserted, the operator inflates the small balloon on the end of the tube with 15 mL of air and the large 100-mL balloon that occludes the pharynx. Then the operator determines whether the tube is in the trachea. If it is, ventilation can be accomplished just as with an endotracheal tube.

If the tube is in the esophagus, ventilation can be accomplished through the other opening. The esophagus

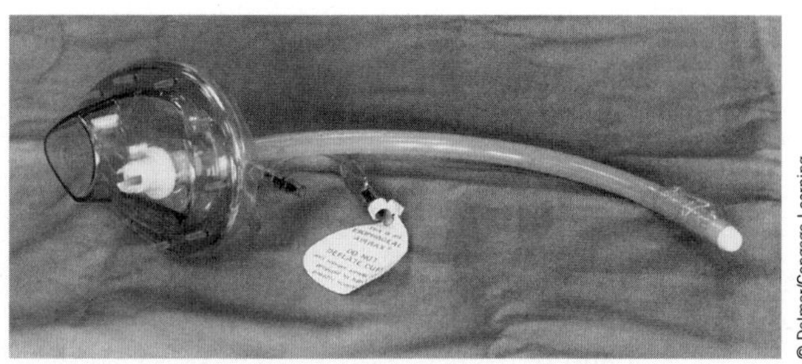

FIGURE 31-12 Esophageal obturator airway.

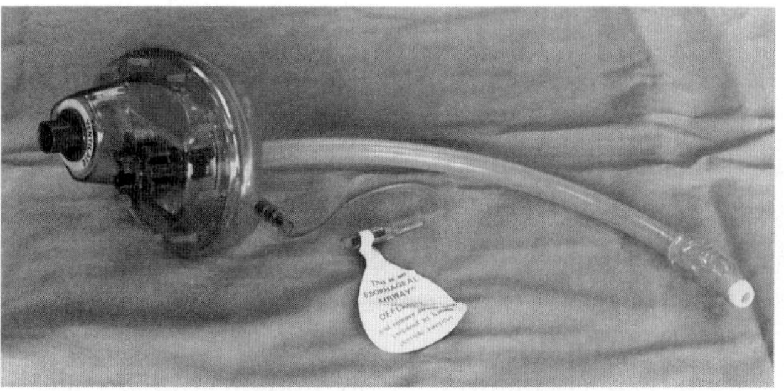

FIGURE 31-13 Esophageal gastric tube airway.

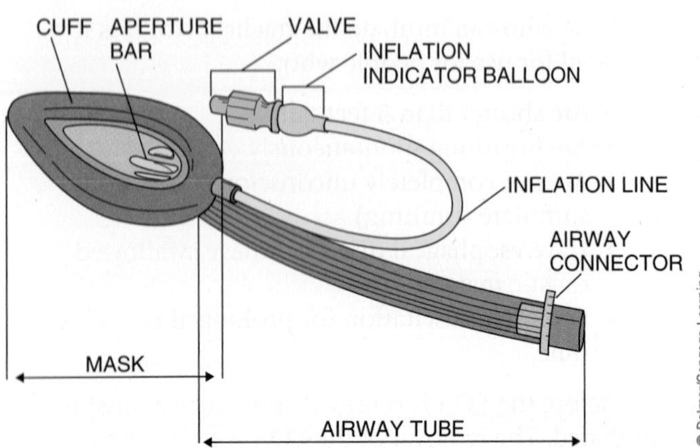

FIGURE 31-14 Laryngeal mask airway.

is sealed by the smaller balloon, and gastric contents can be evacuated through that lumen. The ETC provides ventilation similar to that provided by an endotracheal tube while preventing the aspiration of gastric contents.

The two major limitations of the ETC are that it comes in only one size (making it not suitable for pediatric use) and that the trachea cannot be suctioned if the tube is in the esophagus.

LARYNGEAL MASK AIRWAY

The **laryngeal mask airway (LMA)** is a device that consists of a small mask with an inflatable rim on the end of a tube (Figure 31-14). It comes in several sizes. It is inserted blindly with the mask facing the tongue until resistance is felt; then the inflatable rim is inflated. If the LMA is in the proper position, the tube will rise about 1 cm as the rim is inflated. The mask covers the opening of the trachea and allows ventilation; however, the therapist must remember that the LMA does not prevent against aspiration. It works well in about 90% of cases including pediatrics.

Several limitations of the LMA need to be kept in mind:

- Ventilation may not be adequate because the cuff fails to seal the larynx; either the tongue has been pushed over the larynx, or the epiglottis has been flipped over the larynx.
- If there is inadequate anesthesia when the mask is inserted or removed, laryngospasm may occur.
- It cannot protect well against aspiration.

Summary

In dealing with a patient emergency, the critical priorities are circulation, airway, and breathing. The new priority in the pulseless patient is compressions. The sequence depends on available resources. If someone is unconscious and unresponsive and the therapist is alone with an AED at hand, he should call 911, perform 5 cycles of 30 compressions and 2 breaths, then attach the AED and evaluate the rhythm and shock as appropriate. If there are two rescuers, one calls 911 and retrieves the AED on the way back from calling 911; the other initiates CPR with compressions. If there are three rescuers, one calls 911, one obtains and applies the AED, and the third begins CPR—and so on.

REVIEW QUESTIONS

1. What is the order of the first three priorities in managing an unconscious person?
2. Other than endotracheal intubation, what methods can the respiratory therapist use to open and maintain someone's airway?
3. What equipment is needed for endotracheal intubation? How is intubation done?
4. What is the proper sequence for managing a VF/pulseless v-tach cardiac arrest?
5. What are the priorities in managing cardiac arrest in a child?
6. How do infant and adult resuscitations differ in terms of their priorities?
7. When would you use a laryngeal mask airway or laryngeal-tracheal combitube instead of an endotracheal tube?

MULTIPLE-CHOICE QUESTIONS

1. Equipment and personnel for neonatal resuscitation should be available:
   a. immediately in the delivery room.
   b. somewhere in the hospital on page.
   c. only if the team anticipates needing them.
   d. to be called in if needed.
2. If an infant does not breathe after birth, bag-and-mask ventilation should be instituted immediately because:
   I. the infant may be in secondary apnea.
   II. the longer the delay, the less likely a favorable outcome when resuscitation is needed.
   III. the infant may have already gone through primary apnea.
   a. I only
   b. II only
   c. I and II
   d. I, II, and III

3. In which of the following situations would immediate cardioversion *not* be indicated?
   a. atrial fibrillation, rate 180, BP 80/40, 3 second capillary refill
   b. supraventricular tachycardia, rate 150, BP 125/75, alert, warm skin
   c. atrial flutter, rate 160, BP 90/60, complaint of shortness of breath
   d. ventricular tachycardia, rate 170, unresponsive, BP 70/40
4. What are the guidelines for giving drugs via endotracheal tube?
   I. The dose should be 2–2.5 times that of the IV dose.
   II. The drug should be flushed in with 20 mL of saline.
   III. Only narcan, atropine, epinephrine, vasopressin (in adults), and lidocaine should be given.
   a. I only
   b. III only
   c. I and III
   d. I, II, and III
5. Why would AEDs be useful in a hospital?
   a. They would reduce the amount of training needed.
   b. They would allow patients on floors to be defibrillated faster.
   c. They would decrease costs for monitor-defibrillators.
   d. They would decrease maintenance required for defibrillators.
6. If using a manual defibrillator, what precautions should the RT take?
   I. Remove any transdermal medication patches.
   II. Be sure no one (including the RT) is touching the bed.
   III. Be sure to utilize some sort of conduction enhancer.
   a. I only
   b. II only
   c. I and II
   d. I, II, and III
7. When giving a fluid bolus of saline or Ringer's lactate, it is necessary to deliver three times the estimated fluid deficit. Why?
   a. Only about one-third of crystalloids actually remains in the vascular space.
   b. The crystalloids are diluted when they mix with the blood.
   c. Crystalloids have one-third the effectiveness of colloids.
   d. The crystalloids are being excreted at a rapid rate.
8. When performing a pediatric resuscitation, what device can provide the therapist with drug dosages, ETT size, and suction catheter size?
   a. PALS pocket handbook
   b. American Heart Association pocket cards
   c. Broselow tape
   d. PDR
9. When an infant is newly delivered, what are the very first priorities?
   a. stimulation, bag-and-mask ventilation, compressions
   b. intubating, cannulating the umbilical vein, determining cardiac rhythm
   c. weighing, confirming name, footprinting
   d. drying, warming, and positioning
10. What advantage does the esophageal-tracheal combitube have over the endotracheal tube?
   a. It requires no other equipment to insert.
   b. It provides better ventilation.
   c. It has fewer hazards.
   d. It is cheaper.

CRITICAL-THINKING QUESTIONS

1. An RT is the first person on the scene with an unconscious, unresponsive person in a shopping mall. Many willing but untrained people are available to help. What duties should the RT assign bystanders? What if someone knows CPR?
2. An RT is the team leader for the anticipated resuscitation of an infant about to be born. How many people should be on the team and what would be their functions? What should be checked in preparation for the delivery?
3. A respiratory therapist is employed in a hospital that does not yet allow RTs with an ACLS course completion card to fully participate in resuscitation. Arriving at a code on a medical-surgical floor, the RT finds a woman already attached to a monitor-defibrillator in pulseless v-tach. Someone is doing compressions; a nurse hands over the bag and mask as the RT goes to the head of the bed. What needs to be done next? Whom can the RT get to do it?
4. A therapist is at the local athletic club playing tennis, and he has an AED in the car, having just taught a CPR course. Someone comes running over to say that a person has a problem on the track. If this person is pulseless, should the RT use the AED? What are the pros and cons of using it in this situation?

Suggested Readings

American Association for Respiratory Care. Clinical practice guideline: resuscitation in acute care hospitals. *Respir Care.* 1993;38,12:1179–1188.

American Association for Respiratory Care. Clinical practice guideline: defibrillation during resuscitation. *Respir Care.* 1995;40,7:744–748.

American Association for Respiratory Care. Clinical practice guideline: management of airway emergencies. *Respir Care.* 1995;40,7:749–760.

American Heart Association. *Advanced Cardiac Life Support.* Dallas, TX: American Heart Association; 2010.

American Heart Association. *BLS for Healthcare Providers.* Dallas, TX: American Heart Association; 2010.

American Heart Association. *Guidelines for Cardiopulmonary Resuscitation.* Dallas, TX: American Heart Association; 2010.

American Heart Association. *Instructor's Manual—Advanced Cardiac Life Support.* Dallas, TX: American Heart Association; 2010.

American Heart Association. *Instructor's Manual—Basic Life Support.* Dallas, TX: American Heart Association; 2010.

American Heart Association. *Instructor's Manual—Pediatric Advanced Life Support.* Dallas, TX: American Heart Association; 2010.

American Heart Association, American Academy of Pediatrics. *Textbook of Neonatal Resuscitation.* Dallas, TX: American Heart Association; 2010.

American Heart Association. *Textbook of Pediatric Advanced Life Support.* Dallas, TX: American Heart Association; 2010.

American Red Cross. *Blood Facts and Statistics.* Washington, DC: American Red Cross; 2010.

Centers for Disease Control and Prevention. Unintentional Drowning Fact Sheet, Washington, DC: Centers for Disease Control and Prevention.

Cummins RO, Graves JR. (1996) *ACLS Scenarios: Core Concepts for Case-Based Learning.* New York, NY: Mosby Lifeline.

Division of Injury Control, Center for Environmental Health and Injury Control, Centers for Disease Control and Prevention. Childhood injuries in the United States. *Am J Dis Child.* 1990;144: 627–646.

Dubin, D. (2000) *Rapid Interpretation of EKG's.* Sixth edition. Tampa, FL: Cover Publishing.

Gant NF, Gilstrap LC. Hypertension in pregnancy. *ACOG Tech Bull.* 1996;219.

Grauer K, Cavallaro D. (2000) *Volume I-ACLS Certification Preparation.* 3rd edition. St. Louis, MO: Mosby-Lifeline.

Grauer K, Cavallaro D. (2000) *Volume II-ACLS A Comprehensive Review.* 3rd edition. St. Louis, MO: Mosby-Lifeline.

Haldane, JS. Symptoms, causes, and prevention of anoxemia. *Br Med J.* 1919;2:65.

Health Consequences of Smoking, The. Cardiovascular Disease. A Report of the Surgeon General, publication DHHS (PHS) 84-50204. U.S. Department of Health and Human Services, Public Health Service, 1983, ppiv, 127–129.

Huff, J. (2005). *ECG Workout- Exercises in Arrhythmia Interpretation.* 5th edition. Philadelphia, PA: Lippincott.

Insurance Institute for Highway Safety. Child Restraint Laws. 2010.

NIH Consensus Conference. Physical activity and cardiovascular health. *JAMA,* 1996;276,3: 738–743.

Scanlan CJ, Wilkins RL, Stoller JK, eds. *Egan's Fundamentals of Respiratory Care.* St. Louis, MO: Mosby; 1999.

United States Department of Health and Human Services. *Physical Activity Guidelines for Americans.* Dallas, TX: American Heart Association; 2008.

CHAPTER 32

Managing Disasters: Respiratory Care in Mass Critical Care

Thomas J. Johnson

OBJECTIVES

Upon completion of this chapter, the reader should be able to:

- Define the levels or tiers of disasters and disaster management.
- Describe the Incident Command System and the National Incident Management System (NIMS).
- Describe the injuries associated with natural disasters.
- Describe the medical management of blast and crush injuries.
- List the differences between a natural biological outbreak and a bioterrorist attack.
- Describe the medical responses to a pandemic influenza or other emerging disease.
- Describe the medical countermeasures to chemical agents.

CHAPTER OUTLINE

KEY TERMS

acute respiratory distress syndrome (ARDS)
anthrax
blast lung injury (BLI)
blast overpressure injuries
bronchopleural fistula
cidofovir
coccidioidomycosis
cytokine storm
diplopia
disseminated intravascular coagulopathy (DIC)
dumbels
dysarthria
dysphagia
dysphonia
emergency mass critical care (EMCC)
epidemic
hemagglutinin
high efficiency particulate air (HEPA)
high-order explosion (HE)
hospital emergency incident command system (HEICS)
incident command system (ICS)
interferon
interleukin-6, 7, 8
lewisite
live attenuated vaccine (LAV)
low-order explosion (LE)
mass casualty incident (MCI)
MetHb
multidrug-resistant tuberculosis (MDRTB)
multiple organ system failure (MOSF)
N-acetyl-l-cystine (NAC)
National Incident Management System (NIMS)
neuraminidase
nitrogen mustard
off-gassing
pandemic
pirfenidone
primary blast injury
Push Packs
quaternary blast injury
racemic epinephrine
ribavirin
secondary blast injury
self-contained breathing apparatus (SCBA)
self-evacuation
spalling
staphylococcal enterotoxin B (SEB)
systemic inflammatory response syndrome (SIRS)
tertiary blast injury
trivalent inactivated vaccine (TIV)
tumor necrosis factor-alpha
zoonotic

Disasters are medical emergencies for which respiratory therapists (RTs) must be prepared. For the American College of Emergency Physicians (ACEP), the definition of a disaster is "when the destructive effects of natural or man-made forces overwhelm the ability of a given area or community to meet the demand for healthcare."[1] The impact of a disaster, or **mass casualty incident (MCI)**, affects communities in a disparate way through differences in social economic status, in cultural norms, and in community infrastructure. Events such as the impact of hurricane Katrina,[2] the anthrax bioterror events,[3] World Trade Center attacks (February 1993 and September 2001), Oklahoma City bombing,[4] SARS,[5] and pandemic influenza[6] have galvanized the health care community and respiratory care professionals to prepare for disasters whether man-made or natural.

To some, disaster preparedness is getting ready for something that has a low-probability of occurrence. The time and dollars spent on training, drills, and equipment are often limited to that mandated by the Joint Commission, whose accreditation for hospitals includes the requirement of a disaster plan. In its prepublication version of its chapter on emergency management, the Joint Commission states: "A disaster is a type of emergency that, due to its complexity, scope, or duration, threatens the organization's capabilities and requires outside assistance to sustain [patient] care, safety or security functions." Yet if one considered the potential for loss of hospital infrastructure and hospital services from a community for an extended period of time, as in post-Katrina New Orleans, then disaster planning is in the best interest of the facility and the community it serves.[7] Loss of electrical, heating-ventilation-air conditioning (HVAC), and water, as occurred in New York City's power blackouts, can affect hospitals in a large and complex region.

Disasters occur in different sizes and in different degrees of severity. Most disasters do not overwhelm the hospital's ability to cope. Multivehicle accidents, aircraft accidents, and train wrecks can trigger the hospital disaster plan or emergency operation plan (EOP), but these can be managed by the staff and supplies on hand at the time. Mass casualty incidents may require the redeployment of staff and resources to emergency departments (EDs) for variable amounts of time. An example of this is the MCI response of Rhode Island Hospital to a nightclub fire that generated 215 victims. The rapid, effective response of Rhode Island Hospital was the result of disaster drills directed by a surgeon. Of the 64 patients admitted to Rhode Island

Hospital, 28 (60%) were intubated for inhalation injuries. A step-down unit and a medical-surgical unit were converted to a 21-bed burn ICU.[8]

Respiratory therapists, regardless of where they are employed, must have a working knowledge of disaster management. The hospital, long-term acute care (LTAC), home care, and skilled nursing facilities all have different needs and priorities. By preparing for disaster, respiratory care professionals mitigate the impact and develop mechanisms for recovery and the resumption of normal operations. Facilities and departments should develop communication and plans with police, fire/rescue, first responders, as well as federal, state, and local/tribal agencies. These plans should incorporate cultural, religious, ethical, and legal considerations.

National Incident Management System

In February 2003, President George W. Bush promulgated the Homeland Security Presidential Directive 5, which created the **National Incident Management System (NIMS)** with a goal of having a standard incident response for all government levels and response agencies. NIMS is intended to be a flexible operational system that facilitates governmental and nongovernmental agencies working together at all levels during all phases of an incident, regardless of its size, complexity, or location.

Incident Command System

Internally hospitals can and should have a **hospital emergency incident command system (HEICS)** or **incident command system (ICS)** to activate and coordinate the hospital's response to an incident. The ICS must have as a first step an *emergency operations plan* (*EOP*) and an alert and notification communication system. This plan must consider staff health and safety as well as legal and ethical issues. The ICS is a command, communication, safety, and operational system that should tie into the NIMS seamlessly. Of course, the ultimate goal of the ICS is the safe, efficient, and effective management of the disaster. Hospitals can expect a total first wave of victims to exceed twice the number admitted during the first hour of the MCI.[9] Once the incident has been managed, then demobilization, recovery, and response evaluation (lessons learned) should occur. For more information, the reader is directed to the Emergency Management Institute's Web site (http://training.fema.gov).

In a 2008 supplement,[10] the journal *Chest* published the findings of the Task Force for Mass Critical Care Summit Meeting (January 26–27, 2007 in Chicago, Illinois). This multidisciplinary group of 37 experts in the fields of bioethics, critical care medicine, disaster preparedness and response reported their recommendations for **emergency mass critical care (EMCC)**. Critical care units can expect both a surge in patients and an acuity level that will be a challenge to meet.

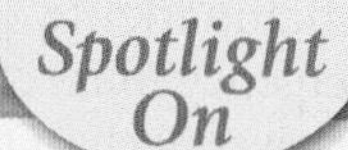

The Logistics Service Branch of the ICS

- *Communication Unit.* Prepares and implements the Incident Communication Plan (ICS-205), distributes and maintains communications equipment, supervises the Incident Communications Center, and establishes adequate communications over the incident.
- *Medical Unit.* Develops the Medical Plan (ICS-206), provides first aid and light medical treatment for personnel assigned to the incident, and prepares procedures for a major medical emergency.
- *Food Unit.* Supplies the food and potable water for all incident facilities and personnel, and obtains the necessary equipment and supplies to operate food service facilities at bases and camps.
- *Supply Unit.* Determines the type and amount of supplies needed to support the incident. The unit orders, receives, stores, and distributes supplies, and services nonexpendable equipment. All resource orders are placed through the Supply Unit. The unit maintains inventory and accountability of supplies and equipment.
- *Facilities Unit.* Sets up and maintains required facilities to support the incident. Provides managers for the incident base and camps. Also responsible for facility security and facility maintenance services: sanitation, lighting, cleanup.
- *Ground Support Unit.* Prepares the Transportation Plan. Arranges for, activates, and documents the fueling, maintenance, and repair of ground resources. Arranges for the transportation of personnel, supplies, food, and equipment.

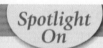

Task Force for Mass Critical Care

In the twentieth century, rarely have mass causality events yielded hundreds or thousands of critically ill patients requiring definitive critical care. However, future catastrophic natural disasters, epidemics or pandemics, nuclear device detonations, or large chemical exposures may change usual disaster epidemiology and require a large critical care response. The Task Force on Mass Casualty Critical Care reviews the existing state of emergency preparedness for mass critical illness and presents an analysis of limitations, which are presented in subsequent articles. Baseline shortages of specialized resources such as critical care staff, medical supplies, and treatment spaces are likely to limit the number of critically ill victims who can receive life-sustaining interventions. The deficiency in critical care surge capacity is exacerbated by lack of a sufficient framework to integrate critical care within the overall institutional response and coordination of critical care across local institutions and broader geographic areas.[11]

Emergency Mass Critical Care

Task Force suggestions: EMCC should include the following: (1) mechanical ventilation, (2) IV fluid resuscitation, (3) vasopressor administration, (4) medication administration for specific disease states (*e.g.*, antimicrobials and antidotes), (5) sedation and analgesia, and (6) select practices to reduce adverse consequences of critical illness and critical care delivery. Also, all hospitals with ICUs should prepare to deliver EMCC for a daily critical care census at three times their usual ICU capacity for up to 10 days.[12]

Hospital Disaster Preparation

In preparing for a disaster, the worst-case scenarios must be evaluated, such as the loss of:

- Structural integrity of the facility.
- Personnel.
- Main oxygen supply.
- Medical air supply.
- Vacuum supply.
- Water supply.
- Food supply.
- Pharmacologic or other consumable supplies or the ability to be resupplied.

Hospitals and departments should develop and promulgate their EOPs that include preparedness, mitigation, response, and recovery. That plan must include preparations for damage/contamination to all or part of the facility and evacuation of all patients, visitors, and personnel. Staff support includes personal protection and vaccination (even for spouses/partners/children), family and pet care, communications, as well as the essential food, water, and personal hygiene. One must expect both active and passive resistance to disaster planning.

The Respiratory Therapist in Response to Multiple Casualty Incidents

For the respiratory therapist in an MCI, the major concerns are oxygen and mechanical ventilation resources. The increase in oxygen consumption may be as much as 200–300% for the duration of an MCI. Cylinder gas is limited by both storage and by the number of regulators for the cylinders. Large H and K cylinders can be used as a manifold for backfeeding a zone of gas outlets.[13]

Mechanical ventilation is the hallmark life support of critical care. So, in emergency mass critical care, RTs can expect a surge in invasive mechanical ventilation with very few, if any reserve ventilators in the hospital fleet. Rental supplies availability may exceed EMCC needs; federal, state, and city stockpiles of ventilators may be delayed or insufficient due to the numbers of casualties. Stockpiled ventilators (Impact Eagle, LP-10, iVent, LTV-1000, LTV 1200, and others) may require training time that is not feasible in the postevent period. Therefore, preparedness training is essential.

Natural Disasters

A natural disaster takes a normal, benign environment and weaponizes it. When nature unleashes its unpredictable, uncontrolled, unpreventable phenomena with ferociousness, humans are among its victims. Earthquakes, tornadoes, hurricanes, floods, and major fires have a regional effect to a degree depending on their intensity, duration, and size. Population density, community infrastructure, and social economics all play a role in the ability to

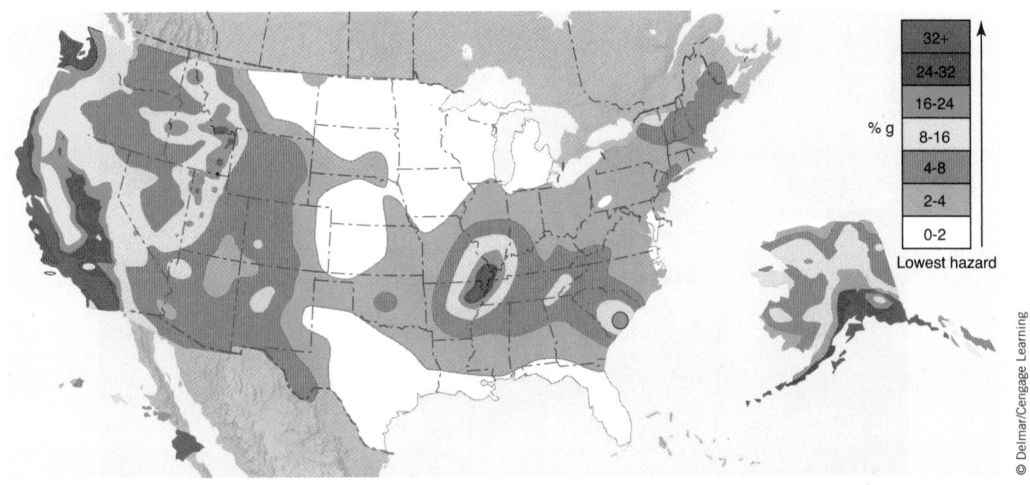

FIGURE 32-1 Seismic map of the United States—'% g' is percentage of seismic field activity.

effectively respond to these incidents. The casualties that result develop in waves:

- The first are the **self-evacuation** victims.
- These are followed by the seriously injured brought in by first responders and by injured first responders.
- Finally, the secondary infections and disease exacerbations follow the primary incident.

EARTHQUAKES

With an increasing population living and working in seismically active regions, the effect of an earthquake of 7 or more on the Richter scale will be devastating (Figure 32-1 and Table 32-1). Although earthquakes do not have a season, they are nonrandom events. Plate tectonics and seismic activity have and will occur in one region more than another. The *epicenter* is the location of the greatest shaking and earth movement, but the seismic energy is felt a significant distance from the epicenter. The destruction of infrastructure and building collapse result in high mortality. In the North Ridge California earthquake in 1994, 15% of the fatal injuries occurred due to collapsing freeways (Figure 32-2).

The most vulnerable of the population affected by earthquakes are the young (<5 years old), old (>65 years old), and those with chronic mental or physical diseases.[14]

The injury patterns range from minor lacerations and injuries to severely traumatic brain injuries and crush injuries. As the name implies, *crush injuries* occur when a body or body part is subject to a high degree of pressure after being squeezed between two or more objects. Crush injuries from entrapment under debris cause ischemia to tissues, resulting in rhabdomyolysis and then in the release of myoglobin, potassium, and phosphate into the circulation. Hyperkalemia results in

TABLE 32-1 **Earthquake Richter scale**

Richter Magnitude	Description
2	Felt by few people; detected by instruments
3	Felt by people indoors with dishes and doors distressed
4	People asleep awakened, walls cracked, and trees damaged
5	People flee buildings; damage to some buildings
6	Moderate to major damage with wall and chimney collapse
7	All buildings damaged, piping broken, landslides possible
8	All structures fall, including bridges, wide ground cracks
>8	Ground surface waves actually seen; destruction of all constructed objects

serious ECG changes such as tall, tented T-waves, prolonged QT intervals, or fatal cardiac dysrhythmias. Crush injuries can lead to kidney failure and require dialysis. All victims of crush injuries with dark, red, or so-called cola urine should have urine analysis for CPK (CK-3) and urine myoglobin and potassium. Severe crush chest injuries and high Injury Severity Scores[15] (ISS >25) are reported to have a mortality rate of 16%.[16] Reported[17] percentages of injuries typically seen after an earthquake include traumatic head injuries (22%), lower extremity injuries (19%), crush syndrome (11%), and upper extremity trauma (10%). Hypothermia, secondary wound infections, gangrene requiring amputation, sepsis, **acute respiratory distress syndrome (ARDS)**, and multiple organ system failure

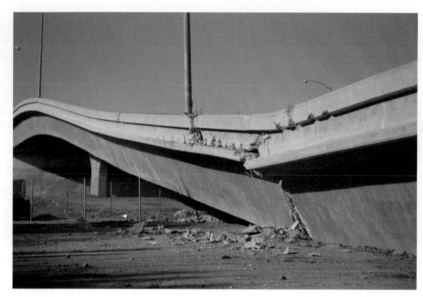

FIGURE 32-2 The collapse of a freeway following an earthquake in California.
Courtesy of Federal Emergency Management Agency

(MOSF) have increased the complexity of care for earthquake victims.

The airborne debris thrown into the atmosphere by earthquakes is of special concern for the respiratory therapist. Dust and contaminants from collapsing structures exacerbate chronic lung disease. Even otherwise healthy search and rescue people may be exposed to asbestos and other native contaminants. The North Ridge earthquake in January 1994 resulted in over 200 cases and 3 fatalities associated with **coccidioidomycosis** infections from the aerosolization of soil in the earthquake region.[18]

An earthquake may be further complicated by landslides, tsunamis, breaching of dams, levies, and water main breaks resulting from the damage of the quake. Gas and electrical supply may be interrupted, and fires can break out.

In the postearthquake period, RTs can expect an increase in respiratory cases from the inhalation of dust, mold spores, asbestos, etc. The stress of an earthquake can be anticipated to cause an upsurge in fatal and nonfatal heart attacks. A significant number of people will self-treat or be treated by neighbors or volunteers who may arrive for care.

Spotlight On

Injury Severity Score

The Injury Severity Score (ISS) is an anatomical scoring system (head, face, chest, abdomen, and extremities including pelvis) that provides an overall evaluation of the trauma patient who has experienced multiple injuries. First, each injured region of the body is assigned an Abbreviated Injury Scale (AIS) score. An AIS score 1–6 (minor, moderate, serious, severe, critical, and unsurvivable) is assigned to the region. Then, the three most severely injured body regions have their score squared, then added together to produce the ISS score. See the on-line resource of Trauma.org (www.trauma.org) for scoring trauma victims.

Source: Baker SP, et al. The Injury Severity Score: a method for describing patients with multiple injuries and evaluating emergency care. J Trauma. *1974;14:187–196.*

Spotlight On

Coccidioidomycosis

Coccidioidmycosis is caused by *Coccidioides immitis*, a soil fungus endemic to California's San Joaquin Valley, southern Arizona, New Mexico, Texas, and northern Mexico. When spores are inhaled, they migrate to the alveoli where they transform into thick-walled spherules that cause granulomas and lung cavitation.

Patients experience weight loss (>10%), night sweats (can be confused with TB), and extreme fatigue. Treatment includes antifungals such as Amphotericin B, which is preferred in pregnancy [0.3–1 mg/kg/IV (adults)]. The precautions are renal and hepatic compromise, bronchospasm, hypoxia, dysrhythmias, and hypotension.[19]

TABLE 32-2 **Classification of tornadoes: Fujita Scale**

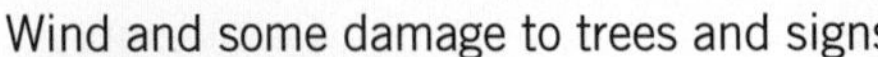

F0 Gale Tornado of 65–85 mph	Wind and some damage to trees and signs 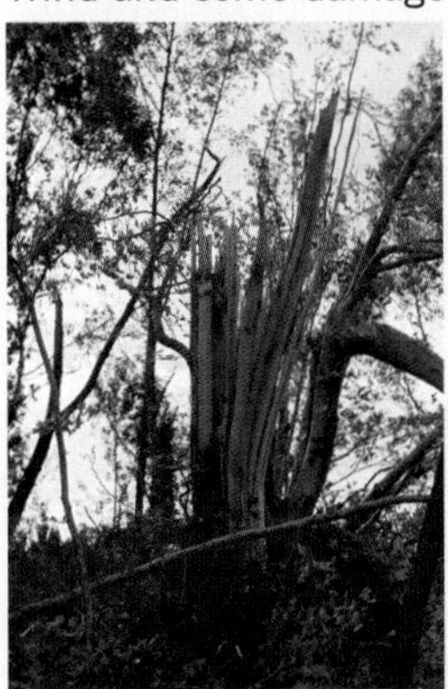	F3 Severe Tornado of 136–165 mph	Trains overturned and roofs and walls torn off well-constructed houses 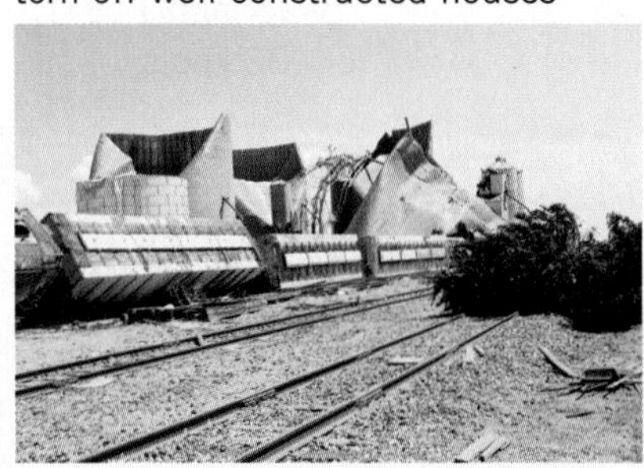
F1 Moderate Tornado of 86–110 mph	Moving cars pushed off roads 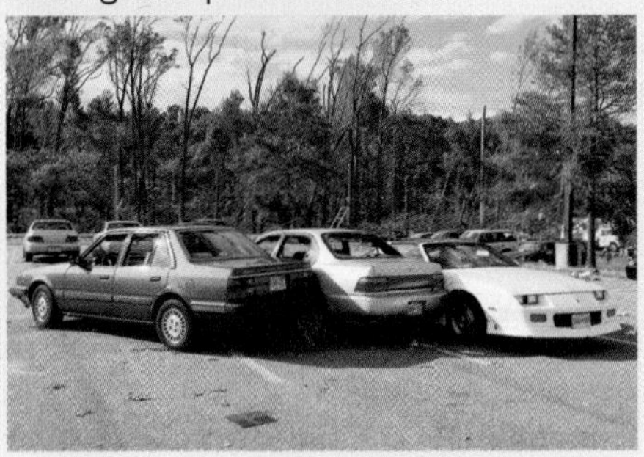	F4 Devastating Tornado of 166–200 mph	Houses leveled 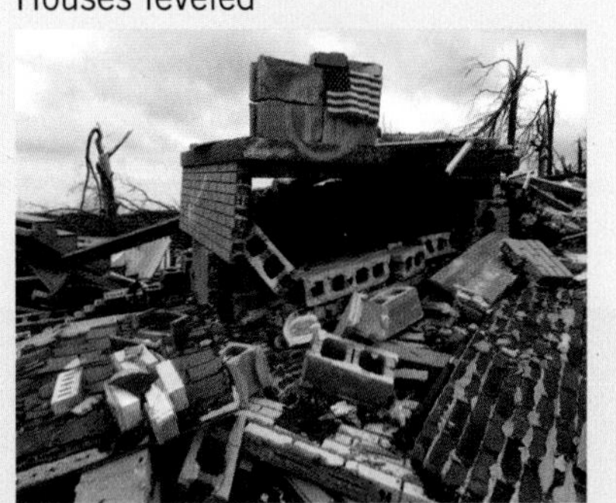
F2 Significant Tornado of 111–135 mph	Roofs torn off, trees snapped or uprooted and cars thrown 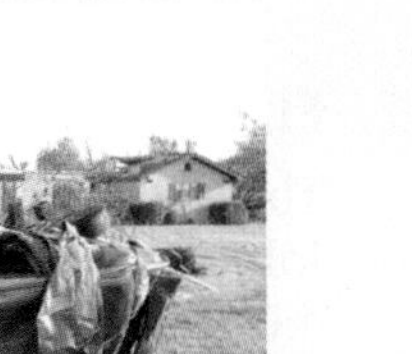	F5 Incredible Tornado of >200	Automobile-size missiles fly in excess of 100 m; entire communities leveled 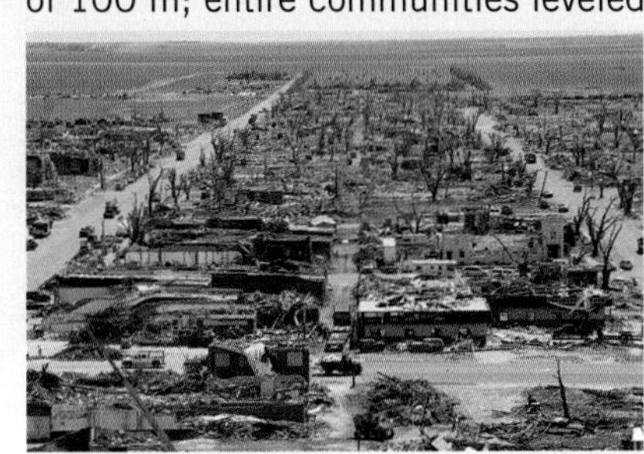

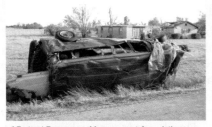

All images are Courtesy of Federal Emergency Management Association

TORNADOES

Tornadoes are relatively brief, violent storms that can occur singly or in clusters. They have been classified by Prof. Theodore Fujita according to wind speed and damage potential (see the Fujita Scale, Table 32-2). The lethality of a tornado varies widely depending on the wind speed, the size of the community it strikes, the structures, the degree of shelter that victims had at the time, and the victims' host factors (victims' ages, physical condition, and ability to react accordingly to the disaster). The May 22, 2011 tornado which extensively damaged Joplin, Missouri killing 159 persons was rated as an F5 incident.

Tornado victims exhibit injuries ranging from minor lacerations to severe penetrating ballistic injuries from debris and crush injuries requiring critical care. As with earthquakes, anticipate exacerbations of chronic diseases and increased incidence of heart attacks.

HURRICANES

Much like tornados, hurricanes are categorized on a numerical scale (Table 32-3). Recent violent and destructive hurricanes have heightened disaster planning. Hurricane Katrina in 2005 had winds of 142 mph and a 20-foot storm surge that killed 2057 (Figure 32-3), and the Galveston Hurricane of 1900 resulted in an estimated 8000 dead. Since hurricanes spawn tornadoes hundreds of miles inland, a hurricane's true path of destruction, injury, and death extend well beyond the coastline.

TABLE 32-3 **Saffir-Simpson Hurricane Scale**

Category	Winds	Storm Surge	Comments
One	75–95 mph/119–153 kph /64–82 knots	4–5 foot	Damage to shrubs, trees
Two	96–110 mph/154–177 kph /83–95 knots	6–8 foot	Window and roofing damage
Three	111–130 mph/178–209 kph/96–113 knots	9–12 foot (evacuation of shoreline areas due to flooding as far as 8 miles inland)	Mobile homes destroyed. *Low-lying escape routes cut 3–5 hours before arrival of the center of the storm*
Four	131–155 mph/ 210–249 kph	13–18 ft (requires evacuation of areas 6 miles or more inland)	Some complete roof failures, doors windows; major damage to structures near shore
Five	>155 mph />249 kph /> 135 knots	>18 foot (requires evacuation of areas 10 miles or more inland)	Major damage to structures; all trees and signs blown down

Source: National Weather Service National Hurricane Center (www.nhc.noaa.gov).

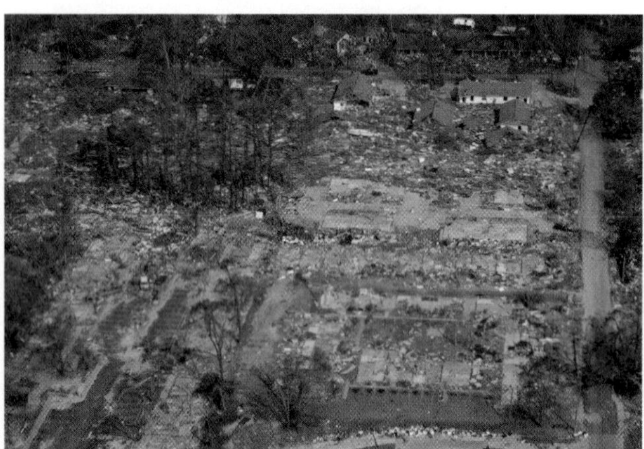

FIGURE 32-3 Aerial shot of the devastation left behind by Hurricane Katrina in the Gulf Coast.
Courtesy of Federal Emergency Management Agency

Hurricanes have destroyed infrastructure, resulting in the loss of power to hospitals and the isolation of the hospital from resupply of liquid oxygen, medical consumables, and food.

The aftereffect of hurricanes can produce injuries and disease.

- Recovery and rescue efforts have resulted in injuries to first responders and to those who are removing downed trees and power lines, as well as to those who are working to reestablish electrical, gas, communication, and road/bridge infrastructure.
- The resulting flooding waters of a hurricane can not only hamper relief efforts but also contain contaminates, toxins, and debris. In the aftermath of the 2005 Hurricane Katrina, the news media reported that the Louisiana American Lung Association had screened approximately 1600 impacted residents and found that 25% had mild to moderate reduction in lung function. Researchers could not determine whether this was the result of breathing mold and dust caused by Katrina, seasonal allergies, or an indicator of a long-term change in respiratory health.

FLOODS

The classic flood disaster in the United States is the Johnstown, Pennsylvania, flood of May 30, 1889. At 4:07 p.m. on that day, a 40-foot wave of water from a dam failure and heavy rain killed an estimated 2200 people. Entire communities may find themselves underwater in the event of a flood (Figure 32-4).

Floods produce casualties similar to those of hurricanes. Stress-related exacerbations of chronic

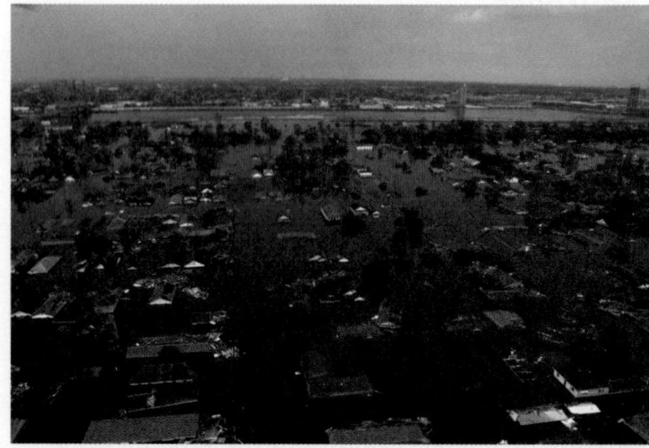

FIGURE 32-4 Flooding can devastate an entire community.
Courtesy of Federal Emergency Management Agency

diseases can be compounded by infections, hypothermia, and psychological stress.

FIRE

Sometimes disasters occur at the same time. The Great Chicago Fire and the lesser known Peshtigo Fire happened at the same hour and the same day: October 8, 1871. The estimated deaths from these two events are probably in excess of the 2400 reported because whole families were wiped out with no one to report their loss. Equally appalling are the fires that raged for 4 days after the San Francisco earthquake, leaving over 250,000 San Franciscans homeless.

Hospital preparedness for an MCI resulting from a fire is exemplified by the Rhode Island nightclub fire that resulted in 215 victims of the 439 patrons of the club. There were 96 deaths at the scene of the fire. Victims were distributed to 16 regional hospitals.[20] Surgical and burn/smoke inhalation medical responses should be part of the EOP.

Man-Made Disasters

Man-made disasters are incidents that overwhelm the health care system's capacity due to a malfunction in something created by another human being or a planned attack devised by human beings. Industrial accidents and terrorist events are classified as man-made disasters.

EXPLOSIONS

Explosions resulting from industrial or transportation accidents, warfare, and terrorism produce similar injuries. The severity of the resulting injuries depends on:

- The type of explosives used.
- The proximity of the victims to the blast.
- The shielding between blast and victim.
- The blast environment (closed place versus open area explosions).

There are two categories of explosions: low-order explosion (LE) and high-order explosion (HE).

Low-order explosions (LE) are the result of a rapid expansion of gases from an ignition. LE creates a subsonic explosion and does not have an over pressurization wave. Examples are pipe bombs, gunpowder, and most pure petroleum-based bombs such as Molotov cocktails. Although an LE may not have the extreme violence of the HE, its lethality is undeniable. An extreme example of a low-order explosion is the one resulting from the impact of fuel-filled aircraft on the World Trade Center and Pentagon buildings, with the horrific damage, deaths, and injuries. The resulting building collapse killed thousands (Figure 32-5).

The collapse of a building results in both crush injuries and relatively few survivors.

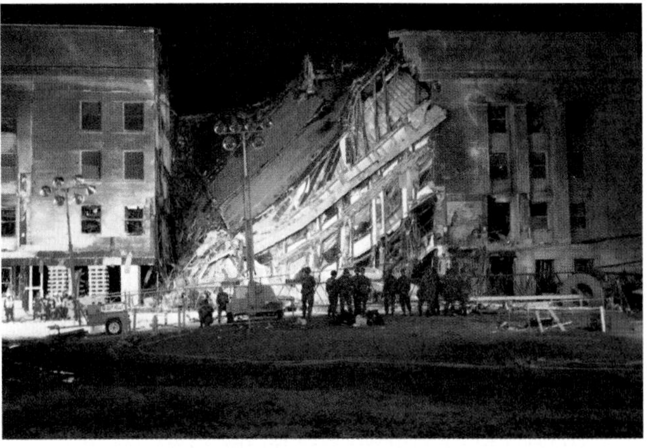

FIGURE 32-5 The collapse of the Pentagon is an example of a low-order explosion.

Courtesy of Federal Emergency Management Agency

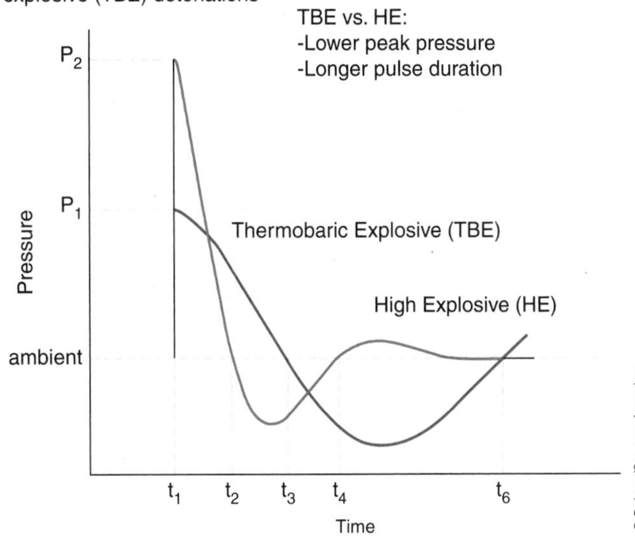

FIGURE 32-6 Pressures associated with high-order explosives.

Terrorists have access to munitions that can produce a **high-order explosion (HE)**, which is an explosion that produces extreme pressure waves traveling faster than the speed of sound (1116 ft/sec or 761 mph) (see Figure 32-6). Examples of materials that produce an HE are:

- TNT.
- C-4.
- Semite.
- Nitroglycerin.
- Dynamite.
- Ammonium nitrate fuel oil

Explosions that occur in closed places, such as cafes, buses, and subways, have a higher mortality (49% mortality) and more severe injuries in survivors than open area bombings, where the mortality rate is about 8%. Even in outdoor explosions, the victims' proximity to the explosion is critical. Victims who are 6 m from the explosion receive 9 times *less* overpressure than those who are only 3 m away. However, all victims within 20 m of the blast should be evaluated for *traumatic brain injury* (*TBI*). If the blast wave is reflected off a surface, then it can be amplified as much as 20 times. The blast wave as it passes through tissue or materials of different density causes **spalling** or shattering, of the inside tissue matrix without penetration. Spalling can result in pneumothorax, bronchopleural fistulas, and acute gas embolism.[21] Spalling also occurs inside vehicles involved in roadside bombing. The vehicle skin is not pierced by the blast, but the materials inside the vehicle spall, or break up, becoming shrapnel that injures or kills the occupants.

The injuries resulting from an HE can be classified as primary, secondary, tertiary, and quaternary.

- **Primary blast injuries**, sometimes called **blast overpressure injuries**, occur only with an HE. Primary blast injuries result from the positive-pressure wave of an HE that rapidly expands to over 20 atm (20 × 760 mm Hg). This is immediately followed by a subambient pressure that exacerbates the blast injury. In addition, the blast wave moves at three to five times the speed of sound! This shock wave travels faster in liquids and solids, rendering the brain, lungs, intestines, and tympanic membrane particularly vulnerable to damage.
- **Secondary blast injuries** are caused by ballistic debris, by shrapnel, by improvised shrapnel such as nails, nuts, and bolts, or even, in the case of a suicide bombing, by bones and body parts. The decontamination of the ballistic debris is an early intervention that is essential for both the patient and the health care provider.
- When the victim's body is thrown by the blast wave, the resulting injuries are **tertiary blast injury**.
- Burns, crush injuries, and toxic inhalations result in **quaternary blast injuries**.[22]

Blast Lung Injuries. The major causes of immediate deaths in explosions are **blast lung injury (BLI)** and air embolism that results from a BLI. *Air embolism* is conjectured to result from cellular damage between the alveoli and pulmonary capillaries.[23] The air embolism of a BLI had been previously thought to be caused by positive pressure; however, a recent study[24] has found that air embolism can occur very early in the event, before positive pressure breathing support. Treatment can be as simple as left decubitus or Trendelenburg positions with high F_IO_2 or very effective hyperbaric oxygen therapy. If hyperbaric oxygen therapy is available for patients with acute gas embolism, it should be initiated with 6 ATA pressure for 15–30 minutes, followed by a decompression with oxygen to 2.8 ATA.[25]

The *blast lung triad* of respiratory distress, hypoxia, and a so-called butterfly or bat wing infiltrate appearance on chest X-ray has been described for over 30 years in the medical literature. Meanwhile, the severity of the BLI can be categorized by P/F ratio, chest X-ray, and the presence or absence of a bronchopleural fistula.[26]

Signs and symptoms are:

- Tachypnea.
- Dyspnea.
- Cyanosis.
- Hemoptysis.
- Decreased level of consciousness.
- Decreased breath sounds with or without fine crackles.

At the same time, diminished heart sounds, low blood pressure with systolic pressure only slightly above diastolic, and distended neck veins (Beck's triad) indicate cardiac tamponade.

The basic ABCDE (airway, breathing, circulation, defibrillation-diagnosis-decontamination, and expose/examine) must be followed.

- Airway compromise is immediately life-threatening.
- Hypopnea and apnea require mechanical ventilation.
- Cardiac status, as determined by heart rate and blood pressure, is vital.
- Defibrillation may not be as prominent, but decontamination of the victim may be. Contamination in wounds can produce sepsis or toxic reactions and can prove fatal in spite of good, aggressive, competent critical care.
- Expose all skin surfaces to examination for evulsions, lacerations, and penetrating injuries. Decontaminate the victim. Monitor the end-tidal CO_2 for increased deadspace due to embolization by clots, air, or fat.

At the first sign of respiratory decompensation:

- Perform rapid-sequence intubation with cervical spine immobilization.
- Mechanical ventilation should be initiated using volume control (6 mL/kg PBW), pressure control with PIP $\leq$ 40 cm H_2O.
- Consider PLVC, IRV, or APRV.
- Start PEEP at 5–14 cm H_2O. If oxygenation does not increase, consider adding inhaled nitric oxide (iNO). Adjust the respiratory rate (*f*) up to 22 to keep the pH $\geq$ 7.20. If the pH cannot be maintained with permissive hypercapnia, then consider HFPPV or HFOV.
- Limit fluid resuscitation to prevent alveolar flooding a worsening P/F.[27]

CASE STUDY 32-1

A bombing in a shopping mall has triggered an MCI alert in the hospital. Initial police and rescue reports indicate that the blast appears to be from a high-grade military weapon—Semtex or C-4.

The first victim arriving by ambulance is a teenaged boy who is cyanotic and coughing up pink frothy secretions. His vitals are HR 130, f 30, B/P 100/70, 36.9ºC with decreased B/S in both lungs. He has shrapnel injuries to his legs and buttocks.

Questions

1. What are the RT's immediate assessment and treatment priorities?
2. What is the value of end-tidal capnography with this patient?
3. What treatment options must be considered for this patient?
4. If intubation and mechanical ventilation is indicated, what settings should be used?
5. If standard mechanical ventilation fails to improve oxygenation and/or ventilation, what alternatives can be used?

CASE STUDY 32-2

The terrorist bombing of the city's power and electrical office building results in a partial building collapse. Nearly 12 hours after the event, a victim is extracted alive and is being transported to the ED. The victim is a woman who has suffered head and chest injuries and who had her left arm pinned under a block of rubble. Paramedics report GCS 10 with occasional loss of consciousness, HR 140, B/P 90/60, and S_pO_2 92%. She has short runs of polymorphic ventricular tachycardia (Torsade de pointes) that resolve spontaneously. The EKG telemetry is:

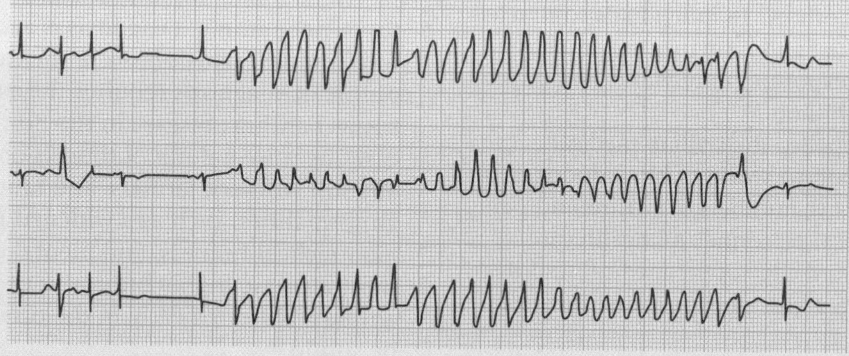

Questions

1. What pathologies are suggested by her history and vital signs?
2. What immediate medical interventions are indicated?
3. What complications can be expected with these types of injuries?
4. What would indicate the need for intubation and mechanical ventilation?
5. What mechanical ventilation strategies can be anticipated?

Psychosocial Issues in the Treatment of Blast Injuries. The long-term sequelae can occur up to 11 months or more after the event.

- Lung function can return to normal or exhibit a mild restrictive defect on pulmonary function test (PFT). Most pulmonary limitations are due to preinjury asthma, COPD, smoking history, and other factors.
- Cultural and language barriers can confound the patient assessment and the recovery.
- Providing "psychological first aid" (e.g., addressing physical needs other than medical care, social support, language and cultural sensitivity,

and a sense of decision making) can be a great help.
- By limiting exposure to the media or media reports of the event, the patient may have the psychological space to develop effective coping mechanisms.
- Post-traumatic stress has not been shown to be reduced consistently by critical incident stress debriefings.

BIOTERRORISM

A biowarfare attack is suggested by an outbreak of a rarely fatal disease that has high virulence and a high mortality rate, such as tularemia. Multiple superinfections that cannot be easily explained suggest a biological attack. Even more alarming would be a single case of smallpox since it has been declared eradicated in 1980 by the World Health Organization. A suicide "bomber" with smallpox could inflict a terrible bioterror event.[28]

The first documented bioterrorist attack occurred in the United States in the fall of 1984. A cult called the Rajneeshee contaminated 10 salad bars in Wasco County, Oregon. Over 700 people were sickened, but there were no fatalities.[29] Other cults/terrorist groups (such as the Aum Shinrikyo (Supreme Truth) that attacked the Tokyo subways with the nerve agent sarin on March 20, 1995) also tried biological agents such as botulinum toxin and even *Ebola*.[30] Fortunately, they were unsuccessful. Then in the aftermath of the tragedy of September 11, 2001, a series of **anthrax** attacks occurred, from Florida to Connecticut.[31] This was the second significant documented bioterror attack in the United States with far-reaching impact. Two branches of the federal government were temporarily shut down, as were several postal offices, 18 individuals contracted anthrax (11 inhalational and 7 cutaneous), more than 33,000 required postexposure prophylaxis, and direct costs approached $3 billion.[32]

These attacks propelled the civilian medical community into the arcane world of bioweapons. With the potential for massive numbers of victims and panic in both lay and medical personnel, all health care personnel at the forward edge of the medical response must have knowledge of this phenomenon. Possible indicators include:

- A disease that either is unusual or does not occur naturally in a given area.
- Multiple disease entities in the same patients.
- Large numbers of casualties inhabiting the same area.
- A massive point-source outbreak.
- An apparent aerosol route of infection.
- Dead sentinel animals.
- The absence of a natural vector in the area.[33]

The bioagents most likely to succeed are:

- Smallpox.
- Anthrax.
- Plague.
- Tularemia.
- Botulinum.
- Mycotoxin.
- Viral hemorrhagic fevers.[34]

However, history has shown that even *Salmonella, Brucellosis*, and others have been weaponized.[35]

The Centers for Disease Control and Prevention (CDC) has organized these agents by priority, ease of dissemination/transmission, mortality and morbidity and major public health impact. Note that, in the CDC's Category C of emerging pathogens is **multidrug-resistant tuberculosis (MDRTB)**. The categories' definitions and a list of these agents may be found in the CDC Web site (http://www.cdc.gov). Interesting also is the fact that the anthrax attacks did not precipitate a declaration of a *local* state of emergency despite the strain and financial burden the attacks placed on the impacted communities.[36]

Anthrax. Anthrax has been a medical problem throughout recorded history. In its spore form, it can survive in the soil for decades. It is primarily a cutaneous disease derived from infected herbivores and occasionally can affect the gastrointestinal tract.[37] Inhalational anthrax is extremely rare. However, once inhaled, the spore is engulfed by alveolar macrophages and carried to the lymph, where it germinates and releases its toxins.

In its inhalational form, anthrax presents like the flu or pneumonia. Diagnosis is accomplished by lab tests and by exclusion. As in the case of a natural outbreak, diagnosis requires the astute clinician to suspect anthrax disease in the non-animal-contact cases because natural outbreaks occur among abattoir workers, farmers, and ranchers. Chest X-ray abnormalities, such as a widened mediastinum, paratracheal fullness, and pleural effusions or infiltrates, are highly indicative of inhalational anthrax, although early in the disease these may be subtle.[38]

Until 2001, surviving inhalation anthrax after the symptoms appeared was virtually unknown. Symptoms of fever, chills, drenching sweats, profound fatigue, chest discomfort, and nausea or vomiting were common findings in the 2001 victims. Rhinorrhea and productive cough were uncommon findings. Arterial blood gases were not highly alarming with pH of 7.45, P_aCO_2 27 mm Hg, P_aO_2 80, and S_bO_2 97% on room air with one anthrax victim.[39]

Treatment has special requirements.

- Decontamination requires standard precautions. Victims' clothing should be bagged, labeled, and held for the FBI because it is evidence. The victims' hair should be washed if it has not been washed since the exposure.
- Early antibiotic chemotherapy is essential, and multidrug resistance must be assumed.
- Pleural effusions can be managed by chest tube thoracostomy. Drainage from the chest tubes or elsewhere can be a route of infection to the therapist, nurse, or physician.[40]

By using routine supportive respiratory care and innovative triple chemotherapy (ciprofloxacin or doxycycline, rifampin, and clindamycin or azithromycin or vancomycin), over 54.5% recovered. The expected survival rate had been less than 15%.[41]

Smallpox. Smallpox was declared eradicated by the World Health Organization (WHO) in 1980, and vaccination programs were terminated. So there is an ever increasing susceptible population. Even a single case of smallpox is a clear indicator of a bioterrorist attack.

A smallpox victim:

- Is febrile, with headache, malaise, back pain, and vomiting.
- Has lesions on the face, limbs, hands and feet, even on the palmar surfaces of the hands and feet, and the lesions are in the same stage of development. The lesions start as papules (2–3 days) and advance to pustular vesicles on the face and extremities (Figure 32-7).

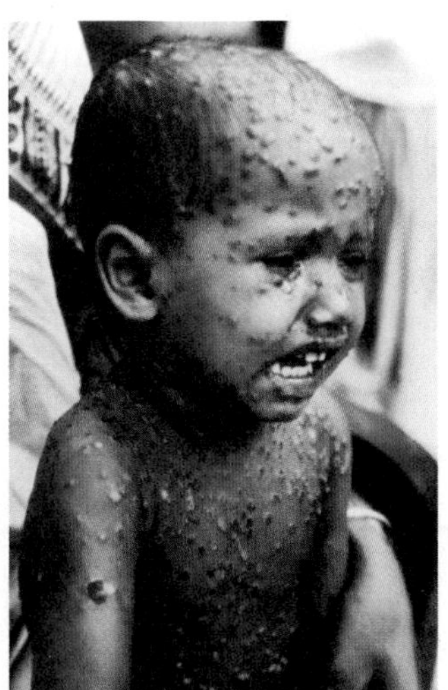

FIGURE 32-7 Child with smallpox.

Courtesy of the Centers for Disease Control and Prevention Public Health Image Library/Dr. Michael Schwartz

If the victim survives, the dried pustules fall off, and they must be considered highly contagious.

Smallpox is highly contagious but not quite as contagious as its viral cousin, chickenpox, a virus of the *Herpes zoster* family. The disease therefore requires respiratory precaution by all.

The Soviets weaponized smallpox and were actively weaponizing it until at least 1990.[42] Smallpox is spread through droplet nuclei with devastating effects. Until 1972, however, smallpox offered the terrorist or rogue government limited effectiveness as a weapon because everyone in the United States over the age of 1 was vaccinated. Nevertheless, these facts created a real concern in the military medical community.[43]

The smallpox vaccine (vaccinia virus) can be administered postexposure, preferably within 7 days. Vaccination is the only effective postexposure treatment, and all other standard treatments are supportive. (In fact, the term "vaccination" comes from the Latin *vacca* meaning "cow," since the Edward Jenner vaccine was derived from cowpox in 1789.)

A recent study reported that the antiviral agents, including ribavirin and cidofovir, could be employed as aerosol therapy for the treatment of victims. Aerosolized **cidofovir (Vistide)** by small particle nebulizer[44] in doses of merely 0.5–5 mg/kg of body weight was more effective against smallpox, cowpox, camelpox, and monkeypox than larger doses or even subcutaneous injection.[45] The respiratory care professional must be prepared to manage these victims.

The Plague. The bubonic plague created a stir in November 2002 when two tourists from New Mexico came down sick with *Yersinia pestis* (originally called *Pasteurella pestis*) in New York City. The news media

Spotlight On

Smallpox

- Incubation Period: 7–17 days
- Droplet and airborne precautions: 17 days
- Presentation: Fever, back pain, vomiting, malaise, headache, rigors; papules (2–3 days) to pustular vessicles face and extremities
- DX: Giemsa or modified silver stain, PCR, and viral isolation IHC
- TX: Immediate vaccination, aerosol cidofovir 0.5–5 mg/kg, and supportive care.

Source: Bray M. Treatment of aerosolized cowpox virus infection in mice with aerosolized cidofovir. Antiviral Research. *2002;54,3: 129–142.*

covered this story avidly.[46] The victims were successfully treated, and their disease was naturally acquired from infected rodents. Both the U.S. and former Soviet military believe that aerosolized *Yersinia pestis* would result in the highly contagious and highly fatal form of the plague, the pulmonic plague.[47] The WHO reported in 1970 that if 50 kg of *Yersinia pestis* were to be released as an aerosol over a city of 5 million, it would cause about 150,000 cases of the pneumonic plague, which would result in 36,000 deaths.[48]

The bubonic plague causes classic lesions called *buboes*, usually in the inguinal area because the flea vector bites the ankles. Although many consider it a disease of only historical interest, the plague still occurs naturally even in the United States. With three clinical presentations, bubonic, primary septicemic, and pneumonic, the gram-negative bacillus *Yersinia pestis* can be identified through laboratory smears of peripheral blood or lymph node needle aspirate.

- The *bubonic* form manifests itself through tender, enlarged (1–10-cm) lymph nodes with surrounding erythema.
- *Septicemic plague* can be a primary infection or the result of hematogenous spread of the bubonic plague. In its primary form, it challenges the clinician since it lacks the plague-related bubo.
- The plague in its *pneumonic* manifestation is the concern of all medical professionals. In the preantibiotic outbreak of the pneumonic plague in Manchuria during 1921, "the expected life of the victim was a mere 1.8 days."[49] Once again, the diagnostic marker of buboes may not appear in the pulmonic plague victim.

The signs and symptoms are as follows:

- The victims present with what appears to be a severe, rapidly progressing pneumonia after an incubation period of 1–6 days.
- They are febrile and short of breath.
- They have chest pain and a cough, which may include hemoptysis.
- At this point, tachycardia, tachypnea, dyspnea, and cyanosis appear.
- Some victims may have cervical buboes.
- The condition can progress to shock.
- **Multiple organ system failure (MOSF)**, **disseminated intravascular coagulopathy (DIC)**, and **acute renal failure (ARF)** are possible.
- Pleural effusions occur in over 50% of the cases.

Patients should be in respiratory isolation until they show clinical improvement for 24 hours.

This bioagent of terror, the pneumonic plague, is contagious and requires respiratory precautions. Even in its bubonic form, the patient may require mechanical ventilation, as in the New York City case. Fortunately, when identified through Gram stain, DNA amplification (polymer chain reaction or PCR), and IHCA, the plague is treated with streptomycin. Yet a misdiagnosis could be fatal. During the last 50 years, 4 of the 7 (57%) victims of the pneumonic plague died.[50] Suctioning, coughing, and draining of tubing require proper barrier precautions. Effective therapies for the bubonic manifestation of the plague include streptomycin, gentamycin, tetracycline, and chloramphenicol. There may also be a role for aerosolized tobramycin.

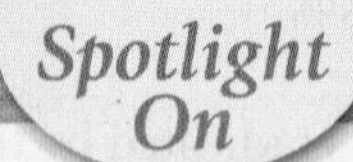

The Pneumonic Plague

- Incubation period: 2–3 days
- Droplet precautions: Respirator and HEPA filtration for ventilators
- Presentation: High fever, chills, hemoptysis, toxemia, shock, stridor, B/S crackles, ARF. *Onset to death is around 36 hrs! There is no time for buboes to appear!*
- DX: Gram stain, C&S, immunoassay for capsulated antigen, DNA amplification (PCR), immunohistochemical stains (IHC)
- TX: Gentamycin 30 mg/kg/day IM; pediatric 2.5 mg/kg/dose (infants and children Q8h) IV or IM

CASE STUDY 32-3

The RT is treating a COPD with CHF, fever, headache, rash, and lesions on the face and limbs in the ED. The examining cardiologist notes Janeway lesions (nontender hemorrhagic lesions) on the palms and soles and says, "She doesn't have bacterial endocarditis."

Questions

1. What is the suspected infection?
2. What precautions are required?
3. What respiratory care is required?
4. What will help confirm the diagnosis?

CASE STUDY 32-4

A 55-year-old male who works in the hospital's shipping-receiving is admitted to the ED. He presents with a nonproductive cough, stridor, and cyanosis: 390C, HR 110, f 28; EKG sinus tachycardia; Lab: Hct 41%, WBC 7500, CK-MB 1; CXR shows lymphoadenopathy and pleural effusions.

Questions

1. What is the suspected infection?
2. What precautions are required?
3. What respiratory care is required?
4. What will help confirm the diagnosis?

Tularemia. *Francisella tularensis*, or tularemia, was first described in 1911 by G. W. McCoy in Tulare County, California. Tularemia causes two forms of the disease in humans: ulceroglandular and typhoidal.

Although noncontagious, tularemia is a bioweapon that causes lesions on the skin and mucus membranes and that is accompanied by fever (85%), chills (45%), cough (38%), and myalgias (31%). Approximately 80% of typhoidal tularemia patients develop pneumonia.[51]

Easily identified by serology, sputum C&S and PCR and IHC, tularemia is treated with gentamycin and streptomycin.[52] **Bronchopleural fistulas** and calcifications can complicate care. Airway care and mechanical ventilation require anticipation of these problems. A restrictive defect and air leaks require careful bedside monitoring.

Botulinum Toxin. Human vanity has brought a toxin, Botox (botulinum), into the chemical cosmetic arena instead of into the emergency room. It is licensed for the treatment of strabismus, blepharospasm, and cervical torticollis.[53] Its licensing may, unfortunately, increase its availability to a terrorist.

Botulinum toxin poisoning can result in a presentation similar to variations of Guillian-Barré syndrome with one important difference: It is a rapidly *descending* paralysis, leading to respiratory failure. It can be confused with myasthenia gravis, tick-borne paralysis, or even nerve agent paralysis. However, miotic pupils and copious respiratory secretions accompany nerve agent paralysis, whereas in botulinum intoxication there is a decrease in secretions. Look for the classic triad of botulinum intoxication:

- Symmetrical, descending paralysis with bulbar palsies of (the so-called 4Ds): **diplopia**, **dysarthria**, **dysphonia**, and **dysphagia**.
- An afebrile patient.
- Clear sensorium.[54]

Airway control is therefore a priority that would not be complicated by bronchorrhea. The RT can expect to mechanically ventilate these patients for extended periods.

Differential diagnosis is vital. By means of serology, toxin assays, and anaerobic cultures, botulism can be identified and readily treated with the pentavalent toxoid vaccine. Standard Universal Precautions suffice because secondary aerosols from patients are not considered hazardous. Botulinum toxin is inactivated by sunlight within 3 hours, and decontamination with soap and water is effective because it is not dermally active. An aerosol attack is the most likely scenario in a botulinum attack; however, it could be used to attack food as well.

Again, the Soviet Union[55] and the Aum Shinrikyo cult[56] both worked avidly to develop Venezuelan equine encephalitis (VEE) and other hemorrhagic viruses (VHF, Hantaan, Marlburg, etc.) into weapons of mass destruction and terror.

- With VEE, the victim presents with a general malaise, labile fever, rigors, headache, and photophobia. The treatment is supportive with standard universal precautions.
- VHF is far more dangerous, with respiratory precautions upgraded to airborne isolation and decontamination with hypochlorite and phenolic disinfectants.
- Interestingly, ribavirin has been demonstrated to be effective in treating the Hantaan virus.[57] The principles of hemodynamic, respiratory, neurologic, and hematologic support apply.
- Intravenous **ribavirin** is effective against Lassa fever with side effects of anemia with reduced oxygen transport. The drug should not be given to pregnant women because it is embryo-lethal.
- Ribavirin has poor *in vitro* and *in vivo activity* against Ebola and Marburg, as well as against dengue and yellow fevers. Human monoclonal antibodies seem to hold the most promise at this time.[58]

Once again, creative use of antiviral agents, such as cidofovir, *as an aerosol* might be critical in saving these victims of bioterror.

Staphylococcal Enterotoxin B. Staphylococcal enterotoxin B (SEB) causes symptoms and toxicity when inhaled in very low doses. Standard Universal Precautions are required. SEB is not dermally active, and secondary aerosols are not a hazard.

Its symptoms include sudden onset of fever, chills, dyspnea, and retrosternal chest pain. Identified by ELISA, or PCR (DNA amplifications), these victims require:

- Intensive respiratory care, including oxygen, BiPAP, or mechanical ventilation with PEEP.
- Close hemodynamic monitoring and excellent fluid management.

A new drug, **pirfenidone**, seems to block the effect of SEB, especially the development of pulmonary fibrosis that complicates ventilator management with a restrictive defect.[59]

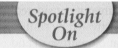

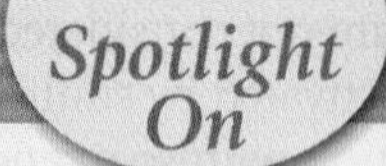

Pirfenidone

- Initial study at the United States Army Medical Research Institute for Infectious Diseases demonstrated effectiveness against SEB (Hale ML, et al. *Infect Immun.* 2002;70:2989–2994).
- In March 2004, the Food and Drug Administration classifies pirfenidone as an *orphan drug* for idiopathic pulmonary fibrosis (Nagai S, et al. *Intern Med.* 2002;41,12:1118–1123).
- Several studies demonstrate effectiveness in bleomycin lung fibrosis (Kakugawa. *Eur Resp J.* 2004), oleic acid ALI (Mei SJ. *Pharmacl Exp Ther.* 2004), kidney fibrosis, and multiple sclerosis (Bowen JD. *Mult Scler.* 2003).

CASE STUDY 32-5

The therapist is called to the ED for intubation and mechanical ventilation of a 30–year-old GBS or MG patient. He has ptosis, diplopia, difficulty speaking, and upper body paralysis. His wife reports that the symptoms started last night with nausea, constipation, and difficulty urinating.

Questions

1. What other diagnosis should be considered?
2. What precautions are required?
3. What respiratory care is required?
4. What will help confirm the diagnosis?

Impact of Bioterrorism on the Health Care Community. Bioterror attacks present the health care community with two unique problems for which it must be prepared: mass casualties requiring effective management and ventilatory support by medical personnel who are burdened with existing patients and a diagnostic blizzard of genuine and psychogenic casualties. In addition, bioterrorism presents the medical professions and especially respiratory care with unique challenges and learning.

- Manual resuscitators can manage respiratory support initially; however, the respiratory and nursing staffs will be quickly overwhelmed.
- **HEPA (high-efficiency particulate air)** filtering of exhalate from manual resuscitators may well forestall the risk to therapists, nurses, and physicians caring for biocasualties.
- In the chaos of the attack, roads, bridges, tunnels, and airports may be closed, as they were on September 11, 2001. Rental ventilators may not arrive in time. The government **Push Packs** may not arrive for 12 hours or 10 days after the disaster has been identified.

Yet this threat presents the profession with an outstanding opportunity to clearly demonstrate its vital importance to hospitals, the public health, and the American public. As more is learned about the agents of bioterror, it becomes obvious that respiratory care can play a significant role in the diagnosis, initial care, management, and follow-up care of the victims of bioterror. The opportunities for expansion of the scope of practice are legion. The unfortunate reality that bioterror will occur again demands that respiratory care professionals be prepared.

Zoonotic Disease. Diseases that are caused by host animals are called **zoonotic**, and they almost always occur in humans who have close contact with the host animal. Even in most farming communities, these zoonotic diseases rarely occur. However, if urban office workers come down with brucellosis, glanders, or tularemia, then a terrorist release should be seriously considered.

Differentiating Epidemics, Pandemics, and Seasonal Disease from Bioterrorism. Differential diagnosis is difficult. Differentiating naturally occurring disease from bioterrorism is challenging and requires the clinician to have a high index of suspicion. Naturally occurring diseases and climatic events can further confound the situation.

- Pandemics start with one or more index cases; then there is a logarithmic growth in the number of victims, perhaps partly due to a seasonal surge.

- Bioterrorism produces a large number of victims in a very short time. These victims have a common geographic point where the terrorists released the agent. On the other hand, natural outbreaks from contaminated water, food, or drink can have single geographic point source too.

Infection Control in Biological Events. *Infection control* is an evolving science that requires frequent updates and training. Emerging diseases such as severe acute respiratory syndrome (SARS), avian influenza, and others require early epidemiologic identification and implementation of infection control (IC) to reduce their spread by means of the infection of other patients and the staff.

The two forms of disease transmission that are of most concern are contact and airborne transmission.

- In *skin-to-skin contact*, transmission occurs when the therapist touches patients to assess, turn, or position them. Contact transmission can occur through contaminated hands and fomites.
- *Airborne* transmission occurs via droplet nuclei containing the infectious agent, such as TB.[60]

The respiratory therapist must be aware that aerosol-generating procedures such as nebulizer treatments, suctioning, intubation, and bronchoscopy have a real potential for disseminating droplet nuclei. In the Canadian SARS experience, viral transmission from the patient to health care personnel occurred during an intubation procedure. Consider additional precautions for hospital personnel or reducing aerosol-generating procedures to only those essential for patient care.

Environmental and administrative controls other than Universal Standard Precautions should be established as early in a biological event as possible.

- The early detection of infectious disease, the vaccination of health care personnel, pharmaceutical prophylaxis, and isolation or cohorting of infectious patients are all essential.
- Emergency departments and clinics should promote the use of masks by symptomatic persons or patients during transport.
- Guidance in the use of personal protective equipment (PPE), the cleaning of equipment, handling lab specimens, and postmortem care must be preestablished.
- There is some evidence to show that the use of ultraviolet light can lower transmission rates.[61]

Respiratory therapists engaged in home care should follow the Standard and the Droplet Precautions when entering a home to provide services to an infectious patient. Professional judgment determines whether a surgical N95 respirator should be worn upon entering the patient's home. Good hand hygiene has been cited as the single most important practice in infection control.[62]

CHEMICAL WEAPONRY

A 1969 United Nations report defined *chemical warfare agents* as "[c]hemical substances, whether gaseous, liquid or solid, which might be employed because of their direct toxic effects on man, animals and plants." The use of chemicals in our daily lives requires bulk shipments by rail, truck, or ship and the large volume storage, all of which subject to accidental release into the air, as in the Bhopal incident of 1984. Perhaps a more alarming event was the sarin nerve agent release by an apocalyptic cult, the Aum Shinrikyo, in the Tokyo subway system in March of 1994, which resulted in 5000 casualties and 12 deaths.[63]

The history of poison gas warfare (i.e., chemical warfare) is not confined to the battlefields of World War I, where it is the most infamous. During the Ethiopian campaign in 1935–1941, the Italian Army used mustard agents (vesicants/blister agents) on the Ethiopians. More recently, Iraq used lethal combinations of nerve and mustard agents against both the Iranians (Iran-Iraq War) and Iraqi Kurdish populations. Some nations considered chemical warfare agents as a "poor man's nuclear weapon." Table 32-4 summarizes categories of chemical agents.

The possible indicators of a chemical release or attack are as follows:

- Are there mass casualties/fatalities with minimal or no physical trauma?
- Are first responders casualties?
- Are there dead animals and/or vegetation in the area?

TABLE 32-4 **Basic categories of chemical agents**

Pulmonary Agents: chlorine, phosgene, cyanide
Vesicant Agents: Lewisite and the nitrogen mustard agents
Nerve Agents: Tabun (GA), Sarin (GB), and VX
Lachrymators: CN (Mace), CS
Insecticides: Malathion, parathion, and sevin
Defoliants: Agent Orange, Round-up, etc.

- Are there reports of unusual odors, smoke, or vapor clouds? (If *you smell* it, then you are a victim too! A phenomenon of off-gassing occurs when chemicals on a victim vaporize and affect rescuers or health care professionals.)

Note: Most military-grade chemical weapons have no smell associated with them.

Chemical Warfare/Terrorism Nerve Agents: Sarin (GB), Soman (GD), Tabun (GA), or VX.

Nerve agents are chemically related to organophosphate insecticides. Sarin and Tabun were developed by German scientists (hence the "G" prefix to its abbreviation) who were working on controlling mites on plants. At the end of World War II, the Soviet Army captured the German chemical munitions plant and thus acquired these agents. The United States countered with its own research and produced the highly lethal, VX. A droplet of VX on the skin is fatal in seconds to minutes. Nerve agents penetrate clothing to produce symptoms or even death and can be effective even through heavy winter clothing.

All of these agents cause a cholinergic crisis by blocking anticholinesterase. Victims exhibit signs and symptoms within a minute or sooner after exposure. In some, the first signs might be seizures and death. Since these agents have volatility similar to water or motor oil, vaporization may be limited.

Victims of nerve agent toxicity have the following signs and symptoms:

- Headache
- Blurred vision from pinpoint pupils (miosis)
- Tight chest (smooth muscle constrictions) with bronchospasm and copious secretions
- Diaphoresis
- Lacrimation
- Salivation
- Unexplained runny nose

The treatment of these victims is time-sensitive, requiring the administration of both atropine (2 mg/IM) and pralidoxime (2-PAM), both of which are in the Mark 1 Nerve Agent Antidote Kit (NAAK) autoinjectors that can be administered through heavy clothing.

Atropine should be administered first. Intramuscular injection into the thigh muscle (vastus lateralis or rectus femoris muscles) can reverse muscarinic effects of nerve agents (i.e., bronchospasm, bradycardia, and excessive secretions). Think dumbels for muscles for muscarinic. (See the Spotlight On Mnemonic for Muscarinic Signs—Dumbels.) Atropine can be instilled via an endotracheal tube if necessary.

Next, *pralidoxime* is administered via autoinjector. Pralidoxime chloride is a cholinesterase reactivator. Nerve agent victims with myasthenia gravis require very close monitoring when pralidoxime is used. Conscious patients should be informed that mild to moderate pain may be felt at the injection site. In an organophosphate pesticide or nerve agent, toxidrome pralidoxime is potentially curative.[64]

Patients should be monitored for a reduction or elimination of symptoms in 5–10 minutes. If symptoms

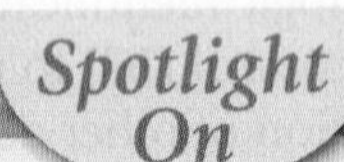

The Nerve Agent–Poisoned Child

Pralidoxime:

- Pediatric dosage:
  - 20–40 mg/kg IV over 10 minutes
  - 5–10 mg/kg/h for 24 hours after initial bolus
- *Route:*
  - IV preferred
  - IM possible (Mark I kits)

Atropine:

- Range: 0.01–0.04 mg/kg
  - Never give less than 0.1mg!
- 0.02 mg/kg, IV every 5 minutes
  - Until bronchorrhea, bronchospasm, and hemodynamically significant bradycardia are controlled

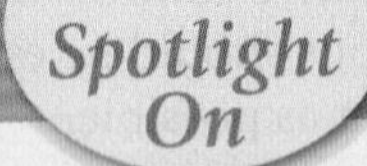

Mnemonic for Diagnosing Nerve Agent Exposure

Mnemonic for Muscarinic Signs—**Dumbels**

- **D**iarrhea
- **U**rination
- **M**iotic pupils
- **B**ronchospasm, bronchorrhea, bradycardia*
- **E**mesis
- **L**acrimation
- **S**alivation

**Bradycardia was not present in the victims of Tokyo sarin attack.*

TABLE 32-5 Chemical agent targets of toxicity

Toxic Agent	Target(s)
Nerve agents (Sarin, VX, etc.)	Airways, breathing, disability (NMJ)
Cyanides (asphyxiants)	Breathing (cellular)
Pulmonary agents (phosgene)	Airway, breathing (alveolar level)
Riot control	Airway, breathing
Insecticides (organophospates)	Airways, breathing, disability (NMJ)
Herbicides	Airway, disability (Carcinogenic)

persist, then a second administration of atropine and pralidoxime should be administered. A total of 3 doses of the drugs may be required. In the Tokyo event, most victims responded to single doses of atropine and pralidoxime.

Table 32-5 lists targets of toxicity involving exposure to chemical agents.

Blister Agents (Vesicants). In this category, the chemical rapidly binds with proteins, including DNA, to produce damage. **Nitrogen mustard** and **lewisite**, for example, were intended to bypass gas mask defense by attacking exposed skin.

"Depending on the vesicant, clinical effects may occur immediately (as with phosgene oxime or lewisite) or may be delayed for 2 to 24 hours (as with mustards). Following exposure, the most commonly encountered clinical effects include dermal (skin erythema and blistering), respiratory (pharyngitis, cough, dyspnea), ocular (conjunctivitis and burns), and gastrointestinal (nausea and vomiting)."[65]

Treatment must be quick.

- The early and gentle decontamination (ideally within minutes of exposure) *reduces* damage.
- Cut off clothing rather than pulling over the head or over uncontaminated skin.
- **Racemic epinephrine** aerosol is effective for stridor.
- **N-acetyl-l-cystine (NAC)** by aerosol may provide some amelioration of inhalation injuries; however, research is still being conducted.

Note: there is no antidote for mustard poisoning; treatment is similar to that for a burn injury.

Vesicant toxidrome can result in:

- Leukocytopenia.
- Decreased RBC (decreased oxygen transport).
- Decreased platelets.
- Sepsis.
- Airway obstruction.
- Atelectasis.
- Disseminated intravascular coagulopathy (DIC).
- Multiorgan system failure (MOSF).

Close monitoring of the victims' airway status is vital since airway compromise can occur at any degree of injury.

Cyanide. Severe cyanide intoxication results in:

- A brief period of hyperpnea.
- Seizures.
- Hypopnea.
- Dysrhythmias.
- Apnea and death.

In mild exposures, only nauseam vertigo, dyspnea, and muscle weakness occur.

The symptoms are a result of the fact that cyanide stops the cellular oxidative process by blocking cytochrome a,a_3 and dramatically reducing the production of ATP. The effect is lactic acidemia and tissue death. Therefore, oxygen consumption is severely reduced in affected cells. Mixed venous (pulmonary artery) blood oxygen levels can have saturations above 76% and partial pressures in excess of 46 mm Hg.

Before treatment of *dermal exposure* cases:

- Remove all the victim's clothing, jewelry, and shoes.
- Bag-and-tag all personal possessions.
- Wash affected areas with large quantities of water and mild liquid detergent, paying attention to skin in skin folds.

With *aerosol exposures*, remove clothing that might have trapped or adsorbed vapors. If the patient is asymptomatic, washing is usually unnecessary, but if in doubt, decontaminate the victim.

Treatment requires the removal of cyanide from the cytochrome a, a_3 by methemoglobin by administering the antidote sodium nitrite. Sodium nitrite oxidizes hemoglobin's $Fe+2$ to produce methemoglobin's $Fe+3$ (**MetHb**). MetHb results in "chocolate brown blood" appearance. This permits the resumption of cytochrome activity and the production of ATP. Sodium thiosulfate accelerates the catabolism of displaced cyanide by the liver.

Personal protection includes:

- HVAC to control the **off-gassing** that occurs when chemicals vaporize from a victim's body or clothing.
- Butyl rubber gloves with Teflon, Responder, or Tychem Protective clothing.
- In some severely contaminated cases, **self-contained breathing apparatus (SCBA)** to provide clean pressurized air to emergency personnel.

The medical management of the cyanide victim includes:

- Administration of 10 ml of 3% sodium nitrate IV over 5–15 minutes while monitoring blood pressure for sodium nitrate–induced hypotension.
- That is followed by 50 ml of 25% sodium thiosulfate IV over 10 minutes.
- Keep MetHb levels below 35% (low Hb) and 45% (normal Hb/Hct level).
- In poorly responding patients, a second half-dose of both sodium nitrate and sodium thiosulfate may be administered.
- Determine the victim's Hb level! If MetHb >30/35% (adult) or >25% (children), treat it with 1–2 mg/kg IV methylene blue.
- Vitamin B_{12} can provide excellent therapeutics with minimal side effects, especially for pregnant women and children.
- Oxygen theoretically should not help; however, early use of high F_IO_2 has good outcomes.
- Also recommended but possibly not feasible with an MCI is hyperbaric oxygen.

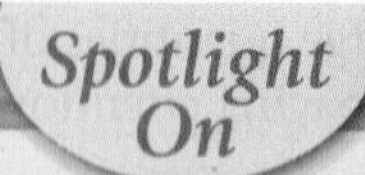

Managing the Cyanide-Poisoned Child

- 100% oxygen
- IV 0.33 mL/kg sodium nitrite
- 1.65 mL/kg of 25% sodium thiosulfate* (Adjust the dose for Hb level** and keep MetHB <30%.)
- Repeat at half dose if symptoms persist.
- Vitamin B_{12} can reverse cyanide toxicity. Watch for anaphylactoid reactions!

**Isom GE, Johnson JD. Sulphur donors in cyanide intoxication.* Clinical and Experimental Toxicology. *1987.*

***Berlin CM. Treatment of cyanide poisoning in children pediatrics. 1970;46:793.*

Phosphene. The onset of symptoms can vary from 2 to 6 hours, and some victims can be asymptomatic for 48 hours. *All exposed victims must be observed for 48 hours!* Children are more vulnerable to phosgene.

The signs and symptoms of phosgene intoxication include:

- Hoarseness.
- Stridor.
- Laryngospasm.
- Wheezing (reactive airways disease syndrome or RADS).
- Cyanosis and fine crackles of noncardiogenic pulmonary edema.

Laboratory evidence of phosgene exposure includes:

- Anemia.
- Evidence of hemolysis.
- Increased bilirubinemia and/or MetHb.
- Decreased P/F ratio or increased $P_{A\text{-}a}O_2$.

Treatment for phosgene exposure includes:

- Oxygen.
- Aerosolized bronchodilators.
- CPAP/Bi-level pressure support (start with 4/8).

All ED personnel should wear protective eye wear and gloves, especially with liquid phosgene exposure.

Pharmacologic therapy includes:

- Leukotriene receptor-blockers.
- Methylprednisolone.
- Ibuprofen.
- N-acetylcystine (NAC) lavage to mitigate lung injury.

Children's stridor responds very well to racemic epinephrine via aerosol 0.25–0.75 ml of 2.25% Q 20 min.[66]

Chlorine. A dense yellow-green gas with a pungent odor, chlorine was the ideal killer in the trenches of World War I. Being heavier than air, it sought out victims in deep trenches and bunkers. Even in industrial or rail accidents, chlorine seeks low ground and basements.

The signs and symptoms are as follows:

- Immediately upon contact, eye and URT irritation (a burning and choking sensation) ensues.
- It is often followed by nausea, vomiting, and dyspnea on exertion (DOE).
- Cough and then hoarseness.
- Pulmonary edema follows in as little as 30 minutes or up to 2–24 hours.

Survivors may have permanent reactive airways disease (RAD) and either restrictive or obstructive PFT defects.

Treatment is as follows:

- Thorough decontamination with soap and water is required, ideally before the victims arrive in the ED.
- Administer nebulized beclomethasone (20 mcg/kg)[67] or budesonide[68] as soon as possible to improve compliance and P/F.
- Therapists should consider racemic epinephrine for stridor, Bi-level (APRV) pressure support, and intubation MV. Inhalation injury should resolve in 3–5 days.

Note: Nebulized $NaHCO_3$ for neutralizing HCL resulting from chlorine intoxication is unproven.

CASE STUDY 32-6

The therapist is paged to the ED STAT. There are 55 adults and children from the neighborhood that was being sprayed for West Nile virus mosquitoes. The RT is ordered to treat the ones with hoarseness and paroxysmal cough. While auscultating one of the victims, she observes that the patient and others have runny noses and are tearing. Their facial and hand skin appears reddened. She smells garlic.

Questions

1. What agent or agents could be responsible?
2. What PPE level is required?
3. What immediate treatment must be rendered?

CASE STUDY 32-7

The respiratory therapist is called to the ED STAT. Upon arrival, he sees six patients who have arrived simultaneously via car. Two have lost consciousness, one is convulsing, and three are tachypneic (f 34), reporting severe headaches. SpO_2 ~90%. A nurse remarks that the victim's venous blood looks almost as red as your ABG on one victim.

Questions

1. What agent or agents could be responsible?
2. What PPE level is required?
3. What immediate treatment must be rendered?

CASE STUDY 32-8

Some 35 people from the airport are in the ED. There was one death in the ED, and one DOA. There is no apparent physical trauma. Paramedics report several immediate deaths at the airport. Several have lost consciousness, are convulsing, and are virtually apneic. Others are vomiting, drooling, and tearing; several have uncontrollable diarrhea and shortness of breath.

Questions

1. What agent or agents could be responsible?
2. What therapeutics must be taken immediately?
3. What are the RT's priorities?

Disease

Outbreaks of disease can at times overwhelm the health care system and have devastating effects on entire populations.

- An **epidemic** affects a large number of people in a given population or community. AIDS is an example of an epidemic that hit the United States in the 1980s.
- A **pandemic** effects a wide geographic location and an exceptionally high proportion of people. The H1N1 influenza of 2009 is an example of a pandemic. Confirmed cases affected 214 countries and overseas territories.

INFLUENZA

The CDC reports that annually an average of 36,000 Americans die of influenza and that an average of 226,000 hospitalizations result from seasonal influenza (during late fall to early spring). Annual influenza vaccination is strongly recommended with:

- Either **trivalent inactivated vaccine (TIV)** for people over 6 years or in a high-risk group.
- Or the **live attenuated influenza vaccine (LAIV)** for healthy, nonpregnant persons.[69]

It is prudent for respiratory therapists to protect themselves with the vaccine.

Influenza viruses are transmitted from person to person via large particle droplets (greater than 5 microns) from coughs and sneezes as well as from hand to nose. Large droplets have a range of less than 1 m and remain airborne for a very short time and can be a source of surface contamination leading to the hand-nose route of transmission. However, droplets less than 5 microns, as might result from the use of small volume nebulizers, can remain suspended in the air for a considerable amount of time.

The typical incubation period is 1–4 days; however, the adult patient is shedding viruses *before symptoms appear.* Children can shed the virus before they are ill and for more than 10 days after symptoms appear. Influenza deaths are low among children less than 5 years of age, as compared to adults over 65 (0.4 deaths compared to 98.3 deaths per 100,000 persons).[70]

Influenza results in:

- Fever.
- Myalgias.
- Headache.
- Malaise.
- Nonproductive cough.
- Sore throat and rhinitis.
- Exacerbation of preexisting cardiac or pulmonary diseases.
- Secondary bacterial infection.

There are two types of influenza viruses: A and B. These are further subtyped by their surface antigens: hemagglutinin and neuraminidase.

- **Hemagglutinin** permits the virus to bind with and to enter the cell to be replicated. Hemagglutinin, a protein, has 16 types; types H5 though H7 are the most dangerous.
- **Neuraminidase** facilitates the release of newly replicated viruses to escape the cell and to infect other cells. There are 9 versions of the N protein with the N1 being the most dangerous.

The variations in paring of H and N proteins permit a *possible 144 versions of the Type A influenza virus alone!*

Pandemic Influenza. Starting in April–May 1918 and resuming in the fall 1918 and well into February 1919, the so-called Spanish Flu (AH5N1) raged around the world. The bodies of the victims of the 1918–1919 pandemic buried in the permafrost of Alaska and Siberia provided the DNA of the virus. The 1918–1919 pandemic provides a template for diagnosis. The AH5N1 infection was characterized uniformly by fevers of 102°F (38.9°C), bronchial pneumonia, septicemia, and CNS involvement with the highest attack rate in persons between 14 and 40 years of age. In an era where travel was slow, Eskimo villages were wiped out, and the island of Fiji suffered 8000 deaths. There were an estimated 20–40 million deaths worldwide.[71] Some survivors suffered from residual postinfluenza encephalitis.

In 1957 another pandemic, the AH2N2 (Asian flu) resulted in 70,000 deaths in the United States. In the Asian flu pandemic, the highest mortality was in the school age and elderly populations. The AH2N2 pandemic of 1969 had a much lower fatality rate. As seen in these pandemics, the virus can share genetic material and mutate, thus frustrating vaccine development and requiring annual inoculation.

In 2009, the most recent flu pandemic from the H1N1 virus resulted in over 25,000 deaths worldwide.

When a pandemic strikes, several aspects of hospital policy and EOP must be preestablished.

- First heating-ventilation-air conditioning (HVAC) must have an excess of 6 air exchanges per hour and filtered.
- Flu shots must be administered to all staff as early in the flu cycle as practicable.
- An adequate supply of gowns and N95 masks must be in the hospital's stock.
- Aerosols and aerosol therapy must be reduced or eliminated.
- All exhalation from mechanically ventilated patients must be filtered using a **high efficiency particulate air (HEPA) filter**.
- The staff should decontaminate or shower and change clothes before going home.

The AH5N1 or a similar influenza virus triggers a **cytokine storm** (releasing **tumor necrosis factor-alpha**, **interleukin-6, 7, 8,** and **interferon**), an immunological overreaction that leads to ARDS. The strong immune response to viral infections results in a high mortality rate.[72] The severity of the ARDS is indicted by:

- A P/F ratio of less than 200.
- Blood lactate greater than 2.2 mmol/L.
- Pulmonary infiltrates on chest films.

Therefore proinflammatory cytokines seem to be the culprit that results in ARDS, **SIRS (systemic inflammatory response syndrome)**, and multiorgan system failure (renal failure, disseminated intravascular coagulopathy, and respiratory failure). Complicating the situation is renal impairment with decreased urine output (requiring careful fluid management), creatinine > 100, urea > 6, and uric acid >400. Lymphocytes can decrease to 0.04 and monocytes to 0.03.[73]

Bird Flu, a Zoonostic Variant. Close contact among humans, birds, and pigs can have the unfortunate result of sharing viruses. The contact creates the optimal environment for viruses to share proteins and emerge as a pandemic. During 2004, Vietnam reported

22 cases and 15 deaths from avian H5 strain. Later, Thailand reported 12 cases with 8 deaths. This mortality rate was 67–68% with a potential to be ten times more lethal than the 1918–1919 pandemic.

Suggested Medical Management of the Pandemic Victim.

- First, scrupulous infection control procedures must be taken. Vaccination with even standard influenza vaccines is prudent until a specific vaccine can be developed, manufactured, and distributed.
- Treating the cytokine storm requires 200 mg hydrocortisone, 10 mg chlorpheniramine, 0.5–3.0 mg metaraminol in divided doses and titrated for effect, and 1 gm acetaminophen—all intravenously.
- In previous cases, neither bronchospasm nor laryngeal edema was evident; therefore bronchodilators may not be necessary. If they become necessary, then minimize the use of aerosol. Consider the use of MDI with a spacer, even with mechanical ventilators. Nebulized particles of less than 5 microns remain suspended in the breathing environment for a considerable period of time.
- In SARS and in some Avian flu cases, patients responded to bilevel pressure with supplemental oxygen. However, there are concerns for the virus being spread via the patient's exhalate.

Mechanical ventilation of patients should fall under the ARDSnet recommendations because the P/F ratios will be in the ALI (<300) or ARDS (<200) range. Ventilation with tidal volumes of 6 ml/kg PBW using assist-control mode is a good starting point. PEEP levels are conventionally 5–12 cm H_2O; however, the positive effects of PEEP on oxygenation (P_aO_2, S_bO_2, and C_aO_2) must be weighed against the negative effects on blood pressure and cardiovascular function.[74] "Drying" the lung with conservative fluid administration and aggressive use of diuretics and/or dialysis has been shown to help reduce the duration of mechanical ventilation in ARDS patients.[75]

Summary

Disasters of any cause or size require a coordinated, prepared response if both the victims and the hospital are to survive. The NIMS and the hospital's ICS are the command and control elements of disaster response. Most disasters are Tier 1 and can be managed by prepared and drilled staff.

Standard Precautions, aerosol protection, and patient decontamination are more important in an MCI because of the many unknowns as the event unfolds. By establishing an early diagnosis and providing prompt, prepared aggressive care, the worst case can be forestalled. Accurate record keeping and the bagging and tagging of victims' personal possessions assist in the investigation that will follow the event.

The regular use of surge ventilators purchased by state or local governments for EMCC precludes or reduces training time. Among the ventilators purchased by state and local governments are the Viasys-Pulmonetics LTV 1200 and the Versamed iVent. Both are excellent volume-pressure-cycled ventilators with PEEP and oxygen options and an internal battery with about 1 hour's worth of use. However, both require annual servicing by company-certified technicians, mandatory battery recharge, and temperature-humidity-controlled storage.[76]

The federal government's emergency National Strategic Stockpile **Push Packs** are 2-ton preloaded and prepositioned supply containers of medicines, equipment, and ventilators (no oxygen) that can be at a site within 12 hours of an emergency. Push Packs include the LP-10 and the Impact Eagle754 transport ventilator which, while easy to operate, still requires in-service education that must be accomplished prior to a disaster of either natural causes or of human intent. The Eagle754 is a touch screen operation ventilator with internal battery (rechargeable) and compressor; it is therefore ideal for emergency situations. With an automatic pressure transducer, the 754 can support patients to an altitude of 25,000 feet. It is approved for use with adults and pediatric patients, including infants. Additionally, the Impact Eagle provides the intensive care–level of mechanical ventilation that nurses, respiratory therapists, and intensivists have come to expect from their ventilators: alarms and graphics display.[77]

Medicine and respiratory care in particular are constantly evolving sciences with new research and clinical experience that constantly broaden knowledge, skills, and pharmacologic treatment. They require respiratory therapists to maintain and update their knowledge and proficiency. The reader is strongly encouraged to confirm information contained in this chapter for updates, evidence-based studies, and clinical competencies.

Study Questions

REVIEW QUESTIONS

1. What is the difference between a natural and a human-made disaster?

2. List at least five biological and five chemical agents that can be used in a terrorist attack and the physiological effects that each produces.
3. What is the role of the respiratory therapist on a disaster response team?

MULTIPLE-CHOICE QUESTIONS

1. Several adult victims of a cyanide terrorist attack have MetHb levels of greater than 35%. Which of the following is the best treatment option?
   a. Administer 100% oxygen via bilevel pressure 4/8.
   b. Administer a half dose of sodium nitrate and sodium thiosulfate.
   c. Administer vitamin B_{12} intravenously.
   d. Administer methylene blue IV until MetHb is less than 30%.
2. Primary blast injuries are the result of which of the following?
   a. shrapnel or suicide bomber's body parts causing penetrating injuries
   b. violent pressure wave of HE
   c. burns or crush injuries from explosions
   d. blast victim being thrown by the blast wave
3. The most important practice to reduce the transmission of infectious agents is:
   a. hand hygiene.
   b. use of ultraviolet lights.
   c. HVAC with 6 to 10 air exchanges per hour.
   d. use of N-95 masks.
4. The care of a patient with inhalation anthrax requires the use of:
   a. droplet precautions.
   b. Standard Precautions.
   c. biohazard level IV controls.
   d. cidofovir aerosol.
5. In a mass casualty incident (MCI), which of the following are the major concerns of the respiratory care service?
   a. oxygen therapy supplies and mechanical ventilators
   b. a stockpile of gowns, masks, and gloves
   c. a stockpile of aerosol bronchodilators
   d. cancellation of elective surgery and PFTs
6. While crush injuries are common in earthquakes, for what type of pathologies must a respiratory therapist prepare?
   a. blast lung injuries
   b. infections, asthmatic, and heart attacks
   c. near drowning injuries
   d. a and c
7. Victims of HE who are 3 m from the explosion are likely to suffer which of the following injuries?
   a. TBI, pneumothorax, bronchopleural fistulas, and acute gas embolism
   b. mold, bacterial, and fungal infections
   c. hypobaric or decompression injuries
   d. none of these
8. A large number of people have been seeking care in your hospital for Guillian-Barré syndrome (GBS). What may be occurring?
   a. an unusual outbreak of the disease
   b. the effect of the flu vaccination program
   c. a bioterror event, not GBS
   d. a mass hysteria event
9. Several ED patients report the symptoms of blurred vision and difficulty with speaking, enunciating, and swallowing. What do their symptoms suggest?
   a. botulinum intoxication
   b. cyanide intoxication
   c. myasthenia gravis crisis
   d. food poisoning with salmonella
10. Twenty patients from this morning's commuter train are in your ED. They exhibit tearing, rhinorrhea, drooling, and excessive productive cough. Several are vomiting. On examination, they have pinpoint pupils, wheezing, and low heart rates. What do their symptoms suggest?
    a. pandemic influenza outbreak
    b. bioterrorist use of tularemia
    c. terrorist use of a nerve agent
    d. terrorist use of a blister or vesicant agent

CRITICAL-THINKING QUESTIONS

1. What can the respiratory therapist do to assure that culturally sensitive situations can be avoided even during a mass casualty event?
2. What is the role of the respiratory therapist in a dual-agent bioterror attack?
3. What actions can the nurse–respiratory therapist perform to successfully manage pediatric casualties of a disaster?
4. What are the difficulties to be expected with the pregnant/elderly/disabled/chronically ill in a mass casualty incident?

References

1. American College of Emergency Physicians. Disaster Medical Services–Policy #400053.
2. American Hospital Association. www.aha.org/aha/content/2005/pdf/2005octbehupdate.pdf

3. Federal Bureau of Investigation. "Amerithrax or anthrax investigation." www.fbi.gov/anthrax/amerithraxlinks.htm
4. Oklahoma State Department of Health. "Oklahoma City bombing." http://www.ok.gov/health/Disease,_Prevention,_Preparedness/Injury_Prevention_Service/Oklahoma_City_Bombing/index.html
5. Centers for Disease Control and Prevention. "Severe acute respiratory syndrome (SARS)." http://www.cdc.gov/ncidod/sars/
6. Centers for Disease Control and Prevention. "CDC resources for pandemic flu." http://www.cdc.gov/flu/Pandemic/
7. Farmer JC, Carlton PK. Providing critical care during a disaster: the interface between disaster response agencies and hospitals. *Crit Care Med.* Supp. 2006;34:S56–S59.
8. Mahoney EJ, Harrington DT, Biffl WL. Lessons learned from a nightclub fire: institutional disaster preparedness. *J Trauma.* 2005;58:487–491.
9. Centers for Disease Control and Prevention. "Mass casualties predictor." http://www.bt.cdc.gov/masscasualties/predictor.asp
10. Devereaux A, Christian MD, et al. Summary of suggestions from the Task Force for Mass Critical Care Summit January 26–27, 2007. *Chest.* 2008; 133:S1–S7.
11. Ibid.
12. Rubinson L, et al. *Chest.* "Definitive Care for the Critically Ill During a Disaster: A Framework for Optimizing Critical Care Surge Capacity from a Task Force for Mass Critical Care Summit Meeting, January 26–27, 2007, Chicago, IL." http://www.chestjournal.org/cgi/content/abstract/133/5_suppl/18S
13. Swift D. Planning for disaster–a starting guide respiratory therapy. 2008;3,4:36–39.
14. Chou YJ , Huang N, Lee CH, Tsai SL, Chen LS, Chang HJ. Who is at risk of death in an earthquake? *Am J Epidemi.* 2004;160,7:688–695;doi: 10.1093/aje/kwh270.
15. Baker SP, et al. The Injury Severity Score: a method for describing patients with multiple injuries and evaluating emergency care. *J Trauma.* 1974;14:187–196.
16. Toker A, Isitmangel T, Erdik O, Sancakli I, Sebit S. Analysis of chest injuries during the 1999 Marmarra earthquake. *Surg Today.* 2002;32,9:769–771.
17. Naghii MR. Public health impact and medical consequences of earthquakes. *Rev Panam Salud Publica.* 2005;18,3:216–221.
18. Schneider E, Hajjeh RA, et al. A coccidioidomycosis outbreak following the Northridge, Calif, earthquake. *JAMA.* 1997;19;277,11:904–908.
19. eMedicine. "Coccidioidomycosis." http://www.emedicine.com/derm/topic742.htm
20. Mahoney EJ, Harrington DT, Biffl WL. Lessons learned from a nightclub fire: institutional disaster preparedness. *J Trauma.* 2005;58:487–491.
21. Bridges EJ. Blast injuries: from triage to critical care. *Crit Care Nurs Clin N Am.* 2006;18:333–348.
22. Centers for Disease Control and Prevention. "Explosions and blast injuries: a primer for clinicians." http://www.bt.cdc.gov/masscasualties/explosions.asp
23. Mayorga MA. The pathology of primary blast overpressure injury. *Toxicology.* 1997;121:17–28.
24. Tsokos M, Paulsen F, Petri S, et al. Histological, immunohistochemical and ultrastructural findings in human blast injury. *AJRCCM.* 2003;168: 549–555.
25. Heurer AJ, Scanlan CL. Medical gas therapy. In: Wilkins RL, Stoller JK, Kacmarek RM, eds. *Egan's Fundamentals of Respiratory Care.* 9th ed. St. Louis, MO: Mosby, 2009:893.
26. Pizov R, Oppenheim-Eden A, Matot I, et al. Blast lung injury from an explosion on a civilian bus. *Chest.* 1999;115:165–172.
27. Avidan A, Herch M, Armon Y, Spira R, Aharoni D, Reissman P, Schecter WP. Blast lung injury: clinical manifestations, treatment, and outcome. *Am J Surg.* 2005;190:945–950.
28. USAMRIID Medical Management of Biological Casualties Course 04 Feb 2001;Washington, DC.
29. Torok TJ, Tauxe RV, Wise RP, Livengood JR, Sokolow R, Mauvais S, Birkness KA, Skeels MR, Horan JM, Foster LR. A large community outbreak of salmonellosis caused by intentional contamination of restaurant salad bars. *JAMA* 1997;278,5:389–395.
30. Centers for Disease Control and Prevention. Olson KB. Aum Shinrikyo: once and future threat? www.cdc.gov/ncidod/EID/vol5no4/olson.htm
31. Heyman D. Lessons from the anthrax attacks, implications for U.S. bioterrorism preparedness April 2002. Defense Reduction Agency DTRA Contract Number DTRA01-02-0013;1–2
32. Ibid., vii.
33. Weiner SL, Barrett J. Biological warfare defense. In: *Trauma Management for Civilian and Military Physicians.* Philadelphia, PA: WB Saunders;1986: 508–509.
34. Franz DR, Jahrling PB, Friedlander AM, McClain DJ, Hoover DL, Bryne WR, Pavlin JA, Christopher GW, Eitzen EM. Clinical recognition and management of patients exposed to biological warfare agents. *JAMA.* 1997;278,5:399–411.
35. Johnson TJ. 2,000 years of biowarfare. *Military History.* 2002;19,3:24, 74–77.
36. Heyman D Lessons. From the Anthrax Attacks, Implications for U.S. Bioterrorism Preparedness

April 2002. Defense Reduction Agency DTRA Contract Number DTRA01-02-0013;9.
37. Morens DM. Epidemic anthrax in the eighteenth century, the Americas. *Emerg Infec Dis.* 2002;288, 17:1160–1162.
38. Centers for Disease Control and Prevention. "Clinical issues in the prophylaxis, diagnosis, and treatment of anthrax." www.cdc.gov/ncidod/EID/vol8no2/01-0521.htm
39. Mayer TA, Bersoff-Matcha S, Murphy C, Earls J, Harper S, Pauze D, Nguyen M, et al. Clinical presentation of inhalation anthrax following bioterrorism exposure, report of 2 surviving patients. *JAMA* 2001;286:2549–2553.
40. Cuneo BM. Inhalational anthrax. In: Moores LK, ed. *Respiratory Care Clinics of North America.* 2004;10,1:79–81.
41. Kortepeter MG. Anthrax and anthrax vaccine. Presented in Bioterrorism, Medical Issues and Response at ROA Mid-Winter Conference. Washington, DC: February 4, 2001.
42. Alibek K, Handelman S. *Biohazard.* New York: Dell Publishing; 1999:107–122.
43. Kortepeter MG, Cieslak TJ, Eitzen EM. Bioterrorism. *Envir Health.* 2001; 21–24.
44. Bray M, Martinez M, Kefauver D, West M, Roy C. Treatment of aerosolized cowpox virus infection in mice with aerosolized cidofovir. *Antiviral Research.* 2002;54,1:129–142.
45. DeClerq, et al. *Antiviral Research.* 2002;55,1:1–13.
46. Albin S. Plague victims slowly recovering. *New York Times.* January 17, 2003:B5.
47. Inglesby TV, Dennis DT, Henderson DA, Bartlett JG, Ascher MS, Eitzen E. Plague as a biological weapon, medical and public health management. *JAMA.* 2000;283:2281–2290.
48. Ibid., 2281.
49. Ziegler P. *The Black Death.* Wolfeboro Falls, NH: Alan Sutton Publishing, Inc; 1969:17.
50. FDA. *Biological Warfare and Terrorism, Medical Issues and Response.* Student material booklet. September 26–28, 2000:35–40.
51. Evans ME, Friedlander AM. Tularemia. In: *Textbook of Military Medicine.* Washington, DC: Office of the Surgeon General, Department of the Army, 1997:Chapter 24.
52. FDA. *Biological Warfare and Terrorism, Medical Issues and Response.* Student material booklet. September 26–28, 2000:35–40.
53. Arnon SS, Schechter R, Inglesby TV, Henderson DA, Bartlett JG. Botulinum toxin as a biological weapon, medical and public health management. *JAMA.* 2001;285:1059–1070.
54. Ibid.
55. Alibek K, Handelman S. *Biohazard.* New York: Dell Publishing; 1999:123–133.
56. Kaplan, M. *The Cult at the End of the World.* New York: Crown Publishing; 1996:87–88, 102, 213–214, 216.
57. Severson WE, Schmaljohn CS, Javadian A, Jonsson CB. Ribavirin causes error catastrophe during hantaan virus replication. *J Virol.* 2003;77,1: 481–488.
58. Parren PW, Geisbert TW, Mauryama T, Jahrling PB, Burton DR. Pre- and post-exposure prophylaxis of ebola virus infection in an animal model by passive transfer of a neutralizing human antibody. *J Virol.* 2002;76,12:6408–6412.
59. Hale MI, Margolin SB, Krakauer T, Roy C, Stiles BG. Pirfenidone blocks the in vitro and in vivo effects of staphylococcal enterotoxin. *B. Infect Immun.* 2002; 70,6:2989–2994.
60. National Tuberculosis Curriculum Consortium. http://ntcc.ucsd.edu/
61. U.S. Department of Health & Human Services. "HHS pandemic influenza plan." http://www.hhs.gov/pandemicflu/plan/
62. Centers for Disease Control and Prevention. "Hand hygiene in healthcare settings." http://www.cdc.gov/handhygiene/pressrelease.htm
63. Kaplan DE, Marshal A. *The Cult at the End of the World.* New York: Crown Publishers, 1996.
64. Drugs.com. "Pralidoxime Chloride." http://www.drugs.com/pro/pralidoxime-chloride.html
65. Centers for Disease Control and Prevention. "Vesicant/blister agent poisoning." http://www.bt.cdc.gov/agent/vesicants/tsd.asp
66. Guo, et al. *J. Appl. Physio.* 1990; Diller J. *Occup Envir Med.* 2001; Sciuto J. *Am J Resp CCM.* 1995; Sciuto J. *Appl Tox.* 1996; Scuito J. *Exp Lung Res.* 1998.
67. Gunnarsson, et al. *J Trauma.* 2000.
68. Wang , et al, *Intensive Care Med.* 2002.
69. MMWR *Early Release* July 17, 2008/57 (Early Release):1–60.
70. Ibid.
71. World Health Organization. "Pandemic preparedness." http://www.who.int/csr/disease/influenza/pandemic/en/
72. Osterholm MT. Proposed mechanism of the cytokine storm evoked by influenza virus. *NEJM.* 2005;352;18.
73. Suntharalingam G, Perry MR, Ward S, Brett SJ, Castello-Cortes A, Brunner MD, Panoskaltsis N. Cytokine storm in a phase 1 trial of the anti-CD28 monoclonal antibody TGN1412. *NEJM.* 2006;355,10:1018–1028.
74. Brower RG, Lanken PN, MacIntyre N, et al. Higher versus lower positive end-expiratory pressures in

patients with the acute respiratory distress syndrome. *NEJM*. 2004;351:327–336.

75. Wheeler AP, Bernard GR, et al. Comparison of two fluid-management strategies in acute lung injury. *NEJM*. 2006;354:2564–2575.
76. VanPutte W, et al., Evaluation of two mechanical ventilators for use in U.S. Army combat support hospitals. USAISR Technical Report. 2004. http://handle.dtic.mil/100.2/ADA424230
77. Impact Instrumentation, Inc. http://www.impactinstrumentation.com

Resources

Biomedtraining.org. www.biomedtraining.org (Domain is for sale.)

Centers for Disease Control and Prevention. www.bt.cdc.gov

United States Army Medical Research Institute of Chemical Defense (USAMRICD), http://chemdef.apgea.army.mil

U.S. Public Health Service Office of Emergency Preparedness. www.ndms.dhhs.gov

CHAPTER 33

Adult Critical Care

Ken D. Hargett and Joy Kraus Hargett

OBJECTIVES

Upon completion of this chapter, the reader should be able to:

- Identify assessment criteria for patients entering into a critical care unit.
- Understand admission and severity scoring guidelines utilized for patient assessment.
- Understand the role of the respiratory therapist in the critical care unit.
- Understand the opportunities for respiratory care involvement in the critical care unit.
- List special procedures that affect the care of the patient in the critical care unit.

CHAPTER OUTLINE

KEY TERMS

care plans
clinical practice guidelines
critical paths
multidisciplinary competencies
severity scoring guideline
therapist-driven protocol (TDP)

The arena of critical care medicine is an ever changing specialty, particularly as it relates to respiratory care. As technology continues to advance and research provides new alternatives to treatment, respiratory therapists (RTs) must be prepared to always be improving their care and acting as an integral part of the patient care team. This chapter evaluates the expectations of the respiratory therapist who is assigned to work with adult patients in critical care. This chapter reviews:

- The assessment of patients admitted to the critical care area, the monitoring of them during their stays in the critical care unit, and the variety of special procedures performed in that unit.
- Intensive care unit (ICU) design and function, to give the respiratory care department members ideas and information on which to base their activities as fully integrated players on the ICU-oriented health care team.
- Tools that assist respiratory therapists or respiratory care departments to provide value to the intensive care unit.
- The various body system functions that affect the patient's care and that have implications for respiratory therapists and the care they render.

Note: In this chapter, the terms "critical care unit," "intensive care unit," and "ICU" are used synonymously.

Entry of the Patient into the Critical Care System

A patient entering the critical care unit of a hospital is a common but still tense situation for the health care provider, whether one is a novice or a seasoned caregiver. Good critical thinking skills, judgment, and experience are important qualities for the health care provider, including the respiratory therapist, to have in order to be successful in caring for the critical care patient.

ASSESSMENT AND STABILIZATION OF THE PATIENT

Assessment of the patient entering the critical care system is essential to providing the right care, regardless of patient origination:

- The emergency department.
- Surgery (which includes planned or unplanned surgical procedures).
- Other diagnostic or treatment procedures (cardiac catheterization laboratory, noninvasive cardiology, chemotherapy, or radiation procedures, etc.).
- Current hospital patients with worsening health conditions.

In the initial patient assessment, the respiratory therapist must quickly ensure that the patient is being treated safely. For example, patients who have been received from the operating room must be evaluated for the return of normal vital signs and, if they are not present, supported with the appropriate interventions until normal vital signs return. Patients appearing with a depressed respiratory rate or tidal volume should be evaluated for mechanical ventilation via invasive or noninvasive means.

Appropriate respiratory care should always be assessed upon the patient's entry into the critical care unit. The basic components of a respiratory assessment are:

- Vital signs (heart rate, respiratory rate, pulse oximetry).
- Breathing pattern [depth of respirations, chest movement (symmetrical/asymmetrical), breath sounds].
- Skin color.

CASE STUDY 33-1

C. C. is a 72-year-old, 70-kg male brought to the ICU postcoronary artery bypass surgery. He was still heavily sedated with a propofol drip and placed on mechanical ventilation in the SIMV mode with a rate of 10, tidal volume 700 cc, F_IO_2 0.6, pressure support of 5 cm H_2O, and PEEP of 5 cm H_2O. The patient has a history of COPD. Bedside report from the anesthesiologist indicated that the patient was slightly fluid overloaded with bounding pulses, as evidenced by a prominent PMI on the chest.

An immediate ventilator check shows the following:

Exhaled V_T	675 cc
PIP	32 cm H_2O
PEEP	5 cm H_2O
Flow	70 Lpm
Total rate	30
Sensitivity	1
Spontaneous rate	20
Spontaneous exhaled volume	50 cc

Questions

1. How would the RT determine whether the ventilator is autocycling?
2. What is the most likely cause of the autocycling?
3. How would the RT correct the autocycling?

- Level of consciousness.
- Airway status.
- Cardiovascular status.

This rapid initial assessment ensures the respiratory therapist that the patient is safe and that immediate needs are addressed as the patient settles into the unit, detailed assessments (discussed later in this chapter) require more time but allow the respiratory therapist to develop the most appropriate care plan.

UNIT ADMISSION AND SEVERITY SCORING GUIDELINES

Usually, a patient is admitted to an intensive care unit because of the ICU's advanced technology or specialty care capability. Some institutions have criteria to determine whether a patient should be admitted into the intensive care unit or to ascertain the patient's acuity level. These rating systems may be foreign to respiratory therapists because this practice is not often used in determining respiratory care workloads. The rating systems may be in the form of a **severity scoring guideline** or severity rate scale, which evaluates the level of care required for the patient and to determine the nurse-to-patient ratio or how many patients the nurses may care for.

Several rating systems have been developed and studied for their effectiveness. Scoring systems are commonly used in research protocols to validate the equality of patient populations or as predictors of outcomes. For the general adult ICU patient, severity scoring systems are available:

- Simplified Acute Physiology Score (SAPS)
- Acute Physiology and Chronic Health Evaluation (APACHE)
- Sequential Organ Failure Assessment (SOFA)
- Mortality Probability Model (MPM)

Other systems are available for pediatrics, cardiac surgery, or trauma patients.

Some of the commonly used systems are as follows:

- A very common public domain rating scale, the *APACHE II* system, evaluates 12 physiological variables (APS) and determines outcomes based on an evaluation of the patient's health status. Each of these parameters has a rated score based on the degree of deviation from normal physiological values. The total score indicates the severity of illness or acuity of the patient.
- The *APACHE III and IV* are proprietary versions and have more parameters.
- The *SOFA* score utilizes the evaluation of 6 systems (respiratory, cardiovascular, hepatic, coagulation, renal, and neurologic) to predict the probability of mortality.[1]

Regardless of the systems used, the intent is to quantitate the severity of illness.[2]

Although these systems may work well for determining nursing ratios, they may not be well suited for respiratory care departments in determining therapist-to-patient ratios. Many respiratory care departments have developed a numerical type of rating system that counts the numbers of tasks that the respiratory therapist has to perform. The RT is then assigned work based on the number of tasks that can be completed in a given time period.

As is the case in many hospitals, respiratory therapists may be assigned to take care of several critically ill patients in one area. In some cases, critically ill patients may require less respiratory care intervention than more stable intensive care patients. This does not preclude the possibility that a very unstable patient may require the extensive involvement of both the nurse and the respiratory therapist to be stabilized. The degree of RT involvement therefore depends on the types of services provided by the respiratory care department. For example, if the respiratory care department is responsible for hemodynamic monitoring, blood gas sampling, blood gas and electrolyte analysis, and advanced airway care procedures (intubations, tracheostomy tube changes, etc.), the therapists may be more involved with higher-level tasks than those working for departments that do not provide such services. Stable intensive care patients being weaned from the mechanical ventilator generally require more RT involvement in such procedures as ventilator weaning or discontinuance, airway management, and psychological support and encouragement.

ESTABLISHING APPROPRIATE RESPIRATORY CARE

To support the patient in the recovery process, it is important to establish the appropriate respiratory care for patients as soon as possible after admission into the critical care unit. Often, respiratory therapists who work in the ICU have very busy days, providing many levels of care to patients. Day-to-day respiratory care duties include basic respiratory care procedures, such as:

- Oxygen administration.
- Aerosolized medication therapy.
- Other treatment modalities, such as chest physical therapy, intrapulmonary percussive ventilation, and incentive spirometry.

More advanced respiratory care procedures may include:

- Mechanical ventilation (including assessments made for weaning).
- Physiological monitoring (pulse oximetry, end-tidal CO_2 monitoring, invasive and noninvasive hemodynamic monitoring).
- Specialized procedures (ventilator patient transports, tracheostomy care, airway care, metabolic monitoring, invasive blood gas and electrolyte monitoring, blood gas punctures, and analysis).

Because these duties require expertise and adequate time to perform, therapists need support in determining the appropriate care for patients.

Patient **care plans** are useful tools in establishing appropriate respiratory care. They are used in many circumstances, and the respiratory care world should be no exception. Whether written or computerized, care plans help therapists organize the shift, so that, on any given day, they know what each patient requires, as well as which practitioners will take care of the patient during the patient's stay in the ICU.

- Care plans can be general or specific. For example, a *general* care plan for ventilated patients can be utilized throughout many intensive care units. However, *specific* criteria can be included for the patient's particular disease process.
- Care plans can incorporate protocols (discussed later in the chapter).
- The information on the care plan should take into consideration the direction that the medical staff or physician feels the patient is moving toward.
- Care plans can be incorporated into documentation that therapists already provide, such as a ventilator flow sheet (Figure 33-1).

As the patient's stay in the intensive care unit continues, therapists should be aware of the long-term goals of the medical plan established for the patient. A

Best Practice

Department Standards

Departments should develop standards for determining the appropriate assignment of daily activities for the respiratory therapist based on the number of interventions that the therapist has to make with the patients. The departments should also have provisions for immediate adjustments of workload to ensure appropriate coverage of needed patient care.

RESPIRATORY CARE DEPARTMENT
Respiratory Critical Care Flow Sheet

Patient Management Section:

Shift 1 Weaning Assessment:

Time/Initials:

Reason Not to Wean:

None Medical Nursing Nutrition Activity Anxiety Rest

Plan of Care (SHIFT 1)

Ventilation Phase(Phase I)
Stage 1: Ventilate
Stage 2: Convert CMV/AC to SIMV
or Decrease SIMV Rate
Weaning Phase (Phase II)

Weaning Strategy: Trach Mask/T-Tube CPAP/PS

Stage 3: Weaning 0-6 hours
Stage 4: Weaning 6-12 hours
Stage 5: Weaning 12-24 hours
Stage 6: DC Ventilator
Other:
O2 Wean: Titrate FIO2 to maintain SpO2 of ___

Gas Flow/WOB

Respiratory: Rate:	<10 20-30	10-15 30-35	15-30 >35
Breath: Sounds:	Clear Crackles Wheezing	Not Decreased Rales Absent	Decreased Rhonchi
Secretions:	Minimal Thin Clear Yellow	Moderate Thick White Brown	Large Tenacious Green Bloody
Neuromuscular:	Not impaired	Semi-Impaired	Impaired

Airway Clearance

Cough:	Good	Adequate	Weak
Swallowing:	Good	Adequate	Weak

Shift 1 Weaning Assessment:

Time/Initials:

Reason Not to Wean:

None Medical Nursing Nutrition Activity Anxiety Rest

Plan of Care (SHIFT 2)

Ventilation Phase (Phase I)
Stage 1: Ventilate
Stage 2: Convert CMV/AC to SIMV
or Decrease SIMV Rate
Weaning Phase (Phase II)

Weaning Strategy: Trach Mask/T-Tube CPAP/PS

Stage 3: Weaning 0-6 hours
Stage 4: Weaning 6-12 hours
Stage 5: Weaning 12-24 hours
Stage 6: DC Ventilator
Other:
O2 Wean: Titrate FIO2 to maintain SpO2 of ___

Gas Flow/WOB

Respiratory: Rate:	<10 20-30	10-15 30-35	15-30 >35
Breath: Sounds:	Clear Crackles Wheezing	Not Decreased Rales Absent	Decreased Rhonchi
Secretions:	Minimal Thin Clear Yellow	Moderate Thick White Brown	Large Tenacious Green Bloody
Neuromuscular:	Not impaired	Semi-Impaired	Impaired

Airway Clearance

Cough:	Good	Adequate	Weak
Swallowing:	Good	Adequate	Weak

FIGURE 33-1 Care plan incorporated into ventilator flow sheet.

thorough review of the medical record is essential. This review should include physician orders, history and physical examination, nurses' notes, and diagnostic findings. These care plans can guide the respiratory therapist in determining the type of care activities required by the patient and enable the practitioner to progress the patient through the process in an organized fashion.

Documentation on a critical care flow sheet for mechanical ventilation is essential in providing information to respiratory therapists, physicians, nurses, and other health care providers, whether for the current management of the patient or for use in quality enhancement projects. A ventilator flow sheet, which includes the care plan, minimizes document duplication. Ventilator flow sheets, along with other types of medical record documentation, can be computerized, thus enhancing communication and accessibility to patient information by a number of health care professionals.

DETAILED ASSESSMENTS

Respiratory therapists can offer their expertise to enhance patient care in several ways, such as:

- Assessment of chest X-rays (CXR).
- Acid-base balance.
- Readiness for weaning.
- Metabolic monitoring.

Chest X-Rays. CXRs are one of the most useful clinical assessment tools available in the intensive care unit. Few bedside caregivers, with the exception of the physician, are as adept in reviewing radiological findings found on the CXR as the respiratory therapist. As a bedside caregiver in the unit, the therapist should be one of the first individuals to view the CXR and should be able to recognize immediate problems (incorrect tube placement, pneumothorax, lung consolidation, etc.). Respiratory therapists must become skilled at identifying straightforward but important medical conditions.[3] With good critical thinking skills, RTs can relate the patient's symptoms with CXR findings to determine problematic situations. This is an invaluable service in medical treatment and patient outcome.

> *Best Practice*
>
> ### Ventilator Flow Sheets
>
> Ventilator flow sheets should be more than a place to record ventilator settings. The flow sheet should be the resource where the patient status is reviewed and on which the results of various indicators of the patient's respiratory status can be recorded for reference. A well designed flow sheet can facilitate weaning or document the failure to progress. When properly used, the flow sheet can help maintain the continuity of care from shift to shift and assist in the implementation of protocols. Documentation is also a key safeguard in the event of a legal question.

Acid-Base Balance. The arterial blood gas is essential in the diagnosis and treatment of oxygenation and acid-base balance. The respiratory therapist is the ideal health professional to evaluate a patient's acid-base balance and to be the expert in arterial blood gas punctures, arterial blood gas analysis and quality control, and acid-base interpretation. Many of the skills needed are taught extensively in respiratory care education programs throughout the country. Respiratory therapists have authored several textbooks on acid-base balance and arterial blood gases. A survey of respiratory care departments in 1992 showed that 83% of respiratory care departments provided blood gas analysis.[4] Acid-base and arterial blood gases are discussed in Chapter 16.

Readiness to Wean. The respiratory therapist is the best practitioner for determining a patient's readiness for weaning. The therapist's daily duties in the intensive care unit are directly related:

- Mechanical ventilation
- Pulmonary function testing
- Pulmonary mechanics
- Airway care such as suctioning or tracheostomy care
- Aerosolized medication treatments
- Weaning trials

Often during these procedures, the therapist assesses the patient's status and documents the observations. This documentation, like the ventilator flow sheet, can assist the respiratory therapist in determining the weaning activities that are beneficial to the patient.

Metabolic Monitoring: Nutritional Assessment. Patients in the ICU, especially mechanically ventilated patients, are at risk for malnutrition. Many of the clinical conditions that present in the ICU cause numerous disturbances in the normal metabolism. Clinicians in the ICU often find it difficult to determine the correct amount and type of nutrients that patients need during their clinical course.

The relationship of improper feeding with poor outcomes, such as increased length of stay, mortality, and morbidity, have been reported in numerous articles.[5] The effect of poor nutritional status on a patient's ability to wean from mechanical ventilation has also been reported.[6] With the continued development of accurate bedside instruments, more and more ICUs have started programs in nutritional assessment to guide the feeding of most patients.

Typically, the caloric requirements of a patient are calculated by means of the *Harris-Benedict equation*. For men, the equation is:

$$66.5 + (13.75 \times \text{weight}) + (5.003 \times \text{height}) - (6.775 \times \text{age})$$

For women, it is:

$$655.1 + (9.563 \times \text{weight}) + (1.85 \times \text{height}) - (4.67 \times \text{age})$$

These formulas are used to approximate the patient's daily requirement in kilocalories (Kcal) per 24 hours. A patient's clinical condition is then taken into account to adjust the calculation. Many clinical factors, such as elective surgery, trauma, and burns, have all been shown to increase metabolic demand by as much as 150%. Sepsis also increases metabolism by as much as 200%.[7] Daily activities in the ICU also have a significant effect on caloric requirements.

The Harris-Benedict equation, developed in 1919, has been shown to be very inaccurate in determining the actual patient's requirements. Hess and colleagues reported that the actual measured requirements of a specific patient population were as much as 60% greater than the calculation.[8] Other studies have indicated that the calculated value is very inaccurate in specific patient conditions.[9] The incorrect use of the Harris-Benedict equation often results in severe under- or overfeeding of the patient.

Malnourishment of the ventilated patient has significant consequences.

- Underfeeding results in the patient's inability to generate adequate diaphragm strength to sustain respiration. Table 33-1 indicates the possible consequences to underfeeding the ventilated patient in the ICU.
- In addition, an increase in infections, particularly pneumonia, is seen in patients who are inadequately nourished.

Overfeeding, especially with a high carbohydrate formula, results in the production of excessive amounts of carbon dioxide. Excess carbon dioxide production, especially in COPD patients who are already susceptible to CO_2 retention, makes weaning from the ventilator difficult.

The following lists show the hazards associated with overfeeding and underfeeding the ventilated patient. The possible hazards of overfeeding are:

- Increased CO_2 production.
- An increase in the necessary level of ventilator support.
- A potential increase in incidence of barotraumas.
- An increase in the work of breathing.

CASE STUDY 33-2

E. H. is a 40-year-old female 15 days post-MVA with a closed head injury and resolved lung contusion. She was trached at day 10 and remains in a coma on ventilatory support. A size 8 Shiley low-pressure disposable inner cannula tracheostomy tube is in place. She is on SIMV of 8, pressure support of 15, F_IO_2 of 0.3, and PEEP of 5 cm H_2O.

The therapist in the neurosurgery unit who is going off duty tells the incoming RT that he has just completed suctioning and trach care on Ms. H. The new RT is called to the room by the nurse because of a continuous ventilator alarm. The alarms that are activated are the low-pressure disconnect, the low exhaled tidal volume, and the low exhaled minute volume alarm. The patient has a pulse oximeter reading of 84% and a falling heart rate.

Questions

1. What are the possible causes of the alarms?
2. What is the first action the RT should take?
3. If adequate ventilation cannot be restored through the tracheostomy tube, what actions should be taken?

Best Practice

All alarms should be responded to immediately. There is no such thing as a "false alarm."

TABLE 33-1 **Respiratory quotient**

RQ > 1.00	Lipogenesis or hyperventilation
RQ 0.90	Primary carbohydrate oxidation
RQ 0.85	Fat, protein, and CHO oxidation
RQ 0.80	Primary protein oxidation
RQ 0.70	Primary fat oxidation
RQ < 0.70	Ketogenesis, alcohol oxidation

The value of the measured respiratory quotient is indicative of the substrates being metabolized. Generally, an RQ of > 1 indicates overfeeding and an RQ < 0.70 indicates starvation.

The possible respiratory consequences of malnutrition are:

- Diaphragm and other muscle weakness.
- Impaired response to hypoxemia and hypercarbia.
- An increase in respiratory infections.
- An increase in atelectasis.
- A decrease in weaning capabilities.
- An increased chance of pulmonary edema.

Metabolic monitoring is accomplished with an instrument called an *indirect calorimeter*. Several versions are on the market. The device consists of:

- A high-speed, very accurate oxygen analyzer.
- A volume measuring device.
- And a carbon dioxide analyzer.

The device measures oxygen consumption ($\dot{V}O_2$) and CO_2 production. From these values the respiratory quotient can be calculated.

$$\text{Respiratory Quotient} = \frac{CO_2 \text{ Produced}}{\text{Oxygen Consumed}}$$

The normal values are a CO_2 production of 200 mL/min and an oxygen consumption of 250 mL/min. This gives us a normal RQ (respiratory quotient) of 0.8. The RQ is related to the amounts of fat and carbohydrate that are being metabolized by the patient. Table 33-1 shows the substrates that are mostly metabolized by the patient at various measured RQs.

If the nitrogen excretion is known from a 24-hour urine sample, then the actual caloric requirement of the patient can be calculated by means of the *Weir formula*. The *resting energy expenditure* (*REE*) is computed, utilizing the oxygen consumption ($\dot{V}O_2$), the carbon dioxide production ($\dot{V}CO_2$), and the urinary nitrogen (UN), as follows:

$$\text{REE (kcal/24 hours)} = [3.94(VO_2) + 1.1(VCO_2)] \times 1.44 - 2.17(UN)$$

As denoted by its name (resting energy expenditure), REE requires that the patient is at rest for the monitoring period, which usually requires about 20 minutes. Another important aspect of obtaining accurate results is that the patient must reach a condition called *steady state*. This is the period during the data collection when oxygen consumption becomes stable, indicating that a patient's minimal activity level and ensuring that the accurate collection of all exhaled gas can be made.

Many benefits have been derived from well implemented metabolic monitoring programs. Decreased length of stay and decreased utilization of very expensive hyperalimentation and enteral feedings have been demonstrated.[10] Additionally, metabolic monitors have been used to determine both oxygen consumption during various modes of mechanical ventilation and oxygen delivery.[11,12]

Intensive Care Unit Design and Function

The ICU is structured to provide a higher level of management and surveillance than the normal floor patient receives. ICUs may be open, closed, or comanaged.

- *Open units* have all qualified staff physicians admit and care for their patients, with consults only as requested. The primary care/admitting physician directs the care to their patients. A medical director or ICU team may handle such issues as triage decisions due to increased census or decreased staff availability.
- In a *closed unit*, the medical director and ICU team are responsible for the admission, discharge, and total care of the patient. Care for the patients is formally turned over to the medical director and associates, who assume responsibility.
- A *comanaged unit* is a blend that allows the primary care physician to utilize the ICU physician team to assist in the management of the patient.

A recent movement has been for patients in the ICU to be managed by physicians with specialized training. These board-certified *intensivists* may have medical, surgical, or anesthesia backgrounds. Organizations like the Leapfrog Group, which is a consortium of insurance purchasers, recommend intensivist coverage for all ICUs.[13] However, recent data support that the closed unit model results in better outcomes and reduced mortality.[14]

A number of characteristics make an ICU functional.

- The care should be multidisciplinary, and teamwork is highly important.
- Caregivers should work in a coordinated manner to ensure the best possible care.
- The unit must be able to support a wide range of medical issues, including mechanisms to treat ventilatory, circulatory, renal, gastrointestinal, hematological, and neurological failure.
- There should be appropriate monitoring and supportive equipment.
- Administrative, technical, and clerical support are necessary.
- On-going training and quality monitoring are essential.
- The medical staff should provide coverage 24 hours per day, whether directly or in a consulting role.

With respect to this last point, telemedicine, or the utilization of long-distance physician coverage, is utilized in some hospitals. Telemedicine physicians provide consults to the physician staff at a time when an attending physician may not be on site. This tool can provide intensive care expertise in hospitals where services are limited, such as in some rural locales. It may also provide access to new or developing medical fields where expertise is limited. In some institutions, residents may provide some of the coverage. Nurse-to-patient ratios should be developed according to standards or needs.

DEPARTMENT ORGANIZATION

The respiratory care department must take an active role in the new health care environment and provide customer-focused patient care.[15] The respiratory care department should be organized so that respiratory therapists are involved in the direct day-to-day patient care activities (previously discussed in the chapter), as well as other projects.

Depending on the department structure and on fluctuations in the day-to-day respiratory care activity, some respiratory therapists may provide high-level activities. These employees may hold titles such as clinical respiratory care supervisors, clinical respiratory care specialists, or respiratory care liaisons. Whatever the title, placing highly trained therapists with excellent critical thinking skills in key positions helps the department prove its worth. These activities can include:

- Patient care rounds with physicians or other multidisciplinary groups.
- Discharge planning rounds.
- Development of care plans.
- Respiratory therapy education and competency verification.
- Resident or medical student teaching.
- Patient and family education.

PERSONNEL CONSIDERATIONS

Personnel orientation and training are essential to the success of the respiratory therapist in the critical care unit. In some institutions, therapists may work only in intensive care units, some may rotate between the acute care areas and the intensive care units, while others work strictly in acute areas. Depending on the size of the institution and the number of critical care areas available, the appropriate number of staff have to be trained. Some institutions have many intensive care units that may be similar or dissimilar in nature. The organization of the department should allow for cross-training of therapists throughout all work areas while placing key practitioners in specific areas. Besides excellent clinical and critical thinking skills, respiratory therapists who are successful in the ICU environment have the following qualities:

- Rapport with other health care providers.
- Eagerness to work in the area.
- Eagerness to take on new projects. Willingness to learn.
- Compassion and empathy for the patients.

Some institutions with centralized respiratory care departments choose to provide a unit-based practitioner model, in which a select number of practitioners are permanently or semipermanently assigned to a specific ICU. This is similar to respiratory therapists who work directly for the ICU, such as in a hospital with a decentralized department. In a model utilized at St. Luke's Episcopal Hospital in Houston, Texas, therapists are assigned to work zones to a particular "zone," or area of the hospital, for a given number of weeks or months. The zone may be an acute care floor or ICU. The therapist works in the zone for that time period. Respiratory therapists are effective in the various work areas based on:

- Their clinical skills (decision making and critical thinking).
- Their rapport with other health care providers (nurses, physicians).
- Their desire to work in the area.
- The contributions they are able to make.
- Their interdependence with other bedside clinicians.[13]

Another model, used at The Methodist Hospital in Houston, Texas, places department therapists in a service line structure. Therapists may work for the medicine or surgical service line, but all therapists work under a centralized respiratory care department. The therapists in the service line work both on the floors and in the ICUs where those patients are housed; however, they work primarily in the service line to which they are assigned.

Depending on the duties and functions of the respiratory therapy department, some specialty areas such as a cardiovascular recovery room or pulmonary ICU, may have therapists zoned in the area for more than their designated time frames or permanently. Utilizing a zoned approach requires the department to establish rotation time frames that work best for them.

Following are advantages of zoning respiratory therapists:

- Uniformity in day-to-day patient care
- Completion of research or educational projects specific to that unit

- Expertise in specific competencies required for the area
- Rapport with other members of the health care team assigned to the unit
- Familiarity with the patients who remain in the unit for a length of time

Rotation out of the area, however, is essential to provide sufficient staff coverage in times of vacation or illness or to give primary respiratory therapists the chance to work in other areas of the system in response to their request or to departmental needs. Rotating unfamiliar people to an area new to them may cause stress; however, this can be alleviated with a good orientation program or an opportunity to work in the area on a regular or occasional basis.

Therapists can also provide clinical leadership activities owing to their educational training. Due to their scientific background, RTs are the logical caregivers to become experts in:

- Modes of ventilation.
- Alternative gas therapy (nitric oxide, heliox).
- Permissive hypercapnia.
- Prevention of ventilator-associated pneumonia and acute lung injury.
- Tracheal gas insufflation.[16]
- Ventilator graphical analysis.[17]

Respiratory therapists are certainly the experts in the areas of oxygen therapy, aerosol therapy, pulse oximetry, and mechanical ventilator management. In these modalities, respiratory therapists can be the educators of other health care professionals. Though fairly mundane to the respiratory therapist, simple respiratory care must often be taught to nurses and physicians. This may be in the form of formal cross-training programs or simple in-service educational classes.

Respiratory therapists may also add value by contributing to formal educational training programs that are attended by nurses and physicians preparing for advanced credentials. Intensive care nurses may prepare for such specialty examinations as the CCRN (critical care registered nurse) examination. This examination encompasses a large number of respiratory and pulmonary questions. The respiratory therapist is the ideal person to teach pulmonary anatomy and physiology, acid-base balance, pulmonary function, and respiratory care procedures. Therapists can offer these types of services to physicians, medical students, and residents. Respiratory therapists can also serve as instructors for classes and coordinate advanced cardiac life support (ACLS) programs.

The cross-training of therapists in traditional nursing duties may be an option at some institutions. However, new roles should be ones that enhance quality and provide value to the institution. Because of the educational training development received by respiratory therapists, they are an ideal caregiver to take on high-level tasks. Their cross-training into nursing roles and nurses into traditional therapists' roles can maximize services provided for the patient.

In many institutions, the number of respiratory therapists employed is greatly less than the number of nurses employed. Also, respiratory therapists assigned to the critical care area might not always be matched to the number of nurses. Some suggestions on cross-training follow, tailored for adult intensive care circumstances:[17]

Respiratory Therapist Only

- Respiratory management of mechanically ventilated patients
- CPAP, IPPB
- Arterial puncture
- Arterial line insertions
- Aerosolized medication delivery to mechanically ventilated patients
- Endotracheal intubation
- Intrahospital transport of ventilated patients
- Administration of exotic gases and drugs by inhalation: nitric oxide, heliox, surfactant, ribavirin
- Continuous inhaled bronchodilators
- Bronchoscopy assist
- Indirect calorimetry

Shared Cross-Training (Respiratory Therapist and Registered Nurse)

- Assisting with insertion of chest tubes, central lines, arterial lines, intubations and extubations, tracheostomies
- Pulmonary assessment
- Phlebotomy
- Cardiac output determination
- Aerosolized medication delivery to nonmechanically ventilated patients
- Suctioning
- Chest physical therapy
- Weaning
- CVVH and CVVHD
- 12-lead ECG
- IV starts
- Troubleshooting biomedical equipment (e.g., monitors, ECG machines)
- IABP
- Oxygen setup
- ECLS
- Cuff pressures
- Vital signs
- Baths

Registered Nurse Only

- Admissions
- Blood and medication administration

Tools for Success in the Intensive Care Unit

A variety of tools are available to ensure that the respiratory therapist can be a welcomed addition to the health care team in the ICU.

CLINICAL PRACTICE GUIDELINES

Policies and procedures, developed by the respiratory care department or by the critical care unit, should guide departments in establishing appropriate respiratory care activities. A good starting place in the development of the appropriate policies is in the use of the **clinical practice guidelines** (CPGs). CPGs used in respiratory care were developed under the direction of the American Association for Respiratory Care (AARC) and are based on scientific research and levels of evidence. Evidence-based medicine is essential in providing appropriate care to patients. Research and publications are graded according to the level of evidence they represent.

- *Level I* is a double-blinded placebo-controlled, multicenter trial.
- *Level II* is peer-reviewed nonrandomized, concurrent or cohort investigations.
- *Level III* is peer-reviewed state-of-the-art review articles, surveys, meta-analysis, or substantial case series.
- *Level IV* is nonpeer reviewed opinions, anecdotal information, or official statements of organizations.

CPGs are employed to provide assistance to respiratory care departments in standardizing respiratory care procedures and in developing or refining policy and procedure. CPGs can also be used as monitors for effectiveness of care. Standardization of care also can provide assistance in the development of training or competency verification programs. These programs, whether for the therapist only or for a multidisciplinary group of health care providers, can be taught effectively if standards of care are set up appropriately.[18]

THERAPIST-DRIVEN PROTOCOLS

The **therapist-driven protocol (TDP)** can enhance departmental efficiency and operation in the critical care unit. The respiratory therapist–driven protocol is a method to provide a particular service (such as oxygen therapy) in a predesigned algorithm or decision matrix. Successful TDP implementation takes its cue from the use of AARC clinical practice guidelines.

By utilizing the CPGs, a best practice model can be developed. However, best practice may require institutions to individually assess programs for success, because sometimes research shows that the same outcomes can be based on different approaches. For example, in 1994 and 1995, two landmark articles on the gradual withdrawal of mechanical ventilator support appeared in the literature.[19,20] These techniques were different from each other, each showing an effective weaning technique. Because conflicts are seen in the literature from time to time, institutions may need to establish their own best practice model that fits well into their organization with its specific patient population.

A source for clinical practice guidelines from the AARC is available from the *Respiratory Care Journal* Web site (www.rcjournal.com). These guidelines and those from related health care organizations have been organized into one Internet Web site: the National Guideline Clearinghouse. These guidelines were also published in the *Federal Register* on April 13, 1998.[21] Due to the number of guidelines available (more than 500 as of October 1999), respiratory therapists now have access to guidelines that have been established by other professional organizations.

QUALITY IMPROVEMENT ACTIVITIES

It is increasingly imperative to balance improvements in clinical effectiveness with the availability of resources.[22] Quality improvement projects are generally useful in demonstrating the effects that respiratory therapists can have on patient outcomes. Such projects may include, for example (discussed later in this chapter):

- Reducing hospital-acquired pneumonia and the implementation of ventilator bundles.
- The use of ventilator weaning protocols.
- Joint Commission preparation.

Respiratory care departments need to become an integral part of these types of clinical and quality improvement activities so that RT-related standards, such as the CPGs, are utilized to their fullest extent. Also, engaging the respiratory care departments in a quality project initiative at its very start can ensure the department's involvement and enhance the role of the therapist as a patient advocate.

Reducing Hospital-Acquired Pneumonia. *Ventilator-associated pneumonia* (*VAP*) has been the focus of hospital-associated pneumonia for some time. In 2002, the CDC's National Nosocomial Infection Surveillance System (NNIS) reported VAP rates ranging from 2 to

15%, depending on the type of patient and medical issue surrounding that patient. This results in:

- Increased mortality rates.
- Increased length of stay and consumption of resources.
- Increased cost of care, estimated at approximately $40,000 more for patients who acquire VAP compared to those who do not.

To avoid this significant detriment to patient care, the Institute for Healthcare Improvement (IHI) has described components of the Ventilator Bundle, which is aimed at preventing ventilator-associated pneumonias. According to IHI, implementing these components together helps in achieving better outcomes for patients. The four components are:

- Elevation of the head of the bed.
- Daily sedation "vacations" and assessment of extubation potential.
- Peptic ulcer disease prophylaxis.
- Deep venous thrombosis prophylaxis.[23,24]

Ventilator Weaning Protocols. Ventilator weaning protocols have been used extensively throughout the United States and reported in the literature.[25–28] Many of the ventilator weaning protocols have had a positive effect on the reduction of intubation times, length of stay, and patient outcomes. These activities have caught the attention of the medical community, and more medically directed ventilator weaning projects are being initiated. A recent project underwritten by the Society of Critical Care Medicine (SCCM), called Project Impact, has reported a decrease in ventilation times with physician-directed protocols, as compared to RN/RRT protocols. Information on this project can be found at the Society for Critical Care Web site (www.sccm.org).

More recent approaches to ventilator weaning include the utilization of *spontaneous breathing trials* (*SBTs*) instead of the gradual withdrawal of ventilator support. This approach has been shown to decrease the length of mechanical ventilation. The technique involves placing all eligible patients ($F_IO_2 < 0.6$, PEEP <8, hemodynamically stable) in a spontaneous breathing mode and monitoring the *rapid shallow breathing index* (*RSBI*). Patient pass if their RSBI stays less than 105 for 30–90 minutes. If they pass, patients should be extubated.[29]

Joint Commission Preparation Teams. The respiratory care department can be engaged in Joint Commission preparation at the grassroots levels. The involvement of respiratory therapists on the hospital core Joint Commission team keeps the department informed of hospital accreditation activities, provides information on enhancements that need to occur in quality activities, and assists in policy and procedure development. There is a great deal of information available on the Joint Commission Web site (www.jointcommission.org).

Best Practice

Quality Improvement

Respiratory care needs to become a part of the solution instead a part of the problem. Integration of the RC department as part of the quality improvement team lends credibility and legitimacy to the respiratory care department as a whole.

MULTIDISCIPLINARY COMPETENCIES

The respiratory care department can flourish in quality improvement activities. In turn, multidisciplinary projects can enhance the performance of the department as well as that of the intensive care unit. One such project reported was a multidisciplinary joint competency program in caregiver performances in code blue situations.[30] Although not specific to an intensive care unit, this program can enhance the skill of any practitioner. The program, initially developed by the nursing service, was designed to give nurses an opportunity to practice code blue skills (beyond that of basic CPR procedures) annually in a controlled setting.

Because personnel other than nurses attend code blue procedures in the hospital, other disciplines needed to be involved in the competency training as well. Therefore, the respiratory care and pharmacy departments, which participate in cardiopulmonary resuscitation procedures in the hospital, were invited to join the group. The respiratory care department is responsible for the ACLS program coordination and training in the hospital and could help ensure that appropriate ACLS guidelines are utilized. The special expertise of the pharmacy department on medication administration was also beneficial to the program's success. Participation of all these disciplines was essential in providing a quality educational program utilizing a team approach.

Programs such as this one provide an individual handbook to each participant, an open-book test, an ECG test, and hands-on validation, which is monitored by instructors. The instructors are nurses, respiratory therapists, and pharmacists. Respiratory therapists may teach essential tasks such as emergency airway management to nurses and pharmacists. Nurses or pharmacists may conduct the review for respiratory therapists on crash cart items.

To make revisions for the following year, after the annual program is complete, the team members review the program's strengths and weaknesses, as reported by the trainers and attendees. This joint program measures the competency of many individuals in an institution and can lead to the development of **multidisciplinary competencies**, which are standards or competency verification activities that are or can be used by multiple groups, such as nursing and respiratory care departments. Multidisciplinary competencies can lead to the establishment of institutional standards of competency verification. This activity is a great indicator for Joint Commission team activities.

One such idea for multidisciplinary competency verification is in the area of specimen sampling. With the current trend toward more bedside sampling and point-of-care testing, individuals need to be trained to use new equipment, and their performance needs to be verified. Pathology departments have traditionally been responsible for much of the laboratory testing in hospitals and are the experts in testing. At the same time, many respiratory care departments provide blood gas analysis in the hospital. These departments can be great resources and developers of testing, training, and competencies, which have moved out of the laboratory and to the bedside.

SHARED POLICIES AND PROCEDURES

Because a variety of professionals often share many tasks, policy and procedural activities have to be considered. If disciplines share responsibilities, such as suctioning or ABG sampling, the policy and procedures for each discipline should duplicate each other. Accreditation agencies such as the Joint Commission examine the consistency of policies between departments, and standards of care should be uniform throughout the hospital. Working through this process may be time-consuming and may take a great deal of coordination, but it is well worth the effort during surveys by accreditation agencies. Having one area responsible for the content of the policy, with review from other disciplines, might facilitate and ease the integration of policies. Having multiple reviewers is important to enhance the effectiveness of the policy and procedure program and to provide timely updates of information and expertise relative to each of the disciplines.

CRITICAL PATHS

Critical paths, otherwise known as care paths or pathways, can act as a consistent mechanism in which to treat patients with similar diagnoses. The critical path, a management tool used for almost 30 years, mixes clinical practices and time guidelines into a coordinated plan for care.[31] Given their expertise, respiratory therapists should become involved in the development of pathways, which target respiratory patients. Paths that involve respiratory diagnoses (asthma, COPD, pneumonia, trached ventilator-dependent patients) or patients with potential pulmonary problems (postoperative patients, for example) should incorporate the AARC CPGs if possible. One such critical path is shown in Figure 33-2.

Reports in the literature have shown that therapist-driven protocols incorporated into a critical path can decrease hospital cost and length of stay.[32] Pathways may also lead to the development of order sets or standard orders, which should enhance the functionality of the respiratory care department in the appropriate administration of therapy, patient billing, and charge capture. An example is found in Table 33-2.

COST CONTAINMENT IDEAS

Cost containment efforts are essential in curtailing costs in a very expensive health care environment. In 2007, total health care spending represented 17% of the United States gross domestic product (GDP). Total spending was $2.4 trillion, or nearly $8000 per person.[33] The current climate in health care stresses that intensive care units function at high efficiency and optimize quality while decreasing risks and expenditures.[2] Mechanisms to identify which patients might be able to be moved through the system quickly or which may have potential complications are keys to moving intensive care patients into more appropriate levels of care. These mechanisms should be in place before or at the time of admission. Multidisciplinary cooperation is key to successful patient care management. For example, one cost savings idea might be to schedule multidisciplinary rounds in the ICU, allowing caregivers from a variety of disciplines to provide input into progressing the patient through the system. Cost savings have also been reported by utilization of respiratory care protocols.[28,34]

Cost containment ideas can be incorporated from studies in the literature. According to one report, an area of consideration is the use of inhaled bronchodilators during mechanical ventilation.[35] Cost comparisons have been made that evaluate the costs of utilizing a metered-dose inhaler (MDI) versus a small-volume nebulizer (SVN) therapy.[35–37] However, departments should determine their own individual costs to ascertain whether this is a justified project. Individual institutional costs, such as labor and cost of materials, may vary significantly among institutions.[35]

As health care institutions strive to control costs, reports are beginning to surface that describe the use of products beyond the suggested life of the products, which is generally specified by the manufacturer. Some health care organizations are challenging these claims

PRIVILEGED AND CONFIDENTIAL MEDICAL PEER REVIEW COMMUNICATION GENERATED
PURSUANT TO AD HOC REVIEW UNDER V.A.T.S. 4495b, SEC.5.06; T.R.C.P. 166b(3)(d)

Addressograph

Initial intubation date:_____ CV Surgery this admit?_____
Reintubation (Y/N)____ number of times:_____ Previous CV surgery?_____
Trach date:____ Percutaneous trach?____ Pulmonologist & consult date_____
Smoker?____ Active Smoker____ Quit?____ When?____
(Check all that apply): History of : COPD ____Asthma ___CAD ___ EF < 40%___
Diabetes___ HTN ___ Depression ____Antidepress. RX ?__________________
Anxiety____ Anti-anxiety RX ? (specify)__________________ ETOH use ______

ST. LUKE'S EPISCOPAL HOSPITAL
Ventilator Dependent: Trach or ET Tube
DRG 483/475

Addressograph

	PHASE I ACUTE VENTILATORY SUPPORT	PHASE II VENTILATORY SUPPORT	PHASE III WEANING	PHASE IV RESOLUTION
CONSULTS	**Pulmonologist consult if patient still intubated after 48 hrs or reintubation required.** Nutritional Support Dietitian PT/OT consult: Mobility Protocol	Speech Pathologist Consult: Dysphagia monitoring per protocol		
DIAGNOSTIC	ABG PRN vent changes or change in clinical status → → Pulse Oximetry → → CXR daily SMA-7, CBC daily Sputum C&S / GS after 48 hrs. of ETT Pre-albumin prn recommendation of Dietitian . Phosphorus QOD X 1 week if pt. On TPN or TF	Pulmonary mechanics daily CXR PRN → →	Pulmonary mechanics daily → → → →	Pulse oximetry prn → → → →
TREATMENTS	Mechanical ventilation: For persistent profound hypoxia or **greatly** ↑ peak airway pressure, consider sedation and paralytics. Respiratory TXs → → Secretion management → → Tracheostomy after ETT in place X 7 - 10 days GI protection with carafate / histamine blockers	→ → →	→ → →	Trach collar or decannulate or extubate or continue vent management and slow wean.
INTERVENTIONS	Daily weight Foley → Suction prn I&O hourly → Specialty bed if meets criteria Social Services: Supportive counseling/crisis intervention.	If patient on specialty bed, reassess need per policy Tracheostomy care Refer to Mechanical Ventilation Weaning protocol	Dysphagia monitoring per protocol. Evaluate need for PEG and permanent IV access. Refer to Mechanical Ventilation Weaning Protocol	→
ACTIVITY	Activity: Physical Therapy per Mobility Protocol →	→ Activity per Mobility Protocol	→ Activity per Mobility Protocol	→ Activity per Mobility Protocol
NUTRITION	Nutritional intervention: TPN/TF* ***Attempt tube feeds to preserve gut integrity; Aspiration precautions when TF instituted. Insert small bore feeding tube ASAP.***	If patient on TPN, transition to tube feedings. Ensure optimal nutritional intake per Dietitians recommendations.	Transition to PO diet if no dysphagia. → →	Continued PO diet or tube feedings. → →
TEACHING	Orient patient/family to ICU: visiting policy, tests, procedures, disease process, changes in care. Establish a communication mode with patient. →	Educate patient/family regarding changes in care, procedures, and improvements/changes in patient's condition. →	Educate patient/family regarding weaning process. →	Educate patient/family regarding DC plan, any new equipment or procedures.
D/C PLANNING	Social Services: High risk screening and initiate assessment or resources. Care Coordinator: Assessment of provider benefits and options. →	**Discharge plan documented before day 20 of mechanical ventilation.**	Social Services & Care Coordinator: evaluate patient for placement options; make initial discharge referrals.	Social Services: finalize arrangements for transportation to D/C destination, equipment, Home Health.
OUTCOMES	Patient/family verbalizes knowledge of surroundings, tests, visitation policy and disease process. Patient demonstrates understanding of need for ETT, suctioning, and alarms.	Patient demonstrates improved/stable ventilatory status as evidenced by CXR, ABGs, pulse oximetry.	Patient demonstrates improved ventilatory status as evidenced by decreased ventilatory support and increased activity without signs and symptoms of respiratory compromise.	Patient family verbalizes knowledge of DC plans, follow-up care and all new equipment, procedures, and medications.

FIGURE 33-2 Ventilator-dependent critical path. (*continues*)

PRIVILEGED AND CONFIDENTIAL MEDICAL PEER REVIEW COMMUNICATION GENERATED
PURSUANT TO AD HOC REVIEW UNDER V.A.T.S. 4495b, SEC.5.06; T.R.C.P. 166b(3)(d)

Addressograph

Total TPN days____________________

Total enteral days____________________

Total days underfed____________________

Total days NPO____________________

Wean off vent? (Y/N) ______ Date vent DC'd________

Dates of central line changes;________________________________

Required permanent IV access? (Y/N) _________

Discharged on TPN? (Y/N)________

Discharged on enteral feedings? (Y/N)_________

Total ventilator days____________

Dysphagia diagnosed? (Y/N)_______ Date:_______

Required PEG or PEJ? (Y/N)________ DOI________

Renal Failure this admit? (Y/N)______ Requires HD? (Y/N) _____

IV line sepsis? (Y/N) _____ Organism:______________________

PHASE I: Acute ventilatory support: Hemodynamically unstable, refractory hypoxemia, acute respiratory failure.	PHASE II: Ventilatory support, hemodynamically stable, insufficient weaning parameters.	PHASE III: Weaning; NIF >-20; RR <24; VC 12-15ml/kg; tolerates trend in vent. support.	PHASE IV: Resolution: weaning successful, or discharge to subacute/other facility with continued ventilatory support or death/dying.

Potential Patient Variances

1. **CVA diagnosed**
2. **Invasive procedure (explain)**
3. **Underfed: < / = 85% protein needs (determined by Dietitian**
4. **Interrupted nutrition due to interventional procedures**
5. **Interrupted nutrition due to unstable condition**
6. **Alteration in GI function (specify)**
7. **Skin breakdown (site & stage)**
8. **Decreased physical endurance**
9. **Anxiety** (DKP define)
10. **Agitation**
11. **Delirium**
12. **Lack of discharge plan (specify)**
13. **Delayed discharge, needs PEG or PEJ**
14. **Delayed discharge, needs permanent IV access**
15. **Delayed discharge, other (specify)**
16. **Nosocomial pneumonia**
17. **Other (specify)**

DATE	PHASE	UNIT	VARIANCE #'S	ACTION TAKEN/OTHER	SIGNATURE

c:\data\wp\dkp\vent-dep.cp

8 St. Luke's Episcopal Hospital, 1996

FIGURE 33-2 (*continued*)

TABLE 33-2 **Example of standardized order sets for respiratory care services**

COPD ADMISSION ORDERS—
RESPIRATORY CARE ORDERS
ABG now, if not done in ER
Pulse oximetry spot check on admission
Titrate F_IO_2 for O_2 saturation ____%
Oxygen therapy via O_2 @ ___liters per nasal cannula or O_2 @ ___ % per venti-mask
Medications:
Respiratory care to assess patient for use of MDI protocol
Bronchodilators metered-dose inhaler with spacer (Please refill for take-home use.)
____Albuterol (Ventolin, Proventil) ___puffs q ___ hours
____Ipratropium (Atrovent)____ puffs q ____ hours
If patient is unable to use MDI, then handheld nebulizer with
____Albuterol 2.5 mg/3.00 NS q ___ hours while awake
____Albuterol 2.5 mg/3.00 NS q ___ hours around the clock
____Ipratropium 0.5 mg/3.00 NS q ___ hours while awake
____Ipratropium 0.5 mg/3.00 NS q ___ hours around the clock

and doing clinical studies to support their efforts. One product under recent consideration for so-called off-label use is the closed system suction catheter. Studies have been done on extending the time period between replacements beyond the manufacturer's recommended time period.[38–40] These studies describe the time extension of the change intervals, which appear to lead to no increase in ventilator-associated pneumonia rates or decrease in functionality of the device. Other reports suggest that ventilator circuits may be changed at a reduced frequency without an increase in hospital acquired pneumonia rates.[40] This practice has been implemented in a number of institutions throughout the country.

In any event, the legal ramification of utilizing a product beyond its suggested life is an important consideration. The risk management department has to be contacted regarding such activities. Also, the infection control department should offer advice on using direct patient care products with a potential for infectious disease. Other departments where changes are likely to have a direct effect should also be contacted, such as the purchasing department, which obtains the product, or patient care supply department, which supplies the product.

INFORMATION SYSTEMS, DATA MANAGEMENT, AND COMPUTERIZED PATIENT RECORDS

Information systems or data management systems are playing an important role in providing timely data collection in the ICUs. *Respiratory care information systems* (*RCIS*) have been in use for several years and have provided mechanisms that allow the caregiver to spend more time at the patient bedside.[15] With the RCIS, in the number of manual data entries is reduced. Respiratory therapists have reported that documenting in a clinical information system in an ICU can produce the time savings and uniformity of charting that is not seen when utilizing manual charting systems.[41]

The RCIS can also be used for research applications, productivity, and billing activities. Depending on the capabilities of the health care information system, the RCIS may be able to be integrated into the hospital system. Maximizing productivity from integration of individual systems is essential to prevent the loss of patient information.[42] Capturing ventilator data directly from the ventilator and integrating them into a cardiac monitor or hospital information system can provide a more accurate medical record, which allows review of medical care during selected time periods. This computerized patient record is the wave of the future. It can improve decision-making activities, based on retrospective and concurrent data. In addition to functioning as a data reporting tool, it can assist in quality monitoring, which in turn can lead to quality improvement activities. Computerized patient records may also improve documentation in terms of medical-legal activities.[43]

Management of the ICU Patient

A patient in critical care has many medical needs that require vigilant monitoring and management. These patients may have conditions that affect multiple systems and may require medical or surgical procedures for care and treatment.

SURGICAL CONSIDERATIONS

A variety of new surgical procedures are announced in the news daily. As new techniques and procedures are developed, the challenge for the bedside caregivers is to continue to provide the best care possible as the patient recovers. Although providing details of the latest surgical enhancements is beyond the scope of this chapter, the following considerations should be made.

- Respiratory therapists need to pay particular attention to patients who have undergone surgical procedures, owing to the possible decline in pulmonary function.[44] This decline may extend past the actual surgical procedure and be related to other causes, such as the delivery of anesthesia, surgical wound dressings, postoperative pain and analgesia, and patient immobilization. Individuals with preexisting lung disease may be particularly susceptible, owing to their decreased lung function, and they may require a higher level of respiratory care than patients without lung disease.[45]
- Surgical procedures that involve the thoracic and upper abdominal areas have the most significant effect on pulmonary function and cause more severe respiratory complication.[45]
- The reason for surgery—whether planned or unplanned (trauma or cardiac arrest, for example)—dictates the evaluation of the patient before surgery. Patients with existing lung disease often have pulmonary function testing or other evaluations before surgery to enhance anesthesia delivery and assist in the care plan afterward.

Other areas to consider include:

- Postoperative changes in lung volume.
- Changes in gas exchange abnormalities.
- Breathing patterns.
- The assessment of pulmonary function, such as vital capacity measurements, acid-base balance, and breathing patterns.
- The aggressive treatment of other complications, such as aspiration, hypothermia, and hemodynamic instability.

Respiratory therapists should be adept at assessment and critical thinking skills in order to manage this type of patient.

MEDICAL CONSIDERATIONS

Equally as challenging to manage as the surgical patient is the medical patient. Patients can be admitted into the ICU for a variety of reasons; however, respiratory therapists are most often involved with specific pulmonary disease entities. Acute respiratory failure in COPD patients or patients admitted in status asthmaticus often end up in the ICU. Often, these patients require some type of mechanical ventilation, by either invasive or noninvasive means. Many patients who have COPD are elderly and also have special age-related needs.

CARDIOVASCULAR CONSIDERATIONS

The heart receives oxygen via the coronary blood flow. Due to its mechanics, the heart uses most of the oxygen available in the coronary circulation and little reserve exists. Because of this phenomenon:

- Patients with coronary artery disease or heart failure usually require supplemental oxygen therapy in the intensive care unit.

CASE STUDY 33-3

Critical Care Management of the COPD Patient

S. S. is a 68-year-old male with severe COPD 2 days postlung volume reduction surgery. He was in the surgical ICU and had been on a PB 7200 ventilator since his surgery. He was hemodynamically stable and still has bilateral chest tubes with minimal air leak. He had been progressing well and was being weaned off the ventilator from assist control to SIMV with pressure support.

The physician ordered the rate on the ventilator to be decreased to 6 breaths per minute and to add 20 cm H_2O pressure support. Immediately after making the ventilator changes, the therapist noticed that the exhaled volume widely fluctuated and read much lower than expected. The therapist also noticed that the spontaneous breaths inspiratory time seemed very long. The chest tube bubbling was now much greater. The patient's pulse oximeter saturations did not change, but the end-tidal CO_2 was much lower than previously.

Questions

1. What is the most probable cause related to the activation of pressure support?
2. How can a chest tube air leak be quantified?
3. Why would the patient's oxygenation not change but the end-tidal CO_2 reading drop?

- After open-heart surgery, such as coronary artery bypass or heart valve replacement, patients require mechanical ventilatory support and oxygen therapy after extubation until pulmonary status is normalized.
- Some patients require extensive support, such as intra-arterial balloon pump (IABP) or left ventricular assist devices (LVAD) in order to support the actions of the heart and may also need advanced respiratory modalities, such as mechanical ventilation.[46]

RENAL CONSIDERATIONS

Mechanical intervention can affect renal function and fluid balance. Mechanical ventilation can cause reductions in atrial natriuretic peptide (ANP) and an increase in plasma antidiuretic hormone (ADH), which ultimately affect urine output and fluid retention. Mechanical ventilation, which decreases cardiac output and blood pressure, may cause a decrease in renal perfusion, which ultimately decreases urine output.[45]

Best Practice

Utilizing CPGs in Lung Inflation Therapy

Postoperative care may include therapies ranging from supplemental oxygen to mechanical ventilation. After extubation, some type of lung inflation therapy is usually indicated. Physician practice or preference or regional practices may dictate the particular type of lung inflation therapy utilized in a hospital. In any event, if protocols are not in place, therapist-directed protocols that address lung inflation techniques are of benefit. The AARC has developed several therapist-driven protocols that may benefit lung inflation. Often many surgical patients who do not progress through the system in the expected manner become patients with a variety of medical issues. Utilizing the following CPGs enhances best practice.

- Incentive spirometry (*Respiratory Care*, 1991)
- Postural drainage therapy (*Respiratory Care*, 1991)
- Use of positive airway pressure adjuncts to bronchial hygiene therapy (*Respiratory Care*, 1993)

NEUROLOGICAL OR NEUROMUSCULAR CONSIDERATIONS

Many patients in intensive care may have disorders of the neurological or neuromuscular system. Spinal cord trauma may result in paralysis depending on the extent and location of injury. Injury above the third cervical segment leads to respiratory muscle paralysis and death unless immediate resuscitative actions (ventilation) occur.[39]

The Glasgow Coma Scale (GCS) is used to assess unconscious. This widely accepted standardized tool assesses the level of consciousness, based on patient responses to eye opening and verbal and motor skills. The score ranges from 3 to 15, with 15 being considered normal.[46]

Summary

The critical care environment is a challenge for any caregiver. With new technologies arriving daily, keeping up is hard. Caregivers who accept new challenges well should survive in this environment. Respiratory therapists are trained to function in the critical care environment and should flourish in the setting.

Study Questions

REVIEW QUESTIONS

1. What qualities are important for respiratory therapists who desire to work in intensive care units?
2. What clinical practice guidelines address lung inhalation techniques?
3. How does an information system enhance patient care?
4. How can respiratory therapists provide benefits to the health care organization in the intensive care setting?
5. What role do respiratory therapists play in cost containment?

MULTIPLE-CHOICE QUESTIONS

1. Which is not an advantage of zoning therapists to selected work areas?
   a. uniformity in patient care on a day-to-day basis
   b. completion of research or educational projects specific to that unit
   c. no expertise required in specific competencies for the area
   d. rapport with other members of the health care team assigned to the unit

2. Which of the following is not a feature of care plans?
   a. They can guide the respiratory therapist in determining the type of care activities required by the patient.
   b. They allow the practitioner to progress the patient through the process in an organized fashion.
   c. They do not assist respiratory therapists in any way.
   d. They are also used by nurses and other health care providers.
3. A well designed ventilator flow sheet can do all the following except:
   a. assist the respiratory therapist in determining the weaning activities.
   b. be used in providing information for respiratory care.
   c. be used for the current management of the patient.
   d. be used in quality enhancement projects.
4. The possible effects of overeating include:
   a. diaphragm and other muscle weakness.
   b. impaired response to hypoxemia and hypercarbia.
   c. increase in respiratory infections.
   d. increase in weaning capabilities.
5. Which surgical procedures have the most significant effect on pulmonary function and cause more severe respiratory complications?
   a. cranial areas
   b. lower extremity surgery
   c. lower abdominal areas
   d. thoracic and upper abdominal areas
6. Which of the following do ventilator weaning protocols not have positive effects on?
   a. length of stay
   b. patient outcomes
   c. intubation time
   d. respiratory infections

CRITICAL-THINKING QUESTIONS

1. What criteria should be assessed for patients entering the critical care system?
2. How does zone scheduling of therapists enhance productivity?
3. What multidisciplinary competencies enhance the workplace?

References

1. Ceriani R. Mazzoni M, Bortone F, et al. Application of the sequential organ failure assessment score to cardiac surgical patients. *Chest*. 2003;123:1229–1239.
2. Garland A, Paz H. *Principals of Critical Care*. 2nd ed. New York: McGraw-Hill; 1999:25–34.
3. Doorley P, Durbin C. Thoracic imaging in the intensive care unit: improving clinical skills and access means better patient care. *Respir Care*. 1999;44:1015–1016.
4. Mishoe S, MacIntyre N. Expanding professional roles for respiratory care practitioners. *Respir Care*. 1997;42:71–86.
5. Robinson G, Goldstein M, Levine G. Impact of nutritional status on DRG length of stay. *JPEN. J Parenter Enteral Nutr.* 1987;11:9–51.
6. Shikora S, Bistrian B, Borlase B, et al. Work of breathing: reliable predictor of weaning and extubation. *Crit Care Med*. 1990;18:157–162.
7. Kreymann G, Grosser S, Buggisch P, et al. Oxygen consumption and resting metabolic rate in sepsis, sepsis syndrome and septic shock. *Crit Care Med*. 1993;21:1012–1019.
8. Hess D, Daugherty A, Large E, Agarwal N. A comparison of four methods of determining caloric requirements of mechanically ventilated patients. *Respir Care*. 1986;31:1197–1203.
9. Weissman C, Kemper M, et al. Resting metabolic rate of the critically ill patient: measured versus predicted. *Anesthesiology*. 1986;64:673–679.
10. Makk L, McClave S, et al. Clinical application of the metabolic cart in the delivery of total parental nutrition. *Crit Care Med*. 1990;18:1320–1327.
11. Lewis W, Chwals W, et al. Bedside assessment of the work of breathing. *Crit Care Med*. 1988;16:117–122.
12. Shoemaker W, Appel P, Kram H. Oxygen transport measurements to evaluate tissue perfusion and titrate therapy: dobutamine and dopamine effects. *Crit Care Med*. 1991;19:672–688.
13. Birkmeyer J, Birkmeyer C, Wennberg D, et al: Leapfrog Safety Standards: Potential benefits of universal adoption. Washington DC: The Leapfrog Group; 2000.
14. Treggiari M, Martin D, Yanez D, et al. Effect of intensive care unit organization model and structure on outcomes in patients with acute lung injury. *Am J Resp Crit Care Med*. 2007;176:685–690.
15. Sabo J. *Respiratory Care in the 1990s: Respiratory Care: A Guide to Clinical Practice*. Philadelphia, PA: Lippincott; 1997:27–60.
16. Hess D. The role of the respiratory therapist in the intensive care unit. *Respir Care*. 1997;42:116–126.
17. Nilsestuen J, Hargett K. Managing the patient-ventilator system using graphic analysis: an overview and introduction to Graphics Corner. *Respir Care*. 1996;41:1105–1122.

18. Opus Communications. Get ready for key changes in 2000. *Briefings on JCAHO*. 1999;10:1–3.
19. Brochard L, Rauss A, Benito S, et al. Comparison of three methods of gradual withdrawal from ventilatory support during weaning from mechanical ventilation. *Am J Respir Crit Care Med*. 1994;150: 896–903.
20. Esteban A, Frutos F, Tobin MJ, et al. A comparison of four methods of weaning patients from mechanical ventilation. *N Engl J Med*. 1995;332:345–350.
21. Bunch D. AARC clinical practice guidelines posted on National Guideline Clearinghouse Web Site. *AARC Times*. 1999;23:28–31.
22. Sibbald W. The "whys" and "wherefores" of measuring outcomes in respiratory critical care. *Respir Care*. 1998;43:1092–1098.
23. Centers for Disease Control and Prevention. Guidelines for preventing health-care associated pneumonia, 2003:7.
24. Institute for Healthcare Improvement. Implement the Ventilator Bundle. 2008. www.ihi.org
25. Sabau D, Sabo J. Weaning protocol evaluation in the cardiovascular recovery room [abstract]. *Respir Care*. 1992;37:1285.
26. Wood G, MacLeod B, Moffatt S. Weaning from mechanical ventilation: physician-directed vs. a respiratory-therapist-directed protocol. *Respir Care*. 1995;40:219–224.
27. Marini J. Weaning techniques and protocols. *Respir Care*. 1995;40:233–238.
28. Kollef M, Shapiro S, Silver P, et al. A randomized controlled trial of protocol-directed versus physician-directed weaning from mechanical ventilation [abstract]. *Respir Care*. 1996;41:948.
29. MacIntyre N. Evidence-based guidelines for weaning and discontinuing ventilatory support. *Respir Care*. 2002;47:1:69–90.
30. Kraus J, Bearden E. Preparing for code blue. *Adv Manage Respir Care*. 1999;8:54–58.
31. Di Guillo N. Introduction to critical pathways: what every RCP should know. *AARC Times*. 1995;19:24–29.
32. Hargett K, Meents C, Wheeler D, Hale K. Integration of therapist driven protocols into a critical pathway: the effect on cost and reduction in length of stay [abstract]. *Respir Care*. 1996;41:949.
33. National Coalition on Healthcare. Health insurance costs. www.nchc.org
34. Reid R, Evey L. Cost savings associated with implementation of a chest physiotherapy (CPT) protocol [abstract]. *Respir Care*. 1999;44:1265.
35. Hess D. Inhaled bronchodilators during mechanical ventilation: delivery techniques, evaluation of response, and cost-effectiveness. *Respir Care*. 1994; 39:105–122.
36. Fuller H, Dolovich M, Posmituck G, et al. Pressurized aerosol versus jet aerosol delivery to mechanically ventilated patients: comparison of doses to the lungs. *Am Rev Respir Dis*. 1990;41:440–444.
37. Hughes M, Saez J. Effect of nebulizer mode and position in a mechanical ventilator circuit on dose efficiency. *Respir Care*. 1987;32:1131–1135.
38. Kollef M, Prentice D, Shapiro S, et al. A prospective randomized trial of mechanical ventilation with daily in-line suction catheter changes versus no routine in-line suction catheter changes [abstract]. *Respir Care*. 1996;41:938.
39. Orens D, Arroliga A, Fatica A. Weekly versus daily changes of in-line suctions catheters: impact on rate of ventilator-associated pneumonia and associated costs [abstract]. *Respir Care*. 1999;44:1263.
40. Goode C, Piedalus F. Evidence-based clinical practice. *J Nurs Adm*. 1999;29:15–21.
41. Irving F. Capturing data under critical conditions. *Adv Health Inf Exec*. 1999;3:47–50.
42. Hewlett Packard Technology White Paper. *Communication Standards in the Clinical Setting: The Hewlett Packard Solution*. Palo Alto, CA: Hewlett Packard; 1998.
43. Sabo J, Williams W. *Information Management Systems, Respiratory Care Equipment*. Philadelphia, PA: Lippincott Williams and Wilkins; 1999: 667–698.
44. Luce J. Clinical risk factors for postoperative pulmonary complications. *Respir Care*. 1984; 29:484–495.
45. Burton G, Hodgkin J, Ward J. *Respiratory Care: A Guide to Clinical Practice*. Philadelphia, PA: Lippincott Williams and Wilkins; 1997:27–60, 611–641, 1141–1156.
46. Alspach J. *Core Curriculum for Critical Care*. Philadelphia, PA: WB Saunders; 1998:144–243, 339–399, 715–716.

Suggested Readings

Branson RD, Hess DR, Chatburn RL, eds. *Respiratory Care Equipment*. Philadelphia, PA: Lippincott Williams and Wilkins; 1999.

Marini J. Weaning Techniques and Protocols. *Respir Care*. 1995;40:233–238.

Scott F. Cost cutting strategies in the ICU. *Adv Manage Respir Care*. 1997;6:39–44.

Sibbald W. The "whys" and "wherefores" of measuring outcomes in respiratory critical care. *Respir Care*. 1998;43:1092–1098.

Society of Critical Care Medicine Coalition for Critical Care Excellence. *ICU Cost Reduction Practical Suggestions and Future Considerations*, Vol. 2. Mount Prospect, IL: Society of Critical Care Medicine, 1995.

CHAPTER 34

Subacute and Long-Term Care

Kathleen S. Wyka

OBJECTIVES

Upon completion of this chapter, the reader should be able to:

- List the care elements of a subacute care program.
- List three groups of respiratory patients accepted into the subacute care setting.
- List three elements of admission for access to the subacute care setting.
- Identify four ventilators that may be used in the subacute setting.
- Identify the two accrediting agencies in subacute care.
- Identify the two tools that determine the daily rate that a subacute facility may earn from CMS.
- Define long-term care (LTC).
- Differentiate the various long-term care facilities on the basis of the patient care provided.
- Explain the reimbursement mechanism for long-term care.

CHAPTER OUTLINE

Definition of Subacute Care
Core Elements of an Ideal Subacute Care Program
Accreditation and Regulation of Facilities
- Respiratory Therapist's Involvement in Subacute Care

Respiratory Care Acuity Levels and Modalities
- Patient Selection
- Patient Evaluation
- Specialized Ventilator Care Facilities

Weaning
Discharge Planning
Reimbursement
Current Practices in View of PPS
Long-Term Care
- Long-Term Care Facilities
- Respiratory Care Personnel

Reimbursement

KEY TERMS

assisted living
capitated care
case management
critical pathway
diagnosis-related group (DRG)
length of stay (LOS)
long-term care (LTC)
managed care organizations (MCOs)
minimum data set (MDS)
postacute care
resource utilization group (RUG-III)
subacute care

In the past, acute care was clearly differentiated from long-term and home care. Patients stayed in the hospital until they were well enough to go home on their own or be transferred to a long-term care facility. Long-term care and home care required very little technical or complicated patient care. The introduction of new health care delivery systems, such as managed care and prospective payment systems, however, encouraged hospitals to discharge patients sooner and with more technical or complicated care needs than in the past ("quicker and sicker"). These needs could not be met by existing long-term and home care programs; therefore a new category of care arose: **Subacute care** usually refers to low-technology, uncomplicated inpatient care, but the term is sometimes used synonymously with **postacute care**, which includes all care given after the acute care stay, no matter where the care occurs. The field of subacute care has experienced rapid growth since the middle of the 1980s. This growth seems to be fueled partly by changes in health care payment systems (see Chapter 1) and partly by the rapid growth of the aging population.

Definition of Subacute Care

The term "subacute" care was formerly used to describe hospitalized patients who failed to meet established criteria for a medically necessary acute stay but who were not stable enough to go either home or to a nursing home. Now the phrase is used almost exclusively to refer to patients treated in any setting other than an acute care bed. So subacute, or postacute, care is nothing new; rather, it is a discrete classification on the continuum of care. It is "a level of care—skilled care for patients with complex needs—that some nursing facilities, home care providers and others have been providing for years under a variety of different names."[1] Subacute care can be classified as the traditional high-end skilled nursing care that was formerly done in the hospital but is now done in an alternative site. It serves patients who require less intensive care than the traditional acute care but more attention than traditional nursing home care.

The Joint Commission has established accreditation criteria and standards for subacute care facilities. The American Health Care Association in Washington, D.C., and The Joint Commission have jointly approved the following definitive definition of subacute care.

> Subacute care is goal-oriented treatment rendered immediately after, or instead of, acute hospitalization to treat one or more specific active complex medical conditions or to administer one or more technically complex treatments, in the context of a person's underlying long-term conditions and overall situation.
>
> Generally, the individual's condition is such that the care does not depend heavily on high-technology monitoring or complex diagnostic procedures. Subacute care requires the coordinated services of an interdisciplinary team including physicians, nurses, and other relevant professional disciplines who are trained and knowledgeable to assess and manage these specific conditions and perform the necessary procedures. Subacute care is given as part of a specifically defined program, regardless of the site . . . It requires frequent . . . patient assessment and review of the clinical course and treatment plan for a limited. . . time period, until the condition is stabilized or a predetermined treatment course is completed.[2]

According to this definition, subacute care can take place just about anywhere, from acute care or specialty hospitals to skilled nursing facilities (SNFs) and from rehabilitation programs to outpatient programs and home care settings. The definition allows for a wide range of patients, for almost all age brackets, and for many traditionally acute care procedures, including infusion therapy, respiratory care, cardiac services, wound care, rehabilitation services, postoperative recovery programs for knee and hip replacements, and cancer, stroke, and AIDS care.[3]

Core Elements of an Ideal Subacute Care Program

In a report to the federal government entitled *Subacute Care: Policy Synthesis and Market Area Analysis,* Manard and coworkers listed four core elements of an ideal subacute care program but pointed out that the field is evolving daily and the core elements may change. The first ideal core element is organization:

> First, ideal subacute care is an organized program. It is more than any type of care provided to high-end Medicare patients. Some programs are organized around specific disease categories (e.g., stroke or cancer); others are organized around specific interventions (e.g., pain management or wound care), and some are organized around other more or less homogeneous patient characteristics (e.g., pediatrics or medically complex). In general, providers tend to distinguish between rehabilitation subacute patients, which include conditions such as hip replacement, spinal cord injuries, and brain injuries. These patients tend to require more rehabilitation services such as physical, occupational, and speech therapies. Conversely, medical

> subacute patients tend to have conditions that require intensive medical and nursing care, but fewer other therapies. This group of patients includes those with cardiovascular diagnoses, cancer, ventilator care, wounds, and IV therapy.[4]

Long-term care facilities often provide rehabilitation subacute care, and hospitals and nursing homes most often provide medical subacute care. Respiratory care obviously has a place in medical subacute care because of respiratory therapists' ability to assess and treat complex cardiopulmonary problems and their knowledge of cardiopulmonary physiology. Since the time the Manard report was written (1995), respiratory care has also found a place in the rehabilitative subacute care area (see Chapter 36).

The second core element of subacute care is focus on outcomes:

> In the ideal, a subacute care program is intensely focused on achieving specified, measurable outcomes. The outcomes or goals may. . . vary for each patient (e.g., healing a wound or restoring the patient to a particular level of functioning) . . . . Subacute programs in the ideal stress . . . achieving outcomes in a particularly efficient and lower cost manner.[4]

With regard to the efficiency and cost, the American Association for Respiratory Care (AARC) has emphasized the need to educate ourselves to the language of managed care. **Managed care organizations (MCOs)** (organizations that provide health care coverage) want positive patient outcomes at the lowest possible cost. Respiratory therapists have traditionally provided positive patient outcomes at a low cost but have failed to adequately measure the costs. Measurement of patient outcomes and the documentation of costs enable respiratory therapists to help subacute care facilities maintain efficient and effective utilization of resources.

The third core element of subacute care is special resources:

> Special resources . . . generally include physical plant features such as a distinct unit . . . and more and better trained staff [than in a traditional nursing facility], especially physicians and nurses.[4]

The AARC research initiative demonstrated that respiratory therapists are "better trained" than traditional nursing facility staff in cardiopulmonary patient assessment and treatment and can provide quality care with positive outcomes at a lower cost.[5]

The fourth core element of subacute care is

> a set of techniques thought essential to achieving stated goals. These techniques include the use of interdisciplinary teams to plan and provide patient care and case managers, whose jobs involve both resource use monitoring and more traditional care-coordination activities. Care techniques . . . also include the use of Acare maps™ and/or critical pathway protocols, program evaluation based on measured outcomes, and an emphasis on continuous quality improvement.[4]

In skilled nursing facilities, on-site case managers who are highly trained, skilled clinical professionals are vital for coordinating the efforts of physicians, clinical team members, patients, and family. (**Case management** is a method of medical management in which a person is assigned patients with the same types of problems to standardize care.) Respiratory therapists are logical case managers for a subacute care unit that is organized around the specific intervention dealing with cardiopulmonary disease or a unit that is devoted to ventilator care. Managed care organizations are pressing for **critical pathways** as a technique for timing the sequence of interventions in the care plan of the patient to achieve positive outcomes. Respiratory care, again with the leadership of the AARC, has provided thorough cardiopulmonary clinical practice guidelines, which are the cornerstone of critical pathways and protocols. Many of the AARC guidelines can be found in the References and Suggested Readings throughout this book.

Many health care workers claim that managed care has been the single most important driving force to alternative site care, such as subacute care. The introduction of **capitated care**, which limits the amount of health care dollars that can be paid over a patient's life, to both institutions and physicians has generated the

Spotlight On

Cost Effectiveness of Respiratory Therapy

The Muse report indicates that respiratory therapists provide high-quality care with definite positive patient outcomes. Using data from 1996, the report demonstrates that persons who receive treatments from respiratory therapists tend to have more positive outcomes and lower costs (i.e., use fewer health care services) than those who do not receive care from respiratory therapists.

Source: Muse & Associates. A Comparison of Medicare Nursing Home Residents Who Receive Services from a Respiratory Therapist with Those Who Do Not. *Washington, DC: Muse & Assoc; July 1999.*

aggressive search for less expensive health care. The financial pressures of capitated care have fueled the search for improvements in two aspects of subacute care: lower cost and higher quality. Capitation has moved into the Medicaid market, and managed care organizations understand that money can be made if the patient is kept out of the acute care hospital. Keeping patients in an acute care setting when they do not require acute care is a waste of money, but sending the patient home too early may result in readmission. Discharging patients to subacute care facilities instead of to their homes can help prevent costly readmissions as long as the subacute care institutions provide quality care.

The health care industry continues to move toward integrated health networks, which offer certain financial advantages to acute care facilities. Acute care facilities that cannot convert beds into subacute care often form alliances with existing facilities that do have subacute care beds. Since hospitals have a much higher cost base because of the needs of acute care patients, the ability to move stable patients to a subacute care facility, such as a nursing home, can save hospitals money. Current trends show that managed care companies, in an effort to contain costs, are shifting increasing numbers of hospital patients into subacute care beds in nursing homes.

For common **diagnosis-related group (DRG)** procedures, subacute care can save thousands of dollars.[6] In addition, increased revenue can be generated by charging for the subacute care. Management companies contract with hospitals and skilled nursing facilities to convert skilled nursing beds to subacute care beds. The management company provides the expertise on subacute care reimbursement and regulations that may be lacking from the partner institutions.

Before any new subacute care facilities are built, most states require that a *certificate of need* (*CON*) be obtained. Currently only 14 states do not require one. A CON is a requirement that a facility must file with its respective state's department of health to receive authorization to institute a particular service or level of care. As an example, in New Jersey, a bill was passed in 1996, allowing hospitals to either convert or designate as subacute up to 7% of the total medical-surgical beds or 12 beds, whichever is greater (NJ Senate Bill No. 368, 1996). The rationale is that the institution is not adding any beds; it is only converting existing beds to a lower level of acuity.

SNFs are highly regulated health care entities; however, the regulations are not specifically tailored to subacute care. Rather the regulations used are for hospitals and nursing homes. Nursing homes and managed care companies find some of these requirements unreasonable. For instance, nursing home providers of subacute services want to eliminate the requirement that subacute care patients undergo a 3-day hospital stay before being transferred to a subacute facility. This requirement comes from the Social Security Act definition of posthospital extended care services: "extended care services furnished an individual after transfer from a hospital in which he was an inpatient for not less than 3 consecutive days."[7] Managed care companies also want to eliminate this requirement. For example, "some large, fully capitated medical groups that contract to staff hospital emergency rooms have directives to transfer any patient who doesn't require acute care services—invasive procedures or complex diagnostics, for example—directly from the ER to a subacute unit."[8]

Accreditation and Regulation of Facilities

Subacute facilities may be accredited by the Joint Commission or the Commission for Accreditation of Rehabilitation Facilities (CARF). The Joint Commission is a private not-for-profit organization that evaluates and accredits more than 17,000 health care organizations and programs, including home care providers and subacute care facilities.[9]

Subacute care facilities gain Joint Commission accreditation by being scored on sets of standards. Standards cover all areas of the subacute care facility, from nursing care to laundry services and from the physical plant to spiritual services. If a facility complies with all related standards a 3-year accreditation is granted. Facilities not in full compliance are awarded either conditional accreditation (deficiencies require remediation or corrective action) or no accreditation. CARF focuses on accrediting agencies and organizations providing a variety of rehabilitation services. Three subcategories were developed, taking into account the different levels and types of rehabilitation (acute or subacute), the location (hospital or SNF), and patient outcome goals.[10]

The National Committee for Quality Care (NCQA), another accrediting body, was formed to ensure quality in managed care organizations. If subacute care organizations or their parent organizations under which they operate wish to contract with MCOs, they must be aware of the NCQA standards and how to meet them.[10]

Federal and state governments have always regulated subacute care facilities and will continue to do so as the field grows. By regulating subacute care, the state has the opportunity to control growth surges, thereby preventing excessive numbers of subacute care beds. Each state incorporates its own policies on regulating subacute care centers.

Best Practice

Accreditation

Even though accreditation by The Joint Commission (TJC) is optional, it is to the advantage of the subacute care facility to be accredited because many managed care organizations (MCOs) look for this accreditation. The Joint Commission is becoming the standard for most MCOs.

RESPIRATORY THERAPIST'S INVOLVEMENT IN SUBACUTE CARE

Different levels of subacute care have implications for respiratory care. Table 34-1 shows four levels along with the respiratory therapist's involvement.

Respiratory Care Acuity Levels and Modalities

Subacute respiratory care generally follows three basic acuity levels, each with its own appropriate level of respiratory therapist and equipment commitments: airway management patients (basic), complex respiratory patients (intermediate), and ventilator-dependent patients (the highest acuity level). All of these patients require frequent respiratory assessment to ascertain the need for such respiratory procedures as bronchodilator therapy, oxygen therapy, bronchopulmonary hygiene, and airway management.

The subacute setting uses many of the same respiratory care modalities as the acute care setting. These modalities range from routine bedside respiratory care to care for the ventilator-dependent patient. Certain subacute facilities may accept only specific types of respiratory patients. These respiratory patients may be classified into three distinct groups depending on the level of respiratory care they need:

- Basic respiratory care
- Intermediate respiratory care
- Ventilatory care

Basic respiratory care includes modalities such as:

- Oxygen therapy.
- Bland aerosol administration.
- Delivery of aerosols to the upper airway.
- Intermittent positive pressure breathing (IPPB).
- Postural drainage.

Patients at this level may be admitted to the subacute facility to continue with the rehabilitation process before being discharged to their home. Most patients requiring basic respiratory care traditionally are taken care of by RNs and LPNs.

Patients in the *intermediate respiratory care* group may have a tracheostomy requiring care and may require aerosol administration. These patients may also be admitted to the subacute facility to continue with weaning trials from the tracheostomy tube, eventually leading to decannulation. Patients who are admitted to subacute facilities with tracheostomies are often cared for by respiratory therapists.

Specific bedside respiratory care modalities for basic and intermediate-level patients in the subacute setting include:

- Oxygen therapy.[11]
- Nasotracheal suctioning.[12]
- Postural drainage therapy.[13]
- Delivery of aerosols to the upper airway.[14]
- Assessing the response to bronchodilator therapy.[15]
- Directed cough.[16]
- Selection of an appropriate aerosol delivery device.[17]
- Bland aerosol administration.[18]
- Incentive spirometry.[19]
- Intermittent positive pressure breathing.[20]
- Use of positive airway pressure adjuncts to bronchial hygiene therapy.[21]

TABLE 34-1 **Four levels of subacute care and respiratory therapist involvement**

	Traditional	General	Chronic	Long-Term Transitional
Location	Within hospital or freestanding	Nursing home	Chronic care facility	Long-term care facility
Respiratory therapist involvement	High: provides same level as acute care, with interdisciplinary teamwork and patient education	Teaching and training functions; can be extended to long-term or home when patient problem leaves	Consultant role to nurses	More intensive than acute care; most patients have some type of respiratory therapy

Source: From Bunch D. Phenomenal growth of subacute care offers new opportunities for RCPs. AARCTimes. *March 1996:48.*

Patients in the *ventilatory care* group may be admitted to the subacute facility for extended weaning from mechanical ventilation or for long-term mechanical ventilation. Any subacute care facility that accepts ventilator patients should have respiratory therapists on staff. Acute care facilities manage patients with an average **length of stay (LOS)** of 4–7 days, whereas subacute facilities focus on longer stays, with an average LOS of 60–90 days.

Specific procedures related to ventilatory support in the subacute setting include:

- Endotracheal suctioning of mechanically ventilated patients.[22]
- Humidification during mechanical ventilation.[23]
- Patient-ventilator system checks.[24]
- Transport of the mechanically ventilated patient.[25]
- Providing patient and caregiver training.[26]
- Discharge planning for the respiratory care patient.[27]

PATIENT SELECTION

When looking at prospective patients for the subacute setting, the admissions team must look at the following elements of admission:

- Evaluation of the patient for the appropriateness of care
- Formulation of an admissions plan and a potential discharge plan
- Determination that financial resources are adequate

PATIENT EVALUATION

Many of the patients discharged from an acute to a subacute facility have a multitude of medically complex problems, including respiratory-related complications. An example of this type of patient is a 75-year-old male who was admitted to the acute care setting with a history of chronic obstructive pulmonary disease (COPD) and a primary admitting diagnosis of a fractured hip. Surgery was performed to repair the fractured hip, and the patient completed a normal postoperative course while in the acute care setting. The time had come for discharge from the acute care setting, but the patient could not be discharged home because of his inability to ambulate. The decision was made to transfer the patient to a subacute facility where he could continue the rehabilitation process. At the same time, he would receive respiratory care to keep his COPD under control.

The admissions team of a subacute facility, especially one that accepts ventilator-dependent individuals, should be multidisciplinary and have a respiratory therapist. The balance of the admissions team should consist of a nurse, a case manager, a physical therapist, an admissions coordinator, and a social worker. The respiratory therapist needs to complete an initial assessment form to gather all the information needed to prepare for the possible admission of this patient to the facility.

The subacute facility should be ready to accept any patient who requires a multitude of services to progress and prepare for discharge to the home or to the long-term setting. Some of the most common diagnoses encountered in the subacute setting are:

- Spinal cord injuries.
- Joint replacements.
- Femur fractures, including hip fractures.
- Major multiple trauma.
- Congenital anomalies.
- Traumatic brain injury (TBI).
- Strokes or cerebral vascular accidents (CVAs).
- Neurological disorders, including multiple sclerosis, motor neuron disease, muscular dystrophy, polyneuropathy, and Parkinson's disease.

Common services needed to accommodate these patients are:

- Physical, occupational, and speech therapy.
- IV therapy; wound care.
- Cardiac rehabilitation.
- Ventilator and pulmonary rehabilitation.
- Pain management.
- Dialysis.
- Chemotherapy.

SPECIALIZED VENTILATOR CARE FACILITIES

The highest level of subacute respiratory care is offered in a specialized ventilator care facility. Some facilities accept only long-term ventilator patients; others may accept long-term as well as weaning ventilator patients.

Best Practice

Preadmission Evaluation

The nurse case manager and the respiratory therapist need to perform an on-site evaluation of any patient being considered for a subacute-based ventilator unit. At this stage, the patient has already exhausted his or her stay in the acute care facility and probably has failed all ventilator weaning attempts. In the preadmission on-site evaluation, the team must gather all the information needed to portray a complete picture of the patient.

Most long-term ventilator patients can be managed on portable positive pressure ventilators such as the Phillips Respironics PLV Continuum ventilators (Figure 34-1), Nellcor Puritan-Bennett Achieva (Figure 34-2), and 540 Portable ventilators. Patients who are admitted to weaning ventilator care facilities may use units such as Nellcor Puritan-Bennett (740, 760, and 7200 series) ventilators the Bird T-Bird AVS/VSO2/VS Series ventilators (Figure 34-3), and the Pulmonetic LTV 1000, 1150 and 1200 ventilators (Figure 34-4). Of these ventilators, all are portable except the Nellcor Puritan-Bennett 740, 760, and 7200 series. Portable ventilators are compact, can be battery operated (internal and external), and can be transported with the patient. Nonportable ventilators are AC power dependent.

Best Practice

All professional personnel working with ventilator patients should be aware of the battery life of both internal and external batteries used to power the ventilator. Additionally, these personnel should also ensure that both audio and visual alarms are functional and at proper volume to assure that alarms will be heard by appropriate personnel.

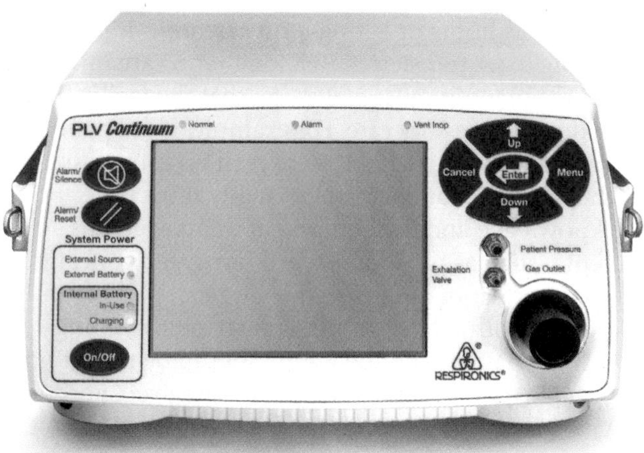

FIGURE 34-1 Continuum ventilator.

Courtesy of Philips Respironics

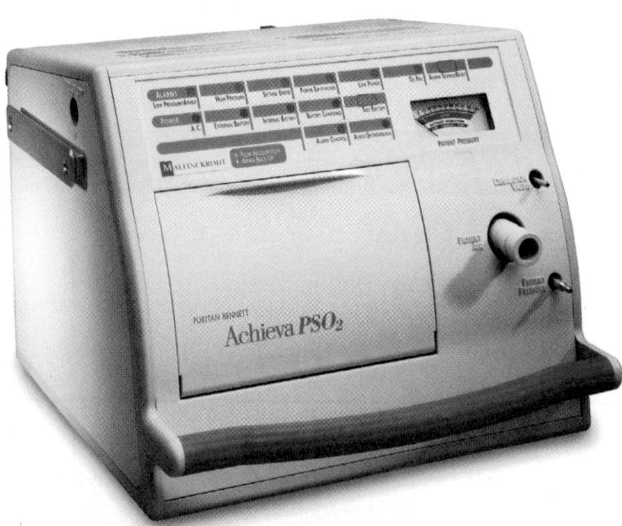

FIGURE 34-2 Achieva ventilator.

Image used by permission from Nellcor Puritan Bennett LLC, Boulder, Colorado, doing business as Covidien.

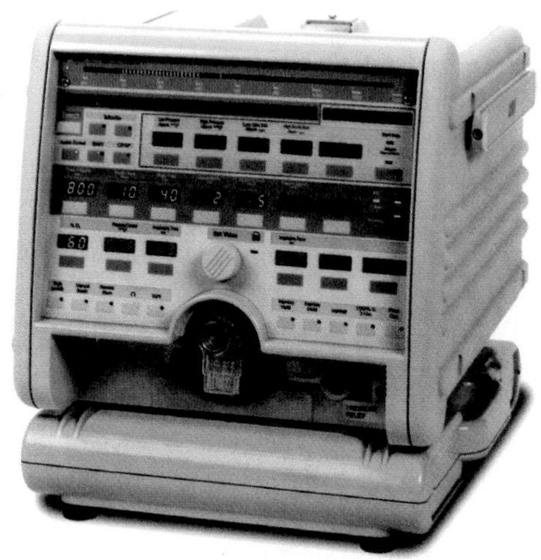

FIGURE 34-3 T-Bird AVS/VSO2/VS Series ventilators.

Courtesy of Bird Products Corporation

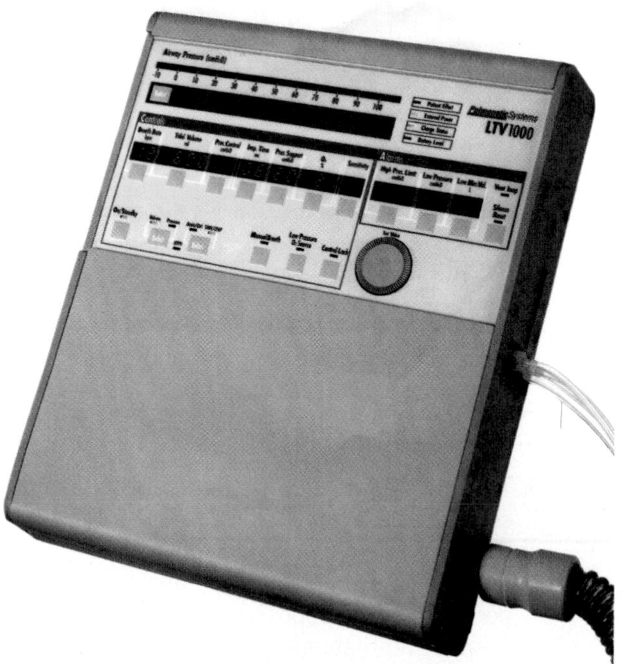

FIGURE 34-4 Pulmonetic Systems LTV 1000 mechanical ventilator.

Courtesy of Pulmonetic Systems

Weaning

With the advent of portable ventilators that can provide synchronized intermittent mandatory ventilation (SIMV), pressure support ventilation, and continuous positive airway pressure (CPAP), many of the same weaning modalities that are used in the acute setting can be continued in the subacute setting. Monitoring techniques such as pulse oximetry, capnography or capnometry during mechanical ventilation, and sampling for arterial blood gas analysis are all accurate methods of evaluating the progress of the weaning patient in the subacute setting.

A typical weaning scenario might progress as follows:

1. Patient is admitted on continuous mechanical ventilation on assist-control.
2. Weaning parameters are performed, indicating that the patient may be strong enough to tolerate SIMV.
3. SIMV and pressure support ventilation are initiated.
4. SIMV rate and pressure support ventilation are titrated as tolerated.
5. Once SIMV4 and pressure support are tolerated, CPAP or tracheostomy collar trials can begin.
6. If tracheostomy collar trials are tolerated during the day, the patient may need to be rested on the ventilator during sleep.
7. Once the patient is able to tolerate a tracheostomy collar for 24 hours, the size of the tracheostomy can be reduced and a fenestrated tube can be used.
8. Institute capping trials to lead to decannulation of the tracheostomy tube.
9. Once the patient is decannulated, begin nasal oxygen to keep the arterial saturation at an acceptable level.

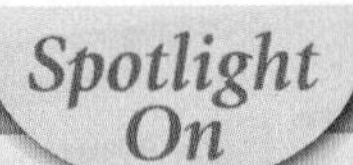

Costs of Ventilator Weaning

Some of the health care costs associated with ventilator weaning in the subacute facility can be lowered with the following:

- Performing fewer arterial blood gas analyses and using pulse oximetry and capnography more. The cost of arterial blood gas analyses is reduced by not having to incur the cost of a full laboratory analysis.
- Typical ventilators in the subacute setting cost anywhere from $6000 to $18,000. These ventilators provide SIMV, CPAP, and pressure support in a compact and portable size as opposed to the larger hospital ventilators, which cost more than $20,000.

Discharge Planning

The respiratory therapist can have an integral role in discharge planning at the subacute level. The respiratory therapist needs to be involved in the discharge process from the day of admission to the day of discharge.

Once patients reach their maximum potential in the subacute setting, arrangements need to be made for their anticipated discharge to the next level of care, whether it is home or a long-term care unit. If patients are going to be transferred to a long-term care unit, the discharge planner must make sure that the facility can provide the necessary care. For example, if the patient has a tracheostomy with 40% oxygen via an aerosol trach collar, the long-term care facility must have the knowledge and the equipment to manage this patient—such as piped-in oxygen or oxygen concentrators, compressors, and oxygen analyzers.

On the other hand, if the same patient is going home, the patient and the family should be taught how to provide the care. The patient and caregivers need to be given a structured, written education program that they can easily understand. Written material can be assembled in a complete, easy-to-read manual. Any education presented to the patient or caregivers must be documented in the medical record on a form such as a Resident Education Flow Sheet.

Best Practice

Plan of Care

The first 48 hours after admission are crucial in the discharge process. During this time, all the disciplines are required to submit their care plans after performing careful evaluations of the patient. The respiratory therapist must also formulate a care plan after reviewing such information as past health history, past hospitalizations, social history, and the wishes of the family to bring their family member home.

Successful Patient Education

The respiratory therapist should present the education to the patient and caregivers in different formats, such as written material, videotape presentations, and hands-on demonstration. All the material must be specific to the age of the caregivers and the patient and must be easy to understand for all involved. The subject and results of these sessions should be recorded in the patient's chart or record.

Once all educational objectives have been accomplished, the patient and the caregivers must be able to demonstrate what they have learned. The respiratory therapist can then develop a complete list of equipment and supplies needed to take care of the patient at home. The interdisciplinary team then meets again to review the final discharge plan, including equipment, caregivers, and transportation on the day of discharge.

Reimbursement

Medicare, Medicaid, private insurers, health maintenance organizations (HMOs), and preferred provider organizations (PPOs) all cover services offered at the subacute level. The HMOs and other managed care organizations are using subacute care facilities because

CASE STUDY 34-1

J. is a 63-year-old Hispanic male who was admitted to the subacute facility after a 4-month stay in an acute care hospital. His admitting diagnosis was respiratory failure secondary to COPD and pneumonia. J. was admitted with a Foley, gastrostomy, and tracheostomy tube in place, and his skin was intact. Physical, occupational, speech, and respiratory therapists evaluated him, and a care plan was initiated. The assessments were as follows:

PT: Patient was unable to ambulate and required maximum assist for transfers.

OT: Patient required maximum assist with dressing, bathing, and grooming as well as all ADLs.

ST: Patient required speech training using a Passy Muir speaking valve and dysphagia studies in an effort to increase his oral nutritional intake.

RT: Patient tolerated increased CPAP trials while on the ventilator. His ventilator settings were: CPAP @ 0, PS +10 cm H_2O, F_IO_2 0.35 (8 a.m.–10 p.m.) and assist/control @ 10, V_t 700 cc, F_IO_2 0.35 (10 p.m.–8 a.m.).

He was doing so well that, within 2 days, he progressed to a trach collar during the day and was maintained on A/C at night so that he could rest. After the third day, he tolerated the trach collar so well that it was not necessary to return him on the ventilator at night. By the twelfth day, his tracheostomy tube was changed to a fenestrated tube to facilitate capping and eventual decannulation. By day 14, J. was on nasal oxygen, which was discontinued 2 days later because he was able to maintain an oxygen saturation of 95%.

During the course of ventilator weaning, all therapists worked with J. to facilitate increased muscle strength, increased oral nutritional intake, and training in activities of daily living. On day 21, he was transferred to the hospital for removal of the tracheostomy and gastrostomy tubes. Two days later, he came back to the subacute facility for the continuation of his rehabilitation program and completion of his discharge plan to home. Within 6 days, he was discharged home with the services provided by a local home health agency.

Questions

1. During on-site evaluation in the acute setting, what was the best method for the respiratory therapist to determine J.'s needs before admitting him to the subacute setting?
2. What monitoring techniques could be used to measure respiratory fatigue during the weaning process of mechanical ventilation in the subacute setting?
3. How would the interdisciplinary team determine a game plan for J.?

their costs are lower than they would be in the acute care setting. Typically, the subacute costs are 40–60% less than the hospital-related acute care costs. In addition, subacute care may generate more income than other nonacute care settings. Reimbursement for a typical nursing home bed may be $150 a day or more depending on region or facility, whereas reimbursement for a bed in a subacute facility may cost up to $800 a day or more, depending on the services needed, such as ventilator care, IV therapy, or specialized wound care.

In the past, respiratory care in the subacute setting was reimbursed in one of two ways.

- The most popular method was for the subacute care facility to have a transfer agreement with a hospital to obtain Medicare reimbursement. The respiratory care staff was then provided to the subacute facility by that transfer hospital.
- In the other method of payment for respiratory care services, the subacute care facility contracted with an outside management company, which would provide the respiratory therapists, equipment, supplies, and policies and procedures to run the respiratory care department. The facility then reimbursed the management company on either a per diem rate or any other rate as set forth on their contract.

In 1998, the Centers for Medicare & Medicaid Services (CMS) cut reimbursement in the subacute care arena, adversely affecting payment for respiratory care. CMS changed from a cost-per-charge reimbursement system to a prospective payment system (PPS). With this transition, the transfer agreement was eliminated. PPS rates consist of a federal rate and a facility-specific rate. The federal payment rate covers all costs of furnishing covered skilled nursing services with the exception of educational costs. This includes Part B services furnished under an arrangement with the subacute facility to subacute inpatients. Therefore, except for physician's services and other practitioners exempted under the law, the unbundling of services allowed under the previous payment mechanism are no longer permitted.

The **resource utilization group (RUG-III)** case-mix classification system consists of 44 categories that capture resource use (nursing and treatment time) of subacute patients and is intended to provide an improved method of tracking the quality of care. The 44 RUG categories are classified from the most clinically complex to the least complex groups. RUG-III groups are used in determining the payment scheme (Figure 34-5).

Patient assessment plays a crucial role in determining the case mix. The assessment process uses a standardized *resident assessment instrument* (*RAI*) called the **minimum data set (MDS)** (Figure 34-6). Over 100 assessment items are used to provide information on the patients' nursing care needs, therapies, medical diagnoses, cognitive status, behavioral problems, and activities of daily living (ADL) impairments. Subacute facilities must prepare the MDS clinical assessment by day 5 of a patient's admission to the facility and must perform ongoing assessments within certain time frames. The patient data gathered on the MDS are analyzed to determine the appropriate RUG-III category for the patient and therefore the per diem rate the facility will receive during the patient's stay.

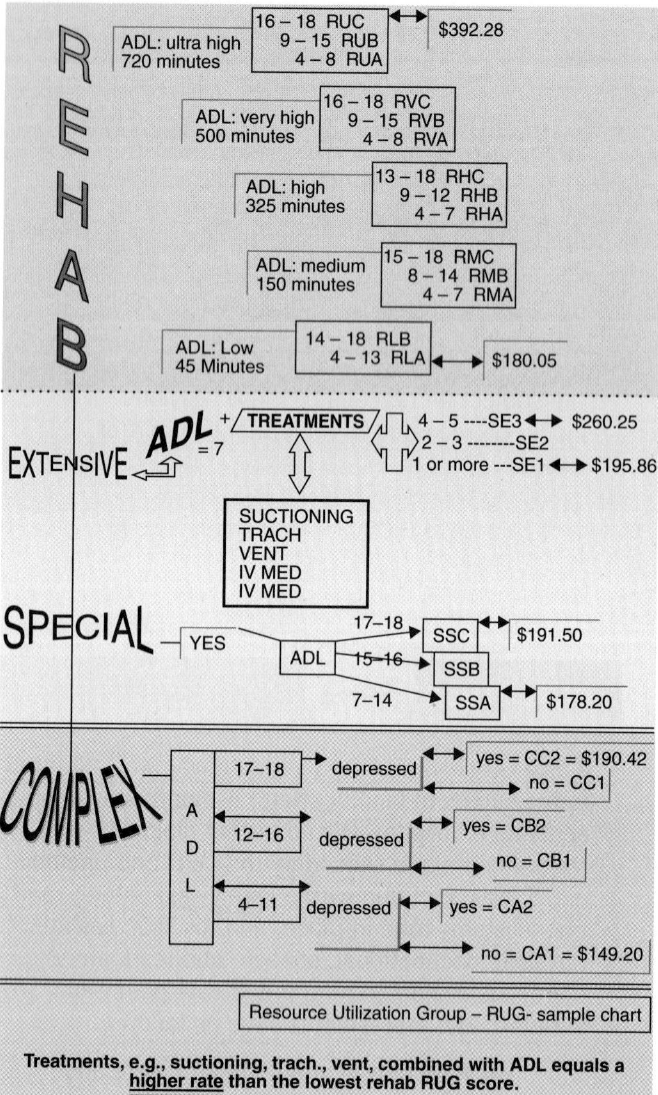

FIGURE 34-5 Resource utilization group (RUG-III) case mix classification system.

Courtesy of Gerry Cannon, RN, BS, Hospicomm Inc., Quality Assurance

Numeric Identifier________________

MINIMUM DATA SET (MDS) — *VERSION 2.0*

FOR NURSING HOME RESIDENT ASSESSMENT AND CARE SCREENING

BASIC ASSESSMENT TRACKING FORM

SECTION AA. IDENTIFICATION INFORMATION

1.	RESIDENT NAME ⊛	(Exactly as appears on Medicare Card) a. (First) b. (Middle Initial) c. (Last) d. (Jr./Sr.)
2.	GENDER ⊛	1. Male 2. Female
3.	BIRTHDATE ⊛	*(Complete all four digits)* Month – Day – Year
4.	RACE/ ⊛ ETHNICITY	1. American Indian/Alaskan Native 2. Asian/Pacific Islander 3. Black, not of Hispanic origin 4. Hispanic 5. White, not of Hispanic origin
5.	SOCIAL ⊛ SECURITY AND ⊛ MEDICARE NUMBERS [C in 1st box if non Med. no.]	a. Social Security Number b. Medicare number (or comparable railroad insurance number)
6.	FACILITY PROVIDER NO. ⊛	a. State No. *(Facility Medicaid Provider number)* *(Facility Medicare Provider number)* b. Federal No.
7.	MEDICAID NO. ["+" if pending, "N" if not a Medicaid ⊛ recipient]	*(Resident Medicaid number)*
8.	REASONS FOR ASSESS-MENT ⊛ *Use 8a if NOT Medicare covered, leave 8b blank. Use 8a & b if Medicare covered.*	[Note—Other codes do not apply to this form] a. Primary reason for assessment 1. Admission assessment (required by day 14)-may be 2. Annual assessment 3. Significant change in status assessment-may be 4. Significant correction of prior full assessment-may be 5. Quarterly review assessment 10. Significant correction of prior quarterly assessment 0. NONE OF ABOVE b. **Codes for assessments required for Medicare PPS or the State** *1. Medicare 5 day assessment* *2. Medicare 30 day assessment* *3. Medicare 60 day assessment* *4. Medicare 90 day assessment* *5. Medicare readmission/return assessment* *6. Other state required assessment* *7. Medicare 14 day assessment* *8. Other Medicare required assessment*
9.	SIGNATURES OF PERSONS COMPLETING THESE ITEMS:	

a. Signatures Title Date

b. Date

⊛ = Key items for computerized resident tracking—Key Field errors may be corrected by submitting a "Key Change Request" to the State.

■ = Medicare covered care

□ = Medicare noncovered care

□ = When box blank, must enter number or letter

a. = When letter in box, check if condition applies

Code "—" if information unavailable or unknown

GENERAL INSTRUCTIONS

Complete this information for submission with all full and quarterly assessments (Admission, Annual, Significant Change, State or Medicare required assessments, or Quarterly Reviews, etc.).

For MDS section AA8 use the following schedule for newly admitted and readmitted residents expected to be covered by Medicare during the first 30 days.

Day 0 = Period prior to admission.

Day 1 = Resident admission day.

Day 1-8 = Reference date for the Medicare 5 day assessment (3 grace days available if not designated as initial admission assessment.)

Day 11-19 = Reference date for the Medicare 14 day assessment (no grace days available if designated as initial admission assessment.)

RAPS MUST BE COMPLETED WITH THE 5 OR 14 DAY ASSESSMENT, WHICHEVER IS DESIGNATED AS INITIAL ADMISSION ASSESSMENT

Day 21-34 = Last day for assessment reference date for Medicare 30 day assessment (RAPs not required unless significant change in status occurred).

Day 50-64 = Last day for assessment reference date for Medicare 60 day assessment (RAPs not required unless significant change in status occurred).

Day 80-94 = Last day for assessment reference date for Medicare 90 day assessment (RAPs not required unless significant change in status occurred).

Day 100 = Last possible day of Medicare coverage.

RETURN TO THE STATE REQUIRED OR CLINICAL MDS ASSESSMENT SCHEDULE.

MDS RUG III CASE MIX GROUPS

- RU = Rehabilitation Ultra High
- RV = Rehabilitation Very High
- RH = Rehabilitation High
- RM = Rehabilitation Medium
- RL = Rehabilitation Low
- SE = Extensive Services
- SS = Special Care
- CC, CB, CA = Clinically Complex

THESE GROUPS ARE CONSIDERED SKILLED CARE COVERED BY MEDICARE FOR ELIGIBLE RESIDENTS.

DOCUMENTATION REQUIRED TO JUSTIFY SKILLED CARE

- IB, IA = Impaired Cognition (NOT AUTOMATIC MEDICARE SKILLED LEVEL OF CARE)
- BB, BA = BEHAVIOR ONLY (NOT AUTOMATIC MEDICARE SKILLED LEVEL OF CARE)
- PE, PD, PC, PB, PA = Physical Function Reduced (NOT AUTOMATIC MEDICARE SKILLED LEVEL OF CARE)

TRIGGER LEGEND

1 - Delirium
2 - Cognitive Loss/Dementia
3 - Visual Function
4 - Communication
5A - ADL-Rehabilitation
5B - ADL-Maintenance
6 - Urinary Incontinence and Indwelling Catheter
7 - Psychosocial Well-Being
8 - Mood State
9 - Behavioral Symptoms
10A - Activities (Revise)
10B - Activities (Review)
11 - Falls
12 - Nutritional Status
13 - Feeding Tubes
14 - Dehydration/Fluid Maintenance
15 - Dental Care
16 - Pressure Ulcers
17 - Psychotropic Drug Use
17* - For this to trigger, O4a, b, or c must = 1-7
18 - Physical Restraints

Form 1728EHH R398

1 of 9 MDS 2.0 1/30/98

FIGURE 34-6 First page of the minimum data set (MDS) form.

Courtesy of Briggs Corporation

Current Practices in View of PPS

The PPS changes in reimbursement mechanisms have resulted in the dissolution of many respiratory programs in the subacute setting because respiratory care is not individually recognized as a reimbursable therapy. Instead it is included within the extensive services and special care groups. Some subacute facilities have eliminated their respiratory care staff and are using specially trained nursing staff to care for their patients. Subacute facilities that accept ventilator patients are still employing respiratory therapists to facilitate the weaning process. These facilities will continue to be the forerunners in subacute respiratory care with more and more referrals of the compromised pulmonary patient.

Long-Term Care

Long-term care (LTC) is defined as a broad scope of medical and nonmedical services that are provided to individuals with a chronic illness or disability. These individuals cannot care for themselves over extended periods of time. LTC may also involve custodial and nonskilled care that includes assistance with normal activities of daily living such as bathing, dressing, and use of the bathroom. The most common form of long-term care is found in the home where either family members or caregivers are available to assist the individual on a daily basis. It is also provided in the community at specialized centers (**assisted living** facilities) and in nursing homes.

LTC can be delivered to patients of any age, but the majority of patients receiving this type of care are elderly.

The Centers for Medicare & Medicaid Services (CMS) reported that in 2006, 9 million men and women in the United States over the age of 65 years needed some type of long-term care. By 2020, this number, according to CMS, will increase to 12 million older Americans. Most of these individuals (an estimated 70%) will be cared for in the home by family members and/or caregivers. The U.S. Department of Health and Human Services (DHHS) also estimates that people 65 years and older will have a 40% chance of entering a nursing home and that approximately 10% of the people entering a nursing home will reside there for 5 or more years.[28]

LONG-TERM CARE FACILITIES

Long-term care is often thought of as being delivered in a facility or institution, including the following:

- *Adult care homes.* Residences for elderly and disabled adults who require 24 hour supervision and assistance with activities of daily living and personal care needs. These facilities were formerly called domiciliary, family care, or rest homes. These homes vary in size from more than 100 residents to smaller ones caring for 2–6 residents.
- *Assisted living.* A living residence for group housing and services for 2 or more unrelated adults that makes available at least one meal per day, housekeeping services, and personal care. Individuals in this type of residence may obtain respiratory care equipment such as compressor/nebulizers, oxygen systems, or positive airway pressure (PAP) therapy devices from a home care company. However, depending on facility regulations and/or state law, residents must be able to safely use and maintain this equipment. Assistance may be provided by properly trained staff members, and home care respiratory therapists may visit, assess the individual, and provide follow-up care. Health insurance payors, including Medicare, reimburse the home care company directly for equipment provided in assisted living arrangements. Some states recognize different types of assisted living residences that include adult care homes, group homes for developmentally disabled adults, and multiunit assisted housing with services. Facilities providing assisted living are usually private pay and may cost an individual $35,000 or more per year, depending on the residence.
- *Continuing care retirement communities (CCRC).* Residences typically providing independent accommodations that include full apartments, efficiency apartments, villas, or cluster homes. A variety of services are provided such as community dining, recreation, social events, housekeeping, transportation, and health-related services (testing and treatment). An entrance fee may be charged along with a monthly fee. The entrance fees may or may not be refundable. The majority of CCRCs are private pay, although some may offer subsidized units.
- *Nursing homes.* Facilities that provide nursing or convalescent care for a specified number of persons unrelated to the licensee. Nursing homes provide long-term care of chronic conditions or short-term convalescent or rehabilitative care for which medical and nursing types of care are indicated. Most residents of nursing homes need long-term care; however, some are admitted for shorter stays following hospitalization for convalescent or rehabilitative care. Nursing homes must be state licensed, and Medicaid pays for certain health care services and nursing home care for older persons in most states. Eligibility, however, is based on income and personal resources.

- *Long-term care ventilator units.* These facilities provide long-term ventilatory care for patients who are not able to be weaned from ventilatory support and who do not have family or caregivers that are able to provide this level of care in the home setting. Specialized units throughout the United States provide care for pediatric, adult, and elderly patients in need of long-term, high-technology respiratory care.

RESPIRATORY CARE PERSONNEL

Respiratory therapists (RTs) working in long-term care do so on either a full-time, part-time, or consulting basis. Many facilities involved in LTC rely on outside vendors to provide diagnostic tests and other related services. Unless the facility specializes in long-term ventilatory support, respiratory care equipment usually has limited availability; most use portable oxygen systems and suction units. RTs tend to work independently with minimal supervision but with a heavy emphasis on patient care planning. In terms of documentation, LTC, as with subacute care, requires initial justification, ongoing follow-up, and detailed financial recordkeeping. Long-term care facilities are state licensed and accredited. RTs on staff are often called on to assist with any licensing and accrediting processes as part of the interdisciplinary, professional team that provides care at the facility.

Reimbursement

There are a variety of ways to pay for long-term care. However, the individual must think ahead and plan accordingly. Many people enroll in long-term care insurance policies that help to pay future long-term care expenses such as those for a nursing home. Premiums can be expensive. Private insurance plans are available, but individuals need to consider enrollment earlier on in life. Normally, the younger people are when they first enroll, the lower their premiums will be. Generally, Medicare does not pay for long-term care. Medicare pays only for a medically necessary skilled nursing facility or home health care, and the person must qualify for this type of care. Medicaid, on the other hand, pays for certain health services and nursing home care for elderly people with low incomes and limited assets. Medicaid is a state and federal government program, and, as such, payment varies from state to state.

Summary

With the advent and proliferation of subacute care, we have found that the respiratory therapist definitely has a role. Many specialty units, such as ventilator care units, require the respiratory care practitioner to be able to work independently. RTs can be successful in their facility by setting up a program that fits well with the needs of surrounding area hospitals. These programs need to accept both weaning and long-term ventilator patients.

Many managed care organizations are constantly seeking specialty ventilator units to contract with in an effort to reduce the overall health care costs to their subscribers. Managed care organizations are also looking for facilities that are accredited by the Joint Commission as a sign of excellence. Because the field of subacute care continues to grow, there will continue to be changes in regulation and reimbursement. Finally, with the growing aging population in the United States, there has been an increasing need for long-term care (LTC). Although LTC can be provided to individuals of any age, most recipients of LTC are elderly and are cared for in the home, assisted living residences, specialty units, and nursing homes. The respiratory therapist can provide care in any of these venues and becomes a valuable member of the interdisciplinary team.

Study Questions

REVIEW QUESTIONS

1. What are the three groups of respiratory patients accepted into the subacute setting?
2. What are the three elements of admission for access to the subacute setting?
3. List some of the ventilators that may be used for long-term and weaning ventilator patients.
4. What are the two accrediting agencies in subacute care?
5. What are the two tools that determine the daily rate that a subacute facility may earn from CMS?
6. What is long-term care and where can it be provided?

MULTIPLE-CHOICE QUESTIONS

1. Which of the following is not used by the respiratory therapist in the subacute setting?
   a. initial assessment form
   b. pulse oximeter
   c. transfer agreement
   d. MDS assessment
2. Subacute facilities are regulated by all of the following agencies except which?
   a. state departments of health
   b. TJC
   c. CORF
   d. ACHMS

3. All of the following ventilators can provide portability in the subacute setting except which?
   a. Pulmonetics LTV 1000
   b. Nellcor Puritan-Bennett 7200
   c. Bird TBird
   d. Nellcor Puritan-Bennett Achieva
4. Which of the following is not a member of the interdisciplinary team in the subacute setting?
   a. respiratory therapist
   b. nurse
   c. occupational therapist
   d. medical laboratory technician
5. Subacute care facilities are accredited by:
   a. state departments of health.
   b. sponsoring hospitals.
   c. TJC.
   d. ACHMS.
6. Ventilator weaning modalities in subacute care facilities may include all of the following except which?
   a. pressure support
   b. CPAP
   c. SIMV
   d. volume control
7. MDS stands for which of the following?
   a. medical delivery standard
   b. maximum data set
   c. minimum data set
   d. Medicare deviation standard
8. The MDS is used:
   a. for assessment and care screening.
   b. to establish minimum standards of care.
   c. to establish maximum standards of care.
   d. to determine discharge criteria.
9. A classification system that sets the per diem rate that the facility is paid by Medicare for treating a particular patient is termed:
   a. RUG.
   b. DRG.
   c. PPS.
   d. MDS.
10. Which of the following is a predetermined method of payment based on diagnostic-related groups regardless of the amount of care given?
    a. RUG
    b. DRG
    c. PPS
    d. MDS
11. Which one of the following is not a long-term care facility?
    a. the home
    b. nursing home
    c. assisted living facility
    d. continuing care retirement community
12. Long-term care is generally not paid for by:
    a. Medicaid.
    b. private long-term care insurance policies.
    c. Medicare.
    d. private pay.

CRITICAL-THINKING QUESTIONS

1. How are ventilators in the subacute setting, such as the Nellcor Puritan-Bennett 7200 and the Bird TBird, different from ventilators in the acute care setting?
2. What is the role of the respiratory therapist as an interdisciplinary team member in a subacute program?
3. How does weaning a ventilator patient in the subacute setting differ from weaning in the acute care setting?
4. What methods could respiratory therapists use to "sell" themselves to subacute and long-term care programs that do not employ RTs in their facilities?

References

1. Shriver K. What's new in subacute care? *Modern Healthcare*. January 1995;26:34–38.
2. Buttaro T., et al. *Clinical Management of Patients in Subacute and Longterm Care Settings*. St. Louis: Elsevier; 2006:2.
3. Tokarski C. Riding the express. *Hospitals Health Networks*. July 1995; 69:20–23.
4. Manard B, et al. *Subacute Care: Policy Synthesis and Market Area Analysis*. Fairfax, VA: Lewin-VHI; 1995.
5. Muse & Associates. *A Comparison of Medicare Nursing Home Residents Who Receive Services from a Respiratory Therapist with Those Who Do Not*. Washington, DC: Muse Assoc; 1999.
6. Epstein J. License to steal. *Finan World*. September 1995;164:34–35.
7. Post-hospital extended care services. Social Security Act. Sec.1861. [42 U.S.C. 1395x(h)] http://www.socialsecurity.gov
8. Maher L. Is subacute care worth your money? *Busin Health*. July 1995;13:18–24.
9. http://www.jointcommission.org/AboutUs/Fact_Sheets/joint_commission_facts.htm
10. Pratt, JR. *Long-Term Care, Managing Across the Continuum*. Sudbury, MA: Jones & Bartlett; 2010:112.
11. American Association for Respiratory Care. AARC clinical practice guideline: oxygen therapy in the home or extended care facility. *Respir Care*. August 2007;52(1):1063–1068.
12. American Association for Respiratory Care. AARC clinical practice guideline: nasotracheal suctioning. *Respir Care*. September 2004;49,9:1080–1084.

13. American Association for Respiratory Care. AARC clinical practice guideline: postural drainage therapy. *Respir Care.* December 1991;36: 1418–1426.
14. American Association for Respiratory Care. AARC clinical practice guideline: bland aerosol administration. *Respir Care.* May 2003;48,5:529–533.
15. American Association for Respiratory Care. AARC clinical practice guideline: assessing response to bronchodilator therapy at point of care. *Respir Care.* December 1995;40:1300–1307.
16. American Association for Respiratory Care. AARC clinical practice guideline: directed cough. *Respir Care.* May 1993;38:495–499.
17. American Association for Respiratory Care. AARC clinical practice guideline: selection of a device for delivery of aerosol to the lung parenchyma. *Respir Care.* July 1996;41,7:647–653.
18. American Association for Respiratory Care. AARC clinical practice guideline: bland aerosol administration. *Respir Care.* May 2003;48,5:529–533.
19. American Association for Respiratory Care. AARC clinical practice guideline: incentive spirometry. *Respir Care.* December 1991;36: 1402–1405.
20. American Association for Respiratory Care. AARC clinical practice guideline: intermittent positive pressure breathing. *Respir Care.* May 2003;48, 5:540–546.
21. American Association for Respiratory Care. AARC clinical practice guideline: use of positive airway pressure adjuncts to bronchial hygiene therapy. *Respir Care.* May 1993;38:516–521.
22. American Association for Respiratory Care. AARC clinical practice guideline: endotracheal suctioning of mechanically ventilated adults and children with artificial airways. *Respir Care.* May 1993;38, 5:500–504.
23. American Association for Respiratory Care. AARC clinical practice guideline: humidification during mechanical ventilation. *Respir Care.* August 1992(8);37:887–890.
24. American Association for Respiratory Care. AARC clinical practice guideline: patient-ventilator system checks *Respir Care.* August 1992;37,8:882–886.
25. American Association for Respiratory Care. AARC clinical practice guideline: in-hospital transport of the mechanically ventilated patient. *Respir Care.* June 2002; 47,6:721–723.
26. American Association for Respiratory Care. AARC clinical practice guideline: providing patient and caregiver training. *Respir Care.* July 1996;41,7: 658–663.
27. American Association for Respiratory Care. AARC clinical practice guideline: discharge planning for the respiratory care patient. *Respir Care.* December 1995;40,12:1308–1312.
28. Centers for Medicare and Medicaid Services. U.S. Department of Health and Human Services. Annual cost of long term care survey (conducted by Genworth Financial). 2007.

Suggested Readings

Argondezzi T. Long term care: finding the perfect fit. *Ad Respir Care Pract.* August 1998;11:20–21.

Krachman SL. Initiating weaning: appropriate measures promote successful extubation. *Adv Manag of Respir Care.* June 1999;8:24–25.

Lewis DL. Transfer agreements. *Adv Manag Respir Care.* March 1997;6:35–38.

Taraszewski R. Subacute respiratory care. *Adv Manag Respir Care.* March 1996;5:30–33.

Wiseman L. *MDS, RUGs and PPS Clinical and Financial Strategies.* Wilmington, NC: Professional Education Seminars; 1998.

CHAPTER 35

Respiratory Home Care

Kathleen S. Wyka and David A. Gourley

OBJECTIVES

Upon completion of this chapter, the reader should be able to:

- Identify the major factors leading to the growth of home respiratory care.
- Describe the responsibilities of the key members of the discharge planning team.
- List the Medicare guidelines for reimbursement of oxygen therapy equipment.
- Differentiate the three systems for home oxygen therapy.
- List the diagnoses of patients successfully managed in a home ventilator program.
- List the basic equipment and supplies needed for a home ventilator patient.
- Define a technology-dependent child.
- List the indications for home apnea monitoring.

CHAPTER OUTLINE

(continues)

(continued)

Clinical Respiratory Services

Assessment

Patient Assessment

Environmental Assessment

Patient Education

Disease Management

Care Planning

Reimbursement

Payors

Regulatory Bodies, Accreditation, and Licensure

Accreditation

KEY TERMS

apparent life-threatening event (ALTE)
care planning
Centers for Medicare & Medicaid Services (CMS)
clinical respiratory services
cuirass
exsufflation
Health Care Financing Administration (HCFA)
home medical equipment (HME) companies
noninvasive positive pressure ventilation (NPPV)
oxygen concentrator
oxygen-conserving device (OCD)
pneumocardiogram (PCG)
technology-dependent children

The dynamics of the health care delivery system in the United States over the past two decades has led to an increasing focus and emphasis on home health care services. The specific delivery of home respiratory care and equipment has grown exponentially during this time. Respiratory care is a highly technical field, dealing with complex and sophisticated medical equipment. Home care is no exception. Therefore, most of this chapter focuses on equipment used to provide respiratory care in the home care setting.

There must be a support system to provide this equipment to patients at home and to ensure that patients or caregivers are properly and appropriately educated. Also, because patients are being cared for in an uncontrolled environment and health care professionals are usually not the primary caregivers, some aspects of the home care environment that are not applicable in other care settings are of extreme importance. Lastly, law and regulation significantly make an impact on the provision of home respiratory care services. All of these subjects are covered as they apply to respiratory therapists and their role in the delivery of home care services.

In 1990, the Council on Scientific Affairs defined home health care as "the provision of services and equipment to the patient in the home for the purposes of restoring and maintaining his or her maximum level of comfort, function, and health." This includes medical and health-related services or care provided in the home and implies that any procedure can be delivered, performed, or administered to a patient at home, providing the patient is willing and capable of receiving the care or that adequate family or professional support for the patient exists.[1]

Traditional home health care services are typically provided by home health agencies. The services of these agencies include:

- Professional nursing visits for skilled care,
- Home health aides,
- Homemaker services,
- Physical therapy.

Owing to reimbursement issues, the respiratory therapist is not usually part of these services. Respiratory care equipment and services are usually provided by **home medical equipment (HME) companies**, sometimes referred to as *durable medical equipment (DME) companies*. This structure for the delivery of home respiratory care will apparently continue in the foreseeable future.

History and Evolution

Several factors have had a significant impact on the evolution of home respiratory care and the dramatic increase in today's demand for these services. The respiratory therapist (RT) must know about them in order to understand the current structure, environment, and delivery of home respiratory care. These factors are:

- Advances in technology.
- Health care economics.
- Changing demographics of the critically ill.

AARC Position Statement Home Respiratory Care Services

Home respiratory care is defined as those prescribed respiratory care services provided in a patient's personal residence. Prescribed respiratory care services include, but are not limited to, patient assessment and monitoring, diagnostic and therapeutic modalities and services, disease management, and patient and caregiver education. These services are provided on a physician's written or verbal order and practiced under appropriate law, regulation, and medical direction. A patient's place of residence may include, but is not limited to, single-family homes, mobile homes, multi-family dwellings, assisted living facilities, retirement communities, and skilled nursing facilities. The goal of home respiratory care is to achieve the optimum level of patient function through goal setting, education, the administration of diagnostic and therapeutic modalities and services, disease management, and health promotion.

It is the position of the American Association for Respiratory Care that the respiratory therapist—by virtue of education, training, and competency testing—is the most competent health care professional to provide prescribed home respiratory care. The complexities of the provision of home respiratory care are such that the public is placed at a significant risk of injury when respiratory care services are provided by unqualified persons, either licensed or unlicensed, rather than by persons with appropriate education, training, credentials, and competency. Therefore, the AARC recommends that practitioners who are employed to provide home respiratory care possess the Certified Respiratory Therapist (CRT) or Registered Respiratory Therapist (RRT) credential awarded by the National Board for Respiratory Care, as well as state licensure or certification where applicable. In addition, the AARC supports efforts to improve access to home respiratory care through improvements in public and private insurance coverage, state and federal reimbursement programs, and enhancement of services in provider models.

Source: Reprinted from AARC Times, *May 2001;25:77. Courtesy of AARC, Dallas, Texas, 2000.*

Advances in technology were certainly one of the most important factors in the early development of home respiratory care. Before 1970, most respiratory equipment was pneumatic, rendering it difficult, if not impossible, for home use.[2] The equipment was developed for use by health care professionals and therefore was usually complex. The development of compact, portable equipment that was simple enough to be operated by patients and caregivers of all ages and educational levels increased its availability and acceptance for use in the home.

Health care economics has also played a significant role in the growth of home respiratory care. In 1965, the federal government enacted legislation creating Medicare and Medicaid benefits. The benefits included reimbursement for durable medical equipment, including respiratory equipment, in the home. This created a rapid growth in the number of HME companies nationwide. Within 10 years, HME companies began providing not only respiratory equipment, but also the care and services of the respiratory therapist as an adjunct to equipment use.

In 1983, the **Health Care Financing Administration (HCFA)**, now known as the **Centers for Medicare & Medicaid Services (CMS)**, introduced a prospective payment system for the reimbursement of hospitals called *diagnosis-related groups* (*DRGs*). Under the DRG system, hospitals are reimbursed at a fixed rate for each of 485 specific diagnoses. This system discourages overutilization of services and encourages early discharge from the acute care hospital—"quicker and sicker." This system has directly increased the number of patients requiring continued care after discharge, including many respiratory care modalities. The increase in managed care and capitation in the 1990s has driven the movement to provide health care in the least costly setting. Patients requiring high-tech care and services may initially be discharged to subacute care facilities, then moved into the home environment where these services are routinely provided.

A third factor behind the growth of home respiratory care is the *changing demographics of the chronically ill population*. Increasing the number of patients needing continuing care and services at home are such forces as:

- The increase in chronic pulmonary disease as a result of cigarette smoking and environmental factors.
- The growth of the elderly population with ongoing health care needs.
- The improved survival rates of patients with pulmonary disorders.

These services are necessary to prevent hospitalization and to improve the function and quality of life. With the Baby Boomer generation reaching retirement age, the predictions are for continued significant growth of this population segment and therefore increased demand for home respiratory services.

SELECTING PATIENTS FOR HOME CARE

The success of providing respiratory care in the home depends on appropriate patient selection and a planned and coordinated discharge. This is more accurately viewed as the admission process to the home care provider. The provider sets specific criteria for admission, which include the patient's home care needs, caregiver support, geographical location, reimbursement, and the home environment.

If a patient is currently in a health care facility, a discharge planner or case manager is usually the first member of the home care team to identify the patient as an appropriate candidate for discharge. The choice of home care may be based on patient diagnosis or therapy required. Tables 35-1 and 35-2 include these selection criteria.

To facilitate a successful, coordinated discharge, the appropriate members of the discharge planning team should meet and begin the plan for the patient's discharge. Table 35-3 identifies the key members of the discharge planning team and their responsibilities.

TABLE 35-1 **Selection criteria for home care by patient diagnosis**

Obstructive Pulmonary Disease:
Chronic obstructive pulmonary disease
Pulmonary emphysema
Chronic bronchitis
Bronchial asthma
Bronchiectasis
Acute bronchitis
Bronchiolitis
Restrictive Pulmonary Disease:
Pulmonary fibrosis
Sarcoidosis
Cystic fibrosis
Pneumoconiosis (occupational lung conditions)
Tuberculosis
Pneumonia, including pneumocystis carinii
Lung cancer
Neuromuscular paralysis and related anomalies, including myasthenia gravis, poliomyelitis, and amyotrophic lateral sclerosis (ALS)
Skeletal abnormalities involving the bony thorax, such as kyphoscoliosis
Severe obesity
Cardiovascular Conditions:
Congestive heart failure
Postmyocardial infarction
Atypical Conditions:
Sleep apnea syndrome
Sudden infant death syndrome (SIDS)
Bronchopulmonary dysplasia (BPD)
Migraine headaches
Ulcerative conditions involving the skin

TABLE 35-2 **Selection criteria for home care based on therapy**

Oxygen Therapy:
Oxygen concentrator
Liquid oxygen (LOX)
Compressed gas
Portable oxygen systems
Oxygen conserving device
Transtracheal oxygen therapy
Hyperbaric oxygen (HBO)
Aerosol Therapy and Tracheobronchial Toilet:
Metered-dose inhaler (MDI)
Small volume nebulizer
Continuous aerosol
IPPB
Exsufflator
Suction
Tracheostomy care
Chest physical therapy (CPT)
Sleep Apnea Therapy:
Nasal CPAP
Bilevel therapy
Neonatal or Pediatric Modalities:
Apnea monitoring
Oximetry monitoring
Mechanical Ventilation:
Positive pressure
Invasive
Noninvasive positive pressure
Negative pressure

TABLE 35-3 **Key members of the discharge team and their responsibilities**

Team Member	Responsibilities
Utilization review board member	Documents patient's in-hospital care and recommends discharge when appropriate.
Physician	Initiates discharge and prescribes home care therapy.
Social worker	May include discharge planning or community health department. Usually functions as team coordinator. Organizes and coordinates all prescribed patient home care. Contacts all team members and outside resources and ensures patient can be discharged safely and properly.
Case manager	Acts as gatekeeper while ensuring continuity of patient care. Grants authorization for purchasing costly equipment or services and reviews outpatient or home care procedures.
Registered nurse	Develops home care plan, provides necessary follow-up, and evaluates patient status and response to prescribed home care. Can function as team coordinator.
Respiratory therapist	Recommends respiratory home care based on patient condition and need and may set up home care equipment and therapy as required. Evaluates home care environment and patient response to therapy. Can function as team coordinator.
HME provider	Provides prescribed home care equipment and supplies and possibly respiratory therapists for equipment setup and scheduled follow-up. Handles all emergencies involving equipment.
Clinical psychologist	Evaluates patient's emotional status and provides counseling as necessary.
Physical therapist	Recommends and provides all forms of prescribed physical therapy.
Occupational therapist	Recommends and provides all forms of prescribed occupational therapy.
Dietitian or nutritionist	Evaluates patient's nutritional needs and prepares dietary plan. As necessary, arranges meal delivery.
Family or caregiver	Implements patient home care daily and notifies team members of any changes in patient status or condition.

The discharge plan should include the following elements:

- Therapeutic needs
- Equipment needs
- Caregiver needs
- Reimbursement
- Patient and/or caregiver education and training
- Assessment of home environment
- Establish time frame for discharge

When the discharge plan is completed, the patient is ready for admission to the home care organization. The respiratory therapist and HME provider subsequently must develop the home care plan to address the initial and ongoing problems and needs of the patient. (This process is discussed later in this chapter.)

The American Association for Respiratory Care (AARC) developed a clinical practice guideline (CPG) in 1995 on discharge planning for the respiratory care patient. The CPG outlines the procedure for the development and implementation of a comprehensive plan for the safe discharge of the respiratory care patient from a health care facility and for continuing safe and effective care at an alternate site. The CPG includes the method for discharge planning as well as patient evaluation, site evaluation, personnel, financial resources, and education and training.[3]

Oxygen Therapy

Home oxygen therapy, which began with the delivery of oxygen cylinders in the home, is the most common modality provided by respiratory therapists in the home today. In 1980, the *nocturnal oxygen therapy trial* (*NOTT*) documented the long-term survival of the COPD patient using *long-term oxygen therapy* (*LTOT*).[4] LTOT has also been demonstrated to improve nocturnal oxygen saturation, reduce pulmonary arterial pressure, and lower pulmonary vascular resistance. In 2000 Petty and Bliss revisited the NOTT study and found that patients who were highly ambulatory and on continuous oxygen therapy (COT) had a 50% higher survival rate than low ambulatory patients and a 40% higher survival rate than high ambulatory patients using only nocturnal oxygen.[5]

In 1985, CMS developed criteria for reimbursement of oxygen therapy equipment by Medicare in order to reduce the indiscriminate ordering of oxygen equipment. CMS requires that patients meet specific diagnosis criteria and have a hypoxemia documented by arterial blood gas analysis or pulse oximetry as depicted in Table 35-4. The physician must prescribe the specific oxygen flow rate (F_IO_2), duration of usage, oxygen system, and route of administration. PRN orders are not acceptable.

TABLE 35-4 Medicare guidelines for reimbursement of oxygen therapy equipment in the home

Acceptable Diagnoses:
Severe lung disease, including chronic obstructive pulmonary disease, diffuse interstitial lung disease, cystic fibrosis, bronchiectasis, and widespread pulmonary neoplasm
Hypoxia related symptoms or findings that have an expected improvement with oxygen therapy, including pulmonary hypertension, recurring congestive heart failure, chronic cor pulmonale, erythrocytosis, impairment of the cognitive process, nocturnal restlessness, and morning headaches
Nonqualifying Diagnoses:
Angina pectoris in the absence of hypoxemia
Severe peripheral vascular disease
Terminal illnesses without lung involvement
Acceptable Blood Gas or Oxygen Saturation Values:
Arterial PO_2 at or below 55 mm Hg
S_pO_2 at or below 88%
Provisional Coverage:
Arterial PO_2 between 56 and 59 mm Hg or S_pO_2 at 89% with a secondary diagnosis, including any of the following conditions:
Dependent edema, suggesting congestive heart failure
Cor pulmonale
Erythrocythemia with a hematocrit of 57% or higher
Nonqualifying Conditions:
Arterial PO_2 60 mm Hg or greater
S_pO_2 90% or greater

Three systems are available for delivery of oxygen in the home.

- *Oxygen concentrators* are the most commonly used system.
- *Liquid oxygen* is a frequently used modality and preferred by some physicians and patients. However, due to reimbursement issues, liquid oxygen use has declined somewhat in recent years.
- *Compressed gas cylinders* are used in specific situations (discussed later in this chapter).

Table 35-5 compares the three home oxygen systems, including the advantages, disadvantages, and safety measures to be followed.

In 1992, the AARC developed a CPG for oxygen therapy in the home and revised it in 2007. The CPG is specific to oxygen administration in the home or alternate site health care facility, and outlines indications, precautions, assessment of need, resources, monitoring, and infection control.[6]

OXYGEN CONCENTRATORS

The **oxygen concentrator** is an electrically powered device that physically separates oxygen from the nitrogen in room air. Initially there were two types of oxygen concentrators:

- Membrane oxygenators, also called oxygen enrichers, are no longer used by HME providers.
- Molecular sieves are the most common type of concentrator used.

Membrane oxygenators (oxygen enrichers) use a plastic membrane approximately 1 micron thick. Oxygen and water vapor diffuse easily across the membrane, providing an enriched output of approximately 40% oxygen at flows up to 10 Lpm. To compensate for this lower concentration, flows approximately three times that of a normal oxygen source must be used.

The *molecular sieve* concentrator operates with an air compressor, delivering room air to one of two sieve beds. The sieve beds contain zeolyte pellets made of sodium aluminum silicate. The pellets absorb nitrogen, carbon dioxide, carbon monoxide, and water vapor. Oxygen and a small amount of argon flow through the sieve beds and are stored in an accumulator until delivered to the patient through a flowmeter. The sieve beds alternate between pressurization to produce oxygen and depressurization to purge the waste gases by what is called the *pressure swing cycle*. Figure 35-1 is a schematic of a typical molecular sieve oxygen concentrator.

Oxygen concentrators can produce an oxygen purity level of up to 98% at flows of 1–2 Lpm. The oxygen purity level (F_IO_2) decreases as the liter flow increases. The highest liter flow available from oxygen concentrators today is 10 Lpm. Oxygen concentrators are the most appropriate for low-flow oxygen therapy via nasal cannula or for titration into other systems, such as high-humidity tracheostomy collars, CPAP units, and portable ventilators. Each oxygen concentrator manufacturer has specific purity levels for each liter flow. These data must be available when performing operational verification on the equipment. The frequency of this verification is also specified by the manufacturer and is usually every 90 days.

Most concentrators manufactured today include a built-in oxygen sensor that monitors the oxygen purity level. The concentrator has an audible and visual alarm that will alert the patient or caregiver if the purity level drops below a predetermined level, usually 90%. The

TABLE 35-5 **Comparison of home oxygen systems**

System	Advantages	Disadvantages	Safety Measures
Oxygen concentrator	Low-pressure system. Does not require deliveries. Can be easily moved. Economical.	Requires electrical power. Requires backup cylinder for power failures. Has limited flow rate capabilities. Oxygen purity level decreases at higher flow rates.	Do not place unit on its side.
Liquid oxygen	No need for electric power. Low-pressure system. Large quantities of oxygen in a relatively small container. Can refill portable unit from reservoir.	Evaporates if not routinely used. Can cause burns if mishandled. Requires periodic deliveries.	Do not tip reservoir or place portable on its side. Fill portable unit carefully. Do not keep portable in heat.
Compressed gas	No loss of supply when not in use. No need for electric power.	Is heavy and cumbersome. Requires frequent deliveries. High pressure unit can be hazardous if dropped.	Secure cylinders with base or cart. Do not lubricate regulator with oil. Do not keep near sources of heat or cold.

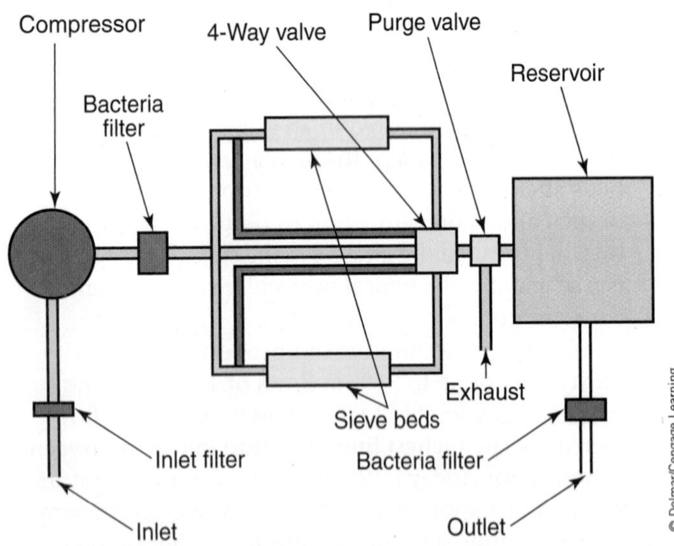

FIGURE 35-1 Schematic of a typical molecular sieve oxygen concentrator.

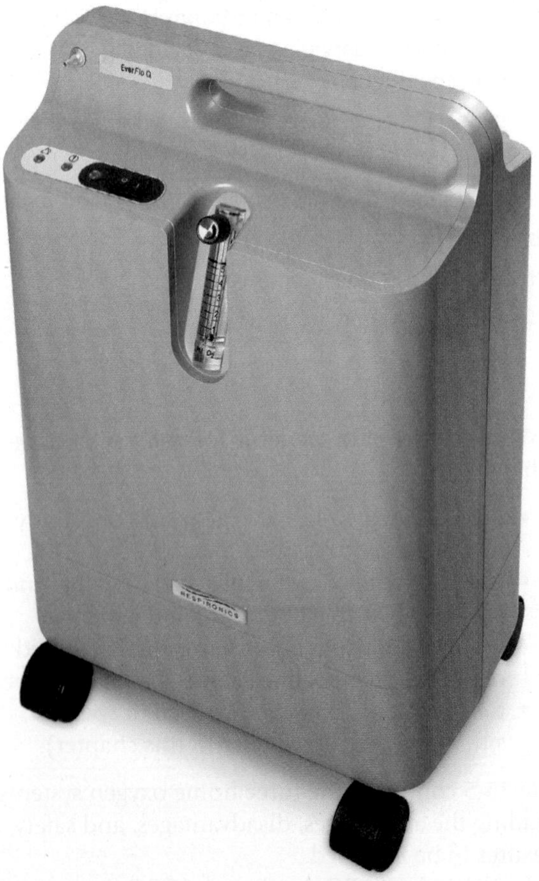

FIGURE 35-2 Everflo Oxygen concentrator.
Courtesy of Philips Respironics, Murrysville, Pennsylvania

alarm eliminates the need for frequent home visits to verify equipment operation and ensures equipment operation between service calls.[2,7] Figure 35-2 is an example of a commonly used oxygen concentrator.

Oxygen concentrators that can transfill portable compressed gas cylinders directly from the concentrator have been developed. These units include a concentrator as the stationary oxygen system for use by patients at home and a mechanism that enables them to fill their portable oxygen cylinder from the stationary system. Patients can control their own portable oxygen supply according to their needs. The units have easy-to-use connections and an automatic shutoff to prevent overpressurization. This system decreases the need for frequent delivery of portable cylinders, and, with the increasing cost of deliveries, it is gaining widespread acceptance.

LIQUID OXYGEN SYSTEMS

The home *liquid oxygen system*, or reservoir, resembles a thermos bottle. A vacuum separates the inner container of the thermos, which holds the liquid oxygen, from the outer container. The vacuum prevents heat transfer and evaporation of the liquid oxygen. In a liquid state, liquid oxygen is at or below −297°F (−147°C). In the reservoir, oxygen is in a gaseous state above the liquid at a pressure of 20–25 pounds per square inch (psi). Figure 35-3 is a schematic of a liquid oxygen system. When the flowmeter is opened, oxygen travels through warming coils, vaporizes into gas, and is delivered to the patient. Because gaseous oxygen occupies approximately 860 times the space of liquid oxygen, the duration of these systems is much greater than compressed gas cylinders. Liquid oxygen systems are capable of delivering up to 8 Lpm.

Numerous liquid oxygen systems are available. Depending on the size of the reservoir, the unit holds 18–40 L (45–100 pounds). The reservoir needs to be periodically refilled by the HME supplier. Liquid oxygen slowly evaporates, even when the unit is not in use, due to ambient heat. Refills are typically performed weekly if the oxygen is being used at 2 Lpm.

A major advantage of liquid oxygen systems is the availability of a portable liquid oxygen unit that can be transfilled directly from the base reservoir by the patient or caregiver. This permits active or ambulatory patients to use the oxygen with relative ease when they are away from home. The transfilling procedure takes approximately 2 minutes to complete. Patients and caregivers must exercise caution when transfilling to avoid burns from the liquid oxygen due to its extremely cold temperature. The portable units weigh 5–15 pounds and can last up to 8 hours at 2 Lpm. With the high efficiency liquid oxygen system (Helios™) that uses conserving technology (see oxygen-conserving devices in this chapter) portables weigh 3.6 pounds and can last up to 7–10 hours depending on the setting and respiratory rate of the user.

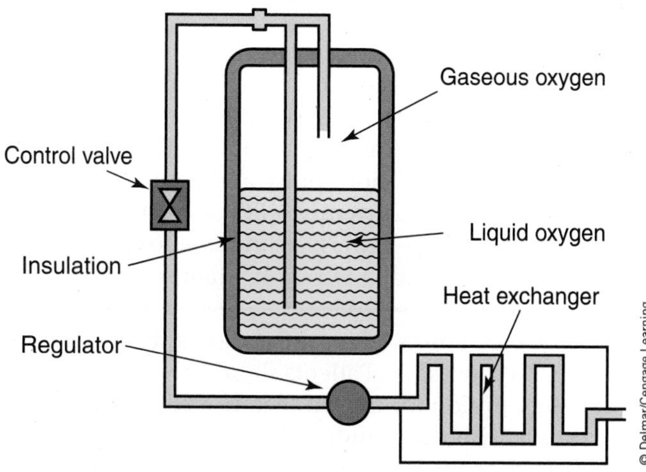

FIGURE 35-3 Schematic of a typical home liquid oxygen (LOX) system.

Innovation. A liquid oxygen system that converts gaseous oxygen from any *oxygen-sensing device (OSD) concentrator* into a supply of liquid oxygen has been developed. The VIAspire Liquefier (Inspired Technologies) allows patients to fill liquid portables in the home. The liquefier runs 4–6 hours per day and liquefies up to 2 L of oxygen per day.[8,9] That is equivalent to 3–4 fills in a day and about 12–16 hours' worth of supply. Two sizes of transfillable portables are available: the VIAspire 300 weighing 4 pounds when full and the 600 weighing 6 pounds.

COMPRESSED GAS CYLINDERS

Compressed gas cylinders, although not preferred for continuous oxygen therapy, play an important role in home oxygen therapy. Due to their relatively low volume, weight, bulkiness, and inherent dangers, compressed gas cylinders are not recommended for the continuous oxygen user. However, they are routinely provided to oxygen concentrator patients as a backup system. The cylinders are used as a safety precaution in the event of a power failure or mechanical breakdown of the concentrator.

Portability is the other major reason compressed gas cylinders are used. Patients who use oxygen concentrators as their stationary source of oxygen frequently need a portable system for ambulation and activities outside the home. D or E cylinders are commonly provided to patients for this purpose. The increased use of oxygen-conserving devices, which provide a demand flow to the patient, has increased the use of much smaller cylinders.

OXYGEN-CONSERVING DEVICES

Portability and duration have been concerns of both patients and HME providers. The availability of several **oxygen-conserving devices (OCDs)**, which provide oxygen to the patient only during the inspiratory

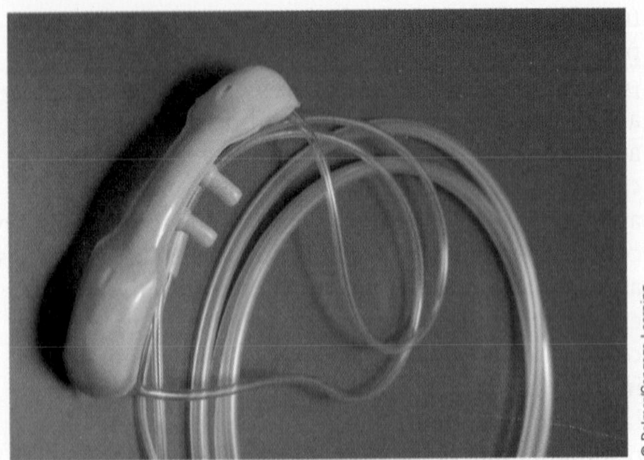

FIGURE 35-4 Mustache or reservoir cannula.

phase, significantly increases the duration of portable oxygen systems.

- The original and least expensive OCD is the *reservoir*, or *mustache*, *cannula* (Figure 35-4). The reservoir cannula functions by storing a small volume of oxygen in the reservoir during exhalation. This oxygen is added to the next inspiration, thereby increasing the volume of oxygen delivered and decreasing the oxygen flow required to achieve the desired F_IO_2. Oxygen flow rates can be reduced to one-third to two-fifths of the flow required for a standard nasal cannula.[2]
- The *pendant cannula* is similar to the reservoir cannula, except that the reservoir pendant hangs below the neck and can be covered with clothing (Figure 34-5). This feature makes the pendant cannula more aesthetically pleasing and more accepted by patients, which leads to greater patient compliance.

Intermittent Flow OCDs are the most commonly used conserving devices. There are three types: demand, pulse, and hybrid.[10]

- *Demand flow* delivers the oxygen, usually at flows of 2–4 Lpm, for most of the inspiratory phase including the dead space volume. No oxygen is delivered during the expiratory phase.
- *Pulse dose* delivers oxygen in the first part of inspiration (0.2–0.4 sec.) at flows that may reach 8–12 Lpm. No oxygen ends up in the dead space.
- *Hybrid* is a combination of the demand and pulse dose delivery systems. Oxygen is delivered at high flow during the first part of inspiration and continues at a lower flow during the remainder of the inspiratory phase.[10]

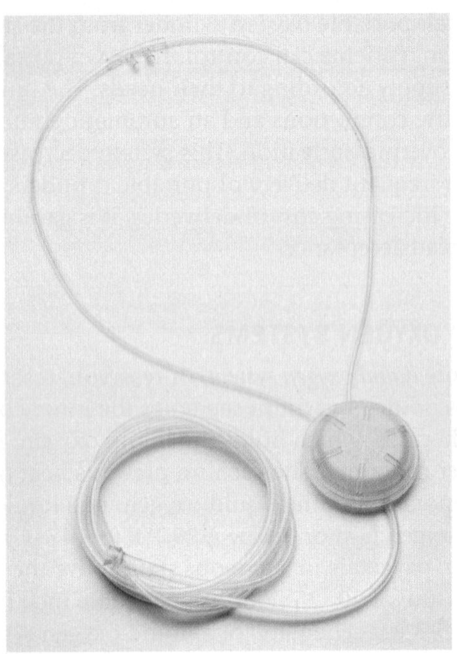

FIGURE 35-5 Pendant oxygen cannula.
Courtesy of Chad Therapeutics

Table 35-6 shows the different models and respective features of some OCDs.

OCDs can be either pneumatically driven or battery operated.[10] Regardless, they sense inspiration and open a valve in the regulator to deliver oxygen; they are either pressure or time cycled. Some devices require the use of a dual lumen nasal cannula. One side of the cannula senses inspiration, and the other side delivers the oxygen. If the nare is blocked on the sensing side, it may not sense inspiration and fail to trigger the delivery of oxygen. Most conservers use traditional single-lumen cannulas.

Innovation. *Portable oxygen concentrators* (*POCs*) are now commonly used, and all employ a pulse dose delivery system. Pulse dose settings range from 1 through 6 depending on the model. The Sequal Eclipse™ can deliver both pulse and continuous flow up to 3 Lpm. Currently 6 POCs are available. All use lithium ion battery technology for portability and come with a D/C volt adapter for use in a car.

POCs are approved for use aboard aircraft, making airline travel possible. Patients should always carry their prescription for oxygen therapy with them and check with their mode of transport—airplane, train, ship, or bus—prior to travel for any specific requirements.

TABLE 35-6 **Comparison of oxygen conserving devices**

Model	Manufacturer	Weight	Hours of Supply	Comments
HomeFill II O_2 concentrator system+	Invacare	ML4: 3.6 pounds ML6: 4.3 pounds ML9: 6.0 pounds	ML4: 4.5 hours at 20 BPM and 2 setting ML6: 5.2 hours at 20 BPM and 2 setting ML9: 7.9 hours at 20 BPM and 2 setting	Also has a continuous flow option at 2 LPM M2 cylinder is now available weighing 2 pounds and can provide 2 hours of O_2 at 20 BPM and 2 setting
HELios*	Puritan Bennett	3.6 pounds 5.5 pounds (Marathon)	8–10 hours/20 hours at 20 BPM and 2 setting	High efficiency LOX system
Pulse-Dose system+	Sunrise Medical	6 pounds with M6 tank	4–6 hours depending on setting and RR	Requires battery for operation
Oxymatic OM-400+	Chad Therapeutics	6 pounds with M6 tank	4–6 hours depending on setting and RR	Requires battery for operation
Easy Pulse 5+	Precision Medical	6 pounds with M6 tank	4–6 hours depending on setting and RR	No battery needed
CR-50 regulator*	Puritan Bennett	6 pounds with M6 tank	4–6 hours depending on setting and RR	No battery needed
O_2 XPRESS regulator*	Salter Labs	6 pounds with M6 tank	4–6 hours depending on setting and RR	No battery needed
SAGE O_2 therapeutic device+	Chad Therapeutics	7 pounds with M6 tank	5–7 hours depending on setting and RR	SMART sensor technology conserves O_2

Key: + pulse dose
* demand flow

CASE STUDY 35-1

R. T. is a 68-year-old male. He has lived in rural Kentucky his entire life. He has worked as a coal miner since he was 22 years old. He smoked 1.5–2 packs of cigarettes per day since he was 15. He quit smoking 2 years ago when the doctor diagnosed his chronic pulmonary disease. He lives with his wife, who is his primary caregiver.

Mr. T. was admitted to the local community hospital 6 months ago with exacerbation of COPD and pneumonia. His ABG on the day before discharge, performed on room air, was pH, 7.34; PCO_2,68; PO_2, 49; HCO_3, 33; and SO_2, 81.5%. The hospital respiratory therapist reported this to the physician, and the physician ordered nasal O_2 at 1.5 Lpm continuously via an oxygen concentrator.

The equipment was set up by the respiratory therapist from the local HME company. Mr. and Mrs. T. were educated in the use and maintenance of the equipment. The respiratory therapist has made a routine visit to Mr. T. every 3 months to perform equipment maintenance procedures. Mr. T. has been compliant with his oxygen usage, and he uses an E cylinder for portability when leaving his home.

Questions

1. Mr. T. complained to his respiratory therapist that it is difficult to carry his portable E cylinder when away from home. What alternatives can the respiratory therapist recommend to the physician and still maintain Mr. T.'s time away from home?
2. What document must the physician complete for Medicare to reimburse for the home oxygen equipment?
3. Which oxygen system is an appropriate alternative to Mr. Turner's oxygen concentrator?

Basic Respiratory Equipment

The respiratory therapist in home care is responsible for providing the common respiratory modalities found in a hospital. All types of aerosol therapy are required in the home setting. In addition, a variety of devices for airway clearance and maintenance are commonly found in home care. The basic respiratory equipment is now described in further detail.

AEROSOL THERAPY

Historically, aerosol therapy has always been a major part of the respiratory therapist's responsibilities. The increase in COPD, asthma, and other pulmonary disorders has created an ongoing need for aerosol therapy in the home. Several different pieces of equipment are currently available to meet the individual needs of the patients.

Metered-Dose Inhalers. Although not usually provided by the respiratory therapist, *metered-dose inhalers* (*MDIs*) are a common mode of administration of respiratory medications in the home care setting. MDIs are small canisters of medication using haloflouroalka (HFA) as a propellant; they are used to deliver bronchodilators, anticholinergics, and steroids. The patient depresses the canister in an actuator, which releases a specific dose of medication and propellant. A significant portion of medication is deposited in the upper airway and gastrointestinal tract. Patient inhalation technique is the most important factor influencing medication deposition. Inhalation accessory devices, such as spacers and holding chambers, are recommended for use with MDIs to increase the deposition of medication in the lower airway and to eliminate the need for accurate patient coordination while activating the MDI and initiating inspiration. When activated, the medication from the MDI is discharged into the spacer or chamber, which serves as a reservoir until the patient inhales the medication from the device. However, larger particles of medication may be removed from suspension in the spacer by gravity and inertia, thereby decreasing the amount of medication that is deposited in the upper airway.[11]

Dry Powder Inhalers. *Dry powder inhalers* (*DPIs*) are actuated by the patient's inspiratory effort. A small capsule of powdered medication is inserted into the device. The DPI container breaks the capsule so that, when patients put it in their mouths and begin to inhale, they receive the medication. Patients must be able to generate enough inspiratory flow to get delivery of the medication. Spacers are not necessary or available for use with DPIs.

MDIs and DPIs are easy to operate and compact. Ehen MDIs are used with a spacer; they have an efficacy comparable to handheld nebulizers. All of these features have led to widespread acceptance of MDIs and DPIs as the primary method for administration of aerosolized medications in the home care setting.

Small Volume Nebulizers. Delivery of aerosolized medication is also achieved with the use of a handheld, or *small volume nebulizer* (*SVN*). The SVN is usually operated with an electrically powered air compressor. These units are available through many manufacturers. The compressors are easy to operate and extremely dependable, and they require minimal ongoing maintenance. The SVN should be cleaned according to the manufacturer's specifications and replaced as needed.

Battery-operated compressors are also available if portability is desired or necessary. These units have an internal battery that must be periodically recharged from a standard 110 VAC outlet. They may also have accommodations for use with a 12-V automobile battery using an automobile's electrical outlet. Most insurances pay for the SVN but do not cover the cost of the battery, which can be costly.

The need and desire for portability have encouraged the development of ultrasonic nebulizers for delivery of aerosolized bronchodilators and other medications. These units are battery operated, lightweight, and operate quietly, unlike the air compressor units. Cost and ongoing maintenance have prevented widespread acceptance of the units.

Continuous Aerosol Therapy. The delivery of a continuous or intermittent bland aerosol is occasionally required in the home care setting, frequently for patients with tracheostomies. The air compressor used for this function is a diaphragm compressor. These units operate by drawing air into a cylinder through an intake valve. Within the cylinder, a rod moves the diaphragm upward and downward. Air then exits the cylinder through an exhaust valve. The compressor must be capable of achieving a maximum pressure of 50 psi. A large-volume nebulizer is attached to the compressor for aerosol delivery. The air compressor usually has a pressure adjustment valve to control flow to the nebulizer, or a flowmeter may be attached to the compressor for this purpose.

INTERMITTENT POSITIVE PRESSURE BREATHING

The use of *intermittent positive pressure breathing* (*IPPB*) in home care continues on a very limited basis nationwide. The electrically powered Bennett AP-5 is the most common device for delivering IPPB. Although it is used for the delivery of aerosolized medication, it is usually used to assist patients with ventilatory insufficiency. The respiratory therapist must set an appropriate inspiratory pressure to ensure delivery of an adequate tidal volume. The prevalence of bilevel therapy and other noninvasive ventilatory assist devices makes these the preferred mode of therapy instead of IPPB.

SUCTION UNITS

Airway maintenance and clearance are essential parts of the management of many home care patients. Basic suction equipment is available to meet these needs. Commonly, patients with tracheostomies or disorders preventing adequate airway clearance, such as patients with cerebrovascular accident (CVA), neuromuscular disease, or terminal cancer, require this equipment. Electrically powered units are the most commonly provided. These units operate from any standard 110 VAC outlet and require minimal maintenance, except for frequent emptying of the suction canister to prevent inadvertent aspiration of secretions into the suction pump. This usually disables the suction unit. Portable units are also available. They usually operate on AC current, on DC current from a automobile outlet adapter, or with a rechargeable internal battery. These units are used for portability and as backup equipment in case of electrical outages. Both of these units are relatively basic to operate.

The AARC developed a CPG on suctioning of the patient in the home. The CPG includes nasal, oral, and endotracheal suctioning techniques and protocols.[12]

PERCUSSORS

Mechanical devices have become an important adjunct to postural drainage and chest physical therapy, owing to the tiring effect on the respiratory therapist from performing manual percussion and vibration. Mechanical percussors can provide consistent rates, rhythms, and vibration. Mechanical percussors are available in electrically powered and pneumatically powered models. The electrically powered units are the preferred models for home use.[11]

The Flimm Fighter is an electrically powered unit designed for home use. The unit enables the patient to self-administer therapy by applying the percussor with a Velcro pad and strap. The only control on the unit is the power switch. Figure 35-6 shows the Flimm Fighter.[11] Several other percussors are available but cannot be self-administered.

DEVICES FOR COUGH ASSISTANCE

Patients who experience difficulty in producing an adequate cough may benefit from one of several cough assistance devices available in lieu of tracheal suctioning. For this purpose, mechanical exsufflation, positive expiratory pressure (PEP) therapy, and high-frequency chest wall oscillation (HFCWO) are available to the home care patient.

Mechanical **exsufflation** was first widely used in the 1950s in all care settings, but its use diminished with the increased use of tracheostomies and suctioning. Because of renewed interest in this procedure in the 1990s, its usage has increased, especially in conjunction with **noninvasive positive pressure ventilation (NPPV)**. The insufflator/exsufflator provides the patient with a mechanical inspiration through a facemask, mouthpiece, or tracheostomy tube. It may also be performed via tracheostomy. The inspiration is followed by a negative pressure, forcing exhalation. This creates a mechanical cough and is very successful for secretion removal. Figure 35-7 illustrates a mechanical insufflator/exsufflator.

Positive expiratory pressures (*PEP*) devices were developed in the 1970s and are effective in the

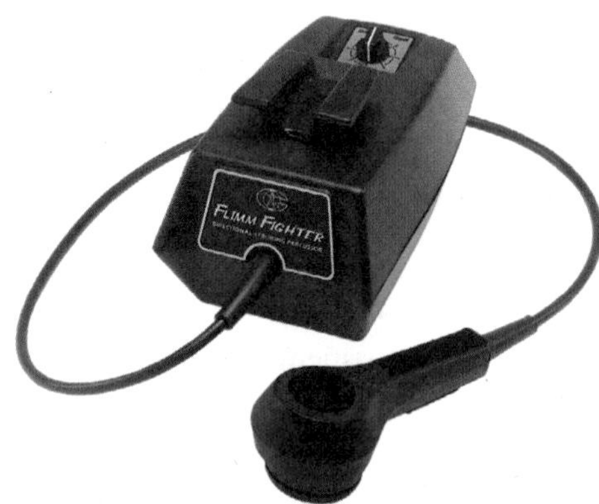

FIGURE 35-6 Flimm-Fighter percussor.
Courtesy of General Physiotherapy, Inc.

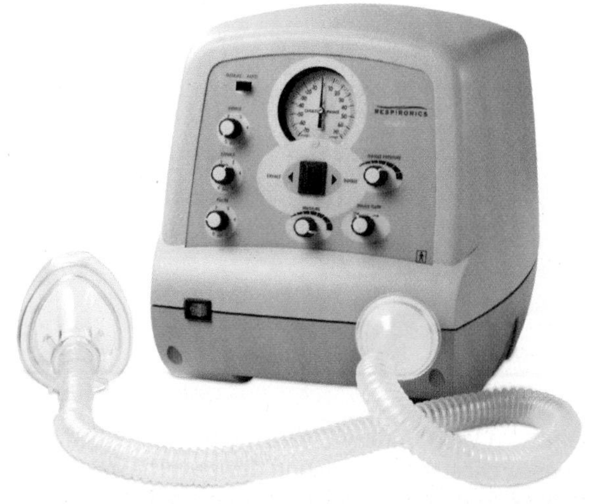

FIGURE 35-7 CoughAssist®, a mechanical insufflation/exsufflation device.
Courtesy of Philips Respironics

mobilization of retained secretions. When using this technique, the patient exhales through a flow resistor, which maintains a positive pressure of 10–20 cm H_2O. The patient repeats this up to 8 times in a 10–20-minute session. The positive pressure reduces airway collapse and air trapping. The patient performs forced or so-called huff coughing after the session, resulting in greater secretion expectoration.

Another option for patients having difficulty mobilizing secretions is *high-frequency chest wall oscillation* (*HFCWO*). This therapy can be self-administered and eliminates the need for chest physical therapy (CPT). High-frequency compression pulses are applied to the chest wall via an air-pulse generator and inflatable vest or chest wrap. The pulses generate temporary increases in airflow at low lung volumes, repetitive coughlike shear forces, and decreased viscosity of secretions. The resulting mobilization of secretions is significantly improved compared to CPT. The HFCWO is pictured in Figure 35-8. (For more information, refer to Chapter 23.)

Intrapulmonary percussive ventilation (*IPV*) is another high-frequency device used for airway clearance. It can be administered simultaneously with an aerosol breathing treatment and delivers high flow rate bursts of gas into the lungs at 100–300 cycles per minute.[13,14] It is especially useful in the home care setting.

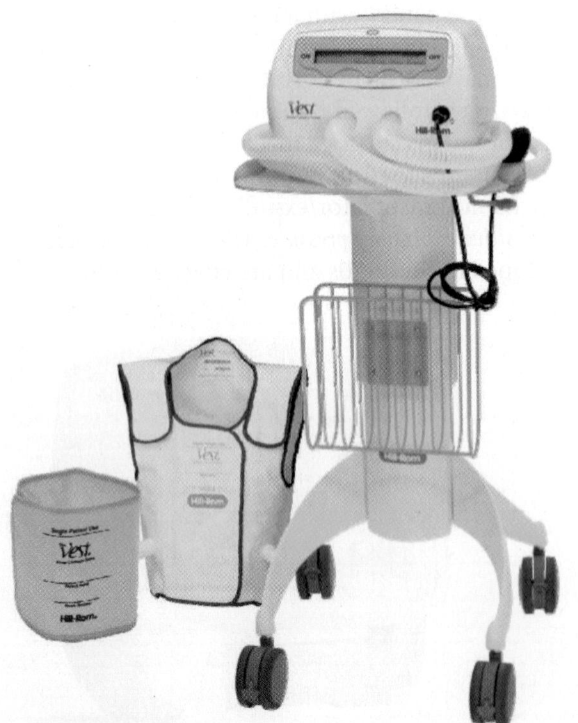

FIGURE 35-8 Vest® Airway Clearance System, a high-frequency chest wall oscillation device. (The Vest® Airway Clearance System is a registered trademark of Hill-Rom Services, Inc.)

Sleep Apnea Therapy

The prevalence of *obstructive sleep apnea* (OSA), increased public awareness, and availability of polysomnography have created a rapid growth in sleep apnea therapy. It is currently estimated that up to 20% of the population may suffer from OSA. In the early 1980s, continuous positive airway pressure (CPAP) was developed as a viable alternative to tracheostomy or uvulo-palato-pharyngoplasty (UPPP) in the treatment of OSA. CPAP was pioneered by Dr. Mark Sanders, and Respironics introduced the first home CPAP unit. See Chapter 18 for further information regarding sleep disorders.

NASAL CONTINUOUS POSITIVE AIRWAY PRESSURE

Nasal CPAP is the primary therapy for OSA. Numerous manufacturers produce nasal CPAP units. The operation of these units is essentially the same.

- The basic unit is a flow generator that is set to a prescribed pressure, usually between 4 and as high as 25 cm H_2O depending on the unit, and that is verified with an external manometer.
- The unit is connected to the patient with smooth, wide-bore tubing and a nasal interface held in place by Velcro straps. The interface can be a nasal mask, nasal prongs, a full-face mask, or a hybrid version, which is a combination nasal prong–mouth seal. If there are excessive air leaks intermittently through the patient's mouth, a chinstrap may be employed.
- The nasal interface includes small openings that allow for exhalation and that prevent rebreathing of carbon dioxide.
- The units usually include a ramp feature, or timer, which gradually increases pressure to the prescribed level over a preset period. This time frame usually does not exceed 45 minutes.
- Many units now employ a setting for expiratory pressure relief (EPR) that enables the patient to start the exhalation phase more comfortably.

These features enhance patient acceptance and tolerance.

Long-term compliance with CPAP is an ongoing problem. Statistics show that the national average for noncompliance is about 50%. The most common causes of noncompliance include acclimating to the interface and/or pressure, feelings of claustrophobia, aesthetic concerns, nasal drying, and improper follow-up by the home care company or treating physician. During the initial setup, proper fitting using a template is essential to prevent complications and to increase patient compliance. Nasal drying may be corrected with the use of a passover humidifier or a heated humidifier. Desensitization techniques may be used to acclimate to the interface and pressure. A program by the HME company for continued follow-up has also been shown to improve compliance with therapy; most insurance companies, as well as Medicare, now require documentation of compliance for reimbursement. Most units now have the capability to record and download or transmit data to substantiate compliance.

BILEVEL THERAPY

Bilevel therapy was introduced for use in patients using high levels of CPAP or for those unable to tolerate CPAP. The bilevel units incorporate an inspiratory positive airway pressure (IPAP) and an expiratory positive airway pressure (EPAP). The EPAP is set lower than the IPAP, allowing the patient to exhale more easily. Bilevel units have enhanced patient acceptance and tolerance.

Bilevel units are available with a timed respiratory rate setting function as *respiratory assist devices* (*RADs*), similar to pressure-limited ventilators. However, the FDA has not approved these units to be used for life support or for patients with tracheostomies. Their use has expanded beyond the original home care role for OSA and now includes acute care and subacute care for a variety of diagnoses. A bilevel unit is illustrated in Figure 35-9.

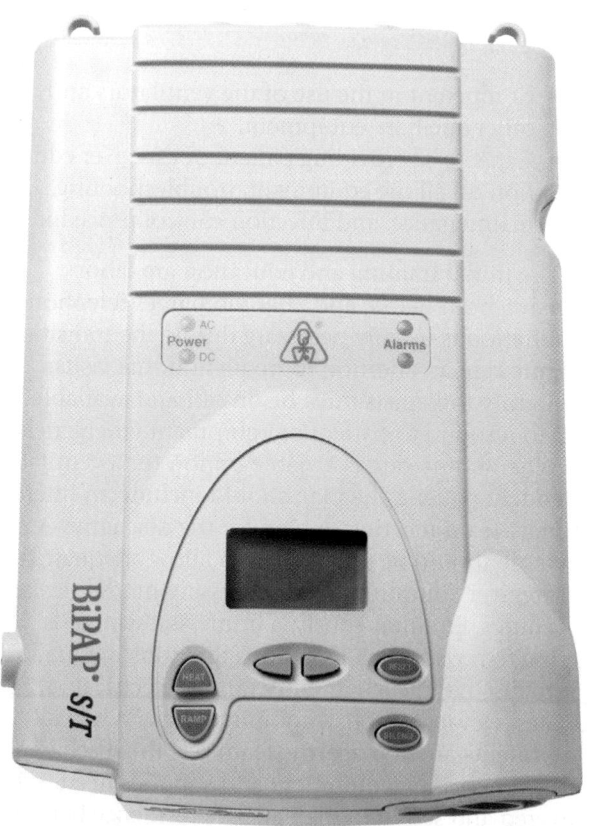

FIGURE 35-9 The BiPap® ST ventilatory support system, shown with an integrated humidifier.

Courtesy of Philips Respironics, Inc.

Home Polysomnography

Home sleep studies have been provided as initial screening studies, in diagnostic testing, and for patient follow-up. They are less expensive than a laboratory-based polysomnogram but are controversial among sleep professionals. Home studies are recommended for patients unable to get to a sleep facility such as for diagnoses of morbid obesity and paralysis.

The study consists of the monitoring of numerous parameters: heart rate, respiratory rate, oximetry, nasal airflow, snoring, and chest and abdominal impedance. If the study is unattended, the clinician instructs the patient or family member on the application of these devices. The clinician returns the following morning to pick up the equipment and the test recording. The recording is downloaded by the HME company or sleep lab and then reviewed and interpreted by the sleep physician or health care provider.

In 2008, CMS approved home studies using type II, III, and IV devices; however, in the same year they proposed and opened for comment in the federal register a regulation prohibiting home care companies from doing both the sleep study and then the setup and implementation of the therapeutic device (CPAP/Bilevel). As mentioned, testing is still controversial, and individuals considering this service should perform adequate research before purchasing the expensive systems needed to perform home polysomnography as the reimbursement mechanism is changing and remains questionable.

Home Mechanical Ventilation

Home mechanical ventilation offers the respiratory therapist the greatest challenges and opportunities in the home care setting. The decision to discharge ventilator-dependent patients to the home setting began in the 1950s as a result of the polio epidemic. Due to the lack of hospital space and qualified personnel, patients were discharged to home and to long-term care facilities in iron lungs. Eventually, compact positive pressure ventilators were developed for home use. During the 1970s and 1980s, portable ventilators were refined, and placement of ventilator-dependent patients into the home care setting became relatively common.

COMPONENTS OF A SUCCESSFUL PROGRAM

The success of a home ventilator program begins with admission criteria to ensure appropriate patient selection. The basic elements to begin the discharge planning of a ventilator-dependent patient are that:

- The patient is clinically stable.
- An adequate number of competent caregivers are available.

CASE STUDY 35-2

A. D. is a 46-year-old male. He is moderately obese. His wife complained for years about his snoring, but he ignored her complaints until he fell asleep while driving home from work one day and hit a parked car. Luckily, Mr. D. was not injured. He saw his primary care physician, who referred him for a polysomnogram.

Mr. D. had his sleep study performed at a hospital-based sleep lab and it was determined that he had obstructive sleep apnea. The physician recommended nasal CPAP at 12 cm H_2O pressure and contacted an HME company that is a preferred provider for Mr. D.'s HMO.

The respiratory therapist from the HME company visited Mr. D. at his home and set up the CPAP unit at 12 cm H_2O pressure with the nasal mask that the sleep lab had indicated. Mr. D. was instructed on the use and maintenance of the CPAP unit and accessories.

Questions

1. After the first night of CPAP usage, Mr. D. complained of air blowing into his eye and of eye irritation. What are two probable causes, and how can the respiratory therapist rectify the problem?
2. Three weeks after initiation of CPAP, Mr. D. called the respiratory therapist and complained of his nose feeling very dry and of several nosebleeds since starting CPAP usage. What can the respiratory therapist recommend to correct this situation?
3. One year after Mr. D. was set up on CPAP, the respiratory therapist was notified that he stopped using the CPAP unit 3 months earlier. He stated that he felt short of breath when he stared using the CPAP and had difficulty exhaling. What are two possible solutions to this problem?

- Reimbursement for services is adequate.
- The home environment is safe and appropriate.

The patient must be free of any cardiopulmonary dysfunction, multisystem failure, or acute infections. Table 35-7 outlines the diagnoses that are most successfully managed in a home ventilator program.

TABLE 35-7 **Diagnoses which are successfully managed in a home ventilator program**

I. Ventilatory Neuromuscular Dysfunction:
Amyotrophic lateral sclerosis (ALS)
Muscular dystrophy (MD)
Multiple sclerosis (MS)
Poliomyelitis
Diaphragmatic paralysis
Guillain-Barré syndrome
Spinal cord injury
Spinal Muscular Atrophy (SMA)
II. Central Hypoventilation Syndromes:
III. Restrictive Lung Disease:
Kyphoscoliosis
Diffuse pulmonary fibrosis
IV. Obstructive Lung Disease:
Chronic obstructive pulmonary disease (COPD)
Bronchopulmonary dysplasia (BPD)

The HME supplier must have an adequate number of appropriately trained respiratory therapists for the program to succeed and grow. Respiratory therapists must be:

- Competent in the use of the ventilators and other ancillary equipment.
- Capable of providing patient or caregiver education on all the equipment, troubleshooting, maintenance, and infection control procedures.

The initial training and education are labor intensive, both before and after discharge. Telephone consultation is usually necessary during the transition to home care, in addition to frequent home visits. Respiratory therapists must be on call and available 24/7 to respond to patient or equipment emergencies.

When home care is a viable option for a ventilator-dependent patient, the plan should include an interdisciplinary team meeting to plan for the discharge. A timetable should be established to allow adequate time for caregiver education on all necessary modalities and procedures. Simultaneously, a home assessment is needed to reveal any adaptations that must be made before discharge, such as entry ramps, electrical updates, elevators, or bathroom redesign. When all components are in place, the team sets the discharge date. All necessary equipment and supplies need to be delivered and set up in the patient's residence before discharge.

In addition to the ventilator, other home medical equipment and supplies are required for the ongoing care of the ventilator patient. Table 35-8 lists the common equipment and supply needs for the patient.

Just prior to discharge, the HME supplier should notify the local telephone company, utilities company, and the police, fire, and emergency medical services (EMS).These agencies are then able to place the patient on a priority list for service. Written backup plans for typical scenarios should be developed and kept in a prominent place for patient and caregiver reference.

CURRENT EQUIPMENT

The home ventilator patient needs a variety of equipment. The few most common discussed in this section are by no means an exhaustive list that the home respiratory therapist might encounter.

TABLE 35-8 Basic equipment and supply needs of the home ventilator patient

Ventilator	*Oxygen Source*
Primary ventilator	Concentrator or liquid system
Secondary ventilator	Portable cylinder
Ventilator circuit	Backup cylinder
Ventilator filters	*Suction Equipment:*
External 12-V battery, cable, and charger	Electrically powered unit
Humidifier or heat moisture exchangers	Battery-powered unit
Manual resuscitator	Spare suction canisters
Tracheostomy Supplies:	Suction connecting tubing
Spare tracheostomy tubes	Suction catheters
One spare tube, one size smaller	Gloves
Tracheostomy dressings	*Aerosol Therapy:*
Trach care kits	Compressor or nebulizer
Disposable inner cannulas	Compressor, 50 psi
Water soluble lubricant	Large-volume nebulizer
Syringe (10 mL)	Tracheostomy masks
Tracheostomy ties	Wide-bore tubing
Sterile gloves	*Miscellaneous:*
Speaking valve	Hospital bed
Solutions:	Overbed table
Sterile water (1000 mL)	Air mattress
Sodium chloride (1000 mL)	Trapeze bar
Unit dose saline	Bedside commode
Hydrogen peroxide	Walker
	Wheelchair
	Pulse oximeter

Positive Pressure Ventilation. Portable ventilator equipment is manufactured by several companies to meet the variety of needs of the ventilator-dependent patient. The most common type of ventilator for home use is the positive pressure ventilator. Currently, the following positive pressure ventilators are available for home use:

- Nellcor Puritan-Bennett (Achieva)
- Respironics/Lifecare (PLV-100 series and Continuum)
- Newport Medical (HT 50)
- Bird (TBird Legacy)
- Pulmonetics (LTV Series)
- Versamed (iVent 201 HC)

All of the positive pressure ventilators are electrically powered by standard AC current. They also have the capability of being operated on a 12-V deep-cycle external battery, which may power the ventilator for up to 24 hours. They also may be operated by an internal battery, which may provide 1–10 hours of operation depending on the make and model. Table 35-9 compares the features of positive pressure ventilators.

The positive pressure ventilator is most commonly used with a tracheostomy; however, the use of NPPV is increasing. Numerous nasal interfaces and mouthpieces are commercially available to provide NPPV. The advantages of NPPV are:

- Decreased infection rates.
- Improved quality of life.
- Normal coughing.
- The ability to communicate normally.

The disadvantages are:

- Difficulty achieving an airtight seal.
- Skin irritation
- Gastric distension.[1]

NPPV has been successfully employed in the COPD population, but, because of its increase in use, Medicare implemented stringent guidelines. Currently, for COPD patients to qualify for NPPV, certain requirements must be met:

- Obstructive sleep apnea with CPAP treatment has been ruled out.
- Either an arterial P_aCO_2 from a blood gas is equal to or greater than 52 mm Hg done while the patient was awake and breathing their usual F_IO_2.
- Or an oxygen saturation is equal to or less than 88% during sleep for at least 5 continuous minutes while breathing their usual F_IO_2 or 2 Lpm, whichever is higher.

TABLE 35-9 **Comparison of the features of current positive pressure ventilators**

Feature	iVent	PLV-102	HT-50	Legacy	Pulmonetics	Achieva
Control	No	Yes	No	Yes	Yes	No
Assist/Control	Yes	Yes	Yes	Yes	Yes	Yes
SIMV	Yes	Yes	Yes	Yes	Yes	Yes
CPAP	Yes	No	Yes	Yes	Yes	No
Pressure cycled	Yes	No	Yes	No	Yes	Yes
Pressure support	Yes	No	Yes	Yes	Yes	Yes
Breath rate	1–80	2–40	1–99	2–80	1–80	1–80
Tidal volume	50–2000	50–3000	100–2200	50–2000	50–2000	50–2200
Peak flow	1–180	10–120	6–100	10–140	—	—
Inspiratory	0.3–3.0 seconds	—	0.1–3.0 seconds	—	0.3–9.9 seconds	0.2–5 seconds
Sensitivity	−0.5 to −20 cm/ 1–20 Lpm	−6 to +18 cm	−9.9 to 0 cm H_2O	1–8 Lpm	1–9 Lpm	−1 to −15 cm
PEEP/CPAP	Yes	No	0–30	0–30	0–20	0–30
Sigh	Yes	Yes	Yes	Yes	No	No
High-pressure	Yes	5–95	4–99	5–120	5–100	2–80 limit
Low-pressure	Yes	2–50	3–98	2–60	1–60	1–59 limit
Alarm silence	Yes	Yes	Yes	Yes	Yes	Yes
Weight	22 pounds	29.9 pounds	15 pounds	43 pounds	12.6 pounds	32 pounds
50 psi O_2 inlet	Yes	Yes	No	Yes	Yes	Yes
O_2 reservoir	Yes	No	Yes	No	No	No

All criteria must be present before NPPV can be initiated.

The use of NPPV in other patient populations, such as postpolio and muscular dystrophy, has been the standard of practice for several decades. Medicare has also implemented criteria for these and any restrictive thoracic disorders:

- Documentation of the progressive neuromuscular disease or severe thoracic cage abnormality.
- COPD does not contribute to the patient's pulmonary limitation.
- Patients must exhibit either an arterial P_aCO_2 equal to or greater than 45 mmHg done while awake and breathing their usual F_IO_2 or an oxygen saturation equal to or less than 88% during sleep for at least 5 continuous minutes while breathing their usual F_IO_2.
- For diagnoses of progressive neuromuscular diseases, they must demonstrate either a maximal inspiratory pressure less than −60 cmH_2O or a forced vital capacity (FVC) less than 50% of predicted value. Refer to Table 35-10.

Even with these restrictions, the use of NPPV has become a popular modality for use in the home.

Negative Pressure Ventilation. Negative pressure ventilation (NPV), a less frequently used technique of noninvasive ventilation, involves generating a negative, or subatmospheric, pressure outside the patient's chest. This negative pressure is then transmitted through the thorax, causing a drop in alveolar pressure, which causes a pressure gradient making airflow into the lungs. Time and pressure limits can be set on the ventilator. NPV was commonly used during the polio epidemic in the 1950s. Hospital wards were set up with iron lungs to ventilate numerous patients suffering from polio. Negative pressure ventilation has been successfully used on patients with neuromuscular or skeletal disease and central hypoventilation syndromes since the 1950s.[15]

Negative pressure ventilation includes a ventilator, which can produce a negative pressure, and a patient attachment that encloses the thorax.

- The *iron lung*, for example, encases the entire body except the head.
- The **cuirass**, or chest shell, fits over the chest or chest and abdomen. In home care, the cuirass is the more commonly used method of negative

TABLE 35-10 Medicare criteria for respiratory assist devices

Criteria for respiratory assist devices (RADs). Medicare pays for a bilevel positive pressure (BiPAP™) unit if the patient has one of the following diagnoses and related qualifying criteria:

Restrictive thoracic disorder

Documented progressive neuromuscular disease (e.g., ALS) or severe thoracic cage abnormality (e.g., post-thoracoplasty or TB)

and

COPD contribute significantly to the patient's pulmonary limitation

and

Patient exhibits any one of the following:

An arterial P_aCO_2 from a blood gas $\geq$ 45 mm Hg, done while the patient was awake and breathing usual F_IO_2

or

An oxygen saturation $\leq$ 88% during a sleep oximetry for at least 5 continuous minutes while breathing usual F_IO_2 or 2 L/min

Applicable for progressive neuromuscular diseases only:

The maximal inspiratory pressure < -60 cm H_2O

or

The forced vital capacity (FVC) <50% of predicted value

Severe COPD:

The arterial P_aCO_2 from a blood gas $>$ 52 mm Hg, done while the patient was awake and breathing usual F_IO_2

and

An oxygen saturation $\leq$ 88% during a sleep oximetry for at least 5 continuous minutes while breathing usual F_IO_2 or 2 Lpm, whichever is higher

and

Obstructive sleep apnea (OSA), with CPAP treatment, ruled out

Central Sleep APNEA:

A complete facility-based, attended polysomnogram performed prior to initiating therapy establishing a diagnosis of central sleep apnea

and

If the patient has OSA, CPAP been ruled out as ineffective

and

OSA is not the predominant cause of sleep-associated hypoventilation

and

A significant improvement of sleep-associated hypoventilation with use of BiPAP™ or BiPAP™ S/T on the setting that will be prescribed for initial use at home while breathing usual F_IO_2

Obstructive Sleep APNEA:

A complete facility-based, attended polysomnogram performed, establishing a diagnosis of OSA

and

CPAP tried and proven to be ineffective

and

The apnea/hypopnea index (AHI) $\geq$15

or

If the AHI was 5–14, did the patient have either excessive daytime sleepiness, cognition problems, history of stroke, or ischemic heart disease?

BiPAP™ S/T is covered after the first 2 months (61 days) of therapy with compliant use of the BiPAP™ and the following:

- Arterial blood gas performed on day 61 or later showing a $P_aCO_2 \geq$ 52 mm Hg
- Sleep oximetry performed on day 61 or later demonstrates an oxygen saturation that is $\leq$ 88% for 5 continuous minutes while using the BiPAP™ at usual F_IO_2 or 2 Lpm, whichever is higher
- Signed and dated physician statement indicating patient was compliant but did not benefit
- Signed and dated statement by patient indicating compliant use of BiPAP for 61 days

Note: All BiPAP™ and BiPAP™ S/T patients must be reevaluated by their physician between day 61 and day 90 of therapy. The patient's record must document progress and compliance with prescribed therapy. Patient must use the device 4 hours per night for 4 days per week. Home care provider must have signed documentation from the physician and patient in the chart with regard to these criteria.

pressure ventilation. It is mass-produced in various sizes, but customization may be necessary, owing to anatomical deformities.

- The *pulmowrap* is a poncho that covers a shell-like grid placed over the patient's chest and abdomen. A back plate may be used for support. Velcro straps or drawstrings fit the poncho snugly on the extremities and around the neck. An elastic belt is used on the hips to provide an airtight seal. The pulmowrap does not have to be customized and is easily applied to and removed from the patient. A major problem with the pulmowrap is that it leaks significantly around the hips, especially in thin patients.
- The *pneumosuit* is similar to the pulmowrap, but it has leggings to reduce leaks. The pneumosuit is usually custom made and therefore more costly.[15]

The negative pressure ventilator is actually a generator with several controls, including peak negative pressure, breath rate, and inspiratory time. The Lifecare NEV-100 and the Emerson are the two most commonly used units.

Alternate Ventilatory Methods. Two other alternative methods provide ventilatory assistance for certain home care patients: the pneumobelt and the rocking bed.

- The *pneumobelt* is an inflatable bladder inside a corset placed around the patient's abdomen. The bladder is connected to a positive pressure ventilator that inflates the bladder at a preset rate and pressure. The inflation of the bladder compresses the abdomen, raising the diaphragm, and causing exhalation. When the bladder deflates, the diaphragm descends and inspiration occurs. The pneumobelt is not effective in the supine position. The patient should be sitting in a 75° angle or greater for the pneumobelt to be the most effective.[15] This device is also used in pulmonary rehabilitation to help patients learn diaphragmatic techniques.
- The *rocking bed* is a platformed mattress over a motor, similar to a standard hospital bed placed on top of a motor. The motor moves the platform according to a set rate and pitch. The movement of the bed causes abdominal contents to shift and inhalation and exhalation to occur. This motion also seems to mobilize secretions and reduces the incidence of skin breakdown.[15]

PATIENT AND CAREGIVER EDUCATION

Once home care has been selected as part of the discharge plan for a ventilatory-dependent patient, the education process begins. The time frame may vary, depending on the specific patient, caregiver support, home modifications, and amount of equipment needed. Usually 2 weeks is a realistic goal to complete a successful discharge.

The home care ventilator is brought to the hospital, and the patient is placed on it early in the training process. This gives the patient time to adapt to the new ventilator and gives the caregivers a chance to become familiar with the ventilator. The accompanying Best Practice table identifies the in-hospital education that must be completed before discharge, as needed. This training should be done incrementally so that the patient and/or caregivers do not become overwhelmed by the amount of information. Daily education sessions of 2 hours are recommended. The home care therapist should enlist the help of the facility respiratory department in augmenting and reinforcing the education.

Upon discharge from the hospital, the respiratory therapist continues the education process in the home:

- Reinforcement of equipment operation and troubleshooting
- Responding to alarms
- General patient care
- Fire safety
- Emergency preparedness

As the patient and caregiver become confident and competent with the ventilator care, the respiratory therapist gradually decreases the number of home visits.

During follow-up visits, which occur at least once a month, the RT provides ongoing assessment and education. The respiratory therapist should reeducate the patient and caregiver on important issues during these visits. Even though the education process was completed on discharge, over time, the caregivers forget information or pick up bad habits in patient care. This is why ongoing assessment, education, and care planning are essential.

The AARC has a CPG on long-term invasive mechanical ventilation in the home.

- It describes the application of invasive mechanical ventilation and care of the patient-ventilator system.
- And it outlines goals, indications, contraindications, hazards and complications, assessment, resources, personnel, monitoring, and infection control.[16]

Best Practice

In-Hospital Instruction on Home Ventilator Management

Training should include the following:

- Ventilator care, maintenance, and operation
- Ventilator alarms and troubleshooting
- Basic anatomy and physiology
- Basic understanding of disease state
- Assembly of ventilator circuit
- Suctioning technique
- Tracheostomy care
- CPR
- General nursing care
- Signs of infection
- Use of manual resuscitator
- Use of suction equipment
- Use of oxygen equipment
- Use of other home medical equipment
- Emergency preparedness
- Emergency contact numbers

Pediatric Home Care

Pediatric and neonatal care has experienced some of the most remarkable advances in medical care in recent years. These advances have led to greatly improved survival rates of infants and children who would have died in decades past. The technological advances have allowed chronically ill children to be maintained long term outside of the hospital setting. In the late 1980s, the United States Department of Health and Human Services formed a Task Force on Long-Term Health Care Policies. In April 1988, the Task Force on Technology-Dependent Children, which was part of the Task Force on Long-Term Health Care Policies, recommended the following definition for **technology-dependent children**: "Technology-dependent children are those who require a particular medical device to compensate for the loss of a body function and are in need of substantial and complex daily nursing care to avert death or further disability."[17] Table 35-11 outlines the definition of a technology-dependent child.

Home care is the preferred setting for the technology-dependent child for several reasons:

- The cost of home care is dramatically less than institutional care.
- Home care encourages social interaction and development.

TABLE 35-11 **Definition of a technology-dependent child**

Ages birth to 21 years old
Suffers from chronic disability
Requires routine use of a medical device to compensate for the loss of a life-sustaining body function
Requires daily ongoing care or monitoring by trained personnel or both

CASE STUDY 35-3

J. W. is an 82-year-old female. She was diagnosed with kyphoscoliosis as a teenager. She functioned well her whole life until 10 years ago, when she was diagnosed with COPD. After a difficult and lengthy hospital course, which required tracheostomy, ventilatory support, and supplementary oxygen, Mrs. W. was deemed unweanable. Mrs. W. is a widow, with one daughter who is married with three children. Her daughter chose home care instead of a long-term ventilator unit.

Mrs. W. was provided with a portable ventilator. The physician ordered the following ventilator settings: Mode, Assist-control; Rate, 14; Tidal volume, 650 mL; Peak flow, 60 Lpm; F_IO_2, .30. In addition, routine suctioning is required and aerosolized albuterol is ordered q.i.d. Education and training of Mrs. W.'s daughter and son-in-law began in the hospital, and, after proficiency was determined, a home environmental assessment was completed and Mrs. W. was discharged after several months.

Mrs. W.'s daughter and son-in-law have cared for her since discharge, with support from the respiratory therapists from the HME company and an RN and home health aides from a home health agency.

Questions

1. What actions should the respiratory therapist take to ensure Mrs. W.'s preparedness for emergencies, such as power failures?
2. For three consecutive months, Mrs. W.'s SO_2 is greater than 96% when assessed by the respiratory therapist. What action should the respiratory therapist take?
3. What four elements had to be present to begin discharge planning for Mrs. W.?

AGE-SPECIFIC CRITERIA

The respiratory therapist must realize that caring for an infant or child is not like caring for a little adult. Depending on their age, children can differ significantly, even within the pediatric population. Major anatomical and physiological differences and issues of growth and development must be taken into consideration. There are also different chronic conditions in pediatrics from those seen in adults. Table 35-12 lists some of the chronic pediatric respiratory diseases commonly seen in home care.[18] Parents play a significant role in the care of the child, even when professionals are providing the care. The emotional and psychosocial issues that present themselves must be taken into consideration. Frequently, siblings are experiencing normal growth and development. The parents must work to maintain a normal environment despite the disruption by the technology and personnel.

EQUIPMENT

Much of the equipment used in home care for the adult patient can be adapted to the pediatric patient with little difficulty. Some equipment is manufactured specifically for the pediatric population.

Oxygen therapy equipment is the same for adults as for pediatric patients. Delivery devices, such as nasal cannulas or face masks are available in smaller sizes to fit the pediatric patient. The flowmeter on the oxygen equipment may need to be changed to accommodate lower flow rates when prescribed for pediatric cases. Some patients may require flow rates as low as 1/64 Lpm.

TABLE 35-12 **Chronic pediatric respiratory diseases commonly seen in home care**

Bronchopulmonary dysplasia (BPD)
Cystic fibrosis
Asthma
Congenital central hypoventilation syndrome
Werdnig-Hoffmann syndrome
Bronchomalacia
Tracheomalacia
Tracheal stenosis
Arnold-Chiari deformity
Trisomy 13
Gastroesophageal reflux
Muscular dystrophy
Apnea of prematurity

Aerosol therapy equipment is identical in both the pediatric and adult patient. The delivery device can be adapted to the infant or child. Frequently, older children can use an adult mouthpiece. Younger children and infants may require a pediatric aerosol mask or a blow-by system, using a T-adapter and a flex tube. Most commonly, these patients are being treated for asthma, reactive airways disease, or bronchiolitis.

Pediatric patients with tracheostomies may require aerosol therapy with a tracheostomy mask. Masks are available in a pediatric size. Overhydration is a potential complication of continuous aerosol therapy, particularly if there is a preexisting fluid or electrolyte imbalance. Suction equipment for these patients is also the same as for adult patients, but the catheters are smaller.

Home ventilator care for the pediatric patient is different from that of the adult patient, owing to the many family and psychosocial issues facing the family and the caregivers. The success of the pediatric ventilator discharge depends on the capabilities and willingness of the parents to meet the needs of the child.

The ventilator equipment is the same as for the adult patient. The major differences in provision of care are that PEEP and CPAP are used more frequently, and pressure-limited ventilation in lieu of volume ventilation is commonly employed.

INFANT APNEA MONITORING

Sudden infant death syndrome (SIDS) is the leading cause of death in infants younger than 1 year old. Cardiorespiratory, or apnea, monitors were developed in the 1970s due to the prevalence of SIDS. Apnea monitors measure heart rate and respiratory pattern by impedance pneumonography.

- Two electrodes are placed on the chest of the infant, which detect chest movement and ECG tracings.
- The monitor is equipped with audible and visual alarms for bradycardia, tachycardia, and apnea. If an alarm condition occurs, the audible alarm not only alerts the parents of the event, but also serves as an audible stimulant for the infant and may cause the infant to take a breath.
- Most monitors today are equipped with memory modules that store data on alarm and event conditions and usage of the monitor. The data are periodically downloaded by the respiratory therapist with a laptop computer and a telephone modem.
- The monitors have internal rechargeable batteries that can power the monitor for up to 72 hours.

The National Institutes of Health developed a consensus statement on infant apnea monitoring. (See the next Best Practice for the indications for home apnea monitoring.)[18]

Before prescribing an apnea monitor, physicians commonly order a **pneumocardiogram (PCG)**, which is usually multichannel, to monitor heart rate, respiratory pattern, pulse oximetry, and nasal airflow. Esophageal pH is sometimes monitored and can be diagnostic for esophageal reflux. The respiratory therapist may be responsible for performing these tests, either before discharge from the hospital or in a home care setting.

When an apnea monitor is ordered, the parents or caregivers must be thoroughly instructed on the use of the monitor and response to monitor alarms. The parents or caregivers must be instructed in CPR in order to respond to a true apnea or bradycardia alarm.

Noncompliance with apnea monitor usage is a significant issue. Ongoing assessment by the respiratory therapist and downloading of compliance data are essential to prevent life-threatening events from going undetected.

Best Practice

Indications for Home Infant Apnea Monitoring

Home cardiorespiratory monitoring is medically indicated in certain groups of infants at high risk for sudden death, including the following:

- Infants with one or more severe **apparent life-threatening events (ALTE)** requiring vigorous stimulation, mouth-to-mouth resuscitation, or CPR.
- Siblings of two or more victims of SIDS.
- Preterm infants with apnea of prematurity.
- Infants with conditions such as central hypoventilation or tracheostomy.

It is not clear from existing evidence whether the potential benefits of monitoring outweigh the risks of monitoring for these groups:

- Siblings of one SIDS victim
- Infants with less severe ALTEs
- Infants of opiate- or cocaine-abusing mothers

Cardiorespiratory monitoring is not medically indicated for normal infants or asymptomatic preterm infants.

Source: Developed by the National Institutes for Health (NIH).

Clinical Respiratory Services

The Joint Commission defines *clinical respiratory services* as "services provided for treatment of individuals with disorders of the cardiopulmonary system, including diagnostic testing, therapeutics, and monitoring."[19]

Because respiratory services are usually reimbursed by equipment rental and purchase, **clinical respiratory services** by a qualified respiratory therapist are not universally provided. However, many HME providers decide to include clinical respiratory services as part of their operation for several reasons:

- Physicians may request the services.
- Managed care organizations may require them.
- The provider may have a philosophical reason for providing these additional services.
- Some HME providers see this as an additional marketing tool.

Typically, the respiratory therapist performs a clinical assessment that includes:

- Vital signs.
- Chest auscultation.
- Medical history.
- Medication use and monitoring.
- Pulse oximetry.

The provision of testing and therapeutics, such as chest physical therapy, tracheostomy tube changes, and arterial blood gases, is less frequent.

To provide clinical respiratory services, the HME provider must have an appropriately trained and competent respiratory therapist. The respiratory therapist must have a mechanism to report clinical findings to the physician or other health care professional. A physician's order is required to provide ongoing clinical services. Some patients may need long-term clinical services, while others may receive clinical services during an acute exacerbation and then be discontinued from the clinical services.

Assessment

The foundation to delivering quality care or service is a comprehensive assessment process. In providing home care, the assessment process includes an assessment not only of the patient, but also of external factors affecting the delivery of care or service. Issues such as the home environment, caregiver support, and psychosocial status all are an integral part of a successful home care admission.

According to the Joint Commission, the goal of assessment is to determine the care or services to be provided to meet the patient's needs. To achieve this goal, the HME provider must collect data to assess the patient's needs, analyze the data to decide how to meet the needs, and make decisions regarding care or service based on the analysis of this information.[19]

PATIENT ASSESSMENT

A complete physical assessment of the patient may or may not be performed, depending on the level of care or clinical service by the HME provider. If this is part of the protocol, the assessment may include any or all of the items in Table 35-13.

The physical assessment of the patient may be tailored. As discussed earlier in this chapter, the pediatric patient has unique problems and needs, which must be assessed. This is also true in the geriatric patient and the dying patient.

The data gathered during the assessment must be evaluated in terms of the care or service being provided. The physician may have to be contacted with findings from the assessment, and the care or service may need to be modified to meet the patient's needs.

ENVIRONMENTAL ASSESSMENT

Providing care and service in the home is much different from caregiving in the controlled environment of a hospital. Environmental issues can significantly make an impact on the success of a home care admission. Assessment of the home environment must be conducted initially to identify any safety hazards or other issues that make a negative impact on the patient. Ongoing assessment of the home environment should occur whenever a representative of the HME provider visits the patient's home because home conditions are not static.

A general assessment of the home environment should include the following components:

- Adequate storage space and clear hallways and pathways.
- A check for infestation and architectural barriers or deficiencies.
- Proper utilities management.
- Electrical safety, particularly when installing multiple pieces of medical equipment. Outlets must be grounded and safe to use. Extension cords or octopus plugs should be avoided. Adequate ventilation systems, including heat and air conditioning, as appropriate, must be reviewed.
- A telephone must be accessible to the patient or caregiver.
- Fire safety. Functioning smoke and carbon monoxide detectors should be in place, and a fire extinguisher should be readily available, especially if oxygen is in use. Fire escape routes should be discussed with the patient or caregiver. Fire department notification of the patient's condition may be appropriate.
- Bathroom safety. Facilities must be accessible to the patient. They also must be safe, including grab bars, raised toilet seats, and bath benches, as needed.

Any significant deficiencies identified during the environmental assessment must be discussed with the patient and caregiver. If the issues are serious enough to impede the safe delivery of care or service, the HME provider must document the findings and report them to the physician and/or discharging facility.

TABLE 35-13 **Elements included in the physical assessment of the patient**

Elements
Medical history
Vital signs
Breath sounds
Height and weight
Cough and sputum production
S_pO_2
Psychosocial status
Nutritional status
Medications
Allergies
General appearance
Smoking history
Occupational history
Family support system
Mental status
Functional limitations
Emergency response
Advance directives

Patient Education

The role of the respiratory therapist in home care is primarily patient and caregiver education. Because respiratory therapists usually do not provide hands-on care, they must train the patient or caregiver on how to use the equipment provided. They must possess good interpersonal skills and be able to provide education to people with varied educational levels. The patient or caregiver may have language barriers or other difficulties in learning.

The HME provider must have adequate resources to provide patient education. Such resources include:

- Qualified personnel.
- Teaching materials such as age-appropriate instruction manuals.
- Proper teaching methods.
- Access to other organizations that may supplement the education process.

In addition:

- The patient or caregiver must be thoroughly trained in the use and maintenance of each piece of home medical equipment.
- Verbal instruction should be provided by the respiratory therapist, and the caregiver should a return demonstrate the ability to perform any tasks. (See the next Best Practice.)
- Written or pictorial educational material should be left with the patient or caregiver to use as a reference.

In addition to education on the equipment and home environmental issues, the RT may have to provide education on clinical issues:

- The disease process
- Symptom recognition and management
- Safe and effective use of medications
- Nutritional issues.
- Relating the use of the equipment to the clinical indicators and outcomes

All education should be documented in the patient's home care record. This is also an ongoing process to ensure the success of the home care patient.

Disease Management

In an effort to prevent rehospitalizations, health care providers and managed care payers have formed a partnership in some locations to manage patients more effectively at home. Disease management programs for asthma and COPD are most commonly seen. These management programs include intensive patient education on the disease process, appropriate behavior, community resources, and compliance with the treatment plan. This is an interdisciplinary approach to the patient's ongoing care. Table 35-14, for example, identifies the topics covered in an asthma management program.

Best Practice

Patient Education for Home Care

Patient education should include:

- Basic home safety
- Infection prevention and control
- Emergency preparedness
- Handling of hazardous materials, including oxygen
- Safe and effective use of medical equipment

Care Planning

After the assessment of the patient, the environment and patient education process, the next step is **care planning**, that is, a planned approach to providing care, treatment, or service. The goal of care planning is to increase positive patient outcomes and to assist in interdisciplinary care coordination. The respiratory therapist:

- Reviews and evaluates the data collected during the assessment and patient education process.
- Identifies the specific problems and needs of the individual patient.
- Sets a goal for resolving the problems and needs.
- Implements an action to meet the set goals.

The care plan issues are reviewed on an ongoing basis. Some issues are resolved, others persist or worsen, and new problems and needs are identified. The care plan is revised as needed to meet the ongoing

TABLE 35-14 **Guidelines for the diagnosis and management of asthma**

Definition of asthma
Key points about signs and symptoms of asthma
Characteristic changes in the airways of patients with asthma and the role of medications
Asthma triggers and how to avoid or control them
Treatment
Patient fears concerning medications
Use of written guidelines
Use of written diaries
Correct use of inhalers
Criteria for premedicating to prevent onset of symptoms
Optimal use of home peak flow monitoring
Evaluation of results of treatment plan
Fears and misconceptions
Family understanding and support
Communication with the child's school
Feelings about asthma

goals. The care plan should be reviewed and revised if any of the following items occur:

- Changes in the patient's physical condition or the patient's psychosocial status
- Lack of achievement of previously set goals
- Lack of patient response to care, treatment, or service
- Changes in the prognosis, treatment, equipment, limitations, or precautions.

If none of these occur, the HME provider should set a maximum time frame by which the patient's care plan is reviewed.

Documentation, an important part of the care planning process, ensures continuity of care. HME providers can design their own care plan document. Some organizations use a generic template that is individualized for each patient. Checklists and narrative forms are other examples of care planning documents.

The respiratory therapist must remember that care planning is paramount in the delivery of quality patient care of service. All home care practitioners must be knowledgeable and feel comfortable with the care planning process.

Reimbursement

Health care financing is an issue of utmost importance to the home care respiratory therapist. Whereas the hospital respiratory therapist may never become involved with reimbursement issues, the home care respiratory therapist deals with these issues daily. As health care reimbursement continues to change, HME providers must stay abreast of the latest reimbursement guidelines and issues.

PAYORS

The three major payor sources for HME reimbursement are governmental agencies, private insurance carriers, and patient self-pay.

Governmental programs established for health care financing are the Medicare and Medicaid programs.

The *Medicare* program was established in 1965 to provide medical coverage for the elderly, aged 65 and older. In 1972, the Medicare program began to provide coverage for those under 65 years old who are disabled for two years or longer. Medicare is administered by CMS, an agency of the United States Department of Health and Human Services.

The Medicare benefit includes two programs: Part A and Part B.

- *Part A* covers hospital services, skilled nursing facilities, home health visits, and hospice care.
- *Part B* covers physician services, outpatient therapy, DME, and ambulance services. Although there is no coverage for clinical respiratory services or the professional services of the respiratory therapist, legislation is pending to allow reimbursement for the services of a therapist. HME providers bill Medicare Part B for the rental or purchase of home respiratory equipment according to Medicare guidelines. Under Part B, the beneficiary is responsible to pay a deductible at the beginning of each year and a copayment of 20% of the rental or purchase price for DME. The HME provider must make every effort to collect the copayment from the beneficiary. CMS requires a *certificate of medical necessity* (*CMN*) for most respiratory equipment. This document must be completed by the ordering physician before billing Medicare. Figure 35-10 is the CMN for oxygen equipment.

Medicare now offers an option to beneficiaries to enroll in a health maintenance organization (HMO). This has gained acceptance with many beneficiaries.

Medicaid is a joint federal and state program that provides health care reimbursement for the indigent. Each state develops its own criteria for eligibility and benefits. There is great variance in coverage from state to state. Some states have contracted with HMOs to reduce Medicaid costs. HME providers must be aware of the specific criteria for the Medicaid program in their state. If they serve more than one state, they must be diligent in adhering to each state's guidelines.

Private insurance carriers cover the vast majority of people under 65 years of age. Private insurance coverage occurs in two methods: traditional indemnity plans and managed care.

- *Traditional indemnity plans* pay a fee for service to health care providers. For HME providers, these plans pay a usual and customary fee for home medical equipment. Patients have their choice of HME suppliers.
- *Managed care organizations* were developed in an effort to contain health care costs. Preferred provider organizations (PPO) and HMOs fall under the managed care umbrella. Under these arrangements, the payor usually contracts with providers, such as HME organizations, to provide care or service at a negotiated rate of reimbursement. The providers are usually willing to accept a lower reimbursement level in exchange for guaranteed business.

Last, there are those who *self-pay*. They do not have health insurance and are not eligible for Medicare or Medicaid. This small percentage of the population falls

DEPARTMENT OF HEALTH AND HUMAN SERVICES Form Approved CENTERS FOR MEDICARE & MEDICAID SERVICES OMB No. 0938-0534

DME 484.03

CERTIFICATE OF MEDICAL NECESSITY CMS-484 — OXYGEN

SECTION A Certification Type/Date: INITIAL ___/___/___ REVISED ___/___/___ RECERTIFICATION___/___/___		
PATIENT NAME, ADDRESS, TELEPHONE and HIC NUMBER (___ ___) ___ ___ ___- ___ ___ ___ ___ HICN ____________		SUPPLIER NAME, ADDRESS, TELEPHONE and NSC or applicable NPI NUMBER/LEGACY NUMBER (___ ___) ___ ___ ___- ___ ___ ___ ___ NSC or NPI #________
PLACE OF SERVICE________	HCPCS CODE	PT DOB ___/___/___ Sex ___ (M/F)
NAME and ADDRESS of FACILITY *if applicable* *(see reverse)*	________ ________ ________ ________	PHYSICIAN NAME, ADDRESS, TELEPHONE and applicable NPI NUMBER or UPIN (___ ___) ___ ___ ___- ___ ___ ___ ___ UPIN or NPI #________

SECTION B Information in This Section May Not Be Completed by the Supplier of the Items/Supplies.	
EST. LENGTH OF NEED (# OF MONTHS): ______ 1–99 *(99=LIFETIME)*	DIAGNOSIS CODES (ICD-9): ______ ______ ______ ______
ANSWERS	ANSWER QUESTIONS 1–9. (Circle Y for Yes, N for No, or D for Does Not Apply, unless otherwise noted.)
a)________mm Hg b)__________% c)___/___/___	1. Enter the result of most recent test taken on or before the certification date listed in Section A. Enter (a) arterial blood gas PO2 and/or (b) oxygen saturation test; (c) date of test.
1 2 3	2. Was the test in Question 1 performed (1) with the patient in a chronic stable state as an outpatient, (2) within two days prior to discharge from an inpatient facility to home, or (3) under other circumstances?
1 2 3	3. Circle the one number for the condition of the test in Question 1: (1) At Rest; (2) During Exercise; (3) During Sleep
Y N D	4. If you are ordering portable oxygen, is the patient mobile within the home? If you are not ordering portable oxygen, circle D.
__________LPM	5. Enter the highest oxygen flow rate ordered for this patient in liters per minute. If less than 1 LPM, enter a "X".
a)________mm Hg b)__________% c)___/___/___	6. If greater than 4 LPM is prescribed, enter results of most recent test taken on 4 LPM. This may be an (a) arterial blood gas PO2 and/or (b) oxygen saturation test with patient in a chronic stable state. Enter date of test (c).
ANSWER QUESTIONS 7-9 **ONLY** IF PO2 = 56–59 OR OXYGEN SATURATION = 89 IN QUESTION 1	

FIGURE 35-10 Certificate of medical necessity. (*continues*)

Y N	7. Does the patient have dependent edema due to congestive heart failure?
Y N	8. Does the patient have cor pulmonale or pulmonary hypertension documented by P pulmonale on an EKG or by an echocardiogram, gated blood pool scan or direct pulmonary artery pressure measurement?
Y N	9. Does the patient have a hematocrit greater than 56%?

NAME OF PERSON ANSWERING SECTION B QUESTIONS, IF OTHER THAN PHYSICIAN (Please Print): NAME:

________________________________ TITLE: ____________________ EMPLOYER: ____________________

SECTION C Narrative Description of Equipment and Cost

(1) Narrative description of all items, accessories and options ordered; (2) Supplier's charge and (3) Medicare Fee Schedule Allowance for each item, accessory and option. (See instructions on back.)

SECTION D Physician Attestation and Signature/Date

I certify that I am the treating physician identified in Section A of this form. I have received Sections A, B and C of the Certificate of Medical Necessity (including charges for items ordered). Any statement on my letterhead attached hereto, has been reviewed and signed by me. I certify that the medical necessity information in Section B is true, accurate and complete, to the best of my knowledge, and I understand that any falsification, omission, or concealment of material fact in that section may subject me to civil or criminal liability. PHYSICIAN'S SIGNATURE

____ DATE ____/____/____ **Signature and Date Stamps Are Not Acceptable.**

FIGURE 35-10 *(continued)*

into the self-pay category for reimbursement. These patients are responsible for the payment of all of their health care bills. HME providers usually determine private pay reimbursement rates directly with the patient before admission and the delivery of equipment.

Regulatory Bodies, Accreditation, and Licensure

Numerous regulatory bodies affect the HME industry. Federal regulations are in place through federal agencies. HME providers must stay informed of current regulations and any changes in them.

The *Department of Transportation* (*DOT*) regulates delivery vehicles of 10,000-pound gross vehicle weight or vehicles that carry a combined hazardous material gross weight of 1000 pounds. The DOT requires:

- Proper placards and decals on vehicles.
- An emergency safety kit.
- A fire extinguisher in the driver's compartment.
- Specific driver qualifications.

There are also regulations regarding:

- Preventive maintenance of vehicles.
- Loading and unloading vehicles.
- Proper shipping papers.
- The inspection and testing of compressed gas cylinders.

The *Food and Drug Administration* (*FDA*) is the federal agency responsible for ensuring the quality, purity, and traceability of drug products. The HME provider should be primarily concerned about oxygen.

- HME providers that transfill liquid or gaseous oxygen must be registered with the FDA as a repackager.
- They must have a written recall procedure and maintain an oxygen complaint log. Oxygen batch or lot numbers must be traceable to the receiving patient.
- Testing of liquid and compressed gas must follow FDA specifications.
- Oxygen analyzers need to be calibrated and documented appropriately.

The regulations for oxygen storage, inspection, and use also affect HME organizations.[15]

The *Occupational Safety and Health Administration (OSHA)* was established to ensure employee safety. OSHA requires that:

- Specific documents be maintained.
- Proper postings be made.
- Specific training programs be held.
- The work environment is safe and suitable.
- Employees are provided with proper personal protective equipment.
- ATB risk assessment is made, with TB testing of at-risk employees and offering of the hepatitis B vaccination to appropriate employees.[20]

ACCREDITATION

Accreditation is a process for independent review of a health care organization to ensure compliance with basic quality standards that are recognized in the industry as indicators of quality care. Although still a voluntary process, HME organizations are pressured into seeking accreditation in order to receive and maintain contracts with third-party payors and demonstrate quality care to the marketplace. Accreditation has been a standard for inpatient health care since the 1950s. It is a newer concept for alternate site care, especially home care. Increased pressure from payors and the general public for accountability in health care delivery and the maturation of the home care industry has increased awareness and demand for accreditation. Medicare accreditation has been required for HME companies as of September 30, 2009.

Currently, three organizations accredit home care providers.

- The Joint Commission
- Accreditation Commission for Home Care (ACHC)
- The Community Health Accreditation Program (CHAP)

Joint Commission. The Joint Commission is the largest and most familiar accreditation agency in the health care community. Formed in 1951, the Joint Commission is an independent, nonprofit organization and the predominant health care accreditation body in the United States. The Joint Commission mission is to improve the quality of care provided to the public through the provision of health care accreditation and related services that support performance improvement in health care organizations. The Board of Commissioners for the Joint Commission includes representatives from the American College of Physicians, American College of Surgeons, American Dental Association, American Hospital Association, and the American Medical Association.

In 1988, the Joint Commission initiated its home care accreditation program. Under this accreditation program, the following services are eligible for accreditation:

- Home health agencies
- Hospice
- Personal care and support services
- Home medical equipment (HME)
- Clinical respiratory services
- Home infusion services
- Home rehabilitation services

The Joint Commission has developed standards to reflect important processes for home care providers. These standards are approved by professional and technical leaders in the home care industry. The standards are reviewed every 2 years to ensure applicability to current practices. The standards are divided into two major areas: patient-focused functions and organization functions. Table 35-15 contains the important functions reviewed by the Joint Commission.[21]

In 2002, the Joint Commission also established the National Patient Safety Goals to help accredited organizations address specific areas of this concern (see the next Spotlight On).[22] Home Care organizations should follow these safety goals routinely.

Home care organization surveys are unannounced. Notice is provided only to the HME company stating that the survey is imminent. The Joint Commission survey schedule is triennial; however, it may be conducted as early as 18 months after the last survey.

Accreditation Commission for Home Care (ACHC). The Accreditation Commission for Home Care (ACHC) was founded in 1985 and began offering services

TABLE 35-15 **The Joint Commission functions in the comprehensive accreditation for home care**

Patient-Focused Functions	Organization Functions
Rights and ethics	Improving organizational performance
Assessment	Leadership
Care, treatment, and service	Environmental safety and equipment management
Education	Management of human resources
Continuum of care and service	Management of information surveillance, prevention, and control of infection

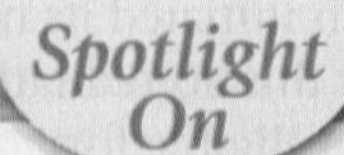

The Joint Commission National Patient Safety Goals for Home Care

- Improve the effectiveness of communication among caregivers.
  - Write down and read back verbal telephone orders.
  - Review the list of abbreviations that are NOT to be used.
  - Timeliness of reporting critical test results i.e. oximetries.
  - Standardized approach to "hand off" communication, including an opportunity to ask questions.
- Reduce the risk of health care-associated infections.
  - Comply with current CDC hand washing guidelines.
- Reduce the risk of patient harm resulting from falls.
  - Complete a home safety assessment and review tripping hazards.
  - Notify your manager if you become aware of a patient falling.
- Encourage patients' active involvement in their own care as a patient safety strategy.
  - Discuss the importance of patient safety and show the patient the information on how they report any concerns about safety. This information can be found in the patient booklet.
- Identify risks associated with long-term oxygen therapy.
  - Make sure that patients' homes are equipped with a fire extinguisher and smoke detector.
  - Educate them on the hazards of open flame devices.
  - No Smoking signs should always be posted.

nationally in 1996. It promotes itself as an alternative to the Joint Commission survey process. The ACHC has introduced five basic accreditation resource manuals:

- Multiservice organizations (Medicare- and non-Medicare-certified home health agencies)
- Home infusion companies
- Home medical equipment suppliers
- In-home aide (including home health aides)
- Hospices[23]

ACHC accreditation has been accepted by several of the larger insurance providers, but many providers are not yet familiar with this accreditation program. ACHC also uses a 3-year accreditation cycle. They announce the survey visit but reserve the right to make unannounced on-site visits at any time during the 3-year period.[23]

Community Health Accreditation Program (CHAP). The Community Health Accreditation Program (CHAP) began in 1965 and has focused on community-based health care instead of inpatient programs. In 1992, CHAP became the first home care accreditation body to receive deemed status by Medicare for home health agencies and then for hospice organizations. In 2006, the organization was granted full deeming authority for HME. Deemed status is granted by CMS to health care providers who are judged to be in compliance with the Medicare Conditions of Participation and CMS has determined the accreditation is equivalent to the standards of the Medicare program.

Although the focus of CHAP is home health services, it currently accredits the following organizations and services:

- Voluntary, nonprofit organizations
- Hospice
- Nursing agencies
- Social work agencies
- Pharmacies
- Durable medical equipment providers and RTs
- Home infusion therapy providers
- Homemakers and home health aides
- Physical, occupational, and speech therapists

CHAP uses a self-study tool to initiate the accreditation process with applicant organizations. The purpose of the self-study is twofold:

- It affords the organization the opportunity to complete a comprehensive internal evaluation and review of their operations in preparation for the site visit.
- It enables the CHAP staff to plan and execute the site visit based on the information submitted to them.

Organizations have the option of using the CHAP Cares Client Portal, which allows them to complete the self-study on-line and upload attachments in interactive on-line sessions.[24]

The accreditation emphasis is on operational management, performance improvement planning, adequate levels of resources, consumer satisfaction and outcomes, and the long-term viability of the organization.[24] Accreditation is granted for a 3-year term, and all site visits are unannounced. Reaccreditation visits take place the year following year 3 of the 3-year cycle.

State governments commonly regulate health care delivery with state licensure for individual practitioners or health care organizations. Respiratory care regulations through licensure, certification, or other legal credentialing are currently in place in all states and Puerto Rico. These regulations affect the HME industry differently from state to state. Providers must be aware of their local respiratory care regulations and their effect on home care practitioners.

There has been interest in licensure for HME companies nationwide as a method to ensure quality. Currently, 12 states have licensure laws in place for home medical equipment companies. This trend may continue as the public and payers demand accountability in health care.

Summary

This chapter has reviewed all the major components of a respiratory home care program, beginning with the discharge planning process. The different modalities and types of equipment were covered in depth. Assessment, patient education, and care planning processes were discussed. These are the foundation for the clinical services of the respiratory therapist. Last, the important issues of reimbursement, regulation, accreditation, and licensure were presented.

The respiratory therapist's role in home care has increased and changed over the last two decades. Today, the respiratory therapist is a respected member of the home care team. The RT's role is based on technology developed for use in the home care setting. New technology, patient education, disease management, and pressure from payers to treat patients in the least expensive setting all cause the respiratory therapist's role in home care to increase. The challenges of reimbursement continue to be a burden for the providers of home care services. Overall, home care continues to be an exciting and challenging setting for the respiratory therapist.

Study Questions

REVIEW QUESTIONS

1. Identify the factors that led to the development and growth of home respiratory care.
2. Identify the key members of the discharge planning team, and describe their responsibilities.
3. List the CMS guidelines for reimbursement of home oxygen equipment by Medicare.
4. List the advantages and disadvantages of each of the three home oxygen systems.
5. Identify the diagnoses of patients most successfully managed in a home ventilator program.
6. List the equipment and supplies most commonly required by a home ventilator patient.
7. Give the definition of a technology-dependent child.
8. List the indications for monitoring an infant with an apnea monitor.

MULTIPLE-CHOICE QUESTIONS

1. Which factor is *not* responsible for the growth of home respiratory care?
   a. technological advances
   b. physician demand
   c. reimbursement for health care
   d. increase in chronic illness
2. Which of the following discharge planning team members may act as team coordinator?
   I. physician
   II. social worker
   III. registered nurse
   IV. respiratory therapist
      a. I and III
      b. III only
      c. II, III, and IV
      d. I only
3. Which of the following elements is *not* commonly included in the discharge plan?
   a. therapeutic needs
   b. equipment needs
   c. reimbursement
   d. physician home visits
4. In 1980, the nocturnal oxygen therapy trial (NOTT) documented which of the following with regard to long-term oxygen therapy?
   a. increased pulmonary artery pressure
   b. improved nocturnal oxygen saturations
   c. higher pulmonary vascular resistance
   d. decreased CO_2 levels

5. Which of the following is a nonqualifying diagnosis under Medicare guidelines for reimbursement of oxygen therapy equipment?
   a. severe peripheral vascular disease
   b. diffuse interstitial lung disease
   c. congestive heart failure
   d. widespread pulmonary neoplasm
6. Which oxygen system is most appropriate for the intermittent oxygen user?
   a. compressed gas cylinders
   b. oxygen concentrator
   c. liquid oxygen
   d. demand flow system
7. Which of the following is *not* a benefit of oxygen-conserving devices?
   a. prolonged duration of portable cylinders
   b. less nasal drying
   c. increased sense of smell and taste
   d. improved oxygen saturations
8. Which of the following are elements to begin the discharge planning of a ventilator-dependent patient?
   I. Patient is clinically stable.
   II. The number of competent caregivers is adequate.
   III. Reimbursement is adequate.
   IV. The home environment is safe.
   a. I, II, and IV
   b. I and IV
   c. II, III, and IV
   d. I, II, III, and IV
9. According to the JCAHO, which service is *not* considered clinical respiratory services?
   a. diagnostic testing
   b. therapeutics
   c. patient monitoring
   d. equipment monitoring
10. Which agency is responsible for the purity of oxygen?
    a. DOT
    b. FDA
    c. JCAHO
    d. OSHA

CRITICAL-THINKING QUESTIONS

1. A primary care physician asks the respiratory therapist what needs to be done to order home oxygen for a patient who is involved in a pulmonary rehabilitation program. What information should the respiratory therapist provide to the physician?
2. A patient with muscular dystrophy is discussing with the physician the option of tracheostomy for nocturnal ventilatory support. What input should the respiratory therapist provide regarding tracheostomy and positive pressure ventilation versus NPPV?
3. In addition to the patient's physical assessment, what other items need to be assessed for the home care patient?

References

1. Wyka K. *Respiratory Care in Alternate Sites*. Clifton Park, NY: Delmar Cengage Learning; 1998:139–151, 154–165, 170–239.
2. Scanlan CL, Wilkins RL, Stoller JK, et al. *Fundamentals for Respiratory Care*. St. Louis, MO: Mosby; 1995:1096–1130.
3. American Association for Respiratory Care. AARC clinical practice guideline: discharge planning for the respiratory care patient. *Respir Care*. 1995a;40: 1308–1312.
4. Nocturnal Oxygen Therapy Trial Group. Continuous and nocturnal oxygen therapy in hypoxemic chronic obstructive lung disease: a clinical trial. *Ann Intern Med*. 1980;93:391–398.
5. Petty TL, Bliss PL. Ambulatory oxygen therapy, exercise and survival with advanced chronic obstructive pulmonary disease (the nocturnal oxygen therapy trial revisited). *Respir Care*. 2000;45,2:204–211.
6. American Association for Respiratory Care. AARC clinical practice guideline: oxygen therapy in the home or alternate site health care facility. *Respir Care*. 2007;52,8:1063–1068.
7. Lucas J, Golish JA, Sleeper G, O'Ryan JA. *Home Respiratory Care*. Norwalk, CT: Appleton & Lange; 1988:50–63.
8. Richardson, Stephanie. Giving COPD patients more options for oxygen therapy. *Focus Journal*. 2008;July–August:52–54.
9. Inspired Technologies, Inc. http://www.inspiredtechnologiesinc.com
10. McCoy, R. Oxygen-Conserving Techniques and Devices. *Respir Care*. 2000;45,1:95–103.
11. White G. *Equipment Theory for Respiratory Care*. Clifton Park, NY: Delmar Cengage Learning; 1996:564–593.
12. American Association for Respiratory Care. AARC clinical practice guideline: suctioning of the patient in the home. *Respir Care*. 1999;44:99–104.
13. Lewarski, Joseph. Notes from the Chair. AARC *Home Care Bulletin* 2002;March/April.
14. Wyka, KA, Mathews, PJ, Clark, WF, et al. *Foundations of Respiratory Care*. Clifton Park, NY: Delmar Cengage Learning; 2002:549–566.
15. Gilmartin M, Make B. *Problems in Respiratory Care, Mechanical Ventilation in the Home: Issues for Health Care Providers*. Philadelphia: JB Lippincott; 1988.
16. American Association for Respiratory Care. AARC clinical practice guideline. Long-term invasive

mechanical ventilation in the home. *Respir Care*. 2007;52(8):1056–1062.

17. Barnhart S, Czervinske M. *Perinatal and Pediatric Respiratory Care*. Philadelphia: WB Saunders; 1995:141–146, 658–679.
18. Dunne P, McInturffs. *Respiratory Home Care: The Essentials*. Philadelphia: FA Davis; 1998:1–11, 43–82, 131–144.
19. Joint Commission on Accreditation of Healthcare Organizations. *Complete Guide to the Survey Process: Home Medical Equipment and Clinical Respiratory Services*. Oakbrook Terrace, IL; Joint Commission; 1999.
20. Sylvia DS. *Fresh Air 2000—A Look at FDA's Medical Gas Requirements*. Rockville, MD: Food and Drug Administration Center for Drug Evaluation and Research; 2000.
21. Joint Commission on Accreditation of Healthcare Organizations. *Comprehensive Accreditation Manual for Home Care*. Oakbrook Terrace, IL; 1999–2000.
22. The Joint Commission. http://www.jointcommission.org
23. Accreditation Commission for Home Care. http://www.achc.org
24. Community Health Accreditation Program. http//www.chapinc.org/process.htm

Suggested Readings

Burton G, Hodgkin J. *Respiratory Care: A Guide to Clinical Practice*. Philadelphia, PA: JB Lippincott; 1997:337–340.

Joint Commission on Accreditation of Healthcare Organizations. *Care Planning: A Guide for Home Care and Hospice Organizations*. Oakbrook Terrace, IL: 1997.

Oakes, Dana, Wyka, A, Wyka, S. *Respiratory Home Care; An On-Site Reference Guide.* Orono, ME: Health Educator Publications; 2006.

Turner J, McDonald GJ, Larter NL, et al. *Handbook of Adult and Pediatric Respiratory Home Care*. St. Louis, MO: Mosby; 1994.

CHAPTER 36

Pulmonary Rehabilitation

Kenneth A. Wyka

OBJECTIVES

Upon completion of this chapter, the reader should be able to:

- Define the term *pulmonary rehabilitation.*
- Differentiate between pulmonary and cardiac rehabilitation.
- Identify the major goal and two principal objectives of pulmonary rehabilitation.
- List at least five patient conditions that would benefit from pulmonary rehabilitation.
- Explain how patients are selected for pulmonary rehabilitation.
- Identify the five key components of a pulmonary rehabilitation program.
- Explain the importance of patient documentation in pulmonary rehabilitation with regard to reimbursement.
- Identify at least three benefits of pulmonary rehabilitation.

CHAPTER OUTLINE

(continues)

(continued)

KEY TERMS

activities of daily living (ADLs)
Borg dyspnea scale (modified Borg dyspnea scale)
cardiac rehabilitation
cardiopulmonary exercise (CPX) evaluation/test
Centers for Medicare & Medicaid Services (CMS)
comprehensive outpatient rehabilitative facility (CORF)
current procedural terminology (CPT) coding
detraining effect
exercise prescription
healthcare common procedure coding system (HCPCS)
HR 6331 (Medicare Improvements for Patients and Providers Act)
International Classification of Diseases, 9th Revision, Clinical Modification (ICD-9-CM)
lung-volume-reduction surgery (LVRS)
maximum oxygen consumption ($\dot{V}O_{2max}$)
metabolic equivalents of energy expenditure (METs)
National Coverage Determination (NCD)
National Emphysema Treatment Trial (NETT)
physical reconditioning
pulmonary rehabilitation
target heart rate

Pulmonary rehabilitation is an area of patient care that continues to receive increased attention. In this discipline respiratory therapists (RTs) can assume considerable responsibility for both organizing and implementing programs. Significant focus has been placed on the rehabilitation and reconditioning of the chronic lung patient, both in the hospital and at alternative care sites. Many of these sites, catering to an ever increasing outpatient population, are now offering pulmonary rehabilitation programs to help meet the needs of a growing population of patients with chronic pulmonary disease. This chapter examines:

- The current concepts of pulmonary rehabilitation.
- The patient selection process.
- Program components.
- Outcomes assessment.
- Operational guidelines essential to the success of any pulmonary rehabilitation endeavor.

Scope and Changing Definitions

- **Pulmonary rehabilitation** is a program of education and exercise that focuses on restoring chronic respiratory patients to the highest functional capacity possible.
- **Cardiac rehabilitation** is a comprehensive education and exercise program designed to improve the cardiovascular fitness of patients with known cardiac dysfunction.

Both pulmonary and cardiac rehabilitation require a stress test to evaluate the patient's condition and status. Both programs are multidisciplinary in approach; both incorporate patient education and physical exercise; and both are reimbursable by insurance. The basic equipment used during exercise sessions—treadmills, exercycles, and arm ergometers—and the space requirements of the two types of rehab are essentially the same.

Pulmonary rehabilitation differs from cardiac rehabilitation with respect to the organ affected and hence to the type of program implemented. Pulmonary patients have exercise limitations due to dyspnea resulting from primary pulmonary impairment and dysfunction. These patients have very low exercise tolerance and, in most cases, demonstrate pulmonary symptoms such as dyspnea, cyanosis, oxygen desaturation, or wheezing with physical activity. Cardiac patients, on the other hand, are able to perform greater amounts of work and are not limited solely by dyspnea.

Other differences center on patient focus and monitoring during exercise.

- Cardiac programs are more concerned with a patient's pulse, blood pressure, and electrocardiogram via telemetry during exercise sessions.
- Pulmonary patients are monitored for pulse rate, respiratory rate, oxygen saturation, and peak flow rates during exercise.

In 1942, the *Council on Rehabilitation of the American College of Chest Physicians* (*ACCP*) defined *rehabilitation* as "the restoration of the individual to the fullest medical, mental, emotional, social, and vocational potential of which he/she is capable."[1] This was a general definition that did not imply any particular dysfunction or impairment. In 1974, the ACCP became more specific and formed the Committee on Pulmonary Rehabilitation, which specified a medical practice that was intended to help pulmonary patients attain their optimum state of heath.

The ACCP definition of pulmonary rehabilitation formed the basis for an official statement on pulmonary rehabilitation that was adopted by the *American Thoracic Society* (*ATS*) Executive Committee in 1981. Pulmonary rehabilitation may be defined as an art of medical practice wherein an individually tailored, multidisciplinary program is formulated which, through accurate diagnosis, therapy, emotional support, and education stabilizes or reverses both the physio- and psychopathology of pulmonary disease and attempts to return patients to the highest possible functional capacity allowed by their pulmonary handicap and overall life situation.[2]

Although many definitions of pulmonary rehabilitation exist today, they all seem to encompass some basic concepts and components, including the following:

- Multidisciplinary approach involving different health specialties
- Essential aim of getting pulmonary patients to function as normally as possible
- Medical direction and involvement
- Multiple forms of treatment and approaches tailored to patients' specific needs

In most instances, pulmonary rehabilitation is aimed at chronic lung patients, in particular those with asthma and chronic obstructive pulmonary disease (COPD), but it is also a viable option for ventilator-dependent and quadriplegic patients. These special cases present enormous challenges to respiratory therapists, who must work effectively within the health care team to help patients who have lost the ability to breathe on their own. Regardless of the type of patient in need of reconditioning, pulmonary rehabilitation involves education, breathing retraining, and physical conditioning through exercise.

In 1977, the *American Association for Respiratory Care* (*AARC*) formed its specialty sections, including one for rehabilitation and continuing care, now referred to as the Continuing Care/Rehabilitation section. Like other specialty sections, it:

- Serves as a consultant to the AARC.
- Provides resource pools for primary and secondary research.
- Acts as a clearinghouse for pertinent information specific to the specialty.
- Plays an integral role in communication and bringing people into the career of respiratory care.[3]

The *American Association of Cardiovascular and Pulmonary Rehabilitation* (*AACVPR*) was incorporated in 1983 to continue the advancement of pulmonary rehabilitation in terms of programs, services, professional practice, networking, and continuing education. With headquarters in Middleton, Wisconsin, it has developed a network of state affiliates. The AACVPR brings both professional and public attention to the importance of pulmonary rehabilitation through its annual national pulmonary rehabilitation week and publications such as the *Journal of Cardiopulmonary Rehabilitation* and the association newsletter, *News and Views*. The AACVPR also maintains a directory of rehabilitation programs throughout the United States.

In 1987, the AACVPR and AARC conducted the first joint national survey to ascertain the extent of pulmonary rehabilitation programs in the United States in terms of numbers, design, and scope. Subsequent surveys have since been conducted, and results continue to demonstrate steady growth in and acceptance of pulmonary rehabilitation as a viable therapeutic modality.

In 2007, the *American College of Chest Physicians* (*ACCP*) and the AACVPR released new evidence-based guidelines recommending pulmonary rehabilitation for patients with COPD indicating that pulmonary rehabilitation can:

- Improve a patient's exercise tolerance.
- Reduce levels of perceived dyspnea.
- Improve health-related quality of life.
- Reduce hospital admissions.
- Reduce the costs of health care utilization.

The guidelines also cited that pulmonary rehabilitation can be beneficial for patients with respiratory-related diseases other than COPD, such as bronchial asthma, interstitial pulmonary fibrosis, and lung cancer.[4,5] These historical developments, along with specific contributions of several key investigators, is presented and summarized in Table 36-1.

TABLE 36-1 **Historical developments in pulmonary rehabilitation**

Date	Development
1942	Council on Rehabilitation of the American College of Chest Physicians (ACCP) presents general definition of rehabilitation.
1951	Barach and associates comments on need for training programs for chronic lung patients.
1962	Pierce and associates publishes study that demonstrated Barach's insight into the value of pulmonary reconditioning.
1964	Paez and associates indicate that reconditioning techniques using both activity and oxygen benefited patients with chronic lung disease.
1968	Christie demonstrates that rehabilitative benefits could be offered on an outpatient basis with minimal supervision.
1974	ACCP forms the Committee on Pulmonary Rehabilitation.
1977	American Association for Respiratory Care (AARC) forms its specialty sections, including the Continuing Care/Rehabilitation section.
1981	American Thoracic Society (ATS) Executive Committee ACCP releases an official statement on pulmonary rehabilitation (based on the ACCP definition).
1983	American Association of Cardiovascular and Pulmonary Rehabilitation (AACVPR) is incorporated to continue the advancement of pulmonary rehabilitation.
1987	AACVPR and AARC conduct the first joint national survey to ascertain the extent of pulmonary rehabilitation programs in the United States.
2007	ACCP and the AACVPR release new evidence-based guidelines recommending pulmonary rehabilitation for patients with COPD.
2008	Medicare approves national coverage policy for beneficiaries enrolled in pulmonary rehabilitation programs [Medicare Improvements for Patients and Providers Act (MIPPA)].

Rationale for Pulmonary Rehabilitation

It is estimated that over 10% of the U.S. population, or close to 26 million Americans, are living with some type of chronic pulmonary disease. Lung diseases, including chronic obstructive pulmonary disease (COPD), now rank as the third leading cause of death in the United States, accounting for approximately 315,000 deaths annually. Direct and indirect expenditures for treating and managing lung disease each year total more than $56 billion.[6] Asthma-related care alone accounts for over $6 billion.[7] By 2020, it is projected that COPD alone will be the third leading cause of death in the United States. In addition, COPD is ranked as the second leading cause of permanent disability in males over 40 years old, resulting in disability payments from Social Security of over $27 billion. Since 1979, the mortality rate for all lung diseases has steadily increased. This increase has also occurred at a faster rate than the other top 10 causes of death, including heart disease and cancer (excluding lung cancer). In fact, during the 1980s, deaths from COPD increased 60%, whereas deaths from heart disease decreased 30%.[8]

In addition, because patients with chronic lung disease tend to be admitted several times during any given year, they tend to significantly strain hospital budgets under the prospective payment system. Keeping patients at home and improving their lifestyle are no longer idealistic goals; they are necessities. Hospitals are now seriously looking at pulmonary rehabilitation programs as a means of achieving these goals.

Patients with chronic lung disease have a variety of physiological and clinical manifestations that need to be addressed as part of any pulmonary rehabilitation effort:

- Increased airways resistance
- Hyperinflation with air trapping
- Decreased lung and chest wall compliance
- Respiratory muscle weakness
- Decreased exercise capacity and endurance
- Significant arterial oxygen desaturation during exercise
- Reduced oxygen consumption (the rate of oxygen uptake, which is a measure of a patient's work capacity)

The overall rationale for pulmonary rehabilitation is to control and perhaps reverse some of these processes, which lead to decreased physical activity. The onset of any one of these processes may trigger a vicious cycle in which dyspnea leads to inactivity, in turn leading to skeletal muscle atrophy, to increased dyspnea, and to further physical inactivity (Figure 36-1). Patients eventually become prisoners in their own homes, confined to a room and then finally to their beds. Some type of intervention is essential to break this vicious cycle. Pulmonary rehabilitation can improve a patient's level of physical activity, reduce dyspnea, and return the patient to a more active life with fewer hospitalizations.

Pulmonary function, cardiovascular function, and skeletal muscle function are integrally related (see Chapters 17 and 19). Each system depends on and affects the others when it develops an abnormality or becomes dysfunctional. When one system falters, the others must compensate, as is especially evident during any substantial physical activity such as exercise. Impaired lungs or ventilatory apparatus do not properly oxygenate the blood or remove carbon dioxide. Cardiovascular problems result in reduced circulation with diminished oxygenation of the blood and body tissues. Poor physical conditioning affects oxygen consumption and the body's acid-base balance; these disturbances place additional demands on the cardiopulmonary system. These relationships highlight the importance of a **cardiopulmonary exercise (CPX) evaluation/test** in differentiating between pulmonary, cardiac, and physical conditioning reasons for dyspnea and the inability to physically perform, thus identifying the need for some type of rehabilitation program.

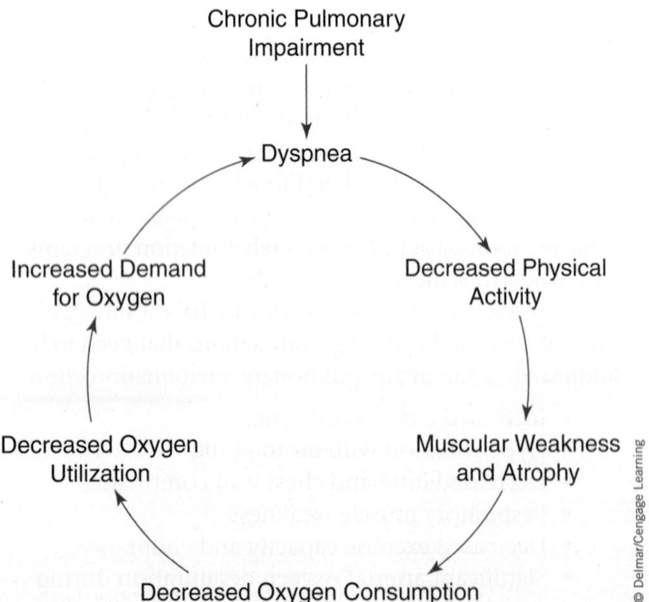

FIGURE 36-1 This vicious cycle is a consequence of inactivity produced by dyspnea resulting from chronic pulmonary disease.

Goals and Objectives of Pulmonary Rehabilitation

The major goal of pulmonary rehabilitation is to restore the patient to the highest possible functional capacity, given the patient's degree of pulmonary impairment and overall life situation. This goal implies specificity on the part of each patient and suggests that pulmonary rehabilitation should be tailored to meet the needs of the individual patient. Two principal objectives of pulmonary rehabilitation are designed to help achieve this major goal:

- To control and alleviate as much as possible the symptoms and pathophysiologic complications of respiratory impairment.
- To teach patients how to achieve optimal capability for carrying out their **activities of daily living (ADLs)**.[9]

Properly structured and administered pulmonary rehabilitation programs can help reverse some of the problems associated with dyspnea and inactivity and thereby help patients cope with their overall pulmonary and physical impairment. The four pillars of pulmonary rehabilitation that help patients understand the concept of pulmonary rehabilitation are:

- Education (information to help patients comprehend the scope of their dysfunction and what measures can be employed to improve their condition).
- Breathing techniques (pursed-lip, diaphragmatic, and inspiratory resistive breathing).
- **Physical reconditioning** (exercises to improve muscle tone, oxygen consumption, and overall exercise tolerance for both upper and lower body).
- Strategies for conserving energy and pacing activities.

Basis for Patient Selection

Impairments in the cardiopulmonary system can diminish the capacity to exercise in four major ways:

- Abnormal pulmonary mechanics—namely, changes in compliance and airway resistance.
- Abnormal gas exchange resulting in hypoxemia and arterial desaturation.
- Impaired cardiac output.
- Sensation or perception of dyspnea.

Abnormal pulmonary mechanics often results in increased respiratory muscle work for a set level of ventilation. This increase in the work of breathing may be due to increased airway resistance (R_{aw}), to hyperinflation, or to decreases in lung or chest wall compliance. Consequently, respiratory muscle fatigue is sometimes the result of an impaired ability to ventilate adequately. This impairment results in a sensation of dyspnea, along with abnormalities in gas exchange.

Gas exchange abnormalities are manifested in hypoxemia with arterial desaturation, reduced delivery of oxygen to the tissues, and lactic acidosis. Arterial desaturation also occurs during activity, especially exercise, in patients with chronic obstructive pulmonary disease (COPD). In fact, hypoxemia during exercise is common in COPD patients. The work of breathing increases as a result of the greater level of ventilation required to compensate for the drop in pH. Patients sense this as dyspnea, which limits their level of work or physical activity.

Cardiac dysfunction frequently follows chronic lung disease as a result of the effects of hypoxemia on the cardiovascular system. COPD patients with normal cardiac function at rest may develop pulmonary hypertension and cor pulmonale (elevated right atrial pressures) during exercise. This may lead to a reduction in cardiac output for some of the following reasons:

- An elevated right atrial pressure can produce a drop in the gradient for venous return to the heart, which diminishes cardiac output.
- In addition, if right ventricular hypertrophy is present, elevations in left ventricular filling pressure are evident, resulting in pulmonary vascular congestion and an interference with cardiac output.
- Finally, in patients with increased airway resistance, decreased compliance, or hyperinflation, pleural pressure can become more negative. This more negative pleural pressure, in turn, increases the pressure gradient against which the heart must pump, limiting the amount of blood ejected from the left ventricle. Pulmonary vascular congestion and trans-vascular fluid filtration follow, resulting in dyspnea and tightness in the chest.

TESTING REGIMENS

Because of these clinical manifestations, patients seek help from their physicians, and physicians often consider the potential benefits of pulmonary rehabilitation. The first step in the process is patient identification and evaluation using a testing regimen that includes:

- Chest X-ray.
- Arterial blood gas (ABG) analysis.
- Pulmonary function testing (PFT).
- Cardiopulmonary exercise (CPX) testing.

Before any testing is performed, a complete patient workup should be completed. This includes:

- A complete patient history consisting of medical/surgical, occupational, family, and social (outside activities plus any smoking and alcohol consumption) components.
- Physical examination.
- Laboratory testing (complete blood count, blood chemistry, theophylline level, and alpha-1 antitrypsin titer).
- Electrocardiogram and chest X-ray.

Both the patient and the health care provider should complete self-assessment scores, patient evaluation tools, **Borg dyspnea scale**, and COPD disability scale—all useful in classifying and categorizing a patient's level of physical activity and degree of dyspnea.[9] This information, in conjunction with appropriate cardiopulmonary function testing, enables the physician and rehabilitation specialist to evaluate the type and degree of impairment present and to tailor a pulmonary rehabilitation routine best suited for the patient's particular needs.

Pulmonary Function Test. The standard *pulmonary function test* (*PFT*) consists of:

- Pre- and postbronchodilator spirometry with a timed forced vital capacity (FVC) and flow volume loop.
- Maximum voluntary ventilation (MVV) maneuver.
- Lung volume and capacity determination using a helium equilibration or nitrogen washout technique.
- Diffusing capacity of the lung (DL_{CO}) using the single-breath method.

PFTs:

- Allow for the differentiation between obstructive and restrictive disease.
- Establish a baseline for the patient.
- Determine the extent of pulmonary impairment present.
- Identify the degree of reversal produced by bronchodilator therapy.

Arterial Blood Gas Analysis. *Arterial blood gas* (*ABG*) *analysis*, commonly performed during the PFT, identifies any hypoxemia, carbon dioxide retention, and acid-base imbalance. At this point, it is not certain to what extent pulmonary rehabilitation improves the patient's overall pulmonary function, but it is advisable to perform PFTs and ABGs at the beginning for patient tracking and the determination of overall patient progress. Pulse oximetry (S_pO_2) is also used to determine a patient's level of oxygenation. However, this technique is more useful in serial determinations to determine the degree of arterial desaturation with physical activities, such as walking or stair climbing.

Cardiopulmonary Exercise Testing. The most important aspect of patient evaluation and testing before any pulmonary rehabilitation effort is the *cardiopulmonary exercise* (*stress*, or *CPX*) *test*. This is the most complex test but the most important in terms of the patient data and information it provides. It is indispensable because it:

- Allows for the differentiation between pulmonary and cardiac causes of dyspnea.
- Determines the degree of oxygen desaturation and hypoxemia that occurs with physical exertion.
- Establishes a baseline for each patient's level of physical conditioning.
- Determines each patient's **target heart rate**, which is used in the **exercise prescription** (amount and intensity of exercise recommended) and physical reconditioning program. A target heart rate approximates the actual heart rate at 65–75% of the maximum oxygen consumption. It is the heart rate at which the patient achieves maximum physical and cardiovascular conditioning with exercise.
- Enables physicians and practitioners to track and document patient progress.
- May be used to exclude patients from pulmonary rehabilitation.

The interdependency of lung, heart, and skeletal muscle establishes an essential basis for the CPX test. This interdependency is the reason that individuals, especially cardiopulmonary patients, experience dyspnea during exercise or, in some cases, even during minimal physical activity. The CPX test is the best tool for testing the integrity of the vital relationships among the pulmonary system, cardiovascular system, and muscle performance. The American Association for Respiratory Care has published a clinical practice guideline (CPG) specifically outlining exercise testing for the evaluation of hypoxemia and desaturation. This CPG examines key components, such as:

- Definition and description.
- Indications.
- Contraindications.
- Precautions and possible complications.
- Procedural limitations.
- Assessment of need and test quality.
- Essential resources.
- Recommendations regarding monitoring.
- Infection control measures.[10]

Actual indications and contraindications for a CPX test vary from general to specific, depending on the underlying pulmonary or cardiovascular condition. Major indications for testing include:

- Patient assessment and evaluation.
- Differentiating between pulmonary or cardiac dysfunction and overall poor physical conditioning.

The main contraindications involve acute electrocardiographic changes associated with serious cardiac dysrhythmias and angina.

The two basic components of the CPX test or evaluation are regimens determining lung function and those measuring cardiovascular function. Components of the exercise evaluation to assess *lung function* include determinations of all of the following:

- Respiratory rate (RR or *f*; breaths per minute)
- Tidal volume and minute ventilation (V_T and $\dot{V}_E$)
- Oxygen saturation via pulse oximetry (S_pO_2)
- Oxygen uptake or consumption ($\dot{V}O_2$) and **maximum oxygen consumption ($\dot{V}O_{2max}$)**
- Carbon dioxide production ($\dot{V}CO_2$)
- Respiratory quotient (RQ, the ratio of carbon dioxide production to oxygen consumption)
- **Metabolic equivalents of energy expenditure (METs)** or oxygen consumption during exercise as compared with the resting level, at which all patients are at 1.0 MET (By definition, 1 MET equals approximately 3.5 mL of oxygen consumption per kilogram of body weight per minute.)
- Anaerobic threshold (AT, where carbon dioxide production equals oxygen consumption)
- Deadspace to tidal volume ratio (V_D/V_T)
- Breathing reserve determined as $1 - [\dot{V}_{Emax}/MVV]$

Components to assess or measure *cardiovascular function* are:

- Heart rate or pulse (HR)
- Blood pressure (BP)
- Electrocardiogram (ECG)
- O_2 pulse (oxygen consumption per heartbeat)
- Cardiac output (CO, or $\dot{Q}$)
- Heart rate reserve determined as $1 - (HR_{max} - HR_{rest}/HR_{pred.max} - HR_{rest})$

The CPX evaluation must be conducted with a physician or health care provider in attendance and is usually performed on a treadmill or an ergometer (electromechanical cycle). It follows any number of exercise protocols, depending on the nature and extent of each patient's ability.

During the test, all of the components previously listed are constantly measured and monitored. In particular, metabolic, pulmonary, and cardiovascular parameters are analyzed by both the computerized equipment and the testing personnel. Changes in the patient's workload with regard to ventilation, oxygen consumption, carbon dioxide production, and cardiac output (heart rate and stroke volume) reflect a definite response to the exercise demands placed on the patient. Figures 36-2, 36-3, and 36-4 illustrate, respectively, the changes in metabolic, pulmonary, and cardiovascular parameters during exercise testing. These invaluable data are then interpreted, allowing for a precise evaluation of the patient and determination of the type and extent of any reconditioning program needed.

The inability to tolerate exercise may be related to a number of factors, including pulmonary and cardiovascular disorders or just to poor physical conditioning. Table 36-2 examines CPX test results on the basis of these three factors.

Best Practice

CPX Test

A CPX test should last about 10–12 minutes or 6 minutes if the patient is elderly. However, the CPX test may be terminated for a number of other reasons, including:

- Equipment or monitoring-system failure.
- Patient fatigue.
- Clinical signs and symptoms of physiological distress (vertigo, pallor, or headache).
- Significant hypoxemia.
- Major cardiac arrhythmias.
- Or substantial changes in blood pressure.

Source: From Madama V. Pulmonary Function Testing and Cardiopulmonary Stress Testing. *Clifton Park, NY: Delmar Cengage Learning; 1998:435; Zavala DC.* Manual on Exercise Testing: A Training Handbook. *Iowa City, IA: Press of the University of Iowa; 1986:30–32.*

CRITERIA FOR PATIENT INCLUSION

Patients should be placed in a pulmonary rehab program for many subjective reasons. However,

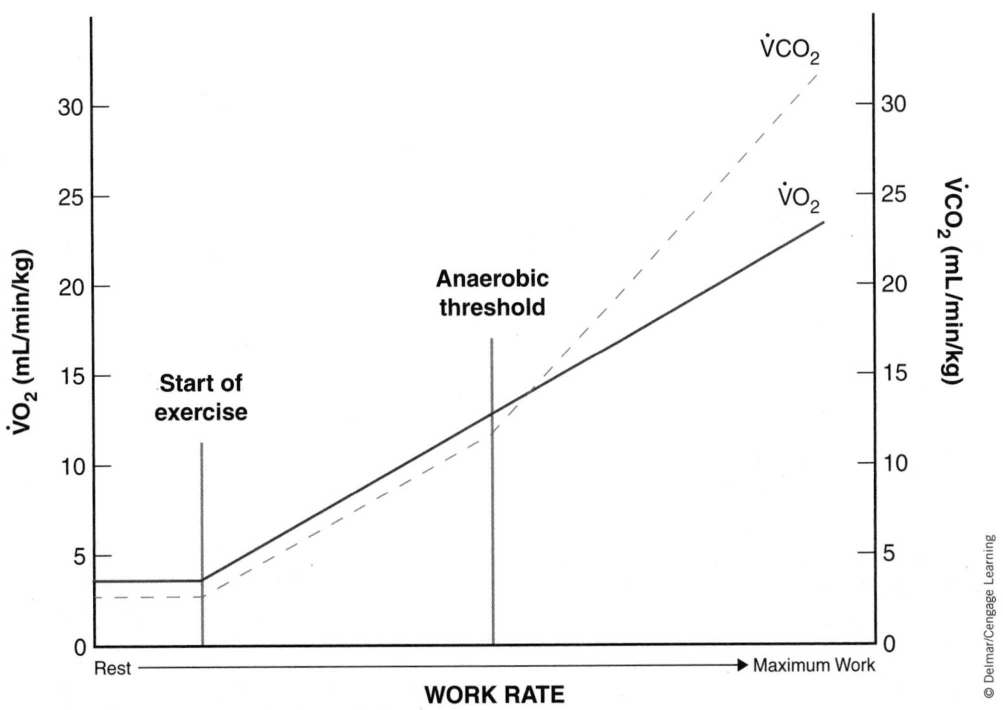

FIGURE 36-2 Key changes in metabolic parameters, namely oxygen consumption ($\dot{V}O_2$) and carbon dioxide production ($\dot{V}CO_2$), take place during exercise. Observe what occurs when the anaerobic threshold is reached.

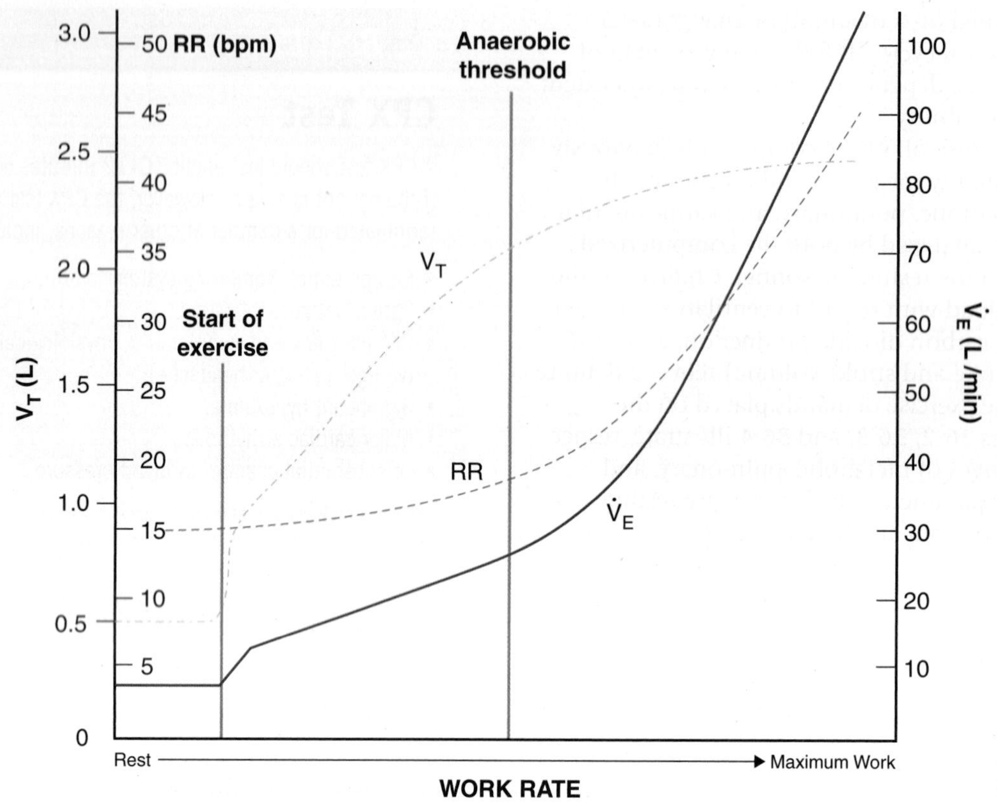

FIGURE 36-3 Key changes in pulmonary parameters, such as respiratory rate (RR), tidal volume (V_T), and minute ventilation ($\dot{V}_E$), occur during exercise.

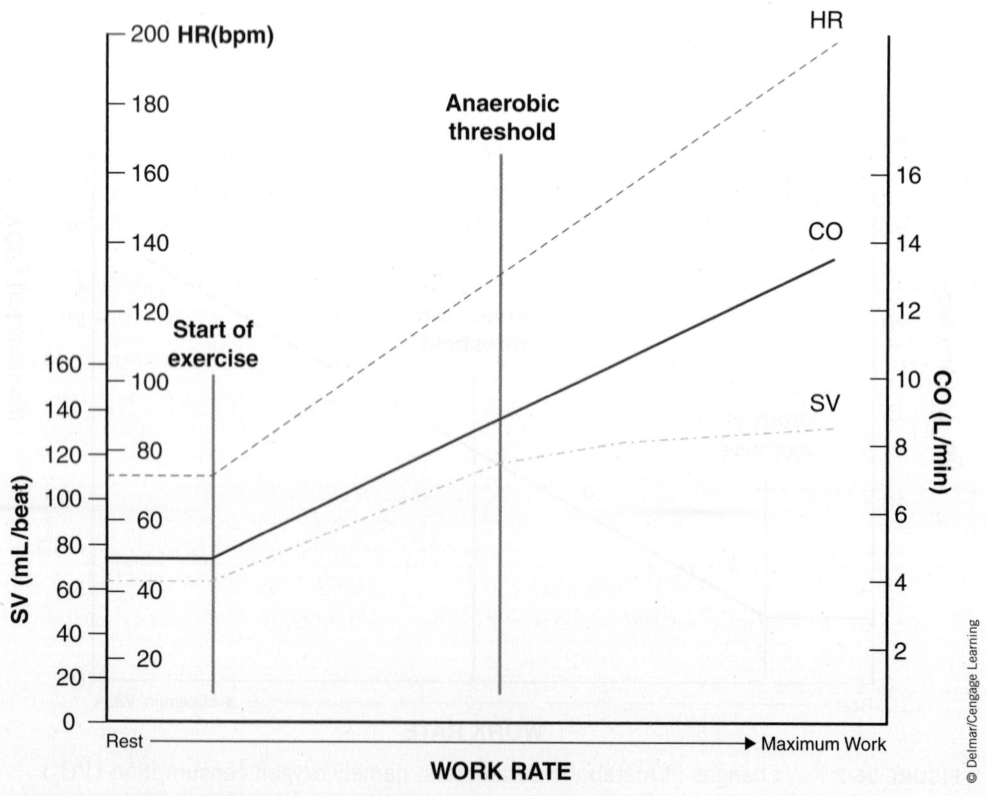

FIGURE 36-4 Key changes in cardiovascular parameters, including heart rate (HR), stroke volume (SV), and cardiac output (CO), occur during exercise.

TABLE 36-2 **Effects of poor physical conditioning, pulmonary disorders, and cardiovascular disorders on stress-testing parameters**

Parameters at Maximum Exercise	Poor Conditioning*	Pulmonary Disorders*	Cardiovascular Disorders*
$\dot{V}O_{2max}$	Low	Low	Low
METs	Low	Low	Low
$\dot{V}_{Emax}$	Low	High	Low
O_2 saturation	Normal	Low	Normal
V_D/V_T	Normal	Normal or high	Normal
HR_{max}/workload	High	Normal	High (with corresponding ECG arrhythmias)
O_2 pulse	Normal	Normal	Low

**Low, measured value is less than normal; high, measured value is greater than normal; normal, measured value is within the normal range.*

objective criteria are more reliable and more useful in substantiating the benefits and value of pulmonary rehabilitation and physical reconditioning. For inclusion in a pulmonary rehabilitation program, patients with primary respiratory limitation to exercise should fulfill one of the following criteria:

- Demonstrate a respiratory limitation to exercise that results in termination of exercise stress testing at a level of <75% of the predicted $\dot{V}O_{2max}$
- Demonstrate significant, irreversible airway obstruction with an $FEV_1 < 2.0$ L or an FEV_1/FVC ($FEV_{1\%}$) < 60%
- Show significant restrictive lung disease with a total lung capacity (TLC) <80% of predicted value and a single-breath carbon monoxide diffusing capacity (DL_{CO}) of <80% of predicted
- Show pulmonary vascular disease where the DL_{CO} using the single-breath method is <80% of predicted value or exercise is limited to <75% of the predicted $\dot{V}O_{2max}$

Use of this type of criteria in the patient selection process ensures patient safety during exercise sessions and provides a degree of objectivity when tracking patient progress or when determining patient outcomes.

CRITERIA FOR PATIENT EXCLUSION

Objective criteria are also useful in excluding patients from pulmonary rehabilitation. A patient who exhibits one of the following criteria is excluded:

- Does not fulfill the criteria for inclusion.
- Has a significant cardiovascular component to exercise limitation (excluding patients with pulmonary vascular disease).
- Demonstrates an adverse cardiovascular response to exercise, such as major arrhythmia or significant change in blood pressure and requires cardiovascular monitoring during rehabilitation.

Exclusionary criteria differentiate between primary cardiac and pulmonary defects and dysfunction. They also help ensure patient safety and that only patients who can benefit from the program are selected to participate.

SPECIFIC PATIENT CONDITIONS

After proper testing and evaluation, patients are prescribed by their physician to attend pulmonary rehabilitation on either an inpatient or an outpatient basis. Although any chronic pulmonary patient may meet the inclusionary criteria, some specific conditions appear to be more appropriate than others for pulmonary rehabilitation and physical reconditioning. These conditions may be categorized as follows:

- *Chronic obstructive pulmonary diseases.* Pulmonary emphysema, chronic bronchitis, bronchial asthma, bronchiectasis, cystic fibrosis
- *Restrictive lung diseases.* Sarcoidosis, pulmonary fibrosis, kyphoscoliosis, occupational lung diseases (pneumoconioses), adult respiratory distress syndrome (ARDS), obesity, poliomyelitis
- *Atypical conditions.* Lung resection, lung transplantation, pulmonary vascular disease, obstructive sleep apnea (OSA)

Of special interest is the group of patients with nonsurgical obstructive sleep apnea (OSA) who may meet the parameters for and benefit from pulmonary rehabilitation. Studies have suggested that these patients have significantly improved after having

CASE STUDY 36-1

M. M. is a 66-year-old white male diagnosed with chronic obstructive pulmonary disease who becomes very dyspneic with moderate physical activity. His expiratory flow rates show no improvement after bronchodilation. No hypoxemia is evident at rest. The indications for an exercise study were to determine whether cardiac or pulmonary factors limited patient activity and to evaluate the level of physical fitness so that a safe and effective reconditioning program can be prescribed.

A CPX test was performed using a cycle ergometer. The total duration of the test was 6 minutes; the test was terminated because of dyspnea and fatigue. The results showed a $\dot{V}O_{2max}$ of 40% of predicted value. The anaerobic threshold was reached after 4 minutes, and the maximum METs was 3.6. In addition, oxygen saturation dropped from 94% to 86%, and the respiratory rate at the end of the study was 40, with a reduction in the respiratory reserve. The heart rate reserve was within normal limits, the peak heart rate was 93% of the maximum predicted heart rate, and blood pressure rose throughout the test. The heart rate at 65% of VO_{2max} was 116 beats per minute (bpm). The ECG showed no major arrhythmias or ST-T wave changes.

These results demonstrated that the limiting factor to physical activity was pulmonary disease with significant physical deconditioning. This patient was referred to a pulmonary rehabilitation program with a specific exercise prescription.

Questions

1. Did this patient meet the criteria for inclusion in a pulmonary rehabilitation program? Why?
2. Why should supplemental oxygen be prescribed for this patient during exercise?
3. What target heart rate should be prescribed for this patient during exercise, and why is it a safe and effective value?

completed a program focusing on weight loss (nutrition and exercise) and sleep position training. Other aspects of pulmonary rehabilitation—including increased contact with health care providers, behavior modification, and compliance with prescribed therapeutic regimens—should also prove helpful in the overall management of sleep apnea syndrome.[11]

Note: Most of the current knowledge of physical reconditioning has been obtained from patients with the intrinsic lung diseases identified here. Very few data exist regarding rehabilitation and reconditioning in patients with degenerative neuromuscular diseases such as amyotrophic lateral sclerosis (ALS), multiple sclerosis, or other similar conditions with symptomatic pump failure. Physical training and exercise may worsen, not improve, the overall condition of these patients. Breathing retraining may help as long it does not place an extra workload or burden on already weakened respiratory muscles. It is believed that ventilatory assistance and rest may be more beneficial to the patient with pump failure than exercise. More research is required in this area.[12]

Program Formats

Pulmonary rehabilitation may be conducted in several formats: closed-format, open-format, individual, and group programs.

CLOSED-FORMAT PROGRAMS

The *closed format* is more traditional than the open format. It uses a set period of time with a designated number of class sessions and a specific end date. Sessions may be conducted once, twice, or three times a week for anywhere from 6 to 16 weeks. Closed-format programs are usually introductory in nature; they address the key concepts of breathing retraining, physical conditioning, ADLs, administration of medications, use of respiratory home care, and aspects of a healthy lifestyle. At the program's conclusion, patients are instructed to continue individually the breathing and exercise routines they learned in the program. Follow-up may be standard for the program, or it may simply depend on each patient's condition and ability to comply with the exercise prescription.

OPEN-FORMAT PROGRAMS

Open-format programs, on the other hand, have no designated number of class sessions or specific end dates. Patients continue in the program and progress at their own pace until they achieve specific objectives and attain prescribed performance levels. These programs are ongoing, and participants meet regularly.

Practitioners should not refer to this type of rehabilitation as a maintenance program because Medicare and other payors do not reimburse for maintenance programs. According to Medicare, therapy services are covered only when performed with the expectation of restoring the level of function lost or reduced. Therapy performed repetitively to maintain a level of function is not eligible for reimbursement. Maintenance begins either when the therapeutic goals of a treatment plan have been achieved or when no additional progress is expected. It consists of activities that preserve a patient's level of function and prevent regression.[13] Once a patient is at a maintenance level, Medicare perceives that rehabilitation is no longer necessary. Patients who are in continual need of rehabilitation, however, are eligible for reimbursement. Most patients who continue pulmonary rehabilitation on a maintenance basis often pay a small out-of-pocket fee for each session attended.

Open-format programs recognize the continual need for physical reconditioning. In the absence of full recovery, chronic lung patients, whose conditions almost always seem to fluctuate, are in perpetual need of some type of pulmonary rehabilitation. Table 36-3 examines the advantages and disadvantages of open-format and closed-format programs.

INDIVIDUAL SESSIONS

Pulmonary rehabilitation may be conducted individually or within a group. *Individual sessions*, which may be conducted in the hospital, at the patient's home, or at the rehab facility, require less equipment and personnel than do group sessions. The individual program is geared specifically to each patient's condition and needs, making implementation both easier and more effective than a group program.

Individual programs are especially effective for ventilator-dependent patients who are being weaned from ventilatory support or for those with neurological disorders. This type of program is also helpful to patients with spinal cord injuries who are learning to breathe on their own. One type of breathing retraining method takes the form of *glossopharyngeal*, or *frog, breathing*. This technique enables patients to remain off ventilatory support for minutes to hours at a time. RTs involved in this type of rehabilitation must properly teach and coach these patients to gulp or swallow air into the lungs using their tongue, pharynx, and larynx. The breathing motion is similar to that observed in frogs. Glossopharyngeal breathing also allows for some increase in vital capacity and a more forceful cough, resulting in more effective removal of secretions and less frequent infections.[14]

Individualized programs may be implemented in the patient's home. Homebound patients include:

- Those with severe chronic pulmonary disease.
- Ventilator-dependent patients.
- Individuals who are so debilitated that out-of-house activities are simply out of the question.

TABLE 36-3 **Advantages and disadvantages of open-format and closed-format pulmonary rehabilitation programs**

Format	Advantages	Disadvantages
Open	Provides ongoing rehabilitative therapy and services.	Patients do not know when program will end.
	Allows for achievement of personal rehabilitation objectives.	Need or reimbursement for program may be questioned.
	Allows personal performance goals or targets to be attained.	May exhaust limits of available resources.
	Allows patients to proceed at their own pace and level of comfort.	Patients may become bored with routine of program.
	Allows patients to drop or continue program on an as-needed basis	
	Allows for continual reinforcement of key concepts.	
Closed	Definite time frame for program is established.	May not allow enough time for achievement of rehabilitation objectives.
	Patients know what to expect from program.	May not allow enough time for performance goals to be attained.
	Allows for predictable budgeting and use of resources.	Program may be too dilute or too concentrated for patients' needs.
	Establishes an introduction or orientation to rehabilitation.	May not allow for patients to proceed at their own pace or level of comfort.
	At completion, patients may continue with reconditioning on their own or in an open-format program.	

Home programs can be designed to cover the same material and allow for similar breathing retraining and physical reconditioning as programs conducted at hospitals or outpatient centers. There is, however, more emphasis on patient and family education, home care equipment use, and infection control measures. Programs that include practitioner home visits on a regular basis may contribute significantly to a patient's recovery both physically and psychologically, resulting in increased physical ability, self-confidence, and self-esteem, as well as fewer hospitalizations.[15] Ultimately, patients may progress enough to be able to continue their reconditioning as an outpatient.

Patients who live in a rural area or who have transportation difficulties can also benefit from individual programs. In these cases, one or two sessions can be given to initiate the reconditioning process. These sessions usually include breathing retraining and an exercise prescription to gradually enhance the physical condition of the patient. Follow-up and reinforcement of principles are done on an as-needed basis, often depending on the patient's ability to obtain transportation.

GROUP SESSIONS

Group sessions involve classes of 4–12 patients, depending on space, equipment, personnel, and the number of patients who qualify. Group programs are more cost-effective than individual sessions. Many patients attend rehabilitation programs more for psychosocial than for physical reasons. Group support usually enhances the progress of people coping with any physical problem. Members of the group tend to strengthen and sustain each other because of their common difficulties, in this case, a chronic respiratory disease with dyspnea resulting from some degree of pulmonary impairment. Table 36-4 lists the major advantages and disadvantages of group and individual rehabilitation.

TABLE 36-4 **Advantages and disadvantages of individual and group pulmonary rehabilitation programs**

Type of Session	Advantages	Disadvantages
Individual	Easy to implement and follow patient's progress.	Is not the most efficient use of available resources.
	Allows for personalized instruction and therapy.	May require extensive travel to patient's home.
	Focuses on patient's specific rehabilitation objectives.	Allows no social interaction with other patients.
	Meets patient's specific needs in terms of time and travel.	Fewer patients are cared for on a daily or weekly basis.
	Allows rehabilitation to be delivered in the home setting.	May pose scheduling difficulties.
	Is better than group for patients being weaned or learning specialized breathing techniques.	May result in decreased revenue for department or facility.
	May be the only way a program can be implemented.	
	Reduces chance of spread of infection.	
Group	Allows for more efficient use of available resources.	More difficult to tailor program to meet individual needs.
	Allows for social interaction between patients.	Requires a central location and adequate space.
	Enhances learning and reconditioning by offering moral support.	Depending on group size, more equipment may be needed.
	More patients can be rehabilitated on a daily or weekly basis.	Scheduling difficulties may occur with larger groups.
	Can increase revenue basis for department or facility.	More chance for spread of infection.

Program Components

The key elements of designing a pulmonary rehabilitation program are:

- Location.
- Space.
- Equipment.
- Supplies.
- Personnel.
- Resources.

These are all dependent on the program design and format. Group sessions, conducted in either closed- or open-format, require substantially more space and equipment than do individual sessions. Personnel requirements depend on the number of patients, regardless of design or format, and on how detailed the sessions are.

LOCATION

Location is the first concern. Pulmonary rehabilitation can be conducted on either an inpatient or an outpatient basis. Because inpatient pulmonary rehabilitation is conducted in the hospital or facility, location is not a concern. However, most pulmonary rehabilitation is implemented on an outpatient basis, with patients visiting the facility (hospital or center) weekly or more often.

Facilities that offer outpatient pulmonary rehabilitation must address patient needs in terms of accessibility, parking, and mass transit.

- A central location or one close to major access roads and mass transportation makes it relatively easy for patients to attend regularly scheduled sessions.
- Facilities must also be wheelchair accessible with ramps and elevators.
- The facility should be not too far away, be near mass transportation, and have parking space that is not too expensive or too far from the building.

To overcome parking problems, a number of options are available.

- Where possible, parking should be adjacent to the facility's entrance.
- If parking near the entrance is not feasible, valet parking might be considered.
- The services of any available community or hospital-based coach service could be employed.

Valet parking or the use of a community coach or van transportation service not only attends to patients' transportation needs but can also be used in marketing and advertising the program.

SPACE

Facilities must have enough space to comfortably accommodate patient seating and physical activities and to ensure adequate room for equipment and the storage of supplies. If the only available space for a rehabilitation program is in the basement of a building, special care should be taken that it is free of mold and mildew. The ideal facility has:

- A ground floor area.
- A patient reception area or waiting room with television or music.
- A secured area for coats and belongings.
- An office where appointments are made and records are kept.
- A classroom with audiovisual aids.
- An exercise area.
- An equipment and supply storage space.
- Adequate ventilation.
- Windows and wall mirrors for a sense of openness and roominess, reducing any claustrophobic sensations.
- Restrooms. Having separate shower rooms for males and females, with lockers for personal effects, is ideal but not necessary.

The amount of actual space, in terms of square footage, depends on available space, projected class size, and budgetary and financial considerations. For an average class of 8–12 patients, a classroom that is 12 feet by 16 feet (192 square feet) is adequate, and an exercise area approximately twice that size (up to 400 square feet) should suffice.

EQUIPMENT

The equipment used depends on:

- The program or facility's operating budget.
- Available space.
- Patient numbers.
- The focus and extent of the reconditioning program.

Patient assessment and evaluation during and after physical exercise are imperative. Most patient monitoring is accomplished through pulse oximetry, simple spirometry, and blood pressure determinations. For this type of monitoring, any standard pulse oximeter with finger and ear probes, basic spirometer, and sphygmomanometer with stethoscope suffices. The number of oximeters, spirometers, and blood pressure cuffs needed depends on how many patients are scheduled for any one session and on how many practitioners are going to be doing the monitoring. The minimum requirements are one oximeter, one spirometer, and one blood pressure cuff.

Patients must be able to use a combination of aerobic or isotonic and isokinetic exercise routines to enhance the strength and stamina of the arms and legs. The exercise equipment for rehabilitation classes should be varied and durable, yet affordable. Programs that include combinations of the following are recommended:

- Standard exercycles or bicycle ergometers (at least one for every two patients) with adjustable seat, tension control, and speedometer/odometer (Some cycles also come equipped with pulse monitoring systems.)
- Automated treadmill with timer and speed and elevation controls (at least one for every two patients)
- One or two rowing machines with timer and counter
- One or two low-impact stepping units or stair simulators with timer and counter
- Four arm ergometers with accompanying worktables
- One or two wall pulley units with adjustable weights
- Several sets of freehand weights ranging from 1- to 10-pound (0.5–4.5 k)
- Two to four floor mats for floor exercises

In addition, the program should have the following medical equipment:

- Oxygen concentrator and/or portable oxygen cylinders with regulators, carts, and/or carrying packs for patient use (number dependent on class size and patient need)
- At least one compressor/nebulizer unit

Where space and cost are considerations, a floor pedal exerciser such as the Pedlar (Battle Creek Equipment) is an option to more expensive exercycles. This device is simple and inexpensive, and it allows patients to pedal easily and safely from any sitting chair. It comes equipped with a tension control but does not have any speedometer or odometer. It can also be used as an arm ergometer if placed on a desk or table. Although a floor pedal unit can be used as an alternative for cycling at pulmonary rehabilitation facilities, any standard exercycle with adjustable seat, odometer, speedometer, and tension control is much more practical and useful, given the patient performance data it can provide. Floor pedal units are more appropriate for patient purchase and home use.

Other equipment, such as NordicTrack walking and skiing units, Lifecycles, and universal-type gyms, may be too difficult or complicated for patient use in pulmonary rehab. In particular, the total body workouts resulting from this type of equipment require simultaneous arm and leg motion, placing excessive physical demands on most pulmonary patients. The increased demand for oxygen by the affected muscle groups reaches a level that some patients find difficult to support. As a result, dyspnea and fatigue limit the exercise sessions with little or no physical conditioning to show for them.

Many manufacturers currently market a wide variety of exercise apparatus. Battle Creek Equipment, Burdick, Monark, Quinton Instrument, and Precor USA are among the more popular suppliers of exercise and rehabilitation equipment. To obtain a more detailed listing of these manufacturers and their products, refer to one of the many buyers' guides published periodically by professional and trade journals. These guides offer valuable information regarding the exercise equipment available for either program or patient home use.

Besides specific exercise apparatus, other room accessories are helpful:

- Television
- Video cassette/DVD player
- Audio tape/CD player
- Radio
- Wall screen
- Flipchart or chalkboard
- Computer with PowerPoint projector
- Overhead projector
- Wall charts depicting cardiopulmonary anatomy and breathing techniques
- Motivational posters
- File cabinets
- Wall clocks
- Comfortable chairs
- Worktable
- Water cooler
- Refrigerator

When equipment and accessories are not in use, they are best stored in closets adjacent to either the classroom or the exercise area. Only equipment believed to be absolutely essential should be purchased in the beginning of the program, with additional expenditures as needs dictate.

SUPPLIES

Supplies vary from program to program but should include items such as:

- A bag-valve-mask unit.
- Nasal cannulas and oxygen masks.
- Nebulizer sets.
- Bronchodilator medications (in unit-dose and metered-dose form).
- Incentive spirometers.
- Inspiratory resistance breathing devices.

- Mouthpieces.
- Simple refreshments such as cookies and juices.
- Batteries.
- Tissues.
- Cups.
- Patient booklets and handouts.
- Writing pads, pens and other writing utensils.

Supplies can be conveniently stored in closets or supply rooms close to the area where class sessions are held.

PERSONNEL

Any credentialed or licensed respiratory therapist with training and experience in pulmonary rehabilitation should be able to design, organize, and conduct individual and group sessions. The input and involvement of other medical personnel are not only helpful but essential, especially if insurance reimbursement is an issue. Pulmonologists with expertise in pulmonary rehabilitation are best suited for these programs. Experience in performing and interpreting CPX test results is definitely advantageous.

Besides a respiratory therapist and a physician, other personnel who may be involved with the implementation of pulmonary rehabilitation are:

- A nurse with rehab experience.
- A physical therapist.
- An occupational therapist.
- A dietitian.
- A pharmacist.
- A clinical psychologist.
- An office manager.

All members of the team must be familiar with the goals and objectives of the program and have a thorough understanding of pulmonary disorders.

Program Content

A pulmonary rehabilitation session can follow any effective format. A typical group session should be approximately 2 hours long, whereas individual sessions can range from a half hour to an hour. A basic format follows an outline with the following components:

- Review of patient activities since the last session
- Patient education: topic presentation with questions and discussion
- Patient exercise
- Assessment by physician (can be pre- or postexercise)
- Establishment of objectives and activity plan for next session

PATIENT EDUCATION

The patient education portion of a pulmonary rehabilitation program covers topics deemed important to the patient's conditions and needs. Individual patient sessions can follow a topic outline similar to that for groups. Some areas covered are:

- The concept and goals of pulmonary rehabilitation.
- Cardiopulmonary anatomy, physiology, and pathology.
- Breathing techniques.
- Stress management.
- Medications.
- Nutrition.
- Chest physiotherapy.
- ADLs.

Normally, 30–60 minutes of each session can be devoted to patient education. Table 36-5 lists topics that can be covered.

Patient education can take other forms:

- Booklets and handouts help the patient learn. Printed information is available commercially or through the AARC, the American Lung Association, and other health-related organizations. Offer a few well written and descriptive booklets and pamphlets to complement the topics covered.
- Select educational materials on the basis of patient need, relationship to stated objectives, and overall cost to the facility. These materials serve as the "course text" for the program.
- A patient manual or log should also be distributed and used by each patient as both a program syllabus and a record of daily exercise activities performed at home.
- Every new program should begin with an orientation on the concept and goals of pulmonary rehabilitation.
- A patient consent form should be completed and signed by each patient during the initial session. This form should specify the types and frequency of exercise required for each patient, possible complications that may occur, the extent of supervision and monitoring that will take place and by whom, and the anticipated duration of the program. Each patient and a witness should read, date, and sign a consent.

Nicotine intervention, although not an integral part of pulmonary rehab since most enrolled patients are no longer smoking, should be available to patients still addicted to nicotine. Methods of smoking cessation include use of the nicotine patch or nasal spray in conjunction with counseling sessions either

TABLE 36-5 **Topics and issues for a pulmonary rehabilitation program**

Presentation Topic	Key Issues to Be Considered
Cardiopulmonary anatomy and physiology	Structure of the heart and lungs and how they work in supplying the body with oxygen and removing carbon dioxide
Cardiopulmonary pathophysiology	Major differences between obstructive and restrictive lung diseases, with specific examples; an explanation of how chronic lung disease can bring about cardiac dysfunction
Breathing techniques and retraining	Diaphragmatic and pursed-lip breathing techniques, inspiratory resistance breathing, basal expansion exercises, and sustained maximal inhalation through incentive spirometry for patients with restrictive lung disease
Stress management and relaxation	Ways to cope with stress, proper breathing techniques, avoidance of panic breathing, and relaxation methods
Physical reconditioning	Ways to exercise properly to promote agility, strength, and endurance using aerobic and isokinetic techniques and calisthenics
Pharmacology	Major cardiopulmonary medications and their effects on the body; proper use of metered dose and dry powder inhalers
Respiratory home care	Use of oxygen in the home; use of other respiratory care devices including small-volume nebulizers and patient monitoring systems
Chest physiotherapy	Postural drainage positions and techniques for percussion, vibration, coughing, and bronchial hygiene, including use of Flutter device and other similar breathing adjuncts
Nutrition and diet	Key elements of good nutrition and weight control with focus on ways of avoiding dyspnea after eating, the right food groups to eat, and trouble foods to avoid
Activities of daily living (ADLs)	Vocational counseling focusing on activities that promote a more active, productive life

individually or in groups, cold turkey, gradual weaning, use of medications, and hypnotism. Preferably, patients enroll in and complete a nicotine intervention program before they enroll in pulmonary rehabilitation.

Each session should begin with a welcoming remark followed by the patients' comments on their progress. The formal presentation can then be delivered and followed by patient questions and discussion. Lectures should focus on and augment or explain material covered in any booklets used in the program. Audiovisuals, charts, demonstrations, and appropriate handout materials should be used to increase the impact of the presentation.

The final session of any program should be reserved for graduation, with:

- Awarding of certificates.
- Summary of all concepts and techniques covered.
- Plans for continuing the rehabilitative process.
- Program evaluation.
- An assessment of patient outcomes.

PATIENT EXERCISES

To physically recondition patients and increase their exercise tolerance, the following goals need to be accomplished:

- Overall oxygen utilization must be improved.
- Essential muscle groups must be strengthened.
- The cardiovascular response to exercise must be enhanced.

Achieving these goals requires that patient exercises be varied, focused, and performed during every class session and regularly at home. In addition, three principles of exercise training must be followed to ensure the desired results: specificity of training, overload, and reversibility.[16]

- *Specificity of training* is founded on observations that programs can be designed to achieve specific goals and objectives and that exercising muscles is beneficial only to the targeted group. In other words, specific muscles or groups of muscles must be targeted to achieve beneficial results.[12]

Age-Specific Competency

Communicating with Elderly and Pediatric Patients

Many elderly chronic pulmonary patients have difficultly hearing.

- Speak slowly and clearly, but not excessively loudly.
- Avoid using complicated terms.
- Repeat information as necessary.
- Use audiovisuals.
- Handouts are useful, but avoid using blues with greens or reds with oranges on any printed materials. Elderly patients may have difficulty distinguishing colors in these combinations. Vivid contrasts on any handouts are definitely better.

For pediatric patients in pulmonary rehabilitation:

- Try to keep activities brief and interesting. Young patients usually have a short attention span.
- Avoid using complicated or confusing terminology.
- Use games and projects to get your point across.
- Encourage participation in each session.

Best Practice

Fostering Compliance

When conducting a session, always maintain eye contact with members of the group, and occasionally ask questions to ensure that the group is following the presentation. Encouraging patients to ask questions and to become involved in any discussion fosters participation. Belief in the rehabilitation process must also be established. Participants must feel an air of trust between practitioner and patient. Patients are more willing to comply with the rigors of the program if they perceive any tangible benefits and the dedication of the rehabilitation team. Their compliance is essential if the program is to have any hope of success.

- The principle of *overload* contends that muscles must be forced or pushed beyond a certain level of activity to produce a training effect.
- The principle of *reversibility*, or **detraining effect**, implies that the benefits of exercise are transient and persist only as long as exercise is continued. Patients who stop exercising quickly lose any exercise-induced changes or benefits.[16]

Specific exercises used in pulmonary rehabilitation can be grouped into two major categories: breathing retraining and physical reconditioning.

Breathing Retraining. Breathing retraining techniques for both chronic obstructive and restrictive lung patients include specific methods, such as:

- Diaphragmatic breathing with pursed lips.
- Incentive spirometry.
- Inspiratory or flow-resistive breathing.
- Threshold loading.

These techniques can produce profound benefits by helping patients control their breathing, improve ventilatory muscle endurance and strength, and reduce the work of breathing and dyspnea.

Diaphragmatic breathing with pursed lips is considered to be the cornerstone of breathing retraining for COPD patients in pulmonary rehabilitation. Pursed-lip breathing (PLB) comes naturally to many patients. By adjusting the size of the orifice created by their lips, patients can vary the degree to which they can retard expiration. Retarding expiration:

- Slows their respiratory rate.
- Reduces the work of breathing.
- Creates a back pressure that prevents collapse of the smaller airways.
- Lessens the probability of air trapping.
- Promotes more effective ventilation.

Diaphragmatic breathing, on the other hand, is more difficult to master. Patients must practice this technique daily, first in a recumbent position and then in sitting, standing, and walking positions. The time spent on diaphragmatic breathing depends on the patient's available time. Practice time can range from 15 to 30 minutes a day and, in most instances, can be performed in conjunction with other types of breathing exercises. It may take 6–8 weeks before some patients breathe diaphragmatically, but the results are worth it, with reduced work of breathing, greater tidal volume, and more effective ventilation.

Incentive spirometry using any currently available disposable device, is far more beneficial in treating restrictive lung disease than COPD. Patients with sarcoidosis, pulmonary fibrosis, or any occupational lung disease should be considered candidates for this type of breathing exercise. Breathing retraining employing sustained maximal inspiration with an incentive spirometer, should be performed for up to 15 minutes, three or four times a day on a regular basis to be effective.

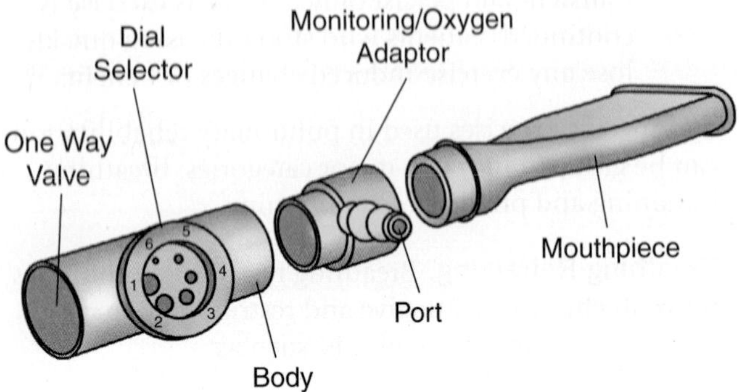

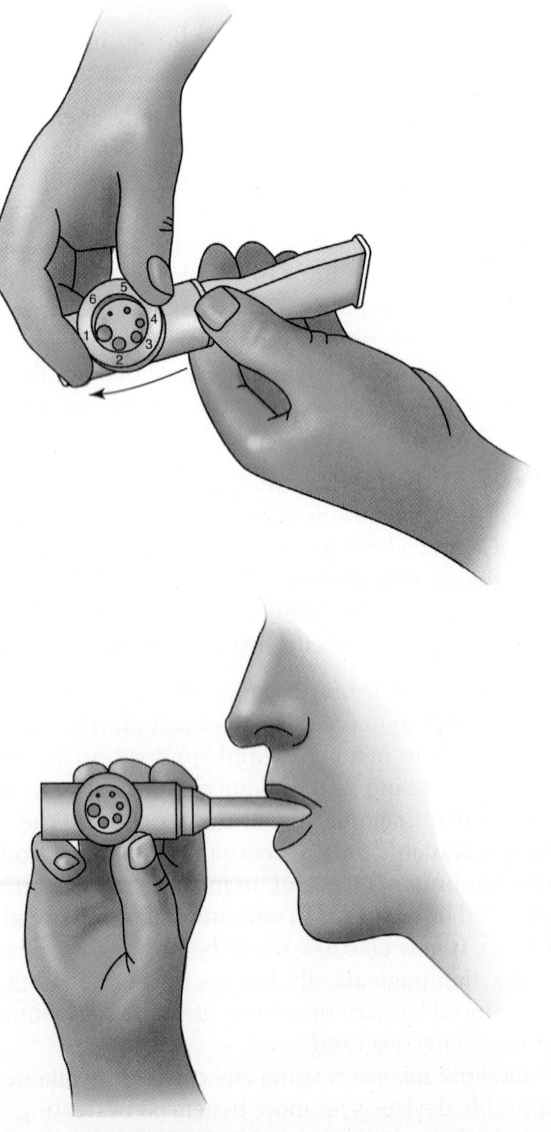

FIGURE 36-5 PFlex® device for inspiratory resistive breathing exercises.

Courtesy of Philips Respironics, Pittsburgh, Pennsylvania

Respiratory dysfunction associated with COPD can be managed *with inspiratory muscle training* (IMT), using either inspiratory or flow-resistive breathing or threshold loading. Inspiratory or flow-resistive breathing is accomplished with a device such as the PFlex illustrated in Figure 36-5. This device uses decreasing hole sizes numbered 1–6. These hole sizes set the inspiratory training load as long as rate, tidal volume, and inspiratory time remain constant. Training begins at hole size number 1 for up to 30 minutes a day. When training at this level is easily tolerated, patients proceed to hole size number 2, and so on until they reach their highest inspiratory resistance level.

Threshold loading is achieved with the Threshold IMT device, shown in Figure 36-6. This apparatus uses a spring-loaded valve mechanism to provide a consistent inspiratory pressure training load, independent of inspiratory flow rate. The breathing pattern is not as critically important as with inspiratory resistive breathing.[10] The manufacturer recommends that the training load be set at approximately 30% of the patient's maximal inspiratory pressure (PI_{max}) and that training sessions increase gradually from 10–15 minutes a day to 20–30 minutes a day.

Other devices used in pulmonary rehabilitation are positive expiratory pressure (PEP) units or devices such

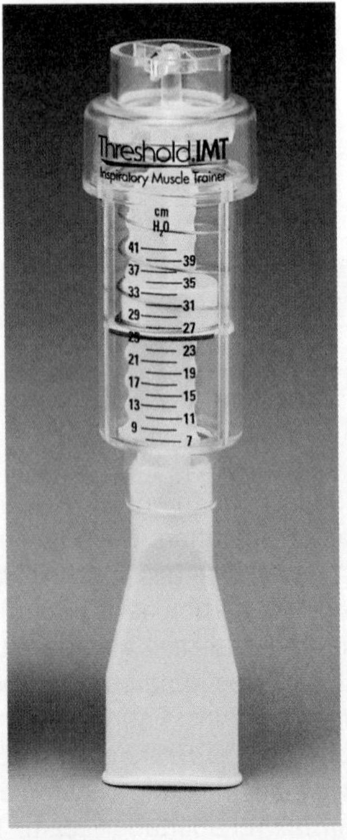

FIGURE 36-6 Threshold® IMT device for inspiratory resistive breathing exercises.

Courtesy of Philips Respironics, Pittsburgh, Pennsylvania

as the Flutter valve that produces an oscillating PEP and Acapella devices to assist patients with the expectoration of secretions. These units are discussed in more detail in the Chapter 23 that deals with pulmonary hygiene.

The results of breathing techniques and retraining in pulmonary rehabilitation have been favorable. In one study, COPD patients who received breathing retraining along with physical reconditioning exercises did better than a group receiving breathing retraining only or a group who performed no exercises at all.[17] Table 36-6 examines the major breathing techniques used in pulmonary rehabilitation programs.

Although it seems logical that increases in strength and endurance following ventilatory muscle training should enhance respiratory muscle function, it appears unlikely that this type of training has any impact on overall physical exercise performance. In fact, the current consensus downplays the overall importance and impact of breathing retraining during pulmonary rehabilitation. The emphasis is on exercise and physical reconditioning. Research has demonstrated that exercising peripheral muscles through low-level intensity conditioning and training helps to increase exercise tolerance and breathlessness in COPD patients.[18] However, breathing retraining is essential and important for a patient's ability to cope with and handle increased ventilatory loads resulting from any acute disease exacerbations.[12]

Physical Reconditioning. The second category of exercises, physical reconditioning, consists of four basic types: aerobic or isotonic conditioning,

TABLE 36-6 **Types of breathing techniques for pulmonary rehabilitation**

Technique/ Exercise	Focus or Rationale	Applications
Pursed-lip breathing	To slow rate of breathing while creating back-pressure to maintain airway patency, thereby preventing airway collapse and air trapping. Pursed lips or cupped hands can be used to retard expiratory airflow.	Used during walking or any type of physical activity, especially stair climbing, bending, and lifting. Most effective in patients with COPD and during panic breathing.
Diaphragmatic breathing (abdominal breathing)	Abdominal muscles promote diaphragmatic excursions, resulting in more effective ventilation and reducing use of accessory muscles.	Constant use is advised to ensure an adequate level of ventilation. Helpful in panic breathing. Most effective in COPD patients.
Segmental breathing	Promotes and maintains chest wall mobility by having patients breathe against hand pressure applied over localized areas of the chest wall.	Useful after thoracic or abdominal surgery, and for neurological and musculoskeletal conditions, asthma, and COPD.
Inspiratory resistance (flow resistance)	A flow-resistive device uses inspiratory load to strengthen ventilatory muscles, promoting ventilatory muscle endurance.	Improves ventilatory muscle endurance in patients with COPD.
Threshold loading	A threshold-loading device uses inspiratory pressure as a prescribed load to strengthen ventilatory muscles, promoting ventilatory muscle endurance.	Improves ventilatory muscle endurance in patients with COPD.
Incentive spirometry (sustained maximal inspiration or SMI)	Inspiratory capacity maneuver with breath-hold at the end of inspiration (sustained maximum inspiration) promotes lung expansion.	Improves overall ventilatory efficiency and effectiveness in patients with restrictive lung disease or conditions.
Glossopharyngeal breathing (frog breathing)	Use of glossopharyngeal muscles promotes capture and swallowing of air, resulting in some increase in vital capacity.	Useful for ventilator-dependent or spinal cord injury patients who are able to come off ventilatory support for brief periods. This is both an exercise and a breathing technique.

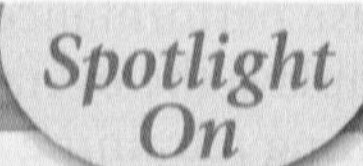

Breathing Retraining

Although not exactly a method for breathing retraining, the Flutter device (Axcan Scandipharm, Inc. Birmingham, Alabama) is effective in the removal of mucus from the airways of patients with cystic fibrosis, chronic bronchitis, and bronchiectasis. It is a small, handheld, pipelike device, made out of hard plastic, containing a small stainless steel ball. As the patient exhales into the unit, this steel ball moves up and down, producing oscillations in expiratory pressure and airflow. This movement creates a fluttering sensation and vibrations in the airway. The frequency of these oscillations ranges between 6 and 20 Hz, corresponding to the range of human pulmonary resonance frequencies. In principle, the Flutter device can vibrate the airways, intermittently increase endobronchial pressure, and accelerate expiratory airflow. Thus it facilitates the upward movement of mucus and its expectoration.

Another technique is positive expiratory pressure (PEP) therapy using the TheraPEP (DHD Healthcare, Wampsville, NY). This device has a highly visible pressure indicator with six fixed orifice options providing different flow resistance levels. According to the manufacturer, TheraPEP enables COPD patients to master PEP therapy quickly, resulting in improved airway opening, enhanced clearance of secretions, and reduced need for postural drainage.

Acapella (Smiths Medical, Dublin, OH), still another device for pediatric and adult patients, is available in several models, including one that allows concomitant delivery of an aerosolized medication. This device also assists in secretion removal and breathing retraining.

These three therapeutic modalities actually fall under chest physiotherapy and bronchial hygiene, but, since they involve breathing maneuvers, they have been covered here.

isokinetic exercises, isometric exercises, and calisthenics.

- Exercises that combine low resistance or low tension with movement or repetition over a long duration overload enzymes of the tricarboxylic acid cycle (TCA, or Krebs, cycle) and electron transport system, resulting in increased endurance and stamina. This is *aerobic or isotonic conditioning*. Walking on level ground and cycling without tension are excellent ways to achieve this type of conditioning.
- Conversely, exercises that combine high resistance or high tension with movement or repetition over a short duration are *isokinetic* and produce increased muscle tone and strength. Cycling with tension applied is one example of an isokinetic activity.
- *Isometric exercises* employ tension with muscle contraction but without any movement of joints or limbs. Pressing two hands together with periods of rest produces the isometric effect, resulting in an increase in muscle tone and strength.
- *Calisthenics*, which encompass stretching and bending exercises, enable patients to develop flexibility and gracefulness in movement.[12]

Table 36-7 lists the focus and specific examples of these physical conditioning exercises.

Allot 15–45 minutes for group or individual exercises, depending on patients' ability, available equipment, and group size. Exercise sessions should gradually increase in duration and intensity as the program progresses. Music with a lively beat to which patients can exercise is recommended. A typical group exercise session is depicted in Figure 36-7.

Patients should be encouraged to reach their target heart rate during each exercise activity. There appears to be a threshold of exercise activity for the induction of training effects beneficial to the muscles and cardiovascular system. This threshold, or target, as determined during the CPX test, represents the heart rate at 50–70% of the $\dot{V}O_{2max}$.[19] Many

Best Practice

Target Heart Rate

To ensure proper physical conditioning during exercise, patients should reach their target heart rates. This target is normally the heart rate at 75% of each patient's maximum oxygen consumption, as determined during the prerehabilitation CPX test. The target heart rate ensures that physical exercise is being conducted safely and properly and that the program will conclude successfully.

TABLE 36-7 **Types of exercises for physical reconditioning**

Type of Exercise	Focus	Examples
Aerobic or isotonic conditioning (movement without resistance or tension)	To increase stamina and endurance, improve cardiovascular status, and increase maximum oxygen consumption	Walking, cycling without tension, running in place, swimming, dancing
Isokinetic techniques (movement with resistance or tension)	To increase muscle strength and tone for both upper and lower body	Cycling with tension, walking with weights, weight lifting
Isometric exercises (resistance or tension without movement)	To increase muscle strength and tone	Pressing hands together, pushing down on floor with feet, pushing against wall or other immovable object
Calisthenics (stretching and bending)	To increase flexibility, agility, and strength	Modified and alternate toe touching, lateral bending and stretching, arm and leg lifts, controlled body movements, such as Tai Chi

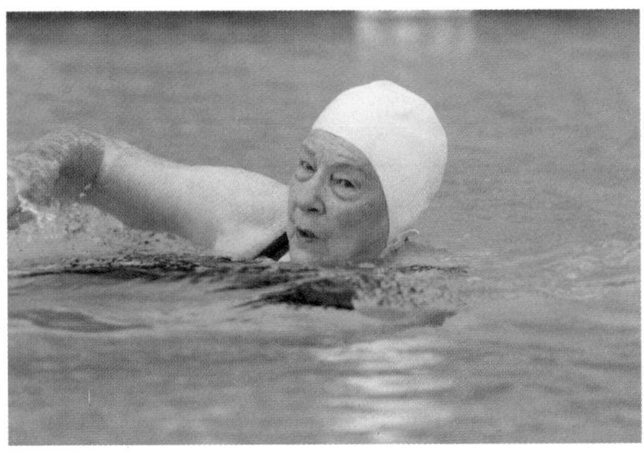

(A)

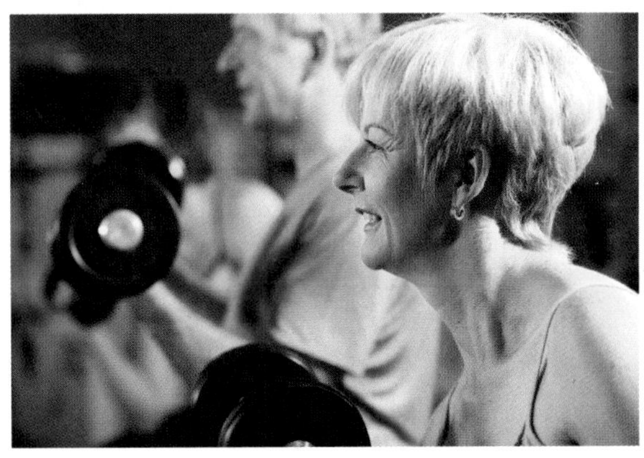

(B)

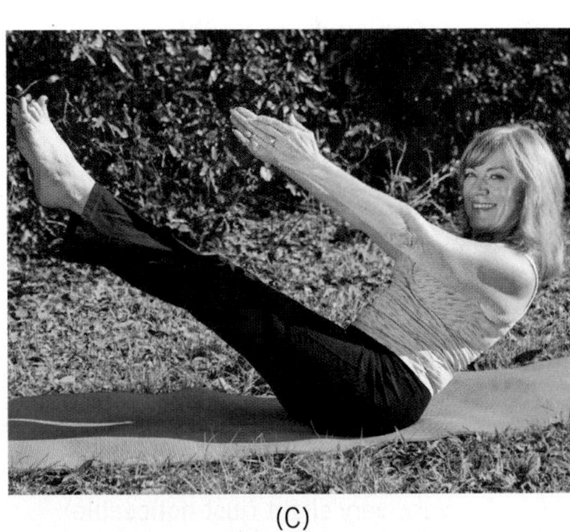

(C)

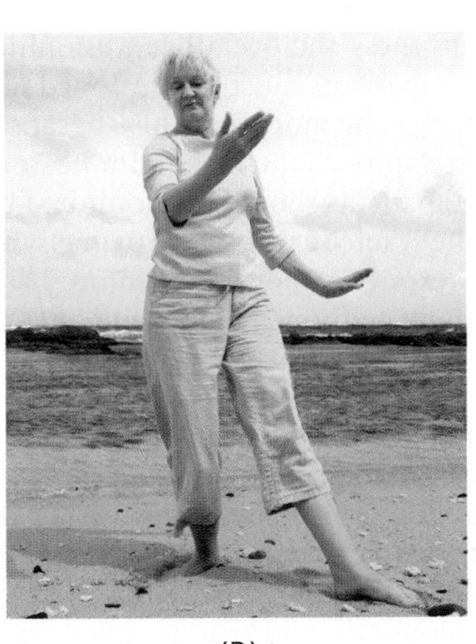

(D)

FIGURE 36-7 Exercise is an important part of pulmonary rehabilitation: (A) Aerobic exercise can be achieved by swimming. (B) Weight training increases muscle strength and tone. (C) Isometric exercises also increase strength and tone. (D) Calisthenics increases flexibility and agility.

(A) © iStock/Lisa Kyle Young, (B) © iStock/kzenon, (C) © iStock/Lisa F. Young, (D) ©iStock/Ashok Rodrigues

PULMONARY REHABILITATION EXERCISE FORM

Patient Name ______________________ I.D. ________ Physician ______________________

Target Heart Rate ________ Insurance ______________ Therapist ______________________

DATE	PRE-	STEPPER	TREADMILL	ROWING	PULLEYS	BIKE	POST-
SpO_2	____	____	____	____	____	____	____
Pulse	____	____	____	____	____	____	____
B/P	____						____
ACTIVITIES PERFORMED:		____ min	____ min	____ min	____ min	____ min	
		____ steps	____ miles	____ strokes	____ reps	____ miles	
		____ tension	____ speed	____ tension	____ weight	____ tension	
TOTAL TIME: ____							
OTHER ACTIVITIES:						____ speed	

FIGURE 36-8 A patient exercise record to document patient activities and progress during pulmonary rehabilitation.

Courtesy of Lung Diagnostics, Glen Ridge, New Jersey

programs have since found 65%–75% of the $\dot{V}O_{2max}$ to be a safe and effective target because it reflects two-thirds to three-fourths of a patient's maximum capability. When the target heart rate is achieved, cardiovascular fitness and overall conditioning take place. However, patients must be cautioned not to exceed their targets by more than 10% because this level begins to approach the maximum heart rate.

As a result, patients should be monitored before, during, and after exercise with pulse oximetry. Blood pressure, peak expiratory flow rates, and/or basic spirometry can be performed before and after an exercise session. Levels of activity or performance and monitored parameters should be documented in each patient's rehab record. The design of this record may vary from program to program, but the content probably does not. Consistency is ensured by documentation of what was done, of how long each activity lasted, and of each patient's observed and monitored response. The Borg or modified Borg Dyspnea scale can also be used to document a patient's perceived degree of dyspnea during each activity performed, and this should also be noted in the patient's record. An example of a patient attendance and exercise record is presented in Figure 36-8, and the modified Borg Dyspnea Scale is shown in Figure 36-9.

Score	Dyspnea Description
10	Maximal (worst possible you can imagine)
9	Very, very severe
8	
7	Very severe
6	
5	Severe
4	Somewhat severe
3	Moderate
2	Slight
1	Very Slight
0.5	Very, very slight (just noticeable)
0	None at all

FIGURE 36-9 Modified Borg Dyspnea Scale.

Patients are instructed to carry on their exercises at home between sessions or group meetings. The types of physical activities that can be conducted depend on each patient's financial resources, available space at home, and ability to use equipment properly and safely. Most patients can perform breathing exercises, walking activities, and basic calisthenics at home because these activities require little or no equipment. On the days they exercise at home, patients are usually required to perform:

- 3–5 minutes of warm-up calisthenics.
- 15–30 minutes of breathing exercises using an inspiratory resistive device or incentive spirometer.
- 6–12 minutes of walking and cycling with gradual increases in duration and tension.

Walking is recognized as a safe and effective physical conditioning technique requiring only a measured indoor area (outdoor if weather conditions allow). Naturally, a treadmill can also be used, but this requires space and an additional expense. The 12-minute walk is a standard in many rehabilitation programs. It represents a *finite parcel of activity* that most chronic pulmonary patients should be able to perform. Since their physical activity is limited by dyspnea, it is unrealistic to require them to walk for up to an hour or for 2–3 miles, as is required of cardiac patients. Depending on patient condition and ability, a 6-minute walk may be used instead. As pulmonary patients perform a daily 6- or 12-minute walk, they should note the total distance traveled and the number of stops made. (*Note*: Time does not stop if this activity is interrupted for any reason.) As patients improve physically and develop greater levels of endurance and exercise tolerance, they make fewer stops and travel greater distances at a faster pace.

In addition, patients who have a stationary bicycle or a floor pedal unit are prescribed daily *cycling*, which is also possible for most rehab patients. They can use a standard exercycle or a floor pedal unit such as Battle Creek Equipment's Pedlar, which can also be used as an arm ergometer on the table. Most cycles used in the home are inexpensive, and arrangements can be made for delivery and assembly. The cycling usually begins at a minimal level with no tension or resistance and increases gradually each week to a maximum of 30 minutes a day with tension by the end of the program.

If patients are unable to cycle, additional walking or other physical activities, including *swimming and aquatic exercises*, can be recommended. Swimming, however, requires regular access to a swimming pool.

The specific duration for each exercise, as noted in the exercise prescription, can be adjusted on the basis of patient objectives and overall condition. The actual level of performance for each activity, along with physiological responses in terms of heart rate, respiratory rate, and peak flow, should be documented in the daily log or record. Patients must be aware of their target heart rate and how to modify their intensity levels once the target has been reached. Therefore, patients should be instructed on how to determine their pulse rate correctly.

Patients should exercise no more than 5 days each week, including group and home exercise sessions. Two nonconsecutive days of rest each week allow muscles to repair and provide each patient with a respite from the daily physical routine. Patients must also be advised to:

- Premedicate with aerosolized bronchodilators (as prescribed).
- Ensure adequate intake of fluids, electrolytes, and vitamins.
- Stop exercising if they experience angina, constant cough, extreme dyspnea, or excessive diaphoresis.
- Not to exercise if they experience fever, vertigo, or headache.
- Document any untoward reactions to physical activity in the daily record and report them to the attending physician or health care practitioner.

Patients who carry out their prescribed exercise routine regularly will begin to note some overall improvement after a few weeks in the program. As they progress in the program, they become more tolerant to greater levels of exercise intensity and duration. A patient progress report similar to the one in Figure 36-10 should be completed periodically to document patient performance and improvement. These reports should be placed in each patient's rehabilitation record, and a copy should be sent to the referring physician.

To avoid any loss of conditioning or physical benefit, patients must be encouraged not to stop their exercise regimen unless enforced inactivity is medically necessary. This detraining effect, or reversibility, has been observed in patients who discontinue their physical reconditioning routine. Positive results can be lost in a few weeks. To regain what was lost will take almost 2 months through gradual increases in exercise duration and progressive resistance.[12]

NICHOLAS MARTINI PULMONARY CENTER - REHABILITATION PROGRESS REPORT

PATIENT NAME: ____________________

	WEEK # ______ DATE ______	WEEK # ______ DATE ______	WEEK # ______ DATE ______
BIKE:	Duration:____ min ____tension Distance:____ km SpO_2:______ HR:____ Comments:____________	Duration:____ min ____tension Distance:____ km SpO_2:______ HR:____ Comments:____________	Duration:____ min ____tension Distance:____ km SpO_2:______ HR:____ Comments:____________
TREADMILL:	Duration:____ min ____mph Distance:____ miles SpO_2:______ HR:____ Comments:____________	Duration:____ min ____mph Distance:____ miles SpO_2:______ HR:____ Comments:____________	Duration:____ min ____mph Distance:____ miles SpO_2:______ HR:____ Comments:____________
ARM ERGOMETER:	Duration:____ min Revs: ______ SpO_2:______ HR:____ Comments:____________	Duration:____ min Revs: ______ km SpO_2:______ HR:____ Comments:____________	Duration:____ min Revs: ______ km SpO_2:______ HR:____ Comments:____________
OTHER:	P-Flex: Level _____ Time_____ Peakflow: Pre _____ Post _____	P-Flex: Level _____ Time_____ Peakflow: Pre _____ Post _____	P-Flex: Level _____ Time_____ Peakflow: Pre _____ Post _____
COMMENTS:	____________	____________	____________

Therapist: ____________________

M.D.'S COMMENTS: _____Continue as prescribed M.D. SIGNATURE: ____________ DATE: ____________

_____Changes: ____________________

FIGURE 36-10 Pulmonary rehabilitation report form for documenting a patient's activity and progress.

Courtesy of the Nicholas Martini Pulmonary Center, St. Mary's Hospital, Passaic, New Jersey

PATIENT TREATMENT PLAN

The treatment or care plan must be tailored for each patient in the program to achieve individual goals. This plan:

- Aids in monitoring patient progress and confirms that goals and objectives have been met.
- Identifies which patient education topics must be covered, which breathing retraining techniques and exercises are best suited for each patient, and what physical exercises should be promoted in the form of an exercise prescription.

An example of a treatment plan, identifying specific short- and long-term patient objectives, is shown in Figure 36-11.

EXERCISE PRESCRIPTION

A key component of any patient treatment plan is the exercise prescription. The physician or health care practitioner overseeing the medical aspects of the program must complete this plan for each patient before the start of rehabilitation. Integral to an exercise prescription are the following elements:

- *Mode* is the type of physical activity performed by the patient, such as walking, stair climbing, cycling, or weight lifting to increase upper body strength.
- *Duration* depends on a patient's level of fitness. Very deconditioned patients should start with short intervals of exercise, according to their tolerance, with brief rest periods as needed. As

PATIENT THERAPEUTIC OBJECTIVES AND TREATMENT PLAN

Patient ______________________ Patient I.D. ____________
Diagnosis ______________________ Target Heart Rate _______
Physician ______________________ Date _________________

Short-term patient therapeutic objectives are as follows (check all that apply):

__ demonstrate the following breathing techniques
  __ pursed-lip breathing
  __ diaphragmatic breathing
__ manage stress and avoid panic breathing
__ enhance activities of daily living (ADL) indoors
  __ washing and personal hygiene _ performing household chores
  __ dressing _ bending, reaching for, and lifting objects
  __ meal preparation _ climbing stairs
__ improve or promote cough and expectoration
__ promote proper use of aerosolized medications with deeper deposition
__ promote upper extremity conditioning
__ promote lower extremity conditioning
__ improve exercise endurance and tolerance
  __ increase duration and intensity of physical activities performed by __%
  __ improve maximum oxygen consumption up to __%
__ improve nutritional status
__ manage weight effectively
__ quit smoking
__ other: ____

Long term-patient therapeutic objectives are as follows (check all that apply):

__ complete breathing retraining program
  __ improve ventilatory muscle strength
  __ improve ventilatory muscle endurance
__ enhance activies of daily living (ADL) outdoors
  __ yard work _ attend social functions
  __ increase walking ability _ participate in social activities
  __ perform shopping routine _ travel
__ continue to increase upper extremity conditioning
__ continue to increase lower extremity conditioning
__ continue to improve exercise endurance and tolerance
  __ increase duration and intensity of physical activities performed by __%
  __ improve maximum oxygen consumption up to __%
__ improve arterial oxygenation

FIGURE 36-11 A patient treatment plan for pulmonary rehabilitation includes both short- and long-term therapeutic objectives and treatment regimens. This form must be completed by a physician, with input from the rehabilitation team.

Courtesy of Lung Diagnostics, Glen Ridge, New Jersey

conditioning increases, the duration of exercise should be increased 1–2 minutes a day with a goal of having patients perform 20–30 minutes of continuous exercise daily.

- *Frequency,* if continuous exercise is less than 15 minutes a day, should be two or three times a day, 5 days a week. If continuous exercise is greater than 20 minutes a day, frequency should be once a day, 3–7 days a week.
- *Intensity* depends on a patient's fitness level, health status, and program goals. The intensity of exercise is usually based on the results of the CPX test and is increased gradually according to a patient's tolerance.

Intensity may be determined on the basis of the target heart rate, as previously discussed, or on the basis of metabolic equivalents of energy expenditure

CASE STUDY 36-2

M. B. is a 68-year-old white male diagnosed with severe chronic obstructive airways disease. His resting S_pO_2 was 94% but decreased to 89% during walking activities and other forms of physical exertion. His CPX evaluation demonstrated that dyspnea resulting from his pulmonary disease was the limiting factor to physical activity. A target heart rate of 120–130 beats per minute was deemed safe and effective. Concerned about his deteriorating respiratory condition and on recommendation from his physician, he willingly agreed to participate in a pulmonary rehabilitation program for 12 weeks.

During this period, the patient actively participated in group sessions and exercises. He mastered diaphragmatic breathing and learned how to use his inhaled medications more effectively while discovering ways to cope with anxiety and panic. At home, he reported that he performed inspiratory resistive breathing daily for 30–45 minutes. In addition, he reported a daily 12-minute walk, noting the distance and number of stops. He also cycled, gradually increasing the time to 30 minutes a day with varying degrees of resistance. Calisthenics and stretching exercises for about 5 minutes a day were also done but not routinely. Most exercises were performed four or five times a week.

As the weeks passed, he demonstrated a lower resting pulse rate and blood pressure. During physical exercises, which included walking, stair climbing, and cycling, he achieved and maintained his target heart rate while exhibiting a lesser degree of desaturation, as evidenced by S_pO_2 monitoring. At the end of each exercise session, his heart rate returned to its resting level in shorter periods of time. Subjectively, he experienced less dyspnea, felt he had a greater exercise tolerance, and found himself participating in more physical activities both at home and in the community.

Questions

1. What factors indicate that this patient actually performed the assigned physical activities and exercises at home?
2. What indicator was used to verify improved recovery at the end of each exercise session?
3. What accounted for the motivation of this patient?

or oxygen consumption (METs). To prescribe exercise for a patient on the basis of METs, the therapist must determine the desired range of energy expenditure (usually 60–85% of maximal functional capacity), expressed in METs. Activities known to require this energy expenditure are then prescribed. Figure 36-12 presents a suggested format for an exercise prescription.

DOCUMENTATION

Both program personnel and patients enrolled in the pulmonary rehabilitation program must keep records of patient activity, response to therapy, and progress in the program. Records should be kept during every rehabilitation session, and patients should be encouraged to maintain a log of all exercise activities performed at home. Figure 36-13 illustrates a simple patient log that can be used to track and monitor patient activities at home. All patient records should be kept on file in the program office for medical-legal reasons, for use in any program accrediting endeavor and for insurance purposes, including any audit of program and patient activities.

Outcomes Assessment

Outcomes assessment, another important facet of pulmonary rehabilitation, can be accomplished in a variety of ways. Regardless of the method or methods used, assessment is essential to patient care, protection,

Best Practice

Documentation

For both medical-legal and billing purposes, practitioners should get into the habit of documenting every patient activity, response, and overall progress. Specific forms can be designed and used for patient records. Some of the more important areas to document are patient objectives, treatment plan, responses to therapy, and progress notes. Physician or health care practitioner input in all of these areas is essential. And, for purposes of insurance reimbursement for pulmonary rehabilitation, the practitioner must document, document, document!

PATIENT EXERCISE PRESCRIPTION

Patient name ______________________ Patient I.D. __________

Diagnosis ______________________ Target Heart Rate ________

Patient to perform the following physical activities, as prescribed, on the following basis:

_______ daily _______ every other day or _______ times per week

_______ Oxygen to be used at _______ Lpm during prescribed physical activities.

All physical activities performed must be recorded in each patient's daily log.

PHYSICAL ACTIVITY	INITIAL	INCREASE WEEKLY
Cycling (exercycle)	Distance_____ miles or Duration _____ minutes Tension _____	Distance_____ miles or Duration _____ minutes Tension _____
Twelve-Minute Walk	Note distance and number of stops during this activity.	Note distance and number of stops during this activity. Increase walking speed on a weekly basis.
Arm Ergometry	Duration _____ minutes Tension _____	Duration _____ minutes Tension _____
Inspiratory Resistance Device: ___________	Level or Setting _______ Duration _____ minutes	Increase level of setting ____ weekly ____ biweekly ____ as tolerated Duration _____ minutes
Stair Climbing	Number of Stairs_______ Duration _____ minutes	Number of Stairs_______ Duration _____ minutes
Other Activities (identify)		

PRESCRIBING PHYSICIAN ______________________ DATE __________

FIGURE 36-12 The exercise prescription is a key part of a patient treatment plan.

Courtesy of Lung Diagnostics, Glen Ridge, New Jersey

PATIENT ACTIVITY LOG Week Number_____

Patient Name________________________ Target H.R._______

Date	PFlex / Threshold	12-Minute Walk	Exercycle	Other Activity	Assessment
	Setting____ Minutes____	Distance ____ No. of Stops _ Pre-H.R. ____ Post-H.R. ____	Distance ____ Duration ____ Pre-H.R. ____ Post-H.R. ____		
	Setting____ Minutes____	Distance ____ No. of Stops _ Pre-H.R. ____ Post-H.R. ____	Distance ____ Duration ____ Pre-H.R. ____ Post-H.R. ____		
	Setting____ Minutes____	Distance ____ No. of Stops _ Pre-H.R. ____ Post-H.R. ____	Distance ____ Duration ____ Pre-H.R. ____ Post-H.R. ____		
	Setting____ Minutes____	Distance ____ No. of Stops _ Pre-H.R. ____ Post-H.R. ____	Distance ____ Duration ____ Pre-H.R. ____ Post-H.R. ____		
	Setting____ Minutes____	Distance ____ No. of Stops _ Pre-H.R. ____ Post-H.R. ____	Distance ____ Duration ____ Pre-H.R. ____ Post-H.R. ____		

Specific Patient Observations:

FIGURE 36-13 The patient activity log can be used to monitor patient exercise progress at home.

and reimbursement for services rendered. With Medicare and other third-party payor reimbursement tightening, demonstrating to the medical and payor communities that pulmonary rehabilitation works is increasingly important. To verify these benefits and the overall value of pulmonary rehabilitation, practitioners must continually perform outcomes assessment by documenting progress and reporting results using appropriate measurement tools.

Outcomes assessment should be an ongoing process that looks at both subjective and objective program results. It offers insight into how a program may be improved or modified to operate more efficiently and effectively. In its simplest form, subjective patient surveys can tell whether a program was beneficial. Patients often relate anecdotally a number of subjective benefits derived from the education, breathing retraining, and physical reconditioning associated with rehabilitation. However, practitioners involved in pulmonary rehabilitation need to be more objective. Objective measurements tend to be more reliable indicators of actual patient outcomes and any patient benefits realized.

Outcomes assessment is a process that should start with identifying and addressing patient expectations and should conclude with responses to the following questions:

1. In what ways did the patient make progress?
2. In what aspects of the program was patient participation most essential?
3. Which patient population seemed to derive the greatest benefit?

Improving the quality of pulmonary rehabilitation depends on how effectively patient expectations are met and how completely those three questions are answered.[20]

BENEFITS OF PULMONARY REHABILITATION

Controversy continues regarding the actual benefits of pulmonary rehabilitation. As research in this area continues in conjunction with the refinement of reconditioning methods and techniques, the real benefits of pulmonary rehabilitation should become more apparent. It is now becoming evident that patients who finish comprehensive pulmonary rehabilitation programs tend to have fewer infections and hospitalizations, experience less dyspnea, and lead more active and productive lives than patients who do not participate in or complete rehabilitation programs. Besides breathing retraining and physical reconditioning, these programs cover all facets of care for the respiratory patient, including ADLs, medication use, and nutrition. There is now substantial evidence that pulmonary rehabilitation is beneficial for patients with COPD and other chronic pulmonary diseases and a body of scientific knowledge now validates this conclusion.[21–32]

Benefits stemming from or associated with pulmonary rehabilitation may be grouped according to those that are accepted, those that are possible, and those that are unlikely.

Accepted Benefits. Chronic obstructive pulmonary disease (COPD) patients who complete a program of pulmonary rehabilitation are able to demonstrate three major accepted benefits, all of which can account for the reduction in respiratory symptoms and lessened degrees of dyspnea they claim to experience.

- *Increased endurance and exercise tolerance*
- *Increase in maximum oxygen consumption*
- *Increase in physical performance*, as evidenced by decreased ventilation, oxygen consumption, and heart rate and increased anaerobic threshold[33]

The postrehabilitation cardiopulmonary exercise (CPX) test is useful in illustrating these accepted benefits, but only if one was performed as part of the program admission. A comparison of the pre- and postprogram CPX studies indicates any degree of improvement in terms of exercise tolerance, maximum oxygen consumption, and physical performance.

Possible Benefits. Several possible benefits from pulmonary rehabilitation have been demonstrated through program evaluations.

- *Subjectively*, there may be an increased sense of well-being, less anxiety and depression, and a better quality of life.
- *Objectively*, there may be an increased hypoxic drive and increased left ventricular function.

Most of these benefits are observed in patients other than those with obstructive airways disease.[33] Possible benefits tend to be less objective than accepted benefits and do not require pre- and post-CPX testing.

Unlikely Benefits. Several benefits from pulmonary rehabilitation remain unlikely or unknown. Some of these questionable benefits are:

- Increased longevity.
- Improved pulmonary function tests (PFTs).
- Improved arterial blood gases (ABGs).
- Changes in muscle oxygen extraction.
- Changes in step desaturation.
- Fewer episodes of apnea.[33]

Table 36-8 lists all of the accepted, possible, and unlikely benefits of pulmonary rehabilitation.

TABLE 36-8 **Accepted, possible, and unlikely or debated benefits of pulmonary rehabilitation**

Accepted Benefits	Possible Benefits	Unlikely Benefits
Increased exercise tolerance and endurance	Increased sense of well-being with less anxiety and depression	Increased longevity and survival
Increased maximum oxygen consumption	Better quality of life	Improvement in PFT
Increased physical performance (with decreased ventilation, oxygen consumption, and heart rate and increased anaerobic threshold)	Ability to be more active and enhanced ability to carry out ADLs	Improvement in ABGs
	Increased mucociliary clearance	Lowered pulmonary artery pressure
	Fewer infections and hospitalizations	Improved blood chemistry, including blood lipids
	Increased hypoxic drive	Change in muscle oxygen extraction
	Increased left ventricular function	Change in step oxygen desaturation and apnea

METHODS OF MEASURING AND ASSESSING OUTCOMES

There are a number of ways to measure and assess patient outcomes in pulmonary rehabilitation. Although subjective assessment is relatively easy to obtain by surveying patients, objective measurements provide more reliable assessment. Five basic steps can be used for the assessment process:

1. Create a focused clinical question.
2. Systematically search the literature.
3. Assess the validity of all studies identified.
4. Apply the results to area of practice.
5. Evaluate targeted performance.[34]

Laboratory evaluations such as pulmonary function tests and arterial blood gas analysis provide limited information regarding the benefits of pulmonary rehabilitation, but the CPX evaluation provides the most objective data.

The CPX Evaluation. The CPX test is essential not only for identifying and admitting patients into pulmonary rehabilitation, but also in measuring and assessing patient outcomes and overall improvement. Recall that the accepted benefits of pulmonary rehabilitation and physical reconditioning are determined on the basis of positive changes observed between pre- and postexercise studies, particularly in the areas of work performance and maximum oxygen consumption. Most postrehabilitation CPX testing is done at the conclusion of the program and should be repeated once every 3 years thereafter or more frequently if warranted by a patient's condition.

In most instances, changes or increases in postrehabilitation CPX testing parameters by 15% or more suggest significant improvement. Parameters that deserve special attention or consideration, because they indicate specific changes or improvement in patient condition, include the following:

- Duration of test
- Highest workload or capacity (in watts) attained
- Maximum oxygen consumption
- Amount of time needed for patient to reach anaerobic threshold
- METs (metabolic equivalents of energy expenditure or oxygen consumption) achieved
- Oxygen saturation at maximum
- Maximum ventilation
- Maximum heart rate
- Maximum blood pressure
- ECG results
- Reasons for terminating test

Other Laboratory Studies. Patients may also be evaluated after pulmonary rehabilitation using standard pulmonary function testing, arterial blood gas analysis, chest radiographs, blood chemistries, and dyspnea indices. Improvement in any of these is not always evident and appears to be unlikely in some cases. Nevertheless, results are related to each patient's overall condition, and this type of information may prove invaluable during any retrospective studies and should therefore remain a part of the medical record.

Patient Surveys. Postprogram surveys that include patient comments, along with a comparison of their physical activities at the beginning and at the end of the program, provide information useful in appraising patient performance and progress made. Patient rehabilitation records and daily log sheets should be used to verify this information because it is recorded on each patient's survey form. All daily log sheets should be collected at the end of the program and placed in each patient's pulmonary rehabilitation record. A section of this survey should also allow patients the opportunity to comment on the overall program in terms of expectations met.

Some patients may require assistance in completing these forms. However, practitioners should not volunteer information, coach patients in their responses, or unwittingly suggest answers or responses. Information obtained from these evaluations should be tabulated, analyzed, and used in modifying or revising affected portions of the program.

An important part of any evaluation process is to ascertain the degree of patient satisfaction. Particular areas include:

- Room comfort.
- Scheduling.
- Time allotted for sessions.
- Competency and skills of the health care providers conducting sessions.
- Available equipment.
- Scope of the program.

Many managed care organizations (MCOs) are interested in patient comments and may require patient satisfaction survey data if a rehabilitation facility is applying for acceptance into any health care provider networks.

Reimbursement for Pulmonary Rehabilitation

Patients can be charged only for the sessions they attend. Fees should be structured in such a way as not to discourage a patient from attending. Many patients

CASE STUDY 36-3

Five patients completed a closed-format pulmonary rehabilitation program of 12 weeks. Sessions were conducted weekly and lasted approximately 2 hours each. At home, each patient kept a daily log of exercise activities, which included cycling on a stationary bicycle, a 12-minute walk, calisthenics, and breathing retraining using inspiratory resistance and diaphragmatic breathing with pursed lips. At the facility, patients cycled, walked, and used arm ergometry for upper extremity conditioning and were monitored accordingly. Physician/health care practitioner follow-up was biweekly. The pulmonary rehabilitation was comprehensive, and patients also received instruction in:

- Breathing techniques.
- Stress management.
- Relaxation.
- Exercise routines.
- Medication delivery.
- Respiratory home care equipment and therapy.
- Nutrition.
- Secretion clearance.
- Personal hygiene.
- ADLs.

At the conclusion of the program, these patients completed evaluation surveys and postrehabilitation CPX testing. The pre- and postrehabilitation results of this testing were as follows:

Patient	Age	Sex	Duration of Test (min:sec)	Workload at Max (watts)	S_pO_2 at Max	$\dot{V}O_{2max}$	METs
R. A.	68	F	4:25/6:30	65/90	94%/95%	805/1110	3.5/4.8
P. C.	74	M	5:15/7:45	75/120	93%/94%	775/1080	3.2/4.5
K. C.	61	F	3:30/5:10	55/80	91%/93%	638/902	2.9/4.1
C. M.	58	F	6:10/7:50	95/120	95%/95%	1200/1425	4.8/5.7
K. W.	73	M	4:00/5:30	70/95	91%/94%	529/1058	2.3/4.6

Questions

1. Of the five patients who completed pulmonary rehabilitation, which one demonstrated the greatest degree of improvement, and on what basis is this determination made?
2. On the basis of this data, which patient was in the "best" condition upon entering the program? On what basis is this determination made?
3. What additional information would have been helpful in assessing the outcomes of this program?

are on fixed incomes and may elect not to attend if they consider session or program fees are excessive. In addition, Medicare providers and other insurance carriers may also cap payments for rehabilitative services received by a patient, including pulmonary rehabilitation. Any capped payments must be taken into consideration when planning program schedules and fees. The actual charge per session depends on what was done in terms of patient education, monitoring, and therapy. Current nationwide charges range from \$60 to more than \$200 per session. If health insurance paid 80% of these charges, patients would be responsible for the remaining 20%, or approximately \$12 to \$40 per session. Grants or scholarships from health-related companies or health organizations such as the American Lung Association may be available to help patients who need to participate in pulmonary rehabilitation.

At the present time, most insurance payors, including Medicare, do not have a blanket code for pulmonary rehabilitation. In 2007, the **Centers for Medicare & Medicaid Services (CMS)** released an official statement that it would not issue a **National Coverage Determination (NCD)** for outpatient pulmonary rehabilitation. In addition, insurance payors often limit the number of sessions a patient can attend during a given year. Insurance reimbursement for pulmonary rehabilitation has always been vague and problematic. Providers have been forced to seek other ways for obtaining payment for services rendered, including charging for each therapeutic and monitoring procedure performed during class sessions. However, this changed significantly with the passage of **HR 6331 (Medicare Improvements for Patients and Providers Act)** on July 15, 2008, which enabled Medicare to issue an NCD for outpatient pulmonary rehabilitation. The change allows programs to bill for 36 pulmonary rehabilitation sessions (usually 3 sessions per week for 12 weeks) plus an additional 36 sessions if continuation of pulmonary rehabilitation is deemed necessary for the patient by the prescribing health care provider.

PATIENT CHARGES AND BILLING PRACTICES

Obtaining reimbursement for pulmonary rehabilitation requires that a specific patient treatment plan be devised and implemented. A physician or health care practitioner involved with the case should authorize the plan and exercise prescription with a signature. These services should be provided two or three times a week for 6–8 weeks, resulting in 12–18 therapeutic sessions. Most patients requiring rehabilitation should be able to exhibit some degree of improvement over this period. An intensity or frequency of less than twice a week implies that a patient is not that ill or is not in dire need of any therapy or rehabilitation. Periodic assessment of patient progress by a physician is also recommended.[13]

Prior to 2008, there was no blanket code for pulmonary rehabilitation even though it was recognized as a therapeutic service. Reimbursement could be obtained from Medicare and other third-party payors for pulmonary rehabilitation in several legitimate ways:

- Charge sessions as physical therapy exercises for patients with COPD. Because physical therapy is being billed, the services of a licensed physical therapist may be required.
- Charge sessions as office visits with therapeutic exercises.
- Charge sessions as physician's office visits.

In addition, patient monitoring procedures may have been considered reimbursable, such as end-tidal CO_2 measurements, spirometry, and serial pulse oximetry determinations. However, providers were cautioned to become thoroughly familiar with and observe all Medicare policies pertaining to any reimbursement for pulmonary rehabilitation service components. This all changed as a result of Congress passing HR 6331 in July 2008, which included provisions for a national coverage policy for pulmonary rehabilitation under Medicare Part B. Patients are now provided with a payment mechanism for pulmonary rehabilitation along with greater access to respiratory therapists, both inside and outside the hospital, who are involved in conducting pulmonary rehabilitation programs.

CODING SYSTEMS

Billing for any pulmonary diagnostic, therapeutic, or rehabilitative services must meet certain requirements, including a correctly coded patient diagnosis in accordance with the fourth edition of the ***International Classification of Diseases, 9th Revision, Clinical Modification (ICD-9-CM)***. This classification system is recommended for use in all clinical settings but is required for reporting diseases and diagnoses to the federal government, in particular to the U.S. Public Health Service (USPHS) and CMS [formerly the Health Care Financing Administration (HCFA)]. Actual patient billing revolves around a system of approved procedural coding from the American Medical Association (AMA) and CMS. Medical procedures are listed in the AMA's **current procedural terminology (CPT) coding**, and medical equipment and supplies used by patients are listed under the CMS **healthcare common procedure coding system (HCPCS)**.

In 1992, there was a proposal to promote cross-coding between the HCPCS codes and CPT coding. However, there appears to be little need for cross-coding between the two systems because CPT coding focuses mainly on procedures and services whereas HCPCS codes focus on equipment and supplies. Instead, a method of cross-referencing is used to avoid confusion between the two systems. For example, when a procedure or service is assigned a CPT code, the HCPCS system deletes it but still refers the individual to the CPT system. The following section briefly describes the three major coding systems in terms of design and scope.

ICD-9-CM. The *International Classification of Diseases, 9th Revision, Clinical Modification*, or *ICD-9-CM*, is published by the U.S. Department of Health and Human Services, through its Public Health Service, in recognition of its responsibility to circulate this classification throughout the country for morbidity or disease coding. The *International Classification of Diseases, 9th Revision* (*ICD-9*), published by the World Health Organization (WHO), is the foundation for the *ICD-9-CM*, which is now in its fourth edition with updates issued annually. It consists of three volumes:

- Tabular list of diseases
- Alphabetic index
- Disease classification

A basic disease or diagnostic code consists of a three-digit rubric that represents a specific disease classification. Subclassifications referring to either a specific anatomical site or a variation of the disease in the body are coded with a fourth or fifth digit or with both. For example, the general diagnostic code for asthma is 493. Asthma, without mention of status asthmaticus, is coded 493.00, whereas asthma with status asthmaticus is 493.01. Extrinsic asthma is 493.0, and intrinsic asthma is coded 493.1. Procedure classifications, on the other hand, use four-digit rubrics or code headings.

The *ICD-9-CM* is recommended for use in all clinical settings and is required when reporting to either the U.S. Public Health Service or CMS. For obtaining reimbursement, a properly coded diagnosis is essential, especially when billing Medicare for any diagnostic or therapeutic service rendered.[35]

CPT Coding. The *Physicians' Current Procedural Terminology* manual is published annually by the AMA, with input from many individuals and organizations, including national medical specialty societies, state medical associations, professional health care organizations, health insurance organizations and agencies, and CMS. It contains a listing of descriptive terms and codes used in reporting medical services and procedures. This CPT coding and related terminology act as a uniform language that accurately depicts medical, surgical, and diagnostic procedures and services and therefore serve as an effective means for reliable communication among physicians, patients, and third parties. CPT coding is related specifically to procedures and services performed by physicians and health care practitioners. Any patient charge must be properly designated with a CPT code, which consists of a five-digit identifying code number and a descriptor for that specific procedure or service. For example, the code and descriptor for procedures related to chest percussion are "94667 Manipulation chest wall, such as cupping, percussion, and vibration to facilitate lung function; initial demonstration and/or evaluation."[36]

In addition, when a service or procedure has been altered by some circumstance but not changed in definition or code, a modifier is employed. This is used when billing for procedures that are separate but necessary, as when performing multiple spirometries or flow volume loops before and after a CPX test to determine the presence of any exercise-induced asthma (EID).

The manual is available at the end of each year, but its listed codes do not take effect until January 1 of the new year. In the event that any procedures are added or revised during the course of a year, a newsletter is published and sent to all subscribers advising them of the changes. However, procedural coding usually changes on an annual basis, as reflected in each year's manual.

Program administration and personnel, especially those in the billing office, must be completely knowledgeable about CPT coding and any changes either that are proposed or that have been adopted because of the effect coding has on reimbursement policies and practices. What is reimbursable one year may be excluded the next. Like disease coding, CPT coding must be performed correctly and consistently.

HCPCS. CMS also publishes annually its *Healthcare Common Procedure Coding System* manual, which outlines reimbursable items, including durable medical equipment (DME), oxygen, and related respiratory equipment and services, such as patient transportation.[37] HCPCS coding is most frequently used by hospitals, physician's offices, and home care companies supplying DME and oxygen and related forms of respiratory care equipment.[38]

The AARC continues to work with CMS regarding proposed coding revisions, especially in the sections of the HCPCS coding system pertaining to Supplies for Oxygen and Related Respiratory Equipment and Durable Medical Equipment. AARC's active role in this process is deemed an important move by the respiratory care profession into procedural coding.[39] Other than portable oxygen for ambulation and some respiratory home care modalities, however, HCPCS has little application to pulmonary rehabilitation.

Table 36-9 reviews the three coding systems presented in this section.

THIRD-PARTY REIMBURSEMENT

Payment by insurance carriers for pulmonary rehabilitation remains a controversial issue. Programs can exist by billing for:

- Pre- and postprogram patient testing and evaluation.
- And for the actual components of physical reconditioning and patient monitoring.

TABLE 36-9 **Coding systems for pulmonary rehabilitation**

System	Purpose	Example	Description
ICD-9-CM	Codes diagnosis	492.8	Emphysema
CPT	Codes procedures and services	94760	Noninvasive ear or pulse oximetry for oxygen saturation, single determination
HCPCS	Codes equipment and supplies	E0431	Portable gaseous oxygen system, rental; includes regulator, flowmeter, humidifier, cannula or mask, and tubing

This issue was resolved, in part, with the passage of HR 6331, Medicare Improvements for Patients and Providers Act (MIPPA) in July 2008, which included provisions for a national coverage policy for pulmonary rehabilitation. This legislation enabled pulmonary rehabilitation to become a fully accepted and recognized clinical modality with its own standard codes.

By properly identifying and utilizing recognized diagnostic and therapeutic procedures, along with related coding systems such as the *ICD-9-CM* and CPT, programs should be able to bill and receive payment for services delivered. Payment for services is essential for program continuance and viability and for patients afflicted with chronic pulmonary disease. The following section examines how Medicare, Medicaid, and private and commercial insurance carriers view pulmonary rehabilitation and reimburse for these services.

Medicare. According to CMS, claims for Medicare patients should be submitted to Medicare Part A for any component of a pulmonary rehabilitation performed during a hospital stay. Conversely, claims for rehabilitation components performed on an outpatient basis must be submitted to Medicare Part B. For reimbursement, Medicare requires:

- Documentation by the attending physician or health care practitioner of the patient's diagnosis.
- An individualized treatment plan containing therapeutic objectives.
- An exercise prescription that specifies type, amount, duration, and frequency of services.
- A plan for periodic patient review and assessment.

Prior to 2008, CMS allowed Medicare intermediaries to interpret CMS policy regarding pulmonary rehabilitation, but there was no consistency in reimbursement by Medicare from state to state. Providers had to be familiar with the policies of their Medicare intermediary.[40] For example, several office-based programs have reported that Medicare was not accepting diagnosis codes that include emphysema, chronic bronchitis, COPD, or interstitial pulmonary disease for billing components of pulmonary rehabilitation. Instead, these outpatient programs have been using the *ICD-9-CM* code 799.3 for debility (general or unspecified). This diagnostic coding has been accepted by Medicare, resulting in reimbursement for patient procedures and activities related to pulmonary rehabilitation.[41]

On July 15, 2008, President George W. Bush vetoed HR 6331. On the very same day, Congress voted to over ride this veto, thus making the bill law. As a result, provisions for a national coverage policy under Medicare Part B for pulmonary rehabilitation was established, along with a blanket code for pulmonary rehabilitation. This law eliminated the need for programs to bill for individual components of pulmonary rehabilitation as programs did in the past.

In addition, the Medicare provision that authorized reimbursement for outpatient services provided by a respiratory therapist are found in the regulations for **comprehensive outpatient rehabilitative facility (CORF)**, released in December 1982. CORFs were the best sites for reimbursement for pulmonary rehabilitation because the roles and responsibilities of respiratory therapists involved in pulmonary rehabilitation at CORFs were clearly defined.[42]

Medicaid. Medicaid is federally mandated and funded by state governments. It currently provides health care to almost 39 million low-income Americans, including women and children and those who are elderly, blind, or disabled. Medicaid appears to be the fastest growing component of state budgets and the second largest state expense after education. As a result, a number of proposals have been made to restructure Medicaid to give those enrolled greater access to health care while reducing the growth in state spending for the program.[43]

There is a rehabilitation category under Medicaid, and payment for pulmonary rehabilitation services exists, but it varies greatly from state to state. These differences are related to the type and degree of state control and to the amount of reimbursement allotted for pulmonary rehabilitation. Both inpatient and outpatient services have been defined, along with a competitive fee schedule resulting from contracts with providers of rehabilitation services. However, some programs may be reluctant to accept Medicaid patients into pulmonary rehabilitation if they think the established fees are too low.

Private and Commercial Insurance Carriers. Most private and commercial insurance carriers have requirements similar to those of Medicare: patient diagnosis and treatment plan and physician authorization. However, a predetermination, preauthorization, or other related documentation may be necessary before a patient receives approval to begin. A managed care plan, such as a health maintenance organization (HMO), may also require that a pulmonary rehabilitation provider be a member of its network before any patient is admitted into a program and allowed to participate. Many plans also limit the number of sessions a patient can attend. Some plans allow up to 36 rehabilitation sessions during any given calendar year. The passage and implementation of HR 6331 in July 2008 allows Medicare to cover up to 36 sessions with an additional 36 sessions if medically necessary for the patient.

PROBLEMS WITH REIMBURSEMENT

Pulmonary rehabilitation programs conducted for hospital inpatients or for outpatients either through a hospital or at a comprehensive outpatient rehabilitative facility (CORF) experience little difficulty with insurance reimbursement. In these cases, Medicare covers correctly structured pulmonary outpatient rehabilitation programs. Furthermore, the *Medicare/Medicaid Coverage Manual* defines the role of respiratory care in a hospital, in addition to describing outpatient hospital services, outpatient therapeutic services, and instructional and home care patient education programs. The manual also indicates that respiratory therapy can entail pulmonary rehabilitation techniques that include (1) exercise conditioning, (2) breathing retraining, and (3) patient education regarding the management of the patient's respiratory problems.[44]

However, other outpatient programs at non-CORF facilities, especially those offered at private, free-standing clinics or centers or physician offices, had encountered more obstacles and had greater difficulty in receiving payment for services rendered. Some insurance carriers, in particular Medicare intermediaries, had denied payment for pulmonary rehabilitation services conducted at these outpatient facilities. These difficulties remain even though pulmonary rehabilitation is now viewed by the medical and health care communities as an integral component of sound, comprehensive patient care.[45]

REASONS FOR REIMBURSEMENT DIFFICULTIES

Initially, the lack of professional licensure was an issue because many insurance carriers reimbursed only the medical procedures provided by licensed personnel. Every state has passed some form of respiratory care licensure or credentialing measure. However, for several reasons, CMS and other insurance carriers appeared to be hesitant about clarifying coverage and reimbursement policies for outpatient pulmonary rehabilitation:

- Time and staff to process claims are lacking.
- Outlining what a pulmonary rehabilitation program should consist of increases reimbursement because more programs would come into existence.[44]
- Most carriers are trying to reduce health care costs, not increase them.
- Proper documentation describing patient activities, progress, and benefit are lacking.
- Insurance carriers hold the traditional conviction that only physical therapists are trained and qualified to conduct pulmonary rehabilitation programs.

Programs may experience meaningful results, and patients may perceive significant benefits from pulmonary rehabilitation. However, if nothing has been documented, carriers will continue to deny payment to the facility or provider. Every program must be able to document:

- Patient assessment and evaluation.
- Short- and long-term patient goals.
- The patient treatment plan, including exercise prescription.
- Patient activity records (program and home).
- Routine physician assessment of patient progress.
- Follow-up assessment and evaluation at the end of the program.

This documentation in patient records has helped demonstrate the benefits of pulmonary rehabilitation and thereby strengthened the argument for insurance coverage. To this end, the **National Emphysema Treatment Trial (NETT)** was conducted and has definitely helped to further change the perspective of third-party payors, including Medicare, regarding reimbursement for pulmonary rehabilitation. This study embraced pulmonary rehabilitation as a primary treatment modality for patients with COPD. It involved 17 clinical centers throughout the United States, along with satellite facilities. NETT protocols include three phases: prerandomization, postrandomization, and long-term or follow-up care. The prerandomization phase had four components:

- Initial evaluation
- Core rehabilitation for 5 days
- Continued rehabilitation for 5–9 weeks
- Reevaluation

Patients were then randomized into either medical or surgical groups with supervised rehabilitation training for up to 9 weeks. The long-term and follow-up care phase lasted for up to 5 years for those in the medical group. Patients in the surgical group underwent **lung-volume-reduction surgery (LVRS)** with 8 weeks of follow-up care.

CMS funded this NETT study in an effort to determine whether pulmonary rehabilitation is a viable treatment modality. Findings from this initiative have had a positive affect on third-party reimbursement and on the role RTs play in pulmonary rehabilitation, as evidenced by the passage of HR 6331 in July 2008.[46–48]

Summary

Pulmonary rehabilitation is a challenging specialty that is rapidly growing. The respiratory therapist who wants to enter this field must be knowledgeable about various aspects of pulmonary rehabilitation, including definition and scope, patient evaluation and selection, required resources, program design and implementation, assessment and documentation of patient outcomes, and methods of obtaining reimbursement for the care provided.

Pulmonary rehabilitation, though in existence since the 1950s, is actually in its infancy. Acceptance of this methodology of care for chronic lung patients is becoming an integral part of continuing respiratory care, especially at alternative sites of care. Studies have indicated the potential benefits of pulmonary rehab, yet much more needs to be done. Practitioners must continue to document the benefits of pulmonary rehabilitation in order to establish a more effective reimbursement mechanism. The CMS-funded NETT study should provide interesting results regarding the validity of pulmonary rehabilitation and reimbursement for it. In the meantime, practitioners need to work closely with their colleagues to design and implement more patient-specific and effective rehabilitation programs. With ever increasing recognition, pulmonary rehabilitation seems to be headed on a course that will make it an essential part of long-term patient care.

Study Questions

REVIEW QUESTIONS

1. What is meant by the term *pulmonary rehabilitation?*
2. What are the major differences between pulmonary and cardiac rehabilitation?
3. State the major goal of pulmonary rehabilitation and its two principal objectives.
4. Identify five patient conditions that would benefit from pulmonary rehabilitation.
5. How are patients selected for pulmonary rehabilitation?
6. What are the five key components of a pulmonary rehabilitation program?
7. Explain the importance of patient documentation in pulmonary rehabilitation with regard to reimbursement.
8. What are three accepted benefits of pulmonary rehabilitation?
9. What are some possible and some debated benefits of pulmonary rehabilitation?

MULTIPLE-CHOICE QUESTIONS

1. Which of the following did the American Thoracic Society Executive Committee not identify as a major component of pulmonary rehabilitation in 1981?
   I. use of a multidisciplinary approach
   II. stabilization or reversal of both the physio- and psychopathology of pulmonary disease
   III. goal of restoring patients to the highest functional capacity possible
   a. III only
   b. I and III
   c. I and II
   d. I, II, and III
2. Which of the following distinguishes cardiac rehabilitation from pulmonary rehabilitation?
   I. focus on improving physical fitness
   II. limitations to exercise
   III. need for a stress test to qualify for rehabilitation
   a. II only
   b. I and II
   c. I and III
   d. I, II, and III

3. The major goal of pulmonary rehabilitation is to:
   a. educate patients about their pulmonary disability.
   b. teach patients how to breathe correctly and more effectively.
   c. reduce hospitalizations and medical costs incurred by each patient.
   d. restore patients to the highest functional capacity possible.
4. The cardiopulmonary exercise (CPX) evaluation is indispensable in which of the following ways?
   I. differentiates between pulmonary and cardiac causes of dyspnea
   II. establishes a baseline for each patient's level of physical conditioning
   III. can be used to include or exclude patients from pulmonary rehabilitation
   a. III only
   b. I and III
   c. I and II
   d. I, II, and III
5. Which of the following parameters are low or reduced in cases of poor conditioning, pulmonary disorders, and cardiovascular disorders?
   I. O_2 pulse
   II. METs
   III. maximum oxygen consumption
   a. III only
   b. I and III
   c. II and III
   d. I, II, and III
6. Patients may be included in pulmonary rehabilitation when they terminate an exercise evaluation at a level less than what percentage of their maximum oxygen consumption?
   a. 75%
   b. 85%
   c. 90%
   d. 95%
7. Group sessions are effective because they address which major patient need?
   a. psychosocial
   b. physiological
   c. educational
   d. financial
8. Which of the following types of exercise employs movement without resistance or tension and results in improved patient stamina and endurance?
   a. isometric
   b. isokinetic
   c. aerobic
   d. anaerobic
9. Which of the following terms implies that the benefits of exercise are transient and persist only as long as exercise is continued?
   a. detraining effect
   b. overload
   c. reinforcement
   d. specificity of training
10. The most effective breathing technique a patient with chronic obstructive pulmonary disease can acquire is which of the following?
    a. inspiratory resistive breathing
    b. sustained maximum inspiratory breathing
    c. diaphragmatic breathing with pursed lips
    d. segmental breathing
11. Patients in pulmonary rehabilitation should exercise to a target heart rate approximating their heart rate at what percentage of their maximum oxygen consumption?
    a. 40–50%
    b. 65–75%
    c. 80–90%
    d. 100%
12. Which of the following are requirements for reimbursement for a pulmonary rehabilitation plan of treatment?
    I. an estimate of cost of treatment
    II. a reasonable estimate of when program goals will be reached
    III. an exercise prescription
    a. II and III
    b. III only
    c. I and II
    d. I, II, and III
13. Which of the following is the most objective way to assess the results of pulmonary rehabilitation?
    a. written surveys and evaluation tools
    b. a cardiopulmonary exercise (CPX) test
    c. serial pulmonary function testing
    d. arterial blood gas analysis
14. After a 16-week pulmonary rehabilitation program, a patient's maximum oxygen consumption increased from 650 mL/min to 780 mL/min and METs increased from 2.5 to 3.5. The postrehab cardiopulmonary exercise (CPX) test lasted 2 minutes longer, and the patient was able to perform at 80 watts versus only 50 watts during the initial study. How would you interpret these results?
    a. no demonstrated improvement
    b. insignificant improvement
    c. significant improvement
    d. further exercise needed

15. Which one of the following is an unlikely benefit of pulmonary rehabilitation?
    a. better quality of life
    b. fewer infections and hospitalizations
    c. improvements in pulmonary function and arterial blood gases
    d. increased oxygen consumption
16. To obtain a diagnostic code for a patient's condition, a practitioner refers to which of the following coding systems?
    a. *ICD-9-CM*
    b. CPT
    c. HCPCS
    d. CORF
17. Which of the following coding procedures is the most useful in obtaining reimbursement for pulmonary rehabilitation procedures performed?
    a. *ICD-9-CM*
    b. CPT
    c. HCPCS
    d. CORF
18. Which of the following is/are true?
    I. Medicare Part A covers in-hospital care.
    II. Medicare Part B covers outpatient care.
    III. CORFs experience fewer difficulties in obtaining reimbursement for pulmonary rehabilitation.
        a. III only
        b. I and II
        c. I and III
        d. I, II, and III

CRITICAL-THINKING QUESTIONS

1. What has brought about the current surge in interest in pulmonary rehabilitation?
2. What attributes make the respiratory therapist the health care practitioner of choice to implement and oversee a pulmonary rehabilitation program?
3. How can chronic respiratory patients be made more receptive to the benefits of pulmonary rehabilitation?
4. How can pulmonary rehabilitation programs become more cost-effective?
5. What can the respiratory care profession do to further legitimize pulmonary rehabilitation in order to secure recognition and reimbursement from Medicare and other third-party insurance carriers?

References

1. Council on Rehabilitation. *Definition of Rehabilitation*. Chicago: American College of Chest Physicians, Council on Rehabilitation; 1942.
2. American Thoracic Society Executive Committee. Pulmonary rehabilitation—an official statement of the American Thoracic Society. *Am Rev Respir Dis*. 1981;124:663–666.
3. Eiserman J. AARC specialty sections. *AARC Times*. 1987;11:22–23.
4. Ries AL, Bauldoff GS, Carlin BW, Casaburi, R, Emery CF, Mahler DA, Make B, Rochester CL, ZuWallach R, Herrerias C. Pulmonary rehabilitation executive summary: joint American College of Chest Physicians/American Association of Cardiovascular and Pulmonary Rehabilitation evidence-based clinical practice guidelines. *Chest*. 2007;131:1S–3S.
5. Ries AL, Bauldoff GS, Carlin BW, Casaburi, R, Emery CF, Mahler DA, Make B, Rochester CL, ZuWallach R, Herrerias C. Pulmonary rehabilitation: Joint ACCP/AACVPR evidence-based clinical practice guidelines. *Chest*. 2007;131:4S–42S.
6. Cathcart M. Other drivers of change deserve consideration. *AARCTimes*. 1995;19:36–37.
7. Kallstrom T. Asthma significantly affects health care expenditures. *AARCTimes*. 1995;19:38.
8. American Lung Association. *Lung Disease Data 1996*. New York: American Lung Assoc; 1996:1–3.
9. Hodgkin JE, Connors GL, Bell CW. *Pulmonary Rehabilitation—Guidelines to Success*. 2nd ed. Philadelphia: JB Lippincott; 1993:6–9, 53–54, 59–60.
10. American Association for Respiratory Care. AARC Clinical Practice Guideline. Exercise testing for evaluation of hypoxemia and/or desaturation. *Respir Care*. 1992;37:907–912.
11. Goren SM. Moving OSA patients into pulmonary rehabilitation. *RT, J Respir Care Pract*. 1996;9: 25–26.
12. Celli BR. Physical reconditioning of patients with respiratory diseases: legs, arms and breathing retraining. *Respir Care*. 1994;39:482–483, 488–491.
13. Xact Medicare Services. *Medicare Medical Policy Bulletins*. Bulletin No. Y-1C, Revision 006. 1995; 7-53–7-54.
14. Burton GG, Gee GN, Hodgkin JE. *Respiratory Care—A Guide to Clinical Practice*. Philadelphia: JB Lippincott 2007.
15. McMahon P. The hospital-based pulmonary rehab home care program. *AARCTimes*. 1988; 12:50–51.
16. Faulkner JA. New perspectives in training for maximum performance. *JAMA*. 1968;205:741.
17. Weiner P, Azgad Y, Ganam R. Inspiratory muscle training, combined with general exercise reconditioning in patients with COPD. *Chest*. 1992;102,5:1351–1356.

18. Clark CJ, Cochrane L, Mackey E. Low intensity peripheral muscle conditioning improves exercise tolerance and breathlessness in COPD. *Eur Respir J.* 1996;9:2590–2596.
19. Bellman MJ, Wasserman K. (1982). Exercise training and testing in patients with chronic obstructive pulmonary disease. *Basics of RD.* Monograph published by the American Thoracic Society.
20. Peske GW. The power of outcomes research. *RT, J Respir Care Pract.* 1995;8:18–19.
21. Ries AL, Kaplan RM, Limberg TM, et al. Effects of pulmonary rehabilitation on physiologic and psychosocial outcomes in patients with chronic obstructive pulmonary disease. *Ann Intern Med.* 1995;122:823–832.
22. Bendstrup KE, Ingemann Jensen J, Holm S, et al. Outpatient rehabilitation improves activities of daily living, quality of life and exercise tolerance in chronic obstructive pulmonary disease. *Eur Respir J.* 1997;10:2801–2806.
23. O'Donnell DE, McGuire M, Samis L, et al. The impact of exercise reconditioning on breathlessness in severe chronic airflow limitation. *Am J Respir Crit Care Med.* 1995;152:2005–2013.
24. Vale F, Reardon JZ, ZuWallack RL. The long-term benefits of outpatient pulmonary rehabilitation on exercise endurance and quality of life. *Chest.* 1993;103:42–45.
25. Griffiths TL, Burr ML, Campbell IA, et al. Results at one year of outpatient multidisciplinary pulmonary rehabilitation: a randomized clinical trial. *Lancet.* 2000;355:362–368.
26. Finnerty JP, Keeping I, Bullough I, et al. The effectiveness of outpatient pulmonary rehabilitation in chronic lung disease: a randomized controlled trial. *Chest.* 2001;119:1705–1710.
27. Troosters T, Gosselink R, Decramer M. Short and long-term effects of outpatient rehabilitation patients with chronic obstructive pulmonary disease: a randomized trial. *Am J Med.* 2000;109:207–212.
28. Lacasse Y, Goldstein R, Lasserson TJ, et al. Pulmonary rehabilitation for chronic obstructive pulmonary disease. *Cochrane Database Syst Rev.* 2006,4:CD003793.
29. Porszasz J, Emtner M, Whipp BJ, et al. Endurance training decreases exercise-induced dynamic hyperinflation in patients with COPD. *Eur Respir J.* 2003;22:205s.
30. Ferreira G, Feuerman M, Spiegler P. Results of an 8 week outpatient pulmonary rehabilitation program on patients with and without chronic obstructive pulmonary disease. *J Cardiopulm Rehabil.* 2006;26:54–60.
31. Guell R, Casan P, Belda J, et al. Long-term effects of outpatient rehabilitation of COPD: a randomized trial. *Chest.* 2000;117:976–983.
32. Rossi G, Florini F, Romagnoli M, et al. Length and clinical effectiveness of pulmonary rehabilitation in outpatients with chronic airway obstruction. *Chest.* 2005;127:105–109.
33. Hughes RL, Davison R. Limitations of exercise reconditioning in COLD. *Chest.* 1983;83:242.
34. Sibbald WJ. The whys and wherefores of measuring outcomes in respiratory critical care. *Respir Care.* 1998;43:1093, 1095.
35. U.S. Public Health Service. *International Classification of Diseases, 9th Revision, Clinical Modification.* Washington, DC: U.S. Department of Health and Human Services; 1991. Publication No. (PHS) 91-1260, Vol. 1:iii, xiii–xvi, xxiii, 419–420.
36. American Medical Association. *Physicians' Current Procedural Terminology (CPT 2007)* Standard ed. Chicago: American Medical Assoc, Dept of Coding and Nomenclature; 2007.
37. Health Care Financing Administration. *HCFA Common Procedure Coding System (HCPCS 1995).* Washington, DC: U.S. Dept of Health and Human Services; 1995:56–57.
38. Molle CJ. More than Morse . . . procedure coding for the respiratory cryptographer—Part II: HCPCS coding. *AARCTimes.* 1993;17:52–55.
39. Molle CJ. More than Morse . . . procedure coding for the respiratory cryptographer—Part II: update on HCPCS coding recommendations. *AARCTimes.* 1994;18:18–21, 23–26.
40. Connors G, Hilling L, Morris KV, Hodgkin JE, Duckett D. Obtaining third-party reimbursement for pulmonary rehabilitation. *AARCTimes.* 1992;16:50–51.
41. American Medical Association. *International Classification of Diseases, 9th Revision, Clinical Modification 1999.* Vol. 2. Dover, DE: Medicode Inc; 1998:78.
42. American Association for Respiratory Care. CORF regulations released. *AARCTimes.* 1983; 7:40–52.
43. Eicher J. The nation's governors propose plan to restructure Medicaid. *AARCTimes.* 1996;20:8.
44. Brown C. Washington overview. *AARCTimes.* 1988;12:22.
45. American Thoracic Society. Pulmonary rehabilitation–1999. *Am J Respir Crit Care Med.* 1999;159:1666–1682.
46. Varnell M. Therapists may benefit from NETT's rehab project. *Ad J Respir Care Pract.* 1999;12:7.
47. National Emphysema Treatment Trial Research Group. A randomized trial comparing lung-volume-reduction surgery with medical therapy for

severe emphysema. *N Engl J Med*. 2003;348: 2059–2073.

48. National Emphysema Treatment Trial Research Group. Cost-effectiveness of lung-volume-reduction surgery for patients with severe emphysema. *N Engl J Med*. 2003;348:2092–2102.

Suggested Readings

American Association for Respiratory Care. AARC clinical practice guideline: pulmonary rehabilitation. *Resp Care*. 2002;47,5:617–625.

Anthonisen NR, Skeans MA, Wise RA, et al. The effects of a smoking cessation intervention on 14.5 year mortality. *Ann Int Med*. 2005;142:233–239.

Hodgkin JE, Celli BR, Connors GL. *Pulmonary Rehabilitation-Guidelines to Success*. 4th ed. St. Louis: Mosby Elsevier; 2009.

Jones AY, Dean E, Chow CC. Comparison of the oxygen cost of breathing exercises and spontaneous breathing in patients with stable chronic obstructive pulmonary disease. *Phys Ther*. 2003;83:424–431.

Jones NL. *Clinical Exercise Testing*. 4th ed. Philadelphia: WB Saunders Co; 1997.

Lorenzi CM, Cilione C, Rizzardi R, et al. Occupational therapy and pulmonary rehabilitation of disabled COPD patients. *Respiration*. 2004;71:246–251.

Lotters F, Van Tol B, Kwakkel G, et al. Effects of controlled inspiratory muscle training in patients with COPD: a meta-analysis. *Eur Respir J*. 2002;20: 570–576.

Morris KV, Hodgkin JE. *Pulmonary Rehabilitation Administration and Patient Education Manual*. Gaithersburg, MD: Aspen Publishers; 1996.

Parker L, Walker J. Effects of a pulmonary rehabilitation program on physiologic measures, quality of life, and resource utilization in a health maintenance organization setting. *Respir Care*. 1998;43,3: 177–182.

Scala E, Rocca J, Marrades RM, et al. Effects of endurance training on skeletal muscle bioenergetics in chronic obstructive pulmonary disease. *Am J Respir Crit Care Med*. 1999;159:1726–1734.

Tiep BL. Disease management of COPD with pulmonary rehabilitation. *Chest*. 1997;112,6: 1630–1656.

Weber KT, Janicki JS. *Cardiopulmonary Exercise Testing: Physiologic Principles and Clinical Applications*. Philadelphia: WB Saunders Co; 1986.

Wilkins RL, Stoller JK, Kacmarek RM. *Egan's Fundamentals of Respiratory Care*. 9th ed. St. Louis: Mosby Elsevier; 2009.

Wyka KA. *Respiratory Care in Alternate Sites*. Clifton Park, NY: Delmar Cengage Learning; 1998.

CHAPTER 37

Patient Transport in Respiratory Care

Albert J. Heuer

OBJECTIVES

Upon completion of this chapter, the reader should be able to:

- Describe general considerations relevant to patient transport.
- Summarize the prerequisites and contraindications for patient transport.
- Review the main factors in a pretransport patient assessment.
- Identify members of the transport team, including their respective roles.
- Describe the equipment used in patient transport.
- Discuss major age-specific and other special conditions.
- Differentiate among the modes of external transport (e.g., ground or air).
- Summarize special considerations, including the effects of air transport.

CHAPTER OUTLINE

KEY TERMS

bends decompression sickness
Boyle's law
Dalton's law
hypobaric condition
intrahospital transport
Society of Critical Care Medicine (SCCM)
thermoregulation

Typically, patients are transported within a hospital because they require diagnostic testing, such as an X-ray or a CT scan, or are scheduled for a surgery or other therapeutic procedures. Likewise, patients may be transferred to a different health care facility because their condition has changed or they require medical services not available at the original site. Many transported patients are clinically stable and/or do not require specialized equipment; they do *not* need a respiratory therapist, nurse, or other health professional to be present. However, a respiratory therapist may well be needed when during the transport of many critically ill and unstable patients, particularly those on life-support equipment, such as mechanical ventilation. The focus of this chapter is on the essentials of transporting such patients.

Whether the transport is intrahospital or external via land or air, the main focus is on ensuring patient safety during transport. For the most part, this is accomplished through appropriate planning and proper execution by competent staff utilizing all the necessary equipment and medication.

Note: The respiratory care concepts related to patient transport, as covered in this chapter, are relevant to many other aspects of respiratory care, including airway management, oxygen cylinder duration of flow, and infection control. These concepts are covered in more detail elsewhere in this text.

General Considerations for Patient Transport

Many steps are required for a successful patient transport, specifically planning, assessment, communication, equipment, and identification of hazards.

PLANNING THE PATIENT TRANSPORT

The first step in all forms of patient transport is advance planning. This means maintaining a constant level of readiness with regard to personnel, equipment, and mode of transportation. For example:

- All transport personnel should be experienced clinicians with the appropriate skill set and credentials, such as the Advanced Cardiac Life Support (ACLS) certification.
- Equipment, including transport bags and portable ventilators, should be maintained and checked regularly.
- Reliable channels of communication should be in place among transport team members as well as between the sending and receiving areas.
- In addition, it is generally preferable for multiple modes of transportation to be available for moving the patient outside the hospital.

PRETRANSPORT ASSESSMENT

Another essential consideration when preparing to transport critically ill patients within or outside the hospital is establishing that they are stable enough to be moved. This pretransport assessment should include:

- Vital signs.
- Hemodynamic values.
- Oxygenation.
- Ventilation.
- Any other relevant clinical parameters.

According to the American Association for Respiratory Care (AARC), patient transport is contraindicated when any one of the following cannot be reasonably met during transport:[1]

- Provision of adequate oxygenation and ventilation
- Maintenance of acceptable hemodynamic performance
- Adequate monitoring of the patient's cardiopulmonary status
- Maintenance of airway control

When evaluating a patient's ability to tolerate being moved within or to another health care facility, consider the impact of the likely additional stress on the patient from being moved. The stress may include excessive vibration, motion, and noise, as well as temperature variations. Age or clinical status may make some patients especially susceptible to such stressors. Because certain stressors have been shown to increase morbidity, especially in neonates and pediatric patients, anticipate and address such concerns. For ill neonates, specially designed isolettes have been shown to reduce noise and vibration and to maintain a neutral thermal environment. Measures such as proper positioning and monitoring can benefit all critically ill patients during transport.[2]

ELEMENTS OF THE PATIENT TRANSPORT

Once it has been determined that the patient is sufficiently stable and special needs have been considered, prepare for the move. According to the **Society of Critical Care Medicine (SCCM)**, the planning and execution of the patient transport must address the following four areas: communication, personnel, equipment, and monitoring.

Communication. The SCCM recommends the following:

- Members of the transport team should communicate with the team at the receiving location.
- Before transport, the receiving location confirms that it is ready to receive the patient.
- Members of the health care team are notified as to the timing of the transport and needed equipment.
- Documentation includes the physician's order, indications for transport, and patient status throughout.

Personnel. The SCCM recommends that at least two people accompany all critically ill patients: usually a critical care nurse and a respiratory therapist. An ACLS-trained physician should also accompany unstable patients.

Equipment. The SCCM recommends the following equipment to support the patient during transport:

- Blood pressure monitor (or standard blood pressure cuff)
- Pulse oximeter
- Cardiac monitor/defibrillator
- Equipment for airway management and secretion clearance (appropriately sized)
- O_2 source with sufficient duration of flow, plus a 30-minute reserve
- BVM (with mask) or portable ventilator
- Basic resuscitation drugs, including epinephrine and antiarrhythmic agents

Age-Specific Competency

Transporting Neonates and Infants

In addition, all equipment and medications must be age-specific. For example, when transporting critically ill neonates, an infant intubation box and manual ventilator are a must, along with age-appropriate flow meters, suction equipment, and appropriately sized oxygen delivery devices. Capabilities for dosing and administering medications should also be anticipated. Medication administration, including age-adjustment of dosages and modes of administration, are discussed in more detail in Chapter 29 of this text.

- Supplemental medications, such as sedatives and narcotic analgesics
- Ample supply of appropriate IV fluids and medications
- Fully charged, battery-operated infusion pump

Basic quality assurance demands that all equipment is checked for proper operation prior to transport.

- In terms of *airway management*, the position of the patient's ET tube should be noted and resecured before transport.
- In regard to support for *ventilation*, hospital protocols usually dictate whether you use a BVM portable transport ventilator. If you use a transport ventilator, it must be capable of providing 100% O_2 and PEEP. It must also have both disconnect and high-pressure alarms, as well as sufficient portable power supply for the duration of transport. An HME generally is satisfactory for providing humidification via the ventilator circuit.
- As for *oxygenation*, unless precise $F_I O_2$ levels are required, you should default to providing 100% O_2 during transport.

Note: If the patient being transported requires a ventilator mode or settings that a portable ventilator cannot duplicate, ensure that the parameters to be used during transport are well tolerated by the patient by a trial run in the originating unit.

Monitoring. Basic physiologic monitoring during transport should, to the extent possible, duplicate that provided for the patient in the originating unit and include at least the following:

- Continuous ECG monitoring
- Continuous pulse oximetry
- Periodic measurement of blood pressure, pulse rate, and respiratory rate
- Periodic assessment of breath sounds

TRANSPORTING MECHANICALLY VENTILATED PATIENTS

If the patient is receiving ventilatory support during transport, airway pressures (PIP, PEEP) and tidal volumes should be monitored. If using a BVM, this may require attaching a pressure manometer and respirometer. According to the SCCM, some patients being transported also may require monitoring of expired CO_2 (capnography), as well as intra-arterial blood pressure and ICP.[3]

The AARC has issued guidelines for transporting mechanically ventilated patients within a health care facility.

Best Practice

In-Hospital Transport of the Mechanically Ventilated Patient—2002 Revision & Update (Excerpt)

1.0 Procedure: Transportation of a mechanically ventilated patient for diagnostic or therapeutic procedures.

2.0 Description/Definition: Transportation of mechanically ventilated patients for diagnostic or therapeutic procedures is always associated with a degree of risk.(1-9) Every attempt should be made to assure that monitoring, ventilation, oxygenation, and patient care remain constant during movement. Patient transport includes preparation, movement to and from, and time spent at destination.

3.0 Settings: This guideline is intended for the critical care and acute care inpatient setting.

4.0 Indications: Transportation of mechanically ventilated patients should only be undertaken following a careful evaluation of the risk-benefit ratio.

5.0 Contraindications: Transportation of the mechanically ventilated patient should not be undertaken until a complete analysis of potential risks and benefits has been accomplished.

5.1 Contraindications include

5.1.1 inability to provide adequate oxygenation and ventilation during transport either by manual ventilation, portable ventilator, or standard intensive care unit ventilator,

5.1.2 inability to maintain acceptable hemodynamic performance during transport,

5.1.3 inability to adequately monitor patient cardiopulmonary status during transport,

5.1.4 inability to maintain airway control during transport,

5.1.5 transport should not be undertaken unless all the necessary members of the transport team are present.

6.0 Hazards & Complications: Hazards and complications of transport include the following:

6.1 Hyperventilation during manual ventilation may cause respiratory alkalosis, cardiac dysrhythmias, and hypotension.

6.2 Loss of PEEP/CPAP may result in hypoxemia or shock.

6.3 Position changes may result in hypotension, hypercarbia, and hypoxemia.

6.4 Tachycardia and other dysrhythmias have been associated with transport.

6.5 Equipment failure can result in inaccurate data or loss of monitoring capabilities.

6.6 Inadvertent disconnection of intravenous access for pharmacologic agents may result in hemodynamic instability.

6.7 Movement may cause disconnection from ventilatory support and respiratory compromise.

6.8 Movement may result in accidental extubation.

6.9 Movement may result in accidental removal of vascular access.

6.10 Loss of oxygen supply may lead to hypoxemia.

6.11 Ventilator-associated pneumonia has been associated with transport.

7.0 Limitations of Method: The literature suggests that nearly two thirds of all transports for diagnostic studies fail to yield results that affect patient care.

8.0 Assessment of Need: The necessity and safety for transport should be assessed by the multidisciplinary team of health care providers, e.g., respiratory therapist, physician, nurse. The risks of transport should be weighed against the potential benefits from the diagnostic or therapeutic procedure to be performed.

9.0 Assessment of Outcome: The safe arrival of the mechanically ventilated patient at his/ her destination is the indicator of a favorable outcome.

10.0 Resources:

10.1 Equipment

10.1.1 Emergency airway management supplies should be available and checked for operation before transport.

10.1.2 Portable oxygen source of adequate volume;

10.1.3 A self-inflating bag and mask of appropriate size;

10.1.4 Transport ventilators have been shown to provide more constant ventilation than manual ventilation in some instances. If a transport ventilator is used, it should:

10.1.4.1 have sufficient portable power supply for the duration of transport;

10.1.4.2 have independent control of tidal volume and respiratory frequency;

Best Practice

(continued)

10.1.4.3 be able to provide full ventilatory support as in assist-control or intermittent mechanical ventilation (not necessarily both);

10.1.4.4 deliver a constant volume in the face of changing pulmonary impedance;

10.1.4.5 monitor airway pressure;

10.1.4.6 provide a disconnect alarm;

10.1.4.7 be capable of providing PEEP;

10.1.4.8 provide an FIO_2 of 1.0.

10.1.5 A pulse oximeter is desirable.

10.1.6 Appropriate pharmacologic agents should be readily available.

10.1.7 Portable monitor should display ECG and heart rate and provide at least one channel for vascular pressure measurement.

10.1.8 An appropriate hygroscopic condenser humidifier should be used to provide humidification during transport.

10.1.9 Stethoscope

10.1.10 Hand-held spirometer for tidal volume measurement

10.2 Personnel: All mechanically ventilated patients should be accompanied by a registered nurse and a respiratory therapist during the entire transport.

10.2.1 At least one team member must be proficient in managing the airway in the event of accidental extubation.

10.2.2 At least one team member should be proficient in operating and troubleshooting all of the equipment described in Section 10.1.

11.0 Monitoring: Monitoring provided during transport should be similar to that during stationary care.

11.1 Electrocardiograph should be continuously monitored for heart rate and dysrhythmias.

11.2 Blood pressure should be monitored continuously if invasive lines are present. In the absence of invasive monitoring, blood pressure should be measured intermittently via sphygmomanometer.

11.3 Respiratory rate should be monitored intermittently.

11.4 Airway pressures should be monitored if a transport ventilator is used.(24)

11.5 Tidal volume should be monitored intermittently to assure appropriate ventilation.(25)

11.6 Continuous pulse oximetry is appropriate during transport of all mechanically ventilated patients.

11.7 Breath sounds should be monitored intermittently.

13.1 Universal Precautions should be observed.

13.2 All equipment should be disinfected between patients.

Source: Excerpted from American Association for Respiratory Care. AARC clinical practice guideline: in-hospital transport of the mechanically ventilated patient. Respir Care. Revision and update *2002;47:721–723.*

HAZARDS DURING TRANSPORT

There are many hazards and complications to be on guard for during patient transport. These problems may involve equipment misuse or malfunction or a change in patient status. Equipment misuse or malfunction includes:

- Hyperventilation associated with overzealous manual BVM ventilation.
- Accidental extubation.
- Loss of IV access.
- Loss of PEEP/CPAP.
- Loss of O_2 supply.
- Ventilator, monitor, or IV pump failure.

You can avoid most of these problems by:

- Proper preplanning (including equipment prechecks).
- Always having a backup BVM with mask and PEEP/CPAP valve ready to go.
- Carefully monitoring the patient and "plumbing" during movement or position changes.

Ensuring proper preplanning and the provision of appropriate equipment, supplies, and support personnel is also the best way to address any potential changes in patient status during transport.

Cross-contamination, another hazard associated with all forms of patient transport, is latent and may not be immediately apparent. Many patients being transported are either colonized with a microbe or have an active infection. Transporters therefore must guard against the spread of infection to health care providers or other patients by strict adherence to infection control techniques. Hence, Universal Standard Precautions should be observed at all times:

- Frequent hand washing and/or the use of antimicrobial solutions.
- Appropriately using gloves, gowns, and masks.
- Disinfecting all equipment or discarding disposable equipment between patients.

Also, the Centers for Disease Control and Prevention recommendations related to tuberculosis and droplet nuclei are to be implemented when a patient is:

- Known or suspected to be immunosuppressed.
- Known to have tuberculosis.
- Has other risk factors for the disease.

These measures include using N-95 masks and the appropriate expiratory filters on the exhalation port of transport ventilators used for such patients.[4]

External Patient Transport

Many special considerations pertain to transporting critically ill patients outside the hospital. Some are similar to those for **intrahospital transport**, such as the need to ensure that the patient is stable enough to be moved, the training and personnel involved, the need for good preplanning and communication, as well as equipment issues, including an adequate O_2 supply.

However, ground and air transport entails unique considerations, most of which fall into the following categories:

- Choosing among ground and air transport modes
- Managing increased patient movement and stimulation
- Accommodating the need for special personnel and equipment
- Addressing the effects of altitude on P_aO_2 and closed air spaces

CHOOSING THE MODES OF TRANSPORT

Once equipment and personnel have been selected, consider the most appropriate mode of ground or air transport. With the possible exception of transporting very unstable patients, including trauma victims, most transports of less than 100 miles are best handled by ground via ambulance. However, in addition to distance being traveled, other factors are involved in selecting the mode of external transportation:

- The condition of the patient.
- Input from medical personnel.
- The availability of ambulance or aircraft.
- Weather conditions.

Table 37-1 summarizes the major advantages and disadvantages of transporting patients via ground, helicopter, and fixed-wing aircraft, all of which need to be considered when choosing the mode of transportation.

MANAGING MOVEMENT AND STIMULATION

Once the mode of transport is selected, secure the patient and all equipment to prevent unwanted movement. Be aware that patient overstimulation and stress can occur during ground transportation, due to the frequent stops, starts, turns, bumps, and road noise. Air transport also can stress a patient, especially when there is excessive vibration and/or insufficient temperature control during flight. These problems are particularly serious when transporting infants and children, who are the most vulnerable to such stimuli. For these reasons, all patients being externally transported should be properly positioned and secured, with appropriate sound protection and temperature control.

In addition, closely monitor the vital signs and general clinical status of all patients being transported so that any untoward distress can be quickly identified and addressed. Due to the high background noise in some aircraft, an automated noninvasive system may be needed to monitor blood pressure, as well as an amplified stethoscope to listen to breath sounds. Moreover, because most audible medical equipment alarms cannot be heard in noisy aircraft, transporters often have to depend on visual alarms and diligent patient assessment.

SPECIALIZED PERSONNEL AND EQUIPMENT

As with intrahospital transport, highly skilled clinicians and appropriate equipment are essential. The air/land transport team commonly includes a physician, nurse or paramedic, and a respiratory therapist. In combination, these personnel should have:

- The applicable advanced life support certification and experience.
- Proficiency in administering IV, intramuscular (IM), subcutaneous (SC), and inhaled medications.
- Competency in artificial airway management and mechanical ventilation.[5]

The respiratory therapist on the team is responsible for ensuring that properly functioning and age-specific

TABLE 37-1 **Advantages and disadvantages of patient transport via ground and air**

Mode	Advantages	Disadvantages
Ground/ ambulance	1. Generally most efficient within 100-mile distance 2. Often usable when inclement weather (fog) prevents air travel 3. Provides more work area for transport team 4. Less vibration and noise than in a helicopter 5. Usable in the absence of landing sites for air travel	1. Generally slower than air travel 2. Not practical in difficult terrain
Helicopter	1. Most efficient for distances between 100–250 miles 2. Faster than ground methods 3. May be faster for short distances in difficult terrain 4. Does not require landing strip and often can land near hospital	1. High noise and vibration resulting in overstimulation 2. May be grounded in inclement weather 3. Small work area 4. Expensive to maintain and operate 5. Hypobaric effects, which must be understood by crew
Fixed-wing aircraft	1. Fastest and most efficient for distances in excess of 250 miles 2. Less vibration and noise than helicopter 3. Able to travel at high altitudes, perhaps over inclement weather	1. May be grounded in inclement weather 2. Must be landed at an airport, requiring further patient transport 3. Small work area 4. Expensive to maintain and operate 5. Hypobaric effects, which must be understood by crew

equipment is available during transport. The equipment needs for air and land transport are essentially the same as those previously described for intrahospital transport. However, external transport entails certain special considerations:

- Ideally, the transport ventilator should be able to function using either 110-volt AC (supplied by a generator or inverter in the ambulance or aircraft) or 12-volt DC power (the typical voltage provided by a vehicle battery/alternator).
- If the portable ventilator is to be used for air transport, its volume, pressure, and flow settings should be adjustable either manually or automatically for variations in altitude and barometric pressure.
- Also needed are a calibrated polarographic or fuel cell O_2 analyzer and an ample supply of applicable medications for inhalation (e.g., bronchodilators, racemic epinephrine).
- Even patients who normally don't need supplemental O_2 may become hypoxic at altitude—commercial aircraft pressurize to between 8,000 and 10,000 ft altitude at barometric pressures 565 mmHg and 526 mmHg respectively.

Best Practice

All US airlines and many international airlines allow use of portable O_2 concentrators on board the plane. However, not all concentrators are approved for this function. Check with the airline prior to the flight where possible to avoid problems.

Air Transportation

Air transportation involves its own conditions, which must be factored into patient care. Altitude and pressure are different in flight than on the ground, and these conditions have an impact on oxygenation, volume, and pressure ventilation.

EFFECTS OF ALTITUDE ON OXYGENATION

During air transport, altitude affects oxygenation and closed air spaces. As a transport helicopter or airplane climbs to cruising altitude, the atmospheric and cabin

TABLE 37-2 **Effect of altitude on oxygenation with $F_IO_2 = 0.21$**

Altitude (feet)	P_b*	P_IO_2	P_aO_2	P_aO_2**
0	760	160	100	95
2000	706	148	88	80
5000	632	133	73	68
8000	565	119	59	54
10,000	523	110	50	45

*All pressures in torr/mm Hg.
** Assumes a $P(A - a)O_2$ of 5 torr and no compensation.

pressures decrease. As demonstrated in Table 37-2, in unpressurized cabins this creates a **hypobaric condition**, which lowers the inspired, alveolar, and arterial partial pressure of oxygen. At 2000 feet, the reduction in partial pressures is minimal, but at altitudes above 5000 feet, even a patient with normal lung capacity can suffer hypoxemia unless supplemental O_2 is provided.[6]

To compute a patient's equivalent F_IO_2 needs at cruising altitude compared with sea level, apply the following formula (based on **Dalton's law**):

$$F_IO_2 \text{ at altitude} = F_IO_2 \text{ at sea level} \times \frac{760}{P_B \text{ altitude}}$$

where P_B altitude equals the barometric pressure in torr at the cruising altitude used for transport. For example, a transported patient is receiving 50% at sea level in an airplane that will be cruising at 8000 feet (P_B = 565 torr). To compute the needed F_IO_2:

$$F_IO_2 \text{ at altitude} = 0.50 \times \frac{760}{565} = 0.67$$

At 8000 ft or higher, an F_IO_2 equivalent to 0.80 or more at sea level cannot be provided. For this reason, patients requiring 80% or more oxygen at sea level either have to be placed on PEEP/CPAP or have their PEEP levels raised to ensure adequate oxygenation.

Some transport aircraft provide pressurized cabins (especially some fixed-wing jets). However, most pressurized cabins are maintained at only about 75% sea level pressure, which is nearly the same as being in an unpressurized cabin at 8000 feet. In these cases, compute an equivalent F_IO_2 but substitute the known cabin pressure for the P_b at altitude.

Of course, the goal of O_2 supplementation should always be to achieve an S_pO_2 of 90% or greater, regardless of F_IO_2 or altitude. Fortunately, pulse oximetry readings are not affected by altitude and should therefore be the final criteria for judging the adequacy of patient oxygenation during transport.

Aircraft humidity tends to be much lower than sea level normal due to both altitude and the drying effects of compressors used to extract gas from the external atmosphere. Supplemental humidity may be needed especially for long flights.

EFFECTS OF ALTITUDE ON VOLUME AND PRESSURE

A second factor to consider during air transport is the relationship between gas volume and pressure. This effect is well-known to all those who have flown on a commercial airline and felt their inner ears pop as the plane climbs or descends. The principle involved is **Boyle's law**, whereby the volume of a gas varies inversely with its pressure. Based on this principle, as altitude increases and atmospheric pressure drops, gas volume increases, and vice versa. Consequently, a few special measures need to be taken, especially with mechanically ventilated patients. These include:

- Changing the set tidal volume, pressure limit, and/or PEEP to maintain proper ventilation and lung expansion.
- Adding or removing air from the ET or tracheostomy tube cuff to maintain a proper seal without damaging the tracheal mucosa.

In terms of cuff pressures, as altitude increases, so too does the volume of gas in the cuff. Because the tube cuff is restricted in its ability to expand within the trachea, a small increase in volume can result in a large increase in pressure. Indeed, some studies have reported a doubling of cuff pressures at altitudes as low as 3000 feet. The only good way to accommodate these changes (and those associated with descent from altitude) is to readjust the cuff pressure using the minimal-leak or occluding-volume technique every few minutes when the altitude is changing.[5]

A more difficult problem is when using a transport ventilator that cannot be adjusted to compensate for changes in altitude and barometric pressure. The difficulty arises from the fact that ventilators perform differently at altitude. For example:

- Volume-limited ventilators that use turbines or blowers tend to deliver *lower* than set volumes at altitude.
- Pneumatically powered systems that use differential pressure transducers to measure flow tend to deliver *higher* than set volumes at altitude.

There are several approaches to this problem with microprocessor-controlled ventilators:

- Temporarily disconnect the patient (and support with BVM + O_2) and recalibrate the device once you reach cruising altitude.
- Another solution is to follow the ventilator manufacturer's recommendation for adjusting settings at various barometric pressures.

Age-Specific Competency

Maintaining a Neutral Thermal Environment

Special sound-reducing incubators, combined with minimal handling and opening of incubator doors, also helps in maintaining a neutral thermal environment and in reducing the likelihood of stress from overstimulation.

- Last, empirically adjust delivered volume or pressure according to end-tidal CO_2 levels, as monitored by capnography. Unfortunately, capnometers also are affected by altitude, with the $P_{et}CO_2$ reading directly proportional to the barometric pressure (causing a falsely low $P_{et}CO_2$ reading at altitude). This error can be overcome by recalibrating the capnometer's high reading at the cruising altitude with a standard known concentration of CO_2 (usually 5%). Unfortunately, this adds equipment and weight to the aircraft, which may not be desirable.

SPECIAL CONSIDERATIONS

In addition to the preceding procedures and guidelines, factors related to the patient's age or clinical condition should be considered.

Neonates. Because of stress imposed on them from overstimulation and difficulties with **thermoregulation**, neonates are perhaps the most vulnerable to complications associated with transport. In addition, most neonates requiring transport suffer from lung disease secondary to prematurity and other factors. As a result, special attention relating to this group of patient is often required. To assist with thermoregulation, the following items may be used during transport:

- Incubators
- Warmed IV bags and blankets
- A head cap
- Commercially made chemical heating pads
- Plastic shields and aluminum wraps to reduce radiant and convective heat loss

Trapped Gas Volume Changes. For patient of all ages, other complications are associated with trapped gas volume changes—that is, gas in an enclosed space that cannot equilibrate with the ambient pressure. This is a common problem in patients with a pneumothorax and/or excessive gas in the stomach or bowel. However, it can also occur after skull trauma or neurosurgery (pneumocephalus) or penetrating eye wounds (intraocular gas). Such problems should be identified and managed prior to transport, specifically, via the insertion of a chest or nasogastric tube.

The Bends. If a patient suffering from **decompression sickness** (the **bends**) has to be transported to a hyperbaric facility, try to ensure that the cabin pressure is maintained as near to sea level as possible. In this condition, the lower the ambient pressure, the worse the morbidity and mortality.[3]

Summary

When transporting critically ill patients, safety is paramount. However, many patients are transported within or between health care facilities because they are critically ill and need special services or procedures. The additional stress that may be imposed on such patients can be clinically challenging. However, through proper planning and execution and follow-up, these risks can be minimized. By following the procedures outlined in this chapter, including maintaining a state of readiness, properly prescreening patients, selecting the most appropriate means of transportation, and ensuring the proper personnel and equipment in place, potential complications can be avoided and patient safety can be maximized during transporting.

Study Questions

REVIEW QUESTIONS

1. Describe the main focus of any patient transport.
2. List the contraindications to patient transport.
3. List the four areas that must be addressed in planning and executing a patient transport.
4. Describe the physiologic monitoring that must be in place when transporting critically ill patients.
5. Summarize the major advantages and disadvantages of each form of external transport.
6. Describe the major effects of hypobaric conditions on oxygenation and ventilation of mechanically ventilated patients.

MULTIPLE-CHOICE QUESTIONS

1. All of the following are required when transporting critically ill patients, *except* which?
   a. adequate oxygenation and ventilation
   b. acceptable hemodynamic performance
   c. airway maintenance
   d. transport of family members

2. What is the term for the atmospheric conditions in an unpressurized aircraft that result in a lower barometric pressure and that generally require adjustments to ensure adequate oxygenation and ventilation?
   a. hyperbaric conditions
   b. thermoregulation
   c. the bends
   d. hypobaric conditions
3. Additional stress may be imposed on patients being transported as a result of all of which of the following factors?
   I. vibration
   II. noise
   III. motion
   IV. temperature variations
      a. I and II
      b. I, II, III, and IV
      c. I and IV
      d. I, II, and III
4. It is recommended that all of the following equipment accompany all critically ill patients on transport, *except* which?
   a. oxygen source with sufficient duration of flow
   b. cardiac defibrillator
   c. manual resuscitator bag and mask
   d. cardiac pacemaker
5. In an unpressurized aircraft, it is often necessary to make adjustments to patients being ventilated through cuffed artificial airways. In addition to closely monitoring such patients' ventilation and oxygenation status, it is commonly necessary to:
   a. add air to the cuff.
   b. remove air from the cuff.
   c. use an uncuffed airway.
   d. use a fenestrated airway.

CRITICAL-THINKING QUESTIONS

1. A critically ill but stable pediatric patient must be transported from one hospital to another, which is located in a rural area 200 miles away. If given the choice, what mode of transport would the respiratory therapist recommend and why?
2. A respiratory therapist is asked to assist in a mechanically ventilated patient via an unpressurized aircraft. What are the major factors to consider regarding the oxygenation and ventilation of such a patient?
3. Describe two conditions that would warrant special considerations when transporting such patients via ground or air. Summarize at least two specific measures to take for each to ensure their safety during the transport.

References

1. American Association for Respiratory Care. AARC clinical practice guideline: in-hospital transport of the mechanically ventilated patient. *Respir Care.* Revision and update 2002;47:721–723.
2. Warren J, Fromm RF, Orr RA, Rotello IC, Horst HM. Guidelines for the inter- and intrahospital transport of critically ill patients. *Crit Care Med.* 2004;32:56–62.
3. Whitaker K. *Comprehensive Perinatal & Pediatric Respiratory Care.* 3rd ed. Clifton Park, NY: Delmar Cengage Learning; 2001.
4. Dooley Jr SW, Castro KG, Hutton MD, Mullan RJ, Polder JA, Snider Jr DE. Guidelines for preventing the transmission of tuberculosis in health-care settings, with special focus on HIV-related issues. *MMWR Recomm Rep.* 1990; 391–392.
5. Voigt LP, Pastores SM, Raoof ND, Thaler HT, Halpern NA. Intrahospital transport of critically ill patients: outcomes, timing, and patterns. *J Intensive Care Med.* 2009;31:72–78.
6. Shepard MV, Trethewy CE, Kennedy J, Davis L. Helicopter use in rural trauma. *Emerg Med Australia.* 2008;20,6:494–499.

Suggested Readings

Andrews PJ, Piper IR, Dearden NM, Miller JD. Secondary insults during intrahospital transport of head-injured patients. *Lancet.* 1990;335,8685:327–330.

Braman SS, Dunn SM, Amico CA, Millman RP. Complications of intrahospital transport in critically ill patients. *Ann Intern Med.* 1987;107,4:469–473.

Branson RD. Intrahospital transport of critically ill, mechanically ventilated patients. *Respir Care.* 1992;37,7:775–795.

Hurst JM, Davis Jr K, Johnson DJ, Branson RD, Campbell RS, Branson PS. Cost and complications during in-hospital transport of critically ill patients: a prospective cohort study. *J Trauma.* 1992;33,4:582–585.

Smith I, Fleming S, Cernaianu A. Mishaps during transport from the intensive care unit. *Crit Care Med.* 1990;18,3:278–281.

SECTION VI

Miscellaneous Applications

CHAPTER 38

Protecting the Patient and the Health Care Provider

Patricia L. Carroll

OBJECTIVES

Upon completion of this chapter, the reader should be able to:

- Describe the elements of the chain of infection.
- Outline proper hand hygiene procedures.
- Discuss the proper use of barrier personal protective equipment (PPE).
- Determine which protective actions are necessary for each type of precautions.
- List ways to reduce the risk of needlestick injury.
- Identify approaches to reduce the risk of latex allergy symptoms.
- Explain how microbial resistance occurs and how drug resistance affects the patient and health care worker.
- Describe how to get the most updated information on care of patients exposed to bioterrorism agents and pandemic influenza.

CHAPTER OUTLINE

KEY TERMS

Airborne Precautions
airborne transmission
antimicrobial-resistant microorganisms
carrier
case
chain of infection
clean
colonization
common vehicle transmission
Contact Precautions
contact transmission
direct contact
Droplet Precautions
droplet transmission
fomite
hand hygiene
health care-associated infection
high-efficiency particulate air (HEPA) filter
indirect contact
infectious agent
Isolation Precautions
latex allergy
method (mode) of transmission
multidrug-resistant microorganism (MDRM)
needlestick injuries
pathogen
personal protective equipment (PPE)
portal of entry
portal of exit
reservoir
resident flora
Standard Precautions
sterile
surgical hand scrubbing
susceptible host
transient flora
Transmission-Based Precautions
vector
vector-borne transmission

More than 100 years ago, special hospitals were set up for patients with infections. Not much was known then about how diseases were transmitted, but health care workers realized that diseases could be passed from patient to patient and, in some cases, from patients to health care providers. Around the end of the nineteenth century, textbooks began to include information about medical asepsis.

Infection control practices continued to evolve until 1985, when the Centers for Disease Control and Prevention established practices called Universal Precautions in response to the emergence of HIV disease. Since then, great attention has been given to two aspects of infection control: how to reduce the spread of disease between and among patients and how to protect health care workers from acquiring diseases in the workplace.

Each year, hundreds of millions of patients who require inpatient care worldwide are diagnosed with a **health-care-associated infection** that was not present on admission. Not only do these infections increase morbidity and mortality and lengthen stay, but they also cost the health care system hundreds of millions of dollars each year and increase the burden on an already stressed system of care.[1] If health-care-associated infections could be reduced, recovered resources could be used to improve the health of citizens worldwide.

Each health care worker has a personal responsibility for following guidelines for reducing infection transmission among patients and between patients and their caregivers. Infection prevention is a key element of safe patient care.

Chain of Infection

The spread of infectious disease requires six elements, called the **chain of infection**. If any link in the chain is broken or missing, infectious disease transmission does not occur (Figure 38-1). The six elements are:

- The infectious agent (also called the causative microorganism or agent).
- The reservoir (or source).
- The portal of exit (from reservoir).
- The method of transmission.
- The portal of entry (to the host).
- A susceptible host. (1,16)

Special strategies applied at each link of the chain make the links easier to break. Whether a link is successfully broken is often determined by the attention that health care workers pay to proper infection control practices.

INFECTIOUS AGENT

The **infectious agent**, sometimes called the causative microorganism, agent, or **pathogen**, is a microorganism that can cause disease. The most common agents are bacteria, viruses, fungi, and protozoa. One of these agents must be present for disease to spread.

The characteristics of the organism can help determine how *pathogenic*, or disease-producing, the organism is. This is one of the concerns about the potential for an avian influenza pandemic. To infect humans, the virus has to mutate, and in mutation, it can become highly pathogenic, meaning a tiny amount of virus exposure can cause illness.

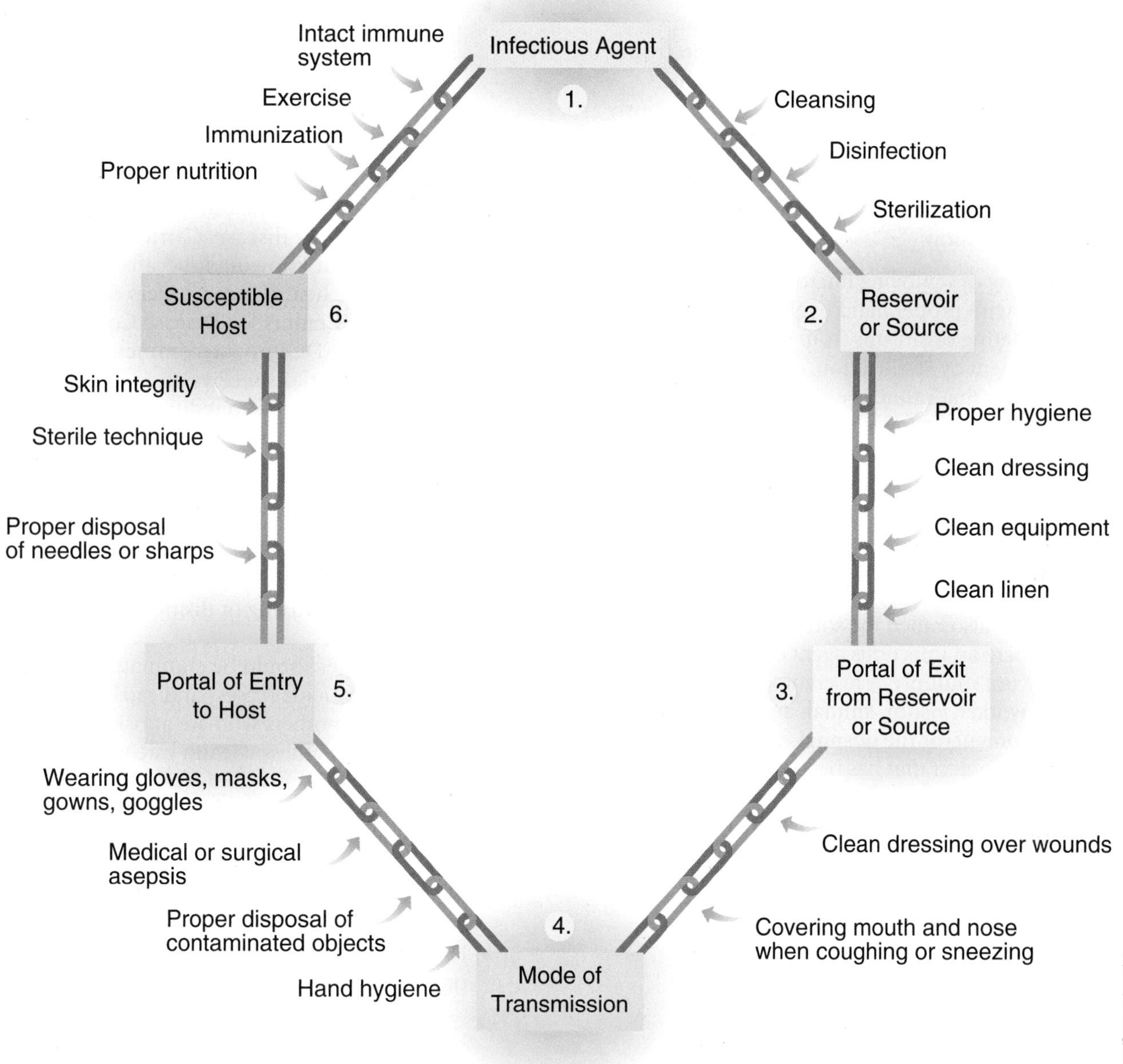

FIGURE 38-1 Chain of infection and methods of breaking the links.

Another issue is bacterial mutation. Bacteria exposed to antibiotics can change their structure so that common antimicrobials no longer kill them. Drug resistance is an emerging health threat, because these new so-called *superorganisms* cause infections that are extremely hard to treat. This is a particular problem with multi-drug-resistant tuberculosis and other increasingly common infections such as those caused by methicillin-resistant staph (MRSA) (see Drug-Resistant Pathogens in this chapter).

Many experts attribute this growth of resistant organisms to the overuse of antimicrobials in the hospital. Recommendations today are to:

- Limit the use of antimicrobials to known infections in which the organism has been identified and that sensitivity tests have

determined to be the most effective antimicrobials to fight that organism.
- Use the lowest-strength narrow-spectrum drug, saving the more potent, broad-spectrum antimicrobials for more serious infections.[2]
- Use antimicrobials prudently and continuously monitor patients in all acute care settings for infection.

Even before disease can spread, health care workers can stop transmission:

- Reducing or removing microbes from their hands with proper hand hygiene.
- Eliminating organisms from surfaces and equipment by sterilization.
- For items that cannot be sterilized, such as floors and furniture, remove some or all of the pathogenic organisms with disinfectants.
- Employ isolation practices to contain the causative agent.

RESERVOIR

The **reservoir**, also called the source of the infection, identifies where an infectious agent can survive but may or may not multiply. A reservoir can be a patient, health care worker, visitor, animal, an inanimate object such as equipment, or the hospital environment itself. A **fomite** is an object that has become contaminated with material that contains a pathogenic microbe. Fomites usually come into direct contact with secretions or excretions from a patient. Common fomites are:

- Bedpans.
- Tissues.
- Linens.
- Bed rails.
- Bed controls.
- Equipment such as nebulizers.
- Containers for laboratory specimens such as sputum.

In hospitals, standing water can also act as a reservoir. Standing water poses a particular risk for transmission of *Legionella pneumophila*, the bacterium responsible for Legionnaire's disease, a form of pneumonia. This organism thrives in standing water and is transmitted to people when infected water becomes aerosolized and the aerosol containing the organism is inhaled. Outbreaks can occur from exposure in buildings where the contaminated water (often from roofs) is transmitted through air-conditioning systems. In addition, in hospitals, contaminated water can be aerosolized in patient showers.[3]

There are two types of human reservoir:

- A **case** is a person who is symptomatic with an illness, for example, a person with pneumonia. Cases are relatively easy to identify because they are visibly sick. From an epidemiologic perspective the first case is called the 'index" case or "patient one."
- A **carrier** is a person who is infected with and can transmit a disease but has no signs or symptoms of the disease. Carriers can transmit illness without knowing it because they are not sick. Because health care workers can be carriers, the Centers for Disease Control and Prevention (CDC) now recommends that all health care workers receive an influenza vaccination each fall to reduce the risk of transmitting the virus to vulnerable patients.[4]

The reservoir link in the chain of infection can be broken in several ways.

- Fomites should be eliminated by properly disposing of contaminated objects, such as tissues, and sterilizing or disinfecting reusable objects.
- Standing water should be eliminated.
- Infectious patients (cases) and carriers should be isolated from others who are at risk for contracting infectious illness. Health care workers who are sick should stay out of work in the clinical setting until they are no longer contagious. Regular screening of health care workers, such as through tuberculosis (TB) skin testing, helps in identifying those who might have been significantly exposed and thus might be infectious.
- Hand hygiene and strict adherence to the principles of asepsis are critical.

PORTAL OF EXIT

The **portal of exit** is the pathway by which an infectious agent leaves the reservoir. This term is most often used to describe how pathogens leave a human reservoir. Common portals of exit are:

- Sputum.
- Blood.
- Saliva.
- Stool.
- Drainage from contaminated wounds.

This link in the chain of infection can be broken by containing the microbes. Ask patients to cover their nose and mouth when they cough or sneeze, to cough into tissues or a covered specimen cup, and to dispose of the tissues in a receptacle at the bedside.

Best Practice

Portal of Exit

Keep in mind that patients' hands can become contaminated by handling used tissues; patients should wash their hands frequently. Hand hygiene interrupts the transmission by eliminating the pathogens. Health care workers should also wash their hands frequently and wear appropriate personal protective equipment, dictated by the risk of exposure (see Standard Precautions).

METHOD OF TRANSMISSION

The **method** (or **mode**) **of transmission** is the way an infectious agent moves from a reservoir to a susceptible host. There are three main methods of transmission: airborne, contact, and droplet. Two less common methods are vector-borne and common vehicle.

Airborne transmission occurs when the pathogens are tiny and lightweight. These microscopic particles remain suspended in the air and move with the air currents, or they become trapped in dust, which is carried through the air and eventually inhaled. *Mycobacterium tuberculosis,* a bacterium, and *Aspergillus* spp spores, a mold fungus, are transmitted this way. Organisms can travel over long distances and infect people without face-to-face contact with the infected patient.[5] Special precautions must be taken to prevent the spread of these organisms, particularly in congregate living situations such as homeless shelters, prisons, and health care facilities.

Contact transmission occurs in two ways.

- **Direct contact** is from person to person, such as when one person's body fluids enter another's body through a break in the skin or through mucus membranes. This is how HIV, hepatitis, and other bloodborne pathogens are transmitted—through fluid passed directly from one person to another.
- **Indirect contact** occurs when a person becomes infected from a contaminated intermediate object or person. Health care workers' contaminated hands are the most common means of indirect contact transmission of disease.[5] In addition, workers' clothing or equipment (such as a stethoscope) may become contaminated during patient care, and the pathogens can be transferred as the health care worker cares for another patient. Contaminated environmental objects also contribute to disease transmission in this way. In pediatric settings, contaminated toys can spread infections, particularly respiratory syncytial virus. This method of disease transmission is particularly troublesome in hospitals because patients are usually hosts with decreased immune response and thus are highly prone to becoming infected with transmitted pathogens. *Clostridium difficile* disease, a serious bacterial intestinal infection, is transmitted through indirect contact and is an increasing problem in health care facilities.

Droplet transmission is considered technically a form of contact transmission. This occurs when pathogens are spread by mucus and other large drops from a patient's respiratory tract directly to the mucus membranes of the recipient. They can be transmitted up to 3 feet when the patient coughs, sneezes, or talks, and during procedures such as airway suctioning, endotracheal intubation, and cardiopulmonary resuscitation.[5] The distance of 3 feet is based on epidemiologic studies; however, in recent years, more evidence shows that droplet transmission can occur over as much as 6 feet. The distance depends on the velocity and mechanism by which the droplets leave the source, droplet size, environmental temperature and humidity, and the ability of the organism to maintain infectivity over distance. Thus the CDC recommends wearing a mask for exposure within 6–10 feet or when entering the patient's room. Pathogens transmitted in this way include *Bordetella pertussis,* influenza virus, adenovirus, rhinovirus, *Mycoplasma pneumoniae,* and SARS-associated coronavirus (SARS-CoV)

Two less common modes of transmission are vector-borne and common vehicle.

- In **vector-borne transmission**, a vector carries the pathogen from one person to another. A **vector** is any organism that carries a pathogen from one host to another. For example, ticks are the vectors of Lyme disease, and mosquitoes are the vectors of malaria and West Nile virus.
- **Common vehicle transmission** is the term used for infections caused by contaminated items such as food, water, or medications or any substance to which many people are exposed. Diseases spread by common vehicle transmission are cholera, salmonellosis, and botulism poisoning. From time to time, liquid medications are recalled by the manufacturer when contamination occurs during the manufacturing process or when multiuse vials are contaminated during use.[6]

Table 38-1 summarizes these transmission methods.

TABLE 38-1 **Methods of transmission of infectious agents**

Airborne Transmission:
Pathogens carried by moisture or dust particles in air; can be carried long distances
Droplet Transmission:
Droplet spread within approximately 3–10 feet (no personal contact) of infected person by:
Coughing
Sneezing
Talking
Laughing
Singing
Contact Transmission:
Pathogen spread by direct contact with infected person:
Touching
Sexual contact
Blood
Body fluids (drainage, urine, feces, sputum, saliva, vomitus)
Pathogen spread by indirect contact with infected person:
Clothing
Dressings
Equipment used in care and treatment
Bed linens
Personal belongings
Specimen containers
Instruments used in treatment
Food
Water
Vector-Borne Transmission:
Pathogen carried from one organism to another by a third organism
Common Vehicle Transmission:
Pathogen carried by a substance used by many people, such as water supply or multiuse drug vial

A number of actions can break the method of transmission link of the chain of infection.

- Airborne and droplet transmission can be reduced by wearing proper masks and isolating patients.
- Direct contact transmission of pathogens can be significantly reduced by following appropriate barrier precautions, particularly gloves.
- Indirect contact transmission can be limited by meticulous attention to hand hygiene, disinfecting surfaces and sterilizing equipment and by using bags or covered containers to separate and contain contaminated materials.
- Vectors can be reduced in the community through public health measures and proper sanitation.
- Common vehicle pathogen transmission can be minimized through the proper handling of food (particularly adequate, timely refrigeration), water, and medications.

PORTAL OF ENTRY

The **portal of entry** is the path by which an infectious agent enters a susceptible host. The most common portals of entry are:

- The respiratory, gastrointestinal, and genitourinary tracts.
- The circulatory system.
- Intact mucus membranes and breaks in the skin.

To break this link in the chain of infection:

- Wear gloves when coming into contact with body fluids and sterile gloves before performing any invasive procedures.
- Use aseptic technique when indicated.
- Change gloves when they become contaminated, and practice proper hand hygiene technique.
- All persons entering rooms in which patients with suspected or confirmed infectious TB disease are being isolated must wear approved respirator masks. [For the most current guidelines on respirator use for health care workers, check the Web sites for the National Institute for Occupational Safety and Health (http://www.cdc.gov/niosh/) and the Occupational Safety and Health Administration (http://www.osha.gov/SLTC/respiratoryprotection/index.html).][7]

SUSCEPTIBLE HOST

The final link of the chain of infection is the **susceptible host**. All of the other links may be intact, but no illness occurs if the host (the target of the pathogens) is not susceptible to the infection. People are exposed to pathogens daily, particularly in a hospital. However, an infection occurs only if a person's immune system is sufficiently weakened or overwhelmed to allow the pathogen to enter the body, begin to multiply, and damage the host. Table 38-2 lists factors that make a patient prone to infection. The CDC also identifies:

- Agent-host interaction as a significant element, including pathogenicity (the agent's capacity to cause disease or damage).

TABLE 38-2 **Factors that make a patient susceptible to infection**[8]

Factor
Exposure
Attendance at child daycare
Institutional or congregate living
Inpatient care
Personal hygiene ability
Occupation
Sexual activity
School attendance or employment
Travel
Illness and severity
Age (the very young and the elderly)*
Immune status*
Gender (for certain conditions)
Lack of (or expired) immunizations
Poor nutritional status
Medications (particularly immunosuppressive therapy including corticosteroids and antibiotics)
Preexisting diseases such as diabetes, HIV/AIDS, malignancy, COPD, alcoholism, and post-transplant
Coexisting infections
Radiation therapy
Use of artificial airway, urinary catheter, vascular access catheter
Pathogen virulence, dose, duration of exposure, and antibiotic resistance
Surgery
Burns
Genetics
Stress (emotional and physiological)
Sleep deprivation

** These two factors are key in determining the likelihood of illness and its severity.*

- Virulence (the disease-producing potential of a particular agent).
- Antigenicity (the ability of the agent to produce a systemic or localized reaction in the host).[6,5]

The susceptible host link in the chain of infection can be broken by several measures that enhance the host's ability to fight off infection.

- Vaccines—such as hepatitis B and influenza (particularly for health care workers), pneumococcus for all persons over age 65 and those at risk for pneumonia, and the *Haemophilus influenzae* type B (Hib) vaccine in children—all reduce the incidence of infection.
- Public health measures, including proper nutrition, clean water, and community health education (such as smoking cessation programs) reduce host susceptibility in the community.
- In the hospital, careful attention to patients' nutrition (particularly during lengthy stays in critical care), preventing pressure ulcers, and minimizing the use of urinary and vascular access catheters also reduce risk for infection.
- Antimicrobials should be used only when clearly indicated.
- Protective isolation measures may be required for hospitalized patients who are severely immunosuppressed—most commonly persons being prepared for or those who have received tissue or organ transplant and cancer patients with neutropenia. These patients must be separated from others with active infections.[5]

Health Care Setting

The CDC identifies health care settings with particular risks for health-care-associated infections (HAI). (20)

- *Intensive care units* (*ICUs*) have a small proportion of hospitalized patients and a large proportion of the infections. ICU patients are the most physiologically compromised, and they have the most invasive procedures. They also have the longest contact with health care professionals and the greatest exposure to antimicrobial therapy.
- *Burn units* present special risk because the patients' compromised skin integrity removes a protective barrier to infection. Care practices to reduce the risk of infection are continually evolving, and there is little evidence to recommend specific patient care practices in this setting.
- In *pediatrics*, health care workers have more intense contact with patients, particularly infants, who are held for many care procedures. Siblings who visit may bring common communicable diseases to inpatients, and open playrooms with shared toys present a clear avenue for pathogenic organism transmission through indirect contact. In addition, children are not as likely to follow infection control practices as well as adults do.
- *Long-term care* (*LTC*) settings house persons who are not able to care for themselves due to changes in physical or cognitive ability. Most are elderly, and many are colonized with various organisms. Most in residential care depend on

health care workers for personal hygiene and mobility. Many LTC residents are frequently hospitalized, increasing the transfer of pathogenic organisms from the LTC facility to the acute care hospital and back again.

Hand Hygiene

According to the World Health Organization, there is convincing evidence that appropriate hand hygiene reduces the frequency of HAI. (25) Many health care workers think they do not have much to learn about hand hygiene because the procedure seems so simple. But following very specific steps increases the effectiveness of hand hygiene while reducing pathogen transmission and the resultant infections in the health care setting.[5,1]

In 2007, the CDC published new guidelines for preventing transmission of infectious agents in health care settings. (20) For the first time, the term "hand hygiene" is used instead of handwashing because the guidelines support the use of hand sanitizers as a supplement to—and in some cases to replace—handwashing.

Hand hygiene is important because many pathogens are normally found on the hands. There are two categories of microbe:

- **Transient flora** describes microorganisms that live and multiply on the skin's surface but are not consistently on the hands of most people. They may be living freely on the skin or loosely attached to dirt particles and skin secretions. These microbes can easily be transmitted to other people and are important causes of HAI. In fact, the common cold is most often transmitted through hand-to-hand contact after the infected person wipes or scratches his nose. Transient flora can easily be removed by hand hygiene. The friction applied to the hand surfaces with a hand rub, as well as during washing with soap and water, serves to eliminate transient flora.
- **Resident flora**, microorganisms consistently present on the skin of most people, are also known as *normal flora* or *endogenous flora*. They are normally shed with old skin cells but are more adherent than transient flora and are not readily removed with simple friction, soap, and water. They are rarely transmitted to patients except when introduced during invasive procedures without proper barrier precautions.[9]

There are two types of hand care.

- Basic **hand hygiene** includes handwashing and using hand sanitizers. Most hand sanitizers are alcohol-based hand rubs, but other agents are being developed. Hand hygiene removes soil and transient flora by the combination of friction, soap or detergent, and water. Hand sanitizers remove transient flora by combining friction with the antimicrobial properties of the sanitizer's active ingredient.
- **Surgical hand scrubbing** removes or destroys transient flora and is the only technique that reduces resident flora. Surgical hand scrubbing requires an antimicrobial soap or detergent preparation, a brush, and a significantly longer period of washing than routine hand hygiene. Published guidelines do not recommend the routine use of antimicrobial soap outside of surgical hand scrubbing.[5,1]

Hand hygiene should be performed:[1]

- Before and after direct patient contact.
- After removing gloves.
- Before handling an invasive device (regardless of whether gloves are used).
- After contact with body fluids or excretions, mucus membranes, nonintact skin, or wound dressings.
- If moving from a contaminated body site to a clean body site during patient care.
- After contact with objects (including medical equipment) in the patient's room.
- Before handling patient medications or preparing food.

Unless hands are visibly soiled, hand sanitizers are preferred over hand hygiene because of superior microbicidal activity, reduced skin drying, and convenience, which increases compliance.[5] Wash hands if they are visibly soiled or if they came into contact with body fluids.

HAND HYGIENE TECHNIQUE

An effective hand hygiene procedure requires some forethought.

- Be sure of an adequate supply of soap for washing and paper towels for drying the hands at the end of the procedure.
- Never stack paper towels on the side of the sink. They can become contaminated from splash from the sink and then contaminate freshly washed hands during drying.
- Avoid multiple-use cloth towels; they can harbor microorganisms.

Best Practice

Hand Hygiene

Hand hygiene is the single most important action health care workers can take to stop the spread of infection. It can break five of the six links in the chain of infection.

- Warm air machines achieve the greatest reduction of flora on the hands but are impractical in health care settings because they are noisy, take longer than paper towels to dry the hands, and are limited to use by one person at a time.
- Liquid soaps are preferable to bar soaps because bar soaps can easily become contaminated. The liquid should be stored in and dispensed from a closed, disposable container. The container should be emptied before more liquid soap is added.

Once the supplies are in order, follow these steps:

1. Turn on the water and wet hands in running water.
2. Apply approximately 3–5 mL of soap.
3. Thoroughly distribute the soap over all hand surfaces, paying special attention to the back of the hands and under the nails.
4. *Vigorously rub* the hands together for at least 10–15 seconds, generating friction on all surfaces, particularly the sides of the fingers.
5. Wash all surfaces, including the whole thumb, between the fingers, and the back of the hands. Remove debris from beneath the fingernails. (The duration of the hand hygiene procedure is key to providing friction for an adequate time to physically remove microbes from all surfaces of both hands.)
6. Thoroughly rinse hands, with the fingertips pointed down into the sink. Do not shake the hands to remove water.
7. *While the water is still running,* dry the hands thoroughly with a paper towel.
8. Use the paper towel to turn off the faucet. (Contaminated hands touched the faucets at the beginning of the procedure. If the paper towel is not used, clean hands instantly become contaminated at the end of the procedure.)

Best Practice

When to Perform Hand Hygiene

A good rule of thumb is to perform hand hygiene whenever doing so seems necessary, especially:

- Before and after patient contact.
- After contact with a source of microorganisms.
- After removing gloves.
- When the hands are visibly soiled.
- After using bed controls.
- After opening exterior or interior door.
- After opening bedside tables or storage units (door handles are seldom cleaned and sanitized).

Skin damage can alter the types of microbial flora present on the skin, resulting in an increased prevalence of clinically important microorganisms that could result in HAI.[10] Hand sanitizers contain emollients that help protect the skin. Frequent water exposure during hand hygiene removes natural oils and increases skin drying. Lotion may be used to keep hands from drying out and cracking as a result of frequent hand hygiene.[1] However, even lotion can become contaminated, particularly if all unit or department staffers use one bottle. Ideally, each health care worker should have a small personal bottle or tube of lotion for use over a short time.

BARRIERS TO HAND HYGIENE

Health care workers do not wash their hands properly or as frequently as they should for many reasons.

- One reason is the physical layout of the workplace. If health care workers must walk some distance from the bedside to a sink, they are much less likely to wash their hands than if sinks are handy and easy to find.

Best Practice

Hand Lotions

Hand lotions that contain petroleum or other oil-based emollients may affect the integrity of latex gloves. Use a water-based lotion or cream. This problem has not been reported with vinyl or nitrile gloves, but it is best to check with the manufacturer before using non-water-based products.

Theoretically, the need for hand hygiene depends on:

- The intensity of contact with a patient or fomite.
- The degree of contamination likely to occur with the contact.
- The susceptibility to infection.
- The procedure being performed.

For example, if a respiratory therapist goes into a patient's room to check the liter flow of oxygen going to a nasal cannula, sees that it is correct, and does not touch anything in the room, hand hygiene is not required as long as the patient is not on special isolation precautions. But if the respiratory therapist has to reposition the patient's nasal cannula or handle other items in the room, hand hygiene is needed.

- When staffing is reduced, people feel they don't have the time to wash their hands after each patient contact because providing care is prioritized over hand hygiene.
- Many people find that frequent hand hygiene dries out and irritates their hands, sometimes resulting in redness and cracking. Hand sanitizers eliminate these barriers. The solution can be carried in the practitioner's pocket or dispensed in the room or hallway just outside the door. Dispensers are rarely more than a few steps away. Using hand rub takes less time, and the solutions actually protect the skin.[5,1]

Standard Precautions

In 1996, the CDC established a system to minimize the risk of transmitting pathogens, **Standard Precautions**.[5] These guidelines were developed after several years of research on and development of the best ways to protect health care workers, patients, and visitors from a wide range of diseases. The guidelines are designed to be epidemiologically sound, to provide comprehensive protection, and to be easy to understand and to use. For Standard Precautions to be effective, however, all health care workers must use them correctly and consistently. Precautions should be used for any contact with blood, moist body substances (except sweat), mucus membranes, or nonintact skin of any patient, as well as contact with any bedside items or equipment that may be contaminated with body fluids.[11,5] Standard Precautions for infection control are shown in Figure 38-2.

Two keys to Standard Precautions are hand hygiene and the use of **personal protective equipment (PPE)**. Personal protective equipment includes gloves, gown, mask and goggles, or face shield.

GLOVES

Gloves can reduce or prevent the spread of disease.

- **Clean** gloves may have pathogens on them but not enough to cause disease.
- **Sterile** gloves have no microorganisms on them. (For more on disinfection and sterilization, see Chapter 5.)

Most patient care procedures, such as assisting a patient to cough sputum into a tissue, drawing a blood gas, or intubating a patient, can be done with clean gloves. More invasive procedures require sterile gloves. For respiratory therapists, sterile gloves are used:

- When they are suctioning an artificial airway with an open suction catheter.
- When the glove touches the catheter that is inserted into the airway.

When used correctly, gloves:

- Protect the patient from organisms on the health care worker's hands.
- Protect the health care worker from picking up pathogens from patients.
- Prevent pathogens from being carried from one patient to another.
- Do not protect against needlesticks or injuries from sharp instruments; these penetrate glove material.
- Can provide adequate barrier protection when they fit and are free from cuts, tears, cracks, or holes.

For general use, latex, vinyl, or nitrile gloves are available powdered or nonpowdered. Powdered gloves are easier to put on, but the powder may cause significant skin irritation and can bind with latex allergens. The CDC recommends latex or nitrile for procedures requiring manual dexterity and those that involve more than brief patient contact.[5] Otherwise, vinyl gloves can be used. Gloves must be provided for health care providers in various sizes for reasonable fit. Some facilities have removed all latex products, including latex gloves because of the risk of latex allergy. If other barrier protective equipment is used, gloves are put on last and over the gown cuffs.

Although gloves minimize the risk of a pathogen contaminating a health care provider's hands, the gloves themselves, if not used correctly, transfer organisms. Perform hand hygiene before putting gloves on and immediately after removing them. Do not wash your hands with the gloves on; doing so can damage the gloves and allow microbes to pass through to your hands. Since gloves are often contaminated during patient care, different activities with the same patient may require changing gloves multiple times so that cross-contamination does not occur. For example, if the respiratory therapist assists a patient with coughing and handles tissues filled with sputum, the gloves must be removed and hand hygiene performed before applying clean gloves to draw a blood gas. Table 38-3 lists situations that require a change of gloves. Clean gloves must be applied immediately before touching the mucus membranes of the patient's mouth and upper airway.

Remember that *anything* touched with a contaminated glove becomes contaminated too. A common mistake is opening doors with a contaminated glove; then the door hardware is contaminated for the next person. The same principle applies to other objects in the patient's room, such as bed rails, the controls that raise and lower the bed, the television control, and the patient call bell. Once a glove has been contaminated,

STANDARD PRECAUTIONS

FOR INFECTION CONTROL

Assume that every person is potentially infected or colonized with an organism that could be transmitted in the healthcare setting.

Hand Hygiene

Avoid unnecessary touching of surfaces in close proximity to the patient.

When hands are visibly dirty, contaminated with proteinaceous material, or visibly soiled with blood or body fluids, wash hands with soap and water.

If hands are not visibly soiled, or after removing visible material with soap and water, decontaminate hands with an alcohol-based hand rub. Alternatively, hands may be washed with an antimicrobial soap and water.

Perform hand hygiene:

Before having direct contact with patients.
After contact with blood, body fluids or excretions, mucous membranes, nonintact skin, or wound dressings.
After contact with a patient's intact skin (e.g., when taking a pulse or blood pressure or lifting a patient).
If hands will be moving from a contaminated body site to a clean body site during patient care.
After contact with inanimate objects (including medical equipment) in the immediate vicinity of the patient.
After removing gloves.

Personal protective equipment (PPE)

Wear PPE when the nature of the anticipated patient interaction indicates that contact with blood or body fluids may occur.

Before leaving the patient's room or cubicle, remove and discard PPE.

Gloves

Wear gloves when contact with blood or other potentially infectious materials, mucous membranes, nonintact skin, or potentially contaminated intact skin (e.g., of a patient incontinent of stool or urine) could occur.

Remove gloves after contact with a patient and/or the surrounding environment using proper technique to prevent hand contamination. Do not wear the same pair of gloves for the care of more than one patient.

Change gloves during patient care if the hands will move from a contaminated body site (e.g., perineal area) to a clean body site (e.g., face).

Gowns

Wear a gown to protect skin and prevent soiling or contamination of clothing during procedures and patient-care activities when contact with blood, body fluids, secretions, or excretions is anticipated.

Wear a gown for direct patient contact if the patient has uncontained secretions or excretions.

Remove gown and perform hand hygiene before leaving patient's environment.

Mouth, nose, eye protection

Use PPE to protect the mucous membranes of the eyes, nose and mouth during procedures and patient-care activities that are likely to generate splashes or sprays of blood, body fluids, secretions and excretions.

During aerosol-generating procedures wear one of the following: a face shield that fully covers the front and sides of the face, a mask with attached shield, or a mask and goggles.

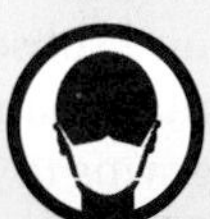

Respiratory Hygiene/Cough Etiquette

Educate healthcare personnel to contain respiratory secretions to prevent droplet and fomite transmission of respiratory pathogens, especially during seasonal outbreaks of viral respiratory tract infections.

Offer masks to coughing patients and other symptomatic persons (e.g., persons who accompany ill patients) upon entry into the facility.

Patient-Care equipment and instruments/devices

Wear PPE (e.g., gloves, gown), according to the level of anticipated contamination, when handling patient-care equipment and instruments/devices that are visibly soiled or may have been in contact with blood or body fluids.

Care of the environment

Include multi-use electronic equipment in policies and procedures for preventing contamination and for cleaning and disinfection, especially those items that are used by patients, those used during delivery of patient care, and mobile devices that are moved in and out of patient rooms frequently (e.g., daily).

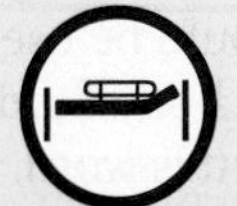

Textiles and laundry

Handle used textiles and fabrics with minimum agitation to avoid contamination of air, surfaces and persons.

FIGURE 38-2 Standard Precautions.

Courtesy of Brevis Corporation, Salt Lake City, Utah

TABLE 38-3 Situations that require a change of gloves

Situations that require a change of gloves
Before beginning patient care
After giving patient care
Immediately before touching mucus membranes
Immediately before touching nonintact skin
Immediately after touching secretions or excretions, before touching another part of the body or environmental surface
Immediately after touching blood or body fluids, before touching another part of the body or environmental surface
After touching contaminated environmental surfaces or equipment
Any time gloves are visibly soiled
Any time gloves are torn or the barrier is broken

TABLE 38-4 Situations that do not routinely require gloves

Situations that do not routinely require gloves
Turning a continent patient
Assisting a patient with walking
Touching clean, intact skin
Measuring blood pressure, pulse, and respirations
Handling clean equipment, supplies, and linens
Handling a clean bag with a specimen inside

remove it as soon as possible, perform hand hygiene, and apply new gloves. Never touch a computer keyboard or other electronic device with gloves used in patient care.

Wearing gloves for all patient care is not necessary; doing so can send patients the message that they are dirty and cannot be touched. Table 38-4 lists procedures that do not routinely require gloves unless special precautions are needed.

GOWNS

With Standard Precautions, gowns protect the arms, exposed body areas, and clothing when soiling from or splashing of blood, body fluids, and other potentially infectious material (OPIM) is likely, such as during trauma resuscitation. Gowns are made of moisture-resistant material and are either disposable or washable. Gowns are also worn when there is a great risk of contamination by direct contact with a patient. For example, a respiratory therapist needs a gown when providing care to a patient who is infected with vancomycin-resistant enterococcus (VRE) or *C. difficile* and the patient is incontinent of stool. The organism is present in the stool, and the respiratory therapist may be exposed when touching the patient and items in the room. Lab coats and other coverings do not meet the criteria for a protective barrier.

Remove a gown in the area or room in which it was worn; do not wear it outside that room. If a gown is needed, gloves are also required; hand hygiene is done right after removing the protective attire. In addition to Standard Precautions, gown and gloves are required to enter the room when patients are on Contact Precautions. They are also used when environmental contamination is likely and organisms, such as *Clostridium difficile* and *Methicillin-resistant staphylococcus aureus* (MRSA), can be easily spread. The gown and gloves protect the health care provider and subsequent patients from environmental contaminants.[5] There is no evidence that routine use of gowns to enter specific patient care areas, such as the ICU, has any benefit.

FACE MASK, GOGGLES, AND FACE SHIELD

With Standard Precautions, either the basic face mask and goggles or a face shield is used. These devices are designed to protect the mucus membranes in the health care worker's eyes, nose, and mouth. This protection is important because pathogens can be transmitted to health care workers through the mucus membrane. The equipment should be used whenever splashing or spraying of blood, body fluids, or OPIM is possible and whenever a gown is worn, except when a gown is used for direct contact protection. (These are simple face masks; special respirators that cover the face and mouth are discussed under airborne precautions.[5])

Best Practice

Gloves

Wear gloves when:

- Cleaning supplies and equipment.
- The skin on your hand is broken (cuts, cracks, or open areas).
- Contact with a patient's mucus membranes (eyes, nose, mouth) or genital area is possible.
- Contact with blood, body fluid, excretions, or secretions is possible.
- Caring for a patient with broken skin.
- Contact with an object or environmental surface that is possibly contaminated with the patient's blood, body fluid, secretions, or excretions is expected.

Face masks are used for three purposes in health care:

- To protect personnel from contact with infectious material from patients.
- To protect a sterile field when worn by a health care professional.
- To protect others in the environment when placed on a coughing patient.

A face mask should completely cover the health care worker's nose and mouth. Use a mask only one time and then discard it. Never wear the mask around the neck for later reuse. Handle the mask only by the ties and change it if it becomes moist. Exhaled breath can make the mask moist or wet if it is worn for a long time; when wet, the mask no longer acts as a protective barrier.

Goggles protect the eyes. In addition to protection from spray and splashing, they also protect against inadvertent touching by contaminated hands. Goggles are always worn with a face mask since a situation requiring eye protection also puts the mucus membranes of the nose and mouth at risk for contamination. This combination led to the development of face shields, devices that combine a mask with a plastic shield that also covers the eyes and provides protection from the chin to the top of the head.

A common misconception is that health care workers who wear eyeglasses do not need goggles or a face shield. Regular eyeglasses do not cover the whole eye area and do not provide critical side protection. Goggles or a face shield should be placed over personal eyeglasses.

To achieve optimal protection, apply the mask before applying eye protection. The eye protection should cover the top of the mask over the bridge of the nose. Table 38-5 recommends a sequence for applying and removing PPE.

Note: The CDC recommends the use of full barrier protection: mask, eye protection or face shield, gown and gloves for endotracheal intubation, especially in emergent circumstances. Although the patient may not be initially diagnosed with an infectious disease, infectious organisms, such as tuberculosis, meningitis, and SARS-CoV may still be present.[5]

TABLE 38-5 **Sequence for applying and removing PPE**

Applying PPE	Removing PPE
Wash hands	Gloves
Mask	Gown
Gown	Goggles/face shield
Goggles/face shield	Mask
Gloves	Wash hands

Best Practice

Eyeglasses and Goggles

Even if health care workers wear eyeglasses, they must also don protective eyewear, either goggles or a face shield over eyeglasses.

RESPIRATORY HYGIENE AND COUGH ETIQUETTE

In late 2003, Standard Precautions were updated after the experience with SARS-CoV earlier that year. The first elements were directed at patients and their families to inform them of their role in reducing the spread of infectious diseases (Figure 38-3). There are four components:[5]

- Information through visual alerts—posters and other informative materials—should be available at the first point of contact with the health care system such as ambulatory care, emergency departments, and any waiting area. Patients should be informed to cover the nose and mouth when coughing or sneezing, to use tissues to contain secretions and place them in designated receptacles, and to perform hand hygiene after contact with respiratory secretions.
- Health care facilities must provide no-touch receptacles for tissue disposal, as well as hand sanitizer or sinks for hand hygiene.
- Patients should be informed that, if respiratory symptoms are present, they should wear a mask that the health care facility will provide. If there is enough room, patients with these symptoms should sit at least 3 feet apart from others.
- Health care providers should observe droplet precautions when examining a person with respiratory symptoms, particularly if fever is present.

An additional recommendation is to cough into the crook of the elbow instead of into the hand to reduce the risk for spread by contact, either with another person or with objects in the environment.

GUIDELINES FOR TRANSMISSION-BASED PRECAUTIONS

The Standard Precautions discussed apply to general patient situations. A second tier of precautions, called **Transmission-Based Precautions**, applies to patients with specific infections.[5] They are used *in addition to Standard Precautions* for specific patients. The type of precautions required is determined by how the infection is spread. The three categories are airborne,

RESPIRATORY HYGIENE/COUGH ETIQUETTE

VISITORS

Please immediately inform healthcare personnel if you have a cold or other respiratory infection.

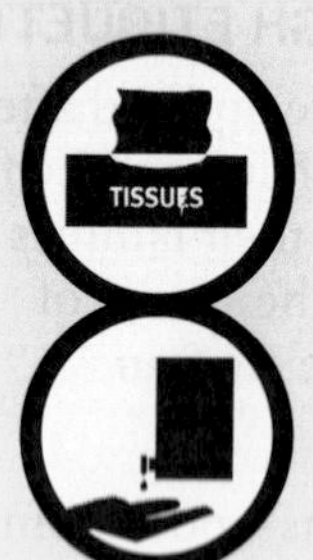

Respiratory Hygiene/Cough Etiquette

All individuals with signs and symptoms of a respiratory infection should:

1. Cover the nose and mouth when coughing or sneezing.
2. Use tissues to contain respiratory secretions. Dispose of used tissues in a waste receptacle.
3. Use proper hand hygiene after contact with mucus and contaminated objects.

Proper hand hygiene consists of:

a. Hand washing with plain soap and water—or
b. Alcohol-based hand rub—or
c. Antiseptic handwash.

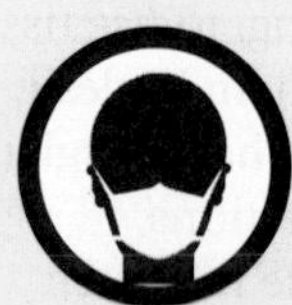

Masking and Separation of Persons with Respiratory Symptoms

Offer masks to persons who are coughing. Masks with ear loops or with ties may be used to contain respiratory secretions. Encourage coughing persons to sit at least three feet away from others.

Droplet Precautions

Advise healthcare personnel to observe Droplet Precautions (i.e., wearing a surgical or procedure mask for close contact), in addition to Standard Precautions, when examining a patient with symptoms of a respiratory infection, particularly if fever is present.

RHC7 · ©2007 Brevis Corporation · www.brevis.com

FIGURE 38-3 Respiratory Hygiene and Cough Etiquette.
Courtesy of Brevis Corporation, Salt Lake City, UT

droplet, and contact. Table 38-6 lists examples of infections in each category.

Airborne Precautions. Airborne Precautions are used to protect against the transmission of disease by pathogens that are small, lightweight, suspended in the air, or attached to dust particles in the air. Sneezing, talking, and coughing can release these pathogens into the air, where they can remain suspended for hours. Air currents can carry the pathogens from room to room and even from floor to floor through a building's ventilation systems. A person is infected by inhaling the pathogen.

- Tuberculosis (TB) is the most important airborne illness in health care settings.
- Serious varicella (chicken pox) infection should be isolated as well in both out- and inpatient areas.

TABLE 38-6 Some airborne, droplet, and contact infections[20]

Airborne	Chickenpox (varicella)
	Measles (rubeola)
	Smallpox (variola)
	Tuberculosis
Droplet	Group A streptococcus
	Influenza
	Mycoplasma pneumonia
	Neisseria meningitidis
	pertussis
	SARS-CoV
Contact	*C. difficile*
	Herpes simplex virus (HSV)
	Methicillin-resistant Staphylococcus aureus infection (MRSA)
	Respiratory syncytial virus
	S. aureus

These recommendations from CDC; hospitals may increase level of precautions depending on circumstances.

- Measles is also transmitted through the airborne route, but people with measles are rarely hospitalized. Measles outbreaks are most common where people live in close contact, such as in college dormitories. Smallpox (variola virus) is another pathogen that can be spread by airborne transmission and for which airborne precautions are needed.[5]

Patients on Airborne Precautions must be placed in a private, negative-pressure room called an *airborne infection isolation room* (*AIIR*). Air is drawn into the room when the door is opened so that airborne pathogens are pulled back into the room, rather than being released into the hallway. Air leaves the room through a special exhaust system directly to the outside where it is dispersed so that it cannot circulate within the building. The door must remain closed, except to let health care workers in and out, and the patient stays in the room. If an AIIR room is not available, CDC guidelines state the patient must be transferred to a facility with one available. (20) A patient who needs to go to another area outside the AIIR, such as medical imaging, must wear a surgical mask at all times. Figure 38-4 summarizes Airborne Precautions.

All health care providers entering the room of a patient under Airborne Precautions with infectious pulmonary or laryngeal tuberculosis or smallpox must wear a fit-tested CDC/NIOSH-approved N95 or higher-level respiratory mask. Fit testing of different mask sizes and types ensures the practitioner that a seal is achieved, based on individual facial structure. Facial-seal leakage is the greatest limit in the effectiveness of respiratory protection.[7] In health care settings, most respirator masks are disposable. The health care facility determines the type of respiratory protection used, as well as which health care providers are included in the respiratory protection program, while meeting CDC/NIOSH regulations.

This mask must also be worn when patients have other forms of tuberculosis and therapy or treatment (such as wound care) could aerosolize organisms. CDC does not have adequate evidence for recommendations regarding the level of respiratory protection required when caring for patients with other conditions that place them under airborne precautions.[5] During transport, health care providers do not need to wear masks as long as the patient is wearing a surgical mask and any infectious lesions are covered.

Droplet Precautions. **Droplet Precautions** are used when a patient has a disease that can be spread by large droplets in the air. Unlike airborne pathogens, which can float in the air, droplets generally do not travel more than 3–10 feet from the source. Patients can spread droplets from the respiratory tract by coughing, talking, and sneezing.

Droplet transmission can occur during procedures such as suctioning and bronchoscopy. A standard surgical mask provides adequate protection for health care providers because the pathogens are too large to pass through the mask.

Ideally, patients should be in private rooms. Patients with the same disease can share a room, but they should be kept at least 3 feet apart with the curtains pulled around the bed. The door may be open, and no special ventilation is required. During transport, the patient should wear a surgical mask. Figure 38-5 summarizes Droplet Precautions.

Contact Precautions. **Contact Precautions** are used for patients with infections that are spread by direct contact (touching of the skin or infected material) or by touching contaminated objects (indirect contact). These precautions protect the health care worker from disease and reduce pathogen transmission from one patient to another.

Two particularly problematic illnesses in health care facilities are methicillin-resistant *Staphylococcus aureus* (MRSA) and *Clostridium difficile* colitis. MRSA is commonly found in infected wounds and pressure ulcers; *C. difficile* causes diarrhea after infecting the bowel. Because these strains have become resistant to antimicrobials, they are particularly difficult to kill. In pediatrics, respiratory syncytial virus is managed with contact precautions.

AIRBORNE PRECAUTIONS

(in addition to Standard Precautions)

STOP **VISITORS:** Report to nurse before entering.

Use Airborne Precautions as recommended for patients known or suspected to be infected with infectious agents transmitted person-to-person by the airborne route (e.g., M. tuberculosis, measles, chickenpox, disseminated herpes zoster).

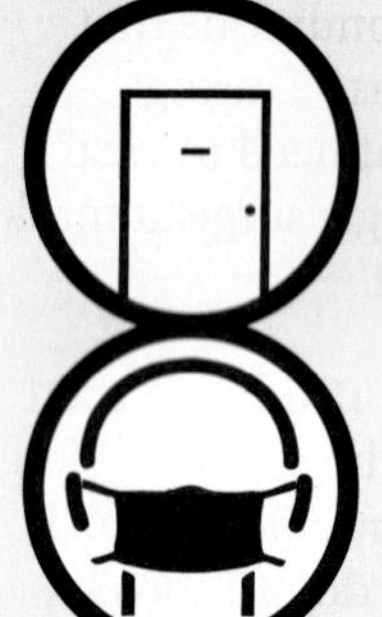

Patient Placement
Place patients in an **AIIR** (Airborne Infection isolation Room).
Monitor air pressure daily with visual indicators (e.g., flutter strips).

Keep door closed when not required for entry and exit.

In ambulatory settings instruct patients with a known or suspected airborne infection to wear a surgical mask and observe Respiratory Hygiene/Cough Etiquette. Once in an AIIR, the mask may be removed.

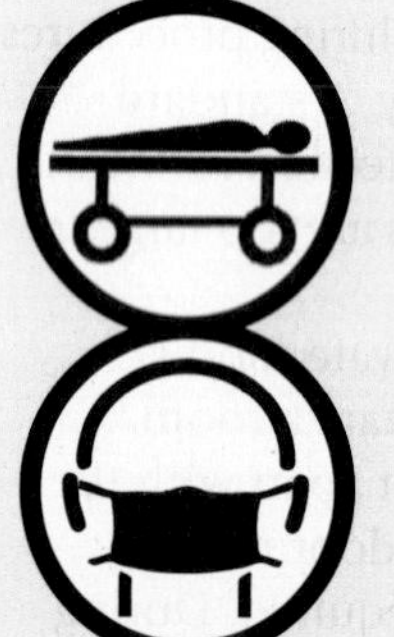

Patient Transport
Limit transport and movement of patients to **medically-necessary purposes.**

If transport or movement outside an AIIR is necessary, instruct patients to **wear a surgical mask,** if possible, and observe Respiratory Hygiene/Cough Etiquette.

Hand Hygiene
according to Standard Precautions

Personal Protective Equipment (PPE)
Wear a fit-tested NIOSH-approved **N95** or higher level respirator for respiratory protection when entering the room of a patient when the following diseases are suspected or confirmed: Listed on back.

FIGURE 38-4 Airborne Precautions.

Courtesy of Brevis Corporation, Salt Lake City, Utah

DROPLET PRECAUTIONS

(in addition to Standard Precautions)

VISITORS: Report to nurse before entering.

Personal Protective Equipment (PPE)

Don a mask upon entry into the patient room or cubicle.

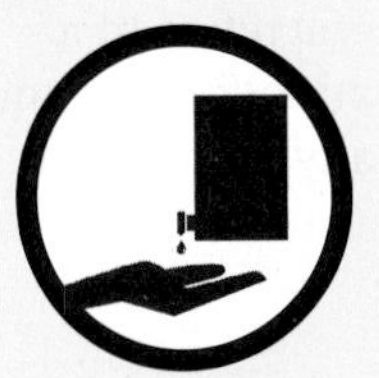

Hand Hygiene

according to Standard Precautions.

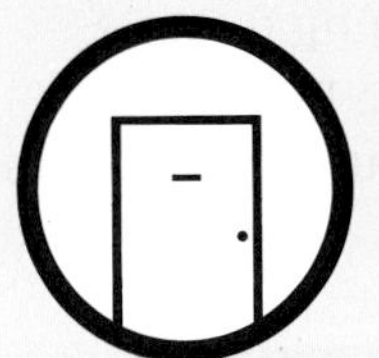

Patient Placement

Private room, if possible. Cohort or maintain spatial separation of 3 feet from other patients or visitors if private room is not available.

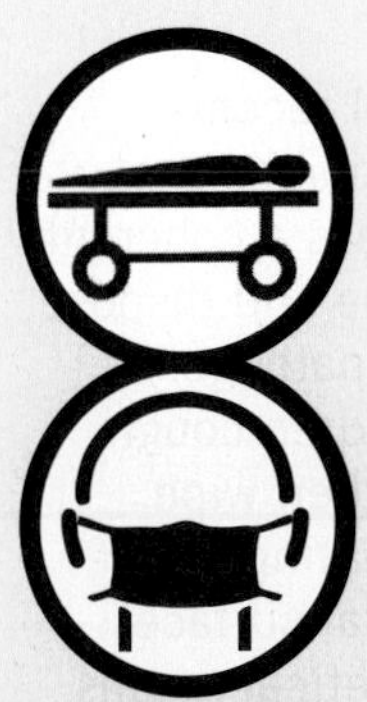

Patient Transport

Limit transport and movement of patients to **medically-necessary purposes.**

If transport or movement in any healthcare setting is necessary, instruct patient to **wear a mask** and follow Respiratory Hygiene/Cough Etiquette.

No mask is required for persons transporting patients on Droplet Precautions.

FIGURE 38-5 Droplet Precautions.

Courtesy of Brevis Corporation, Salt Lake City, Utah

A common pattern of contamination occurs this way:

- A health care worker empties a commode or cleans an incontinent patient who is infected with *C. difficile*.
- Not realizing the gloves have become contaminated, the worker goes on to take the patient's blood pressure while wearing the same gloves. The blood pressure cuff is now contaminated.
- The respiratory therapist comes along later and takes the patient's blood pressure during a treatment. The RT's hands were not near contaminated stool, but because the blood pressure cuff was contaminated, the RT's hands are now contaminated.
- Then, using the stethoscope to listen to breath sounds without changing gloves, the therapist has inadvertently contaminated the stethoscope simply by touching it.
- If the RT then goes to another patient and uses the same stethoscope, the pathogen can be transmitted to the second patient by indirect contact.

Therefore, whenever a patient is on Contact Precautions:

- Equipment should be dedicated to that room. Stethoscopes, pulse oximeters, and ventilators cannot be moved out of the room until they have undergone thorough cleaning and disinfection.
- Patients should be in a private room if possible. If not, they should be paired with another patient with the same infection (called *cohorting*).
- Gloves and gowns must be worn for any patient contact or contact with environmental surfaces (for example, checking a ventilator).
- Gloves must be changed after any potential contact with the pathogen—primarily stool, wound drainage, or respiratory secretions in children who are too young to practice proper respiratory hygiene.
- The gown and gloves must be removed before leaving the room, and hand hygiene must be performed immediately after glove removal.
- After removing protective attire, do not touch anything else in the room.
- To be safe, use a paper towel to open the door to the room; the inside doorknob or handle is almost always inadvertently contaminated. After the door is open, discard the paper towel in the room before you walk out the door.

Figure 38-6 summarizes Contact Precautions.

Although respiratory diseases are not typically transmitted through direct or indirect contact, respiratory therapists care for patients who have infections transmitted this way. Careful attention to proper infection control procedures is critical because the RT cares for many patients and can easily carry pathogens from one patient to the next.

Table 38-7 summarizes precautions for airborne, droplet, and contact transmission, and Table 38-8 describes the type of precautions indicated for selected pulmonary infections.

Isolation Precautions. In some cases, patients' signs and symptoms suggest an infectious disease, but the diagnosis is delayed while culture and sensitivity tests are done. For some conditions, **Isolation Precautions** are required if the infection is suspected. If the disease turns out not to be highly infectious, Isolation Precautions can be discontinued. If a different infection is identified, precautions can be modified. Table 38-9 lists CDC recommendations for empiric Isolation Precautions.[5] (*Empiric* refers to a reasonable suspicion based on the patient's signs and symptoms, history of exposure, and any patterns of illness in the community.)

REMOVING GLOVES AND GOWNS

Wearing appropriate PPE is critical to safe practice regardless of what level of precautions must be followed. Just as critical is how the PPE is taken off. Specific techniques for removing PPE keep health care workers from contaminating themselves

Age-Specific Competency

Infection Control Measures in Children

In the care of children, traditional recommendations for appropriate infection control precautions may not apply. Whereas a coherent adult is able to cough into a tissue and dispose of it properly, thereby containing pathogens, a child usually is not as tidy. Children cough and sneeze into their hands and then wipe their hands everywhere, contaminating themselves, clothing, and environmental surfaces. Therefore, regardless of the theoretical means of transmission, many children with infectious respiratory diseases are placed on Contact Precautions.

CONTACT PRECAUTIONS

(in addition to Standard Precautions)

VISITORS: Report to nurse before entering.

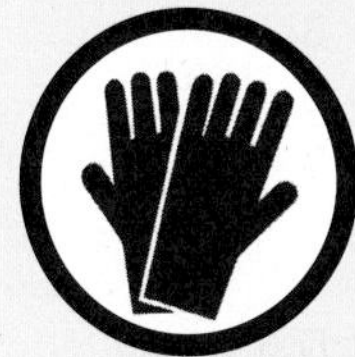

Gloves
Don gloves upon entry into the room or cubicle.
Wear gloves whenever touching the patient's intact skin or surfaces and articles in close proximity to the patient.
Remove gloves before leaving patient room.

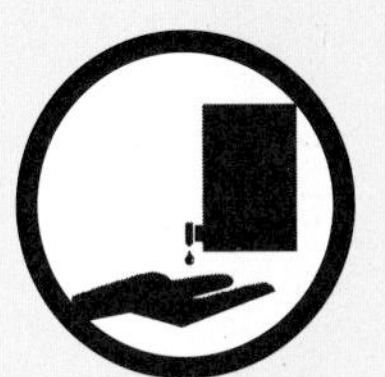

Hand Hygiene
according to Standard Precautions

Gowns
Don gown upon entry into the room or cubicle.
Remove gown and observe hand hygiene before leaving the patient-care environment.

Patient Transport
Limit transport of patients to medically necessary purposes.
Ensure that infected or colonized areas of the patient's body are contained and covered.
Remove and dispose of contaminated PPE and perform hand hygiene prior to transporting patients on Contact Precautions.
Don clean PPE to handle the patient at the transport destination.

Patient-Care Equipment
Use disposable noncritical patient-care equipment or implement patient-dedicated use of such equipment.

FIGURE 38-6 Contact Precautions.

Courtesy of Brevis Corporation, Salt Lake City, Utah

TABLE 38-7 **Precautions based on method of transmission**

Transmission Method	Patient Placement	Precautions
Airborne	Airborne infection isolation room (AIIR)	CDC/NIOSH approved N95 or higher-level respirator mask or respirator mask
	Keep door closed	Surgical mask on patient for transport
Droplet	Private room or share with patient with same infection	Mask when within 3 feet
	Separate from other patients by at least 3 feet	Mask on patient for transport
	Door may be open	
	No special airflow	
Contact	Private room	Gloves when entering room
		Frequent glove changes
		Gown for contact with patient or environmental surfaces

or their environment. Figure 38-7 shows the proper technique for removing gloves, and Figure 38-8 shows the proper technique for removing gowns.

Preventing Needlestick Injuries

Another important aspect of Standard Precautions is protection from **needlestick injuries** (injuries caused by sharp objects or needles). Approximately 972,000 needlestick injuries to health care workers are reported each year in the United States, or about one injury every 30 seconds. However, the reporting system is voluntary, and it is estimated that up to 53% of all needlestick injuries go unreported, bringing the actual total number of annual injuries closer to 2 million. The CDC considers occupationally acquired HIV/AIDS as *seroconversions* in which there is a documented exposure to an HIV-positive source and

TABLE 38-8 **Type of precautions indicated for selected pulmonary infections**[5]

Type of Infection	Precaution*
Pneumonia:	
Adenovirus	D, C
Bacterial, general (including gram-negative)	S
Burkholderia cepacia in cystic fibrosis, including respiratory colonization	C
Chlamydia	S
Fungal	S
Haemophilus influenzae	
Adults	S
Infants and children	D
Legionella pneumophilia	S
Meningococcal	D
Multidrug-resistant	
General	C
Pneumococcal	S
Mycoplasma	D
Pneumocystis carinii	S
Staphylococcus aureus	S
Streptococcus, group A	
Adults	D
Infants and young children	D
Viral	
Adults	S
Infants and young children	C
C Respiratory syncytial virus	
Tuberculosis	A
Anthrax, pulmonary	S
Bronchiolitis	C
Coccidiomycosis pneumonia	S
Epiglottitis hib	D
Influenza	D
MDRO	S/C
Pertussis	D
Pneumococcal pneumonia	S/D
Pneumonic plague	D
SARS CoV	A/D/C
Varicella	A

Source: From Centers for Disease Control and Prevention. Guideline for Isolation Precautions in Hospitals, Appendix A. Copyright 1996 by Public Health Service, U.S. Department of Health and Human Services, Centers for Disease Control and Prevention.

**D, Droplet; C, Contact; S, Standard; A, Airborne.*

TABLE 38-9 **Clinical presentations requiring empiric isolation precautions until definitive diagnosis**[20]

Condition	Potential Pathogen	Precautions
Cough, fever, upper lobe pulmonary infiltrate in an HIV-negative patient or a patient at low risk for HIV	Mycobacterium tuberculosis Respiratory viruses, *S. pneumonia*, *S. aureus*, MRSA	Airborne Contact
Cough, fever, pulmonary infiltrate in any lung location in an HIV-infected patient or a patient at high risk for HIV infection	Mycobacterium tuberculosis Respiratory viruses, *S. pneumonia*, *S. aureus*, MRSA	Airborne Contact
Paroxysmal or severe persistent cough during periods of pertussis activity (outbreak)	Bordetella pertussis	Droplet
Respiratory infection, particularly bronchiolitis and pneumonia in infants and small children	Respiratory syncytial or parainfluenza virus Adenovirus Influenza virus	Contact
Cough/fever/pulmonary infiltrate in any lung location in a patient with a history of recent travel (10–21 days) to countries with active outbreaks of SARS, avian influenza	Mycobacterium tuberculosis SARS-CoV Avian influenza	Airborne Contact Eye protection

These may be modified or adapted based on local conditions and circumstances.

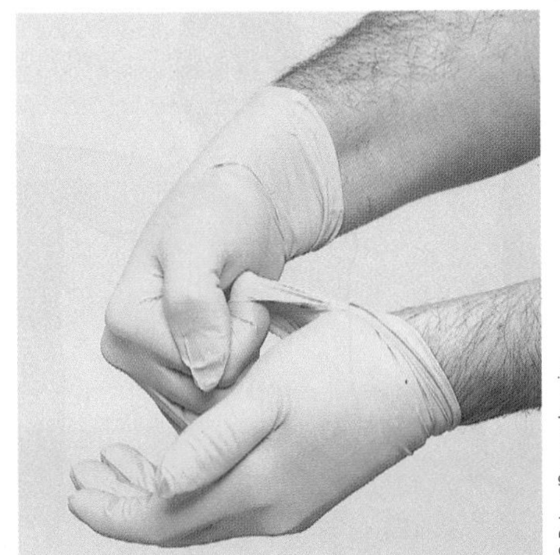

(A)

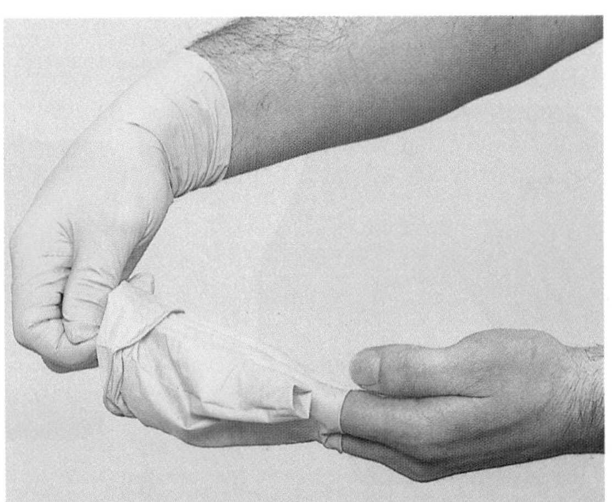

(B)

(C)

FIGURE 38-7 Proper technique for removing gloves: (A) Grasp the palm or outside cuff of the left glove with the gloved right hand. (B) Pull the left glove toward the fingertips. The glove should turn inside out as it is removed. (C) Hold the removed glove in the still-gloved right hand. Insert the thumb of the ungloved left hand under the cuff of the right glove, carefully avoiding any contaminated areas. Pull the right glove toward the fingertips, turning it inside out as it is removed. The soiled left glove should remain in the palm of the right glove as it is removed.

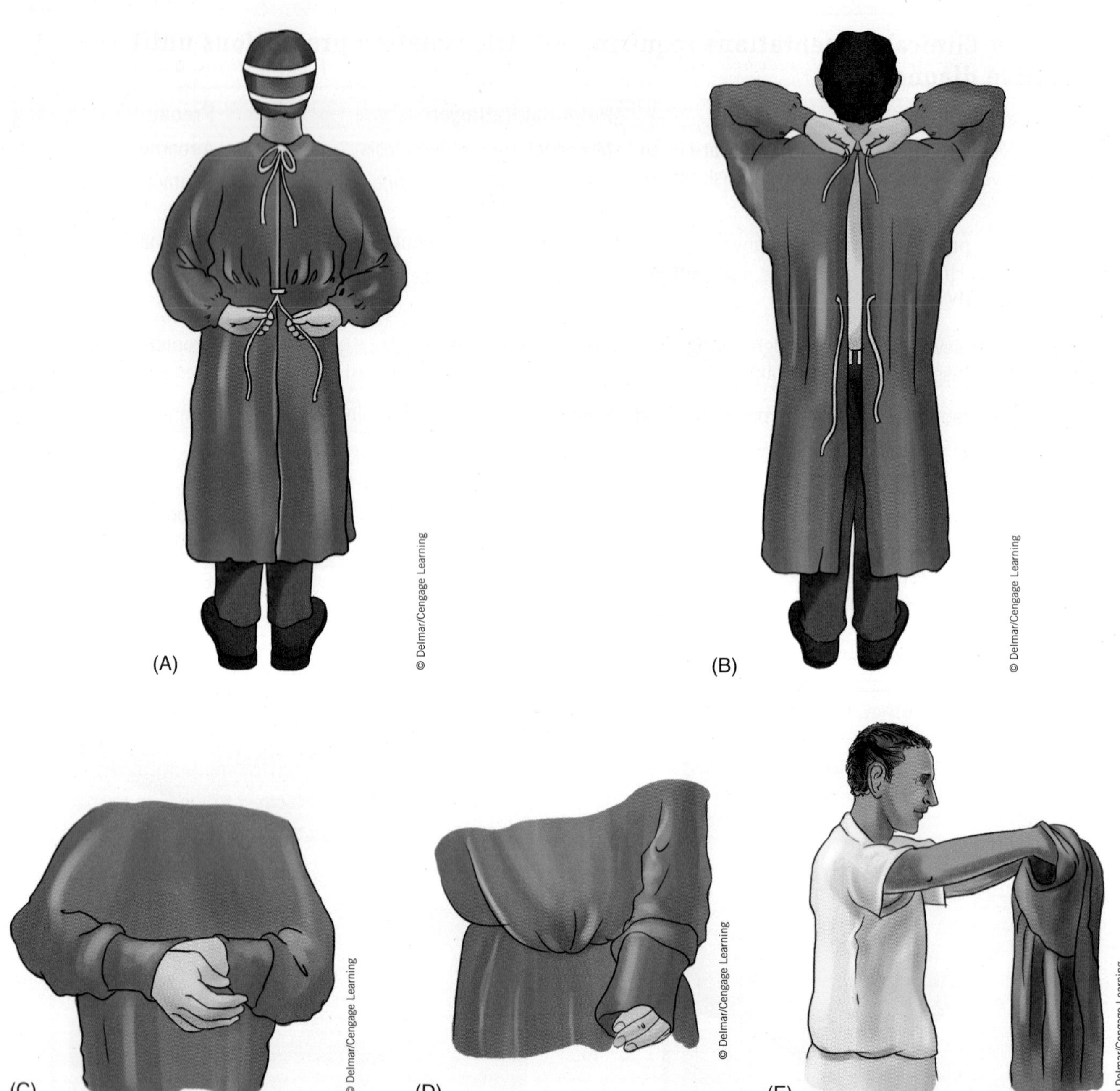

FIGURE 38-8 Proper technique for removing a gown: (A) Untie waist of gown. (B) Untie neckties of gown. (C) Slip fingers of one hand inside cuff of the other hand. Pull gown down over the hand. Do not touch the outside of the gown with either hand. (D) Using the gown-covered hand, pull the gown down over the other hand. (E) Pull the gown down off the arms, being careful that the hands do not touch the outside of the gown. Hold the gown away from your uniform and roll it up with the contaminated side inside. Place the disposable gowns in the receptacle for contaminated trash. Place nondisposable gowns in laundry hamper for contaminated items.

the worker has no nonoccupational risk factors for the disease.

As of December 2006, there were 57 documented seroconversions between 1981 and 2006 following occupational exposures. Eighty-four percent resulted from skin punctures or cuts, 9% were from mucus membrane and/or skin exposure, and 4% had both exposures. Four percent had an unknown exposure. Of the 57 workers, 49 had exposure to HIV-infected blood, 3 to concentrated virus in a laboratory, one to bloody fluid, and 4 to an unspecified body fluid. The most cases were in 1992, with none in 1996 and 1997. The last case reported to CDC and confirmed was in 2000.[12] Nurses represented the most documented cases, with 24 of the 57. Next are clinical laboratory workers with 16, nonsurgical physicians with 6, and nonclinical laboratory workers with 3. One respiratory therapist became HIV-positive as a result of a work-related exposure between 1991 and 1997 with none since.[12]

The risk of contracting HIV infection from a needlestick is 0.0000128%. For a needlestick from a patient known to have HIV infection, the risk is 0.3%. Although health care workers are usually most concerned about acquiring HIV infection, more than 20 pathogens can be transmitted through blood. The two most common are hepatitis B (HBV) and hepatitis C (HCV). The risk of acquiring HBV from all possible exposures is as high as 30%, and the risk of HCV infection from a needlestick is 1.8%. HBV is 10 times more infectious than HIV. However, for persons who have received the HBV vaccine, there is virtually no risk for infection after exposure.[13]

The most risky exposure is when a health care worker is stuck with a hollow-core needle filled with the patient's blood, such as a needle used to draw blood. Other sharps, such as the lancet used to pierce an infant's heel to draw capillary blood, are less risky. The lancet may have blood on it, but it is not filled with blood that can enter the health care worker's bloodstream. There is virtually no risk of infection if the respiratory therapist is stuck with a needle before it is used on a patient; however, even this injury should be reported because broken skin provides a potential portal of entry for other microorganisms.

The risk of needlestick injuries can be reduced through careful handling of sharps and using equipment designed to minimize handling used syringes. Most needlestick injuries occur when health care workers dispose of needles, administer injections, draw blood or start IVs, recap needles, and handle trash or dirty linens that contain improperly discarded needles or sharps.

Therefore, to minimize risk, the health care worker must follow proper needle disposal practices.

- Needles and syringes should never be laid on a bed or stretcher or on a table beside the bed where they could be left behind and injure another person.
- When drawing blood, workers should have a sharps container nearby so that they do not have to walk any distance with a used needle in hand.
- Never bend or break a needle.
- Do not recap a used needle unless absolutely necessary.
- If recapping, never hold the cap in one hand while directing the needle toward the hand holding the cap. Instead, use the *one-handed technique* (Figure 38-9).
  Place the cap on a hard, steady surface.
  Place the needle with syringe in your dominant hand.
  Place your nondominant hand behind your back so that you won't be tempted to use it.
  Gently ease the needle into the cap.
  Once the needle is partway in the cap, tilt the needle so it points toward the ceiling. The cap will slide down and cover the needle
- Never push the cap onto the syringe. However, if the cap has to be secured to remove the needle, then, and only then, use the nondominant hand to pull the cap down and secure it at the base of the needle. Never push down on the cap at the tip; the needle can sometimes puncture a cap that is not on perfectly straight.

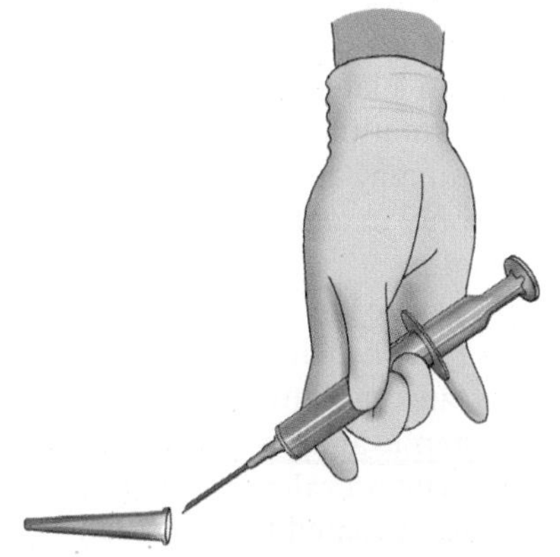

1. Scoop into cap using one hand. Do not touch the cap with the other hand.

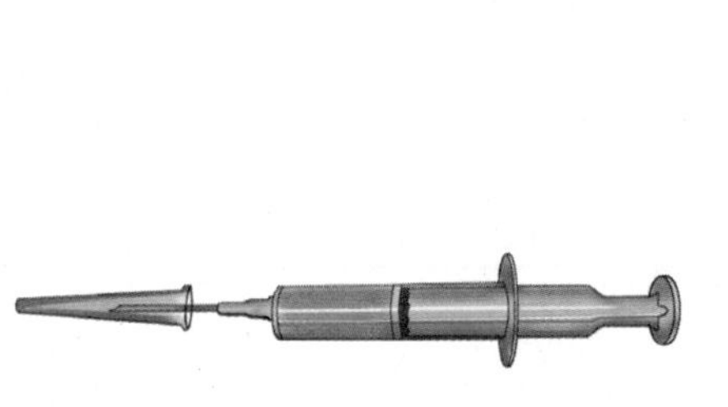

2. Slide needle into cap resting on table.

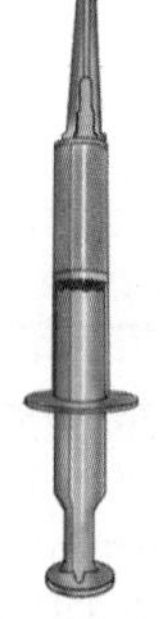

3. Holding the barrel of the syringe in one hand, carry to the sharps container. Do not push the cap onto the syringe.

FIGURE 38-9 One-handed needle recap technique.

Safety devices should be used whenever they are available. These engineering controls consist of needle-less systems (particularly for intravenous therapy), recessed needles, needle guards, and other protective devices. Some safety syringes have a plastic sheath covering the syringe. After the needle with syringe is used, the plastic sheath is pulled down over the needle, making it virtually impossible for the needle to cause injury. Health care workers need to know what devices are available in their practice setting, know how they work, and be diligent about using them whenever needles are required for a procedure.

All sharps must be discarded by the person who uses them; they should never be left on a procedure tray. Scalpel blades, suture needles, and other sharps must be removed by the user rather than being left on the tray to be cleaned up by someone else who may not be aware of their presence.

Best Practice

Sharps Disposal

When a needle with syringe is placed in a sharps disposal container, it should drop freely into the container. Do not try to force it into the disposal container; forcing it increases the risk for injury. Containers should be replaced when they are one-half to three-quarters full.

Spotlight On

Needle Safety Devices

Over the past 10 years, legislation has been enacted requiring the use of needle safety devices, and manufacturers have developed products that help protect health care workers. To keep up-to-date with regulations and safety products available, visit the Web site for the International Health care Worker Safety Center at the University of Virginia Health System. The center maintains a database on occupational exposures to bloodborne pathogens, a list of available safety devices, and other resources (www.healthsystem.virginia.edu/internet/epinet/about_center.cfm).

Special Issues in Infection Control

In addition to understanding the chain of infection, proper hand hygiene techniques, and Standard Precautions for preventing pathogen transmission, the respiratory therapist must also be aware of special issues in infection control:

- The increased occurrence of latex reactions and allergies
- The growing problem of **antimicrobial-resistant microorgamisms**
- Care of persons exposed to bioterrorism agents and pandemic influenza

LATEX ALLERGY

Since barrier precautions were initiated, latex glove use in health care settings has increased dramatically. Today, the main occupational use of latex is in gloves. However, in health care, latex may be found in other items:

- Stethoscope tubing
- Masks and manual resuscitation bags
- ECG electrodes
- Oral and nasopharyngeal airways
- Bite blocks
- Endotracheal tubes (particularly double-lumen)
- Cuffs on plastic endotracheal tubes
- Syringes
- Stoppers in medication vials
- Blood pressure cuffs
- Tourniquets
- Injection ports in intravenous tubing
- Adhesive tape

There are two types of immune-system reactions to latex.

- *Type IV* reactions are simple cell-mediated reactions to the chemical additives in the latex, not to latex proteins. More properly classified as a rubber allergy than a latex allergy, the reactions result in contact dermatitis caused by delayed hypersensitivity and may appear hours to days after contact and only in areas with direct contact with the latex.
- *Type I* immediate, severe reactions to latex proteins occur in persons who have developed IgE antibodies to latex protein. When activated, they can cause systemic anaphylaxis and be life-threatening.[14] The prevalence of latex allergy in the workplace is estimated to be as high as 17% in health care workers, food handlers, and hairdressers. Unfortunately, there is no standard definition for **latex allergy**; so research studies may use different criteria under the same classification.

Latex allergies affect both patients and their care providers. Many health care organizations have voluntarily created latex-free environments, but there is no requirement to do so. For organizations still using latex, the Royal College of Physicians (RCP) in London published the first evidence-based guideline providing recommendations for occupational latex use in 2008.[14]

Using powder-free, low-protein latex gloves instead of powdered gloves significantly reduces the incidence of latex allergy. Although powder makes gloves easier to put on and is not allergenic itself, it binds with the latex proteins and releases them into the air when gloves are applied and removed. Workers with reactions to latex need latex-free gloves; this is also an OSHA requirement.[15] Allergic signs and symptoms decrease in latex-sensitive employees whether coworkers use powder-free, low-protein gloves or latex-free gloves. And there have been no reports of latex allergy development in health care workers using the low-protein, powder-free gloves. The RCP notes that the evidence does not support a complete ban on the use of latex gloves in the workplace.[14] However, health care organizations must have latex-free materials for patients with a history of type IV reactions to the substance.

To reduce the risk of developing latex allergy or exposing a patient unnecessarily, respiratory therapists can take these steps:

- Select powder-free latex, nitrile, or vinyl gloves whenever possible.
- Dry hands thoroughly before applying gloves.

If using powdered latex gloves:

- Carefully apply and remove gloves to minimize airborne distribution of powder.
- Do not snap gloves on and off.
- Wash hands thoroughly after glove use to remove all powder residue. Do not touch anything before washing hands because powder can be transferred to another surface.

Report any hand irritation or rashes associated with gloves to the infection control team for monitoring.

Best Practice

Latex-Free Equipment

Each health care facility should have a cart stocked with latex-free or latex-safe equipment that can be rolled to the bedside of any patient with true latex allergy. Respiratory therapists should be familiar with latex-free equipment that can be used for these patients.

Age-Specific Competency

Latex Allergies

Infants and children are especially at risk for latex allergies because of an undeveloped or weakened immune system. Many pediatrics departments are trying to eliminate the use of all types of latex and are using vinyl and other synthetic gloves instead.

Spotlight On

Gloves

Gloves can be made of many substances other than latex. The barrier to the widespread use of these other materials is usually the cost. Materials used to make gloves are:

- Neoprene (polychloroprene polymer)
- Styrene butadiene block polymer
- Styrene ethylene butadiene co-polymer
- Nitrile (butadiene copolymer)
- Polyvinyl chloride
- Nitrile

Source: Siegel JD, Rhinehart E, Jackson M, Chiarello L, Healthcare Infection Control Practices Advisory Committee. Guideline for isolation precautions: preventing transmission of infectious agents in healthcare settings 2007. (http://www.cdc.gov/hicpac/2007IP/2007isolationPrecautions.html; NHS Plus RCoP, Faculty of Occupational Medicine). Latex allergy: occupational aspects of management. A national guideline. 2008.

DRUG-RESISTANT PATHOGENS

When antimicrobials were first introduced in the 1940s, the decrease in mortality and morbidity rates was remarkable. Clinicians finally had a weapon to fight infections, and the world of medicine changed. However, since the 1990s there has been a significant increase in the number of **multidrug-resistant microorganisms (MDRMs)**. These pathogens have an altered genetic structure and can survive even when the infected patient is treated with antibiotics designed to kill them. CDC defines MDRO as microorganisms that are resistant to one or more classes of antimicrobial agents. The number of persons affected and the type of organism varies with location in the United States and the care setting, as well as host factors including age and preexisting health conditions.[2]

Infectious organisms can be cultured from persons who are not ill. This is called **colonization**. Pathogens are present, but the body has been able to fight infection. Colonization is a key concept in MDRO because patients and health care workers can be colonized with these organisms and can pass them on to more compromised patients whose immune systems are not able to fend off infection.

Two common MDRO organisms are *vancomycin-resistant enterococcus* (*VRE*) and *methicillin-resistant Staphylococcus aureus* (*MRSA*). MRSA was first identified in the United States in 1968. By the early 1990s, it made up 20–25% of all hospital-cultured *S. aureus* infections, and by 2003, 60% of *S. aureus* infections in ICUs were MRSA. Between 1990 and 1997, VRE rose from a presence in less than 1% of hospitalized patients to 15%; by 2003, VRE accounted for 29% of enterococcus infections in ICUs. Organisms that cause pneumonia, such as *Klebsiella pneumoniae, Streptococcus pneumoniae,* and *Pseudomonas aeruginosa* have also evolved multidrug resistant strains. Research has shown the incidence of infections in hospitalized patients, particularly those in ICU, rises significantly when other patients are colonized with these organisms.[2]

MDRO are transmitted in hospitals on the hands of health care workers. Following Standard Precautions is a key element in reducing the number of MDRO infections. Other important practices are:

- Reducing the time indwelling urinary and vascular catheters are used.
- Preventing pneumonia in ventilated patients.
- Careful use and monitoring of antibiotic prescribing practices in hospitals.

The CDC further recommends using Contact Precautions for patients in acute care hospitals who have been previously identified as being colonized with MDRO.[2]

Emergence of Drug-Resistant Microorganisms. Antimicrobials rely on several specific strategies for eradicating pathogens (see Chapter 5), and the pathogens have some way of defending against each one. Essentially, bacteria can use seven mechanisms to become drug resistant, as shown in Table 38-10.

Spread of Resistant Organisms. Once a resistant strain of microorganism has emerged, it can pass along the resistance to offspring and to other species, compounding the problem. One example of a drug-resistant pathogen is *Streptococcus pneumoniae,* the most common cause of community-acquired pneumonia. This type of infection is acquired from the environment; it is distinguished from hospital-acquired pneumonia by the types of organisms involved. *Streptococcus pneumoniae* can also cause bacteremia, meningitis, and acute otitis media. Patients younger than 2 years and older than 70 years are at increased risk for infection with this organism. Older people, HIV-positive people, immune-suppressed transplant patients, and radiation therapy patients can prevent infection by getting a pneumococcus vaccine. Infections caused by other drug-resistant pathogens are not as easy to prevent.

In the past, clinicians relied on pharmaceutical companies to develop new antimicrobials by the time bacteria became resistant to current drugs. Today, resistance is emerging much more quickly; so this approach no longer solves the problem.

Antimicrobials are used in one of three ways.[2]

- In *prophylactic* prescribing, an antimicrobial is prescribed to prevent infection in an at-risk patient.
- In *empiric* prescribing, the clinician uses clinical judgment to determine the most likely infecting organism and prescribes antimicrobials on the basis of this best guess. This approach should be

TABLE 38-10 **Mechanisms for bacterial resistance to antimicrobials**

1. *Enzymatic inhibition.* Bacteria synthesize enzymes that destroy the antimicrobial or modify it so that it does not kill them.
2. *Altering bacterial membranes.* Bacteria change the cell membrane, making it impermeable to antimicrobials.
3. *Promoting antimicrobial efflux.* Bacteria generate an inner membrane protein that resists antimicrobials.
4. *Altering ribosomal target sites.* Many antimicrobials work by binding on bacterial ribosomes. If the bacteria alter the target sites, the antimicrobial cannot kill the bacteria.
5. *Altering cell wall precursor targets.* Bacteria prevent the antimicrobial from being incorporated into the cell wall.
6. *Altering target enzymes or overproduction of target enzymes.* Bacteria alter or overproduce enzymes that antimicrobials target. Both mechanisms keep the bacterial enzyme functional but insensitive to the antimicrobial.
7. *Bypassing antimicrobial inhibition.* Bacteria develop mutant strains, called *auxotrophs,* that allow bacteria to grow despite the antimicrobial's growth-inhibiting enzymes.

Source: Tenover FC. *Mechanisms of antimicrobial resistance in bacteria.* Am J Med. *2006;119,6A:S3–S10.*

limited to patients ill enough to need treatment while waiting for culture and sensitivity testing results. However, empiric prescribing is also used when antimicrobials are prescribed over the phone and a specimen for culture and sensitivity testing has not been obtained. This practice is strongly discouraged. Once a specimen has been obtained and culture and sensitivity results are available, the antimicrobial may need to be changed.

- In *therapeutic* prescribing, the choice of antimicrobial is based on laboratory culture and sensitivity testing that identifies the microorganism and tests that antimicrobials kill the organism in vitro. (For details on specimen collection, culturing, and sensitivity testing, see Chapter 5.)

Several factors must be considered before a specific antimicrobial is chosen.

- One is the *site* of the infection. Some antimicrobials work better than others in a particular area of the body; the options are particularly limited in the treatment of central nervous system infections because not all medicines cross the blood-brain barrier. Some antimicrobials penetrate abscesses better than others.
- *Patient* factors must be considered as well, including renal and hepatic function (which affect excretion of the drug) and a history of allergic reactions (which can prevent the use of entire classes of antimicrobials).
- Finally, the clinician considers how to *administer* the drug. In the hospital, intravenous administration is convenient; this route may not be available to all outpatients, who may have to be treated with oral therapy instead.

Using antimicrobials to kill bacteria is like waging a war. The antimicrobials are the army, and the bacteria are the enemy. As in any war, the army has greater success if the enemy is caught by surprise. The less often pathogens are exposed to a particular antimicrobial, the more likely it is that the antimicrobial will kill a given microorganism.

In the outpatient setting, antimicrobial resistance occurs when people do not complete prescriptions for antimicrobials; they take some of the pills, but not all that were prescribed. This partial treatment of infections exposes bacteria to antimicrobial agents but does not kill them all. The exposed but unkilled bacteria can develop resistance. This mechanism is a particular concern in multidrug-resistant tuberculosis (MDR-TB). Patients who have no health insurance and cannot pay for medication are likely to only partially treat their infection. Other people stop taking the medication because they feel better, they forget about it, or they have unpleasant side effects. Making sure people take all of their antimicrobial therapy is a new challenge for all public health and health care professionals.

There is no doubt that the widespread use (some experts say overuse) of antimicrobials has fostered the emergence and spread of resistant bacteria. Today, infection control professionals are trying to establish guidelines for the use of antimicrobials in the hospital to try to reduce the development of resistant bacterial strains. For years, physicians were free to prescribe any antimicrobial at any time in the hospital, but not all physicians are experts at choosing appropriate antimicrobial therapy. Now, many institutions require that prescribing clinicians consult with infection control teams before using certain antimicrobials. Some facilities have developed standard protocols for treating specific diseases such as community-acquired pneumonia, and many have set up audit teams to review hospital-wide antimicrobial prescribing patterns. National guidelines have been established by the Centers for Disease Control and Prevention (CDC), but experience has shown that medical practice is guided much more by local practice; that is, systems set up by individual hospitals and health care systems, rather than by national guidelines.[2] The CDC maintains a Web page containing current information on appropriate antibiotic use (http://www.cdc.gov/getsmart/specific-groups/healthcare-providers.html).

Ideally, narrow-spectrum antimicrobials should be prescribed to treat infections caused by specific microorganisms. The general use of broad-spectrum antimicrobials that are effective against many bacterial species can contribute to resistance, and their use should be carefully monitored. These drugs, such as vancomycin, should be used only for therapeutic prescribing, not for prophylactic or empiric prescribing.

Reducing the factors that contribute to the development of microbial resistance is largely the responsibility of prescribing clinicians. Limiting the spread of these dangerous organisms is *every* health care worker's responsibility, through careful attention to Standard Precautions and specific Isolation Precautions.

AGENTS OF BIOTERRORISM

The CDC defines a bioterrorism attack as the deliberate release of microorganisms with the intent to cause illness or death. Agents are divided into three categories:

- *Category A* agents pose the highest risk to the public and national security because they can be easily spread from person to person, result in high death rates, have the potential for a major impact on public health and safety, and require

CASE STUDY 38-1

H. E. was admitted to the hospital on March 14 after he came to the emergency department with shortness of breath, fever, purulent sputum, night sweats, and recent weight loss. He was isolated empirically. A definitive diagnosis of tuberculosis was made on the basis of his test results.

Mr. E. was hospitalized, placed in AIIR, and treated with appropriate antimicrobial therapy based on culture results. His condition was stabilized, and he was prepared for discharge 6 weeks after admission. He was given prescriptions for antimicrobials and taught how important it was for him to take his pills every day and to return to the clinic for follow-up care. He said he understood and left the hospital.

However, Mr. E. had lost his job as a result of his hospitalization. He had no health insurance and very little money in the bank. He took the prescriptions to the pharmacy, but when he learned that a one-month supply would cost $49, he walked out without his medicine.

The microorganisms responsible for Mr. E.'s infection had been exposed to antimicrobial therapy for 6 weeks. This is not enough time for all of the pathogens to be killed by drug therapy, but it is long enough for the bacteria to begin to change their structure to fight off the antimicrobials. If Mr. E. spreads the infection to others, the drugs used in his care may not be as effective on these newly infected people. Over time, this pattern results in an organism that has developed enough changes in its makeup that none of the common antituberculosis medications will kill it.

Questions

1. What follow-up resources are available in your community that would have helped Mr. E. obtain his medication?
2. How can public health systems monitor people infected with TB to ensure they take the proper medicine every day?
3. In some communities, people infected with TB have been hospitalized or jailed against their will for failing to take their medication as prescribed. Do you agree or disagree with this approach? Why or why not?
4. How could the situation described in this case study have been prevented?

special action for emergency preparedness (see Chapter 32). The CDC has identified microorganisms that cause anthrax, smallpox, plague, tularemia, viral hemorrhagic fevers, and botulism as category A.

- *Category B* agents are moderately easy to spread, have low mortality rates, result in moderate illness rates, and require specific enhancements at CDC and enhanced disease monitoring. Agents causing brucellosis, salmonellosis, psittacosis, Q fever, and food- and waterborne microorganisms *E. coli* 0157:H7, *shigella*, and *Cryptosporidium* are in category B.
- *Category C* agents are emerging pathogens that could be engineered for mass spread and include Hantavirus and MDR-TB.

All health care providers need to stay up-to-date on emerging threats for bioterrorism because they are the first to identify patterns of signs and symptoms that could indicate that an attack has occurred in patients coming to the emergency department and being admitted to the hospital.

The United States government has established the Web site Ready.gov as a means to communicate about a variety of hazards to the general public. The section on biological agents is at http://www.ready.gov/america/beinformed/biological.html.

The CDC has a comprehensive Web repository containing first-line actions for identifying and responding to a biological attack, as well as for health threats relating to chemical and radiation emergencies, mass casualty events, and natural disasters (http://www.bt.cdc.gov/). This site is updated as new information is learned and one that health care workers should check regularly.

PANDEMIC INFLUENZA

Unlike seasonal influenza, a pandemic influenza is a severe outbreak of a new virus that rapidly affects all parts of the world and to which persons have little or no natural immunity. Pandemic outbreaks can occur at any time of the year and have high mortality rates in otherwise healthy, young people. The last great pandemic began in 1918 and killed 50 million people

Bioterrorism

Information about agents of bioterrorism, emerging infectious diseases, and related emergency preparedness is continually updated. In the event of an attack or outbreak, respiratory therapists need to know the very latest information about the threat and guidance on how to manage it. Check these Web sites:

Emergency preparedness:

- Agency for Healthcare Research and Quality. Public health emergency preparedness. www.ahrq.gov/prep
- Centers for Disease Control and Prevention. Clinician outreach and communication activities. www.emergency.cdc.gov/coca
- Johns Hopkins Center for Public Health Preparedness. Online courses. www.jhsph.edu/preparedness/training/

Bioterrorism:

- Centers for Disease Control and Prevention. Emergency preparedness and response. www.bt.cdc.gov/bioterrorism

Pandemic influenza:

- U.S. Department of Health and Human Services. Flu.gov. www.pandemicflu.gov
- World Health Organization. Avian influenza. www.who.int/csr/disease/avian_influenza/en

worldwide and at least 675,000 in the United States. A pandemic in 1957–1958 took 1–2 million lives worldwide with at least 70,000 deaths in the United States, and in 1968, the Hong Kong influenza pandemic had a death toll of approximately 700,000 worldwide and 34,000 in the United States, which is consistent with the number of annual seasonal influenza deaths in the United States.[16–18]

Avian influenza is an infection caused by bird flu viruses. The viruses naturally occur in birds, and wild birds worldwide carry them in their intestines without ever getting sick. However, when the infected birds shed the virus in their saliva, nasal secretions, and feces, susceptible birds get sick after coming into contact with these substances,

The terms "avian influenza virus" and "A(H5N1)" typically refer to a type A influenza virus commonly found in birds; however, human cases have been reported since 1997. Human cases have been reported in Asia, Europe, the Near East, and Africa with outbreaks studied in Thailand, Vietnam, and Indonesia. Through 2008, the World Health Organization (WHO) has confirmed 395 cases with 250 deaths in 15 countries.[19]

At this point, human infection has occurred in situations in which there was very close contact with sick or dead infected poultry (chicken, ducks, and turkeys). Apparently, the virus has been spread from the person in contact with the bird to another person, but it has not spread farther than one person from contact with the source infection. Epidemiologists are concerned that a small mutation in the virus could produce a strain that is easily spread to and among humans with a high mortality.[17,19]

The World Health Organization recommends Standard Precautions when caring for A(H5N1) patients, with Airborne Precautions instituted when there is a risk for aerosolization of secretions. When available, **high-efficiency particulate air (HEPA) filters** should be attached to the expiratory ports of ventilators, and a closed tracheal suction system should be used. The WHO guidelines also describe modifying an N95 respirator mask to function as a nonrebreathing mask for oxygen administration.[20]

For the latest information on avian influenza, visit the Web sites of the World Health Organization (http://www.who.int/csr/disease/avian_influenza/en/) and the U.S. Health and Human Services (http://www.pandemicflu.gov/index.html). Both sites are regularly updated and provide many links to additional information. Both are key sources of information in the case of a pandemic influenza outbreak.

Summary

Many of the microorganisms in the health care setting do not cause respiratory illness. However, respiratory therapists encounter them regularly in patients with traditional and drug-resistant infections who also have respiratory disease that requires treatment or in critically ill patients who need mechanical ventilatory support for respiratory failure. Thus a thorough understanding of the chain of infection and Standard Precautions is an essential element of every RT's practice. In modern practice, the RT does not focus on respiratory disease alone. Respiratory therapists often care for patients with multisystem involvement, which, more often than not, includes infectious disease. Because critically ill patients are compromised hosts and are likely to undergo invasive procedures, such as endotracheal intubation, their risk of developing infections is extremely high.

Each RT must make a commitment to follow all infection control procedures and to keep up-to-date as recommendations change. Only a multidisciplinary effort by all members of the health care team can keep infectious diseases under control and protect patients and health care workers.

Study Questions

REVIEW QUESTIONS

1. Describe the elements of the chain of infection.
2. Outline the proper hand hygiene procedure.
3. Discuss the proper use of personal protective equipment (PPE).
4. List ways to reduce the risk of needlestick injury.
5. Explain how antimicrobial resistance occurs.

MULTIPLE-CHOICE QUESTIONS

1. Which element of the chain of infection describes how likely a person is to contract an infectious disease?
   a. reservoir
   b. susceptible host
   c. causative agent
   d. mode of transmission
2. Which form of precautions is used for patients with tuberculosis?
   a. contact
   b. droplet
   c. airborne
   d. respiratory
3. Which of the following statements is true regarding the use of personal protective equipment (PPE)?
   a. Goggles are not required for a health care worker who wears eyeglasses.
   b. Gloves are required for any procedure that involves touching a patient.
   c. In some circumstances, goggles may be required when a mask is not.
   d. In some circumstances, a gown may be required when a face shield is not.
4. Which of the following statements best describes Droplet Precautions?
   a. A mask is required when working within 3 feet of the patient; the patient should wear a surgical mask for transport.
   b. A respirator mask is required at all times; the door to the room must remain closed; the patient should wear a surgical mask for transport.
   c. A mask, goggles, gown, and gloves are required when there is the potential for exposure to blood.
   d. Gloves are required when entering the room; a gown is required for touching the patient or environmental surfaces; dedicated equipment should stay in the patient's room.
5. A needlestick injury would put a health care worker at greatest risk for infection by which pathogen?
   a. HIV
   b. hepatitis A
   c. hepatitis B
   d. hepatitis C
6. A needlestick would pose the greatest risk of disease transmission if the needle had been used to
   a. draw an arterial blood gas.
   b. suture a wound.
   c. draw medication from a multiuse vial.
   d. give an intramuscular injection.

CRITICAL-THINKING QUESTIONS

1. How do patients in critical care units become more susceptible to infections?
2. How would the respiratory therapist learn which type of precautions are needed before caring for a patient?
3. How can respiratory therapists reduce the transmission of infection throughout the hospital?
4. What actions can RTs take to reduce the occurrence of latex allergies?

References

1. World Health Organization. WHO guidelines on hand hygiene in health care (Advanced Draft). 2005. http://www.who.int/patientsafety/information_centre/ghhad_download_link/en/
2. Siegel JD, Rhinehart E, Jackson M, Chiarello L, Healthcare Infection Control Practices Advisory Committee. Management of multidrug-resistant organisms in healthcare settings, 2006.
3. Goetz AM, Stout JE, Jacobs SL, et al. Health care-associated infection: Legionnaires' disease discovered in community hospitals following cultures of the water system: seek and ye shall find. *American Journal of Infection Control.* 1998;26:8–11.
4. Pearson ML, Bridges CB, Harper SA. Influenza vaccination of health-care personnel. *MMWR.* 2006;55,RR02:1–16. http://www.cdc.gov/mmwr/preview/mmwrhtml/rr5502a1.htm
5. Siegel JD, Rhinehart E, Jackson M, Chiarello L, Healthcare Infection Control Practices Advisory Committee. Guideline for isolation precautions: preventing transmission of infectious agents in

healthcare settings 2007. 2007. http://www.cdc.gov/hicpac/2007IP/2007isolationPrecautions.html

6. Vonberg R, Gastmeier P. Hospital-acquired infections related to contaminated substances. *Journal of Hospital Infection.* 2007;65(1):15–23.
7. Jensen PA, Lambert LA, Iademarco MF, Ridzon R. Guidelines for preventing the transmission of *Mycobacterium tuberculosis* in health-care settings, 2005. *MMWR.* 2005;54,RR-17.
8. Osterholm MT, Hedberg CW. Epidemiologic principles. In: Mandell GL, Bennett JE, Dolin R, eds. *Principles and Practice of Infectious Diseases.* 6th ed. Philadelphia: Churchill Livingstone; 2006.
9. Edmond MB, Wenzel RP. Isolation. In: Mandell GL, Bennett JE, Dolin R, eds. *Principles and Practice of Infectious Diseases.* 6th ed. Philadelphia: Churchill Livingstone; 2006.
10. Larson EL, Hughes CA, Pyrek JD, Sparks SM, Cagatay EU, Bartkus JM. Changes in bacterial flora associated with skin damage on hands of health care personnel. *American Journal of Infection Control.* 1998;26:513–521.
11. Bell M. HICPAC isolation guideline: infection control on the horizon: Association for Professionals in Infection Control (APIC); 2007.
12. Centers for Disease Control and Prevention. Surveillance of occupationally acquired HIV/AIDS in healthcare personnel, as of December 2006. 2007.
13. Centers for Disease Control and Prevention. Updated U.S. Public Health Service guidelines for the management of occupational exposures to HIV and recommendations for postexposure prophylaxis. *MMWR.* September 30 2005; 54,RR-9.
14. NHS Plus RCoP, Faculty of Occupational Medicine. Latex allergy: occupational aspects of management. A national guideline. 2008. http://www.nhsplus.nhs.uk/web/public/default.aspx?PageID=478
15. Occupational Safety & Health Administration. 10/23/1995—Bloodborne pathogens and the issue of latex allergy and latex sensitivity. *Standard Interpretations, Standard.* 1995;1910–1930.
16. Centers for Disease Control and Prevention. Key facts about avian influenza (bird flu) and avian influenza A (H5N1) virus. 2006.
17. Centers for Disease Control and Prevention. Avian influenza A virus infections of humans. 2008. http://www.cdc.gov/flu/avian/gen-info/avian-flu-humans.htm
18. Treanor JJ. Influenza virus. In: Mandell GL, Bennett JE, Dolin R, eds. *Principles and Practice of Infectious Diseases.* 6th ed. Philadelphia: Churchill Livingstone; 2006.
19. World Health Organization. Cumulative number of confirmed human cases of avian influenza A(H5N1) reported to WHO. Table. 2009. http://www.who.int/csr/disease/avian_influenza/country/cases_table_2009_01_27/en/index.html
20. World Health Organization. Clinical management of human infection with avian influenza A(H5N1) virus. 2007. http://www.who.int/csr/disease/avian_influenza/guidelines/clinicalmanage07/en/index.html

CHAPTER 39

Health Promotion

Bill Galvin

OBJECTIVES

Upon completion of this chapter, the reader should be able to:

- Describe the general principles and concepts associated with health, to include related terms, models of health, dimensions of health, philosophies of health, historical factors affecting health in the United States, and determinants of health status.
- Compare and contrast the leading causes of death in the United States in 1900, 1990, and 2005 in terms of the actual diseases or conditions as well as their behavioral causes.
- Draw, label, and describe the illness and wellness continuum.
- List and describe the general components of an individual health promotion process and the action steps employed in the implementation stage of the process.
- Briefly describe selected models of community-based health promotion.
- Identify and describe the significant reports published by the federal government that address the issue of health promotion in the United States.
- Explain the role of the respiratory therapist in the health promotion movement.

CHAPTER OUTLINE

(continues)

(continued)

Leading Causes of Death
Behavioral Causes of Death
Determinants of Health Status
- Heredity
- Environment
- Health Care System
- Lifestyle

Continuums
Health Promotion Process
- Individual or Personal Wellness
- Community or Organizational Wellness

Role of the Federal Government
- Healthy People: The Surgeon General's Report on Health Promotion and Disease Prevention
- Promoting Health/Preventing Disease: Objectives for the Nation
- Healthy People 2000
- Healthy People 2010
- Healthy People 2020

Role of Respiratory Therapist in Health Promotion

KEY TERMS

average life span
cultural norms
disease prevention
environmental model
health
health promotion
holistic model
life expectancy
lifestyle behavior
locus of control
medical model
morbidity
mortality
primary prevention
secondary prevention
tertiary prevention
wellness

Health promotion is not a new term that was recently discovered by the health care professionals. It is also more than a fashionable idea that has found favor in the news media or a popular craze that has caught on to the health conscious and fitness zealots in society. It is a concept, a process, a way of life that has become popular and attractive because of emerging and convincing evidence to support its acceptance and adoption as a valuable means to curtail health care cost and to improve people's health and well-being.

Numerous studies, articles, and reports by employer groups, by the federal government, and by professional organizations are finding that the adoption of certain basic tenets and principles has a lasting and profound effect in improving the health and quality of life of the general public. The overwhelming support for their adoption comes in many forms, most notably in the form of:

- Decreased absenteeism from work and school.
- Increases in productivity.
- The reduction of **morbidity** and **mortality**.
- The enhancement in longevity and quality of life.

Respiratory care professionals need to:

- Be aware of the basic principles and concepts of health promotion.
- Understand the issues related to **life expectancy**, longevity, and life span.
- Be familiar with the factors that have made an impact on health care in the United States over the past 100 years.
- Know the leading causes of death and the fact that five of these top ten killers are cardiorespiratory in nature.
- Recognize the behavioral causes of death, such as smoking, excessive dietary intake, seat belt disuse, sedentary lifestyle, and other unhealthy lifestyle behaviors.
- Understand that these lifestyle behaviors lead to increased morbidity and mortality and a compromised state of well-being.
- Know the health promotion process for individual wellness as well as the health and well-being of a community, a group, or an organization.
- Master the steps involved in the development, design, and implementation of a health promotion program.

- Appreciate the role of the federal government in fostering and supporting the health promotion movement.
- Most importantly, know and understand that they have a vital role to play in this emerging and evolving component of health care.

Very clearly, the health care system will more openly endorse the concepts and practices of health promotion in the not too distant future. Health promotion is clearly a concept whose time has come. And its acceptance and practice will undoubtedly go a long way in resolving a significant portion of the health care problems in this country. For respiratory therapists (RTs) to maintain a prominent place in health care delivery of the future, they must be well versed in all aspects of this discipline and welcome the opportunity to be viewed as key players in incorporating and promoting the related principles and practices. This chapter is written for this purpose and with the hope that all respiratory therapists will readily adopt, endorse, and foster the role of health care educator in their daily practices and routines.

General Principles and Concepts of Health

Historically, health in the United States has generally been perceived rather narrowly. Many people have considered **health** as the absence of disease. In other words, in the absence of significant signs or symptoms, a person is considered healthy. Respiratory therapists are no different because they too view health in a rather limited therapeutic context. This context is reflected in their role, duties, and responsibilities as RTs and is expressed by their day-to-day functions and interactions with their patients. These day-to-day functions and interactions consist of such tasks and procedures as:

- Listening to breath sounds.
- Evaluating a chest radiograph.
- Performing an arterial blood gas.
- Administering an aerosol treatment.
- Interpreting a pulmonary function study.
- Initiating and adjusting a mechanical ventilator.
- In general, making decisions and judgments regarding the appropriate care and treatment of patients.

Such procedures, techniques, and practices are the norm for respiratory therapists and certainly considered their standards of care and professional practice.

However, over the years, health has been redefined and reevaluated. Back in 1947, the very year that the respiratory care profession was incorporated and formally established, the World Health Organization came out with a revised and more comprehensive definition of health, defining it as *"a state of complete physical, mental, and social well-being and not merely the absence of disease or infirmity."*[1] Although this certainly is far better than the previous and very limited definition of health as the absence of disease, many still view it as less than satisfactory and somewhat limited in scope. The more contemporary thinking is to expand the "treatment and curative" definitions of health to something more comprehensive, something more all-inclusive, something that goes beyond the limits of curation and addresses the critical issues of disease prevention and health promotion.

Confounding the problem of this narrow definition are the complicated issues of defining health in light of genetically or environmentally determined physical, social, psychological, vocational, or intellectual limitations. For example, if someone is born with a benign and relatively harmless disorder such as webbed toes, is this person any less healthy than others? Or suppose someone sustained a serious motor vehicle accident 10 or 15 years ago and has obviously adapted to his physical limitations, is participating in a loving relationship, is actively and productively engaged in a meaningful vocation, and is a prominent and contributing member of his community. In short, he has a purposeful and productive existence in society. Is he any less healthy? Suppose someone is financially successful with a six-figure salary, driving a Mercedes Benz, a true up-and-comer in her company, with lots of friends, and the envy of her peers and middle management. Yet she is miserably unhappy with her personal life. What is her level of health? Clearly, the meaning of the term "health" is quite complex. The word has numerous definitions and is viewed from a variety of perspectives. At times it lacks clarity, is subjective, arbitrary, ambiguous, controversial, and highly debatable. A universally accepted definition is not likely to exist. Nonetheless, health care professionals should attempt to bring some degree of clarity and precision to its meaning and interpretation.

Health as the absence of *physical* disease was often discussed and evaluated quantitatively and described in terms of vital statistics. Some of the more commonly cited vital statistics were life expectancy or longevity, life span, infant mortality, the leading causes of death, and issues of morbidity and mortality. *Life expectancy*, or *longevity*, is considered to relate to the estimated number of years of life remaining to a living organism, usually determined by comparing the organism's current age to the average age at death of other members of the species during a fixed period.[2] More simply stated, it is the average length of time that members of a population can expect to live. Life expectancy in the

United States has changed drastically over the last 100 years. In 1900, life expectancy was approximately 47. Today life expectancy in the United States is 80.4 years for women and 75.2 years for men, yielding an average of approximately 77.8 years of age.

Although a long life may appear to be desirable, comparing these figures with those of other industrialized countries demonstrates a rather dismal picture because there are almost four dozen countries ahead of us. Leading the list are Macau, Andorra, Japan, Singapore, San Marino, Hong Kong, Australia, Canada, France, Sweden, and Switzerland, to name some. Table 39-1 depicts life expectancy figures for approximately 25 selected countries. Those at the top of the list have average life expectancy figures that approximate 80 years of age and yet represent significantly lower per-capita expenditures for health than in the United States. The undeveloped countries of Africa (Zambia, Angola, and Swaziland) are at the bottom of the list with average life expectancy figures averaging below 37 years of age.[3]

Another way to measure and explain the health of a nation is to express it in the form of *infant mortality*. Once again, the statistics are rather dismal. When the U.S. infant mortality is compared to that of other nations, the United States is positioned 42 out of the 222 countries cited in the statistics, with an infant mortality rate of 6.30 per 1000. Singapore has a 2008 estimated infant mortality rate of 2.30, followed by Sweden, Japan, and Hong Kong at 2.75, 2.80, and 2.93, respectively. Table 39-2 depicts the infant mortality rates of selected countries.[4]

Another fascinating way to quantitatively measure health is to look at the maximum or optimum life span and the average life span.

TABLE 39-1 **Rank order of life expectancy at birth in selected countries (2008 estimated)**

Rank	Country	Life Expectancy at Birth
1	Macau	84.33
2	Andora	82.67
3	Japan	82.07
4	Singapore	81.89
5	San Marino	81.88
6	Hong Kong	81.77
7	Australia	81.53
8	Canada	81.16
9	France	80.87
10	Sweden	80.74
11	Switzerland	80.74
12	Guernsey	80.65
13	Israel	80.61
14	Iceland	80.55
15	Anguilla	80.53
16	Cayman Island	80.32
17	New Zealand	80.24
18	Italy	80.07
19	Gibraltar	80.06
20	Monaco	79.96
46	United States	78.14
221	Zambia	38.59
222	Angola	37.92
223	Swaziland	31.99

Source: Based on data compiled from CIA, The World Fact Book *(Washington, DC: Office of Public Affairs; 20505). https://www.cia.gov/library/publications/the-world-factbook/rankorder/2102rank.html*

TABLE 39-2 **Rank order of infant mortality in selected countries (2008 estimate and reported per 1000 live births)**

Rank	Country	Infant Mortality
1	Singapore	2.3
2	Sweden	2.75
3	Japan	2.8
4	Hong Kong	2.93
5	Macau	3.23
6	Iceland	3.25
7	France	3.36
8	Finland	3.50
9	Anguilla	3.54
10	Norway	3.61
11	Andorra	3.68
12	Malta	3.79
13	Czech Republic	3.83
14	Germany	4.03
15	Switzerland	4.23
16	Spain	4.26
17	Israel	4.28
18	South Korea	4.29
19	Slovenia	4.30
20	Denmark	4.40
42	United States	6.30

Source: Based on data compiled from CIA, The World Fact Book *(Washington, DC: Office of Public Affairs; 20505).*

Maximum or *optimum life span* is defined as the theoretical maximum number of years that individuals of a species can live. This term is not without some controversy; different authors have provided contradictory values. Theodore Reiff has expressed a view that the maximum or optimum life span is approximately 120 years of age.[5] He feels that from a purely physiological point of view, the human body has the potential to achieve the age of 120 before significant degeneration of body parts occurs. In other words, if all factors are optimized to their full potential, organ systems can sustain themselves until the age of 120. Numerous examples and citations are found to support this view.

The oldest verified case of a human living beyond 120 years of age is a French woman by the name of Jeanne Calmet, who reportedly lived to be 122 years of age.[6] She entered the world in 1875 before the invention of the telephone and automobile and before the birth of Albert Einstein, Pablo Picasso, and Joseph Stalin. She rode a bike until the age of 100, and it has been speculated that her longevity was linked to her genes as well as to her lifestyle. Her father lived to the age of 94 and her mother to 86. She died in 1997. Another source indicated that one of the oldest human beings was Shigechiyo Izumi of Japan who reportedly died on June 19,1984 at the age of 119.[7]

Other citations speak of increased life span among isolated agrarian societies, such as the Soviet Georgians, who also live to be 100 or more years of age. Common findings among this agrarian group suggest that certain variables may have a bearing on longevity:

- Primary source of food consisting of whole grains, vegetables, and very little red meat.
- Vigorous work patterns that continue into old age.
- A strong social support system consisting of family and friends.

What is especially interesting to note is that they attain these extremely old ages in the absence of sophisticated medical care.[8]

Additionally, two highly significant research studies addressed the issues of longevity among centenarians. The first was a case study research conducted over a 40-year period in the 1940s and entailed over 12,000 centenarians. The results indicated that family, self, work ethic, and social relationships were repeatedly identified as the "reasons for ongoingness."[9] The second was initiated by Poon in 1988 and was known as the Georgia Centenarian Study.[10] It was an investigation of adaptational characteristics of long-lived persons and identified the following four common characteristics of centenarians: optimism, flexibility, commitment, and engagement in some activity. Although no strong agreement exists regarding common universal factors underlying increased longevity, several additional factors have been identified throughout the literature:[11]

- Genetic influences
- Nutritional factors
- Moderate alcohol consumption
- Physical activity throughout life
- Sexual activity into advanced years
- Environmental influences
- Psychosocial factors
- Laughter
- Low ambitions
- Daily routines
- Belief in God
- Close family ties
- Freedom and independence
- Organized purposeful behavior
- A positive view of life

Although attainment of this optimum or maximal life span is quite fascinating and certainly a desirable quest, accidents, diseases, and various other medical conditions often prevent this theoretical or idealized situation from occurring. Thus, a more realistic and valuable term to express longevity and life span would be the term *average life span*. **Average life span** is the age at which half the members of a population have died.[1] The maximum average life span is approximately 85–90 years of age, a figure that the insurance industry and the government have determined. The insurance industry is capable of compiling large volumes of data on actual populations and using these data to determine insurance premiums for various genders and ages throughout life. The government has been able to perform statistical studies and estimate how many additional years of life can be added if major diseases were eliminated. For example, if all cancers could be cured or prevented, about three years of life would be added. If all heart disease could be eliminated, an additional 14 years could be added.[12] This is indeed a fascinating issue because the average life span in the United States has increased dramatically in the last century and certainly will have significant implications on society and health in the future.

Other terms used to measure the relative health of a population are morbidity and mortality.

- *Morbidity* is defined as the ratio of persons who are diseased to those who are well in a given community.[1]
- *Mortality* is defined as the number of deaths per unit of population in a specific region, age range, or other group.[1]

Mortality rates have dropped precipitously since 1900 with the 1900 figure estimated at 17.2 per 1000 and the 2005 figure standing at 8.2 per 1000.

In the mid-1960s, health began to take on a different meaning in society. Broader definitions and interpretations of health became popular. In 1967, Halbert Dunn, from the Wellness Institute at the University of Wisconsin in Stevens Point, expressed it as "an integrated method of functioning which is oriented toward maximizing the potential of which the individual is capable."[13] He indicated that "it requires that the individual maintain a continuum of balance and purposeful direction with the environment where he/she is functioning."[13] Health was described as an interrelationship and a unity of mind, body, and spirit. With this movement came a multidimensional perspective of health that entailed the practice of positive health traits and characteristics and that became synonymous with the term "wellness."

Wellness has been expressed as "an approach to personal health that emphasizes individual responsibility for well being through the practice of health-promoting **lifestyle behaviors.**"[2] It is considered a dynamic rather than a static process that takes into account all decisions people make daily. These decisions entail activities and practices such as what people eat and drink, the amount of regular exercise, driving habits and seat belt usage, smoking habits, alcohol use, and other activities of daily living. The decisions entail choice, not chance, and choice is a decision to move toward optimal health. Wellness is a way of life, a lifestyle designed to achieve a person's highest potential for well-being.

Whereas health was considered a state, and in many cases a passive state, wellness is a process, a developing awareness that there is no end point but rather that health and happiness are possible in each moment, here and now. It is an efficient channeling of energy—energy received from the environment, transformed within an individual, and sent to affect the world outside. It is the integration of body, mind, and spirit. It is the appreciation that everything a person does and thinks and feels and believes has an impact on his or her state of health. Wellness is defined as a process of developing patterns of behavior that lead to improved health and heightened satisfaction.[8]

Models of Health

Just as there are different definitions for health, the underlying beliefs and attitudes acting as the core principles or foundations of health have more than one definition. Some people have expressed this foundation of core beliefs in the form of different models. There are three different models for health:

- The medical model
- The environmental model
- The holistic model

TABLE 39-3 **The characteristics of the three models of health**

Model	Characteristics
Medical	Biologically/physiologically based Quantitatively/statistically driven Treatment oriented
Environmental	Ecosystem based Environmentally adapted Psychologically/culturally sensitive
Holistic	Multidimensional (whole person) Disease prevention oriented Health promotion focused

Source: Based on data compiled from Edlin G, Golanty E, McCormack Brown K. Health and Wellness. *6th ed. Sudbury, MA: Jones & Bartlett Publishers; 1999:4–6.*

Table 39-3 identifies the three models and their more prominent characteristics.

MEDICAL MODEL

The **medical model**[1] is based almost exclusively on biological explanations of illness and disease. Virtually every illness and disease is interpreted in terms of cellular abnormality, organ dysfunction, or some other biological system failure. It is perhaps the closest to the traditional and pure definition of health as the absence of disease by which a person is considered to be in the best attainable state of health whenever sickness is absent. One author has expressed the model in terms of the absence of one or more of the following five Ds: death, disease, discomfort, disability, and dissatisfaction.[1] It entails assessing the population in the form of vital statistics where the number of deaths (mortality) and the presence of illness or disease (morbidity) is reported and compared to previous years. This purely quantitative approach is rather sterile and void of any social or psychological factors and thus is considered by many to be of limited value.

Reliance is solely on biological processes, curing the disease or problem, and restoring the damaged part. It does not focus on the psychosocial aspects of health and thus does not take into account the influence of family, friends, and personal interactions and relationships. Additionally, it does not reflect the influence of culture, beliefs, attitude, or values and the power that these factors have on one's state of health and well-being. Success lies in the ability to describe, diagnose, and treat disease. There is little emphasis in fostering health and preventing disease. It is an excellent way to gather data and vital statistics and to quantify and measure disease. However, quality issues cannot be factored into the equation, and hard-core number crunching does not reflect the importance of preventative measures and the reversal of unhealthy lifestyles and destructive behaviors.

ENVIRONMENTAL MODEL

The **environmental model**[1] evolved from modern analysis of ecosystems and environmental risks, and it focuses on the person's adaptation to the environment as conditions change. It includes the effects on personal health of such issues as socioeconomic status, education, and multiple environmental factors. It focuses on conditions outside the individual, which include the quality of air and water, living conditions, exposure to harmful substances, socioeconomic conditions, social relationships, and the health care system. It has also been associated with ancient Eastern cultures and Native American philosophies that stress health as being related to harmony and harmonious interactions. In essence, such cultures and philosophical beliefs indicate that, as the environment changes, so too must the individual.

HOLISTIC MODEL

The **holistic model**[1] is defined in terms of the whole person rather than in terms of a disease state. It has also been expressed as a state of optimal or positive wellness. It is a comprehensive approach to health and encompasses the physiological, mental, emotional, social, spiritual, and environmental aspects of the individual. Additionally, it entails the community and focuses on optimizing health, preventing disease, and fostering positive mental and emotional health for both the individual and the population as a whole. It has been criticized as being too idealistic; however, it has gained considerable credibility, acceptance, and notoriety in recent years.

Dimensions of Health

The current view of health is more comprehensive, taking into account the issues of **disease prevention** and health promotion.

In U.S. culture, modern medicine emphasizes a growing interest in striving toward an optimum state of health. In fact, the old English root for the word health is "wholeness." This optimum state of health should take into account the whole person, and the whole person consists of more than the body. It should also entail the mind, the spirit, the family, the community, and the country, the job, education, and beliefs. Viewing health from this perspective clearly demands a multidimensional approach and view of the interrelatedness of all these components. These components are listed as the six dimensions of wellness:[14]

- *Physical.* The physical dimension encourages cardiovascular endurance, flexibility, and strength, and it encourages regular physical activity. Physical development encourages knowledge about food and nutrition and discourages the use of tobacco, drugs, and excessive alcohol consumption. It encourages activities that contribute to high-level wellness, including medical self-care and the appropriate use of the medical system.
- *Occupational.* The occupational dimension involves preparing for work in which a person gains personal satisfaction and enrichment. Occupational development is related to an individual's attitude about work.
- *Intellectual.* The intellectual dimension encourages creative, stimulating mental activities. An intellectually well person uses the resources available to expand knowledge, improve skills, and increase the potential for sharing with others. Intellectually well people use the intellectual and cultural activities in and beyond the classroom, combined with the human and learning resources available within their community.
- *Social.* The social dimension encourages contributing to the human and physical environment for the common welfare of the community. It emphasizes the interdependence with others and nature, and it includes the pursuit of harmony within your family.
- *Spiritual.* The spiritual dimension involves seeking meaning and purpose in human existence. It includes the development of a deep appreciation for the depth and expanse of life and natural forces that exist in the universe. It also involves developing a strong sense of personal values and ethics.
- *Emotional.* The emotional dimension emphasizes an awareness and acceptance of feelings. Emotional wellness includes the degree to which people feel positive and enthusiastic about themselves and life. It includes the capacity to manage feelings and related behaviors, including the realistic assessment of your limitations, development of autonomy, and ability to cope effectively with stress. The emotionally well person maintains satisfying relationships with others.

PHYSICAL DIMENSION

The physical dimension deals with the functional operation of the body and how it responds to damage and disease. To be in good physical condition, people must care for their physical dimension. The physical dimension consists of physical fitness as well as the appropriate use of medical care. Physical fitness encompasses muscular strength, muscular endurance, flexibility, and body composition. In this context, one could certainly ask the question, "Who is the most physically fit—Frank Shorter, Nadia Comaneci, or Arnold Swartzenegger?" Obviously all three are physically fit in their own right. However, maintaining a balance among the three components of flexibility, strength, and endurance is critical for optimum physical fitness.

Additionally, this dimension also involves other elements:

- Dietary habits and the partaking of the right foods—a balanced diet of protein, fats, and carbohydrates and the maintenance of desirable weight.
- Getting sufficient sleep.
- Avoiding drugs and excessive alcohol.
- Using the medical system appropriately for routine medical checkups, timely vaccinations, proper use of medications and, in general, taking the necessary and appropriate measures when one is ill.

OCCUPATIONAL DIMENSION

The occupational dimension involves deriving satisfaction and pleasure in one's job. Does the individual enjoy and look forward to getting up and going to work every day? Does work provide stimulation, creativity, social interaction, and a sense of fulfillment? Is the individual happy with the working conditions, the salary, the growth potential, the mobility? Are there advancement, leadership, autonomy, and camaraderie?

Or does she simply punch a clock five days a week and live for the weekends? A happy medium should exist between work life and leisure life. Much of life is spent at work, and a person has to choose a vocation that provides meaning and enjoyment. If someone is not happy with an occupation, the discontent spills over to the family and circle of friends, ultimately affecting the individual's entire well being.

INTELLECTUAL DIMENSION

The intellectual dimension involves the use of the mind. Contrary to popular belief, this dimension is not limited to formal education but rather extends to the lifelong attainment of knowledge, education, and experiences. Curiosity and learning should never stop. Reading, writing, and keeping abreast of current events are intellectual pursuits. And although intellectual development varies from one person to the next, a person still has to engage in stimulating and creative mental exercises. Intellectual growth also includes the acquisition and evaluation of information for the purpose of developing or deterring alternatives and arriving at appropriate and logical decisions. Someone who is intellectually well seeks new experiences, challenges, and opportunities.

This inquisitiveness generally encourages a richness of intellect and a rewarding sense of fulfillment.

SOCIAL DIMENSION

The social dimension refers to one's ability to fulfill one's role as a husband, wife, son, daughter, parent, friend, neighbor, or citizen. Each of these roles requires a certain expectation and a give-and-take in any relationship.

- Individuals are not islands unto themselves. They must exist in harmony with others. There is always an interdependence among people. Being able to maintain appropriate relationships is crucial to one's existence. Being a team player and able to work with a group is a much sought-after and frequently rewarded trait in today's society.
- The social dimension also implies appropriate expressions of friendship, companionship, justice, honesty, loyalty, care, love, and intimacy.
- It also entails the ability to master social graces.

The highly technical world of medicine is replete with situations calling for quick and demanding responses to emergent circumstances. In such an environment, health care providers need to demonstrate warmth, care, compassion, and sensitivity in their interactions with patients.

SPIRITUAL DIMENSION

Spiritual wellness is not always synonymous with religion. It need not identify a god, a creator, or a theological belief. Spiritual wellness is someone's inner belief and is made up of that person's interpretation of the meaning and purpose of existence. Everyone needs purpose and direction in life. Their spiritual dimension provides this force. This sense of purpose can be expressed:

- In nature as the awe and beauty of the surroundings.
- In science as one views their relationship with the universe.
- In religion as an expression of deeply held religious beliefs and convictions.

Spiritual wellness involves the development of the inner self and soul. It is a way of living that views life as meaningful, purposeful, and pleasurable. It is characterized by faith, optimism, peace, and an undaunted comfort with life and its outcome. Individuals who are spiritually well can generally see beyond isolated events and envision the whole picture. They are able to identify true sources of joy, pleasure, and fulfillment in their lives.

EMOTIONAL DIMENSION

The emotional dimension reflects a person's feelings toward self, situations, and other people. It entails understanding and accepting these feelings as well as one's capabilities and limitations. Of considerable importance is the ability to cope with emotions as well as change. Health care is an incredibly dynamic and volatile environment, and the health care worker's ability to cope with the ever increasing and constant change is a tremendous challenge. Stress management is a vital component of the emotional dimension and of critical importance to today's health care provider. Being able to identify the stressors, to understand the stress response, and to employ appropriate stress-reduction strategies and techniques can aid immeasurably in coping with the trials and tribulations of today's fast-paced and hectic health care delivery system. The hallmark of emotional wellness is a deep and abiding sense of contentment and happiness, and it generally involves one's ability to laugh, to enjoy life, to adjust to change, to cope with stress, and to maintain appropriate relationships.

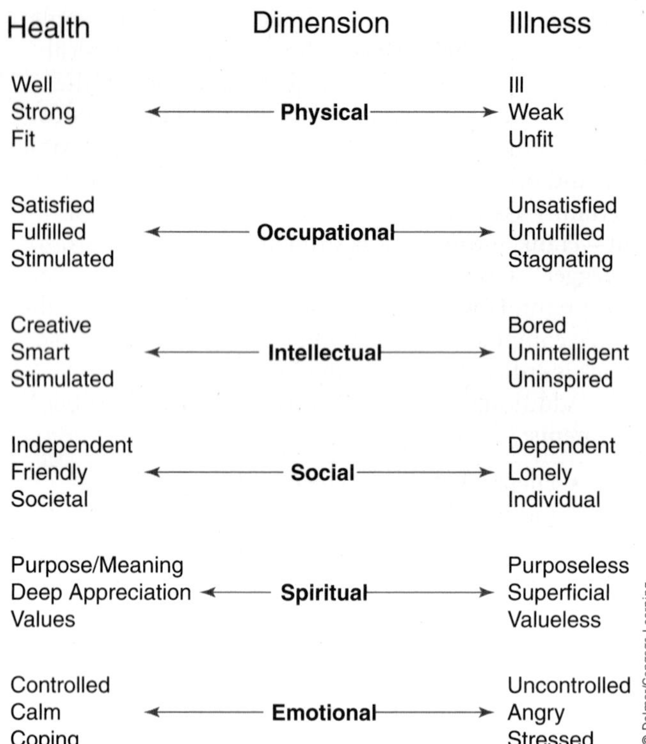

FIGURE 39-1 Continuums for the six dimensions of health.

MAINTAINING BALANCE

Figure 39-1 reflects a continuum of the different dimensions of health. Each dimension must be as fully developed as possible for inadequate development of any dimension can create a condition of imbalance. A simple analogy clarifies this point. In Figure 39-2, each dimension is viewed as a spoke to a wheel. If one of the spokes (a dimension) is inadequately developed (shorter than other spokes), a state of imbalance exists. This imbalance can be converted to life events such that one's travels through life can be either smooth (balanced and concentric wheel) or rocky (undeveloped dimension and unbalanced wheel). This simple analogy makes the point that complete or holistic health requires the development of the whole person. No single dimension may exist in isolation; each and every dimension must be maximized.

Philosophy of Holistic Health

The word "holistic" comes from the Greek word *holos*, meaning "whole." The notion of wholeness came from some of the early civilizations that viewed health and disease as a combination of mind and body or mind and matter. The term "holism" was actually coined by a South African named Jan Smuts,[7] who used the term to refer to the tendency in nature to synthesize and organize toward greater wholes. He wrote that the meaning of the whole organism was greater than the sum of its parts. He suggested thinking of the human organism not as separate parts, such as the cells or organs, but rather as the sum of all its parts, meaning the physical, occupational, psychological, social, and spiritual. He suggested that health entailed the healing of the whole person and every aspect of being. Many followers have offered many variations of this theme; however, in short, it became the notion that holistic health consists of treatment, prevention, and promotion.[7] Treatment consisted of the traditional Western notion of doctors using techniques and procedures to diagnose, medicate, and perform surgical interventions for the purpose of treating the physical components of disease and illness. Although these treatments brought with them many successes and advancements, they were nonetheless somewhat limited because they merely addressed the reactive portion of the problem. Treatment entails the use of medical care and begins with the sick and seeks to keep them alive, make them well, or minimize their disability. What is missing in this perspective of health

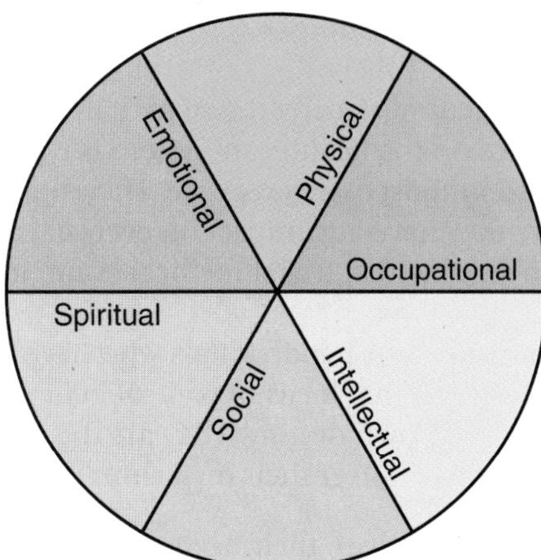

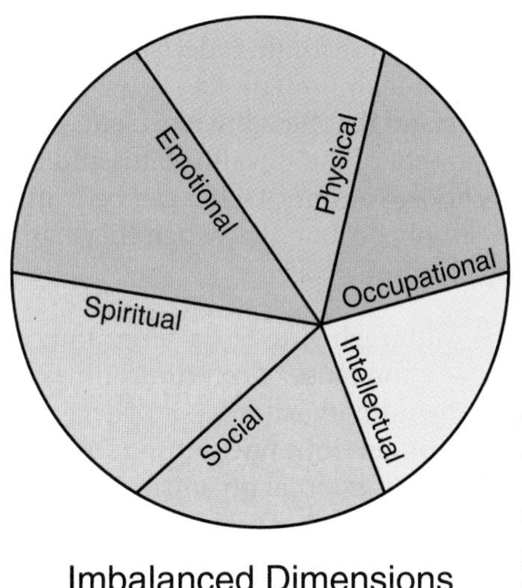

FIGURE 39-2 The balanced and imbalanced dimensions of health.

is the proactive position, and this is where the concepts of prevention and promotion come into play.

DISEASE PREVENTION

Where treatment begins with the sick, disease prevention begins with people who are exposed to a threat to their health and strives to protect them from the harmful and deleterious effects of the threats.[15] *Prevention of disease* means inhibiting the development of disease and interrupting or slowing its progression after it has started. It can be grouped into three distinct categories: primary prevention, secondary prevention, and tertiary prevention.[16]

- **Primary prevention** involves activities that prevent a disease or condition from occurring in the first place. Examples of primary prevention are the conscious decision to significantly curtail the eating of saturated fats or to eliminate cigarette smoking. The result of reducing saturated fats is the prevention of heart disease; the elimination of smoking reduces the likelihood of developing emphysema or other pulmonary conditions.
- **Secondary prevention** involves activities that detect a disease condition early in the process so that its duration and severity can be shortened or halted. Screening for cancers, such as a breast self-examination or testicular self-examination, are examples because both are a means for early detection of cancerous lesions and potentially prevent the long-term consequences of breast and testicular cancer. Inherent in this definition is the fact that, no matter what lifestyle changes are employed, a person may still develop a major chronic disease at some stage in life. Being able to identify signs and symptoms early enables the person to secure appropriate and timely therapeutic intervention.
- **Tertiary prevention** is best represented by rehabilitative measures that aid an individual who has already contracted a disease process but that prevent it from reoccurring or becoming exacerbated. Pulmonary rehabilitation for a patient with emphysema is a clear example of tertiary prevention. Tertiary prevention is designed to lessen or eliminate the sometimes serious consequences of the condition. An overwhelming body of evidence suggests the tremendous value of preventive measures. One such landmark study indicated that preventable illness makes up approximately 70% of the burden of illness and the associated costs.[17]

HEALTH PROMOTION

Health promotion focuses on people who are basically healthy and seeks to develop the community and individual lifestyle measures that maintain and enhance a state of well-being.[15] The philosophy of health promotion was initiated by the Carter administration[7] in 1980 when the United States Department of Health and Human Services published its landmark report identifying health goals for the nation. (This report is addressed in considerable detail later in the chapter.) The focus of the report and the movement was on informing the public of risky lifestyle behaviors with the intention of motivating them to change these behaviors.

Health promotion has been defined in numerous ways.

- It was expressed as a movement in which knowledge, practices, and value stances are transmitted to people for their use in lengthening their lives, reducing the incidence of illness, and feeling better.[18]
- The American Hospital Association has defined it as the process of fostering awareness, influencing attitudes, and identifying alternatives so that individuals can make informed choices and change their behavior in order to achieve an optimum level of physical and mental health and improve their physical and social environment.[19]
- It has also been expressed as the application of wellness principles and as a systematic effort by an organization to enhance the wellness of its members through education, behavior change, and cultural support.[8]

Opatz has also indicated that wellness entails two critical themes: individual responsibility for one's actions and the influence of cultural norms.

Individual Responsibility. Individual responsibility for one's actions or self-responsibility[20] has four components: the recognition of your own power, conscious commitment, making choices, and understanding limitations. These four factors center on the concept known as locus of control. **Locus of control** entails the perception as to whether a person believes she has control or influence over the circumstances, situations, or people around her. It entails a deep-seated belief that she can make an impact on these variables. The continuum represents two extremes: an external locus of control and an internal locus of control.[21] Essentially, the individual can perceive a range of empowerment from complete control to virtually no control over these variables.

If people have an *external* locus of control, they believe that they have little or no control over the events or circumstances that shape their lives. They are at the whim of others, and life is essentially governed by fate or luck. They are said to be *other-controlled* as opposed to *self-controlled*.

In the area of health care, other-controlled individuals are likely to believe that "That is simply the way it is." They cannot do anything to change things. It is the hand they are dealt, and nothing they do can change the outcome. These persons are likely to rely heavily on the health care system and, when illness strikes, depend heavily on the actions of their physician or other health care providers. They may even believe that they can persist in unhealthy behaviors, such as excessive alcohol consumption or overeating, and then, when misfortune strikes, they can go to their physician for a pill or medical remedy that makes them all better. Their reliance on the health care system is typically extreme and in most cases excessive. They simply do not believe they have any impact on eventual outcomes and, when faced with a trivial medical event, look for the quick medical fix.

On the other hand, individuals who have a strong and dominant internal locus of control believe that they control their own destiny. They are the masters of their fate, and they "steer their own ship." They:

- Know themselves, their needs, and their preferences.
- Have an active sense of accountability and assume responsibility for their health by taking ownership for the cause and effect of their actions.
- Are responsible for their decision making and recognize their limitations.
- Understand that heredity represents only one component of their health status and that they can choose to control what can be controlled and simply deal or cope when they have little or no control.

For example, although viruses, bacteria, and other parasites can be the cause of infectious illnesses, not everyone in the military barracks or college dormitory catches a cold or develops pneumonia when outbreaks occur. Although an external organism clearly has a role in determining illness, that role is incomplete and limited.

Individuals with an internal locus of control recognize their power, understand their limitations, and make conscious commitments and decisions to behave healthily. For example, they practice effective hand washing and avoid direct inhalation of microorganisms from airborne contaminants to control the disease process. To prevent heart disease, they make a conscious decision to avoid fatty foods and adopt a highly active physical exercise program. In addition to avoiding heart disease, they are certainly more likely to be physically fit, feel better, and live a longer and more satisfying existence.

None of this means that they do not use the health care system. They are responsible enough to seek appropriate medical attention and avoid frivolous or unnecessary trips to the doctor. They do not take the position that coronary artery surgery is a means to permit them to engage in sedentary lifestyle replete with a diet high in cholesterol and fatty foods. For them, life consists of choices over which they have considerable control. They simply make choices that direct them to assume a greater degree of responsibility for their actions. Their stance is to make something happen rather than simply to let it happen to them. Theirs is not a fatalistic posture of throwing up one's arms and lamenting that they just cannot do anything about their health. For them, life events are not predetermined, and they believe that they have considerable ability to change the course and sequence of events.

Years ago, humankind was considered to be at the mercy of the environment and was essentially other-controlled. During this same time period, the major killers were the infectious diseases, which were characterized as diseases over which there was little or no control and for which there was little or no cure or treatment. Modern medicine has virtually eliminated this problem, at least to a large extent, and today's leading killers are categorized as lifestyle diseases. With lifestyle diseases comes the potential for humans to better control their behavior and thus their destiny. In other words, no bacterium causes heart disease, our number one killer. And although heredity plays a part in its development, experts have clearly identified the major determinants as unhealthy lifestyle behaviors: a sedentary lifestyle, high blood pressure, and a diet rich in saturated fats, to name but a few. The point is that individuals must understand and believe that they have considerable control over their health. The body of evidence to support this position and the numerous studies have unequivocally demonstrated the strong influence that a sense of control can aid in stress reduction, blood pressure problems, minimal use of painkiller and sedatives, and many other medical interventions.

Cultural Norms. Although the influence of individual responsibility for one's actions is paramount to the promotion of heath and well-being, the influence of cultural norms is also quite significant. **Cultural norms**[22] are the collection of shared practices, rules, values, and beliefs of a large group of people. Examples of cultural norms that most Americans share are such practices as driving on the right-hand side of the road, the sharing of a turkey dinner with family at Thanksgiving, and tolerating religious diversity. Cultural norms are also subject to change. For example, smoking in the United States was once considered socially acceptable. Now, studies regarding the ill effects of passive or second-hand smoke have changed this cultural view, and many states and municipalities have laws prohibiting smoking in public places.

Cultural norms can be subtle or very obvious.

- Regrettably, some individuals view a wedding reception, New Year's Eve celebrations, Super Bowl parties, and other such social occasions as a time to drink a lot of alcohol. For some, these events have connotations and premeditated plans to get inebriated and "tie on a load." These individuals literally equate these events with acceptable excessive alcohol use. Not drinking heavily is an exception; it even raises questions as to whether the nondrinkers are not feeling well.
- Another example is the overt and open support of increased sugar consumption by children and significant others. At various times of the year—Halloween and Valentine's Day—children are provided with bags of chocolate, candy bars, and other sweet treats. Sweethearts are given that heart-shaped box of chocolate.
- The tan look is often equated with wealth and health. The well-tanned body is the envy of many. Often the well tanned person is perceived to be full of life and vigor and even perceived to be wealthy. Yet the excessive exposure to ultraviolet rays has serious health consequences and has recently catapulted skin cancer to the top of the list with the highest incidence of newly reported cancers in the country.
- The couch potato is another example. Virtually every household in America has numerous television sets that are cable driven and all remote controlled!

At least in the American culture, an expectation and an acceptance support unhealthy lifestyle practices.

Herein lies the problem. Some of the best intentioned individuals contemplate a change in behavior and firmly commit to make the change stick. However, their willingness and commitment to change are undermined by society—by the culture. As a medical example, suppose an individual contemplates and later commits to lose 15 pounds. She exercises over the weekend and is vigilant in what she eats. When she arrives at work at the Monday morning meeting, she is greeted with scrumptious-looking creamed-filled and chocolate-covered eclairs. Her decision to refrain from taking an eclair is met with considerable resistance and even an insistence by her peers to join in and enjoy the tasty treats. In such a situation, the well intentioned healthful behavior is met with tremendous peer pressure to partake of an accepted office ritual and may well become virtually impossible to resist.

The peer group has incredible power. Many parents have done an admirable job of raising their children, having had them avoid the excessive and adverse behaviors of smoking, alcohol consumption, and sexual promiscuity, only to find their children engaging in such rituals during their later years in college. That is the power and influence of the culture—of the accepted practices and expectations of society—at work. Such an influence is ever present and elusive in our culture, and, despite the best of intentions, it is likely to wear down even the most persistent and ardent supporter of desirable health practices.

John Knowles was a physician and former president of the Rockefeller Foundation. In 1975, he convened a proceeding of prominent physicians, scientists, administrators, and health care leaders and later published a book titled, *Doing Better and Feeling Worse: Health in the United States.*[23] Dr. Knowles made a rather profound statement that speaks to this issue:

> The cost of sloth, gluttony, alcoholic intemperance, reckless driving, sexual frenzy, and smoking is now a national, and not an individual, responsibility. This is justified as individual freedom—but one man's freedom in health is another man's shackle in taxes and insurance premiums. I believe the idea of a "right" to health should be replaced by the idea of an individual moral obligation to preserve one's own health—a public duty if you will. The individual then has the "right" to expect help with information, accessible services of good quality, and minimal financial barrier.

Dr. Knowles indicates that the initiative should come from the individual and that health should be regarded as not only a right but also a responsibility.

Factors Affecting Health Care in the United States in the Twentieth Century

Life expectancy back in the 1900s was approximately 47 years. In 1950, it was approximately 68, and in 2005 it was up to 78 years of age. If one were to plot the age-adjusted number of deaths per year for a somewhat similar span of time, it would extend from a high of approximately 17 per 1000 in 1900 to a low of approximately 8 per 1000 in 2005. An interesting and fascinating perspective regarding health in the United States over the past 100 or so years is reflected in this continuous decline in the death rate. When one looks at this decline and plots these changes with the significant medical discoveries, advances, and health practices of the past century, an interesting picture unfolds. Figure 39-3 depicts this decline and has been categorized into four separate and distinct eras: [8]

- The era of public health improvements
- The era of drug and chemical discoveries
- The era of medical and technological advances
- The era of lifestyle

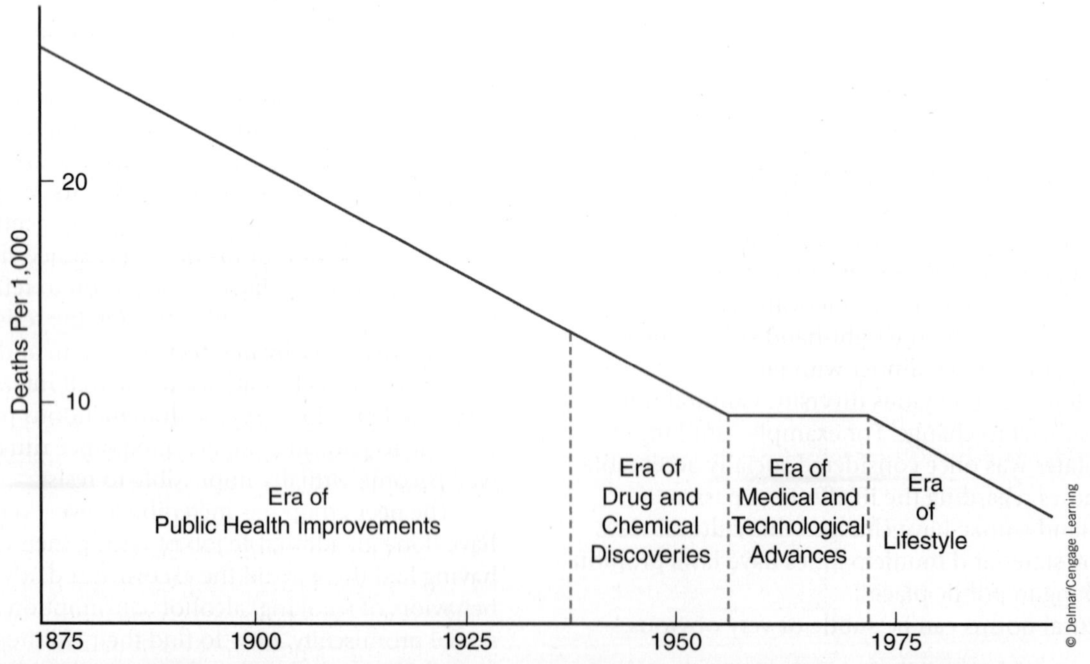

FIGURE 39-3 Factors affecting health care in the United States. (Adapted from mortality data from National Center for Health Statistics: Health, United States. Public Health Service, 1983. In Opatz, J. A. *A Primer of Health Promotion: Creating Healthy Organizational Cultures.* Washington, DC: Oryn Publications; 1985:3–6, 7–9, 11.)

ERA OF PUBLIC HEALTH IMPROVEMENTS

The era of public health improvements is represented by the time span from the mid-1800s to approximately 1920. It was characterized by:

- The establishment of the first State Board of Health in 1855.
- The introduction of antiseptic surgery in 1867.
- The establishment of the United States Marine Hospital Service (the forerunner of the Public Health Service) in 1870.
- The establishment of city health departments in the late 1880s and 1890s.
- The practice of pasteurization of milk in the early 1900s.
- Massive public health campaigns in the 1920s.

In short, it was a period of tremendous improvement in the death rate from over 20 per 1000 to approximately 12 per 1000, all because of public health improvements. The public health improvements had their greatest impact on deaths from infectious disease and infant mortality. The reason was not the improvement projects themselves but rather that people simply paid greater attention to personal hygiene, improved sanitation conditions, reduced the overcrowding conditions, fluorinated the water, and paid more attention to nutrition.

ERA OF DRUG AND CHEMICAL DISCOVERIES

This era of public health improvements was followed by what was called the era of drug and chemical discoveries, extending from the mid-1920s through the mid-1950s. The era was characterized by rather significant drug and chemical discoveries. Cleanliness and improved sanitation were effective. However, infectious diseases such as pneumonia and tuberculosis were still prevalent, and efforts were directed at identifying chemical agents that could be used to combat them. Specific discoveries and accomplishments were:

- The discovery of sulfa drugs in the late 1930s and early 1940s.
- The discovery and use of penicillin in the late 1940s.
- The discovery and use of antituberculosis and polio medications in the early 1950s.

Once again, the death rate declined to an all-time low of fewer than 10 per 1000. Obviously tremendous progress was being made in health care, and this was an exciting time for medical advances.

ERA OF MEDICAL AND TECHNOLOGICAL ADVANCES

An interesting phenomenon occurred in the late 1950s and early 1960s. A plateau effect occurred in the death rate, which did not change for 10–12 years. During this time, a number of medical advances and technologies were practiced and employed. Open-heart surgery was instituted on a fairly large-scale basis. The coronary care unit was showcased. Heart transplants were first performed, and coronary artery surgery was being employed. This era became known as the era of medical and technological advances. Some of these advances formed the basis for the practice of respiratory care. Although this was indeed an exciting time for the health care system, a tremendous amount of money and resources was devoted to the industry with little improvement in the death rate. This interesting phenomenon raised some serious and controversial questions regarding the role and value of technology.

ERA OF LIFESTYLE

This relative standstill in the death rate existed until the early 1970s. Given the historical events occurring in society at this time, a rather significant emphasis was being placed on health and fitness. It seemed that Americans went into a health craze: Fitness centers proliferated. Spas became popular. There was a tremendous interest in weight reduction, healthy eating, and the incorporation of healthy lifestyle practices. Companies such as Jenny Craig, Weight Watchers, and NutriSystems were commonly viewed on commercial television. The running shoe business became a multimillion-dollar industry, and people purchased separate shoes for running, walking, playing tennis, and playing basketball. There was even a cross-training shoe that was worn for multiple sports. Aerobic centers sprang up across the country and workout tapes by Jane Fonda, Richard Simmons, and others became popular. In short, people became obsessed with health and fitness, and there was tremendous interest in caring for one's body.

This era appears to be continuing to this day and is often cited as the era of lifestyle. It is characterized by an unprecedented interest in taking control and responsibility for caring for one's health and well-being. Although the final verdict is still pending, there appears to be compelling evidence to suggest that the death rate decline to approximately 8 in 2005 may well be due to this focus on healthy lifestyle practices and behaviors.

Watching the trend over these four eras makes for a rather strong and convincing argument that Americans may be reaching a point of diminishing returns, a point where any truly significant curtailment in death rate may occur only through personal and individual lifestyle interventions. Public health improvements and improvements associated with drug and chemical discoveries unquestionably had a profound effect on the death rate. During the era of medical and technological advances, the effect was lessened. Yet improved lifestyle behaviors have had a marked effect on the death rate. The ability to identify, treat, and cure disease may come not from the medical community but from us. Health promotion, disease prevention, and wellness practices may hold a key to resolving much of the future's health care woes.

Leading Causes of Death

Table 39-4 provides a complete listing of the top 10 leading causes of death in the years 1900, 1990, and 2005. Although the shift from 1900 to 1990 was significant, there was no shift in the top five and only some shifting in the remaining five leading killers over the 15-year period from 1990 to 2005. Why?

The leading causes of death at the turn of the century were largely infectious diseases, such as tuberculosis, pneumonia, enteritis, and diphtheria. With the advent of modern medicine came the discovery of effective chemical agents, which essentially eradicated deaths from infectious disease. While infectious diseases persist, their prominence has been replaced by a group of conditions known as the lifestyle diseases:

- At the top of this more contemporary list is heart disease. Heart disease consists of coronary and other cardiac ailments that account for a significant number and percentage of all leading causes of death. The number of reported cases in 2005 was 652,091.
- Heart disease is followed by cancer, which accounted for 559,312 reported cases in 2005. The National Center for Health Statistics' figures reveal that lung cancer leads the list of sites for both men and women at 159,292, with men representing a figure of 90,187 and women representing over 69,000 deaths in 2005. Among men, lung cancer is followed by prostate cancer, which is a rather distant second, with almost 29,000 deaths. Among women, breast cancer is second to lung cancer and represents approximately 41,000 deaths per year.
- Third on the list of leading killers is another heart-related condition: stroke. Although the relative percentage of deaths attributed to strokes is significantly lower than the figures for heart disease and cancer, strokes continue to represent a sizable percentage of all deaths in the United States, representing 143,579 deaths in 2005. High blood pressure is considered to be the primary culprit and plays a role in at least 70% of all strokes. Given that the risk factor can be largely controlled by diet and the large array of highly effective antihypertensive medications, there is obviously considerable room for improvement.

Some shifting has occurred at the lower end of this list of leading killers.

- HIV/AIDS, suicide, and homicide have recently dropped off the list, replaced by Alzheimer's disease, nephritis, and septicemia.
- Alzheimer's is perhaps reflective of the shifting population trends and the aging of the Baby Boomer generation.
- Nephritis is an indicator of excessive alcohol use.
- Additionally, pneumonia/influenza and septicemia reflect infectious agents.
- Diabetes has moved up the list, reflective of the recent increase in obesity.

TABLE 39-4 **Ten leading causes of death in the United States (1900, 1990, 2005)**

1900	1990	2005
1. Tuberculosis	1. Heart disease	1. Heart disease
2. Pneumonia	2. Cancer	2. Cancer
3. Diarrhea and enteritis	3. Cerebrovascular disease	3. Cerebrovascular disease
4. Heart disease	4. COPD	4. COPD
5. Liver disease	5. Accidents	5. Accidents
6. Injuries	6. Pneumonia and influenza	6. Diabetes
7. Stroke	7. Diabetes	7. Alzheimer's Disease
8. Cancer	8. HIV/AIDS	8. Pneumonia and influenza
9. Bronchitis	9. Suicide	9. Nephritis
10. Diptheria	10. Homicide	10. Septicemia

Source: Adapted from Kung HC, Hoyert DL, Xu JQ, Murphy SL. Deaths: Final Data for 2005. National Vital Statistics Reports. *Vol. 56 no. 10. Hyattsville, MD: National Center for Health Statistics. 2008. http://www.cdc.gov/nchs/data/nvsr/nvsr56/nvsr56_10.pdf*

A considerable number of publications have been devoted to discussion and analysis of this topic. The obvious and most apparent conclusion lies in the high association that virtually every leading killer has with environmental and lifestyle factors. Heredity and genetic predisposition have a relationship to many items on the list; however, clearly lifestyle and environmental factors and their control have a prominent presence. Two profound points have to be made with regard to the leading causes of death in the United States.

- First, individuals must take responsibility for their day-to-day activities of daily living and better control the risk factors associated with these menacing conditions.
- Second, the respiratory therapist should recognize that 5 of the 10 leading causes of death are *directly* related to the cardiorespiratory system. Thus, there should be little doubt about the critical role that the respiratory care profession plays in the prevention and treatment of these conditions.

Behavioral Causes of Death

Beyond the statistics, facts, figures, and hard data related to the leading causes of death in the United States, there are the causative agents, substances, activities, and practices associated with death and disease. Table 39-5 presents the causative factors and the incredibly high number of preventable deaths in the United States in 2000.[24] In essence, the table reflects the behaviors attributed to the diseases and certainly provides rather striking and compelling evidence for the role that lifestyle plays.

- Number one on the list is the use of *tobacco* products. Tobacco use was considered to be responsible for more than 435,000 deaths in the United States in 2000. This is an absolutely astounding figure, given the absolutely overwhelming evidence associating smoking with heart disease, cancer, and COPD.
- Tobacco use is closely followed by *diet and activity patterns*, which provide 365,000 deaths per year. At issue is the tremendous amount of saturated fats and high levels of cholesterol ingested by the American public. When the dietary problem is coupled with a reduced level of physical activity and sedentary lifestyle, it is clear how these factors can play such a significant role in the attainment of disease.
- *Drug and alcohol misuse and abuse* are of growing concern to the medical community. Alcohol abuse and misuse are responsible for over 85,000 deaths per year, and the illicit use of drugs another 17,000. Regrettably, alcohol toxicity has become rampant among American youth, especially on college campuses.
- When driving *an automobile at excessive speeds* is factored in, another 43,000 deaths per year can be added to the list.
- *Promiscuity and unprotected sex*, which raise the risk of sexually transmitted disease, accounted for approximately 20,000 deaths.
- *Firearm-relate deaths* are also quite high on the list, representing approximately 29,000 deaths per year.
- *Microbial and toxic agents* combine to represent approximately 3.1% of total preventable deaths and reflect a combined figure of 75,000 deaths per year.

The point to be made is that approximately half (48.2%, or 1.159 million) of the 2.4 million deaths per year in the United States are due to lifestyle behaviors and are largely preventable.[24]

TABLE 39-5 **Actual causes of death in the United States in 2000 (behavioral causes of death)**

Cause	Estimated Number	Percentage of Total Deaths
Tobacco	435,000	18.1%
Diet/activity patterns	365,000	15.2%
Alcohol	85,000	3.5%
Microbial agents	75,000	3.1%
Toxic agents	55,000	2.3%
Motor vehicles	43,000	1.8%
Firearms	29,000	1.2%
Sexual behavior	20,000	0.8%
Illicit use of drugs	17,000	0.7%
Total	1,159,000	48.20%

Source: From Mokdad AH, et al. Actual causes of death in the United States, 2000. JAMA. *2005;293,3:293. http://jama.ama-assn.org/cgi/content/full/291/10/1238*

Determinants of Health Status

What factors determine the state of someone's health? What variables are ultimately responsible for whether we consider ourselves ill or well?

Numerous epidemiologic studies have been performed over the years in an attempt to identify the major determinants of health status. Perhaps two of the most prominent were the Canadian National Government Study and the Framingham Heart Study. The Canadian National Government Study was conducted by the Ministry of Health and Welfare, under Minister Marc Lelonde, and was entitled, "A New Perspective on the Health of Canadians: A Working Document." The study entailed a conceptual framework that was called the "Health Field Concept."[25] The purpose of the study was to identify the causes of death and sickness throughout the country and ultimately provide information regarding the determinants of Canadians' health status.

It identified four contributing elements:

- Inadequacies in the existing health care system
- Behavioral factors or unhealthy lifestyles
- Environmental hazards
- Human biological factors

Interestingly, similar studies were conducted in this country that paralleled the work of the Canadian National Government, of which the most comprehensive and widely known was the Framingham Heart Study. This study is considered one of the greatest and perhaps most elaborate efforts in the history of public health to get at the issue of the rising concern for heart disease in this country. It was a long-term study started in 1948 in a small town in Massachusetts called Framingham. Conducted by the New England Research Institute and supported by grants from the National Institutes of Health, it was an ongoing effort to study geographically circumscribed men. The study consisted of 5209 individuals between the ages of 28 and 62 who were retrospectively studied to determine the specific factors responsible for premature death associated with cardiovascular disease. The information was continually updated through surveillance of hospital records and biennial examinations. The results of this study produced similar results to those of the Canadians. The Framingham Study was supportive in identifying the following four factors as major determinants of our health status:

- Human biology or heredity
- The environment
- The health care organization
- Lifestyle

The relative weight of influence for each of these four factors on all causes of death in this country was identified by the United States Department of Health and Human Services, Public Health Service in a landmark report, which is presented in Figure 39-4.[26]

The following subsections elaborate on the four factors addressed in the Canadian National Government Study.

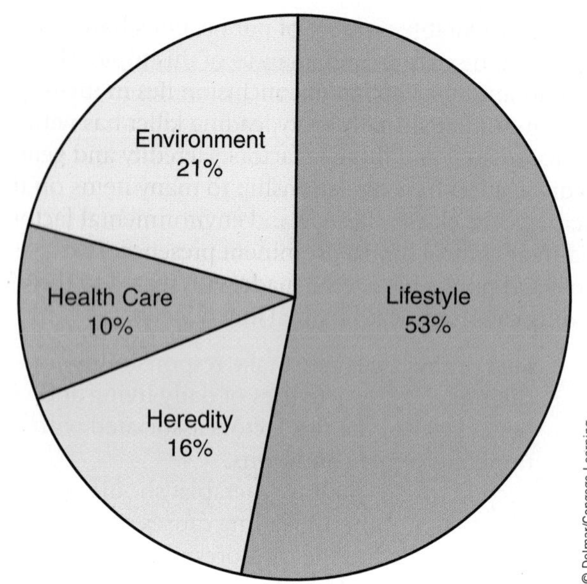

FIGURE 39-4 Determinants of health status. (Data compiled from U.S. Department of Health, Education, and Welfare. Ten *Leading Causes of Death in the United States, 1975*. Atlanta, GA. Public Health Service, CDC, Bureau of State Services, Health Analysis and Planning for Preventive Services:46.)

HEREDITY

This first factor, heredity, covered all aspects of health that were endogenous to the individual: genetic inheritance, the aging process, the metabolic processes, and overall processes of maturation. Heredity, or genetic predisposition as it was expressed in the United States study, simply meant that individuals were predisposed to health or well-being by virtue of their genes, by their genetic makeup. Individuals were at the mercy of their ancestors, their grandparents, their parents, as to whether they would develop heart disease, cancer, familial emphysema, diabetes, or some other condition. This is even more profoundly displayed by such conditions as sickle cell anemia, Tay-Sachs disease, Down syndrome, and cystic fibrosis.

In other words, an individual is likely to succumb to these dreaded diseases through little or no control but merely by virtue of being born into a particular family. Clearly, acceptance of this fact reflects an external locus of control because the individual unfortunately cannot change or influence the outcome. It is simply in the genes. Unless medical research makes significant strides to alter DNA and other genetic material, the individual is destined to live with the ill effects of the disease or condition.

ENVIRONMENT

The second determinant of health status is the environment, which can be either conducive or detrimental to health status. The environment is a very broad category and entails any condition in the societal and physical environment of the individual that can affect health. It can encompass the obvious issues of pollution, such as the water we drink, the food we eat, and the air we breathe. It can also entail the not so obvious, such as noise, trash, land abuse in the form of exposure to toxins and chemical spills, crowded and densely populated regions, and, in general, the stresses of urban life. Although many profits-driven corporations have regrettably created and generated significant problems for the environment, a large number of interest groups work diligently to promote a healthy environment. Organizations and interest groups, such as Green Peace, the Clean Air Council, the American Lung Association, and the Sierra Club, are advocacy groups and organizations that lobby on behalf of the environment and attempt to combat those insensitive to natural resources and the beauty of our surroundings.

HEALTH CARE SYSTEM

The medical or health care system, perhaps the most entails the quantity, quality, arrangement, nature, and relationship of people to health resources, facilities, technology, and personnel. It includes hospitals, extended care facilities, public health and community health centers, ambulances, physicians, etc. It also involves more than the resources, facilities, technology, and personnel; it entails their access and utilization. The ability to access and use health care is tied not only to the ability to purchase appropriate health care benefits but also to attitudes, values, and beliefs regarding the health care system and the role people play in maintaining health.

In 2005, the National Coalition of Health Care estimated that approximately 47 million people are uninsured in the United States. In addition, significant numbers of people simply do not use the system because of denial, religious beliefs, or cultural attitudes. Regrettably, some cultures perceive a hospital as a place that one goes to die. With such perceptions and beliefs, there is little wonder why individuals do not partake of a service that could clearly aid in the elimination or improvement of unhealthy conditions.

There are also individuals who take little or no responsibility for their health. Either they seek inappropriate advice and attention from the health care system or request quick-fix remedies, such as a pill, from the physician for conditions or maladies that are frivolous or over which they have considerable control. Their expectation is that, if they get sick, the health care system will fix them; they have no control over their actions and behaviors and take no responsibility for them. These other-controlled individuals take the posture that they can engage in excessive and unhealthy lifestyle behaviors because the system will correct the situation when called on to do so. Acting passively and helplessly, they expect too much of the health care system, which they view as having all the answers to the ills of society.

The question is whether the health care system is the primary means to a healthy existence by curing and treating disease, or are people the primary means by living health lives and fending off illness.

LIFESTYLE

Lifestyle entails activities of daily living and regular, day-to-day routines or habits. Lifestyle is perhaps the least understood and the least appreciated factor related to health status. Lifestyle behaviors affect the food we eat, the level of physical activity and exercise, sleeping habits, the use of tobacco, alcohol, and drugs, and our use or disuse of seat belts, to name but a few. It was identified in both the Canadian National Government Study and the Framingham Heart Study as having the greatest impact on health care status. Numerous citations in the literature support the profound effect that this category has on determining health status.

Perhaps the most compelling and convincing evidence linking health and lifestyle comes from the work of N. Belloc and L. Breslow.[27] Their research entailed a 5.5-year study of over 7000 people that identified 7 distinct habits associated with life expectancy and health:

- Eating three meals a day at regular intervals instead of snacking
- Eating breakfast every day
- Engaging in moderate exercise two or three times a week
- Getting adequate (7–8 hours per night) sleep
- Not smoking
- Maintaining moderate weight
- Consuming little or no alcohol

Obviously, attention to these factors entails rather modest changes in lifestyle. Yet incorporation of these practices can go a long way in substantially reducing the long-term consequences of illness and disease. Bill Hettler, one of the foremost experts in wellness and a distinguished member of the Wellness Institute at the University of Wisconsin in Stevens Point, is quoted as saying, "one of my frustrations in medicine was having people come to me expecting way too much of me and not expecting anything of themselves."[14] He goes on to say that Americans still look to the physician community to keep them well. In fact, if we lump all the causes of death together, physicians can help approximately 10% of the time. The other 90% are outside of the control of the physician. They are the result of lifestyle abuse, heredity, and environment.[14]

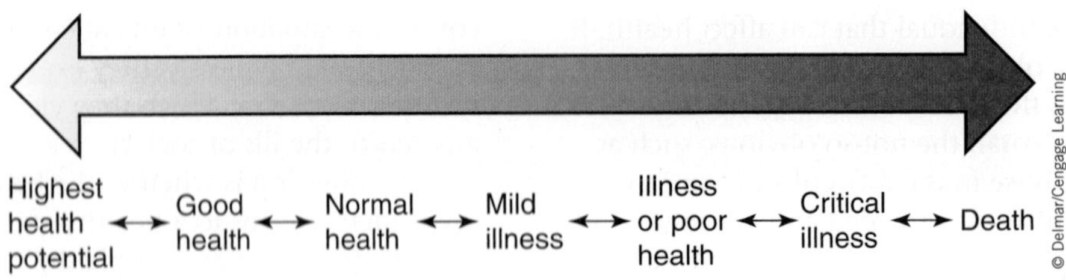

FIGURE 39-5 Health continuum.

Continuums

Perhaps one of the more effective ways to view health is by means of a graphic display known as a *continuum*. Of the numerous models with various points of emphasis, two displays are presented here: The health continuum is traditional in nature and more representative of the traditional view of health; the illness and wellness continuum is an expanded and more contemporary model that incorporates some of the more recent thinking about health and wellness.

- *Health continuum*. The health continuum is shown in Figure 39-5. It is a rather simple model that depicts health from a perspective of death on the one extreme and health on the other. On the far left is health, or what was traditionally viewed as the absence of disease. As people become less healthy, they traverse to the right and go through various levels of illness from a mild to a severe level.
- *Illness and wellness continuum*. This more contemporary view or model[28] consists essentially of two views of health: the traditional view and the wellness model. The traditional view of health is limited to a health care system that activates resources that address the specific medical problem once it has occurred. In this sense, the best that traditional health care can do is to bring the individual back to the center of the continuum where there is no discernible disease. The other side of the illness and wellness continuum represents wellness or health promotion and disease prevention. The key values on this side of the continuum are awareness, education, motivation, behavior change, and high-level wellness.

Health Promotion Process

It is one thing to talk about the principles and concepts of health and its associated terms or to argue for incorporating a holistic approach to health that emphasizes components that clearly are more proactive and self-management oriented. However, to adopt these more contemporary concepts of wellness, people need the tools, the means, or, better yet, a process to follow to make a transition from the traditional to the holistic model. Respiratory therapy health educators may be asked to advise, counsel, and guide patients through the process of modifying an unhealthy lifestyle behavior, such as smoking. Additionally, they may be called on to put together a full-blown and comprehensive smoking cessation program or pulmonary rehabilitation program, which is targeted to the local community or to a selected group or population. This section explains:

- The process that enables individuals to achieve individual wellness.
- The process of developing programs for community or organizational wellness.

INDIVIDUAL OR PERSONAL WELLNESS

Individual or personal wellness programming can be extremely difficult and complex. Numerous authors have written about this subject and numerous models have been suggested. Despite the extensive number of models and their variations, adapting a health promotion philosophy, with its view toward healthy lifestyle behavior, means making choices. Having individuals make a choice about their health requires them to:

- Have appropriate health knowledge and information.
- Comprehend the motivations for change.
- Understand the factors impacting their health behavior.
- Appreciate the value and role of social supports and a nurturing and supportive environment.

Excluding any of these variables only results in a less than successful intervention.

Equally important and critical, any effort to adopt a healthy lifestyle behavior has to entail a *systematic strategy*. Individuals can take three steps toward this end:

- *Commitment (buying into the process)*. Such a strategy includes making a commitment, assessing the current situation, and developing an action plan.[16] Making a commitment to change is more than a simple statement not to smoke a cigarette or to lose weight. It takes self-management, self-responsibility, self-respect, and, critically, assuming individual responsibility for their actions. Taking responsibility is the most essential component of the process; without it, any effort at change is likely to fail.

- *Wellness inventory and health risk assessment.* Individuals need to take the time to identify their own personal health practices with the view to identifying the health behaviors that need to be added, eliminated, or modified.
- *Comprehensive and personal plan of behavior change.* The implementation of an action plan entails more detailed coverage of the steps needed to make the process more effective.

Respiratory therapists working with their patients to assist them in adopting a health promotion philosophy need to take these three general points and express them in a more specific and comprehensive manner. Presumably, the individual has already taken the first two general steps: making the conscious decision and commitment to change unhealthy health practices and assessing the need by means of a health assessment inventory. So the only step remaining is to develop an action plan.

Action Steps for Individual or Personal Wellness. Development of the action plan is essentially addressing specific action steps that make up the individual health promotion process. The action steps are: goal identification, record keeping, making an individual action plan, building commitment, and maintaining the new behavior.

Goal identification is the crucial first step in the process. It should include looking at the results of the wellness survey or health assessment inventory and identifying a single goal or lifestyle behavior to work on or to develop. This may seem obvious and perhaps even oversimplified; however, goal development should not be taken lightly and should include a goal statement that is SMART:

- *Specific.* Avoid general statements, such as to lose weight. Although this may sound fine, it is far too general a statement and needs clarification and refinement.
- *Measurable.* Measurability helps significantly because the individual can specify the amount of weight, say 15 pounds.
- *Attainable.* A person should not specify a goal that is unattainable, such as the loss of 15 pounds if the individual is already at the desirable weight of, say, 105.
- *Realistic.* Equally unwise is to strive for something that is unrealistic, such as the loss of 100 pounds in a week.
- *Trackable.* The goal statement should specify a time line. Depending on the behavior or lifestyle, it may be a good idea to have terminal time lines as well as periodic time lines. Periodic time lines allow for assessment at periodic intervals and a more gradual achievement of the desired outcome.

The second step in the health promotion process, *record keeping*, can be as simple as a log sheet kept throughout the day. For example, many smoking cessation programs use this tactic because they require the individual to document their smoking patterns for periods of time and to indicate the antecedent (trigger) of a behavior as well as its consequences. This methodology can be exceedingly valuable in determining any associations to the behavior and in addressing the next step, namely, development of a plan.

Developing an *individual action plan* is the actual intervention strategy employed in modifying the behavior. Behavior modification experts frequently use such strategies as:

- Eliminating the antecedent.
- Anticipating and preparing for the antecedent.
- Substituting behaviors.
- Breaking or scrambling the behavior chain.
- A reward system.
- A support system.

Once again, the elimination of smoking in someone's normal routine can be achieved or modified by substituting gum for a cigarette or by closely monitoring the sequence of events that precede the lighting up of the cigarette. Rewarding yourself by going to a movie or having a family member or close friend aid in your effort can be a powerful and effective means to curtail this dangerous habit.

Building commitment entails strengthening your resolve to adhere to the positive lifestyle and to avoid the negative behavior. This step can be quite difficult. However, listing the positive effects of the behavior, enlisting others as support systems, or making a monetary investment in a positive aspect of the behavior can all aid in this effort. For example, purchasing a membership to a health club can strengthen the commitment to a physical fitness program. Visualizing an improved physique, a more attractive appearance, and gaining of new friendships can all serve as ways to strengthen and build the commitment to joining a health club.

The last component of the process is *maintaining the new behavior*. In the case of smoking, for example, individuals can focus on the positive aspects of not smoking, concentrate on the number of smoke-free days and applaud themselves for the success. Additionally, they can identify factors that cause them to regress, as well as the strategies to overcome lapses. In the case of smoking, they can ascertain what worked and what was responsible for their digression. Was it because of association with a particular person or group? Or was it due to a stressful event? If so, then stress management may be an appropriate intervention. Just a temporary avoidance of a person may be suitable until the undesirable behavior is changed and replaced with a positive behavior that is deeply implanted in your daily routine. Maintenance of a new behavior is always difficult because it often entails unlearning and relearning behaviors. One should always be reassessing goals, monitoring behavior, reviewing strategies, and acknowledging successes. A final strategy may be to employ a written contract. An example of such a contract appears in Figure 39-6 and should include some of the variables already discussed as well as a list of rewards and obstacles and a means to evaluate and reevaluate progress.

The respiratory therapist must keep in mind that individual health promotion activities should be embedded in the normal day-to-day activities of the respiratory therapist. RTs have numerous opportunities throughout the day to impart knowledge and information to their patients. These opportunities have been referred to as *teaching moments*, and respiratory therapists should not take these opportunities lightly. To capitalize on these opportunities, the RT is encouraged to employ a systematic approach that includes the steps of assess, plan, implement, and evaluate.

COMMUNITY OR ORGANIZATIONAL WELLNESS

In addition to individual or personal health promotion, the respiratory therapist may be asked to initiate or participate in a community or organizational health promotion program. Although there is considerable similarity between health promotion activities for an individual and those of an organization- or community-based effort, there are differences. Virtually every model follows the standard assess, plan, implement, and evaluate steps This section presents two models: the PRECEDE-PROCEED model[29] and the 4Ds model.[30]

PRECEDE-PROCEED Model. Perhaps the most popular and most often used community-based health promotion model is the *PRECEDE-PROCEED model*.

- PRECEDE is an acronym for *p*redisposing, *r*einforcing, and *e*nabling *c*onstructs in *e*ducation/environmental *d*iagnosis, and *e*valuation.

I (*your name*), ______________________________

hereby agree to (your personal behavior to be changed) ______________

____

____

____

I will achieve this goal by (date) ______________________

I will employ the following action steps (plan) ______________

____

My motivators are ______________________________

My perceived obstacles are ______________________

____

My solutions to these obstacles are ______________

____

Signature ______________ Date ______________

Support person ______________ Date ______________

FIGURE 39-6 Sample contract.

- PROCEED is an acronym for *p*olicy, *r*egulatory, and *o*rganizational *c*onstructs in *e*ducational and *e*nvironmental *d*evelopment.

This model is well received and well utilized by the health education community because it is theoretically grounded and comprehensive in nature. The PRECEDE portion of the model deals with the multiple factors that shape health status and helps the planner arrive at targets for intervention. Additionally, it deals with the writing of objectives and the development of criteria for evaluation. PROCEED is an elaboration of PRECEDE and was a result of its developers' involvement in national policy initiatives and community-based health promotion programs.[29] The model has nine phases that address the diagnostic components, that entail the social, epidemiologic, behavioral, environmental, educational, organizational, administrative, and policy-related diagnostic features. This is indeed quite elaborate and provides an extensive information base for the other phases, which deal with planning, evaluation, process, impact, and outcome.

The 4Ds Model. The *4Ds model* entails diagnosis, development, delivery, and determination.[30] These four major components are further broken down into the following steps:

- *Diagnosis*
  Sensing
  Securing leadership commitment
  Developing a master plan
  Designing an evaluation mechanism
- *Development*
  Determining staffing needs
  Selecting professional staff
  Teaching professional staff
  Developing the leadership committee
  Selecting and training vendors
  Acquiring lifestyle modules
  Planning facilities
  Developing ways to increase participation
- *Delivery*
  Promoting organizational health
  Promoting individual health
  Modifying the environment
- *Determination*
  Collecting the data
  Analyzing the data
  Writing the report
  Recycling the process

Following is an overview of the steps:

- *Diagnosis* is comprised of those elements essential to diagnosing the behavioral issue under study. Diagnosis entails sensing, securing leadership commitment, developing a master plan, and designing an evaluation mechanism.
- *Development* consists of determining staffing needs, selecting professional staff, teaching professional staff, developing the leadership committee, selecting and training vendors, acquiring lifestyle modules, planning facilities, and developing ways to increase participation.
- *Delivery* includes promoting organizational health, promoting individual health, and modifying the environment.
- *Determination* is made up of collecting the data, analyzing the data, writing the report, and recycling the process.

Based on this model, there are 20 skills for successful and effective health promotion program design. Respiratory therapists interested and likely to get involved in community- or organizational-based programming are advised to secure the resource materials listed in the References at the end of the chapter. Addressing the health promotion needs of a large community and doing so on a large scale requires considerable preparation, planning, and expertise. The evolving role and extensive background of respiratory therapists makes them a likely candidate for future involvement in this area.

Role of the Federal Government

The federal government has taken a position of leadership with regard to health promotion and disease prevention. It has embarked rather aggressively on health promotion initiatives that have led to a number of significant publications, which have been instrumental in furthering the health promotion and disease prevention movement in this country. Three out of the five publications noted here come under the appropriate title of "Healthy People" and all piggyback on each other in driving the movement to a credible and prominent place in health care delivery:

- *Healthy People: The Surgeon General's Report on Health Promotion and Disease Prevention*[15]
- *Promoting Health/Preventing Disease: Objectives for the Nation*[31]
- *Healthy People 2000*[32]
- *Healthy People 2010*[33]
- *Healthy People 2020*[34]

The following section briefly examines each of these publications.

HEALTHY PEOPLE: THE SURGEON GENERAL'S REPORT ON HEALTH PROMOTION AND DISEASE PREVENTION

On July 26, 1979, Joseph A. Califano Jr, then secretary of the now defunct Department of Health, Education, and Welfare, wrote the foreword to the first of four government publications on health promotion and disease prevention titled *Healthy People: The Surgeon General's Report on Health Promotion and Disease Prevention*.[15] In it he expressed enthusiasm and excitement for what he considered the second public health revolution in the history of the United States. This enthusiasm stemmed from mounting and emerging consensus among scientists and health care providers calling for a health strategy to shift its emphasis from treatment and curation to promotion of healthy lifestyle behaviors and prevention of insidious and preventable diseases. Califano indicated that the consensus was as strong as that voiced in the 1964 *Surgeon General's Report on Smoking and Health* and also as prominent and critical as that displayed in the nation's first public health revolution that attacked the eradication of infectious diseases.

The report went on to address what has been expressed throughout this chapter of the text, namely, that the leading causes of death in this country are highly preventable. It addressed these leading killers in considerable detail and spoke to the shift that has occurred from infectious diseases, such as influenza, pneumonia, diphtheria, tuberculosis, and gastrointestinal infections, to today's killers: heart disease, cancer, stroke, chronic lung disease, accidents, and the like. There was a strong outcry from all sectors of the health care delivery system that significant efforts must be taken to arrest and reverse the trend toward allowing preventable diseases to kill people.

The report went on to say that people are literally killing themselves by means of careless habits, by carelessly polluting the environment, and by permitting harmful social conditions, such as poverty, hunger, and ignorance, to persist and destroy our health and well-being. The report raised the consciousness of the nation to the notion that we need to exercise the personal discipline and political will to solve these menacing health problems. Califano has been quoted on numerous occasions for stating that "you, the individual, can do more for your health and well-being than any doctor, any hospital, any drug, any exotic medical device."

Clearly, the theme and strategy of the report were to recast emphasis on preventing disease and promoting healthy lifestyles. The report further stated that scientific research had clearly revealed that the key to a long life versus a premature death was taking control of one's actions. The report stated, "It is the controllability of many risks—and, often, the significance of controlling even only a few—that lies at the heart of disease prevention and health promotion." The report alluded to simple measures that, if practiced, could greatly enhance the prospect of good health. The report went on to say that adherence to these simple measures resulted, on average, in 11 years of longer life compared with those who did not practice any of the measures. These simple measures are:

- Elimination of cigarette smoking
- Reduction of alcohol misuse
- Moderate dietary changes to reduce intake of excess calories, fat, salt, and sugar
- Moderate exercise
- Periodic screening (at intervals determined by age and sex) for major disorders such as high blood pressure and certain cancers
- Adherence to speed laws and use of seat belts[15]

What brought considerable clarity and weight to this report was the identification of five public health goals that were measurable and achievable. There was one goal for each age group in our society, and the intention was to assess the progress of their attainment in the year 1990. The five goals appear in Table 39-6. In

TABLE 39-6 **U.S. health goals set in 1979 surgeon general's report, *Healthy People***

Age Group	Goals	Focus
Healthy infants (birth–age 1)	35% fewer deaths	Reduction of number of low birth weights
		Reduction of number of birth defects
Healthy children (ages 1–14)	20% fewer deaths	Enhancement of growth and development
		Reduction of accidents and injuries
Healthy adolescents/young adults (ages 15–24)	20% fewer deaths	Reduction of number of fatal motor vehicle accidents
		Reduction of ETOH (ethyl alcohol) and drug abuse
Healthy adults (ages 25–64)	25% fewer deaths	Reduction of number of heart attacks and strokes
		Reduction of number of deaths from Ca (cancer)
Healthy older adults (age 65+)	20% fewer sick days	Increase of number of functioning independently
		Reduction of number of premature deaths from influenza and pneumonia

Source: Based on data compiled from U.S. Department of Health, Education and Welfare. Healthy People: The Surgeon General's Report on Health Promotion and Disease Prevention. *Washington, DC: U.S. Government Printing Office; 1979:xi–xii.*

short, this first and original report on the topic of health promotion and disease prevention was grounded in the notion that establishing national health goals and monitoring our progress could lead to action to improve the nation's health.

PROMOTING HEALTH/PREVENTING DISEASE: OBJECTIVES FOR THE NATION

This second government report was a sequel to the first and released in 1980.[31] The emphasis of this document was that it expanded the 5 goals and 15 priority areas to 226 specific objectives. The 15 priority areas are:

- High blood pressure control
- Family planning
- Pregnancy and infant health
- Immunization
- Sexually transmitted diseases
- Toxic agent control
- Occupational safety and health
- Accident prevention and injury control
- Fluoridation and dental health
- Surveillance and control of infectious diseases
- Smoking and health
- Misuse of alcohol and drugs
- Nutrition
- Physical fitness and exercise
- Control of stress and violent behavior

In each of the 15 priority areas, the nature and extent of the problem (including health implications, status, and trends), prevention and promotion measures, specific national objectives, principal assumptions, and data necessary for tracking progress were outlined and discussed.

HEALTHY PEOPLE 2000

Healthy People 2000[32] was released in September 1990 and consisted of 3 broad goals, 22 priority areas, and 319 national objectives. Central to this document were the three broad goals that called for:

- Increasing the length of healthy life for Americans.
- Reducing health disparities among Americans.
- Achieving access to preventive health services for all Americans.

This report was much more comprehensive than the previous ones and was built on the efforts of more than 10,000 individuals and organizations. It was essentially an attempt to rectify the shortcomings of the previous documents, but, perhaps more important, it was geared to taking the goals, priorities, and objectives to the grassroots level.

What seemed to be lacking in the previous two reports was the public's ownership of the process. This document was targeted to the state and local levels, and thus buy-in and accountability were to be encouraged at a grassroots level. A significant means to better ensure attainment of this buy-in was through the ongoing involvement of the Healthy People Consortium, which was an alliance of 350 national membership organizations and 300 state health, mental health, substance abuse, and environmental agencies.

A mid-decade account of *Healthy People* demonstrated a high degree of success with more than two-thirds of the national objectives for which data were available being met. In short, this mid-decade report demonstrated that a partnership between state and local levels of the government as well as the private sector proved to have a positive influence on the ultimate goals of the report. Despite these very promising preliminary signs, much still needs to be done in terms of low-income, disabled, and minority groups in order to reverse the disproportionate share of poor health outcomes. The three broad goals of *Healthy People 2000* are:[32]

- Increasing the length of healthy life for Americans.
- Reducing health disparities among Americans.
- Achieving access to preventive health services for all Americans.

Table 39-7 shows the 22 priority areas broken into the 5 general categories of health objectives.

HEALTHY PEOPLE 2010

Healthy People 2010 [33] was released in November 2000. It was an ambitious effort to address the recent advances in preventive therapies, the advances in pharmaceuticals and vaccinations, computerization, the heightened awareness and demand for preventive services, the changes in demographics, science, technology, and disease transmission throughout the world.

The report is attuned to the shrinking of the world and the interdependence that exists among cultures and nations. It entails a collaborative and cooperative arrangement and alliance between American health care and the World Health Organization. It has engaged focus group sessions, public meetings, and a Web site and as such has allowed people from across the country to make their voices heard.

HEALTHY PEOPLE 2020

The most recent effort on the part of the federal government to address the issues of health promotion and disease prevention is *Healthy People 2020: The Road Ahead.*[34] This initiative is currently under way and is designed to be highly inclusive and collaborative. The process strives to maximize transparency, public input, and stakeholder dialogue to ensure that it is relevant

TABLE 39-7 **Twenty-two priority areas of *Healthy People 2000***

Area	Components
Health promotion	1. Physical activity and fitness 2. Nutrition 3. Tobacco 4. Alcohol and other
Drugs	5. Family planning 6. Mental health and mental disorders 7. Violent and abusive behavior 8. Education and community-based programs
Health protection	9. Unintentional injuries 10. Occupational safety and health 11. Environmental health 12. Food and drug safety 13. Oral health
Preventive services	14. Maternal and infant health 15. Heart disease and stroke 16. Cancer 17. Diabetes and chronic debilitating disease 18. HIV infection 19. Sexually transmitted diseases 20. Immunization 21. Clinical preventive services
Surveillance data systems	22. Surveillance and data systems

Source: From U.S. Department of Health, Education and Welfare. Healthy People 2000. *Washington, DC: U.S. Government Printing Office; 1990:76.*

to diverse public needs. It provides a framework to address risk factors and determinants of health and the diseases and disorders that affect our communities.

Healthy People 2020 was released in two phases. Phase 1, released in 2009, outlined the framework (the vision, mission, goals, focus areas, and criteria for selecting and prioritizing objectives). Phase 2 was released in 2010 with the 2020 objectives along with guidance for achieving the new 10-year targets.[34]

Role of Respiratory Therapist in Health Promotion

The traditional role of the respiratory therapist has been that of a technician, diagnostician, and clinician. The respiratory care profession had its origins in the technical area of oxygen transport and administration. From this technical role of the so-called oxygen jockey came expansion into the areas of intermittent positive pressure breathing, aerosol administration, chest physical therapy, and continuous mechanical ventilation. This therapeutic role was later enhanced to include the diagnostic. The performance of such procedures as pulmonary function studies and the procurement and processing of arterial blood gases were added to the armamentarium of procedures and techniques. While RTs continue to provide all of these services, their technical and diagnostic roles have been overshadowed and surpassed by a role that now places greater emphasis on clinical bedside assessment.

Obviously, respiratory therapists must possess superior clinical assessment skills to practice in today's health care environment. Assessment skills have become indispensable. The respiratory care curriculum has been expanded and enhanced to include didactic, laboratory, and clinical expertise and experiences that have positioned the respiratory therapist as the foremost nonphysician expert in the bedside assessment and management of the respiratory-impaired patient. This role of expert clinician is absolutely critical and essential to the future of a cost-effective and competent health care system.

Considerable advancements in technologies added speed, precision, efficiency, and effectiveness to virtually every aspect of respiratory care. Simultaneously, there has been increased emphasis on the implementation of cost-cutting measures to better control and reduce spiraling health care costs. Continuous efforts to reduce the cost of health care have placed more and more pressure on a system that is already financially fragile and on practitioners who are already overextended. Of course, whenever such economic constraints are exercised, there is a risk that the recipient of care, namely the patient, can be compromised and consequently receive less than optimal care. Such a situation demands that respiratory therapists be vigilant in their effort to ensure the provision of high-quality and appropriate care. Thus respiratory therapists of the future must continue to assume the role of patient advocate and serve as watchdogs and gatekeepers of appropriate, essential, and timely respiratory care.

Although the technical, diagnostic, clinical, and advocacy roles of the respiratory therapist are apparent, perhaps not so obvious is the innovative role of the respiratory therapist as health care educator. Respiratory therapists must try to teach people healthful behaviors, regarding both themselves and their children, for whom they have responsibility. For adults, the behaviors are best described as heart healthy behaviors and address those cardiac risk factors that can be modified. Such a role has considerable merit for a number of reasons. Respiratory therapists possess the knowledge, skills, and abilities to impart disease-specific information to the patients, but more importantly their daily presence at the bedside makes them uniquely positioned to engage in such a role. During the course of treatment, the patient is a captive audience for meaningful and targeted education, counseling, and advice. This therapist-patient interaction could address issues related to asthma, chronic lung disease, pneumonia, and many other cardiorespiratory conditions. It could be as rudimentary as a basic discussion of the disease process, the signs and symptoms of the disease, medication use, or therapeutic measures to be employed during crisis intervention for the life-threatening exacerbation of the disease.

Such interactions could also consist of discussions regarding disease prevention and health promotion. Respiratory therapists are already uniquely qualified to address the issues of tobacco use and its relationship to chronic lung disease. RTs are already at the bedside and thus with some basic training in counseling techniques could easily transition into the role of health counselor and educator. Also, if facilitation and marketing skills and techniques are added to the list, the respiratory therapist could engage in community, organizational, or group sessions and provide an extensive array of offerings related to cardiopulmonary health and wellness. Obvious on the list of offerings is smoking cessation programs, asthma education programs, and cardiopulmonary rehabilitation offerings, to name but a few. The main cause of coronary artery disease (CAD) is smoking; cessation of smoking by adults would probably have the most significant effect on the rate of CAD in the United States of any behavior. As respiratory therapists, helping people stop smoking should be high on the priority list.

Hypertension is another cause of CAD. Respiratory therapists' first step in controlling blood pressure is knowing what theirs is. And an easy way to have blood pressure taken several times a year is to donate blood! One can donate blood every 56 days. RTs could have their blood pressure taken in a relatively nonstressful environment as many as seven times each year while performing a significant public service. Continuing to take prescribed medication is the most important step in controlling hypertension. Of course, if people do not feel ill, they frequently stop taking prescribed medication.

Obesity is another treatable cause of CAD. Pediatricians feel that lifelong eating habits are established in early childhood. Perhaps hundreds of thousands of people each year learn how hard it is to alter those long-standing eating patterns. Nonetheless, decreasing the amount of cholesterol in the diet and keeping calories provided by fat at less than 30% of the total daily intake are the two mainstays of the heart healthy diet. Planning meals using the food pyramid (with five servings of fruits and vegetables, high intake of complex carbohydrates, and minimal intake of red meats and food containing fats) further enhances health. Furthermore, parents can help their children by inculcating healthy eating habits from the beginning and ensuring that the children are not obese; a large proportion (as high as 75%) of those who are obese as children are obese as adults.

Besides being a risk factor itself for CAD, obesity promotes hypertension, diabetes, and physical inactivity. The lack of physical activity is another modifiable cause of CAD. The physical activity does not have to be exhausting, prolonged, or organized in a gym to provide health benefits. To achieve cardiovascular conditioning, exercise (not including stretching and warmup and cool-down afterward) should be of 30–45 minutes long, 3–4 times per week, to at least 60% of predicted maximum heart rate (calculated as 220 - age in years). One can also accrue the disseminated benefits of exercise by taking the stairs instead of the elevators, for example. Exercise can also consist of home maintenance activities, such as mowing the lawn, raking leaves, or carpentry.

Regardless of the depth and breadth of the offering, the respiratory therapist has to be intimately involved in the health promotion and disease prevention (HP/DP) movement. Respiratory therapists have the skill mix as well as the opportunity to participate in such interactions. With a deep and rich appreciation of the importance of HP/DP, as well as an understanding of health promotion program development, design, and delivery, respiratory therapists can clearly make a contribution to improving the heath and well-being of patients. Following is the AARC position statement on health promotion.[35]

> The American Association for Respiratory Care (AARC) submits this paper to identify and illustrate the involvement of the respiratory care practitioner in the promotion of health and the prevention of disease and supports these activities.
>
> The AARC realizes that respiratory care practitioners are integral members of the healthcare team, hospitals, home healthcare settings, pulmonary laboratories, rehabilitation programs, and all other environments where respiratory care is practiced as outlines in the AARC Statement of Principles.
>
> The AARC recognizes that education and training of the respiratory care practitioner is the best method by which to instill awareness of the opportunity to improve the quality and length of life, and that such information should be included in their formal education and training.

Age-Specific Competency

Preventing Injury and Death

Even more than for adults, for children, the key to minimizing injury and death is prevention.

- Because motor vehicle trauma causes nearly half of all pediatric injuries and deaths each year, it behooves adults to use appropriate restraints when children are in the car. Children should be buckled into an age-specific car seat that is properly fastened to the car. (Proper fastening of a child or infant seat may include a strap that fastens to the car floor.) They should also be seated in the rear seat to avoid injury from air bags.
- Children should be properly supervised and educated regarding walking and playing near streets. When they are riding bicycles, children should be wearing an approved helmet, which can prevent the vast majority of head and brain injuries.
- Because drowning is a major cause of death in the younger population of children, adults should supervise these children closely when they are near water. Children should know how to swim and what to do in an emergency around water. Even such a seemingly innocuous "body" of water as a 2-gallon bucket can be fatal to the unsupervised child.
- Adults have the responsibility to minimize the danger from house fires, which result in the overwhelming majority of burns. Having a smoke detector on each floor of the house and, better yet, one in each bedroom would be a good first step.
- Last but not least concerning prevention, especially in the light of recent events, is firearm safety. At the least, the firearms should be secured, unloaded, and separate from ammunition; there should also be trigger locks on all guns.

The AARC recognizes the respiratory care practitioner's responsibility to participate in pulmonary disease training, smoking cessation programs, pulmonary function studies for the public, air pollution alerts, allergy warnings, and sulfite warnings in restaurants, as well as research in those and other areas where efforts could promote improved health and disease prevention.

Furthermore, the respiratory care practitioner is in a unique position to provide leadership in determining health promotion and disease prevention activities for students, faculty, practitioners, patients, and the general public.

The AARC recognizes the need to provide and promote consumer education related to the prevention and control of pulmonary disease to establish a strong working relationship with other health agencies, educational institutions, federal and state government, business, and other community organizations, and to monitor such.

Furthermore, the AARC supports efforts to develop personal and professional wellness models and action plans that will inspire and encourage all members and non-members alike to cooperate on health promotion and disease prevention.

Summary

This chapter on health promotion provided an overview of the general concepts and principles associated with health promotion. It presented the various models of health, the dimensions of health, the underlying philosophy of health promotion, and the major role played by the individual and by society. It also presented a brief historical account of the factors that have affected health over the past century. This chapter identified and discussed the leading causes of death, but more importantly it identified and discussed the behaviors responsible for these leading killers. It identified the determining factors that render people ill or healthy and stressed the critical importance of lifestyle. It also presented a health continuum that was expanded and enhanced to depict both a traditional perspective as well as a health promoting perspective. Compelling evidence was offered to support the incorporation of health promotion and disease prevention principles and practices into today's health care delivery system.

Clearly, there is much to be gained by engaging in healthy lifestyle behaviors. Health maintenance organizations and managed care groups have affirmed the value of such practices and have endorsed the principles in their mission statements.

Employers and insurers have identified the economic rewards of such practices. The federal government has vigorously embarked on four separate initiatives targeting Healthy People as a major goal of the future. It is equally obvious that respiratory therapists possess the clinical expertise to participate in this new and evolving component of health care. They are pivotally positioned every day at the bedside to provide the knowledge and skills requisite for respiratory health.

Respiratory therapists are clearly capable of engaging in community and organizational health promotion programming. Their stature, expertise, and knowledge in the art and science of cardiopulmonary care enable them to be major players in this movement. Health promotion is simply good medicine and certainly has a complementary role in the health care system of the future. It will certainly continue to evolve, and respiratory therapists should welcome the opportunity to assume the role of health educator and to share their knowledge, skills, and abilities with the respiratory-impaired patient whom they serve.

Study Questions

REVIEW QUESTIONS

1. List and explain the three models of health.
2. List and explain the six dimensions of health.
3. Compare and contrast the 10 leading causes of death in the United States in 1900, 1990, and 2005.
4. Identify and explain the four determinants of health status.
5. Draw, label, and describe the illness and wellness continuum.
6. Explain the role of the respiratory therapist in the health promotion movement.

MULTIPLE-CHOICE QUESTIONS

1. According to the author, the *average life span* in the United States is considered to be between the ages of:
   a. 60 and 70.
   b. 70 and 80.
   c. 80 and 90.
   d. 90 and 100.
2. Morbidity is defined as:
   a. the number of deaths per unit of population.
   b. the ratio of persons who are diseased to those who are well.
   c. the frequency at which a disease occurs.
   d. the predominance of a disease.
3. The obvious two leading causes of death in the United States in 2005 were heart disease and cancer. What are the third, fourth, and fifth (in their proper order)?
   a. pneumonia, accidents, stroke
   b. stroke, COPD, accidents
   c. COPD, stroke, accidents
   d. COPD, pneumonia, stroke
4. Approximately what percentage of all deaths every year in the United States are due to lifestyle?
   a. 30%
   b. 40%
   c. 50%
   d. 70%
5. Which of the following is the number one preventable cause of death in the United States?
   a. tobacco
   b. diet
   c. microbial agents
   d. firearms
6. Which of the following surgeon general's reports specifically dealt with reducing health disparities among Americans?
   a. *Surgeon General's Report on Smoking*
   b. *Surgeon General's Report on Health Promotion and Disease Prevention*
   c. *Promoting Health/Preventing Disease: Objectives for the Nation*
   d. *Healthy People 2000*
7. Which of the following models of health was based almost exclusively on cellular abnormality, organ dysfunction, or biological system failure?
   a. medical model
   b. holistic model
   c. lifestyle model
   d. wellness model
8. Which dimension of health is best characterized in making informed and responsible decisions and seeking medical attention when appropriate?
   a. physical
   b. social
   c. emotional
   d. spiritual
9. The largest percentage of our health care status is determined by which variable?
   a. medical system
   b. lifestyle
   c. heredity
   d. environment
10. What two factors were identified as the basic principles for health promotion?
    a. heredity and social status
    b. individual responsibility and cultural norms
    c. education and motivation
    d. peer pressure and values and attitudes

11. Which of the following had the greatest impact in curtailing the death rate in the United States over the past 100 years?
    a. public health improvements
    b. drug discoveries
    c. advances in medical technology
    d. healthy lifestyle practices
12. Which term best describes activities that detect a disease condition early in the process so that the duration and severity of the condition can be shortened or eliminated?
    a. primary prevention
    b. secondary prevention
    c. tertiary prevention
    d. curation
13. Factors that contribute to health behavior can be categorized into which major categories?
    I. predisposing
    II. enabling
    III. reinforcing
    IV. causative
    a. I, II, and III
    b. I, II, and IV
    c. I, III, and IV
    d. II, III, and IV
    e. I, II, III, and IV
14. Which of the following steps are employed in the process of initiating health promotion programs?
    I. assessment
    II. planning
    III. implementing
    IV. evaluating
    a. I, II, and III
    b. I, II, and IV
    c. I, III, and IV
    d. II, III, and IV
    e. I, II, III, and IV
15. For respiratory therapists to assume a more prominent position in the practice of health promotion, which set of skills do they need to enhance?
    a. assessment skills
    b. technical skills
    c. diagnostic skills
    d. education skills

CRITICAL-THINKING QUESTIONS

1. What do you think will be the leading causes of death in the United States in the next 10 years, 20 years, 50 years, 100 years? Will heart disease and cancer still be at the top of the list? What other diseases or conditions will emerge? What diseases or conditions are likely to disappear?
2. The definition of health has shifted from the absence of disease to a multidimensional focus. Aside from the dimension addressed in the text, should other dimensions be considered? Will there be any additional dimensions in the future? How will this definition change in the future?
3. Can humans live beyond the age of 125? If so, what will be the optimum or maximum age? What will humans need to do to prolong life? Will this simply be an issue of increased quantity of years, or will there be a real improvement in the quality of life?
4. The globalization of the world has exposed the West to the East, with all the differences in cultures and beliefs. What has the Western world gained from the East and vice versa?
5. The factors that contribute to health behavior have been addressed extensively in this chapter. Have others not been addressed? What factors will emerge in the future? What can society do to aid individuals in modifying unhealthy lifestyle behaviors?
6. Do you think the health care reimbursement system in this country supports disease prevention and health promotion initiatives? How can the health care reimbursement system be manipulated to better support and encourage health promotion?
7. Will there come a time when significant and substantial economic incentives will be employed on the health care system? Will the United States ever adopt rationing measures in its practice of health care delivery?
8. What additional activities and involvements do you feel your professional organization can engage in that would further the efforts of the health promotion movement?
9. Discuss the future role of the federal government, employers, health care organizations, and educational institutions in the health promotion movement.

References

1. Edlin G, Golanty E, McCormack K. *Health and Wellness*. 6th ed. Sudbury, MA: Jones & Bartlett: 1998:4–6, 293.
2. Hurley JS, Schlaadt R. *Wellness: The Wellness Life-Style*. Guilford, CT: Duskin Publishing Group; 1992:4, 11.
3. CIA. *The World Factbook*. Washington, DC: Office of Public Affairs: 2010. https://www.cia.gov/library/publications/the-world-factbook/rankorder/2102rank.html
4. CIA. *The World Factbook*. Washington, DC: Office of Public Affairs: 2010. https://www.cia.gov/library/publications/the-world-factbook/rankorder/2091rank.txt

5. Reiff T. An overview of human aging. In: Opatz J, ed. *Wellness Promotion Strategies*. Dubuque, IA: Kendall/Hunt; 1984:73–93.
6. Bernstein A. France's Doyenne of Humanity. Outlook section—people in the news. *US News and World Report*. August 18, 1997;123:9.
7. Smith S, Smith C. *Personal Health Choices*. Boston: Jones & Bartlett; 1990:2–3, 5, 470.
8. Opatz JP. *A Primer of Health Promotion: Creating Healthy Organizational Cultures*. Washington, DC: Oryn Publications; 1985:3–6, 7, 9, 11.
9. Beard BB. *Centenarians: The new generation*. Wilson NK, Wilson, AJE, eds. New York: Greenwood; 1991:247.
10. Poon, LW, Johnson MA, Martin P. The Georgia Centenarian Study. *Int J Aging and Hum Dev*. 1993:324:1–17.
11. Pascucci MA, Loving GL. Ingredients of an old and healthy life: a centenarian perspective. *J of Holistic Nurs*. 1997:15:199–213.
12. Hayflick L. *How and Why We Age*. New York: Balantine Books; 1994.
13. Dunn HL. *High Level Wellness*. Arlington, VA: R W Beatty; 1961.
14. Hettler B. *Six Dimensions of Wellness*. National Wellness Institute. Stevens Point: University of Wisconsin–Stevens Point; 1979.
15. U.S. Department of Health and Human Services. *Healthy People: The Surgeon General's Report on Health Promotion and Disease Prevention*. Washington, DC: Public Health Service; 1979:119, 219.
16. Mullen K, Gold R, Belcastro P, McDermott R. *Connections for Health*. Dubuque, IA: Wm. C. Brown; 1990:7, 28–29, 661.
17. Fries J, Koop CE, Beadle CE. Reducing health care costs by reducing the need and demand for medical services. *N Engl J Med*. 1993;329:321–325.
18. Hahn D, Payne WA. *Focus in Health*. St. Louis, MO: Mosby-Yearbook; 1991:2.
19. Chatham MAH, Knapp BL. *Patient Education Handbook*. Bowie, MD: Robert J. Brady;1982:7.
20. Robbins G, Powers D, Burgess S. *A Wellness Way of Life*. Dubuque, IA: William C Brown; 1991:8, 23, 25. [Now in its 6th edition, published 2005]
21. Hafen B, Hoeger W. *Wellness: Guidelines for a Healthy Lifestyle*. Englewood, CO: Morton; 1994:97. [Now in its 4th edition, published 2007]
22. Bruess C, Richardson G. *Decisions for Health*. Dubuque, IA: Brown and Benchmark; 1995:1–10, 1–11, 1–22.
23. Knowles J. *Doing Better and Feeling Worse: Health in the United States*. Dallas, TX: Daedalus; 1977:59.
24. Ali H. Mokdad, et al. Actual causes of death in the United States, 2000. *JAMA*. 2005; 293,3:293. http://jama.ama-assn.org/cgi/content/full/291/10/1238
25. Lalonde M. *A New Perspective on the Health of Canadians—A Working Document*. Ottawa, Canada: Office of the Canadian Minister of National Health and Welfare; 1974.
26. U.S. Department of Health, Education and Welfare. *Ten Leading Causes of Death in the United States, 1975*. Atlanta, GA: Public Health Services, CDC, Bureau of State Services, Health Analysis and Planning for Preventative Services; 46.
27. Belloc N, Breslow L. Relationship of physical health status and health practices. *Prev Med*. 1972;1:409–421.
28. Travis J, Ryan RS. *The Wellness Workbook*. 2nd ed. Berkeley, CA: Ten Speed Press; 1981:1988. [Now in its 3rd edition, published 2004]
29. McKenzie J, Smeltzer J. *Planning, Implementing and Evaluating Health Promotion Programs: A Primer*. 2nd ed. Boston: Allyn & Bacon; 1997:11–14.
30. Bellingham R, Tager M. *Designing Effective Health Promotion Programs: The 20 Skills for Success*. Chicago: Great Performances; 1986:i, 2.
31. U.S. Department of Health and Human Services. *Promoting Health/Preventing Disease: Objectives for the Nation*. Washington, DC: Public Health Service; 1980.
32. U.S. Department of Health and Human Services. *Healthy People 2000*. Washington, DC: Public Health Service; 1992.
33. U.S. Department of Health and Human Services. *Healthy People 2010: Understanding and Improving Health*. 2nd ed. Washington, DC: U.S. Government Printing Office; 2000.
34. U.S. Department of Health and Human Services. *Healthy People 2020: The Road Ahead*. Washington, DC: Office of Disease Prevention & Health Promotion; 2008.
35. *AARC Position Statement on Health Promotion*. Dallas, TX: American Association for Respiratory Care; 1986.

Suggested Readings

Anderson G. In search of value: an international comparison of cost, access and outcomes. *Health Affairs*. November/ December 1997;163–170.

Vital Statistics. *U.S. Department of Health and Human Services*. Washington, DC: Public Health Service, 2005.

Wallis C. How to live to be 120. *Time*. March 6,1995:85.

CHAPTER 40

Fundamentals of Patient Education

Gail A. Watkins Varcelotti

OBJECTIVES

Upon completion of this chapter, the reader should be able to:

- Define and identify the modalities in learning.
- Define and write a sample goal in patient education.
- Define and write a sample objective in patient education.
- Define and assess a sample outcome in patient education.
- Describe the stages of learning.
- List the components of interpersonal communication.
- Define patient compliance.
- Describe the purpose of clinical practice guidelines.
- Identify sites for patient education.
- Develop a sample patient education program.
- Discuss predicted changes to reimbursement for respiratory therapists performing patient education.

CHAPTER OUTLINE

KEY TERMS

communication
compliance
education
goal
modality
objective
outcome
training

Education is . . . hanging around till you catch on.
—Robert Frost

Although Robert Frost's quote on education is quite humorous, this cannot be the case when dealing with patient education in health care. Patient education is a vital and important part of health care and disease management, although the luxury of time is frequently not available. The goals of patient education typically are to promote healthy behavior and involvement of patients in their own care and decisions about their care. Unfortunately, owing to the frequent acuteness of most patient situations, an educational project must be effective and timely. With that in mind, respiratory therapists (RTs) have a vital role as educators, which includes educating themselves, their peers, other health care practitioners, and, most importantly, the patients. The educator is the individual who must assess programs and activities, develop program goals, allocate resources, prioritize educational needs, and provide the actual education. Anyone taking on the process of education and **training** must realize that what may appear as a complex situation can frequently be placed into a simple format with the correct amount of planning and implementation. The terms "education" and "training" are used synonymously and although much has been written on what to's and why to's in education, the process is not as well-defined as one would expect. D. Falvo[1] summarizes that, before education can be said to be complete, a change in behavior, skill, or attitude must take place. Therefore, patient **education** is the process of influencing patient behavior and producing the changes in knowledge, attitudes, and skills required for maintaining and improving health.

Almost all types of education involve the same basic building blocks, which can be manipulated to obtain specific set goals and objectives for patient education to be effective.

According to D. Falvo,[1] the patient educator should be able to:

- Build a rapport with the patient.
- Assess the patient's learning readiness, skills, and abilities that can help or hinder the learning process.
- Organize teaching in a way best suited to the patient's needs.
- Communicate clearly and effectively.
- Identify and appropriately utilize teaching resources for facilitating the learning process.
- Assess potential barriers to carrying out treatment recommendations.
- Problem-solve with the patient to reach solutions.

The patient education process is more than just providing material to the patient. It is a process rather than an individual segment in the total health care plan. As the concept of patient education continues to gain acceptance and credibility in the health care system, respiratory therapists should give patient education more than just a thought or a nod. Involvement in the stepwise progression permits RTs to meet the future challenges and to guide patients through what may be a difficult adaptation to illness and therapy.

This chapter identifies the basic building blocks while providing ideas and examples of how respiratory therapists can develop the different facets of education they may be faced with during their career.

> *Best Practice*
>
> **Patient Education**
>
> When starting any type of educational endeavor, remember this: The learner learns *what* the learner wants to learn *when* the learner *wants* to learn it.
>
> Any learner can be placed into a learning environment, but without the correct preparation and facilitation the endeavor is wasted.

The Educational Process

Learning, in most environments, is a natural yet necessary characteristic of human nature. The desire to learn can be fueled by self-fulfillment or simply by need. The true test of learning is whether the education process accomplishes the goal set by both the learner and the educator. That is why it is so important for an educator to look at the basic levels of learning before developing any kind of instruction. By acknowledging patient learning modalities, the respiratory therapist can better assess the needs of the patient.

MODALITIES OF LEARNING

A **modality** is any type of route where an individual can receive and retain information. In the fundamentals of basic learning, there are three basic keys or modalities: sensation, perception, and memory. These modalities can be further defined and specifically made relevant to patient education by relating them to visual, auditory, and kinesthetic modalities. Each modality identifies specific types of learning that a learner may experience or require in different educational settings or experiences. The visual and auditory modalities relate to seeing and hearing, while the kinesthetic modality involves the use of muscles and tactile (touch) abilities. When placed in a learning situation, patients may exhibit a predominant or preferred modality. The success of their ability to process information is affected by this dominant modality. But that is not to say that they cannot have mixed modality preferences.

Most educational programs are designed to include at least two modalities, thus permitting an educator to adopt initial strategies. Follow-up strategies that incorporate other modalities may be required to deal with the learner who has difficulty grasping the initial concepts. This difficulty may be due to literacy or cultural differences. Modality-based instruction can occur at all levels of learning, and it is of greatest value in teaching basic skills. Therefore, this type of instruction can be of great value in instructing patients. Because modality-based instruction is strength oriented, any instructor can expect the learner to learn rapidly and enjoy doing the learning. A benefit of modality-based instruction is that separate and unrelated skills are eliminated, and application rather than just understanding is emphasized.

When patient groups or individuals are identified for instruction or education of some sort, performing a basic assessment of modality strengths is ideal. Understanding the patients' needs and abilities are key to developing effective and efficient programs of learning. Table 40-1 is helpful in identifying observable indicators of modality strength. Questioning the patient, questioning the patient's family or caregivers, and reviewing the patient chart all prove to be worthwhile in determining the characteristics that indicate modality strengths.

Once the learning modality of a patient is ascertained, an educational program can be developed or tailored to suit the ability of the learner. When developing a program, beware of using the *broad-spectrum approach*, which combines types of multisensory information in one unit. For example, an educational class combines small portions of lecture, videos, and manual practice all at the same time for the same skill. Many educators and textbooks use this technique to be able to provide a little of everything to the learner. Although this may seem to accomplish a lot, many learners with strong predominate modalities do not benefit from this type of experience. Because patient education is so vital in the managed care approach to disease, a more helpful style of education program is the *menu approach*. This approach permits the educator to provide instruction that stresses one modality and

TABLE 40-1 **Selected observable characteristics indicative of modality strengths**

	Visual	Auditory	Kinesthetic
Learning style	Learns by seeing; watching demonstration	Learns through verbal instructions from others or self	Learns by doing, direct involvement
Memory	Remembers faces; forgets names; writes things down, takes notes	Remembers names; forgets faces; remembers by repetition	Remembers best what was done, not what was seen or talked about
Problem solving	Deliberate; plans in advance; organizes thoughts by writing them; lists problems	Talks problems out; tries solutions verbally subvocally, talks self through problem	Attacks problems physically; impulsive; often selects solution involving the greatest activity
Responses to new situations	Looks around; examines structure	Talks about situation, pros and cons, what to do	Tries things out; touches, feels, manipulates
Communication	Quiet; does not talk at length; becomes impatient when extensive listening required; may use words clumsily; describes without embellishment; uses words such as "see," "look," etc.	Enjoys listening but cannot wait to talk; descriptions are long but repetitive; likes hearing self and others talk; uses words such as "listen," "hear," etc.	Gestures when speaking; does not listen well; stands close when speaking or listening; quickly loses interest in detailed verbal discourse; uses words such as "get," "take," etc.
General appearance	Neat, meticulous, likes order; may choose not to vary appearance	Matching clothes not so important, can explain choices of clothes	Neat but soon becomes wrinkled through activity

Source: From Barbe WB, Swassing RH. Teaching Through Modality Strengths. *Columbus, OH: Zaner-Bloser; 1988.*

then continue to instruct using other modalities as the patient progresses. For example, the part of an asthma management program dealing with using a metered-dose inhaler (MDI) could consist of:

- *Auditory modality*. Providing a 10-minute discussion on the MDI; confirming understanding through verbal questions and answers.
- *Visual modality*. Showing a video about MDI or having the patient tune into the hospital television system regarding MDI usage.
- *Visual modality*. Provide written materials for the patient and family to read at their leisure. A returnable question form can be collected later to verify understanding.
- *Kinesthetic modality*. Perform the correct use of the MDI for the patient, and then ask the patient to demonstrate its use .

When using the menu format, stressing certain modalities permits the educator to individualize the program of study to each patient's needs.

Age-Specific Competency

Identifying a Patient's Learning Modality

The respiratory therapist in the role of educator needs to be aware that patient settings involve many sites and patients of all ages. The patient educator must give special consideration and take special approaches to address patients according to their age. For example, children may be instructed at one level according to their modality of learning, and the parents may require additional intervention. On the other hand, a geriatric patient may have specific modalities but, due to advancing age, requires assistance to accomplish the educational unit. A good rule of thumb is to consider the varying teaching approaches suggested by D. Falvo when educating the patient.[1]

Life Stage	Approach
Prenatal through infancy	*Patient:* Use open-minded approach with no preconception; be nonjudgmental; give emotional support to both parents; work within parents' framework. *Parents:* Foster security by giving positive feedback regarding parents' ability to care for child; no nagging or lecturing; take what may appear to be small problems seriously.
Toddler	*Patient:* Encourage child in warm, matter-of-fact manner; use no analogies when giving explanations; give explanations in accurate, simple terms. *Parents:* Use nonjudgmental approach; continue support and positive reinforcement.
Preschool	*Patient:* Encourage child to express fear; give no false promises; explain procedures before doing them. *Parents:* Provide guidance and encouragement.
Later Childhood	*Patient:* Give explanations in simple, logical way; approach child in confident, optimistic manner. *Parents:* Continue guidance and support.
Young Adult	*Patient:* Be empathetic, have a nonjudgmental attitude.
Middle Years	*Patient:* Be empathetic, have a nonjudgmental attitude.
Later Years	*Patient:* Approach patient as unique, not stereotyping because of age; keep awareness that aging is a multidimensional process in which multiple factors affect function; capitalize on patient's strengths; refrain from using first names unless invited to do so; speak clearly and concisely; avoid patronizing patient.

CASE STUDY 40-1

V. A. is a 64-year-old female who has been admitted several times over the past year complaining of shortness of breath and weakness. She has since been diagnosed as having chronic obstructive pulmonary disease through pulmonary function and laboratory studies. She uses metered-dose inhalers and oral bronchodilators. Due to documented chronic hypoxemia, her physician has now ordered her to receive 2 Lpm of oxygen via a nasal cannula at home. Due to the lack of patient compliance with previous medical orders, the physician wants the respiratory care department to provide instruction at the hospital on using and caring for a nasal cannula. The respiratory care department usually relies on the home care service to provide this type of instruction and therefore does not have educational materials ready. The supervisor has requested you to develop an educational program to prepare this patient to go home on oxygen therapy.

Questions

1. To begin preparing learning materials, the RT interviews the patient to discover which learning modality to use. What questions should the RT ask the patient and the patient's family?
2. List the types of materials the RT should try to use to complement each type of modality (visual, auditory, kinesthetic).

Best Practice

Helpful Hints in Writing Goals

- A goal implies some achievement as a result of doing something.
- A goal should relate to a single end result.
- The measurement of the completion of the goal should be as simple as possible.
- The goal should specify when the end result is achieved.

GOALS, OBJECTIVES, AND OUTCOMES

Most clinicians are goal and objective oriented owing to the education and clinical process they have experienced while learning their profession.

- A **goal** is general statement of purpose, and it is usually a simple item that may be measured to determine the success of a plan.
- An **objective** is a declarative statement that directs the learner's action toward a specific goal. Typically, several objectives are attached to a single goal. Many educators mix these terms up when developing an instructional unit.
- **Outcomes** are the end products. Assessment assists in determining the outcome of any situation, whether it is educational or therapeutic.

The process of developing goals, objectives, and outcomes may seem tedious, but once the educator is provided with simple definitions and examples, they are actually fun to create and write.

Goals. The goals of patient education are designed to include the control of symptoms, the promotion of wellness and health, and the improvement of patient knowledge, all of which can reduce patient anxiety.

Some examples of goals in respiratory care could include the following:

- The educational program will instruct the learner in the use of a peak flowmeter.
- The patient will be instructed on how to use the BiPAP unit in the home.

Initially when writing goals, the statement typically comes from a general idea of what needs to be accomplished, what the learner already knows, and how the learning will be approached (i.e., lecture, handout material, and demonstration). Most of the initial process is in the mind of the educator, and the ultimate statement of what will be accomplished is written as the goal.

Objectives. Educational objectives can improve the method of teaching. They guide the educator in thinking and planning the learning experiences. Objectives help select and develop the techniques and materials that produce the proposed learning. Objectives are defined as the behaviors and processes that learners are expected to acquire or master by the end of a learning unit. Some guidelines to consider when writing objectives that will develop health education methods and materials are as follows:

- Set realistic objectives.
- To change health behaviors, focus on behaviors and skills.
- Present context first (before giving new information).
- Partition complex instructions.
- Make it interactive.

As an educator develops objectives, an effort should be made to create clear objectives, which enable the educational process to be a smooth transition between learning units. The objective should clearly outline what is expected of the learner when the instructional units have been completed. Each statement should include an action verb to identify what the learner must do to be successful in learning. For example, an educator has determined the need to teach a patient about metered-dose inhalers. One segment of the learning unit is to instruct the patient how to use the MDI. The objective could be written as follows: "The patient will be able to demonstrate how to properly use the MDI after receiving instruction and handout for steps on using the inhaler" (Figure 40-1). The objective statement is very clear about what the educator expects the learner to be able to do after being instructed. The word "demonstrate" tells exactly what the learner must do to successfully complete the learning unit, while the rest of the statement informs the learner what items to use in completing the objective.

The following action verbs are categorized according to what the learner has to demonstrate:

- *Knowledge:* cite, define, identify, label, list, name, recall, recite, state
- *Comprehension:* describe, tell, explain, summarize
- *Using Ideas:* demonstrate, prepare, show, use, solve, utilize
- *Evaluation:* write, compare, evaluate, judge
- *Response:* answer, consent, respond, communicate

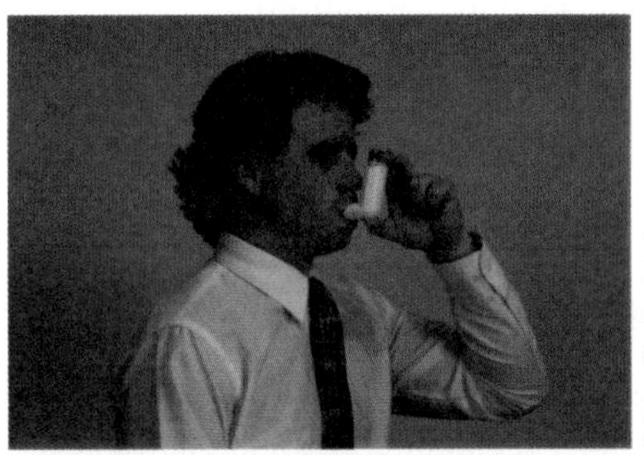
© Delmar/Cengage Learning

(A)

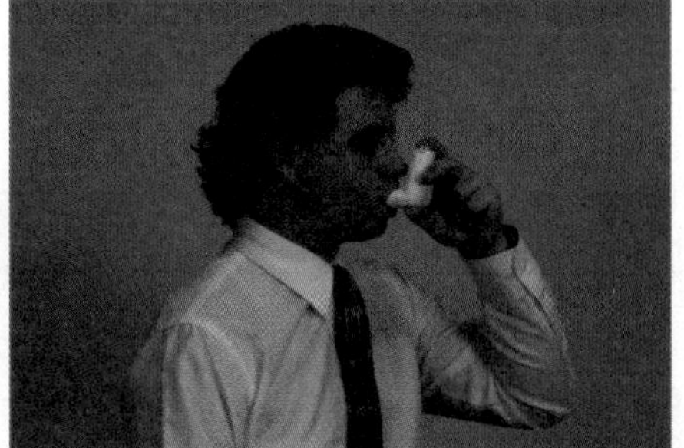
© Delmar/Cengage Learning

(B)

FIGURE 40-1 Self-administration with a metered-dose inhaler: (A) Insert mouthpiece into mouth, forming a tight seal with the lips. (B) Push the cylinder down and inhale.

- *Attitude:* seek, choose, adjust
- *Perception:* detect, feel, hear, listen, observe, recognize, see, smell, taste

After writing the objectives for a learning unit, the educator should ask whether the action can be assessed either by seeing it or hearing it. If it cannot be assessed, the objective writer should seek another action verb for the objective statement

Outcomes. The end process of education is assessment to determine whether the goal was achieved—whether the process caused a patient's behavior or attitude to change. With outcomes, educators need to identify what they are trying to assess. Learning outcomes demonstrate patient achievement through interests and attitudes that the educator wants to see developed. When determining outcomes, educators should:

- Reflect on their own learning experiences.
- Consider how instructors make an impact on learning.
- Analyze their own beliefs about training and learning.
- Identify the method of learning required for the situation.

An outcome can be measured, formally and informally, in many ways.

- *Informally*, the educator can simply ask questions that address the expectations for the patient after the learning process is completed.
- More *formally*, many predeveloped assessment forms are available for use by someone providing patient education. The next Best Practice provides an example of a patient education list for a learning module about oxygen concentrators. It can be used in verifying the learning process simply by using it as a checklist for patient understanding. The respiratory therapist can direct questions from this form to the patient or to the family to verify that they understand. The form is used after the patient has received instruction and demonstration of the device. The assessment can be performed at any predetermined time to verify patient understanding and effectiveness of the original instruction.

Most outcomes can be measured in an intelligent yet informal way, but some educators desire a more detailed system that involves scientific and objective data. This type of formal assessment usually involves explicit statements of judgment and decisions and includes measures based on those statements. Because patient education is usually done in the hospital or home care setting, formal assessment is not usually required. That type of assessment for outcome is accomplished when a clinical study is being performed.

COMMUNICATION SKILLS

Communication should receive high priority in patient education. "We can't afford to get in such a hurry that we allow our communication skills to atrophy," says Frederic Platt, regional consultant for the Bayer Institute for Health Care Communication and clinical professor of internal medicine at the University of Colorado in Denver. "The time we spend with patients is limited, so we must approach our interactions with even more care."

Communication in patient education is predominately interpersonal in nature. It involves a series of behaviors that are specifically verbal and nonverbal and that stimulate personal inquiry between two or more persons. Good communication requires the educator to have skills that include:

- Attending behavior.
- Active listening.
- Reflection and inventory questioning.
- Encouraging alternative behaviors.

Attending Behavior. *Attending behavior* includes the use of nonverbal and verbal gestures that involve eye contact, facial and body gestures, and brief verbal communication. It helps in demonstrating empathy and concern for what a learner has said to the educator. It reassures patients that their feelings and thoughts are being considered and heard. Some attending behavior examples could include the listener leaning slightly forward while the speaker is explaining a symptom, slightly touching the patient's hand, and verifying with brief phrases such as, "I understand."

Active Listening. *Active listening*, on the other hand, includes being able to differentiate between the intellectual and emotional content of a conversation. Any type of conversation has both types of content, and an educator must develop the skill to differentiate the two. Information of a more personal nature is frequently revealed when the listener attentively follows the speaker's verbal and nonverbal cues. To help in differentiating, the listener should ask questions and try and direct the conversation content to become more objective, thus keeping the subjective content separate. Examples of questions could include:

- *Objective question, specific number sought in this question.* "How many times do you awaken at night because you are short of breath?"

Best Practice

Patient Instruction Checklist

Oxygen Concentrator Therapy—Instructions

Cautions:

1. Do not smoke, and stay at least 5 feet from open flames while using your oxygen (flame on gas stove, fireplaces, candles, etc.).
2. Oxygen is a drug; use it as ordered by your physician. Too much or too little may be harmful to your health.
3. Keep your concentrator at least 6 inches from walls or curtains. Do not allow the inlet filter to become blocked.
4. Keep your concentrator away from heaters or heating ducts.
5. Use a 110-V electrical outlet, and try not to have any other household appliances attached to the outlet.
6. If an electrical power outage occurs, turn off your concentrator. This turns off the alarm. Use your backup oxygen cylinder as instructed.

Procedure:

1. Connect the humidifier to the screw-adapter on the front panel of the concentrator.
2. Fill the jar (to the designated line) of the humidifier with distilled water.
3. Connect your nasal cannula or oxygen mask (use whatever device is ordered by your physician) to the humidifier.
4. Plug in the concentrator and turn the concentrator on. Be sure that the flow reads __________ liters per minute (use exactly what was prescribed by your physician).
5. If you do not think that oxygen is coming through the cannula, use the following steps:
   a. Be sure all connections between the humidifier and concentrator are straight and tight.
   b. Look for bubbling in the humidifier.
   c. Place the cannula in a glass of water and check for bubbles.
   d. If you have performed all the above and still have a problem, call _______________ for assistance.
6. Follow the cleaning and maintenance instructions provided with the concentrator.

- *Subjective, leaves a lot of opportunity for patients to tell you about themselves and their problems.* "How do you sleep at night?"

Reflecting and Inventory Questioning. *Reflecting and inventory questioning* permits educators to direct feedback to learners regarding how their messages are being received. The educator may mirror or question the learner to ultimately see how the learner's behavior has changed and then assess the effectiveness of the behavior. These skills may assist in showing the discrepancies between the actual and desired behavior being sought during the education process. For example, after listening to a patient who has been receiving home oxygen tell about his or her daily activities post–oxygen use, the listener could return a question. The inquiry could be "So I understand, then, that you are not getting out of the house at all because you are so short of breath." The speaker might then respond, "No, my shortness of breath is better now: The reason I don't get out of the house is because there is no one to drive me." The listener has then learned more about the speaker's behavior.

Encouraging Alternative Behaviors. *Encouraging alternative behaviors* encourages an exploration of behaviors. Learners can:

- Practice a behavior change, such as techniques to stop smoking cigarettes.

CASE STUDY 40-2

The supervisor of the department has requested the RT to assist in developing an instructional unit to help W. C., a 62-year-old female, with her metered-dose inhaler. She has had the inhalers for several years but seemed to get little relief when at home. During her hospital stays, she insisted that the respiratory therapists and nurses administer the inhaler. Her physician was convinced that she did not know how or did not remember how to do the maneuver required for metered-dose inhaler delivery. She wanted the respiratory care department to develop an instructional course for Mrs. C. and other patients.

Questions

1. Write a goal for the program.
2. Write two objectives for the program.
3. What outcome assessment form could be developed to demonstrate success in the program?

Best Practice

Developing Materials for Educational Use

To demonstrate the ability to develop materials for educational use, a patient educator needs to write the general goal, develop several objectives to support the goal, and determine how to assess the outcome of the educational process after patient delivery has been accomplished. Practice the process of development with as many tasks or skills as possible. Practice enables the writer to become more skilled in the development process, which, after a period of time, becomes second nature. In other words, practice, practice, practice.

- Determine how it makes them feel.
- Then continue to develop the behavior change until they no longer have a sense of change.

In a manner of speaking, the interpersonal skills are a format in which the educator becomes the facilitator of change via communication.

Nonverbal Cues. In addition to the preceding interpersonal communication measures, educators should be aware of some simple rules regarding nonverbal cues.

- When making eye contact with the learner, be aware of the effect that eye-to-eye contact may have with some people. You may need to adjust your direct eye contact when learners are particularly sensitive to this type of focus and shy away from it.
- Facial expression (or the lack of it) gives feedback to learners. Educators may convey something that they do not mean to convey.
- Body posture is also vital when speaking or listening to someone. Try to maintain a comfortable yet professional pose; be wary of pointing fingers and crossed arms because they are frequently construed as aggressive or hostile.
- Pay attention to the body posture of the learner; it may assist in determining the mood of the environment during the learning session.
- Physical space is often not thought of and is actually very valuable in the communication process. An 18-inch distance between two people speaking is typically thought to be an *intimate space*. A distance of 18 inches to 4 feet is considered *personal space*, and a distance 4–12 feet is called *social distance*. Anything beyond 12 feet is

called *public space*. When you are speaking or listening, consider the connotation of the space between two people; the effectiveness of the communication may be dramatically affected if the distance is too great or too small. When trying to relay something of great importance it may be essential to decrease the distance between the speaker and the listener.
- Nonverbal eye contact and space constraints vary by culture. These variations can cause misinterpretations, and the RT should consider and research them before dealing with patients with whom they are likely to occur.

Verbal Cues. *Verbal cues* validate and encourage improved communication. These cues include silence, brief verbal acknowledgments, and subsummary.

- *Silence* can be very effective to relay reflection or, in other words, an opportunity for either party to think about what was just said. Many educators and learners are uncomfortable with pauses, but they are important to good communication.
- The same can be said about *brief verbal acknowledgments*, because they assist in moving a conversation or topic along and express interest and concern to the conversation. A simple "I see" or "How interesting" may assist in understanding or refocus the conversation between two or more persons.
- Subsummaries become important when several sentences or topics have been communicated. This technique permits the educator or the learner to validate the intent of the communication.

An example of such a conversation might go as follows:

Listener: So, how did your visit to the doctor go last week?

Patient: It was terrible. He was late and then he rushed me and then I didn't get to ask him my list of questions.

Listener: [after a brief pause] Hmmm, that was probably very frustrating. How about if we look at your questions and see if I can help you in any way, and then let's write down the questions you still have left and you can take them during your next visit.

PATIENT READINESS

Usually the recipients of education in health care are adults who require education about their illness or that of a loved one, medical equipment, or therapy procedure. Consequently, the educator should consider the principles of adult learning, that, according to M. S. Knowles, constitute "the foundation stones of modern adult learning theory":[2]

- Adults are motivated to learn as they experience needs and interests that learning will satisfy; therefore, these needs and interests are appropriate starting points for organizing adult learning activities.
- Adult orientation to learning is life centered; therefore, the appropriate units for organizing adult learning are life situations, not subjects.
- Experience is the richest resource for adult learning; therefore, the core methodology of adult education is the analysis of experience.
- Adults have a deep need to be self-directing; therefore, the role of the educator is to engage in a process of mutual inquiry rather than to transmit knowledge to them and then evaluate their conformity to it.
- Individual differences among people increase with age; therefore, adult education must make optimal provision for differences in style, time, place, and pace of learning.

Change is a process, not an event in a patient's care plan. It is a personal experience, and the individual

Best Practice

Improving Communication Skills

When educators are trying to develop improved communication skills, a self-assessment is extremely helpful in correcting weaknesses. By simply asking themselves the following questions, they can begin an improvement pattern by becoming aware of items being done wrong. Ask:

- If they had direct eye contact with the learner, what type of facial expressions did they make during the conversation?
- What was their body posture?
- Did they permit periods of silence or provided brief verbal acknowledgments?

If they cannot answer these questions or are unsure of how their interpersonal skill came across, they should ask someone to observe them and comment. When teaching, educators must critique themselves and strive for improvement in areas that may be weak. The benefit of the critique is being able to conduct ever more effective teaching sessions.

needs to be the focal point. Learner readiness is essential in having a successful educational program. In 1985, J. O. Prochaska and C. C. DiClemente stated that patients go through a variety of stages when learning.[3] The stages permit them to gradually adopt new beliefs and behaviors. The stages are:

- *Precontemplative.* The patient may not be aware or even considering a change.
- *Contemplative.* The patient begins thinking about changes but is not yet taking any action.
- *Action.* The patient has begun to make changes to behavior and is now practicing them.
- *Maintenance.* The patient has retained the behavior either by learning or via reinforcement.
- *Termination.* Intervention for the patient has ended, and the behavior has become a way of life and is no longer visualized by the patient as a change.

It is vital to consider the patient's state of readiness. Otherwise, a great deal of time and energy is spent, and the patient does not obtain anything, even when a great deal may have been presented. The patient education process should be flexible enough to adapt to potential unwillingness or the lack of readiness.

To address the patient's readiness when dealing with the home care situation after an acute care stay, the *predischarge process* is helpful. The patient and family might note the following benefits associated with providing predischarge education:

- The patient and family are more comfortable with the equipment or procedure at home for the first time.
- The patient has time to formulate questions in the hospital, before being left alone with the equipment.
- The patient has time to decide where the equipment is best placed in the home before arriving there.
- Fears concerning therapies or equipment can be discussed and minimized while in the hospital.

Predischarge training allows the home care personnel to use their time for reinforcement and reassurance.

PATIENT COMPLIANCE

Compliance is simply when the patient does as instructed, the patient's behavior has changed, and the change is helping the health care plan. The lack of compliance is an interesting area to deal with in patient education. With noncompliance, the patient is not doing as instructed or ordered, the behaviors being sought are not accomplished, and the lack of compliance actually begins to hinder the health care plan. Noncompliance is frequently overlooked because most educators seem not to want to recognize that all of their effort has been done for nothing. To deal with this situation, the educator needs to examine the source or sources of the problem. When addressing the issue of noncompliance, it may be helpful to ask the following questions:

- How is the patient reacting to the illness or therapy? Many patients have great difficulty coping with their problems and actually behave in ways that hinder their care. The use of facilitative behaviors[1] is encouraged when dealing with patient compliance and conducting patient education. Coping styles are defenses patients use to protect themselves from threats, either real or imagined.
- Has the RT taken into consideration all of the cultural or social issues that the patient may be encountering? The issues may include language barriers, illiteracy, lack of familial support, lack of financial assistance, and the like.
- Have some environmental issues not been addressed? These are frequently not noticed because the educator may be hospital based and items are not discovered until the home care educator arrives.

In addition, educators must:

- Recognize that patients' reactions to their condition and recommendations are determined by a combination of personal characteristics, learning history, and current circumstances.
- Avoid stereotyped approaches to the patient or to the content of information presented. Even patients with the same conditions do not adapt and react in the same way.
- Recognize that the timing of the teaching intervention is important to the patient's readiness to learn and to work toward established goals. If a good relationship has not previously been established, suggesting that the patient change may lead to rejection of other education efforts.
- Lay a foundation for effective teaching later with empathetic understanding.
- Acknowledge and accept the patient's fears, frustrations, and other reactions in an understanding way.
- Give sensitive support that recognizes the stress the patient feels.
- In instances of denial or other coping styles that appear to be having a detrimental effect, gently and gradually confront the patient with reality.
- Avoid agreeing with patients' statements that do not appear to be accurate representations of fact; do not reinforce patients' negative beliefs.
- If the coping style is not interfering with the patient's conditions or treatment, leave it alone.

The Respiratory Therapist as the Educator

As already stated, the respiratory therapist is not only a clinical caregiver but also an educator. This is an essential role that needs to be developed further to meet the demands of the future of health care. The ability to assume the role of educator lies with the respiratory therapist's willingness and motivation to engage in the education process. Once the RT assumes the role, research is required to determine the patient education site, the resources, and the actual ability to perform and succeed in the education process.

PATIENT SITES

The respiratory therapist provides patient education on a daily basis. Educational programs for patients may be found in acute care, subacute care, chronic care, rehabilitative care, and home care delivery sites. The type of education provided in each type of site varies according to the clientele and can be adapted from site to site. The initiation of patient teaching may be either informal or formal, depending on the purpose. When teaching is a routine part of care due to therapy or a visit to a laboratory, patient education becomes a normal communication skill between patient and therapist. A formal approach may require more preparation and therefore guidelines, because the development of this type of education may be a matter of departmental policy and procedure in a variety of patient sites.

To start actual development of education setups in a patient site, the American Association for Respiratory Care (AARC) has two specific clinical practice guidelines that are extremely helpful in the development of informal and formal educational programs:

- Training the Health Care Professional for the Role of Patient and Caregiver Educator[4]
- Providing Patient and Caregiver Training[5]

Once developed, these programs promote interactive communication among the practitioner, patient, and patient's family.

WITHIN THE COMMUNITY

Another arena for the respiratory therapist serve as educator is in the community. No one can relay information about health care issues of the cardiopulmonary system and the profession as well as a respiratory therapist can. Many ongoing educational programs are currently being delivered in the community by a variety of organizations, and the number of community health education programs is ever increasing. The programs are typically designed to educate individuals or groups of individuals and usually target patients, their friends, relatives, and coworkers with a variety of education, prevention, and cessation programs. Most programs include activities, various media materials, and messages. Involvement in programs by a respiratory therapist may range from voluntary or actual employment in the programs. Typically, they have been developed to mass market the product (the education) and have several steps in the education process.

The mission statement of most programs is to support and educate the patients and families. The increase in the number of programs is due to a global health care goal of prevention rather than intervention. What this means is promoting understanding of health behaviors, supporting recovery, and returning the patient to active daily life.

Some examples of community programs are:

- Asthma education programs
- COPD support groups
- Cancer support groups
- Smoking cessation programs
- General health awareness
- Support groups for cardiopulmonary disorders

A good example of how a program develops is one designed for an individual who wants to quit cigarette smoking. Common learning objectives used in developing a community smoking cessation program could include the following:

- Discuss the incidence of smoking in the United States. Include in the discussion the prevalence of smoking, the trends among adults, and the characteristics of beginning smokers.
- Discuss why people start to smoke.
- Discuss the problems associated with stopping smoking.
- Identify the methods used to stop smoking and their relative success rates.
- Identify the programs available nationally (and locally) to smokers who want to quit.
- Explain the role of the respiratory therapist in helping patients stop smoking.
- Identify the criteria that can be used to match patients with the program most likely to help them succeed in stopping smoking.
- Explain why many people gain weight when they quit smoking. Identify what can be done to prevent this weight gain.
- Cite the prerequisites necessary to be present for a successful attempt at stopping smoking.
- Explain why the programs with higher success rates use multiple strategies.
- Explain why a program's stated success rate should be questioned. How do the programs differ in their calculations of success rate?

IN THE HEALTH CARE FACILITY

Many patient education modules are developed within a health care facility itself. These programs are usually designed out of need and are offered either free or for a nominal fee to the public. The education department of a health care facility is typically responsible for the development and administration of educational programs and is usually community driven in their planning. Activities used in patient and family education typically address the following processes:

- Improve patients' understanding of and coping with their health status.
- Promote interactive communications between patient and provider.
- Encourage patients' participation in their care and decision making.
- Increase patients' compliance and self-involvement in their care plans.
- Promote healthy lifestyles.
- Provide patients with the financial implications of care.

Although the creation of patient education projects requires time and skill by the educator, these projects became very marketable in the 1990s, and they should be developed with a long-range plan in mind.

The resources to complete such projects are abundant (see the resources for patient education materials and ideas listed at the end of this section). Many educational items are willingly shared by professionals and should not be overlooked by the health care educator.

However, be cautious about using prepared or printed educational materials. While prepared patient education materials can be very useful and time-saving tools, they can also be ineffective or even counterproductive if they confuse patients or disagree with what you say. The American Association of Family Practice Publications Division suggests evaluating all patient education materials for the following when the material is either prepared by your facility or purchased from an outside source:

- *Reading level.* Newspapers and other commonly read materials are written on the sixth- to eighth-grade level. Even patients who normally read at a higher level appreciate receiving information that is simple and to the point. When the educator is writing the material, here are some tips:

  Keep things to one or two syllables per word, one idea per sentence, one concept per paragraph, no more than five key points per handout.

  Avoid medical terminology whenever possible. If it can't be avoided, the terms should be carefully defined. For example, shortness of breath should be used rather than dyspnea. Because there is no "lay" term for bronchiectasis, the material should try to explain how to pronounce the word and what the condition involves.

  Keep the terminology consistent.

  Use analogies, simple punctuation, contractions, and even slang if they increase patient understanding.
- *Design.* The type font should be big enough to be read easily. Avoid fancy typefaces and long stretches of text in italic type or all in capital letters. Readability is increased with white space (generous margins, blank lines between sections, etc.) and subheadings. A ragged right margin is usually more readable than an even one.
- *Illustrations.* Illustrations usually help those with poor reading skills and are generally easier to remember than text. But a bad illustration can wreck an otherwise excellent patient education handout. The words in the illustration must match the words in the written material. The reader should be able to understand the illustrations without having to read the written material. Illustrations should be simple and suited to your target audience
- *Content.* Simply put, content must be accurate, up-to-date, and consistent with what is being taught. When you are reviewing or writing the materials ask yourself these questions:
  - Is the benefit of the information clear to the reader?
  - Is too much detail provided or too little?
- *Patient management.* Make sure the materials always include specific advice to help patients understand when they should (and should not) seek medical attention.
- *Balance.* Ask yourself whether the content respects diverse cultural and religious views and avoids bias. Does it present information about treatment objectively, address both sides of controversial issues, and explain positive and negative aspects of procedures?
- *Source.* Review how the material content might have been influenced by its source. Look into who funded the piece, who endorsed it, and whether there is commercial interest in its content. If the information is not copyrighted, you can adapt the content to fit your needs. However, it is advisable to cite all sources and to give appropriate attribution when the origin of idea, concept, or material is not yours. Educators must always be cognizant of possible plagiarism, copyright infringement, and violation of intellectual property even when a copyright is not apparent. It is better to be safe than sorry.

A benefit of providing education in the health care facility is that patients are introduced to the programs either as inpatients or as visitors, thus promoting the wellness goal that is typically aimed for in a health care facility's doctrine of care.

The value of a respiratory therapist's involvement in patient education is now being demonstrated with the 2011 push for acceptance and passage of the Medicare Respiratory Therapy Initiative (S 343/HR 941). This bill, once passed, will revise the Medicare law to permit qualified respiratory therapists to provide certain services, such as smoking cessation, asthma management, medication education, and inhaler training. These services will be provided to asthma, COPD, and other respiratory patients under the general supervision of a physician, but without the doctor present under Part B Medicare law

Inservice education is another avenue for the respiratory therapist as an educator. Most departments do not have the financial support to employ an individual to provide ongoing inservice education. This form of education is important to a progressive respiratory care department. By providing education within the department, practitioners can continually update their knowledge and perform at their highest levels of performance. In addition, many states require continuing education credits on an annual or biannual basis, and inservice education may assist respiratory therapists in meeting the requirements if they use the AARC's continuing education system. Also, agencies for accreditation of health care facilities (e.g., Joint Commission) and home care services typically require ongoing and documented continuing education. Inservice education should include, yet not be limited to, continuing education regarding:

- Technological advances
- New equipment
- Therapeutic advances
- Patient education materials
- Professional development
- Current safety standards and regulations
- Cost effectiveness

Programs for inservice education are designed the same way as patient education. The same AARC clinical practice guidelines noted earlier in this chapter are excellent resources for providing education within the department. The human resources for providing inservice education are vast and should include the medical director, department supervisors and therapists, and other health care professionals. Many respiratory therapists are fearful of providing education, yet it is a central part of their work on a daily basis. The fear typically comes from two sources:

- The belief that the educational process is too time-consuming and therefore impossible to get done.
- The lack of knowledge on how to provide patient education.

More and more educational programs now incorporate training development segments and educational practices for students; so the majority of respiratory therapists at least have the basic principles accomplished or available.

Another facet of inservice education is to include opportunities for respiratory therapists to become involved in teaching other areas of patient care as well. Respiratory therapists should actively educate other health care professions to improve others' understanding of patient procedures and to improve working relationships among all patient care areas. For example, instruction to radiologic technologists about oxygen administration may decrease the number of times patients wind up off their required oxygen. This approach can ultimately improve patient education because the other health care professionals can champion the therapeutic modalities patients might receive during their care.

PATIENT EDUCATION RESOURCES

Table 40-2 shows contact information for organizations with a great variety of educational materials available. In addition to this list, an educator can locate multiple organizations by searching the Internet for specifics. Do not hesitate to contact these organizations because they have many resources and materials already developed and ready to incorporate into any program.

Best Practice

Promoting Inservice Education

To promote inservice education within a respiratory care department, a committee should be formed to review the types of education provided in the past and to ascertain whether the education accomplished any goals. For each instructional unit, goals and objectives should be developed and an assessment verifying that learning took place. Delegating topics among peers is bound to produce involvement and interest. Additionally, if therapists are fearful, bring in an educator from a local college to present topics to allay fears and to promote sound educational presentations.

TABLE 40-2 Resources for patient education materials

American Association for Respiratory Care
Phone: (972) 243-2272
Internet address: http://www.aarc.org

American Association of Cardiovascular and Pulmonary Rehabilitation
Phone: (312) 321-5146
Internet address: http://www.aacvpr.org

American Association of Critical Care Nurses
Phone: (949) 362-2050
Internet address: http://www.aacn.org

American Cancer Society
Phone: (404) 320-3333
Internet address: http://www.cancer.org

American College of Allergy, Asthma, and Immunology
Phone: (800) 842-7777
Internet address: http://www.acaai.org

American College of Chest Physicians
Phone: (847) 498-1400
Internet address: http://www.chestnet.org

American Health Care Association
Phone: (202) 842-4444
Internet address: http://www.ahca.org

American Heart Association
Phone: (214) 373-6300
Internet address: http://www.americanheart.org

American Lung Association
Phone: (800) LUNG USA
Internet address: http://www.lungusa.org

American Medical Association
Phone: (312) 464-5000
Internet address: http://www.ama-assn.org

American Public Health Association
Phone: 202-789-5600
Internet address: http://www.apha.org

American Sleep Apnea Association
Phone: (202) 293-3650
Internet address: http://www.sleepapnea.org

American Sleep Disorders Association
Phone: (507) 285-4386
Internet address: http://www.asda.org

American Thoracic Society
Phone: (212) 315-8700
Internet address: http://www.thoracic.org

Asthma and Allergy Foundation of America
Phone: (800) 7-ASTHMA
Internet address: http://www.aafa.org

Center for Health Promotion and Education
Centers for Disease Control
Phone: 404-639-3311
Internet address: http://www.cdc.gov

Foundation for Hospice and Home Care
Phone: (202) 547-7424
Internet address: http://www.nahc.org

Gerontological Society of America
Phone: (202) 842-1275
Internet address: http://www.geron.org

The Institute for Healthcare Advancement
Phone: (800) 434-4633
E-mail address: info@iha4health.org

The Joint Commission
Phone: (630) 792-5000
Internet Address: http://www.jcaho.org

National Association for Home Care
Phone: (202) 547-7424
Internet address: http://www.nahc.org

National Asthma Education and Prevention Program
Phone: (301) 251-1222
Internet address: http://www.nhlbi.nih.gov/about/naepp

National Council of Patient Information and Education
Phone: 202-347-6711
Internet address: http://www.talkaboutrx.org/about_mem_app.jsp

National Heart, Lung, and Blood Institute
Phone: (301) 251-1222
Internet address: http://www.nhlbi.nih.gov

National Long-Term Care Resource Center
Phone: (612) 624-5171
Internet address: http://www.nccnhr.org/

National Lung Health Education Program
Phone: 972-910-8555
Internet address: http://www.ncbi.nlm.nih.gov/pubmed/15165302

Office of Disease Prevention and Health Promotion
Phone: (202) 205-8611
Internet address: http://odphp.oash.dhhs.gov

Tobacco Information and Prevention Source
Centers for Disease Control and Prevention
Phone: (770) 488-5705
Internet address: http://www.cdc.gov/tobacco

Summary

When properly developed and delivered, patient education is a valuable tool that may reduce a patient's length of hospitalization and number of hospital stays, improve the quality of life, and increase the knowledge level of the patient and the respiratory therapist. Although the process may be complex, respiratory therapists should involve themselves in assessing patient needs, developing educational materials, providing support to patients, and assessing the success of intervention. Falvo summarizes patient education as being a patient right as well as a professional responsibility.[1] Educational materials developed with patient interest at heart and with the ideology of changing behaviors can deliver results in overall improvement in health care.

Study Questions

REVIEW QUESTIONS

1. What are the three components in the educational process?
2. Write a simple goal for educating a patient about a pulse oximeter.
3. What type of verb is essential for objective writing? Discuss why.
4. List three components important to communication.
5. Describe two reasons a patient may not be compliant after receiving instruction.
6. List the sites where a respiratory therapist may take on the role of a patient educator.
7. What are the AARC clinical practice guidelines that are useful in patient education?

MULTIPLE-CHOICE QUESTIONS

1. Patient education can be defined as:
   a. providing instruction to a patient.
   b. a change in patient behavior, attitude, or knowledge.
   c. developing goals and objectives for instruction.
   d. an individual process of learning.
2. Modalities specifically relevant to education are:
   I. auditory
   II. visual
   III. psychic
   IV. kinesthetic
   a. I, II, and IV
   b. II, III, and IV
   c. I, II, and III
   d. I, III, and IV
3. When developing objectives, action verbs help determine what the learner is to accomplish by the end of a learning unit. Which of the following is not classified as an action verb?
   a. demonstrate
   b. define
   c. think
   d. list
4. What is a goal?
   a. a set of objectives
   b. a measurement used to signal completion of a task
   c. a complex list of instructions
   d. a single end result
5. What is an objective?
   a. a single end result
   b. a declarative statement used to measure the success of a plan
   c. a declarative statement that directs learners toward a specific goal
   d. a nonsubjective way to evaluate a patient
6. Which of the following are true about learning outcomes?
   I. They demonstrate patient achievement.
   II. Measurement of outcomes can occur at any predetermined time.
   III. They verify patient understanding.
   IV. They help in determining the effectiveness of the original instruction.
   a. I, II, III, and IV
   b. I, II, and IV only
   c. II and III only
   d. I, II, and III only
7. The stage of learning where the patient may not be aware or even considering a change is called:
   a. contemplative.
   b. action.
   c. maintenance.
   d. precontemplative.
8. Which of the following is *not* considered a general goal of patient education?
   a. control of symptoms
   b. promotion of health and well-being
   c. reduced anxiety
   d. eliminate physician office visits

CRITICAL-THINKING QUESTIONS

1. A patient is constantly being admitted for reversible bronchospasm. This patient has received patient education about peak flowmeters and metered-dose inhalers, yet he does not seem to understand the concept. The physician would like

the RT to instruct the patient again. How might the RT deal with this patient scenario?

2. What steps might an RT take to develop a program for children with asthma for a health fair?
3. How would a respiratory therapist determine the modalities of his or her peers for inservice education?

References

1. Falvo DR. *Effective Patient Education: A Guide to Increased Compliance.* 3rd ed. Sudbury, MA: Jones & Bartlett Publishers; 2004.
2. Knowles MS. The modern practice of adult education: Pedagogy to andragogy. Boston: Cambridge Books; 1988.
3. Prochaska JO, DiClemente CC. Towards a comprehensive model of change. In: Miller WR, Heather N, eds. *Treating Addictive Behaviors—Process of Change*. New York: Plenum Press; 1986;3–27.
4. American Association of Respiratory Care. Clinical practice guidelines: providing patient and caregiver training. *Respir Care.* 1996;41:658–663.
5. American Association of Respiratory Care. Clinical practice guideline, training the health-care professional for the role of patient and caregiver educator. *Respir Care.* 1996;41:654–657.

Suggested Readings

Abbott S. The benefits of patient education. *Gastroenterol Nurs*. 1998;21:207–209.

Abbott S. A patient education notebook. Caregiver resources. *Home Care Provid*. 1998;3:258–259.

Aldridge MD. Writing and designing readable patient education materials. *Nephrol Nurs J*. 2004;31,4: 373–377.

Barbe W, Swassing R. *Teaching Through Modality Strengths*. Columbus, OH: Zaner-Bloser; 1988.

Bastable, SB, *Essentials of Patient Education: A Practical Approach*. Sudbury, MA: Jones & Bartlett Learning; 2006.

Bateman W, ed. *Patient and Family Education in Managed Care and Beyond: Seizing the Teachable Moment*. New York: Springer; 1999.

Bee HL. *The Journal of Adulthood*. 3rd ed. Englewood Cliffs, NJ: Prentice Hall; 1996.

Belda T. Computers in Patient Education and Monitoring. *Respir Care*. 2004;49(5):480–487.

Bergeron B. Where to find practical patient education materials. Empowering your patients without spending a lot of time and money. *Postgrad Med*. 1999; 106:35–38.

Blonshine S. Patient education: the key to asthma management. *Home Care Provid*. 1998;3:153–159.

Brown A. Improving patient and family education through diagnosis-driven protocols and documentation. *Nurs Qual Connect*. 1995;5:28–29.

Burton GG, Hodgkin JE, Ward J, eds. *Respiratory Care: A Guide to Clinical Practice.* 4th ed. Philadelphia: Lippincott Williams & Wilkins; 1997.

Campbell A, Iacono J, Aleksandrowicz A. *Patient and Family Education: The Compliance Guide to the JCAHO Standards.* Marblehead, MA: Opus Communications; 1997.

Clay J, Wyatt L, Norris G. Patient and family education: an interdisciplinary process. *Medsurg Nur.* 1996;5:333–338, 354.

Coates VE. *Education for Patients and Clients (Routledge Essentials for Nurses)*. New York: Routledge; 1999.

Cook L, Castrogiovanni A, David D, Stephenson DW, Dickson M, Smith D, Bonney A. Patient education documentation: is it being done? *Medsurg Nurs.* 2008 Oct;17,5:306–10.

Curtis M. Commentary: patient education presentations. *Am J Med Qual*. 1998;13:164–165.

Davidhizar R, Bechtel G, Dowd S. Patient education: a mandate for health care in the 21st century. *J Nucl Med Techno*. 1998;26:235–241.

Day J. Why should patients do what we ask them to do? *Patient Educ Couns*. 1995;26:113–118.

Desmond J. Copeland L. *Communicating with Today's Patient: Essentials to Save Time, Decrease Risk, and Increase Patient Compliance*. Hoboken, NJ: Jossey-Bass; 2000.

Di Lima SN, ed. *Chronic Disease Patient Education Manual*. Greenwood Village, CO: Aspen; 1998.

Doak CC, Doak LG, Root JH. *Teaching Patients with Low Literacy Skills.* 2nd ed. Philadelphia, PA: Lippincott Williams & Wilkins; 1995.

Dolinar RR, Kumar V, Coutu-Wakulczyk G, Rowe B. Pilot study of a home based asthma health education program. *Patient Educ Couns*. 2000;40:93–102.

Fink J. Identifying asthma patient education materials that support National Heart, Lung and Blood Institute guidelines. *Chest*. Supp. 1999;116, 1:195S–196S.

Fisher E. Low literacy levels in adults: implications for patient education. *J Contin Educ Nurs*. 1999; 30:56–61.

Gallefoss F, Bakke P. How does patient education and self-management among asthmatics and patients with chronic obstructive pulmonary disease affect medication? *Am J Respir Crit Care Med*. 1999;160:2000–2005.

Gallefoss F, Bakke P, Rsgaard P. Quality of life assessment after patient education in a randomized controlled study on asthma and chronic obstructive pulmonary disease. *Am J Respir Crit Care Med*. 1999;159:812–817.

Gershenson T, Quon H, Somerville S, Cohn E. Tilling the soil: nurturing the seeds of patient and family education. *J Nurs Care Qual.* 1999;13:83–91.

Gulledge J, Beard S, eds. *Asthma Management: Clinical Pathways, Guidelines, and Patient Education* (Aspen Chronic Disease Management Series). Greenwood Village, CO: Aspen; 1999.

Haworth K, ed. *Patient Teaching Made Incredibly Easy!* Springhouse, PA: Springhouse; 1998.

Hutchings D. Partnership in education: an example of client and educator collaboration. *J Contin Educ Nurs.* 1999;30:128–131.

It's on paper, but do they understand it? *RN.* 1999;62:24.

Jones M. *Asthma Self-Management Patient Education. Respir Care.* 2008;53,6:778–784.

Kanzer-Lewis G. *Patient Education: You Can Do It!* Alexandria, VA: American Diabetes Association;2003.

Lawrence KE, Di Lima SN, Niemeyer S, eds. *Home Health Care Patient Education Manual.* Greenwood Village, CO: Aspen; 1994.

Leaffer T, Gonda B. The Internet: an underutilized tool in patient education. *Computer Nursing.* 2000;18:47–52.

London F, Miller CJ. *No Time to Teach! A Nurse's Guide to Patient and Family Education.* Philadelphia, PA: Lippincott, Williams & Wilkins; 1999.

Longe M, Thomas K. *Consumer Health Resource Centers: A Guide to Successful Planning and Implementation.* Chicago, IL: American Hospital Association; 1998.

Lorig K. *Patient Education: A Practical Approach.* Thousand Oaks, CA: Sage; 2004.

McConnell E. Myths and facts about adult patient education. *Nursing.* 1999;29:81.

Meyers D. *Client Teaching Guides for Home Health Care.* 2nd ed. Greenwood Village, CO: Aspen; 1997.

Muma RD, Lyons BA, Newman T, contributor. *Patient Education: A Practical Approach.* New York: McGraw-Hill; 1996.

Murtagh J. *Patient Education.* 5th ed. Macquarie Park, N.S.W.: McGraw-Hill; 2008.

Myerscough P, Ford M. *Talking with Patients: Keys to Good Communication.* 3rd ed. New York: Oxford University Press; 1996.

Neitch S, ed. *Becoming a Clinician: A Primer for Students.* New York: McGraw; 1998.

Palmerini J, Jasovsky D. Patient education: a guide for success. *Nurs Manager.* 1998;29:45–46.

Patient Education (Healthcare Professional Guides). Springhouse, PA: Springhouse; 1997.

Patient education program. *Can Fam Physician.* 1998.

Patyk M, Gaynor S, Verdin J. Patient education resource assessment: project management. *Nurs Care Qual.* 2000;14:14–20.

Pestonjee SF. *Nurse's Handbook of Patient Education.* Springhouse, PA: Springhouse; 1999.

Peyrot M. Behavior change in diabetes education. *Diabetes Educ.* Supp. 1999;25,6:62–73.

Ragland G. *Instant Teaching Treasures for Patient Education.* St. Louis, MO: Mosby-Yearbook; 1996.

Rankin S, Stallings K. *Patient Education: Issues, Principles, Practices.* Philadelphia, PA: Lippincott, Williams & Wilkins; 1996.

Redmond B. Advances in Patient Education. New York City: Springer; 2004.

Redman BK, ed. *Measurement Tools in Patient Education.* New York: Springer; 1997.

Redman BK. *The Practice of Patient Education.* 8th ed. St. Louis, MO: Mosby-Yearbook; 1996.

Rice R. Implementing patient education in the home: concepts and teaching strategies. *Geriatr Nurs.* 1999;20:110, 112.

Sheldon J. Patient education: adding to quality of care. *Am J Hosp Palliat Care.* 1998;15:239–242.

Smith S. Patient education for decision making: more important now than ever! *Insight. 1998;*23:41–42.

Sparks-Langer G, Pasch M, Starko A, Moody A. *Teaching as Decision Making: Successful Practices for the Secondary Teacher.* Upper Saddle River, NJ: Prentice Hall; 1999.

Tomita M, Takabayashi K, Honda M, et al. Computer assisted instruction on multimedia environment for patients. *Medinfo.* 1995;2:1192.

Wilson, M. Readability and patient education materials used for low-income populations. *Clin Nurse Spec.* 2009;23,1:33–40.

CHAPTER 41

Management of Respiratory Care Services

George W. Gaebler

OBJECTIVES

Upon completion of this chapter, the reader should be able to:

- Identify typical management principles as they apply to respiratory care.
- Describe the various management and leadership roles in respiratory care.
- Explain the diversity of services provided by respiratory care departments.
- Identify the normal patterns of work typical of the modern respiratory care department.
- Understand the basic concepts of budgeting and financial operation for respiratory care.
- Understand the basic concepts of human resource management, recruitment, interviewing, evaluation, and retention of respiratory care personnel.
- Identify the basic reporting standards and benchmarking used in health care management.
- Identify computer applications commonly used in department operations.
- Define basic reimbursement terms and methods common to health care.

CHAPTER OUTLINE

(continues)

(continued)

KEY TERMS

capital budget
diagnosis-related groups (DRGs)
human resource management
interdisciplinary
managed care
medical director
operational budget
performance improvement
resource utilization groups (RUGs)
staffing
uniform reporting standards

Management and leadership activities for respiratory care are among the most dynamic and challenging found in management science. Reasons for the dynamic nature of all health care management are related to reimbursement, controversies in health policy, relationship of physicians to operations, and the changing scope of services found in the respiratory care arena.

Respiratory care began as small groups of patient care providers who were first designated as inhalation therapists. This title persisted as a designation until the early 1970s when the professional designation was changed to respiratory therapy. During the 1980s the designation changed again to respiratory care. Respiratory care departments with such names as cardiopulmonary or cardiorespiratory care usually include cardiology diagnostic activities within the department's scope of responsibility. The profession's name changes were necessitated by the ever evolving nature of patient care activities under the responsibility of the typical respiratory care department.

This chapter identifies the operational responsibilities, reporting relationships, financial relationships, multidisciplinary nature of contemporary respiratory care, and the common management techniques found to coordinate these activities. In addition, this chapter covers some of the contemporary information management activities typically found in today's respiratory care department. Maybe most important to the current respiratory care student, however, is the discussion of professional and personal responsibilities that should be the model for the everyday activities of the current respiratory care professional. The role and history of the growth of the profession can be directly attributed to activities related to the American Association for Respiratory Care (AARC), which is the organization built by, and for, the profession of respiratory care (see Chapter 1).

Key Definitions, Concepts, and Professional Standards

This section introduces key definitions and concepts.

HUMAN RESOURCE MANAGEMENT

Human resource management activity creates the human resource that provides direct and indirect patient care in the profession. Effective recruitment, retention, education, evaluation, motivation, and reward systems in respiratory care human resource management provide the lifeblood for all sites of practice.

MEDICAL DIRECTION OR MEDICAL DIRECTOR

The profession of respiratory care has consistently been practiced under the guidance of physicians with specific interests in the art, science, and management of respiratory diseases. The **medical director** is the individual who has direct responsibility for the quality of patient care. Typically, the respiratory care medical director is from a subspecialist group in internal medicine known as *pulmonary physicians* or *pulmonologists*. However, the respiratory care medical director could be from several other areas of medical practice including anesthesia, critical care medicine, internal medicine, pediatrics, or surgery, provided there is a special interest in respiratory disease and treatment.

CLINICAL TIME STANDARDS

Sometimes called **uniform reporting standards** or benchmark standards, *clinical time standards* are the normal timed work units assigned to various activities performed by respiratory care departments. These standards are developed by direct observation of the average amount of time required to perform respiratory care duties with attention to a high degree of detail and accuracy. The significance of these standards is usually denoted by **staffing** plans that are tied directly to the number of timed work units performed in the average reporting period.

PERFORMANCE IMPROVEMENT

Performance improvement activities, commonly denoted by total quality management (TQM) or continuous quality improvement (CQI), are the quality measures used to track consistency and quality in the practice of respiratory care. True quality improvement functions denote systematic monitoring of high use and high morbidity activities with the intent to incrementally improve the quality over a period of time. Therefore, there is no right amount of quality. Professionals should continuously strive to improve systems and practices using a multidisciplinary format.

A recent development in this area is the use of Core Measures by the Centers for Medicare & Medicaid Services (CMS) as a direct measuring tool to compare care from organization to organization. By setting the expectations of, say, smoking cessation instruction and counseling by CMS for certain diagnoses such as acute myocardial infarction, there is new emphasis on quality in respiratory care departments. They are being compared to one another across regions and states. Similarly, the Joint Commission has moved to patient safety goals that measure certain expectations of care across all organizations to which they award accreditation.

INTERDISCIPLINARY

Interdisciplinary is the term referring to the use of professional and nonprofessional stakeholders in teams to make an impact on systems and practice. *Stakeholders* are those impacted by or involved with the commission of the team. The use of diverse or interdisciplinary teams of individuals to provide and analyze practice activities usually ensures better attention to all aspects of patient care.

AMERICAN ASSOCIATION FOR RESPIRATORY CARE

The AARC functions on a national and state level (in the form of chartered affiliates) to enhance, govern, guide, and nurture the practice of respiratory care. In addition, the AARC has several medical sponsors such as the American College of Chest Physicians, the American Society for Anesthesiology, the Society for Critical Care Medicine, and the American Thoracic Society. Many of the physicians currently practicing as medical directors for respiratory care come from one of these groups. Every respiratory therapist (RT) should consider membership in the AARC as a precursor to practice and evidence of dedication to the ideals of quality respiratory care practice.

CLINICAL PRACTICE GUIDELINES

The AARC develops and provides clinical practice guidelines (CPGs),[1] which are used throughout the profession for the provision for quality respiratory care. Nearly all clinical patient care providers are using evidence-based practice to reexamine their approaches. Evidence-based practice requires the weighting and grading of research literature to provide increased emphasis on systematically controlled studies that are randomized with little or no false positive or negative results.

History, Professional, and Community Involvement in Respiratory Care

The dominant reason for the growth of the profession has been the presence of a solid base of operations in the form of the American Association for Respiratory Care and its leading members. For more than 50 years, the AARC has provided the leadership, guidance, public forum, and example for new members in the profession. The AARC has been a solid contributor to the profession's growth because of the quality of the members who serve the profession in tireless pursuit of excellence in education, research, leadership, and clinical patient care. The AARC has provided the professional medium to guide the profession, but only through continuous development of new voluntary leaders who guide the profession from year to year. The future growth of the profession depends on the entry of new professional volunteers who can perpetuate legacy of the pioneers in the profession.

It has been shown repeatedly that professional respiratory therapists who are involved in the activities of their profession find solutions to patient care and educational dilemmas that others do not. Respiratory therapists should consider membership in the AARC and therefore in their local state society as an essential ingredient for their professional maturation and growth. Furthermore, membership should always be accompanied by volunteered time and expertise to service in the local, state, and national portions of the association. The profession is not old historically; however, its long-term sustained growth may be directly attributed to pioneer respiratory therapists who gave their time on weekdays, weeknights, and weekends to attend to the legislative, educational, political, and research activities of the association. Without this long-term tireless activity, the profession may have been consumed by an onslaught of other areas seeking portions of the respiratory care function. Only a short time ago, the first state-chartered affiliate announced that licensure had become a reality. Today, professional initiatives have succeeded in bringing about professional licensure for 49 states and territories of the United States.

Many new respiratory care professionals explain that they are not involved as volunteers because they feel they have nothing to contribute. Nothing could be further from the truth. The profession continues its sustained growth only when newcomers become involved and learn the attributes that they sense they do not have early in their careers. The state and national presenters or leaders who many view with high regard were once new graduates.

Attendance at professional seminars for continuing respiratory care education should be considered not only when an employer pays, but also as a normal sacrifice for the personal growth in career and knowledgeability.

COMMUNITY INVOLVEMENT

Respiratory care professionals should also extend their professional activity to the community, even after the work shift is completed. Many RTs have indicated that social services such as respiratory care carry a different level of dedication for success and the satisfaction of a job well done. Respiratory care has always carried a higher responsibility in the form of off-shift, weekend, and holiday workdays that most never endure in their chosen profession. It requires dedication to and a central focus on the professional ideals of service and dedication to patients. Respiratory care professionals should be involved in community health and wellness activities that allow them to offer public service beyond the work site. New respiratory care professionals may be homegrown through volunteer activities such as the Boy Scouts of America Coed Explorer Program, which introduces highly motivated high school students to health professions. In New York, the Board of Cooperative Education has a special program, called New Visions, that allows high school seniors the opportunity to spend most of their last year before college in the hospital, nursing home, and home care environments. This allows motivated students the opportunity to study possible professional careers from a shadowing first-hand perspective. Check your home state for similar opportunities to introduce future colleagues to the profession.

Other community activities include health fairs and not-for-profit groups, such as the American Heart Association, that contribute to awareness of health issues. Respiratory therapists may become CPR instructors who volunteer time to teach groups in their hometown, thereby strengthening the tie to the profession and the community. The list of possible activities is limited only by the imagination.

Merriam-Webster's Collegiate Dictionary defines "profession" as "a calling requiring specialized knowledge and often long and intensive academic preparation."[2] This definition seems to sum up the need for continuous, career-long growth of the RT's command of the field.

Departmental Structure

The typical respiratory care department generally consists of a vertical management structure that includes overall reporting through a medical director and administrator who may have a designation of vice president for patient care or professional services. The direct, or line, responsibility for daily activities is through the vice president. Clinical reporting for quality of care is generally through the medical director for respiratory care. Respiratory care may be centralized, quasidecentralized, or decentralized under a service or product line structure.

- *Centralized* means the respiratory care department is an autonomous department within the hospital or nursing home.
- *Quasidecentralized* denotes that the department has a reporting structure that is in a centralized or matrix format with a strong professional identity for the autonomy of the department. The matrix format allows input to the respiratory care department for performance measurement of its staff.

- *Decentralized* denotes a structure whereby the respiratory care personnel report directly to a patient care area such as a nursing unit. This structure experienced growth in the early 1990s but declined in the late 1990s because the loss of professional identity resulted in a decrease in quality care provision. Cost issues were not a factor.

The quasidecentralized structure is preferred because it blends interdisciplinary patient care with a strong sense of professional identity. This structure is associated with a strong patient focus on customer service while maintaining a streamlined departmental structure that provides the highest quality for the lowest cost per timed work unit of care.

Most respiratory care departments are led by a manager, usually called the *technical director for respiratory care*, a title that reflects the difference between the medical director and this position. Larger departments in university or other large hospitals may have:

- An assistant director and several clinical supervisors to administer the day-to-day operations of the department.
- An equipment manager whose responsibility lies in the timely procurement, delivery, and availability of equipment and supplies for respiratory care.

Staff therapists report and are aligned under the clinical supervisors who provide the clinical guidance and expertise to the overall staff.

Most of the hospitals nationwide are found in the community hospital designation. Usually there are only:

- A technical director.
- One or no clinical supervisor.
- Clinical staff.

In a quasidecentralized department, the service line personnel may have input into the evaluation of therapists assigned to a particular area. In larger departments, clinical care teams may have been formed of which the respiratory therapist is a member. Whoever provides the patient care area with management and leadership may have a role in therapist evaluation through a matrix reporting structure.

COMMUNICATIONS

Communications are perhaps the most important aspect of any structural design, and the respiratory care department promotes extensive communications with other departments. The current trend toward interdisciplinary teams requires open, constant communications by and between departments. Regardless of the type of organizational structure, communications remain very important for the day-to-day operations of the organization.

Diversity of Respiratory Care Services

The education and technical know-how of the average respiratory therapist has led to a great deal of diverse responsibilities. Many sources cite that respiratory care departments have the department designation of cardiopulmonary or cardiorespiratory in more than 50% of all departments found in U.S. hospitals. Furthermore, in addition to hospitals, the site for respiratory care may include the home care setting, nursing homes, physicians' offices, clinics, and other sites. Expanding roles include asthma management through alternative sites that could be considered nontraditional for respiratory care personnel.[3] Additionally, some innovative respiratory care leaders have seized the opportunity to add highly skilled procedures such as arterial line insertion, thereby increasing the prestige for the respiratory therapist and sometimes improving outcomes as well.[4]

Respiratory care usually includes:

- Ventilator management.
- Oxygen.
- Hyperinflation.
- Aerosol and percussion or drainage therapies.
- Diagnostics, such as pulmonary function and arterial blood gas analysis.
- Blood chemistry where some departments use instrumentation with multiple functions.

In addition to respiratory care procedures, the cardiopulmonary designation usually means the addition of cardiology diagnostics such as:

- Electrocardiograms (ECGs).
- Echocardiography.
- Noninvasive vascular studies.
- Cardiac stress testing.
- To a lesser extent, angiocatheter and electrophysiology (EP) laboratories and electroencephalographic (EEGs) activities.

Increasingly, respiratory care personnel are involved with sleep medicine both in diagnostic laboratories and in treatment interventions such as continuous positive pressure ventilation (CPAP) or bilevel ventilation for use in the home care sector.

Home respiratory care activities usually entail the assessment, treatment, maintenance, and provision of various interventions outside the hospital or nursing home setting. The home care setting requires a completely different equipment design because of the absence of centralized oxygen delivery found in many nursing homes and all hospitals. Oxygen concentrators, oxygen cylinders, and liquid oxygen systems are employed in homes, depending on the required liter flow for the patient's needs.

In physician practice and clinic settings, respiratory care takes the form of disease management, most prominently asthma care. Continued growth is expected in disease management activities where respiratory therapists are becoming involved with managed care companies for the these purposes. See Appendix A for further discussion of this topic.

Operational Issues

The respiratory care department manager has to address a number of operational issues every day. Most of these issues involve the daily work assignment, using either a manual or automated information system, and departmental performance and productivity. Communications by and among respiratory therapists and other departments, such as nursing, have changed in many hospitals. Many still use pagers to communicate. However, there is growing use of hands-free communication devices such as those provided by companies like Vocera. These devices allow direct, fast, two-way communications between one or more individuals at the same time.

DAILY WORK ASSIGNMENT

Data-driven daily work assignments can be done by two means: manual paper systems and automated information system-driven assignments. Either type of system requires having a manual template. That template is best formed using a department work team comprised of individuals from management, staff, and clerical positions—a department-specific multidisciplinary team representing all the departments' staff. These teams are designed to brainstorm a manual system so that implementation of the automated system works effectively. In the design of that template, the team should use uniform reporting standards, such as those published by the AARC. Several consulting agencies use the AARC *Uniform Reporting Manual* as the basis for their timed work units also.[5] When these standards are combined with the AARC clinical practice guidelines, the quality of care and efficiency are addressed simultaneously, thereby accommodating the real needs of the current respiratory care department to document quality. The AARC CPGs are available through the AARC as well as through the National Guideline Clearinghouse (http://www.guideline.gov).[6]

PLANNING THE MANUAL SYSTEM

To create a manual system, a master file, such as in a database or spreadsheet program, is needed containing information as outlined in Figure 41-1. The reason is that, the main purpose of patient work assignment systems is to accurately predict the workload that may be expected to be accomplished in a prescribed period of time. The subsequent tracking of this data through information systems serves to legitimize staffing and productivity levels. Once a manual template is designed and accepted for use, a *manual assignment system* can be started up by determining the maximal workload for both 8- and 12-hour shift patterns. An example of the equation to determine potential productive work time for an 8 hour-shift without a paid lunch or dinner break is shown in Figure 41-2. In that example, all tasks assigned to each therapist per shift have to total 7.5 hours per scheduled shift for 8.5 hours, assuming 100% productivity. However, some time is always wasted time during a shift, such as travel time to and from work areas and moving contaminated

Modality	Department Timed Work Units	AARC Uniform Reporting Standard
Aerosol therapy initial		
Aerosol therapy subsequent		
Mechanical ventilator per shift		
Mechanical ventilator initiate		
Oxygen therapy per shift		
Oxygen therapy initiate		
Aerosol mist tent initiate		
Aerosol mist tent per shift		
Chest PT/PD initial		
Chest PT/PD subsequent		

FIGURE 41-1 Sample manual workload tool.

Shift Hours	−	Hospital Lunch Break	−	Hospital Mandatory Break	−	Report Activities	=	Maximum Productive Hours
8.5	−	0.5	−	0.25	−	0.25	=	7.5 hours per shift

Productive Hours	×	60 Minutes/Hour	×	90% Productivity	=	Maximum Timed Work Units Possible
7.5	×	60	×	90%	=	405 TWU possible per hour

FIGURE 41-2 Determination of potential productive time in an 8-hour shift.

equipment back to the decontamination area. Therefore, most departments plan for about 85–90% productivity as a benchmark target for department-wide function, as shown in the second example in Figure 41-2.

Given the type of information reflected in Figure 41-2, a *manual assignment form* is created that uses the maximal productive work time as a starting point and that keeps track of each patient assignment work unit prediction. The aim is to come to a reasonable work assignment for each therapist on each shift. Refer to Figure 41-3 for an example workload assignment with a maximum productivity of 90%. The work assignment example in Figure 41-3 has a few more work units than 90% productivity. However, the assignment is probably typical because the work units rarely come out right on the productivity target.

AUTOMATED INFORMATION SYSTEMS ASSIGNMENT DEVELOPMENT

The planning team prepares templates such as the examples in Figure 41-3 for a manual system. Once the manual templates are complete, functional members of the information system implementation team sets up the configuration, following the program's manufacturer requirements.

The planning team configuration data for a system such as MediLinks from MediServe Inc. allow the automatic printing of work assignments by the supervisor at the beginning of each shift. This is a large time-saving tool. In addition, the staff and supervisor may print new assignments every four hours or set up alert systems that indicate when new patient tasks being added to a therapist are exceeding work capacity and impossible to accomplish with the expected degree

Therapist Name	**Work Area**	**Date**	**Shift**	**Supervisor**	**Total Possible TWU**
Susan Thomas	IMCU	9/30/11	3-11	McDonald	405
Patient Name	**Room #**	**Treatment**	**Frequency**	**TWU**	**Total Time Required**
Sandra Smith	IMCU 1	Aer Ther Albuterol	q.4h	14	28 min
Sue Jones	IMCU 2	Aer Ther Albuterol	q.2h	14	56 min
James Stith	IMCU 4	Aer Ther Albuterol	q.6h	14	14 min
Monty Python	IMCU 5	Ventilator SIMV 800 × 11, PEEP +12, F_IO_2 .60, Press Support 8	Continuous	56	56 min
		Aer Ther Albuterol	q.3h	12	36 min
		Chest PT/PD	q.3h	17	51 min
Mina Murray	IMCU 6	Ventilator SIMV 650 × 14, PEEP +16, F_IO_2 .60, Press Support 6	Continuous	56	56 min
		Aer Ther Albuterol	q.4h	12	24 min
		Chest PT/PD	q.4h	17	34 min
Sherry Johnson	IMCU 7	Aer Ther Albuterol	q.2h	14	56 min
				Total Assigned TWU 411	

FIGURE 41-3 Sample workload assignment worksheet.

of accuracy and quality. (The sophistication of today's specialized respiratory care information systems is discussed later in the chapter.)

Clinical Competencies. State and national accrediting agencies, such as the Joint Commission, require written initial and periodic assessments of personnel work activities to ensure that therapists are performing their job duties in a safe and consistent manner. Consequently, there must be an assessment that an individual performs procedures consistently with policies specific to each work site, regardless of credentials and education. This oversight makes sense, because, for example, a newly hired therapist who is registered with 10 years of experience may know how to do the procedure at the last work site; however, entering a new institution may require familiarization with equipment with which the therapist may not be familiar.

Interdisciplinary Teams. Interdisciplinary teams are used in all contemporary health care organizations to perform many duties related to planning and quality improvement. The use of diverse professional and nonprofessional personnel to brainstorm ideas and to create new and more effective policies and procedures is a mainstream method of choice at present.

In the making of the team, diverse personalities need to be included, as well as differing backgrounds, to ensure that one or more individuals do not unduly influence the outcome or output of the group. The inclusion of many contributors to a team usually diminishes concerns that may arise about turf-related issues.

The leader of an interdisciplinary team may or may not be a member of management and leadership, depending on the target subject. The role of the team leader is to facilitate the process but not control either the process or outcome. The leader's role in a meeting may include:

- Assignment or transcription of meeting minutes.
- Timekeeping.
- Redirection when the group strays from the goal.
- Setting agenda and next meeting times.

In reality, anyone may become an informal leader for a meeting due to expertise or experience and then go back to a secondary role for the next meeting because of lack of knowledge or input on the new topic. Informal leaders are individuals whom the groups recognize as having the abilities to move a process forward regardless of their position in the organization. This style of team meetings for process and quality improvement is very common and desired because the output and outcome have a much broader perspective in the planning phases. This usually translates to a higher degree of success in implementation.

A major use of interdisciplinary teams is the planning of controversial change processes. Having many representatives of diverse groups allows the inclusion even of individuals who may be an impediment to the implementation of new ideas or policies. Inclusion of those with contra opinions enables them to be a part of the planning, and they usually support the new activity, outcome, or change in policy because of their involvement. Those who fail to support change diminish their credibility with their peers; including them is a widely used management and leadership tool in the change process, which usually follows the Lewin model, a popular change model consisting of three steps:

- Step 1: Unfreezing the individuals who are affected by leading them to recognize the need for change.
- Step 2: Implement the change so that it becomes part of the normal system.
- Step 3: Refreeze the process with the newly implemented change as the norm and reinforce where necessary.[7]

Interdisciplinary teams whose goal is creating major changes in process may also use a technique known as *force-field analysis*, described simply as the elimination of the forces against a process change while simultaneously tipping the scales toward the forces that favor the change.[7] Force-field analysis may be accomplished in teams through process improvements to a policy, procedure, or method that decrease concerns expressed in the feedback process of quality improvement. This may sound very involved, but it really is quite simple. Feedback mechanisms such as questionnaires may provide a multitude of clues about what should be addressed, thereby eliminating objections to the change.

Fiscal Issues

Two of the primary fiscal issues needing consideration are operating budget and capital budget.

OPERATING BUDGET

The operating budget in most respiratory care work environments is derived from historical data from previous fiscal years. The fiscal managers of any given health care work environment have the option of using *zero-based budgeting* or *historical trended budgeting* as a basis for the construction of the next fiscal year's budget. [Zero-based budgeting is where expense and income are balanced. Historical trended budgeting looks at past trends. At times, expenses and income do not match or balance, and budgets (usually on a quarterly basis) are designed to address these variations.] It may be assumed that most fiscal managers would prefer zero-based budgets because the department manager is forced to assume a starting position for all operational costs of zero, including all staffing models.

Strictly defined, the **operational budget** consists of all categories of expenses that are for nondepreciable items such as employee salaries, benefits, medical supplies, repairs, educational travel, and books. A department manager might want to track many different categories; so the variability of expense categories changes from organization to organization. An example of the cardiology section of a respiratory therapy budget summary is shown in Figure 41-4.

Staffing Plans. The staffing plan for a respiratory care work site should be derived from the management information system either in manual form or directly from the hospital or respiratory care specific system of timed work units (TWUs). Therefore, the staffing budget is derived based on the number of *full-time equivalents* (*FTEs*) that are required to provide care multiplied by the salaries for each individual providing that care. An example is shown in Figure 41-5.

Salaries are a significant portion of the typical respiratory care budget. As a general rule, manpower costs are 65–70% of all operating costs, including benefits.[7] Benefit costs vary from institution to institution, but they are generally 22–33% of salaries depending on the type of institution. A state institution is generally on the high end due to state subsidies, whereas a small community hospital may be on the low end due to a lack of subsidies. Obviously, pressures to hold costs at reasonable levels usually center on salaries, because so much of the overall cost of operations are found in this one area of the budget.

Another observation from Figure 41-5 is the variation in increases that must be budgeted for each individual. The variation in percentage is due to the reality that each employee receives an increase at a different month; so the effect may vary on overall salary increases. In the example, the reader may assume that each employee is going to receive a 4% increase but budgets at 2% of salary because the increase is scheduled for six months into the fiscal year.

Supply Costs. *Supply costs* are all other usual budget items except capital that are found in respiratory care budgets. Medical supplies budgeting benefits greatly from trended information: the previous year's costs, the current fiscal year's year-to-date costs, and the projected patient care days or admissions. The finance department provides all of this information based on assumptions that the administration has derived from other statistical indicators of the operations of the hospital or other work site.

The two basic methods of tracking non-salary-operating expenses are based on the organization's philosophy of a higher or lesser degree of detail. The more expense categories in the budget, the more easily the manager can track variations in specific costs. Some organizations find the detail cumbersome, however, and may track on only a macro level with general categories. This variation should be expected from one organization to another. A supplies budget example is found in Figure 41-6.

Management needs to describe why actual cost variances exceed expected costs when projecting the budget as well as why current year-to-date costs are far ahead of the previous fiscal year. An example from Figure 41-6 is the office supplies amount, which is running ahead of the previous year's. This sort of activity might be related to increased computer usage and therefore increased paper and printing cartridge costs. Recently, new methods of comparison use cost-per-unit as a method for comparison of costs over time. This allows a manager to divide total procedures by total salary and benefit costs and get a quick snapshot of human resource costs over time. The same can be used for costs associated with supplies.

CAPITAL BUDGET

Capital budgets account for items that are stationary, like buildings or renovations, and for fixed and movable large equipment, such as ventilators and pulmonary function systems, that have a useful life of greater than 5 years. Therefore, an organization might define all equipment that costs over $500 and has a useful life of more than 5 years as capital equipment. Capital equipment costs are not contained in the operating budget. In reality, for accounting purposes, all permanent equipment like oxygen regulators and carts could be put in the capital budget because they are used for a number of years before replacement. The level of the budget's specificity depends greatly on the philosophy of the organization and probably its financial leadership personnel. Capital equipment has some advantage over operational equipment due to complex reimbursement formulas that are beyond the scope of this chapter. The major point is that, in general terms, a health care organization such as a hospital or nursing home seeks to capitalize as much equipment as possible for finance purposes.

Purchasing Groups. Many health care organizations belong to purchasing groups that have greater buying

University Hospital
Anywhere, USA
Respiratory Therapy
3630
Budget Summary

	Actual 2007/2008	Actual 2008/2009	Budget 2009/2010	Annualized Actual 2009/2010	Budget Projection 2010/2011	% Variance
Statistical Summary:						
IP Statistic	365,331	287,259	372,217	298,447	**372,217**	24.7%
OP Statistic	3,349	2,749	3,543	2,479	**2,479**	0.0%
Total Statistic	368,680	290,008	375,760	300,926	**374,696**	24.5%
IP Statistic - Departmental	0	0	0	0	**0**	0.0%
OP Statistic - Departmental	0	0	0	0	**0**	0.0%
Total Statistic - Departmental	0	0	0	0	**0**	0.0%
Gross Revenue:						
IP Revenue	($6,793,238)	($5,516,024)	($7,163,938)	($5,865,336)	**$7,163,938**	0.0%
OP Revenue	(73,230)	(58,938)	(75,376)	(51,667)	**(51,667)**	0.0%
Other Revenue	0	0	0	0	**0**	0.0%
Total Gross Revenue	($6,866,468)	($5,574,962)	($7,239,314)	($5,917,003)	**$7,112,271**	0.0%
Expenses:						
Salaries and Wages	$1,609,446	$1,655,606	$1,754,016	$1,796,479	**$1,978,663**	10.1%
Employee Benefits	525,680	490,434	519,192	541,998	**596,963**	10.1%
Professional Fees	4,873	1,192	3,996	4,724	**4,724**	0.0%
Medical and Surgical Supplies	126,328	152,139	165,984	132,735	**132,735**	0.0%
Nonmedical Supplies	71,943	149,632	74,999	110,641	**110,642**	0.0%
Purchased Services	26,897	171,154	42,078	61,346	**42,078**	−31.4%
Other Expenses	6,430	7,779	13,320	16,976	**16,976**	0.0%
Leases/Rentals	1,277	1,304	4,500	4,722	**4,722**	0.0%
Interest	0	0	0	0	**0**	0.0%
Total Expenses	$2,372,874	$2,629,241	$2,578,085	$2,669,622	**$2,887,502**	8.2%
Hours/FTEs:						
Total Paid Hours	88,881	90,885	106,580	85,144	**109,879**	29.1%
Total FTEs	42.7	43.7	51.2	40.9	**52.8**	29.1%
Authorized Signature:						

FIGURE 41-4 Sample respiratory care budget.

Staff Name	Title	FTE	Salary	Expected Increase	Total Salary
Jill Jones	Manager	1.0	$47,474	3.0%	$48,898
Malmud Singh	Staff Ther.	1.0	$33,129	4.0%	$34,454
Bonnie McClusky	Staff Ther.	1.0	$34,152	3.0%	$35,177
Heather Ryan	Staff Ther.	1.0	$27,399	2.0%	$27,947
Sam Killias	Staff Ther.	0.5	$14,873	4.0%	$15,468
Pam Howard	Staff Ther.	0.4	$13,980	3.0%	$14,399
Joe Fellows	Clerk	1.0	$18,341	2.0%	$18,708
Totals		**5.9 FTEs**	**$189,348**	**3.0%**	**$194,051**

FIGURE 41-5 Sample salary worksheet.

Non-Salary Expenses	YTD 2009	2010 Actual	Projected Increase	2011 Projection
Medical Supplies	$112,454	$144,577	4%	$155,936
Repairs	$8,372	$12,131	4%	$11,609
Office Supplies	$1,233	$1109	4%	$1,644
Education/Travel	$3,167	$4,190	4%	$4,223
Books/Magazines	$438	$521	4%	$584
Totals	**$125,664**	**$162,528**	**4%**	**$173,996**

FIGURE 41-6 Sample supplies budget.

power than a single organization does. Entry into purchasing groups may be through local or state hospital association groups or through membership in for-profit or not-for-profit hospital councils. Purchasing groups generally require membership dues that are paid to buy group rights and thereby guarantee savings that more than offset the cost of the dues. In addition, the purchasing groups may offer rebate programs:

- By pooling product purchase and offering additional savings in the form of steeper discounts.
- For equipment and supplies based on purchasing levels.

The latter form of purchasing inducement is fairly common in respiratory care purchasing groups. To secure rebates, the purchaser usually has to declare purchasing levels that must be achieved to meet quotas based on lower contract pricing. The hospital receives lower up-front costs for goods such as medical equipment through the purchasing group's contract pricing structure. At the end of each reporting period, the manufacturer reports the rebate dollars available to the hospital or nursing home based on the previous year's purchase levels. The institution may then use the rebate money to purchase products like oximeters at list price.

Figure 41-7 shows an example of a rebate profile. The more a facility purchases in the example in Figure 41-7, the higher the rebate it is entitled to. In reality, the dollar break levels shown in Figure 41-7 for different percentage rebates are probably higher. For

Contract Purchasing Rebate Profile		
$ 0–5,000 per year	=	0.5% rebate
$ 5,001–10,000 per year	=	1% rebate
$10,001–15,000 per year	=	1.5% rebate
$15,001–20,000 per year	=	2% rebate
$20,000–25,000 per year	=	3% rebate
$25,001–30,000 per year	=	4% rebate

FIGURE 41-7 Sample rebates for contract purchasing.

example, the rebate calculation for purchases of \$28,970 are \$28,970 × 0.04 = \$1,158.80. The purchasing hospital may purchase \$1,158.80 from the company in goods or services without an exchange of dollars due to the applied rebate. Thus, the normal purchasing creates more buying power through applied rebates.

Still another savings mechanism is the application of higher contract discount percentages as the buying increases. In the example shown in Figure 41-7, there may be increasing discounts on the purchased products in addition to higher rebates for higher volumes of sales.

Capital budget planning involves short- and long-range planning in the form of one-year purchase requests and a 2- to 5-year purchasing plan that would vary based on updates each successive year. Considerations about many costs and projections of care changes should occur before any equipment is considered. The purchase requests for year one require justification that should include those shown in Table 41-1.

TABLE 41-1 **Capital considerations**

Cost Considerations	Technology Advances
Cost savings	Patient care time savings
Increased revenues	Increased effectiveness
Lower operating costs	New tests
Lower life cycle costs	Portability
Company viability projections	New procedures
Software upgrade costs	Long-range technology changes
Service contract costs	Time before obsolete
Parts costs	
Repair costs	
Implementation costs	
Staff education costs	

In Figure 41-8, budget years 2 and 3 are for forecasting only, to be used by the finance department for planning purposes based on equipment obsolescence and increasing technology advancements. Also, note that in year 3, flowmeters do not cost more than \$500 for each unit; however, many times these types of equipment are aggregated to break the capital budget threshold.

Reimbursement

Payment for health care services has changed significantly since the 1980s. Some of the major developments regarding reimbursement for the delivery of health care include prospective payment through diagnostic-related groups (DRGs) or resource utilization groups (RUGs) and the advent of managed care. The manager of any respiratory care service should be thoroughly familiar with these and other reimbursement systems.

DIAGNOSIS-RELATED GROUPS AND RESOURCE UTILIZATION GROUPS

In the hospital and nursing home area of respiratory care management, there are fixed payment systems called **diagnosis-related groups (DRGs)** for hospitals and **resource utilization groups (RUGs)** for nursing homes. At present, these payment systems are only for inpatient activities; however, the Centers for

Capital Budget

Year 1 Requests:

1. 2 Hamilton Galileo Ventilators @ \$26,000 = \$52,000
2. 4 Wright Respirometers @ \$900 = \$3,600
3. 2 Ohmeda Pediatric Aerosol Tents @ \$3,000 = \$6,000
4. 2 Nellcor Puritan Bennett Oximeters @ \$1,200 = \$2,400

Long-Range Capital Budget

Year 2:

1. 2 Hamilton Galileo Ventilators
2. 1 ABL Blood Gas Instrument
3. 2 Nellcor Puritan Bennett Oximeters

Year 3:

1. 2 Hamilton Galileo Ventilators
2. 2 Ohmeda Pediatric Aerosol Tents
3. 1 Sensormedics PFS system
4. 25 Timeter Oxygen Flowmeters

FIGURE 41-8 Sample capital budget.

Medicare & Medicaid Services (CMS) is currently in the process of converting outpatient care reimbursement to a prospective or capped payment system based on historical trends gathered from past activity. The introduction of these payment methodologies has caused most respiratory care work sites to view operations as an added patient care expense, not as a revenue producer.

All these changes have taken place since 1983 when the DRG system for Medicare payment went into effect nationwide. The DRG system for prospective payment was developed in response to health care costs that escalated faster than inflation for many years in the Medicare system. There are many reasons for cost growth rates that exceeded inflation, but in simple terms the design of the original program promoted growth in programs in hospitals with reimbursement based on overall spending. This reimbursement methodology actually promoted increased costs and therefore faster growth in costs to the Medicare system.

In New York, for example, the state government has adopted an all-payer DRG system whereby insurance and managed care payments are derived by the Medicare payment schedules. Even patients who self-pay their entire bill are not paying the charges on the bill but instead a derived figure, based on the all-payer DRG system. This was done in part through a waiver for the Medicare system that allowed states to follow the Medicare system but also to exceed Medicare initiatives to curb spending. Each state has the option of requesting a waiver or using the Medicare DRG system.

MANAGED CARE

Managed care usually takes the form of health maintenance organizations (HMOs). HMOs are an insurance derivative that provide health care insurance to individuals and families at lower costs through the prevention and limiting of care through different mechanisms. The process for cost controls is usually related to the elimination of the fee-for-service payments to providers, which, as described by Erman, causes the structure of "services and payments to be turned upside down."[8] The use of services is decreased so that utilization and efficiency, not the use of technology and more care, can decrease costs compared to the fee-for-service payment system.

Some of the most common methods to control health care expenditures used by HMOs are:

- *Decreased hospitalized days*. Most activities occur outside the hospital setting. According to one study, hospitalized days for general insurance patients average 692 per 1000 insured lives whereas the HMO industry generally averages about 390 hospitalized days per 1000 insured lives.[9] This amounts to a huge cost savings per insured life.
- *Gatekeeping*. Gatekeeping is a practice whereby the HMO restricts the patient's access to specialists, who always have higher prevailing fees when compared to the general population of family practice physicians. HMOs generally use family practice physicians who have a group of nurse practitioners and physician assistants working with them to see large numbers of patients. This system of access to patient care creates a gate that the patient must pass through before contact with a specialty physician. In addition, these gatekeepers may be housed in an urgent care center that acts as a low-level emergency room in the hospital setting. The use of an off-site emergency center further decreases costs because the patients usually have to go through a prior approval process to use emergency rooms in hospitals, which are the highest-cost access points to health care in the industry. The common urgent care type center is usually located in an easily accessed area, such as along a busy shopping area.
- *Capitation*. Capitation refers to a payment methodology that allows an HMO to contract with a physician or other provider at a capitated maximum rate for each insured life.[8,9] An HMO may pay physicians $10 per month to cover all of the care for each patient insured by the HMO. So, if patients are seen regularly and taken care of, the physician probably has lower costs owing to a lack of hospitalizations and other urgent care. Prevention initiatives have grown greatly in the last 3–5 years; however, most providers have lost large sums of money through capped fees, which are inadequate to cover reasonable costs of care. Therefore, the trend has been to move away from these models.

Some common types of HMO groups are outlined in Table 41-2. Note that HMO types are based on geography, physician models, and patient choice of physician.

PRIVATE PAY

The *private pay* group includes any individuals who lack conventional health insurance or a membership in a managed care plan, such as an HMO. The group includes two categories: those who are very rich and therefore able to pay health care bills themselves and those who cannot afford health insurance in any form (the medically indigent). Of course, very few patients have such large financial resources as to pay their own

TABLE 41-2 **HMO types**

HMO Type	Geography	Physician Configuration	Patient/Physician Choice
Staff model	Small area	Salaried small group	Smallest
Group model	Small but larger than staff model	Contracted fee-for-service multispecialty group	Small but larger than staff model
Network mode	Moderate size multicounty area	Contract fee-for-service; capitation or others using two or more multispecialty practices	Larger, owing to more than one multispecialty practice
Independent practice association (IPA)	Could be a state or more	Usually fee schedule with many multispecialty and sole practice physicians	Large, with this group making up 60% of all HMO subscriber groups
Point of service (POS)	Huge; could be states or national	Fee schedule	Largest, even nonparticipating may be used by paying copay

medical bills. This group usually carries some sort of major medical insurance at least to cover catastrophic health care problems such as cancer. These self-payers must identify the plan covering the state where they reside. New York, for example, has the all-payer DRG system; so that even private pay patients are able to pay hospital and health care bills that are far less than would have been charged on a fee-for-service basis.

At the other end of the health care spectrum, the majority of Americans who lack any health insurance are the working class individuals, usually in the nonskilled service industries. They usually have hourly incomes at or just above minimum wage and therefore cannot afford health insurance, which averages $600 per month or more for a typical family coverage plan.[9] This rate is based on simple coverage, not coverage that includes dental and other supplemental coverage. The majority of Americans without health insurance are working full time is usually surprising to those conducting studies about health insurance. Many states have adopted programs during the Bill Clinton and George W. Bush presidencies that include subsidized children's health insurance coverage. In New York, for example, the program called Child Health Plus covers children whose parents have incomes that exceed Medicaid eligibility levels but also have incomes that fail to provide for the "luxury" of health insurance.

With more than 45 million Americans currently estimated to be uninsured, there certainly is a gap between those with coverage (which is usually related to employment and socioeconomic level) and those without coverage.[9] The reality of becoming uninsured, for example, is usually a surprise to most new college graduates. Insurance laws prohibit coverage of individuals under their parents' plans after age 23 or beyond graduation from college.

Human Resource Management

Staffing involves a seven-step process that follows the planning function already described using manual and information systems functions that predict staffing needs:[7,10,11]

- Recruitment
- Selection and placement
- Orientation
- Compensation
- Training and development
- Performance appraisal
- Employee discipline

RECRUITMENT

Success in the recruitment of respiratory care staff involves several facets that must be continuously considered.

The manager must develop and pay attention to *staffing trends* for pay rates and benefits. Successful management of this function includes attention to trends in the employment market so that the manager advocates for higher salaries and benefits when the market dictates upward trends. Failure to attend to this responsibility results in attrition of highly qualified staff because they have the greatest potential for mobility. The manager should keep track of advertisements of competitors to make changes as they arise when advertising is needed.

Although advertising is a frequent first response to staffing needs, staying involved in *professional activities* provides a network that may be tapped when staff is needed.

- Managers may offer to provide panel discussions or clinical training for local respiratory care

programs, thereby keeping their institutions on the minds of future graduates.
- They can be involved in high school activities such as the Explorer Program sponsored by the Boy Scouts of America. The national Explorer Program involves high school seniors who have interests in health care careers, and these students spend a significant portion of their senior year participating at their local hospital.
- In New York, a program called New Visions is provided by the Board of Cooperative Educational Services (BOCES). This program involves high school seniors with high grade point averages who intend to pursue health care careers after graduation. These students spend most of the senior year in the hospital setting learning about potential career opportunities in the professions. Managers should offer to have these students perform rotations in the respiratory care area to promote the profession and because managers may recruit a future employee as well. Managers who locate these programs in their hospital also promote the return of these students to the community and may provide long-term employees for their department.
- One of the best recruiting tools may be having your institution be a clinical training site for the local RT school. This offers the hospital staff and managers to get a look at the upcoming future graduates and gives the students a chance to observe the culture and workings of the institution.

SELECTION AND PLACEMENT

The selection and placement process involves the selection of an individual for the position being recruited for, using the job description and needs of the position. Managers should consider current employees and determine which of them fits the needs most closely. For successful recruiting, the concept of seeking diversity in race, heritage, religion, lifestyle, and personality cannot be stressed enough. The manager knows the strengths of the current staff; so the search is for an individual whose strengths fill in the gaps. Managers must seek the right individual, not hire a so-called warm body just because a position is open. Failure to heed this caution usually yields a marginal employee and, in the long run, a staff that questions the leader's recruiting abilities. Always seek the best potential employee the first time and avoid the temptation to hire when someone to fill the role is available.

ORIENTATION

Orientation is the introduction of the new employee to the practice of the work site. The mission, vision, and departmental philosophy should be provided in writing to the new employee to aid in assimilation into the institution. Orientation must cover:

- Benefits.
- Departmental policies and procedures.
- Safety.
- Quality improvement.
- Increasingly, customer service.

The new employee usually attends a formal, institution-specific orientation program of a day or two in length. Then the department or work site must provide the specific orientation that enables the individual to provide safe and effective care. Depending on the state and the Joint Commission, one must also provide some mandated orientation activities. Examples of mandatory orientation programs are:

- Safety education.
- Infection control procedures.
- TB control procedures.
- Back safety education.

COMPENSATION

Compensation consists of all benefits that make an employee want to stay in the work site. Pay and institutional benefits make up only part of the package needed to keep high-quality employees. According to nearly every human resource study, pay is usually near the middle of a top 10 list of important issues to employees, especially professional employees such as those found in respiratory care.[10]

- Items such as release time and reimbursement for seminars and external education in the form of tuition reimbursement are very important. Considering that most new respiratory care graduates arrive with an associate's degree, tuition reimbursement is obviously high on a wish list for these new graduates.
- Flex staffing, such as 8- and 12-hour shift patterns, are also desired by many new staff members. Several new studies surmise that the generation of 20- to 30-year-olds, who make up the majority of new graduates, seek flexible staffing patterns as maybe their most important option when seeking employment.
- Recently, higher scales for pay associated with bachelor's degree respiratory therapists have come into use.

TRAINING AND DEVELOPMENT

The area of training and development goes beyond the orientation program and includes:

- Periodic reorientation.
- Access to learning new procedures.

- Inservice education.
- Input from a multidisciplinary group of presenters.

The respiratory care medical director should be included in inservice education when possible to give a medical perspective to new procedures and trends in health care. Providing education by means of teleconferences, videotapes, and other creative methods is needed to keep new and seasoned staff under employment.

PERFORMANCE APPRAISAL

Performance appraisal is among the most neglected tool a manager has to bring about behavioral change in staff. Scored, logic-based appraisal tools that also serve as the job description are very valuable in keeping new and existing employees. Consistency of appraisal from employee to employee is perhaps the single most important tool a manager has to promote harmony and motivation in a work site. Staff seeks out managers and leaders who treat all members in a fair and equitable manner at all times.

However, fair treatment does not always mean equal treatment. Managers and highly effective leaders use continuous assessment to be sure decisions are not arbitrary. However, some situations demand a different approach when feedback indicators and the specific situation warrant a change. Managers must be careful to ensure that variations are for unusual situations and that these changes from customary practice are available to all staff.

Performance appraisals should be set up in advance, and ideally the employee should perform a self-appraisal using the same tool the manager use's. A point scale system is beneficial because the employee understands that normal practice is meeting standards.

The comparison of best performance with one's own performance and therefore objective rating of exceeding or failing to meet standards is more obvious to employees when this sort of tool is used. The current Joint Commission standards for human resource management requires that the job description and subsequent performance appraisal tool be competency based. This approach alleviates some of the possibility of characterizing personality traits instead of the consideration of competent performance of an employee's work duties. Successful ongoing communications with employees should provide that the performance appraisal be a focused and relaxed discussion because employees are and have been aware of expectations and how they have been performing all during the reporting period. Performance appraisal meetings with employees should never be used for disciplinary activity, nor should any discussion or written information be a surprise to the employee being evaluated. It is always desirable to have the appraisal meeting as free from interruption as possible. This allows the leader to concentrate on the individual employee as a positive process even when the appraisal is not as stellar as that of other coworkers.

The objective nature of this tool provides that employees who consider themselves seriously and objectively probably give themselves a lower score on average than the appraiser might. This author has held many performance appraisal conferences at which the self-appraisal's and the manager appraisal's overall scores have varied by only one or two points. This sort of performance appraisal conference is usually quite at ease after the first couple of minutes, which nearly always contain some apprehension on the part of employees. Use the appraisal process to praise and develop goals for the next reporting period for both improvement and professional growth.

EMPLOYEE DISCIPLINE

The discipline of employees is highly important to the successful manager and leader because the process reinforces the need for employees to follow standards. It deals with employees who fail to meet expectations, and it helps in motivating employees who always perform to the best of their ability. In fact, the failure to discipline employees might be the fastest route to demotivation and the loss of talented staff. The constructive use of discipline reinforces the concepts of quality and conformity for all employees. The failure to perform this process usually causes all employees to perform at a lower level, thereby creating a staff of mediocre productivity and quality.

A frequent area of discussion involves time and attendance issues. Failure to apply disciplinary measures to offenders usually results in substandard attendance and tardiness problems with many staff members. Employees sink or rise to the prevailing level of expectations; so only high levels of expectation must be communicated.

Manager Accountability

The responsibilities of managers working in the respiratory care areas are related to administration, medical direction and leadership, and staffing.

ADMINISTRATIVE ACCOUNTABILITY

Administrative accountability has varied for respiratory care almost in a cycle over the past 15 or so years.

In the early 1980s, respiratory care department leaders typically reported through a vice president for patient services or assistant administrator. In some cases these administrators had a primary clinical or nursing background. As time passed, many hospitals moved the professional ancillary departments together because many of the issues of reimbursement and the like had common elements. These department groups were usually respiratory care, medical laboratory, radiologic technology, nuclear medicine, physical therapy, occupational therapy, and others, depending on the work site.

During the mid- to late 1990s, there was a transition back to a patient services structure because many hospitals rearranged their services into product or service lines. This philosophic behavior caused respiratory care to move typically back under a vice president with a primary nursing or other clinical background.

In some areas, this activity has included decentralizing the respiratory care departments into service lines, in many cases only to be partially recentralized over the last couple of years. The AARC has a large volume of data that support the move back to a quasidecentralized department structure. This hybrid department structure contains a centralized department that allows maintenance of professional identity while providing therapists to work on teams in the service line structure. This structure leads to a dual identity for therapists: the respiratory care department and the service line where they typically perform their therapy. Thus the therapists themselves engage in quality improvement activities on their service line. This has been a major change in activity in the 1990s.

A significant outcome of these decentralized or quasidecentralized structures may be a matrixed form of evaluation for respiratory care staff. "Matrix" in this context means that respiratory therapists may have evaluations that contain direct input from the service line component; that usually means nursing and other clinical disciplines. These types of quasidecentralized structures are positive work environments for therapists. After all, the typical respiratory therapist has a high-level patient care background that is more like nursing compared to almost any other professional staff. Nearly all of a respiratory therapist's activity occurs in the patient's room, which is precisely where nurses perform their care. Most other professional ancillary departments have the patient brought to their departments for either care or diagnostic activities.

The respiratory care director was replaced with a nurse in many fully decentralized departments. Most of the impetus for decentralization activities is a direct result of hospitals and nursing homes seeking methods to curb costs during the 1990s. The means for these changes involved consultants brought in to suggest areas where costs could be curtailed. One of the primary reasons that respiratory care has frequently been a target for cost-cutting activities may be traced directly to the reimbursement—or the lack of it—for direct provision of respiratory care services. As of this writing, some improvements are occurring in this area. Over a period of years, total decentralization usually leads to:

- The loss of professional identity.
- High staff turnover rates.
- Quality problems

These are the major reasons why many fully decentralized respiratory care functions have at least partially or fully recentralized in the last several years.

Accountability for respiratory care also resides at least partially with the financial and information systems administrative personnel (discussed later in this chapter). Furthermore, the technical director has direct responsibilities for quality activities in concert with the medical director. Most surveillance, data retrieval systems design, and continuous activity for departmental quality fall in the realm of the technical director's responsibilities. Therefore, the technical director has direct accountability through the quality management function of administration.

In the nursing home or home care industry, respiratory care personnel typically work in the nursing service structure, because these industries have regulations that call for patient care providers to work under the direction of a nurse. As an example, New York State requires that certified home health or licensed home health agencies be managed by a nurse. Similar health department regulations may well be found when research in this subject is done in various states.

MEDICAL DIRECTION

The title for the leader of a typical respiratory or cardiopulmonary department usually contains the word "technical" to denote the difference between the full directorship of a department and the medical direction. Requirements from the Joint Commission and most state health departments mandate that respiratory care personnel and their leadership have reporting mechanisms that include medical leadership. An example of an organizational chart is found in

Figure 41-9. An example is found in the application for AARC membership where applicants working in a hospital setting are expected to identify their respective medical directors when applying for active membership in the AARC.

The dominant function of the respiratory care medical director is for consultation and professional input for the operations of the department. Stoller further describes "four arenas that the Respiratory Care Medical Director should actively participate that include: Administrative and Supervisory, Educational, Clinical and Investigational."[12] The medical director may initiate the development of protocols, monitor the appropriateness of respiratory care, and aid in the allocation of respiratory care services.[12] One of the major activities related to medical direction involves intervention when therapists believe that care is being compromised by decisions made by other professionals or physicians. For this reason, respiratory care departments should have a medical director and assistant medical director so that the staff always has the ability to contact one of them in case their intervention is needed. Respiratory care medical directors should be involved and provide consistent in-service education to respiratory care staff, as well as provide medical guidance for trends in patient care. In most cases, the respiratory care medical director is directly responsible for the quality practice of the department.[12]

Quality improvement programs usually describe the respiratory care medical director as the main professional entity responsible for quality care outcomes. Obviously most of these activities are delegated to the manager; however, the medical director should provide continuous input to the practice and quality activities for the department.

More than 2000 respiratory care medical directors belong to the National Association of Medical Directors for Respiratory Care (NAMDRC). If the new medical director is not a member of this organization, suggesting membership is advisable because the organization keeps its members abreast of the trends and issues related to the profession of respiratory care.

STAFFING ACCOUNTABILITY

The respiratory care staff also has accountability for the direct involvement in patient care as well as quality improvement activities in their practice setting. The respiratory care technical director has

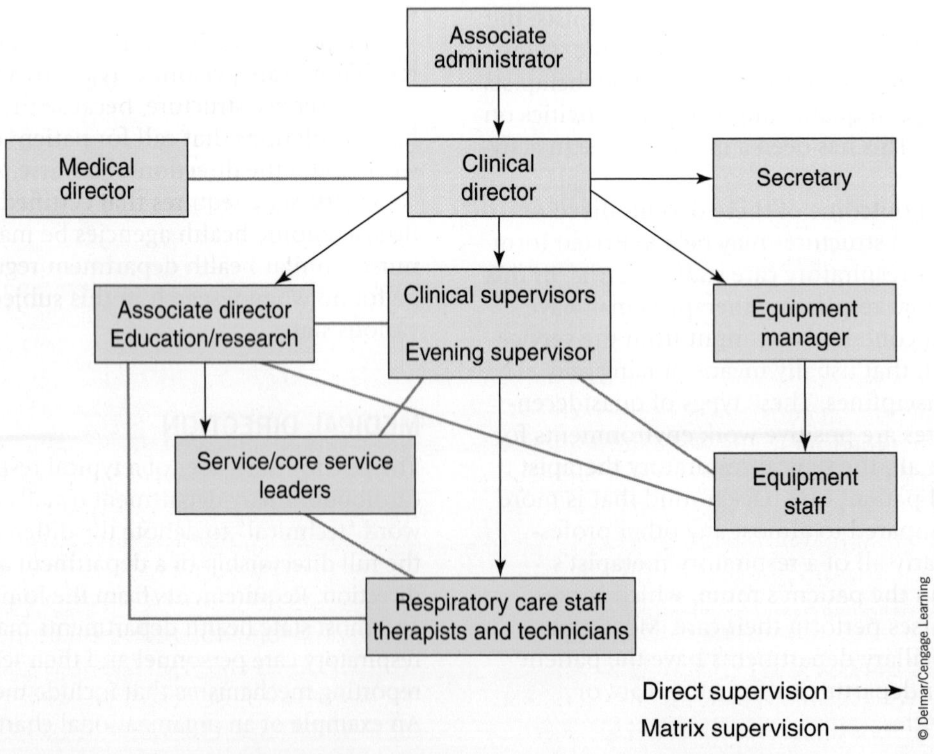

FIGURE 41-9 Sample organizational chart.

CASE STUDY 41-1

R. M., a new respiratory care manager in a typical community hospital, began to analyze recruitment and retention of professional staff in her department for the previous 24 months.

The hospital is located in a rural small city of about 25,000 people, 30 miles from a city of 80,000 people. The larger city has a large private university of 14,000 students, whereas the small city where the hospital is located has a state university with about 6000 students. There is a community college in the large city with an associate degree program in respiratory care that typically produces about 24 graduate respiratory therapists per year.

Most of the graduates recruited in the past have left employment or are considering other employment after about a year of service. A small core group of staffers in the respiratory care department have long-term service records. Pay rates for the staff therapists are found to be just above the median for the region.

Questions

1. List some of the possible causes for the failure to retain staff that could be related to the human resource management of the department or hospital.
2. Using this book as a reference, list the possible corrections for the answers to question 1.

accountability to lead the staff in a way that is always ethical, professional, and up-to-date with the latest and most acceptable practice patterns for care. Respiratory care leaders must provide guidance and motivation for their staff. Failure of RC managers to attend to these important issues usually results in departments that are behind in current practice and that lack a professional identity in the work site. One of the results of the failure to stay current is detrimental when consultants arrive and are able to prove to senior administration that the respiratory care area could operate better without the current leader. This behavior may be described as the "manager has quit and stayed."

Staff also has a personal responsibility to be professionally involved, attending seminars even when the employer does not fund their attendance, as well as striving for best practices in all their activities.

Computer Applications

Respiratory care involvement in applying computers to care usually involves financial and quality functions. In some cases computers may be interfaced with ventilators or pulmonary functions systems, thereby decreasing documentation of patient bedside documentation because the information is available online.

When possible, the respiratory care department should have a dedicated information system for respiratory care services. Most hospital information systems, such as Meditech or Siemans, have only partial applications for the needs of our professional specialty. In most cases, a hospital information system with applications for respiratory care have adapted a nursing clinical module for respiratory care documentation. Financial applications are designed for one-time activities, such as those found in radiology or the medical laboratory.

Respiratory care, however, has most of its activities in continuous modes of care such as mechanical ventilation and therapies that continue on a regular basis until the patient's condition improves. Under these assumptions, a mainframe hospital information system is woefully inadequate for the day-to-day operation of the RC department.

Given the current trends toward a quasidecentralized setting, the therapist needs practice resources that allow for constant contact and ease of use for documentation and charging for services. This patient care need necessitates the use of a *point-of-care access* (e.g., a handheld computer for documentation at the bedside) for:

- Documentation.
- Patient charges.
- Quality improvement data input.
- Communications with the department and patient care area.

Point of care denotes that testing is done and records are generated at the patient beside systems such as what have been described here only exist in add-on information systems specific for respiratory or cardiopulmonary care activities.

Several manufacturers—CliniVision by Tyco, MediServe Inc., and Tenet—offer systems with many of the attributes described as mandatory for a successful respiratory care information system.

Clearly, the advent of outcome measurement as a tool for financial and clinical management necessitates the automation of information in ways not required for departmental management in the past. Tools such as those described in this chapter make automation and retrieval of longitudinal data much more realistic. Bunch[13] quotes Long-Goding in her description of the typical formulation of outcome data measurement with the requirement of a clear research question that may focus on a simple problem. The ability to log this sort of data when documenting the results of therapy creates a constant stream of relevant information for the measurement of outcomes.[13] Nearly all quality improvement initiatives from the Joint Commission involve movement toward outcome measurement. Information systems designed for use specifically for respiratory care are most effective in implementing this sort of accountability.

A VENDOR-SPECIFIC APPLICATION EXAMPLE

MediLinks (MediServe Inc.) is one of the oldest and most widely used respiratory care clinical information systems in the industry. The use of the MediLinks system requires each user to configure it in order to customize its usefulness to the hospital based on current methods and practices. Customization offers the ability to create outcomes assessment and procedure data that the therapist may provide with no specific extra effort because the pathways for the data retrieval have been built into the background using the MediLinks configuration system. The development of protocols through the use of the AARC CPGs and uniform reporting standards creates a seamless system that is user-friendly and cost-effective for patient care.

The use of a customized clinical information system brings all of the components of quality, cost accounting, outcomes measurement, and documentation into one tool that the therapist may use at the bedside using a radio frequency–activated system, such as that available through MediServe. This method of quality and efficiency measurement is ideal for activities such as those described by Miranda in quantifying caregiver workload in the ICU setting.[14] Although some measurement tools do not cover all of the caregiver's activities, MediLinks provides the normal process of patient care documentation that yields all of the needed data for these functions with no extra work by the respiratory therapist. This supplies the leadership of respiratory care with the data needed to effectively function in today's challenging health care financial climate. MediLinks provides patient charges, productivity data, quality data, and a means of patient care documentation free from the constraints of handwritten notes and manual charging systems found in most hospitals today. Every time an RT documents work with a handheld computer, all of the streams of data are generated without thought because the backbone was built during the configuration phase of installation. The usefulness of systems such as MediLinks arises from the user's configuration, which may be adapted as ongoing changes are needed, thus serving as a respiratory care information system that permits growth as advances in the profession occur.

Summary

Managers must follow continuous quality improvement tenets to improve their work sites' effectiveness; however, managers or leaders must assume that continuous growth in their personal knowledge is an inherent responsibility of the professionals they lead. Individuals who hold leadership positions have described the growth of the respiratory care profession in Chapter 1 as directly dependent on activity levels in the profession. *Management* by definition is the concept of getting things done through others. The ability of respiratory therapists to perform management functions effectively may be learned and practiced during their career. Leadership, on the other hand, is the innate ability to convey a vision to others of how they should act or perform. Leadership is not so easily learned. This chapter contains information on management philosophy, management science, leadership characteristics, and operational methods for the day-to-day guidance of respiratory care professionals in their respective work sites. The concepts of leadership defy easy description or definition, although most people would say that they know a good leader when they see one.

A simple characteristic of accomplished leaders is that they provide consistent ethical and moral guidance to their charges, even when there are easier ways to accomplish a task. Effective communications abilities, both written and verbal, characterize managers and leaders that moreover move their areas of responsibility to a higher level of effectiveness.

Study Questions

REVIEW QUESTIONS

1. Explain the four functions of management science.
2. Describe the attributes of successful staffing and human resource management.
3. Describe the characteristics of quality improvement.
4. List some of the attributes for tracking productivity and efficiency in respiratory care.
5. Plot a typical departmental organization chart with roles and responsibilities listed with their reporting responsibilities.
6. Describe the blossoming role of clinical competency in the evolution of the respiratory care profession.

7. List briefly the typical descriptions of operational budget expenses that may be expected in the respiratory care profession.
8. Define and describe items that might be included in a capital budget.
9. Define the role responsibilities of a respiratory care therapist for reporting and accountability in a hospital.
10. List some of the attributes that a management information system must have for the proper operation of a respiratory care work site.
11. Describe the personal role that RTs should aspire to achieve with respect to the profession and their own personal involvement.
12. List two possible community activities that RTs may be involved in that are important to growth and lay knowledge of the profession.

MULTIPLE-CHOICE QUESTIONS

1. Management functions in the health care setting are some of the most difficult in the management profession because:
   a. they are static and unchanging.
   b. there is no specific style needed for health care management.
   c. they are dynamic and change daily.
   d. they are impossible to resolve.
2. The participation of all respiratory therapists in AARC is important to all in the profession because:
   a. participation in the profession of respiratory care as AARC members enhances growth in the science, technology, and education of the profession.
   b. participation decreases lobbying strength for the profession.
   c. active membership takes the place of continuing education by individual therapists.
   d. active membership results in higher salaries.
3. Capital budgets usually denote items that exceed what in cost?
   a. $1 million
   b. $500
   c. $10 million
   d. $150
4. Which of the following is *not* a skill that all levels of management must possess to be effective in the highest degree?
   a. technical skills
   b. leadership skills
   c. communication skills
   d. financial skills
5. The use of a dedicated information management system improves tracking and data retrieval for the financial and quality management of respiratory care departments because:
   I. information is gathered at the point of care.
   II. information is more easily stored and aggregated for a specific department like respiratory care.
   III. quality improvement activities and data generation may be built into normal documentation activities for all patient care activities.
   a. I only
   b. I and III
   c. II and III
   d. I, II, and III

CRITICAL-THINKING QUESTIONS

1. Why are most respiratory care managers salaried and not reimbursed on an hourly basis?
2. What is the single most challenging issue facing respiratory care managers today? Why?
3. Would you want to be a respiratory care department manager someday? Why? Why not?

References

1. American Association for Respiratory Care. *Clinical Practice Guidelines*. Dallas, TX: American Association for Respiratory Care; 2001. www.aarc.org
2. Merriam-Webster. *Merriam-Webster's Collegiate Dictionary*. 11th ed. Springfield, MASS: Merriam-Webster; 2006.
3. Thornton E. Asthma management program provides special services to impoverished families. *AARC Times*. 1999;23:32–38.
4. Bunch D. Therapists at Satilla regional demonstrate value by performing arterial line insertions. *AARC Times*. 1999b;23:14–17.
5. American Association of Respiratory Care. *Uniform Reporting Manual*. 3rd ed., revised. Dallas, TX: American Association for Respiratory Care; 1993.
6. Bunch D. AARC clinical practice guidelines: posted on National Guideline Clearinghouse web site. *AARC Times*. 1999a;23:28–31.
7. Griffin R. *Management*. Boston, MA: Houghton Mifflin; 1987.
8. Erman MK. The impact of managed care on the practice of sleep disorders medicine. *Respir Care*. 1998;43:401–407.
9. Raffel MW, Raffel NK. *The U.S. Health Care System*. 5th ed. Clifton Park, NY: Delmar Cengage Learning; 2008.

10. Haimann T. *Supervisory Management for Health Care Organizations*. St. Louis, MO: The Catholic Health Association of the United States; 1984.
11. Stevens GH. *The Strategic Health Care Manager: Mastering Essential Leadership Skills*. San Francisco: Jossey Bass; 1991.
12. Stoller JK. Medical direction of respiratory care: past and present. *Respir Care*. 1998;43: 217–223.
13. Bunch D. Using data to improve outcomes. *AARC Times*. 1999c;23:18–22.
14. Miranda DR. Quantitating care giver workload in the ICU: the therapeutic intervention scoring system. *Respir Care*. 1999;44:70–72.

Suggested Readings

American Association for Respiratory Care. AARC Ethics Statement. Dallas, TX: American Association for Respiratory Care. Effective December 1994; revised July 2009.

Kovner AR, Neuhauser D. *Health Services Management, A Book of Cases*. 6th ed. Ann Arbor, MI: Health Administration Press; 2004.

Redican KJ, Baffi C, Wessel T. *Dimensions of Consumer Health*. 4th ed. Englewood Cliffs, NJ: Prentice Hall; 1994.

Williams SJ, Torrens PR. *Introduction to Health Services*. 7th ed. Albany, NY: Delmar; 2007.

APPENDIX A

The Respiratory Therapist in Nontraditional Roles

Anthony Everidge

It is no doubt or surprise that the world has radically changed over the years. The affects of these widespread changes have touched every aspect of the world, including health care. As a result, it is apparent that the roles of the respiratory care practitioner are evolving also. Managed care, as well as changes to the Medicare system and the U.S. health system, contributes to these changes, along with a natural evolving and expansion of the role of the respiratory care practitioner. These changes and reforms are lending to the opportunity and the creation of more and more nontraditional roles for the respiratory care practitioner.

Traditionally, the respiratory therapist has worked in the hospital setting. The therapist has worked under the department's umbrella covering all hospital areas as well as pulmonary functions. These areas have been the standard for respiratory care workers for decades and will continue to be so. With these changes in our world and U.S. health systems, and the unique set of skills held by the respiratory care practitioner, it has become obvious that the respiratory care practitioner can utilize these skills in expanding roles.

Expanding Roles of Respiratory Therapists

Therapists of today have the opportunity to add to their already broad base of clinical knowledge by adding extra certifications to the CRT/RRT national certification, thereby furthering the opportunity for advancing career opportunity. These credentials can include:

- Neonatal/Pediatric Specialty (NPS) certification.
- Asthma Educator–Certified (AE-C) certification.
- Sleep Disorders Specialty certification.
- Certified Pulmonary Function Technologist (CPFT).
- Registered Pulmonary Function Technologist (RPFT).

According to an article in *RT for Decision Makers*,[1] a new program has been designed for respiratory care practitioners at the Texas Children's Hospital. Respiratory care practitioners were identified as a population of clinical workers that possessed wide and varied skills as well as a professional license, enabling the practitioner to act independently and to serve in nontraditional roles. Cost reduction as well as providing quality care to the patient population was a major factor in the process of determining and creating new roles for the RT.

According to the article, these roles were created to work in accordance with a Family Centered Health Care Delivery Model. This model, according to The Medical College of Georgia, states, "Patient and family-centered care is an approach to the planning, delivery and evaluation of health care providers, patients, and families. It redefines the relationships between and among consumers and health providers."[2] A few of the key concepts noted for the model are respect, choice, information, collaboration, and empowerment. The overall plan enables the patient and the staff to act in collaboration to provide the best service with the best patient outcome in the most cost-effective manner. This model and the recognized skills of the respiratory care practitioner create the nontraditional roles to follow.

The roles developed at Texas Children's Hospital were tooled and designed for respiratory care practitioners (RCPs) based on clinical depth and ability. These roles were:

- Administrator for transport services and specialist.
- Assistant vice president (hospital).
- Pulmonary research director.
- Asthma-cystic fibrosis specialist.
- Discharge facilitator.
- Operating room-advanced care practitioner.
- Special projects and research coordinator.
- Staff development and education.

The implementation and design of these nontraditional roles show the need for respiratory care practitioners to be effective in their clinical roles as well as to display broad clinical skills. The need for these practitioners to be critical thinkers is also a major factor. The therapist of the new millennium has to be able to think outside of the box and to show the ability to turn their thinking into action. The ability to be effective in these new roles depends greatly on the practitioner being able to move smoothly among departments of the organization. Practitioners must be well versed in respiratory care as it applies to the patient population that their role applies to. The practitioner needs to possess excellent written and verbal communication skills and be able to build a supportive and expert networking base. These roles present different and unique challenges for the practitioner, but they advance the roles of the RCP into areas that typically have not been filled by respiratory therapists (RTs). As the business environment takes more control to the areas of cost-effective treatment of the patient population and as changes in the health care system progress, these nontraditional roles will become more abundant and require well trained and educated practitioners.

Home Care

Another area of somewhat nontraditional work roles is home care. The home care field has been a part of respiratory care for decades now. With the technical advancements in respiratory care, the opportunity for different roles other than oxygen administration has arisen. The system today requires that patients return home much sooner than in the past. As RCPs enter the home care field, they must be aware that, upon working in the patient's home, a whole different set of parameters come into focus for the practitioner. The RCP must be aware of the patient's condition, how this condition factors into the patients treatment, and what effects the practitioner may expect to see with this patient, negative or positive.

With the advent of more seriously ill patients returning home and with the use of more highly technical equipment, the RCP has to stay current with new technology and be able to operate this equipment. Home care therapists must take it upon themselves to be dedicated to pursuing current modalities of therapy and being able to offer the best clinical practice of these modalities in the patient's home. These home RTs must research new devices that may not be so common in the home place, as well as be well versed in the more common modalities of oxygen administration, such as portable nebulizers in the home. The RT must also be knowledgeable in both noninvasive and home mechanical ventilation. The home care RCP must also be aware of regulatory requirements and be familiar with patient safety goals as they relate to the Joint Commission (TJC) and regulatory reimbursement programs through governmental agencies.

The home care RCP also must act as the eyes of the physician. In acting as the conduit between patient and physician, the RCP must demonstrate excellent clinical knowledge and be able to communicate any findings, normal or abnormal, to the physician. This interaction requires that the RCP possess excellent interpersonal and communication skills. This nontraditional role of home care does not allow the home therapist the luxury of daily interaction with the physician and staff in the hospital. This reinforces the need for the therapist to stay current with patient and equipment education. This can be accomplished through annual conferences, state society meetings, and respiratory affiliated agencies that sponsor continuing education in the field. Home care therapists need to be sharp in their presentation skills and spend time with respiratory colleagues to discuss and educate themselves on new or standard issues that affect the home care industry. This knowledge enforces the education base of the home therapist as well as enables the therapist to provide cutting-edge technological service to the patient and thus improve positive patient outcome.

The home care field also offers the opportunity for the RCP to engage in the marketing aspect of the agency he/she works for. Typically this calls for the therapist to engage in a meeting with the physician and the office staff to make the staff and physician aware of what services the company the therapist represents has available. This end of the home care field requires that the RCP has excellent interpersonal skills as well as outstanding verbal and written communication skills. The RCP engaged in the marketing aspect of home care spends a great majority of time speaking to groups as well as presenting information in regard to current technology, as well as future and new technology to health care providers.

As with all the other nontraditional roles, this role requires the RCP to:

- Have excellent clinical knowledge.
- Be able to think in a clinically critical mode.
- Present complex technology in a fashion that makes it clear and concise on the modality being presented.

The ultimate goal is once again to offer the most effective patient care, both from a clinical basis and cost basis. This results in the most positive patient outcome in the home care setting.

Sleep Medicine

The home care setting has also seen a boom due to sleep medicine, which has become a leading factor in the diagnosis and treatment of sleep apnea. Sleep medicine has also unveiled connections between a host of medical conditions connected to sleep apnea. It is estimated that upward of 40 million adults suffer with sleep apnea. This has resulted in the development of numerous freestanding sleep labs, as well as sleep labs opened by hospitals. These hospital-based sleep labs may operate on- or off-site.

The RCP who seeks to work in a nontraditional role can find a wide-open field for both work and study in the sleep field. The RCP who seeks work in the sleep area can expect to work in several different capacities.

RCPs working in sleep can seek to further prove their expertise by seeking advanced certifications. The designation of Registered Polysymnographic Technologist (RPSGT) is available through the Board of Registered Polysymnographic Technologists, as well as a designation of Sleep Disorder Specialty through the National Board of Respiratory Care. These designations are available by provision of the required education as well as passing standardized testing.

The RCP involved in sleep study becomes familiar with the placement of EEG leads, as well as proper analysis and interpretation of EEG results. The area of sleep medicine provides a natural segue for the RCP, as administration and titration of positive pressure, both CPAP and BiPap devices, are required. The typical sleep study may be conducted in either two separate studies or a split study conducted in one night. The study consists of first analyzing percentages of sleep stages, measuring sleep latency indexes, and monitoring and recording sleep apneas and hypopneas—this all leading to a breakdown of incidence of apnea to include both obstructive and central or combined. The next phase of the testing involves the RCP titrating positive pressure to the patient either via continuous positive pressure or bilevel positive pressure. The RCP uses clinical knowledge of positive pressure to apply enough pressure to overcome the obstructive events to maintain an open and patent airway, while not overpressuring the patient. The goal is to maintain minimal pressures to provide maximum benefit to the patient while eliminating obstructive events and clearing the apneic episodes.

RCPs can also further their role in sleep medicine by progressing to the position of reading, scoring, and interpreting sleep studies. This position makes itself available typically after several years of performing sleep studies and applying positive pressure to overcome sleep obstruction. The RCP also has the opportunity to advance as sleep center director in freestanding locations, as well as department manager in hospital-based programs. These nontraditional roles require excellent clinical skills, as well as the ability to think critically and in ways that may require additional skills to more traditional roles of the RCP.

Asthma Educator

Another nontraditional role has been emerging with the advent of the AE-C (Asthma Educator–Certified). The designation of AE-C shows a proficiency in both the understanding of the asthma disease process and treating it. The asthma educator is considered an expert in counseling and educating people with asthma. The AE-C is also responsible for educating families with the proper knowledge and skill that are required to treat asthma and to help to decrease the debilitating effects of asthma. The RCP with the designation has seen nontraditional roles of work developing as purveyors of this knowledge. These roles have manifested themselves in the both clinical and educational areas.

Clinical programs have been developed under the umbrella of respiratory departments, with opportunities for the RCP to administer treatment to patients in both hospital and clinical settings, while dispensing education to patients and families on how best to control the disease process.

The educational aspect of the AE-C has presented itself in several areas. The education aspect is more community based. Many programs have been supported and funded by government agencies. These government sponsorships provide financial grants for the RCP with the AE-C designation to take the message to the community, typically via school-based programs. These programs, given via both print and presentation, enhance the public knowledge of the disease and provide education to teachers and school health personnel. Families of students with asthma, as well as those generally interested or possibly acquainted with a friend or relative, are also invited to attend. The idea is to disseminate as much information regarding asthma to as many people as possible. The spreading of information via the community leads to further education and control of the disease. In turn, this leads to better management of the disease and to better treatment, both prophylactically and in the acute and chronic stages. The greater understanding and treatment result in less time and expense for treatment, as well as better positive patient outcomes.

The RCP that chooses the area of AE-C has to be extremely educated in the clinical area of disease process. The RCP, AE-C who decides to go into community-based program education also has to develop very good communication skills, both verbal and written. Public speaking is a necessity, and practitioners have to hone their skills in presenting smoothly and deliberately. The practitioner has to tailor the information delivered so that it meets the need of the audience being addressed.

All of these nontraditional roles require practitioners to possess a broad base of clinical skills and to be well organized. They must be critical thinkers with the ability to use their unique set of skills possessed by RCPs. Those very skills made these nontraditional roles possible.

Certification for Nontraditional Roles

Many nontraditional roles require extra certifications and thus more education. Studies have concurred that education is a crucial aspect of both creating nontraditional roles for the RCP and putting the roles into action. Studies suggest that advanced degrees were preferred for RCP's acting as managers, clinical specialists, educators, and supervisors. This education is very important to the RCP that is working with the public and patient population. Furthering the education of the RCP not only enforces the practitioner's knowledge base, but also provides the community and patient population with the confidence and security that the practitioner is well versed on the topic being presented and the therapy being performed. RCPs engaged in nontraditional roles have to commit themselves to be lifelong learners. For these roles to not only survive but flourish, RCPs must bring all their clinical talents and skills as decision makers as well as educators to create a progressive, positive outcome-based result.[3]

Staff Developers and Clinical Educators

Roles as staff developers and/or clinical educators have also been on the increase in the respiratory field. The goal of corporate organizations, whether hospital based or private sector based, is to run smoothly and efficiently, and that goal requires a positive environment that produces positive results. These positive results are an outcome of great employees that perform at maximum levels. Hospitals also subscribe to this theory. Hospitals strive for positive patient outcome and to provide excellent service to the patient population—cost-effectively. This is where the staff educator and/or clinical educator comes into play. The RCP in this role is typically responsible for the education, accountability for standards of care, and the promotion of respiratory practice changes through educational development. The RCP in this role provides oversight for clinical education and competency for the respiratory department. The staff/clinical educator is also primarily responsible for orienting and integrating new employees and for supporting the advancement of both new and current therapists.

For the organization, this role helps greatly in achieving the goal of running effectively and financially efficiently. Employee education and retention are very big cost factors for an organization. The staff educator is responsible for ensuring that the proper education and tools are given to the staff employees and new employees to perform their duties at the highest level and with the highest amount of efficiency. Doing so enables the greatest possibility for positive patient outcomes and ensures the satisfaction of the employees. With both employee satisfaction and positive patient outcomes, the organization runs effectively and financially efficiently.

Conversely, if employees are not provided with the best tools and education, they may become dissatisfied or frustrated and seek employment elsewhere. This type of loss leads to staffing issues, shortages, and high turnover. Before long, patients are dissatisfied, and positive patient outcomes decrease, thus causing a fracture in efficiency and leading to negative financial outcomes for the organization.

Proper staff development is crucial, and failure to bring employees along can be costly in the future. The RCP as staff educator is responsible for ensuring a consistent interface between practitioners and clinical areas. This position is responsible for the presentation and implementation of the educational and clinical skills needed to run a forward-thinking and progressive respiratory department.

The traditional role of the RCP is always going to be present. The areas that have always been present in the world of respiratory care are going to not only remain but to expand. The population is ever aging and swelling in number with ever growing life expectancies. Regardless of the blurred boundary between financing and the delivery of health services, the fact remains that as a society we are aging, and we are creating the need for more health care. This health care must be delivered in an efficient and cost-effective manner. This very dilemma has created a new and golden opportunity for respiratory care practitioners.

Summary

RCPs who are willing to be visionary can see the opportunity that lies ahead. Those who are dedicated to the respiratory field and committed to interfacing with all aspects of the educational and clinical areas will see abundant chances to practice respiratory care in an ever increasing pool of nontraditional roles.

RCPs who choose this venue need to possess the skills that make them successful in this arena. One such skill is a vast and broad clinical base. This clinical base has to be combined with extraordinary communication skills and the ability to express these skills both verbally and in writing. RCPs also need to display the desire not only personally to provide the best service possible, but to educate all those in contact with them to be the most informed.

The cause and effect in a changing world and the reforms to the health care system provide RCPs—new graduates and experienced practitioners—the opportunity to participate in these exciting times and to contribute both knowledge and experience in the respiratory field. Whether the RCP chooses to enter the roles mentioned in this chapter as an educator, a clinical specialist, research specialist, or the ever expanding roles in the sleep medicine world or home care, the opportunities will continue to grow and to evolve into even more future potential for the eager and educated RCP.

References

1. Creative Visions Foundation. RT for Decision Makers in Respiratory Care. http://www.rtmagazine.com/issues/articles/1999-12_13.asp
2. Medical College of Georgia. MCG Health System. http://www.mcg.edu/aafairs/associate/familycenteredcare/INDEXfamilyANDpatients.htm
3. Becker EA. Respiratory care managers' preferences regarding baccalaureate and masters degree education for respiratory therapists. *Respir. Care.* 2003;48,9:840–858.

Abbreviations

AACVPR	American Association of Cardiovascular and Pulmonary Rehabilitation
AAP	American Academy of Pediatrics
AARC	American Association for Respiratory Care
AAT	alpha-1 antitrypsin
ABG	arterial blood gas
A/C	assist/control (mode)
ACB	active cycle of breathing
ACCP	American College of Chest Physicians
ACE	angiotensin-converting enzyme
ACHC	Accreditation Commission for Home Care
ACLS	advanced cardiac life support
ACS	American Cancer Society
ACT	airway clearance technique
ADLs	activities of daily living
AED	automatic external defibrillator
AFB	acid-fast bacilli
AG	anion gap
AHA	American Heart Association or American Hospital Association
AHI	apnea/hypopnea index
AIDS	acquired immunodeficiency syndrome
AIP	acute interstitial pneumonia
ALA	American Lung Association
A-line	arterial line
ALS	amyotrophic lateral sclerosis
ALTE	apparent life-threatening event
AMA	American Medical Association
AMD	age-related macular degeneration
AMP	adenosine monophosphate
ANS	autonomic nervous system
ANSI	American National Standards Institute
A-P	anterior-posterior (diameter)
APACHE	acute physiology and chronic health evaluation
APM	airway pressure monitor
APRV	airway pressure release ventilation
APS	acute physiology score
ARDS	adult respiratory distress syndrome
ASA	American Society of Anesthesiologists
AT	anaerobic threshold
ATP	adenosine triphosphate
ATPS	atmospheric (ambient) temperature and pressure, saturated
ATS	American Thoracic Society
AV	atrioventricular (node)
AVPU	alert, responds to voice, responds to pain, unresponsive (scale)
AZT	zidovudine
BAL	bronchoalveolar lavage or blood alcohol level
b.i.d.	twice daily
BiPAP	bi-level positive airway pressure
BLS	basic life support
BOOP	bronchiolitis obliterans organizing pneumonia
BP	blood pressure
BPD	bronchopulmonary dysplasia
BTPS	body temperature and pressure, saturated
BUN	blood urea nitrogen

CAD	coronary artery disease
cAMP	cyclic adenosine monophosphate
C_aO_2	content of oxygen in arterial blood
CAP	community acquired pneumonia
CARF	Commission for Accreditation of Rehabilitation Facilities
CAT	computerized axial tomography (scan)
CBNT	continuous bronchodilator nebulization therapy
CCU	cardiac care unit
CDC	Centers for Disease Control and Prevention
CF	cystic fibrosis
CGA	Compressed Gas Association
CHAP	Community Health Accreditation Program
CHF	congestive heart failure
CI	cardiac index
CISD	critical incident stress debriefing
CLD	chronic lung disease
CLIA	Clinical Laboratory Improvement Amendments
CLRT	continuous lateral rotation therapy
CMI	cell-mediated immune (system)
CMN	certificate of medical necessity
CMS	Centers for Medicare & Medicaid Services
CMV	continuous mechanical ventilation or cytomegalovirus
CNS	central nervous system
CO	cardiac output or carbon monoxide
CoARC	Committee on Accreditation for Respiratory Care
COHb	carboxyhemoglobin
CON	certificate of need
COP	colloidal oncotic pressure
COPD	chronic obstructive pulmonary disease
CORF	comprehensive outpatient rehabilitation facility
Co-Ox	co-oximeter
CPAP	continuous positive airway pressure
CPG	clinical practice guideline
CPR	cardiopulmonary resuscitation
CPT	chest physical therapy or current procedural terminology
CPX	cardiopulmonary exercise test or evaluation
CQI	continuous quality improvement
CSF	cerebrospinal fluid
CT	computerized tomography (scan)
CVA	cerebrovascular accident
C_vO_2	content of oxygen in mixed venous blood
CVP	central venous pressure
CXR	chest X-ray
DHHS	Department of Health and Human Services
DIP	desquamative interstitial pneumonia
***D*LCO**	diffusing capacity of the lung using carbon monoxide
DME	durable medical equipment
DNA	deoxyribonucleic acid
DNR	do not resuscitate
DOT	Department of Transportation (Also "Directly observed treatment" in TB control)
DPG	diphosphoglycerate (usually noted as 2,3 DPG)
DPI	dry powder inhaler
DRG	diagnosis-related group or dorsal respiratory group
Dx	diagnosis
EA	esophageal atresia
ECG	electrocardiogram (also expressed as EKG)
ECF	extracellular fluid
ECMO	extracorporeal membrane oxygenation
EDD	esophageal detector device
EDS	excessive daytime sleepiness
EEG	electroencephalogram
EGTA	esophageal gastric tube airway
ELISA	enzyme-linked immunosorbent assay
EMD	electromechanical dissociation
EMG	electromylogram
EOA	esophageal obturator airway
EOG	electrooculogram
EPAP	expiratory positive airway pressure
EPT	exhalation port test

ER emergency room

ERV expiratory reserve volume

ETC esophageal-tracheal combitube

$ETCO_2$ end-tidal carbon dioxide

ETO ethylene oxide

ETT endotracheal tube

EWNP exsufflation with negative pressure

FBA foreign body aspiration

FBAO foreign body airway obstruction

FDA Food and Drug Administration

FDG fluorodeoxyglucose

$FEF_{\%}$ forced expiratory flow rate expressed as a percentage of the FVC

$FEF_{200-1200}$ forced expiratory flow rate from 200 to 1200 mL

FET forced exhalation technique

FEV_t forced expiratory volume over a period of time (in seconds)

FEV_t/FVC ratio of FEV_t to FVC (expressed as a percentage: e.g., $FEV_{60\%}$)

F_IO_2 fractional concentration of inspired oxygen

FLV full liquid ventilation

FPOL fluorescence polarization

FRC functional residual capacity

FVC forced vital capacity

G_{AW} airway conductance

GI gastrointestinal

HAFOE high air flow with oxygen entrainment

HbA adult hemoglobin

HbCO carboxi hemoglobin

HbF fetal hemoglobin

HBO hyperbaric oxygen

HCFA Health Care Financing Administration

HCH hygroscopic condenser humidifier

HCO_3^- bicarbonate ion

HCP healthcare provider or handicap

HCPCS HCFA common procedure coding system

HEENT head, eyes, ears, nose, and throat

HEPA high-efficiency particulate air (filter)

HFA hydrofluoroalkane

HFCWC high-frequency chest wall compression

HFCWO high-frequency chest wall oscillation

HFJV high-frequency jet ventilation

HFOV high-frequency oscillation ventilation

HFV high-frequency ventilation

HIV human immunodeficiency virus

HME home medical equipment or heat and moisture exchanger

HMO health maintenance organization

HR heart rate

HR_{max} maximum heart rate

HRCT high-resolution computerized tomography (scan)

Hx history

Hz hertz

IA intra-arterial

IABP intra-arterial balloon pump

IADLs instrumental activities of daily living

IC inspiratory capacity

ICD-9-CM international classification of diseases, 9th revision, clinical modification

ICF intracellular fluid

ICU intensive care unit

ID internal diameter

IDDM insulin-dependent diabetes mellitus (type I)

IDM infants of diabetic mothers

Ig immunoglobulin (denoted as classes G, M, A, D, and E)

ILD interstitial lung disease

IM intramuscular

IMV intermittent mandatory ventilation

INH isoniazid

INO inhaled nitric oxide

IPA independent practice association

IPAP inspiratory positive airway pressure

IPPB intermittent positive pressure breathing

IPV intrapulmonary percussive ventilation

IRDS infant respiratory distress syndrome

IRV inspiratory reserve volume or inverse ratio ventilation

IS	incentive spirometry
ISE	ion-specific electrode
ISO	International Standards Organization
IT	implantation tested or inspiratory time
IV	intravenous
IVC	inferior vena cava
IWL	insensible water loss
JCAHO	The Joint Commission on Accreditation of Healthcare Organizations
JVD	jugular vein distention
JVP	jugular venous pressure
LEAN	lidocaine, epinephrine, atropine, Narcan
LIP	lymphocytic interstitial pneumonia
LMA	laryngeal mask airway
LOC	level of consciousness
LOS	length of stay
LOX	liquid oxygen
L/S	lecithin to sphingomyelin (ratio)
LTB	laryngotracheobronchitis
LVAD	left ventricular assist device
LVN	large-volume nebulizer
LVRS	lung volume reduction surgery
MAC	*Mycobacterium avium* complex
MAS	meconium aspiration syndrome
MCO	managed care organization
MD	muscular dystrophy or medical doctor
MDI	metered-dose inhaler
MDR-TB	multidrug-resistant tuberculosis
MDS	minimum data set
MEP	maximum expiratory pressure
MetHb	methemoglobin
METS	metabolic equivalents of energy expenditure or oxygen consumption
MI	myocardial infarction
MKSD	meter, kilogram, second, degree
MMAD	mass median aerodynamic diameter
MMV	mandatory minute ventilation
MOTT	mycobacteria other than tuberculosis
MPM	mortality probability model
MRI	magnetic resonance imaging
MRSA	methicillin-resistant *Staphylococcus aureus*
MS	multiple sclerosis
MSLT	multiple sleep latency test
MVV	maximum voluntary ventilation
MWT	maintenance of wakefulness test
NAEPP	National Asthma Education and Prevention Program
NAMDRC	National Association of Medical Directors for Respiratory Care
NBRC	National Board for Respiratory Care
NETT	national emphysema treatment trial
NFPA	National Fire Protection Association
NICU	neonatal intensive care unit
NIH	National Institutes of Health
NIOSH	National Institute for Occupational Safety and Health
NOTT	nocturnal oxygen therapy trial
n.p.o.	nothing by mouth
NPPRA	noninvasive positive pressure respiratory assist
NPPV	noninvasive positive pressure ventilation
NPV	negative pressure ventilation
NREM	nonrapid eye movement (sleep)
NRP	neonatal resuscitation program
NSAID	nonsteroidal anti-inflammatory drug
NSCLC	non-small-cell lung cancer
NSCPT	National Society for Cardiopulmonary Technology
NTE	neutral thermal environment
NTM	nontuberculous mycobacterial (infection)
OD	outside diameter or overdose
O_2Hb	oxyhemoglobin
OLB	open lung biopsy
OSA	obstructive sleep apnea
OSHA	Occupational Safety and Health Administration
P-A	posterior-anterior (view)
PALS	pediatric advanced life support
PAP	positive airway pressure or pulmonary artery pressure

P_B barometric pressure

PCG pneumocardiogram

PCO_2 partial pressure of carbon dioxide (usually in either arterial blood, P_aCO_2, or mixed venous blood, $P_{\bar{v}}CO_2$)

PCP *Pneumocystis carinii* pneumonia

PCV pressure-controlled ventilation

PCWP pulmonary capillary wedge pressure

PDA patent ductus arteriosus

PDPV postural drainage, percussion, and vibration

PE physical examination or pulmonary embolism

PEA pulseless electrical activity

PEEP positive end-expiratory pressure

PEFR peak expiratory flow rate

PEP positive expiratory pressure

PERRLA pupils equal, round, and reactive to light and accommodation

PET positron emission tomography (scan)

$P_{et}CO_2$ end-tidal carbon dioxide

$P_{et}O_2$ end-tidal oxygen

PFC persistent fetal circulation

PFT pulmonary function test

pH hydrogen ion concentration

PH_2O water vapor pressure

PICU pediatric intensive care unit

PIE pulmonary interstitial emphysema

PIF peak inspiratory flow

PIP peak inspiratory pressure

pK denotes a constant equal to 6.1 in the Henderson-Hasselbach equation

PLMS periodic limb movements in sleep

PLV partial liquid ventilation

PMI point of maximal impulse

PNS peripheral nervous system

p.o. by mouth (oral)

PO_2 partial pressure of oxygen (usually in either alveolar air, P_AO_2, arterial blood, P_aO_2, or mixed venous blood, $P_{\bar{v}}O_2$)

POC point of care

POMR problem-oriented medical record

POS point of service

PPD purified protein derivative

PPE personal protective equipment

PPHN persistent pulmonary hypertension of newborns

PPO preferred provider organization

PPS prospective payment system

PPV positive pressure ventilation

PS pressure support

PSG polysomnography

PSV pressure support ventilation

PSVT paroxysmal supraventricular tachycardia

PTCA percutaneous transluminal coronary angioplasty

PVC premature ventricular contraction or polyvinyl chloride

PVR pulmonary vascular resistance

QA quality assurance

QC quality control

q.h. every hour (or hourly as noted: e.g., q4h)

q.i.d. four times a day

$\dot{Q}_S/\dot{Q}_T$ ratio of shunted blood flow to total blood flow (shunt fraction)

RAD respiratory assist device

R_{AW} airway resistance

RBC red blood cell

RCIS respiratory care information system

RDI respiratory disturbance index

RDS respiratory distress syndrome

REE resting energy expenditure

REM rapid eye movement (sleep)

RHb reduced hemoglobin or deoxyhemoglobin

RLS restless legs syndrome

RNA ribonucleic acid

ROP retinopathy of prematurity

ROSC	return of spontaneous circulation
RQ	respiratory quotient
RR	respiratory rate
RSV	respiratory syncytial virus
RUG	resource utilization group
RV	residual volume
SA	sinoatrial (node)
S_aO_2	oxygen saturation in arterial blood
SAPS	simplified acute physiology score
SAR	surfactant/albumin ratio
SBTP	standard body temperature and pressure
SCLC	small-cell lung cancer
sd	standard deviation
SG_{AW}	specific airway conductance
SI	standard international (unit) or Système International
SICU	surgical intensive care unit
SIDS	sudden infant death syndrome
SIMV	synchronized intermittent mandatory ventilation
SMI	sustained maximum inflation
SNF	skilled nursing facility
SOAP	subjective, objective, assessment, and plan
SPAG	small-particle aerosol generator
S_pO_2	oxygen saturation obtained via pulse oximetry
SR_{AW}	specific airway resistance
SREMs	slow rolling eye movements
SRSA	slow-reacting substance of anaphylaxis
SRT	surfactant replacement therapy
S/T	spontaneous/timed
S/T-D	spontaneous/timed with diagnostic package
STPD	standard temperature and pressure, dry
SulfHb	sulfhemoglobin
SV	stroke volume
SVC	slow vital capacity or superior vena cava
SVN	small-volume nebulizer
SVR	systemic vascular resistance
SVT	supraventricular tachycardia
TB	tuberculosis
TBB	transbronchial needle biopsy
T_cCO_2	transcutaneous (partial pressure of) carbon dioxide
T_cO_2	transcutaneous (partial pressure of) oxygen
TDP	therapist-driven protocol
TEF	tracheo-esophageal fistula
t.i.d.	three times a day
TLC	total lung capacity
TQM	total quality management
TTNB	transient tachypnea of the newborn
TTOT	transtracheal oxygen therapy
TU	tuberculin unit
UIP	usual interstitial pneumonia (idiopathic pulmonary fibrosis)
USN	ultrasonic nebulizer
V_A	alveolar volume
$\dot{V}_A$	alveolar minute ventilation
VAP	ventilator-associated pneumonia
VATS	video-assisted surgery
VC	vital capacity
V_D/V_T	deadspace volume to tidal volume ratio
$\dot{V}_E$	minute volume or ventilation
$\dot{V}_{Emax}$	maximum minute volume or ventilation
VF	ventricular fibrillation
$\dot{V}O_{2max}$	maximum oxygen consumption
$\dot{V}/\dot{Q}$	ventilation to perfusion ratio
VRE	vancomycin-resistant enterococcus
VRG	ventral respiratory group
V_T	tidal volume (also TV)
V_{TG}	thoracic gas volume (also TGV)
VTLB	video-thorascopic lung biopsy
WBC	white blood cell
WHO	World Health Organization
WOB	work of breathing
YTD	year-to-date
Z79	committee of the American Materials Standards Institute

Routes for Entry-Level (CRT) Practice and Registry-Level (RRT) Practice

CRT Entry-Level Admission Requirements

1. Applicants shall be 18 years of age or older.
2. Applicants shall satisfy ONE of the following educational requirements:
   a. Applicants shall have a minimum of an associate degree from a respiratory therapist education program 1) supported or accredited by the Commission on Accreditation for Respiratory Care (CoARC), or 2) accredited by the Commission on Accreditation of Allied Health Education Programs (CAAHEP) and graduated on or before November 11, 2009.
   b. Applicants enrolled in an accredited respiratory therapy program in an institution offering a baccalaureate degree may be admitted to the CRT Examination with a "special certificate of completion" issued by a sponsoring educational institution. The CoARC will authorize such institutions to issue the "special certificate of completion" at the advanced-level following completion of the science, general academic and respiratory therapy coursework commensurate with the requirements for accreditation.

RRT Registry-Level Admission Requirements

1. Applicants shall be 18 years of age or older.
2. Applicants shall satisfy ONE of the following educational requirements:
   a. Be a CRT having earned a minimum of an associate degree* from a respiratory therapist educational program 1) supported or accredited by the Commission on Accreditation for Respiratory Care (CoARC), or 2) accredited by the Commission on Accreditation of Allied Health Education Programs (CAAHEP) and graduated on or before November 11, 2009. *Graduates of accredited 100-level respiratory therapist education programs are not eligible for admission to the RRT Examination under this admission provision.*

      OR

   b. Be a CRT having been enrolled in an accredited respiratory therapy program in an institution offering a baccalaureate degree offering a "special certificate of completion" issued by a sponsoring educational institution. The CoARC will authorize such institutions to issue the "special certificate of completion" at the advanced level following completion of the science, general academic and respiratory therapy coursework commensurate with the requirements for accreditation.

      OR

   c. Be a therapist Certified (CRT) by the NBRC who has four years* of full-time clinical in respiratory therapy under licensed medical supervision following Certification and prior to applying for the Registry Examination. In addition, the applicant shall have at least 62 semester hours of college credit from a college or university accredited by its regional association or its equivalent. The 62 semester hours of college credit must include the following courses: anatomy and physiology, chemistry, microbiology, physics, and mathematics.

      OR

   d. Be a CRT having earned a minimum of an associate degree from an accredited entry-level respiratory therapist educational program with two years of full-time, clinical experience in respiratory care under licensed medical supervision following Certification and prior to applying for the examination.

      OR

   e. Be a CRT with a baccalaureate degree in an area other than respiratory care, including college credit level courses in anatomy and physiology,

*Individuals certified (CRT) prior to January 1, 1983, are required to complete only three years of clinical experience.

chemistry, mathematics, microbiology and physics. In addition, they shall have two years of full-time clinical experience* in respiratory care under licensed medical supervision following Certification and before applying for the examination. In addition, the applicant shall have at least 62 semester hours of college credit from a college or university accredited by its regional association or its equivalent.

CRT to RRT Admission Requirements

The NBRC continually receives inquiries regarding the "Entry-Level-to-RRT" provision of the admission policies for the Registry Examination. Below are answers to the most commonly asked questions relating to this alternative route to the RRT Examination. If you have questions which are not answered below, or if you need further clarification of this admission policy, please contact the NBRC Executive Office.

The CRT-to-RRT provision is as follows:

Be a CRT with four years** of full-time clinical in respiratory therapy under licensed medical supervision following Certification and prior to applying for the Registry Examination. In addition, the applicant shall have at least 62 semester hours of college credit from a college or university accredited by its regional association or its equivalent. The 62 semester hours of college credit must include the following courses: anatomy and physiology, chemistry, microbiology, physics, and mathematics.

OR

Be a CRT with a baccalaureate degree in an area other than respiratory therapy, including college-level courses in anatomy and physiology, chemistry, microbiology, physics, and mathematics. In addition, the applicant shall have two years of full-time clinical experience in respiratory therapy under licensed medical supervision following Certification and before applying for the examination.

OR

Be a CRT with two years of full-time clinical experience in respiratory therapy under licensed medical supervision following Certification and prior to applying for the Registry Examination and hold a minimum of an associate degree in respiratory therapy from an accredited entry-level respiratory therapy education program.

Clinical experience for both of the above categories is interpreted as a minimum of 21 hours per week, following Certification. Clinical experience must be completed before applying for the Registry Examination.

Semester Hour Requirements for the Basic Science Courses

The Board of Trustees has not established any minimum hour requirement for the required basic science courses. A minimum of 62 semester hours of college credit must be completed; within the 62 hours, a minimum of one course must be completed in each of the following areas: anatomy and physiology, chemistry, microbiology, physics, and mathematics.

The reason semester hour requirements were not established for the basic science courses is because of the lack of uniformity in semester hours (or quarter hours) awarded for similar courses by various colleges or universities across the country. For example, some colleges combine anatomy and physiology, and some colleges offer the two courses separately. Semester hours are awarded by some colleges, while others award credit in quarter hours. Completion of the courses themselves is more important than the number of hours awarded for the required courses.

The NBRC suggests students complete more than the minimum one course in mathematics and the basic sciences, because the more knowledge accumulated in these areas, the better the chance for success on the Registry Examination. No laboratory is required for the basic science courses, if the college or university offers the courses for credit without a laboratory requirement. Many colleges will not offer chemistry, physics, microbiology, etc., without a laboratory portion of the course.

Transcript Requirements

1. CRTs with four years of experience following Certification: Official transcripts must be submitted with a Registry application and fee at the time of application under this provision. A minimum of one course in anatomy and physiology, chemistry, microbiology, mathematics, and physics must appear, by name, on the official transcripts. It must be apparent from the transcript that these courses have been completed. If any of the courses do not appear on the transcripts, by these names, the applicant must obtain a course description from the college catalogue for any course(s) in question and submit each course description(s) to the Admission Committee,

---

*Clinical experience in respiratory care under licensed medical supervision is interpreted as a minimum of 21 hours per week. Clinical experience must be completed before the candidate applies for this examination.

**Individuals certified (CRT) prior to January 1, 1983, are required to complete only three years of clinical experience.

in care of the NBRC, for review and final determination.

2. CRTs with a baccalaureate degree (other than in respiratory therapy) and two years of clinical experience following Certification:
   a. Proof of completion of a baccalaureate degree must be submitted in the form of either official college transcripts or a notarized copy of your baccalaureate degree. Official transcripts verifying completion of the basic sciences and mathematics must also be submitted with a Registry application and fee.
   b. A minimum of one course in anatomy and physiology, chemistry, microbiology, physics, and mathematics must appear, by name, on the official transcript. It must be apparent from the transcript that these courses have been completed. If any of the courses do not appear on the transcript by these names the applicant must obtain a course description from the college catalogue. For any course(s) in question, submit course description(s) to the Admission Committee, in care of the NBRC, for final determination.

College Level Examination Program (CLEP)

Courses challenged through the College Level Examination Program (CLEP) will be accepted toward the 62 semester hours and basic science courses required, provided transferable college credit is awarded by an accredited college or university for each course completed by CLEP examination. The courses attempted through the CLEP program and the credit awarded must be recorded on an official transcript.

Courses Completed at Foreign Colleges or Universities

Courses taken at a foreign college or university do not satisfy the NBRC's requirement of 62 semester hours of college credit. Foreign programs are not "accredited by their regional association or its equivalent." Persons who attended a foreign college should contact an accredited college to have transfer credit awarded for the training they have received. The NBRC will accept transfer credit for foreign courses if an accredited United States college or university is willing to award transfer credit. A letter sealed by the Registrar indicating the courses and hours for which transfer credit is awarded may be accepted in lieu of official college transcripts.

Training Completed at Hospital-Based Nursing or other Health-Related Programs

If you completed courses at a hospital-based nursing or other educational program not accredited by its regional association or its equivalent, the course work will not be accepted unless transfer credit for the courses is awarded from an accredited college or university. A letter sealed by the Registrar indicating the courses and hours for which transfer credit is awarded may be accepted.

Selected Diagnostic Studies

Test	Explanation/Normal Values	Health Care Team Responsibilities
Arterial blood gases (ABGs)	Direct measurement of the pH, P_aO_2, and P_aCO_2 and calculated measurement of HCO_3^- and SaO_2 from samples of arterial blood. pH expresses the acidity or alkalinity of the blood. P_aO_2 = partial pressure of oxygen in the blood. P_aCO_2 = partial pressure of carbon dioxide in the blood. S_aO_2 = arterial oxygen saturation. HCO_3^- = bicarbonate ion concentration in the blood. C_aO_2 = oxygen content of arterial blood expressed as a percentage of the oxygen-carrying capacity of the blood. Normal: pH: 7.35–7.45 P_aO_2: 80–100 mm Hg P_aCO_2: 35–45 mm Hg S_aO_2: > 95% (at sea level) HCO_3^-: 22–26 mEg C_aO_2: 19.8 mL/dL	Explain that an arterial sample of blood is required. Arterial punctures cause more discomfort than venous. Instruct the patient not to move. Assess the adequacy of collateral circulation. Draw the blood sample in a syringe containing heparin. After the specimen has been obtained, rotate the syringe to mix the blood and heparin. Place the blood sample on ice and take it immediately to the lab. Apply pressure to the arterial site for 3–5 minutes or 15 minutes if patient is on an anticoagulant. Assess site for bleeding.
Bronchoscopy	Direct visual examination of the bronchi through a fiberoptic scope. Used to remove foreign bodies, for aggressive pulmonary cleansing, and to obtain sputum and tissue specimens.	Explain the procedure to the patient: that the patient must be n.p.o. for at least 6 hours before the test; that, if ordered, preprocedure sedation is administered; that an IV access will be obtained and sedation given during the procedure via this route. Following the procedure, frequently assess vital signs and respiratory status. Assess the patient for unusual amounts of bleeding. Inform the patient that sputum may be blood tinged initially after the procedure. Maintain the patient in a side-lying position until the gag reflex returns. Withhold all food and fluids until the patient is fully awake and has a gag reflex. Obtain written informed consent per facility policy.

Test	Explanation/Normal Values	Health Care Team Responsibilities
Chest X-ray	Provides a two-dimensional image of the lungs without using contrast media. Used to detect the presence of fluid within the interstitial lung tissue or the alveoli; tumors or foreign bodies; and the presence and size of a pneumothorax. The size of the heart can also be determined by chest X-ray.	Explain the test to the patient. If appropriate, inquire whether the patient may be pregnant, to prevent exposure of the fetus to X-rays. The patient is generally required to stand for various views; if the patient is unable to stand, views may be obtained with the patient in a sitting position, or a portable X-ray may be obtained. Instruct the patient to inspire deeply and hold the breath. Instruct the patient to remove all metal objects from the chest and neck area and to don a hospital gown that does not have snap closures.
Computerized tomography (CT) scan	Provides a three-dimensional cross-sectional view of tissues. Computer-constructed picture interprets densities of various tissues. Useful for viewing tumors in the chest and abdominal cavity.	Explain the procedure to the patient. Obtain informed consent. Initiate n.p.o. status 8 hours before scan. Assess for iodine allergy. Observe for signs of anaphylaxis, if dye is used. Check for claustrophobia. Inform the patient that the test will take approximately 45 minutes to 1 hour. The patient must lie still on a hard, flat table and will be put through a large machine. Because barium will interfere with the test, schedule tests using barium either after or 4 or more days before the scan.
Hemoglobin (Hb)	Measures the oxygen-carrying capacity of the blood. Normal: Male: 14–18 g/dL Female: 12–16 g/dL Critical value: <5 g/dL	The patient is not required to fast for the test. Sample may be drawn from a finger of a child or the heel of an infant.
Magnetic resonance imaging (MRI)	Uses magnetic field and radio waves to detect edema, hemorrhage, blood flow, infarcts, tumors, infections, aneurysms, demyelinating disease, muscular disease, skeletal abnormalities, intervertebral disc problems, and causes of spinal cord compression. Provides greater tissue discrimination than do chest X-ray or CT scans. Performed by qualified technologist. Takes approximately 1 hour.	Assess the patient for the presence of metal objects within the body (e.g., shrapnel, cochlear implants, pacemakers). Explain the procedure to the patient: that the patient will be required to lie still for up to 20 minutes at a time; that the patient will be placed within a scanning tunnel; that sedation may be required if the patient has claustrophobic tendencies; that the magnet will make a loud thumping noise as images are obtained (provide earplugs as necessary). Because the test may require up to 2 hours to perform, have the patient void before entering the scanning tunnel. Obtain informed written consent per facility policy.
Pulmonary angiography	Assesses the arterial circulation of the lungs. Most often used to detect pulmonary emboli.	Explain the procedure to the patient. Assess for allergy to iodine or shellfish. Inform the patient that an arterial puncture is required, usually of the femoral artery, and that the injection of the dye may cause a flushing or warm sensation due to vasodilation. After the study, assess the arterial puncture site frequently for evidence of bleeding. Assess vital signs and respiratory status. The patient may be required to lie flat for up to 6 hours if the femoral artery is used for access. Obtain informed consent per facility policy.

Test	Explanation/Normal Values	Health Care Team Responsibilities
Pulmonary function tests (PFTs)	A group of studies used to evaluate ventilatory function. Measurements are obtained directly via spirometer or are calculated from the results of spirometer measurements. Bronchodilators may be used during the study. Measurements included are: Tidal volume: the amount of air inhaled and exhaled during a normal respiration. Inspiratory reserve volume: the maximum amount of air inspired at the end of a normal inspiration. Expiratory reserve volume: the maximum amount of air expired after a normal expiration. Residual volume: the amount of air left in lungs after maximal expiration. Vital capacity: the total volume of air that can be expired after maximal inspiration. Total lung capacity: the total volume of air in the lungs when maximally inflated. Inspiratory capacity: the maximum amount of air that can be inspired after normal expiration. Forced vital capacity: the capacity of air exhaled forcefully and rapidly after maximal inspiration. Minute volume: the amount of air breathed per minute.	Explain the procedure to the patient. PFTs should not be done within 1–2 hours after a meal. After the test, monitor respiratory status. Advise the patient to avoid activity and to rest after the test, as fatigue may result.
Pulse oximetry	A noninvasive procedure. A transdermal clip is placed on a finger or earlobe to detect the arterial oxygen saturation (S_pO_2). Normal: >95% (at sea level)	Explain the procedure to the patient. Assess peripheral circulation, as this may alter results. Place the sensor on the earlobe, fingertip, or pinna of the ear. Keep the sensor intact until a consistent reading is obtained. Observe and record readings. Report measurements below 95%.
Sputum analysis	Sputum samples are examined for the presence of bacteria, fungi, molds, yeasts, and malignant cells. Appropriate antibiotic therapy is determined via culture and sensitivity studies.	Explain the procedure and its purpose to the patient. Obtain specimens early in the morning to prevent contamination via ingested food or fluids. Instruct the patient to breathe deeply and cough, so as to facilitate collection of a specimen originating from the lower respiratory tract. If necessary, pulmonary suctioning may be used to obtain such a specimen. Instruct the patient to expectorate sputum into the appropriate container. Deliver specimens to the laboratory as soon as possible.

Test	Explanation/Normal Values	Health Care Team Responsibilities
Thoracentesis	Removal of fluid for diagnostic purposes. Also used to obtain biopsy, instill medications, and remove fluid for patient comfort and safety.	Explain the procedure to the patient. Obtain informed consent. Position the patient in an upright sitting position, leaning forward. Have patient rest the arms on an overbed table to facilitate this position. Explain to the patient that the area will be anesthetized before the procedure. Instruct the patient to hold as still as possible during the insertion of the thoracentesis needle. Assist the physician during the procedure. Deliver the specimen to the laboratory as soon as possible. Observe the thoracentesis site for bleeding after the procedure. Assess breath sounds before and after the procedure. Report absent breath sounds immediately.
Ventilation-perfusion scan abbreviation = $\dot{V}/\dot{Q}$	Assesses ventilation and perfusion of the lungs. Most often used to detect the presence of pulmonary emboli.	Assess for allergy to iodine and shellfish. Explain the procedure to the patient: that a radioactive contrast media will be introduced via an IV access and inhalation of radioactive gas and that the patient will be required to hold the breath for short periods as images are obtained. Obtain informed written consent per facility policy.

APPENDIX E

Arterial Blood Gases: Normal Values

Measurement in Blood	Normal Value
Acidity or alkalinity (pH)	7.35–7.45
Arterial oxygen saturation (S_aO_2)	95% (at sea level)
Bicarbonate ion (HCO_3^-)	22–26 mm Hg
Oxygen content (C_aO_2)	19.8 mL/dL
Partial pressure of carbon dioxide (P_aCO_2)	35–45 mm Hg
Partial pressure of oxygen (P_aO_2)	80–100 mm Hg

Characteristics of Adventitious Breath Sounds

Breath Sound	Respiratory Phase	Timing	Description	Clear with Cough	Etiology	Conditions
Fine crackle (rale)	Predominantly inspiration	Discontinuous	Dry, high-pitched crackling, popping, short duration; roll hair near ears between your fingers to simulate this sound	No	Air passing through moisture in small airways that suddenly reinflate	COPD, congestive heart failure (CHF), pneumonia, pulmonary fibrosis, atelectasis
Coarse crackle (coarse rale)	Predominantly inspiration	Discontinuous	Moist, low-pitched crackling, gurgling; long duration	Possibly	Air passing through moisture in large airways that suddenly reinflate	Pneumonia, pulmonary edema, bronchitis, atelectasis
Sonorous wheeze (wheeze)	Predominantly inspiration	Continuous	Low-pitched; snoring	Possibly	Narrowing of large airways or obstruction of bronchus	Asthma, bronchitis, airway edema, tumor, bronchiolar spasm, foreign body obstruction
Sibilant wheeze (wheeze)	Predominantly expiration	Continuous	High-pitched; musical	Possibly	Narrowing of large airways or obstruction of bronchus	Asthma, chronic bronchitis, emphysema, tumor foreign body obstruction
Plerual friction rub	Inspiration and expiration	Continuous	Creaking, grating	No	Inflamed parietal and visceral pleura can occasionally be felt on thoracic wall as two pieces of dry leather rubbing against each other	Pleurisy, tuberculosis, pulmonary infarction, pneumonia, lung abscess
Stridor	Predominantly inspiration	Continuous	Crowing	No	Partial obstruction of the larynx, trachea	Croup, foreign body obstruction, large airway tumor

Note: The red markings on the inspiratory and expiratory "waveforms" indicate which part of the respiratory cycle the sounds are generally heard.

Source: From Estes MEZ. Health Assessment & Physical Examination. *2nd ed. Clifton Park, NY: Delmar Cengage Learning; 2002.*

absolute humidity (AH) The actual amount of water vapor present in a given volume of gas, expressed as the mass of water in a given volume of gas (mg/L or g/m^3).

ACE inhibitors ACE is an abbreviation of angiotensin converting enzyme; first-line drugs used in the treatment of hypertension and congestive heart failure; lower arteriolar resistance and increase venous capacity, increase cardiac output, lower kidney resistance, and increase $Na+$ excretion by the kidney; suppress the renin-angiotensin-aldosterone system (RAAS), which is activated in response to hypotension, decreased sodium in the distal tubule of the nephron, decreased cardiac output, and renal sympathetic nerve stimulation.

acrocyanosis A condition in the newborn characterized by a cyanotic discoloration of the hands and feet; also known as peripheral acrocyanosis of the newborn.

action potential One electrical cycle of depolarization and repolarization within a single cell.

active cycle breathing The combination of forced exhalation technique (FET) with thoracic expansion exercises and diaphragmatic breathing.

active exhalation An exhalation valve that allows spontaneous exhalations.

active listening Verbal and nonverbal techniques to indicate interest and comprehension.

activities of daily living (ADLs) Basic self-care activities such as dressing, bathing, grooming, toileting, and eating.

acuity level A measure of the overall level of acuity among patients.

acute respiratory distress syndrome (ARDS) The most severe form of acute lung injury caused by a variety of direct or indirect insults to the lung; characterized by inflammation of the lung parenchyma leading to oxygenation failure; can be fatal and usually requires admission to the intensive care unit and mechanical ventilation.

acute shunt An area of pulmonary perfusion with no ventilation; refractory to oxygen therapy. *Also known as* absolute shunt.

additive effect The effect when two or more drugs are administered with the same effect on the body; an exaggerated response.

adherence The degree to which a patient follows a therapeutic regimen.

adjuvant therapy Treatment used in addition to the main treatment, usually in reference to chemotherapy, radiation therapy, or immunotherapy, added after surgery to increase the chances of curing the disease or keeping it in check.

administrative law Rules and regulations developed and implemented by agencies of the government.

adrenergic Nerve fibers that release norepinephrine when stimulated. *Also known as* sympathetic.

advanced cardiac life support (ACLS) An algorithm-driven system based on cardiac rhythm to treat cardiac emergencies in adults.

adventitious breath sounds Sounds that are not usually heard in the lungs, such as wheezing and crackles.

aerosol Any liquid or solid particle that is suspended in a gas; a substance that contains solid or liquid particles.

afterload The resistance against which the myocardium must work to pump blood to the lungs and systemic circulation.

air bronchogram In a chest X-ray, the visible outline of bronchi caused by pulmonary infiltrates.

airborne precautions Practices used to protect against the transmission of disease by pathogens that are small, lightweight, suspended in the air, or attached to dust particles in the air.

airborne transmission A method of infectious agent transmission that occurs when the pathogens are tiny and lightweight and can move with air currents or become trapped in dust and then carried through the air.

airway conductance (G_{aw}) A measure of the ease with which air passes through the conducting airways of the pulmonary system; the reciprocal of airway resistance; calculated by dividing the flow produced by the driving pressure (the difference between atmospheric pressure and mouth pressure).

airway obstruction The occlusion of the airway, either partially or completely.

airway resistance (R_{aw}) *See* transairway resistance.

airway suctioning The removal of secretions from the airway with suction devices.

Allen's test (modified) A clinical assessment of the presence and degree of collateral circulation provided to the hand by the ulnar artery.

alveolar recruitment maneuver A procedure that converts collapsed alveoli into open ventilated alveoli and increases lung volume.

alveolar-capillary membrane The interface between alveoli and capillaries where gas exchange via diffusion takes place, with a total surface area of about 75 m^2.

American Association for Respiratory Care (AARC) Professional organization that develops, organizes, and represents the activities of respiratory therapy.

amyloidosis A rare clinical disorder caused by extracellular deposition of an insoluble fibril protein in various tissues and organs; results in end-organ damage (typically the kidney, liver, spleen); occurs with various chronic inflammatory disorders such as rheumatoid arthritis, alkylosing spondylitis, Crohn's disease, tuberculosis, and some neoplasms such as multiple myeloma.

anaerobic threshold (*AT*) During exercise, the point at which oxygen delivery is not sufficient for the tissues to metabolize aerobically and they switch to anaerobic metabolism.

analyte A substance being analyzed; a parameter tested by an analyzer; one of a battery of substances or values measured, such as pH in a blood gas.

anaplastic carcinoma Cancer in which cells have lost specialized characteristics, including physical placement.

anergic An immunological term that refers to diminished immediate hypersensitivity or to diminished delayed hypersensitivity or to both.

angiogram A radiograph of blood vessels made after injection of a radiopaque substance.

angiotensin receptor blockers (ARBs) Medications that block the action of angiotensin II, a potent vasoconstrictor, used in the treatment of hypertension and congestive heart failure; similar in action to ACE inhibitors and often used when patients do not tolerate an ACE inhibitor.

anion gap (AG) The mathematical difference between the cations and anions in the blood plasma.

antagonism The result when two drugs have the opposite effect.

anthrax An infectious disease caused by bacteria called *Bacillus anthracis.*

antibody A protein substance that develops in response to a specific antigen and interacts with it; the antigen-antibody reaction forms the basis for immunity.

antibody titer The reciprocal of the highest dilution of the patient's serum in which antibody is detectable.

anticholinergic A drug that is antagonistic to or blocks the action of parasympathetic or other cholinergic sites. *Also known as* parasympatholytic.

antigen A substance such as pollen, bacteria, a toxin, or foreign blood cell that induces the formation of antibodies that interact specifically with it.

antigenic drift Small changes in the virus that happen continually over time; produces new virus strains that may not be recognized by the body's immune system.

antigenic shift A major modification of the genetic makeup of a virus or bacteria that occurs approximately three times per century and causes major pandemics of infection with high mortality rates.

antimicrobial-resistant microorganisms Pathogens that have altered genetic structure and can survive even when the patient they have infected is treated with a drug designed to kill them.

antiseptic A chemical substance that prevents or inhibits the growth of microorganisms and that is safe to use on the skin.

aortic insufficiency (AI) The incomplete closure of the aortic valve during diastole, resulting in aortic backflow of blood into the left ventricle; may result from a congenitally defective valve, rheumatic heart disease, or syphilis. *Also known as* aortic regurgitation.

aortic stenosis (AS) The obstruction of blood flow across the aortic valve; can ultimately cause congestive heart failure; caused by congenital deformity, rheumatic fever, and degenerative calcific changes of the valve.

APGAR score A means of evaluating newborns that is typically performed at 1 min and 5 min after birth. The following five categories are evaluated and given a rating of 0–2 (the total can thus range from 0 to10): Appearance (pink = 2, acrocyanosis = 1, cyanosis, pale or gray = 0); Pulse (>100 = 2, <100 = 1, absent = 0); Grimace (grimace and cough or sneeze = 2, grimace = 1, absent = 0); Activity (active motion = 2, some flexion of limbs = 1, limp = 0); Respiration (good, strong cry = 2, slow, irregular, weak cry = 1, absent = 0).

aphasia The inability to communicate via speech or impairment of any language modality.

apnea Absence of airflow for greater than of 10 seconds.

apnea/hypopnea index (AHI) Sum of apnea and hypopnea episodes divided by the total sleep time.

apparent life-threatening event (ALTE) An episode experienced by an infant that is characterized by some combination of apnea, color change, marked change in muscle tone, choking, or gagging.

arterial blood gases (ABG) A clinical test to determine the partial pressures of oxygen and carbon dioxide and the pH of an arterial blood sample.

arteriogram A radiograph of an artery made after injection of a radiopaque substance.

artifact Extraneous electrical activity that alters or obscures the biological signal being measured.

artificial airway A device placed in the normal airway to either protect it, keep it patent, and/or afford a route for artificial ventilation.

asphyxia Severe hypoxia that leads to hypoxemia, hypercapnia, acidosis, and eventual death if not corrected.

assault Threatening harm or wrong and the ability to inflict such harm or wrong.

assisted living A facility where patients live independently but receive a limited amount of health-related and daily living assistance as needed.

asthma A chronic inflammatory disorder of the airways in which many immunological cells play a role.

asystole Complete absence of ventricular electrical activity; generally a confirmation of death rather than a rhythm to be treated.

atelectasis Airlessness of a pulmonary segment; the collapse of a lung or a position of a lung.

atopy A genetic predisposition toward an immediate hypersensitivity reaction when exposed to specific antigens.

auscultation The act of using a stethoscope to listen to sounds from a patient.

autocycling Ventilator autocycling occurs if the sensitivity is improperly set or if a gas leak exists in the respiratory system, which creates a negative change in proximal airway pressure resulting in the ventilator cycling prematurely.

autogenic drainage A sequenced pattern of breathing in phases at three increasing lung volumes to enhance movement of secretions to larger airways.

automatic external defibrillator (AED) A device that analyzes the patient's EKG rhythm and that can deliver a shock to the heart.

automaticity The property of the heart that allows it to initiate its own beat without outside stimulation.

autonomic nervous system (ANS) Regulates involuntary functions of the heart, smooth muscle, and glands; impulses from the two divisions, sympathetic and parasympathetic, result in airway smooth muscle tone.

autonomy The ability of an individual to make un-coerced decisions.

auto-PEEP Gas trapped in alveoli at end expiration, due to inadequate time for expiration, bronchoconstriction or mucus plugging. This gas is not in equilibrium with the atmosphere, and it exerts a positive pressure that results in increased work of breathing.

autotitrating CPAP A system for adjusting continuous positive airway pressure automatically through monitoring of various indices of obstruction.

AV dissociation A clinical condition that occurs during any rhythm in which separate pacemakers control the atria and the ventricles.

average life span The age at which half the members of a population have died.

bacteria Unicellular, microscopic organisms classified as Prokaryotae, usually lacking a nuclear membrane and other organelles such as mitochrondria.

barotrauma Damage caused by excessive pressure.

baseline pressure Airway pressure at end-exhalation; either zero, without PEEP, or the PEEP/CPAP level.

basement membrane A thin membrane made up of proteins held together by type-IV collagen that is a vital component of the extracellular matrix.

basic life support (BLS) A system for evaluating and supporting life during a cardiopulmonary emergency following the basics of airway, breathing, and circulation—in infants, children, and adults—with minimal or no adjunctive equipment.

battery Intentional touching of another person without that person's consent.

bends Condition occurring when gas leaves the blood and enters body cavities and spaces because of rapid depressurization. *Also known as* caisson worker's disease but it is not the same as rapture of the deep or nitrogen narcosis.

beneficence The duty to do good and avoid doing harm.

benign tumor An abnormal growth that is not cancer and that does not spread to other areas of the body.

bias flow Background flow that starts when the patient's expiratory flow is complete.

bicarbonate buffer system A buffer system consisting of the bicarbonate–carbonic acid pair; buffers a noncarbonic acid or base.

bicycle ergometer A stationary bicycle that can be programmed to alter the resistance to pedaling or workload for the user; used in cardiovascular or pulmonary diagnostic laboratories to provide a controlled change in workload during exercise stress tests.

bi-level positive airway pressure (BiPAP™) A variation of continuous positive airway pressure that delivers separate levels of positive pressure during inspiration and expiration.

biofeedback The provision of visual or auditory information about physiologic functions.

blast lung injury (BLI) The major cause of immediate deaths in explosions along with the presence of an air embolism that results from a BLI.

blast overpressure injuries *See* primary blast injury.

blind nasotracheal intubation Intubation performed without the use of lyrngeal or fiberoptic scopes.

body humidity (BH) The water vapor content required to fully saturate alveolar air at normal body temperature; expressed as a percentage.

body plethysmography A method for measuring changes in pressure and volume in the thorax.

body temperature pressure saturation (BTPS) The condition of fully saturated alveolar air at normal body temperature (37°C) and at barometric (atmospheric) pressure (760 mm Hg); 100% relative humidity in the body.

Bohr effect The increased oxygen release by hemoglobin in the presence of elevated carbon dioxide levels.

Borg scale A validated linear numerical score – usually from 0–10 and sometimes label 0 = none 10 = most that can be used to assess patient's level of pain, dyspnea, anxiety almost any subjective symptom. *See also* Modified Borg Dyspnea Scale.

Boyle's law The principle that, at constant temperature, the pressure of a gas varies inversely with its volume.

brachytherapy Internal radiation treatment given by placing radioactive seeds or pellets directly into the tumor or close to it.

bradycardia An abnormally low heart rate.

bradypnea An abnormally low breathing rate.

bronchopleural fistulas An abnormal connection between the tracheobronchial tree (bronchi and bronchioles) and the lining of the lung or pleura, producing air leaks.

bronchoprovocation A testing regimen used to detect airway hyperreactivity or exercise-induced asthma.

bruit Noise auscultated over an artery narrowed by vascular disease; caused by turbulence generated by the obstruction. (Normally one cannot hear anything when auscultating over an artery.)

bulla An air- or fluid-filled cyst in the lung tissue (plural, bullae).

calibration A test to determine the accuracy of measuring equipment.

cancer A group of diseases that cause cells in the body to change and grow out of control, in most cases forming a lump or mass, called a tumor, which, in turn, can invade and destroy healthy tissue.

cancer susceptibility genes Genes inherited from one's parents that greatly increase the risk of a person developing cancer. About 5–10% of all cancers are caused by these genes.

capital budget The budget formed for equipment with a useful life longer than 5 years and usually a unit cost of over $500.

capitated care A method for controlling the cost of health care by setting a total amount to be spent on a patient over his or her lifetime.

capnogram The graphic representation of the carbon dioxide percentages in expired gas throughout the respiratory cycle, as opposed to a simple display of numeric values.

capnometer A device that collects and measures exhaled carbon dioxide and displays the numeric value as a percentage.

carbogen A therapeutic mixture of carbon dioxide and oxygen.

carcinogen Any substance that causes cancer or helps it grow, such as tobacco smoke, which contains many carcinogens that greatly increase the risk of lung cancer.

carcinoid tumors Tumors that develop from neuroendocrine glands, usually digestive tract, lung, or ovary. The cancer cells from these tumors release certain hormones into the bloodstream, which are sometimes high enough to cause symptoms.

carcinoma in situ A premalignant neoplasm in which the tumor cells are confined to the epithelium of origin and have not invaded the basement membrane.

cardiac cycle One complete heartbeat, including atrial and ventricular systole and diastole.

cardiac markers Enzymes (e.g., creatinine kinase-MB isoforms, cardiac troponins, and myoglobin) released from damaged heart muscle following a heart attack or myocardial infarction (MI); important chemistry tests to diagnose an acute MI; The best markers depend on the time from onset of symptoms: earliest, myoglobin and CK-MB isoforms; 6–24 hours, troponins and CK-MB.

cardiac output (CO) The amount of blood ejected by each ventricle each minute.

cardiac rehabilitation A program of education and exercise that focuses on restoring cardiac patients to the highest possible functional capacity; patients are monitored for pulse rate, blood pressure, and cardiac function.

cardiac tamponade A condition in which a large volume of fluid in the pericardium causes compression of the heart.

cardiogenic shock A type of shock manifested by a decreased pumping ability of the heart, causing global hypoperfusion; commonly associated with acute myocardial infarction; diagnosis based on clinical signs of oliguria (<30 mL/h), altered mental status, hypotension (systolic pressure < 90 mm Hg lasting more than 30 minutes), with evidence of tissue hypoperfusion with adequate left ventricular filling pressure and cold peripheries (extremities colder than core).

cardiopulmonary exercise (CPX) evaluation/test Diagnostic evaluation involving measurement of pulmonary and cardiac function during exercise. *Also known as* stress test.

cardioversion The delivery of electrical energy to the heart synchronized to the R-wave to convert a rapid rhythm (atrial fibrillation, atrial flutter, supraventricular tachycardia, ventricular tachycardia [with a pulse]) to a more effective perfusing rhythm.

care plan (planning) A planned approach to providing care that is designed to identify problems and needs, set goals, and take actions in order to improve outcomes.

Carlen's tube A double lumen endobrochial tube used for independent lung ventilation.

carrier A person who is infected with and can transmit an illness but has no signs or symptoms of it.

case A person who is symptomatic with an illness.

case law Law resulting from judicial interpretations of statutes.

case management A method of medical management in which a person is assigned patients with the same types of problems to standardize care.

caseous necrosis A form of tissue necrosis in which the tissue is converted into a dry, amorphous mass that resembles cheese or curd.

castle port A circular opening in the connector between the circuit tubing and the patient interface. Gas flow out of this opening constitutes a consistent leak and serves to flush the patient's exhalation out of the circuit.

cataplexy A sudden decrease in muscle tone precipitated by anger, laughter, or other types of emotion; a predominant finding in narcolepsy.

catheter whip Excessive movement of the catheter tip, causing an erratic pressure curve in heart cauterization and arterial pressure monitoring.

centenarian An individual who is 100 years old or older.

Centers for Medicare & Medicaid Services (CMS) Federal administrative agency charged with primary responsibility for Medicare and the federal portion of the Medicaid programs; formerly the Health Care Financing Administration (HCFA).

central cyanosis Blueing of the central mucous membranes such as the lips and gums, indicating a decrease in hemoglobin saturation; most likely caused by hypoxemia.

central sleep apnea Complete cessation of airflow due to loss of neural drive.

centriacinar emphysema A type of emphysema in which the respiratory bronchioles are affected but the alveolar ducts and alveoli are not.

chain of infection The elements that must be present for infectious disease transmission to occur.

Charles's law The principle that, at constant pressure, the volume of a gas is directly proportional to its absolute (Kelvin) temperature.

chemotherapy Treatment with drugs to destroy cancer cells; often used either alone or with radiation and surgery, to treat cancer that has spread or come back or when there is a strong change of recurrence. *Also known as* chemo.

chronic Term meaning long term, or lasting longer than 3 months; the opposite of acute or sudden.

chronic disease An illness that lasts for more than 3 months.

cidofovir (Vistide) An antiviral agent (Vistide) that can be delivered by a small particle nebulizer or aersol generator.

clean refers to removal of surface debris but does not infer destruction of microbes.

clinical practice guidelines (CPGs) Systematically developed statements to assist practitioner and patient decisions about appropriate health care for specific clinical circumstances.

clinical respiratory services Services provided for treatment of individuals with disorders of the cardiopulmonary system, including diagnostic testing, therapeutics, and monitoring.

coagulopathy A disorder in the blood's clotting systems.

coccidioidomycosis A fungal infection caused by *Coccidioides immitis*, a soil fungus endemic to California's San Joaquin Valley, southern Arizona, New Mexico, Texas, and northern Mexico. Inhaled spores migrate to the alveoli, where they transform into thick-walled spherules that cause granulomas and lung cavitation.

code of ethical conduct A statement of values and precepts under which a profession conducts itself and to which its members adhere.

coefficient of variance (CV) The standard deviation expressed as a percentage of the mean.

cohort A group of individuals having a statistical factor in common in a demographic study.

collateral ventilation The entrance of air through channels between adjacent airways or alveoli, allowing for ventilation around obstructed airways.

colonization Infectious organisms cultured from persons who are not ill.

Committee on Accreditation of Respiratory Care (CoARC) The entity that accredits respiratory care education programs.

common law Law that is in effect through custom precedent and history.

common vehicle transmission A method of infectious agent transmission in which many people use the same substance, such as contaminated food, water, or medications.

communication A series of behaviors that are specifically verbal and nonverbal and that stimulate personal inquiry between two or more persons.

community-acquired infection/pneumonia *See* hospital-acquired infection/pneumonia.

comorbid Refers to coexisting disease processes.

compensatory pause A prolonged period of time between a premature ventricular contraction and the next normal QRS beat.

compliance A patient's following the health plan; also, the volume change per unit pressure change across the lung.

comprehensive outpatient rehabilitative facility (CORF) Outpatient rehabilitation programs that meet certain criteria as prescribed by Medicare for the implementation of physical reconditioning, including pulmonary rehabilitation for chronic lung patients.

computerized (axial) tomography (CT or CAT) A radiographic method that projects radiation in an axial plane and processes continuous measurements to create a two-dimensional or a three-dimensional image.

conditional variable The variable that determines a change in ventilation; if a certain situation occurs, then the ventilator will change ventilation in some manner.

conducting zone Region of the tracheobronchial tree that does not participate in gas exchange; serves as a conduit for gases to the respiratory zone; extends from the trachea and includes the terminal bronchioles (generations 0 through 19).

conduction Occurs when the newborn's skin comes in direct contact with objects that are lower than body temperature.

confidentiality Keeping the privacy of information.

conjugate pair A pair consisting of a weak acid and a weak base that make up a buffer system.

constitutional law The segment of public law that deals with the organization, its granted powers, and the framework of government; sets limits on what federal and state governments may do.

constrictive pericarditis A rare condition when a thickened fibrotic pericardium impedes normal diastolic filling; usually involves the parietal pericardium and sometimes the visceral pericardium; prognosis determined by the underlying disease; may be idiopathic or caused by infections such as tuberculosis, postsurgical, radiation induced, and end-stage renal failure.

contact precautions Practices used to protect against pathogen transmission when a patient has an infection that can be spread by direct or indirect contact.

contact transmission A method of infectious agent transmission that can be direct (person to person, usually resulting from improper handwashing or contact with contaminated fluid) or indirect (touching a contaminated object, then touching a person and transmitting the pathogen).

continuous lateral rotation therapy (CLRT) A method of providing constant turning of patients who have decreased mobility and who are unable to reposition themselves.

continuous mandatory ventilation (CMV) All breaths are mandatory in that the machine triggers *and/or* cycles the breath.

continuous positive airway pressure (CPAP) A form of therapy, first described in 1981, in which a positive pressure, established in the patient's airway, acts as a pneumatic splint to prevent the airway from collapsing; the primary treatment option for obstructive sleep disordered breathing.

continuous spontaneous ventilation (CSV) All breaths are spontaneous in that the patient must trigger and cycle the breath.

contractility The force produced by myocardial muscle fibers as they shorten.

contrast Use of a substance that alters the density of a structure or its surrounding space to make that structure visible in a radiographic study.

convection The principle by which heat is transferred from food in a refrigerator or freezer. As cool air is circulated around the food, heat is transferred from the warmer food to the cooler air.

co-oximetry The measurement of oxyhemoglobin species or types by near infrared light wave spectrometry; an advanced form of oxyimetry.

coulometric-amperometric method An analytical technique based on the measuring of electrical current through an electrochemical cell while a constant electrical potential is applied to the electrodes.

cricothyrotomy A surgical or manual puncture through the skin and membrane separating the cricoids and thyroid cartilages of the trachea to provide an opening between the trachea and the atmosphere. *Also known as* cric.

critical path A management tool that was developed in the 1950s that guides and coordinates patient care to ensure quality; mixes processes and time limits to set appropriate length of stay to reduce costs. *Also known as* critical pathway.

CT angiogram (CTA) The standard for the diagnosis of pulmonary embolism (noninvasive, fast, able to depict thrombi from first- to fourth-order vessels); able to see associated lung findings (infarcts, collapse consolidation, and pleural effusion, central pulmonary artery emboli that are adherent to vessel walls).

cuff A balloonlike structure attached above the patient end of a tracheostomy or endotracheal tube to create an airtight seal between the outer walls of the tube and the inner wall of the trachea.

cuirass A device used in negative pressure ventilation that fits snugly over the patient's chest or chest and abdomen. It is attached to a negative pressure ventilator and produces a negative extrathoracic pressure, causing inspiration.

cultural norms The expected practices, rules, values, and beliefs of a large group of people.

cumulative effect The effect when doses of the same drug are administered before inactivation and removal from the body takes place, especially if the drug has a long half-life (time required to metabolize 50% of the drug administered); an exaggerated response and possibly toxic situation.

current procedural terminology (CPT) coding Medical procedure coding system maintained and published by the American Medical Association (AMA).

cycle The variable on a mechanical ventilator that ends an inspiration; time, volume, flow, or pressure.

cytokine storm The release of tumor necrosis factor-alpha, interleukin-6, 7, 8, and interferon; an immunologiocal overreaction that leads to acute respiratory distress syndrome (ARDS).

cytology The branch of science that deals with the structure and function of cells; also, testing to diagnose cancer and other diseases by looking at cells under the microscope.

Dalton's law The principle that the total pressure of a mixture of gases equals the sum of the individual pressures.

damped pressure curve A low, rounded pressure curve, without distinct characteristics, usually due to air bubbles in the extension tubing or fibrin collecting at the tip of the arterial or cardiac pressure catheter.

decompression sickness A condition arising from dissolved gases coming out of solution into bubbles inside the body on depressurization. *Also known as* the bends or caisson worker's disease.

decortication The removal of part or all of the outer surface of an organ.

defamation An injury to a person's reputation or character caused by false statements made by another to a third party.

defendant The person or agency who allegedly has done wrong or harm to another.

defibrillation Unsynchronized delivery of electrical energy to the heart to convert either ventricular fibrillation or pulseless ventricular tachycardia to a perfusing rhythm.

delayed hypersensitivity reaction An immunological reaction that is initiated by sensitized (antigen-reactive) T-cells reacting with specific antigens.

demand flow system A portable oxygen device that provides a bolus of oxygen in response to the patient's inspiration, eliminating the need for continuous oxygen flow on portable oxygen cylinders.

depolarization A change in transmembrane potential from negative toward positive that occurs inside cardiac cells.

deposition The depositing of an aerosol particle that has fallen out of solution on to a surface.

derived units Scientific measures that are results of combinations of other derived or measured units.

detraining effect The loss of physical conditioning that results when patients cannot continue their exercise prescription.

diagnosis-related groups (DRGs) Designations of diagnoses used for reimbursement purposes by Medicare.

diaphragmatic hernia A birth defect in which there is an abnormal opening in the diaphragm.

diaphoresis Profuse sweating resulting from hyperthyroidism, shock, stimulants, acute myocardial infarction, and infections and accompanying fever and/or chills.

diastasis A period of cessation of ventricular filling in the diastolic phase of the cardiac cycle.

diastole The period of the cardiac cycle in which the ventricles relax and fill with blood.

diastolic dysfunction A type of heart failure in which changes in ventricular diastolic properties have an adverse effect on stroke volume; a combination of impaired ventricular relaxation and a decrease in passive ventricular distensibility; in the ICU, commonly caused by ventricular hypertrophy, myocardial ischemia, and positive pressure ventilation.

diastolic gallop A third or fourth heart sound that sometimes sounds like the gait of a horse; due to rapid ventricular filling in early diastole, causing high-pitched vibrations of the ventricular wall as the blood abruptly stops; signifies serious heart disease or decompensation and is associated with coronary, hypertensive, rheumatic, and congenital cardiac disease. *Also known as* gallop rhythm.

differential pressure pneumotachometer A device used to measure flow rate by measuring the difference in pressure from one side of a resistive element to the other side as air flows through the resistive element.

difficult airway An airway that is not easily visualized or manipulated due to physical deformaties or tramatic injury to the mouth, nose, and/or throat.

diffusing capacity The rate at which a gas (oxygen) diffuses from the alveoli into the capillaries.

diffusion The movement of gas molecules from an area of relatively high concentration to lower concentration, which continues until all of the gases reach equilibrium.

dimensional analysis The examination and reduction of the units of measure calculated in mathematical or scientific equations.

dimensionless number A derived number whose solution has no unit value owing to the cancellation process of mathematics.

diplopia Seeing double or double vision.

direct contact Person-to-person contact with the possibility of contamination.

direct cost Value of health-care resources devoted to the diagnosis and management of a disease, including hospitalization, drug therapy, rehabilitation; costs generally reimbursed by health insurance.

discovery The fact-finding period, before trial, in a lawsuit.

disease prevention Activities undertaken to decrease the likelihood of the occurrence of a disease, to detect disease as early as possible, or to rehabilitate people when disease occurs.

disinfectant A chemical substance that prevents or inhibits the growth of microorganisms and that is too harsh to use on the skin.

disinfected Refers to an item that has been treated in such a way as to reduce the number of pathogens to the point where they pose no danger of disease.

disinfection The process of inhibiting or killing vegetative cells or microorganisms, in which some organisms may not be destroyed.

disphonia *See* dysphonia.

disseminated intravascular coagulopathy (DIC) A pathological activation of coagulation (blood clotting) mechanisms that happens in response to a variety of diseases.

distant metastasis Cancer that has spread to organs or tissues that are far away from the original site; for example, the spread of lung cancer to the liver or bone. (Pleural: metastases)

distending pressure The pressure required to expand the volume of a distensible object by a given amount.

divine command ethics A system of ethics based on the belief in either divine or exemplary individuals; generally characterized by a no exception clause, either explicit or implicit.

Doppler sonography The ultrasound techniques that involve a shift in the frequency of sound waves.

double effect A situation in which an action can have both a good and a bad effect.

doubling time The time it takes to double in size or number.

droplet precautions Practices used to protect against pathogen transmission when a patient has an infection that can be spread by means of droplets in the air.

droplet transmission A method of infectious agent transmission that occurs when the pathogens are spread by mucus and other droplets from a patient's respiratory tract.

ductus arteriosus The vascular channel that connects the pulmonary artery to the descending aorta in fetal circulation.

ductus venosus The vascular channel in the fetal circulation that passes through the liver and connects the umbilical vein to the inferior vena cava.

dumbbels The symptoms of a cholinergic toxidrome; mnemonic for diarrhea, urination, miosis/muscle weakness, bronchorrhea, bradycardia, emesis, and lacrimation.

dynamic compliance The value of lung compliance (C_L) estimated during breathing by dividing the tidal volume by the difference in instantaneous transpulmonary pressures at the end inspiration, when flow in the airway is momentarily zero.

dysarthria A motor speech disorder resulting from neurological injury, characterized by poor articulation.

dyshemoglobins Variants of hemoglobin that do not contribute to the transport of oxygen: methemoglobin, sulfhemoglobin, and carboxyhemoglobin.

dysphagia Difficulty in swallowing.

dysphonia A disorder of the voice; an impairment in the ability to produce voice sounds using the vocal organs. *Also spelled* disphonia.

echocardiography A specialized form of ultrasound used to image the heart in motion.

eclampsia Hypertension accompanied by seizures or coma unrelated to any underlying neurologic conditions.

education The process of influencing behaviors, producing changes in knowledge, attitudes, and skills required to maintain a state; sometimes used synonymously with training and teaching.

elastance The change in pressure per change in volume; the natural ability of an object to return to its original size and shape after an external force is removed.

elastic recoil The tendency to return to original size or shape after expansion.

elasticity A physical property of mucus that allows it to return to its original size and shape after being stretched.

electroencephalogram (EEG) A recording of the electrical activity of the brain.

electrolyte Anion or cation circulating in body fluids.

electromyogram (EMG) A recording of electrical activity from muscles, frequently from the chin and leg muscles during polysomnography.

electrooculogram (EOG) A recording of voltage changes that occur between the back and front of the eye as the eye moves.

emergency mass critical care (EMCC) The surge in patients and acuity levels that will challenge the resources on hand during an emergency or disaster.

empirical Referring to decisions made with knowledge gained through clinical experience.

empyema The presence of pus in the pleural space.

endemic Belonging exclusively or confined to a particular place or people.

endogenous Produced or originating from or within the body.

endotracheal intubation An artificial airway inserted into the trachea for the purpose of maintaining a patent airway.

environmental model Modern analyses of ecosystems and environmental risks to health, such as socioeconomic status, education, and various environmental factors that affect health.

epidemic An unusually high incidence of a disease in a community.

epithelium Lining of the respiratory system from the trachea to the respiratory bronchioles; consists of ciliated and nonciliated cells, many of which contain mucus-producing goblet cells.

epoch A standard page on a polysomnogram, typically with a 30-second time interval.

Esen % The adjustable cycle flow rate for pressure-support and volume-support breaths on the PB-840 ventilator. Called Inspiratory Cycle-off % on the Servo^{i} ventilators.

esophageal gastric tube airway (EGTA) A modification of the EOA with a central lumen that allows passage of a gastric tube to decompress the stomach, which has had gas insufflated during bag-mask ventilation.

esophageal obturator airway (EOA) A device that is inserted blindly into the esophagus to prevent gastric insufflation and regurgitation of gastric contents during artificial ventilation. *See also* esophageal gastric tube airway (EGTA).

esophageal tracheal combitube (ETC) A dual-lumen tube with a small cuff (about 10 mL) around the end and a large cuff (about 100 mL) farther up.

ethics The critical reflection about morality and the rational analysis of it.

etiology The cause of a disease.

evaporation A natural cooling mechanism by which sweat and other liquids on the surface of the skin transition from liquid to the vapor phase, absorbing heat as they do.

excessive daytime sleepiness (EDS) Difficulty maintaining alertness during the day. Also known as hypersomnolence.

exercise prescription The amount and intensity of exercise recommended for patients in rehabilitation and physical reconditioning programs.

expiratory pause Exhalation valve closes (and inspiratory valve remains closed) at end exhalation. Ventilator pressure measures alveolar pressure during the pause. Expiratory pause pressure will detect auto-PEEP or intrinsic-PEEP.

expiratory positive airway pressure (EPAP) The level of CPAP in spontaneous modes or the level of PEEP in timed modes.

exponent A power of 10.

exsufflation Mechanical production of a negative pressure to the patient's airway in order to stimulate a cough and expectoration.

extracellular matrix All the connective tissues and fibers that are not part of a cell but that provide support. The extracellular matrix includes the interstitial matrix and the basement membrane.

extrathoracic Outside or around the thorax.

exudate Fluid with a high concentration of protein that has accumulated in a body space or cavity.

FAARC Fellows of the AARC

false imprisonment The unlawful restriction of another's freedom.

fee-for-service A type of payment system in which each activity is charged individually.

fellowship The fellowship program of the Society of Critical Care Medicine (SCCM). The American College of Chest Physicians (ACCP) or other professional societies.

felony A major crime; a serious breach of law punishable by death or imprisonment in a state or federal penitentiary.

fertilization The union of a male gamete and a female gamete to form a zygote, from which the embryo develops.

fiberoptic intubation Intubation using a lighted fiberoptic tube, which allows direct visualization of the oral and tracheal airways.

fibrinolysis Primary fibrinolysis refers to the normal breakdown of clots. In secondary fibrinolysis, a fibrin clot is broken down due to a medical disorder, a fibrinolytic drug, or other cause. Clot dissolution leads to circulating fibrin clot fragments that are cleared by other enzymes, the kidney, or the liver.

fiduciary relationship A legal relationship that requires the provider to act in the best interests of the receiver.

flail chest A condition in which two or more fractures in two or more adjacent ribs cause inappropriate movement of a segment of the chest wall.

flow The volume of a liquid or gas moved per time period.

flow-volume loop A graphically depicted display of the rate of airflow on the *y*-axis and the total volume inspired or expired on the *x*-axis of a two dimensional *x*-*y* plot.

fluid physics The study of the physical properties of matter and energy as applied to materials that flow.

fluoroscopy An imaging method that displays an X-ray image on a video monitor in real time rather than on a photographic plate.

fomite An inanimate object that carries viable pathogenic microorganisms.

fontanelle The space on a newborn's cranium between the cranial bones, covered by a tough membrane.

foramen ovale An opening in the septum separating the atria of the heart in fetal circulation.

fraction of inspired oxygen (F_IO_2) The oxygen concentration of inspired air, technically expressed as a decimal.

fractional concentration In a gas mixture, the percent composition, by material, expressed in a percentage of the total.

fractional saturation A measure obtained when four wavelengths of light are used to compare oxyhemoglobin with total hemoglobin; obtained by co-oximetry.

Frank-Starling principle An expression of the relationship between ventricular preload and cardiac output; "more in, more out."

fremitus Vibrations transmitted through the skin.

functional residual capacity (FRC) The total amount of gas remaining in the lungs after exhaling to the normal resting level.

functional saturation A measure obtained when two wavelengths of light are used to compare oxyhemoglobin with reduced hemoglobin; obtained by pulse oximetry.

fungi Microscopic plants that lack chlorophyll and are filamentous in structure.

gallop rhythm An abnormal sequence of heartbeats that sounds like a horse galloping.

Gay-Lussac's law Principle that, at a constant volume, the temperature of a gas will change in the same direction as a change in temperature.

geriatrics A specialized branch of medicine that deals with the diseases of later life and the provision of health care for older people.

Ghon complex An isolated calcified density that appears in the middle or lower lung zones and that is the result of fibrosis and calcification of the layers of the tuberculous granulomata; seen on the chest X-rays of people with primary tuberculosis infection.

glossopharyngeal breathing A method of increasing the lung volume at end-inspiration. *Also known as* frog breathing or glossopharyngeal insufflation.

glycolysis The series of reactions that convert one molecule of glucose into two molecules of pyruvic acid; the first stage of cellular respiration of a molecule of glucose, releasing a small amount of energy in the form of ATP.

goal A general statement of purpose that is usually a simple item and that may be measured to determine the success of a plan to achieve it.

granulomatous Term describing a lung disease that results in the formation of pulmonary nodules of inflammatory cells, such as macrophages surrounded by a rim of lymphocytes; a chronic inflammatory response initiated by various infectious and noninfectious agents.

gray hepatization stage The third stage of the pneumonic consolidation process; occurs 4–5 days postinfection; lung is yellow-gray and looks similar to the liver; the alveoli fill with polymorphonuclear leukocytes.

Haldane effect The effect of changes in oxyhemoglobin saturation based on the relationship of carbon dioxide content to PCO_2.

hand antisepsis The removal or destruction of transient flora through the use of antimicrobial soap, detergent, or an alcohol-based hand scrub.

hand hygiene Handwashing and other related measures to control microbial growth and transmission.

handwashing The removal of soil and transient flora by the combination of friction, plain soap or detergent, and water.

harm principle Principle that health-care providers must report information that is necessary to protect others who are vulnerable to grave health and safety risks in order to prevent greater harm.

health A state of complete physical, mental, and social well-being, not merely the absence of disease or infirmity.

Health Insurance Portability and Accountability Act (HIPAA) Legislation designed to encourage the use of electronic transmission of health information (to assist in cost containment) and to provide new safeguards to protect the security and confidentiality of the information.

health promotion Activities geared toward enhancing the quality of life and preventing disease and disability.

healthcare common procedure coding system (HCPCS) The Health Care Financing Administration coding system for reporting outpatient health care services provided to Medicare beneficiaries.

health-care-associated infection Any infection associated with a medical or surgical intervention; replaces "nosocomial," which is limited to adverse infectious outcomes occurring in hospitals.

heliox A therapeutic mixture of helium and oxygen.

hemagglutinin A substance that causes red blood cells to agglutinate, a spike-shaped protein that extends from the surface of the virus; one of the reasons that influenza virus is so effective.

hemoglobin buffer system A buffer system consisting of the $HHb–Hb^-$ and $HHbO_2–Hb_2^-$ pairs.

hemothorax Extravascular blood in the pleural space.

hepatojugular reflux The distention of the jugular vein from elevation of the venous pressure induced by applying manual pressure over the liver; suggestive of right heart dysfunction.

high-efficiency particulate air (HEPA) filter A special filtering mask designed to block particles smaller than 10 μm; must be fit-tested to each individual by a qualified tester.

high-flow oxygen system An oxygen delivery system that meets the entire peak inspiratory flow requirements of the patient; F_IO_2 is fixed.

high-frequency chest wall oscillation (HFCWO) Pulsation of air at frequencies between 5 and 25 Hz applied to a vest worn by the patient, producing transient increase in airflow and shear forces that alter the physical properties of mucus and increase mucus mobilization.

high-frequency filter A component of the polygraph that allows for the attenuation of a high-frequency artifact obscuring a biological signal.

high-frequency oscillation (HFO) The vibration of air in the airways at frequencies of 6–20 Hz to loosen secretions.

high-frequency ventilation (HFV) Respiratory rates that greatly exceed the rate of normal breathing. Three principal types of HFV: high-frequency positive pressure ventilation (HPPV, rate 60–150/minute); high-frequency jet ventilation (HFJV, rate 100–600); high-frequency oscillatory ventilation (HFOV, rate 300–3000/minute).

high-order explosion (HE) An explosion that produces extreme pressure waves traveling faster than the speed of sound (1116 ft/sec or 761 mph); produced by TNT, C-4, Semtex, nitroglycerin, and dynamite.

holistic model Encompasses the physiological, mental, emotional, social, spiritual, and environmental aspects of health.

Homan's sign Any condition causing signs and symptoms of deep venous thrombosis may cause a positive Homan's sign; with the patient's knee in the flexed position, the examiner forcibly and abruptly dorsiflexes the calf.

home medical equipment (HME) companies Providers of medical equipment and supplies for use in the home care setting. Previously referred to as durable medical equipment (DME) companies.

homeostasis A state of relatively constant conditions in a changing environment.

honeycomb lung A lung in end-stage pulmonary fibrosis.

Hooke's law Rule governing elastance; within the elastic limits of an elastic structure, the amount of stretch is directly and linearly proportional to the force exerted on the object.

hospital emergency incident command system (HEICS) An internal emergency incident command system (HEICS) or incident command system (ICS) that hospitals should have and be ready to activate in order to coordinate the hospital's response to an incident.

hospital-acquired infection An infection acquired in a hospital or other medical facility. *Also known as* nosocomial infection.

hospital-acquired pneumonia A pneumonia acquired in a hospital or other medical facility. *Also known as* nosocomial infection.

hot-lighting Use of a high-intensity light to enhance contrast when reading and interpreting radiographic films.

HR 6331 (Medicare Improvements for Patients and Providers Act) The act that enabled Medicare to issue an NCD for outpatient pulmonary rehabilitation, allowing programs to bill for 36 pulmonary rehabilitation sessions (usually 3 sessions per week for 12 weeks) plus an additional 36 sessions if continuation of pulmonary rehabilitation is deemed necessary for the patient by the prescribing healthcare provider.

human resource management The management of staff in any organization.

humidifier A device designed to add molecular water to the surrounding gas.

humidity The amount of water present in gaseous form being transported by air or other gases; water in its molecular form.

humidity deficit The difference between the body humidity and absolute humidity of inspired gas.

hydrostatic pressure The pressure at any given point of a nonmoving (static) fluid. The average capillary hydrostatic pressure is determined by arterial and venous pressures and by the ratio of postcapillary to precapillary resistances.

hygrometer An instrument used to measure humidity in the atmosphere.

hygroscopic Refers to a substance that absorbs moisture from the surrounding environment.

hyperbaric oxygen therapy (HBO) Exposing a patient to a pressure greater than 1 atmosphere while breathing 100% oxygen continuously or intermittently.

hypercapnea An increased P_ACO_2; commonly accepted as a P_ACO_2 above 45 mm Hg.

hyperinflation Inflation to a volume above normal; inspiration to nearly maximal levels to inflate collapsed alveoli.

hypertonic Refers to a substance that contains greater concentration of solute than body fluids with a greater tendency to absorb water.

hypnagogic Occurring during the transition from wakefulness to sleep.

hypnogogic Occuring during the transition from sleep to wakefulness.

hypobaric condition State in which barometric pressure is lower than ambient at sea level or <760 torr.

hypopnea An episode of reduced airflow for at least 10 seconds.

hypotonic Refers to a substance that has a less of a tendency than body fluids to absorb water.

hypoxemia A low level of oxygen in the arterial blood.

hypoxia A low level of oxygen at the tissue level.

hypoxic drive The stimulus to breathe when the P_AO_2 falls below 60 mm Hg; activation of peripheral chemoreceptors.

I/E ratio The proportion of inspiratory time to expiratory time: $E = T_e/T_i$.

iatrogenic Refers to diseases or symptoms induced, intentionally or unintentionally, by healthcare providers examinations or treatments, including adverse drug reactions.

idiopathic Arising from a obscure or unknown cause, used to describe some diseases whose root causes are unknown.

idiopathic hypersomnia A condition of excessive daytime somnolence that has no known cause.

incentive spirometry (IS) The use of a device that provides visual feedback regarding the achievement of a predetermined goal for inspiration; incentive spirometers are generally used in conjunction with sustained maximal inflation (SMI).

incident command system (ICS) *See* hospital emergency incident command system (HEICS).

indirect contact Contact that occurs when a person becomes infected from a contaminated intermediate object or person.

indirect cost Monetary consequences of disability, missed work, premature death, and the caregiver or family costs resulting from the illness; costs that reflect the shortened contribution of the afflicted individual to society and the burden on the family.

inductance plethysmography Methodology for measuring thoracic and abdominal effort.

infectious agent A microorganism that can cause disease; the most common infectious agents are bacteria, viruses, fungi, and protozoa. *Also known as* pathogen.

inflammatory stage The first stage in the pneumonic consolidation process; occurs in the first 12–24 hours following infection; characterized by marked inflammatory pulmonary edema with engorgement of capillaries and exudation of acellular serous fluid into the alveolar spaces.

informed consent A patient's autonomous authorization of medical intervention.

inotrope A drug that can affect the contractility (or force of contraction) of the myocardium. A positive inotrope increases contractility; a negative inotrope decreases contractility. If it is not specified, positive is implied when referring to inotropes because there are no therapeutic indications for decreasing the contractility of the heart.

inspection A process by which a practitioner observes a patient's outward appearance for positive and negative signs and symptoms.

inspiratory capacity (IC) The maximum amount of air that can be inhaled from the resting end-expiratory level or FRC. *Also means* the inspiratory center in the brain.

inspiratory cycle off (usually inspiratory cycle off %) Determined when the ventilator flow cycles from inspiration to expiration based on a given variable (time, pressure, or volume).

inspiratory pause The interval from the end of inspiratory flow to the start of expiratory flow; used only in the volume control mode. The operator can prolong inspiration by not allowing inhaled air to be exhaled. It may be used therapeutically to improve distribution of air in the lungs, or it may be used diagnostically to determine static compliance.

inspiratory positive airway pressure (IPAP) The pressure support level in spontaneous modes or the pressure control level in timed modes.

inspiratory rise time (IRT) Determines the time to reach the selected airway pressure; the rate at which airway pressure rises during the beginning of inspiration.

inspiratory time (T_i) Total cycle (respiratory) time/$(I + E)$ or T_i = VT/Peak flow for rectangular flow waveforms; does not include pause time (no flow during pause); does include pause time if set.

instrumental activities of daily living (IADLs) Self-care activities that require cognitive and physical ability, such as shopping, cooking, using the telephone, and taking medications.

interdisciplinary Term used to describe a process that involves a number of health-care disciplines or professions for the purpose of working together and achieving stated goals and objectives, usually for the benefit of the patient

interferon Any of a group of glycoproteins produced by different cell types in response to various stimuli, such as exposure to a virus.

interleukin-6, 7, 8 Cytokines that participate in the regulation of immune responses and that mediate communication between cells.

intermittent positive pressure breathing (IPPB) The use of positive pressure on inspiration of significant magnitude to inflate the lungs to greater than the inspiratory capacity that the patient can achieve unassisted.

International Classification of Diseases, 9th Revision Clinical Modification (ICD-9-CM) Coding mechanism for classifying disease entities.

interrogatory A series of questions, usually in writing, asking for statements of fact regarding an incident.

intimate space An individual's comfort zone in a group.

intra-alveolar pressure Pressure within the alveoli.

intrahospital transport The movement of patients within the hospital.

intraosseous A means of access to the venous system in a child 6 years of age or less through the flat anteromedial surface of the tibia just below the tibial tuberosity; using a special needle, the therapist enters the bone marrow cavity, which connects with the tibial vein. Can be used for drugs usually given IV and also fluid administration.

intrapleural pressure (IPP) The pressure difference between the lungs and the pleural cavity of the lungs; the pressure within the pleural space.

intrapulmonary percussive ventilation (IPV) A form of physical therapy that administers high-frequency oscillation and continuous positive pressure to the airways during inhalation.

intrapulmonary shunting Pulmonary blood flow while the V/Q ratio equals 0; calculated by comparing the oxygen contents in arterial blood, mixed venous blood, and pulmonary capillary blood. *Also known as* venous admixture.

intrinsic PEEP *See* auto-PEEP.

invasion of privacy The publicizing of or wrongful intrusion into one's private activities.

inverse square law The magnitude of the influence caused by one event is inversely related to the square of the distances between the original event and the point at which the effect is noted.

ionized calcium Calcium in plasma that is not bound to proteins or diffusible ligands.

ionized magnesium Magnesium existing free (approximately 55% of total plasma magnesium); not bound to proteins (albumin) or complexed to anions.

ion-specific electrode (ISE) Electrode containing a biological membrane that allows for selective permeability of certain ions (usually smaller ions) and impermeable to larger ions such as protein ions. *Also known as* ion-selective electrode.

isohydric principle The principle that all buffer pairs in a physiological system are in equilibrium, having the same hydrogen ion concentration.

Isolation Precautions Airborne, droplet, and contact precautions.

isotonic Refers to a substance that neither gains nor loses water.

J-type juxtapulmonary receptors Lung receptors attached to unmyelinated afferent fibers found close to the pulmonary capillaries; stimulated by the increase in the interstitial fluid volume and in pulmonary blood flow. Their stimulation is postulated to be involved in the dyspneic sensations associated with pulmonary edema and diffuse parenchymal lung disease.

justice The principle that deals with issues of fairness, just desserts, and entitlements.

Kerley's lines Thin horizontal lines caused by engorged lymphatic channels that drain to the lateral pleural surfaces; seen on the chest radiograph in interstitial pulmonary edema. These are described as Kerley A, B, or C lines depending on their location and orientation relative to the CXR. Kerley B lines are most commonly identified.

kyphoscoliosis An abnormal anteroposterior (forward) and lateral curvature of the spine; a combination of kyphosis and scoliosis.

kyphosis An abnormal anteroposterior (forward) curvature of the spine.

laryngeal mask airway (LMA) A small, flexible oval mask with an inflatable rim, which is attached to a tube.

lateral decubitus The patient is placed on a table or cart, lying with the affected side down.

latex allergy An allergic reaction to the latex in gloves or other equipment; reactions can range from hives and itching to difficulty breathing to death from shock and total airway obstruction.

law A statement of scientific fact that has never been proven wrong.

Leland-Clark electrode A PO_2 electrode consisting of a platinum cathode and an Ag/AgCl anode in a phosphate buffer.

length of stay (LOS) The number of days a patient spends in a health-care setting.

lewisite A chemical blister agent (vesicant) that rapidly binds with proteins, including DNA, to produce damage.

liability Responsibility or obligation as defined by law.

libel False or malicious writing that is intended to defame or dishonor another.

life expectancy The estimated number of years of life remaining to a living organism, usually determined by comparing the organism's current age to the average age at death of other members of the species during a fixed period.

life span Longevity; usually measured in years.

lifestyle behavior Individual practices and habits that one adopts and that often affects health status and wellness.

limit A variable on a mechanical ventilator that is not exceeded during the inspiratory phase but that does not end inspiration; does not refer to alarm settings, which are sometimes called limits.

live attenuated vaccine (LAIV) A vaccine created by reducing the virulence of a pathogen, while keeping it viable or "live."

locus of control The perception of whether one believes one has control or influence over the circumstances, situations, or people.

long-term care (LTC) A type of care where patients are managed on a chronic or long-term basis, usually for longer than 90 days.

loop diuretics Potent diuretics that act on the ascending loop of Henle in the kidney; used to treat hypertension and edema seen in congestive heart failure or renal insufficiency.

lordosis An abnormal posteroanterior (backward) curvature of the spine.

lower airways The portion of the respiratory system below the larynx.

low-flow oxygen system An oxygen delivery system that does not meet the entire inspiratory flow demand of the patient; the patient entrains an uncontrolled amount of room air; F_IO_2 is variable.

low-frequency filter A component of a polygraph that allows for the attenuation of a low-frequency artifact obscuring a biological signal.

low-order explosion (LE) The result of a rapid expansion of gases from a subsonic explosion (e.g., a pipe bomb); does not have an overpressurization wave.

lung capacities The sum of two or more lung volumes: inspiratory, functional residual, vital, and total lung capacities.

lung compliance A measure of the ease with which the combined lung tissue and the chest wall expand on inspiration; the volume inhaled divided by the intrathoracic pressure required to make that volume change.

lung volumes The four segments into which the amount of air moving into and out of the lungs is divided: tidal, inspiratory reserve, expiratory reserve, and residual volume.

lung-thorax relationship The natural tendency for the lungs to recoil and for the thorax (chest wall) to expand upward and outward; together, these tendencies create a slight subatmospheric pressure within the pleural cavity.

lung-volume-reduction surgery (LVRS) The resection of the most severely affected areas of a diseased lung.

lupus erythematosus A group of connective tissue disorders primarily affecting young women; clinical forms include chronic cutaneous lupus, complement deficiency syndromes, drug-induced lupus erythematosis, neonatal lupus erythematosis, and systemic lupus erythematosis.

magnetic resonance imaging (MRI) An imaging method that creates images based on the behavior of hydrogen nuclei (protons) in a magnetic field.

malignant tumor A mass of cancer cells that may invade surrounding tissues or spread (metastasize) to distant areas of the body.

managed care A type of health-care plan or service in which the cost of quality care is reduced by preventive services and volume purchasing.

managed care organizations (MCOs) Organizations that provide health care coverage.

mass casualty incident (MCI) The impact of a disaster on a community and its infrastructure.

mathematical coupling A principle that the effects of an error made early in a series of mathematical calculations will be magnified at each subsequent step in the series.

maximum oxygen consumption ($\dot{V} \cdot O_{2max}$) The maximum amount of oxygen consumed during strenuous physical activity; indicates the level of physical conditioning.

maximum voluntary ventilation (MVV) The maximum amount of air a subject can move into and out of the lungs in 1 minute.

mean airway pressure (MAP) The average level of positive pressure throughout a breathing cycle; equals mean alveolar pressure if the inspiratory and expiratory airway resistances are approximately the same; directly related to alveolar distending volume and functional residual volume.

mechanism of action The means by which a drug effect is produced in the body, such as direct stimulation, blockade, or inhibition.

meconium Contents of the fetus's lower intestinal tract, which can be expelled into the amniotic fluid if the infant undergoes hypoxic stress during delivery; must be suctioned out of the upper and lower airways as soon as possible after birth.

mediator antagonist A drug that competes for a receptor site and prevents a subsequent response to a stimulus.

Medicaid A federally mandated, state-run program that provides health-care financing for the poor and disabled.

medical director The physician director who monitors, provides expertise, and enhances the practice of respiratory care.

medical model A model that interprets health in terms of the absence of disease and illness.

Medicare A federal program that provides health-care financing for the elderly and persons with disabilities and certain diseases.

metabolic acidosis A condition caused by the excessive production of organic acids that exceeds the rate of elimination, by the reduced excretion of acids, or by the excessive loss of bicarbonates.

metabolic alkalosis A condition resulting from a decrease in hydrogen ion concentration or an excess of bicarbonate and/or other conjugate bases.

metabolic equivalents of energy expenditure (METs) One MET equals approximately 3.5 mL of oxygen consumption per kilogram of body weight per minute.

metabolism The sum of all chemical and physical changes that take place in an organism; all the energy and material transformations that take place in a living cell.

metastasis Cancer cells that have spread to one or more sites elsewhere in the body, often by means of the lymph system or bloodstream. *See also* distant metastasis, regional metastasis.

MetHb An abnormal form of hemoglobin affecting the transport of oxygen within the body. Hemoglobin's $Fe+2$ is oxidized, producing methemoglobin's $Fe+3$ and resulting in chocolate brown blood. *Also known as* methemoglobin.

method of transmission The way in which an infectious agent moves from a reservoir to a susceptible host. *Also known as* mode of transmission.

miliary tuberculosis A fulminant type of tuberculosis that occurs most commonly in children.

minimal mandatory ventilation (MMV) The patient breathes spontaneously until minute volume falls below preset value. Ventilator delivers mandatory breaths until the minute volume is 10% greater than the preset value (indicating the patient is contributing 10%).

minimum data set (MDS) A clinical assessment tool to gather data on patients, in subacute facilities, which is then analyzed to determine the RUG-III category for that patient.

misdemeanor A minor crime punishable by less than a year incarceration.

mitral regurgitation Regurgitation during systole of some blood from the left ventricle through the partially open mitral valve back into the left atria; commonly caused by a mitral valve prolapse (a mitral valve leaflet is displaced into the left atrium during systole).

mitral stenosis Narrowing of the inlet valve into the left ventricle, preventing the proper opening during diastolic filling. Patients with mitral stenosis have mitral leaflets that are thickened, commissures that are fused, and/or chordate tendineae that are thickened and shortened. Commonly caused by rheumatic fever.

mixed apnea Cessation of airflow initially without evidence for central respiratory effort, followed by increasing respiratory effort.

MKSD Meter-kilogram-second-degree system; a system of measurement. *Also known as* the metric system.

modality Any type of learning channel (visual, auditory, kinesthetic) where an individual can receive and retain information from education.

Modified Borg Dyspnea Scale A simplified variation of the Borg Scale used to assess severity of dyspnea.

morals What people believe to be right and good.

morbidity The ratio of persons who are diseased to those who are well in a given community.

mortality The number of deaths per unit of population in a specific region, age range, or other group.

mucociliary escalator The transport of mucus by cilia toward the larynx for expulsion by coughing or swallowing.

mucokinesis The movement of mucus.

mucolytic A drug that reduces the viscosity of mucus by chemically disrupting the long mucopolysaccharide chains.

mucostasis The stagnation of mucus.

multidisciplinary competencies Testing of abilities and skills to perform tasks or procedures that encompass several areas of expertise.

multidrug-resistant organisms (MDRO) Microorganisms which are resistant to the antimicrobial action of more than one antibiotic or anti viral drug.

multidrug-resistant tuberculosis (MDRTB) A strain of *Mycobacterium tuberculosis* that is resistant to at least one antimicrobial agent that would normally be effective in controlling the infection.

multiple organ system failure (MOSF) A quantitative degree of organ dysfunction in six organ systems, resulting in the inability of host defense mechanisms to maintain homeostasis. *Also known as* multiple systems organ failure.

murmur An abnormal sound heard over the heart that indicates the flow of blood through a valve.

mycelium A fungal mat of long, branching, filamentous tubes containing cytoplasm; the individual filaments that make up the mycelium are called hyphae.

myocardial scintigraphy A nuclear imaging technique for evaluating coronary blood.

n-acetyl-l-cysteine (NAC) An agent undergoing research as an aerosol that could result in improvement in inhalational injuries.

nasal mask A mask that covers the entire nose or a minimask that fits under the nose, flush to the nares.

nasopharyngeal airway A soft, flexible tube, beveled at one end and flared at the other; inserted into the nare after being lubricated with sterile, water-soluble lubricant. *Also known as* nasal trumpet.

National Board for Respiratory Care (NBRC) The organization that develops and conducts the respiratory care credentialing system.

National Coverage Determination (NCD) A nationwide determination of whether Medicare will pay for an item or service.

National Emphysema Treatment Trial (NETT) A CMS-funded initiative at 17 nationwide clinical centers to validate that pulmonary rehabilitation is a viable treatment modality for COPD patients.

National Incident Management System (NIMS) The agency that follows a standard incident response for all government levels and response agencies.

nebulizer A device designed to produce an aerosol, using baffling to control particle size, and project it into a gas stream.

needlestick injury An injury to health care workers from sharp objects; most common cause of occupational exposures to bloodborne pathogens.

negative pressure ventilation (NPV) Lung inflation by the application of subambient pressure applied to the body surface.

negligence The causing of harm without an intent to harm.

neonatal A newborn of less than 28 days.

neonatal resuscitation program (NRP) A joint program of the American Heart Association and the

American Academy of Pediatrics to teach a systematic means of assessing and resuscitating the newborn.

nephrotic syndrome A nonspecific kidney disorder in which the kidneys are damaged, causing them to leak large amounts of protein (>3.5gm/day/1.73m^2 BSA from the blood) into the urine; characterized by proteinuria, hypoalbuminemia, hyperlipidemia, and edema.

nephrotoxicity A kidney disorder resulting from ingestion of a toxic substance or drug that damages kidney tissue.

neuraminidase Glycoside hydrolase enzymes (EC 3.2.1.18) that cleave the glycosidic linkages of neuraminic acids.

neutral thermal environment For neonates and infants, an environment that does not cause the infant to lose heat; generally requires heating via a radiant warmer or maintaining a closed environment, such as an isolette.

nitrogen mustard A chemical blister agent (vesicant) that rapidly binds with proteins, including DNA, to produce damage.

noninvasive positive pressure ventilation (NPPV) Positive pressure ventilation applied to the patient by a nasal or oronasal mask, nasal pillows, lip seal, or mouthpiece.

nonmalfeasance The duty to do no harm.

nonrapid eye movement (NREM) sleep The portion of a complete sleep period during which phasic eye movements are absent and muscle tone is present.

nonvolatile acid Noncarbonic, or fixed, acid, such as hydrochloric, lactic, and acetoacetic acids.

normative elements Ideal rules of conduct, as found in rules of professional etiquette, legal requirements, and ethical codes.

nosocomial infection *See* hospital-acquired infection.

nosocomial pneumonia *See* hospital-acquired pneumonia.

objective A declarative statement that directs the learner's action toward a specific goal.

obstructive lung disease A lung disease characterized by an inability to exhale as quickly as normal.

obstructive sleep apnea (OSA) Cessation of airflow due to obstruction of the upper airway, with continued respiratory efforts to breathe.

obstructive sleep disordered breathing (OSDB) A sleep disorder characterized by the repetitive reduction or cessation of airflow due to obstruction of the upper airway.

off-gassing Gases that occurs when chemicals vaporize from a victim's body or clothing.

oncotic pressure A form of osmotic pressure exerted by proteins in the blood plasma; tends to pull water into the circulatory system from the interstitial space. *Also known as* colloid osmotic pressure.

open pneumothorax When the pleural cavity is in direct communication with the atmosphere through a penetrating chest wound.

operational budget The budget projections for nondepreciable expenses such as costs of day-to-day salaries, benefits, and supplies.

opportunistic Term used to describe an infection occurring because of the opportunity afforded by an altered physiological state of the host.

oronasal mask A mask that covers both the nose and the mouth.

oropharyngeal airway A curved plastic tube available in several sizes for assisting in maintaining an open airway during bag-mask ventilation.

osmolality Concentration of osmotically active particles in solution expressed as osmoles per kilogram of solvent.

ototoxicity A toxicity affecting the ears or hearing.

outcome The end product assessment that assists in determining the outcome of any type of situation, whether it is educational or therapeutic.

outcome-oriented essentials A system that evaluates educational programs and that is focused on the achievement of targeted goals.

overwedging An artificially elevated pulmonary capillary wedge pressure tracing caused by overinflation of the balloon tip.

oxygen concentrator A device used for oxygen administration in the home setting that entrains room air, physically separates the oxygen from other room air gases, and supplies the oxygen directly to the patient.

oxygen conserving device (OCD) A device that is either pneumatic or electrically powered and that delivers oxygen to the patient only during the inspiratory phase by patient demand, resulting in greater efficiency and longer duration of use from an oxygen cylinder.

oxygen content The total amount of oxygen in the blood.

oxyhemoglobin The molecule formed by the chemical binding of oxygen to hemoglobin.

palliative Treatment that relieves symptoms, such as pain, but that is not expected to cure the disease, usually to improve the patient's quality of life.

palpation The act of using touch to perform a physical examination of a patient.

palpitations An unpleasant awareness of the beating of the heart, as if the heart is pounding or racing.

panacinar emphysema An emphysematous condition in which the entire acinus of the pulmonary parenchyma is abnormally and permanently enlarged. *Also known as* panlobular emphysema.

pandemic A worldwide epidemic.

paraneoplastic syndromes Manifestations of extrapulmonary, remote effects of lung tumors.

paraseptal emphysema Emphysema involving the alveolar ducts and sacs while sparing the respiratory bronchioles.

parasympathetic blockade The parasympathetic nervous system decreases heart rate by its effect on the SA node. Blocking its action with drugs allows the resumption of normal cardiac rhythm.

paroxysmal nocturnal dyspnea The sensation of air hunger that develops during sleep, wakes one up, and often produces panic such that the patient sits on the side of the bed or rushes to a window for air.

pathogen An organism capable of producing disease in humans.

pathogenesis The origination and development of a disease.

pathogenicity The ability of an organism to cause disease.

patient assessment A review of body systems to determine the clinical status of a patient.

patient calibration Procedure in a sleep study in which recorded biological signals are checked for appropriate response to specific changes induced in the signals.

PC-CMV Time- or flow-triggered, pressure-limited, time-cycled continuous mandatory ventilation with set point control.

peak inspiratory pressure (PIP) The highest positive pressure level achieved during a mechanically supported inspiration.

peak pressure The highest airway pressure occurring during a mandatory inspiration.

pectus carinatum An abnormal protrusion of the sternum.

pectus excavatum An abnormal depression of the sternum.

pediatric Relating to children; from the Greek *pais* for "child" and *iatreia* for "treatment."

pediatric advanced life support (PALS) A system for treating cardiac emergencies in infants and children that is less algorithm driven than ACLS; emphasizes prevention and BLS when prevention fails.

percussion (1) The process by which a practitioner can assess areas of a patient with gentle tapping to produce vibrations. (2) Application of mechanical energy through the chest wall to enhance movement of secretions, used with segmental drainage positions.

performance improvement The monitoring of activities with focus plan-do-check-act cycles that seek to improve systems of care.

perfusion pressure The driving pressure of blood that is the difference between the mean blood pressure and the vascular resistance or the systolic diastolic BP difference.

pericarditis Inflammation of the pericardium; may lead to constriction of the myocardium, thereby reducing ventricular filling.

periodic limb movements in sleep (PLMS) Stereotyped movements of the arms and/or legs that occur during sleep; a characteristic feature of restless legs syndrome.

peripheral cyanosis Blueing of the fingers or the fingernail beds, indicating a decrease in hemoglobin saturation; most likely caused by decreased circulation.

personal protective equipment (PPE) Gloves, gowns, masks, goggles, and face shields, worn to protect health care workers, patients, and visitors from pathogens.

personal space Distance of $1\frac{1}{2}$–4 feet between the patient and the practitioner varies with culture and ethnicity.

pH The negative log of the hydrogen ion concentration.

pharmaceutical phase The method by which a drug is administered; commonly referred to as the route of administration.

pharmacodynamic phase The mechanism of action by which a drug causes its therapeutic effect in the body.

pharmacodynamics A drug's mechanism of action.

pharmacokinetic phase The time required for drug absorption, action, distribution in the body, metabolism, and elimination.

pharmacokinetics The body's absorption, distribution, hepaticmetabolism, and renal clearance of a drug.

phlogiston theory An early theory of the makeup and function of our atmosphere, according to which phlogiston was thought to be an invisible gas released by burning materials.

phosphate buffer system A buffer system consisting of the $H_2PO_4^-$–HPO_4^{2-}= pair.

physical examination A thorough examination of the patient for all positive and negative medical conditions.

physical reconditioning Process of improving a patient's level of fitness through a program of exercise and physical activity.

physics The scientific discipline that studies the relationships between matter and energy.

physiological acid A substance that can donate electrons in a living physiological system.

physiological base A substance that can accept electrons in a living physiological system.

physiological buffer A substance that resists changes of hydrogen ion concentrations in living organisms such as mammals.

Pirfenidone A new drug that seems to block the effect of SEB, especially the development of pulmonary fibrosis, which complicates ventilator management with a restrictive defect.

plaintiff The person or agency bringing legal action in a civil lawsuit, claiming damage or harm.

plateau pressure ($P_{plateau}$) The airway pressure during an inspiratory pause; equal to the alveolar pressure.

plethysmography The study of changes in the shape or size of an organ; one of the principles of pulse oximetry.

pleural effusion An accumulation of fluid in the pleural space.

pleural pressure The pressure in the pleural space.

Pneumatic Institute The first institution (Bristol, England) designed specifically for the delivery of oxygen as a therapeutic material.

pneumocardiogram (PCG) A study performed on infants to record heart rate, respiratory pattern, oximetry, and nasal airflow in order to identify and predict respiratory abnormalities.

pneumotachometer A device used to measure flows.

pneumothorax The accumulation of air or gas in the pleural space.

Poiseuille's law The principle that resistance to flow is directly related to the length of a tube and inversely related to the fourth power of the tube's radius.

polycythemia An excess or increased number of red blood cells.

polygraph An instrument used to measure and record multiple physiological variables during sleep.

polymicrobial Referring to infections that involve more than one species of microorganism.

polypharmacy The use of multiple medications.

polysomnogram A continuous recording of physiological variables during sleep used for diagnosing sleep disorders.

polysomnography (PSG) The art of recording, analyzing, and interpreting multiple physiological parameters obtained during sleep.

portal of entry The path by which an infectious agent enters a susceptible host.

portal of exit The pathway by which an infectious agent exits or leaves a reservoir.

positive airway pressure (PAP) The generation of positive pressure in the airways, either on inspiration, expiration, or over the entire breathing cycle.

positive end-expiratory pressure (PEEP) An airway pressure that is kept above atmospheric pressure at the end of expiration and maintained during the entirety of exhalation.

positive pressure ventilation (PPV) A type of mechanical ventilation in which a positive transrespiratory pressure is generated by increasing airway opening pressure above body surface pressure.

positron emission tomography (PET) A nuclear imaging technique in which emitted photons are used to form images.

postacute care Any care given after the acute care stay, no matter where the care occurs.

potentiation The effect when two drugs produce an effect that is greater than what they usually produce when given alone or when one drug enhances the effect of another.

P-R segment The portion of an electrocardiogram that represents the delay of depolarization at the AV node.

practice acts Statuatory laws that seek to regulate practice in a certain field, such as medicine, nursing or respiratory care.

pre-eclampsia Hypertension or increase of 30 mm Hg systolic or 15 mm Hg diastolic accompanied by proteinuria, edema, or both.

preload The stretch exerted on the myocardial fibers before ventricular contraction.

pressure gradient The actual difference in pressure between the peak and baseline pressure. Pressure gradient is what causes flow thus driving gas into the lungs.

pressure support (PS) A pressure-targeted mode of ventilation in which the patient's effort must trigger inspiration.

pressure transducer A device used to measure the pressure of a liquid or a gas.

pressure ventilation The use of positive pressure to support ventilation.

pressure-volume loop Compliance (change in volume for a given change in pressure) over time or a single breath cycle.

primary blast injury Injuries that result from a high-order explosion. The positive-pressure wave rapidly expands to over 20 atm (20 × 760 mm Hg) and then immediately drops to a subambient pressure level, exacerbating the blast injury. *Also known* as blast over-pressure injuries.

primary infection tuberculosis The initial process of infection with the organism *Mycobacterium tuberculosis* and the body's response to it.

primary prevention Activities that prevent a disease or condition from occurring in the first place.

principle A statement of perceived truths about a defined situation.

private law Law that is concerned with the definition, regulation, and enforcement of rights in cases in which both the parties involved are private citizens; civil law.

problem-oriented medical record (POMR) A system of interdisciplinary documentation in which all practitioners document according to specified patient problems.

product-oriented essentials Evaluation measures based on the quality of the product.

proprioceptive Sensation of a stimulus arising within one's self.

prospective payment system (PPS) A health-care reimbursement system in which payments based on the projected use of services are made before services are rendered.

protein buffer system A buffer system consisting of the protein macromolecule Pr^-–Pr pair. The most important protein buffer in the physiological pH range consists of the imidazole group of histidine.

proteinuria The presence of protein in the urine; an abnormal finding in anyone and one of the signs of pre-eclampsia.

public law Law that deals with the relationships between private parties and the government; criminal law.

pulmonary edema A pathological condition wherein there is excess lung water accumulation in the interstitial space and ultimately alveolar flooding; commonly caused by the failure of the L ventricle with elevation of the L atrial pressure.

pulmonary hypoplasia An abnormal underdevelopment of the pulmonary tree, often caused by a space-occupying lesion such as diaphragmatic hernia, which does not allow the lungs to develop normally.

pulmonary rehabilitation A program of education and exercise that focuses on restoring chronic respiratory patients to the highest possible functional capacity; patients are monitored for pulse rate, respiratory rate, oxygen saturation, and peak flow rate (OPVR).

pulmonary shunting The part of cardiac output that enters the left side of the heart without having exchanged gases with alveoli.

pulmonary surfactant A substance that lowers alveolar surface tension, thereby maintaining alveolar stability.

pulmonary vascular resistance The force the right ventricle must overcome to maintain pulmonary blood flow.

pulse pressure The difference between the systolic blood pressure and the diastolic blood pressure.

pulseless electrical activity (PEA) The presence of organized electrical activity on the EKG with no palpable pulse. *Previously called* electromechanical dissociation (EMD), now considered a subset of PEA.

pulsus alternans A condition in which the arterial blood pressure varies, alternating high and low, with a regular cardiac rhythm.

pulsus bisferiens A condition in which the arterial pressure curve displays two systolic peaks.

pulsus paradoxus A condition in which the arterial systolic pressure falls by more than 10 mm Hg during spontaneous inspiration, despite a regular heart rate.

pulsus parvus A condition in which there is a low arterial blood pressure with a weak pulse.

P-wave The portion of an electrocardiogram that represents atrial depolarization.

QRS complex The portion of an electrocardiogram that represents ventricular depolarization.

quantity equations Equations that show numerical solutions for physics problems.

quaternary blast injury A type of trauma that results in burns, crush injuries, and toxic inhalations.

racemic epeinephrine An isomeric form of epinephrine or adrenalin that has a bronchodilator and vasoconstrictive effect within the body; used in treating stridor.

radiation therapy Treatment with high-energy rays (such as X-rays) to kill or shrink cancer cells.

radiodensity The degree of resistance to the passage of radiation.

radiograph An image produced by radiant energy, such as an X-ray.

radiology The study of the use of radiant energy, such as X-rays, in the diagnosis and treatment of disease.

radiopaque Impenetrable by radiation.

Ranke complex A lesion in a *Mycobacterium tuberculosis* infection that includes the Ghon complex and the patient's calcified hilar pulmonary lymph nodes.

rapid eye movement (REM) The portion of a complete sleep period characterized by decreased or absent muscle tone, phasically occurring rapid eye movements, and a low-amplitude, mixed-frequency EEG.

reactivation tuberculosis Tuberculosis that occurs when the individual's previously contained endogenous tuberculosis recurs. *Also known as* postprimary tuberculosis.

red hepatization stage The second stage of the pneumonic consolidation process; occurs 24–72 hours postinfection; lung has a deep red liverlike appearance; alveolar spaces are full of coagulated exudate containing fibrin, red blood cells, polymorphonuclear leukocytes, and the causative organism and mononuclear cells.

reflex irritability (crying, cough or sneeze = 2, grimace = 1, absent = 0); activity (active flexion of extremities = 2, some flexion = 1, flaccid = 0) respirations (crying, vigorous = 2, weak or gasping = 1, absent = 0). A score of <3 indicates the need for resuscitation, but the therapist should begin resuscitation if needed before the 1-min Apgar score is determined.

refractory period The portion of the cardiac cycle during which cardiac muscle cells are resistant to electrical stimulation.

regional or local metastasis Cancer that has spread to the lymph nodes, tissues, or organs close to the primary site.

relative humidity (RH) Comparison of the actual amount of water present in a given volume of gas (AH) at a given temperature with the amount the gas is capable of holding at that temperature; expressed as a percentage.

REM latency The interval from initial sleep onset to the first occurrence of REM sleep.

repolarization A change in transmembrane potential from positive toward negative that occurs inside the cardiac cell.

res ipsa loquitor The thing speaks for itself. A legal premise that some things are self evident.

reservoir A location where an infectious agent can survive but may or may not multiply; can be a patient, health-care worker, visitor, animal, or inanimate object such as equipment.

resident flora Microorganisms consistently found on the skin of most people.

resistance (R_{aw}) Airway resistance = (Peak − Plateau)/Peak flow in L/s for volume control ventilation with a rectangular flow waveform.

resistant A condition in which a microorganism does not respond to treatment with a particular anti-infective agent or technique.

resolution stage The final (healing) phase of the pneumonic process; alveolar fibrinous exudate is liquefied by the enzymes liberated from the leukocytes; phagocytes reabsorb the liquid; the atelectatic lung starts to reinflate.

resource utilization group (RUG) A classification that sets the prospective per diem rate that a facility is paid by Medicare for treating a particular patient in subacute case settings.

respiration The interchange of gases between an organism and the medium in which it lives; specifically, the taking in of oxygen, its use by the tissues, and the giving off of carbon dioxide.

respiratory acidosis An increase in carbonic acid and in PCO_2 resulting from the lung's inability to adequately exhale CO_2.

respiratory alkalosis An increase in the rate of CO_2 loss and a decreased PCO_2 resulting from an excessive ventilation.

respiratory care practitioner (RCP) A person specializing in the delivery of respiratory care. *Also known as* respiratory therapist.

respiratory disturbance index (RDI) The number of apnea and hypopnea episodes per hour of sleep time; used to describe the severity of sleep disordered breathing.

respiratory therapist (RT) A person specializing in the delivery of respiratory care. *Also known as* respiratory care practitioner.

respiratory zone Region of the tracheobronchial tree that allows gas exchange between alveoli and capillaries; extends from the respiratory bronchioles to the alveoli (generations 20 through 28).

respondeat superior The legal doctrine that holds employers responsible for their employees' actions.

restless legs syndrome (RLS) A neurological disorder characterized by an urge to move the legs.

restrictive lung disease A lung disease characterized by an inability to inhale normally.

Reynolds number A dimensionless number, describing flow, based on density, viscosity, and velocity of a fluid and the inertial force applied on the fluid.

rheologic The term used to describe the ability to flow or be deformed.

rheology The ability to be deformed or to flow.

ribivarin An antiviral agent that is used in the treatment of viral infections and that can be administered via aerosol or intravenous routes.

rise time percentage A ventilator control that lengthens the time required to reach the set IPAP pressure by reducing the maximal flow rate allowed initially; its purpose is to increase patient comfort by reducing the initial blast of airflow.

role duty A duty that exists owing to a person's job or position.

S/T mode A mode on the BiPAP S/T-D that allows a backup respiratory rate to be set to provide timed-triggered pressure ventilation in the event of apnea; inspiration is flow cycled.

SA node The sinoatrial node is the primary pacemaker for the heart; comprised of specialized tissue that depolarizes faster than any other in the heart.

sarcoidosis A systemic granulomatous disease that commonly involves the lungs and lymph nodes; unknown etiology.

scalar A graph depicting a single variable against time; represented by position on a scale or line.

scientific notation Mathematical and scientific shorthand notation for large and small quantities.

scoliosis A lateral curvature of the spine.

scope of practice The list of functions performed or provided by an occupational group.

scoring Process of extracting information from the physiological variables recorded on a polysomnogram.

secondary blast injury An injury caused by ballistic debris, by shrapnel, by improvised shrapnel such as nails, nuts, and bolts, or even, in the case of a suicide bombing, by bones and body parts.

secondary prevention Activities that detect a disease condition early in the process so that the duration and severity of the condition can be shortened or eliminated.

secondary spontaneous pneumothorax A type of pneumothorax that results from the spontaneous entrance of air into the pleural cavity of individuals with chronic diseases that promote the development and sudden rupture of of blebs or bullae.

self-contained breathing apparatus (SCBA) Equipment that provides clean, pressurized air to emergency personnel.

self-evacuation The ability to remove oneself from an endangered area or emergency situation.

Sellick maneuver The application of posterior pressure on the cricoid ring to move the larynx in a posterior direction and either (1) facilitate direct laryngoscopy during intubation or (2) occlude the esophagus to prevent insufflation of air into the stomach during positive pressure ventilation to the face (such as mouth-to-mouth or bag-mask ventilation) or to prevent gastric contents from moving into the pharynx and then possibly into the lungs.

sensitivity The change in airway pressure or base flow that must be generated by the patient in order to initiate an inspiration from the ventilator.

sentinel lymph node biopsy A relatively new procedure that might replace standard lymph node dissection. Blue dye and/or a radioisotope tracer is injected into the tumor site at the time of surgery and the first (sentinel) node that picks up the dye is removed and biopsied. If the node is cancer-free, fewer nodes are removed.

severity scoring guideline A standardized rating scale that evaluates the level of care required for a patient.

shape signal Graphic representation of the patient's actual ventilatory flow pattern.

shunt effect A condition of perfusion in excess of ventilation (low $\dot{V}/\dot{Q}$).

shutter In a body plethysmograph, a device used to completely occlude the tube through which the subject is breathing; located distal to the pressure transducer.

sinus venosus The embryologic structure in the fetal heart that eventually becomes the inferior and superior venae cavae and a portion of the right atrium.

slander False statements spoken in the presence of a third person that injure the character or reputation of another: the spoken form of defamation.

sleep apnea *See* sleep disordered breathing (SDB).

sleep architecture The distinct cycling of sleep stages.

sleep deprivation Sleep that is not of a sufficient duration.

sleep disordered breathing (SDB) A sleep disorder characterized by abnormal breathing patterns resulting from upper airway obstruction or loss of central respiratory neural drive. *Also known as* sleep apnea or hypopnea syndrome.

sleep fragmentation Decreased consolidation of sleep as a result of frequent arousals and/or awakenings.

sleep histogram A plot of the progression of sleep stages throughout the sleep period. *Also known as* sleep hypnogram.

sleep latency The duration of time between lights out and the onset of sleep. *Also known as* sleep onset latency.

sleep paralysis The inability to move the body during the transition from sleep to wakefulness; frequently associated with narcolepsy.

slow-wave sleep A term used to signify sleep characterized by greater than 20% delta waves; frequently used to designate stages 3 and 4 sleep. *Also known as* delta sleep.

SOAP An acroynm for subjective, objective, assessment, and plan—a method of documentation.

social space Distance of 4–12 feet between the patient and the practitioner.

Society of Critical Care Medicine (SCCM) The organization that oversees the professional activities and direction of practitioners providing critical care medicine to their patients; the largest multiprofessional organization dedicated to ensuring excellence and consistency in the practice of critical care.

source-oriented charting method A system in which the medical chart was divided into various departments and each department documented in its separate section.

spalling The shattering of the inside tissue matrix without penetration; can result in a pneumothorax, bronchopleural fistulas, and acute gas embolism.

specific gravity (SG) The ratio of the density of one substance to the density of a standard substance; the standard for gases is air; the standard for solids and liquids is water.

spectrophotometry The generation of light at a known intensity going into a solution and the measurement of the intensity of light leaving the solution; one of the principles of pulse oximetry.

sphygmomanometer A device for measuring blood pressure noninvasively.

spinnability The physical property of mucus related to its capacity to form threads under traction.

spirometry A test that measures changes in lung volumes and flows.

S_pO_2 Oxygen saturation as measured by a pulse oximeter.

spontaneous mode A patient-triggered, pressure-targeted, and patient-cycled mode. The patient's breathing effort must create the change from inspiration to exhalation and from exhalation to inspiration.

spontaneous or timed (S/T) mode Mode where patient can breathe either spontaneously or if a spontaneous breath does not occur, the unit will deliver a breath to the patient at a pre-set rate.

S-T segment The portion of an electrocardiogram that represents the refractory period of a cardiac cycle.

stability In aerosol therapy, the ability of an aerosol to remain suspended in a gas; influenced by particle size, particle activity, and concentration of particles.

staffing The activities associated with provision of staff to provide respiratory care.

standard deviation (SD) A measure of the dispersion of values around the mean for a set of data.

Standard Precautions Guidelines established by the Centers for Disease Control and Prevention (CDC) to minimize the risk of infectious agent transmission.

staphylococcal enterotoxin B (SEB) A potential terror bioagent that causes symptoms (sudden onset of fever, chills, dyspnea, and retrosternal chest pain) and toxicity when inhaled in very low doses; not dermally active; secondary aerosols are not a hazard; identified by ELISA or PCR (DNA amplifications). Standard Universal Precautions are required.

stare decisis "Let the decision stand"; principle of using rulings made in previous cases to rule on a matter.

static compliance The compliance measured when there is no gas flow into or out of the lung; the pressure required to maintain a given volume of inflation.

statutory law Collective term for laws passed or enacted through the legislative process.

sterile The state of an item that has been treated in such a way that no microorganisms are on it.

sterilization The killing all microorganisms, including spore forms.

stress test *See* cardiopulmonary exercise (CPX) evaluation/test.

stroke volume (SV) The volume of blood ejected by each ventricular contraction.

strong acid An acid that is almost completely ionized in a water solution.

stylette A flexible yet rigid metal rod placed inside an endotracheal tube to provide rigidity or shape in order to facilitate endotracheal intubation

subacute care Comprehensive inpatient care designed for patients who do not depend on high-technology monitoring or complex diagnostic procedures. *Also known as* postacute care.

subcutaneous emphysema Air under the skin.

sublimation The direct transition of a solid into the vapor or gaseous state.

Sugarloaf Conference A consensus conference held in the 1970s at which the scientific basis of respiratory therapy practices was first examined.

summary judgment A judgment made by the judge without trial.

surface tension The intermolecular forces on the surface of a liquid that tend to make the surface as small as possible. In the lung these forces, which exist in the alveoli, are countered by surfactant, which acts to reduce surface tension.

surfactant A combination of lipoproteins found in mature alveoli that reduces the surface tension of the pulmonary fluids.

surgical hand scrubbing Scrubbing that removes or destroys transient flora and reduces resident flora; requires an antimicrobial soap or detergent, a brush, and a longer period of washing than do handwashing and hand antisepsis.

susceptible host A person whose immune system is sufficiently weakened to allow a pathogen to enter the body, multiply, and cause illness.

sustained maximal inflation (SMI) A breathing maneuver for which patients are coached to inhale from the normal end-exhalation level (FRC) up to or near maximal inflation (TLC). The maximal inflation is held for a period of time (sustained) to allow for the distribution of air to collapsed or underinflated areas of the lungs.

Swan-Ganz catheter A specialized type of intervascular catheter that is threaded into the heart from a peripheral vessel; used to measure heart pressures and resistance to blood flow.

synchronized intermittent mandatory ventilation (SIMV) The SIMV rate or frequency sets the number of machines breaths per minute. Patient-triggered breaths over that frequency are spontaneous and usually pressure- or volume-supported or CPAP.

synergy The effect when two or more drugs produce an effect or response that neither could produce alone.

Système International d'Unités (SI system) A universally used system of measures and appropriate abbreviations.

systemic inflammatory response syndrome (SIRS) An inflammatory state affecting the whole body and frequently a response of the immune system to either trauma, infection, or burn.

systemic vascular resistance (SVR) The force the left ventricle must overcome to maintain systemic blood flow.

systole The period of the cardiac cycle in which the ventricles are contacting and ejecting blood into the great vessels.

systolic dysfunction Low cardiac output caused by disease of the L ventricular myocardium; most commonly caused by ischemia or infarction.

tachycardia An abnormally high heart rate.

tachyphylaxis The rapid development of drug tolerance.

tachypnea An abnormally high breathing rate.

target heart rate Heart rate at which a patient exercises to achieve maximum physical and cardiovascular conditioning.

technology-dependent children Children suffering from a chronic disability who require a medical device to compensate for a loss of a life-sustaining function.

tertiary blast injury An injury produced when the victim's body is thrown by the blast wave.

tertiary prevention Rehabilitative measures that aid an individual who has already contracted a disease process but prevent it from reoccurring or exacerbating to a full-blown stage.

theory A statement of probable fact that has not been completely proven to be irrefutable.

therapeutic index (TI) The ratio of the lethal dose (LD_{50}, the dose that would be lethal to 50% of the test population) to the effective dose (ED_{50}, the dose that would be effective for 50% of the test population).

therapist-driven protocol (TDP) A method used to perform a procedure in a standardized manner.

thermal pneumotachometer A device that measures flow by measuring the difference between two sides of a heated element as air passes by the heated element.

thermoregulation The regulation of temperature both ambient and within a controlled environment.

thoracentesis The introduction of a large-bore needle into the pleural space to retrieve fluids for diagnostic testing or to alleviate patient symptoms.

tight intracellular junctions Tight intracellular bridges on the alveolar side of the capillary endothelium that prevent alveolar flooding in early cardiac failure and direct the capillary leak into the pulmonary interstitium.

time constant The mathematical product of respiratory system resistance and compliance; used to determine the time required for the lungs to passively inflate or deflate: 1 time constant represents filling or emptying of 63% of the volume. Approaching 100% of the volume passively inhaled or exhaled requires 5 time constants.

tolerance The effect when increased amounts of a drug are needed to produce the desired effect.

tonicity The tendency of a substance to absorb water.

tort A legal wrong committed on a person or property independent of contract.

total cycle time T_{ct} in seconds = 60 breaths/min or 60 frequency or 60 rate. The time allowed for one inspiration and exhalation.

total lung capacity (TLC) The total amount of gas in the lungs after a maximal inhalation or inspiration.

trachea The windpipe; beginning of the tracheobronchial tree.

tracheobronchial tree The series of airway branchings, 28 generations, from the trachea to the alveolar level.

tracheostomy tube The artificial airway placed in the trachea through the opening.

training The application of information to performance and doing what was learned (the psychomotor domain). *See also* education.

transairway resistance A measure of the difficulty with which air passes through the conducting airways of the pulmonary system; calculated by dividing the driving pressure (the difference between atmospheric pressure and mouth pressure) by the flow produced. *Also known as* airway resistance.

transcutaneous monitoring A method of measuring the partial pressures of oxygen and carbon dioxide diffusing through the skin.

transcutaneous pacing The delivery of electrical energy to the myocardium through the skin in a rhythmic fashion to cause depolarization and then contraction; used in asystole and in symptomatic bradycardias in adults.

transducer A device that converts one form of energy to another and back again.

transient flora Microorganisms on the hands (for example, common cold germs) that are not consistently present on most people.

transmission-based precautions A second tier of precautions that applies to patients with specific infections and that depend on the specific infection; used in addition to Standard Precautions for specific patients.

transpulmonary pressure The difference in pressures between the pleural space and the alveoli.

transthoracic pressure (TTP) The pressure in the pleural space measured relative to the pressure of the ambient atmosphere outside the chest; the transmural (across the wall) pressure across the chest wall.

transudate A fluid that passes through a membrane that filters out much of the protein and cellular elements to yield a watery solution; fluid with a low concentration of protein that passes through capillary walls and can accumulate in a body space or cavity.

tricarboxylic acid (TCA) cycle The main biochemical pathway of terminal oxidation; a complex series of reactions involving the oxidative metabolism of pyruvic acid and the release of energy. *Also known as* Krebs cycle.

trigger The signal on a mechanical ventilator that initiates an inspiration; patient-triggered breaths are flow- or pressure-triggered; mandatory breaths are time-triggered.

trigger-timeout The adjustable apnea interval for spontaneous breaths in Automode.

triple point The temperature-pressure point at which a substance can exist with all three states of matter at equilibrium.

trivalent inactivated vaccine (TIV) A vaccine that contains three strains of inactivated (killed) virus (usually A/H1N1, A/H3N2, and B); may be administered intramuscularly (IM) or by nasal spray or mist (LAIV).

true shunt An area of pulmonary perfusion with no ventilation; refractory to oxygen therapy. *Also known as* absolute shunt.

tumor necrosis factor-alpha (TNF-a) A cytokine involved in systemic inflammation and required in the protective immune response against infection. *Also known as* cachexin or cachectin.

T-wave inversion An ECG T-wave that has negative amplitude in the leads that are typically positive (leads I, II, and V_3–V_6) and that are symmetrical and sharply pointed; commonly observed in myocardial ischemia.

T-wave The portion of an electrocardiogram that represents ventricular repolarization.

ultrasonic pneumotachometer A device that measures flow by the amount of turbulence created by an obstruction inside a tube through which air is flowing; the turbulence is measured by an ultrasonic beam as it passes through the turbulent air.

ultrasound An imaging method based on the different propensities of body tissues to transmit, absorb, or reflect high-frequency sound waves.

uniform reporting standards Timed work unit standards developed from input from a large number of respiratory care providers.

upper airway The portion of the respiratory system above the larynx, including the nose, oral cavity, and pharynx.

utilitarianism The belief that good resides in the promotion of happiness or the greatest net increase in pleasure over pain; the basis of consequence-oriented ethics.

vagal tone The state of hyperexcitability of the parasympathetic nervous system; the vagus nerve is the parasympathetic nerve that inhibits heart rate by its effect on the SA node and conduction of the electrical impulses through the AV junction.

valsalva maneuver The tight closing of the larynx during exhalation, with an increase in pressure in the lungs; used in lifting, coughing, vomiting, and defecating.

vascular system The system containing blood vessels; the overall vascular system has two divisions: systemic and pulmonary.

vector (1) Direction, as in the vector of force. (2) An organism that transmits a pathogen to an individual.

vector-borne transmission A method of infectious agent transmission in which the pathogen is carried from one host to another by an organism of a different species from the hosts.

ventilation The gross mechanical movement of air into and out of the lungs.

ventilation/perfusion ($\dot{V}/\dot{Q}$) scan A test in which radioactive tracers are used to determine the ratio of ventilation ($\dot{V}$) to perfusion ($\dot{Q}$) in the lungs.

ventricular afterload The force the ventricles must produce to eject blood.

ventricular fibrillation (v fib) Chaotic, uncoordinated depolarization of the ventricular muscle, resulting in no effective cardiac output.

ventricular preload The amount the ventricle is stretched with blood before the next contraction.

ventricular tachycardia (v tach) Three or more premature ventricular contractions (PVCs) in a row; may result in pulse and blood pressure, probably depending on rate.

veracity Truth telling.

vibration The application of mechanical energy to the chest wall to enhance movement of secretions, used with segmental bronchial drainage positions.

vibrissae Coarse hairs in the nasal vestibules.

video-assisted thoracoscopic surgery (VATS) An operative procedure that is replacing surgical procedures previously performed by open thoracotomy; performance of a minithoracotomy with the aid of a videoscope device.

virtue ethics Moral reasoning that focuses on the intent of the person doing an action rather than on the person's duty or the consequences of the action.

virulence The degree to which a microorganism has the capacity to produce disease.

virus An obligate intracellular parasitic microorganism smaller than a bacterium.

viscosity A physical property of mucus related to the internal friction between molecules that gives mucus its sticky or gelatinous character.

voice sounds Vibrations of spoken letters or words heard by the practitioner via auscultation of the chest.

volume support Assisted flow-triggered, pressure-limited, flow-cycled continuous spontaneous ventilation with adaptive control.

volume targeted PC Time- or flow-triggered, pressure-limited, time-cycled continuous mandatory ventilation with adaptive control. *Also known as* adaptive pressure control (APC–CMV).

volume ventilation A mode of positive pressure ventilation in which the volume delivered on each breath is the same (constant) and pressure is variable.

volutrauma A complication from mechanical ventilation in which the lung parenchyma sustains injury from alveolar overexpansion and shear stress.

water vapor content The amount of water vapor present in a gas; expressed as mg/L or g/m^3.

water vapor pressure The amount of pressure exerted by molecules of water in a gas, expressed as mm Hg.

weak acid An acid that is only slightly ionized in a water solution.

wellness An approach to personal health that emphasizes individual responsibility for well-being through the practice of health-promoting lifestyle behaviors.

Westermark's sign A radiographic sign in chest X-rays that shows large sections of lung on one side or the other without vascular markings; usually indicative of a sizable pulmonary infarction from embolus.

zoonotic Term used for diseases caused by host animals.

INDEX

Page numbers followed by T indicate tables; those in *italics* indicate figures.

C

N

S

T

V

W

X

Y

Z